The
MOLECULAR
BASIS
of
BLOOD
DISEASES

GEORGE STAMATOYANNOPOULOS, M.D., Dr. Sci.

Professor of Medicine and Genetics
Division of Medical Genetics
University of Washington School of Medicine
Seattle, Washington

ARTHUR W. NIENHUIS, M.D.

Director, St. Jude Children's Research Hospital
Memphis, Tennessee

PHILIP W. MAJERUS, M.D.

Professor of Medicine and Biological Chemistry
Division of Hematology-Oncology
Washington University School of Medicine
St. Louis, Missouri

HAROLD VARMUS, M.D.

American Cancer Society Professor of Molecular Virology
Departments of Microbiology and Immunology and of Biochemistry and Biophysics
University of California, San Francisco
San Francisco, California

The
MOLECULAR
BASIS
of
Second Edition
BLOOD
DISEASES

W.B. SAUNDERS COMPANY

A Division of Harcourt Brace & Company

PHILADELPHIA, LONDON, TORONTO, MONTREAL, SYDNEY, TOKYO

W.B. SAUNDERS COMPANY
A Division of Harcourt Brace & Company

The Curtis Center
Independence Square West
Philadelphia, PA 19106

Library of Congress Cataloging-in-Publication Data

The Molecular basis of blood diseases / George Stamatoyannopoulos . . . [et al.].—2nd ed.

    p. cm.

Includes bibliographical references and index.

ISBN 0–7216–4735–9

1. Blood—Diseases—Molecular aspects.   I. Stamatoyannopoulos, George.   [DNLM: 1. Hematologic
  Diseases.   2. Molecular Biology.   WH 100 M718]

RC636.M57   1994   616.1'5071—dc20

DNLM/DLC   92–48879

The Molecular Basis of Blood Diseases   ISBN 0–7216–4735–9

Printed in the United States of America.

Last digit is the print number: 9   8   7   6   5   4   3   2

CONTRIBUTORS

TED ABEL, M. Phil.

Graduate Student, Department of Biochemistry and Molecular Biology, Harvard University, Cambridge, Massachusetts.

Mechanisms of Eukaryotic Gene Regulation

GROVER C. BAGBY, Jr., M.D.

Professor of Medicine and Medical Genetics, Oregon Health Sciences University; Head, Division of Hematology and Medical Oncology, Oregon Health Sciences University and Veterans Affairs Medical Center, Portland, Oregon.

Hematopoiesis

EDWARD J. BENZ, Jr., M.D.

Jack D. Myers Professor and Chairman, Department of Medicine, and Professor of Molecular Genetics and Biochemistry, University of Pittsburgh School of Medicine; Adjunct Professor of Biological Sciences, Carnegie Mellon University; Attending Physician, University of Pittsburgh Medical Center, Pittsburgh, Pennsylvania.

The Erythrocyte Membrane and Cytoskeleton: Structure, Function, and Disorders

ERNEST BEUTLER, M.D.

Chairman, Department of Molecular and Experimental Medicine, The Scripps Research Institute, La Jolla; Clinical Professor of Medicine, University of California, San Diego; Senior Consultant, Division of Hematology-Oncology, The Scripps Clinic and Research Foundation, La Jolla, California.

The Molecular Biology of Enzymes of Erythrocyte Metabolism

GEORGE J. BROZE, Jr., M.D.

Professor of Medicine, Cell Biology, and Physiology, Washington University School of Medicine; Attending Physician, Barnes and Jewish Hospitals, St. Louis, Missouri.

Regulation of Blood Coagulation by Protease Inhibitors

H. FRANKLIN BUNN, M.D.

Professor of Medicine, Harvard Medical School; Research Director, Hematology/Oncology Division, Brigham and Women's Hospital, Boston, Massachusetts.

Sickle Hemoglobin and Other Hemoglobin Mutants

DÉSIRÉ COLLEN, M.D., PhD.

Professor of Medicine, University of Leuven; Adjunct Head of Clinic, University Hospitals, Leuven, Belgium.

Fibrinolysis and the Control of Hemostasis

JOHN T. CURNUTTE, M.D., Ph.D.

Associate Member, Department of Molecular and Experimental Medicine, The Scripps Research Institute, La Jolla, California.

Genetic Disorders of Phagocyte Function

BJÖRN DAHLBÄCK, M.D., Ph.D.

Professor of Blood Coagulation Research, Department of Clinical Chemistry, Lund University, Malmö General Hospital; Senior Physician, Department of Clinical Chemistry, Malmö General Hospital, Malmö, Sweden

Vitamin K–Dependent Proteins; The Protein C Anticoagulant System

EARL W. DAVIE, Ph.D.

Professor of Biochemistry, University of Washington School of Medicine, Seattle, Washington.

Hemophilia A, Hemophilia B, and Von Willebrand Disease

JEFFREY E. DeCLUE, Ph.D.

Senior Staff Fellow, Laboratory of Cellular Oncology, National Cancer Institute, National Institutes of Health, Bethesda, Maryland.

Molecular Aspects of Oncogenesis

STEPHEN M. DENNING, M.D.

Assistant Professor of Medicine, Duke University School of Medicine; Staff, Division of Cardiology, Duke University Medical Center, Durham, North Carolina.

Lymphopoiesis

MARY C. DINAUER, M.D., Ph.D.

Associate Professor of Pediatrics and of Medical and Molecular Genetics, Indiana University School of Medicine; Staff, Herman B. Wells Center for Pediatric Research, James Whitcomb Riley Hospital for Children, Indiana University Medical Center, Indianapolis, Indiana.

Genetic Disorders of Phagocyte Function

RUSSELL F. DOOLITTLE, Ph.D.

Professor of Biology and Chemistry, University of California, San Diego, San Diego, California.

The Molecular Biology of Fibrin

EDWARD F. FRITSCH, Ph.D.

Vice President, Product Development, Genetics Institute, Andover, Massachusetts.

Methods of Molecular Genetics

JOE B. HARFORD, Ph.D.

Director of Biochemistry and Cell Biology, RiboGene, Inc., Hayward, California

Molecular Mechanisms of Iron Metabolism

BARTON F. HAYNES, M.D.

Frederic M. Hanes Professor of Medicine, Department of Medicine, Duke University School of Medicine; Chief, Division of Rheumatology and Immunology, and Director of the Duke University Arthritis Center, Duke Hospital, Duke University Medical Center, Durham, North Carolina.

Lymphopoiesis

HELMUT A. HUEBERS, M.D., Ph.D.

Professor, University of Saarland, Saarland, Germany

Molecular Mechanisms of Iron Metabolism

ILAN R. KIRSCH, M.D.

Section Chief, National Cancer Institute; Attending Physician, Pediatric Branch, National Cancer Institute Clinical Center, National Institutes of Health, Bethesda, Maryland.

Gene Rearrangements in Lymphoid Cells

RICHARD D. KLAUSNER, M.D.

Chief, Cell Biology and Metabolism Branch, National Institute of Child Health and Human Development, National Institutes of Health, Bethesda, Maryland.

Molecular Mechanisms of Iron Metabolism

W. MICHAEL KUEHL, M.D.

Chief, Section on Molecular Biology of Differentiation, National Cancer Institute— Navy Medical Oncology Branch, National Institutes of Health, Bethesda, Maryland.

Gene Rearrangements in Lymphoid Cells

H. ROGER LIJNEN, Ph.D.

Associate Professor of Medicine, University of Leuven, Leuven, Belgium.

Fibrinolysis and the Control of Hemostasis

JOHN B. LOWE, M.D.

Associate Professor of Pathology, University of Michigan Medical School; Associate Investigator, Howard Hughes Medical Institute, Ann Arbor, Michigan.

Red Cell Membrane Antigens

DOUGLAS R. LOWY, M.D.

Chief, Laboratory of Cellular Oncology, National Cancer Institute, National Institutes of Health, Bethesda, Maryland.

Molecular Aspects of Oncogenesis

PHILIP W. MAJERUS, M.D.

Professor of Medicine and Biochemistry, Washington University School of Medicine; Physician, Barnes Hospital, St. Louis, Missouri.

Platelets

TOM MANIATIS, Ph.D.

Professor of Biochemistry and Molecular Biology, Harvard University, Cambridge, Massachusetts

Mechanisms of Eukaryotic Gene Regulation

MALCOLM A. MARTIN, M.D.

Chief, Laboratory of Molecular Microbiology, National Institute of Allergy and Infectious Diseases, National Institutes of Health, Bethesda, Maryland.

The Molecular and Biological Properties of the Human Immunodeficiency Virus

ARTHUR W. NIENHUIS, M.D.

Chief, Clinical Hematology Branch, National Heart, Lung, and Blood Institute, National Institutes of Health, Bethesda, Maryland.

Hemoglobin Switching

STUART H. ORKIN, M.D.

Professor, Department of Pediatrics, Harvard Medical School; Investigator, Howard Hughes Medical Institute, Boston, Massachusetts.

Genetic Disorders of Phagocyte Function

ROGER M. PERLMUTTER, M.D., PH.D.

Professor, Departments of Immunology, Biochemistry, and Medicine, University of Washington School of Medicine; Investigator, Howard Hughes Medical Institute, Seattle, Washington.

Antigen Processing and T-Cell Effector Mechanisms

TRACEY A. ROUAULT, M.D.

Senior Scientist, Cell Biology and Metabolism Branch, National Institute of Child Health and Human Development, National Institutes of Health, Bethesda, Maryland.

Molecular Mechanisms of Iron Metabolism

J. EVAN SADLER, M.D., PH.D.

Professor of Medicine, Washington University School of Medicine; Associate Investigator, Howard Hughes Medical Institute; Associate Attending Physician, The Jewish Hospital of St. Louis, and Assistant Physician, Barnes Hospital, St. Louis, Missouri.

Hemophilia A, Hemophilia B, and Von Willebrand Disease

GEORGE STAMATOYANNOPOULOS, M.D., DR. SCI.

Professor of Medicine and Genetics, and Head, Division of Medical Genetics; Director, Markey Molecular Medicine Center,

University of Washington School of Medicine, Seattle, Washington.

Hemoglobin Switching

JOHAN STENFLO, M.D., PH.D.

Professor of Clinical Chemistry, Department of Clinical Chemistry, Lund University, Malmö General Hospital; Senior Physician, Department of Clinical Chemistry, Malmö General Hospital, Malmö, Sweden.

Vitamin K–Dependent Proteins; The Protein C Anticoagulant System

THOMAS P. STOSSEL, M.D.

American Cancer Society Professor of Medicine, Harvard Medical School; Senior Physician, Brigham and Women's Hospital, Boston, Massachusetts.

The Molecular Basis of White Blood Cell Motility

BILL SUGDEN, PH.D.

Professor of Oncology, McArdle Laboratory for Cancer Research, University of Wisconsin, Madison, Wisconsin.

Viral Pathogenesis of Hematological Disorders: Herpesviruses

DOUGLAS M. TOLLEFSEN, M.D., PH.D.

Professor of Medicine, Division of Hematology-Oncology, Washington University School of Medicine; Physician, Barnes Hospital, St. Louis, Missouri.

Regulation of Blood Coagulation by Protease Inhibitors

D. J. WEATHERALL, M.D., F.R.S.

Regius Professor of Medicine, University of Oxford; Honorary Director, Institute of Molecular Medicine, John Radcliffe Hospital, Oxford, United Kingdom.

The Thalassemias

OWEN N. WITTE, M.D.

Professor, Microbiology and Molecular Genetics, and Investigator, Howard Hughes Medical Institute, University of California, Los Angeles, Los Angeles, California.

Mechanisms of Leukemogenesis

JOHN M. WOZNEY, PH.D.

Director, Bone Research, Genetics Institute, Inc., Cambridge, Massachusetts.

Methods of Molecular Genetics

MITSUAKI YOSHIDA, Ph.D.

Professor, Institute of Medical Science, The University of Tokyo, Tokyo, Japan.

Viral Pathogenesis of Hematological Disorders: Retroviruses

NEAL S. YOUNG, M.D.

Chief, Hematology Branch, National Heart, Lung, and Blood Institute, National Institutes of Health, Bethesda, Maryland.

Viral Pathogenesis of Hematological Disorders: Introduction; B19 Parvovirus

PREFACE

Molecular biology has revolutionized hematology research. The first edition of this book, published in 1987, was among the first texts to examine the impact of molecular biology on disease mechanisms. In the intervening six years, the body of knowledge about proteins, cells, and organisms gained by manipulation and characterization of DNA and RNA has grown exponentially. The challenge now is not only to understand disease mechanisms but also to apply this new knowledge to find more effective therapies.

Virtually all facets of hematology have now been subjected to study by molecular genetic techniques. Most inherited and many acquired diseases are now at least partially understood at the molecular level. Fundamental cellular mechanisms such as transcriptional regulation, signal transduction, antigen processing, and cell motility are coming to be understood. Our purpose with this second edition remains the same, namely to assemble this body of knowledge about gene structure, function, and organization and about disease mechanisms that form the basis for a molecular approach to hematology. The growth in information and our desire to provide a comprehensive exposition of principles has resulted in substantial increase in size of this second edition. Again we have relied on experts with broad perspective to write chapters related to their own areas of expertise.

The knowledge acquired by molecular techniques has broadened the scope of this edition of "The Molecular Basis of Blood Diseases." However, it, like the first edition, is not a textbook of hematology. No effort has been made to describe diseases for which molecular biological and sophisticated cell biological approaches have not yet yielded relevant information about disease mechanisms.

The book begins with a section, "Basic Concepts," that contains three chapters of broad relevance. An understanding of methods remains essential to comprehend the body of knowledge acquired by molecular techniques. Accordingly, Chapter 1 provides a general description of the methodology of molecular biology and serves as an introduction to gene structure and function. The mechanisms by which regulatory proteins interact with one another and with nucleic acids to regulate gene expression in determining patterns of cellular differentiation is addressed in Chapter 2. Blood-forming tissues are a dispersed hematopoietic organ that respond to microenvironmental influences including cytokines, negative regulators, and cytoadhesive molecules to achieve controlled production of red cells, lymphocytes, phagocytic cells including neutrophils, and platelets. Thereby the number of these elements remain fairly constant in circulating blood. Chapter 3 provides a comprehensive introduction to hematopoietic mechanisms.

Several chapters are included in the section on red cells. Effective treatment of sickle cell anemia and severe β thalassemia could be achieved if the fetal to adult switch during the perinatal period that initiates disease manifestations in affected individuals were reversed. Progress toward this goal achieved by application of molecular and cellular techniques provides a paradigm for understanding regulation of gene expression during development. Knowledge of the thalassemias, disorders reflecting deficient globin synthesis, illustrates the level of understanding about disease manifestations that can be achieved by consistent application of molecular methods. Sickle cell anemia, the first molecular disease for which the amino acid and nucleotide substitutions were known, remains challenging with respect to the pathophysiology of disease causing vaso-occlusive episodes. Since the first edition, there has been substantial progress in defining the structure of membrane proteins and surface antigens and mutations that lead to membrane dysfunction. Red cell enzyme defects, defined by classic biochemical techniques, have now come to be defined at the molecular level. New chapters on each of these topics have been included. Much progress has also been achieved in understanding how cells control iron uptake and storage to ensure availability for critical functions as described in the final chapter in this section.

Consideration of immunoglobulin and T-cell receptor gene rearrangements, lymphopoiesis, and the effector arm of the immune response has been expanded in Section III. These chapters are meant to provide a comprehensive account of important principles that have emerged as molecular knowledge about the immune system has grown. The function of phagocytic cells including endocytosis, the oxidative burst, and cell motility required much expanded consideration in the two chapters of Section IV.

Much progress has also been achieved in the study of hemostasis and its pathological counterpart, thrombosis, by application of molecular methods. The genes for the proteins involved in hemostasis and thrombosis have been characterized and mutations identified in individuals with deficiencies providing insights into protein structure and function. There is now a better understanding of the fibrinolytic mechanism and new therapies have been applied. Many new platelet functions have been characterized and these cellular fragments continue to provide novel insights into signaling mechanisms and cellular activation. The several chapters in Section V are designed to capture these new developments.

Neoplasms have come to be understood as acquired diseases with gene defects. Chromosome rearrangements create novel oncoproteins, and point mutations, gene amplification, or gene deletion either activate, increase or decrease critical cellular proteins. Each neoplastic cell has several mutations that interact in causing uncontrolled growth. Our approach, in Section VI, has been to emphasize important principles with representative examples providing the framework to allow the interested reader to learn details through further reading.

Viruses manage to evade the immune system in establishing and maintaining infection, thereby creating disease by unique mechanisms. Section VII has been expanded to provide a comprehensive chapter on AIDS and a second chapter that covers other viruses that may invade and cause disease in both normal and immunocompromised individuals.

The size and weight of this book is one testimony to the impact of molecular biology on our understanding of the fundamental properties of the blood, bone marrow, and lymphoid organs and the elucidation of hematological diseases. What about therapy? Coagulation factor replacement, use of cytokines to stimulate hematopoiesis, and various fibrinolytic agents are current products of the molecular biological revolution. In the future, one hopes that pharmaceutical agents that target specific defective gene products or cellular functions will be discovered based on an appreciation of the molecular basis of blood diseases. The use of genes as investigative or therapeutic agents is already a clinical reality. Our decision not to cover this emerging area of research reflects the current status in which most research has focused on developing methodology and testing vectors in animal models. Undoubtedly future editions of this book will contain many examples of the successful use of gene therapy and other therapeutic approaches derived from molecular knowledge.

We hope that individuals of diverse backgrounds will find this book useful. For the serious student of hematology, whether medical student, resident or fellow, it will serve as a supplement to standard textbooks. Individuals engaged in the practice or teaching of hematology should find the book useful in learning and applying the principles of molecular biology in their discipline. The text should also be valuable to the graduate student, postdoctoral fellow, or established scientist with a working knowledge of molecular biology who desires to learn about the molecular basis of various blood diseases.

GEORGE STAMATOYANNOPOULOS

ARTHUR W. NIENHUIS

PHILIP W. MAJERUS

HAROLD VARMUS

CONTENTS

SECTION II
RED CELLS AND ERYTHROPOIESIS

8

RED CELL MEMBRANE ANTIGENS 293

John B. Lowe

9

THE MOLECULAR BIOLOGY OF ENZYMES
OF ERYTHROCYTE METABOLISM 331

Ernest Beutler

10

MOLECULAR MECHANISMS OF IRON METABOLISM 351

Joe B. Harford
Tracey A. Rouault
Helmut A. Huebers
Richard D. Klausner

15

THE MOLECULAR BASIS OF WHITE BLOOD CELL MOTILITY 541
Thomas P. Stossel

SECTION V
HEMOSTASIS

16

VITAMIN K–DEPENDENT PROTEINS 565
Johan Stenflo
Björn Dahlbäck

17

THE PROTEIN C ANTICOAGULANT SYSTEM 599
Björn Dahlbäck
Johan Stenflo

SECTION VI
MOLECULAR ONCOLOGY

SECTION VII
VIRUSES

SECTION I

BASIC CONCEPTS

Methods of Molecular Genetics

Edward F. Fritsch and John M. Wozney

INTRODUCTION

In the 6 years since the first edition of this book, there has been a tremendous explosion in the techniques of molecular biology and especially in the application of these techniques to solve fundamental problems in biology. The quintessential spirit of that growth is aptly represented by the acceptance and initiation of the Human Genome Project, a project of monumental proportion and significance. Nonetheless, despite this growth, the fundamental targets of analysis—DNA, RNA, and protein—have remained the same, and the approaches are conceptually unaltered. Identification and isolation of genes, analysis of gene structure, and detection and characterization of expressed RNA molecules continue to be the primary activities of molecular biologists interested in the flow of genetic information in normal cellular processes and in disease. What has changed has been the rapid advances in improvements in the fundamental tools used in molecular analysis and the widespread distribution of those tools and techniques to biological researchers in all fields.

This chapter is aimed at the reader who has not yet been pulled deeply, by necessity, into the fields of molecular cloning and gene analysis. It emphasizes both the fundamental technologies that have been the lifeblood of molecular genetics over the past 15 years and the elegant ways in which molecular technologies can and have been utilized to increase our basic understanding of biological processes. The remaining chapters of this book are testimony to the power and success of that technology in the field of hematology. We hope that this chapter provides a solid basis for a better understanding of the technologies used in the experiments described later, as well as a reference document. A more detailed description of many of these molecular techniques and a complete list of references can be found in *Recombinant DNA—A Short Course* by James Watson, John Tooze, and David Kurtz[1]; *Molecular Biology of the Cell*, second edition, by Bruce Alberts et al.[2]; and *Molecular Cloning—A Labo-*

3

ratory Manual, first and second editions, by Joe Sambrook, Ed Fritsch, and Tom Maniatis.[3, 4]

BASIC PRINCIPLES OF MOLECULAR CLONING

Central to the following discussion is molecular cloning technology because of the important role cloning has had and continues to have in formulating and approaching many molecular problems. In simplest terms, the process of molecular cloning consists of joining two DNA molecules: the DNA molecule that we wish to study and a DNA molecule known as a vector, which is capable of replicating in a suitable host, usually a bacterium. Following the introduction of this hybrid DNA into the host and the identification and selection of those cells containing the DNA molecule of interest, a large quantity of the DNA can be easily prepared for detailed structural and functional analysis. This technology was initially built upon and continues to be improved by important advances in the areas of enzymology of restriction endonucleases and other DNA- or RNA-modifying enzymes, the genetics and biochemistry of bacteria and their viruses, and the molecular biology of bacterial plasmids. These advances have led to the construction of suitable vectors, the development of efficient methods for manipulating DNA and RNA molecules, the methods for introducing purified DNA into host cells, and the techniques for identifying and characterizing recombinant clones. In this section, we describe how these fundamental tools are utilized to produce recombinant clones in bacteria.

Restriction Endonucleases and DNA- or RNA-Modifying Enzymes

A variety of enzymes that act on DNA, RNA, or their precursors are essential in the analysis and manipulation of DNA and RNA. Principal among these enzymes have been the type II restriction endonucleases. Type II restriction endonucleases are enzymes that recognize specific sequences in double-stranded (and sometimes single-stranded) DNA and that result in specific cleavage of the DNA within or very near the recognition site.

For example, the recognition sequence for the type II restriction endonuclease *Eco*RI is the following:

$$5' \ldots pG \downarrow pApApTpTpC \ldots 3'$$
$$3' \ldots pCpTpTpApAp \uparrow Gp \ldots 5'$$

The enzyme will nick the DNA at the positions of the two arrows, resulting in the following fragments:

$$5' \ldots G\text{–}OH(3') \ (5')pApApTpTpC \ldots 3'$$
$$3' \ldots CpTpTpApAp(5') \ (3')HO\text{–}Gp \ldots 5'$$

Other restriction endonucleases recognize different sequences of nucleotides. Almost all restriction enzymes have recognition sites that consist of 4, 5, or 6 nucleotides (nt), although several have the desirable feature of recognizing as many as 8 base pairs (bp). This latter property is especially useful in many cloning operations and in long-range gene analysis by providing tools that recognize sequences infrequently in most DNAs (see below). Most recognition sequences are palindromic (palindromic sequences have the same order of bases when reading either strand in the 5′ → 3′ direction), although interrupted palindromes and non-palindromic recognition sequences are known.

The number of times a given enzyme cuts within a DNA fragment is in most cases inversely related to the number of nucleotides in the recognition site; it also depends, to an extent, on base composition and sequence of the DNA. For example, even though the enzyme *Msp* I recognizes only four bases, $5' \ldots$ CpCpGpG $\ldots 3'$, *Msp* I rarely cuts in most mammalian DNAs because the dinucleotide CpG is underrepresented in mammalian DNA.

The specificity as well as utility of restriction endonucleases has been extended in several important and clever ways. Most type II restriction endonucleases have a corresponding methylase that modifies the recognition sequence at one or more bases, rendering it resistant to cleavage. The discovery and availability of such modification enzymes have provided the opportunity to alter the specificity of restriction endonucleases by blocking digestion of a subset of the possible sequences. For example, any *Bam*HI site, $5' \ldots$ pGpGpApTpCpC $\ldots 3'$, that is preceded by a $5' \ldots$ pCpC $\ldots 3'$ or followed by a $5' \ldots$ pGpG $\ldots 3'$ will generate a site for modification by the modification enzyme *M.Msp* I, which has the recognition sequence $5' \ldots$ pCpCpGpG $\ldots 3'$. This enzyme methylates at the 5′-cytosine, resulting in modification of the internal cytosine of the *Bam*HI recognition sequence:

$$5' \ldots pCpC\mathbf{pGpGpApTp}{^m}\mathbf{5CpC}pCpGpG \ldots 3'$$

This modified sequence is resistant to cleavage by *Bam*HI; thus, the modification enzyme was able to provide added specificity by preventing digestion at a subset of *Bam*HI sites.

Cleavage of a DNA molecule with a restriction endonuclease is used to fragment the DNA in a characteristic fashion, depending on the location of cleavage sites. The fragments produced by cleavage can then be efficiently separated by agarose or acrylamide gel electrophoresis and accurately sized by comparison with known markers. Through the use of many restriction endonucleases, a "map" of the cleavage sites within a DNA segment can be generated, which is of significant value in gene characterization.

A second useful property of most restriction endonucleases is that all fragments produced by the enzyme can be joined through the action of another enzyme known as DNA ligase. For example, the ends created by *Eco*RI can reform transiently through complementary base pairing to form the following:

$$5' \ldots G\text{–}OH \ pApApTpT\text{---}p \ \ C \ldots 3'$$
$$3' \ldots Cp\text{---} \ \ TpTpApAp \ HO\text{–}G \ldots 5'$$

DNA ligase can then reseal the phosphodiester

bonds between the G—OH and pA to yield the unbroken duplex:

$$5' \ldots \text{pGpApApTpTpC} \ldots 3'$$
$$3' \ldots \text{CpTpTpApApGp} \ldots 5'$$

All DNA molecules digested with *Eco*RI produce identical 4 nt single-stranded tails independent of the flanking sequence. Thus, any two DNA molecules that have been digested with *Eco*RI can be conveniently joined through transient annealing of the single-stranded tails and resealing of the phosphodiester bonds with DNA ligase.

Almost all restriction endonucleases result in ends that can be joined through the action of DNA ligase. Many of the restriction endonucleases are similar to *Eco*RI in that a single-stranded tail with a length of 1 to 4 nt is produced by digestion. However, digestion of DNA by some restriction endonucleases results in ends in which the last nucleotide in each strand is base paired. Such ends are termed blunt ends, and these ends can also be joined through the action of DNA ligase. For example,

HaeIII
$$5' \ldots \text{pGpGpCpC} \ldots 3' \rightarrow 5' \ldots \text{pGpG—OH} + \text{pCpC} \ldots 3'$$
$$3' \ldots \text{CpCpGpGp} \ldots 5' \leftarrow 3' \ldots \text{CpCp HO–} \quad \text{GpGp} \ldots 5'$$
DNA Ligase

More than 125 restriction endonucleases have been identified, most of which are commercially available and have distinct recognition sequences.[5] Moreover, more than a dozen modification enzymes are available to further enhance the utility of a subset of those restriction endonucleases. Thus, restriction endonucleases and modifying enzymes provide powerful and specific tools both to cut a DNA segment into one or more specific fragments and, in conjunction with DNA ligase, to splice together DNA fragments for cloning or other purposes.

A variety of other DNA- or RNA-modifying enzymes also available for the analysis of gene structure and expression are listed in Table 1–1. These enzymes function in a number of very specific ways, including synthesis of DNA or RNA, controlled degradation of single- or double-stranded DNA or RNA, and site-specific methylation of DNA. As is observed later in this chapter and throughout this book, these enzymes have significant utility in cloning procedures, in preparation of hybridization probes, in characterization of isolated genes, and in DNA sequencing.

Vectors

A vector is a DNA molecule that is capable of replicating in a bacterial cell and that can be readily isolated in pure form from bacterial cells. Insertion of a foreign DNA fragment into a vector, using restriction endonucleases and DNA- or RNA-modifying enzymes, as previously described, results in replication of the inserted fragment along with the vector and eventual isolation in pure form of the DNA fragment of interest.

TABLE 1–1. DNA- AND RNA-MODIFYING ENZYMES

ENZYME	FUNCTION
DNA polymerase I	1. Template-dependent synthesis of DNA in the 5′→3′ direction 2. 5′→3′ degradation of double-stranded DNA 3. 3′→5′ degradation of single- or double-stranded DNA
DNA polymerase I, large (Klenow) fragment	Same as (1) and (3) for DNA polymerase I
T4 DNA polymerase	Same as DNA polymerase I, large fragment
Sequenase (T7 DNA polymerase-modified)	Same as (1) for DNA polymerase I
Taq DNA polymerase	1. Same as (1) for DNA polymerase I 2. Optimal incorporation at 75–80°C
RNA-dependent DNA polymerase (reverse transcriptase)	Template-dependent synthesis of DNA in the 5′→3′ direction; RNA or DNA can be used as a template
T4 polynucleotide kinase	Transfer of the γ-phosphate of ATP to a 5′—OH group on DNA or RNA
Alkaline phosphatase (*E. coli* or calf intestine)	Removal of 5′-phosphate from DNA or RNA
*Bal*31	Exonucleolytic degradation of both the 5′ and 3′ termini of DNA
Nuclease S1	Endonuclease that is specific for single-stranded DNA or RNA or single-stranded regions in DNA or RNA
Mung bean nuclease	Similar to nuclease S1
SP6 RNA polymerase	Template-dependent synthesis of RNA in the 5′→3′ direction from a double-stranded DNA template containing an SP6 promotor
T7 RNA polymerase	Similar to SP6 RNA polymerase except it requires a T7 promotor
Ribonuclease A	An endoribonuclease that cleaves RNA on the 3′ side of pyrimidine (C or U) residues, leaving a 3′-phosphate
Ribonuclease T1	Similar to ribonuclease A except that cleavage occurs on the 3′ side of G residues
Terminal deoxynucleotidyl transferase	Template-independent synthesis of DNA in the 5′→3′ direction
*Eco*RI methylase	Methylates the *Eco*RI recognition sequence, thus preventing cleavage by *Eco*RI

Four broad classes of vectors are used for cloning in *Escherichia coli*. These include plasmids, single-stranded bacteriophage, bacteriophage λ, and cosmids. Each type of vector system has particular features that are advantageous for certain situations. In the following sections, we present the important aspects of each vector system and describe how each system can be used.

Plasmids

Plasmids are closed circular double-stranded DNA molecules that are capable of extrachromosomal replication in bacterial cells. Plasmids can vary in size from several hundred base pairs to several hundred kilobase pairs (kb; a kilobase pair represents 1000 base pairs). Plasmid cloning vectors are specially designed small plasmids with three essential features:

1. An origin of DNA replication.
2. A selectable marker (usually an antibiotic resistance gene).
3. Suitable sites for cloning.

The replication origin is a DNA sequence that is necessary for replication of the plasmid in the bacterial cell, usually independent of replication of the cellular DNA. The replication origin thus confers the property of replication to high copy number on the plasmid and also provides a mechanism for maintenance of the plasmid sequence in the bacterial cells.

The selectable marker on a plasmid is used to provide a substantial selective advantage to cells that contain the plasmid over cells that do not and thus aids in selecting cells that have stably incorporated plasmids. Most useful selectable markers on plasmid cloning vectors are bacterial genes specifying resistance to one or more antibiotics through a variety of mechanisms. As a tool for molecular cloning, selectable markers provide a simple means to identify bacterial cells containing sequences derived from the parent vector plasmid and also a way to ensure that a plasmid is not lost from a bacterial cell population by supplying a continual selection for those cells containing a plasmid.

Finally, to insert a foreign DNA fragment easily into a plasmid, there must be at least one region in the plasmid that is non-essential for plasmid growth or selection and that can be modified by insertion. This insertion is greatly facilitated through the use of restriction endonucleases, and many plasmid vectors have been highly engineered so that the number and location of restriction endonuclease cleavage sites permit easy introduction and excision of foreign DNA into the plasmid.

Beyond these essential plasmid components, many vectors have incorporated additional sequences that confer novel capabilities on plasmids. These components include the following:

1. **Multiple restriction endonuclease sites** arranged in tandem, known as polylinkers, that provide target sites for incorporation of DNA fragments generated by a variety of restriction endonucleases and facilitate the excision and/or analysis of the inserted fragment.

2. **Replication origins for single-stranded phage** so that the plasmid DNA can be easily converted into a single-stranded DNA form, analogous to the DNAs of single-stranded cloning vectors (see below).

3. **Cloning sites within the coding region of a protein** so that a fusion protein is produced. Such a fusion protein can be used to identify the gene of interest through screening for the fused protein (see below).

4. **Recognition sites for RNA polymerases** that can be used to produce RNA copies of part or all of the inserted gene.

A diagram of a prototypical plasmid cloning vector is shown in Figure 1–1. This plasmid, known as pUC119,[6] has a *col*E1-type origin of replication (which permits replication to high copy number in a cell), with the antibiotic resistance gene conferring ampicillin resistance, a polylinker sequence containing recognition sequences for 13 restriction endonucleases and capable of incorporating DNA digested with any of a vast number of different individual restriction endonucleases alone and in combination, and the origin of single-stranded DNA replication from the filamentous phage M13, which is capable of generating single-stranded DNA. This plasmid is representative of a wide variety of plasmid cloning vectors now available that have greatly simplified many basic cloning operations and have made possible more complex operations; a complete listing is beyond the scope of this chapter. The entire DNA sequence of PUC119 and most other useful plasmid cloning vectors is known. This information is useful in the precise characterization of newly isolated plasmids.

A crucial step in the use of plasmids as cloning vectors was the development of techniques for the introduction of in vitro–modified DNA into single bacterial cells. The method most extensively used is to expose the cells to one or more divalent cations under the appropriate conditions. This treatment renders the cell "competent" to take up extracellular DNA and express this exogenous genetic information. Following exposure of competent cells to DNA and a brief period of recovery, a selective agent can be used to identify those cells expressing the selectable marker. More

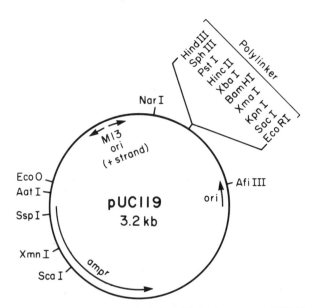

FIGURE 1–1. The prototypical plasmid cloning vector pUC119.

recently, exposure of bacterial cells to DNA in a pulsed, high electric field environment (electroporation) has been shown to be a highly efficient means of introducing DNA into bacterial cells.

A diagram depicting the important features of cloning in plasmids is shown in Figure 1–2. The plasmid vector is digested with the appropriate restriction endonuclease (or endonucleases), which will result in linearization of the circular plasmid DNA and which will leave ends compatible with the ends of the DNA fragment to be cloned. The DNA to be cloned is digested with an endonuclease, mixed with the digested plasmid vector DNA at the appropriate ratio and concentration, and ligated. From among the various ligation products that are possible, a closed circular DNA with a single vector and a single insert molecule will be generated. This DNA is then used to "transform" competent bacterial cells, and the resulting cell population is spread on an agar plate containing one or more antibiotics. Those cells that have incorporated the circular recombinant molecule,

which still contains the selectable marker, will be capable of growth, forming a bacterial colony. All other cells that have not incorporated a circular plasmid molecule will not grow or will be killed in the presence of the antibiotic. Plasmid DNA from those colonies that do form can then be further analyzed to verify that the desired product has been obtained.

Single-Stranded Phage Cloning Vectors

M13 and F1 are bacteriophages that produce particles containing circular single-stranded DNA.[7] During the life cycle of these viruses (Fig. 1–3), phage particles containing circular single-stranded DNA enter the cell, and the single-stranded DNA is converted to a circular double-stranded form called a replicative form (RF), identical in structure to plasmid DNA. This RF replicates until other viral gene products shift the replication to the production of single-stranded progeny virion DNA later in the cycle. This DNA is unique in

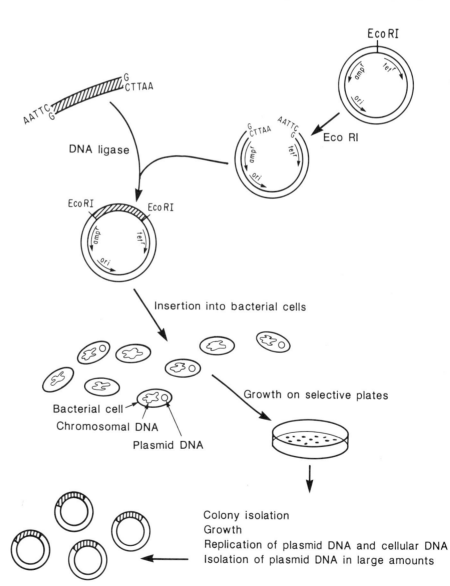

FIGURE 1–2. The process of cloning a DNA fragment into a plasmid cloning vector.

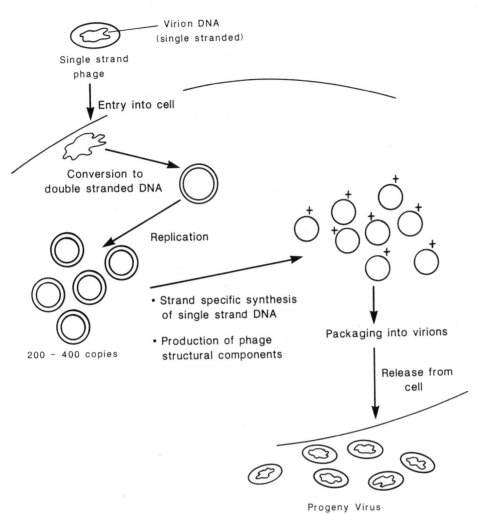

FIGURE 1–3. The life cycle of a single-stranded phage.

that it represents only one of the two possible complementary DNA (cDNA) strands.

Cloning in such phages utilizes the intracellular double-stranded RF DNA for manipulations, in a manner analogous to cloning in plasmids. First, the M13 or F1 origin of replication serves a function analogous to the plasmid origin of replication. Second, the function of the selectable markers is replaced by the characteristic growth of the phage on a bacterial lawn, resulting in easily recognizable areas of slow bacterial growth, or "plaques." Third, multiple cloning sites have been built into highly engineered forms of the vector. In the most common type of single-stranded cloning vector (the "M13mp" series), the polylinker is engineered into a portion of the β-galactosidase gene. Insertion of a foreign DNA fragment into this gene usually results in inactivation of the β-galactosidase gene and a characteristic and easily recognizable phenotype of white plaques on special indicator plates containing a chromogenic substrate. This feature makes identification of recombinants in M13 very simple.

Cloning in M13 is facile owing to similarity to cloning in plasmids as well as to simple procedures for preparation of large quantities of DNA. However, the primary advantage of cloning in single-stranded phage vectors is that progeny-virus DNA represents only one of the two DNA strands, as previously noted. Which of the two strands is produced depends on the orientation of the insert in the cloning sites and can be easily determined. This single-stranded DNA has many useful applications, such as DNA sequencing, probe preparation, and mutagenesis. Some of these applications are presented later.

The prototypical single-stranded phage cloning vector M13mp8 is shown in Figure 1–4.

As noted above, plasmids containing the origin region from a single-stranded phage have been constructed. These are frequently known as "phagemids." These phagemids have a useful property in that infection by a single-stranded helper phage of cells containing such plasmids results in the production of virion particles containing single-stranded DNA derived from the plasmid DNA (the superinfecting phage is engineered to be non-productive in the plasmid-containing cell). The orientation of the insert in the cloning vector determines which of the two insert strands is produced. Such vectors maximize the simplicity and stability of cloning in plasmids and the utility of single-stranded DNA phage.

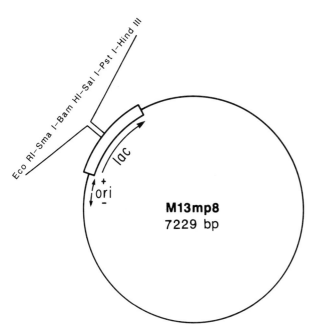

FIGURE 1–4. The prototypical single-stranded phage cloning vector M13mp8.

Bacteriophage λ

One of the earliest, most widely used vectors for cloning large mammalian genes was bacteriophage λ. This large (50,000 bp) double-stranded DNA-containing virus had been intensively studied for many years, and a considerable background on the understanding of the molecular genetics, biochemistry, and structure of bacteriophage λ has developed. In addition, it has been known for many years that the central third of the genome can be removed and replaced by fragments of *E. coli* DNA. An analysis of the bacteriophage λ map (shown in Fig. 1–5) reveals how and why λ can be used as a cloning vector. The gene functions in λ are located on the physical map in functional clusters that reflect the two pathways of replication possible with λ. In the lytic pathway, the infecting virus replicates to produce more infectious virus, ultimately killing the cell and releasing viral particles following lysis. For lytic growth, only the genes located between 0 and 20 kb and 40 and 50 kb are required. These

genes code for replicative and structural components of the virus. By contrast, during lysogenic growth, the genes between 0 and 20 kb and 41 and 50 kb are not expressed, and the genes located between 21 and 40 kb are used to insert the infecting λ genome into the *E. coli* chromosome and to maintain it in that form, replicating within the cellular DNA. Bacteriophage λ as a cloning vector is most frequently used as a lytic virus, although there are instances in which lysogenic growth is exploited.

To understand how λ is used as a cloning vector (and also cosmids, as discussed below), it is necessary to examine certain details of normal λ lytic growth. The mature λ genome (as isolated from infectious phage) contains at each end a 12 nt single-stranded tail, or "sticky end." The sticky ends at the left and right ends are complementary to each other, and following infection of a bacterial cell with a λ phage particle, these ends ligate, forming a circular λ genome. During replication of this circular DNA via a "rolling circle" mechanism, a long concatemer of λ monomers is produced. The sticky end sequence and adjacent sequences (known together as the COS sites) then form the recognition sites for cleaving this long concatemeric DNA into unit-length monomers during the normal morphogenesis of infectious λ particles that occurs in infected cells (known as DNA packaging). This cleavage regenerates the sticky ends, and the mature phage DNA is then inserted into an empty phage head, forming an infectious phage particle, thereby completing the cycle.

Recombinant λ phage DNA can enter this cycle by preparing DNA similar in structure to the concatenated λ DNA in vitro, using fragments of λ DNA, the foreign DNA to be inserted, and DNA ligase. This in vitro assembled DNA is then incorporated into viable phage particles using the procedure known as in vitro packaging. This procedure relies on the observation that the normal morphogenesis of an infectious λ particle occurring in a bacterial cell can be made to occur in vitro. By using a variety of genetic and physiological tricks, cell "extracts" can be prepared that can be used to insert ("package") any intact or recombinant λ genomes into viable phage particles, which can then be used to infect cells efficiently. The structure of the bacteriophage λ DNA to be packaged

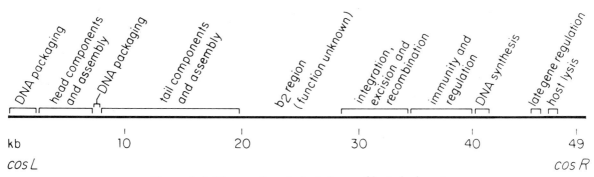

FIGURE 1–5. The genetic and physical map of bacteriophage λ.

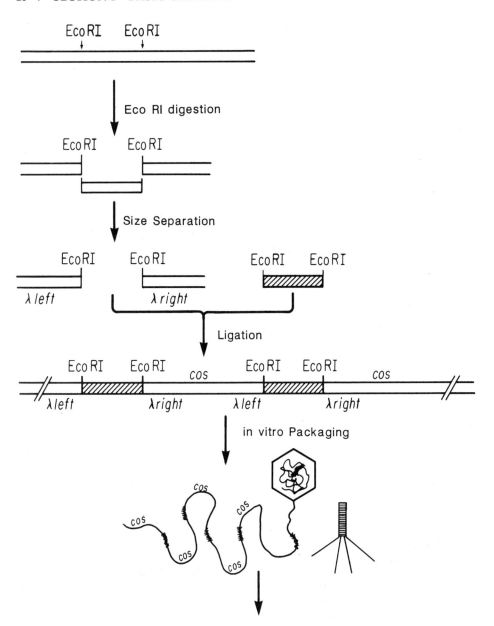

FIGURE 1–6. Cloning in bacteriophage λ vectors.

is important in obtaining optimal efficiency and should resemble as closely as possible the in vivo substrate, concatemeric bacteriophage λ DNA.

The original process of cloning large DNA in λ is diagrammed in Figure 1–6.[8] The vector is designed to contain one or more restriction endonuclease cleavage sites that separate the central replaceable region from the 0 to 20 kb and 40 to 50 kb regions (usually referred to as the λ left and λ right "arms") essential for lytic λ growth. Digestion with the appropriate enzyme, followed by size fractionation, results in the preparation of the vector arms. The fragment of interest is cleaved with the same (or compatible) restriction endonuclease and is ligated to the purified vector arms. Because the λ left and λ right sticky ends will also ligate to each other at the appropriate con-

centration of vectors and insert, concatemers will form, some of which have the structure shown in Figure 1–6. This concatemeric molecule can then be packaged in vitro to produce an infectious recombinant phage particle containing the desired insert fragment.

Vectors for Cloning Large DNA Fragments

As a practical matter, it is difficult to clone fragments larger than about 10 to 15 kb in plasmids owing to difficulties in generating large circular DNAs in vitro and inefficiencies in the uptake of large circular DNA into bacterial cells by standard transformation protocols. Moreover, there is an upper limit (20 to 24 kb) on the size of DNA that can be cloned in bacteriophage λ because of size limitations on the amount of DNA that can be incorporated into a bacteriophage head and the genes necessary for lytic growth of λ. These size limitations on cloning in plasmid or λ vectors are restrictive, and efficiency could be gained and some experiments made possible if vectors that accept larger DNA inserts were available. The original solution to this problem was the development of cosmid cloning vectors. Cosmids are cloning vectors designed to incorporate up to 45 kb of foreign DNA. More recently, bacteriophage P1 cloning vectors that can incorporate up to 100 kb have been utilized, as well as yeast artificial chromosomes, which can incorporate several hundred kilobases. These cloning systems are described in more detail below.

Cosmid vectors accomplish the cloning of large DNA fragments by combining the small size of a plasmid vector with the limited requirements for packaging DNA into a bacteriophage λ infectious particle.[9] A cosmid vector and the cloning process are outlined in Figure 1–7. Like plasmids, cosmid vectors have a plasmid replication origin, a selectable marker, and cloning sites. From bacteriophage λ, cosmid vectors have utilized the COS site, the region in λ that is recognized during cleavage of the intracellular concatemeric λ DNA into DNA monomers for insertion into the phage head.

To clone a large fragment in a cosmid vector, the vector is first linearized with a restriction endonuclease and then ligated at high concentration to the large DNA fragment to produce concatemers of the cosmid vector and insert, some of which have the following structure:

ori	amp	ori	amp

COS   45 kb   COS

→   →

| ←   COSMID   → |

The only requirements for packaging of DNA into bacteriophage λ particles is the presence of two COS sites in the proper orientation separated by 38 to 52 kb. Thus, the concatemer shown above can be packaged into a phage particle and, during the process, is cleaved within each COS region to produce the characteristic λ sticky ends. Following infection of a bacterial cell, the DNA then circularizes via the sticky ends and forms a large plasmid, complete with replication origin and selectable marker.

Bacteriophage P1 offers an alternative approach for cloning large fragments that is very similar in principle to cosmid cloning but is based on bacteriophage P1 instead of λ.[10] P1 is a bacteriophage containing a double-stranded DNA genome that can be as large as 110 kb. The genomic DNA contains specialized genes and sequences for specific cleavage of the DNA during the packaging process (known as pacase and the pac site) as well as sequences (loxP) and genes (Cre, or recombinase) for circularization of the genome within the newly infected cell. The pac site is the sequence that the pacase cleaves to initiate the process of inserting DNA into the bacteriophage head. After approx-

imately 100 to 110 kb of DNA is inserted into the head, another enzyme cleaves the DNA to complete the DNA insertion process, and the remainder of the infectious phage is then assembled. Upon infection of the host cell by these phages, the linear DNA is injected into the cell, and the product of the Cre gene (the recombinase) recognizes loxP sites arranged in the same orientation on a DNA molecule and generates a circular DNA molecule by stimulating recombination at the loxP sites. The phage DNA then replicates as a circular DNA and goes on to produce progeny phage. Vectors have been designed with these sequences, and specialized hosts or bacterial packaging strains have been generated with the particular genes; in combination, these vectors and hosts have been utilized for cloning large fragments, as outlined in Figure 1–8. The vector is designed so that the polylinker cloning site (for accepting 100 kb fragments of DNA) and a plasmid replication origin and selectable marker are located between two loxP sites. Any DNA located between these sites will, upon transfection into an appropriate host, be converted into a circular DNA molecule through the action of the Cre gene on the loxP sites. The plasmid replication origin and selectable marker on the vector permit the maintenance of this circular DNA within the host cell, generating a stable recombinant.

Finally, a system that is capable in principle of cloning even larger fragments of DNA has been developed in yeast.[11] This approach is based on recent understanding of the cis-acting sequence elements required for chromosome stability in yeast, including centromeric sequences (the sequences required for chromosome segregation at mitosis), telomeres (the sequences that define the ends of the yeast chromosome), and origins of replication (known as ARS for autonomously replicating sequences) as well as methods to introduce DNA into yeast more efficiently. Vectors have been designed with these sequences (as well as with sequences needed for growth of the vector in bacteria) and multiple cloning sites; these vectors have been successfully used to clone fragments larger than 500 kb. These vectors are known as YAC (yeast artificial chromosome) vectors.

Construction of Gene Libraries

The most commonly used and most successful approach to the primary isolation of a particular gene begins with the construction of a set of recombinant clones from some source known to contain the sequence of interest. This collection of clones is usually termed a "library" and, in principle, contains all sequences represented in the source nucleic acid. Clones of interest can then be isolated from the library, using any of a variety of screening techniques, as is discussed in a subsequent section. Libraries can be divided into two categories: cDNA libraries, which represent DNA copies of the mRNA population within a cell, and genomic libraries, which are derived from the genomic

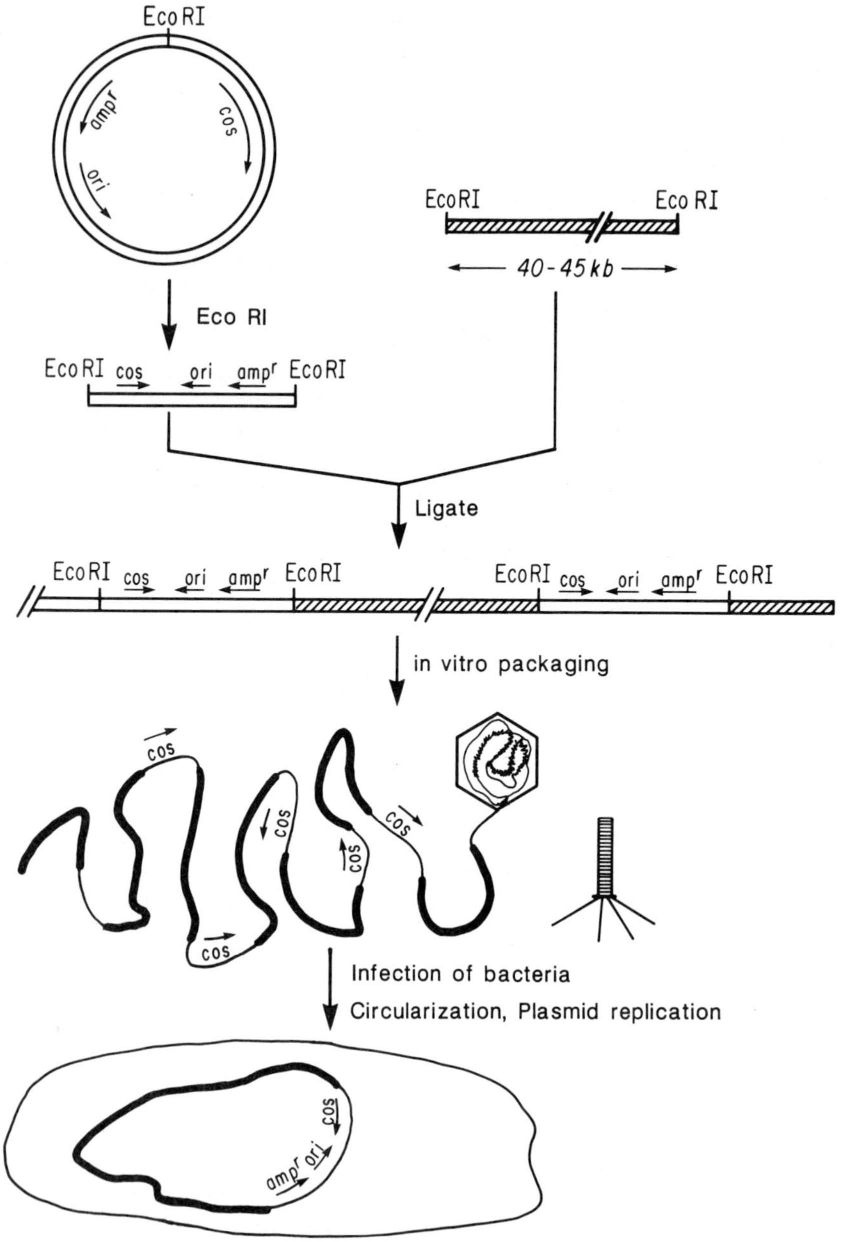

FIGURE 1–7. Cloning in a cosmid vector.

DNA of an organism. The methods of construction and the utility of each type of library are different and are discussed in the following sections.

cDNA Cloning

The messenger RNA (mRNA) population within a cell is unique in two respects. First, mRNA in a given cell type represents a specific subset of the total genetic information of the organism. In highly specialized cells, such as the red cell, the mRNA consists of nearly a single message—globin. In most cell types, however, there are some mRNAs unique to that particular cell and others that are in common with many or most other cell types. Thus, mRNA provides the possibility for focusing on the narrowly defined set of genes that are expressed in a particular type of cell. Cellular

mRNA in eukaryotes is also unique in that it represents a continuous coding strand for its protein product. This is in contrast to the corresponding genomic DNA, in which the coding strand is usually interrupted by one or more introns.

Since no methods exist for cloning mRNA directly and because methods for detailed structural and sequential characterization of RNA are inadequate, techniques were developed to synthesize and to clone DNA copies of mRNA (cDNA). Critical to the development of these techniques were the identification and isolation from retroviruses of the enzyme RNA-dependent DNA polymerase (reverse transcriptase). This enzyme has the helpful property of using RNA as a template and of synthesizing a DNA strand. Like all DNA polymerases, reverse transcriptase requires a primer to initiate DNA synthesis. Most commonly, the small

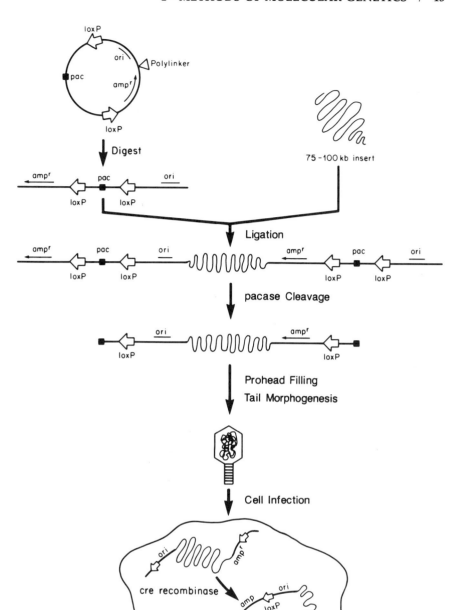

FIGURE 1–8. Cloning in a P1 vector.

homopolymer oligo dT_{12-18} is used as a primer to make cDNA. The oligo dT is annealed to the poly A tail on the mRNA, and under the appropriate conditions, the entire mRNA is copied and the cDNA strand is produced (Fig. 1–9). Any of several methods are then used to convert the single-stranded cDNA/mRNA hybrid into a double-stranded molecule.

Today, the most commonly used approach to convert the single-stranded cDNA/mRNA hybrid into a double-stranded DNA is by replacement synthesis[12] (see Fig. 1–9). With use of the enzymes *E. coli* RNase H (an enzyme that produces nicks and gaps in the RNA strand of an RNA/DNA hybrid) and *E. coli* DNA polymerase I, the RNA strand of the hybrid gets nicked by RNase H, and these nicked sites serve as primers for initiation of DNA synthesis to fill in the gaps. Eventually, most of the strand has been copied in pieces to second-strand cDNA, and DNA ligase is used to seal the fragments into an intact second strand.

Insertion of this double-stranded DNA into a vector then requires modification of the ends of the cDNA and the vector so that the cDNA can join to the vector. Originally, complementary homopolymeric tails (e.g., poly dC and poly dG) were added to the ends of the cDNA and vector using the enzyme terminal transferase and one deoxyribonucleotide triphosphate substrate. The tailed vector and cDNA were then annealed and inserted into a cell. Although the procedure was successful, the efficiency was low and the resulting cDNA clones were difficult to analyze. Most cDNA cloning now is done using synthetic linkers (see Fig. 1–9). These small synthetic duplex fragments

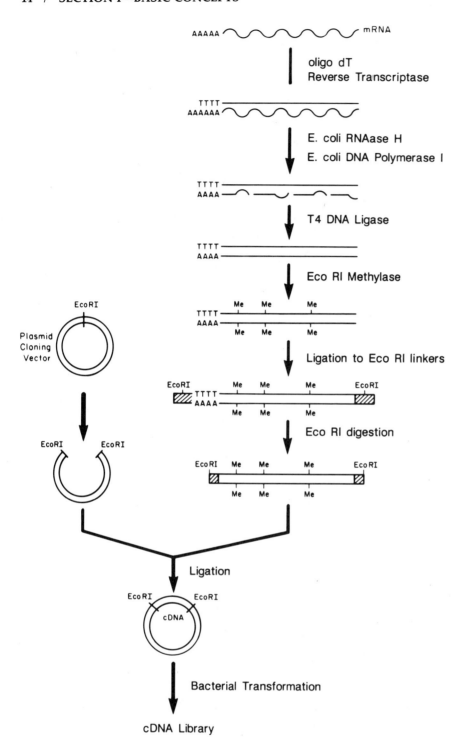

FIGURE 1–9. cDNA cloning utilizing replacement synthesis and synthetic linkers.

consist of 8 to 20 bp segments that contain the sequence of a restriction endonuclease cleavage site. Ligation of the linkers to both ends of the cDNA and digestion produce cDNA molecules with single-stranded tails specific for the restriction endonuclease used. Digestion of recognition sites that might be present in the cDNA can be prevented by treating the cDNA (before linker addition) with a methylase specific for the chosen recognition site (see Table 1–1). In the example shown in Figure 1–9, *Eco*RI methylase specifically methylates 1 nt in the recognition site and

prevents cleavage by the complementary restriction endonuclease. These modified cDNAs can now be ligated to the appropriate vector DNA molecule. A variety of linkers (and corresponding methylases) can now be used. One useful variation on this approach includes the use of specialized oligonucleotides as primers of first-strand cDNA synthesis containing oligo dT linked to the sequence of a rare cutting restriction endonuclease (e.g., *Not* I). When cDNA is constructed with this primer for first strand, the 3' end of the cDNA will contain the recognition sequence for *Not* I, whereas the 5' end will contain the sequence specified by the linker/methylase/endonuclease combination. This cDNA is now "directional," having a different cleavage site at each end, and can be inserted into a vector in a specific orientation. This modification is particularly useful when attempting to express the resulting cDNAs in the host cells; specifying the orientation reduces by 50 per cent the number of clones that need to be constructed or screened.

A variety of cloning vectors are available for cDNA cloning. Classically, plasmid vectors were used; almost any plasmid vector can be used, although a number have been designed specifically for this purpose. More recently, though, bacteriophage λ has become a vector of choice for constructing large libraries of cDNA clones. This shift was based on the development of λ vectors (the "gt" series) that readily accept small (0 to 7 kb) inserts of DNA and that have selection schemes for enrichment of those phage-containing inserts.[13] The use of these vectors coupled with the high efficiency of introducing recombinant DNA into bacteria through in vitro DNA packaging has immensely improved the efficiency of most cDNA cloning procedures. For certain purposes, such as for screening by expression, particular plasmid or phage λ vectors containing transcription and translation signals adjacent to the cloning site have been developed.

The complexity of the mRNA population determines the complexity of the resulting cDNA. A population of cDNA clones that are derived from the mRNA of a particular cell or tissue type is usually referred to as a cDNA library. The construction, amplification, and storage of a high-quality cDNA library has the obvious advantage of representing continuing access to a set of cDNA clones for all the genes being expressed in a cell in a particular stage of development or differentiation.

Once constructed, a cDNA library must be screened to identify the clone of interest, using any of several methods described below. Obviously, the level of difficulty of this task depends on the abundance of the mRNA in the cell, the quality of the library, and the method of screening. Particularly important are the construction of full-length cDNA clones, especially if an expressed biological activity is to be measured, and the number of clones in the library, especially for rare mRNAs. There must, on average, be enough independent clones in the library to ensure that one or more copies of the desired clone are present.

Fractionation of the mRNA or other enrichment procedures prior to cloning can significantly reduce the number of clones to be screened. These enrichment procedures usually depend on having two closely related but non-identical cell types available. A large excess of synthesized single-stranded cDNA or single-stranded DNA from a library prepared in a single-stranded cloning vector from one cell type is used to hybridize to mRNA or first-strand cDNA from the second related cell type. Those sequences that hybridize are enriched for sequences in common, whereas those that do not hybridize are enriched for unique sequences. This approach is particularly useful in identifying rare and cell-specific genes.

Genomic Cloning

A detailed analysis of the structure and function of the chromosomal DNA of an organism is crucial to understanding the complex expression of genetic information during development and differentiation. One of the most useful approaches for gathering detailed information on gene structure is the cloning of genomic DNA.

Just as for cDNA cloning, cloning of genomic DNA is accomplished most efficiently through the construction of a collection of recombinant clones that together contain most of the sequences found in the DNA of an organism. This collection of clones is termed a genomic library and is constructed as shown in Figure 1–10. High molecular weight genomic DNA is first partially digested with a restriction endonuclease that cuts frequently, such as *Sau*3AI. *Sau*3AI recognizes the four-base sequence 5' . . . GATC . . . 3' and should produce fragments of 256 bp (4^4) on average. However, the extent of digestion is controlled, so that the average size of the DNA products is approximately 20,000 bp. Optimally, though not necessarily, the DNA is then fractionated by size (e.g., by agarose gel electrophoresis), and DNA in the range of 18 to 20 kb is selected. In this manner, a near-random collection of large, uniformly sized DNA fragments from the genome is produced. A bacteriophage λ vector is then chosen based on the presence of a cloning site compatible with the partially digested genomic DNA and the ability to accept inserts of 18 to 20 kb. For example, to clone genomic DNA that has been digested with *Sau*3AI, a vector containing *Bam*HI cloning sites is used. *Bam*HI is chosen because the single-stranded terminus left following *Bam*HI digestion (below)

$$5' \ldots \text{pGpGpApTpCpC} \ldots 3'$$
$$3' \ldots \text{pCpCpTpApGpG} \ldots 5' \quad \rightarrow \quad 5' \ldots \text{pGpApTpCpC} \ldots 3'$$
$$\text{HO–G} \ldots 5'$$
$$\textit{Bam}\text{HI}$$

is the same (and therefore complementary because it is palindromic) as the single-stranded terminus produced by *Sau*3AI:

$$5' \ldots \downarrow \text{pGpApTpC} \ldots 3'$$
$$3' \ldots \quad \text{CpTpApGp} \uparrow \quad \rightarrow \quad 5' \ldots \text{pGpApTpC} \ldots 3'$$
$$\text{HO} \ldots 5'$$
$$\textit{Sau}\text{3AI}$$

The two types of ends can therefore ligate together. Following digestion with *Bam*HI, the left and right phage fragments (or "arms") are purified, usually by agarose gel electrophoresis or another sizing method. As discussed earlier, at the appropriate concentrations of vector and insert fragments, ligation results in long concatemeric molecules that are efficiently recognized in an in vitro packaging system and can be inserted into a phage head, forming an infectious phage particle. The object of this is to produce enough independent recombinant phage to ensure that nearly all

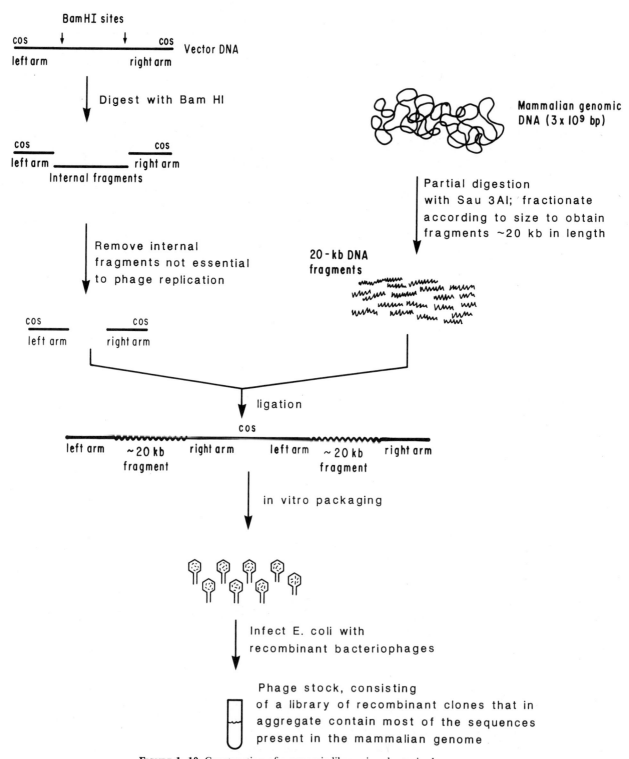

FIGURE 1–10. Construction of a genomic library in a bacteriophage vector.

sequences in the genome will be present. For example, for a typical mammalian genome (3×10^9 bp), approximately 7×10^5 recombinants with an average size of 20 kb are required to have a 99 per cent probability that any DNA sequence will be present in the library. This large collection of phage can be amplified and stored, forming a "permanent" genomic library. This library can then be used multiple times to isolate many different genes.

Similar methods are used to prepare libraries in cosmid, bacteriophage P1, or YAC vectors. In these cases, the partial digestion of genomic DNA is adjusted so that the average size is approximately 40 to 45 kb (for cosmids), 90 to 100 kb (for P1), or more than 250 kb (for YACs). For cloning in cosmids and P1, it is usually desirable to purify the DNA with this size range; it is impractical to purify the DNA of more than 250 kb for cloning into YACs. The primary advantage of cloning in cosmid, P1, or YAC vectors rather than λ vectors is the much larger sizes of inserts that can be accommodated. Thus, fewer clones are required for a "complete" library. However, this feature can be a disadvantage in that some large eukaryotic fragments are not stable in bacteria and rearrangements can occur.

Construction of partial digest libraries by limited digestion of genomic DNA with enzymes that recognize many sequences in the genome produces a series of overlapping clones covering the genome. Thus, once a given gene or portion of a gene is isolated, it is possible to "walk" along the chromosome to adjacent sequences by a continual process of selecting overlapping clones. In this way, entire gene clusters can be obtained.

Identification of Recombinant Clones

Once recombinant DNA has been inserted into bacterial cells as a plasmid or as a growing phage, it is important to be able to identify and to isolate specifically the desired recombinant. The complexity of this process depends on the abundance of the desired recombinant in the population of cells or viruses to be examined and on the means by which the correct clone can be identified. In the simplest situations, the desired clone can be identified by direct DNA sequencing (e.g., more than 50 per cent of cDNA clones from red cell mRNA are globin clones). More commonly, though, one of several screening approaches needs to be utilized before sequencing is possible. The most common screening approach is based on using nucleic acid hybridization with ^{32}P-labeled DNA or RNA probes specific for the sequence of interest. Methods for preparation of ^{32}P-labeled probes are described in the following text.

To detect specific plasmid DNAs in bacterial colonies (colony hybridization), bacteria are spread over the surface of a culture dish at low density and incubated until colonies appear (Fig. 1–11). A piece of nitrocellulose filter paper is then gently placed over the colonies on the surface of the culture dish and removed after 10 to 30 seconds. Most of each colony is removed with the filter paper, forming a replica of the colonies on the dish. This replica can then be treated with NaOH to lyse the bacteria and denature the DNA; the single-stranded DNA is fixed to the filter paper by baking at 80°C. Hybridization of this replica with ^{32}P-labeled probes under conditions in which only exact or nearly exact complementary sequences will hybridize, followed by washing and autoradiographic detection, results in an autoradiographic signal indicating the position of the desired recombinant. The viable cell is then recovered from the culture dish and purified. A similar procedure is available for screening bacteriophage λ plaques.

^{32}P-labeled probes can be prepared by a variety of methods from existing cloned DNAs: nick-translation, M13 synthesis, and SP6 RNA synthesis. (See Preparation of Radiolabeled Probes, below.) The probe must have the features that make it single stranded in at least the region that will hybridize to the sequence of interest and that give it enough ^{32}P atoms per molecule (i.e., specific activity) to ensure that a signal can be detected following hybridization and autoradiography. DNA from which a probe is prepared could represent a portion of, or a form of, the desired clone, an analogous clone from a related species, or a partially related gene. The conditions used for hybridization thus depend on the relation of the probe to the desired sequence. In many cases the ^{32}P-labeled probe is a synthetic oligonucleotide with a sequence deduced from the partial amino acid sequence of a purified protein, as shown in Figure 1–12. By using hybridization conditions in which only perfectly matched oligonucleotides will hybridize, high specificity can be achieved. This technique has proved invaluable in the isolation of both cDNA and genomic clones for many proteins that can be purified in only small amounts.

A second means of clone identification for genes that code for proteins is to attempt direct expression of a cDNA copy of the mRNA in *E. coli* (Fig. 1–13). Several vectors, both plasmid and bacteriophage λ, have been designed for this purpose. Usually, the protein produced is a fusion protein between a specific bacterial gene (such as β-galactosidase) and a portion of the gene encoded by the inserted cDNA. The objective is to synthesize in the bacterium one or more antigenic determinants of the sought-for protein and to identify the bacterial colonies containing such an antigen by specific binding of a polyclonal or monoclonal antibody.[14]

Another type of expression approach to clone identification is to attempt expression of a biologically active protein and to use some biological assay for identification. This type of approach can be particularly useful in the isolation of genes for polypeptides with high biological specific activity, such as polypeptide hormones and growth factors. In some cases, if mutant strains are available, a simple complementation assay can be used (e.g., the isolation of a gene that can correct an auxotrophic mutation). In other cases, the

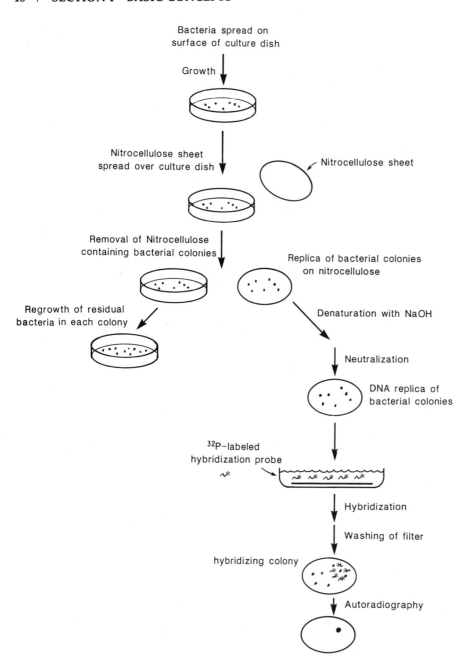

Bacteria spread on
surface of culture dish

Growth

Nitrocellulose sheet
spread over culture dish

Nitrocellulose sheet

Removal of Nitrocellulose
containing bacterial colonies

Replica of bacterial colonies
on nitrocellulose

Regrowth of residual
bacteria in each colony

Denaturation with NaOH

Neutralization

DNA replica of
bacterial colonies

^{32}P–labeled
hybridization probe

Hybridization

Washing of filter

hybridizing colony

Autoradiography

FIGURE 1–11. Identification of plasmid clones by colony hybridization.

desired gene product imparts a new property to the cell that can be easily identified (e.g., transformation by an oncogene and subsequent loss of growth control or expression of a cell surface molecule [such as a growth factor receptor or surface ligand] that can be detected by radiolabeled ligand binding, fluorescence-activated cell sorting [FACS], or binding to plates coated with antibody). Finally, as shown in Figure 1–14, polypeptides could be expressed in and secreted from cells transformed by the cloned DNA and the medium harvested. A sensitive biological assay is then used to determine whether the biological activity is present. By repeating this procedure on smaller and smaller groups of clones, the correct clone can be eventually identified.

Finally, the use of the polymerase chain reaction (PCR) has added a significant new approach to gene identification that can be used independently or in combination with gene libraries. This technique is discussed separately below.

In summary, a variety of approaches are available to identify recombinant clones containing specific gene sequences. The strategic decision regarding which approach to use depends on the availability of reagents (e.g., antibodies, related gene probes) and assays for the gene of interest, as well as the type of libraries that have been prepared. Table 1–2 summarizes the commonly used alternate strategies and how each can lead to the clone of interest. Of course, each gene will require its own strategy, and no predictions can be made regarding which strategy or strategies will ultimately be successful.

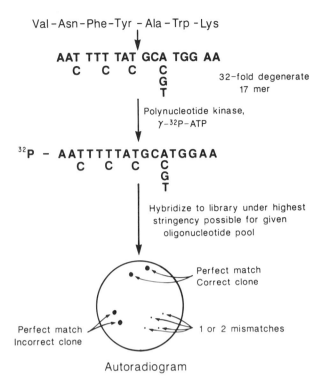

Val-Asn-Phe-Tyr-Ala-Trp-Lys

↓

AAT TTT TAT GCA TGG AA
 C   C   C   C
                 G
                 T

32-fold degenerate
17 mer

↓ Polynucleotide kinase,
γ-32P-ATP

32P - **AATTTTTATGCATGGAA**
     C   C   C   C
                   G
                   T

↓ Hybridize to library under highest
stringency possible for given
oligonucleotide pool

Perfect match
Correct clone

Perfect match
Incorrect clone

1 or 2 mismatches

Autoradiogram

Number of positives and range of intensities dependent on size and degeneracy of oligonucleotide, hybridization and washing conditions, and complexity of library being screened.

Figure 1–12. Screening cloned libraries with mixed-sequence oligonucleotide probes based on partial amino acid sequence analysis.

It should be appreciated that many of the techniques and reagents used in the cloning and identification of a particular gene are also helpful in subsequent characterization, once the desired clone is available. Some other uses of this technology are discussed in the next section.

Polymerase Chain Reaction

Probably the most important advance in molecular biological methods in the past decade has been the application of the PCR for the chemical amplification of nucleic acid sequences.[15] With this technique, undetectable and virtually unmanipulable levels of nucleic acids are transformed to detectable and biochemically manipulable levels. Similar in principle to molecular cloning techniques that use biological amplification, PCR has revolutionized the way in which molecular genetic studies are done.

Amplification in PCR arises from multiple cycles of a simple set of reactions. In each cycle (Fig. 1–15A), the double-stranded DNA template is first denatured with heat. After cooling, specific oligonucleotide primers designed to flank the DNA region of interest anneal to the template strands. A DNA polymerase is then used to copy the two DNA strands beginning at the oligonucleotide primers. The result is two double-stranded copies of the particular DNA region. By repeating this cycle, using the products of one cycle

as templates for the next, this region is exponentially amplified during each subsequent cycle (Fig. 1–15B). Thus, after 30 cycles, 2^{30} or 10^9 DNA fragments are generated from each initial template; starting with 1 μg of total mammalian genomic DNA, a 1 kb gene fragment, which represents only 0.3 pg of DNA, can be amplified to microgram levels.

Two advances allowed the PCR reaction to become practical for widespread use. The first is the inclusion of *Taq* polymerase in the reaction. Whereas most enzymes are inactivated upon heating and thus would have to be added at each cycle following the thermal denaturation step, *Taq* polymerase, isolated from the thermophilic bacterium *Thermus aquaticus,* is capable of retaining its full activity even after multiple cycles at high temperatures. The second advance is the design of instruments, called thermocyclers, which are capable of programmable rapid cycling between the various temperatures required for the PCR. With the use of these thermocyclers, a complete 30 cycle reaction can be completed in a matter of hours.

The desired PCR product is generally detected by gel electrophoresis of the total reaction products, which separates DNA fragments on the basis of size. Since the oligonucleotide primers are designed to be a particular distance apart, the size of the product can be predicted. Although certain applications make use of PCR alone, PCR is often combined with molecular

TABLE 1–2. STRATEGIES TO CONSIDER IN GENE CLONING

REAGENT OR INFORMATION AVAILABLE	APPROACH
Cloned DNA from related gene	1. Low-stringency hybridization screen of cDNA or genomic library 2. PCR with partially degenerate primers
Partial amino acid sequence analysis	1. Construction of oligonucleotide probes based on genetic code and screening of cDNA or genomic library 2. Synthesis of peptide fragment, immunization, isolation of specific polyclonal or monoclonal antisera, and screening by expression in *E. coli* 3. PCR with degenerate primers
Specific polyclonal or monoclonal antisera	1. Screening by expression in *E. coli* 2. Fractionation of mRNA, in vitro translation, and identification of enriched mRNA by immunoprecipitation 3. Hybrid selection of mRNA, using DNA from pooled cDNA clones and identification of pools containing correct cDNA by immunoprecipitation
Biological assay for protein of interest	Transform mammalian cells with cDNA or genomic library in appropriate vector and examine cells for desired phenotypic change or harvest supernatant media and assay biological activity

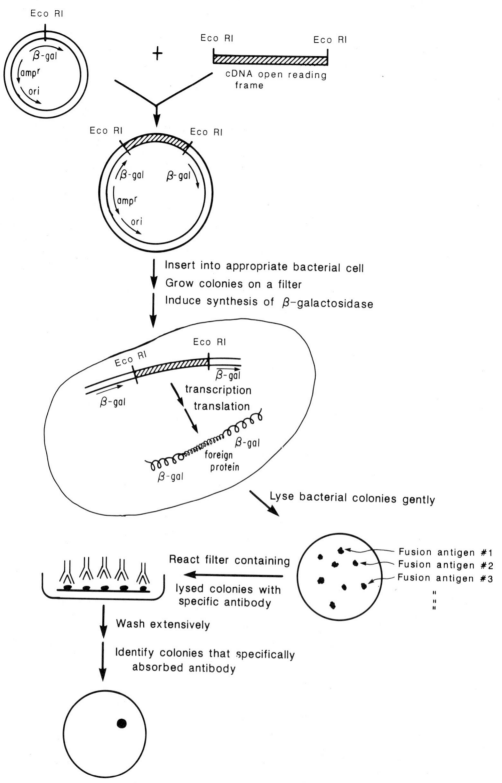

FIGURE 1–13. Cloning by expression in *Escherichia coli* and antibody screening.

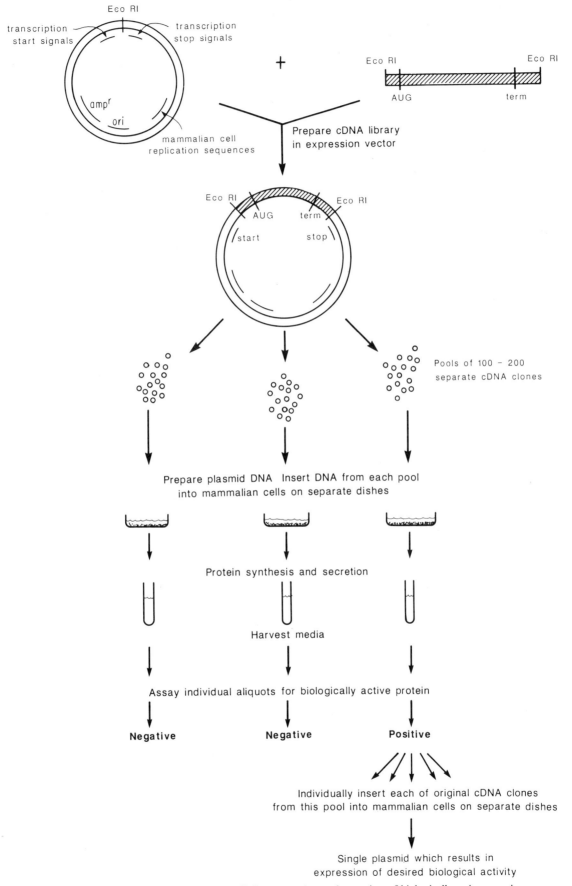

FIGURE 1–14. Cloning in mammalian cells by expression and secretion of biologically active protein.

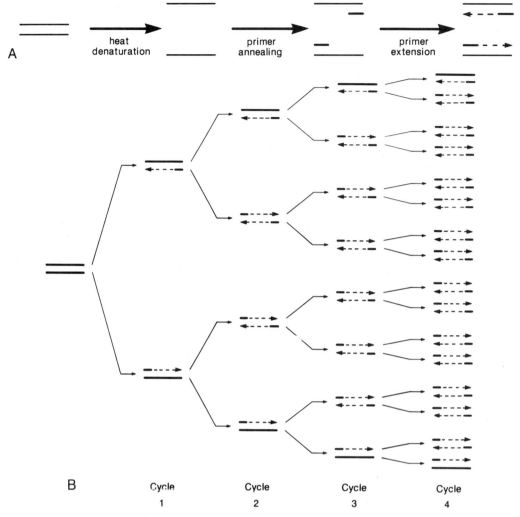

FIGURE 1–15. *A* and *B,* DNA amplification by polymerase chain reaction (PCR).

cloning. This combining is easily accomplished by the inclusion of the nucleotides for a restriction site at the ends of the primer oligonucleotides (Fig. 1–16). Although these sequences are not homologous to the original PCR template, the reaction products will con-

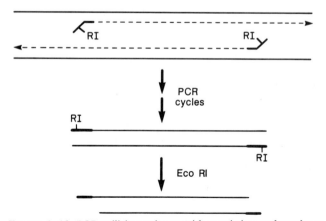

FIGURE 1–16. PCR utilizing primers with restriction endonuclease cleavage sites.

tain the primer oligonucleotide sequences at their ends, and virtually all products will contain these restriction enzyme sites. The PCR product can thus be digested with the corresponding restriction enzyme and easily cloned in a vector.

As with any technique, PCR does have certain pitfalls. Probably the most frequently encountered problem is reamplification of previous PCR products or other contaminating DNAs. Because PCR is so incredibly sensitive and able to detect and amplify single DNA molecules, minute contaminants from reagents, instruments, clothing, or the air can become major components of the reaction product. Techniques are now available whereby products from previous PCR can be destroyed and therefore made unavailable for further amplification. Misincorporation of nucleotides is also often encountered in PCR, probably owing in part to the fact that *Taq* polymerase does not contain a 3' to 5' exonuclease proofreading activity. Because of the nature of the reaction, a single misincorporation in one cycle is amplified throughout the reaction. Although adjustments to the reaction conditions have decreased this problem, care still must be exercised in the interpretation of single base pair changes relative to the expected product. Another problem intrinsic to PCR can be alleviated by isolation of the desired product after gel electrophoresis. Because the primer annealing step is not entirely specific under the conditions of the annealing, the primers sometimes bind to the incorrect sequence, and alternative or additional products are generated, especially when the template DNA is of high complexity. Since statistically these products are of random size or of a size different from that of the desired product, they can be separated and detected by gel electrophoresis. Aberrant product generation can also be decreased with the use of nested primers. In this instance, one set of primers is used for a first set of PCR reactions, and then another set of primers that lie inside the sequences used for the primary PCR is used. In this manner, only the correct sequences will be amplified in the second round. Another limitation of PCR is the size of the fragments that can be amplified. Although fragments as large as 10 kb can be amplified, in practical terms the specificity and efficiency of the reaction decrease dramatically at such sizes.

The uses of PCR appear to be limitless. PCR and subsequent recloning of known sequences have now become simple. Oligonucleotide primers of unique sequence can be synthesized based on the known sequence and used to create PCR products from a variety of sources, including genomic DNA, cDNA derived from mRNA, and cloned DNAs. This feature makes PCR particularly helpful in detecting mutations or polymorphisms within genes, and it has even been successfully used in such situations as amplification of DNA sequences from mummies, in which little intact DNA remains. The ability of oligonucleotide primers of inexact matching sequence to prime can be exploited in a number of applications. Deriving probes or clones of a specific gene from additional species is easily accomplished using primers based on the DNA sequence of a gene from a single species. This feature has allowed the rapid cloning of the same gene from multiple species for evolutionary examination. Site-directed mutagenesis can also be accomplished using PCR by incorporating the desired nucleotide change into one of the primers. New related genes have also been identified and isolated by using PCR. In this case, multiple oligonucleotide primers (degenerate primers) are designed to encode a small series of amino acids conserved between different members of a family of proteins. By this method, new members of the family containing these same conserved peptide regions will be amplified.

ANALYSIS OF GENE STRUCTURE AND EXPRESSION

Once a gene or a portion of a gene has been isolated, a variety of techniques can be used to obtain structural and functional information about that gene or gene family. DNA sequencing, isolation of corresponding genes for other species, Southern blotting, and RNA transcript analysis are the most commonly used procedures; these are discussed in the following sections.

DNA Sequencing

One of the most precise ways of characterizing a region of DNA is to obtain the DNA sequence. Such a sequence can yield important information about the structure of the DNA, the protein encoded (if any), and the relation of the isolated sequence to other genes. Two methods are commonly used for determining a DNA sequence: the chemical method of Maxam and Gilbert[16] and the chain-termination method of Sanger.[17] Both methods rely on three features:

1. Base specificity.
2. Partial reactions.
3. Accurate size discrimination from a fixed end by gel electrophoresis.

Today, most routine sequencing of cloned DNA is done by the chain-termination method. The chain-termination method of DNA sequence analysis utilizes enzymatic synthesis to produce a ladder of products terminating in a specific base. In the most commonly used variation, dideoxynucleotide triphosphates are utilized as the reagents that cause chain termination, since such nucleotide analogues lack the $3'-OH$ group on the sugar and thus prevent subsequent elongation. This method is shown in Figure 1–17.

A single-stranded DNA containing the gene to be sequenced is used as the template for a DNA polymerase. In most cases, the template is prepared in a single-stranded vector such as M13, although denatured double-stranded DNA from circular plasmids can also be used. A specific oligonucleotide primer is then annealed to the template, and DNA synthesis is initiated in four separate reactions, each including three normal deoxyribonucleotide triphosphates and a mixture of normal and dideoxynucleotide triphosphate for the fourth nucleotide. Incorporation occurs from the primer through the sequence until a dideoxynucleotide is incorporated, which stops the elongation of the chain owing to the absence of the $3'-OH$ group. Each position along the chain specified by a particular base will be a position at which some of the growing chains will stop synthesis because of incorporation of the dideoxynucleotide. Usually, a [32]P- or ^{35}S-labeled deoxynucleotide is included in the reaction or is incorporated as a $5'$ end label on the primer; this radiolabel provides the method of detection for each chain. The reaction thus yields a set of labeled molecules, with the length of each molecule identifying the position in the chain of the base specified by the dideoxynucleotide. The reaction products are then separated by high-resolution denaturing acrylamide gel electrophoresis, yielding a ladder of autoradiographic signals. The sequence can be easily read from this ladder.

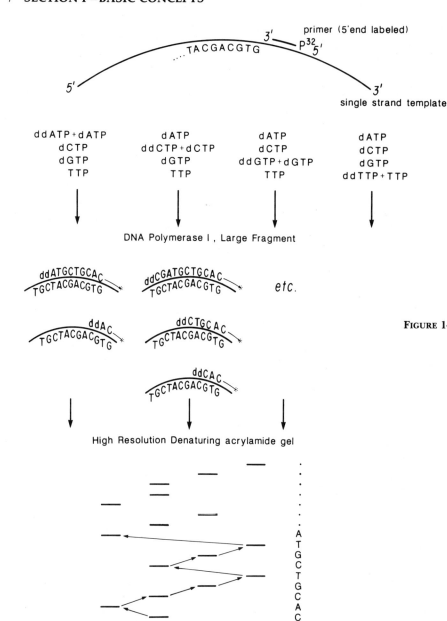

FIGURE 1–17. Sanger dideoxy sequencing.

Various modifications of this procedure and well-controlled reactions permit the sequencing of 5000 to 10,000 nt per day with only a handful of personnel. Combined with computer data bases (NIH Genbank and EMBL data base) for DNA sequences, useful comparisons of DNA sequences of newly isolated genes can be rapidly and efficiently obtained. Currently, more than 50,000 separate gene sequences are in these data bases. The Human Genome Project will likely result in further improvements in both the technology for DNA sequencing and the computer software for data handling and comparative analysis for maximizing the value of this enormous amount of information.

Southern Blotting

One of the first important advances in the development of techniques to characterize DNA accurately was a method that combined high-resolution gel electrophoresis of restriction endonuclease fragments of DNA and the use of specific hybridization probes.[18] In this method, commonly known as Southern blotting (named after Ed Southern, who developed the technique), DNA fragments produced by digestion with one or more restriction endonucleases are separated by gel electrophoresis. The DNA in the gel is then denatured to separate the strands, neutralized, and transferred to a sheet of nitrocellulose filter paper. The most common method for transferring DNA to the nitrocellulose is to place the nitrocellulose between the gel and a stack of absorbent towels and to allow the flow of fluid through the gel and nitrocellulose to move the DNA out of the gel (Fig. 1–18). Nitrocellulose membranes have the convenient but poorly understood property of binding single-stranded DNA. This initial binding can be made more "permanent" by baking the filter in vacuo after the transfer. The

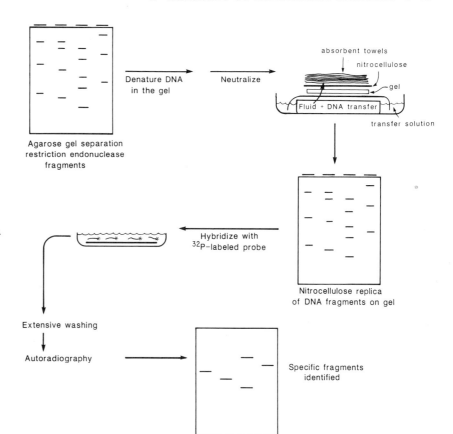

FIGURE 1–18. Southern blot technique.

DNA on the filter after this procedure is available for hybridization. Recent modifications of the procedure include the development of alternate membranes and an electrophoretic transfer procedure.

The importance of this procedure is that the high-resolution pattern of the DNA molecules separated by agarose or acrylamide gel electrophoresis is faithfully transferred to the filter in a form that is still available for hybridization. Thus, by using ^{32}P-labeled DNA or RNA (see the following discussion) as a hybridization probe, specific sequences can be identified on the filter, and important size and structural information can be obtained. For example, with this approach, a small gene can be easily localized in a large fragment of cloned genomic DNA. This localization greatly simplifies the detailed analysis of the gene. The technique is sensitive enough (in combination with appropriate hybridization probes) to detect single-copy genes in genomic DNA. Prior to more detailed analysis by cloning, such "genomic blotting" could yield important structural information about a gene (or genes). Such analysis has been and continues to be one of the most common approaches to identifying gene defects in abnormal chromosomes, as is discussed in subsequent chapters. In many situations, the information desired can be obtained by genomic blotting alone, without the need for cloning. In this case, large numbers of samples containing small quantities of DNA can be rapidly processed. Such procedures are of significant value in population studies of genetic diseases.

An important advance over the past several years has been the development of gel systems capable of resolving DNA fragments in the 50 to 5000 kb range that can be readily subjected to Southern blotting. This technology, known as pulse-field gel electrophoresis (PFGE)[19] allows large DNA fragments to be separated in agarose gels that are easily handled; prior to this approach, the separation of large DNA fragments was limited by the pore size of the gel, which resulted in using very porous and extremely fragile gels for large fragments. In PFGE, DNA migrates through the gel in response to alternating orthogonal electric fields. One field drives the DNA forward in the gel. The other field forces the DNA to reorient itself along the direction of this second field, the length of the DNA being a key determinant in how long it takes to reorient itself. The net result is that very large fragments of DNA migrate through the gel at a rate inversely proportional to their length. This approach has resulted in the design of many apparati and is successful in effectively separating fragments larger than 5000 kb. A key factor in being able to utilize this technology has been the identification of restriction endonucleases or methylase/endonuclease combinations that recognize sites in mammalian DNA infrequently (see above). These advances, coupled with the use of cloning vectors that accept large DNA inserts, have significantly extended the range of gene mapping studies with specific probes so that long-range chromosome maps can now be prepared, revealing linkage between genes or DNA sequences and providing further insights into the arrangement of complex DNAs.

Nick-Translation

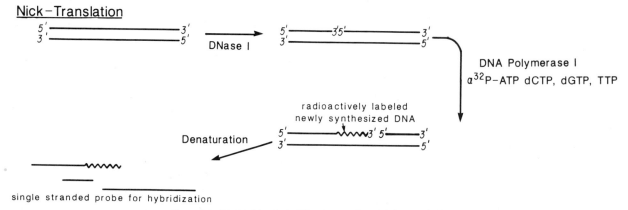

FIGURE 1-19. Making hybridization probes. Nick-translation.

Preparation of Radiolabeled Probes

Various methods for incorporating ^{32}P-labeled ribonucleotides or deoxyribonucleotides into a probe are available. Three of the most common approaches are shown in Figures 1–19 to 1–21. In nick-translation (Fig. 1–19), a double-stranded plasmid DNA or a purified restriction fragment containing the gene of interest is partially nicked by a deoxyribonuclease. These nicks then serve as primer sites for DNA polymerase I, which simultaneously extends the 3' end of the nick and degrades the 5' end of the nick, thus moving ("translating") the nick along the DNA strand. If ^{32}P-labeled deoxyribonucleotide triphosphates are included as substrates, the ^{32}P label is incorporated into the molecule. Following completion of the reaction and denaturation of the DNA, a ^{32}P-labeled single-stranded hybridization probe can be prepared. A disadvantage of this type of probe is that both strands of the desired sequence are present in the probe. Thus,

hybridization of the complementary probe strands in solution can occur as a reaction competing with hybridization of the probe to the filter. Such probes are, however, sensitive enough for genomic blotting and for Northern blotting (see below) of rare mRNAs.

Single-stranded DNA probes can be prepared from sequences cloned in a single-stranded vector such as M13 (Fig. 1–20). In this reaction, a specific primer is used to initiate DNA synthesis on the template and to synthesize the complementary strand through the gene of interest, incorporating ^{32}P-labeled nucleotides. Following synthesis, the DNA is digested with a restriction endonuclease that has a cleavage site located downstream of the desired probe, and a pure single-stranded ^{32}P-labeled fragment can be easily isolated by gel electrophoresis. Such probes are as sensitive or more sensitive than nick-translated probes and do not have the competing strand present to reduce hybridization efficiency.

Synthetic oligodeoxyribonucleotides are now com-

M13 Probes

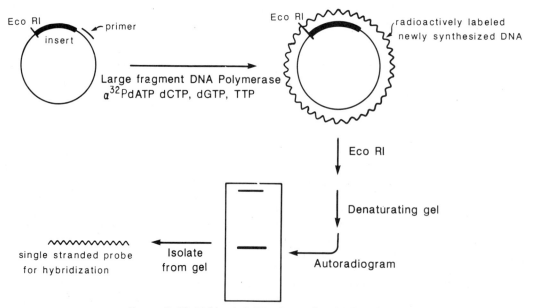

FIGURE 1-20. Making hybridization probes. M13 probes.

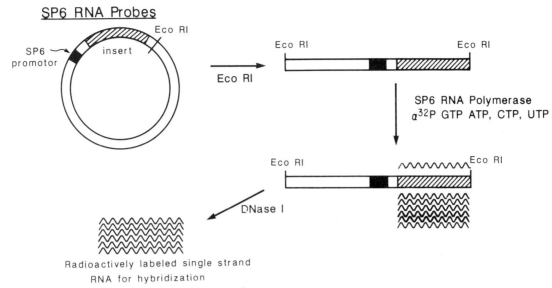

FIGURE 1–21. Making hybridization probes. SP6 RNA probes.

monly used DNA hybridization probes. These probes can be prepared in large quantities with any desired sequence in lengths of 10 to 100 nt. In addition, mixed-sequence oligonucleotide probes can be prepared that are extremely useful in the isolation of genes based on partial amino acid sequence information (see preceding discussion). These probes can be easily labeled with ^{32}P by using polynucleotide kinase and γ-^{32}P-ATP (see Fig. 1–12). This reaction transfers the terminal (γ) phosphate from the labeled ATP to the 5′–OH of the oligodeoxyribonucleotide. The hybridization and washing conditions are critical for efficient use of small oligonucleotide probes, and several guidelines for their use have been published. A number of advances in the use of oligonucleotide hybridization probes have now been widely utilized. The first is the use of quaternary ammonium salts (such as tetramethylammonium chloride), which permit specification of the hybridization temperature based on the length of the oligonucleotide, independent of base composition.[20] This method is used most commonly when all possible coding combinations are included in the probe based upon the known amino acid sequence. Second, oligonucleotides can be synthesized with a "neutral" base, such as inosine, which adequately pairs with more than one base. Such probes allow better assignment of hybridization conditions, since the range of temperatures around which that neutral base pairs with each of the other bases is smaller than the range would be if there were mismatched normal bases. Finally, longer oligonucleotides that have limited the degeneracy by selecting only one or two of the possible codons at each position based on "rules" such as codon preference or CpG bias (such oligonucleotides are referred to as "guessmers") are easy to prepare and have been used, very often successfully.[21, 22]

^{32}P-labeled RNA probes can also be prepared using vectors that contain initiation sites for specific RNA polymerases. The two systems that have been developed to date utilize the RNA polymerase from the bacteriophage SP6 and its promoter or T7 RNA polymerase and its promoter (Fig. 1–21).[23] Specific RNAs are synthesized by first cloning the desired DNA in the proper orientation adjacent to the transcription start site. The plasmid is then linearized at some restriction site within or downstream of the cloned insert. In the presence of ribonucleotide triphosphates and reaction buffer, RNA polymerase will initiate transcription at the proper transcription start site and will synthesize RNA until the end of the template is reached, producing a discrete RNA molecule. Multiple initiations can occur on a single DNA template, producing large quantities of RNA for use as a probe. Because the melting temperature of a DNA/RNA hybrid is higher than that for the corresponding DNA/DNA hybrid, higher hybridization or washing temperatures, or both, can be used, resulting in lower backgrounds.

Recently, systems for preparing DNA or RNA probes with enzymatic or fluorescent, rather than radioactive, tags have been designed. One commonly used system utilizes incorporation of a biotinylated nucleotide into a probe DNA strand. After hybridization, the probe is detected by treatment of the filter with avidin bound to a fluorophore for direct detection or to an enzyme for detection following enzymatic turnover of substrate into a detectable product. In general, non-radioactive probes can be prepared well in advance and in large quantities, are safer to use than radioactive probes, and offer the potential for high sensitivity because of high enzyme turnover.

GENE EXPRESSION AND FUNCTION

Isolation of a gene and characterization of gene structure constitute the first step in understanding gene expression and ultimately function. Addressing these questions requires technologies to qualitatively and quantitatively monitor RNA produced from these genes as well as controlled systems for carrying out experiments to ask defined questions. The remainder of this chapter discusses these technologies and recently developed model systems. Much of the remainder of this book will then expand on the application of these methods.

Transcript Mapping

Detailed analysis of gene structure and function necessitates techniques that analyze the nuclear and cytoplasmic RNAs for these genes with a level of precision similar to that obtained with sequence analysis for DNA. Such information is necessary to characterize initiation, termination, and processing sites for transcription. Combined with DNA sequence analysis of the corresponding cDNA clones and partial sequence analysis of genomic clones, a very detailed description of the synthesis and processing of a given mRNA can be achieved. The three most common approaches to obtaining such information are RNA blotting, S1 nuclease mapping, and primer extension analysis.

RNA blotting (sometimes referred to as Northern blotting) is a procedure in which cellular RNA is size fractionated by agarose gel electrophoresis and transferred to nitrocellulose paper, using only slight modifications of the procedures developed for DNA. RNA molecules that are homologous to specific probes are then identified by hybridization analysis. RNA blotting of mRNAs thus provides a sensitive method to determine the presence or absence of specific mRNAs in a tissue or cell sample and can be used to analyze the size or cell distribution of related mRNA transcripts. More recently, PCR technology has replaced or complemented Northern blotting as the method of choice to determine whether a cell or tissue type produces mRNA from a given gene.

S1 mapping and primer extension analysis focus on providing detailed information on the number and size of exons in the genes, the exact locations of the splicing sites, the extent of alternate splicing, and the exact 5' end of the mRNA.[24] S1 nuclease is an endonuclease that exhibits substantial preference for single-stranded DNA or RNA molecules compared with molecules that are base paired. One way in which S1 nuclease is used to characterize an RNA molecule is shown in Figure 1–22. A single-stranded DNA probe is first prepared, usually by uniformly internally labeling a fragment of genomic DNA that is partially coextensive with the RNA. Hybridization of the RNA to the DNA probe results in formation of an RNA/DNA hybrid in the regions of the RNA and DNA, which are homologous. Following digestion by S1 nuclease to remove the unhybridized portion or portions of the probe, the resulting fragments are separated by gel electrophoresis and detected by autora-

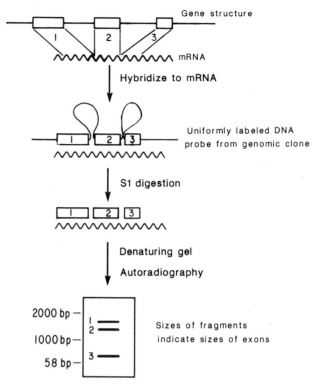

FIGURE 1–22. S1 mapping. Exon sizing.

diography. The number and size of such protected fragments indicate the number and size of exons contained within the DNA probe. Variations of this technique can permit exact identification (to the nucleotide) of the splicing positions or of the 5' or 3' end of the mRNA. The identification of the 5' end of the mRNA is especially valuable for two reasons. First, most cDNA cloning protocols do not result in cDNA clones that extend to the penultimate 5' nucleotide of the mRNA. Second, there are, as of now, no general rules by which transcription start sites can be accurately predicted based on DNA sequence analysis of the gene.

S1 mapping techniques can also be used as a quantitative method to measure the mRNA content of particular cells. Quantification by S1 analysis is more reproducible and more sensitive than similar analysis by RNA blotting, since the variabilities in transfer and hybridization capacity inherent to RNA blots are eliminated.

Retroviral Vectors

Analogous to the bacteriophage systems for introducing cloned DNA into bacteria, retroviral vectors provide a biological method for introducing DNA into mammalian cells.[25] These vector systems are often used when other techniques such as transfection or electroporation are not efficient enough, or to introduce DNA into cells within an adult animal. A retroviral virion consists of two copies of a single-stranded RNA genome and an RNA-dependent DNA polymerase (reverse transcriptase), surrounded by a capsid and envelope, which consist of virally encoded proteins and host cell membrane components. In its life cycle, the retrovirus first binds specifically to the host cell and introduces its RNA genome and reverse transcriptase into the cell. The reverse transcriptase transcribes the viral RNA genome into double-stranded DNA, which then integrates stably into the host cell DNA. This integrated proviral genome contains two long terminal repeats (LTRs) at its ends, which contain the viral promoter, enhancers, and polyadenylation signals. Between the LTRs lies a sequence necessary for packaging the viral RNA into virions (the "packaging sequence"), as well as the *gag, pol,* and *env* genes. The *gag* and *env* genes encode structural proteins of the core and outer envelope, respectively, whereas the *pol* gene encodes the reverse transcriptase. The envelope proteins control the host range of the retrovirus: Ecotropic viruses are able to infect cells of only the same species, whereas amphotropic viruses can also infect cells of other species.

The most commonly used retroviral vectors have been derived from the murine viruses Moloney murine leukemia virus, Harvey murine sarcoma virus, murine mammary tumor virus, and murine myeloproliferative sarcoma virus and from the chicken viruses Rous sarcoma virus and reticuloendotheliosis virus. For ease of manipulation, the double-stranded DNA version of a retroviral genome is transferred into a bacterial plasmid. In the simplest vector constructs, the structural genes of the virus (i.e., *gag, pol,* and *env*) are replaced in vitro by the gene one wishes to transfer. In this case, transcription can be directed by the regulatory machinery present on the viral LTR. More commonly, a selectable marker is also incorporated into the expression vector. In this case, the expression of the selectable marker can be driven by the viral LTR, and internal promoters are used independently to regulate transcription of the gene of interest. Figure 1–23 is a diagram of a typical retroviral vector.

Once a gene has been transferred into a retroviral expression vector using recombinant DNA techniques, this DNA construct must be converted into a viable virus particle. This is accomplished through the use of a special cell line known as a packaging cell line, which provides the *gag, pol,* and *env* structural gene products in *trans*. The most commonly used lines have been created by transfecting separate plasmids encoding *gag/pol* and *env* into a fibroblast cell line such as NIH3T3. The retroviral vector plasmid DNA is then transfected into this packaging cell line, and the RNA generated from the plasmid will be packaged into virions using the structural components provided by the packaging cell line. These virions can then be used to infect suitable susceptible cells and thus transfer the gene of interest into the genomic DNA of that target cell.

Identification of Regulatory Proteins

The regulation of eukaryotic gene expression is accomplished on the molecular level through the interaction of a variety of proteins with specific DNA sequences. These protein-DNA interactions may positively or negatively affect the transcription of the gene where they occur. Thus, the identification of the various DNA-binding proteins and an analysis of the sequences with which they interact are major thrusts in current molecular biology research.[26]

DNA-binding proteins can be detected in crude cellular extracts, using polyacrylamide gel electrophoresis. This technique, known as a "gel-shift" assay, relies on the different electrophoretic mobility of a DNA-protein complex relative to free DNA. A cloned or synthetic DNA sequence containing the regulatory region of interest is radiolabeled and incubated with extracts of nuclei from cells containing the presumed regulatory proteins. The reaction products then undergo electrophoresis on a polyacrylamide gel, and the position of the DNA-containing bands is visualized using autoradiography (Fig. 1–24). If protein has bound to any of the DNA, the protein will retard the mobility of the DNA, so that the DNA-protein complex appears as a discrete new band. Since many proteins can interact with DNA, additional steps are typically

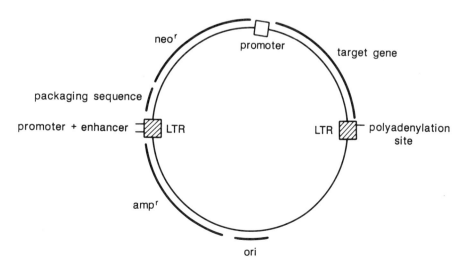

FIGURE 1–23. Essential features of a retroviral cloning vector.

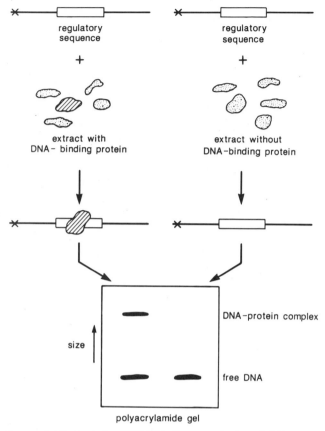

size

DNA-protein complex

free DNA

polyacrylamide gel

FIGURE 1–24. Analysis of DNA-binding proteins by gel-shift assay.

taken to characterize further the specificity of the DNA-protein interaction. These include introducing mutations into the probe DNA or using specific DNA sequence competitors to demonstrate loss of the observed interaction.

Another technique that can be used to identify a regulatory protein as well as its site of interaction with DNA is footprinting. In this technique, the protein-DNA complex is first formed and then exposed to a chemical or enzymatic agent that directly or indirectly is capable of cleaving the DNA. The protein bound to DNA protects the DNA from either cleavage by the enzyme (DNase) or modification by the chemical agent. Protected DNA fragments are again detected by gel electrophoresis. The base-specific reactions utilized in chemical DNA sequencing techniques, including genomic sequencing, can be modified to incorporate footprinting; modification of the bases will be prevented in regions where a DNA-binding protein interacts with the DNA, and following chemical cleavage, these regions of interaction will be detected as a gap in the DNA sequencing ladder.

Several techniques for the purification of regulatory proteins are available. Traditional purification can be done using the gel-shift technique as an assay. A more direct method is the use of affinity chromatography. A DNA regulatory sequence of interest having been identified, multiple DNA copies of this sequence are made either by molecular cloning or by polymerization

of oligonucleotides. This DNA is then coupled to a column chromatography resin to create an affinity column. To decrease isolation of non-specific DNA-binding proteins, cellular extracts are first reacted with a non-specific DNA (e.g., *E. coli* DNA) or passed over an affinity column containing this non-specific DNA. These extracts are then put on the affinity column with the sequence of interest. Molecules with specificity for this sequence will bind, and others will pass through the column. The proteins that have been bound can then be eluted and characterized.

Another method for identifying regulatory proteins is to clone the genes (or cDNAs) encoding them. The most direct method is similar to expression cloning using antibody probes, except that the antibody probe is replaced with a DNA sequence probe. A bacterial expression library is created, in which each clone expresses a particular protein. An oligonucleotide containing the regulatory sequence of interest is synthesized and radiolabeled. The expression library is then screened with this oligonucleotide. Binding of the probe DNA to proteins with which it interacts is used to identify clones encoding those proteins.

Transgenic Mice

The ability to change the genetic makeup of living animals has provided a powerful tool for molecular genetics.[27-31] With these systems, genes can be manipulated in vitro using all the available molecular biology techniques, and the biological effects of these manipulations can be assessed by transfer of the genes back into an animal. Mice have typically been used as the recipient host, owing to the available genetic knowledge about the animal, the relatively short generation time, and the ease of using in vitro culture systems for murine cells.

Several methods have been used for the reintroduction of DNA into the mouse. The first method is the microinjection of recombinant DNA into one of the pronuclei of a fertilized egg. The egg is then reimplanted into a pseudopregnant female mouse; about 20 per cent of the implanted eggs will develop into a living embryo. During this process, the DNA can stably integrate into a chromosome; again, this event occurs only in approximately 1 of 10 viable embryos. When the recombinant DNA integrates, it does so at a random chromosomal location, apparently as multiple copies of the injected DNA arranged in a head-to-tail fashion. Although this results in stable integration of the injected DNA, the process of this integration usually results in rearrangements of the host DNA around the integration site. DNA can also be introduced into mice with the use of retroviruses. DNA can be cloned in a retroviral expression vector (see previous section), and the derived viral stocks can be used to infect mouse embryos. As with injected DNA, the retroviral DNA containing the DNA of interest stably integrates in the mouse genome. In this case, however, a single copy of the DNA is integrated, and major rearrangements of the host DNA around the integration site do not occur. Disadvantages of this system include uncontrolled effects of the site of insertion on gene expression, as well as effects of the regulatory elements of the virus on the genes of interest.

A more recently developed method, and one that probably represents the method of choice for the future, makes use of mouse embryonic stem (ES) cells. ES cells are totipotent cells capable of differentiating into various cell lineages and giving rise to all tissues of the adult animal. These cells can be maintained and manipulated in culture and then transferred into a mouse. Recombinant DNA can be introduced into ES cells in culture, using transfection techniques or retroviral vector–mediated infection. Vectors containing markers that allow selection in vitro can be used, and ES cell clones can be examined in vitro for those that carry integrated copies of the gene of interest. These cells are then injected into mouse blastocysts, the stage of development in which the embryo consists of a single layer of cells surrounding a cavity. As the embryo develops, the ES cells carrying the transgene contribute to the production of various tissue types. The resulting adult mouse is therefore chimeric, some cells being normal, since they were contributed by the host blastocyst, and others being transgenic, since they were contributed by the manipulated ES cells. In some fraction of these animals, the ES cells colonize the germ cells and therefore can be transmitted to the next generation. Cross-breeding of these animals thus can result in progeny that are homozygous for the transgene and consequently contain it in all tissues. An advantage to the ES cell system is that it allows replacement of a particular cellular gene with a modified one, rather than simply introduction of an extra gene. With the use of homologous recombination along with complex selection techniques, DNA with homology to a cellular gene can be introduced into ES cells. Since these cells can be carried in culture, rare cells can be identified in which the introduced DNA has recombined with its cellular homologue and replaced it.

Transgenic mice are a powerful system for the examination of genes and gene regulation. A major area in which transgenic mice have been useful is the examination of tissue-specific gene regulation and the understanding of normal development. The role of various *cis*-regulatory elements in a gene can be examined by either mutation or deletion, often by transferring these elements to direct expression of a marker gene. The roles of protein products themselves can be examined by altering their expression temporally or spatially during development, by increasing their expression using regulatable promoters, or by introducing so-called dominant negative mutations that abolish their functional expression. Retrovirus insertion into a chromosome has also been used to obliterate expression of the gene in which it inserts to correlate phenotype with the expression of a particular gene. Finally, transgenic mouse technology can be used to derive animal models of human disease; that is, once the genetic defect is known in a human condition, that same mutation can be introduced into an animal.

ACKNOWLEDGMENTS: We wish to thank Flo Smith for typing the manuscript and H. Jane Anthony and Kevin J. Porter for the illustrations.

REFERENCES

1. Watson, J. D., Tooze, J., and Kurtz, D. T.: Recombinant DNA— A Short Course. New York, W. H. Freeman & Co., 1983.
2. Alberts, B., Bray, D., Lewis, J., Raff, M., Roberts, K., and Watson, J.: Molecular Biology of the Cell. 2nd ed. New York, Garland Publishing, 1989.
3. Maniatis, T., Fritsch, E., and Sambrook, J.: Molecular Cloning— A Laboratory Manual. Cold Spring Harbor, N.Y., Cold Spring Harbor Laboratory, 1982.
4. Sambrook, J., Fritsch, E., and Maniatis, T.: Molecular Cloning— A Laboratory Manual. 2nd ed. Cold Spring Harbor, N.Y., Cold Spring Harbor Publications, 1989.
5. Roberts, R. J.: Restriction enzymes and their isoschizomers. Nucleic Acids Res. (Suppl.) 16:271, 1988.
6. Vierra, J., and Messing, J.: Production of single-stranded plasmid DNA. Methods Enzymol. 153:3, 1987.
7. Messing, J.: New M13 vectors for cloning. Methods Enzymol. 101:20, 1983.
8. Maniatis, T., Hardison, R. C., Lacy, E., Lauer, J., O'Connell, C., Quon, D., Sim, G. K., and Efstratiadis, A.: The isolation of structural genes from libraries of eukaryotic DNA. Cell 15:687, 1978.
9. Bates, P. F., and Swift, R. A.: Double cos site vectors: Simplified cosmid cloning. Gene 26:137, 1983.
10. Sternberg, N., Ruether, J., and deRiel, K.: Generation of a 50,000-member human DNA library with an average DNA insert size of 75–100 kbp in a bacteriophage P1 cloning vector. New Biologist 2:151, 1990.
11. Burke, D. T., Carle, G. F., and Olson, M. V.: Cloning of large segments of exogenous DNA into yeast by means of artificial chromosome vectors. Science 236:806, 1987.
12. Gubler, U., and Hoffman, B. J.: A simple and very efficient method for generating cDNA libraries. Gene 25:263, 1983.
13. Huynh, T. V., Young, R. A., and Davis, R. W.: Constructing and screening cDNA libraries in lambda gt10 and gt11. *In* Glover, D. M. (ed.): DNA Cloning: A Practical Approach. Vol. 1. Oxford, England, IRL Press, 1985, p. 49.
14. Mierendorf, R. C., Percy, C., and Young, R. A.: Gene isolation by screening lambda gt11 libraries with antibodies. Methods Enzymol. 152:548, 1987.
15. Erlich, H. A., Gelfand, D., and Sninsky, J. J.: Recent advances in the polymerase chain reaction. Science 252:1643, 1991.
16. Maxam, A., and Gilbert, W.: A new method for sequencing DNA. Proc. Natl. Acad. Sci. USA 74:560, 1977.
17. Sanger, F., Nicklen, S., and Coulson, A. R.: DNA sequencing with chain terminating inhibitors. Proc. Natl. Acad. Sci. USA 74:5463, 1977.
18. Southern, E. M.: Detection of specific sequences among DNA fragments separated by gel electrophoresis. J. Mol. Biol. 98:503, 1975.
19. Schwartz, D. C., and Cantor, C. R.: Separation of yeast chromosome-sized DNAs by pulsed field gradient gel electrophoresis. Cell 37:67, 1984.
20. Jacobs, K. A., Rudersdorf, R., Neill, S. D., Dougherty, J. P., Brown, E. L., and Fritsch, E. F.: The thermal stability of oligonucleotide duplexes is sequence independent in tetraalkylammonium salt solutions: Application to identifying recombinant clones. Nucleic Acids Res. 16:4637, 1988.
21. Jaye, M., de la Salle, H., Schamber, F., Balland, A., Kohli, V., Findeli, A., Tolstoshev, P., and Lecocq, J.-P. Isolation of a human anti-hemophilic factor IX cDNA clone using a unique 52-base synthetic oligonucleotide probe deduced from the

amino acid sequence of bovine factor IX. Nucleic Acids Res. 11:2325, 1983.

22. Anderson, S., and Kingston, I. B.: Isolation of a genomic clone for bovine pancreatic trypsin inhibitor by using a unique-sequence synthetic DNA probe. Proc. Natl. Acad. Sci. USA 80:6838, 1983.

23. Melton, D. A., Krieg, P. A., Rebagliati, M. R., Maniatis, T., Zinn, K., and Green, M. R.: Efficient in vitro synthesis of biologically active RNA and RNA hybridization probes from plasmids containing a bacteriophage SP6 promotor. Nucleic Acids Res. 12:7035, 1984.

24. Favaloro, J., Treisman, R., and Kamen, R.: Transcription maps of polyoma virus–specific RNA: Analysis by two-dimensional nuclease S1 gel mapping. Methods Enzymol. 65:718, 1980.

25. McLachlin, J. R., Cornetta, K., Eglitis, M. A., and Anderson, W. F.: Retroviral-mediated gene transfer. Prog. Nucleic Acid Res. Mol. Biol. 38:91, 1990.

26. Johnson, P. F., and McKnight, S. L.: Eukaryotic transcriptional regulatory proteins. Annu. Rev. Biochem. 58:799, 1989.

27. Landel, C. P., Chen, S., and Evans, G. A.: Reverse genetics using transgenic mice. Annu. Rev. Physiol. 52:841, 1990.

28. Palmiter, R. D., and Brinster, F. L.: Transgenic mice. Cell 41:343, 1985.

29. Jaenisch, R.: Transgenic animals. Science 240:1468, 1988.

30. Hanahan, D.: Transgenic mice as probes into complex systems. Science 246:1265, 1989.

31. Hanahan, D.: Transgenic mouse models of self-tolerance and autoreactivity by the immune system. Annu. Rev. Cell Biol. 6:493, 1990.

2

Mechanisms of Eukaryotic Gene Regulation

Ted Abel and Tom Maniatis

INTRODUCTION

The development of eukaryotic organisms involves the growth and differentiation of functionally distinct cell types in a precise spatial pattern. The morphological and functional specialization of differentiated cells is achieved by cell- or tissue-specific gene expression. Only a fraction of the hundreds of thousands of genes contained within each human cell are expressed. Many "housekeeping" genes, such as those encoding ubiquitous cytoskeletal components like actin, are on in all cells at all times. In contrast, differentiated cells pro-

duce large quantities of specialized gene products. Differential gene expression also plays a central role in physiological homeostasis. Many genes are activated in response to metabolic changes and to environmental stresses such as heat shock or infection by virus or bacteria. Inappropriate gene expression can have dire consequences, as illustrated by the fact that many forms of human cancer and some genetic diseases are the consequence of abnormal gene expression. Finally, it seems likely that the function of the human brain and the storage of information involve differential gene expression. Thus, an understanding of the mechanisms involved in gene regulation is a central problem in human biology and medicine.

Developmental biologists discovered that the diversity of gene expression in somatic cells is not due to the irreversible loss or change of genetic material.[1] As it became possible to study the pattern of transcription in individual cell types, it became clear that differential gene expression is controlled at the level of transcriptional initiation. Thus, at a deeper level, the classical problems of cell specialization, differentiation, and the intricate responses of cells to extracellular inducers are the problems of differential gene expression: That is, what mechanisms act to turn the transcription of eukaryotic genes on and off?

The development of techniques to clone and characterize genes provided the opportunity to study these transcriptional mechanisms at the molecular level. The initial analysis began with the identification of the *cis*-acting DNA sequences required for gene regulation by introducing mutations into cloned genes and then analyzing their effects on expression in vivo or in vitro. The realization that these *cis*-acting DNA motifs served as binding sites for sequence-specific DNA-binding proteins led to the purification and cloning of many transcriptional regulatory factors. By using the techniques of molecular biology to produce modified forms of these transcription factors, it became clear that these proteins are surprisingly modular in nature. This modularity allows for the exchange of DNA-binding domains and transcriptional activation domains between proteins of diverse function from various species. The current challenges are to determine the detailed molecular mechanism by which these transcriptional regulatory proteins act to modulate transcription, to understand how specific protein-DNA and protein-protein interactions are integrated into the overall pattern of gene regulation within the cell, and to explore how these regulatory factors are able to function in a eukaryotic nucleus in which DNA is packaged into chromatin. In this chapter, we review the identification and characterization of the *cis*-acting DNA sequences and the *trans*-acting protein factors involved in transcriptional regulation, and we discuss the information available regarding the mechanisms of gene regulation at the level of transcriptional initiation in higher eukaryotes.

The exploration of the anatomy of eukaryotic protein-encoding genes became possible with the establishment of molecular cloning techniques and the advent of Northern and Southern blotting technology. The first thing that became apparent was that most, but not all, eukaryotic genes, unlike their prokaryotic counterparts, are not colinear with their protein products. Rather, intervening sequences (introns) are found between the regions of DNA that code for proteins (exons). The initial transcript, called the pre-messenger RNA (pre-mRNA), contains the entire gene and is found in a population of RNAs termed heterogeneous nuclear RNAs (hnRNAs).

By a process known as pre-mRNA splicing (described in detail below), the introns are precisely re-moved, generating the mature mRNA. The exact role of introns and their evolutionary significance have been the source of much speculation. The correlation in some genes between protein domains and exons led to the postulate that exon shuffling may provide for the rapid evolution of novel protein functions.[2] Further, the existence of introns provides additional mechanisms for regulation through processes such as alternative splicing. Recent studies have led to significant new insights into the complex mechanisms involved in "constitutive splicing" and in regulated alternative splicing. The best example of the latter is sex determination in the fruit fly *Drosophila*, which involves a cascade of regulated alternative pre-mRNA processing events. We will review our knowledge of basic splicing mechanisms and discuss current ideas about the mechanisms that underlie alternative splicing events.

PROKARYOTIC PROMOTER STRUCTURE AND FUNCTION

The activity of a gene is controlled in large part at the level of initiation of transcription, and this initiation by RNA polymerase can be controlled in two distinct ways: by altering the site of initiation and by modulating the frequency of initiation. In *Escherichia coli*, the organization of regulatory elements appears to be relatively straightforward. RNA polymerase complexed with its associated σ factor (usually a protein with an apparent molecular mass of 70 kDa, called σ^{70}) binds specifically to the promoter region, recognizing conserved sequences that are located about 10 base pairs (bp) (the Pribnow box; Fig. 2–1) and about 35 bp upstream (5') of the initiation site.[3] Operator sequences that mediate negative or positive regulation are located within about 50 bp of the constitutive promoter elements. In positive regulation by proteins such as λ repressor or catabolite activator protein (CAP), an activator protein recognizes a specific DNA sequence in the upstream promoter region. From this site, the activator protein acts to stimulate transcription via a mechanism that may involve direct contact with RNA polymerase.[4]

In negative regulation, a repressor binds to operator sites that often overlap the binding site for RNA polymerase. Occupancy of this site by a repressor molecule inhibits transcription. Initially, repressors were thought to act by directly occluding RNA polymerase binding. It is interesting that one well-studied negative regulatory protein, Lac repressor, can coexist with RNA polymerase in a joint non-productive complex on the promoter.[5] Recent experiments have revealed that Lac repressor acts by preventing the escape of RNA polymerase from the initial transcribing complex, thus preventing elongation of the transcript.[6]

EUKARYOTIC GENE TRANSCRIPTION

Transcription in eukaryotic cells involves three classes of RNA polymerase. Genes fall into one of

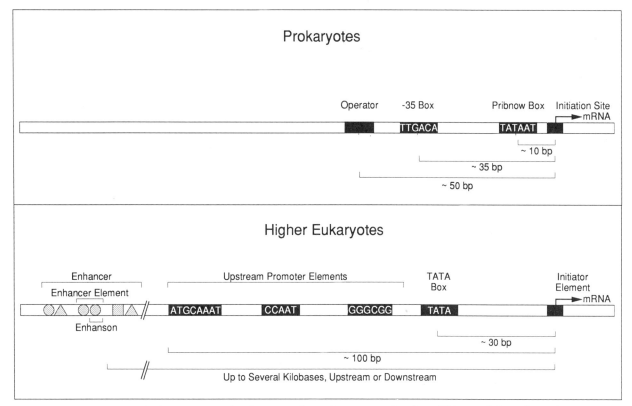

FIGURE 2–1. A typical promoter region from a prokaryotic gene contains the −35 box and the Pribnow box, which interact with RNA polymerase, as well as an operator region to which activators or repressors bind. A typical promoter region for a protein-encoding gene in eukaryotes has a TATA box and is regulated by upstream promoter elements as well as enhancers. Three examples of upstream promoter elements are shown. Enhancers, which are capable of functioning over large distances either upstream or downstream of the gene, are composed of enhancer elements, which in turn contain enhansons. Enhansons are usually the binding sites for regulatory proteins.

these classes on the basis of the type of promoter that regulates their expression. The large ribosomal RNA (rRNA) precursor is transcribed by RNA polymerase I, messenger RNAs by RNA polymerase II, and transfer RNAs (tRNAs) and other small RNAs by RNA polymerase III. These polymerases are traditionally defined by their differential sensitivity to various inhibitors of transcription, such as α-amanitin, which most effectively inhibits RNA polymerase II. Each class of genes has a distinct promoter that contains characteristic sets of conserved sequences that are recognized by the appropriate group of transcription factors and RNA polymerase.

It is important to note one major difference between prokaryotic and eukaryotic RNA polymerases. In prokaryotes, the RNA polymerase holoenzyme itself recognizes promoter sequences with selectivity and specificity. Transcription factors, which bind to operator sequences, then act to modulate the activity of the polymerase. In contrast, eukaryotic RNA polymerases must be assisted by other factors (the so-called general transcription factors, which are discussed below for RNA polymerase II) in order to recognize the promoter specifically. In this chapter, we discuss the regulation of transcription directed by RNA polymerase II, which is responsible for the synthesis of protein-encoding transcripts. Other reviews have discussed RNA polymerase III and its regulatory factors[7] and RNA polymerase I and its regulatory factors.[8, 9]

Eukaryotic Promoter Structure and Function

In eukaryotes, the promoter region spans about 100 to 200 bp of DNA around the initiation site and includes areas that interact with RNA polymerase, the general transcription machinery, and regulatory factors. The original work that has shaped most of our ideas about how RNA polymerase II promoters are organized derives from the study of several viral promoters, particularly those of the herpes simplex virus *thymidine kinase (tk)* gene and the simian virus 40 (SV40) early transcription unit.[10, 11] The functional dissection of the *tk* gene promoter by McKnight and his colleagues was the first detailed demonstration of the crucial components of a eukaryotic promoter (see Fig. 2–1). These studies were carried out by introducing *tk* genes containing modified promoters into either frog oocytes or mouse fibroblasts and assaying the expression of *tk* mRNA in the absence of any other genes from the virus. Deletion mutagenesis experiments established the boundaries of a control region

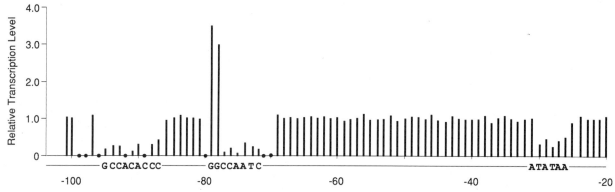

FIGURE 2–2. The effect of specific point mutations in the mouse β globin gene promoter on the level of transcription. Each line represents the transcriptional level of a mutant promoter determined relative to the wild-type promoter. Dots represent nucleotides for which no mutations were assayed. Shown below are the TATA box and the two upstream promoter elements. (From Myers, R.M., Tully, K., and Maniatis, T.: Fine structure genetic analysis of a β globin promoter. Science 232: 613–618, 1986; with permission. Copyright 1986 by the AAAS.)

located within 100 bp of the start site of transcription.[12] This study provides a basis for the working definition of the term promoter: Promoters for genes transcribed by RNA polymerase II are typically about 100 bp long and located immediately upstream of the start site of transcription. This small region was subsequently studied in detail by the use of "linker-scanning" mutagenesis, a technique developed by McKnight that allows small clusters of base substitutions to be introduced in a site-directed manner. By testing the effects of 18 of these mutations on expression in the frog oocyte microinjection assay, the control region of the *tk* gene was dissected into three domains: the proximal signal (ps), which contains a TATA homology (the "TATA box"); the first distal signal (dsI), which contains a GC hexanucleotide; and the second distal signal (dsII), which contains two sequence elements, a "CCAAT homology" and a GC hexanucleotide.[13]

One of the first cellular gene promoters to be extensively dissected was the mammalian β globin gene promoter (Fig. 2–2). Deletion analysis had shown that the first 100 bp preceding the initiation site were sufficient for the correct initiation of β globin gene transcription by RNA polymerase II.[14] This analysis was extended by using a novel procedure for saturation mutagenesis of the region between −101 and +24 of the mouse β globin gene promoter.[15] With this method, it was possible to delineate precisely the *cis*-acting DNA sequences required for accurate and efficient initiation of β globin gene transcription in vivo. More than 130 single-base substitutions were generated within this region and assayed by transfecting the cloned mutant genes on plasmids containing an SV40 enhancer (see below). In most cases, mutating a base in the 5′ region did not affect the efficiency of β globin gene transcription. Clusters of mutations in three regions of the promoter, however, did significantly reduce the level of transcription: the CACCC region located between −87 and −95; the CCAAT upstream promoter element located between −72 and −77; and the TATA box located between −26 and −30 (see

Fig. 2–2). In our brief consideration of the *tk* and β globin gene promoters, we can see that promoters share common elements. The CCAAT and TATA elements are found in many eukaryotic promoters.[16] In contrast, the CACCC sequence is found predominantly in erythroid cell–specific promoters. It is interesting that a naturally occurring mutation in the CACCC sequence in the human β globin gene promoter causes reduced levels of β globin gene transcription, thus leading to β thalassemia.[17] This juxtaposition of ubiquitous promoter elements with gene-specific modules is a common theme found in many promoters. Thus, each promoter has a unique collection—a promoter-specific collection—of upstream elements. The combinatorial interactions between the factors bound to each of these promoter elements result in a gene-specific pattern of transcriptional activity (Fig. 2–3).

Combinatorial Regulation

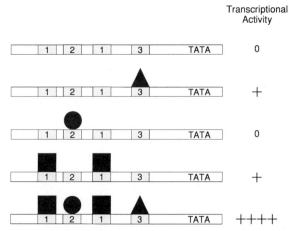

FIGURE 2–3. The combinatorial nature of gene regulation. Individual factors may have little effect on transcription when present in isolation. In the presence of multiple factors, however, high levels of transcription are achieved.

These detailed genetic analyses have led to the view that promoters are composed of discrete functional modules, each approximately 7 to 20 bp in size. These modules are the recognition sites for transcriptional regulatory proteins (see below) as first revealed by Dynan and Tjian[18] in their studies of the binding of Sp1 to the 21 bp, GC-rich repeats within the promoter for the SV40 early transcription unit.

At least one of the modular elements present in each promoter functions to accurately position the start site for RNA synthesis. In most cases, this function is fulfilled by the TATA box, which is usually located about 30 bp upstream from the start site of transcription. Some promoters, such as the promoter for the mammalian terminal deoxynucleotidyl transferase gene, lack a TATA box. In this case, a discrete initiator element overlaps the start site itself and helps to fix the place of initiation.[19]

Upstream promoter elements, such as the CCAAT box and the CACCC motif described above, are each specifically recognized by DNA-binding proteins that then act to regulate the frequency of transcriptional initiation. Typically, these modules are located 30 to 110 bp upstream of the start site, although in some cases they can be located downstream of the start site as well.[20] Depending on the promoter, these modules can function in either a cooperative or an independent manner to activate transcription. In general, the spacing between these modules is relatively flexible. The spacing between the two distal signals in the *tk* promoter, for example, can be increased by about 45 bp before activity begins to decline.[21]

Enhancer Structure

The detailed mutagenesis of viral promoters initially explored the regulatory potential of the region just upstream of the transcriptional start site, and the conclusions of this analysis were very much in line with the predictions made by studies of prokaryotic gene regulation, with the marked exception of the role of the TATA box in selecting the start site of transcription. A puzzling observation, which was not expected from studies in other organisms, was made by Grosschedl and Birnstiel[22, 23] in their study of the expression of the cloned sea urchin histone genes after injection into *Xenopus* oocytes. They found that sequences located more than 200 bp upstream of the initiation site of a histone H2A gene could act in either orientation to promote efficient transcription. Thus, this element exhibits orientation independence, even though it does not possess dyad symmetry.

In parallel with these studies on histone gene expression, studies of the regulation of SV40 early gene expression led to the discovery of enhancers in several laboratories.[24–26] In these experiments, sequences located about 200 bp upstream of the early promoter of the SV40 were found to increase transcription of a linked β globin gene by two to three orders of magnitude. Remarkably, these sequences, referred to as enhancers, could act over distances greater than 3000 bp, when present in either orientation or even from a position downstream of the gene.[25] This ability to function over large distances had no precedent in studies of prokaryotic transcriptional regulatory components.

The initial localization of the SV40 enhancer revealed that it spanned a region of the genome containing two 72 bp repeats.[25] Both repeats are necessary for proper viral growth, but a 100 bp region containing only one copy of the 72 bp repeat is active in stimulating the transcription of a linked gene.[27] The systematic mutagenesis of this 100 bp region revealed that it contained multiple sequence motifs,[27] many of which appear to represent binding sites for *trans*-acting protein factors.[10] Thus enhancers, like promoters, consist of a collection of elements, each of which is specifically recognized by a set of regulatory proteins. In the SV40 enhancer, these elements reside within functional domains. Zenke and associates[27] identified two such functional domains, A and B (Fig. 2–4). Mutation of either A or B results in a significant decrease in transcription in vivo, but the A and B domains have little activity when present in isolation. The duplication of either domain, either separately or in combination, however, results in high levels of transcriptional stimulation. Further, it is important to note for the discussion below that the effect of duplicating A or B or both is independent of their relative position or orientation.[27]

An elegant genetic analysis undertaken by Winship Herr and colleagues underscores the importance of multiple elements for enhancer activity.[28, 29] For these experiments, certain SV40 enhancer elements were mutated, thus reducing the activity of the region below that necessary for the proper growth of the virus. They then isolated growth revertants and analyzed the enhancer region present in these viral genomes. In almost every case, revertants were found to contain duplications of the remaining enhancer elements.[28, 29] This genetic analysis suggested that the SV40 enhancer consisted of three functional units, each 15 to 20 bp long, called by these authors A, B, and C (see Fig. 2–4). As with the study by Chambon's group,[27] full enhancer activity requires a minimum of two wild-type enhancer elements.

It is interesting that each of these enhancer elements displays a unique pattern of cell type–specific activity,[30, 31] and the mutagenesis of different sequence motifs within the enhancer has distinct effects on expression in different cell types.[32] Different sequence motifs within the SV40 enhancer are recognized by different factors present in HeLa and B-cell nuclear extracts. Sequences specifically bound by HeLa cell factors are necessary for in vivo enhancer function in HeLa cells but not in B cells. Similarly, regions protected by factors present in B-cell nuclear extracts are necessary for expression in B cells.[32] The complex organization of these viral enhancer elements may serve to extend the host cell range of the virus by making it highly active in a wide variety of cell types.

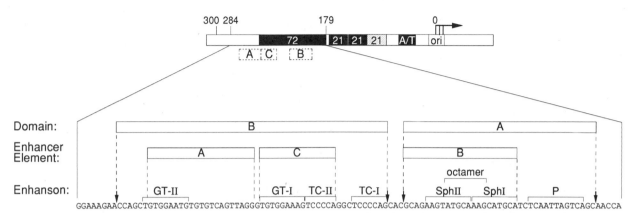

FIGURE 2–4. Organization of the SV40 enhancer. The upper line shows the SV40 early promoter region containing only one copy of the 72 bp repeat. The locations of the 21 bp repeats and the 72 bp repeat are shown. Below is an expanded view of the detailed composition of the region of the 72 bp repeat. This region contains two enhancer domains, each of which contains enhancer elements. These enhancer elements, in turn, consist of enhansons, which represent the binding sites for regulatory proteins.

Detailed analysis of the regulatory regions within enhancers revealed that each element could be further subdivided into short DNA sequences that appear to be the basic units of enhancer structure.[33] These subunits are called enhansons, and they correlate with the sequence motifs first observed in the early studies of the SV40 enhancer (see Fig. 2–4). Enhancer elements are bipartite, containing two enhansons, each one probably corresponding to the binding site for a transcriptional activator protein. By mixing various oligonucleotides containing these enhansons, Ondek and associates[33] demonstrated that these subunits could be duplicated or combined with heterologous enhansons to create new enhancer elements. In contrast to the flexibility observed when combining enhancer elements, strict limitations are placed on the spacing between adjacent enhansons. This factor could be explained by the stringent requirement for protein-protein interactions between factors bound to adjacent enhansons in order to form a functional enhancer element. The regulatory structure of enhancers is thus binary and hierarchical: At least two enhancer elements come together within about 100 bp of each other to create an enhancer, whereas each enhancer element in turn is composed of two enhansons located within 5 bp of each other.

Our discussion of enhancers and promoters has revealed that they are similarly organized: Both consist of multiple modular elements that function as recognition sites for regulatory factors, each with a specific function. This modularity provides a combinatorial mechanism that allows the transcriptional machinery to gather and integrate information from various sources, thus enabling a gene to be regulated in a developmental, tissue-specific, and/or inducible fashion (see Fig. 2–3). The novel juxtaposition of two elements can create a unique expression pattern, thus allowing for a greater degree of transcriptional regulation with a limited number of transcription factors. The existence of these promoter and enhancer modules, then, provides the building blocks for evolutionary change.

How, then, do enhancers and promoters differ? The distinction between enhancers and promoters is in large part operational. Enhancers activate transcription from a great distance and are therefore stronger elements, consisting of multiple domains. Promoters, on the other hand, must include one or more elements that can function to direct the initiation of RNA synthesis at a particular site and in a particular orientation. Outside of these few operational distinctions, promoters and enhancers appear to be homologous entities that may function through the same fundamental mechanisms to activate transcription. Indeed, certain sequence elements, such as the immunoglobulin octamer motif, are found in both enhancers and promoters.[34]

Mechanisms of Enhancer Action

The startling discovery of enhancers led to much speculation about how these elements function to enhance transcription in such a novel fashion. Initial work by Treisman and Maniatis revealed that enhancers act by increasing the density of RNA polymerase II over a linked gene, thus leading to a high rate of transcription.[35] These authors also explored the role of promoter elements in mediating transcriptional activation by the SV40 enhancer. Their conclusion, consistent with more recent observations in many other systems, was that enhancers require intact promoter elements located near the transcription start site in order to activate transcription from a distance.

Several mechanisms of enhancer action have been postulated, and these models have been classified into several groups: the topological, the scanning, and the looping models.[36] The topological model postulates that enhancers might act as binding sites for a sequence-specific topoisomerase that could function to introduce negative supercoils into the DNA and in so doing perhaps increase the rate of transcriptional initiation. Alternatively, enhancer sequences might be regions of intrinsically altered DNA structure. In an elegant experiment, Plon and Wang[37] constructed a "tailed circle" in which the SV40 enhancer formed a hairpin protruding from an otherwise intact circle containing a human β globin gene. In this configuration, the enhancer is topologically uncoupled from the promoter, yet it still functions to activate transcription. Thus, enhancers do not appear to act by changing the topological state of the DNA.

The second class of models has been referred to as the scanning, or the entry site, model. On the basis of the observation that the enhancer region of SV40 was a nucleosome-free region,[38] a number of investigators speculated that the enhancer may serve as an entry site for RNA polymerase II (or a transcription factor). After binding, this factor slides in either direction along the DNA until it reaches proximal promoter elements, where it acts to facilitate the formation of a transcriptional initiation complex.[26] The strongest support for the scanning model came from the experiments of Brent and Ptashne.[39] Working in yeast, they found that the bacterial repressor LexA would act to strongly inhibit transcription when its operator site was placed between the upstream activator sequence UAS_G and the TATA box. Experiments by Courey and his colleagues[40] have also provided support for the sliding model. They found that psoralen-modified DNA inserted between the SV40 enhancer and the human β globin gene inhibited the enhancer effect in vivo. Although these observations are consistent with the sliding model, they do not rule out the looping model discussed below, since looping could be prevented by a protein bound between the enhancer and the promoter.

The looping model has a precedent in several cases in prokaryotic gene regulation, including the cooperative binding of λ repressor over a distance, site-specific recombination, and DNA replication.[41] In eukaryotes, the support for DNA looping comes from the observation of cooperative action or binding of transcription factors over a distance.[42, 43] The self-association of DNA-bound eukaryotic transcriptional regulatory proteins has been observed in the electron microscope.[44, 45] For one of these activator proteins, Sp1, in vivo activation of transcription correlates with DNA looping in vitro.[45] The looping model predicts that enhancers and upstream promoter elements need not necessarily be covalently linked to the gene in order to function; that is, they may be able to function in trans. Indeed, the strongest evidence in favor of the looping model was the demonstration that the SV40 enhancer could stimulate the transcription of the rabbit β globin gene in vitro even when linked to its promoter via the protein streptavidin or avidin. Al-

though there remains no decisive evidence against the possibility that a sliding mechanism is operating in vivo, most of the available evidence favors the DNA looping model of enhancer action. In this model, proteins bound to sites on the DNA separated by a large distance come together to form a complex that, in turn, acts to stimulate transcription. This model underscores the importance of protein-protein interactions between DNA-bound transcription factors, a theme that we return to below in our discussion of transcriptional regulatory factors.

THE TRANSCRIPTIONAL MACHINERY

RNA Polymerase II

RNA polymerase II has been purified from a wide variety of organisms, including yeast, *Drosophila*, plants, and mammals. The holoenzyme, which usually contains 9 or 10 subunits, has an evolutionarily conserved multisubunit architecture, and the amino acid sequence identity between subunits from different organisms is between 40 and 50 per cent.[46, 47] The enzyme contains two large subunits. One, about 220 kDa in size, has an apparent DNA-binding site. The binding site for the toxin α-amanitin, which permits initiation of RNA chains but blocks their elongation, appears to be on this large subunit, since α-amanitin–resistant mutants of *Drosophila* and *Saccharomyces cerevisiae* map to this gene. The other large subunit, about 140 kDa in size, binds nucleotide substrates. Both the 220 kDa and 140 kDa subunits appear to contribute to the active site for catalysis.

In support of early work that described the immunological cross-reactivity of the three RNA polymerases found in eukaryotic cells, the molecular analysis of their subunits has revealed a close structural and chemical similarity between the two largest subunits found in all these enzymes. Each of these large subunits bears sequence similarity to its *E. coli* counterpart, β′, which functions to bind DNA, or β, which binds nucleotide triphosphate substrates.[48] Further, RNA polymerase II shares three smaller subunits with the two other classes of RNA polymerases; the remaining five subunits are unique to RNA polymerase II. This structural similarity between the different RNA polymerases suggests that they may also share some elements of the general transcriptional machinery that is described below for RNA polymerase II.

Much attention has been focused on the detailed genetic and biochemical analysis of the largest RNA polymerase II subunit of 220 kDa. All 10 subunits of the yeast RNA polymerase II have been cloned and sequenced,[47] and thus studies have focused on this organism. Biochemically, the most striking feature of the 220 kDa subunit is that it is highly phosphorylated in vivo on serine and threonine residues. A role for this extensive phosphorylation in transcription is suggested by the observation that the phosphorylated form is found actively transcribing in vivo. In addition, the phosphorylated form of the enzyme is considerably more active than the unphosphorylated form when tested in vitro using the adenovirus major late promoter as a template.[49]

The most striking aspect of the sequence of the 220 kDa subunit of RNA polymerase II from yeast, mouse, *Drosophila, Arabidopsis,* and *Caenorhabditis elegans* is the presence of multiple tandem repeats of a heptapeptide, Tyr-Ser-Pro-Thr-Ser-Pro-Ser.[49–51] The number of repeats in this carboxy-terminal domain (CTD) varies from 26 in yeast to 52 in mice. This repeated "tail," which is unique to eukaryotic RNA polymerase II, is essential for enzyme function in vivo. Yeast cells containing RNA polymerase II large subunits encoding fewer than 10 repeats are non-viable, while 13 or more repeats allow for wild-type growth at all temperatures. Cells containing RNA polymerase II subunits encoding between 10 and 12 repeats are sensitive to heat and cold, and they exhibit a variety of other phenotypes. Young and his coworkers[52] have shown that the ability of these partial deletion mutants of RNA polymerase II to respond to signals from certain upstream activating sequences, such as those bound by the activator GAL4 (see below), is impaired. These results have also been observed in vitro where the progressive truncation of the CTD of yeast RNA polymerase II leads to the progressive loss of activator-dependent transcription.[53] Thus, at least for certain promoters in yeast, an intact CTD is necessary for proper transcriptional regulation. Additional evidence in support of a regulatory role for the CTD comes from the observation that the deletion of the SIN1 gene, which codes for a protein functioning as a negative regulator of transcription of certain genes, suppresses the lethality and phenotypic characteristics of certain CTD truncations.[54]

The presence of multiple serine and threonine residues in the CTD suggested that the repeat may be phosphorylated. Indeed, the CTD is the site of multiple phosphorylations, and it appears that these repeats are the target of the phosphorylation events described above, which may serve to regulate the transcriptional activity of RNA polymerase II.[49] The phosphorylation of the CTD appears to be highly dependent on the formation of the preinitiation complex, and it may be concomitant with the initiation of transcription.[55] In support of this, the purification of RNA polymerase II initiation factors from yeast has revealed a CTD kinase activity that is associated with a nearly homogeneous general initiation factor.[56] Thus, the phosphorylation of the CTD may be an integral part of the process of transcriptional initiation.

The exact function of the C-terminal repeats of the large subunit of RNA polymerase II remains unclear, although they are necessary for transcriptional initiation in vivo. One possibility is that this domain functions through direct interaction with DNA, as was suggested by the observation that the peptide Tyr-Ser-Pro-Thr-Ser-Pro-Ser can bind DNA.[57] The CTD may play a regulatory function, perhaps dependent on its phosphorylation state. It is particularly attractive to speculate that regulatory proteins may interact specifically with the different repeats of the CTD,[58] although other intermediate factors may be involved. Thus, this domain may provide a central switch for gene expression, with its repetitive nature allowing for the integration of multiple, simultaneous signals.

General Transcription Factors

Purified RNA polymerase II will not accurately initiate transcription in vitro without the addition of protein factors present in nuclear extracts. Accurate initiation can be reconstituted using partially purified fractions of nuclear extract, and this fractionation has revealed that at least six distinct general transcription factors (TFs) are required, designated TFIIA, TFIIB, TFIID, TFIIE, TFIIF, and TFIIH. Fundamental to the process of initiation is the ordered addition of factors during the assembly of the preinitiation complex. The combination of these fractions with RNA polymerase II results in accurate initiation from a minimal promoter containing only a TATA box and a start site.[59, 60] By using these fractions and a native gel electrophoresis DNA-binding assay, a model for the interactions of these components during the initiation of transcription has been proposed[61, 62] (Fig. 2–5). DNase I protection experiments were used to determine the relative positions of each factor in the initiation complex.

The first step in promoter activation involves the binding of TFIID to the TATA box. This step, which plays a major role in the formation of a template-committed complex at the promoter, may be aided by the TFIIA.[63] TFIID is the only fraction that binds DNA specifically, and the interaction of TFIID with DNA is stable only in the presence of TFIIA or its recently discovered functional substitute, TFIIG.[64] Next, TFIIB binds to the complex. DNase I protection experiments indicate that TFIIB extends the footprint of TFIID, and it appears that TFIIB may act as a "bridge" between the polymerase and the initiation site. RNA polymerase in the presence of TFIIF can

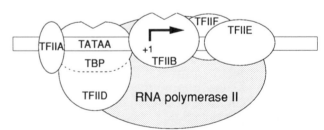

Figure 2–5. The preinitiation complex contains RNA polymerase, TFIIA, TFIIB, TFIID, TFIIE, and TFIIF. The assembly of this complex begins with the sequence-specific interaction between the TATA box–binding protein (TBP) and the TATA box. TBP is a component of the TFIID fraction. The complete preinitiation complex is assembled by the sequential addition of TFIIA, TFIIB, RNA polymerase, TFIIE, and TFIIF. The relative position of TFIIH in the complex is not known and is therefore not indicated in this figure.

then bind to this D-A-B complex. Next, TFIIE enters the complex, perhaps by directly contacting RNA polymerase, TFIIF, and/or DNA. TFIIE extends the footprint of the complex into the +20 to +30 region of the promoter. Finally, TFIIH associates with the complex, perhaps by interacting with TFIIE, to form the stable preinitiation complex.[62]

RNA polymerase II has an energy requirement for the initiation of transcription, and the addition of ATP alters the footprinting pattern and gel mobility of the preinitiation complex.[61] This complex thus appears to undergo isomerization, as has been observed for *E. coli* RNA polymerase.[65, 66] TFIIF appears to contain a DNA-dependent ATPase activity, which may be the helicase activity essential for unwinding the DNA helix and generating the energy required for transcription to occur. Once the preinitiation complex is assembled, transcription may begin with the formation of the first phosphodiester bond of RNA. Following initiation, TFIIE and TFIIF may dissociate from the activated transcription complex.

One of the major goals of studying the basic transcriptional machinery is to reconstitute the transcriptional machinery from proteins produced from cloned genes. To accomplish this, the nuclear activities described above have to be purified to homogeneity, the protein sequence has to be obtained, and the complementary DNAs (cDNAs) have to be isolated. TFIID can be regarded as a commitment factor whose binding to the TATA box region is a prerequisite for assembly of the initiation complex and a kinetically limiting step in this assembly. The purification and cloning of TFIID, therefore, took on extraordinary significance in our understanding of the mechanisms of transcriptional initiation. Further, unlike with the other components of the basic transcriptional machinery, a DNA-binding assay could be used to study TFIID.

The purification of human TFIID, or actually the component of the TFIID fraction that bound DNA (called the TATA-binding protein [TBP]), proved to be difficult. A critical advance in the isolation of TBP came from studies of the yeast transcriptional machinery, which demonstrated that the yeast TFIID fraction would complement a TFIID-depleted HeLa nuclear extract. Yeast TFIID thus binds specifically to a mammalian TATA box and interacts with mammalian RNA polymerase.[67] By using this assay, it proved possible to purify yeast TBP, obtain the N-terminal amino acid sequence, and isolate the cDNA encoding this protein.[68, 69]

Yeast TBP binds specifically to TATA sequences and potentiates basal level transcription in a HeLa cell reconstituted system, but it is unable to support activated transcription by regulators such as the human GC box–binding factor Sp1. Using this yeast TBP sequence as a basis for the design of oligonucleotide probes, several groups isolated a cDNA clone encoding the human TBP.[68] TBP has been cloned now from many organisms, including *Drosophila*.[70] A comparison of the protein sequences of TBP from yeast, humans, and *Drosophila* reveals a bipartite organization.[68, 69] A highly conserved (about 80 per cent identical in all organisms) C-terminal domain binds the TATA box specifically and activates basal transcription. This DNA-binding domain contains two 66 or 67 amino acid repeats that flank a basic region. TBP binds DNA as a monomer, so each of the two repeats likely contacts a part of the TATA box.[71] Also within this C-terminal domain is a region with homology to the portion of bacterial σ factors known to interact with the −10 element (consensus TATAAT) of bacterial promoters (see Fig. 2–1).[71]

The amino-terminal region of TBPs from different species varies greatly in size and amino acid composition. This variability raises the possibility that the N-terminal tail could have evolved to satisfy functions specific to each species. Thus, this domain could be responsible for interacting with transcriptional regulatory factors. A series of experiments, which are described below in our discussion of activation domains, has led to the conclusion that this is the case.

The important distinction to make here is the difference between TFIID, an activity contained within an impure fraction of HeLa nuclear extract, and TBP, a pure protein produced from a cDNA clone. Indeed, TFIID from HeLa cells has an apparent molecular mass of between 300 and 700 kDa, substantially greater than the 38 kDa TBP.[72] Thus, TBP associates with a variety of proteins, and the identification and cloning of these TBP-associated factors (TAFs) are now of great interest.[73] In this context, it is interesting that there is only one human gene encoding a single TBP polypeptide, despite the presence of variant TATA sequences in promoters and the involvement of TFIID in initiation from TATA-less promoters.[74] The interaction of TBP with a variety of other proteins provides a potential source of this heterogeneity. The recent identification of two functionally distinct forms of mammalian TFIID indicates the biological importance of the interactions between TBP and other protein components of the TFIID activity.[72]

Some promoters have an additional basal element, the pyrimidine-rich initiator element, which overlaps the transcription start site. This element can function together with or independently of a TATA element. Recent biochemical studies have shown that a novel factor, TFII-I, binds specifically to the initiator element and functions to support basal transcription from promoters containing an initiator element.[75] The interactions between TFII-I and other basal transcription factors or upstream activators have yet to be characterized in detail.

The general transcription factor TFIIB associates with the TFIID-TFIIA complex, and this complex is then recognized by RNA polymerase. On the basis of this information, it has been postulated that TFIIB may serve as a molecular bridge between the DA complex and RNA polymerase. It may be a "molecular ruler" that determines the distance between the TATA box and the start site of transcription.[61] Recently, TFIIB has been purified to homogeneity and found to consist of a single polypeptide chain of 33 kDa. A cDNA encoding this protein has been isolated, and recombinant TFIIB produced in bacteria substitutes for all the functions attributed to the human TFIIB protein.[76] The sequence of TFIIB contains a motif similar to that found in the DNA-binding domain of the prokaryotic σ factors, although TFIIB has not been shown to bind double-stranded DNA.

TFIIF is a heteromeric transcription factor that joins the initiation complex along with RNA polymerase II. TFIIF contains two subunits with relative molecular masses of 30 kDa and 74 kDa and has also been called RAP30/74.[77] Preparations of TFIIF bind RNA polymerase and have an associated ATP-dependent DNA helicase activity, which probably functions to melt the DNA at the site of transcriptional initiation. The gene encoding RAP30 has been cloned, and it contains a region of homology to bacterial σ factors. This region of homology lies in the portion of σ that is thought to contact RNA polymerase, consistent with the function of TFIIF.[77] Recombinant RAP30 produced in *E. coli* binds to RNA polymerase II and prevents RNA polymerase II from binding non-specifically to DNA in a manner analogous to bacterial σ factors. Thus, RAP30 functions in part by preventing non-specific transcription by RNA polymerase II.[78] A cDNA encoding RAP74 has recently been isolated. Bacterially produced RAP30 and RAP74 associate in vitro, and together they complement a TFIIF-depleted nuclear extract.[79, 80]

Human TFIIE has been purified to homogeneity and shown to consist of two subunits with relative molecular masses of 56 kDa and 34 kDa. TFIIE forms a heterotetramer ($\alpha_2\beta_2$), and both subunits are required to reconstitute basal transcriptional activity. The genes encoding both of these subunits have been cloned, and recombinant proteins produced from these clones complement TFIIE-depleted extracts for transcription in vitro.[62, 81, 82] These subunits contain regions homologous to several structural motifs (such as the zinc [Zn] finger and leucine zipper) and sequence similarities to bacterial σ factors. The functional analysis of these proteins is necessary to explore the role of these domains in the process of transcriptional initiation.

The cloning of several general transcription factors has, then, led to the interesting possibility that the functional domains of bacterial σ factors may be distributed among several proteins in higher eukaryotes: TBP may have maintained the portion of σ responsible for promoter recognition, whereas TFIIF (RAP30) contains the function domain responsible for interaction with RNA polymerase. The heteromeric TFIIE appears to contain many regions homologous to several distinct domains of σ. This partitioning of functional domains may provide for the greater complexity and control mechanisms characteristic of eukaryotes.

DNA-BINDING DOMAINS OF TRANSCRIPTION FACTORS

Although much progress has been made in the characterization of the general transcriptional machin-ery, an even greater effort has been made in the investigation of how promoters and enhancers work. When eukaryotic promoters and enhancers were first characterized, little was known about how they functioned, beyond the observation that they consisted of small, discrete regions. An important advance in our understanding came from the observation that the transcription factor Sp1 binds avidly to a motif repeated five times in the promoter of the SV40 early transcription unit. This DNA-binding protein was then shown to activate transcription when bound to these sites.[18] This early work represented the first demonstration outside of bacteria that regulatory elements of genes could be controlled by the proteins bound to them. In addition, it provided the foundation for the current view that the frequency of transcriptional initiation ultimately depends on factors that interact with specific DNA elements found in enhancers and promoters.

Several sensitive techniques have been developed to detect factors in cell extracts that bind to *cis*-acting DNA elements, including gel retardation assays[83] and DNase I footprinting.[84] These factors can be purified from extracts using conventional chromatography as well as sequence-specific DNA affinity chromatography[85, 86] in amounts sufficient to obtain material for biochemical assays and protein sequencing. This protein sequence can then be used as the basis for cloning the gene encoding the factor of interest. Cloning strategies have also been devised to screen expression libraries for cDNA clones encoding DNA-binding proteins of a certain sequence specificity.[87, 88]

Transcription factors perform at least two functions: They bind specifically to DNA, and they promote transcription initiation. The methods described above have led to the cloning of many genes encoding transcription factors, and the functional dissection of these proteins has provided several generalizations about the organization of eukaryotic transcriptional regulatory factors. The first essential conclusion is that transcriptional regulatory proteins are modular in nature. Independent domains mediate DNA binding and transcriptional regulation. This idea was first developed in structural and biochemical studies of λ repressor, whose N-terminal DNA-binding domain and C-terminal oligomerization domain are separable,[89] and has since been extended to many eukaryotic transcriptional activator proteins.[90] The implication of this modular structure is that these domains represent independently folding structures that can be exchanged between proteins. The first demonstration of this sort of swap experiment was the creation of a hybrid eukaryotic transcriptional activator containing a DNA-binding domain from the prokaryotic repressor LexA fused to a portion of the yeast transcriptional activator GAL4. This hybrid protein activates transcription in yeast from a *lexA* operator.[91] The second major point about eukaryotic transcriptional activators, which was discovered as a direct extension of the investigation of their modularity, is the fact that in many cases these activators can function across species.

Thus, the yeast transcriptional activator GAL4 can activate transcription in mammalian, insect, and plant cells.[92]

Given the modularity of these transcriptional regulatory proteins, we first turn our attention to DNA-binding domains. The study of these domains had its beginnings in the structural analysis of the bacteriophage λ cro and repressor proteins as well as the *E. coli* catabolite activator protein[93] and has recently been extended to higher eukaryotic proteins. These studies[94, 95] have led to general ideas about how proteins interact with specific DNA sequences. All DNA-binding domains fold in such a way as to present a protruding surface or a flexibly extended structure in order to contact the DNA base pairs. Often, this structure is an α helix, which fits snugly into the major groove of B-DNA. The side chains of amino acids within this helix can then interact with the exposed surfaces of the base pairs via both hydrogen bonds and non-polar van der Waals interactions. In this context, it is important to note that there is no simple code that dictates that certain DNA base pairs are recognized by certain amino acids. Indeed, an individual amino acid can contact more than one kind of base and vice versa. Interactions also occur between amino acids and the sugar-phosphate backbone of DNA. These electrostatic interactions provide much of the interaction energy that stabilizes the DNA-protein complex. In the general case, DNA remains in its classic B conformation, although in some cases local perturbations in the structure are seen. In the dramatic case of the CAP-DNA complex, for example, the DNA is bent by 90°.[96] Some mammalian regulatory proteins are also known to bend DNA upon binding.[97]

The Helix-Turn-Helix and Homeodomains

The helix-turn-helix (HTH) is the best characterized structural motif for DNA binding. It was first identified in λ cro and repressor proteins, and most prokaryotic transcriptional regulatory proteins fall into this group, as do the eukaryotic homeodomain proteins.[98] One major difference between these classes of proteins is that most of the prokaryotic HTH proteins bind to palindromic sites as dimers, whereas homeodomain proteins bind as monomers.

The HTH is generally regarded as a 20 amino acid domain that contains two α helices that cross at an angle of 20° (Fig. 2–6), but this motif is found buried in a larger domain. The second helix of the HTH lies in the major groove, and its side chains make contacts with the exposed surfaces of a stretch of base pairs. Thus, this helix is called the "recognition helix." When residues that reside on the outer surface of this helix are modified, the DNA-binding specificity of the resultant protein is altered.[99] The exact alignment of this helix in the major groove, as well as which residues make contacts with the base pairs, differs from protein to protein. The first helix of the HTH lies along the

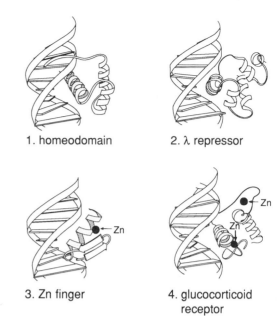

1. homeodomain   2. λ repressor

3. Zn finger   4. glucocorticoid receptor

FIGURE 2–6. A diagram of the crystal structures of DNA-binding domains complexed with DNA. Structures of the homeodomain (from the *Drosophila* engrailed protein), λ repressor, the Zn finger (from the *Xenopus* protein Xfin), and the glucocorticoid receptor are shown. In each case, the recognition helix that lies in the major groove and makes sequence-specific contacts with the base pairs is shaded. (From Harrison, S.: A structural taxonomy of DNA-binding domains. Reprinted by permission from Nature, Vol. 352, pp. 715–719. Copyright © 1991 Macmillan Magazines Ltd.)

DNA backbone and makes contacts with the sugar-phosphate backbone.[98]

The homeodomain is of particular interest to developmental biologists because proteins containing this 60 amino acid sequence are involved in regulating a variety of developmental decisions in many organisms. This motif, termed the homeobox, was initially found in *Drosophila* homeotic genes.[100] These genes function to specify segment identity in the developing *Drosophila* embryo, and related genes have been found in worms, frogs, mice, and humans.[101] The yeast α2 repressor, which is the product of the MATα2 gene, specifies cell identity in yeast, and it is a member of the homeodomain family. In all cases, then, the general view is that these genes perform lineage-determining functions.

Determination of the structure of the homeodomain was thus a particularly important goal, and several structures have now been ascertained. Two crystal structures of homeodomain proteins complexed with DNA (the engrailed homeodomain–DNA complex[102] and the MATα2 homeodomain–DNA complex[103]) have been solved. In these structures, the positioning of the homeodomain HTH on DNA is quite different from that found in prokaryotic HTH proteins (see Fig. 2–6). A major difference is the presence of an extensive set of side-chain contacts with the sugar-phosphate backbone in the segments that flank the place where the recognition helix lies in the major groove. These contacts maintain the proper "docking" arrangement of the HTH on the DNA. In addition, an N-terminal arm extends into the adjacent minor groove, making additional DNA contacts. These structural results are consistent with mutagenesis studies, which indicate that the ninth recognition helix residue has a role in specifying the base "X" of a TAATX-binding site.[104]

The recognition helix within the homeodomain is not always the sole determinant of binding site specificity. This is the case for the POU domain proteins, a novel subclass of homeobox proteins. This domain, originally found in the pituitary-specific transcription factor Pit-1/GHF-1, the octamer-binding proteins, and the *C. elegans* cell lineage control gene *unc-86*, consists of an 80 amino acid POU-specific domain and a 60 amino acid POU homeodomain.[105] The entire POU domain is involved in DNA binding, and the POU-specific domain carries much of the binding specificity. All POU domain proteins have a cysteine residue at position 9 of the recognition helix, so this residue is not as crucial as in other homeodomain proteins. Indeed, the transfer of only the POU-specific domain from one protein to another is sufficient to alter binding specificity.[106] The determination of the structure of the POU domain and the analysis of its interaction with DNA will reveal how the POU-specific domain modifies the recognition of specific binding sites by the homeodomain.

Zn-Binding Domains

The second group of DNA-binding domains is defined by their structural requirement for zinc (Zn). This group was discovered by analysis of the amino acid sequence of TFIIIA, one of the factors required for 5S rRNA gene transcription in *Xenopus*. This original "Zn finger" motif (referred to as a class I Zn domain[95]) is a sequence motif of 30 residues that is repeated consecutively nine times in TFIIIA. In each of these modules, one Zn ion is liganded by two cysteines and two histidines.[107] The second class of Zn-binding domains is defined by the receptor proteins of the steroid and other related hormones. In this 70 amino acid domain, the metal ligands are exclusively cysteine, with two Zn ions tetrahedrally liganded by four cysteines.[108] The third class of Zn domains, which contains two Zn ions sharing six cysteines, is found in a group of yeast transcriptional activators that includes GAL4.[109]

The class I Zn-binding domain, or Zn finger, is found in more than 200 proteins, including general transcription factors, proto-oncogenes, and proteins induced by mitotic signals. These proteins define a consensus sequence motif: ϕ-X-Cys-X_{2-4}-Cys-X_3-ϕ-X_5-ϕ-X_2-His-X_{3-4}-His-X_{2-6}, where ϕ is a hydrophobic amino acid and X is any amino acid.[110] Most proteins containing this motif have three or more fingers repeated one after the other. The structure of the Zn finger from several proteins has been determined, and in one case the crystal structure of a Zn finger–DNA complex has been solved.[95, 111] Essentially as predicted by Jeremy Berg,[112] each individual finger independently folds into a compact unit that consists of a 12-residue helix packed against two β strands that are arranged in a hairpin structure (see Fig. 2–6). The two invariant cysteines, located on each side of the turn in the hairpin, and the two invariant histidines, which are on the inward-facing side near the C-terminus of the helix, coordinate a central Zn ion, thus forming a compact globular domain.

The crystal structure of three Zn fingers from Zif268 complexed with DNA reveals that the Zn fingers bind in the major groove of DNA, with the N-terminus of each helix lying closest to the edges of the bases.[111] Each domain is connected to the adjacent domain in such a way as to allow the protein to wrap around the DNA. Each finger makes its primary contacts with 3 bp. The structure thus exhibits periodicity, with neighboring fingers contacting adjacent 3 bp subsites. Base pair contacts are made by the residue immediately preceding the helix and the residues in the amino-terminal portion of the helix itself. One of the β strands contacts the sugar-phosphate backbone along one strand of the DNA, making ionic and hydrogen bond interactions. One noteworthy interaction is a hydrogen bond between the first Zn-chelating histidine in each finger and a DNA phosphate. This histidine is invariant, and its interaction with the DNA suggests that most Zn fingers may bind DNA in the same way.

The structure of a class II Zn-binding domain (the C_2C_2 Zn finger) from the glucocorticoid receptor complexed with DNA has been determined.[108, 113] This domain contains two loop-helix elements, each containing a Zn ion coordinated to two cysteines in the loop and two cysteines at the N-terminus of the helix (see Fig. 2–6). The first helix lies in the major groove of DNA, and side chains from the second and third turn of this helix make sequence-specific contacts with the DNA bases. The initial loop and the second loop-helix element make contacts with the DNA sugar-phosphate backbone, thus positioning this first helix properly in the major groove. Proteins of this class bind DNA as dimers, and this dimerization is mediated by contacts between residues in the second loop.

The third class of Zn domains is exemplified by the yeast transcriptional activator GAL4, which binds to a twofold symmetric site as a dimer. The 74 amino acid DNA-binding domain of GAL4 contains six cysteines and binds two Zn ions.

The Importance of Dimerization: The Leucine Zipper and Helix-Loop-Helix

The CCAAT/enhancer-binding protein (C/EBP), a protein originally isolated on the basis of its ability to bind to the regulatory region of the herpes simplex virus *tk* gene, was the founding member of the leucine zipper (or bZIP) family of transcriptional regulatory proteins.[114] This family includes the yeast transcriptional activator GCN4, the serum-inducible genes *fos* and *jun*, and the cyclic AMP (cAMP) response element–binding protein (CREB). These proteins bind DNA as dimers, and their DNA-binding domain is bipartite[115] (Fig. 2–7). The bZIP domain consists of a basic region that contacts DNA directly adjacent to a heptad repeat of leucine residues (the "leucine zipper"), which mediates dimerization. Dimerization is an absolute requirement for DNA binding, and the leucine zipper of GCN4 can be replaced by a disulfide bond.[116] Thus, the basic region of GCN4 is sufficient for sequence-specific DNA binding, and the major function of the leucine zipper is simply to mediate protein dimerization.

A "scissors-grip" model for the interaction between the bZIP domain and DNA has been proposed on the basis of available biochemical information.[117] In this model, the domain is entirely α-helical, with the basic region located in the major groove of DNA. At least one kink in this extended helix is necessary so that the basic region can make contacts in the major groove extending over a distance of 10 bp. An interesting feature of bZIP proteins that has emerged from physical studies is that the basic regions assume a stable α-helical structure only when bound to a specific DNA site. Thus, binding induces a coil-to-helix transition in the protein, a conformational change that may be crucial if the basic region is to form a molecular clamp that encircles the DNA.[118]

In an elegant series of experiments, Peter Kim and his colleagues established that a 30 amino acid peptide containing the leucine zipper of the yeast transcriptional activator GCN4 forms a stable dimer of α helices in solution.[119] This interaction has the characteristics of a coiled-coil, a classical interface for protein-protein interaction whose existence was first predicted by Francis Crick in 1953.[120] The coiled-coil is formed by the "knobs into holes" packing of the side chains protruding from the two helices. This model was confirmed by the recently determined X-ray structure of the GCN4 leucine zipper.[121] It underscores the importance of the 4,3 hydrophobic repeat that lies along one face of the α helix and shows that the two helices interact extensively.

The bZIP proteins do not dimerize randomly: GCN4, C/EBP, and CREB form homodimers, whereas Fos and Jun participate in heteromeric complexes. Short peptides containing the leucine zipper regions

FIGURE 2–7. *A,* bZIP proteins contain a bipartite DNA-binding domain, which includes a basic region and a leucine zipper. *B,* Leucine zippers associate to form a parallel coiled-coil. This dimerization interface brings into juxtaposition two basic regions, which function to contact DNA. (From Abel, T., and Maniatis, T.: Action of leucine zippers. Reprinted by permission from Nature, Vol. 341, pp. 24–25. Copyright © 1989 Macmillan Magazines Ltd.)

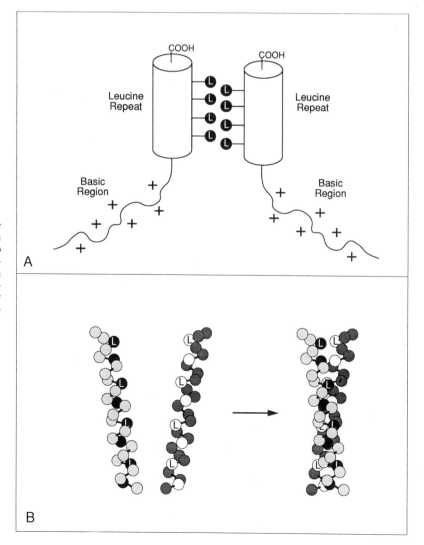

of Fos and Jun preferentially form heterodimers of parallel α helices, demonstrating that the leucine zipper region specifies dimerization. The molecular basis of this specificity may not lie at the hydrophobic interfaces between the two helices in the coiled-coil. Rather, heterodimeric specificity may be the result of interhelical ion pairing between side chains protruding from the helix.[122]

The study of the bZIP family of DNA-binding proteins has done much to emphasize the importance of protein-protein interactions in transcriptional regulation.[123, 124] Heterodimer formation could lead to novel DNA recognition properties or to different regulatory activities, thus expanding the repertoire of a finite number of transcriptional activators. All heterodimers formed between the bZIP proteins studied thus far do not recognize a novel DNA sequence. The demonstration that a heterodimeric repressor protein can bind to a hybrid operator sequence[125] is a precedent for the idea that a heterodimer can bind a sequence not recognized by either homodimer.

An additional possibility is that different protein complexes could display distinct transcriptional regulatory activities. For example, Fos can act as a positive or negative regulatory protein in different DNA sequence contexts. The Fos protein acts to stimulate transcription when bound to an AP-1 or a tetradecanoyl phorbol acetate (TPA)–responsive element (TRE) but acts as a negative factor when bound to an adipocyte-specific regulatory element. Also, Fos acts to negatively regulate its own expression.[126, 127]

A second bipartite DNA-binding/dimerization motif, the basic helix-loop-helix (bHLH), has been described.[128] This family includes E12 and E47, which bind a specific DNA sequence found in immunoglobulin κ chain enhancers[128]; the proteins MyoD1, Myf-5, and myogenin, which play crucial roles in muscle determination[129]; and a number of Drosophila genes that regulate the development of the peripheral nervous system, such as achaete-scute and daughterless.[130] Like the bZIP proteins, the bHLH proteins interact to form homodimers and heterodimers. The HLH region, which has conserved sequence characteristics suggesting that it may form two short amphipathic helices, mediates dimerization, whereas the basic region contacts DNA.[131, 132]

A striking example of how dimerization can regulate the activity of a protein is provided by the discovery of Id, a protein that contains the consensus HLH motif but lacks an adjacent DNA-binding domain.[133] Indeed, Id does not bind DNA, but it can efficiently dimerize with either MyoD1, E12, or E47. These heterodimers containing the Id protein fail to bind DNA. Thus, Id provides a natural form of a dominant negative mutation.[134] When Id levels are high, this protein acts to block the function of positively acting factors such as MyoD1, E12, and E47.

Our discussion of the cis-acting sequences that regulate gene expression revealed the combinatorial nature of transcriptional regulation. The study of transcriptional regulatory proteins, particularly the bZIP

and bHLH families, has demonstrated that trans-acting factors can also function in a combinatorial fashion. At least two members of the bHLH family, E12[128] and myogenin,[135] also contain a heptad repeat of leucine residues. This interesting observation raises the possibility that interfamily dimerization may occur. Novel protein-protein interactions, made possible by the dimerization of regulatory proteins, thus greatly increase the regulatory possibilities available in the eukaryotic cell.

Recently, the study of the myc family of oncogenes and the cloning of several new transcriptional regulatory proteins have led to the discovery of a new family of transcription factors, the bHLH-ZIP family. Members of this family bind DNA as homodimers and heterodimers, and they contain an HLH domain and bZIP domain immediately adjacent to a single basic region. This family includes c-, L-, and N-myc,[136] USF,[137] and AP-4.[138] The Myc protein binds DNA only weakly on its own, but the complex between Myc and another bHLH-ZIP family member, Max, binds DNA in a sequence-specific manner. DNA binding depends on the integrity of the basic, HLH, and zipper regions of each partner.[136] On the basis of the presence of two potential dimerization domains, one would expect that these proteins would form tetramers, and this has been shown to be the case for two proteins, Myc[139] and TFEB.[140] It appears, however, that it is the dimer form that actually binds DNA.[137, 140] In general, bHLH-ZIP proteins will only selectively heterodimerize with other bHLH-ZIP proteins, and they do not cross-dimerize with bHLH or bZIP proteins. In one striking example, however, a bHLH-ZIP protein, FIP, has been shown to dimerize with Fos.[141] Thus some, albeit limited, cross-dimerization between families may occur.

Although we have discussed several DNA-binding motifs, a number of well-characterized DNA-binding proteins, such as heat shock factor,[142] serum response factor,[143] NF-κB,[144, 145] and TFIID,[71] do not fall into any of the groups described above. One major group of DNA-binding proteins that we have not discussed is the β ribbon group. This domain has been found only in prokaryotic DNA-binding proteins (as exemplified by the Arc[146] repressor), and it will be interesting to see if this motif is found in eukaryotic DNA-binding proteins as well.

TRANSCRIPTIONAL ACTIVATION DOMAINS

Transcriptional activator proteins possess at least two functional domains: One tethers the protein to DNA, and the other serves to activate transcription of the linked gene. The DNA-binding domain, as we have just described, is usually well defined, and the interaction between the protein and DNA depends on precise and relatively invariant contacts between amino acid side chains and functional groups on the DNA. Transcriptional activation can be attributed to certain regions of each protein, but the boundaries and sequences of most activation domains are considerably less well defined. In addition, factors often have more than one activation domain.

The analysis of transcriptional activation had its beginnings, as did much of the work described in this chapter, with the studies of bacteriophage λ. The λ repressor protein functions as both a positive and a negative regulator of gene transcription. Specifically, repressor bound at O_R2 acts to stimulate its own transcription from P_{RM}.[147] The detailed mutagenesis of λ repressor led to the isolation of positive-control mutants that bind operator DNA sequences and mediate negative control but that are deficient in the positive regulatory function. Three different positive-control mutants have been isolated, and they all lie in the HTH region of repressor, but outside the recognition helix.[4] Thus, they do not influence DNA binding. Model building studies and X-ray crystallographic analysis have led investigators to propose that these residues lie on the surface of repressor, in a region that may directly contact RNA polymerase. Repressor functions in a positive manner, then, by snuggling with RNA polymerase, thereby leading to an increase in the rate of transcriptional initiation. In this context, it is important to observe that this postulated direct contact between an activator protein and RNA polymerase depends on the precise positioning of the activator site, and it has been proposed only for *E. coli* promoters that use a specific σ factor, σ^{70}. Although σ^{70} is used by the majority of *E. coli* promoters, some use a different factor, termed σ^{54}. The characteristics of the σ^{54} system resemble those of RNA polymerase II more closely than those of σ^{70} initiation. In particular, the σ^{54} system involves activation from distant sites in a manner analogous to enhancer action in higher eukaryotes.[66]

Identification of Activation Domains

The first defined activation domains in eukaryotic transcription factors were identified in studies of the yeast activators GAL4 and GCN4.[148, 149] The activation domains of these factors, which are 80 to 110 amino acids in length, share two features: They are regions with a relative abundance of negatively charged (acidic) amino acids, with overall charges of −7 to −16, and they can form amphipathic α-helical structures. GAL4 contains two such acidic activation domains. Each of these activating regions retains significant activity when fused to a heterologous DNA-binding domain. These fusion proteins are capable of activating the transcription of a reporter gene containing a binding site for the heterologous DNA-binding domain in yeast and a variety of higher organisms. These acidic activators, which can even be constructed from random segments of *E. coli* proteins containing a high proportion of acidic amino acids,[150] are thus termed "universal activators."[92, 151]

Deletion analysis of the human GC box–binding protein, Sp1, has uncovered four separate domains of the protein that contribute to transcriptional activation.[152, 153] The two most potent regions are highly enriched in the amino acid glutamine. These glutamine-rich activation regions are typically about 25 per cent glutamine and have very few charged amino acids. Glutamine-rich regions are also found in the *Drosophila* Antennapedia, Ultrabithorax, and zeste proteins and in some mammalian transcriptional activators. Experiments in which these domains have been swapped between proteins or fused to heterologous DNA-binding domains have demonstrated that they function as activation domains, although they share little primary sequence similarity beyond their high glutamine content.[154]

The dissection of CTF/NF-1 has revealed a third class of activation domains, the proline-rich domain.[155] This domain, which contains about 20 to 30 per cent proline residues, also activates transcription when fused to a heterologous DNA-binding domain. Proline-rich regions are found in several other eukaryotic transcriptional activator proteins, but their function has not been investigated in all cases.[154]

Although our discussion has focused on activator proteins that contain two functional domains within a single polypeptide, activators can be assembled from two separate proteins. In this case, an acidic activation region and a DNA-binding surface are carried on separate molecules. An example of this is provided by the herpes simplex virus VP16 gene product. VP16 contains a strong transcriptional activation domain but has no intrinsic DNA-binding activity. When the acidic activation domain of VP16 is fused to a heterologous DNA-binding domain, the resultant hybrid protein is a potent transcriptional activator.[156] In the cell, VP16 forms a complex with the ubiquitous octamer-binding protein Oct-1 and perhaps other cellular factors. Oct-1 lacks an acidic activation domain and functions by contacting DNA. It is thought that Oct-1 is the primary determinant of DNA binding in this complex, but the Oct-1/VP16 complex protects a larger DNA sequence from chemical modification than does Oct-1 itself, suggesting that some other component of the complex may contribute to DNA binding.[157, 158] It is interesting that the Oct-1/VP16 interaction site maps to the POU domain of Oct-1, underscoring the idea that DNA-binding domains can serve other functions.[159] In the absence of cellular factors, VP16 can recognize the Oct-1 homeodomain, and the region of VP16 involved in this interaction has been mapped to a 33 amino acid region near the acidic activation domain.[160]

Two important conclusions have come from the study of VP16: The acid-rich activation domain of VP16 has provided the "gold standard" in the field, and it has been used in many studies that have explored the mechanism of transcriptional activation. The detailed dissection of this domain has revealed that negative charge contributes to, but is not sufficient for, transcriptional activation. In particular, a single phenylalanine to proline alteration within the acidic domain renders VP16 inactive.[161] Using GAL4-VP16 fusion proteins as well as the intact GAL4 protein, investigators have discovered that acidic activation domains, in contrast to the glutamine-rich and proline-rich activation domains,[92, 151] function "universally" in eukaryotes. Further, analysis of the Oct-1/VP16 interaction has highlighted the importance of protein-protein interactions in transcriptional activation. In this case, the activity of Oct-1 at particular promoters depends on another factor, VP16. VP16 thus provides a means of differentiating among DNA-binding proteins that recognize similar sequences. Of the many members of the octamer family, only Oct-1 interacts with VP16. Another example of the assembly of a transcriptional activator from multiple subunits is provided by the HAP2/3/4 complex, which functions to activate transcription of the *S. cerevisiae* CYC1 gene.[162]

Mechanisms of Transcriptional Activation

Recently, attention has turned to the identification of targets for transcriptional activation domains. A hypothesis being actively pursued is that the DNA-bound transcriptional activator interacts with some component of the general transcriptional machinery, causing this component to bind DNA or change its conformation or both.[92] This event results in the modification of the "preinitiation" complex, thus leading to the formation of a complete active initiation complex containing RNA polymerase II and its ancillary factors, which were discussed above[61] (see Fig. 2–5).

TFIID appears to be a pivotal factor in the assembly of the basal apparatus, and thus the idea that it served as the target for activators was particularly attractive.[69] TFIID is a commitment factor whose interaction with the TATA box is a prerequisite for the assembly of the general transcriptional machinery. This interaction with DNA represents the only sequence-specific protein-DNA interaction in the assembly of the initiation complex. A variety of upstream activating factors, including ATF and GAL4, change the footprint made near the TATA box by a partially purified TFIID fraction from mammalian cells,[163, 164] thus suggesting that one function of transcriptional activators may be to modify the interaction of TFIID with DNA (Fig. 2–8).

Direct support for this notion comes from the demonstration that the acidic activating region of VP16 interacts directly with TFIID.[165] Stringer and colleagues have shown that the proteins retained on an affinity column bearing VP16 will restore activity to a HeLa cell extract lacking TFIID activity. In addition, this column retains recombinant yeast TBP produced in bacteria. The functional importance of this interaction is underscored by the observation that mutants in the acidic activation domain of VP16 that fail to activate transcription in vivo[161] also fail to bind yeast TBP in vitro.[166]

In our discussion above, we emphasized the difference between TBP, which has been cloned from many species, and TFIID, a partially purified protein fraction.

Activation

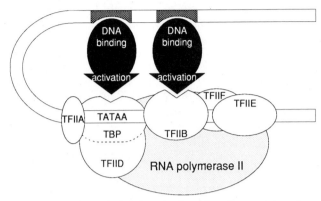

FIGURE 2–8. Transcriptional activation domains are thought to function by contacting two components of the preinitiation complex, TFIID and TFIIB.

tion. It is important to reconsider this distinction in light of our knowledge of transcriptional activation domains. In their studies of the interaction between Sp1 and the basal transcriptional machinery, Pugh and Tjian[167] found that Sp1 stimulates transcription in vitro from promoters containing a TATA box in the presence of partially purified TFIID fractions from either human or *Drosophila* cells. In contrast, Sp1 is unable to stimulate transcription when this fraction is replaced by purified, cloned *Drosophila*, human, or yeast TBP.[68, 167] Thus, the interaction between Sp1 and the basal machinery requires novel activities present in the partially purified TFIID fractions. These activities have been termed coactivators. In addition, studies with truncated versions of TBP have demonstrated that these coactivators function through the N-terminal tail of TBP. The sequence of this region is highly variable between species, and indeed, the coactivator-TBP interactions are species specific. Future work will be directed toward purifying these coactivators, and progress has been made in that direction, with the chromatographic separation of the TBP and coactivator activities.[73, 168]

Although we have emphasized TFIID as the target within the basal transcriptional machinery, two lines of evidence suggest that multiple targets may exist. The first is the observation of synergy between bound transcriptional activators containing similar or distinct types of activation domains.[169–171] In these experiments, multiple activators are able to stimulate transcription to levels that greatly exceed the additive effect of each individual activator. Second, particular activation domains are able to inhibit ("squelch"[172]) the activity of some, but not all, kinds of activation domains.[173, 174]

Activators in bacteria are known to function in distinct ways, some by aiding the binding of RNA polymerase to the promoter and others by aiding RNA polymerase in the melting of DNA necessary for the initiation of transcription.[69] In eukaryotes, there are several molecular ways in which activators could stimulate transcription. The simplest scenario to envision is that distinct coactivators present in the TFIID fraction may mediate activation by distinct activation domains. Evidence to support this notion is provided by the observation that a coactivator fraction can restore activation by proline-rich (CTF) and glutamine-rich (Sp1) domains, but not acidic (VP16) domains.[168]

Evidence for another target of transcriptional activators comes from attempts to reconstitute the basal transcriptional machinery from purified components. Addition of an activator to reactions containing highly purified basal factors results in only a two- to fivefold stimulation of transcription. In contrast, the addition of the same transcription factor to a reaction containing total nuclear extract results in the same 100-fold transcriptional enhancement observed in vivo.[175] Thus, there appears to be some other component missing from the reconstituted activity. One candidate for this component is histone H1, a protein that interacts with the nucleosome and with the linker DNA present between nucleosomes. The addition of histone H1 to a nuclear extract depleted of this protein leads to a repression of basal levels of transcription. Addition of an activator protein (e.g., GAL4-VP16) can relieve this repression. In the presence of histone H1, then, transcriptional activation is increased about 20-fold.[176]

In a series of experiments, Workman and colleagues have shown that transcription in vitro is suppressed if nucleosomes are reconstituted on the DNA template.[177] When partially purified TFIID, or bacterially produced yeast TBP, is prebound to the promoter, repression by nucleosomes is prevented.[178] GAL4-VP16, perhaps by enhancing the action of TBP, can also function to prevent repression by nucleosomes. Under conditions in which nucleosome assembly is carried out in the presence of an acidic activator, the addition of basal fractions leads to a 50-fold increase in transcription.[177] When histone H1 is added to these chromatin templates, activation by GAL4-VP16 goes up 200-fold.[179] Thus, in addition to the basal transcriptional machinery, nucleosomes and histone H1 may play a role in the process of transcriptional activation.[180]

Recent studies of transcription complexes purified at various stages of assembly in the presence of an acidic activator provide evidence that TFIIB, rather than TFIID, may be the primary target of acidic activators.[181] TFIIB is the factor that associates with the TFIID-DNA complex prior to the binding of RNA polymerase to the preinitiation complex. In protein affinity chromatography experiments, TFIIB activity is retained on a column containing an immobilized form of VP16.[181] This experiment monitors only TFIIB activity, but recombinant TFIIB produced in E. coli also binds directly to the acidic region of VP16[182] (Fig. 2–8). These data are in apparent contradiction with the results obtained using a similar assay, which showed that VP16 interacts with TFIID.[165] However,

this apparent discrepancy may be due to differences in the sensitivity of the complexes to salt, since the TFIID-VP16 complex is much more sensitive to monovalent cations than is the TFIIB-VP16 complex. The ability of an acidic activator to interact with two general transcription factors, TFIID and TFIIB, provides a possible explanation for the observed synergistic activation by multiple, DNA-bound acidic domains.

MECHANISMS OF TRANSCRIPTIONAL REPRESSION

Initially, investigation of eukaryotic gene regulation focused on positive control mechanisms, owing in large measure to the early discovery of enhancers, which function as powerful positive regulators of transcription. This observation was surprising, since negative control mechanisms were shown to play a very important role in prokaryotic gene regulation. However, as eukaryotic regulatory elements were studied in more detail, numerous examples of negative control were discovered.[183, 184] In fact, the genetic and biochemical dissection of the hierarchy of regulatory events during early Drosophila development has demonstrated that both positive and negative regulation is necessary for the proper spatial expression of developmental control genes (see below). Negative regulatory elements also appear to be responsible for extinguishing the expression of tissue-specific genes in inappropriate tissues.[185] Moreover, inducible gene expression depends on mechanisms that rapidly repress expression once the inducing stimulus is removed and on mechanisms that maintain the gene in an inactive state in the absence of inducer.[186] Three types of negative control mechanisms have been proposed (Fig. 2–9): (1) steric interference with the binding of transcriptional activators; (2) silencing of transcriptional activators by repressor bound at some distance from the activator binding site and the promoter; and (3) inhibition of transcriptional activation by direct protein-protein interactions between the activator and repressor.

Steric Interference

In prokaryotes, the most frequent mode of repression is the direct competition between a DNA-binding repressor and the general transcriptional machinery. Repressors, as exemplified by λ repressor, block the interaction of RNA polymerase with the promoter by binding to an operator sequence that overlaps the binding site for RNA polymerase.[147] In eukaryotes, this type of repression appears to explain the negative effect that the SV40 T antigen has on its own promoter.[187] Other repressor proteins whose binding sites overlap or are directly adjacent to the TATA box have been described. The binding of these proteins prevents the formation of the initiation complex by block-

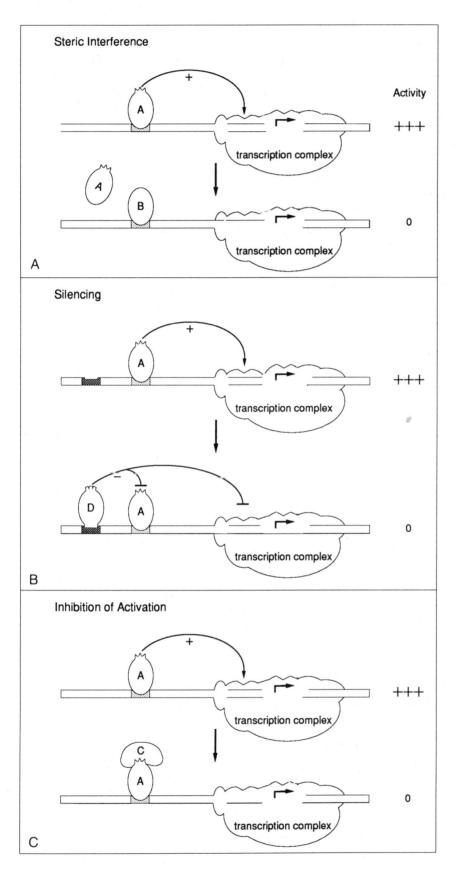

FIGURE 2–9. Transcriptional repressors function through three mechanisms: steric interference, when the repressor blocks the ability of an activator to bind DNA; silencing, in which repressors function over large distances to inhibit activation; and inhibition of transcriptional activators, whereby a repressor interacts directly with an activator, blocking its ability to enhance transcription.

ing the interaction of the general transcription factor TFIID with the TATA box.[188-190]

A transcriptional repressor often functions by competing with a transcriptional activator for binding to identical or overlapping sites. In this case, the binding of the negative regulator is dominant, and thus the repressor displaces the activator. An example of this is the human interferon-β gene promoter, in which two different transcriptional repressors can prevent the binding of transcriptional activators to a critical promoter element.[191]

Although the competitive binding examples we have described involve binding to identical sites, negative regulatory elements are also found overlapping positive sites. In some genes whose expression is repressed by glucocorticoids, the binding site for the glucocorticoid receptor overlaps a binding site for a positive activator.[192] A similar architecture of overlapping sites may exist in the promoter element that is responsible for directing the striped expression of the *Drosophila* pair-rule gene *even-skipped* (see below).[193] The clearest example of steric hindrance by repressor binding to an overlapping site, however, comes from the study of the fat body–specific enhancer of the *Drosophila alcohol dehydrogenase* gene. In this case, the binding site for a Zn finger protein, AEF-1, overlaps the binding site for the activator C/EBP. The binding of AEF-1 leads to the displacement of C/EBP and the repression of transcription.[194]

Silencing

Some sequence-specific DNA-binding repressor proteins are able to function over large distances either upstream or downstream of a promoter. The sequences to which these repressors bind are termed silencers, and they appear to have properties opposite those of a transcriptional enhancer.[195] Although first identified in yeast, silencing (or active repression[196]) has been well characterized in *Drosophila*. Several gene products involved in establishing the segmental body plan of the embryo function as active repressors. Engrailed,[196] even-skipped,[197] and Krüppel[198] have all been shown to function as repressors under appropriate circumstances. The Krüppel protein contains an alanine-rich domain that functions to repress transcription when fused to a heterologous DNA-binding domain.[198] Alanine-rich domains are also found in other active repressors, such as even-skipped. Thus, active repressors, like transcriptional activators, contain two separable domains: one responsible for DNA binding and the other responsible for mediating repression. The target of these repression domains is unknown.

Inhibitory of Transcriptional Activation

The best characterized examples of this class of repressors come from the study of transcriptional regulation in yeast. The MATα2 gene product is a homeodomain protein that is a regulator of cell identity in yeast. The α2 protein is a repressor present in α cells, where it represses **a**-specific genes, and in **a**/α diploids, where it acts in combination with the **a**1 protein to repress the haploid-specific genes.[199] In α haploids, α2 protein blocks the MCM1-mediated activation of **a**-specific genes. A dimer of α2 occupies the two ends of the operator region upstream of **a**-specific genes and straddles the binding site for the ubiquitous activator protein MCM1. It appears that both MCM1 and α2 can occupy DNA simultaneously.[200] The α2 protein must bind DNA to function as a repressor, but the homeodomain is not sufficient to mediate repression. This result suggests that a region near the N-terminus of α2 functions as a repression domain that inhibits the activation function of MCM1.[201]

Repressors need not bind DNA to inhibit activation, as clearly demonstrated by the GAL80 protein of yeast. In the absence of galactose, GAL80 interacts with the C-terminal 30 amino acids of GAL4, forming a complex that is capable of binding DNA but is unable to activate transcription.[202] Thus, GAL80 functions as an inhibitor by directly complexing with an activation domain of GAL4 and masking its activity. Galactose causes GAL80 to dissociate from GAL4, thus leading to transcriptional activation. In higher eukaryotes, the estrogen receptor can also function as a non–DNA-binding repressor.[203]

Other variations on this theme are provided by higher eukaryotes. As we described in our discussion of dimerization domains, a protein containing a mutant DNA-binding domain adjacent to an intact dimerization domain can function as a repressor. Two well-characterized examples of this type of repressor are the Id protein, which forms an inactive heterodimer with bHLH proteins,[133] and the I-POU protein, a POU domain protein that inhibits neuron-specific gene activation by forming a non–DNA-binding heterodimer with the transcriptional activator Cf1-a.[204] Protein-protein interactions can also function to repress transcription by sequestering a transcriptional activator in the cytoplasm. Thus, IκB complexes with the activator NF-κB and maintains NF-κB in an inactive state in the cytoplasm. Only after induction (e.g., by lipopolysaccharide [LPS] or TPA) is the complex between NF-κB and IκB disrupted, thus allowing NF-κB to translocate to the nucleus and activate transcription[205] (Fig. 2–10). Cytoplasmic sequestration is also observed for the steroid receptors. In this case, the glucocorticoid receptor forms a complex with the 90 kDa heat shock protein (hsp90) in the cytoplasm[206] (see Fig. 2–10).

INDUCIBLE GENE EXPRESSION

Steroid Hormone Receptors

Many eukaryotic genes are turned on in response to extracellular signals such as growth factors and

Inducible Gene Expression

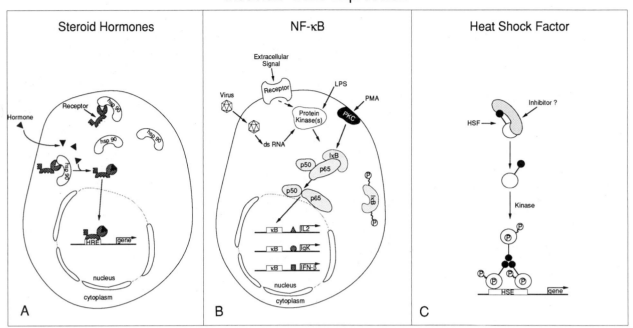

FIGURE 2–10. Inducible gene expression. *A*, The glucocorticoid receptor (GR) is normally present in the cytoplasm as a complex with a 90 kDa heat shock protein (hsp90). In the presence of hormone, the receptor-hormone complex moves to the nucleus, where it binds to regulatory elements and functions to regulate transcription. *B*, NF-κB is a central player in many signal transduction pathways. These pathways all lead to the phosphorylation of the inhibitor IκB. The phosphorylated form of IκB can no longer interact with NF-κB. NF-κB then moves to the nucleus, where it activates expression of a variety of genes. *C*, In response to heat shock, heat shock factor (HSF) is phosphorylated. This phosphorylated form functions as a transcriptional activator of genes containing a heart shock response element (HSE).

hormones or to stresses such as heat shock or virus infection. During the past few years, significant advances have been made in understanding the mechanisms involved in these processes. Perhaps the best understood example of inducible gene expression is the activation of gene expression in response to steroid hormones[207] (see Fig. 2–10). These hormones, which include the glucocorticoids, as well as the reproductive hormones estrogen and testosterone, play a central role in the control of cellular growth and differentiation in higher eukaryotes. The key components of these inducible systems are the hormone receptors, transcription factors located in the cytoplasm of many cell types.[207, 208] In the absence of hormone, these receptors are held in the cytoplasm by their association with an inhibitor protein, hsp90. However, within minutes after the addition of hormone, the receptor binds specifically to the hormone and dissociates from the inhibitor protein. This dissociation leads to the translocation of the receptor from the cytoplasm to the nucleus, where the activated receptor binds specifically to regulatory sequences upstream from hormone-inducible genes and activates transcription. These binding sites for hormone receptors function as inducible enhancer elements, in that they can confer hormone-inducible activation on heterologous promoters.

Like the other transcription factors we have discussed, hormone receptors are modular in their or-

ganization. The N-terminus of the receptor contains an acidic activation domain, the middle of the protein contains a Zn finger DNA-binding domain, and the hormone-binding domain is located near the C-terminus of the protein. As different hormone receptors were cloned and sequenced, it became apparent that they are all members of a large family of proteins that share this tripartite modular organization.[207] Remarkably, the domains can be freely exchanged between different family members, resulting in a change in hormone or gene specificity. For example, if the hormone-binding domain of the glucocorticoid receptor is exchanged for the hormone-binding domain of the progesterone receptor, the hybrid receptor will respond to progesterone but will bind to regulatory sequences normally controlled by the glucocorticoid receptor. In fact, this property has been exploited to identify hormone ligands for "orphan receptors" isolated by virtue of their sequence similarity to known receptors. The strategy is to create a hybrid protein containing the DNA-binding domain of the glucocorticoid receptor and the hormone-binding domain of the unknown receptor. The hybrid protein will then activate promoters containing a glucocorticoid regulatory element, but only in the presence of the appropriate hormone. Candidate hormones are then screened for their ability to activate the hybrid protein. This strategy was used to identify the retinoic acid receptor.[209]

Although hormone receptors were originally characterized as transcriptional activators, they can also function as hormone-dependent repressors. One way in which they function as repressors involves protein-protein interactions with Jun/Fos proteins, another family of transcriptional regulatory proteins.[210] For example, the combination of the glucocorticoid receptor and Jun/Fos heterodimers leads to hormone-dependent repression of certain promoters. In contrast, positive synergistic interactions are observed with the combination of the glucocorticoid receptor and Jun/Jun homodimers on the same promoters. Thus, the activity of hormone receptors depends on the nature of the DNA-binding site, as well as on interactions with other transcriptional regulatory proteins.

NF-κB

Another class of inducible genes comprises those that respond to extracellular signals through membrane-bound receptors. An example of this is the group of genes that are activated in response to phorbol esters that act through the cell surface receptor protein kinase C. At least one mechanism by which kinase C acts to stimulate transcription is through a cytoplasmic complex containing the transcription factor NF-κB, a heterodimer consisting of 50 and 65 kDa subunits (p50 and p65), and a 40 kDa inhibitor protein called IκB, which is bound to NF-κB through the p65 subunit.[205] Activated kinase C is thought to act by phosphorylating the IκB, which leads to its dissociation from NF-κB (Fig. 2–10). The p50/p65 heterodimer then translocates from the cytoplasm to the nucleus, binds to regulatory sequences adjacent to phorbol ester–inducible genes, and activates transcription. When the genes encoding p50 and p65 were cloned, both were found to be members of a family of proteins that includes the c-*rel* oncogene and the *Drosophila* developmental regulatory protein dorsal. As with other families of transcription factors we have discussed, a large number of different heterodimers can be formed between different members of the *rel* gene family, and these heterodimers appear to have distinct regulatory properties.

cAMP Response Element–Binding Protein (CREB)

The kinase A pathway is another example of a signal transduction pathway that involves a membrane-bound receptor. In this case, extracellular inducers activate adenyl cyclase, which leads to an increase in the intracellular levels of cAMP. High levels of cAMP in turn activate protein kinase A, which phosphorylates transcription factors. One of these factors is, in fact, NF-κB, which can respond to a number of different signal transduction pathways. Another kinase A–inducible transcription factor is CREB, which binds to cAMP response elements (CREs) located near cAMP-inducible genes.[211, 212] Unlike the situation with the hormone receptors and NF-κB, the CREB protein is already present in the nucleus in a form capable of binding specifically to the CRE sequence, but it is transcriptionally inactive. Phosphorylation of CREB converts the protein to a transcriptionally active state. The cloning and characterization of CREB cDNAs revealed that the protein is a member of the family of transcription factors containing a leucine zipper and basic region. The transcriptional activation domain of the protein lies in a region containing phosphorylation sites. One of these sites (serine 133) has been shown to be critical for the cAMP-dependent activation of CREB.

Heat Shock Factor (HSF)

Exposure of eukaryotic cells to higher than normal temperatures leads to the activation of a number of genes whose products are involved in coping with the resulting damage. These genes, appropriately known as heat shock genes, are coordinately induced, and the mechanism involves the activation of a transcription factor that binds to regulatory sequences located near each of the heat shock genes. As with the other inducible genes, these regulatory sequences can function as inducible enhancer elements, in that they can confer heat shock induction to heterologous promoters. The transcription factor that binds to these sequences is called heat shock factor (HSF; see Fig. 2–10). In contrast to most transcription factors, which act as monomers or dimers, HSF associates to form protein trimers in solution and when bound to DNA.[142] In fact, HSF can multimerize further to form hexamers capable of interacting with complex arrays of HSF-binding sites present upstream from a number of heat shock genes. The region of HSF required for multimerization is thought to be capable of forming a three-stranded α-helical coiled-coil. The binding of individual subunits of the trimer to adjacent sites on DNA is highly cooperative. The DNA-binding domain of HSF is similar over a short region to the recognition domain of bacterial σ factors but does not resemble any known eukaryotic DNA-binding domain.

The mechanism of HSF activation appears to be different in yeast and higher eukaryotes. In yeast, HSF is bound to the heat shock regulatory sequences prior to induction, and induction involves a phosphorylation-dependent activation of HSF. By contrast, HSF in higher eukaryotes binds to DNA only after induction. However, because HSF in higher eukaryotes becomes highly phosphorylated after heat shock, two steps may be required for HSF activity in these organisms: activation of binding and phosphorylation-dependent activation of the transcriptional activity. A number of observations suggested that HSF may be bound to an inhibitory protein prior to induction and is released upon heat shock. This inhibitor could act by preventing multimerization of HSF. In fact, recent studies in *Drosophila* have verified this hypothesis.[213]

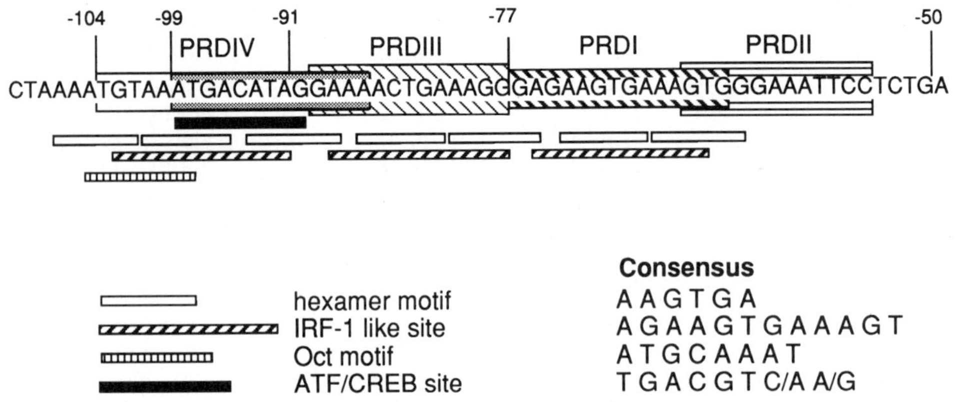

FIGURE 2–11. The virus-inducible interferon-β promoter contains a variety of cis-acting elements, all of which play a role in the induction process. The four boxes indicate the positive regulatory domains (PRDs), and the boxes beneath the promoter denote sequence motifs found in these domains. (From Du, W., and Maniatis, T.: An ATF/CREB binding site is required for virus induction of the human interferon-β gene. Proc. Natl. Acad. Sci. USA 89: 2150, 1992; with permission.)

Prior to heat shock induction, the 104 kDa HSF protein is present in the nucleus in a complex of 220 kDa molecular weight. This complex, which does not bind to DNA, could be a homodimer of HSF incapable of further multimerization, or it could be HSF bound to an inhibitor protein. In any case, upon heat shock the *Drosophila* HSF forms a hexamer, capable of binding DNA.

In summary, the three examples of inducible gene systems that we have discussed appear to be variations on a theme. In each case, the inducible transcription factor is inactive prior to induction, and induction leads to activation, possibly through phosphorylation or some other post-translational modification. In all three examples, gene expression is induced by specific binding of the activated transcription factor to a regulatory sequence adjacent to the gene. In most cases, two or more copies of the regulatory sequence are present.

Induction by a Variety of Stimuli: The Interferon-β Gene

A more complex example of inducible gene expression is provided by the human interferon-β (IFN-β) gene.[214] Interferons are proteins secreted in response to virus infection. These inducible proteins bind to specific cell surface receptors and in so doing activate a large number of interferon-inducible genes that encode antiviral proteins. A number of experiments have shown that the inducer is double-stranded RNA produced during virus infection. Prior to virus infection, the IFN-β gene is tightly repressed, but within minutes after the virus enters the cell the gene is transiently activated at the level of transcription. The level of IFN-β mRNA peaks at around 12 hours and then decreases to low levels by 20 to 24 hours. Inhibition experiments have shown that protein synthesis is not required for the activation of the gene but is required for its postinduction repression. Thus, like the other inducible systems we have discussed, transcriptional activation likely involves the post-translation modification of transcription factors. On the other hand, postinduction repression requires the synthesis of new proteins. In fact, there is evidence that genes

encoding the postinduction repressor are themselves inducible by virus infection.

Detailed studies of the DNA sequence requirements for virus induction and postinduction repression reveal a highly compact and remarkably complex organization of regulatory sequences. As shown in Figure 2–11, the sequences within approximately 100 bp upstream contain at least three distinct positive regulatory sequences and two distinct negative regulatory sequences. Positive regulatory domain I (PRDI) and PRDIII are variations on the same regulatory motif, whereas PRDII and PRDIV are distinct regulatory elements. Negative regulatory domain I (NRDI) and NRDII are distinct negative regulatory sequences, defined by mutations that increase the constitutive level of IFN-β gene expression. A number of proteins that bind specifically to each of the positive regulatory elements have been identified, but similar efforts have yet to identify proteins that bind specifically to the negative regulatory domains. The positive regulatory domains were defined by saturation mutagenesis experiments and by showing that they can confer virus induction on a heterologous promoter when the elements are present in two or more copies. An important point is that none of the positive regulatory domains are sufficient for virus induction of a heterologous promoter when present in one copy. However, two copies of any simple element or a combination of one copy each of two different elements (e.g., PRDI + PRDII) efficiently respond to virus induction. Thus, the IFN-β promoter provides another example of a combinatorial mechanism for gene activation. At least three different factors must be activated by virus induction before the gene is activated.

The best characterized positive regulatory element is PRDII. Surprisingly, the transcription factor involved in PRDII-dependent virus induction appears to be NF-κB. Several lines of evidence are consistent with this possibility. First, PRDII and the original binding site for NF-κB (κB) are functionally interchangeable. That is, two or more copies of PRDII or κB function both as B-cell–specific enhancers and as virus-inducible elements in fibroblasts. Second, both PRDII and κB bind specifically to NF-κB in vitro. Third, mutations in PRDII that interfere with NF-κB binding in vitro also prevent virus induction in vivo.

Fourth, virus infection leads to the activation of the cytoplasmic NF-κB/IκB complex. On the basis of this observation and the fact that NF-κB can be activated by a variety of other inducers, NF-κB has been proposed to act as a "protein second messenger" in signal transduction pathways. Virus-inducible transcription factors that act on PRDI, PRDIII, and PRDIV have yet to be identified.

The role of NF-κB in the expression of the immunoglobulin light chain gene and the IFN-β gene provides an interesting example of the combinatorial mechanism involved in the expression of both genes. Certain types of pre-B lymphoid cell lines have rearranged their endogenous immunoglobulin κ (Igκ) genes, but the genes are not expressed because NF-κB is present in its inactive form. Of course, the endogenous IFN-β gene is also not expressed. However, when the differentiation of the pre-B cells into mature B cells is activated by lipopolysaccharide, NF-κB is activated and the Igκ chain gene is expressed at a high level. However, even though large amounts of NF-κB are present, the endogenous IFN-β gene is not turned on. It is believed this is because the NRDI repressors have not been inactivated and the factors that bind to PRDI and PRDIV have not been activated. Consistent with this possibility, infection of the pre-B cells with virus leads to the activation of not only the IFN-β gene but also the Igκ gene. Presumably, virus infection not only activated NF-κB, which is sufficient to activate the Igκ chain gene in this cell type, but also activated the transcription factors that bind to PRDI and PRDIV. Similarly, treatment of cells with phorbol esters activates NF-κB but does not activate the IFN-β gene. Thus, activation of the IFN-β gene, and probably most other genes, operates on a "fail safe" mechanism. The gene is turned on only after a number of different criteria have been satisfied.

TISSUE-SPECIFIC GENE EXPRESSION

Studies of genes that are expressed in a cell- or tissue-specific manner have revealed that their expression is regulated at the level of transcription. With the discovery of viral enhancers, it seemed likely that similar elements would be involved in the expression of cellular genes. The first such enhancer identified was that of the immunoglobulin heavy chain gene.[215, 216] This enhancer, which is located in the first intron of the gene, has all the characteristics of viral enhancers: It activates transcription of a heterologous gene in an orientation-independent fashion at large distances. The activity of this enhancer, however, is restricted to B lymphocytes. Thus, by using conventional molecular biological techniques and an array of cell lines derived from various tissues, transfection assays have been used to identify cis-acting sequences involved in the cell type–specific expression of many different genes.

In addition to transfection and in vitro transcription experiments, the use of P-element transformation in Drosophila[217, 218] and the generation of transgenic mice[219] have provided the opportunity to investigate the function of cis-acting sequences in vivo. This analysis has led to the identification of many regulatory elements involved in generating tissue specificity and the subsequent isolation and characterization of the trans-acting factors that bind to these sequences. Our discussion of tissue-specific gene expression draws on data from many systems in an attempt to sketch out the strategies used to generate the restricted expression of a gene during development.

Tissue-Specific Expression of Regulatory Factors

The most direct way to generate tissue-specific patterns of gene expression is to restrict the expression of a transcription factor to the cell type in which it regulates transcription. For example, the expression of the prolactin gene specifically in the pituitary gland is due to the pituitary-specific expression of a regulatory factor Pit-1, a POU domain protein.[220, 221] Mutations at the mouse dwarf locus disrupt the development of the anterior pituitary and result in the lack of three pituitary cell types. The demonstration that these mutations lie in the gene encoding Pit-1 provides a direct link between a transcription factor and cell-specific developmental events in mammals.[222]

Among the other transcriptional regulatory proteins that are expressed in a tissue-specific fashion are the following: Oct-2, a member of the family of octamer-binding proteins that is involved in the regulation of B-cell–specific immunoglobulin gene transcription[223]; GATA-1, a factor that recognizes a sequence found in the majority of erythroid-specific regulatory elements and plays a role in the erythroid-specific expression of these genes[224, 225]; and MyoD1, a master regulator whose expression is restricted to skeletal muscle.[129] Regulation at the level of translation is an additional way to generate a limited expression pattern for a regulatory protein, and this mechanism appears to be responsible for the limited tissue distribution of the liver-enriched transcriptional activators LAP[226] and DBP.[227]

A crucial question regarding regulatory proteins expressed in only one cell type is how their expression is accomplished. Thus, one has, in a sense, just moved the regulatory problem back one step. A partial answer to this regulatory regression problem comes from the observation that several of these transcriptional regulatory proteins, including Pit-1,[228] MyoD1,[229] and GATA-1,[230] are known to positively regulate their own expression. This positive feedback loop provides a mechanism for the continuous maintenance of the differentiated state, but it does not explain how expression is turned on in the first place. The dissection of the cis-acting elements governing the expression of these transcription factors is still in its beginning stages, and further study is needed to identify the factors involved in the expression of regulatory proteins.

The MyoD1 protein, a member of the bHLH family of proteins that appears to play a crucial role in the specification of the muscle cell lineage, has become a paradigm for the study of tissue-specific gene expression. The gene encoding MyoD1 was cloned by making use of a cell culture system in which fibroblasts can be converted into myoblasts.[231] By transfection it was demonstrated that MyoD1 could convert a variety of differentiated cell types into muscle. MyoD1 apparently functions to activate myogenesis by directly binding to the control region of muscle-specific genes and activating their expression.[131] MyoD1 is thus thought to be a master regulatory gene that acts to specify the fate of an individual cell. MyoD1 does not, however, function alone. As mentioned above in our discussion of bHLH proteins, MyoD1 forms heterodimers with the ubiquitous bHLH protein E12. These heterodimers have a higher affinity for DNA than do MyoD1 homodimers, and it appears that the heterodimer is the active form in vivo.[132] Further complexity is added by Id, a protein that acts as a dominant negative regulator of MyoD1 activity. Since Id heterodimerizes more readily with E12 than does MyoD1, it appears that Id acts to block muscle-specific gene expression by forming non-productive heterodimers with E12, preventing its interaction with MyoD1.[133] In addition, the existence of other genes, such as myogenin, Myf-5, and MRF4, which perform functions similar to those of MyoD1 in cell culture assays, has led researchers to realize that the story in vivo may be more complex.[129]

The Importance of Combinatorial Regulation

In many cases, the analysis of tissue-specific gene regulation has not identified a "master" regulatory molecule like MyoD1 whose activity is itself tissue specific. In certain cases, the regulatory elements are complex, and expression depends on the interplay of various cis-acting elements. In the case of Drosophila alcohol dehydrogenase (Adh), for example, neither the enhancer nor the promoter alone is sufficient to generate the proper pattern of expression. Rather, the expression of the Adh gene in several tissues is the result of specific interactions between the enhancer and promoter.[232] Similarly, the stage-specific and tissue-specific expression of the chicken β globin gene depends on the interplay between enhancer and promoter elements.[233]

Studies of the liver-specific transcription of genes encoding serum proteins (e.g., albumin and transthyretin) and enzymes (e.g., tyrosine aminotransferase and phosphoenol pyruvate carboxykinase) have provided some of the strongest evidence in support of the importance of combinatorial regulation in gene control.[234] These studies, which have relied primarily on tissue culture transfection experiments using hepatocyte cell lines, have led to three major conclusions.

First, multiple cis-acting sequences, which include both promoter and enhancer elements, contribute to the high level of expression of these genes in hepatocytes. Second, the identification and characterization of the proteins that bind to these elements have revealed that both ubiquitous factors and those with a limited tissue distribution are involved in generating liver-specific gene expression. Four transcriptional activator proteins, all of which are members of families of transcriptional regulatory molecules, are expressed in the liver and have a limited tissue distribution: C/EBP, the prototype leucine zipper protein[235]; HNF-1α, a homeodomain protein (also called LF-B1)[236]; HNF-3, a protein with sequence similarity to the Drosophila homeotic gene fork head[237]; and HNF-4, a member of the steroid hormone receptor superfamily.[238] None of these factors, however, is restricted to the liver, and none plays a dominant role as a master regulator. Rather, the promoter of each liver-specific gene has a unique array of binding sites for liver-enriched and ubiquitous trans-acting factors. It is the combinatorial interactions between these factors that result in liver-specific expression (see Fig. 2–3). The involvement of ubiquitous factors in tissue-specific gene regulation is an important conclusion, and data from other systems have recently indicated that cell type–specific gene regulation can be accomplished by altering the levels of non–tissue-specific factors.[210] Finally, negative regulation appears to be responsible for the silencing of liver-specific genes in other tissues[239] (see below).

The study of the transcriptional regulation of liver-enriched transcription factors has recently led to the discovery of a transcriptional cascade that may play a role in the specification of cell type. Although many tissue-specific regulators are known to regulate their own expression (autoregulation), studies of the HNF-1α promoter have revealed that HNF-4 and HNF-3, two other liver-enriched transcription factors, are essential positive regulators of HNF-1α expression.[240] While transcriptional hierarchies are well known in the study of Drosophila development (see below), this transcriptional hierarchy involved in liver-specific gene expression represents one of the most clearly understood examples in mammalian systems.

Regulation of Transcription Factors by Post-translational Modification

Many of the mechanisms described in our discussion of inducible gene expression appear to be used to generate tissue-specific gene expression. Indeed, several proteins involved in inducible gene regulation also appear to play a role in tissue-specific regulatory mechanisms. CREB, for example, is involved in the regulation of liver-specific[241] (see below) and pituitary-specific[228] gene expression in mammals and fat body–specific gene expression in Drosophila.[242] The best characterized example of overlap between inducible and tissue-specific regulatory proteins is NF-κB. NF-κB specifically interacts with the immunoglobulin κ light chain enhancer and functions to control expression in mature B cells, but not in pre-B cells.[243] As described above, the activity of NF-κB is inhibited by the cytoplasmic protein IκB.

As tissue-specific expression is studied in more detail, many more mechanisms that function to regulate factor activity are discovered. Dimerization is known to play an important role in regulating the activity of DNA-binding proteins. Indeed, heterodimerization appears to play a crucial role in the activity of bHLH family members such as MyoD1. The recent characterization of a cofactor that regulates the dimerization of the liver-enriched homeodomain protein HNF-1α and the demonstration that this factor has a restricted tissue distribution suggest that the regulation of dimerization may contribute to determining tissue-specific patterns of gene expression.[244]

Extinction: The Negative Regulation of Tissue-Specific Gene Expression

Although our discussion has focused thus far on the activator proteins involved in tissue-specific gene expression, negative regulators also play a critical part in some systems. This negative regulation can take two forms: In one mechanism, termed modulation, negative regulators function to decrease expression in the tissue in which the gene is active. This mechanism appears to result from the competitive binding of an activator and a repressor to adjacent or identical sites, and it may play a role in liver-specific gene expression in mammals[245] and fat body–specific expression in Drosophila.[194] The second type of regulation, termed extinction, functions to repress expression of a tissue-specific gene in the inappropriate tissues.[185, 239]

Analysis of the extinction of the tyrosine aminotransferase (TAT) gene in tissues other than the liver has revealed that the mechanism of extinction is indirect, involving not repression but rather a lack of activation.[239] Investigation of the extinction of liver-specific genes was made possible by the observation that fusion of fibroblasts with differentiated rat hepatoma cells leads to the repression of liver-specific genes.[246] The locus responsible for this repression, tissue-specific extinguisher 1 (TSE1), was mapped to mouse chromosome 11. TSE1 was found to repress a group of liver-specific genes, all of which are inducible by glucocorticoids and cAMP.[247] Two groups have recently cloned TSE1, and it encodes R1α, a regulatory subunit of protein kinase A.[248, 249] TSE1 functions by preventing the phosphorylation and activation of CREB, thus leading to the decreased transcription of genes whose expression is normally activated by CREB. Although TSE1 does not provide novel insights into direct mechanisms of negative control, it does resolve the apparent paradox that fibroblasts would have to produce a group of repressors for the entire set of differentiated gene products. Rather, existing mechanisms are recruited to ensure that a gene is not inappropriately expressed in the incorrect cell type.

This example of extinction also serves to emphasize the critical role that ubiquitous factors play in regulating tissue-specific gene expression. Expression of the immunoglobulin heavy chain enhancer is also under negative control in non-lymphoid tissues. Although this system is less well characterized, it appears that repression may be direct, involving a factor present in non-expressing cells that binds to suppressor sites within the enhancer.[250]

TRANSCRIPTIONAL REGULATION IN DROSOPHILA DEVELOPMENT

The genetic and molecular analysis of the early stages of Drosophila embryonic development has advanced dramatically in recent years. Drosophila is a metameric organism composed of serially repeating body segments, and extensive genetic screens have been carried out to isolate mutants defective in this segmentation process.[251] Analysis of these mutants has led to insights into the events of early development. The general mechanism involves the subdivision of the embryo into repeated units, followed by the specification of the fate of each segment[252, 253] (Fig. 2–12).

Even before fertilization, the oocyte is polarized along the anterior-posterior body axis, both morphologically and in the distribution of regulatory molecules. This polarization is in part the result of a concentration gradient of the anterior determinant, bicoid (bcd). Bicoid protein is present at high levels near the anterior pole and is distributed in a gradient, gradually decreasing over about half the egg's length. The posterior determinant, nanos, is sharply localized to the posterior of the embryo. Bicoid and nanos are deposited in the oocyte during oogenesis, and thus this class of genes is referred to as the maternal genes. The products of these genes create a broad distinction between the anterior and posterior regions of the embryo.

The concentration gradients of the maternal gene products lead to the regional expression of the zygotic gap genes. This group of genes includes hunchback (hb), Krüppel (Kr), and knirps (kni). The hb gene is expressed in the region extending from the anterior pole to the middle of the egg and at a lower level at the posterior pole. Kr is expressed in the region just posterior to the anterior domain of hb, and the kni gene is active in the portion of the embryo just posterior to the Kr band (Fig. 2–12). The broad gradient of maternal gene expression is converted into stable regions of gap gene expression as the embryo develops.

The spatial localization of the gap gene products results in the position-specific expression of the next group of genes, the pair-rule genes. These genes, such as even-skipped (eve) and fushi tarazu (ftz), are localized to seven stripes along the anterior-posterior axis. The last step in this hierarchy involves the activation of two sets of genes. The segment polarity genes, such as engrailed (en), are involved in the further subdivision

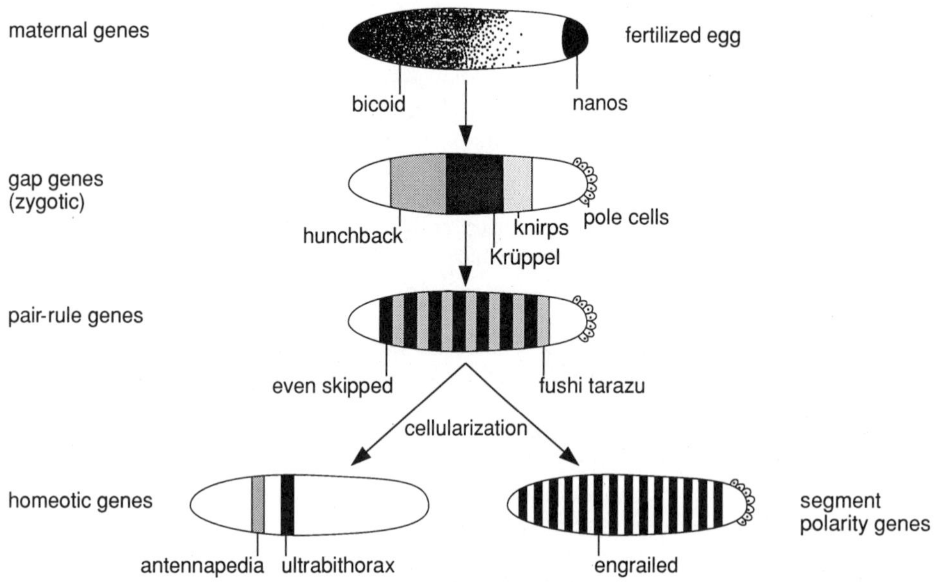

FIGURE 2–12. Segmentation of the *Drosophila* embryo is achieved through a cascade of regulatory events, beginning with a broad, graded distribution of maternal gene products. This hierarchy eventually results in the expression of the pair-rule genes in certain segments and the activation of homeotic genes in the appropriate region of the embryo.

of each segment into anterior and posterior compartments. The identity of each segment is specified by the homeotic genes. These genes, which include *Ultrabithorax* (*Ubx*) and *Antennapedia* (*Antp*), are activated only in certain regions, and they function later in the differentiation process to specify cell fate.

The molecular cloning of a large number of the genes involved in this segmentation hierarchy has revealed that the majority of them encode proteins that contain DNA-binding domains, particularly the Zn finger or the homeodomain.[252, 253] Thus, this genetic hierarchy appears to be a cascade of transcriptional regulation. Subsequent biochemical and molecular characterization of these gene products has shown that they are indeed DNA-binding transcriptional regulatory proteins. Two examples of regulatory events in this hierarchy will serve to illustrate the type of study that is under way to investigate the molecular basis of pattern formation.

Genetically it was known that the gradient of the morphogen bcd plays a crucial role in the early establishment of the anterior-posterior axis of the embryo. Bcd functions as a transcriptional activator, binding to sites located in the promoter of the gap gene *hb*.[254] An analysis of these binding sites and the study of bcd-dependent gene activation have demonstrated that a threshold level of bcd is required for the expression of the *hb* promoter.[255, 256] Bcd thus provides an example of a concentration-dependent transcriptional switch responsible for the activation of gene expression.

A more complex example of gene regulation in the early embryo is provided by analysis of the regulation of the striped expression of the *eve* gene.[257] The *eve* gene is expressed in seven stripes in the embryo, and expression in individual stripes is regulated by separate *cis*-acting elements within the *eve* promoter[258, 259] (Fig. 2–13). A 700 bp region, extending from 1.0 to 1.7 kb upstream of the *eve* gene, is required for expression in stripe 2. Genetic studies, as well as analysis of the expression pattern of maternal and gap

gene products, have suggested that four segmentation genes are involved in regulating the formation of *eve* stripe 2. Three gap gene products—*hb*, *Kr*, and *giant* (*gt*)—as well as the maternal morphogen *bcd* all bind to the element that directs expression in stripe 2.[193] DNA-binding assays, tissue culture cotransfection experiments,[193] and the in vivo analysis of the effect of mutagenesis of the binding sites for these proteins[260] are consistent with the following model. Bcd and hb proteins, both of which are expressed in the region of stripe 2, mediate activation. The proteins gt and Kr are expressed at very low levels in stripe 2, with the region of highest gt expression located anterior to stripe 2 and the region of highest Kr expression located posterior to stripe 2 (see Fig. 2–13). The proteins gt and Kr function as repressors, and they serve to establish the stripe borders. Although the interplay between these activators and repressors on the 700 bp stripe 2 element has not been determined in detail, it is clear that the *eve* stripe 2 element has all the properties of a genetic on-off switch.

In the regulatory hierarchy, the *eve* gene plays a pivotal role in the transition from the gap genes to the segment polarity genes, and this is accomplished through a two-step mechanism of *eve* expression. In the first step, the broad distribution of gap gene products is "read" by the *eve* gene, using stripe-specific regulatory elements. As shown in Figure 2–13, there is a different element for each stripe of *eve* expression, and these elements are activated by the appropriate combination of gap gene products, as described in the example of stripe 2 above. However, once the *eve* gene is activated, it autoregulates its expression through a single element that specifies *eve* expression in all seven stripes. In turn, *eve* regulates the expression of other pair-rule genes and of segment polarity genes. Thus, the initially broad distribution of gap gene signals is converted into seven broad stripes of *eve* expression, followed by refinement into sharp intersegmental boundaries.

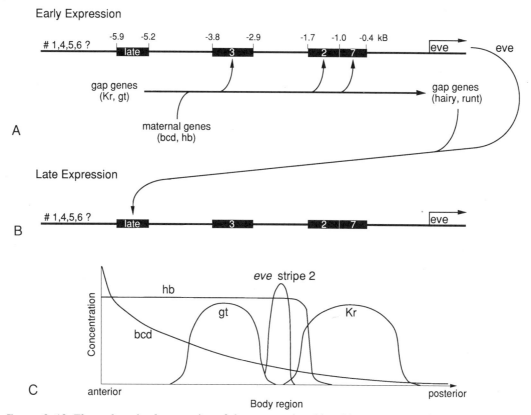

FIGURE 2–13. The early striped expression of the *eve* gene is achieved by separate regulatory elements that mediate expression in each stripe. *A,* Elements for stripes 2, 3, and 7 have been localized, and elements for the other stripes are thought to be located in the region upstream of the late regulatory element. *B,* The late expression of *eve* is driven by an enhancer element, which directs expression in all seven stripes. The pair-rule gene products, including eve itself, regulate this late expression. *C,* Early expression is regulated by the maternal and gap gene products hb, bcd, Kr, and gt. The expression pattern of these proteins in the region of stripe 2 is shown here. (*C* is from Stanojevic, D., Small, S., and Levine, M.: Regulation of a segmentation stripe by overlapping activators and repressors in the *Drosophila* embryo. Science 254: 1385–1387, 1991; with permission. Copyright 1991 by the AAAS.)

RNA PROCESSING

Our discussion has thus far focused on the transcriptional regulation of gene expression. This transcriptional regulation represents a major control point in many systems, but expression can be regulated at other levels. The striking discovery of introns in the genes of higher eukaryotes raised the possibility that expression could be regulated at the level of RNA processing.

Pre-mRNAs are processed and modified in many ways. A 7-methyl-guanosine (m⁷G), which is linked 5′–5′ with the first base of the mRNA, is added cotranscriptionally to the 5′ end of the message.[261] This 5′ cap appears to play a role in translation, since it is known to be necessary for the binding of some mRNAs to the ribosome.[262]

The 3′ termini of most eukaryotic mRNAs (with the notable exception of those messages encoding histones) have a poly (A) tail consisting of approximately 200 adenosine residues. Polyadenylation is an early step in the post-transcriptional maturation of the primary transcript. This process involves two steps. First, the mRNA transcript is cleaved 10 to 25 nucleotides (nt) downstream of the highly conserved sequence element AAUAAA.[263] Then, a specific poly (A) polymerase, which has recently been cloned,[264] catalyzes the sequential polymerization of ATP onto the 3′ end of the message.[265] This poly (A) tail has several biological roles. It acts to increase the stability of the message, plays a role in the export of the mRNA from the nucleus, and, in some cases, may function in translation regulation.[266] Some messages are subject to differential polyadenylation, but only one example is known in which a specific factor has been clearly implicated in the regulation of polyadenylation.[157]

The Mechanism of Pre-mRNA Splicing

In the process known as pre-mRNA splicing, the introns present in the primary transcript are removed, generating the mature mRNA. During the past 5 years, considerable progress has been made in understanding basic splicing mechanisms, and a number of essential RNA- and protein-splicing components have been identified and characterized. Further, studies have begun to describe possible mechanisms responsible for the regulation of alternative splicing events.

Introns can vary in size from 31 bp to well over 10 kilobase pairs (kb), but analysis of the intron sequences has revealed consensus sequences near the exon/intron junctions (Fig. 2–14). The functional significance of these sequences was demonstrated by showing that single-base mutations adversely affect splicing in vivo and in vitro. In addition, natural mutations in these sequences—for example, in the human β globin gene—lead to β thalassemia.[267] The nucleotide sequence at the exon/intron boundary is remarkably conserved in virtually all pre-mRNAs. The first two nucleotides at the 5' end of the intron are almost always GU. The 3' end of the intron invariably ends with an AG, which is preceded by a pyrimidine-rich stretch. An A residue near the 3' splice site is an essential participant in the splicing reaction (see below) but is not found as part of a stringent consensus sequence in mammalian cells. In the yeast *S. cerevisiae*, in which introns are less frequent and the requirements more stringent, this A is part of a branch point consensus sequence that is located between 10 and 60 nt of the 3' splice site.[268]

Exploration of the mechanism of pre-mRNA splicing was facilitated by the availability of cloned genes containing introns. By investigating naturally occurring mutations and constructing novel altered forms of these genes, the structural requirements for accurate and efficient splicing were determined. The most crucial advance, however, was the establishment of nuclear extracts competent to carry out splicing in vitro.[269, 270] This technology, when combined with the ability to transcribe specifically designed DNA templates in vitro,[271] allowed the detailed investigation of splicing mechanisms and the purification of the components of the splicing machinery.[272, 273]

The crucial conceptual problem with splicing is that of splice site selection: How are the multiple introns present in a pre-mRNA spliced accurately to maintain the proper reading frame and so that neighboring

exons are joined to one another? Since it is known that the 5' splice site of one intron can be joined to the 3' splice site of another intron, as occurs in alternative splicing, it is crucial to understand how this is normally prevented during the splicing reaction.

By studying splicing in vitro, the pathway of cleavages and ligations that occur during the reaction has been characterized. Studies by Guthrie and by Cech[274, 275] of the splicing of the intron within the large rRNA subunit from the ciliated protozoan *Tetrahymena* have done much to form our ideas about how splicing occurs. In these pioneering studies, it was demonstrated that this intron is precisely and efficiently excised in vitro in the complete absence of protein.[276] Indeed, the only essential cofactor is guanosine. This novel RNA-catalyzed reaction, which is efficiently catalyzed in part by the precise three-dimensional folding of the intron,[277] occurs via two successive *trans*-esterification events. This reaction, therefore, does not require energy, since the *trans*-esterification mechanism results in no net change in the total number of phosphodiester bonds. Because of the involvement of a guanosine cofactor, the mechanism of splicing of these so-called group I introns differs in its details from that of pre-mRNA splicing (see references 274 and 275 for comparison of these mechanisms). Autocatalytic splicing is not, however, restricted to group I introns. Group II introns, present in yeast mitochondrial pre-mRNAs, also undergo self-splicing in vitro. The mechanism by which this self-splicing occurs involves a lariat intermediate and does not require a nucleoside cofactor.[278] It is thus very similar to pre-mRNA splicing.

Pre-mRNA splicing in higher eukaryotes occurs via a two-step *trans*-esterification mechanism.[272, 279] The first step involves cleavage of the 5' splice site, which is accomplished by the attack of the 2'–OH group of the adenosine residue at the branch point on the guanosine residue at the 5' splice site (see Fig. 2–14). The formation of this 2'–5' phosphodiester bond generates a novel intermediate termed a lariat, which contains the intron and the 3' exon.[269, 270] In the second step, the 3' splice site is cleaved by the 3'–OH on the first exon. The two exons are thus joined together to form the mature RNA and free lariat intron. The existence of the lariat structure was proposed on the basis of the anomalous electrophoretic mobility of the excised intron, its resistance to digestion by some ribonucleases, and a block to reverse transcription near the 3' end of the intron. The isolation of the branched nucleotides confirmed the existence of a 2'–5' diester linkage between the 5'-phosphate of the guanosine at the 5' intron junction and the 2'–OH group of the adenosine residue at the branch point.[279]

Spliceosome Assembly

The splicing of nuclear pre-mRNAs differs from self-splicing in vitro in that it requires multiple nuclear factors. Self-splicing is facilitated by the precise three-

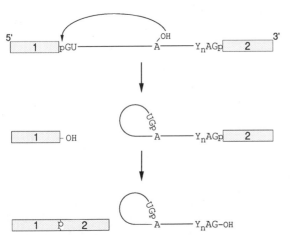

FIGURE 2–14. The mechanism of pre-mRNA splicing. Splicing occurs by two successive *trans*-esterification events and involves the formation of a lariat intermediate. Exons are shown as boxes, and the line indicates the intron. The conserved sequences found in mammalian introns are shown.

dimensional folding pattern of the intron; thus, group I and group II introns carry the structural requirements for their own catalysis. In pre-mRNA splicing, however, a large, multisubunit complex, termed the spliceosome, must be assembled.[280–282] The spliceosome, which contains proteins and small nuclear ribonucleoprotein complexes (snRNPs), is assembled in an ATP-dependent, ordered fashion prior to cleavage of the 5′ splice site.[272]

These snRNPs contain one snRNA molecule, ranging in size from 56 to 217 nt, and a small set of proteins.[274, 283] The major snRNAs found in the mammalian spliceosome are U1, U2, U4, U5, and U6, so named because of their unusually high uracil content. These snRNAs contain a unique trimethylguanosine cap at their 5′ ends, antibodies to which have been used to purify these snRNAs. The snRNPs are associated with a variety of antigens, including the Sm antigen, which are recognized by patients with autoimmune disease.[284] The snRNPs involved in splicing contain a common set of proteins as well as proteins unique to each complex.

The spliceosome assembly pathway (Fig. 2–15) and the role of RNA-snRNA base pairing as well as RNA-protein and protein-protein interactions in this process have been investigated using a variety of techniques.[272] In vitro studies have been aimed at purifying the spliceosome and identifying its components.[285, 286] Sucrose or glycerol density gradients,[282] native gel electrophoresis,[287] and gel filtration[288] have been used to identify intermediates on the spliceosome assembly pathway. The power of yeast genetics has been combined with biochemical analysis to study splicing in *S. cerevisiae*.[268, 289]

The first hint of a role for snRNPs in splicing came from the recognition that the nucleotide sequence at the 5′ end of U1 RNA is complementary to the consensus sequence found at the 5′ splice site. By making compensatory changes in U1 snRNA and the 5′ splice site, it was demonstrated that the U1 snRNP does indeed interact specifically with the 5′ splice site in vitro.[283, 290] The association of the U1 snRNP with the 5′ splice site, which is ATP independent, represents the first step in spliceosome assembly, formation of the E complex.[272, 288]

The second step in spliceosome assembly is the interaction of the U2 snRNP via base pairing with the nucleotide sequence surrounding the branch point adenosine, an interaction that requires ATP hydrolysis and results in the formation of the A complex.[272, 291] The binding of U2 snRNP to the intron is facilitated by interactions with a number of proteins, including U2 snRNP auxiliary factor (U2AF), which binds specifically to the polypyrimidine stretch located immediately upstream of the AG dinucleotide at the 3′ splice site,[292, 293] and by prior binding of U1 snRNP to the 5′ splice site.[272]

A tri-snRNP complex, containing U4/U6 and U5, next associates in an ATP-dependent manner to form the mature spliceosome (see Fig. 2–15, B complex). The first step in the splicing reaction (cleavage at

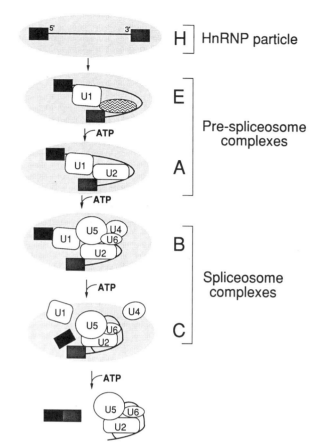

FIGURE 2–15. The process of mammalian spliceosome assembly. Boxes indicate exons, and the line indicates the intron. Interactions between the snRNPs are drawn arbitrarily. The shaded oval represents hnRNP proteins, which associate with the pre-mRNA to form the H complex. At least some of these proteins remain bound throughout the process of spliceosome assembly. (From Michaud, S., and Reed, R.: An ATP-independent complex commits pre-mRNA to the mammalian spliceosome assembly pathway. Genes Dev. 5: 2534–2546, 1991; with permission.)

the 5′ splice site by formation of the lariat intermediate) is not accomplished, however, until U4 is released.[272, 294] Since U4 and U6 are associated via multiple base-pairing interactions,[295] this dissociation is likely to be an active event, perhaps requiring an ATP-dependent helicase.

General Splicing Factors

The spliceosome contains a large number of non-snRNP proteins in addition to the snRNPs described above.[286] Three different mammalian splicing factors, SF2/ASF,[296, 297] U2AF (described above), and SC35,[298] have been purified to homogeneity and shown to be required for the earliest steps of spliceosome assembly. A factor, termed the 88 kDa antigen, has been purified and shown to be necessary for B complex formation.[299]

SF2/ASF, which was simultaneously identified by two groups, is a 33 kDa RNA-binding protein that contains an arginine- and serine-rich region and an RNP-type RNA-binding domain.[300, 301] The purified factor does not bind specifically to U1 snRNP or 5′ splice sites, although it is capable of influencing 5′ splice site selection.[297, 302] Extracts depleted of SF2/ASF are unable to assemble the A complex (see Fig. 2–15), suggesting that this factor plays a role in the initial steps in spliceosome assembly, perhaps by catalyzing RNA-RNA base pairing.[296]

SC35 was identified by raising monoclonal antibodies against partially purified spliceosomes.[298] Like SF2/ASF, SC35 is also required for A complex formation. The recent cloning of a cDNA encoding this protein has revealed that it contains an RNP consensus sequence and a long arginine- and serine-rich region similar to that found in SF2/ASF (X.-D. Fu and T. Maniatis, personal communication). Studies of the function of SC35 have suggested that it may mediate interactions between spliceosomal components and the 5′ and 3′ splice sites of the pre-mRNA.[303] One intriguing aspect of SC35 comes from immunofluorescence studies of the localization of the SC35 protein. Monoclonal antibodies to SC35 show a speckled pattern of staining in the nucleus, similar to that seen with anti-Sm antibodies.[298] This finding has increased interest in the idea that splicing may occur in specific locations within the nucleus. Alternatively, spliceosomes may be assembled in certain subnuclear locales. Both of these possibilities underscore the view that a high degree of structural organization exists within the nucleus.[304]

A number of pre-mRNA processing (PRP) mutants of the yeast *S. cerevisiae* have been identified.[268, 272] Some mutations lie in genes encoding integral components of snRNPs, and others are proteins associated with the spliceosome. Studies of splicing in yeast have complemented and extended many studies of mammalian pre-mRNA splicing, and it appears that many of the fundamental mechanisms are very similar. There are certain differences, however. Yeast has very few introns and no known examples of alternative splicing, and the *cis*-acting sequence requirements are more stringent than in mammalian systems. With these caveats in mind, the study of splicing in yeast can be extraordinarily informative. The cloning and characterization of these PRP genes have shown that many are related to a group of ATP-binding proteins that may be RNA helicases.[305] The founding member of this family, called the DEAD family because their similar regions contain the motif Asp-Glu-Ala-Asp, is the ATP-dependent RNA helicase eIF4a. This homology is of particular interest, since ATP is required for spliceosome assembly in vitro and RNA unwinding is a likely source of this requirement.

The Regulation of Pre-mRNA Splicing

In higher eukaryotes, some pre-mRNAs are alternatively spliced, thus leading in some cases to the production of different proteins from a single pre-mRNA. This alternative exon usage can be regulated temporally or in a tissue-specific fashion.[306, 307] Regulated splicing can also serve as an on-off switch during development if one of the spliced forms of an mRNA lacks an open reading frame.[308] The importance of alternative splicing for achieving genetic diversity in eukaryotes may provide an explanation for why nuclear pre-mRNA splicing requires such complicated machinery, in stark contrast to the simplicity of self-splicing. The structural requirements for self-splicing are stringent and provide little opportunity for regulation. In contrast, the complex mammalian spliceosome frees the intron to diverge in ways that may allow for differential regulation.

Alternative splicing occurs in every conceivable pattern and is sometimes complicated by the use of alternative promoters and/or polyadenylation sites.[306] Recent biochemical and genetic analysis of the mechanisms of alternative splicing has begun to yield insight into these processes.

The SV40 early pre-mRNA is alternatively spliced by the utilization of two different 5′ splice sites and a single 3′ splice site to produce large T and small t mRNAs. Small t mRNA is produced by use of the weaker proximal 5′ splice site, whereas large T mRNA is produced by use of the stronger distal 5′ splice site. Both spliced products are produced in all cell types, but the ratio of small t to large T produced in human embryonic kidney cells is 10 to 20 times higher than that found in other human cells.[297] This observation suggested that a cell-type–specific factor may act to modulate alternative splicing. With use of a complementation assay, this factor, termed ASF, was purified to homogeneity and cloned.[300] ASF, when added to HeLa nuclear extract, promotes the use of a weaker proximal 5′ splice site over a stronger distal 5′ splice site. Intriguingly, it is identical to SF2,[301] which is a general splicing factor. These observations thus suggest that alternative splicing need not be regulated by cell-type–specific factors. Rather, changes in the concentrations of general splicing factors can influence splice site selection.

The study of sex determination in *Drosophila* has highlighted the importance of alternative splicing as a biological regulatory mechanism. In the sex determination pathway, a cascade of alternative splicing events is regulated by specialized proteins that control the splicing of specific pre-mRNAs[309] (Fig. 2–16). *Sex lethal* (*Sxl*), which acts early in the cascade, regulates the choice between a single 5′ splice site and two 3′ splice sites in its own pre-mRNA and the *transformer* (*tra*) pre-mRNA. Sxl appears to act by negative control. Sxl, an RNA-binding protein that is produced only in females, binds specifically to the proximal 3′ splice site, preventing its usage. The use of the distal splice site produces functional tra protein in females.[310] Negative control of splice site selection appears to play a major role in many other examples of alternative splicing.[307]

An example of positive control of pre-mRNA processing comes from the study of other alternative processing events in the *Drosophila* sex determination pathway. The sex-specific splicing and polyadenylation of the final gene in the pathway, *doublesex* (*dsx*), requires

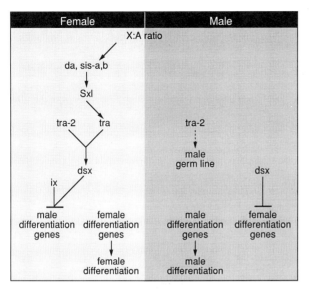

Female	Male

FIGURE 2–16. The cascade of regulatory events involved in somatic sexual differentiation in *Drosophila*. A line drawn from a gene indicates that it is expressed and that its function is required. In females, the X:A (autosome) ratio, sensed by a group of genes that includes *daughterless* (*da*) and *sisterless-a* and *-b* (*sis-a*, *sis-b*), leads to the activation of *Sex lethal* (*Sxl*). Sxl then leads to the female-specific alternative splicing of *transformer* (*tra*), resulting in the generation of functional tra protein. In association with transformer-2 (tra-2), tra leads to the female-specific splicing of *doublesex* (*dsx*). Dsx, in conjunction with *intersex* (*ix*), results in the repression of male differentiation genes. In males, functional Sxl and tra are not produced. A male-specific, alternatively spliced form of tra-2 is produced, and this acts in the male germ line. The male-specific, alternatively spliced form of dsx acts to repress female differentiation genes.

the tra and transformer-2 (tra-2) proteins. The tra-2 protein specifically binds to a site within the female-specific exon of dsx and acts as a positive regulator of dsx pre-mRNA processing.[311]

PERSPECTIVES

During the past decade, our knowledge of eukaryotic gene regulation has progressed tremendously. Gene cloning and DNA transfection methods have led to the identification of *cis*-acting regulatory elements, and many of the genes encoding transcription factors that bind specifically to these DNA sequences have been cloned. At the same time, in vitro transcription procedures have provided functional assays for the identification, the purification, and ultimately the cloning of general transcription factors that are involved in the formation of the preinitiation complex on eukaryotic promoters. In addition, all of the subunits of RNA polymerase II have been purified and cloned. Mechanistic studies have provided a clearer understanding of how transcription factors bound to enhancers located at great distances from promoters can promote transcription initiation. It now seems likely that this is accomplished by interactions between transcription factors bound to enhancers and general transcription factors bound to the promoter. At least two

of these "target" proteins of transcriptional activators have been identified: TFIID and TFIIB. Studies of transcription factors have revealed that they consist of multiple functional domains, one of which is required for specific DNA binding and another that is required for transcriptional activation.

The complex organization of many enhancers and promoters suggests that specificity of activation is achieved in part by synergistic interactions between different transcription factors. A unique set of regulatory sequences and factors therefore appears to be required for the activation of each gene. This combinatorial mechanism for specificity is further amplified by specific protein-protein interactions within and between families of transcription factors. Thus, gene activity appears to be the consequence of the arrangement of regulatory sequences adjacent to the gene, the presence or absence of the appropriate transcription factors, and specific interactions between different transcription factors. In this way, a relatively small number of regulatory sequences and transcription factors appear to be used in a combinatorial mechanism to achieve the incredible specificity required to turn on one out of many tens of thousands of genes in a particular cell during the appropriate stage of development.

In spite of this progress, the relatively crude model systems thus far employed to discern basic transcriptional mechanisms are clearly not adequate for a detailed understanding of regulatory mechanisms. For example, we know little about the mechanisms governing protein-protein interactions in vivo, or how transcription factors interact with DNA packaged into chromatin. It is hoped that some insights into the former problem will come from the use of *Drosophila* genetics and gene knockout experiments in mice. However, the apparent redundancy of gene function suggested by recent knockout experiments may complicate this analysis enormously.

Significant progress in understanding the mechanisms involved in pre-mRNA splicing has also been made, but the complexity of the spliceosome poses a major obstacle to the elucidation of detailed mechanisms. Fortunately, however, a combination of genetic approaches in yeast and biochemical studies in mammals provides the tools for a systematic attack on the problem. Clearly, an understanding of basic splicing mechanisms is a prerequisite for progress in determining how alternative splicing is regulated. The sex determination system of *Drosophila* is the only system in which the regulatory factors have been identified, and an in vitro system has been established. Thus, a reasonable understanding of at least one example each of negative and positive control of splice site selection appears to be near. However, more complex examples of alternative splicing, such as those involved in the production of different isoforms of contractile proteins, will be considerably more difficult. The recent findings that different levels of "general splicing" factor can lead to alternative 5' splice site selection will complicate this analysis and possibly make the establishment of in vitro systems that accurately reflect the situation in vivo quite difficult.

An underlying problem that is shared by tissue-specific and inducible gene expression, and possibly by regulated alternative splicing, is the mechanisms involved in signal transduction. That is, how does the cell interpret extracellular signals and translate these signals into a specific pattern of gene expression? This signal can be transmitted as a diffusible factor, as in the case of morphogens in early development, or as specific cell-cell interactions, as exemplified by cell determination during the development of the eye in *Drosophila*. It seems likely that signal transduction mechanisms employed in gene regulation also function in the control of cell growth and division, and in the uptake and storage of information by the brain. Thus, the investigation of fundamental transcriptional mechanisms as well as the exploration of the connection between signal transduction systems and the regulation of transcription factor activities will do much to further our understanding of many biologically and medically important processes.

REFERENCES

1. Gurdon, J. B.: Adult frogs derived from the nuclei of single somatic cells. Dev. Biol. 4: 256, 1962.
2. Gilbert, W.: The exon theory of genes. Cold Spring Harb. Symp. Quant. Biol. 52: 901, 1987.
3. Siebenlist, U., Simpson, R. B., and Gilbert, W.: *E. coli* RNA polymerase interacts homologously with two different promoters. Cell 20: 269, 1980.
4. Hochschild, A., Irwin, N., and Ptashne, M.: Repressor structure and the mechanism of positive control. Cell 32: 319, 1983.
5. Straney, S. B., and Crothers, D. M.: Lac repressor is a transient gene-activating protein. Cell 51: 699, 1987.
6. Lee, J., and Goldfarb, A.: Lac repressor acts by modifying the initial transcribing complex so that it cannot leave the promoter. Cell 66: 793, 1991.
7. Gabrielson, O. S., and Sentenac, A.: RNA polymerase III and its associated factors. Trends Biochem. Sci. 16: 412, 1991.
8. Jantzen, H.-M., Admon, A., Bell, S. P., and Tjian, R.: Nucleolar transcription factor hUBF contains a DNA-binding motif with homology to HMG proteins. Nature 344: 830, 1990.
9. Sollner-Webb, B., and Tower, J.: Transcription of cloned eukaryotic ribosomal RNA genes. Annu. Rev. Biochem. 55: 801, 1986.
10. Jones, N. C., Rigby, P. W. J., and Ziff, E. B.: *Trans*-acting protein factors and the regulation of eukaryotic transcription: Lessons from studies of DNA tumor viruses. Genes Dev. 2: 267, 1988.
11. McKnight, S. L., and Tjian, R.: Transcriptional selectivity of viral genes in mammalian cells. Cell 46: 795, 1986.
12. McKnight, S. L., Gavis, E. R., Kingsbury, R., and Axel, R.: Analysis of transcriptional regulatory signals of the HSV thymidine kinase gene: Identification of an upstream control region. Cell 25: 385, 1981.
13. McKnight, S. L., and Kingsbury, R.: Transcriptional control signals of a eukaryotic protein-coding gene. Science 217: 316, 1982.
14. Dierks, P., van Ooyen, A., Cochran, M. D., Dobkin, C., Reiser, J., and Weissman, C.: Three regions upstream from the cap site are required for efficient and accurate transcription of the rabbit β-globin gene in mouse 3T6 cells. Cell 32: 695, 1983.
15. Myers, R. M., Tilly, K., and Maniatis, T.: Fine structure genetic analysis of a β-globin promoter. Science 232: 613, 1986.
16. Efstratiadis, A., Posakony, J. W., Maniatis, T., Lawn, R. M., O'Connell, C., Spritz, R. A., DeRiel, J. K., Forget, B. G., Weissman, S. M., Slightom, J. L., Blechl, A. E., Smithies, O., Baralle, F. E., Shoulders, C. C., and Proudfoot, N. J.: The structure and evolution of the human β-globin gene family. Cell 21: 653, 1980.
17. Treisman, R., Orkin, S. H., and Maniatis, T.: Specific transcription and RNA splicing defects in five cloned β-thalassaemia genes. Nature 302: 591, 1983.
18. Dynan, W., and Tjian, R.: The promoter-specific transcription factor Sp1 binds to upstream sequences in the SV40 early promoter. Cell 35: 79, 1983.
19. Smale, S., and Baltimore, D.: The "initiator" as a transcription control element. Cell 57: 103, 1989.
20. Stenlund, A., Bream, G. L., and Botchan, M.: A promoter with an internal regulatory domain is part of the origin of replication in BPV-1. Science 236: 1666, 1987.
21. McKnight, S. L.: Functional relationships between transcriptional control signals of the thymidine kinase gene of herpes simplex virus. Cell 31: 355, 1982.
22. Grosschedl, R., and Birnstiel, M. L.: Spacer DNA sequences upstream of the TATAAATA sequence are essential for promotion of H2A histone gene transcription in vivo. Proc. Natl. Acad. Sci. USA 77: 7102, 1980.
23. Grosschedl, R., and Birnstiel, M. L.: Identification of regulatory sequences in the prelude sequences of an H2A histone gene by the study of specific deletion mutants *in vivo*. Proc. Natl. Acad. Sci. USA 77: 1432, 1980.
24. Fromm, M., and Berg, P.: Simian virus 40 early and late region promoter functions are enhanced by the 72 base pair repeat inserted at distant locations and inverted orientations. Mol. Cell. Biol. 3: 991, 1983.
25. Banerji, J., Rusconi, S., and Schaffner, W.: Expression of a cloned globin gene is enhanced by remote SV40 DNA sequences. Cell 27: 299, 1981.
26. Moreau, P., Hen, R., Wasylyk, B., Everett, R., Gaud, M. P., and Chambon, P.: The SV40 72 bp repeat has a striking effect on gene expression both in SV40 and other chimeric recombinants. Nucleic Acids Res. 9: 6047, 1981.
27. Zenke, M., Grundstrom, T., Matthes, H., Wintzerith, M., Shatz, C., Wildeman, A., and Chambon, P.: Multiple sequence motifs are involved in SV40 enhancer function. EMBO J. 5: 387, 1986.
28. Herr, W., and Gluzman, Y.: Duplications of a mutated simian virus 40 enhancer restore its activity. Nature 313: 711, 1985.
29. Herr, W., and Clarke, J.: The SV40 enhancer is composed of multiple functional elements that can compensate for one another. Cell 45: 461, 1986.
30. Fromental, C., Kanno, M., Nomiyama, H., and Chambon, P.: Cooperativity and hierarchical levels of functional organization in the SV40 enhancer. Cell 54: 943, 1988.
31. Schirm, S., Jiricny, J., and Schaffner, W.: The SV40 enhancer can be dissected into multiple segments, each with a different cell type specificity. Genes Dev. 1: 65, 1987.
32. Davidson, I., Fromental, C., Augereau, P., Wildeman, A., Zenke, M., and Chambon, P.: Cell-type specific protein binding of the enhancer of simian virus 40 in nuclear extracts. Nature 323: 544, 1986.
33. Ondek, B., Gloss, L., and Herr, W.: The SV40 enhancer contains two distinct levels of organization. Nature 333: 40, 1988.
34. Rosales, R., Vigneron, M., Macchi, M., Davidson, I., Xiao, J.-H., and Chambon, P.: *In vitro* binding of cell-specific and ubiquitous nuclear proteins to the octamer motif of the SV40 enhancer and related motifs present in other promoters. EMBO J. 6: 3015, 1987.
35. Treisman, R., and Maniatis, T.: Simian virus 40 enhancer increases the number of RNA polymerase II molecules on linked DNA. Nature 315: 72, 1985.
36. Ptashne, M.: Gene regulation by proteins acting nearby and at a distance. Nature 322: 697, 1986.
37. Plon, S. E., and Wang, J. C.: Transcription of the human β-globin gene is stimulated by an SV40 enhancer to which it

is physically linked but topologically uncoupled. Cell 45: 575, 1986.

38. Saragosti, S., Moyne, G., and Yaniv, M.: Absence of nucleosomes in a fraction of SV40 chromatin between the origin of replication and the region coding for the late leader RNA. Cell 20: 65, 1980.

39. Brent, R., and Ptashne, M.: A bacterial repressor protein or a yeast transcriptional terminator can block upstream activation of a yeast gene. Nature 312: 612, 1984.

40. Courey, A. J., Plon, S. E., and Wang, J. C.: The use of psoralen-modified DNA to probe the mechanism of enhancer action. Cell 45: 567, 1986.

41. Gralla, J.: Bacterial gene regulation from distant DNA sites. Cell 57: 193, 1989.

42. Schule, R., Muller, M., Otsuka-Murakami, H., and Renkawitz, R.: Cooperativity of the glucocorticoid receptor and the CACCC-box binding factor. Nature 332: 87, 1988.

43. Cohen, R., and Meselson, M.: Periodic interactions of heat shock transcriptional elements. Nature 332: 856, 1988.

44. Theveny, B., Bailly, A., Rauch, C., Rauch, M., Delain, E., and Milgrom, E.: Association of DNA-bound progesterone receptors. Nature 329: 79, 1987.

45. Su, W., Jackson, S., Tjian, R., and Echols, H.: DNA looping between sites for transcriptional activation: Self association of DNA bound Sp1. Genes Dev. 5: 820, 1991.

46. Young, R. A.: RNA polymerase II. Annu. Rev. Biochem. 60: 689, 1991.

47. Woychik, N. A., and Young, R. A.: RNA polymerase II: Subunit structure and function. Trends Biochem. Sci. 15: 347, 1990.

48. Allison, L. A., Moyle, M., Shales, M., and Ingles, C. J.: Extensive homology among the largest subunits of eukaryotic and prokaryotic RNA polymerases. Cell 42: 599, 1985.

49. Corden, J. L.: Tails of RNA polymerase II. Trends Biochem. Sci. 15: 383, 1990.

50. Allison, L. A., Wong, J. K.-C., Fitzpatrick, V. D., Moyle, M., and Ingles, C. J.: The C-terminal domain of the largest subunit of RNA polymerase II of *Saccharomyces cerevisiae*, *Drosophila melanogaster*, and mammals: A conserved structure with an essential function. Mol. Cell. Biol. 8: 321, 1988.

51. Corden, J. L., Cadena, D. L., Ahearn, J. M., and Dahmus, M. E.: A unique structure at the carboxy terminus of the largest subunit of eukaryotic RNA polymerase II. Proc. Natl. Acad. Sci. USA 82: 7934, 1985.

52. Schafe, C., Chao, D., Lopes, J., Hirsch, J. P., Henry, S., and Young, R. A.: RNA polymerase II C-terminal repeat influences response to transcriptional enhancer signals. Nature 347: 491, 1990.

53. Liao, S.-M., Taylor, I. C. A., Kingston, R. E., and Young, R. A.: RNA polymerase II carboxy-terminal domain contributes to the response to multiple acidic activators in vitro. Genes Dev. 5: 2431, 1991.

54. Peterson, C. L., Kruger, W., and Herskowitz, I.: A functional interaction between the C-terminal domain of RNA polymerase II and the negative regulator SIN1. Cell 64: 1135, 1991.

55. Arias, J. A., Peterson, S. R., and Dynan, W. S.: Promoter-dependent phosphorylation of RNA polymerase II by a template-bound kinase. J. Biol. Chem. 266: 8055, 1991.

56. Feaver, W. J., Gileadi, O., Li, Y., and Kornberg, R. D.: CTD kinase associated with yeast RNA polymerase II initiation factor b. Cell 67: 1223, 1991.

57. Suzuki, M.: The heptad repeat in the largest subunit of RNA polymerase II binds by intercalating into DNA. Nature 344: 562, 1990.

58. Sigler, P. B.: Acid blobs and negative noodles. Nature 333: 210, 1988.

59. Sawadogo, M., and Sentenac, A.: RNA polymerase II and general transcription factors. Annu. Rev. Biochem. 59: 711, 1990.

60. Roeder, R. G.: The complexities of eukaryotic transcription initiation: Regulation of preinitiation complex assembly. Trends Biochem. Sci. 16: 402, 1991.

61. Buratowski, S., Hahn, S., Guarente, L., and Sharp, P. A.: Five intermediate complexes in transcription initiation by RNA polymerase II. Cell 56: 549, 1989.

62. Peterson, M. G., Inostroza, J., Maxon, M. E., Flores, O., Admon, A., Reinberg, D., and Tjian, R.: Structure and functional properties of human general transcription factor IIE. Nature 354: 369, 1991.

63. Cortes, P., Flores, O., and Reinberg, D.: Factors involved in specific transcription by mammalian RNA polymerase II: Purification and analysis of transcription factor IIA and identification of transcription factor IIJ. Mol. Cell. Biol. 12: 413, 1992.

64. Sumimoto, H., Ohkuma, Y., Yamamoto, T., Horikoshi, M., and Roeder, R. G.: Factors involved in specific transcription by mammalian RNA polymerase II: Identification of general transcription factor TFIIG. Proc. Natl. Acad. Sci. USA 87: 9158, 1990.

65. Wang, W., Carey, M., and Gralla, J. D.: Polymerase II promoter activation: Closed complex formation and ATP-driven start site opening. Science 255: 450, 1992.

66. Gralla, J. D.: Transcriptional control—lessons from an *E. coli* promoter data base. Cell 66: 415, 1991.

67. Buratowski, S., Hahn, S., Sharp, P. A., and Guarente, L.: Function of a yeast TATA element–binding protein in a mammalian transcription system. Nature 334: 37, 1988.

68. Lewin, B.: Commitment and activation at Pol II promoters: A tail of protein-protein interactions. Cell 61: 1161, 1990.

69. Greenblatt, J.: Roles of TFIID in transcriptional initiation by RNA polymerase II. Cell 66: 1067, 1991.

70. Hoey, T., Dynlacht, B. D., Peterson, M. G., Pugh, B. F., and Tjian, R.: Isolation and characterization of the *Drosophila* gene encoding the TATA box binding protein, TFIID. Cell 61: 1179, 1990.

71. Horikoshi, M., Yamamoto, T., Ohkuma, Y., Weil, P. A., and Roeder, R. G.: Analysis of structure-function relationships of yeast TATA box binding factor TFIID. Cell 61: 1171, 1990.

72. Timmers, H. T. M., and Sharp, P. A.: The mammalian TFIID protein is present in two functionally distinct complexes. Genes Dev. 5: 1946, 1991.

73. Dynlacht, B. D., Hoey, T., and Tjian, R.: Isolation of coactivators associated with the TATA-binding protein that mediate transcriptional activation. Cell 66: 563, 1991.

74. Pugh, B. F., and Tjian, R.: Transcription from a TATA-less promoter requires a multisubunit TFIID complex. Genes Dev. 5: 1935, 1991.

75. Roy, A. L., Meisterernst, M., Pognonec, P., and Roeder, R. G.: Cooperative interaction of an initiator-binding transcription initiation factor and the helix-loop-helix activator USF. Nature 354: 245, 1991.

76. Ha, I., Lane, W. S., and Reinberg, D.: Cloning of a human gene encoding the general transcriptional initiation factor IIB. Nature 352: 689, 1991.

77. Sopta, M., Burton, Z. F., and Greenblatt, J.: Structure and associated DNA helicase activity of a general transcription factor that binds RNA polymerase II. Nature 341: 410, 1989.

78. Killeen, M. T., and Greenblatt, J. F.: The general transcription factor RAP30 binds to RNA polymerase II and prevents it from binding nonspecifically to DNA. Mol. Cell. Biol. 12: 30, 1992.

79. Finkelstein, A., Kostrub, C. F., Li, J., Chavez, D. P., Wang, B. Q., Fang, S. M., Greenblatt, J., and Burton, Z. F.: A cDNA encoding RAP74, a general initiation factor for transcription by RNA polymerase II. Nature 355: 464–467, 1992.

80. Aso, T., Vasavada, H. A., Kawaguchi, T., Germino, F. J., Ganguly, S., Kitajima, S., Weissman, S. M., and Yasukochi, Y.: Characterization of cDNA for the large subunit of the transcription factor TFIIF. Nature 355: 461, 1992.

81. Ohkuma, Y., Sumimoto, H., Hoffman, A., Shimasaki, S., Horikoshi, M., and Roeder, R.: Structural motifs and potential σ homologies in the large subunit of human general transcription factor TFIIE. Nature 354: 398, 1991.

82. Sumimoto, H., Ohkuma, Y., Sinn, E., Kato, H., Shimasaki, S., Horikoshi, M., and Roeder, R. G.: Conserved sequence

motifs in the small subunit of human general transcription factor TFIIE. Nature 354: 401, 1991.

83. Fried, M., and Crothers, D.: Equilibrium and kinetics of *lac* repressor-operator interactions by polyacrylamide gel electrophoresis. Nucleic Acids Res. 8: 6505, 1981.

84. Galas, D. J., and Schmitz, A.: DNAse footprinting: A simple method for the detection of protein-DNA binding specificity. Nucleic Acids Res. 5: 3157, 1978.

85. Rosenfeld, P. J., and Kelly, T. J.: Purification of nuclear factor I by DNA recognition site affinity chromatography. J. Biol. Chem. 261: 1398, 1986.

86. Kadonaga, J. T., and Tjian, R.: Affinity purification of sequence-specific DNA-binding proteins. Proc. Natl. Acad. Sci. USA 83: 5889, 1986.

87. Singh, H., LeBowitz, J. H., Baldwin, A. S., and Sharp, P. A.: Molecular cloning of an enhancer binding protein: Isolation by screening of an expression library with a recognition site DNA. Cell 52: 415, 1988.

88. Vinson, C. R., LaMarco, K. L., Johnson, P. F., Landschulz, W. H., and McKnight, S.: *In situ* detection of sequence-specific DNA binding activity specified by a recombinant bacteriophage. Genes Dev. 2: 801, 1988.

89. Pabo, C. O., Sauer, R. T., Sturtevant, J. M., and Ptashne, M.: The λ repressor contains two domains. Proc. Natl. Acad. Sci. USA 76: 1608, 1979.

90. Frankel, A. D., and Kim, P. S.: Modular structure of transcription factors: Implications for gene regulation. Cell 65: 717, 1991.

91. Brent, R., and Ptashne, M.: A eukaryotic transcriptional activator bearing the DNA specificity of a prokaryotic repressor. Cell 43: 729, 1985.

92. Ptashne, M.: How eukaryotic transcriptional activators work. Nature 335: 683, 1988.

93. Pabo, C. O., and Sauer, R. T.: Protein-DNA interaction. Annu. Rev. Biochem. 53: 293, 1984.

94. Steitz, T. A.: Structural studies of protein-nucleic acid interaction: The sources of sequence-specific binding. Q. Rev. Biophys. 23: 205, 1990.

95. Harrison, S. C.: A structural taxonomy of DNA-binding domains. Nature 353: 715, 1991.

96. Schultz, S. C., Shields, G. C., and Steitz, T. A.: Crystal structure of a CAP-DNA complex: The DNA is bent by 90°. Science 253: 1001, 1991.

97. Kerppola, T. K., and Curran, T.: DNA bending by Fos and Jun: The flexible hinge model. Science 254: 1210, 1991.

98. Harrison, S. C., and Aggarwal, A. K.: DNA recognition by proteins with the helix-turn-helix motif. Annu. Rev. Biochem. 59: 933, 1990.

99. Wharton, R. P., and Ptashne, M.: Changing the binding specificity of a repressor by redesigning an α-helix. Nature 316: 601, 1985.

100. McGinnis, W., Garber, R. L., Wirz, J., Kuroiwa, A., and Gehring, W.: A homologue protein-coding sequence in *Drosophila* homeotic genes and its conservation in other metazoans. Cell 37: 403, 1984.

101. Scott, M. P., Tamkun, J. W., and Hartzell, G. W.: The structure and function of the homeodomain. Biochim. Biophys. Acta 989: 25, 1989.

102. Kissinger, C. R., Liu, B., Martin-Blanco, E., Kornberg, T. B., and Pabo, C. O.: Crystal structure of an engrailed homeodomain-DNA complex at 2.8 Å resolution: A framework for understanding homeodomain interactions. Cell 63: 579, 1990.

103. Wolberger, C., Vershon, A. K., Liu, B., Johnson, A. D., and Pabo, C. O.: Crystal structure of a MATα2 homeodomain-operator complex suggests a general model for homeodomain-DNA interactions. Cell 67: 517, 1991.

104. Hanes, S. D., and Brent, R.: A genetic model of interaction of the homeodomain recognition helix with DNA. Science 251: 426, 1991.

105. Ruvkun, G., and Finney, M.: Regulation of transcription and cell identity by POU domain proteins. Cell 64: 475, 1991.

106. Ingraham, H. A., Flynn, S. E., Voss, J. W., Albert, V. R., Kapiloff, M. S., Wilson, L., and Rosenfeld, M. G.: The POU-specific domain of Pit-1 is essential for sequence-specific, high affinity DNA binding and DNA-dependent Pit-1–Pit-1 interactions. Cell 61: 1021, 1990.

107. Miller, J., McLachlan, A. D., and Klug, A.: Repetitive zinc-binding domains in the protein transcription factor IIIA from Xenopus oocytes. EMBO J. 4: 1609, 1985.

108. Schwabe, J. W. R., and Rhodes, D.: Beyond zinc fingers: Steroid hormone receptors have a novel structural motif for DNA recognition. Trends Biochem. Sci. 16: 291, 1991.

109. Pan, T., and Colman, J. E.: Structure and function of the Zn(II) binding sites within the DNA binding domain of the GAL4 transcription factor. Proc. Natl. Acad. Sci. USA 86: 3145, 1990.

110. Jacobs, G., and Michaels, G.: Zinc finger gene database. New Biol. 2: 583, 1990.

111. Pavletich, N. P., and Pabo, C. O.: Zinc finger–DNA recognition: Crystal structure of a Zif268-DNA complex at 2.1 Å. Science 252: 809, 1991.

112. Berg, J. M.: Proposed structure for the zinc-binding domains from transcription factor IIIA and related proteins. Proc. Natl. Acad. Sci. USA 85: 99, 1988.

113. Luisi, B. F., Xu, W. X., Otwinowski, Z., Freedman, L. P., Yamamoto, K. R., and Sigler, P.: Crystallographic analysis of the interaction of the glucocorticoid receptor with DNA. Nature 352: 497, 1991.

114. Landschulz, W. H., Johnson, P. F., and McKnight, S. L.: The leucine zipper: A hypothetical structure common to a new class of DNA binding proteins. Science 240: 1759, 1988.

115. Abel, T., and Maniatis, T.: Action of leucine zippers. Nature 341: 24, 1989.

116. Talanian, R. V., McKnight, C. J., and Kim, P. S.: Sequence-specific DNA binding by a short peptide dimer. Science 249: 769, 1990.

117. Vinson, C. R., Sigler, P., and McKnight, S.: A scissors-grip model for DNA recognition by a family of leucine zipper proteins. Science 246: 911, 1989.

118. Sauer, R. T.: Scissors and helical forks. Nature 347: 514, 1990.

119. O'Shea, E. K., Rutowski, R., and Kim, P. S.: Evidence that the leucine zipper is a coiled-coil. Science 243: 538, 1989.

120. Crick, F. H. C.: The packing of α-helices: Simple coiled-coils. Acta Cryst. 6: 689, 1953.

121. O'Shea, E. K., Klemm, J. D., Kim, P. S., and Alber, T.: X-ray structure of the GCN4 leucine zipper, a two-stranded, parallel coiled-coil. Science 254: 539, 1991.

122. O'Shea, E., Rutkowski, R., Stafford, W. F., and Kim, P. S.: Preferential heterodimer formation by isolated leucine zippers from Fos and Jun. Science 245: 646, 1989.

123. Jones, N.: Transcriptional regulation by dimerization: Two sides to an incestuous relationship. Cell 61: 9, 1990.

124. Lamb, P., and McKnight, S. L.: Diversity and specificity in transcriptional regulation: The benefits of heterotypic dimerization. Trends Biochem. Sci. 16: 417, 1991.

125. Hollis, M., Valenzuela, D., Pioli, D., Wharton, R., and Ptashne, M.: A repressor heterodimer binds to a chimeric operator. Proc. Natl. Acad. Sci. USA 85: 5834, 1988.

126. Curran, T., and Franza, B. R.: Fos and Jun: The AP-1 connection. Cell 55: 395, 1988.

127. Vogt, P. K., and Bos, T. J.: The oncogene *jun* and nuclear signalling. Trends Biochem. Sci. 14: 172, 1989.

128. Murre, C., McCaw, P. S., and Baltimore, D.: A new DNA binding and dimerization motif in immunoglobulin enhancer binding, daughterless, MyoD and myc proteins. Cell 56: 777, 1989.

129. Weintraub, H., Davis, R., Tapscott, S., Thayer, M., Krause, M., Benezra, R., Blackwell, T. K., Turner, D., Rupp, R., Hollenberg, S., Zhuang, Y., and Lassar, A.: The myoD gene family: Nodal point during specification of the muscle cell lineage. Science 251: 761, 1991.

130. Campos-Ortega, J. A., and Knust, E.: Genetics of early neurogenesis in *Drosophila melanogaster*. Annu. Rev. Genet. 24: 387, 1990.

131. Davis, R. L., Cheng, P.-F., Lassar, A. B., and Weintraub, H.: The myoD DNA binding domain contains a recognition code for muscle-specific gene activation. Cell 60: 773, 1990.

132. Murre, C., McCaw, P. S., Vaessin, H., Caudy, M., Jan, L. Y., Jan, Y. N., Cabrera, C. V., Bushkin, J. N., Hauschka, S. D., Lassar, A. B., Weintraub, H., and Baltimore, D.: Interactions between heterologous helix-loop-helix proteins generate complexes that bind specifically to a common DNA sequence. Cell 58: 537, 1990.

133. Benezra, R., Davis, R. L., Lockshon, D., Turner, D. L., and Weintraub, H.: The protein Id: A negative regulator of helix-loop-helix DNA binding proteins. Cell 61: 49, 1990.

134. Herskowitz, I.: Functional inactivation of genes by dominant negative mutations. Nature 329: 219, 1987.

135. Wright, W. E., Sassoon, D. A., and Lin, V. K.: Myogenin, a factor regulating myogenesis, has a domain homologous to MyoD. Cell 56: 607, 1989.

136. Blackwood, E. M., and Eisenman, R. N.: Max: A helix-loop-helix zipper protein that forms a sequence-specific DNA-binding complex with Myc. Science 251: 1211, 1991.

137. Gregor, P. D., Sawadogo, M., and Roeder, R.: The adenovirus major late transcription factor is a member of the helix-loop-helix group of regulatory proteins and binds DNA as a dimer. Genes Dev. 4: 1730, 1990.

138. Hu, Y. F., Luscher, B., Admon, A., Mermod, N., and Tjian, R.: Transcription factor AP-4 contains multiple dimerization domains that regulate dimer specificity. Genes Dev. 4: 1741, 1990.

139. Dang, C. V., McGuire, M., Buckmire, M., and Lee, W. M. F.: Involvement of the "leucine zipper" region in the oligomerization and transforming activity of human cMyc protein. Nature 337: 664, 1989.

140. Fisher, D. E., Carr, C. S., Parent, L. A., and Sharp, P. A.: TFEB has DNA-binding and oligomerization properties of a unique helix-loop-helix/leucine zipper family. Genes Dev. 5: 2342, 1991.

141. Blanar, M. A., and Rutter, W. J.: Interaction cloning: Identification of a helix-loop-helix protein that interacts with cFos. Science 256: 1014, 1992.

142. Sorger, P. K.: Heat shock factor and the heat shock response. Cell 65: 363, 1991.

143. Norman, C., Runswick, M., Pollock, R., and Treisman, R.: Isolation and properties of cDNA clones encoding SRF, a transcription factor that binds to the c-fos serum response element. Cell 55: 989, 1988.

144. Ghosh, S., Gofford, A. M., Riviere, L. R., Tempst, P., Nolan, G. P., and Baltimore, D.: Cloning of the p50 DNA binding subunit of NF-κB: Homology to rel and dorsal. Cell 62: 1019, 1990.

145. Ruben, S. M., Dillon, P. J., Schreck, R., Henkel, T., Chen, C.-H., Maher, M., Baeuerle, P. A., and Rosen, C. A.: Isolation of a rel-related human cDNA that potentially encodes the 65 kDa subunit of NF-κB. Science 251: 1490, 1991.

146. Breg, J. N., van Opheusden, J. H. J., Burgering, M. J. M., Boelens, R., and Kaptein, R.: Structure of Arc repressor in solution: Evidence for a family of β-sheet DNA-binding proteins. Nature 346: 586, 1990.

147. Ptashne, M.: A Genetic Switch: Gene Control and Phage λ. Cambridge, Mass., Cell Press and Blackwell Scientific Publications, 1986.

148. Ma, J., and Ptashne, M.: Deletion analysis of GAL4 defines two transcriptional activating segments. Cell 48: 847, 1987.

149. Hope, I. A., and Struhl, K.: Functional dissection of a eukaryotic transcriptional activator protein, GCN4 of yeast. Cell 46: 885, 1986.

150. Ma, J., and Ptashne, M.: A new class of yeast transcriptional activators. Cell 51: 113, 1987.

151. Ptashne, M., and Gann, A. A. F.: Activators and targets. Nature 346: 329, 1990.

152. Pascal, E., and Tjian, R.: Different activation domains of Sp1 govern formation of multimers and mediate transcriptional synergism. Genes Dev. 5: 1646, 1991.

153. Courey, A. J., and Tjian, R.: Analysis of Sp1 in vivo reveals multiple transcriptional domains, including a novel glutamine-rich activation motif. Cell 55: 887, 1988.

154. Mitchell, P. J., and Tjian, R.: Transcriptional regulation in mammalian cells by sequence-specific DNA binding proteins. Science 245: 371, 1989.

155. Mermod, N., O'Neill, E. A., Kelly, T. J., and Tjian, R.: The proline-rich transcriptional activator of CTF/NF-1 is distinct from the replication and DNA binding domain. Cell 58: 741, 1989.

156. Sadowski, I., Ma, J., Triezenberg, S., and Ptashne, M.: GAL4-VP16 is an unusually potent transcriptional activator. Nature 335: 563, 1988.

157. McLauchlan, J., Simpson, S., and Clements, J. B.: Herpes simplex virus induces a processing factor that stimulates poly (A) site usage. Cell 59: 1093, 1989.

158. O'Hare, P., and Goding, C. R.: Herpes simplex virus regulatory elements and the immunoglobulin octamer domain bind a common factor and are both targets for virion transactivation. Cell 52: 435, 1988.

159. Stern, S., Tanaka, M., and Herr, W.: The Oct-1 homeodomain directs formation of a multiprotein-DNA complex with the HSV transactivator VP16. Nature 341: 624, 1989.

160. Stern, S., and Herr, W.: The herpes simplex virus trans-activator VP16 recognizes the Oct-1 homeo domain: Evidence for a homeo domain recognition subdomain. Genes Dev. 5: 2555, 1991.

161. Cress, W. D., and Triezenberg, S. J.: Critical structural elements of the VP16 transcriptional activation domain. Science 251: 87, 1991.

162. Olesen, J. T., and Guarente, L.: The HAP2 subunit of yeast CCAAT transcriptional activator contains adjacent domains for subunit association and DNA recognition: Model for the HAP2/3/4 complex. Genes Dev. 4: 1714, 1990.

163. Horikoshi, M., Hai, T., Lin, Y.-S., Green, M. R., and Roeder, R. G.: Transcription factor ATF interacts with the TATA factor to facilitate establishment of a preinitiation complex. Cell 54: 1033, 1988.

164. Horikoshi, M., Carey, M. F., Kakidani, H., and Roeder, R. G.: Mechanism of action of a yeast activator: Direct effect of GAL4 derivatives on mammalian TFIID-promoter interactions. Cell 54: 665, 1988.

165. Stringer, K. F., Ingles, C. J., and Greenblatt, J.: Direct and selective binding of an acidic transcriptional activation domain to the TATA-box factor TFIID. Nature 345: 783, 1990.

166. Ingles, C. J., Shales, M., Cress, W. D., Triezenberg, S. J., and Greenblatt, J.: Reduced binding of TFIID to transcriptionally compromised mutant of VP16. Nature 351: 588, 1991.

167. Pugh, B. F., and Tjian, R.: Mechanism of transcriptional activation by Sp1: Evidence for coactivators. Cell 61: 1187, 1990.

168. Tanese, N., Pugh, B. F., and Tjian, R.: Coactivators for a proline-rich activator purified from the multisubunit human TFIID complex. Genes Dev. 5: 2212, 1991.

169. Carey, M., Lin, Y.-S., Green, M. R., and Ptashne, M.: A mechanism for synergistic activation of a mammalian gene by a GAL4 derivative. Nature 345: 361, 1990.

170. Lin, Y.-S., Carey, M., Ptashne, M., and Green, M. R.: How different eukaryotic transcriptional activators can cooperate promiscuously. Nature 345: 359, 1990.

171. Tora, L., White, J., Brou, C., Tasset, D., Webster, N., Scheer, E., and Chambon, P.: The human estrogen receptor has two independent nonacidic transcriptional activation functions. Cell 59: 477, 1989.

172. Gill, G., and Ptashne, M.: Negative effect of the transcriptional activator GAL4. Nature 334: 721, 1988.

173. Martin, K. J., Lillie, J. W., and Green, M. R.: Evidence for interaction of different eukaryotic transcriptional activators with distinct cellular targets. Nature 346: 147, 1990.

174. Tasset, D., Tora, L., Fromental, C., Scheer, E., and Chambon, P.: Distinct classes of transcriptional activating domains function by different mechanisms. Cell 62: 1177, 1990.

175. Sharp, P. A.: TFIIB or not TFIIB? Nature 351: 16, 1991.

176. Croston, G. E., Kerrigan, L. A., Lira, L. M., Marshak, D. R., and Kadonaga, J. T.: Sequence-specific antirepression of histone H1–mediated inhibition of basal RNA polymerase II transcription. Science 251: 643, 1991.

177. Workman, J. L., Taylor, I. C. A., and Kingston, R. E.: Activation domains of stably bound GAL4 derivatives alleviate repression of promoters by nucleosomes. Cell 64: 533, 1991.

178. Meisterernst, M., Horikoshi, M., and Roeder, R. G.: Recombinant yeast TFIID, a general transcription factor, mediates activation by the gene-specific factor USF in a chromatin assembly assay. Proc. Natl. Acad. Sci. USA 87: 9153, 1990.

179. Laybourn, P. J., and Kadonaga, J. T.: Role of nucleosome cores and histone H1 in regulation of transcription by RNA polymerase II. Science 254: 238, 1991.

180. Felsenfeld, G.: Chromatin as an essential part of the transcription mechanism. Nature 355: 219, 1992.

181. Lin, Y.-S., and Green, M. R.: Mechanism of action of an acidic activator in vitro. Cell 64: 971, 1991.

182. Lin, Y.-S., Ha, I., Maldonado, E., Reinberg, D., and Green, M. R.: Binding of general transcription factor TFIIB to an acidic activating region. Nature 353: 569, 1991.

183. Renkawitz, R.: Transcriptional repression in eukaryotes. Trends Genet. 6: 192, 1990.

184. Levine, M., and Manley, J. L.: Transcriptional repression of eukaryotic promoters. Cell 59: 405, 1989.

185. Aamodt, E. J., Chung, M. A., and McGhee, J. D.: Spatial control of gut-specific gene expression during Caenorhabditis elegans development. Science 252: 579, 1991.

186. Goodbourn, S., Burstein, H., and Maniatis, T.: The human β-interferon gene enhancer is under negative control. Cell 45: 601, 1986.

187. Tjian, R.: T antigen binding and the control of SV40 gene expression. Cell 26: 1, 1981.

188. Dostatni, N., Lambert, P. F., Sousa, R., Ham, J., Howley, P. M., and Yaniv, M.: The functional BPV-1 E2 trans-acting protein can act as a repressor by preventing formation of the initiation complex. Genes Dev. 5: 1657, 1991.

189. Kato, H., Horikoshi, M., and Roeder, R. G.: Repression of HIV-1 transcription by a cellular protein. Science 251: 1476, 1991.

190. Kaufman, P. D., and Rio, D. C.: Drosophila P-element transposase is a transcriptional repressor in vitro. Proc. Natl. Acad. Sci. USA 88: 2613, 1991.

191. Harada, H., Fujita, T., Miyamoto, M., Kimura, Y., Maruyama, M., Furia, A., Miyata, T., and Taniguchi, T.: Structurally similar but functionally distinct factors, IRF-1 and IRF-2, bind to the same regulatory elements of IFN and IFN-inducible genes. Cell 58: 729, 1989.

192. Akerblom, I. W., Slater, E. P., Beato, M., Baxter, J. D., and Mellon, P. L.: Negative regulation by glucocorticoids through interference with a cAMP responsive enhancer. Science 241: 350, 1988.

193. Small, S., Kraut, R., Hoey, T., Warrior, R., and Levine, M.: Transcriptional regulation of a pair-rule stripe in Drosophila. Genes Dev. 5: 827, 1991.

194. Falb, D., and Maniatis, T.: A conserved regulatory unit implicated in tissue-specific gene expression in Drosophila and man. Genes Dev. 6: 454, 1992.

195. Brand, A. H., Breeden, L., Abraham, J., Sternglanz, R., and Nasmyth, K.: Characterization of a "silencer" in yeast: A DNA sequence with properties opposite to those of a transcriptional enhancer. Cell 41: 41, 1985.

196. Jaynes, J. B., and O'Farrell, P. H.: Active repression of transcription by the Engrailed homeodomain protein. EMBO J. 10: 1427, 1991.

197. Biggin, M. D., and Tjian, R.: A purified Drosophila homeodomain protein represses transcription in vitro. Cell 58: 433, 1989.

198. Licht, J. D., Grossel, M. J., Figge, J., and Hansen, U. M.: Drosophila Kruppel is a transcriptional repressor. Nature 346: 76, 1990.

199. Johnson, A. D., and Herskowitz, I.: A repressor (MATα2 product) and its operator control expression of a set of cell type specific genes in yeast. Cell 42: 237, 1985.

200. Keleher, C., Goutte, C., and Johnson, A. D.: The yeast cell-type-specific repressor α2 acts cooperatively with a non-cell-type-specific protein. Cell 53: 927, 1988.

201. Hall, M. N., and Johnson, A. D.: Homeo domain of the yeast repressor α2 is a sequence-specific DNA-binding domain but is not sufficient for repression. Science 237: 1007, 1987.

202. Ma, J., and Ptashne, M.: The carboxy-terminal 30 amino acids of GAL4 are recognized by GAL80. Cell 50: 137, 1987.

203. Adler, S., Waterman, M. L., He, X., and Rosenfeld, M. G.: Steroid receptor–mediated inhibition of rat prolactin gene expression does not require the receptor DNA-binding domain. Cell 52: 685, 1988.

204. Treacy, M. N., He, X., and Rosenfeld, M. G.: I-POU: A POU-domain protein that inhibits neuron-specific gene activation. Nature 350: 577, 1991.

205. Baeuerle, P. A.: The inducible transcription activator NF-κB: Regulation by distinct protein subunits. Biochim. Biophys. Acta 1072: 63, 1991.

206. Renoir, J. M., Radanyi, C., Faber, L. E., and Baulieu, E. E.: The non-DNA binding heterooligomeric form of mammalian steroid hormone receptors contains a hsp90-bound 59-kDa protein. J. Biol. Chem. 265: 10740, 1990.

207. Evans, R. M.: The steroid and thyroid hormone receptor superfamily. Science 240: 889, 1988.

208. Beato, M.: Gene regulation by steroid hormones. Cell 56: 335, 1988.

209. Petkovich, M., Brand, N. J., Krust, A., and Chambon, P.: A human retinoic acid receptor which belongs to the family of nuclear receptors. Nature 330: 444, 1987.

210. Diamond, M. I., Miner, J. N., Yoshinaga, S. K., and Yamamoto, K. R.: Transcription factor interactions: Selectors of positive or negative regulation from a single DNA element. Science 249: 1266, 1990.

211. Montminy, M. R., Gonzalez, G. A., and Yamamoto, K. K.: Regulation of cAMP inducible genes by CREB. Trends Neurosci. 13: 184, 1990.

212. Ziff, E. B.: Transcription factors: A new family gathers at the cAMP response site. Trends Genet. 6: 69, 1990.

213. Westwood, J. T., Clos, J., and Wu, C.: Stress-induced oligomerization and chromosomal relocalization of heat-shock factor. Nature 353: 822, 1991.

214. Maniatis, T., Whittemore, L.-A., Du, W., Fan, C.-M., Keller, A. D., Palombella, V. J., and Thanos, D. N.: Positive and negative control of human interferon-β gene expression. In McKnight, S. L. and Yamamoto, K. R. (eds.): Transcriptional Regulation, Part 2. Cold Spring Harbor (NY) Laboratory Press, 1992, pp. 1193–1220.

215. Gillies, S. D., Morrison, S. L., Oi, S., and Tonegawa, S.: A tissue-specific enhancer element is located in the major intron of a rearranged immunoglobulin heavy chain gene. Cell 33: 717, 1983.

216. Banerji, J., Olson, L., and Schaffner, W.: A lymphocyte-specific cellular enhancer is located downstream of the joining region in immunoglobulin heavy chain genes. Cell 33: 729, 1983.

217. Goldberg, D. A., Posakony, J. W., and Maniatis, T.: Correct developmental expression of a cloned alcohol dehydrogenase gene transduced into the Drosophila germ line. Cell 34: 58, 1983.

218. Rubin, G. M., and Spradling, A. C.: Genetic transformation of Drosophila with transposable element vectors. Science 218: 348, 1982.

219. Costantini, F., and Lacy, E.: Introduction of the rabbit β-globin gene into the mouse germ line. Nature 294: 92, 1981.

220. Ingraham, H. A., Chen, R., Mangalam, H. J., Elshotz, H. P., Flynn, S. E., Lin, C. R., Simmons, D. M., Swanson, L., and Rosenfeld, M. G.: A tissue-specific transcription factor containing a homeodomain specifies pituitary phenotype. Cell 55: 519, 1988.

221. Bodner, M., Castrillo, J.-L., Theill, L. E., Deerinck, T., Ellisman, M., and Karin, M.: The pituitary-specific transcription factor GHF-1 is a homeobox-containing protein. Cell 55: 505, 1988.

222. Li, S., Crenshaw, E. B., Rawson, E. J., Simmons, D. M., Swanson, L. W., and Rosenfeld, M. G.: Dwarf locus mutants lacking three pituitary cell types result from mutations in the POU-domain gene pit-1. Nature 347: 528, 1990.

223. Scheidereit, C., Cromlish, J. A., Gerster, T., Kawakami, K., Balamceda, C.-G., Currie, R. A., and Roeder, R. G.: A human lymphoid-specific transcription factor that activates

immunoglobulin genes is a homeobox protein. Nature 336: 551, 1988.

224. Evans, T., and Felsenfeld, G.: The erythrocyte-specific transcription factor Eryf1: A new finger protein. Cell 58: 877, 1989.
225. Tsai, S.-F., Martin, D. I. K., Zon, L. I., D'Andrea, A. D., Wong, G. G., and Orkin, S. H.: Cloning of cDNA for the major DNA-binding protein of the erythroid lineage through expression in mammalian cells. Nature 339: 446, 1989.
226. Mueller, C. R., Maire, P., and Schibler, U.: DBP, a liver-enriched transcriptional activator, is expressed late in otogeny and its tissue specificity is determined posttranscriptionally. Cell 61: 279, 1990.
227. Descombes, P., Chojkier, M., Lichtsteiner, S., Falvey, E., and Schibler, U.: LAP, a novel member of the C/EBP gene family, encodes a liver-enriched transcriptional activator protein. Genes Dev. 4: 1541, 1990.
228. Chen, R., Ingraham, H. A., Treacy, M. N., Albert, V. R., Wilson, L., and Rosenfeld, M. G.: Autoregulation of pit-1 gene expression mediated by two cis-active promoter elements. Nature 346: 583, 1990.
229. Thayer, M. J., Tapscott, S. J., Davis, R. L., Wright, W. E., Lassar, A. B., and Weintraub, H.: Positive autoregulation of the myogenic determination gene MyoD1. Cell 58: 241, 1989.
230. Tsai, S.-F., Strauss, E., and Orkin, S. H.: Functional analysis and in vivo footprinting implicate the erythroid transcription factor GATA-1 as a positive regulator of its own promoter. Genes Dev. 5: 919, 1991.
231. Davis, R. L., Weintraub, H., and Lassar, A. B.: Expression of a single transfected DNA converts fibroblasts to myoblasts. Cell 51: 987, 1987.
232. Fischer, J. A., and Maniatis, T.: Drosophila Adh: A promoter element expands the tissue specificity of an enhancer. Cell 53: 451, 1988.
233. Choi, O.-R. B., and Engel, J. D.: Developmental regulation of β-globin gene switching. Cell 55: 17, 1988.
234. Lai, E., and Darnell, J. E.: Transcriptional control in hepatocytes: A window on development. Trends Biochem. Sci. 16: 427, 1991.
235. Landschulz, W. H., Johnson, P. F., Adashi, E. Y., Graves, B. J., and McKnight, S. L.: Isolation of a recombinant copy of the gene encoding C/EBP. Genes Dev. 2: 786, 1988.
236. Frain, M., Swart, G., Monaci, P., Nicosia, A., Stampfli, S., Frank, R., and Cortese, R.: The liver-specific transcription factor LF-B1 contains a highly divergent homeobox DNA-binding domain. Cell 59: 145, 1989.
237. Lai, E., Prezioso, V. R., Tao, W., Chen, W. S., and Darnell, J. E.: Hepatocyte nuclear factor 3α belongs to a gene family in mammals that is homologous to the Drosophila homeotic gene fork head. Genes Dev. 5: 416, 1991.
238. Sladek, F. M., Zhong, W., Lai, E., and Darnell, J. E.: Liver-enriched transcription factor HNF-4 is a novel member of the steroid hormone receptor superfamily. Genes Dev. 4: 2353, 1990.
239. Weiss, M. C.: Extinction by indirect means. Nature 355: 22, 1992.
240. Kuo, C. J., Conley, P. B., Chen, L., Sladek, F. M., Darnell, J. E., and Crabtree, G. R.: A transcriptional hierarchy involved in mammalian cell-type specification. Nature 355: 457, 1992.
241. Boshart, M., Weih, F., Schmidt, A., Fournier, R. E. K., and Schutz, G.: A cyclic-AMP response element mediates repression of tyrosine aminotransferase gene transcription by the tissue-specific extinguisher. Cell 61: 905, 1990.
242. Abel, T., Bhatt, R., and Maniatis, T.: A Drosophila CREB/ATF transcriptional activator binds to both fat body and liver-specific regulatory elements. Genes Dev. 6: 466, 1992.
243. Sen, R., and Baltimore, D.: Inducibility of κ immunoglobulin enhancer-binding protein NK-κB by a posttranslational mechanism. Cell 47: 921, 1986.
244. Mendel, D. B., Khavari, P. A., Conley, P. B., Graves, M. K., Hansen, L. P., Admon, A., and Crabtree, G. R.: Character-

ization of a cofactor that regulates the dimerization of a mammalian homeodomain protein. Nature 254: 1762, 1991.
245. Descombes, P., and Schibler, U.: A liver-enriched transcriptional activator protein, LAP, and a transcriptionally inhibitory protein, LIP, are translated from the same mRNA. Cell 67: 569, 1991.
246. Schneider, J. A., and Weiss, M. C.: Expression of differentiated functions in hepatoma cell hybrids. I. Tyrosine aminotransferase in hepatoma-fibroblast hybrids. Proc. Natl. Acad. Sci. USA 68: 127, 1971.
247. Lem, J., Chin, A. C., Thayer, M. J., Leach, R. J., and Fournier, R. E. K.: Coordinate regulation of two genes encoding gluconeogenic enzymes by the trans-dominant locus Tse-1. Proc. Natl. Acad. Sci. USA 85: 7302, 1988.
248. Jones, K. W., Shapero, M. H., Chevrette, M., and Fournier, R. E. K.: Subtractive hybridization cloning of a tissue-specific extinguisher: TSE1 encodes a regulatory subunit of protein kinase A. Cell 66: 861, 1991.
249. Boshart, M., Weih, F., Nichols, M., and Schutz, G.: The tissue-specific extinguisher locus TSE1 encodes a regulatory subunit of cAMP-dependent protein kinase. Cell 66: 905, 1991.
250. Scheuermann, R. H., and Chen, U.: A developmental-specific factor binds to suppressor sites flanking the immunoglobulin heavy-chain enhancer. Genes Dev. 3: 1255, 1989.
251. Nusslein-Volhard, C., and Wieschaus, E.: Mutations affecting segment number and polarity in Drosophila. Nature 287: 795, 1980.
252. Akam, M.: The molecular basis for metameric pattern in the Drosophila embryo. Development 101: 1, 1987.
253. Ingham, P.: The molecular genetics of embryonic pattern formation in Drosophila. Nature 335: 25, 1988.
254. Driever, W., and Nusslein-Volhard, C.: The bicoid protein is a positive regulator of hunchback transcription in the early Drosophila embryo. Nature 337: 138, 1989.
255. Driever, W., Thoma, G., and Nusslein-Volhard, C.: Determination of spatial domains of zygotic gene expression in the Drosophila embryo by the affinity of binding sites for the bicoid morphogen. Nature 340: 363, 1989.
256. Struhl, G., Struhl, K., and Macdonald, P.: The gradient morphogen bicoid is a concentration-dependent transcriptional activator. Cell 57: 1259, 1989.
257. Carroll, S. B.: Zebra patterns in fly embryos: Activation of stripes or repression of interstripes. Cell 60: 9, 1990.
258. Goto, T., Macdonald, P., and Maniatis, T.: Early and late periodic patterns of even-skipped expression are controlled by distinct regulatory elements that respond to different spatial cues. Cell 57: 413, 1989.
259. Harding, K., Hoey, T., Warrior, R., and Levine, M.: Autoregulatory and gap response elements of the even-skipped promoter of Drosophila. EMBO J. 8: 1205, 1989.
260. Stanojevic, D., Small, S., and Levine, M.: Regulation of a segmentation stripe by overlapping activators and repressors in the Drosophila embryo. Science 254: 1385, 1991.
261. Rottman, F. A., Shatkin, A. J., and Perry, R. P.: Sequences containing methylated neucleotides at the 5′ termini of messenger RNAs: Possible implications for processing. Cell 3: 197, 1974.
262. Shatkin, A. J.: Capping of eukaryotic mRNAs. Cell 9: 645, 1976.
263. Proudfoot, N.: Poly(A) signals. Cell 64: 671, 1991.
264. Raabe, T., Bollum, F. J., and Manley, J. L.: Primary structure and expression of bovine poly (A) polymerase. Nature 353: 229, 1991.
265. Wickens, M.: How the messenger got its tail: Addition of poly (A) in the nucleus. Trends Biochem. Sci. 15: 277, 1990.
266. Jackson, R. J., and Standart, N.: Do the poly (A) tail and 3′ untranslated region control mRNA translation? Cell 62: 15, 1990.
267. Treisman, R., Proudfoot, N., Shander, M., and Maniatis, T.: A single base change at a splice site in a β⁰-thalassemic gene causes abnormal RNA splicing. Cell 29: 903, 1982.
268. Ruby, S. W., and Abelson, J.: Pre-mRNA splicing in yeast. Trends Genet. 7: 79, 1991.
269. Grabowski, P. J., Padgett, R. A., and Sharp, P. A.: Messenger

RNA splicing *in vitro*: An excised intervening sequence and a potential intermediate. Cell 37: 415, 1984.

270. Krainer, A. R., Maniatis, T., Rushkin, B., and Green, M. R.: Normal and mutant human β-globin pre-mRNAs are faithfully and efficiently spliced *in vitro*. Cell 36: 993, 1984.

271. Melton, D. A., Krieg, P. A., Rebagliati, M. R., Maniatis, T., Zinn, K., and Green, M. R.: Efficient *in vitro* synthesis of biologically active RNA and RNA hybridization probes from plasmids containing a bacteriophage SP6 promoter. Nucleic Acids Res. 12: 7035, 1984.

272. Green, M. R.: Biochemical mechanisms of constitutive and regulated pre-mRNA splicing. Annu. Rev. Cell Biol. 7: 559, 1991.

273. Lamond, A. I.: Nuclear RNA processing. Curr. Opin. Cell Biol. 3: 493, 1991.

274. Guthrie, C.: Catalytic RNA and RNA splicing. Am. Zool. 29: 557, 1989.

275. Cech, T. R.: The generality of self-splicing RNA: Relationship to nuclear mRNA splicing. Cell 44: 207, 1986.

276. Kruger, K., Grabowski, P., Zaug, A., Sands, J., Gottschling, D., and Cech, T.: Self-splicing RNA: Autoexcision and autocyclization of the ribosomal RNA intervening sequence of Tetrahymena. Cell 31: 147, 1982.

277. Bass, B., and Cech, T.: Specific interaction between the self-splicing RNA of Tetrahymena and its guanosine substrate: Implications for biological catalysis by RNA. Nature 308: 802, 1984.

278. Peebles, C., Perlman, P., Mecklenburg, K., Petrillo, M., Tabor, J., Jarrell, K., and Cheng, H.-L.: A self-splicing RNA excises an intron lariat. Cell 44: 213, 1986.

279. Rushkin, B., Krainer, A., Maniatis, T., and Green, M. R.: Excision of an intact intron as a novel lariat structure during pre-mRNA splicing *in vitro*. Cell 38: 317, 1984.

280. Reed, R., Griffith, J., and Maniatis, T.: Purification and visualization of native spliceosomes. Cell 53: 949, 1988.

281. Grabowski, P. J., Seiler, S. R., and Sharp, P. A.: A multicomponent complex is involved in the splicing of messenger RNA precursors. Cell 42: 345, 1985.

282. Brody, F., and Abelson, J.: The "spliceosome": Yeast pre-mRNA associates with a 40S complex in a splicing dependent reaction. Science 288: 963, 1985.

283. Maniatis, T., and Reed, R.: The role of small nuclear ribonucleoprotein particles in pre-mRNA splicing. Nature 325: 673, 1987.

284. Lerner, E. A., Lerner, M. R., Janeway, C. A., and Steitz, J.: Monoclonal antibodies to nucleic acid–containing cellular constituents: Probes for molecular biology and autoimmune disease. Proc. Natl. Acad. Sci. USA 78: 2737, 1981.

285. Krainer, A. R., and Maniatis, T.: Multiple factors including the small nuclear ribonucleoproteins U1 and U2 are necessary for pre-mRNA splicing *in vitro*. Cell 42: 725, 1985.

286. Reed, R.: Protein composition of mammalian spliceosomes assembled *in vitro*. Proc. Natl. Acad. Sci. USA 87: 8031, 1990.

287. Konarska, M. M., and Sharp, P.: Electrophoretic separation of complexes involved in the splicing of precursors to mRNAs. Cell 46: 845, 1986.

288. Michaud, S., and Reed, R.: An ATP-independent complex commits pre-mRNA to the mammalian spliceosome assembly pathway. Genes Dev. 5: 2534, 1991.

289. Seraphin, B., and Rosbash, M.: Identification of functional U1 snRNA–pre-mRNA complexes committed to spliceosome assembly and splicing. Cell 59: 349, 1989.

290. Zhuang, Y., and Weiner, A. M.: A compensatory base change in U1 snRNA suppresses a 5' splice site mutation. Cell 46: 827, 1986.

291. Parker, R., Siliciano, P., and Guthrie, C.: Recognition of the TACTAAC box during mRNA splicing in yeast involved base-pairing with the U2-like snRNA. Cell 49: 229, 1987.

292. Ruskin, R., Zamore, P. D., and Green, M. R.: A factor, U2AF, is required for U2 snRNP binding and splicing complex assembly. Cell 52: 207, 1988.

293. Zamore, P. A., and Green, M. R.: Biochemical characterization of U2 snRNP auxiliary factor: An essential pre-mRNA splicing factor with a novel intracellular localization. EMBO J. 10: 207, 1991.

294. Cheng, S. C., and Abelson, J.: Spliceosome assembly in yeast. Genes Dev. 1: 1014, 1987.

295. Brow, D. A., and Guthrie, C.: Spliceosomal RNA U6 is remarkably conserved from yeast to mammals. Nature 334: 213, 1988.

296. Krainer, A. R., Conway, G. C., and Kozak, D.: Purification and characterization of pre-mRNA splicing factor SF2 from HeLa cells. Genes Dev. 4: 1158, 1990.

297. Ge, H., and Manley, J. L.: A protein factor, ASF, controls cell-specific alternative splicing of SV40 early pre-mRNA *in vitro*. Cell 62: 25, 1990.

298. Fu, X.-D., and Maniatis, T.: Factor required for mammalian spliceosome assembly is localized to discrete regions in the nucleus. Nature 343: 437, 1990.

299. Ast, G., Goldblatt, D., Offen, D., Sperling, J., and Sperling, R.: A novel splicing factor is an integral component of 200S large nuclear ribonucleoprotein (lnRNP) particles. EMBO J. 10: 425, 1991.

300. Ge, H., Zuo, P., and Manley, J. L.: Primary structure of the human splicing factor ASF reveals similarities with *Drosophila* splicing regulators. Cell 66: 373, 1991.

301. Krainer, A. R., Mayeda, A., Kozak, D., and Binns, G.: Functional expression of human splicing factor SF2: Homology to RNA-binding proteins U1, 70K and *Drosophila* splicing regulators. Cell 66: 383, 1991.

302. Krainer, A. R., Conway, G. C., and Kozak, D.: The essential splicing factor SF2 influences 5' splice site selection by activating proximal sites. Cell 62: 35, 1990.

303. Fu, X.-D., and Maniatis, T.: The 35-kDa mammalian splicing factor SC35 mediates specific interactions between U1 and U2 small nuclear ribonucleoprotein particles at the 3' splice site. Proc. Natl. Acad. Sci. USA 89: 1725, 1992.

304. Spector, D. L., Fu, X.-D., and Maniatis, T.: Associations between distinct pre-mRNA splicing components and the cell nucleus. EMBO J. 10: 3467, 1991.

305. Wassarman, D. A., and Steitz, J. A.: Alive with DEAD proteins. Nature 349: 463, 1991.

306. McKeown, M.: Regulation of alternative splicing. Genet. Eng. 12: 139, 1990.

307. Maniatis, T.: Mechanisms of alternative pre-mRNA splicing. Science 251: 33, 1991.

308. Bingham, P. M., Chou, T.-B., Mims, I., and Zachar, Z.: On/off regulation of gene expression at the level of splicing. Trends Genet. 4: 134, 1988.

309. Baker, B.: Sex in flies: The splice of life. Nature 340: 521, 1989.

310. Sosnowski, B. A., Belote, J. M., and McKeown, M.: Sex-specific alternative splicing of RNA from the transformer gene results from sequence-dependent splice site blockage. Cell 58: 449, 1989.

311. Hedley, M. L., and Maniatis, T.: Sex-specific splicing and polyadenylation of dsx pre-mRNA requires a sequence that binds specifically to tra-2 protein *in vitro*. Cell 65: 579, 1991.

3

Hematopoiesis

Grover C. Bagby, Jr.

INTRODUCTION

All mature blood cells have finite life spans, and most of them are completely incapable of replicating. Consequently, neutrophils, erythrocytes, platelets, eosinophils, and basophils are described as "terminally" differentiated. To maintain steady-state blood cell counts, production rates must equal the rate of senescence. Taking into account the stability of blood counts in normal humans and the fact that the bone marrow must produce approximately 10^{10} cells per day to keep pace with normal losses, the control of blood cell production is obviously tightly regulated in the steady state. The hematopoietic system must also respond to a variety of environmental stressors by increasing blood cell counts of specific lineages at various times. For example, erythrocyte production will predictably increase in the setting of hypoxia, but neutrophil production will not. Conversely, in patients who have acquired bacterial infection, neutrophil production will increase but erythrocyte production will not. These lineage-specific responses are governed by three generic categories of cellular competencies: the capacity of hematopoietic stem cells to give rise to progenitors committed to a particular hematopoietic lineage, the capacity of progenitors of a lineage to give rise to differentiated progeny, and the faculty of the organism to perceive environmental stimuli by generating both extracellular and intracellular signals that either permit or repress these pathways of differentiation.

The production of blood cells in hematopoietic tissues involves the establishment, in early embryogenesis, of pluripotential hematopoietic stem cells. These cells are capable of a high degree of self-replication and have not yet committed themselves to the production of any one specific lineage. Hematopoietic stem cells remain in residence in hematopoietic niches for the entire life of the mammal and, in fact, can be removed from the animal and establish hematopoiesis for another lifetime in another lethally irradiated recipient. Therefore, stem cells (1) are pluripotent and (2) can reconstitute the hematopoietic system of lethally irradiated animals because of their capacity for both self-renewal and production of committed progeny.

Although committed progenitor cells cannot be distinguished morphologically (they resemble small lymphocytes), they can be quantified in vitro because in semisolid media (e.g., agar or methylcellulose) they form colonies containing morphologically recognizable, differentiated progeny. Committed progenitors are the immediate precursors of blast forms, the earliest morphologically recognizable precursor cells of the lineages. Progeny of the blasts (e.g., *erythro*blasts in the case of erythroid precursors) can be identified morphologically and undergo predictable phenotypic changes as they progressively acquire more attributes of the functional, terminally differentiated cell (Fig. 3–1).

In the normal adult, all of these steps of replication and maturation take place almost exclusively in the

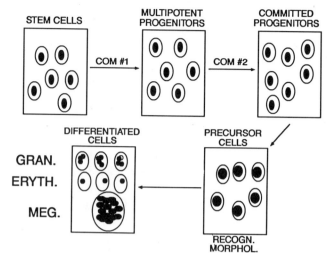

FIGURE 3–1. The five classes of hematopoietic populations. Stem cells are pluripotent and quantified by their capacity to repopulate lethally irradiated animals. Multipotent progenitor cells are daughters of stem cells (commitment step 1 [COM #1]) that have more limited self-replicative capacity yet have retained multipotentiality. The multipotential progenitor cells are quantified by colony assays in vitro. A second commitment step (COM #2) results in the production of daughter cells (also quantified in colony assays in vitro) that are completely committed to a specific lineage. These cells cannot be morphologically recognized but give rise to precursor cells, which can, in fact, be morphologically recognized (RECOGN. MORPHOL.) as belonging to a specific lineage. The replicative capacity of precursor cells (including blast forms and "pro" forms) is limited. The precursor cells replicate a few more times and in doing so give rise to cells that are of intermediate stages of differentiation. These intermediate forms are the immediate precursors of differentiated cells of the granulopoietic (GRAN.), erythroid (ERYTH.), and megakaryocytic (MEG) lineages.

bone marrow, an environment that provides growth factors, growth inhibitory factors, differentiation factors, and adhesion molecules that aid in the retention, survival, and growth of stem cells and progenitors in that particular niche. In the past 30 years, a good number of factors involved in regulating growth and differentiation of hematopoietic cells in the bone marrow have been identified, thanks to contributions from the fields of transplantation biology, in vitro hematopoiesis, protein chemistry, and molecular biology. In the past 8 years, information on the molecular events involved in regulating hematopoiesis in humans has appeared at a remarkable pace. Consequently, this chapter seeks to explicate some common themes in hematopoietic regulation, often using key references or recent reviews on a subject rather than presenting an encyclopedic compilation of the massive literature supporting the models presented. In addition, although this chapter seeks to focus on information derived from studies on human cells, when observations in animal models are critical to the definition of our current hematopoietic paradigm, such studies are included as well. In this regard, it should be recognized that murine models are highly relevant to human physiology. For example, virtually all in vitro assays for human hematopoietic progenitor cells derive from similar methods established using murine cells. In fact, the first clear evidence that hematopoietic stem cells existed derived from the seminal studies of Till and McCulloch.[1]

HEMATOPOIETIC STEM CELLS

Pluripotent Stem Cells

Original Animal Models

During the course of studies on radiation sensitivity of cells of the bone marrow that reconstitute hematopoiesis in lethally irradiated recipient mice, Till and McCulloch noticed that in irradiated mice infused with syngeneic marrow cells, macroscopically visible nodules formed in the spleen and that each nodule was composed of cells of multiple hematopoietic lineages at various stages of differentiation.[1] A wide variety of studies on this phenomenon subsequently demonstrated that each of these spleen colonies derived from a single[2, 3] pluripotent[4] hematopoietic progenitor cell now known as the spleen colony-forming unit, or CFU-S. CFU-S possess high replicative potential. Although the fraction of CFU-S proliferating at a given time is low[5–8] in steady-state bone marrow, the proliferative activity of CFU-S increases during hematopoietic recovery after bone marrow transplantation.[6]

The CFU-S give rise to other progenitor cells that are more "committed" to a given lineage. These committed progenitors can be quantified using in vitro clonal assays. Because CFU-S are multipotential cells with a high self-replicative potential and give rise to committed progenitor cells, they are very likely stem cells. However, some uncertainty remains about whether CFU-S are the most primitive stem cells.[9]

The contribution of hematopoietic stem cells to blood cell production has been studied using some innovative strategies. First, for example, Lemischka and colleagues[10] transplanted irradiated mice with stem cells uniquely marked by randomly integrated (through retroviral-mediated gene transfer) marker genes and demonstrated unambiguously that myeloid and lymphoid lineages evolve from a single cell,[10] thereby validating, using a molecular tactic, the studies of Wu and associates[11] published 20 years earlier. Second, studies described by Weissman and his colleagues (reviewed in reference 12) have permitted the purification of murine hematopoietic stem cells to near-homogeneity. Only about 20 to 30 of these cells are capable of reconstituting the entire hematopoietic system in irradiated mice. Moreover, these cells were fully capable of forming colonies in both the spleen and the thymus. Therefore, it is very likely that the CFU-S or some cell type very much like it is a legitimate pluripotent hematopoietic stem cell. However, the capacity of a cell to form a spleen colony is not the most fundamental definition of "stemness"; rather it is the capacity of a pluripotential cell to undergo repeated rounds of self-replication and give rise to daughter cells committed to multiple lineages.

Surface Antigens of Stem Cells

The capacity to purify murine stem cells using immunological methods has evolved as a result of a large number of studies characterizing the cellular surface antigens of primitive cells (e.g., CD34) and other surface antigens that are found in cells committed to a specific lineage. A battery of antibodies can be used to identify (and select against) cells that express lineage-specific markers (Lin+). This approach, taken by Weissman and his colleagues, has demonstrated that the surface of murine stem cells has low levels of Thy-1.1 antigen and no lineage-specific antigens and that it expresses stem cell antigen (Thy-1.1lo/Lin-/Sca-1+).[13] Validating that a given cell is a human stem cell is a more difficult prospect than it is with murine models. The human stem cell phenotype can be deduced from in vitro studies on colony-forming cells that yield colonies containing a number of blast forms. When these blast colonies are plucked from culture, suspended in medium, and replated in secondary and tertiary cultures, the colonial cells also contain multilineage progenitor cells. Terstappen and coworkers used a variety of monoclonal antibodies in an attempt to identify the phenotype of these blast CFUs and found that the cells were CD34+/CD38−.[14] CD38 is a 45 kDa glycoprotein the function of which is unknown. It is expressed by cells of all hematopoietic lineages.[14] CD34 is a 110 kDa glycoprotein encoded by a gene on human chromosome 1q[15] and is expressed by human hematopoietic progenitor cells and stem cells of non-human primates[16] as well as by capillary endothelial cells.[17] CD34+/CD38− cells from human bone marrow plated at a density of one cell per well gave rise to primitive colonies 28 to 34 days after sorting (after 14 days of culture in medium, erythropoietin, granulocyte-macrophage colony-stimulating factor [GM-CSF], granulocyte colony-stimulating factor [G-CSF], interleukin [IL]-6, and IL-3 were added to the wells). More important, during culture periods of up to 4 months, as many as five sequential generations of clones were seen after replating of the cells from these primitive colonies.[14] There are other promising reagents that may aid in the full characterization of human hematopoietic stem cells, including antibodies to c-kit (for positive selection) and CD33 (for negative selection).[18] Figure 3–2 displays the surface antigen phenotype of stem cells and progenitors and the parent-progeny relationships in hematopoiesis; it also lists the growth factors that exert biological activity within a certain cell population. Table 3–1 defines the progenitor populations in functional terms. Combinations of the immunological approaches to phenotyping and cell isolation described above when combined with other methods (e.g., transgenic and chimeric murine models) now provide investigators with tools powerful enough to test directly, using human cells, a number of theories that evolved from transplantation biology.

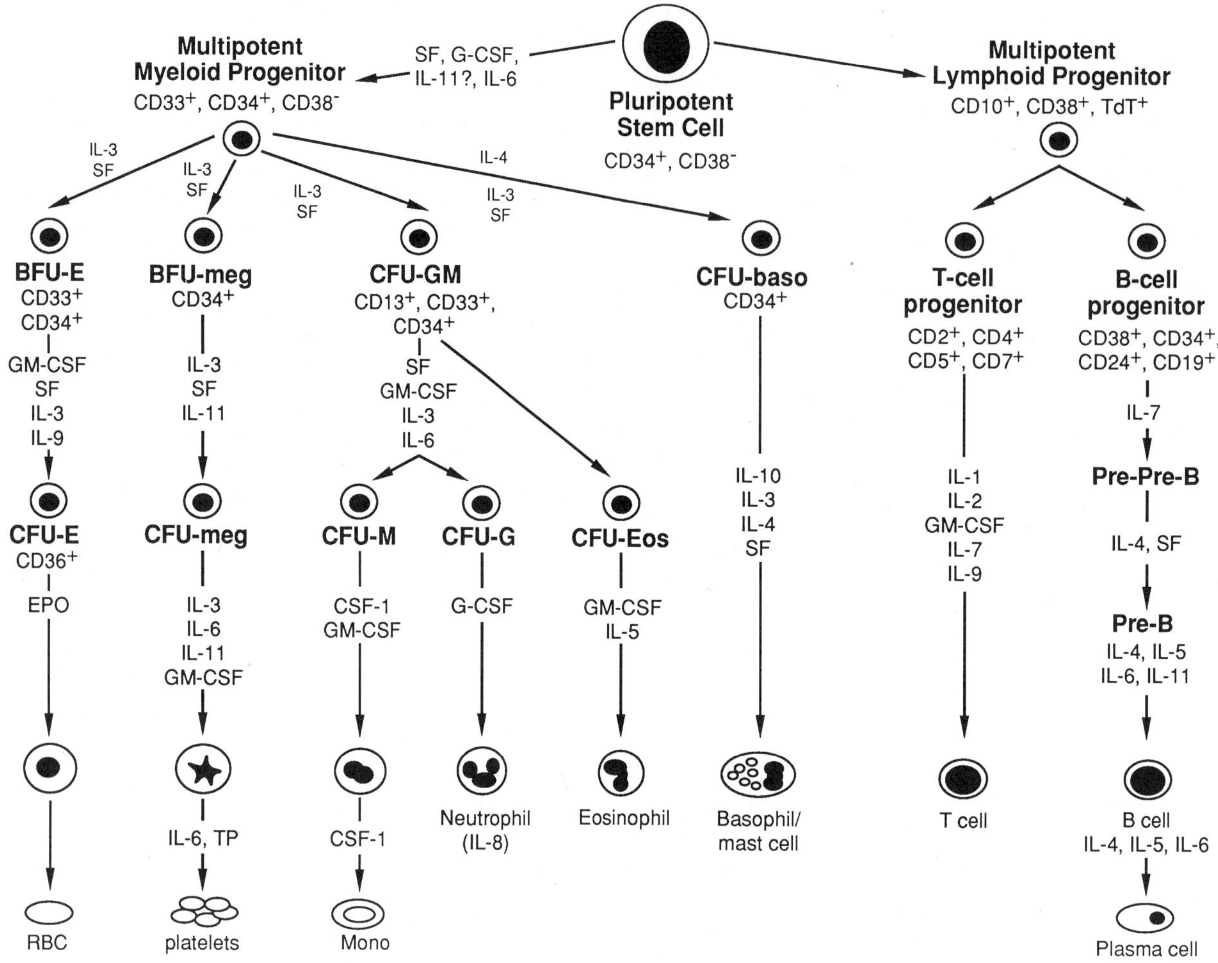

Multipotent Myeloid Progenitor
CD33+, CD34+, CD38−

SF, G-CSF, IL-11?, IL-6

Pluripotent Stem Cell
CD34+, CD38−

Multipotent Lymphoid Progenitor
CD10+, CD38+, TdT+

IL-3 SF

IL-3 SF

IL-3 SF

IL-4 IL-3 SF

BFU-E
CD33+
CD34+

GM-CSF
SF
IL-3
IL-9

CFU-E
CD36+

EPO

RBC

BFU-meg
CD34+

IL-3
SF
IL-11

CFU-meg

IL-3
IL-6
IL-11
GM-CSF

IL-6, TP

platelets

CFU-GM
CD13+, CD33+, CD34+

SF
GM-CSF
IL-3
IL-6

CFU-M

CSF-1
GM-CSF

CSF-1

Mono

CFU-G

G-CSF

Neutrophil
(IL-8)

CFU-Eos

GM-CSF
IL-5

Eosinophil

CFU-baso
CD34+

IL-10
IL-3
IL-4
SF

Basophil/
mast cell

T-cell progenitor
CD2+, CD4+
CD5+, CD7+

IL-1
IL-2
GM-CSF
IL-7
IL-9

T cell

B-cell progenitor
CD38+, CD34+,
CD24+, CD19+

IL-7

Pre-Pre-B

IL-4, SF

Pre-B
IL-4, IL-5
IL-6, IL-11

B cell
IL-4, IL-5, IL-6

Plasma cell

FIGURE 3–2. This diagram illustrates the hierarchical relationship between pluripotent and multipotent progenitor cells of the myeloid and lymphoid lineages, some of the growth factors that influence the growth of cells at these stages of differentiation, and some of the important surface antigens expressed by the stem cells and progenitor cells. TdT = Terminal deoxyribonucleotidyl transferase; SF = Steel factor; EPO = erythropoietin; CSF-1 = M-CSF; TP = thrombopoietin; Mono = monocyte; and RBC = red blood cell.

TABLE 3–1. IN VITRO COLONY-FORMING CELLS

CELL	LINEAGE	OTHER
CFU-B1	Mult	Very primitive; colonial cells are also multipotential in secondary replating experiments; enriched in post–5-FU marrow; can survive (but not replicate) in absence of defined hematopoietic growth factors
CFU-GEMM	Mult	Form multilineage colonies; circulate in peripheral blood like BFU-E (see below)
HPP-CFC₁	Mult	Highly replicative; enriched in post–5-FU marrow; colonies are huge (50,000 cells or more); rhodamine-"dull" CFC are IL-1 responsive and are precursors of rhodamine-"bright" CFC that are not IL-1 responsive[292]
HPP-CFC₂	Mo	Highly replicative macrophage progenitor; may be the same as HPP-CFC₁ but driven to form macrophage colonies by specific growth conditions
BFU-E	E	IL-3, GM-CSF, and Steel factor (SF)–responsive CFU, less responsive to EPO than CFU-E
CFU-E	E	Express both high- and low-affinity EPO receptors
CFU-GM	G/M/Eo	Require GM-CSF, G-CSF, IL-3, or IL-5 for survival; 40% are actively proliferating in a freshly obtained marrow cell population
BFU-Mk	Meg	GM-CSF and IL-3 responsive; give rise to bursts of megakaryocyte colonies
CFU-Mk	Meg	IL-3, GM-CSF, IL-6, and IL-11 responsive; give rise to single small megakaryocyte colonies

Mult = Multilineage; Mo = monocyte/macrophage; E = erythroid; G = neutrophilic leukocyte; Eo = eosinophil; Meg = megakaryocyte; 5-FU = 5-fluorouracil.

Committed Progenitor Cells

Committed progenitor cells, all of which have the capacity to form colonies containing cells of one or more specific hematopoietic lineages in semisolid culture media (see Figs. 3–1 and 3–2), are the progeny of pluripotent stem cells. At least four types of multipotential progenitor cells can also form colonies in vitro. CFU-GEMM (also known as the multipotent myeloid progenitor cell) (see Fig. 3–2) form colonies containing erythroid, myeloid, and megakaryocytic elements. CFU-Blast form colonies of undifferentiated cells that on replating contain committed progenitor cells.[19, 20] The high-proliferative potential colony-forming cell (HPP-CFC) is relatively resistant to the drug 5-fluorouracil, forms macroscopically visible colonies in vitro, and gives rise to multilineage progeny. Although CFU-GEMM are viewed as more committed than CFU-Blast and HPP-CFC, no clear relationship between the latter two has been established. Finally, the long-term culture initiating cell (LTCIC) is capable of "recharging" irradiated hematopoietic stroma in vitro. That is, it accounts for the appearance of multipotential and committed progenitor cells in long-term cultures.[21, 22] The LTCIC is considered the most primitive (the most like the stem cell) of the culturable mammalian cells.[21] Because there is no clonal assay for long-term repopulation, it will be difficult to know whether the LTCIC and the hematopoietic stem cell are identical.

HEMATOPOIETIC GROWTH FACTORS AND THEIR RECEPTORS

Committed progenitor cells form colonies only in the presence of hematopoietic growth factors and, in general, depend on such factors for their survival in vitro. The particular lineage represented in any colony arising in the culture of bone marrow cells depends completely on the nature and activity of the glycoproteins added to the culture system (Fig. 3–3). Genes encoding some of these factors have been cloned and sequenced, and the biological activity of their products assessed comprehensively in vitro and in vivo. Some of the recombinant human factors—specifically, erythropoietin, G-CSF, and GM-CSF—have even been approved for clinical use. More recently, receptors for many of these factors have been characterized as well. Table 3–2 lists the well-defined cytokines with hematopoietic activity, their molecular weights, the location of the gene encoding them on the human chromosome, the cells that express the cytokine genes and factors that induce their expression, as well as the receptor or receptors for the cytokine and their molecular weight and cells of origin.

Some of these factors act directly, whereas others act indirectly. Most factors, however, are capable of acting in both ways. That is, some cytokines with hematopoietic activity directly stimulate growth or differentiation of one or more cell types, but in other

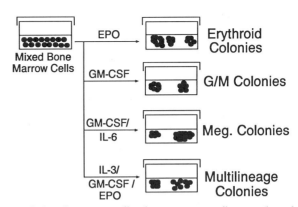

FIGURE 3–3. When mammalian bone marrow cells are cultured in semisolid media for periods of 7 to 21 days in the presence of lineage-specific growth factors, specific cells, known as colony-forming units (CFUs), proliferate and form colonies. In the presence of erythropoietin (EPO), erythroid colonies are produced, whereas in the presence of GM-CSF, granulocyte-macrophage colonies are produced. GM-CSF and interleukin-6 (IL-6) are capable of inducing megakaryocyte colonies, and multilineage colony growth is stimulated, in part, by IL-3, GM-CSF, and EPO.

cells, the same proteins induce expression of other growth factor genes and thus act indirectly as well. GM-CSF, for example, stimulates the growth of progenitors and induces IL-1 expression[23, 24] (this becomes enormously perplexing when one considers the capacity of IL-1 to induce at least seven other direct-acting cytokines [see below]). Attributing to any protein, therefore, a discrete set of biological activities can be exceedingly difficult. Generally, however, four categories of biological activities can be attributed to these growth factors: lineage-specific, multilineage, synergistic, and inductive (see Table 3–3). These arbitrary divisions are conceptually useful and provide a basic working framework for these and any molecules with hematopoietic activity, to be described in the future. It must be emphasized, however, that the activity of some cytokines is such that they fall into more than one category. Because each of the cytokines transduces its signal through a receptor unique to it, it is most appropriate at this point to focus on these receptor molecules.

Hematopoietic Growth Factor Receptor Superfamilies

Receptors with Cytoplasmic Tyrosine Kinase Domains

Amino acid sequence analysis has provided a framework for the categorization of three subclasses of a tyrosine kinase receptor family. Subclass 1 includes the *neu*/HER2 proto-oncogene and epidermal growth factor (EGF); subclass 2 includes the insulin and insulin-like growth factor–1 (IGF-1) receptors; and subclass 3 includes the receptors for macrophage colony-stimulating factor (M-CSF), Steel factor, and platelet-derived growth factor (PDGF). Because this subclass

TABLE 3–2. HEMATOPOIETIC FACTORS AND THEIR RECEPTORS

LIGAND	MW (kDa)	CHROMO-SOME	SOURCE	PHYSIOLOGICAL INDUCTIVE FACTORS	RECEPTOR	MW	EXPRESSED BY	SUBUNIT SHARING	OTHER
EPO	18–32	7q	Renal hepatocyte	Hypoxia	EPO-R	55	E, S, Mg	?	Homodimerization occurs, receptor on chromosome 19p
G-CSF	18–25	17q	Stromal cells and macrophages	IL-1, TNF-α LPS	G-CSF-R	150	N	None	
GM-CSF	14–35	5q	Stromal cells	IL-1, TNF-α LPS	GM-CSF-Rα, GM-CSFβ	80–85 130	M, N, Eo, Er	With IL-3Rα and IL-5Rα	α and β chains dimerize
IL-3	14–28	5q	T lymphocytes	Antigen IgE receptor activation	IL-3Rα, GM-CSFβ	130 130	M, L, N, Eo, Meg, Ba	With IL-5Rα and GM-CSF	α and β chains dimerize
IL-5	40	5q	T lymphocytes	Antigens, mitogens	IL-5Rα, GM-CSFβ	? 130	B, T, Eo	With IL-3Rα and GM-CSF	α and β chains dimerize
IL-6	21–26	7p	Most mesenchymal cells	LPS, TNF, IL-1, mitogens	IL-6Rα, gp 130	80 130	S, Ng, Hep, Ec, B, T, M	gp 130 shared with LIF-Rα	LIF-Rα and gp 130 dimerize and bind oncostatin M as well as LIF
LIF	58	22q	Mononuclear leukocytes and stromal cells	LPS, TNF, IL-1	LIF-Rα, gp 130	130	Mg, Hep, Myo, neu, osteo, M, ES	gp 130 shared with IL-6Rα	LIF-Rα and gp 130 dimerize and bind oncostatin M as well as LIF
M-CSF	40–90	1p	Many mesenchymal cells	GM-CSF, IL-4, IL-3, TNF-α	c-fms	150	M	No	Cytoplasmic region of receptor has tyrosine kinase domains; on chromosome 5q
SF	46 membrane bound; 30 secreted	12q	Ub	Constitutive	c-kit	145	S, BFU-E, HPP-CFC	No	Cytoplasmic region has tyrosine kinase domains; as member of the c-fms PDGF-R subclass; on chromosome 4
IL-1	14–17	2q	Ub	LPS, IL-1, TNF, IL-2	IL-1RI, IL-1RII	87–100 68–80	T, S, Ep, B, M, S	No	
IL-2	23	4q	T lymphocytes	LPS, mitogens, antibodies	p55, p75	55 75	B, T, NK	No	p55 and p 75 dimerize
IL-4	18	5q	T lymphocytes, mast cells, basophils	IgE, substance K, mitogens	IL-4R	140 kDa	M, Ba, B, T	No	Receptors are heavily glycosylated
IL-7	17–25	8q	Stromal cells	?	IL-2R	50–75	B, T, Meg	?	160 kDa receptor may be a homodimer
IL-8	8–9	4q	Stromal cells, macrophages, T cells	LPS, TNF-α, IL-1	IL-8R	58	T, N	No	
IL-10	30–35	1	T cells, macrophages	LPS, mitogens	?	?	?	?	
TNF-α	17	6p	Macrophages, B cells, NK cells	LPS, IL-3, GM-CSF	TNF R-α, TNF R-β	75 55	Ub Ub	No	Each receptor binds to both TNF-α and TNF-β

Ub = Ubiquitous; E = erythroid; S = stromal; Mg = megakaryocyte; M = monocyte/macrophage; N = neutrophil; Eo = eosinophil; Ba = basophil; Ec = endothelial cell; Hep = hepatocyte; neu = neural tissue; osteo = osteosarcoma; ES = embryonal cells; T = T lymphocyte; B = B lymphocyte; NK = natural killer cell; Myo = myocytes; Ep = epithelial cells; LPS = lipopolysaccharide.

includes receptors for hematopoietic growth factors, it is discussed further here.

The c-kit and c-fms genes encode two related hematopoietic growth factor receptors, the ligands for which are Steel factor and M-CSF, respectively (see below). Along with PDGF (A and B) receptors, they constitute a subclass of receptor tyrosine kinases with similar topologies (reviewed in reference 25). All receptors with tyrosine kinase activity possess large glycosylated extracellular domains, a single transmembrane spanning region, and a cytoplasmic domain that contains one or more tyrosine kinase catalytic sites (Fig. 3–4).

Features of the Hematopoietic Growth Factor Receptor Superfamily

The characterization of receptors for many of the growth factors, described in more detail below, has permitted the identification of a receptor family that includes receptors for leukemia inhibitory factor (LIF), IL-1, IL-2, IL-3, IL-4, IL-5, IL-6, IL-7, GM-CSF, G-CSF, erythropoietin (EPO), prolactin, growth hormone, ciliary neurotrophic factor, and c-mpl.[26, 27] As shown in Figure 3–4, a number of repetitive structural and functional themes are included in this unique integral membrane protein superfamily, including (1)

TABLE 3–3. BIOLOGICAL ACTIVITIES OF HEMATOPOIETIC FACTORS

FACTOR	BIOLOGICAL ACTIVITIES
EPO	Stimulates clonal growth of CFU-E and a subset of BFU-E, induces globin synthesis in erythroid cells, stimulates murine megakaryocyte colony growth but has no apparent thrombopoietic activity in vivo
G-CSF	Stimulates clonal growth of CFU-GM and production of neutrophils in vivo, stimulates neutrophil maturation of certain leukemic cells, activates phagocytic function of mature neutrophils, stimulates quiescent pluripotent progenitor cells to enter G_1–S phase, induces migration and proliferation of vascular endothelial cells in vitro; stimulates growth of some cancer cells
GM-CSF	Stimulates growth of CFU-GM and production of monocytes, eosinophils, and neutrophils in vivo; stimulates growth of CFU-GEMM, BFU-E, and CFU-Meg; primes (preactivates) phagocytic and chemotactic function of monocytes and granulocytes, stimulates growth of certain leukemic cells, induces expression of IL-1, TNF-α, and M-CSF by monocytes, and IL-1 production by neutrophils; stimulates functional activation of eosinophils; costimulates T-cell growth with IL-2, stimulates growth of some cancer cells, and induces migration and proliferation of vascular endothelial cells; activates HIV-1 proviral gene expression in latently infected mononuclear phagocytes
IL-3	Stimulates CFU-GEMM and CFU-S growth; stimulates proliferation of HPP-CFC, BFU-E, B lymphocytes, T lymphocytes (synergistically with IL-2), and growth of myeloid leukemic cells; induces macrophages to express M-CSF; stimulates growth of mast cells and pre-B cell lines
IL-5	Activates cytotoxic T lymphocytes, co-induces immunoglobulin secretion, stimulates eosinophil production and activation in vitro and in vivo
IL-6	Synergistic with IL-3 in stimulating CFU-GEMM colony growth, with M-CSF in macrophage colony growth, and with GM-CSF in inducing granulocyte colony growth; synergistic with IL-4 in inducing T-cell proliferation, hematopoietic colony formation by multipotential progenitor cells, and immunoglobulin secretion by B lymphocytes; synergizes with IL-2 and IL-1 in inducing T-cell growth, co-induces B-cell growth, and induces terminal differentiation of certain murine myeloid leukemic cell lines; induces neuronal differentiation in certain pheochromocytoma cell lines, co-induces cytotoxic T cells, stimulates plasmacytoma growth, induces acute phase responses in vivo, induces acute phase protein synthesis in hepatocytes, synergistic with IL-3 in stimulating CFU-GEMM and CFU-Meg colony growth; promotes megakaryocyte maturation in vitro and stimulates platelet production in vivo; activates HIV-1 proviral gene expression
LIF	Enhances efficiency of CFU-S infection by retroviral shuttle vectors; induces differentiation of certain murine and human leukemic cells; inhibits differentiation of embryonal carcinoma cells; stimulates bone resorption; enhances growth of megakaryocytes in vivo; augments proliferation of pluripotent human progenitor cells
M-CSF	Induces monocyte/macrophage growth (murine cells) and differentiation (both murine and human cells); induces phagocytic and secretory function in monocytes and macrophages
SF	Markedly enhances clonal growth of CFU-GEMM, BFU-E, and pre-B cells when combined with direct-acting growth factors, IL-3, EPO, or IL-7; enhances growth of mast cells
IL-1	Induces expression of GM-CSF, G-CSF, IL-6, and IL-1 in stromal cells; induces proliferation of preactivated T cells, induces acute phase protein synthesis, induces fever and sleep, stimulates the release of ACTH, promotes the transendothelial passage of neutrophils, synergizes with IL-3 in stimulating proliferation in primitive hematopoietic progenitor cells, stimulates PGE production in fibroblasts, monocytes, and neutrophils, modulates EGF receptor expression, induces IL-2 receptor number and binding activity, enhances growth of virulent strains of *Escherichia coli*, and induces maturation of pre-B cells
IL-2	Induces proliferation and activation of T lymphocytes, B lymphocytes, and NK cells; induces expression of IL-1 in monocytes and macrophages, co-induces (with IL-1) expression of interferon-γ in T cells; costimulates B-cell differentiation and induces non–MHC-restricted cytotoxic T lymphocyte (CTL) activity
IL-4	Induces proliferation of activated B cells, inhibits IL-2–stimulated proliferation of B cells, co-induces immunoglobulin secretion and isotype switching, co-induces proliferation of T cells and fibroblasts, and co-induces IL-2 receptor expression in T cells; inhibits induction of lymphokine-activated killer cells, inhibits IL-1 synthesis, induces expression of M-CSF and G-CSF genes in monocytes, induces expression of an inhibitor of hematopoiesis by mixed murine marrow stromal cells; enhances murine BFU-E and CFU-E growth (with EPO) and enhances CFU-GM growth (with G-CSF or GM-CSF); stimulates expression of MHC class II antigens on B cells and monocytes
IL-7	Costimulates T cells (with mitogens), enhances growth of allospecific CTLs, induces cytokine secretion by monocytes and macrophages, and induces clonal growth of pre-B cells
IL-8	Induces neutrophil chemotaxis
IL-10	Induces proliferation of B lymphocytes and mast cells; inhibits cytokine production by monocytes, inhibits T-lymphocyte proliferation and IL-2 production, inhibits IL-5–mediated antibody secretion, synergizes with TGF-β and IL-4 to inhibit macrophage cytotoxicity
TNF-α	Induces expression of GM-CSF, G-CSF, IL-6, and IL-1 in fibroblasts and endothelial cells; enhances mitogen-induced GM-CSF expression in T cells, induces release of GM-CSF and M-CSF in vivo, and inhibits replication of certain viruses synergistically with interferons; also induces expression of HIV-1 provirus in vitro; stimulates PGE production in fibroblasts and neutrophils, enhances parasite and tumor cell cytotoxicity of eosinophils and macrophages, inhibits growth of hematopoietic progenitor cells, lymphocytes, and certain leukemic cell lines; mediates the hemodynamic and toxic effects of endotoxin; induces expression of adhesion molecules in myeloid and stroma cells, including endothelial cells, induces expression of IL-8, increases production of plasminogen activator inhibitor in vascular endothelial cells, suppresses transcription of the thrombomodulin gene in endothelial cells, modulates EGF receptor expression, promotes transendothelial passage of neutrophils, activates NF-κB transactivation protein in lymphoid cells (this function probably accounts for the effect of this cytokine on HIV-1 gene activation)

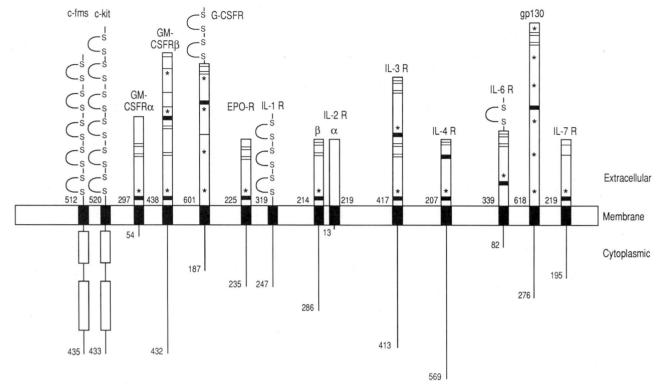

FIGURE 3–4. The structures for a variety of hematopoietic growth factor receptors. The first two molecules on the left, c-*fms* and c-*kit*, are integral membrane proteins with tyrosine kinase domains (shown as *open boxes* in the cytoplasmic portions of the molecules). The other growth factor receptors shown are members of the hematopoietic growth factor superfamily. The extracellular domains include the immunoglobulin-like regions shown as loops above for c-*fms*, c-*kit*, G-CSFR, IL-1R, and IL-6R. The members of the superfamily have conserved cysteines in the extracellular domains (the Cys residues in the extracellular domain are shown as parallel lines). The dark boxes above the membrane region of the receptors represent the WSXWS motif. Stars indicate locations of the fibronectin type III motifs. Tyrosine kinase domains are indicated as cytoplasmic boxes. Two heterodimeric subunits are illustrated: The GM-CSF receptor β-subunit (a subunit it shares with IL-3R and IL-5R) is paired with GM-CSFRα, and the gp130 subunit is paired with IL-6Rα.

four cysteine residues in the extracellular domain, (2) the sequence W-S-X-W-S in the ligand-binding extracellular domain, (3) a capacity for enhanced binding or signal transduction, or both, when the protein is expressed as a heterodimer or homodimer, (4) lack of a known catalytic domain in the cytoplasmic portion of the molecule, and (5) the presence of fibronectin type III domains[28] in the extracellular regions (see Fig. 3–4). Apart from these shared homologous domains, not much sequence homology is found among these receptors, and the size of their cytoplasmic domains (see Fig. 3–4) is enormously variable. Nonetheless, these homologies are likely of substantial functional importance and also give clues to the evolution of this family. For example, that fibronectin type III domains are shared with several cell adhesion molecules suggests that cytokine receptors evolved from ancestral genes whose products functioned largely to facilitate cellular adhesion to both substrates and other cells.

Another interesting feature of some of these receptor molecules is their capacity to share peptide subunits with other receptors. For example, IL-5, GM-CSF, and IL-3 have unique low-affinity (α chain) receptors, but they share the same β chain,[29, 30] and association of the two chains results in the formation of a specific high-

affinity dimer capable of effective signal transduction (Fig. 3–5). Shared subunits have also been identified for high-affinity complexes that serve as receptors for LIF, IL-6, and oncostatin M[31] (Fig. 3–6). In this case, gp130 functions as a signal-transducing component of

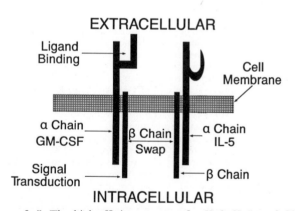

FIGURE 3–5. The high-affinity receptors for IL-3, IL-5, and GM-CSF are each heterodimers consisting of unique chains and a shared β chain. The capacity to compete for a limited number of β chains, shown here as a swap between the α chain of the IL-5 receptor and the α chain of the GM-CSF receptor, accounts for the capacity of one ligand to reduce binding to the receptors for the other two ligands.

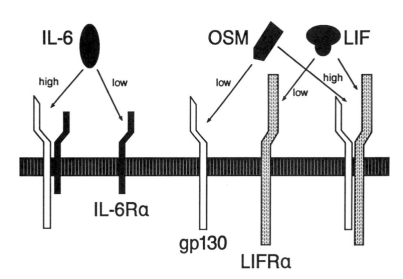

FIGURE 3–6. The receptors for IL-6, oncostatin M (OSM), and leukemia inhibitory factor (LIF) are heterodimers. When IL-6Rα pairs with the signal-transducing gp130 protein, it is converted from a low-affinity monomeric receptor to a high-affinity heterodimeric receptor. gp130 also functions as a low-affinity receptor for OSM, and the low-affinity LIF receptor (LIFRα) functions as a low-affinity receptor for LIF. When these two subunits are combined, the heterodimer binds with high affinity to both OSM and LIF.

the IL-6Rα/gp130 and LIFRα/gp130 complexes. The details of the stimulus-response coupling pathways are not yet known, but it has been reported that gp130 is phosphorylated at tyrosine residues upon stimulation of cells with the ligand.[32]

In many instances, soluble forms of the receptor can be found, sometimes resulting from translation of differentially spliced messenger RNA (mRNA) (summarized below). Soluble forms have been described for IL-4, IL-5, IL-7, G-CSF, Steel factor, EPO, and GM-CSF receptors.[33–37] Although the biological meaning of this phenomenon is not yet fully understood, the soluble forms may act as competitive binding proteins for the ligand and, as is clearly the case for the soluble IL-4 receptor,[37] serve as natural in vivo antagonists for specific cytokines.

Growth Factors and Receptors with Lineage Specificity

Erythropoietin

Erythropoietin is expressed largely by cells in the liver of the fetus[38] and specifically in the kidney[39] in adult life. The production of EPO is induced by reductions of tissue oxygenation,[40] a mechanism that involves the initial activation, by hypoxia,[41] of heme proteins that govern EPO mRNA accumulation. Different *cis*-acting hypoxia-responsive elements account for expression of this gene in liver and kidney.[42]

Erythropoietin stimulates growth and differentiation[43] of erythroid progenitor cells and stimulates proliferation and RNA synthesis in morphologically recognizable erythroid precursor cells[44] (see Table 3–2). Although EPO has been reported to stimulate various levels of megakaryocytopoiesis in vitro and platelet production in experimental animals[45–47] and although high-affinity EPO receptors have been reported in rodent megakaryocytes,[48] the physiological relevance of these observations is unclear. First, this is not an effect seen in serum free cultures[47] or in

cultures of cells enriched for progenitors[49] (and relatively free, therefore, of accessory cells). Moreover, others have failed to observe an effect of EPO on megakaryocyte colony growth in human bone marrow cell cultures, and in clinical trials, recombinant human EPO has shown no consistent effects on platelet counts.

Erythropoietin was the first hematopoietic growth factor to be identified experimentally, and the use of the recombinant protein has been shown to be effective in the management of anemia associated with renal failure. Although EPO receptors seem to be highly expressed by cells committed to erythropoiesis, the receptor is also expressed to some degree on embryonal stem cells and endothelial cells[50, 51] and in IL-3–responsive cell lines that lack erythroid characteristics (but may have erythroid potential), as well as in rodent megakaryocytes.[48]

The murine[52] and human[53] EPO receptors have been cloned and characterized (see Table 3–1). The extracellular domain binds to a carboxy-terminal domain on EPO,[54] and the cytoplasmic portion of the receptor, as is the case with many other hematopoietic growth factor receptors,[26] lacks a tyrosine kinase or other catalytic domain. Therefore, like other members of the growth factor receptor superfamily, EPO likely requires help from a related integral membrane protein cofactor to form a highly functional receptor.[55]

On binding to EPO, the receptor transduces signals that result in an early rise in free intracellular calcium and cytosolic protein phosphorylation.[56, 57] The activation of *raf*-1 is induced by EPO and is an essential mediator of the EPO response. As shown in Figure 3–7, *raf*-1 activation is a coupling step necessary for the transduction of signals through a variety of hematopoietic growth factor receptors.

Granulocyte Colony-Stimulating Factor

The biological activities of G-CSF are reviewed in Table 3–3. The G-CSF receptor has been cloned and characterized as a member of the cytokine receptor superfamily[36, 58, 59] (see Table 3–2). Clear-cut evidence

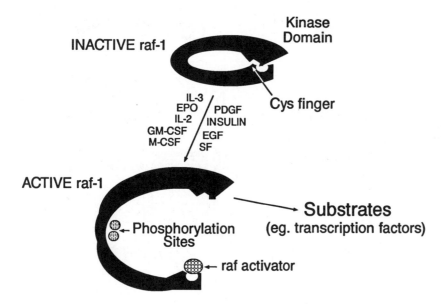

FIGURE 3–7. *Raf*-1 kinase is a serine/threonine kinase whose kinase domain is inactivated by a Cys finger domain located at the other end of the molecule. Stimulation of the cell with a variety of hematopoietic (and other) growth factors results in *raf*-1 phosphorylation, binding of an accessory molecule at the Cys finger site, and subsequent activation (by loss of autoinhibition) of the kinase domain, resulting in substrate phosphorylation on serines and threonines of downstream signaling molecules, including, but not necessarily limited to, transcription factors.

exists that G-CSF enforces the neutrophil differentiation program in primitive factor–dependent cell lines[60] and in certain myeloid leukemia cell lines.[61, 62] When administered to humans, it induces neutrophilic leukocytosis. Therefore, although there is some evidence that G-CSF can exert a degree of synergistic stimulatory effect on multilineage progenitor cells,[63] its most readily quantifiable activity is specific to the neutrophil lineage.

Interleukin-5

The IL-5 gene,[64] along with IL-4, IL-3, GM-CSF, and c-*fms* (the receptor for M-CSF), is located on the long arm of chromosome 5.[65, 66] IL-5 is produced by T lymphocytes induced by antigens, mitogens, and phorbol esters (see Table 3–2). Although IL-5 exerts a synergistic effect on lymphoid differentiation,[67] its impact on non-lymphoid cellular growth and differentiation seems to be specifically on cells of the eosinophil lineage (see Table 3–3). The soluble form of the IL-5 receptor has been cloned and characterized[29] and shares a common β subunit with GM-CSF and IL-3 (see Fig. 3–5), a phenomenon that accounts for the capacity of GM-CSF, IL-5, and IL-3 to cross-compete for surface receptors on selected cell types.[68]

Macrophage Colony-Stimulating Factor

The M-CSF gene encoded by a gene on the short arm of human chromosome 1[69] (see Table 3–2) gives rise to two glycoprotein species (70 to 90 kDa and 40 to 50 kDa) as a result of alternative splicing of pre-mRNA.[70, 71] It binds to a well-characterized receptor, the glycoprotein product of the c-*fms* proto-oncogene, one of the few hematopoietic growth factor receptors with a C-terminal tyrosine kinase domain (see Fig. 3–4).

Interleukin-7

The major biological impact of the 17 kDa IL-7 molecule is on lymphoid cells (see Table 3–3). It has also been reported to induce cytokine secretion by peripheral blood monocytes,[72] but this effect may be mediated by other factors induced by IL-7 in lymphoid cells. The human IL-7 gene product binds to a receptor molecule, a member of the cytokine receptor superfamily,[26, 34] and stimulates phosphoinositide turnover and tyrosine phosphorylation.[73]

Interleukin-2

The bioactivity of IL-2, a 23 kDa protein (see Table 3–3), is exerted largely on growth and differentiation of lymphoid cells, although it also induces expression of IL-1 and tumor necrosis factor–α (TNF-α) in mononuclear phagocytes.[74–76] IL-2 binds to a heterodimeric receptor made up of 75 and 55 kDa subunits (see Table 3–2 and Fig. 3–4) expressed by T lymphocytes, natural killer (NK) cells, and B cells and transduces signals, at least in part, through activation of tyrosine-specific and calmodulin-dependent kinases.[76, 77] Phosphorylation of the serine/threonine kinase *raf*-1 also occurs in response to ligand binding (see Fig. 3–7).[78, 79] A gamma chain of the IL-2 receptor has now been identified.

Multilineage Factors

Multilineage factors either induce replication of multipotential progenitors (CFU-GEMM) or simultaneously stimulate growth of committed progenitors of more than one lineage, or both. They almost always enhance the overall proliferative response of bone marrow cells exposed to lineage-specific factors (see Table 3–3), but as multipotential hematopoietic progenitors differentiate, most of their daughter cells lose the capacity to proliferate in response to multilineage factors.[60, 80, 81]

Granulocyte-Macrophage Colony-Stimulating Factor

Widespread clinical use of GM-CSF has validated the capacity of this molecule to induce neutrophil, monocyte, and eosinophil production (see Table 3–3 for biological activities). The receptor (see Table 3–2 and Fig. 3–3) is a heterodimeric protein made up of a unique α subunit encoded by a gene located on the pseudoautosomal regions of chromosomes X and Y[82] and a β subunit[83] that also serves as the β subunit for the heterodimeric receptors for IL-3 and IL-5.[29] Binding of the ligand to its high-affinity receptor results in immediate membrane depolarization,[84] stimulates protein phosphorylation on tyrosine and serine,[85, 86] and, as is the case with a number of other growth factors, activates *raf*-1 kinase (see Fig. 3–7).[87] Evidence also exists that p21-*ras* is involved in signal transduction via this receptor, an attribute it shares with IL-3 and IL-2, but not IL-4.[88]

Interleukin-3 and Its Receptor

The biological activities of IL-3 (see Table 3–3) derive from direct effects on progenitors as well as from its capacity to induce other cells to produce direct-acting factors. The direct growth-stimulatory effects of IL-3 seem to be limited to the most primitive of the committed progenitors and to cells with multilineage potential. The IL-3 receptor α and β chains[30] transduce signals coupled to the cellular response via activation of p21-*ras*,[88] *raf*-1 kinase,[87] and tyrosine kinases.[86, 89, 90] Human IL-3 DNA (see Table 3–2) resides on the long arm of chromosome 5 only 9 kb upstream of the gene for GM-CSF; however, these two are very differently regulated. GM-CSF is produced by a variety of stromal cells, whereas significant IL-3 gene expression seems to be limited to T lymphocytes (reviewed in reference 91). There is also evidence that IL-3 gene expression and GM-CSF gene expression even in T cells, which express both genes, are regulated independently of each other.[91]

Interleukin-11

The 199 amino acid molecule IL-11,[92] like IL-6, stimulates plasmacytoma cell growth but has other activities as well, including induction of B-lymphocyte differentiation (a T-lymphocyte–dependent activity), synergistic multilineage colony growth activity with IL-4 (an activity shared with G-CSF and IL-6),[93] and induction of megakaryocyte colony formation in collaboration with IL-3.[92]

Synergistic Factors

Individual factors that do not, on their own, induce hematopoietic colony growth can serve to augment the clonal growth of progenitors induced by other growth factors. These "synergistic" factors include IL-1, IL-6, IL-4, and Steel factor.

Interleukin-6

The IL-6 gene is expressed by heterogeneous cell types and is induced by a variety of factors (see Table 3–2), including IL-1, TNF-α,[94] TNF-β,[95] mitogens,[96] and endotoxin. The α chain of the IL-6 receptor, encoded by a gene located on chromosome 1,[97] consists of 468 amino acids, 90 of which are in an immunoglobulin superfamily domain, but as is commonly the case with members of the growth factor receptor superfamily, high-affinity ligand binding and signal transduction require expression of an additional β subunit, gp130, a molecule that also serves as the β subunit of the LIF receptor (see Fig. 3–4). The biological activity of IL-6 is exceedingly broad (see Table 3–3).

Recombinant human IL-6 has no clearly demonstrable direct effect on the proliferation of any human hematopoietic cell, yet it functions synergistically with many direct-acting hematopoietic growth factors (reviewed in references 91 and 98). For example, when combined with IL-3, IL-6 induces proliferation of primitive hematopoietic progenitor cells,[99, 100] including CFU-S.[101]

Steel Factor and Its Receptor

Steel factor (reviewed in reference 102), also known as stem cell factor, c-*kit* ligand, and mast cell growth factor, is a heavily glycosylated protein that exists in at least two integral membrane forms and two soluble forms. The soluble forms result from proteolytic cleavage of the integral membrane forms. As shown in Figure 3–8, major cleavage sites are removed by differential splicing from Steel factor mRNA of exon 6–encoded ribonucleotides, so that unstimulated cells release largely the protein translated from the unspliced mRNA. Another cleavage site involving a domain encoded by sequences downstream of exon 6 has been described,[103] but this is evident only after stimulation of cells with phorbol ester or calcium ionophore. Consequently, cells stimulated with these factors release equivalent amounts of the full-length and truncated forms of the protein.[104] Steel factor exhibits multiple biological activities in development, oogenesis, and hematopoiesis (see Table 3–3).

The cytoplasmic domain of the Steel factor receptor, an integral membrane protein encoded by the c-*kit* proto-oncogene, functions as a tyrosine kinase. Although the complete hematopoietic activities of Steel factor are not yet fully defined, it is clear that it cannot, on its own, induce clonal growth of committed progenitor cells. It does, however, substantially enhance the number and size of colonies that develop in vitro when added to cultures containing IL-3, IL-7, or EPO.

The identification of Steel factor, simultaneously by a number of investigative teams, clarified two genetic disorders of murine hematopoiesis that have been studied for almost 40 years, disorders resulting from mutations at the Steel (Sl) and white spotting (W) loci. Mice with such defects have developmental abnormal-

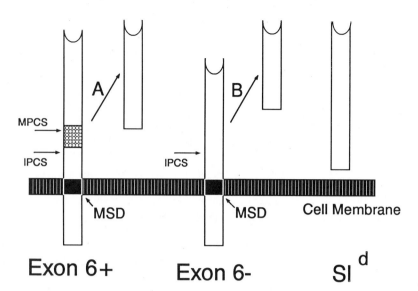

FIGURE 3–8. The three molecular mechanisms by which Steel factor, an integral membrane protein with hematopoietic activity, gives rise to soluble forms. In the first case (A), proteolysis of Steel factor occurs at a major proteolytic cleavage site (MPCS). In this case, proteolysis is constitutive and does not require an induction step. In the second case (B), the removal of exon 6 coding material deletes the MPCS, leaving only a minor cleavage site that is sensitive to cleavage only after stimulation of the cell. Therefore, this site is designated as an inducible PCS (IPCS). In the first two cases, there remains the capacity to retain at least some membrane-bound molecules. This is not the case with the Steel-Dickie mutation, a deletion of the entire membrane-spanning domain (MSD). This truncated molecule is soluble but not membrane bound, and although the soluble molecule is biologically active, the absence of the membrane-bound form results in bone marrow failure in Sl^d mice.

ities of hematopoiesis, hypopigmentation, and gonadal dysgenesis. Homozygous mutations of either gene are often lethal, but compound heterozygotes can reach maturity, notwithstanding the presence of marrow failure. A variety of studies in these mice demonstrated that although stem cell development in both mutant types was impaired, the marrow failure in W mice derived from a functional mutation of hematopoietic stem cells and progenitors, whereas the mutation in Sl mice caused dysfunction of hematopoietic stromal cells (reviewed in reference 105). The identification of both c-*kit* and Steel factor confirmed predictions made more than 21 years ago (based on historical in vitro and transplantation experiments using these models) that the Steel and W loci would prove to be genes encoding complementary receptor molecules.[105]

The membrane form of Steel factor may be of more importance to the maintenance of hematopoiesis in the steady state than is the soluble form. The most suggestive evidence of this is from studies on one Steel factor mutation (Sl^d) that has deleted membrane-spanning and cytoplasmic domains.[106] Although the secreted protein in Sl^d mice has full biological activity, the absence of the integral membrane form of this molecule results in bone marrow failure (Fig. 3–8).

Leukemia Inhibitory Factor (LIF)

Human LIF DNA has been identified as a 7.6 kb clone with three exons, two introns, and a 3.2 kb 3′ untranslated region.[107] The gene product, produced by activated monocytes[108] and human bone marrow stromal cells,[109] is a glycoprotein with 78 per cent amino acid sequence identity with murine LIF. The biological activities of murine and human LIF are similar and are reviewed in Table 3–3.

Interleukin-4

The IL-4 gene, like that of IL-3, resides on the long arm of chromosome 5 and encodes an 18 kDa protein (see Table 3–2). IL-4 is listed as a synergistic factor because lymphoid cells are generally more responsive to IL-4 after they have been primed with other factors. Although it has the capacity to stimulate the growth of mast cells, T cells, and fibroblasts and to induce M-CSF and G-CSF gene expression in human monocytes (see Table 3–3),[110] it also induces expression of TNF-α as well as acts as an inhibitor of hematopoiesis in mixed murine marrow stromal cells.[111] The possibility that IL-4 functions as an inhibitor of hematopoiesis is discussed below.

Indirectly Acting Factors

Some proteins that stimulate hematopoiesis in vivo and in vitro do so indirectly (see Table 3–1) (reviewed in reference 91). That is, they incite bystander (auxiliary) cells to synthesize direct-acting factors.

Interleukin-1

IL-1 exists in two molecular forms (IL-1α and IL-1β), which are encoded by two genes on human chromosome 2. Each of these genes encodes 31 kDa precursor molecules, which are cleaved to 17 kDa peptides (see Table 3–2).[112] IL-1 can be produced by virtually all cells exposed to endotoxin, IL-1, GM-CSF, TNF-α, and IL-2. There are two distinct IL-1 receptors, both of which bind both forms of IL-1. The type I receptor is expressed by T lymphocytes, fibroblasts, and endothelial cells, whereas the type II receptor is expressed by B lymphocytes and myeloid cells[113–115] (see Table 3–2). The bioactivity of IL-1 is tremendously broad, and there is good evidence that it regulates most processes involved in inflammation (see Table 3–3).

The broad bioactivity of IL-1 derives from its ability to induce the expression of other interleukin and CSF genes, which themselves function as subordinate effector molecules in the inflammatory process.[116] The

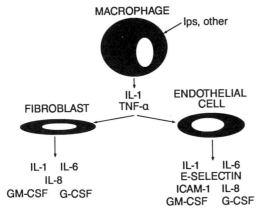

FIGURE 3–9. The hierarchical relationship between the inflammatory cytokines and the initial inductive event is demonstrated, in which a macrophage, exposed to endotoxin (lipopolysaccharide [LPS]) or other inflammatory stimuli, immediately expresses IL-1 and tumor necrosis factor-α (TNF-α) gene products. These proteins are capable of rapidly provoking the production of multilineage hematopoietic growth factors, adhesion molecules, and inflammatory cytokines by stromal cells in any organ. Shown here are some of the molecules known to be induced in fibroblasts and endothelial cells by IL-1 and TNF-α, which, because of these capacities, play an essential role in regulating multiple arms of the inflammatory response. The leukocyte/endothelial cellular adhesion molecule (LEC-CAM2) was also known as ELAM-1 and is now termed, by general agreement, E-selectin.

hierarchical control of IL-1 over a variety of other cytokines is shown graphically in Figure 3–9.

Tumor Necrosis Factor–α

The TNF-α gene, located on chromosome 6 near the major histocompatibility complex (MHC),[117] shares with IL-1 a large number of heterogeneous biological activities (see Table 3–3) and, like IL-1, functions largely to induce the expression of other subordinate genes, which, in turn, function as more specific regulators of hematopoietic and immunological responses to inflammation (see Fig. 3–9). Although TNF-α can directly inhibit progenitor cell growth,[118, 119] the ability of TNF-α to induce expression of other growth factor genes may override its inhibitory activity, at least in lymphopoiesis and granulopoiesis (see Table 3–3).

Common Themes in Growth Factor Biology

Multifunctionality

Virtually all cytokines with hematopoietic activity are multifunctional. Certain of them have a dominant function in cells of a certain lineage, but none have only one single target cell or cell type. G-CSF, for example, has a high degree of specificity for the neutrophil lineage, but there is evidence that it can also influence the replication of primitive precursor cells in vitro.

Effects on Progenitors Correlate with Effects on Progeny

Growth factors for progenitors of a hematopoietic lineage often activate function of the daughter cells of the same lineage. For example, GM-CSF stimulates clonal growth of CFU-GM and also activates most terminally differentiated phagocytes evolving from CFU-GM, including neutrophils, macrophages, and eosinophils (reviewed in reference 91). G-CSF (neutrophil activation), M-CSF (macrophage activation), and IL-5 (eosinophil activation) all function in the same way (reviewed in reference 91). The frequency of this particular theme has a number of implications. For example, expression of all growth factor receptors is not necessarily suppressed as progenitor cells mature, and binding of the ligand transduces an entirely different final response in progenitor cells compared with their more differentiated progeny. Therefore, critical elements of stimulus-response coupling mechanisms are substantially different in undifferentiated and differentiated cells.

Cytokines with Hematopoietic Activity Act Directly, Indirectly, or Both

As described above, hematopoietic factors may bind to receptors on progenitor cells and their daughters to dispatch a biological signal directly. Other factors are also capable of binding to their receptor to induce the target cell to secrete a different cytokine. GM-CSF, for example, induces neutrophils to secrete other cytokines,[24] one of which, IL-1,[120] is capable of inducing expression of a wide variety of additional cytokines. This degree of complexity must be remembered by any scientist attempting to clarify biological activities in vivo. More important, because the induced elaboration of a particular cytokine may be undesirable (e.g., the in vitro and in vivo growth of certain malignancies can be stimulated by some inducible cytokines[121, 122]), this point must be recognized in particular by physicians designing clinical trials in which such factors are to be used.

Synergistic Activities of Hematopoietic Growth and Differentiation Factors

When the biological activity of two factors exceeds the sum of the activities of each factor alone, the factors are said to be synergistic. Some stimuli induce transcription (e.g., endotoxin induces IL-1 gene transcription[123]), some stabilize ordinarily unstable mRNA molecules (e.g., IL-1 prolongs the half-life of GM-CSF and IL-6 mRNA[124, 125]), and others enhance mRNA translation (e.g., endotoxin enhances translation of TNF-α mRNA[126]). Combining two inductive factors that operate by unique inductive mechanisms would give rise to a synergistic response. There are more than 25 examples of cytokine synergy in hematopoiesis (reviewed in reference 91).

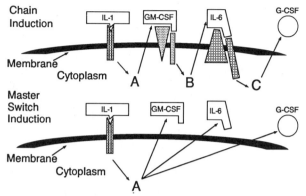

FIGURE 3–10. IL-1 induces the expression of a variety of cytokines, including GM-CSF, IL-6, and G-CSF. The mechanisms by which G-CSF is induced by IL-1 might be complex and depend on the induction of intermediate factors that are secreted by the IL-1–induced cell and subsequently bind to their cognate receptors. The chain induction model, demonstrated in the figure, is one in which IL-1 binds to its receptor, transduces a set of inductive signals (A) that result in the secretion of GM-CSF, which then binds to its receptor and transduces signals (B) that result in the secretion of IL-6, which binds to its receptor and activates the ultimate signal transduction mechanism (C), the step that directly induces G-CSF. The master switch induction model holds that IL-1 simultaneously induces GM-CSF, IL-6, and G-CSF independently of one another. Studies by Segal and colleagues[127, 128] using antisense oligonucleotides to GM-CSF and G-CSF, have ruled out the chain induction model by specifically repressing the early steps of the chain induction model. Specifically, 100 per cent inhibition of GM-CSF production has no impact on the production of G-CSF.

Network Hierarchies

Even when in vitro assays are used, the targets of a given test factor might be either the cell whose function is being observed (the colony-forming cell) or a different cell that can be induced by the test factor to make proteins that directly induce colony growth. Such cells are known as "auxiliary" or "accessory" cells and are almost universally present in most clonal assays. In addition, over time in any in vivo or in vitro assay system, daughters of the progenitors (in vitro daughter cells within the colonies) can become auxiliary cells. A monocyte or promonocyte that appeared in an early macrophage colony, for example, would be capable of being induced to produce G-CSF, M-CSF, IL-1, TNF-α, or IL-6. Therefore, biological effects either in vitro or in vivo are sometimes difficult to decipher, even when the test substance is a recombinant protein.

Fortunately, one element of the network that seems to provide a helpful conceptual framework is that certain cytokine relationships are hierarchical.[116] The central roles of IL-1 and TNF-α in governing hematopoietic responses to inflammatory stimuli serve as particularly obvious examples of this.[91] Both IL-1 and TNF-α genes are expressed early in the inflammatory response. These two gene products induce the expression of a wide variety of subordinate interleukin and growth factor genes and thereby serve to orchestrate the inflammatory response (see Fig. 3–9). The capacity of IL-1 or TNF to induce multiple cytokine genes

does not derive from their capacity to induce expression of only one additional hierarchical factor. For example, IL-1 does not provide the first link in a single chain of dependent molecular events; rather, it simultaneously induces multiple cytokine genes. The clearest evidence of this derives from the use of specific antisense oligonucleotides to break chains of potentially linked inductive molecular events (Fig. 3–10).[127] Antisense strategies are also useful tools for studies on linked versus hierarchical events in the steady state.[128]

Signal Amplification Mechanisms

Certain gene products that appear early in the inflammatory response can induce their own expression. IL-1, for example, enhances IL-1 gene expression (reviewed in reference 91). In addition, IL-1 gene expression is induced by proteins that IL-1 itself induces.[24, 116, 120] Thus, such signal amplification mechanisms can be autocrine, paracrine, or both (Fig. 3–11). Molecular mechanisms by which signal amplification occurs involve both transcriptional and post-transcriptional control points.

Shared Structural Features

CHROMOSOME 5. Many of the growth factors with primary hematopoietic activity are located on the long

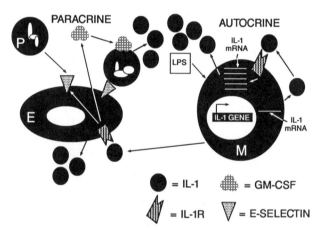

FIGURE 3–11. Amplification of induced signals is common in the cytokine network. In this example, endotoxin (LPS) induces transcription of the IL-1 gene in a macrophage (M), which produces a small quantity of IL-1 mRNA. Because the mononuclear phagocyte also has IL-1 receptors, the IL-1 it releases can bind to this receptor and transduce signals that stabilize IL-1 mRNA, thereby amplifying protein synthesis. Because this mechanism involves only a single cell, it is an example of "autocrine amplification." In vivo, however, the macrophage does not exist in a vacuum. Macrophages regularly influence neighboring cells, in the case illustrated, by inducing other cells to express the IL-1 gene as well ("paracrine amplification"). Here is shown the IL-1 receptor on the surface of endothelial cells (E) binding to IL-1 released by macrophages. IL-1 induces endothelial cells to synthesize IL-1, GM-CSF, and E-selectin, an endothelial-leukocyte adhesion molecule. An additional amplification step occurs when polymorphonuclear leukocytes (P) adhere to endothelial cells (via the adhesion molecule induced by IL-1) and come under the influence of GM-CSF (also induced by IL-1), which stimulates P to express IL-1. Therefore, all cells near the macrophage participate in amplifying IL-1 gene expression.

arm of chromosome 5. Studies using pulsed transverse field electrophoresis[66] have suggested that IL-4, IL-5, IL-3, and GM-CSF are located within 500 kb of each other. IL-3 is only 9 kb upstream of GM-CSF.[129] Other genes involved in hematopoietic growth and differentiation are also located on chromosome 5 (see Table 3–2), including c-*fms* (a cellular proto-oncogene that encodes the M-CSF receptor), the human tyrosine kinase gene *fer*,[130] IL-9,[131] endothelial cell growth factor,[132] the B chain of PDGF receptor,[133] and the monocyte differentiation antigen, CD14.[134] The proximity of these genes is of evolutionary interest and is compatible with the notion that at least some of these functionally related proteins may have evolved from a single ancestral gene. In addition, these related genes may have clinical relevance as well, particularly in patients with the primary clonal hematopoietic disorder known as the "5q minus syndrome," in which some of these genes are deleted from one of the chromosomes 5 in hematopoietic cells.[65, 135] Although it is not yet clear that the loss of one allele is directly related to the abnormalities of growth and differentiation seen in marrow cells of patients with this disorder, a search for inactivating mutations of the remaining alleles (resulting in a reduction to homozygosity) is clearly indicated.

FEATURES THAT INFLUENCE REGULATION OF HEMATOPOIETIC GROWTH FACTOR GENE EXPRESSION. Hematopoietic growth factors and interleukin genes are expressed in many cell types, including T lymphocytes, B lymphocytes, fibroblasts, endothelial cells, and mononuclear phagocytes. Regulation of gene expression in these various cells is accomplished at both transcriptional and post-transcriptional control points.

Transcriptional Control. The complexities of transcriptional control have not been fully elaborated for the hematopoietic growth factor genes. Many factors contain consensus sequences for a variety of transcription factors. Some binding sites are unique to certain families of genes and are shared between cytokines. The IL-6 gene is a good case in point. As shown in Figure 3–12A, sequences necessary for IL-1 to induce IL-6 gene expression are found in the 5' non-coding region. One such sequence, a 14 bp element with dyad symmetry (see Fig. 3–12A), serves as a binding site for the transcription factor nuclear factor (NF)–IL-6.[136]

NF-IL-6 is a cytoplasmic protein that becomes phosphorylated after stimulation of the cell and, within 30 minutes, translocates to the nucleus, where it binds to its recognition site and activates gene transcription. Its capacity to form a heterodimer with NF-IL-6β augments its transcription-inducing activity.[137] NF-IL-6

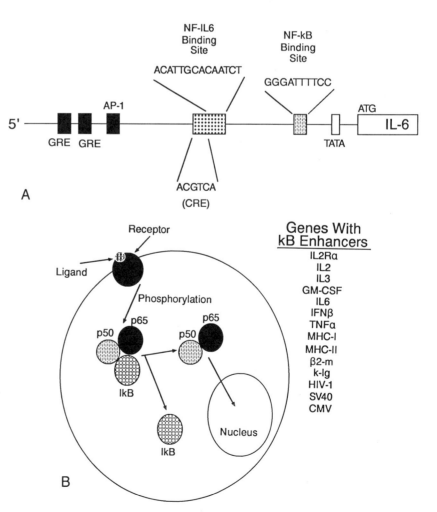

FIGURE 3–12. Transcriptional control of hematopoietic growth factor gene expression. *A*, In addition to the TATA sequence, there are five transcription factor–binding motifs upstream of the IL-6 coding region. Shown are the target binding sites for NF-κB and NF-IL-6, a motif that overlaps with the core cAMP response element (CRE), in which the 3' A of the CRE is the 5' A of the NF-IL-6 site. Two glucocorticoid response elements (GRE) and one AP-1 site are shown as black boxes. *B*, The NF-κB–binding site is an active enhancer element in a variety of genes that participate in the immune response. NF-κB (made up of p50 and p65 subunits) exists as a catalytically inactive cytoplasmic heterotrimeric complex with I-κB. Phosphorylation events evolving from ligand-receptor binding result in the dissociation of I-κB from the p50/p65 complex, which promptly translocates to the nucleus and then binds to its target site (see *A*). Notice that certain viral enhancer elements, including both 5' and 3' regulatory elements of human immunodeficiency virus–1 (HIV-1), also respond to NF-κB.

mRNA is ordinarily undetectable but accumulates in cells stimulated with endotoxin, IL-1, or IL-6. The NF-IL-6 protein also binds to similar consensus sequences found in the 5' non-coding region of the IL-8, G-CSF, and TNF-α genes.[136] This dyad symmetry motif therefore serves as a landmark for a variety of genes activated during the inflammatory response, and the transcription factor NF-IL-6 functions as an important coordinator of that response.

Another transcriptional control mechanism for cytokine gene expression involves NF-κB, originally defined as a factor that binds to enhancer elements found in the immunoglobulin κ chain transcription unit. It exists largely in the cytoplasm of unstimulated cells as a trimeric complex, the first two elements of which, p65 and p50, represent the transcription complex, and the third of which, the inhibitor of κB (I-κB), functions to retain p65/p50 in the cytoplasm (Fig. 3–12B). Upon stimulation of the cell, a variety of phosphorylation events occur; one of the substrates includes I-κB, which, when phosphorylated, dissociates from the p65/p50 complex, allowing it to translocate to the nucleus, bind to its recognition site, and stimulate gene transcription (Fig. 3–12B). A large number of genes involved in regulating the immune response and hematopoiesis are influenced by NF-κB (Fig. 3–12B). An additional feature of interest is the capacity of NF-κB to govern the expression of human immunodeficiency virus (HIV)–1, cytomegalovirus, and SV40 viral gene transcription. In fact, the demonstrated capacity of IL-1 and TNF-α to induce HIV-1 proviral transcription depends on the activation of NF-κB.[138]

Although the molecular details have not yet been clarified, transcriptional control is also a point of inhibition for cytokine gene expression. IL-10, for example, inhibits endotoxin-induced transcription of IL-1, IL-6, TNF-α, IL-8, GM-CSF, and G-CSF in mononuclear phagocytes.[139]

As a cautionary note, the reader should be advised that some studies reporting transcriptional control elements in cytokine genes have relied on the identification of consensus sequences, promoter reporter analysis, and/or gel-shift analyses, all of which, even when combined, are inadequate to formally demonstrate transcriptional control and by themselves can lead to confusion. Before such studies are done, it is important to demonstrate formally—using nuclear runoff analysis, for example—that a given inductive or inhibitory response is truly transcriptionally controlled. The 5' non-coding regions of the G-CSF and GM-CSF genes contain the CK-1 sequence, 5'-GA-GNTTCCAC–3', a motif that may play a role in transcriptional control of IL-3, G-CSF, GM-CSF, and IL-2 gene expression in T lymphocytes stimulated by activation of CD28.[140] In fibroblasts, however, promoter reporter analysis of G-CSF and GM-CSF gene expression induced by TNF-α indicates that CK-1 contributes only to G-CSF gene expression and not GM-CSF gene expression,[141] leading to speculation that a "silencer" element exists upstream of the GM-CSF CK-1 site. In fact, it is just as likely that a "silencer"

element also exists upstream of the site in the G-CSF gene and that in creating the G-CSF promoter-reporter construct, the silencer was excised, thus creating an inducible element that is not functional in nature. Using promoter-reporter assays in diploid fibroblasts, our group has encountered transcriptional control elements in the GM-CSF promoter that "respond" to IL-1 when lifted away from upstream suppressor sequences, but we view these elements as largely irrelevant because IL-1 does not substantially induce GM-CSF gene transcription in nuclear runoff analysis. Excision of undefined suppressons may also explain some of the unexpected results seen with certain transgenic models as well. One candidate example is a report from Liu and colleagues[142] that brain tissue of mice transgenic for the human EPO receptor expressed the human transgene but not the murine gene.

Messenger RNA (mRNA) Catabolism. The expression of many cytokine genes is controlled largely by dynamic alterations in transcript half-life. Several genes encoding interleukins and hematopoietic growth factors have, in their 3' untranslated regions, motifs containing reiterated ATTTA pentamers[143, 144] (Table 3–4). Shaw and Kamen have demonstrated that mRNA molecules containing these AU-rich regions (AURE) can destabilize certain otherwise stable, heterologous mRNAs to which they are attached[143] (Fig. 3–13). Thus transcribed, the 3' AURE somehow targets mRNA for rapid degradation by ribonucleases.

Borrowing on the transferrin receptor model, in which an iron-depleted molecule (IRE-binding protein; see Chapter 10) binds to transferrin receptor mRNA to protect it from ribonucleolytic degradation, several investigators have expected to discover inducible (e.g., by IL-1, a cytokine that stabilizes mRNAs that contain AURE) AURE-binding proteins. Al-

TABLE 3–4. AU-RICH ELEMENTS IN THE 3' UNTRANSLATED REGION OF mRNAs*

mRNA	3' AUUUAs	IL-1 Inducible?
GM-CSF	8	+
G-CSF	6	+
IL-6	6	+
IL-1β	6	+
IL-1α	5	+
IL-8	11	+
E-selectin	9	+
TNF-α	8	+
c-*fos*	5	+
gro/MGSA	4	+
TGF-β	0	–
M-CSF	0	–
γ-Actin	1	–
β-Globin	1	–

*These are found in a number of cytokine and adhesion molecule transcripts. The frequency of AUUUA pentamers and IL-1 inducibility is listed.

The European Molecular Biology Library was searched for the pentameric and octameric sequences. Published sequences were directly examined in the cases of IL-8[293] and E-selectin (also known as LEC-CAM2 and ELAM-1[294]). The numbers of AUUUA pentamers found 3' of the last codon and 5' of the polyadenylation signal are listed above for selected mRNAs known to accumulate in response to IL-1 stimulation. γ-Actin, TGF-β, and M-CSF (CSF-1), known not to be induced by IL-1, are included as well.

FIGURE 3–13. The AU-rich 3′ untranslated region and mRNA catabolism. A number of the cytokine gene and nuclear proto-oncogene transcripts contain homologous AU-rich domains in the 3′ untranslated region. These AU-rich domains commonly contain reiterated sequences of the pentamer AUUUA (see Table 3–4). As shown, the AU-rich element (AURE) in the 3′ untranslated region of GM-CSF mRNA is an element that confers a high degree of instability not only on GM-CSF mRNA but also on heterologous mRNAs, to which this element is experimentally attached. Studies by Shaw and Kamen[143] demonstrate that the attachment of the 3′ untranslated region to β globin cDNA in place of the wild-type globin 3′ untranslated region gives rise to a globin mRNA (GLO-GM) that has a very short half-life. When the inserted element is depleted of AUUUA pentamers by multiple point mutations, it no longer confers a high degree of instability on β-globin mRNA (GLO-GC). GLO/GLO represents wild-type β-globin mRNA.

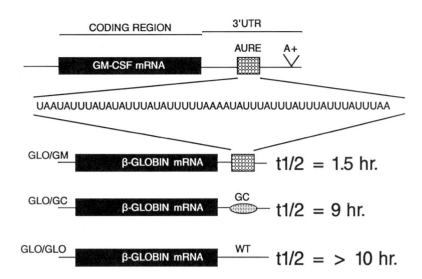

though AURE-binding proteins have been identified,[145–148] their AURE binding is found under conditions of rapid degradation. To date, none stabilize cytokine mRNA. Moreover, it is known that other motifs serve as stabilization response elements. In c-*fos*[149] and c-*myc*[150] transcripts, both of which have 3′ AURE, certain portions of coding regions can function as stability determinants.

Accumulation of GM-CSF, G-CSF, IL-1β, and IL-6 mRNA in endothelial cells and fibroblasts in response to IL-1 results not from transcriptional activation but from stabilization of mRNA.[124, 125, 151] This phenomenon explains some of the biological effects of IL-1, including its breadth of activity, its autocrine amplification loop (an initial stimulus [e.g., endotoxin] stimulates IL-1 gene transcription; IL-1 protein is synthesized; and the IL-1 receptor transduces a signal that stabilizes IL-1 mRNA, thus amplifying IL-1 production[143]), and its ability to synergize with other factors (by inducing production of synergistic growth factors translated from mRNAs bearing the AUUUA motif). Finally, because this mechanism of regulating mRNA content does not necessarily require gene transcription, it is conceivable that this is a regulatory process that has been highly conserved throughout evolution, a mechanism that might even have functioned in an ancient "RNA world."[152]

Production of Isoforms by Alternative Splicing. Cloning of complementary DNAs (cDNAs) of receptors for hematopoietic growth factors has permitted the identification of both soluble and membrane-anchored forms, most of which are generated by alternative splicing. Alternative splicing can result in a soluble form of a receptor in at least two ways (Fig. 3–14). First, differentially spliced forms may include an exon that encodes a proteolytic cleavage site in the extracellular domain, thereby permitting the release of a soluble form by proteolysis. Second, spliced forms may exist that delete an exon that encodes the transmembrane domain, resulting in the release of an obligatory soluble form. Soluble receptor forms have been described for Steel factor (see Fig. 3–8),[103] as well as the receptors for EPO,[52] G-CSF,[36] activin,[153] IL-5, IL-7, IL-6, and IL-4.[32] Complex variations on the theme presented in Figure 3–14 include those found in the case of Steel factor, in which removal of a major

FIGURE 3–14. Production of soluble growth factor receptor molecules. Differential splicing of functionally relevant domains from mRNA molecules can result in the release of receptor molecules from the cell. Shown here are full-length and differentially spliced forms of a theoretical receptor molecule. The full-length mRNA encodes a proteolytic cleavage site (PCS) and a transmembrane domain (TM). As shown in Figure 3–8, soluble receptor molecules can result from regulated extracellular proteolytic cleavage phenomena. Other soluble forms can evolve from mRNAs from which TM domain coding regions have been excised by splicing. Molecules from which PCS coding sequences have been excised by splicing would exist only as obligatory membrane forms.

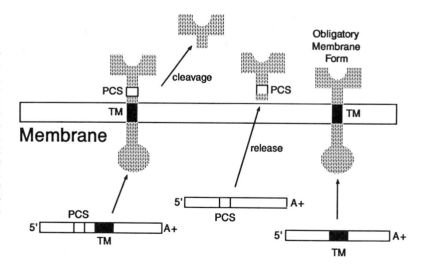

proteolytic cleavage site by differential splicing reduces the susceptibility of membrane-bound Steel factor to constitutive proteolytic degradation (Fig. 3–8) and interdiction of the membrane-associated form by a 3' deletion mutation encompassing the membrane-spanning domain omits the integral membrane form and results in bone marrow failure.

STEM CELL DEVELOPMENT AND DIFFERENTIATION

Development of the Hematopoietic System

The most primitive pluripotent hematopoietic cells are those that represent the first in embryogenesis to commit themselves to the development of the hematopoietic system. These cells arise in mesoderm because virtually all hematopoietic activity is found first in the blood islands of the yolk sac. Specifically at 21 to 28 days of gestation, primitive erythroid cells and undifferentiated blast cells can be found in contact with the endoderm of the yolk sac (reviewed in reference 154). From here the hematopoietic cells migrate to the liver, giving rise to hematopoietic islands by 42 to 44 days of gestation. By the second month, hepatic hematopoiesis dominates, and before the third month, yolk sac hematopoiesis is completely suppressed. By the fifth month of gestation, 80 per cent of hematopoietic activity takes place in the liver and 20 per cent in the spleen. At the same time, the bone marrow begins to exhibit hematopoietic activity and, by the eighth month, becomes the dominant hematopoietic organ (Fig. 3–15).

Multipotent and committed hematopoietic progenitor cells are found in yolk sac and in the liver early in embryogenesis, just as they are in adult marrow,[155] but there seem to be important differences between adult and embryonic progenitor cells. For example, with adult marrow cells, maximal erythroid burst growth (in vitro clones deriving from committed erythroid progenitor cells known as burst-forming units–erythrocytes [BFU-E]) occurs only in the presence of both EPO and a second factor (GM-CSF, IL-3, or Steel factor[156–159]), whereas maximal colony growth of embryonic or fetal liver erythroid progenitors is induced by EPO alone.[18, 160] Other investigators have demonstrated that embryonic BFU-E, unlike those from adult marrow, are resistant to the inhibitory effect of interferon-γ (IFN-γ).[118] Finally, the capacity of Steel factor and EPO to synergistically enhance CFU-GEMM growth in vitro is minimal in adult marrow cell cultures but maximal in cultures of hematopoietic cells derived from fetal liver.[18]

Patterns of gene expression in adult versus embryonic hematopoietic cell differentiation are also clearly different. A variety of genes (e.g., those encoding acetylcholinesterases[161] and enzymes of intermediary metabolism[162]) are expressed differentially during development, but the most extensively studied are the globin genes in developing erythroid cells. The stepwise expression of unique embryonic hemoglobin molecules involves differential transcription of both α and β chain loci (reviewed in Chapter 4).

Microenvironmental influences can be assessed using transgenic models designed to study fetal/adult globin gene switching. Using these models to test the influence of growth factors and integral membrane proteins expressed by auxiliary cells will lead to the identification of a potential role of the niche in the maintenance of a given genetic program. Indeed, studies by Ohneda and colleagues[163] demonstrate that stromal cells can play a permissive role in the expansion of erythroid cells in fetal liver. With such approaches, it is likely that the capacity of any developmental niche (i.e., liver versus bone marrow versus spleen versus thymus) to influence patterns of gene expression in hematopoietic cells can be formally tested and may prove to be distinctly organ specific.

Clonal Succession

Retroviral-mediated gene transfer has significantly aided research on mammalian hematopoietic stem cells. Because proviral DNA integrates randomly, progeny of a single stem cell can be identified in one or more hematopoietic lineages. When stem cells marked with retroviruses are injected into lethally irradiated recipients, the bulk of the hematopoietic

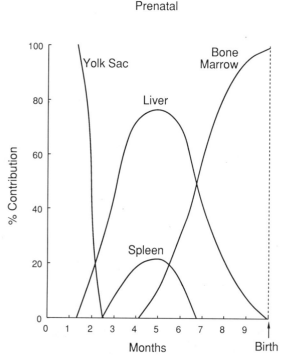

FIGURE 3–15. Dynamic alterations of organ-specific hematopoietic foci during development. Early hematopoiesis occurs in the yolk sac, but by 2.5 months of gestation the most active sites are the liver and spleen. The bone marrow, in which foci of hematopoiesis can be found as early as the fourth month, dominates by the seventh month and beyond, although some foci of hematopoiesis in the liver are regularly present at birth.

system in the recipient is often constituted of only one or two clones.[10, 164] These observations suggest that of the stem cells lodged in a hematopoietic niche, only a few would be "activated" to repopulate the marrow at any given time.[165] This phenomenon, wherein only one or two clones among many are active at any given time and might be followed, later in the life of the animal, by an outgrowth from another newly activated stem cell, is known as clonal succession. In support of this model, observations on long-term hematopoiesis deriving from retrovirally marked transplanted cells have indicated that after 4 to 6 months new clones emerge and contribute virtually 100 per cent to steady-state hematopoiesis,[165] a view compatible with the idea that the new clones may have spent most of their post-transplant period in a strict self-replicative mode.

Although clonal succession clearly occurs in the setting of bone marrow transplantation, there is some debate about the applicability of this model to normal steady-state hematopoiesis (reviewed in reference 12) by investigators who argue that oligoclonal repopulation is due to the small number of genetically marked stem cells injected into recipient mice.[12] This controversy has not yet been resolved, but the innovative retroviral marker strategy[10] demonstrates the capacity of single stem cells to repopulate hematopoiesis entirely.

Commitment and Stem Cell Differentiation

Self-replication of stem cells results in the production of daughter cells both of which retain pluripotentiality. Two other varieties of replicative events can occur in stem cells (Fig. 3–16). Either both daughter cells become "committed" to one lineage or an "asymmetrical" division can occur,[166] giving rise to one committed progenitor and one multipotential progenitor. This phenomenon, known as quantal mitosis, has been validated by the replating studies of Ogawa's group (reviewed in reference 167).

One general model of differentiation holds that stem cells have receptors for only a limited number of growth factors (Steel factor and IL-3, for example), but no receptors for lineage-specific growth factors, and that commitment might actually be defined best by the new acquisition of lineage-specific receptors

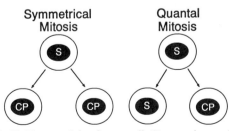

FIGURE 3–16. Two models of stem cell (S) commitment have been described: symmetrical mitosis, in which each daughter cell is a committed progenitor (CP), and quantal mitosis, in which one daughter is committed (CP) but the second daughter cell remains uncommitted (S).

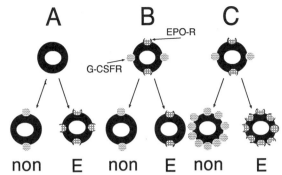

FIGURE 3–17. Models of stem cell commitment, differentiation, and receptor expression. In the model shown, stem cells give rise to an erythroid progenitor (E) and a non-erythroid (non) progenitor cell, the latter of which is committed, in this example, to granulocyte development. A, The receptor expression model holds that lineage-specific receptors (the erythropoietin receptor [EPO-R] and G-CSF receptor [G-CSFR], in this example) are not expressed in pluripotent stem cells and that expression of these receptors (1) in any cell must be mutually exclusive and (2) defines commitment to a particular lineage. B, The receptor exclusion model holds that stem cells have receptors for most growth factors, including those that are generally considered to be lineage specific, and that the exclusion of one type of receptor defines a lineage. C, The hybrid model shown here is closest to biological reality. In this case, stem cells do have low numbers of receptors for a variety of "lineage-specific" growth factor receptors, and commitment involves simultaneous repression of one gene and enhanced expression of the other.

(Fig. 3–17A). Corollaries of this model are that cells committed to granulopoiesis do not express an EPO receptor[50] but will express a G-CSF receptor. Some argue that the biological effects exerted by IL-6 and G-CSF on primitive pluripotent hematopoietic cells (synergistically with IL-3) serve as evidence against this paradigm and that a second model should be considered.

The second model maintains that pluripotent hematopoietic stem cells express, at low levels, receptors for a multitude of multilineage and lineage-specific growth factors and that the commitment process results in the systematic loss of most of these receptors (Fig. 3–17B). Consequently, a stem cell that begins life with a few receptors for virtually all growth factors might terminate its multipotential life by retaining just a few. Theoretically, then, repression of receptors for IL-5, M-CSF, G-CSF, IL-6, and IL-8 and retention of receptors for Steel factor, IL-3, GM-CSF, and EPO would, necessarily, define a BFU-E–, a GM-CSF–, Steel factor–, and IL-3–responsive cell irrevocably committed to the erythroid lineage. Conversely, the repression of receptors for EPO, IL-5, IL-4, and IL-6 would result in a progenitor cell that could respond only to G-CSF, IL-8, and GM-CSF, a de facto definition of a progenitor committed to neutrophil production. This model of repression of multipotential competence has not been formally validated, but it soon can be, using currently available methods of stem cell purification[12, 168] and probes for most of the hematopoietic growth factor receptors.

Neither the first nor the second model withstands the scrutiny engendered by studies using recombinant factors. In the second model, late in the life of a committed erythroid cell, receptors for IL-3, G-CSF, GM-CSF, and Steel factor are repressed (none of these factors have much influence on the proliferation of CFU-E but do profoundly influence the proliferation of BFU-E). In fact, Sawada et al. have formally demonstrated that the BFU-E to CFU-E transition is associated with loss of IL-3 dependence.[169] On the other hand, the receptor exclusion model would predict at least some functional EPO receptors on the surface of BFU-E, yet although there is evidence that more well differentiated daughter cells of BFU-E have EPO receptors, these receptors may be of lower affinity and may not be particularly functional in BFU-E themselves.[160] Accordingly, EPO receptors likely increase in number and/or functionality at the CFU-E stage.[170–172] It is likely, therefore, that commitment of stem cells incorporates elements of both models (Fig. 3–17C) in which multiple receptors are present in low numbers on pluripotent cells and that commitment is characterized both by repression of "wrong lineage" receptors (e.g., EPO receptors in granulocyte progenitor cells) and by amplification of "correct lineage" receptors (e.g., EPO receptors in committed erythroid cells). In fact, studies on lineage-specific expression of the EPO receptor are most compatible with this hybrid model (Fig. 3–17C). In these studies, pluripotent embryonal stem cells and multipotential hematopoietic cells transcribe the EPO receptor gene. Commitment to nonerythroid lineages in these cells is associated with a complete repression of EPO receptor gene expression. However, at the same time, EPO receptor mRNA increases substantially in cells committed to erythropoiesis.[50]

Stochastic and Instructed Models of Differentiation

Until Ogawa and his colleagues actually tested some determinants of commitment in the serial replating analysis,[173] a number of investigators had anticipated that lineage-specific growth factors would play a role in the pattern of commitment of the stem cell pool. It was reasonable to hypothesize that under conditions demanding an increase in red cell mass, pluripotent cells would be "forced" (by exogenous regulatory factors) to give rise to more daughter cells committed to the erythroid lineage. This paradigm of stem cell commitment has been called "instructed." An alternative model, one favored by Ogawa's group, proposes that stem cell commitment may be "stochastic" and that lineage-specific amplifications occur among cells of the committed progenitor cell compartment (arising on demand from an increase in the quantity of lineage-specific growth factors) rather than in the uncommitted population.

The Role of Growth Factors in Differentiation of Hematopoietic Cells

There are at least two potential biochemical explanations for the lineage specificity of hematopoietic growth factors. First, as a kind of variation on the theme presented in Figure 3–17, cells of multiple lineages might express a given receptor, but a lineage-specific repertoire of intracytoplasmic or nuclear events permits only the cells of one lineage to respond. Second, cells of only one lineage may express the gene for a particular growth factor receptor. The importance of this potential mechanism (reviewed in reference 81) is nicely exemplified by the observations of Roussel and her coworkers,[174] in which the receptor for the monocyte/macrophage lineage-specific M-CSF gene is enforced, by transfection of the gene, in fibroblasts (which ordinarily neither express the receptor nor respond to M-CSF). As a result of such "promiscuous" receptor expression, the fibroblasts become capable of proliferating in response to M-CSF. This is clearly not a paradigm for all receptors, however. For instance, fibroblasts infected with a retrovirus carrying a mutant self-activating EPO-receptor does not cause transformation of fibroblasts, but the virus does transform cells of the erythroid lineage.[175] Therefore, in this instance, expression of the receptor is insufficient to transduce a growth signal in heterologous cells because lineage-specific signaling factors are absent in fibroblasts. One reasonable explanation of the differences between the transforming fms gene and the transforming EPO receptor gene might be the general requirement for cofactor interaction for receptor function in the case of EPO,[176] but not for fms, a gene product that has subunits with tyrosine kinase domains.[177]

In normal cells, serial replications of committed progenitor cells proceed hand in hand with reasonably synchronous cellular differentiation. Because these two processes are linked, the capacity of any protein to have an impact on the process of differentiation, per se, is difficult to assess. G-CSF, for example, might directly influence neutrophil differentiation as well as induce growth of progenitors and precursor cells, or it might simply induce growth of committed progenitors, in which the process of differentiation is permitted (because of the permissive effect of G-CSF on survival of only one lineage). The importance of investigating differentiation in normal hematopoietic stem cells cannot be overemphasized. Historically, analyses of hematopoietic cellular differentiation have often relied on the use of transformed or leukemic cell lines or both.[178] Whether leukemic models reveal global truths of hematopoiesis will be unclear until the paradigms established by them are validated in normal cells. Of notable importance is a focus on the capacity of isolated single cells to express specific growth factor receptor molecules.

Nuclear Proto-oncogenes and Differentiation

The c-myc Oncogene

The oncogene c-myc, the cellular homologue of the leukemogenic viral oncogene v-myc, is rearranged in a variety of hematopoietic malignancies. The c-*myc* gene encodes a leucine zipper protein that forms a sequence-specific DNA-binding complex with a helix-loop-helix protein known as *max*.[179] Widely regarded as a gene expressed in proliferating cells, in hematopoiesis it is more likely that the c-*myc* gene product serves to enforce a primitive phenotype. Evidence in support of this view originated in studies on human leukemic cells. Acute myelogenous leukemia is a clonal neoplasm that in its classic form represents a failure of primitive hematopoietic cells to differentiate beyond myeloblasts or progranulocytes. Leukemic myeloblasts express the c-*myc* gene, but neutrophils do not. When leukemic cells are induced to differentiate in vitro, they repress c-*myc* transcription.[180–182] A cause-and-effect relationship between differentiation state and c-*myc* expression is suggested by findings that repression of c-*myc* gene expression is sufficient to induce differentiation in certain leukemic cells.[183] There is also a dose effect of the c-*myc* gene product on the process of erythroid differentiation. Yamamoto and colleagues[184] transfected murine erythroleukemic cells with rat c-*myc* DNA placed under the control of a human metallothionein promoter (Zn^{2+} responsive) and demonstrated an inverse relationship between the concentration of Zn^{2+} in the medium and the proportion of differentiated cells. Consequently, in hematopoietic cells, c-*myc* may function as a generic switch that blocks the development of the differentiated phenotype, and for a cell to undergo terminal differentiation, the c-*myc* gene must be silenced.

The c-myb Oncogene

Expression of the nuclear proto-oncogene c-*myb* in hematopoiesis parallels that of c-*myc*. Messenger RNA transcribed from the c-*myb* gene accumulates in primitive erythroid and myeloid cells as well as in megakaryocytes but is reduced in more differentiated cells.[185, 186] A relationship between c-*myb* expression and differentiation is suggested by experiments showing that overexpression of c-*myb* blocks differentiation of murine erythroleukemia cells[187] and inhibits maturation of mononuclear phagocytes.[188] Other studies have shown that the degree of inhibition of murine erythroleukemic cell differentiation correlates with c-*myb* mRNA content.[189] These findings suggest that c-*myb* repression is an absolute prerequisite for primitive erythroid cells to undergo terminal differentiation.[190]

The c-fos and c-jun Oncogenes

The nuclear proto-oncogene c-*fos* (reviewed in reference 191) encodes a 380 amino acid protein with a molecular weight of 55 kDa. The *fos* protein associates with the c-*jun* gene product to form a sequence-specific heterodimeric DNA-binding protein[192] that binds to the consensus sequence 5′–TGACTCA–3′, originally identified as the consensus binding site for the yeast transcription factor GCN4 and the mammalian factor AP-1.[193] The c-*fos* gene is rapidly inducible by growth-

inductive stimuli[194, 195] in certain cells. In contrast to c-*myb* and c-*myc*, the product of c-*fos* is expressed specifically in later differentiation stages, including neutrophils and monocytes.[186, 196–198] The c-*jun* gene is also highly expressed during hematopoietic cellular differentiation.[199] Since the *jun/fos* heterodimer represses transcription of c-*myc* by binding to a negative regulatory element (positioned at bases $-293/-353$ relative to c-*myc* promoter 1),[200] it is reasonable to speculate that the product of c-*fos* may function with *jun* to induce differentiation programs by repressing genes that maintain such programs.

Homeobox Genes

First described as products of homeotic genes involved in *Drosophila* development, these proteins, now known to exist in multiple mammalian species (reviewed in reference 201), contain homologous domains of approximately 60 amino acids that are involved directly in binding to consensus sequences.[202, 203] The *Hox* family in vertebrates is a group of about 40 genes arranged in four homeobox clusters on four different chromosomes (Table 3–5). Other transcription factors have homeobox homologies. For example, both Oct-1 (a ubiquitous transcription factor that binds the 5′–ATTTGCAT–3′ octameric motif) and Oct-2 (a lymphocyte-specific octamer-binding protein) contain homeobox-like domains.[204–206]

Mammalian homeobox genes are often arranged in clusters reaching from 20 to 100 kb, any one of which might contain from four to eight genes. Because *Hox* clusters are involved in regulating developmental programs, and because of the evidence that human homeobox genes are expressed in embryonic development,[207] some investigators have reasoned that they might also be involved in hematopoietic stem cell differentiation. It has been reported that a human *Hox*-1 homeobox gene is expressed specifically in cells of the myeloid lineage[208] (see Table 3–5) and that certain genes of the human *Hox*-2 cluster, specifically *Hox*-2E, *Hox*-2D, *Hox*-2B, *Hox*-2A, and *Hox*-2G, are expressed in erythroid cell lines, but not in non-

TABLE 3–5. HOMEOBOX GENES EXPRESSED IN HEMATOPOIETIC CELLS

CHROMOSOME	HOX GENE (HUMAN)	HEMATOPOIETIC LINEAGES
7	1J, 1I, 1H	Myeloid
7	1A, 1C	All
7	1F	Erythroid and myeloid
12	3G, 3F, 3H	Erythroid
12	3C, 3D	Erythroid and myeloid
12	3E	Lymphoid
12	3A	All
17	2A, 2B, 2D, 2E, 2G	Erythroid
17	2C, 2F	All
17	2H	Erythroid and myeloid

There is a fourth set of *Hox* genes located on chromosome 2, but to date, none are known to be expressed in hematopoietic cells.

erythroid lines.[209, 210] Other indirect evidence that homeobox genes may be involved in hematopoietic cellular differentiation is found in studies on human hematopoietic cell lines[211] and in reports that selected homeobox genes are deleted in some myeloid leukemias.[212] *Hox*-2 gene expression is induced by IL-2 and IL-1 in NK cells,[213] and HB24 and HB9 are induced by IL-3 and GM-CSF in CD34+ marrow cells.[214] Other experiments have shown that antisense HB24 oligodeoxyribonucleotides inhibit growth-related gene expression (c-*fos*, c-*myc*, c-*myb*, and CDC2) in CD34+ cells and that enforced expression of HB24 inhibits differentiation.[215] The influence of homeobox genes on normal hematopoietic cellular differentiation is currently unknown.

INHIBITION OF HEMATOPOIETIC CELLULAR GROWTH AND DIFFERENTIATION

As is the case with most renewable systems, inhibition of proliferation of hematopoietic cells can be controlled by limiting the production of mitogenic factors or by factors that inhibit cellular growth—a kind of "braking" phenomenon. Some active modulators of hematopoiesis reduce synthesis of mitogenic factors and, at the same time, directly inhibit the proliferation of hematopoietic cells. Members of the transforming growth factor–β (TGF-β) superfamily are excellent examples of such inhibitory factors.

Transforming Growth Factor–β

Five isoforms (60 to 80 per cent amino acid homology) of TGF-β are found in vertebrates, TGF-β1 through TGF-β5 (reviewed in reference 216). Each TGF molecule is a disulfide-linked dimer of two 112 amino acid proteins, each cleaved from a larger 390 amino acid pro-TGF-β molecule. Although each TGF gene is located on a different chromosome (β1 on 19q, β2 on 1q, and β3 on 14q[216]), it is likely that the TGFs arose by duplication of a common ancestral gene. TGF-β is expressed in multiple tissues and organs, and although some exceptions exist, these factors largely function to inhibit cellular growth directly and indirectly. To date, four high-affinity receptors for TGF-β have been identified,[216] one of which is a proteoglycan.

The most well studied of these isoforms—TGF-β1, 2, and 3—exert antiproliferative effects on many cell types, in part[217] by inhibiting phosphorylation of the Rb protein,[218] an event required for progression from the G_1 to the S phase of the cell cycle. TGF-β inhibits lymphoid cell proliferation[219] and inhibits growth of hematopoietic progenitors of all lineages in clonal assays,[220–223] in long-term cultures,[224–226] and in vivo.[227]

Transforming growth factor–β inhibits hematopoiesis in at least two ways. First, the protein directly inhibits proliferation of progenitor cells,[221, 223, 228] mediated, in part, by direct inhibition of Rb protein

phosphorylation[218] and additionally by its capacity to repress the expression of receptors for GM-CSF, G-CSF, and IL-3.[229] Second, TGF-β interrupts the capacity of inductive factors (i.e., IL-1 and TNF-α) to stimulate expression of hematopoietic growth factors by accessory cells, including monocytes,[230] fibroblasts,[231] endothelial cells,[232] and T lymphocytes.[233, 234]

Inhibins and Activins

Inhibins and activins[235] are dimeric proteins of the TGF-β superfamily and share a common subunit.[216] Activins A and B are homodimers of peptide chains $β_A$ and $β_B$, and activin AB is the heterodimer. Inhibins A and B are heterodimers of a separate α chain and one of the two activin chains (reviewed in reference 153). These factors are produced in many tissues and affect an enormous number of biological processes, including the production of follicle-stimulating hormone (FSH), growth hormone, and adrenocorticotropic hormone (ACTH); enhancement of neuron survival in vitro; proliferation of certain cell lines; and promotion of erythroid differentiation in vitro.[236]

To date, five activin A receptors have been found, four of which are isoforms derived from alternative splicing events from a single gene, ActR-IIB.[153] These receptors bind activin A, activin B, and inhibin A with different affinities.[153, 236] The receptors have single membrane-spanning domains, as well as cytoplasmic protein kinase domains predicted to possess serine/threonine specificity.[153, 236]

Although the capacity of activins to regulate erythropoiesis was first reported in 1987,[237] the complexities of the hematopoietic activity of activin A and inhibin A were identified by Broxmeyer and colleagues,[235] who observed that human recombinant activin A enhances clonal growth of CFU-GEMM and BFU-E, but not CFU-GM, and that inhibin A blocks this effect of activin. They also observed that depletion of monocytes and/or T lymphocytes from marrow abrogated the effects of both activin and inhibin in vitro. The mechanisms by which these indirect but progenitor type–specific phenomena occur have not been clarified, nor have in vivo studies yet documented that similar biological effects occur in the intact animal.

Interleukin-4

In addition to the inductive effects of IL-4 on hematopoietic cell growth and differentiation described earlier in this chapter (see page 82), this factor also consistently inhibits expression of granulopoietic inductive factors IL-1 and TNF-α[238] by mononuclear phagocytes, directly inhibits certain proliferative responses induced by mitogenic factors,[239, 240] and inhibits release of mitogenic factors in cells exposed to biologically relevant inductive factors (e.g., IL-1).[241] As is the case with TGF-β, IL-4 inhibits clonal growth of monocytes and macrophages when added to clonal cultures of human marrow cells. However, IL-4 does not inhibit neutrophil colony formation, BFU-E, or CFU-E growth in vitro.[242] Therefore, although the exact role of IL-4 in modulating hematopoiesis has not been developed fully, it is possible that it functions as an in vivo "brake" for production of macrophages and lymphocytes, rather than acting on megakaryocytes and erythroid cells.

Interleukin-10

Interleukin-10, produced by endotoxin-induced monocytes[139] and mitogen-activated CD4+ T lymphocytes,[243] exhibits heterogeneous biological activities. Although IL-10 is a growth factor of B lymphocytes and mast cells,[244, 245] its hematopoietic inhibitory activity is rather broad. IL-10 inhibits cytokine production by mononuclear phagocytes in vitro,[139, 246, 247] inhibits T-cell proliferation and IL-2 production,[248] suppresses IL-5—mediated immunoglobulin secretion induced by T-cell—independent antigens,[249] and synergizes with IL-4 and TGF-β to inhibit the cytotoxicity of activated macrophages.[250] Because it has been identified more recently than many of the other cytokines, its role in the regulation of hematopoiesis in vivo is uncertain.

Prostaglandins

The eicosanoids, lipids that share a common origin from eicosanoic acids (C_{20} polyunsaturated), include prostaglandins, thromboxanes, and leukotrienes. One of the prostaglandins, PGE_2, is known to function both in vitro and in vivo as a suppressor of myelopoiesis, mostly for monocytopoiesis.[251, 252] Administration of PGE_2 to mice recovering from a myelosuppressive dose of cyclophosphamide[251] reduced marrow cellularity and CFU-GM content. In other studies, the administration of indomethacin, a cyclooxygenase inhibitor that reduces prostaglandin biosynthesis, augmented the expansion of CFU-GM in the spleens of mice treated with IL-1.[253] The mechanisms by which PGE_2 mediates its inhibitory effects are not understood, but it has been suggested that PGE_2-mediated inhibition of granulopoiesis requires the participation of a factor produced by CD8+ T lymphocytes.[254]

Interferons

Both IFN-α and IFN-γ indirectly inhibit hematopoiesis in vitro by inducing production of TNF-α (a direct inhibitor of colony growth, especially erythroid) by accessory cells of bone marrow stroma[119, 255] and by inhibiting the expression of IL-1 (an inducer of growth factor gene expression) by mononuclear phagocytes.[256] The capacity of IFN-α to inhibit granulopoiesis and erythropoiesis has been widely validated in vivo owing to the widespread use of IFN-α in clinical practice (reviewed in reference 257). Studies in BALB/c mice have shown that IFN-γ functions as an inhibitor of IL-3 and IL-6 gene expression in vivo.[258]

Lactoferrin

In 1957, Edwin Osgood proposed that normal terminally differentiated cells (e.g., neutrophils) must be able to produce factors that inhibit hematopoiesis to effect feedback regulation.[259] Evidence to support this model was ultimately developed by Broxmeyer and his colleagues, who determined that lactoferrin, an iron-binding glycoprotein found in breast epithelial cells and in the specific granules of neutrophils, was capable of inhibiting hematopoietic progenitor cell proliferation in vitro[252, 260] and in vivo.[261, 262] Initially, it was thought that lactoferrin directly inhibits production of colony-stimulating activities by mononuclear phagocytes,[260] but it now appears that lactoferrin inhibits the expression by monocytes of the indirect inductive factor, IL-1.[263, 264]

Ferritin

Several studies have shown that the heavy chain of ferritin (H-ferritin) inhibits normal progenitor cell growth.[265–268] The inhibitory effect of H-ferritin has been investigated using a large number of mutant molecules. These studies have demonstrated that its capacity to suppress myelopoiesis correlates with its ferroxidase activity (ferroxidase converts Fe^{2+} to Fe^{3+}).[268] Reports that leukemic cells are more resistant to the inhibitory effects of H-ferritin than normal progenitors[269] suggest that this molecule might mediate clonal competition (in favor of the leukemic clone) at some point in the leukemogenic process.

Tumor Necrosis Factor–α

TNF-α, encoded by a gene on chromosome 6[270] near the MHC,[111] inhibits granulocyte colony growth, but this effect is overridden by the capacity of TNF-α to induce production of granulopoietic factors by accessory cells. TNF-α also inhibits erythroid progenitor cell growth[271] and expression of the EPO gene.[272] If these effects are shown to exist in vivo, they could explain the suppression of erythropoiesis in chronic inflammatory diseases.[273]

HEMATOPOIESIS IN CONTEXT: THE FUNCTION OF THE MICROENVIRONMENT

Homing and Adhesion Molecules

For many years, the capacity of stem cells to "home" to the appropriate niche at various times in development has been a wondrous mystery. Following intravenous infusion of bone marrow cells, stem cells traverse the walls of the vascular sinus (endothelium, adventitia, and a basement membrane) to snuggle with stromal cells of the marrow, there to self-replicate and differentiate. No biologically meaningful hematopoietic activity occurs in non-hematopoietic organs in transplant recipients. The capacity of stromal cells to support stem cell growth and differentiation derives from a number of functions owned by the cell. They include the expression of homing receptors, the production of extracellular matrix factors that interact both with growth and differentiation factors and with progenitors themselves, the production of soluble growth and differentiation factors, and the expression of integral membrane proteins that function as juxtacrine factors.

Juxtacrine Molecules

Integral membrane proteins of stem cells bind to membrane proteins expressed specifically by stromal cells in hematopoietic niches. Steel factor and its receptor c-kit, for example, exist as integral membrane proteins of stromal cells and stem cells, respectively. The interaction of these two gene products provides an intercellular binding function as well as a growth-inductive signal. That the microenvironmental defect found in the Steel-Dickie mouse results from a failure to express the membrane-bound form of Steel factor[106] indicates that its membrane location plays a role in its capacity to support stem cell growth and differentiation. This type of cell-cell contact-dependent growth has been termed "juxtacrine," a concept reviewed by Dainiak.[274]

Families of Adhesion Molecules

Stem cells and progenitors may express adhesion molecules that interact with integral membrane proteins of stromal cells. This model of homing is based on studies of the adherence of lymphocytes to high endothelial venules of lymph nodes, a response required to maintain the normal traffic of lymphocytes between lymph vessels and circulating blood. The Hermes antigen (CD44) is a 90 kDa acidic sulfated glycoprotein expressed by lymphoid cells that mediate adhesion to an integral membrane protein (gp58–66) expressed by endothelial cells.[275] Because of its homing target function, the endothelial protein is classified as one of the vascular addressins.[276, 277] Hermes cDNAs were cloned and characterized and interestingly found to share amino acid homology with tandemly repeated domains in the cartilage link protein and proteoglycan monomer, proteins that coordinately bind to hyaluronic acid in cartilage.[278] Other tissue-specific adhesion molecules in lymphocytes have been described (adhesion of B lymphocytes to germinal centers involves at least two specific complexes, VLA-4 and INCAM-110[279]), and with the notable exception of the Hermes molecule, these adhesion molecules are generally members of the immunoglobulin supergene family,

the selectin/LEC-CAM superfamily, or the integrin superfamily (reviewed in reference 280).

The Integrin Family

The integrin family includes surface receptors for adhesion to extracellular matrix molecules and to other membrane proteins. Integrins are membrane glycoproteins usually consisting of α/β heterodimers. The three major subsets of integrins and their subunit structures are presented in Table 3–6. To date, more than 14 different α/β heterodimers made up of 11 α subunits and 6 β subunits have been found. The dimer α^4/β_1 is known as VLA-4 (reviewed in reference 281) and has been the subject of much study because of its emerging role as a regulator of stem cell homing. Williams and colleagues, for example, have demonstrated that day 12 murine CFU-S expresses the VLA-4 integrin receptor and that it serves as a binding site for the C-terminal peptide of fibronectin.[282] It is interesting that this portion of fibronectin also contains a heparin-binding site, a site known to bind to lymphoid cells. Heparin does not, however, block CFU-S adherence, documenting that CFU-S–binding and lymphoid-binding sites are different. Antibodies to VLA-4 inhibit lymphopoiesis and myelopoiesis in murine long-term bone marrow cell cultures.[283] Cell surface receptors for VLA-4 have been identified as well,[283] one of which, VCAM-1, is expressed by cytokine-induced endothelial cells and interacts with a site that differs from the fibronectin-binding site of VLA-4.[284]

Homing is most likely not the only function of VLA-4. Recent evidence suggests that VLA-4 promotes proliferation of T lymphocytes and probably provides similar functions for stem cells and progenitor cells in hematopoietic niches. Because of the evidence that the extracellular matrix may function as a compartment that provides hematopoietic growth factors by its capacity to bind such factors,[285] adhesion molecules, by bringing progenitors into proximity with growth factors, could also serve to enhance their proliferative

TABLE 3–6. THE INTEGRIN FAMILY*

SUBFAMILY	INTEGRIN	SUBUNITS
VLA Proteins	VLA-1	α^1/β_1
	VLA-2	α^2/β_1
	VLA-3	α^3/β_1
	VLA-4	α^4/β_1
	VLA-4	α^4/β_p
	VLA-5	α^5/β_1
	VLA-6	α^6/β_1
	VLA-6	α^6/β_4
LEUCAMS	LFA-1	α^L/β_2
	Mac-1	α^M/β_2
	p150,95	α^X/β_2
Cytoadhesins	gpIIb/IIIa	α^{IIb}/β_3
	VNR	α^V/β_5
	VNR	α^V/β_s

*Integrins are surface receptors for cell-matrix and cell-cell adhesion interactions. The three subfamilies, the names of the specific complexes, and the subunit structure are shown. Notice that VLA-4, VLA-6, and VNR consist of two heterodimeric isoforms each.

potential. The development of stem cell purification techniques[12] will permit a functional analysis of additional adhesion molecules of significance in hematopoiesis.

Provision of Soluble Growth Factors

Marrow stromal cells produce both direct-acting and inductive interleukins and growth factors.[91, 116] Evidence in support of the effects of in situ growth factors has been obtained using time-lapse video microscopy,[286] with which it was observed that granulocyte production occurred beneath stromal "blanket" cells, whereas erythroid development transpired in close contact with macrophage-like cells (these observations are available on a videocassette tape).[286] Extracellular matrix factors produced by these different cells may account for some of their differential supportive effect.

Extracellular Matrix

Proteoglycans, heparan sulfate, fibronectin, and hemonectin are factors present in the hematopoietic stroma that can regulate hematopoiesis in two ways. First, matrix factors such as glycosaminoglycans can bind hematopoietic growth factors and may provide a mechanism by which such factors can be optimally presented to and utilized by progenitors (reviewed in reference 287). Other matrix molecules can bind to inhibitory factors (e.g., fibronectin binds to TGF-β1).[288] Second, some matrix proteins bind directly to hematopoietic progenitor cells. For example, CFU-E bind to fibronectin, and CFU-GM bind to hemonectin.[287]

Is the Stroma Transplantable?

Although there are some experimental models in which hematopoietic stromal cell lines can be transplanted,[289] bone marrow stromal cells from recipients of conventional marrow transplants are largely derived from the marrow of the host.[290] It is important to recognize, however, that because of the well-described intercellular interleukin/CSF network (described above), host stromal cell function can be substantially influenced by the transplantable components of the microenvironment (monocytes, macrophages, and lymphoid cells in the donor marrow and, later, the same cell types evolving from transplanted pluripotential stem cells).[290, 291] Therefore, in both anatomical and functional terms, non-hematopoietic elements of the stroma are inextricably linked with cells derived from hematopoietic stem cells. Recently, in fact, Terstappen's group has identified a single human fetal cell type that is capable of giving rise to both hematopoietic stroma and hematopoietic stem cells, at least in vitro.[295] Whether this cell is found only during development is not yet known.

REFERENCES

1. Till, J. E., and McCulloch, E. A.: A direct measurement of the radiation sensitivity of normal mouse bone marrow cells. Radiat. Res. 14:213, 1961.
2. Becker, A. J., McCulloch, E. A., and Till, J. E.: Cytological demonstration of the clonal nature of spleen colonies derived from transplanted mouse marrow cells. Nature 197:452, 1963.
3. Wu, A. M., Siminovitch, L., Till, J. E., and McCulloch, E. A.: Evidence for a relationship between mouse hemopoietic stem cells and cells forming colonies in culture. Proc. Natl. Acad. Sci. USA 59:1209, 1968.
4. Juraskova, V., and Tkadlecek, L.: Character of primary and secondary colonies of haematopoiesis in the spleen of irradiated mice. Nature 206:951, 1965.
5. Blackett, N. M., Millard, R. E., and Belcher, H. M.: Thymidine suicide in vivo and in vitro of spleen colony forming and agar colony forming cells of mouse bone marrow. Cell Tissue Kinet. 7:309, 1974.
6. Becker, A. J., McCulloch, E. A., Siminovitch, L., and Till, J.: The effect of differing demands for blood cell production on DNA synthesis by hemopoietic colony-forming cells of mice. Blood 26:296, 1965.
7. Rickard, K. A., Shadduck, R. K., Howard, D. E., and Stohlman, F. Jr.: A differential effect of hydroxyurea on hemopoietic stem cell colonies in vitro and in vivo. Proc. Soc. Exp. Biol. Med. 134:152, 1970.
8. Iscove, N. N., Till, J. E., and McCulloch, E. A.: The proliferative states of mouse granulopoietic progenitor cells. Proc. Soc. Exp. Biol. Med. 134:33, 1970.
9. Magli, M. C., Iscove, N. N., and Odartchenko, N.: Transient nature of early haematopoietic spleen colonies. Nature 295:527, 1982.
10. Lemischka, I. R., Raulet, D. H., and Mulligan, R. C.: Developmental potential and dynamic behavior of hematopoietic stem cells. Cell 45:917, 1986.
11. Wu, A. M., Till, J. E., Siminovitch, L., and McCulloch, E. A.: A cytological study of the capacity for differentiation of normal hemopoietic colony-forming cells. J. Cell. Physiol. 69:177, 1967.
12. Spangrude, G. J., Smith, L., Uchida, N., Ikuta, K., Heimfeld, S., Friedman, J., and Weissman, I. L.: Mouse hematopoietic stem cells. Blood 78:1395, 1991.
13. Uchida, N., and Weissman, I. L.: Searching for hematopoietic stem cells: Evidence that Thy-1.1lo Lin-Sca-1+ cells are the only stem cells in C57BL/Ka-Thy-1.1 bone marrow. J. Exp. Med. 175:175, 1992.
14. Terstappen, L. W. M. M., Huang, S., Safford, M., Lansdorp, P. M., and Loken, M. R.: Sequential generations of hematopoietic colonies derived from single nonlineage-committed CD34+CD38− progenitor cells. Blood 77:1218, 1991.
15. Molgaard, H. V., Spurr, N. K., and Greaves, M. F.: The hemopoietic stem cell antigen, CD34, is encoded by a gene located on chromosome 1. Leukemia 3:773, 1989.
16. Berenson, R. J., Andrews, R. G., Bensinger, W. I., Kalamasz, D., Knitter, G., Buckner, C. D., and Bernstein, I. D.: Antigen CD34+ marrow cells engraft lethally irradiated baboons. J. Clin. Invest. 81:951, 1988.
17. Fina, L., Molgaard, H. V., Robertson, D., Bradley, N. J., Monaghan, P., Delia, D., Sutherland, D. R., Baker, M. A., and Greaves, M. F.: Expression of the CD34 gene in vascular endothelial cells. Blood 75:2417, 1990.
18. Papayannopoulou, T., Brice, M., Broudy, V. C., and Zsebo, K. M.: Isolation of c-kit receptor-expressing cells from bone marrow, peripheral blood, and fetal liver: Functional properties and composite antigenic profile. Blood 78:1403, 1991.
19. Nakahata, T., and Ogawa, M.: Identification in culture of a class of hemopoietic colony-forming units with extensive capability to self-renew and generate multipotential hemopoietic colonies. Proc. Natl. Acad. Sci. USA 79:3843, 1982.
20. Rowley, S. D., Sharkis, S. J., Hattenburg, C., and Sensenbrenner, L. L.: Culture from human bone marrow of blast

progenitor cells with an extensive proliferative capacity. Blood 69:804, 1987.

21. Eaves, C. J., Sutherland, H. J., Cashman, J. D., Otsuka, T., Lansdorp, P. M., Humphries, R. K., Eaves, A. C., and Hogge, D. E.: Regulation of primitive human hematopoietic cells in long-term marrow culture. Semin. Hematol. 28:126, 1991.

22. Andrews, R. G., Singer, J. W., and Bernstein, I. D.: Human hematopoietic precursors in long-term culture: Single CD34 + cells that lack detectable T cell, B cell, and myeloid cell antigens produce multiple colony-forming cells when cultured with marrow stromal cells. J. Exp. Med. 172:355, 1990.

23. Sisson, S. D., and Dinarello, C. A.: Production of interleukin-1α, interleukin-1β, and tumor necrosis factor by human mononuclear cells stimulated with granulocyte-macrophage colony-stimulating factor. Blood 72:1368, 1988.

24. Lindemann, A., Riedel, D., Oster, W., Ziegler-Heitbrock, H. W. L., Mertelsmann, R., and Herrmann, F.: Granulocyte-macrophage colony-stimulating factor induces cytokine secretion by human polymorphonuclear leukocytes. J. Clin. Invest. 83:1308, 1989.

25. Ullrich, A., and Schlessinger, J.: Signal transduction by receptors with tyrosine kinase activity. Cell 61:203, 1990.

26. Nicola, N. A., and Metcalf, D.: Subunit promiscuity among hemopoietic growth factor receptors. Cell 67:1, 1991.

27. Bazan, J. F.: Structural design and molecular evolution of a cytokine receptor superfamily. Proc. Natl. Acad. Sci. USA 87:6934, 1990.

28. Patthy, L.: Homology of a domain of the growth hormone/prolactin receptor family with type III modules of fibronectin [letter]. Cell 61:13, 1990.

29. Tavernier, J., Devos, R., Cornelis, S., Tuypens, T., Van der Heyden, J., Fiers, W., and Plaetinck, G.: A human high affinity interleukin-5 receptor (IL5R) is composed of an IL-5–specific α chain and a β chain shared with the receptor for GM-CSF. Cell 66:1175, 1991.

30. Kitamura, T., Sato, N., Arai, K., and Miyajima, A.: Expression cloning of the human IL-3 receptor cDNA reveals a shared β subunit for the human IL-3 and GM-CSF receptors. Cell 66:1165, 1991.

31. Gearing, D. P., Comeau, M. R., Friend, D. J., Gimpel, S. D., Thut, C. J., McGourty, J., Brasher, K. K., King, J. A., Gillis, S., Mosley, B., Ziegler, S. F., and Cosman, D.: The IL-6 signal transducer, gp130: An oncostatin M receptor and affinity converter for the LIF receptor. Science 255:1434, 1992.

32. Taga, T., Hibi, M., Murakami, M., Saito, M., Yawata, H., Narazaki, M., Hirata, Y., Sugita, T., Yasukawa, K., Hirano, T., and Kishimoto, T.: Interleukin-6 receptor and signals. Chem. Immunol. 51:181, 1992.

33. Kuramochi, S., Ikawa, Y., and Todokoro, K.: Characterization of murine erythropoietin receptor genes. J. Mol. Biol. 216:567, 1990.

34. Goodwin, R. G., Friend, D., Ziegler, S. F., Jerzy, R., Falk, B. A., Gimpel, S., Cosman, D., Dower, S. K., March, C. J., Namen, A. E., and Park, L. S.: Cloning of the human and murine interleukin-7 receptors: Demonstration of a soluble form and homology to a new receptor superfamily. Cell 60:941, 1990.

35. Honda, M., Yamamoto, S., Cheng, M., Yasukawa, K., Suzuki, H., Saito, T., Osugi, Y., Tokunaga, T., and Kishimoto, T.: Human soluble IL-6 receptor: Its detection and enhanced release by HIV infection. J. Immunol. 148:2175, 1992.

36. Fukunaga, R., Seto, Y., Mizushima, S., and Nagata, S.: Three different mRNAs encoding human granulocyte colony-stimulating factor receptor. Proc. Natl. Acad. Sci. USA 87:8702, 1990.

37. Fanslow, W. C., Clifford, K. N., Park, L. S., Rubin, A. S., Voice, R. F., Beckmann, M. P., and Widmer, M. B.: Regulation of alloreactivity in vivo by IL-4 and the soluble IL-4 receptor. J. Immunol. 147:535, 1991.

38. Zanjani, E. D., Ascensao, J. L., McGlave, P. B., Banisadre, M.,

and Ash, R. C.: Studies on the liver to kidney switch of erythropoietin production. J. Clin. Invest. 67:1183, 1981.

39. Jacobson, L. O., Goldwasser, E., Fried, W., and Pizak, L.: Studies on erythropoiesis. VII. The role of the kidney in the production of erythropoietin. Trans. Assoc. Am. Physicians 70:305, 1957.

40. Stohlman, F., Jr., Rath, C. E., and Rose, J. C.: Evidence for a humoral regulation of erythropoiesis: Studies on a patient with polycythemia secondary to regional hypoxia. Blood 9:721, 1954.

41. Goldberg, M. A., Dunning, S. P., and Bunn, H. F.: Regulation of the erythropoietin gene: Evidence that the oxygen sensor is a heme protein. Science 242:1412, 1988.

42. Semenza, G. L., Koury, S. T., Nejfelt, M. K., Gearhart, J. D., and Antonarakis, S. E.: Cell-type–specific and hypoxia-inducible expression of the human erythropoietin gene in transgenic mice. Proc. Natl. Acad. Sci. USA 88:8725, 1991.

43. Browne, J. K., Cohen, A. M., Egrie, J. C., Lai, P. H., Lin, F-K., Strickland, T., Watson, E., and Stebbing, N.: Erythropoietin: Gene cloning, protein structure and biological properties. Cold Spring Harbor Symp. Quant. Biol. 51:693, 1986.

44. Stohlman, F., Jr.: Some aspects of erythrokinetics. Semin. Hematol. 4:304, 1967.

45. McDonald, T. P., Cottrell, M. B., Clift, R. E., Cullen, W. C., and Lin, F. K.: High doses of recombinant erythropoietin stimulate platelet production in mice. Exp. Hematol. 15:719, 1987.

46. Ishibashi, T., Koziol, J. A., and Burstein, S. A.: Human recombinant erythropoietin promotes differentiation of murine megakaryocytes in vitro. J. Clin. Invest. 79:286, 1987.

47. Clark, D. A., and Dessypris, E. N.: Effects of recombinant erythropoietin on murine megakaryocytic colony formation in vitro. J. Lab. Clin. Med. 108:423, 1986.

48. Fraser, J. C., Tan, A. S., Lin, F. K., and Berridge, M. V.: Expression of specific high-affinity binding sites for erythropoietin on rat and mouse megakaryocytes. Exp. Hematol. 17:10, 1989.

49. Lu, L., Bruno, E., Briddell, R. A., Graham, C. D., Brandt, J. E., and Hoffman, R.: Effects of hematopoietic growth factors on in vitro colony formation by human megakaryocyte progenitor cells. Behring Inst. 83:181, 1988.

50. Heberlein, C., Fischer, K.-D., Stoffel, M., Nowock, J., Ford, A., Tessmer, W., and Stocking, C.: The gene for erythropoietin receptor is expressed in multipotential hematopoietic and embryonal stem cells: Evidence for differentiation stage-specific regulation. Mol. Cell. Biol. 12:1815, 1992.

51. Anagnostou, A., Lee, E. S., Kessimian, N., Levinson, R., and Steiner, M.: Erythropoietin has a mitogenic and positive chemotactic effect on endothelial cells. Proc. Natl. Acad. Sci. USA 87:5978, 1990.

52. D'Andrea, A. D., Lodish, H. F. M., and Wong, G. G.: Expression cloning of the murine erythropoietin receptor. Cell 57:277, 1989.

53. Winkelmann, J. C., Penny, L. A., Deaven, L. L., Forget, B. G., and Jenkins, R. B.: The gene for the human erythropoietin receptor: Analysis of the coding sequence and assignment to chromosome 19p. Blood 76:24, 1990.

54. Fibi, M. R., Stüber, W., Hintz-Obertreis, P., Ljüben, G., Krumwieh, D., Siebold, B., Zettlmeissl, G., and Kjüpper, H. A.: Evidence for the location of the receptor-binding site of human erythropoietin at the carboxyl-terminal domain. Blood 77:1203, 1991.

55. Atkins, H. L., Broudy, V. C., and Papayannopoulou, T.: Characterization of the structure of the erythropoietin receptor by ligand blotting. Blood 77:2577, 1991.

56. Bailey, S. C., Spangler, R., and Sytkowski, A. J.: Erythropoietin induces cytosolic protein phosphorylation and dephosphorylation in erythroid cells. J. Biol. Chem. 266:24121, 1991.

57. Miller, B. A., Scaduto, R. C., Jr., Tillotson, D. L., Botti, J. J., and Cheung, J. Y.: Erythropoietin stimulates a rise in intracellular free calcium concentration in single early human erythroid precursors. J. Clin. Invest. 82:309, 1988.

58. Fukunaga, R., Ishizaka-Ikeda, E., Seto, Y., and Nagata, S.:

Expression cloning of a receptor for murine granulocyte colony-stimulating factor. Cell 61:341, 1990.

59. Fukunaga, R., Ishizaka-Ikeda, E., Pan, C. X., Seto, Y., and Nagata, S.: Functional domains of the granulocyte colony-stimulating factor receptor. EMBO J. 10:2855, 1991.

60. Valtieri, M., Tweardy, D. J., Caracciolo, D., Johnson, K., Mavilio, F., Altmann, S., Santoli, D., and Rovera, G.: Cytokine-dependent granulocytic differentiation: Regulation of proliferative and differentiative responses in a murine progenitor cell line. J. Immunol. 138:3829, 1987.

61. Yamasaki, Y., Izumi, Y., Sawada, H., and Fujita, K.: Probable in vivo induction of differentiation by recombinant human granulocyte colony stimulating factor (rhG-CSF) in acute promyelocytic leukaemia (APL). Br. J. Haematol. 78:579, 1991.

62. Nicola, N. A., and Metcalf, D.: Binding of the differentiation-inducer, granulocyte-colony-stimulating factor to responsive but not unresponsive leukemic cell lines. Proc. Natl. Acad. Sci. USA 81:3765, 1984.

63. Ikebuchi, K., Clark, S. C., Ihle, J. N., Souza, L. M., and Ogawa, M.: Granulocyte colony-stimulating factor enhances interleukin 3–dependent proliferation of multipotential hemopoietic progenitors. Proc. Natl. Acad. Sci. USA 85:3445, 1988.

64. Campbell, H. D., Tucker, W. Q. J., Hort, Y., Martinson, M. E., Mayo, G., Clutterbuck, E. J., Sanderson, C. J., and Young, I. G.: Molecular cloning, nucleotide sequence, and expression of the gene encoding human eosinophil differentiation factor (interleukin 5). Proc. Natl. Acad. Sci. USA 84:6629, 1987.

65. Sutherland, G. R., Baker, E., Callen, D. F., Campbell, H. D., Young, I. G., Sanderson, C. J., Garson, O. M., Lopez, A. F., and Vadas, M. A.: Interleukin-5 is at 5q31 and is deleted in the 5q − syndrome. Blood 71:1150, 1988.

66. Van Leeuwen, B. H., Martinson, M. E., Webb, G. C., and Young, I. G.: Molecular organization of the cytokine gene cluster, involving the human IL-3, IL-4, IL-5, and GM-CSF genes, on human chromosome 5. Blood 73:1142, 1989.

67. Purkerson, J. M., Newberg, M., Wise, G., Lynch, K. R., and Isakson, P. C.: Interleukin 5 and interleukin 2 cooperate with interleukin 4 to induce IgG1 secretion from anti-Ig–treated B cells. J. Exp. Med. 168:1175, 1988.

68. Lopez, A. F., Vadas, M. A., Woodcock, J. M., Milton, S. E., Lewis, A., Elliott, M. J., Gillis, D., Ireland, R., Olwell, E., and Park, L. S.: Interleukin-5, interleukin-3, and granulocyte-macrophage colony-stimulating factor cross-compete for binding to cell surface receptors on human eosinophils. J. Biol. Chem. 266:24741, 1991.

69. Morris, S. W., Valentine, M. B., Shapiro, D. N., Sublett, J. E., Deaven, L. L., Foust, J. T., Roberts, W. M., Cerretti, D. P., and Look, A. T.: Reassignment of the human CSF1 gene to chromosome 1p13-p21. Blood 78:2013, 1991.

70. Le Beau, M. M., Pettenati, M. J., Lemons, R. S., Diaz, M. O., Westbrook, C. A., Larson, R. A., Sherr, C. J., and Rowley, J. D.: Assignment of the GM-CSF, CSF-1, and FMS genes to human chromosome 5 provides evidence for linkage of a family of genes regulating hematopoiesis and for their involvement in the deletion (5q) in myeloid disorders. Cold Spring Harbor Symp. Quant. Biol. 51:899, 1986.

71. Ralph, P., Warren, M. K., Nakoinz, I., Lee, M. T., Brindley, L., Sampson-Johannes, A., Kawasaki, E. S., Ladner, M. B., Strickler, J. E., Boosman, A., et al.: Biological properties and molecular biology of the human macrophage growth factor, CSF-1. Immunobiology 172:194, 1986.

72. Alderson, M. R., Tough, T. W., Ziegler, S. F., and Grabstein, K. H.: Interleukin 7 induces cytokine secretion and tumoricidal activity by human peripheral blood monocytes. J. Exp. Med. 173:923, 1991.

73. Dibirdik, I., Langlie, M.-C., Ledbetter, J. A., Tuel-Ahlgren, L., Obuz, V., Waddick, K. G., Gajl-Peczalska, K., Schieven, G. L., and Uckun, F. M.: Engagement of interleukin-7 receptor stimulates tyrosine phosphorylation, phosphoinositide turnover, and clonal proliferation of human T-lineage acute lymphoblastic leukemia cells. Blood 78:564, 1991.

74. Economou, J. S., McBride, W. H., Essner, R., Rhoades, K., Golub, S., Holmes, E. C., and Morton, D. L.: Tumour necrosis factor production by IL-2–activated macrophages in vitro and in vivo. Immunology 67:514, 1989.

75. Hancock, W. W., Muller, W. A., and Cotran, R. S.: Interleukin 2 receptors are expressed by alveolar macrophages during pulmonary sarcoidosis and are inducible by lymphokine treatment of normal human lung macrophages, blood monocytes, and monocyte cell lines. J. Immunol. 138:185, 1987.

76. Kovacs, E. J., Brock, B., Varesio, L., and Young, H. A.: IL-2 induction of IL-1β mRNA expression in monocytes: Regulation by agents that block second messenger pathways. J. Immunol. 143:3532, 1989.

77. Saltzman, E. M., Thom, R. R., and Casnellie, J. E.: Activation of a tyrosine protein kinase is an early event in the stimulation of T lymphocytes by interleukin-2. J. Biol. Chem. 263:6956, 1988.

78. Zmuidzinas, A., Mamon, H. J., Roberts, T. M., and Smith, K. A.: Interleukin-2–triggered Raf-1 expression, phosphorylation, and associated kinase activity increase through G1 and S in CD3-stimulated primary human T cells. Mol. Cell. Biol. 11:2794, 1991.

79. Turner, B., Rapp, U., App, H., Greene, M., Dobashi, K., and Reed, J.: Interleukin 2 induces tyrosine phosphorylation and activation of p72-74 Raf-1 kinase in a T-cell line. Proc. Natl. Acad. Sci. USA 88:1227, 1991.

80. Lopez, A. F., Dyson, P. G., To, L. B., Elliott, M. J., Milton, S. E., Russell, J. A., Juttner, C. A., Yang, Y.-C., Clark, S. C., and Vadas, M. A.: Recombinant human interleukin-3 stimulation of hematopoiesis in humans: Loss of responsiveness with differentiation in the neutrophilic myeloid series. Blood 72:1797, 1988.

81. Metcalf, D.: The molecular control of cell division, differentiation commitment and maturation in haemopoietic cells. Nature 339:27, 1989.

82. Gough, N. M., Gearing, D. P., Nicola, N. A., Baker, E., Pritchard, M., Callen, D. F., and Sutherland, G. R.: Localization of the human GM-CSF receptor gene to the X-Y pseudoautosomal region. Nature 345:734, 1990.

83. Hayashida, K., Kitamura, T., Gorman, D. M., Arai, K., Yokota, T., and Miyajima, A.: Molecular cloning of a second subunit of the receptor for human granulocyte-macrophage colony-stimulating factor (GM-CSF): Reconstitution of a high-affinity GM-CSF receptor. Proc. Natl. Acad. Sci. USA 87:9655, 1990.

84. Sullivan, R., Fredette, J. P., Leavitt, J. L., Gadenne, A.-S., Griffin, J. D., and Simons, E. R.: Effects of recombinant human granulocyte-macrophage colony-stimulating factor (GM-CSF_rh) on transmembrane electrical potentials in granulocytes: Relationship between enhancement of ligand-mediated depolarization and augmentation of superoxide anion (O_2^-) production. J. Cell. Physiol. 139:361, 1989.

85. Evans, J. P. M., Mire-Sluis, A. R., Hoffbrand, A. V., and Wickremasinghe, R. G.: Binding of G-CSF, GM-CSF, tumor necrosis factor-α and gamma-interferon to cell surface receptors on human myeloid leukemia cells triggers rapid tyrosine and serine phosphorylation of a 75-Kd protein. Blood 75:88, 1990.

86. Kanakura, Y., Druker, B., Cannistra, S. A., Furukawa, Y., Torimoto, Y., and Griffin, J. D.: Signal transduction of the human granulocyte-macrophage colony-stimulating factor and interleukin-3 receptors involves tyrosine phosphorylation of a common set of cytoplasmic proteins. Blood 76:706, 1990.

87. Kanakura, Y., Druker, B., Wood, K. W., Mamon, H. J., Okuda, K., Roberts, T. M., and Griffin, J. D.: Granulocyte-macrophage colony-stimulating factor and interleukin-3 induce rapid phosphorylation and activation of the proto-oncogene Raf-1 in a human factor–dependent myeloid cell line. Blood 77:243, 1991.

88. Satoh, T., Nakafuku, M., Miyajima, A., and Kaziro, Y.: Involvement of ras p21 protein in signal-transduction pathways from interleukin 2, interleukin 3, and granulocyte/

macrophage colony-stimulating factor, but not from inter-leukin 4. Proc. Natl. Acad. Sci. USA 88:3314, 1991.

89. Murata, Y., Yamaguchi, N., Hitoshi, Y., Tominaga, A., and Takatsu, K.: Interleukin 5 and interleukin 3 induce serine and tyrosine phosphorylations of several cellular proteins in an interleukin 5–dependent cell line. Biochem. Biophys. Res. Commun. 173:1102, 1990.

90. Whetton, A. D., Monk, P. N., Consalvey, S. D., Huang, S. J., Dexter, T. M., and Downes, C. P.: Interleukin 3 stimulates proliferation via protein kinase C activation without increasing inositol lipid turnover. Proc. Natl. Acad. Sci. USA 85:3284, 1988.

91. Bagby, G. C., and Segal, G. M.: Growth factors and the control of hematopoiesis. In Hoffman, R., Benz, E. J., Shattil, S. J., Furie, B., and Cohen, H. J. (eds.): Hematology. Basic Principles and Practice. New York, Churchill Livingstone, 1991, pp. 97–121.

92. Paul, S. R., Bennett, F., Calvetti, J. A., Kelleher, K., Wood, C. R., O'Hara, R. M., Jr., Leary, A. C., Sibley, B., Clark, S. C., and Williams, D. A.: Molecular cloning of a cDNA encoding interleukin 11, a stromal cell–derived lympho-poietic and hematopoietic cytokine. Proc. Natl. Acad. Sci. USA 87:7512, 1990.

93. Musashi, M., Clark, S. C., Sudo, T., Urdal, D. L., and Ogawa, M.: Synergistic interactions between interleukin-11 and in-terleukin-4 in support of proliferation of primitive hema-topoietic progenitors of mice. Blood 78:1448, 1991.

94. Walther, Z., May, L. T., and Sehgal, P. B.: Transcriptional regulation of the interferon-β2/B cell differentiation factor BSF-2/hepatocyte-stimulating factor gene in human fibro-blasts by other cytokines. J. Immunol. 140:974, 1988.

95. Akashi, M., Loussararian, A. H., Adelman, D. C., Saito, M., and Koeffler, H. P.: Role of lymphotoxin in expression of interleukin 6 in human fibroblasts. Stimulation and regula-tion. J. Clin. Invest. 85:121, 1990.

96. Horii, Y., Muraguchi, A., Suematsu, S., Matsuda, T., Yoshi-zaki, K., Hirano, T., and Kishimoto, T.: Regulation of BSF-2/IL-6 production by human mononuclear cells: Macro-phage-dependent synthesis of BSF-2/IL-6 by T cells. J. Immunol. 141:1529, 1988.

97. Szpirer, J., Szpirer, C., Riviëre, M., Houart, C., Baumann, M., Fey, G. H., Poli, V., Cortese, R., Islam, M. Q., and Levan, G.: The interleukin-6–dependent DNA-binding protein gene (transcription factor 5: TCF5) maps to human chro-mosome 20 and rat chromosome 3, the IL6 receptor locus (IL6R) to human chromosome 1 and rat chromosome 2, and the rat IL6 gene to rat chromosome 4. Genomics 10:539, 1991.

98. Arai, K., Lee, F., Miyajima, A., Miyatake, S., Arai, N., and Yokota, T.: Cytokines: Coordinators of immune and inflam-matory responses. Annu. Rev. Biochem. 59:783, 1990.

99. Ikebuchi, K., Wong, G. C., Clark, S. C., Ihle, J. N., Hirai, H., and Ogawa, M.: Interleukin 6 enhancement of interleukin 3–dependent proliferation of multipotential hemopoietic progenitors. Proc. Natl. Acad. Sci. USA 84:9035, 1987.

100. Leary, A. G., Ikebuchi, K., Hirai, Y., Wong, G. G., Yang, Y.-C., Clark, S. C., and Ogawa, M.: Synergism between interleukin-6 and interleukin-3 in supporting proliferation of human hematopoietic stem cells: Comparison with inter-leukin-1α. Blood 71:1759, 1988.

101. Suzuki, C., Okano, A., Takatsuki, F., Miyasaka, Y., Hirano, T., Kishimoto, T., Ejima, D., and Akiyama, Y.: Continuous perfusion with interleukin 6 (IL-6) enhances production of hematopoietic stem cells (CFU-S). Biochem. Biophys. Res. Commun. 159:933, 1989.

102. Witte, O. N.: Steel locus defines new multipotent growth factor. Cell 63:5, 1990.

103. Huang, E. J., Nocka, K. H., Buck, J., and Besmer, P.: Differ-ential expression and processing of two cell associated forms of the Kit-ligand: KL-1 and KL-2. Mol. Biol. Cell 3:349, 1992.

104. Flanagan, J. G., Chan, D. C., and Leder, P.: Transmembrane form of the kit ligand growth factor is determined by

alternative splicing and is missing in the Sl^d mutant. Cell 64:1025, 1991.

105. Metcalf, D., and Moore, M. A. S.: Genetic defects in haemo-poiesis. In Neuberger, A., and Tatum, E. L. (eds.): Haemo-poietic cells. Amsterdam, North-Holland Publishing Co., 1971, pp. 488–535.

106. Brannan, C. I., Lyman, S. D., Williams, D. E., Eisenman, J., Anderson, D. M., Cosman, D., Bedell, M. A., Jenkins, N. A., and Copeland, N. G.: Steel-Dickie mutation encodes a c-Kit ligand lacking transmembrane and cytoplasmic do-mains. Proc. Natl. Acad. Sci. USA 88:4671, 1991.

107. Stahl, J., Gearing, D. P., Willson, T. A., Brown, M. A., King, J. A., and Gough, N. M.: Structural organization of the genes for murine and human leukemia inhibitory factor. Evolutionary conservation of coding and non-coding re-gions. J. Biol. Chem. 265:8833, 1990.

108. Anegon, I., Moreau, J.-F., Godard, A., Jacques, Y., Peyrat, M.-A., Hallet, M.-M., Wong, G., and Soulillou, J. P.: Pro-duction of human interleukin for DA cells (HILDA)/leukemia inhibitory factor (LIF) by activated monocytes. Cell. Immunol. 130:50, 1990.

109. Wetzler, M., Talpaz, M., Lowe, D. G., Baiocchi, G., Gutterman, J. U., and Kurzrock, R.: Constitutive expression of leukemia inhibitory factor RNA by human bone marrow stromal cells and modulation by IL-1, TNF-α, and TGF-β. Exp. Hematol. 19:347, 1991.

110. Wieser, M., Bonifer, R., Oster, W., Lindemann, R., Mertels-mann, R., and Herrmann, F.: Interleukin-4 induces secre-tion of CSF for granulocytes and CSF for macrophages by peripheral blood monocytes. Blood 73:1105, 1989.

111. Peschel, C., Green, I., and Paul, W. E.: Interleukin-4 induces a substance in bone marrow stromal cells that reversibly inhibits factor-dependent and factor-independent cell pro-liferation. Blood 73:1130, 1989.

112. Dinarello, C. A.: Interleukin-1 and interleukin-1 antagonism. Blood 77:1627, 1991.

113. Chizzonite, R., Truitt, T., Kilian, P. L., Stern, A. S., Nunes, P., Parker, K. P., Kaffka, K. L., Chua, A. O., Lugg, D. K., and Gubler, U.: Two high-affinity interleukin 1 receptors represent separate gene products. Proc. Natl. Acad. Sci. USA 86:8029, 1989.

114. Boraschi, D., Rambaldi, A., Sica, A., Ghiara, P., Colotta, F., Wang, J. M., De Rossi, M., Zoia, C., Remuzzi, G., Bussolino, F., Scapigliati, G., Stoppacciaro, A., Ruco, L., Tagliabue, A., and Mantovani, A.: Endothelial cells express the interleukin-1 receptor type I. Blood 78:1262, 1991.

115. Bomsztyk, K., Sims, J. E., Stanton, T. H., Slack, J., McMahan, C. J., Valentine, M. A., and Dower, S. K.: Evidence for different interleukin 1 receptors in murine B- and T-cell lines. Proc. Natl. Acad. Sci. USA 86:8034, 1989.

116. Bagby, G. C.: Interleukin 1 and hematopoiesis. Blood Rev. 3:152, 1989.

117. Spies, T., Blanck, G., Bresnahan, M., Sands, J., and Stromin-ger, J. L.: A new cluster of genes within the human major histocompatibility complex. Science 243:214, 1989.

118. Migliaccio, A. R., and Migliaccio, G.: Human embryonic hem-opoiesis: Control mechanisms underlying progenitor differ-entiation in vitro. Dev. Biol. 125:127, 1988.

119. Cannistra, S. A., Groshek, P., and Griffin, J. D.: Monocytes enhance gamma-interferon–induced inhibition of myeloid progenitor cell growth through secretion of tumor necrosis factor. Exp. Hematol. 16:865, 1988.

120. Lindemann, A., Riedel, D., Oster, W., Meuer, S. C., Blohm, D., Mertelsmann, R. H., and Herrmann, F.: Granulo-cyte/macrophage colony-stimulating factor induces interleu-kin 1 production by human polymorphonuclear neutrophils. J. Immunol. 140:837, 1988.

121. Levy, Y., Tsapis, A., and Brouet, J.-C.: Interleukin-6 antisense oligonucleotides inhibit the growth of human myeloma cell lines. J. Clin. Invest. 88:696, 1991.

122. Segawa, K., Ueno, Y., and Kataoka, T.: In vivo tumor growth enhancement by granulocyte colony-stimulating factor. Jpn. J. Cancer Res. (Gann) 82:440, 1991.

123. Donnelly, R. P., Fenton, M. J., Kaufman, J. D., and Gerrard,

T. L.: IL-1 expression in human monocytes is transcriptionally and posttranscriptionally regulated by IL-4. J. Immunol. 146:3431, 1991.

124. Bagby, G. C., Shaw, G., Heinrich, M. C., Hefeneider, M., Brown, M. A., DeLoughery, T. G., Segal, G. M., and Band, L.: Interleukin-1 stimulation stabilizes GM-CSF mRNA in human vascular endothelial cells: Preliminary studies on the role of 3′ AU-rich motif. In Daniak, N. (eds.): Biology of Hematopoiesis. New York, Wiley-Liss, 1990, pp. 233–239.

125. Elias, J. A., and Lentz, V.: IL-1 and tumor necrosis factor synergistically stimulate fibroblast IL-6 production and stabilize IL-6 messenger RNA. J. Immunol. 145:161, 1990.

126. Han, J., Brown, T., and Beutler, B.: Endotoxin-responsive sequences control cachectin/tumor necrosis factor biosynthesis at the translational level. J. Exp. Med. 171:465, 1990.

127. Segal, G. M., Smith, T., Heinrich, M. C., Ey, F. S., and Bagby, G. C.: Specific repression of granulocyte-macrophage and granulocyte colony-stimulating factor gene expression in interleukin-1–stimulated endothelial cells with antisense oligodeoxynucleotides. Blood 80:609, 1992.

128. Segal, G. M., Fenton, L., Williamson, W., and Bagby, G. C.: Selective inhibition of interleukin-1 (IL-1)–induced granulocyte-macrophage colony stimulating factor (GM-CSF) gene expression in endothelial cells (ECs) by antisense oligonucleotides: Expression of GM-CSF and G-CSF are not linked. Blood 72:133a, 1988.

129. Yang, Y.-C., Kovacic, S., Kriz, R., Wolf, S., Clark, S. C., Wellems, T. E., Nienhuis, A., and Epstein, N.: The human genes for GM-CSF and IL3 are closely linked in tandem on chromosome 5. Blood 71:958, 1988.

130. Morris, C., Heisterkamp, N., Hao, Q. L., Testa, J. R., and Groffen, J.: The human tyrosine kinase gene (FER) maps to chromosome 5 and is deleted in myeloid leukemias with a del(5q). Cytogenet. Cell Genet. 53:196, 1990.

131. Mock, B. A., Krall, M., Kozak, C. A., Nesbitt, M. N., McBride, O. W., Renauld, J.-C., and Van Snick, J.: IL9 maps to mouse chromosome 13 and human chromosome 5. Immunogenetics 31:265, 1990.

132. Jaye, M., Howk, R., Burgess, W., Ricca, G. A., Chiu, I. M., Ravera, M. W., O'Brien, S. J., Modi, W. S., Maciag, T., and Drohan, W. N.: Human endothelial cell growth factor: Cloning, nucleotide sequence, and chromosome localization. Science 233:541, 1986.

133. Kobilka, B. K., Dixon, R. A., Frielle, T., Dohlman, H. G., Bolanowski, M. A., Sigal, I. S., Yang-Feng, T. L., Francke, U., Caron, M. G., and Lefkowitz, R. J.: cDNA for the human beta 2-adrenergic receptor: A protein with multiple membrane-spanning domains and encoded by a gene whose chromosomal location is shared with that of the receptor for platelet-derived growth factor. Proc. Natl. Acad. Sci. USA 84:46, 1987.

134. Goyert, S. M., Ferrero, E. N., Rettig, W. J., Yenamandra, A. K., Obata, F., and LeBeau, M. M.: The CD14 monocyte differentiation antigen maps to a region encoding growth factors and receptors. Science 239:497, 1988.

135. Le Beau, M. M., Westbrook, C. A., Diaz, M. O., Larson, R. A., Rowley, J. D., Gasson, J. C., Golde, D. W., and Sherr, C. J.: Evidence for the involvement of GM-CSF and FMS in the deletion (5q) in myeloid disorders. Science 231:984, 1986.

136. Akira, S., Isshiki, H., Sugita, T., Tanabe, O., Kinoshita, S., Nishio, Y., Nakajima, T., Hirano, T., and Kishimoto, T.: A nuclear factor for IL-6 expression (NF-IL6) is a member of a C/EBP family. EMBO J. 9:1897, 1990.

137. Kinoshita, S., Akira, S., and Kishimoto, T.: A member of the C/EBP family, NF-IL6β, forms a heterodimer and transcriptionally synergizes with NF-IL6. Proc. Natl. Acad. Sci. USA 89:1473, 1992.

138. Osborn, L., Kunkel, S., and Nabel, G. J.: Tumor necrosis factor α and interleukin 1 stimulate the human immunodeficiency virus enhancer by activation of the nuclear factor kappa B. Proc. Natl. Acad. Sci. USA 86:2336, 1989.

139. De Waal Malefyt, R., Abrams, J., Bennett, B., Figdor, C. G., and De Vries, J. E.: Interleukin 10(IL-10) inhibits cytokine synthesis by human monocytes: An autoregulatory role of IL-10 produced by monocytes. J. Exp. Med. 174:1209, 1991.

140. Fraser, J. D., Irving, B. A., Crabtree, G. R., and Weiss, A.: Regulation of interleukin-2 gene enhancer activity by the T cell accessory molecule CD28. Science 251:313, 1991.

141. Kuczek, E. S., Shannon, M. F., Pell, L. M., and Vadas, M. A.: A granulocyte colony-stimulating factor gene promoter element responsive to inflammatory mediators is functionally distinct from an identical sequence in the granulocyte-macrophage colony-stimulating factor gene. J. Immunol. 146:2426, 1991.

142. Liu, Z. Y., Schechter, A. N., and Noguchi, C. T.: Expression of the human erythropoietin receptor gene in transgenic mice. Clin. Res. 40:350A, 1992.

143. Shaw, G., and Kamen, R.: A conserved AU sequence from the 3′ untranslated region of GM-CSF mRNA mediates selective mRNA degradation. Cell 46:659, 1986.

144. Caput, D., Beutler, B., Hartog, K., Thayer, R., Brown-Shimer, S., and Cerami, A.: Identification of a common nucleotide sequence in the 3′ untranslated region of mRNA molecules specifying inflammatory mediators. Proc. Natl. Acad. Sci. USA 83:1670, 1986.

145. Malter, J. S.: Identification of an AUUUA-specific messenger RNA binding protein. Science 246:664, 1989.

146. Brewer, G.: An A+U−rich element RNA-binding factor regulates c-myc mRNA stability in vitro. Mol. Cell. Biol. 11:2460, 1991.

147. Gillis, P., and Malter, J. S.: The adenosine-uridine binding factor recognizes the AU-rich elements of cytokine, lymphokine, and oncogene mRNAs. J. Biol. Chem. 266:3172, 1991.

148. Bohjanen, P. R., Petryniak, B., June, C. H., Thompson, C. B., and Lindsten, T.: An inducible cytoplasmic factor (AU-B) binds selectively to AUUUA multimers in the 3′ untranslated region of lymphokine mRNA. Mol. Cell. Biol. 11:3288, 1991.

149. Shyu, A.-B., Belasco, J. G., and Greenberg, M. E.: Two distinct destabilizing elements in the c-fos message trigger deadenylation as a first step in rapid mRNA decay. Genes Dev. 5:221, 1991.

150. Bernstein, P. L., Herrick, D. J., Prokipcak, R. D., and Ross, J.: Control of c-myc mRNA half-life in vitro by a protein capable of binding to a coding region stability determinant. Genes Dev. 6:642, 1992.

151. Yamato, K., El-Hajjaoui, Z., and Koeffler, H. P.: Regulation of levels of IL-1 mRNA in human fibroblasts. J. Cell. Physiol. 139:610, 1989.

152. Joyce, G. F.: RNA evolution and the origins of life. Nature 338:217, 1989.

153. Attisano, L., Wrana, J. L., Cheifetz, S., and Massague, J.: Novel activin receptors: Distinct genes and alternative mRNA splicing generate a repertoire of serine/threonine kinase receptors. Cell 68:97, 1992.

154. Metcalf, D., and Moore, M. A. S.: Embryonic aspects of haemopoiesis. In Tatum, E. L., and Neuberger, A. (eds.): Haemopoietic Cells. Amsterdam, North-Holland Publishing Co., 1971, pp. 172–271.

155. Migliaccio, G., Migliaccio, A. R., Petti, S., Mavilio, F., Russo, G., Lazzaro, D., Testa, U., Marinucci, M., and Peschle, C.: Human embryonic hemopoiesis. Kinetics of progenitors and precursors underlying the yolk sac–liver transition. J. Clin. Invest. 78:51, 1986.

156. Broxmeyer, H. E., Hangoc, G., Cooper, S., Anderson, D., Cosman, D., Lyman, S. D., and Williams, D. E.: Influence of murine mast cell growth factor (c-kit ligand) on colony formation by mouse marrow hematopoietic progenitor cells. Exp. Hematol. 19:143, 1991.

157. Williams, D. E., Eisenman, J., Baird, A., Rauch, C., Van Ness, K., March, C. J., Park, L. S., Martin, U., Mochizuki, D. Y., Boswell, H. S., Burgess, G. S., Cosman, D., and Lyman, S. D.: Identification of a ligand for the c-kit proto-oncogene. Cell 63:167, 1990.

158. Copeland, N. G., Gilbert, D. J., Cho, B. C., Donovan, P. J., Jenkins, N. A., Cosman, D., Anderson, D., Lyman, S. D., and Williams, D. E.: Mast cell growth factor maps near the

steel locus on mouse chromosome 10 and is deleted in a number of steel alleles. Cell 63:175, 1990.

159. Zsebo, K. M., Williams, D. A., Geissler, E. N., Broudy, V. C., Martin, F. H., Atkins, H. L., Hsu, R.-Y., Birkett, N. C., Okino, K. H., Murdock, D. C., Jacobsen, F. W., Langley, K. E., Smith, K. A., Takeishi, T., Cattanach, B. M., Galli, S. J., and Suggs, S. V.: Stem cell factor is encoded at the *Sl* locus of the mouse and is the ligand for the c-*kit* tyrosine kinase receptor. Cell 63:213, 1990.

160. Valtieri, M., Gabbianelli, M., Pelosi, E., Bassano, E., Petti, S., Russo, G., Testa, U., and Peschle, C.: Erythropoietin alone induces erythroid burst formation by human embryonic but not adult BFU-E in unicellular serum-free culture. Blood 74:460, 1989.

161. Garre, C., Ravazzolo, R., Ajmar, F., and Bruzzone, G.: Electrophoretic difference between fetal and adult acetylcholinesterase of human red cell membranes. Cell Differ. 9:165, 1980.

162. Chen, S. H., Anderson, J. E., Giblett, E. R., and Stamatoyannopoulos, G.: Isozyme patterns in erythrocytes from human fetuses. Am. J. Hematol. 3:23, 1977.

163. Ohneda, O., Yanai, N., and Obinata, M.: Microenvironment created by stromal cells is essential for a rapid expansion of erythroid cells in mouse fetal liver. Development 110:379, 1990.

164. Snodgrass, R., and Keller, G.: Clonal fluctuation within the haematopoietic system of mice reconstituted with retrovirus-infected stem cells. EMBO J. 6:3955, 1987.

165. Jordan, C. T., and Lemischka, I. R.: Clonal and systemic analysis of long-term hematopoiesis in the mouse. Genes Dev. 4:220, 1990.

166. Osgood, E. E.: The etiology of leukemias, lymphomas and cancers. Geriatrics 29:208, 1961.

167. Ogawa, M.: Hemopoietic stem cells: Stochastic differentiation and humoral control of proliferation. Environ. Health Perspect. 80:199, 1989.

168. Smith, L. G., Weissman, I. L., and Heimfeld, S.: Clonal analysis of hematopoietic stem-cell differentiation *in vivo*. Proc. Natl. Acad. Sci. USA 88:2788, 1991.

169. Sawada, K., Krantz, S. B., Dai, C. H., Sato, N., Ieko, M., Sakurama, S., Yasukouchi, T., and Nakagawa, S.: Transitional change of colony stimulating factor requirements for erythroid progenitors. J Cell Physiol. 149:1, 1991.

170. Broudy, V. C., Lin, N., Brice, M., Nakamoto, B., and Papayannopoulou, T.: Erythropoietin receptor characteristics on primary human erythroid cells. Blood 77:2583, 1991.

171. Landschulz, K. T., Noyes, A. N., Rogers, O., and Boyer, S. H.: Erythropoietin receptors on murine erythroid colony-forming units: Natural history. Blood 73:1476, 1989.

172. Wickrema, A., Bondurant, M. C., and Krantz, S. B.: Abundance and stability of erythropoietin receptor mRNA in mouse erythroid progenitor cells. Blood 78:2269, 1991.

173. Suda, T., Suda, J., and Ogawa, M.: Disparate differentiation in mouse hemopoietic colonies derived from paired progenitors. Proc. Natl. Acad. Sci. USA 81:2520, 1984.

174. Roussel, M. F., Dull, T. J., Rettenmier, C. W., Ralph, P., Ullrich, A., and Sherr, C. J.: Transforming potential of the c-*fms* proto-oncogene (CSF-1 receptor). Nature 325:549, 1987.

175. Longmore, G. D., and Lodish, H. F.: An activating mutation in the murine erythropoietin receptor induces erythroleukemia in mice: A cytokine receptor superfamily oncogene. Cell 67:1089, 1991.

176. Krantz, S. B.: Erythropoietin. Blood 77:419, 1991.

177. Sherr, C. J., Borzillo, G. V., Kato, J., Shurtleff, S. A., Downing, J. R., and Roussel, M. F.: Regulation of cell growth and differentiation by the colony-stimulating factor 1 receptor. Semin. Hematol. 28:143, 1991.

178. Fibach, E., and Sachs, L.: Control of normal differentiation of myeloid leukemic cells. IV. Induction of differentiation by serum from endotoxin treated mice. J. Cell. Physiol. 83:177, 1974.

179. Blackwood, E. M., and Eisenman, R. N.: Max: A helix-loop-helix zipper protein that forms a sequence-specific DNA-binding complex with *myc*. Science 251:1211, 1991.

180. Gowda, S. D., Koler, R. D., and Bagby, G. C.: Regulation of c-*myc* expression during growth and differentiation of normal and leukemic human myeloid progenitor cells. J. Clin. Invest. 77:271, 1986.

181. Tobler, A., Miller, C. W., Johnson, K. R., Selsted, M. E., Rovera, G., and Koeffler, H. P.: Regulation of gene expression of myeloperoxidase during myeloid differentiation. J. Cell. Physiol. 136:215, 1988.

182. Sawyer, S. T., Krantz, S. B., and Luna, J.: Identification of the receptor for erythropoietin by cross-linking to Friend virus-infected erythroid cells. Proc. Natl. Acad. Sci. USA 84:3690, 1987.

183. Holt, J. T., Redner, R. L., and Nienhuis, A. W.: An oligomer complementary to c-*myc* mRNA inhibits proliferation of HL-60 promyelocytic cells and induces differentiation. Mol. Cell. Biol. 8:963, 1988.

184. Yamamoto, T., Masuko, K., Takada, S., Kume, T. U., and Obinata, M.: A balance between self-renewal and commitment in the murine erythroleukemia cells with the transferred c-*myc* gene: An in vitro stochastic model. Cell Differ. 28:129, 1989.

185. Kirsch, I. R., Bertness, V., Silver, J., and Hollis, G. F.: Regulated expression of the c-*myb* and c-*myc* oncogenes during erythroid differentiation. J. Cell. Biochem. 32:11, 1986.

186. Gonda, T. J., and Metcalf, D.: Expression of myb, myc and fos proto-oncogenes during the differentiation of a murine myeloid leukemia. Nature 310:249, 1984.

187. Clarke, M. F., Kukowska-Latallo, J. F., Westin, E., Smith, M., and Prochownik, E. V.: Constitutive expression of a c-*myb* cDNA blocks friend murine erythroleukemia cell differentiation. Mol. Cell. Biol. 8:884, 1988.

188. Yanagisawa, H., Nagasawa, T., Kuramochi, S., Abe, T., Ikawa, Y., and Todokoro, K.: Constitutive expression of exogenous c-*myb* gene causes maturation block in monocyte-macrophage differentiation. Biochim. Biophys. Acta 1088:380, 1991.

189. McClinton, D., Stafford, J., Brents, L., Bender, T. P., and Kuehl, W. M.: Differentiation of mouse erythroleukemia cells is blocked by late up-regulation of a c-*myb* transgene. Mol. Cell Biol. 10:705, 1990.

190. Todokoro, K., Watson, R. J., Higo, H., Amanuma, H., Kuramochi, S., Yanagisawa, H., and Ikawa, Y.: Down-regulation of c-*myb* gene expression is a prerequisite for erythropoietin-induced erythroid differentiation. Proc. Natl. Acad. Sci. USA 85:8900, 1988.

191. Ransone, L. J., and Verma, I. M.: Nuclear proto-oncogenes fos and jun. Annu. Rev. Cell Biol. 6:539, 1990.

192. Neuberg, M., Adamkiewicz, J., Hunter, J. B., and Muller, R.: A fos protein containing the Jun leucine zipper forms a homodimer which binds to the AP1 binding site. Nature 341:243, 1989.

193. Rauscher, F. J., Sambucetti, L. C., Curran, T., Distel, R. J., and Spiegelman, B. M.: Common DNA binding site for Fos protein complexes and transcription factor AP-1. Cell 52:471, 1988.

194. Lin, J.-X., and Vilcek, J.: Tumor necrosis factor and interleukin-1 cause a rapid and transient stimulation of c-*fos* and c-*myc* mRNA levels in human fibroblasts. J. Biol. Chem. 262:11908, 1987.

195. Nishikura, K., and Murray, J. M.: Antisense RNA of proto-oncogene c-*fos* blocks renewed growth of quiescent 3T3 cells. Mol. Cell. Biol. 7:639, 1987.

196. Tsuda, H., Neckers, L. M., and Pluznik, D. H.: Enhanced c-*fos* expression in differentiated monomyelocytic cells is associated with differentiation and not with the position of the differentiated cells in the cell cycle. Exp. Hematol. 15:700, 1987.

197. Muller, R., Curran, T., Muller, D., and Guilbert, L.: Induction of c-*fos* during monomyelocytic differentiation and macrophage proliferation. Nature 314:546, 1985.

198. Mitchel, R. L., Zokas, L., Schreiber, R. D., and Verman, I. M.: Rapid induction of the expression of proto-oncogene c-*fos*

during human monocytic cell differentiation. Cell 40:209, 1985.

199. Larsson, L.-G., Anton, R., Ivhed, I., Öberg, F., Pettersson, U., and Nilsson, K.: c-*jun* is induced to high continuous expression during differentiation of hematopoietic cells and is regulated independently from c-*fos*. Leuk. Lymphoma 4:193, 1991.

200. Hay, N., Takimoto, M., and Bishop, J. M.: A *FOS* protein is present in a complex that binds a negative regulator of *MYC*. Genes Dev. 3:293, 1989.

201. Johnson, P. F., and McKnight, S. L.: Eukaryotic transcriptional regulatory proteins. Annu. Rev. Biochem. 58:799, 1989.

202. Levine, M., and Hoey, T.: Homeobox proteins as sequence-specific transcription factors. Cell 55:537, 1988.

203. Treisman, J., Gönczy, P., Vashishta, M., Harris, E., and Desplan, C.: A single amino acid can determine the DNA binding specificity of homeodomain proteins. Cell 59:553, 1989.

204. Scheidereit, C., Cromlish, J. A., Gerster, T., Kawakami, K., Balmaceda, C.-G., Currie, R. A., and Roeder, R. G.: A human lymphoid-specific transcription factor that activates immunoglobulin genes is a homeobox protein. Nature 336:551, 1988.

205. Clerc, R. G., Corcoran, L. M., LeBowitz, J. H., Baltimore, D., and Sharp, P. A.: The B-cell–specific Oct-2 protein contains POU box– and homeo box–type domains. Genes Dev. 2:1570, 1988.

206. Mitchell, P. J., and Tjian, R.: Transcriptional regulation in mammalian cells by sequence-specific DNA binding proteins. Science 245:371, 1989.

207. Simeone, A., Mavilio, F., Acampora, D., Giampaolo, A., Faiella, A., Zappavigna, V., D'Esposito, M., Pannese, M., Russo, G., Boncinelli, E., and Peschle, C.: Two human homeobox genes, c1 and c8: Structure analysis and expression in embryonic development. Proc. Natl. Acad. Sci. USA 84:4914, 1987.

208. Lowney, P., Corral, J., Detmer, K., LeBeau, M. M., Deaven, L., Lawrence, H. J., and Largman, C.: A human Hox 1 homeobox gene exhibits myeloid-specific expression of alternative transcripts in human hematopoietic cells. Nucleic Acids Res. 19:3443, 1991.

209. Mathews, C. H., Detmer, K., Boncinelli, E., Lawrence, H. J., and Largman, C.: Erythroid-restricted expression of homeobox genes of the human HOX2 locus. Blood 78:2248, 1991.

210. Magli, M. C., Barba, P., Celetti, A., De Vita, G., Cillo, C., and Boncinelli, E.: Coordinate regulation of HOX genes in human hematopoietic cells. Proc. Natl. Acad. Sci. USA 88:6348, 1991.

211. Shen, W.-F., Largman, C., Lowney, P., Corral, J. C., Detmer, K., Hauser, C. A., Simonitch, T. A., Hack, F. M., and Lawrence, H. J.: Lineage-restricted expression of homeobox-containing genes in human hematopoietic cell lines. Proc. Natl. Acad. Sci. USA 86:8536, 1989.

212. Blatt, C., and Sachs, L.: Deletion of a homeobox gene in myeloid leukemias with a deletion in chromosome 2. Biochem. Biophys. Res. Commun. 156:1265, 1988.

213. Petrini, M., Quaranta, M. T., Testa, U., Samoggia, P., Tritarelli, E., Care, A., Cianetti, L., Valtieri, M., Barletta, C., and Peschle, C.: Expression of selected human HOX-2 genes in B/Y acute lymphoid leukemia and IL-2/IL-1 stimulated NK lymphocytes. Blood (in press).

214. Deguchi, Y., and Kehrl, J. H.: Selective expression of two homeobox genes in CD34-positive cells from human bone marrow. Blood 78:323, 1991.

215. Deguchi, Y., Wilson, G. L., and Kehrl, J. H.: A human homeobox gene, HB24, is important in the proliferation and lineage commitment of hematopoietic progenitor cells. Clin. Res. 40:350A, 1992.

216. Massagué, J.: The transforming growth factor-β family. Annu. Rev. Cell Biol. 6:597, 1990.

217. Zentella, A., Weis, F. M., Ralph, D. A., Laiho, M., and Massagué, J.: Early gene responses to transforming growth

factor–beta in cells lacking growth-suppressive RB function. Mol. Cell Biol. 11:4952, 1991.

218. Laiho, M., DeCaprio, J. A., Ludlow, J. W., Livingston, D. M., and Massagué, J.: Growth inhibition by TGF-beta linked to suppression of retinoblastoma protein phosphorylation. Cell 62:175, 1990.

219. Zhou, D. H., Munster, A., and Winchurch, R. A.: Pathologic concentrations of interleukin 6 inhibit T cell responses via induction of activation of TGF-beta. FASEB J. 5:2582, 1991.

220. Ishibashi, T., Miller, S. L., and Burstein, S. A.: Type beta transforming growth factor is a potent inhibitor of murine megakaryocytopoiesis in vitro. Blood 69:1737, 1987.

221. Ohta, M., Greenberger, J. S., Anklesaria, P., Bassols, A., and Massagué, J.: Two forms of transforming growth factor–β distinguished by multipotential haematopoietic progenitor cells. Nature 329:539, 1987.

222. Hino, M., Tojo, A., Miyazono, K., Urabe, A., and Takaku, F.: Effects of type β transforming growth factors on haematopoietic progenitor cells. Br. J. Haematol. 70:143, 1988.

223. Keller, J. R., Mantel, C., Sing, G. K., Ellingsworth, L. R., Ruscetti, S. K., and Ruscetti, F. W.: Transforming growth factor β1 selectively regulates early murine hematopoietic progenitors and inhibits the growth of IL-3–dependent myeloid leukemia cell lines. J. Exp. Med. 168:737, 1988.

224. Eaves, A. C., and Eaves, C. J.: Maintenance and proliferation control of primitive hemopoietic progenitors in long-term cultures of human marrow cells. Blood Cells 14:355, 1988.

225. Eaves, C. J., Cashman, J. D., Kay, R. J., Dougherty, G. J., Otsuka, T., Gaboury, L. A., Hogge, D. E., Lansdorp, P. M., Eaves, A. C., and Humphries, R. K.: Mechanisms that regulate the cell cycle status of very primitive hematopoietic cells in long-term human marrow cultures. II. Analysis of positive and negative regulators produced by stromal cells within the adherent layer. Blood 78:110, 1991.

226. Cashman, J. D., Eaves, A. C., Raines, E. W., Ross, R., and Eaves, C. J.: Mechanisms that regulate the cell cycle status of very primitive hematopoietic cells in long-term human marrow cultures. I. Stimulatory role of a variety of mesenchymal cell activators and inhibitory role of TGF-beta. Blood 75:96, 1990.

227. Jansen, R., Damia, G., Usui, N., Keller, J., Futami, H., Goey, H., Back, T. T., Longo, D. L., Ruscetti, F. W., and Wiltrout, R. H.: Effects of recombinant transforming growth factor–β1 on hematologic recovery after treatment of mice with 5-fluorouracil. J. Immunol. 147:3342, 1991.

228. Koyasu, S., Miyajima, A., Arai, K., Okajima, F., Ui, M., and Yahara, I.: Growth regulation of multi-factor-dependent myeloid cell lines: IL-4, TGF-β and pertussis toxin modulate IL-3– or GM-CSF–induced growth by controlling cell cycle length. Cell Struct. Funct. 14:459, 1989.

229. Jacobsen, S. E. W., Ruscetti, F. W., Dubois, C. M., Lee, J., Boone, T. C., and Keller, J. R.: Transforming growth factor–β trans-modulates the expression of colony stimulating factor receptors on murine hematopoietic progenitor cell lines. Blood 77:1706, 1991.

230. Musso, T., Espinoza-Delgado, I., Pulkki, K., Gusella, G. L., Longo, D. L., and Varesio, L.: Transforming growth factor β downregulates interleukin-1 (IL-1)–induced IL-6 production by human monocytes. Blood 76:2466, 1990.

231. Elias, J. A., Lentz, V., and Cummings, P. J.: Transforming growth factor–beta regulation of IL-6 production by unstimulated and IL-1–stimulated human fibroblasts [published erratum appears in J Immunol 1991 Aug 15;147(4):1460]. J. Immunol. 146:3437, 1991.

232. Shalaby, M. R., Waage, A., and Espevik, T.: Cytokine regulation of interleukin 6 production by human endothelial cells. Cell. Immunol. 121:372, 1989.

233. D'Angeac, A. D., Dornand, J., Emonds-Alt, X., Jullien, P., Garcia-Sanz, J. A., and Erard, F.: Transforming growth factor type beta 1 (TGF-beta 1) down-regulates interleukin-2 production and up-regulates interleukin-2 receptor expression in a thymoma cell line. J. Cell. Physiol. 147:460, 1991.

234. Espevik, T., Waage, A., Faxvaag, A., and Shalaby, M. R.:

Regulation of interleukin-2 and interleukin-6 production from T-cells: Involvement of interleukin-1 beta and transforming growth factor-beta. Cell. Immunol. 126:47, 1990.

235. Broxmeyer, H. E., Lu, L., Cooper, S., Schwall, R. H., Mason, A. J., and Nikolics, K.: Selective and indirect modulation of human multipotential and erythroid hematopoietic progenitor cell proliferation by recombinant human activin and inhibin. Proc. Natl. Acad. Sci. USA 85:9052, 1988.

236. Mathews, L. S., and Vale, W. W.: Expression cloning of an activin receptor, a predicted transmembrane serine kinase. Cell 65:973, 1991.

237. Yu, J., Shao, L. E., Lemas, V., Yu, A. L., Vaughan, J., Rivier, J., and Vale, W.: Importance of FSH-releasing protein and inhibin in erythrodifferentiation. Nature 330:765, 1987.

238. Essner, R., Rhoades, K., McBride, W. H., Morton, D. L., and Economou, J. S.: IL-4 down-regulates IL-1 and TNF gene expression in human monocytes. J. Immunol. 142:3857, 1989.

239. Jelinek, D. F., and Lipsky, P. E.: Inhibitory influence of IL-4 on human B cell responsiveness. J. Immunol. 141:164, 1988.

240. DeFrance, T., Vanbervliet, B., Aubry, J.-P., and Banchereau, J.: Interleukin 4 inhibits the proliferation but not the differentiation of activated human B cells in response to interleukin 2. J. Exp. Med. 168:1321, 1988.

241. Te Velde, A. A., Huijbens, R. J. F., Heije, K., De Vries, J. E., and Figdor, C. G.: Interleukin-4 (IL-4) inhibits secretion of IL-1β, tumor necrosis factor α, and IL-6 by human monocytes. Blood 76:1392, 1990.

242. Jansen, J. H., Wientjens, G.-J. H. M., Fibbe, W. E., Willemze, R., and Kluin-Nelemans, H. C.: Inhibition of human macrophage colony formation by interleukin 4. J. Exp. Med. 170:577, 1989.

243. Bendelac, A., and Schwartz, R. H.: CD4+ and CD8+ T cells acquire specific lymphokine secretion potentials during thymic maturation. Nature 353:68, 1991.

244. Rousset, F., Garcia, E., DeFrance, T., Peronne, C., Vezzio, N., Hsu, D. H., Kastelein, R., Moore, K. W., and Banchereau, J.: Interleukin 10 is a potent growth and differentiation factor for activated human B lymphocytes. Proc. Natl. Acad. Sci. USA 89:1890, 1992.

245. Thompson-Snipes, L., Dhar, V., Bond, M. W., Mosmann, T. R., Moore, K. W., and Rennick, D. M.: Interleukin 10: A novel stimulatory factor for mast cells and their progenitors. J. Exp. Med. 173:507, 1991.

246. Fiorentino, D. F., Zlotnik, A., Mosmann, T. R., Howard, M., and O'Garra, A.: IL-10 inhibits cytokine production by activated macrophages. J. Immunol. 147:3815, 1991.

247. Ralph, P., Nakoinz, I., Sampson-Johannes, A., Fong, S., Lowe, D., Min, H.-Y., and Lin, L.: IL-10, T lymphocyte inhibitor of human blood cell production of IL-1 and tumor necrosis factor. J. Immunol. 148:808, 1991.

248. Taga, K., and Tosato, G.: IL-10 inhibits human T cell proliferation and IL-2 production. J. Immunol. 148:1143, 1992.

249. Peçanha, L. M. T., Snapper, C. M., Lees, A., and Mond, J. J.: Lymphokine control of type 2 antigen response: IL-10 inhibits IL-5- but not IL-2-induced Ig secretion by T cell–independent antigens. J. Immunol. 148:3427, 1992.

250. Oswald, I. P., Gazzinelli, R. T., Sher, A., and James, S. L.: IL-10 synergizes with IL-4 and transforming growth factor-β to inhibit macrophage cytotoxic activity. J. Immunol. 148:3578, 1992.

251. Gentile, P., Byer, D., and Pelus, L. M.: In vivo modulation of murine myelopoiesis following intravenous administration of prostaglandin E2. Blood 62:1100, 1983.

252. Pelus, L. M., Broxmeyer, H. E., Kurland, J. I., and Moore, M. A.: Regulation of macrophage and granulocyte proliferation: Specificities of prostaglandin E and lactoferrin. J. Exp. Med. 150:277, 1979.

253. Pelus, L. M.: Blockade of prostaglandin biosynthesis in intact mice dramatically augments the expansion of committed myeloid progenitor cells (colony-forming units–granulocyte, macrophage) after acute administration of recombinant human IL-1 alpha. J. Immunol. 143:4171, 1989.

254. Pelus, L. M., Levi, E., and Welte, K.: The response of human

marrow colony-forming units–granulocyte and macrophage to inhibition by prostaglandin E and acidic isoferritins is associated with expression of MHC class II antigens and requires the participation of a CD8+ T lymphokine. J. Immunol. 141:1658, 1988.

255. Pelus, L. M., Ottmann, O. G., and Nocka, K. H.: Synergistic inhibition of human marrow granulocyte-macrophage progenitor cells by prostaglandin E and recombinant interferon-α, -β, and -τ and an effect mediated by tumor necrosis factor. J. Immunol. 140:479, 1988.

256. Danis, V. A., Kulesz, A. J., Nelson, D. S., and Brooks, P. M.: Cytokine regulation of human monocyte interleukin-1 (IL-1) production in vitro. Enhancement of IL-1 production by interferon (IFN)gamma, tumour necrosis factor-alpha, IL-2 and IL-1, and inhibition by IFN-alpha. Clin. Exp. Immunol. 80:435, 1990.

257. Galvani, D. W., and Cawley, J. C.: The current status of interferon α in haemic malignancy. Blood Rev. 4:175, 1990.

258. Ferran, C., Dy, M., Sheehan, K., Schreiber, R., Grau, G., Bluestone, J., Bach, J.-F., and Chatenoud, L.: Cascade modulation by anti-tumor necrosis factor monoclonal antibody of interferon-gamma, interleukin 3 and interleukin 6 release after triggering of the CD3/T cell receptor activation pathway. Eur. J. Immunol. 21:2349, 1991.

259. Osgood, E. E.: A unifying concept of the etiology of the leukemias, lymphomas, and cancers. J. Natl. Cancer Inst. 18:155, 1957.

260. Broxmeyer, H. E., Smithyman, A., Eger, R. R., Meyers, P. A., and de Sousa, M.: Identification of lactoferrin as the granulocyte-derived inhibitor of colony-stimulating activity production. J. Exp. Med. 148:1052, 1978.

261. Gentile, P., and Broxmeyer, H. E.: Suppression of mouse myelopoiesis by administration of human lactoferrin in vivo and the comparative action of human transferrin. Blood 61:982, 1983.

262. Broxmeyer, H. E., Williams, D. E., Cooper, S., Shadduck, R. K., Gillis, S., Waheed, A., Urdal, D. L., and Bicknell, D. C.: Comparative effects in vivo of recombinant murine interleukin-3, natural murine colony-stimulating factor-1, and recombinant murine granulocyte-macrophage colony-stimulating factor on myelopoiesis in mice. J. Clin. Invest. 79:721, 1987.

263. Bagby, G. C., Rigas, V. D., Bennett, R. M., Vandenbark, A. A., and Garewal, H. S.: Interaction of lactoferrin, monocytes, and T-lymphocyte subsets in the regulation of steady-state granulopoiesis in vitro. J. Clin. Invest. 68:56, 1981.

264. Zucali, J. R., Broxmeyer, H. E., Levy, D., and Morse, C.: Lactoferrin decreases monocyte-induced fibroblast production of myeloid colony-stimulating activity by suppressing monocyte release of interleukin-1. Blood 74:1531, 1989.

265. Broxmeyer, H. E., Jacobsen, N., Kurland, J., Mendelsohn, N., and Moore, A. S.: In vitro suppression of normal granulocytic stem cells by inhibitory activity derived from human leukemia cells. J. Natl. Cancer Inst. 60:497, 1978.

266. Broxmeyer, H. E., Grossbard, E., Jacobsen, N., and Moore, M. A. S.: Evidence for a proliferative advantage of human leukemic colony-forming cells in-vitro. J. Natl. Cancer Inst. 60:513, 1978.

267. Broxmeyer, H. E., Bognacki, J., Dorner, M. H., and DeSousa, M.: Identification of leukemia associated inhibitory activity as acidic isoferritins. A regulatory role for acidic isoferritins in the production of granulocytes and macrophages. J. Exp. Med. 153:1426, 1981.

268. Broxmeyer, H. E., Cooper, S., Levi, S., and Arosio, P.: Mutated recombinant human heavy-chain ferritins and myelosuppression in vitro and in vivo: A link between ferritin ferroxidase activity and biological function. Proc. Natl. Acad. Sci. USA 88:770, 1991.

269. Lu, L., Broxmeyer, H. E., Moore, M. A., Sheridan, A. P., and Gentile, P.: Abnormalities in myelopoietic regulatory interactions with acidic isoferritins and lactoferrin in mice infected with Friend virus complex: Association with altered expression of Ia antigens on effector and responding cells. Blood 65:91, 1985.

270. Goeddel, D. V., Aggarwal, B. B., Gray, P. W., Leung, D. W., Nedwin, G. E., Palladino, M. A., Patton, J. S., Pennica, D., Shepard, H. M., Sugarman, B. J., and Wong, G. H. W.: Tumor necrosis factors: Gene structure and biological activities. *In* Molecular Biology of Homo Sapiens. Vol. LI. Cold Spring Harbor, N.Y., Cold Spring Harbor Laboratory, 1986, pp. 597–610.

271. Roodman, G. D.: Mechanisms of erythroid suppression in the anemia of chronic disease. Blood Cells 13:171, 1987.

272. Fandrey, J., and Jelkmann, W. E.: Interleukin-1 and tumor necrosis factor-alpha inhibit erythropoietin production in vitro. Ann. N.Y. Acad. Sci. 628:250, 1991.

273. Moldawer, L. L., Marano, M. A., Wei, H., Fong, Y., Silen, M. L., Kuo, G., Manogue, K. R., Vlassara, H., Cohen, H., Cerami, A., and Lowry, S. F.: Cachectin/tumor necrosis factor-α alters red blood cell kinetics and induces anemia in vivo. FASEB J. 3:1637, 1989.

274. Dainiak, N.: Surface membrane–associated regulation of cell assembly, differentiation, and growth. Blood 78:264, 1991.

275. Streeter, P. R., Berg, E. L., Rouse, B. T. N., Bargatze, R. F., and Butcher, E. C.: A tissue-specific endothelial cell molecule involved in lymphocyte homing. Nature 331:41, 1988.

276. Nakache, M., Berg, E. L., Streeter, P. R., and Butcher, E. C.: The mucosal vascular addressin is a tissue-specific endothelial cell adhesion molecule for circulating lymphocytes. Nature 337:179, 1989.

277. Berg, E. L., Goldstein, L. A., Jutila, M. A., Nakache, M., Picker, L. J., Streeter, P. R., Wu, N. W., Zhou, D., and Butcher, E. C.: Homing receptors and vascular addressins: Cell adhesion molecules that direct lymphocyte traffic. Immunol. Rev. 108:5, 1989.

278. Goldstein, L. A., Zhou, D. F., Picker, L. J., Minty, C. N., Bargatze, R. F., Ding, J. F., and Butcher, E. C.: A human lymphocyte homing receptor, the hermes antigen, is related to cartilage proteoglycan core and link proteins. Cell 56:1063, 1989.

279. Freedman, A. S., Munro, J. M., Rice, G. E., Bevilacqua, M. P., Morimoto, C., McIntyre, B. W., Rhynhart, K., Pober, J. S., and Nadler, L. M.: Adhesion of human B cells to germinal centers in vitro involves VLA-4 and INCAM-110. Science 249:1030, 1990.

280. Long, M. W.: Blood cell cytoadhesion molecules. Exp. Hematol. 20:288, 1992.

281. Hemler, M. E., Elices, M. J., Parker, C., and Takada, Y.: Structure of the integrin VLA-4 and its cell-cell and cell-matrix adhesion functions. Immunol. Rev. 114:45, 1990.

282. Williams, D. A., Rios, M., Stephens, C., and Patel, V. P.: Fibronectin and VLA-4 in haematopoietic stem cell–microenvironment interactions. Nature 352:438, 1991.

283. Miyake, K., Weissman, I. L., Greenberger, J. S., and Kincade, P. W.: Evidence for a role of the integrin VLA-4 in lympho-hemopoiesis. J. Exp. Med. 173:599, 1991.

284. Elices, M. J., Osborn, L., Takada, Y., Crouse, C., Luhowskyj, S., Hemler, M. E., and Lobb, R. R.: VCAM-1 on activated endothelium interacts with the leukocyte integrin VLA-4 at a site distinct from the VLA-4/fibronectin binding site. Cell 60:577, 1990.

285. Gordon, M. Y., Riley, G. P., Watt, S. M., and Greaves, M. F.: Compartmentalization of a haematopoietic growth factor (GM-CSF) by glycosaminoglycans in the bone marrow microenvironment. Nature 326:403, 1987.

286. Allen, T. D., and Testa, N. G.: Cellular interactions in erythroblastic islands in long term bone marrow cultures, as studied by time lapse video. Blood Cells 17:29, 1991.

287. Papayannopoulou, T., and Abkowitz, J.: Biology of erythropoiesis, erythroid differentiation, and maturation. *In* Hoffman, R., Benz, E. J., Shattil, S. J., Furie, B., and Cohen, H. J. (eds.): Hematology: Basic Principles and Practice. New York, Churchill Livingstone, 1991, pp. 252–263.

288. Mooradian, D. L., Lucas, R. C., Weatherbee, J. A., and Furcht, L. T.: Transforming growth factor-β1 binds to immobilized fibronectin. J. Cell. Biochem. 41:189, 1989.

289. Anklesaria, P., Kase, K., Glowacki, J., Holland, C. A., Sakakeeny, M. A., Wright, J. A., FitzGerald, T. J., Lee, C. Y., and Greenberger, J. S.: Engraftment of a clonal bone marrow stromal cell line in vivo stimulates hematopoietic recovery from total body irradiation. Proc. Natl. Acad. Sci. USA 84:7681, 1987.

290. Simmons, P. J., Przepiorka, D., Thomas, E. D., and Torok-Storb, B.: Host origin of marrow stromal cells following allogeneic bone marrow transplantation. Nature 328:429, 1987.

291. Lennon, J. E., and Micklem, H. S.: Stromal cells in long-term murine bone marrow culture: FACS studies and origin of stromal cells in radiation chimeras. Exp. Hematol. 14:287, 1986.

292. Bertoncello, I., Bradley, T. R., Hodgson, G. S., and Dunlop, J. M.: The resolution, enrichment, and organization of normal bone marrow high proliferative potential colony-forming cell subsets on the basis of rhodamine-123 fluorescence. Exp. Hematol. 19:174, 1991.

293. Mukaida, N., Shairoo, M., and Matsushima, K.: Genomic structure of the human monocyte-derived neutrophil chemotactic factor IL-8. J. Immunol. 143:1366, 1989.

294. Bevilacqua, M. P., Stengelin, S., Gimbrone, M. A., and Seed, B.: Endothelial leukocyte adhesion molecule 1: An inducible receptor for neutrophils related to complement regulatory proteins and lectins. Science 243:1160, 1989.

295. Huang, S., and Terstappen, L. W. M. M.: Formation of haematopoietic microenvironment and haematopoietic stem cells from single human bone marrow stem cells. Nature 360:745, 1992.

SECTION II

RED CELLS AND ERYTHROPOIESIS

Hemoglobin Switching

George Stamatoyannopoulos and Arthur W. Nienhuis

INTRODUCTION

Hemoglobin production in humans is characterized by two major "switches" in the hemoglobin composition of red cells.[1–15] During the first 3 months of gestation, human red cells contain embryonic hemoglobins, whereas during the last 6 months of gestation, red cells contain predominantly fetal hemoglobin. The major transition from fetal to adult hemoglobin occurs in the perinatal period, and by the end of the first year, red cells have a hemoglobin composition that subsequently remains stable. In adult red cells, the major hemoglobin is hemoglobin A (Hb A), but there are small amounts of Hb A_2 and Hb F. Only a few species (primates, sheep, goats, and bovids) exhibit embryonic-to-fetal and fetal-to-adult hemoglobin

switches comparable to those found in man. All other species that have hemoglobin as the oxygen-carrying pigment (birds, amphibians, reptiles, and mammals) exhibit only one switch from embryonic to adult hemoglobin.[2]

The general organization of the human globin gene clusters, the genes expressed, and the hemoglobins produced during the embryonic, fetal, and adult developmental periods are shown in Figure 4–1. The globin genes are arranged from 5' to 3' according to the order of their expression during ontogeny. Two genes of the β locus, the $^G\gamma$ and $^A\gamma$, are structurally identical products of gene duplication and gene conversion. The two types of γ chains can be distinguished only at amino acid position 136, where the $^G\gamma$ gene encodes for glycine while the $^A\gamma$ gene encodes

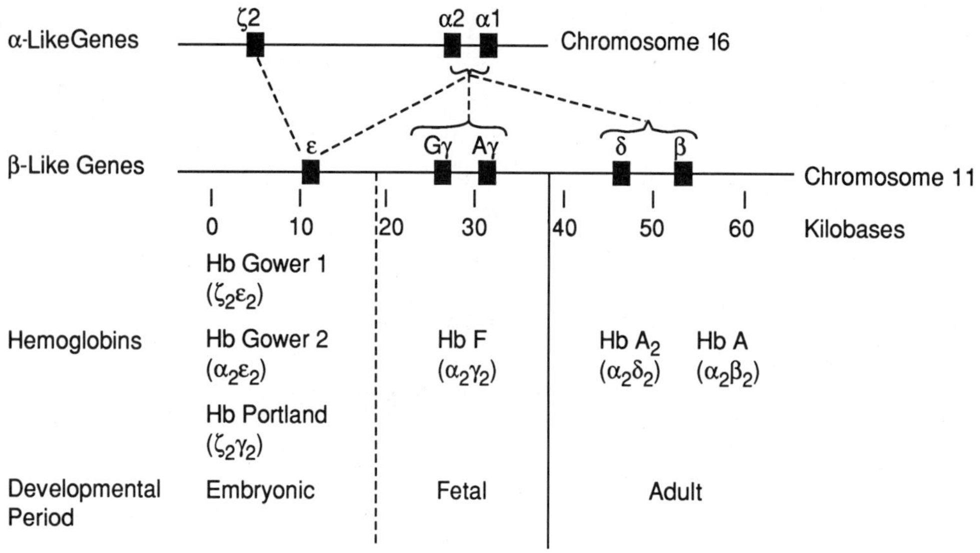

FIGURE 4–1. Organization of the human globin genes and hemoglobins produced during each stage of human development.

for alanine.[16] The relative synthesis of $^G\gamma$ and $^A\gamma$ chains changes during the perinatal switch from fetal to adult hemoglobin; the $^G\gamma/^A\gamma$ ratio of 3:1 found in fetal red cells becomes 2:3 in adult red cells.[17–19] Red cells containing Hb F exhibit a higher oxygen affinity than do cells containing Hb A, mainly because Hb F does not bind 2,3-diphosphoglycerate (2,3-DPG).[11] (See Chapter 6.) The higher oxygen affinity of fetal blood compared with maternal blood may facilitate oxygen transport across the placenta. This differential in oxygen affinity is not obligatory, however, as normal infants have been born of mothers who have a high-affinity hemoglobin variant.[20]

HEMOGLOBIN PRODUCTION DURING DEVELOPMENT

Erythropoiesis in the human begins in the yolk sac, but at about 5 weeks of gestation the site of hematopoiesis changes from the yolk sac islands to the liver. The liver remains the predominant site of erythropoi-esis in the fetus until about the twentieth week of gestation (Fig. 4–2). Hematopoiesis subsequently occurs in the spleen and the bone marrow, and by the time of birth the bone marrow is the main hematopoietic organ.[21–25]

Shifts in the site of erythropoiesis are characteristic during development of all species. In amphibians, the first red cells arise from the ventral blood islands of the embryo. Subsequently, the kidneys become erythropoietically active, and ultimately the liver becomes the main erythropoietic organ in amphibian larvae.[26–29a] In the juvenile frog, the liver is the primary erythropoietic site, whereas in the adult frog erythropoiesis resides in the bone marrow.[28, 29a, 30, 31] In chickens, precursors to the erythroid series are found in the primary mesenchyme, whereas descendants of these precursors become part of the yolk sac; late in embryonic life and after hatching, the bone marrow becomes the predominant site of erythropoiesis.[32, 33]

In all species, the shifting sites of erythropoiesis coincide with changes in the hemoglobin composition of red cells and also with changes in other morpholog-

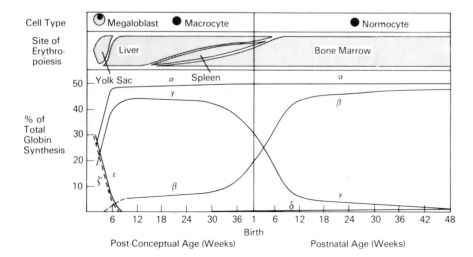

FIGURE 4–2. Changes in globin chain production, sites of hematopoiesis, red cell morphology, and size of erythrocytes during the course of development. (From Wood, D. G.: Haemoglobin synthesis during human fetal development. Brit. Med. Bull. 32:282, 1976; with permission.)

ical and biochemical characteristics. In the human, embryonic erythrocytes are very large nucleated cells (average volume about 200 μ^3). The volume of human fetal red cells is approximately 125 μ^3, whereas adult red cells are significantly smaller,[21, 25] with an average volume of 80 μ^3. The membrane carbohydrate profile also changes strikingly.[34] For example, the unbranched carbohydrate of the i antigenic determinant is found on fetal red cells, whereas adult red cells have the branched structure reflecting the acquisition of a branching enzyme, present in adult red cells but absent from the red cells of the fetus. (See also Chapter 8.) The i antigenic determinant may be detected on adult red cells,[35] but these red cells differ from fetal red cells in that they also fully express the I antigenic determinant. The activity of several glycolytic enzymes is lower in fetal red cells than in those of adult individuals, and characteristic changes in isozyme profiles, such as those exhibited by carbonic anhydrase, may also be observed.[36–38]

In the human, the switch from ε to γ globin production begins very early in gestation, as Hb F is readily detected in 5-week human embryos,[39, 40] and it is completed well before 10 weeks of gestation.[39, 41] Staining of embryonic and fetal erythroblasts from 38 to 60 day human fetuses shows that ε globin expression is restricted in yolk sac cells, whereas both γ and β globins are restricted to erythroblasts of liver origin[42, 42a] β Globin expression starts early in human development, and small amounts of Hb A can be detected by biosynthetic or immunochemical methods even in the smallest human fetuses studied.[42–44] γ Gene expression in the fetus is approximately 50 times higher than β gene expression. Double immunofluorescent staining of erythroblasts and fetal red cells shows that γ and β globin are coexpressed in the same cell.[42a] β Chain synthesis increases progressively during intrauterine development, to approximately 10 per cent of γ chain synthesis by 30 to 35 weeks. Then β chain synthesis increases sharply and γ chain production falls steadily. At birth, Hb F comprises 60 to 80 per cent of the total hemoglobin. In the 16 to 20 week old infant, Hb F constitutes about 3 per cent of all hemoglobin synthesized.[45] It takes about 2 years to reach the level of Hb F that is characteristic of adult red cells.

Only 0.5 to 1 per cent of the total hemoglobin in human adult red cells is Hb F; it is restricted to a few erythrocytes called "F cells" (Fig. 4–3). Approximately 3 to 7 per cent of erythrocytes are F cells, and each contains about 4 to 8 picograms (pg) of Hb F, along with 22 to 26 pg of Hb A.[46, 47] Both the number of F cells and the amount of Hb F in each F cell may be increased in various acquired and genetic conditions characterized by elevated Hb F levels.

The mouse has been used extensively to study the regulation of globin gene expression by creation of transgenic animals. In this species, the embryonic to adult switch takes place at 10½ days of gestation.[48, 49] The yolk sac erythrocytes of the embryo contain ζ and α globin chains, the two embryonic globins—βh1 and

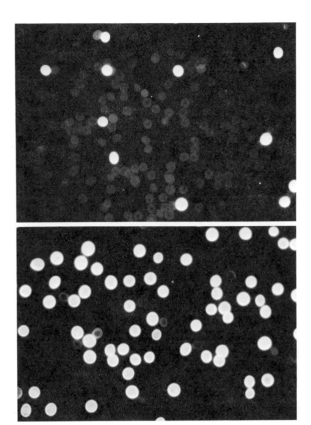

FIGURE 4–3. Detection of F cells in the blood from an adult, using staining with fluorescent anti-γ globin chain monoclonal antibodies. *Upper*, Normal adult. *Lower*, Juvenile chronic myeloid leukemia (CML).

εγ—but no adult β globin chains. The definitive fetal liver erythroblasts of the fetus produce α globin and the two adult-type β globins, β major and β minor. There is no hemoglobin in the mouse expressed with the pattern of human fetal hemoglobin.

MUTATIONS AFFECTING SWITCHING

Many insights into the regulation of hemoglobin switching have been acquired by study of mutations that increase fetal hemoglobin production during adult life. These mutations are clinically relevant, since increased synthesis of Hb F in individuals with sickle cell anemia or β thalassemia reduces disease severity. More than 50 such mutations have been discovered.[50, 51] The phenotypic classification of these mutations will be described briefly (Tables 4–1 to 4–3). Insights that specific mutations have provided into globin gene regulation will be presented in subsequent sections.

Several parameters may be used in classifying these mutations. Many reflect deletion of a portion of the β globin gene cluster, whereas others reflect point mutations within or potentially outside the cluster. These are called "deletion" (see Table 4–2) and "non-dele-

TABLE 4–1. PHENOTYPES OF $^G\gamma^A\gamma$ HPFH AND $^G\gamma^A\gamma$ ($\delta\beta$)^0 THALASSEMIA HETEROZYGOTES

	HPFH	δβ THALASSEMIA
Red cell morphology	Normal	Abnormal
Mean corpuscular hemoglobin (MCH)	Near normal	Decreased
Hematocrit	Normal	Slightly decreased
Hb F (%)	15–35	4–18
Distribution of Hb F in red cells	Pancellular	Heterocellular

tion" (see Table 4–3) mutations, respectively. Among both the deletion and the non-deletion classes are mutations that result in a more or less uniform distribution of Hb F in peripheral blood cells (pancellular) and those that result in a non-uniform increase in Hb F (heterocellular). Mutations that cause a heterocellular increase in Hb F may lead to an increase in the percentage of F cells and/or an increase in the average amount of Hb F per F cell.[52] Some mutations result in

an increase in $^G\gamma$ globin only, others in an increase in $^A\gamma$ globin only, and still others in a more or less equal increase in both globins. Finally, mutations that increase Hb F production may be categorized depending on whether they are characterized by hypochromic, microcytic, or morphologically normal red cells in heterozygous individuals (see Table 4–1). The first are the thalassemia mutations, whereas the second are called the "hereditary persistence of fetal hemoglobin" (HPFH) type of mutations.

Much of the older literature on mutations that increase Hb F synthesis is highly descriptive, with classifications relying on phenotypic features rather than molecular characterization. For example, when the HPFH-type mutations were recognized, an African form[53] and a Greek form[54] were defined. The African variety was subsequently subdivided into a common variant in which both $^G\gamma$ and $^A\gamma$ chains were present and a rare variant exhibiting only $^G\gamma$ chains ($^G\gamma$-HPFH).[55] The Hb F in Greek HPFH contains predom-

TABLE 4–2. DELETION MUTATIONS OF THE β GLOBIN GENE CLUSTER

TYPE	ETHNIC GROUP	Hb F LEVEL IN HETEROZYGOTES (%)	REFERENCES
A. Hereditary persistence of fetal hemoglobin (HPFH)			
1	American black	20–30	59–64
2	Black (Ghana)	20–30	59, 61–66
3	Indian	22–23	66–68
4	Italian	14–30	69
5	Italian	16–20	70
6	Kenyan (Hb Kenya)	5–8	74–77
B. (δβ)^0 thalassemia			
1	Japanese	5–7	85, 86
2	Corfu	<1	87–90
3	Spanish	5–15	59, 81, 82
4	Black	25	83
5	Eastern Europe	13–18	84
6	Laotian	11.5	91
7	Thai	10	94
8	Sicilian	5–15	65, 78–80
9	Macedonian	7–14	92, 93
10	Mediterranean (Hb Lepore)	1–5	95–99
C. ($^A\gamma\delta\beta$)^0 thalassemia			
1	Indian	10–18	100, 101, 104
2	Turkish	10–14	60, 70, 103, 104
3	American black	6–21	65, 102
4	German	10–13	108
5	Belgian	14–15	111
6	Malaysian (1)	Unknown	104
7	Cantonese	19–20	109
8	Malaysian (2)	Unknown	105
9	Yunnanese	9–17	110
10	Thai	17–23	112, 113
11	Chinese	9–20	106, 107
D. ($\gamma\delta\beta$)^0 thalassemia			
1	Hispanic		114
2	English		115
3	Dutch		116–118
4	Anglo-Saxon		60, 117, 119
5	Mexican		120
6	Scotch-Irish		121
7	Yugoslavian		122
8	Canadian		122
E. β^0 thalassemia			
1	Indian	Normal	123–126
2	American black	7.0–7.9	127, 128
3	Dutch	4–11	129, 130
4	Turkish	2.7–3.3	131, 132
	Jordanian		133
5	Czech	3.3–5.7	134
	Canadian		
6	Black		135

TABLE 4–3. NON-DELETION FORMS OF HPFH

TYPE AND RACIAL GROUP	MUTATION IN GLOBIN GENE	% Hb F in HETEROZYGOTES	REFERENCES
$^G\gamma$ HPFH			
Japanese	$^G\gamma$–114 C to T	11–14	136
Black	$^G\gamma$–175 T to C	20–30	137
Sardinian	$^G\gamma$–175 T to C	17–21	138
Black	$^G\gamma$–202 C to G	15–25	139
$^A\gamma$ HPFH			
Georgia	$^A\gamma$–114 C to T	3–6.5	140
Black	$^A\gamma$–114 to –102 deleted	30–32	141
Greek	$^A\gamma$–117 G to A	10–20	54, 142, 143
Sardinian	$^A\gamma$–117 G to A	12–16	144
Black	$^A\gamma$–117 G to A	11–16	145
Black	$^A\gamma$–175 T to C	36–41	146
Brazilian	$^A\gamma$–195 C to G	4.5–7	147
Southern Italian	$^A\gamma$–196 C to T	12–16	148
Chinese	$^A\gamma$–196 C to T	14–21	149, 150
British	$^A\gamma$–198 T to C	3.5–10	151, 152
Black	$^A\gamma$–202 C to T	1.6–3.9	153

inantly $^A\gamma$ chains[56]—hence this variant was named "$^A\gamma$HPFH." The African $^G\gamma^A\gamma$ and $^G\gamma$ variants as well as the Greek $^A\gamma$ variant display a "pancellular" distribution of Hb F, whereas other forms of HPFH display heterocellular distributions.[57] The term "$\delta\beta$ thalassemia" was reserved for the form of thalassemia in which heterozygotes have relatively high levels of Hb F and normal levels of Hb A_2. (See Chapter 5.) Because of its high F phenotype, this condition was initially called "F thalassemia."[58] Subsequent molecular characterization has revealed an extraordinary complexity to these mutations.

Deletion Mutations

Summarized in Table 4–2 and Figures 4–4 and 4–5 are the general features of the deletion mutations of the β globin gene cluster. Also see Chapter 5 and Figure 4–18 with accompanying text for a discussion of these mutations. More detailed consideration of the molecular mechanisms by which these mutations may alter Hb F synthesis is presented in later sections of this chapter.

DELETION HPFH. $^G\gamma^A\gamma$ HPFH is found among individuals of African, Indian, and Italian descent.[59–70]

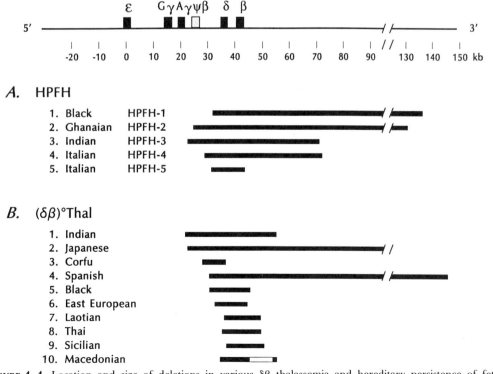

FIGURE 4–4. Location and size of deletions in various $\delta\beta$ thalassemia and hereditary persistence of fetal hemoglobin (HPFH) mutants.

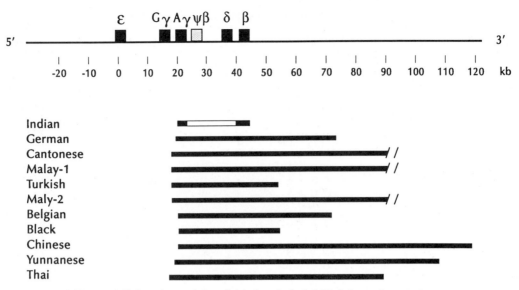

FIGURE 4–5. Location and size of deletions in $^{G}\gamma(^{A}\gamma\delta\beta)^{0}$ thalassemia mutations.

With these mutations, there is total absence of δ and β globin synthesis in *cis* to the HPFH determinant. Both $^{G}\gamma^{A}\gamma$ globins are produced in almost equal proportion. Heterozygotes produce 20 to 30 per cent Hb F and are clinically and hematologically normal. Although homozygotes were found to produce 100 per cent Hb F,[71, 72] their red cells failed to show other properties of fetal erythrocytes. Such individuals are healthy, although their hemoglobin levels and red cell counts are higher than normal, reflecting the increased oxygen affinity of blood in which the red cells contain only Hb F. (See Chapter 6.) The only additional hematological manifestations in homozygotes are microcytosis, hypochromia (mean corpuscular hemoglobin [MCH] of 23 to 37 pg), and an increased α/γ biosynthetic ratio (1.3:1.4).[73] These findings suggest that the γ genes of HPFH deletion mutations are functioning at a lower level than the normal γ genes of the fetus. Structural studies have identified five deletions producing $^{G}\gamma^{A}\gamma$ HPFH phenotypes (see Table 4–2 and Fig. 4–4).

A mutation designated Kenya HPFH reflects an unequal crossing over between the $^{A}\gamma$ gene and the β gene that deletes the $^{A}\gamma$ to β region and leads to the production of a new fusion globin. (See also Chapter 5.) The $(^{A}\gamma\beta)$ chain of Hb Kenya is a fusion protein containing amino acids 1 to 80 of the $^{A}\gamma$ chain and 81 to 146 of the β chain.[74–77] Heterozygotes produce 7 to 25 per cent Hb Kenya and 5 to 15 per cent Hb F; all of the hemoglobin contains $^{G}\gamma$ chains. The Hb F has a pancellular distribution. Red cell morphology and hematological indices are normal.

DELETION THALASSEMIAS. The clinical features of individuals with HPFH may be contrasted with those exhibited by individuals with $(\delta\beta)^{0}$ thalassemia (see Table 4–2 and Fig. 4–4). The most common variant is found in Mediterranean populations.[65, 78–80] Heterozygotes produce from 1 to 2 per cent to 10 to 15 per cent Hb F, which is heterogeneously distributed among the red cells. Heterozygotes also have very mild anemia and abnormalities of red cell morphology. There is total absence of δ and β globin chain production in *cis* to the thalassemia determinant, so that homozygotes produce only Hb F. Hemoglobin levels of homozygotes usually range from 8 to 11 g/dl, and the α/γ biosynthetic ratio averages 2.4:1. The "thalassemic" hematological findings in heterozygotes and clinical manifestations in the homozygotes indicate that production of γ chains is inefficient and cannot fully compensate for the lack of β globin. Two types of δβ thalassemia are distinguished, depending on the types of γ globin chains present in Hb F: $^{G}\gamma^{A}\gamma(\delta\beta)^{0}$ thalassemia, in which both $^{G}\gamma$ and $^{A}\gamma$ globin chains are present in Hb F, usually in a 1:1 ratio; and $^{G}\gamma(^{A}\gamma\delta\beta)^{0}$ thalassemia, in which only $^{G}\gamma$ globin chains are found in Hb F.

Several mutations that cause $(\delta\beta)^{0}$ thalassemia have been analyzed structurally, and an extensive variability in the 5′ and 3′ breakpoints and in the size of deletions has been discovered (see Fig. 4–4). The deletions in the Spanish and Japanese δβ mutants are even larger than those of HPFH-1 and -2, whereas other mutants delete the δ and β genes and limited flanking upstream and downstream sequences. With very few exceptions (see later discussion), neither the size of deletions nor the location of breakpoints has provided clues to why the $^{G}\gamma^{A}\gamma$ HPFH and the $^{G}\gamma^{A}\gamma(\delta\beta)^{0}$ thalassemia deletion mutants produce different phenotypes. There is considerable variation, among mutants, in the level of Hb F production in heterozygotes and in the severity of hematological manifestation in homozygotes, indicating that individual mutations may variably affect the efficiency of γ gene expression in the adult.[78–99]

The $(^{A}\gamma\delta\beta)^{0}$ thalassemias are found in several ethnic groups but are more common among Asiatic Indians and Chinese.[100–113] Heterozygotes produce 5 to 16 per cent Hb F. Homozygotes produce Hb F that contains only $^{G}\gamma$ chains. The 11 mutants that have been characterized so far display considerable variation in both the 5' and 3' breakpoints (see Table 4–2 and Fig. 4–5). There are also differences in the efficiency of γ globin production among mutants. Thus, the Chinese and Yunnanese mutants delete about 100 kilobases (kb) of the β locus. Yet the homozygote for the Chinese mutant presented with severe anemia requiring frequent transfusions and a splenectomy, whereas the homozygote for the Yunnanese mutant had moderate anemia (a hemoglobin value of 10 g/dl), no other clinical manifestations, and no need for transfusions.[110–113]

The (γδβ)⁰ thalassemias are characterized by complete absence of γ and β chain production. Heterozygotes present during the perinatal period with transient hemolytic anemia.[114–123] Subsequently, their red cells have the characteristics found in other individuals with the β thalassemia trait. Presumably, these mutations are lethal to homozygotes in utero. There are two types of (γδβ)⁰ thalassemia mutations: those that have deleted all the genes of the β locus and those that leave all or some β locus genes intact but delete regulatory sequences (see below).

The β⁰ deletion mutations remove all or a portion of the β globin gene.[123–135] Phenotypically, these individuals have β thalassemia trait (see Chapter 5), but their fetal hemoglobin levels are higher than those of most individuals with that condition. As discussed below, in the absence of the β genes, the γ genes may compete more favorably for regulatory sequences.

Non-deletion Mutations

An increase in Hb F without a major deletion in the clusters[54, 136–153] usually reflects a point mutation or small deletion in a promoter of the individual γ globin genes (see Table 4–3), as discussed in later sections. When combined on the same chromosome with a mutation in the β gene that lowers globin production, a δβ thalassemia phenotype is produced. (See Chapter 5.)

Mutations that produce a ${}^G\gamma$ HPFH or ${}^A\gamma$ HPFH phenotype are summarized in Table 4–3. Individuals with these mutations have normal red cell morphology and red cell counts and no clinical abnormalities. There is genetic evidence for both γ and β globin production in *cis* to the African ${}^G\gamma$ HPFH and to the Greek ${}^A\gamma$ HPFH determinants. β Globin expression in *cis*, however, is reduced below the normal levels. Structural analyses have shown that the ${}^G\gamma$ HPFHs have mutations affecting the ${}^G\gamma$ promoter, whereas the mutations in ${}^A\gamma$ HPFH affect the ${}^A\gamma$ promoter (see below). Heterogeneity in γ gene expression is characteristic.

Mutations Outside the Globin Gene Cluster

Certain HPFH variants are characterized by production of low levels of Hb F, characteristically distributed in a heterocellular pattern without an identified mutation in the β globin gene cluster.[154–162] Little is known about the molecular biology of these variants. Initial family studies suggested linkage with the β globin cluster.[156–158, 163] Analyses of other families using restriction enzyme polymorphisms as markers for the β globin gene cluster have suggested free recombination between the HPFH determinant and the globin structural genes.[159–162, 164, 165] This form of HPFH is likely to be genetically heterogeneous and composed of several variants, some of which may be linked to the β cluster and others of which may be found at more distant chromosomal positions.

Clinical Significance

The major clinical significance of mutations that increase Hb F is found in their interactions with the β thalassemia and Hb S genes.[10, 58, 164, 166–170] Compound heterozygotes have a much milder clinical syndrome than do homozygous individuals with either thalassemia or sickle cell anemia. For example, individuals with ${}^G\gamma{}^A\gamma$ HPFH and either a β thalassemia or an Hb S allele are asymptomatic and detected by chance during population screening. The combination of Greek HPFH with β thalassemia produces a hemolytic anemia of mild to moderate severity.[54] Even nondeletion HPFHs that modestly increase Hb F in heterozygotes are thought to have ameliorating effects in individuals homozygous for β thalassemia or Hb S genes.[155, 164, 167–170]

MOLECULAR REGULATION OF THE GLOBIN GENES

The coding portion of each globin gene is contained in three exons separated by two introns.[171] The distribution of codons that specify the 141 or 146 amino acid sequence of the α-like or β-like globin chains, respectively, is shown in Figure 4–6. An effort has been made to correlate distinct function with each of the exons, with some success.[172, 173] Exon 2 encodes for the segment involved in heme binding and α-β dimer formation, whereas exon 3 encodes for many of the amino acids involved in globin subunit interactions required for cooperativity of the hemoglobin tetramer in binding oxygen. (See also Chapter 6.) The intron lengths are variable, but the largest, intron I of the ζ gene, is only 1265 base pairs (bp). Thus, the globin genes of man and most other species are relatively compact in contrast to other genes, for which the coding sequences may be distributed over several hundred kilobases of DNA.

The tissue and developmental specificity of expression of the individual globin genes reflects the interaction of *cis*-active regulatory elements in DNA with *trans*-acting factors. The factors that regulate globin genes are both tissue restricted and ubiquitous with respect to their pattern of expression. Important *cis*-

	Exon 1 Codons	Intron 1 Length	Exon 2 Codons	Intron II Length	Exon 3 Codons
α-Like Genes	1-31	117 bp ($\alpha_1\alpha_2$) 1265 bp (ζ)	32-99	140 149 or ($\alpha_1\alpha_2$) 341 (ζ)	100-141
β-Like Genes	1-30	122-130 bp	31-104	850-904	105-146

FIGURE 4–6. The human globin genes. Indicated are the number of codons or length (in base pairs) of the introns of the various genes.

active elements already defined include the promoters of each gene, a downstream enhancer in the case of the β and perhaps the γ globin gene, a silencer upstream from the ε globin gene, and intragenic sequences within the β globin gene (Fig. 4–7). The β globin gene locus control region (LCR), cis-active regulatory elements distributed between 6 and 19 kb upstream from the ε globin gene, is required for establishment of an active chromatin domain that encompasses and extends beyond the β-like globin gene locus (see Fig. 4–7). This LCR is also responsible for high-level expression of the individual globin genes during the appropriate developmental stages. An LCR of the α globin gene locus seems to be required for high-level expression of α-like globin genes but may not be involved in establishing an active chromatin domain.

Before considering each of the cis-active elements in detail, we will provide a description of trans-acting factors important for erythroid cell development and function that exhibit a tissue-restricted pattern of expression. These include two sequence-specific DNA-binding proteins—GATA-1 and nuclear factor–erythroid 2 (NF-E2)—and stem cell leukemia factor now known as SCL. Information already available has established that these factors, in addition to many ubiquitously expressed DNA-binding proteins, interact in regulating expression of the globin genes.

Erythroid Transcriptional Factors

GATA-1. This transcriptional regulator was recognized as a DNA-binding protein with the consensus binding motif (T/A)GATA(A/G).[174] The "GATA" motif, noted first in the promoters of the chicken globin gene[175] and in the enhancer downstream from the

human β globin gene,[176] was shown to interact with a DNA-binding protein that was apparently erythroid specific. Binding of GATA-1 to a motif in the γ globin gene promoter is altered by the −175 HPFH point mutation,[177, 178] implicating the GATA motif in the increased level of fetal hemoglobin production in adults with this mutation. Subsequent study has localized one or more copies of the "GATA" motif in the regulatory elements of all genes expressed specifically in erythroid cells, attesting to the importance of GATA-1 for red cell development and function.[174] Initially known by a variety of names, including nuclear factor–erythroid 1 (NF-E1), the GATA-1 designation was adopted when the core GATA sequence was fully defined and other members of the GATA family that bind this core (GATA-2, GATA-3, and GATA-4) were discovered.

GATA-1 is a DNA-binding protein of the zinc finger class.[179–182] (See Chapter 2.) Indeed, it has two zinc-binding fingers, stabilized by intramolecular cysteine bonds, that interact with specific nucleotides in the DNA double helix by interdigitating into the major groove. GATA-1 activates minimal promoters containing a GATA motif in non-erythroid cells, establishing its ability to function as a transcriptional activator.[183, 184] The DNA-binding domain by itself is inactive in such assays; the N-terminal and C-terminal domains appear to be required for transcriptional activity.[183–185]

Other members of the GATA family were discovered[186] by using coding sequences for the zinc finger region of GATA-1 as a probe to screen complementary DNA libraries. (See Chapter 1.) The GATA family members share a strong homology in the zinc finger region and bind with high affinity to DNA sequences having the consensus GATA motif.[174] Within a single species, the individual family members diverge outside the DNA-binding domain. With the

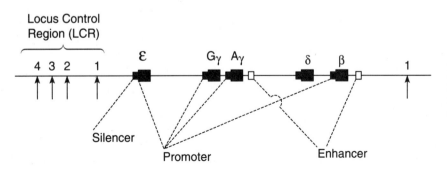

FIGURE 4–7. Regulatory elements within the β-like globin gene cluster. Not shown are potential silencing elements associated with the γ globin genes and an intragenic enhancer within the β globin gene. See text for details.

exception of GATA-1, the individual GATA proteins are conserved by evolution throughout their entire sequence; for instance, GATA-2 of chickens is highly homologous to GATA-2 of humans. Despite the conserved role of GATA proteins in erythroid cell development, there is significant divergence in the GATA-1 proteins of different species (e.g., human, mouse, chicken, and *Xenopus*) outside the DNA-binding domain. Each of the GATA proteins has been shown to function as a transcriptional activator when cotransfected with a reporter gene having a minimal promoter containing the GATA motif. GATA-1 and GATA-4 show the highest activity in this assay.[114]

GATA-1 first seemed to be an erythroid-specific transcriptional factor, but subsequently it was shown to be expressed in multipotential hematopoietic cell lines, mast cells, megakaryocytes, and endothelial cells.[187–191] GATA-2 is expressed in multipotential hematopoietic cell lines, mast cells, megakaryocytes, endothelial cells, and various other cell types, including myeloid cells. GATA-3 is expressed at high levels in lymphoid cells, and indeed there are GATA DNA-binding motifs in the enhancers of the genes encoding components of the T-cell antigen receptor.[192, 193] GATA-2 and GATA-3 are expressed in embryonic brain, but with slightly different timing and anatomical patterns.[194] GATA-4 is expressed at high levels in adult liver (T. Evans, personal communication).

The pattern of expression of the GATA proteins suggests diverse functions in regulating gene expression. Specificity could be achieved by limited accessibility of individual "GATA" motifs by virtue of chromatin structure (active or heterochromatin), the exact nucleotides within the motif and adjacent DNA, the presence of cofactors that interact with DNA sequences and/or domains of individual GATA proteins, and cell type–specific post-translational modification of the individual proteins. In cells in which the GATA proteins are coexpressed, such as GATA-1 and GATA-2 in multipotential hematopoietic cells, mast cells, megakaryocytes, and endothelial cells, the mechanisms noted above may be sufficient to confer specificity at GATA motifs within particular gene regulatory elements.

GATA-1 is absolutely required for erythroid differentiation. The gene for GATA-1 is on the X chromosome, so that only a single active allele needs to be "knocked out" by homologous recombination in embryonic stem cells to test its function. (See Chapter 1.) Chimeric mice developed from such GATA-1–deficient stem cells and from normal embryonic stem cells lack any contribution to the erythroid lineage from the GATA-1–deficient embryonic stem cells.[195] Arrest in differentiation occurs at the stage of the proerythroblast. Indeed, erythropoiesis derived from normal embryonic stem cells appears to be suppressed in chimeric animals by mechanisms that have yet to be defined. Myeloid cells derived from GATA-1–deficient embryonic stem cells are present, but the status of mast cells and endothelial cells in chimeric animals remains to be determined.

In summary, investigation of a seemingly erythroid-specific DNA-binding activity with a consensus motif in globin *cis*-active regulatory elements uncovered a family of transcriptional regulators of the zinc finger class that appear to have diverse functions within the lymphoid and hematopoietic systems. GATA-1 has functions outside the erythroid lineage, but it clearly is a necessary component for erythroid differentiation. To be described below is its diverse roles in LCR, promoter, and enhancer function that contribute to the high levels of globin gene expression characteristic of erythroid cells.

NUCLEAR FACTOR–ERYTHROID 2 (NF-E2). NF-E2 is the second DNA-binding protein, thought initially to be erythroid specific, to be uncovered by identification of its binding motif in regulatory elements of genes expressed in erythroid cells.[188, 196–199] Its antecedent, NF-E1, is now known as GATA-1, making the designation NF-E2 somewhat anachronistic. The consensus binding motif for NF-E2 is (T/C)GCTGA(C/G)TCA(T/C).[200] Within this sequence is the binding motif TGAGTCA, for activating protein-1 (AP-1), a family of heterodimers and homodimers of individual members of the JUN and FOS families of proto-oncogenes. NF-E2 was first identified as a DNA-binding protein that interacts with an AP-1 motif in the porphobilinogen promoter.[196, 197] Its binding to this AP-1 motif was shown to require a G residue 2 nucleotides (nt) upstream from the AP-1 consensus sequence. Subsequent work has defined the extended consensus sequence for NF-E2 shown above. The importance of NF-E2 for globin gene expression was established by demonstration that its binding was required for erythroid-specific, high-level activity of a powerful enhancer within the β globin LCR[198, 199] (see below).

The coding sequences for NF-E2 have been molecularly cloned and sequenced.[200, 201] A basic DNA-binding domain and adjacent leucine zipper within a 45 kDa protein identify NF-E2 as being among the B-zip class of transcriptional activators. As discussed in Chapter 2, a leucine zipper is usually involved in protein dimerization, and indeed the 45 kDa protein has an 18 kDa partner required for NF-E2's sequence-specific DNA-binding activity. The 45 kDa component of NF-E2 has a limited cellular distribution of expression that includes erythroid cells, whereas the 18 kDa protein is thought to be ubiquitously expressed. The mRNA for the 45 kDa component of NF-E2 is found in multipotential hematopoietic cell lines, mast cells, and megakaryocytes. In addition, it is found in the intestine of severely anemic but not normal mice. This observation plus the finding of an NF-E2 motif in the promoter of the chicken ferritin[200, 202] heavy chain suggests that NF-E2 has a role in iron metabolism.

The mk/mk mouse has a severe hypochromic microcytic anemia that is thought to reflect defects in iron metabolism and hemoglobin synthesis.[203] Chromosomal localization of the gene for the 45 kDa component of NF-E2 in the mouse genome established its linkage to the mk locus. Subsequently, the complementary DNA (cDNA) for the 45 kDa component of NF-E2 was cloned from erythroid cells of the mk/mk mouse. This cDNA was shown to contain a missense mutation, and thus it is likely to encode a dysfunctional NF-E2 protein. Globin chain synthesis is balanced in the mk/mk mouse, suggesting a parallel decrease in synthesis of the α and β chains and therefore a role for NF-E2 in both globin gene clusters. As noted above, NF-E2 is required for enhancer activity of the β gene cluster LCR, and indeed there is an analogous NF-E2 site in the enhancer element of the α-globin gene cluster LCR (see below). A role for NF-E2 in iron metabolism is supported by the observation that the mk/mk mouse has a defect in iron absorption that is not corrected by bone marrow transplantation.

NF-E2 has emerged as a major transcriptional activator important in hemoglobin synthesis and iron metabolism. Although consensus binding motifs are found in the cis-active control elements of other erythroid genes, high-affinity binding has been established at only a few sites. These include both the α and β globin gene cluster LCRs,[198, 199, 204, 205] the promoter for the heavy chain of chicken ferritin,[202] the promoter for human ferrochelatase,[206] and the porphobilinogen deaminase promoter.[196, 197]

Of interest is the parallel pattern of expression of GATA-1 and NF-E2. Both are expressed in multipotential hematopoietic cell lines, mast cells, and megakaryocytes in addition to the erythroid lineage.[188, 189] The functional NF-E2 sites that have been defined occur in close proximity to a GATA-1 binding site. These two transcriptional activators may interact in establishing high-level globin gene expression in erythroid cells.[207, 208]

SCL. The SCL (stem cell leukemia) gene encodes a basic helix-loop-helix protein that by analogy to other proteins containing this motif (see Chapter 2) is thought to be a transcriptional activator.[209] SCL was first discovered as a translocation partner of the T-cell receptor δ chain gene in T-cell and stem cell leukemia cell lines containing translocations involving chromosomes 1 and 14.[210] Subsequently, about 30 per cent of T-cell acute leukemias have been shown to have an interstitial deletion of chromosome 1 whereby the SCL coding sequences are put under the control of the promoter of a second gene termed SIL (SCL interrupting locus).[211]

The normal SCL gene is expressed at high levels in cells of the erythroid, megakaryocytic, and mast cell lineages.[212, 213] Chemical induction of erythroid maturation by murine erythroleukemia cell lines is accompanied by a 5- to 10-fold increase in SCL expression.[214] Overexpression of SCL in erythroleukemia cells by transfection of its coding sequences under the control of heterologous transcriptional and RNA-processing signals results in a higher frequency of spontaneous and induced erythroid maturation. Conversely, blocking SCL synthesis or activity by expression of antisense coding sequences or a mutant protein lacking the basic region, respectively, inhibits erythroid maturation in murine erythroleukemia cells. Furthermore, antisense SCL RNA inhibits self-renewal and induces maturation of human erythroleukemia cells.[215] These data suggest an important role for SCL in erythroid cells. Its DNA-binding motif remains to be defined, and it has not yet been shown to have a direct role in globin gene regulation.

The promoter of the SCL gene contains a GATA motif that has been shown to bind both GATA-1 and GATA-2.[214] The SCL promoter efficiently drives a reporter gene when transfected into erythroid cells, but promoter activity is lost when the GATA-binding motif is mutated. Expression of the SCL promoter-reporter gene in non-erythroid (NIH 3T3) cells depends on cotransfection with a GATA-1 vector.[214] These findings suggest that expression of the SCL gene in hematopoietic cells may depend on GATA-1 (or GATA-2).

OTHER ERYTHROID DNA-BINDING PROTEINS. A number of additional binding activities with an apparent restricted cellular distribution that includes the erythroid lineage have been identified during study of various cis-acting regulatory elements. These include a protein designated nuclear factor–erythroid 3 (NF-E3) that binds to the distal γ globin gene promoter[216] and the stage selector element protein that binds just upstream of the TATA box of the γ globin gene promoter.[217] Molecular cloning of the coding sequences for these proteins will be required before their tissue distribution of expression can be fully established and their role in globin gene regulation defined.

Regulatory Elements of the Individual Globin Genes

Each globin gene has regulatory elements, a promoter, an enhancer (or enhancers), and/or a silencer that contribute to high-level, tissue-specific, and developmentally modulated expression (see Fig. 4–7). These elements are thought to interact with the LCR in achieving control of individual globin gene expression (see below). Each regulatory element, whether promoter, enhancer, or individual nuclease-sensitive site within the LCR, contains binding motifs for multiple erythroid-specific and ubiquitously expressed transcriptional activators. The general concept that has emerged is that these individual factors interact with one another and other cofactors that do not directly contact DNA in creating multimeric complexes that influence gene expression. Each globin gene promoter has a "TATA" box onto which the transcription initiation complex assembles. (See Chapter 2.) The frequency of initiation of individual genes is influenced by the interaction of this initiation complex with multimeric protein complexes that assemble on upstream promoter elements, enhancers, or elements of the LCR. Formation of DNA loops is required to bring such protein complexes into the vicinity of the initiation complex in the case of physically distant regulatory elements.

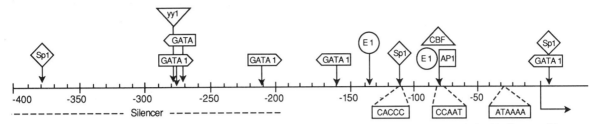

FIGURE 4–8. The ε gene promoter. Shown are the location of the conserved "boxes" and the binding motifs for various proteins. See text for definition of the individual DNA-binding proteins and for further details. The orientation of the "GATA" motifs is indicated by the direction of the arrowhead.

THE ε GLOBIN GENE. Tissue-specific expression of the ε gene is based on promoter sequences that interact with erythroid-specific proteins such as GATA-1[208, 218] and perhaps NF-E2,[218] whereas developmentally restricted expression in embryonic red cells reflects operation of a silencer within the distal promoter (see below). The ε gene promoter has the canonical CAC, CCAAT, and TATA boxes characteristic of globin gene promoters (Fig. 4–8). The CAC motif, which binds Sp1,[219] and a conserved GATA-1 motif at −160 to −166 have been shown to be required for promoter activity.[208, 218] A linked enhancer is also required for high-level expression of the ε promoter; either the chicken β/ε enhancer or the human 5′ HS2 (see below) functions in this capacity. When 5′ HS2 is used as the enhancer, the NF-E2 tandem binding sites are required to stimulate high-level promoter function.[208, 218] These observations are consistent with a model whereby NF-E2 interacts with GATA-1 or Sp1 (or a related GT protein) in establishing a high level of promoter activity.[207, 208]

Expression of the ε globin gene in transgenic mice requires elements from the LCR.[220, 221] This gene exhibits autonomous developmental control in that even without a linked γ or β gene it is expressed in embryonic but not in definitive stage erythroid cells (see below).[220] This turn-off of ε gene expression requires a silencer within the distal promoter[222] that had previously been identified as a negative regulatory element, using transfection assays in cultured cells.[223] The silencer has been mapped to a region between −182 and −467 upstream from the start site of transcription (see Fig. 4–8).[222, 224] Sequences between −250 and −300 contain the binding motif for a ubiquitously expressed zinc finger protein, YY1,[225] that has been shown to act as a repressor in several systems.[226–229] This binding site for YY1 overlaps with tandem inverted GATA-1 sites that also overlap with one another.[225] Point mutations in the overlapping segments of the YY1 and GATA-1 motifs interfere with binding of both proteins. These regulators may compete for binding to this region in vivo in modulating activity of the ε gene silencer. A comparison of the level of expression of GATA-1 and YY1 in embryonic versus definitive stage erythroid cells may be of considerable interest with respect to developmental regulation of ε gene expression.

THE γ GLOBIN GENES. Several local regulatory elements seem to be involved in regulation of the tandemly duplicated γ globin genes. The 300 or so base pairs of DNA that constitute the γ globin gene promoters have been intensely studied in an effort to understand the mechanism of hemoglobin switching and most specifically the nearly complete suppression of γ globin synthesis in adult erythroid cells. At least 15 DNA-binding proteins have been shown to interact with this promoter (Fig. 4–9). Many point mutations that produce the phenotype of HPFH have been identified in the γ promoters (see Table 4–3); most occur in binding motifs for transcriptional regulators. Regulatory mechanisms appear to be redundant, involving promoter function directly and/or indirectly through interaction of the promoter with the LCR and perhaps an upstream silencer. Studies in transgenic mice suggest the existence of this silencer (see p. 126), and phylogenetic footprints,[230] short segments of evolutionary conserved sequence, in the distal γ gene promoters have localized binding sites for the negative regulator, YY1.[226–229] In addition, a regulatory element downstream from the ^Aγ gene, first identified as an enhancer[231] but now thought to act as a nuclear matrix attachment region, may play a role in modulating γ gene expression.

The two γ globin gene promoters are identical in

FIGURE 4–9. The γ globin gene promoter. The disposition of the conserved "boxes" and position of binding motifs for various proteins are shown. See text for definition of the individual proteins and for further details. The direction of the arrowhead indicates the orientation of each "GATA" motif.

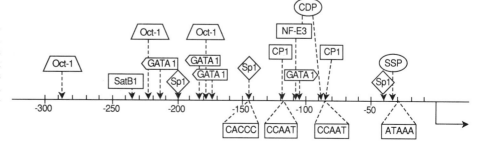

sequence. Each contains a single canonical CAC box, two CCAAT boxes within a duplicated 27 bp segment, and a single TATA box (see Fig. 4–9). As is true for other promoters, the TATA box is the region of assembly of the transcription initiation complex (see Chapter 2); the efficiency of its assembly and therefore the frequency of initiation are influenced by interactions with proteins that bind to several upstream regions. For purposes of discussion, these upstream regions will be considered individually, although the level of promoter activity throughout development is likely to depend on simultaneous, complex interactions of several regions with the initiation complex. The regions will be considered from proximal to distal in the promoter without implying any hierarchy of importance with respect to gene regulation.

The region between −40 and −60 of the γ promoter interacts with two proteins, Sp1 and a DNA-binding activity that has been designated stage selector protein (SSP).[217, 232] The sequence between −53 and −34 of γ gene promoter appears to function as a stage selector element (SSE)[217] analogous to the SSE defined in the chicken β globin gene promoter that captures the β/ε enhancer in adult erythroid cells by mediation of an SSP, designated NF-E4.[233] A phylogenetic footprint between −34 and −50 is conserved in species that express the γ gene in fetal stage cells but diverges in species in which the γ gene homologue is expressed in embryonic red cells.[230]

Two CpG dinucleotides (between −55 and −50) are methylated in adult and embryonic erythroblasts but infrequently methylated in fetal stage erythroblasts.[234, 235] Substantial evidence suggests that methylation may modulate gene activity by influencing binding of transcriptional regulators or other proteins to DNA.[236] Methylation of the CpG residues in the γ promoter causes a 10-fold enhancement of Sp1 binding that occurs at the expense of SSP when the two proteins compete for their overlapping binding sites.[232] Since SSP binding correlates with high promoter activity in the fetal stage environment of human erythroleukemia cells,[217] Sp1 could be acting as a repressor in this context. Methylation may play a secondary role in

modulating γ gene expression, since available data suggest that the gene may be turned off in erythroid cells before these sites become methylated.[237] Nonetheless, the mechanism involving competitive binding of Sp1 and SSP could contribute to developmental silencing of the γ genes. It is to be noted that the hypomethylation of the γ promoter induced by 5-azacytidine administered to patients with either sickle cell disease or thalassemia is accompanied by increased Hb F synthesis (see below).

The CCAAT box region of the promoter interacts with several proteins.[136, 216, 238–240] CP1, a ubiquitously expressed protein, is thought to act as a positive transcriptional activator; it binds to both CCAAT boxes. CCAAT displacement protein (CDP) binds competitively with CP1, interacting with a broad region of DNA that includes both CCAAT boxes. CDP has been molecularly cloned and shown to be a transcriptional repressor.[241] Inducibility of the γ promoter in human erythroleukemia cells depends on the CCAAT region and is associated with a decrease in CDP,[240] although attempts to demonstrate that CDP acts as a repressor of γ globin gene expression have yielded equivocal data. There is a binding site for GATA-1 between the two CCAAT boxes, and a second, apparently erythroid-specific binding activity designated NF-E3 also interacts with a motif in this region.[216, 239]

Several HPFH mutations have been identified in the CCAAT box region (Fig. 4–10). The −117 G to A mutation has been reported to cause a fourfold increase in CP1 binding and a twofold increase in CDP binding but an eightfold decrease in GATA-1 binding and also a decrease in NF-E3 binding.[238, 239] These results obtained by in vitro gel-shift assays (see Chapter 1) are difficult to integrate into a simple functional model. A 13 bp deletion that removes the distal CCAAT box is associated with a 100-fold increase in γ gene expression in adult erythroid cells. It eliminates in vitro binding of CP1, CDP, and NF-E3.[216] These observations led to the suggestion that CDP and NF-E3 may both act as repressors of γ gene expression in adult erythroid cells. Conversely, a substitution at

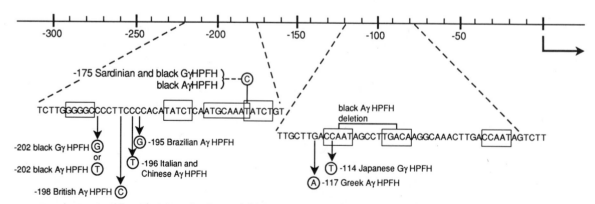

FIGURE 4–10. Point mutations in the γ globin gene promoter that cause HPFH. The enclosed sequences contain conserved sequences or binding motifs for specific transcriptional regulators, as discussed in the text. (Adapted from Bollekens, J. A., and Forget, B. G.: δβ Thalassemia and hereditary persistence of fetal hemoglobin. Hematol. Oncol. Clin. North Am. 5:399, 1991; with permission.)

−114 also associated with HPFH appears to decrease CP1 binding selectively.[136]

The CAC region is required for high-level γ promoter function in various transfection assays.[242] It binds several ubiquitously expressed proteins, most notably Sp1 or a related protein.[242] Although the CAC box is required for high-level expression, no evidence implicating the CAC box in developmental control has been forthcoming.

A T to C substitution at −175 of the γ gene promoter is associated with a 40-fold increase in γ expression in adult erythroid cells.[137, 138, 146] This mutation abolishes a weak binding site for Oct-1, a ubiquitously expressed "octamer" binding protein, and alters the interaction of this region with GATA-1.[177, 243–245] There are two potential GATA-1–binding sites in an inverted orientation flanking the Oct-1–binding site. Although artificial promoter constructs containing this region of the γ promoter with the −175 mutation are much more active than similar artificial promoters with the wild-type sequence,[207, 242] direct correlation of promoter activity with binding affinity of GATA-1 has been problematical, leading to the suggestion that a cofactor may be involved.[242]

The −200 region of the γ promoter is again the site of several individual mutations that cause the HPFH phenotype (see Fig. 4–10). A T to C substitution at −198 increases interaction with Sp1[246]; this Sp1 site has a major effect on γ promoter activity in heterologous expression assays.[247] The −202 C to G substitution creates a new binding site for the SSP, and indeed a 19 bp segment of the −200 region containing this substitution functions as a surrogate SSE in expression assays in human erythroleukemia cells.[232] An alternative model suggests that these and other HPFH point mutations in this region operate by altering the DNA conformation. Indeed, this region of the promoter forms an intramolecular triplex, leaving the −206 to −217 region of the promoter single stranded.[248] The triplex is thought to be the binding site for a repressor in normal cells that is displaced by the HPFH mutations, leading to expression of the γ gene in adult erythroid cells. It is to be noted that the two models, that of increased binding of a transcriptional activator versus displacement of a repressor, are not mutually exclusive. Indeed, these two proposed consequences of individual mutations, such as −202 C to G, could synergize in giving particularly high levels of Hb F in adult red cells.

The −200 to −240 region of the promoter has been shown to interact with several DNA-binding proteins[242, 249] (J. Cunningham and A.W. Nienhuis, unpublished observations). These include Oct-1, GATA-1, and SATB1, a protein involved in nuclear matrix interactions. Gel-shift assays demonstrate the formation of bimolecular and trimolecular complexes involving these proteins. The functional relevance of these interactions remains to be defined. Attempts to demonstrate an influence of this region of the promoter on the level of expression or developmental modulation have been unsuccessful. Perhaps this region functions as a "boundary" or matrix-associating region in regulating gene expression in the normal chromosomal context.

Several DNA-binding proteins have been shown to interact with sequences farther upstream of the γ globin gene promoters. Oct-1 binds between −280 and −300.[250] YY1, the transcriptional repressor, interacts with a phylogenetic footprint at −1250.[230] GATA-1 and Oct-1 bind to a phylogenetic footprint at −810, and several other DNA-binding interactions involving footprints at −930 and −960 have been found. The functional relevance of these protein-DNA interactions remains to be established.

An extensive survey, based on cellular expression assays, for an enhancer activity in the γ globin gene region identified an active 750 bp fragment downstream from the ^{A}γ gene.[231] This region is sensitive to nuclease digestion in nuclear chromatin, supporting this localization of regulatory sequences.[231, 251] Subsequent dissection of this fragment has identified eight footprints, three of which contain binding motifs for GATA-1.[249] Several other transcriptional activators bind to the enhancer fragment. The GATA-1–binding sites appear to be sufficient to account for the weak enhancer activity of this fragment in erythroid cells.[249] Subsequently, the same fragment has been shown to silence expression of a reporter gene containing a globin promoter on induction of human erythroleukemia cells to macrophage differentiation.[252] Furthermore, the so-called special AT binding protein 1 (SATB1)[253] has been shown to bind in two footprinted regions of the "enhancer" fragment. The fragment also binds to the nuclear matrix in a standard in vitro assay. Thus, the function of this "enhancer" remains enigmatic. Most likely, it forms a point of association of the β globin gene cluster domain with the nuclear matrix and as such may act as a boundary sequence.[254] Simultaneous interaction of the promoter through an SATB1 site between −200 and −240 with the nuclear matrix could result in a concentration of activators near the transcription initiation site.

THE β GLOBIN GENE. The promoter, an intragenic enhancer, and a downstream enhancer are likely to interact in controlling β globin gene expression.[255] The promoter exhibits tissue-specific expression; it contains elements that interact with the LCR and others that contribute independently to increased gene expression with erythroid maturation.[256, 257] The enhancers also have the potential to establish tissue and developmental stage specificity of β globin gene expression.[258–262]

Saturation mutagenesis has identified the TATA, CCAAT, and CACC boxes (Fig. 4–11) as being required for high expression of the β globin gene promoter in both non-erythroid and erythroid cells.[263, 264] The CACC box is duplicated, but the proximal box appears to be the most important functionally. Naturally occurring mutations in the TATA and proximal CACC boxes cause the β⁺ thalassemia phenotype (see Chapter 5), supporting a role for these sequences in normal gene function.

The CCAAT-binding protein, CP1, and GATA-1

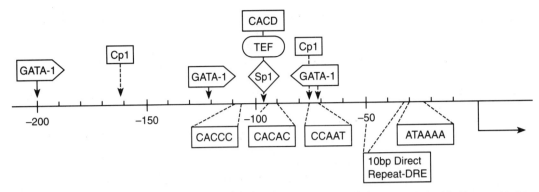

FIGURE 4–11. The β globin gene promoter. The disposition of conserved "boxes" and the binding motifs for functionally important transcriptional activators are shown. See text for definition of the individual factors and for further details. The direction of the arrowhead indicates the orientation of each "GATA" motif.

bind to the CCAAT box region.[255–257] The proximal CACC box binds several transcriptional activators, including Sp1, TEF-2, and CACD.[265] The last-named protein binds with high affinity. Furthermore, a parallel reduction in CACD-binding affinity to promoters with point mutations in the CACC box and a decrease in promoter activity in erythroid cells suggest that CACD may be the relevant CACC-binding protein in vivo. The relationship of CACD to a previously identified erythroid-specific CACC box–binding activity has not been established.[266]

The proximal promoter contains an interesting 10 bp directly repeated sequence between the CCAAT and TATA boxes called the direct repeat element (DRE).[267] The βDRE is highly conserved during evolution. Its position is analogous to that of SSE in the chicken β and human γ globin gene promoters.[216, 233] Mutations in one of the βDRE repeats have no effect on promoter function, but corresponding mutations in each repeat reduce promoter function significantly in erythroleukemia cells that have been induced to undergo erythroid maturation. A DNA-binding activity that interacts with the DRE and increases with erythroid induction has been identified.[268]

Located in the upstream region of the human β globin gene promoter are two binding motifs for GATA-1 (−120 and −200) and a binding motif for CP1 (−160).[256, 257] At least one of the GATA-1–binding sites and the CP1 site appear to be required for inducible promoter activity in erythroleukemia cells.[257] The requirement for these sites is eliminated when the minimal β globin gene promoter (−100) is linked to elements from the LCR.[257] The physiological relevance of these observations to normal β globin gene expression remains to be established.

Within the β globin gene in the region near the junction of intron II and exon 3 is an enhancer that increases expression of a linked heterologous or globin promoter in erythroleukemia cells.[255] This element also extends γ gene expression in transgenic mice, normally restricted to embryonic red cells, into the fetal-adult developmental period.[261] Another enhancer with similar properties is located just downstream from

the β globin gene polyadenylation site.[258–262] The intragenic and downstream regions contain three and four binding motifs for GATA-1, respectively, perhaps accounting for their enhancing activity. Recently, the region containing the intragenic enhancer has been shown to be required for high-level β globin gene expression because of an influence on the efficiency of polyadenylation of the β globin gene transcript.[269]

THE ζ GLOBIN GENE. The promoter is the only regulatory element identified within the ζ globin gene. It has TATA (−28), CCAAT (−66), and CACC (−95) boxes analogous to those found in other globin gene promoters. Mapping of binding motifs for transcriptional activators has identified binding sites for GATA-1, Sp1, and Cp2 between −110 and −60.[270, 271] The GATA-1 and Sp1 sites overlap, and these two proteins bind competitively, with GATA-1 exhibiting higher affinity.[271] Overlapping Sp1 and GATA-1 sites are also present between −250 and 220, and again GATA-1 binds with highest affinity. Thus, the available evidence suggests that GATA-1 may have a critical role in the function and regulation of the ζ gene promoter.

THE α GLOBIN GENE. Several features of the α globin gene are unusual in comparison to other globin genes. Its promoter contains TATA and CCAAT boxes but lacks the CACCC box, although it is generally GC rich. When transfected into erythroid and non-erythroid cells, the α gene is expressed independent of a linked enhancer.[272, 273] Efforts to locate an enhancer within its coding sequences or adjacent DNA have been unsuccessful. Rather, an element within exon 1 appears to function as an activator.[274] This element exerts its positive effect on the α promoter only when it is in its natural orientation and does not enhance the activity of other linked promoters. The α globin gene promoter contains binding motifs for a number of transcriptional activators, including GATA-1 (−185), CP1 (−90), and inverted repeat protein (−70 and −45).[275] It also contains several binding sites for CP2, a novel DNA-binding protein that has recently been cloned.[276] CP2 concentration increases with induced erythroid maturation and may contribute to enhanced α globin gene expression as red cells mature.

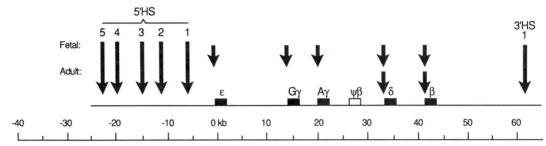

FIGURE 4–12. **Location of nuclease-hypersensitive sites within the β globin gene cluster.** These sites in nuclear chromatin mark the position of nucleosome-free DNase sequences. Developmentally stable hypersensitive sites flank the cluster; 5' HS 1 to 4 are erythroid specific and contain the locus control region (LCR) activity. Each promoter has a hypersensitive site in fetal stage erythroid cells, but only the δ and β genes are nuclease sensitive in adult stage erythroid cells.

The β Globin Gene Cluster Locus Control Region

Attention to the 20 kb region upstream from the ε globin gene was engendered by discovery of erythroid-specific, developmentally stable nuclease hypersensitive sites (HS) in chromatin of this region[251, 277] (Fig. 4–12). The first clue to the existence of important regulatory sequences remote from the individual globin genes was, however, provided by characterization of deletion mutants that removed sequences upstream but left the globin genes intact[278–281] (Fig. 4–13). The Dutch (γδβ)⁰ thalassemia deletion begins 2.6 kb 5' to an intact β globin gene that functions normally in vitro, but this gene is silent and encompassed in inactive chromatin in erythroid cells.[279] Subsequently, the Hispanic deletion that begins 8 kb 5' to the ε globin gene, leaving the entire gene cluster and the first erythroid-specific HS intact, was shown to silence the entire cluster.[282] The seminal observation that conclusively identified the LCR was the demonstration that this region, when linked to a normal β globin gene, conferred integration position–independent, copy number–dependent expression of this gene in

transgenic mice.[283] A large body of data obtained by gene transfer into cultured cells and by creation of transgenic animals has shown that the activities of the LCR are largely encompassed collectively within the 250 to 500 bp of DNA located at each HS in nuclear chromatin.

The β globin gene cluster LCR was the first to be discovered. Subsequently, an extensive search (see below) identified an HS upstream from the α globin gene cluster that is required for α-like globin gene expression.[284] This LCR-like element appears to lack the unique quality of the β globin cluster LCR, namely, the ability to confer integration position–independent, copy number–dependent expression on a linked gene.[285] LCR-like elements have been discovered adjacent to the T-cell–specific CD2 gene[286, 287] within the first intron of the gene for adenosine deaminase[288] and flanking the chicken lysozome gene.[289] Most genes are likely to have regulatory elements that have one or more functions of the LCR.

FUNCTIONS OF THE LCR. The unique property of the LCR that distinguishes it from a classical enhancer is its capacity to confer integration position–independent expression on a linked gene.[283] In earlier studies,

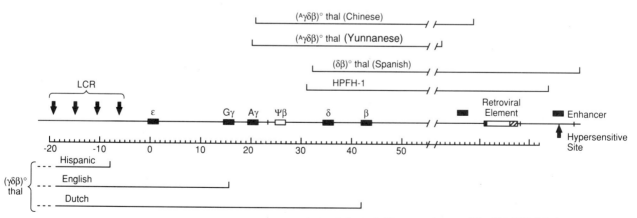

FIGURE 4–13. **Functionally important deletion mutations of the β globin gene clusters.** The 5' (γδβ)⁰ deletions inactivate the remaining intact globin gene as a consequence of loss of the LCR. The higher levels of Hb F observed in heterozygous patients (Table 4–2) with the HPFH-1 and Yunnanese (ᴬγδβ)⁰ thalassemia deletions compared with the Spanish (δβ)⁰ thalassemia or Chinese (ᴬγδβ)⁰ thalassemia deletions, respectively, are thought to reflect juxtaposition of enhancers adjacent to the γ globin genes (see text for details and references).

globin genes without the LCR were expressed in only about 50 per cent of transgenic mouse strains and then only at the level ranging from 0.1 to 3 per cent that of a normal mouse globin gene.[258-262, 290] Variable expression without the LCR was thought to reflect the influence of chromatin structure and nearby regulatory elements at the site where the globin transgene had integrated. The LCR establishes an active chromatin domain regardless of integration position and dominates nearby cis-active elements. In this context, the LCR differs from boundary elements described in Drosophila[254] in that it actively influences gene expression rather than simply insulating the gene from other regulatory influences.

A second important property of the LCR is its ability to confer tissue-specific expression on linked, heterologous promoters.[291] For example, the herpes simplex thymidine kinase gene promoter exhibits erythroid-specific expression in transgenic mice when linked to the LCR, and furthermore, the promoter becomes inducible during erythroid maturation. The human γ and β globin genes by themselves exhibit erythroid-specific and developmentally restricted expression,[258-262, 290] but the LCR is clearly able to complement this inherent specificity in achieving high-level expression.

Elements of the LCR do function as classical enhancers. A tandem NF-E2/Ap-1–binding site in the 5' HS2[198, 199, 292] and an HS from the α globin gene locus[293, 294] (see below) act as erythroid-specific, inducible enhancers when linked to reporter genes assayed in erythroleukemia cells. This enhancer function is clearly separable from the property of conferring integration position–independent expression, although such enhancers undoubtedly contribute to the overall level of gene expression in the normal chromosomal context.

The LCR may also have a role in establishing the pattern of early DNA replication that characterizes the locus in erythroid but not in non-erythroid cells.[295, 296] The entire β locus, with the exception of sites between the two γ globin genes 20 kb 5' to the ε globin gene and 20 kb 3' to the β globin gene, replicates very early in S phase. With the Hispanic (γδβ)⁰ thalassemia deletion mutation, this whole region of DNA is replicated late in S phase.[282]

Each HS encompasses 250 to 500 bp of DNA and contains multiple binding motifs for erythroid-specific and ubiquitously expressed transcriptional activators (see below). The active components of 5' HS2, 5' HS3, and 5' HS4 have been mapped to segments of DNA that coincide with the hypersensitive sequences in erythroid nuclear chromatin.[198, 199, 269, 297-315] All four HS singly have LCR activity in centering integration position–independent, copy number–dependent expression; 5' HS2 and 5' HS3 have about 50 per cent of the activity of all four sites linked together. 5' HS2 as a single copy enhances globin gene expression in cultured cells[316, 317] but does not give integration position–independent expression in transgenic mice,[301] suggesting that individual sites must cooperate in the domain-forming activity of the LCR.

Several models have been developed to explain how the LCR influences gene expression as an enhancer over many kilobases of DNA.[318] Although the effect could be exerted through chromatin structure or DNA conformation or both, the most attractive model envisions loops whereby individual HS of the LCR are brought into close proximity with the individual globin gene promoters.[233, 318, 319] Because the sites act cooperatively to confer normal expression in transgenic animals, multimeric complexes involving proteins that bind at two or more HS may come together to influence, along with proteins bound to the upstream region of the promoter, the frequency of transcription by interaction with the initiation complex on the TATA element.

The LCR HS form in primitive, multipotential hematopoietic cells.[320] Indeed, GATA-1, a protein that appears to play a role in the formation of the individual HS (see below), is expressed in cell populations highly enriched in stem cell–reconstituting activity.[321] With differentiation into the myeloid or monocytic pathways, the individual HS disappear.[320] These data suggest that multipotentiality may reflect the opening of chromatin domains for multiple lineages, with subsequent shutdown of those that contain genes not expressed in particular cell types.

LCR AND CHROMATIN STRUCTURE. Mapping of individual HS has shown that 250 to 500 bp of DNA is exposed to nuclease action at each site.[297-300, 302] Formation of these sites is thought to represent displacement of one or two nucleosomes, the number usually associated with this length of DNA. Each HS contains one or more binding motifs for the two erythroid-restricted transcriptional activators, GATA-1 and NF-E2, and for other ubiquitous DNA-binding proteins, most notably those associated with the CACC/GTGG class of binding motifs (Fig. 4–14) (see below). The segment required for formation of 5' HS4 of the β locus, mapped by deletional and site-directed mutagenesis,[302] contains binding motifs for these proteins (see Fig. 4–14).

DNA-binding proteins can be shown to compete with nucleosomes for binding to DNA fragments that contain their binding motif.[318, 322, 323] Competitive binding of transcriptional activators might allow displacement of nucleosomes in non-dividing cells. An alternative model suggests preemptive binding whereby transcriptional activators gain access to binding motifs during the chromatin disruption associated with DNA replication. Activation of globin genes without DNA replication occurs in fibroblast nuclei, following formation of heterokaryons by fusion of fibroblasts to erythroleukemia cells.[324] However, formation of the active chromatin domain in vivo is likely to occur in proliferating stem and progenitor cells.

Establishment of the HS within the LCR is thought to be the first step in initiating an active chromatin structure throughout the entire β globin gene cluster domain. Transcribed genes have an altered chromatin structure in erythroid cells compared with transcriptionally silent loci.[318, 325, 326] In addition to HS at control

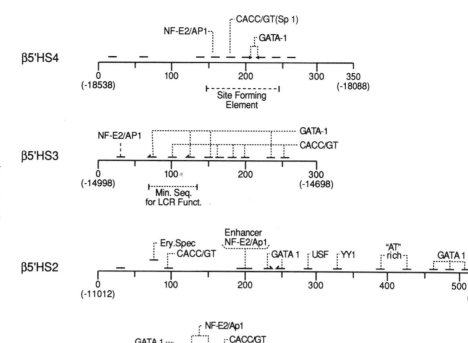

FIGURE 4–14. Disposition of binding motifs for various proteins within individual hypersensitive sites. See text for definition of the individual proteins and for additional details.

elements such as promoters, enhancers, and components of the LCR (see Fig. 4–12), the entire β globin gene cluster has a higher sensitivity to nuclease digestion in erythroid nuclei compared with inactive genes, such as those for the immunoglobulins.[251, 296] This active domain extends from the 5′ LCR beyond the β globin genes; indeed, LCR-dependent HS are found 20 kb[327] and more than 100 kb[328, 329] downstream from the β globin gene. The sequences upstream from the LCR are resistant to nuclease digestion, suggesting that the 5′ end of the domain ends at the LCR. The structural basis for this heightened nuclease sensitivity reflects unraveling of higher order chromatin structure, including, within the transcribed regions, the 30 nM fiber.[318, 325, 326] Nucleosomes in active regions are hyperacetylated; the concentration of histone H1—a protein that is usually associated with the nucleosome spacer region—is decreased, and the high-mobility group proteins 13 and 17 are increased in concentration.

EVOLUTIONARY CONSERVATION OF THE β GLOBIN GENE CLUSTER LCR. Another approach to understanding the LCR and its function has been to compare its structure and organization among species. The LCRs of goat and mouse have been molecularly cloned and sequenced, permitting comparison with the human LCR.[330–334] The general organization and spatial array of the individual sites have been conserved, although the goat genome appears to lack 5′ HS4. The goat and human LCR share 6.5 kb that are approximately 68 per cent conserved; the introns of the β globin genes are only 40 per cent conserved. The homology is between 80 and 90 per cent within and adjacent to the individual HS and specific binding

motifs; for example, the NF-E2 sites in 5′ HS2 are nearly identical.

The mouse and human LCRs have an identical organization, although insertion of repetitive sequences within this region during evolution has altered the exact distances between sites.[330–334] Again, there are extended regions of significant homology, with highest conservation within and adjacent to the individual HS. Overall, the evolutionary comparison suggests that the functionally important sequences extend beyond the minimal segments required for LCR activity in cultured cells and transgenic mice. This inference is consistent with investigation of other LCR in which the active sequences, although circumscribed, are modulated by sequences that are several hundred base pairs to either side of the HS.

The chicken β gene cluster LCR has also been partially characterized. Three upstream HS correspond to 5′ HS1, HS2, and HS4, but the enhancer function of the LCR appears to be contained within an HS between the adult β and the embryonic ε genes.[335–337] This site confers integration position–independent and copy number–dependent expression on a linked human β globin gene in transgenic mice.[336]

THE 3′ END OF THE β GLOBIN GENE CLUSTER DOMAIN. There is an erythroid-specific and developmentally stable HS about 20 kb downstream from the human β globin gene.[327] Sequencing has shown that this site contains binding motifs for GATA-1 and NF-E2. Topoisomerase sites and a nuclear matrix attachment site have also been identified.[327] This HS lacks LCR or enhancer activity in cultured cells and transgenic mice, and thus a function for this site has not yet been defined. One hypothesis is that it is a bound-

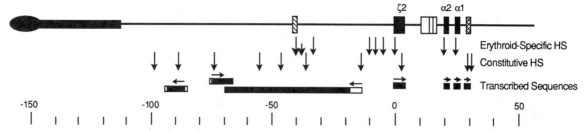

FIGURE 4–15. The α-like globin gene locus. Shown are the disposition of erythroid-specific and constitutive HS and the location of transcribed sequences. The open boxes within the cluster are pseudogenes, and the downstream hatched box represents the θ gene. Shown at position −40 is the enhancer region that is required for α gene expression. (Adapted from Vyas P., et al.: Cis-acting sequences regulating expression of the human δ-globin cluster lie within constitutively open chromatin. Cell 69:781, 1992. Copyright by Cell Press.)

ary sequence, demarcating the end of the active chromatin domain established by the 5′ LCR, but data relevant to this hypothesis are not yet available. Indeed, as noted above, the influence of the 5′ LCR appears to extend beyond 3′ HS1.

A gene and nearby HS have been discovered more than 100 kb beyond the 3′ HS1.[328, 329] This gene and HS became known because they are juxtaposed 3′ to the γ globin genes by HPFH deletion mutations (see earlier section). This gene encodes a membrane protein with multiple transmembrane-spanning domains. It has homology to G protein–type receptors, most specifically the acetylcholinesterase receptor. This gene has an active chromatin structure in erythroid cells, and the nearby HS is erythroid specific.[282, 328] An enhancer within the HS may contribute to the high Hb F phenotype of the HPFH deletion mutations (see Fig. 4–13). This region of DNA is also early replicating in erythroid but not in non-erythroid cells. Each of these features is lost with the Hispanic (γδβ)⁰ deletion mutation that removes the 5′ HS2–4, suggesting that the β globin gene domain under control of the LCR extends far downstream on chromosome 11.[282]

The α Globin Gene Cluster Locus Control Region

Like the individual genes of the β cluster, the α globin genes exhibit tissue-specific and developmentally modulated gene expression. The ζ gene is expressed in embryonic red cells during the first trimester, whereas the α globin genes are expressed in fetal stage cells during the last two trimesters and then in adult red cells. Despite similar tissue restriction and developmental modulation, regulatory mechanisms operative in controlling the α globin gene cluster differ in many significant respects from those that control β gene expression.[272–274]

The α genes are found on the most distal light Giemsa band of the short arm of chromosome 16 (16p31.3). This region, in contrast to the β globin gene cluster, is GC rich, having several CpG islands that are undermethylated.[338, 339] Several constitutively expressed genes are found within the region upstream from the α cluster (Fig. 4–15); the function of their

products has not been established. Several erythroid-specific HS are found upstream from the α globin gene cluster, but these lie within a constitutively active chromatin domain in both erythroid and non-erythroid cells (see Fig. 4–15). Indeed, the one HS that has been shown to be functionally relevant lies within an intron of a constitutively transcribed gene.[284, 285, 338]

Two lines of evidence firmly establish an LCR type of function upstream from the α globin gene locus. Several deletion mutants that remove upstream sequences have been described; these mutants leave the cluster intact but nonetheless silence the linked globin genes.[339–341] Furthermore, the α globin genes alone are not expressed at high levels in either cultured erythroleukemia cells or transgenic mice but are expressed at high levels and with erythroid specificity when linked to elements from the β globin gene cluster LCR.[342, 343] A systematic search for LCR activity in the region upstream from the α gene cluster identified an HS 40 kb (HS-40) 5′ to the ζ globin gene as a powerful erythroid-specific enhancer of linked gene expression.[284, 285, 293, 294] The linked α globin gene is expressed at high levels in all transgenic strains, indicating a degree of integration position independence, but the level of expression declines with development and is not copy number dependent, particularly at high gene copy numbers. The HS-40 appears to function very much like 5′ HS2 of the β gene cluster.[344, 345] Other functions of the LCR region required for β gene expression may be provided in the α globin gene cluster by mechanisms that are not limited to the α globin genes. The function of the other erythroid-specific HS upstream from the α globin genes has not yet been uncovered, if indeed these sites have a role in α globin gene expression.

Structure of Individual Hypersensitivity Sites

Each HS contains binding motifs for several transcriptional activators. These include erythroid-specific and ubiquitous expressed proteins.

One or more GATA-1–binding motifs are found within each HS. The inverted GATA-1 sites in HS4 are required for HS formation.[302] Two of the GATA-1 motifs in HS3, those placed around position 100 on the diagram in Figure 4–14, are required for LCR activity of a minimal HS3 fragment in transgenic mice.[315] Mutagenesis of the GATA-1 sites at position 230 to 250 of HS2 reduces the activity of a minimal fragment of HS2 (approximately 150 to 350) when linked to a β globin gene transferred into mouse erythroleukemia cells.[301] The same mutation has no effect on β gene expression in transgenic mice or on expression of a linked γ globin gene in human erythroleukemia cells.[317] These apparent discrepant results may reflect limitations of current assays. Overall, the data suggest critical roles for GATA proteins in LCR function pertaining both to chromatin structure and to gene activity. Although these roles are generally ascribed to GATA-1, note should be made that GATA-2 is also expressed in primitive hematopoietic cells.

The binding motif for NF-E2 is also found in each of the characterized HS. In β 5′ HS2, tandem motifs are phased at a 10 bp interval, establishing binding sites on successive turns of the DNA double helix.[198, 199, 299, 304, 306, 311–313] These binding motifs for NF-E2 are required for inducible enhancer activity of HS2, as demonstrated both in transient assays and after gene integration in human erythroleukemia cells. Furthermore, NF-E2 binding to these sites is also necessary for full LCR activity of HS2 in transgenic mice.[304, 314] Mutations that eliminate NF-E2 but preserve AP-1 binding markedly reduce HS2 activity in each of these assays. Two closely spaced NF-E2–binding sites in α HS-40[344, 345] (see Fig. 4–14) may have a similar role in the ability of this HS to enhance gene expression, but the relevant data are not yet available. Similarly, the role, if any, of the NF-E2/Ap-1 motifs in β 5′ HS3 and HS4 has not been defined.

Proteins that interact with the general motif, CACC/GT (GT proteins), have also been implicated in LCR function. Each characterized HS has binding motifs of this type.[297, 301] The binding site in β 5′ HS3 near position 100 of the diagram in Figure 4–14 is required for integration position–independent expression of a linked globin gene in transgenic mice.[315] CACC/GT motifs in each HS are protein bound in intact cells, as shown by in vivo footprinting. Sp1, a ubiquitously distributed transcriptional activator, interacts with such motifs. However, the "GT" class of DNA-binding proteins may include several factors,[346] one or more of which could interact functionally with each of the several motifs within the individual HS. Other widely expressed proteins, such as USF and YY1, have been shown to interact with the LCR,[301] but the functional relevance of such interactions has not been defined.

In summary, each HS appears to contain clustered motifs for several DNA-binding proteins. Two transcriptional activators, GATA-1 and NF-E2, with limited cellular distribution of expression that includes red cells, have been directly implicated in the regulation of erythroid cell development and hemoglobin synthesis. Other proteins that interact with the LCR are likely to be ubiquitously expressed. Some protein-

DNA interactions defined primarily by in vitro methods may not be functionally relevant or may not even occur in vivo.

MOLECULAR CONTROL OF SWITCHING

The analysis of developmental expression of human globin genes in transgenic mice has provided many new insights into molecular regulation. In the mouse there is a single switch from embryonic to adult hemoglobin.[48, 49] Embryonic hemoglobins are expressed in the yolk sac, whereas adult hemoglobin production starts in the 10.5 day old fetus when hematopoiesis shifts to liver.

The γ and β genes exhibit both tissue- and developmental stage–specific expression independent of the LCR, whereas the ε, ζ, and α globin genes are not expressed in transgenic mice without elements from the LCR. Less than 50 per cent of transgenic animals created with a DNA fragment containing the γ or β coding sequences with 1 to 2 kb of flanking DNA express the globin transgene at only 0.1 to 3 per cent the level of a normal globin gene.[290, 347] Expression is restricted to erythroid tissues. The β gene is expressed in fetal and adult erythroblasts, whereas the γ gene is expressed in yolk sac–derived erythroblasts,[258–261, 290] indicating that the genes or their flanking sequences contain elements responsible for the developmental specificity of the γ and β globin genes.

With discovery of the LCR, an obvious paradox emerged: How could developmental regulation of the globin genes be accomplished in the presence of such powerful regulatory elements? The analysis of transgenic mice containing the LCR linked to globin genes individually and in combination led to the proposal of two mechanisms of molecular control of switching: gene silencing and gene competition.

Globin Gene Silencing

Transgenic mice produced with a 3.7 kb fragment containing the ε globin gene failed to express ε globin in any developmental stage.[221] The same gene linked to a 2.5 kb fragment containing 5′ HS1, 2, 3, and 4 was expressed at approximately 30 per cent the level of a mouse globin gene in yolk sac–derived erythroblasts.[220] Similar results were obtained when the ε gene was linked to HS2.[221] As described in an earlier section (see Fig. 4–8) a silencer, defined by assays of promoter function in erythroleukemia cells, has been localized to the upstream region of ε promoter.[223–225] Deletion of the putative silencing elements abolished developmental regulation in transgenic mice as ε globin gene expression persisted in definitive erythroid cells.[222] These results proved that the ε globin gene is controlled during development by silencing.

Autonomous control has also been demonstrated for the ζ globin gene. When linked to elements from the β LCR, this gene is expressed appropriately in yolk sac–derived erythroblasts but not in the definitive erythroblasts of fetal liver or adult bone marrow.[348] A 550 bp promoter fragment driving a β-galactosidase reporter gene and linked to the −40 HS from the α globin gene cluster exhibits tissue-specific and developmentally specific expression in transgenic mice.[349] Deletional analyses of the ζ promoter up to −128 failed to localize a silencing element,[350] demonstrating that autonomous control for the ζ globin gene is achieved differently than for the ε globin gene.

The α globin gene requires a linked element from the β LCR or its own positive regulatory element from −40 for expression in transgenic mice. When linked to a 2.5 kb LCR fragment, it behaves autonomously in that expression is restricted to fetal-adult stage erythroblasts even in the absence of a competing gene.[351]

Silencing of the γ globin gene has been more difficult to demonstrate. The $^A\gamma$ gene within a 3.3 kb fragment, when linked to a 2.5 kb LCR fragment containing 5′ HS1 to 4, was expressed in yolk sac, fetal liver, and adult stages of development.[352] Without the LCR, the $^A\gamma$ gene exhibits restricted expression in embryonic red cells. The LCR appeared to override the developmental control of the γ genes, suggesting that regions outside the 3.3 kb $^A\gamma$ gene fragment are involved in silencing the γ genes in adult red cells. Developmental regulation was restored when transgenic mice were produced using a cosmid containing the γ and β genes in their normal chromosomal location, suggesting a model involving competition between genes for the LCR.[352] Similar results were obtained by Behringer and colleagues, who used an 18 kb LCR fragment containing all of the HS in their natural positions linked to an $^A\gamma$ gene fragment.[353] A different conclusion, however, was reached by Dillon and Grosveld, who used the 3.3 kb $^A\gamma$ gene fragment linked to LCR cassettes. Transgenic mice containing one or two copies displayed developmental regulation in that γ globin was expressed in the yolk sac and liver stages of development, but not in the adult stage.[354] These investigators concluded that the γ globin genes were controlled through silencing.

Further insights into the control of the γ globin genes were obtained by examining the effects of γ globin promoter truncations in transgenic mice.[355] Three regulatory elements in the γ promoter, one positive and two negative, were identified. An element with negative effects on gene expression in adult erythroid cells was localized to sequences downstream of −141. Transgenic mice containing the LCR linked to −141 $^A\gamma$ gene expressed this gene in the yolk sac and liver, but not in the adult stage of development. In contrast, transgenic mice produced using a γ gene truncated to −201 displayed high levels of copy number–dependent expression in all stages of development. These results suggest that the region between −141 and −201 contains a positive element that is dominant over the downstream negative element. It was proposed that this positive element is involved in the interaction between γ and the LCR.[355] Extension

of the promoter to −730 revealed another regulatory element between −730 and −382.[355] This element, the function of which appears to be influenced by the integration position, acts as a silencer in the adult stage of development.

Competitive Control

Expression of the adult β globin gene is controlled by a process distinctly different from that which turns off the embryonic globin genes. As noted earlier, constructs containing a human β globin gene but lacking LCR sequences display proper developmental control in transgenic mice: The gene is silent in the yolk sac and active during the definitive stage of erythropoiesis. When the LCR was linked to the β gene, developmental specificity was lost. Only when the β gene was linked to the γ gene in the normal configuration was developmental specificity achieved.[352, 353, 356, 357]

These results led to the proposal of a competitive model for the γ to β switch.[352, 353, 356, 357] The model implies that the probability of LCR interaction with either the γ promoter or the β promoter is primarily determined by the *trans*-acting environment. The gene that successfully competes for the LCR is expressed; the unsuccessful gene is switched off. This model, expanded to explain the ε to γ to β switches, is diagrammed in Figure 4–16. In the embryonic stage, the LCR interacts with the ε globin gene. In the fetus, ε is silenced, and the LCR interacts with the $^G\gamma$ and $^A\gamma$ genes. In the adult, the γ genes are silenced, and the LCR now recognizes β, the last available gene. Such a competition model was originally proposed to explain switching in the chicken globin system by Choi and Engel.[233] Support for the competition model has been obtained by targeted insertion of a heterologous promoter between the LCR and the β globin gene in cultured cells. The β globin gene was silenced while the heterologous promoter was expressed and became inducible.[358]

Another question addressed using transgenic mice was whether the relative distances of the individual globin genes from the LCR were the basis for the temporal sequence of globin gene expression during switching. Data obtained with combinations of tandem globin genes (αβ, βα, γβ, and βγ) linked to the LCR were interpreted as showing that the polar organization of the globin genes relative to the LCR is an important determinant of the sequence of globin gene expression.[357] Experiments using combinations of tandem γ or β globin genes suggested that gene order (relative to LCR) contributes relatively less to developmental regulation than does the *trans*-acting environment.[359]

Transgenic Mice Containing a 248 kb Yeast Artificial Chromosome

The physiological relevance of the gene order experiments mentioned above is questionable, given the

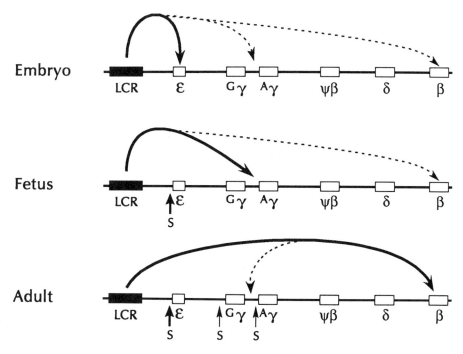

FIGURE 4–16. The competition model of human globin gene switching (see text). The arrows point to locations of *cis* active silencers.

tremendous spatial differences between the tested constructs in the normal locus, especially with regard to the distance of the globin genes from the LCR. This problem has recently been solved by the production of transgenic mice bearing the entire β globin domain as a 248 kb fragment in a yeast artificial chromosome (YAC). The γ globin genes are expressed predominantly in yolk sac cells, at a lower level in the fetal liver, and only minimally in adult mice.[360] β Globin expression is totally absent in embryonic cells and accounts for 99.5 per cent of globin in the adult. This experimental system will permit the facile manipulation of any *cis* sequences of interest, via homologous recombination in yeast and analysis of their expression in transgenic mice. The *cis* control of switching, therefore, can be studied in the context of the whole chromosomal β locus domain.

CELL BIOLOGY OF SWITCHING

The switches in hemoglobin phenotypes during development were known to physiologists working on oxygen transport in amphibians since the 1930s.[361, 362] When, in the 1950s, simple electrophoretic techniques became available, many new observations about the pattern of hemoglobins during the development of various species were made. Questions such as whether switching is controlled by an intrinsic mechanism or by an inductive extracellular environment or whether it relates to changes in hematopoietic cell lineages were addressed by early investigators. These questions were again asked in the 1970s and 1980s, when more sophisticated cell biological techniques were introduced. In this part of the chapter, we will review the

major insights obtained from the studies of the cell biology of switching during the past 20 years.

Globin Gene Switching Is an Intrinsic Property of Hematopoietic Cells

When clonal hematopoietic cell cultures were introduced for the study of erythropoiesis, progenitors from various developmental stages were analyzed to gain insights into the cellular control of hemoglobin switching. The levels of Hb F and Hb A observed in colonies derived from fetal, neonatal, or adult burst-forming units–erythroid (BFUe) were generally the expected ones for the ontogenic stage from which the clones were derived.[363] In cultures of adult BFUe, moderate levels of Hb F are produced, but these are distinctly lower than those observed in cultures of fetal or neonatal progenitors (Fig. 4–17). In adult BFUe colonies, Hb F is restricted to a subset of the total cells within the burst that are distributed in a segmental pattern (Fig. 4–18). In contrast, BFUe from human fetal liver give rise to erythroid colonies that make 90 to 95 per cent Hb F. Intermediate Hb F levels are produced in BFUe colonies of neonates (see Fig. 4–17). Apparently, erythroid progenitors encode developmental programs of globin gene expression that are characteristic for each developmental stage, suggesting that switching is an intrinsic property of hematopoietic cells.

Switching Occurs in Cells of a Single Hematopoietic Cell Lineage

Early models of the control of embryonic to adult globin switch in chickens and in amphibians assumed

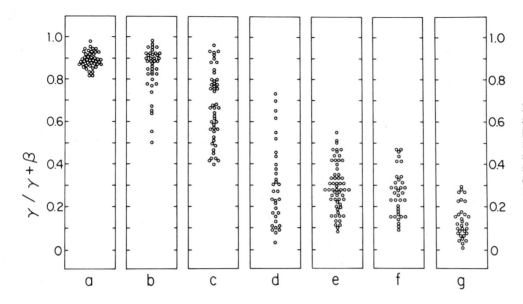

FIGURE 4–17. Proportions of γ and β chains (expressed as γ/γ + β ratios) in erythroid colonies from various developmental stages. Each open circle represents a measurement in a single colony. a, Fetus. g, Adult. b–f, Newborns.

the existence of two hematopoietic cell lineages, primitive and definitive.[364] The primitive lineage was thought to be irreversibly committed to expression of the embryonic globin program, whereas the definitive lineage was thought to be committed to expression of the adult globin program. Hemoglobin switching was attributed to the replacement of the primitive by the definitive hematopoietic cell lineage. The transitions in major erythropoietic sites during ontogeny (see page 108) seem to support this hypothesis.

Several observations argue against the clonal evolution model of switching. The model predicts a restriction of embryonic globins to primitive cells and of adult globins to definitive cells. No such restriction occurs, however. Thus, during switching in chickens, erythrocytes of the definitive erythropoiesis coexpress embryonic and definitive globin chains,[365] whereas in the mouse, primitive erythrocytes of the yolk sac erythropoiesis coexpress embryonic and adult globins.[366] In quail chick chimeras,[367] the yolk sac and intraembryonic stem cells generate erythroblasts containing both embryonic and definitive hemoglobins.[368] In humans, embryonic ζ chains are observed even in erythroid cells of neonates,[369] that is, cells of the definitive hematopoietic lineage.

Evidence against the clonal evolution model has also been obtained with studies in clonal erythroid cell cultures. Each colony originates from a single committed progenitor. If there are separate stem cell lineages, embryonic, fetal, and adult globins should be produced in separate erythroid colonies. However, colonies produced by plating progenitors from early human fetuses coexpress ε and γ globins,[370, 371] indicating that during the ε to γ switch the progenitor cells have a program allowing coexpression of γ and ε genes.

Clonal evolution models based on the existence of separate fetal and adult stem cell lineages were also proposed to explain the γ to β switch.[372–375] Evidence

against these models has been obtained from analyses of globins in single neonatal erythroid colonies. If indeed the γ to β switch were due to the replacement of a fetal stem cell lineage by an adult stem cell lineage, there should be a discontinuous change in the pattern of Hb F synthesis in BFUe-derived colonies during the neonatal period. In contrast, if the erythroid progenitors of the fetal, neonatal, and adult stages derived from a single stem cell lineage, a continuous distribution of Hb F values in erythroid colonies is expected during the switching period. Most experimental data support the latter interpretation. The amounts of Hb F in erythroid burst colonies derived from umbilical cord blood BFUe have a continuous distribution intermediate between the Hb F contents of fetal and adult progenitor-derived colonies[363, 376] (see Fig. 4–17). Although other studies[374, 377] have yielded data interpreted to support the clonal evolution hypothesis, the weight of evidence supports a single stem cell population.

Direct experimental evidence against the clonal evolution model comes from analyses of human globin expression in hybrids produced by fusing human fetal erythroid cells with mouse erythroleukemia (MEL) cells.

HETEROSPECIFIC HYBRIDS. Somatic cell hybrids produced by fusion of MEL cells with human cells inherit the unlimited proliferative potential of MEL cells and the capacity of this cell line to undergo erythroid maturation following exposure to a variety of inducers.[378] There is rapid segregation of human chromosomes following fusion, so that after several generations of growth only a few human chromosomes are retained by the hybrids. A specific human chromosome can be retained if culture conditions that select for hybrids containing that chromosome are used. There is no culture condition that can select hybrids containing human chromosome 11. An alternative system based on immunochemical detection of a chro-

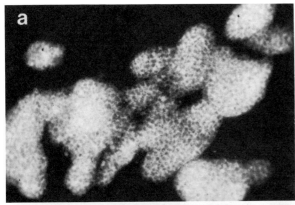

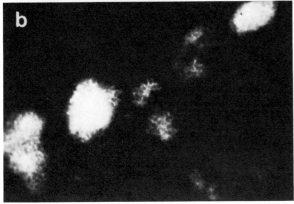

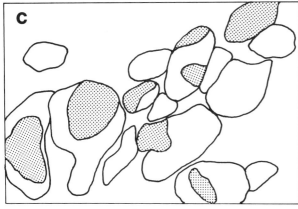

FIGURE 4–18. An adult erythroid colony (an erythroid burst from a plasma clot culture) composed of many subcolonies has been stained with anti-β adult *(a)* and anti-fetal hemoglobin *(b)* fluorescent antibodies. All the subcolonies are homogeneously stained in *a,* whereas only sectors are stained in *b.* In *c,* the sectors expressing fetal hemoglobin are shown. Such data show that F cells and non–F cells are progeny of a single burst-forming unit–erythroid (BFUe).

mosome 11–linked cell surface determinant allows maintenance of chromosome 11–containing hybrids, using immune adherence or cell sorting.[379]

There is an apparent developmental specificity to the complement of *trans*-acting factors present in MEL cells. When the human chromosome 11 transferred into MEL cells is derived from adult erythroid or nonerythroid cells (fibroblasts or lymphoblasts), only the β globin gene is activated[380–384]; the human fetal globin gene is not expressed in these hybrids. There is, however, human γ globin gene expression when the

human chromosome 11 is derived from an erythroleukemia cell producing γ globin.[385] Human γ globin is also produced when the transferred human β locus contains an HPFH mutation.[386] Thus, hybrids that contain a deletion $^A\gamma^G\gamma$ HPFH chromosome produce only γ human globin, whereas those containing a $-117\ ^A\gamma$ HPFH chromosome produce $^A\gamma$ and β globin, as expected from the molecular lesions underlying these mutations.[386]

The most interesting observations have been made when MEL cells were fused with human fetal erythroblasts.[379] Such hybrids produce only fetal or predominantly fetal human globin (Fig. 4–19). Apparently, the human fetal erythroid cell transmits to the hybrids a program, which determines that there will be high γ and low β gene transcription. Whether the hybrids express this program because they inherit from the fetal cells a locus producing a *trans*-acting factor that induces γ gene expression remains to be determined. When these hybrids are propagated in culture, a "switch" from γ to β expression is observed (Fig. 4–20). One interpretation of this switch is that the chromosome containing the locus for the *trans*-acting factor required for γ gene expression is initially present in the hybrids but is subsequently lost by chromosomal segregation. Cytogenetic and restriction fragment length polymorphism (RFLP) studies[387] have failed to support this suggestion, however. Other possibilities are that such a locus is present on chromosome 11 and turns off as culture time advances[379] or that the molecular mechanism that controls switching acts primarily in *cis*.

Each hybrid originates from a single cell. The fact that the γ to β switch occurs during the propagation of single-cell clones (see Fig. 4–20) provides direct evidence that switching occurs in cells of a single lineage.

The Time of Switching Is Determined by the Developmental Maturity of the Fetus

Many observations have been done in human fetuses in order to detect factors that influence switching. It is possible that switching is related to the rate of hematopoietic cell regeneration, which is very high in the fetus and slows down after birth. However, acceleration of erythropoiesis in the fetus has no significant effect on the rate of switching. Thus, infants suffering from hemolytic disease due to blood group incompatibility or newborns with severe hypoxemia secondary to congenital heart disease exhibit a normal switching pattern.[388, 389] A delay in switching is often observed in the presence of placental insufficiency or maternal hypoxia.[390, 391] One cannot conclude that there is a direct relationship between these conditions and switching because infants affected by these conditions exhibit generalized developmental retardation.

The proportion of Hb F in newborns is related to their age from conception rather than to birth itself.[392–394] Premature newborns have very high levels

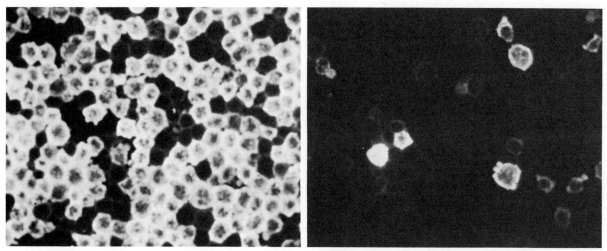

Figure 4–19. Staining of a human fetal erythroid × mouse erythroleukemia (MEL) hybrid with anti-human γ *(left)* and anti-human β *(right)* fluorescent antibodies. Notice the abundance of γ-positive cells on the left and the rarity of β-positive cells on the right. (Reprinted with permission from Papayannopoulou, Th., et al.: Analysis of human globin switching in MEL × human fetal erythroid cell hybrids. Cell 46:469, 1986. Copyright by Cell Press.)

of Hb F; such newborns switch to Hb A at a time corresponding to the end of their normal gestational period.[395] This observation suggests that the switch is developmentally determined independent of the intrauterine or extrauterine status of the individual; rather, the degree of developmental maturity of the fetus determines the rate as well as the timing of γ to β switch.

Switching May Be Controlled by a Developmental Clock

The model of developmental clock assumes that hemoglobin switching represents a developmental progression intrinsic to cells that form the erythroid lineage.[363] The clock is set as embryogenesis begins and proceeds inevitably regardless of external influences. Two sets of observations support this concept.

As described earlier, hybrids produced by fusion of MEL cells with fetal erythroblasts initially produce high levels of fetal globin but several weeks later switch to adult globin synthesis. The rate of the switch of these hybrids correlates to the age of the fetus from which the erythroblasts were derived.[379] Thus, hybrids produced using cells of younger fetuses switch slower than do hybrids produced using cells of older fetuses (Fig. 4–21). It is as if the human fetal erythroid cells

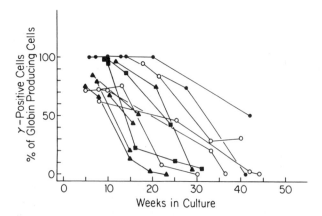

FIGURE 4–20. Time-related switching of human fetal erythroid × MEL hybrids in culture. Proportion of γ globin–positive cells is shown as per cent of total cells expressing human globin. Identical symbols represent different hybrids from the same fusion. These results prove that switching occurs in the cells of a single lineage, perhaps by a developmental clock type of mechanism. (Reprinted with permission from Papayannopoulou, Th., et al.: Analysis of human globin switching in MEL × human fetal erythroid cell hybrids. Cell 46:469, 1986. Copyright by Cell Press.)

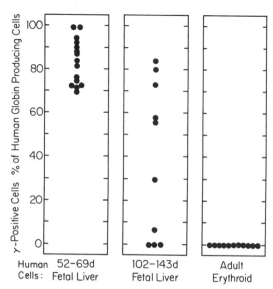

FIGURE 4–21. Rate of switching in hybrids correlates with the developmental age of the human erythroblasts used for hybrid production. (Reprinted with permission from Papayannopoulou, Th., et al.: Analysis of human globin switching in MEL × human fetal erythroid cell hybrids. Cell 46:469, 1986. Copyright by Cell Press.)

"know" whether they belong to an early or to a late developmental time, and they transmit this information into the hybrid cells. The analyses of chromosomal composition of somatic cell hybrids[387] suggest that the developmental clock for switching is located on chromosome 11.

The second line of evidence comes from the results of hematopoietic cell transplantation experiments.

THE TRANSPLANTATION MODEL. These experiments were designed to distinguish between the mechanisms of "developmental clock" and "inductive environment." The model of the inductive environment assumes that hemoglobin switching reflects physiological changes occurring within the fetus. The hematopoietic environment acts on erythroid progenitors and determines the pattern of hemoglobin synthesis in their progeny erythroblasts.[363] Switching reflects changes in the environment to which the erythroid lineage responds.

Adult bone marrow cells injected into fetal sheep in utero resulted in the formation of erythroid cells containing adult-type hemoglobin.[396] This was interpreted as indicating that the fetal environment fails to influence the program of adult cells.

Another experimental approach has been the injection of fetal liver cells into lethally irradiated adult sheep.[397–399] Analogous observations have been made in humans transplanted with fetal liver cells.[400, 401] Initially, in transplanted sheep, Hb F is produced. Subsequently, there is a switch to adult hemoglobin production by the transplanted cells. The rate of the switch is dependent on the gestational age of the donor fetus (Fig. 4–22). The fetal to adult sheep transplantation experiments lead to two conclusions. First, the perinatal switch from fetal to adult hemoglobin synthesis is not dependent directly on changes occurring in the organism at that time. Second, the transplanted fetal stem cells appear to know their developmental age and switch slower or faster, depending on the age of the fetus from which they derive.

The Rate of Switching Can Be Modulated by the Environment

Several observations suggest that the developmental clock of switching can be modulated by the environment. Among the more dramatic changes that occur in the fetus are those of the endocrine system. Fetal thyroidectomy, nephrectomy, adrenalectomy, and hypophysectomy have all been performed in sheep in an

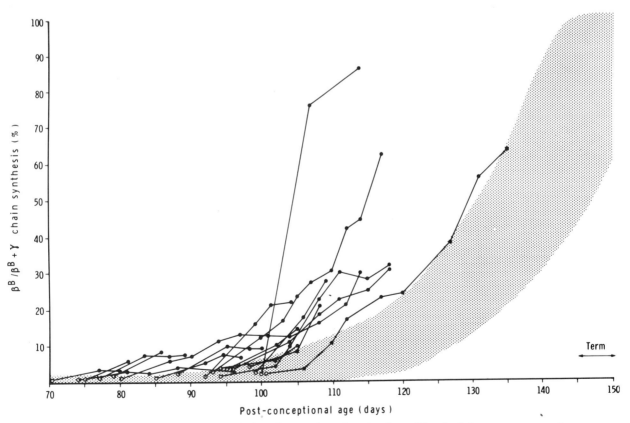

FIGURE 4–22. Fetal to adult hematopoietic cell transplantations in sheep. The shaded area represents the normal range of β/β + γ chain synthesis in peripheral blood reticulocytes of normal sheep fetuses. Open circles are the results from donor reticulocytes at the time of transplantation. Closed circles are the results from bone marrow samples from the transplanted recipient. (Reprinted by permission from Nature Vol. 313, p 320. Copyright © Macmillan Magazines Limited.)

effort to influence the rate of switch.[402, 403] With hypophysectomy, there is general developmental retardation; such abnormal sheep fetuses exhibit a delay in the γ to β switch. Removal of the adrenal inhibits the normal increase in plasma cortisol that precedes birth.[403] The γ to β switch in such adrenalectomized animals is delayed, although the animals are grossly normal with respect to developmental progression.[403] Administration of cortisol to establish levels approximating those found in fetuses with normal adrenals allows the switch to progress with normal kinetics.

FETAL HEMOGLOBIN IN THE ADULT

The γ to β switch is leaky in that low levels of γ globin continue to be produced in the adult stage of development. As described earlier, this γ globin is restricted to a minority of cells, called F cells (see Fig. 4–3). Activation of γ globin expression occurs in several inherited and acquired conditions and in clonal cultures of adult erythroid progenitors.

Hemoglobin F Production Is Consistently Activated by Acute Erythropoietic Stress

Observations in several pathological conditions and physiological states suggest that rapid regeneration of the erythroid marrow induces F-cell production.[404–413] Transient erythroblastopenia of childhood is a condition characterized by an arrest in erythropoiesis. The bone marrow of such children is severely erythroblastopenic but suddenly and spontaneously recovers, and vigorous erythropoiesis appears. This recovery is typically associated with increased F-cell production.[405, 406] Increased F-cell production is also characteristic of bone marrow regeneration following bone marrow transplantation.[407] Induction of Hb F also follows the chemotherapeutic ablation of bone marrow.[408] Enhanced F-cell production may also be observed during expansion of erythropoiesis. For example, in severe, untreated iron deficiency anemia, the levels of F cells are within normal limits; following treatment with iron, there is a sharp reticulocyte response, and during this stage of erythroid expansion, F cells are preferentially produced.[404] Acute hemolysis also results in elevated F-cell production,[406] although acquired or congenital chronic hemolytic anemias are only rarely associated with increased Hb F. A kinetic model based on our knowledge of the regulation of F-cell production during erythroid progenitor differentiation has been developed to account for these observations and will be discussed in a later section.

An increase in F-cell production early during the second trimester of pregnancy is very characteristic.[414, 415] The obvious idea that humoral factors of fetal origin might affect the maternal bone marrow with respect to F-cell production has found no experimental support. Rather, the increase in F cells occurs during a period when the blood volume (and therefore red cell production) in the pregnant woman increases sharply.[10] Hence, the enhanced F-cell production may be analogous to that observed in other situations in which there is acute expansion of erythropoiesis.

The relationship between rapid erythroid regeneration and activation of γ globin expression has been documented experimentally. Acute bleeding in baboons or in humans activates γ globin production.[409–413] The induction of fetal hemoglobin by acute erythropoietic stress has also been reproduced in vivo by administration of high doses of recombinant erythropoietin.[416, 417]

Hemoglobin F in Chronic Anemia

The consistent activation of Hb F in acute erythropoietic expansion should be contrasted to the findings in chronic anemias. With the exception of hemoglobinopathies and congenital hypoplastic anemias, there is no elevation of Hb F in most patients with chronic anemias.[418] Administration of low doses of erythropoietin to baboons increases the hematocrit but fails to induce Hb F.[416] Treatment of patients in renal failure with low doses of erythropoietin induces erythropoiesis but fails to increase F-cell production.[419] Following bleeding there is a surge of F-reticulocyte production, but when chronic anemia is instituted the number of F reticulocytes falls.[411, 413] The difference in the rates of F-cell formation between acute and chronic erythropoietic stress suggests that the *kinetics* of erythroid regeneration influence whether a cell will become an F cell or an A cell.

Among the chronic anemias, fetal hemoglobin is typically increased in individuals with thalassemia or sickle cell syndromes. (See Chapters 5 and 6.) The major factor in the activated production of Hb F is the intense erythropoietic stress of these syndromes. The levels of Hb F in the peripheral blood reflect the increased rate of F-cell production but mainly the preferential survival of erythrocytes containing fetal hemoglobin.

SICKLE CELL SYNDROMES. Several factors account for the striking variation in the amount of Hb F found in the blood of patients with sickling disorders. One significant influence is the heterogeneous distribution of Hb F in the red cells of patients with these disorders. F cells have a lower concentration of Hb S, and furthermore, Hb F inhibits polymerization, directly accounting for the lower propensity of F cells to form intracellular polymer and undergo sickling.[420–424] (See also Chapter 6.) Hence, there is selective survival of sickle red cells containing Hb F, leading to amplification of the F-cell population.[425–427]

There is also marked variability in the intrinsic capacity for Hb F synthesis among individuals with the various Hb S syndromes.[166–170, 428] Co-inheritance of a non-deletion HPFH[155, 167] is likely in many patients who have high levels of Hb F production. Particular chromosomal haplotypes, as defined by restriction enzyme polymorphisms (see Chapter 6), have been associated with relatively high levels of Hb F and a correspondingly mild clinical syndrome in sickle cell anemia patients of diverse ethnic origins.[429–431] A unique chromosomal haplotype is observed in individuals with sickle cell anemia from Saudi Arabia and the subcontinent of India.[431] The Saudi patients have high levels of Hb F and are more or less free of symptoms resulting from vaso-occlusive episodes.[168, 431–433] Although the increase in the amount of Hb F in Saudis with homozygous Hb S disease has a genetic basis, it is exhibited only in the presence of accelerated erythropoiesis.

THALASSEMIA SYNDROMES. Individuals who are homozygous for β thalassemia have a striking increase in Hb F that is of diagnostic significance.[10] The proportion of Hb F in the blood may range from 10 to 98 per cent, depending on whether the patient has inherited thalassemia mutations of the β^+ or β^0 variety. (See Chapter 5.) The amount of Hb F in peripheral blood grossly misrepresents the actual production of γ chains in the patient's bone marrow.[434] Characteristic of the thalassemic marrow is the heterogeneous synthesis of Hb F by erythroid cells. Those erythroblasts lacking capacity for γ chain synthesis are eliminated in the bone marrow because of the toxic effects of excess α chains. Marked ineffective erythropoiesis is characteristic of these disorders. The minority of cells capable of producing γ chains in significant quantity (F erythroblasts) survive preferentially both in the bone marrow and in peripheral blood. (See Chapter 5.) There may be as much as a 40-fold amplification of Hb F levels compared with the intrinsic capacity for γ chain synthesis.

Patients with homozygous β thalassemia may also inherit a determinant that increases Hb F.[10, 156, 164] The same chromosomal haplotypes observed in individuals with a sickle cell syndrome with high Hb F have also been associated with an increased capacity for Hb F production in thalassemic individuals. As outlined in Chapter 5, interaction of the β thalassemia genes with mutations that increase Hb F in compound heterozygotes may give rise to thalassemia syndromes of moderate severity. Hb F and F-cell numbers are also above normal in about 50 per cent of β thalassemia heterozygotes, although the mechanism for this increase is unknown.

CONGENITAL HYPOPLASTIC OR APLASTIC ANEMIAS. Congenital hypoplastic anemia (Diamond-Blackfan syndrome) affects only the erythroid series and occurs as autosomal recessive, autosomal dominant, and sporadic forms.[435] Untransfused individuals with this disorder have elevated Hb F[435–438] that is heterogeneously distributed among red cells. Often these patients improve with corticosteroid treatment and exhibit further increase in Hb F. Hematologically normal parents of patients with the autosomal recessive form of Diamond-Blackfan syndrome have no increase in Hb F. The mechanism of increased γ chain synthesis in these patients may reflect disordered erythroid progenitor maturation.

Pancytopenia is characteristic of Fanconi's anemia,

an autosomal recessive condition that affects all three hematopoietic lineages.[435, 439–442] A defect in DNA repair mechanisms is the likely underlying cause. Hb F may be strikingly elevated. Distortions of cell kinetics early in erythropoiesis might form the basis for increased Hb F synthesis.

Hematopoietic Malignancy Can Induce a Fetal Globin Program

Juvenile chronic myelogenous leukemia (JCML) is characterized by very striking increases in Hb F production[443–445]; Hb F may represent 70 to 90 per cent of the total hemoglobin. In addition, the red cells of these patients exhibit other "fetal" characteristics, such as low glycolytic enzyme activity, the carbonic anhydrase isozyme characteristic of fetal red cell, and the absence of I antigen. Initially, these features suggested a reversion to true fetal erythropoiesis.[443–446] However, careful study of red cell populations has shown that the various "fetal" characteristics are not expressed in a coordinated fashion. Some cells having predominantly Hb F may express the I antigen, whereas other cells lacking Hb F express the i antigen. Apparently, there is a gross distortion in the coordinate regulation of gene expression in this syndrome rather than a simple reversion to fetal erythropoiesis.[447] Occasional patients with a myeloproliferative disorder or a preleukemia syndrome exhibit a striking increase in Hb F production.[448, 449] Their red cells may resemble those found in patients with JCML, with respect to enzyme activity and antigen expression. Rarely, Hb F synthesis may be increased in patients with solid tumors. Choriocarcinomas of the testes or placenta, adenocarcinomas of the lung, and hepatomas are among the tumors in which this phenomenon has been observed.[15, 450–454] An increased capacity for Hb F production, observed in individuals without anemia who are not being treated with chemotherapeutic agents, suggests the production by the tumor of a humoral substance that influences F-cell production. There is no experimental evidence to support this hypothesis, however.

The increase of F cells in hematopoietic malignancy has been attributed to transformation of "fetal stem cells" that happen still to reside in the bone marrow of the patients.[372, 408, 449] In view of the evidence against the existence of separate fetal and adult stem cell lineages summarized earlier in this chapter, other explanations should be considered. It is possible that malignancy per se in some way activates the fetal globin program. Alternatively, these fetal phenotypes may reveal the primitive programs of globin expression that are encoded by the transformed progenitors or the stem cells from which the malignant cell population is derived. This hypothesis has also been proposed to explain why a fetal/embryonic globin program is typical of all the human erythroleukemia lines characterized to date.

HUMAN ERYTHROLEUKEMIA LINES. Fifteen human

TABLE 4–4. HUMAN ERYTHROLEUKEMIA LINES

LINE	GLOBIN PHENOTYPE	REFERENCES
K562	ϵ, γ, δ, ζ, α	455–457
HEL	ϵ, γ, ζ, α	457, 458
KMOE	γ, β	457, 459
OCIM1	γ, α	457, 460
OCIM2	γ, δ, (β), ζ, α	457, 460
RM10	ϵ, γ, δ, ζ†	461
KU-812	γ, β, α	462
CMK	γ†	463
UT-7	γ, (β)†	464, 465
JK-1	ϵ, γ, β, ζ, α	466
MB-02	ϵ, γ, β, α	467
F-36	γ, β, ζ	468
LAMA-84*	γ†	469
MEG-01*	γ†	470, 471
TF-1*	+γ†	472

*Phenotype from published reports only. For the rest of the lines, the data are derived from testing in our laboratory (472).

†These lines have not been analyzed for the presence of the remaining globin species.

() = Barely detectable (472); + = presumed positive but not yet tested in our laboratory (472).

erythroleukemia lines have been established (Table 4–4) by culturing cells of adult patients with hematopoietic malignancies. Typical of all these lines is the expression of a primitive globin program characterized by synthesis of predominantly fetal and some embryonic globin chains. The K562 cells produce $^G\gamma$, $^A\gamma$, and ϵ chains, but no β chains. Human erythroleukemia (HEL) cells produce $^G\gamma$ and $^A\gamma$ chains but no β chains. A variant of the HEL line, HEL-R, shows considerable ϵ gene expression. KMOE cells express mainly γ globin. Predominant γ expression is characteristic of OCI-M1 and OCI-M2 cells. These lines also have multiple myeloid-erythroid-megakaryocytic potentialities. In addition, HEL cells have monocytic/macrophagic properties.

Hemoglobin F Production in Adult Progenitor Cell–Derived Colonies

Application of the clonal hematopoietic culture methodology to the analysis of hemoglobin synthesis in human progenitor–derived colonies immediately identified higher levels of Hb F production in culture than in vivo.[473] As noted earlier, Hb F is not uniformly distributed. Some subclones of the erythroid colonies produce Hb F in all cells, and others have no detectable Hb F, whereas most clones are composed of both F erythroblasts and A erythroblasts. Statistical analyses are compatible with the assumption that expression of Hb F in erythroid progenitors depends on random or stochastic events occurring during the first few cell divisions of the colony progenitor.[474] If the stochastic event occurs with the first cell division, a colony may be formed that is composed of erythroblasts, all or none of which contain Hb F. On the other hand, if stochastic events occur during several subsequent cell cycles, sectoral distribution of Hb F within the ery-

throid burst–derived colony would be predicted, as indeed is observed. It has been proposed that one factor influencing the stochastic process by which F-cell production is determined is the stage at which a progenitor cell enters the erythroblast compartment.[474] A "short circuit" of the normal continuum from BFUe to colony-forming unit–erythroid (CFUe) to proerythroblasts might enhance the probability for F-cell formation (Fig. 4–23).

Stochastic events, although apparently random, are dependent on many parameters. The amount of Hb F in adult human progenitor–derived erythroid colonies may be influenced by conditions within the culture medium. Many of these are poorly defined and undoubtedly account for the different results obtained by various laboratories interested in the switching problem. Other factors that control the amount of Hb F produced in clonal culture without affecting colony development[475] have emerged from well-designed experiments. Sera from sheep fetuses strikingly decrease (or even abolish) fetal hemoglobin in adult or neonatal BFUe-derived colonies.[476–478] A physiological role for this "switching activity" might involve suppression of γ chain synthesis during erythroid maturation; this activity, however, does not affect the pattern of hemoglobin synthesis in fetal BFUe-derived colonies. Presumably, the developmental switch results in the acquisition of sensitivity to the "switching factor." Conversely, fetal calf serum contains inducers of Hb F expression.[479–482] Growth factors such as granulocyte-macrophage colony-stimulating factor (GM-CSF) or stem cell factor have been implicated in γ globin activation in BFUe-derived colonies,[483, 484] although the experimental results have not been consistent.[481]

There Is a γ to β Switch During Erythroid Cell Maturation

Whenever fetal and adult hemoglobins are coexpressed in human cells, they are produced asynchronously during maturation of erythroblasts[485–489] (see Fig. 4–23). Synthesis of γ globin occurs in proerythroblasts and basophilic erythroblasts predominantly, whereas β globin synthesis begins slightly later. Thus, there is a hemoglobin switch within the compartment of erythroblasts. Both globins are produced in the peripheral blood reticulocytes, however.

Models of Cellular Control

The heterocellular distribution of Hb F in normal adults and those with many hematological disorders fostered the notion that F cells and cells lacking Hb F might be derived from different stem or progenitor populations.[372, 374, 375] The finding of F erythroblasts and A erythroblasts (erythroblasts without Hb F) in colonies derived from a single progenitor (see Fig. 4–18) disproves this hypothesis.[490] Further evidence was derived from the study of clonal hematopoietic disor-

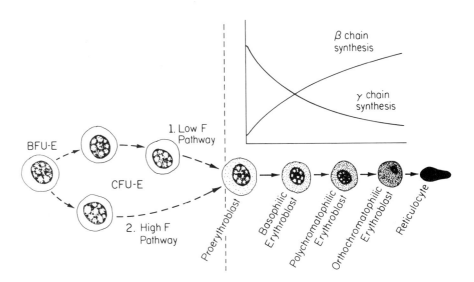

FIGURE 4–23. Model of modulation of Hb F synthesis during erythroid maturation and progenitor cell differentiation. The left diagram illustrates the hypothesis that F cells are formed by a premature commitment of earlier progenitor cells. Pathway 1 is that of normal progenitor differentiation and has a low chance for formation of F cells. In pathway 2, premature commitment or skipping of divisions increases the chance that a cell will become an F cell. The right diagram illustrates the asynchronous synthesis of γ and β globin during the maturation of erythroblasts.

ders such as chronic myelogenous leukemia, polycythemia vera, or paroxysmal nocturnal hemoglobinuria.[491–494] It has been established that these hematopoietic diseases are of single-cell origin. Nonetheless, individuals with these disorders exhibit a heterocellular distribution of Hb F, providing further evidence that determination with respect to this phenotypic characteristic occurs after commitment of progenitors to the erythroid lineage.[491–494]

Another hypothesis on the control of Hb F in the adult assumes that early progenitors encode a program allowing expression of fetal globin genes, but this program is changed to one allowing only adult globin expression during the downstream differentiation and maturation of progenitor cells[490, 495] (Fig. 4–24). Presumably, the earlier cells contain trans-acting factors that favor γ globin expression, whereas the late progenitors have trans-acting factors that favor β globin expression. F cells are produced when earlier progenitors become committed prematurely.[495] The hypothesis predicts that accelerated erythropoiesis will increase the chance of premature commitment of early progenitors, resulting in an increment in production of F cells. In chronic anemia, the kinetics of differentiation are less distorted, recruitment of early forms is diminished, and there is a lower rate of F-cell formation compared with the acute stress.

In support of this hypothesis is the induction of F-cell formation in acute marrow regeneration[404–413] and following administration of high doses of recombinant erythropoietin.[416, 417] Experimental evidence has also been obtained by sequential daily measurements of erythroid progenitor pools in baboons treated with high doses of recombinant erythropoietin.[417] These studies showed that the major effect of Epo is an acute expansion of the late erythroid progenitors and a mobilization of BFUe. An increase in F-programmed CFUe accounts for almost all the expansion of CFUe. The increase in F-CFUe is followed by a striking increase in F-positive erythroid clusters, which precedes the appearance of F reticulocytes in the circulation.

Experiments in culture were interpreted to suggest an inverse relationship between fetal hemoglobin expression and the degree of differentiation of the progenitors that form the colonies,[490, 495] but this issue remains controversial.[496–499] Experimental support for this relationship has been obtained in baboon bone marrow cultures in which BFUe-derived colonies produce the highest levels of fetal globin, whereas the most mature progenitors produce the lowest levels.[500]

Another hypothesis links the control of γ and β genes to the rate of progression through the cell cycle.[363, 413] β Gene expression might depend on the accumulation of rate-limiting trans-acting factors late in G_1. Rapidly dividing cells might accumulate little or no amounts of such factors, whereas adult erythroid cells progressing through the cell cycle more slowly might accumulate an adequate amount to ensure β gene expression. The preponderance of γ chain synthesis in proerythroblasts of adult progenitor origin may reflect the operation of such a mechanism. Only as erythroid maturation proceeds might the trans-acting environment required for β gene expression accumulate in adequate amounts to activate the β gene and secondarily to suppress γ gene expression.

Genetic Control of F Cells

That the F cells of the normal adult are genetically controlled is indicated by the existence of mutants not linked to the β locus that are manifested by increased F-cell numbers.[159–162, 164, 165] Family studies have been done to determine the pattern of inheritance of F-cell numbers[156–158, 163, 501–503]; autosomal[157, 158] or X-linked dominant[502, 503] patterns of inheritance have been proposed. The main argument for X-linked inheritance is that higher levels of F cells are observed in females than in males. However, this finding would be compatible with X linkage only if the locus controlling F-cell numbers escapes X inactivation. It is likely that, as

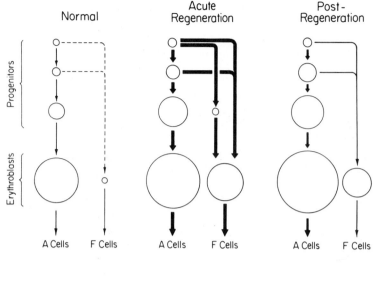

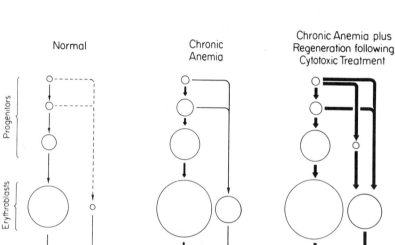

FIGURE 4–24. Model of formation of F cells in the normal adult, in acute erythroid regeneration, in the postregeneration period (or in chronic anemia), and following cytotoxic drug treatment. Normally, only a rare cell becomes an F cell. Acute regeneration forces cells to commit prematurely (in order to meet the peripheral demand); as a result, F cell production is induced. Expansion of erythropoiesis in the postregeneration stage satisfies the peripheral demand with less distortion of differentiation kinetics; fewer F cells (compared with the acute regeneration stage) are formed.

in the case of many other quantitative traits, F cells are determined polygenically.

The ability of individuals to respond with high or low levels of F cells when their erythropoiesis is stressed may also be under genetic control. Genetic control of the degree of F-cell response to stress has been shown in baboons: Animals segregate to either high F-cell responders or to low F-cell responders following an acute erythropoietic stress, and this phenotype is transmitted as a simple mendelian trait.[412] Genetic control of the response to acute stress is also indicated by the differences in F-cell response among species. Baboons usually exhibit striking F-cell increases when their erythropoiesis is stressed,[409–412] whereas monkeys (G. Stamatoyannopoulos, unpublished data) and humans[406] show modest F-cell induction; there is no induction of F-cell production when sheep are submitted to severe erythropoietic stress (W. G. Wood, personal communication).

As described in Chapters 5 and 6, certain β globin locus haplotypes are associated with a higher level of Hb F production in patients with sickle cell anemia or β thalassemia (reviewed in reference 431). A reasonable explanation for this association is that haplotypes are linked to variants of *cis*-acting elements that modulate γ gene expression. Such elements may be located in the γ gene promoters or in other regulatory regions of the β locus. The activation of γ genes by these variants may depend on *trans*-acting factors present in higher concentration during stressed erythropoiesis. This is a necessary assumption because normal persons who carry these haplotypes have normal numbers of F cells. Observations derived from studies of erythroid progenitors of these individuals in clonogenic erythroid cultures[432] are in support of this interpretation.

PHARMACOLOGICAL MANIPULATION OF HEMOGLOBIN F SYNTHESIS

In this chapter the concept has been developed that Hb F synthesis in humans beyond the perinatal period occurs because extinction of γ gene expression is not absolute. Furthermore, the usual low level of Hb F synthesis may be amplified by genetic and acquired factors that affect gene structure and function or perturb erythropoiesis. Pharmacological intervention to alter gene structure and/or erythropoiesis has been successful in inducing Hb F synthesis in experimental animals and in patients with sickle cell anemia or severe β thalassemia (reviewed in reference 504). As summarized earlier, induction of fetal hemoglobin is expected to decrease the probability of in vivo sickling and to decrease the size of ineffective erythropoiesis, improve red cell survival, and ameliorate anemia in the patient with homozygous β thalassemia. Data collected during a large multicenter study of the course of sickle cell disease show that any increase in Hb F synthesis has some beneficial effect on these syndromes.[505]

5-Azacytidine

5-Azacytidine causes DNA demethylation by substituting for cytosine residues in DNA. The incorporated 5-azacytidine inhibits the activity of the methyltransferase that methylates cytosine in newly synthesized DNA.[506, 507] There is a general correlation between cytosine methylation and gene expression; active genes are usually hypomethylated, whereas inactive genes are more frequently methylated. Several exceptions to this rule exist, however. A relationship between globin gene expression and DNA methylation has been established,[234, 235] but as mentioned earlier, DNA methylation does not appear to be a primary mechanism controlling globin gene switching.[237]

The first attempt at pharmacological induction of Hb F synthesis was done by DeSimone and associates,[508] who treated anemic juvenile baboons with escalating doses of 5-azacytidine; a striking augmentation of Hb F production occurred.[508, 509] Anemia was required, suggesting that optimal drug action occurred on an expanded erythron. Subsequently, Ley and colleagues[510] treated a patient with severe homozygous β thalassemia with a 7 day course of 5-azacytidine; a sevenfold increase in γ globin synthesis, a decrease in α chain excess, and a transient increase in hemoglobin concentration were observed. Induction of fetal hemoglobin was subsequently demonstrated in patients with homozygous Hb S or S/β thalassemia who received short courses of the drug or β thalassemia.[510–514] Long-term administration (200 to 500 days) of 5-azacytidine to Hb S homozygotes increased Hb F, decreased hemolysis, and, in one patient, reduced the frequency of vaso-occlusive crises.[512, 513] Because of concerns about risks of carcinogenicity,[515] this compound has been subsequently used only for compassionate treatment of patients with end-stage homozygous β thalassemia. In a patient with severe congestive heart failure due to cardiomyopathy secondary to iron overload, periodic infusion of 5-azacytidine over 2 years reduced ineffective erythropoiesis and increased hemoglobin levels from 6.0 g/dl to 10 to 12 g/dl, allowing the institution of an iron mobilization regimen consisting of chelation and periodic phlebotomies.[516] Another patient who had developed multiple autoantibodies and alloantibodies and severe anemia was treated with 5-azacytidine for 21 months, with substantial hematological improvement.[516]

The mechanism of action of 5-azacytidine has been debated. This cytotoxic compound is expected to kill the most actively cycling erythroid cells. The resulting decrease in late erythroid progenitor cells could trigger rapid erythroid regeneration and induce F-cell formation.[413, 517] Measurements of erythroid progenitor cell pools in baboons treated with 5-azacytidine are compatible with this hypothesis.[517] A direct effect on erythroid progenitors or early erythroblasts is also suggested by studies in culture.[518–520] Recently, the methylation status of CpG dinucleotide in the γ gene promoter has been shown to influence relative binding of transcriptional activities, one of which has been implicated in switching.[232] It is likely that a combined effect on erythropoiesis and on the methylation status of regulatory elements of the β locus is the cause for the superior in vivo induction of Hb F by 5-azacytidine.

Hydroxyurea

The discovery of Hb F induction by hydroxyurea was a consequence of the debate on the mechanism of action of 5-azacytidine. It was argued that if cytoreduction and secondary regeneration are the cause of Hb F induction by 5-azacytidine, other cytotoxic compounds producing similar perturbations of erythropoiesis but not DNA demethylation would also induce F-cell formation.[521, 522] Baboons treated with cytotoxic doses of ara-C responded with striking elevations of F reticulocytes with kinetics indistinguishable from those elicited by 5-azacytidine.[521] Induction of γ globin also occurred in monkeys or baboons treated with hydroxyurea.[522] Vinblastine, an M stage–specific agent that arrests cells in mitosis, also produces perturbations of erythropoiesis and stimulates Hb F synthesis in baboons.[523] Administration of cytotoxic doses of hydroxyurea or ara-C to Hb S homozygotes stimulated γ globin production.[524, 525] Stimulation of Hb F synthesis by cell cycle–specific drugs was transient and associated initially with a reduction and subsequently an expansion of the late erythroid progenitor pools.[521, 525] Following these studies, hydroxyurea, a readily available drug that can be taken orally, that is not carcinogenic, and that has been extensively used in the treatment of myeloproliferative disorders, was used for induction of Hb F in patients with sickle cell disease and β thalassemia. The outcome in β thalassemia patients has been disappointing, but promising results have been obtained in patients with Hb S syndromes[526] (Fig. 4–25).

Various regimens have been used in attempts to define schedules and doses that can produce maximal F-cell stimulation in sickle cell disease.[527–531] The most

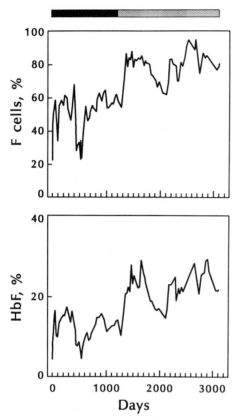

FIGURE 4–25. Induction of fetal hemoglobin in a patient with sickle cell anemia who was treated with hydroxyurea for approximately 10 years. The black bar indicates treatment with 10 to 20 mg of hydroxyurea 3 to 5 days a week (pulse therapy). The hatched bar indicates treatment with 15 to 20 mg of hydroxyurea 7 days a week (daily therapy). (Data from Dr. George Dover, Johns Hopkins Medical School, Baltimore, Maryland.)

effective regimen requires a daily administration of hydroxyurea.[531] Highest levels of Hb F are achieved when myelotoxic doses of the compound are used[530, 531]; myelotoxicity mainly manifests with moderate granulocytopenia and is reversible.[530, 531] There is considerable variation in the maximal tolerated dose of hydroxyurea, ranging from 10 mg/kg to 30 mg/kg. In general, the levels of Hb F achieved correlate with the dose of hydroxyurea tolerated. A few patients fail to respond to hydroxyurea with a significant increase in F cells.[531] A 4 to 12 week lag period between the initiation of treatment and maximal increase in fetal hemoglobin has been observed.[530, 531] In 32 patients participating in a large multicenter, open label, dose escalation trial, fetal hemoglobin increased from a mean pretreatment value of 4 per cent to a mean of 15 per cent at maximum tolerated dose.[531] In some patients, Hb F increased above 20 per cent, the concentration predicted to have a substantial inhibitory effect on in vivo sickling.

Several objective measurements suggest that hydroxyurea treatment is beneficial. A decrease in hemolysis, improvement of red cell survival, decrease in the calculated amount of Hb S polymer in F cells, and virtual disappearance of dense cells from the circula-

tion and of irreversibly sickled erythrocytes from the blood smear have been reported.[530–533] In a multicenter trial, patients were followed up to 24 months. There was a decline in painful crises from 2.1 crises per patient in the first 6 month interval to 0.8 in the fourth 6 month interval.[531] A double-blind multicenter study currently in progress examines whether this clinical improvement is real or a placebo effect due to the better medical care that patients participating in clinical trials are likely to receive.

The induction of F-cell formation by hydroxyurea was expected under the hypothesis linking F-cell induction to erythroid regeneration. The finding that optimal F-cell responses are achieved with myelosuppressive doses of this drug is compatible with this mechanism. Alternatively, hydroxyurea might influence γ gene expression in late cells, such as erythroblasts, and reprogram such cells to express the fetal globin program.[528] However, in vitro studies measuring effects of cell cycle drugs on late progenitors and proerythroblasts failed to demonstrate induction of γ globin by hydroxyurea,[519, 520] although induction of Hb F by 5-azacytidine and ara-C was observed in cultures under identical conditions.[519, 520]

Erythropoietin

Erythropoietin was used to stimulate F-cell production under the hypothesis that this compound will induce rapid erythroid regeneration accompanied by an increase in fetal hemoglobin production. Relatively low doses of Epo failed to induce F cells in baboons.[416] To produce acute regeneration kinetics, high doses of Epo (1500 IU/kg and higher) were used and caused sharp elevations of F reticulocytes.[416] F-reticulocyte induction correlated with the degree of reticulocytosis and the dose of Epo[416, 534] (Fig. 4–26). In contrast to the findings in baboons, erythropoietin produced only minor induction of F cells in patients with sickle cell disease.[535, 536] Patients treated with 800 IU to 1500 IU kg/day responded with twofold to threefold elevation of F reticulocytes.[535] In a double-blind study, the F-cell response to Epo was shown to require iron supplementation. Non-supplemented patients failed to increase the F reticulocytes, whereas F reticulocytes at least doubled in iron-supplemented patients.[536]

Treatment of baboons with Epo and hydroxyurea increases fetal hemoglobin in an additive fashion,[537, 538] suggesting that this combination treatment could increase Hb F levels in patients on lower doses of hydroxyurea or increase F-cell production in patients who responded poorly to hydroxyurea alone. Patients treated with maximally tolerated doses of hydroxyurea and various doses of Epo failed to show F-cell induction by Epo.[533] Another study,[539] however, clearly showed that this combination treatment increases Hb F and F cells above the levels achieved by hydroxyurea alone (Fig. 4–27). The difference between the two studies may be attributed to differences in the degree of marrow perturbation induced by hydroxyurea.

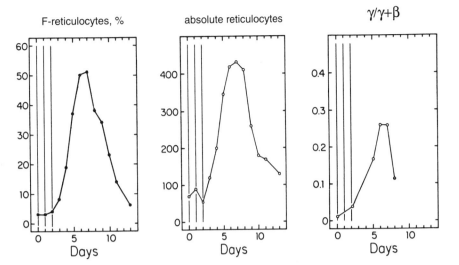

FIGURE 4–26. Induction of fetal hemoglobin in baboons treated with intravenous injection of human recombinant erythropoietin. (Reprinted, by permission, from the New England Journal of Medicine, Vol. 317, p. 415, 1987.)

When this compound produces a maximal F-cell stimulation, Epo may fail to increase F-cell production. When F-cell stimulation by hydroxyurea is suboptimal, Epo may further stimulate erythropoiesis to reach its maximal capacity of F-cell formation.

Administration of other hematopoietins (GM-CSF, interleukin-3 [IL-3], stem cell factor) has failed to induce Hb F in baboons when these compounds were administered alone. A combination treatment of IL-3 and Epo was tried under the hypothesis that IL-3 will expand the early progenitor cell pools on which Epo acts. An increase in the absolute numbers of F reticulocytes was observed, but there was no increase in the percentage of F reticulocytes.[540] Another study showed that a combination of hydroxyurea, IL-3, and GM-CSF induced F cells above the level induced by hydroxyurea alone.[538]

Butyric Acid Analogues

Butyric acid analogues have phenotypic effects on gene expression in many mammalian cell types and are known to induce erythroid differentiation in murine and human erythroleukemia cells.[541–543] In the course of studies of induction of embryonic globin genes by 5-azacytidine, Ginder and associates observed that whereas administration of 5-azacytidine alone in anemic chickens produces only a small induction of the embryonic rho gene, co-administration of 5-azacytidine and sodium butyrate resulted in a 5- to 10-fold increase in the level of embryonic globin mRNA.[544] Bard and Prosmanne[545] and Perrine and associates[546] observed that the γ to β switch is strikingly delayed in infants of diabetic mothers. With experiments in sheep fetuses, Perrine subsequently showed

FIGURE 4–27. Induction of fetal hemoglobin in a patient with sickle cell anemia who was treated with a combination of erythropoietin and hydroxyurea (see text).

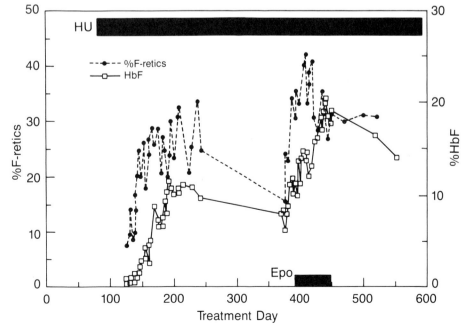

that α-aminobutyric acid, which is elevated in maternal diabetes, is responsible for the delayed γ to β switch.[547] Studies in baboons by Constantoulakis and associates subsequently showed that butyric acid analogues stimulated γ globin production in the adult stage of development, when these compounds are administered with continuous intravenous infusion.[548, 549] Butyric acid analogues also induced γ globin in neonatal erythroid colonies or in colonies formed by erythroid progenitors from adult animals or patients with sickle cell anemia.[548–550] Co-administration of butyrate and erythropoietin in baboons increased fetal hemoglobin in an additive fashion, whereas treatment with 5-azacytidine and butyrate increased fetal hemoglobin in a synergistic fashion.[548, 549, 551]

A phase I to II clinical trial was recently done with three patients with sickle cell anemia and three with severe β thalassemia.[552] Continuous infusion of arginine butyrate (1.5 g to 2.0 g per kilogram of body weight) for 2 to 8 weeks resulted in an impressive induction of γ globin production. A homozygous Hb Lepore patient treated with 2 g/kg of arginine butyrate (arginine is added to adjust the pH of the sodium butyrate solution) for more than 50 days increased the hemoglobin concentration from 4.7 g/dl to 10.2 g/dl. Apparently, γ globin induction had a profound effect on red cell survival and on the ineffective erythropoiesis in that patient. Concerns about the use of high concentrations of this compound were raised by tox-icity studies in baboons. Serious side effects, such as a fulminant multiorgan failure and specific neuropathological lesions,[551] were produced by doses of this compound only fourfold higher than those used in patients. Sickle cell patients have been treated by another butyrate analogue, sodium phenylbutyrate.[553] This drug, used in the treatment of urea cycle disorders, can be taken orally and has not been thus far associated with untoward effects. Five adult Hb S homozygotes responded to this compound with a rapid increase in F reticulocytes (Fig. 4–28).

The best characterized biochemical effect of butyrate is its ability to inhibit histone deacetylase, resulting in hyperacetylation of nucleosomal core histones.[554–556] The relationship of this effect to γ gene induction is unknown. Promoter sequences containing a putative butyrate response element have been identified in the chicken embryonic globin gene.[557] It has also been suggested that butyrate induces γ gene expression by inhibiting the interaction between CAAT box sequences and the CAAT displacement protein.[240] Treatment of transgenic mice carrying various γ gene promoter constructs is compatible with the interpretation that a butyrate response element is located in the distal γ globin promoter (B. Pace and G. Stamatoyannopoulos, unpublished observations).

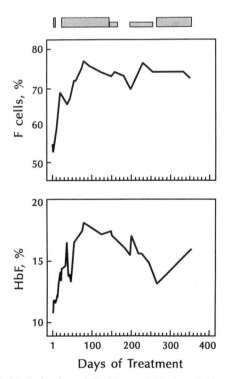

FIGURE 4–28. Induction of fetal hemoglobin in a sickle cell anemia patient treated with sodium phenylbutyrate (SPB) for approximately 1 year. Two doses of SPB were given: 20 g per day (large boxes); 10 g per day (small boxes). Therapy after day 50 was given on an outpatient basis. (Data from Dr. George Dover, Johns Hopkins Medical School, Baltimore, Maryland.)

REFERENCES

1. Stamatoyannopoulos, G., and Nienhuis, A. W.: Cellular and Molecular Regulation of Hemoglobin Switching. New York, Grune & Stratton, 1979.
2. Stamatoyannopoulos, G., and Nienhuis, A. W.: Hemoglobins in Development and Differentiation. New York, Alan R. Liss, 1981.
3. Stamatoyannopoulos, G., and Nienhuis, A. W.: Organization and Expression of Globin Genes. New York, Alan R. Liss, 1981.
4. Stamatoyannopoulos, G., and Nienhuis, A. W.: Globin Gene Expression and Hemopoietic Cell Differentiation. New York, Alan R. Liss, 1983.
5. Stamatoyannopoulos, G., and Nienhuis, A. W.: Experimental Approaches for the Study of Hemoglobin Switching. New York, Alan R. Liss, 1985.
6. Stamatoyannopoulos, G., and Nienhuis, A. W.: Developmental Control of Globin Gene Expression. New York, Alan R. Liss, 1987.
7. Stamatoyannopoulos, G., and Nienhuis, A. W.: Hemoglobin Switching, Part A: Transcriptional Regulation. New York, Alan R. Liss, 1989.
8. Stamatoyannopoulos, G., and Nienhuis, A. W.: Hemoglobin Switching, Part B: Cellular and Molecular Mechanisms. New York, Alan R. Liss, 1989.
9. Stamatoyannopoulos, G., and Nienhuis, A. W.: The Regulation of Hemoglobin Switching. Baltimore, The Johns Hopkins University Press, 1991.
10. Weatherall, D. J., and Clegg, J. B.: The Thalassemia Syndromes. 3rd ed. Oxford, England, Blackwell Scientific Publications, 1981.
11. Bunn, H. F., and Forget, B. G.: Hemoglobins: Molecular, Genetic and Clinical Aspects. Philadelphia, W. B. Saunders Co., 1986.
12. Karlsson, S., and Nienhuis, A. W.: Developmental regulation of human globin genes. Annu. Rev. Biochem. 54:1071, 1985.

13. Collins, F. S., and Weissman, S. M.: The molecular genetics of human hemoglobin. Prog. Nucleic Acid Res. Mol. Biol. 31:315, 1984.
14. Wood, W. G., Clegg, J. B., and Weatherall, D. J.: Developmental biology of human hemoglobins. Prog. Hematol. 10:43, 1977.
15. Weatherall, D. J., Pembrey, M. E., and Pritchard, J.: Fetal haemoglobin. Clin. Haematol. 3:467, 1974.
16. Schroeder, W. A., Huisman, T. H. J., Shelton, J. R., Shelton, J. B., Kleihauer, E. F., Dozy, A. M., and Robberson, B.: Evidence for multiple structural genes for the γ chain of human fetal hemoglobin. Proc. Natl. Acad. Sci. USA 60:537, 1968.
17. Huisman, T. H. J., Harris, H., and Gravely, M.: The chemical heterogeneity of the fetal hemoglobin in normal newborn infants and in adults. Mol. Cell. Biochem. 17:45, 1977.
18. Schroeder, W. A.: The synthesis and chemical heterogeneity of human fetal hemoglobin. Hemoglobin 4:431, 1980.
19. Nute, P. E., Pataryas, H. A., and Stamatoyannopoulos, G.: The Gγ and Aγ hemoglobin chains during human fetal development. Am. J. Hum. Genet. 25:271, 1973.
20. Parer, J. T.: Reversed relationship of oxygen affinity in maternal and fetal blood. Am. J. Obstet. Gynecol 108:323, 1970.
21. Wintrobe, M. M.: Clinical Hematology. Philadelphia, Lea & Febiger, 1961.
22. Bloom, W., and Bartelmez, G. W.: Hematopoiesis in young human embryos. Am. J. Anat. 67:21, 1940.
23. Knoll, W.: Die Blutbildung beim Embryo. In Hirschfeld, H., und Hittmair, A.: Handbuch Der Allgemeinen Haematologie. Vol. 1. Berlin, Urban & Schwarzenberg, 1932, p. 553.
24. Knoll, W., and Pingel, E.: Der Gang der Erythropoese beim Menschlichenembryo. Acta Haematol. 2:369, 1949.
25. Wintrobe, M. M., and Shumacker, H. B., Jr.: Comparison of hematopoiesis in the fetus and during recovery from pernicious anemia. J. Clin. Invest. 14:837, 1935.
26. Hollyfield, J. G.: The origin of erythroblasts in Rana pipiens tadpoles. Dev. Biol. 14:461, 1966.
27. Turpen, J. B., Turpen, C. J., and Flajnik, M.: Experimental analysis of hematopoietic cell development of the liver of larval Rana pipiens. Dev. Biol. 69:466, 1979.
28. Maniatis, G. M., and Ingram, V. M.: Erythropoiesis during amphibian metamorphosis. I. Site of maturation of erythrocytes in Rana catesbeiana. J. Cell. Biol. 49:372, 1971.
29. Broyles, R. H., Johnson, G. M., Maples, P. B., and Kindell, G. R.: Two erythropoietic microenvironments and two larval red cell lines in bullfrog tadpoles. Dev. Biol. 81:299, 1981.
29a. Broyles, R. H.: Changes in the blood during amphibian metamorphosis. In Gilbert, L. I., and Friden, E. (eds.): Metamorphosis: A Problem in Developmental Biology. New York, Plenum Press, 1981, pp. 461–490.
30. Maniatis, G. M., and Ingram, V. M.: Erythropoiesis during amphibian metamorphosis. III. Immunochemical detection of the tadpole and frog hemoglobins (Rana catesbeiana) in single erythrocytes. J. Cell. Biol. 49:390, 1971.
31. Broyles, R. H., Dorn, A. R., Maples, P. B., Johnson, G. M., Kindell, G. R., and Parkinson, A. M.: Choice of hemoglobin type in erythroid cells of Rana catesbeiana. In Stamatoyannopoulos, G., and Nienhuis, A. W. (eds.): Hemoglobins in Development and Differentiation. New York, Alan R. Liss, 1981, pp. 179–191.
32. Ingram, V. M.: Hemoglobin switching in amphibians and birds. In Stamatoyannopoulos, G., and Nienhuis, A. W. (eds.): Hemoglobins in Development and Differentiation. New York, Alan R. Liss, 1981, pp. 147–160.
33. Bruns, G. A. P., and Ingram, V. M.: The erythroid cells and hemoglobins of the chick embryo. Philos. Trans. R. Soc. Lond. (Biol.) 266:225, 1973.
34. Hakomori, S.: Blood group ABH and Ii antigens of human erythrocytes: Chemistry, polymorphism, and their developmental change. Semin. Hematol. 18:39, 1981.
35. Papayannopoulou, Th., Chen, P., Maniatis, A., and Stamatoyannopoulos, G.: Simultaneous assessment of i-antigenic expression and fetal hemoglobin in single red cells by immunofluorescence. Blood 55:221, 1980.
36. Chen, S.-H., Anderson, J. E., Giblett, E. R., and Stamatoyannopoulos, G.: Isozyme patterns in erythrocytes from human fetuses. Am. J. Hematol. 2:23, 1977.
37. Tashian, R. E.: Biochemical genetics of carbonic anhydrase. Hum. Genet. 7:1, 1976.
38. Boyer, S. H., Dover, G. J., Smith, K. D., and Scott, A.: Some interpretations of in vivo studies of globin gene switching in man and primates. In Stamatoyannopoulos, G., and Nienhuis, A. W. (eds.): Hemoglobins in Development and Differentiation. New York, Alan R. Liss, 1981, pp. 225–241.
39. Huehns, E. R., Dance, N., Beaven, G. H., Keil, J. V., Hecht, F., and Motulsky, A. G.: Human embryonic haemoglobins. Nature 201:1095, 1964.
40. Hecht, F., Motulsky, A. G., Lemire, R. J., and Shepard, T. E.: Predominance of hemoglobin Gower 1 in early human embryonic development. Science 152:91, 1966.
41. Gale, R. E., Clegg, J. B., and Huehns, E. R.: Human embryonic haemoglobins Gower 1 and Gower 2. Nature 280:162, 1979.
42. Papayannopoulou, Th., Shepard, T. H., and Stamatoyannopoulos, G.: Studies of hemoglobin expression in erythroid cells of early human fetuses using anti-γ and anti-β-globin chain fluorescent antibodies. In Stamatoyannopoulos, G., and Nienhuis, A. W. (eds.): Globin Gene Expression and Hemopoietic Differentiation. New York, Alan R. Liss, 1983, pp. 421–430.
42a. Papayannopoulou, Th. and Stamatoyannopoulos, G.: Unpublished data.
43. Kazazian, H. H., Jr., and Woodhead, A. P.: Hemoglobin A synthesis in the developing fetus. N Engl. J. Med. 289:58, 1973.
44. Cividalli, G., Nathan, D. G., Kan, Y. W., Santamarina, B., and Frigoletto, F.: Relation of β to γ synthesis during the first trimester: An approach to prenatal diagnosis of thalassemia. Pediatr. Res. 8:553, 1974.
45. Bard, H.: The postnatal decline of hemoglobin F synthesis in normal full-term infants. J. Clin. Invest. 55:395, 1975.
46. Boyer, S. H., Belding, T. K., Margolet, L., and Noyes, A. N.: Fetal hemoglobin restriction to a few erythrocytes (F cells) in normal human adults. Science 188:361, 1975.
47. Wood, W. G., Stamatoyannopoulos, G., Lim, G., and Nute, P. E.: F-cells in the adult: Normal values and levels in individuals with hereditary and acquired elevations of Hb F. Blood 46:671, 1975.
48. Farace, M. G., Brown, B. A., Raschella, G., Alexander, J., Gambari, R., Fantoni, A., Hardies, S. C., Hutchison III, C. A., and Edgell, M. H.: The mouse βh1 gene codes for the z chain of embryonic hemoglobin. J Biol. Chem. 259:7123, 1984.
49. Chada, K., Magram, J., and Costantini, F.: An embryonic pattern of expression of a human fetal globin gene in transgenic mice. Nature 319:685, 1986.
50. Bollekens, J. A., and Forget, B. G.: δβ Thalassemia and hereditary persistence of fetal hemoglobin. Hematol. Oncol. Clin. North Am. 5:399, 1991.
51. Poncz, M., Henthron, P., Stoeckert, C., and Surrey, S.: Globin gene expression in hereditary persistence of fetal haemoglobin and (δβ)⁰ thalassemia. In MacLean, N. (ed.): Oxford Surveys on Eukaryotic Genes. Vol. 5. Oxford, England, Oxford University Press, 1988, pp. 163–203.
52. Weatherall, D. J., Wood, W. G., and Clegg, J. B.: Genetics of fetal hemoglobin production in adult life. In Stamatoyannopoulos, G., and Nienhuis, A. W. (eds.): Cellular and Molecular Regulation of Hemoglobin Switching. New York, Grune & Stratton, 1979, pp. 3–27.
53. Conley, C. L., Weatherall, D. J., Richardson, S. N., Shepard, M. K., and Charache, S.: Hereditary persistence of fetal hemoglobin: A study of 79 affected persons in 15 Negro families in Baltimore. Blood 21:261, 1963.
54. Fessas, P., and Stamatoyannopoulos, G.: Hereditary persistence of fetal hemoglobin in Greece. A study and a comparison. Blood 24:223, 1964.
55. Huisman, T. H. J., Schroeder, W. A., Dozy, A. M., Shelton, J.

R., Shelton, J. B., Boyd, E. M., and Apell, G.: Evidence for multiple structural genes for the γ-chain of human fetal hemoglobin in hereditary persistence of fetal hemoglobin. Ann. N.Y. Acad. Sci. 165:320, 1969.

56. Huisman, T. H. J., Schroeder, W. A., Stamatoyannopoulos, G., Bouver, N., Shelton, J. R., Shelton, J. B., and Apell, G.: Nature of fetal hemoglobin in the Greek type of hereditary persistence of fetal hemoglobin with and without concurrent β thalassemia. J. Clin. Invest. 49:1035, 1970.

57. Boyer, S. H., Margolet, L., Boyer, M. L., Huisman, T. H. J., Schroeder, W. A., Wood, W. G., Weatherall, D. J., Clegg, J. B., and Cartner, R.: Inheritance of F cell frequency in heterocellular hereditary persistence of fetal hemoglobin; An example of allelic exclusion. Am. J. Hum. Genet. 29:256, 1977.

58. Stamatoyannopoulos, G., Fessas, Ph., and Papayannopoulou, Th.: F-Thalassemia: A study of thirty-one families with simple heterozygotes and combinations of F-thalassemia with A₂-thalassemia. Am. J. Med. 47:194, 1969.

59. Feingold, E. A., and Forget, B. G.: The breakpoint of a large deletion causing hereditary persistence of fetal hemoglobin occurs within an erythroid DNA domain remote from the β-globin gene cluster. Blood 74:2178, 1989.

60. Tuan, D., Feingold, E., Newman, M., Weissman, S. M., and Forget, B. G.: Different 3' end points of deletions causing δβ-thalassemia and hereditary persistence of fetal hemoglobin: Implications for the control of γ-globin gene expression in man. Proc. Natl. Acad. Sci. USA 80:6937, 1983.

61. Fritsch, E. F., Lawn, R. M., and Maniatis, T.: Characterization of deletions which affect the expression of fetal globin genes in man. Nature 279:598, 1979.

62. Bernards, R., and Flavell, R. A.: Physical mapping of the globin gene deletion in hereditary persistence of foetal hemoglobin (HPFH). Nucleic Acids Res. 8:1521, 1980.

63. Jagadeeswaran, P., Tuan, D., Forget, B. G., and Weissman, S. M.: A gene deletion ending at the midpoint of a repetitive DNA sequence in one form of hereditary persistence of fetal hemoglobin. Nature 296:469, 1982.

64. Tuan, D., Murnane, M. J., deRiel, J. L., and Forget, B. G.: Heterogeneity in the molecular basis of hereditary persistence of fetal hemoglobin. Nature 285:335, 1980.

65. Henthorn, P. S., Smithies, O., and Mager, D. L.: Molecular analysis of deletions in the human β-globin gene cluster: Deletion junctions and locations of breakpoints. Genomics 6:226, 1990.

66. Kutlar, A., Gardiner, M. B., Headlee, M. G., Reese, A. L., Cleek, M. P., Nagle, S., Sukumaran, P. K., and Huisman, T. H. J.: Heterogeneity in the molecular basis of three types of hereditary persistence of fetal hemoglobin and the relative synthesis of the Gγ and Aγ types of chains. Biochem. Genet. 22:21, 1984.

67. Wainscoat, J. S., Old, J. M., Wood, W. G., Trent, R. J., and Weatherall, D. J.: Characterization of an Indian (δβ)⁰ thalassemia. Br. J. Haematol. 58:353, 1984.

68. Henthorn, P. S., Mager, D., Huisman, T. H. J., and Smithies, O.: A gene deletion ending within a complex array of repeated sequences 3' to the human β-globin gene cluster. Proc. Natl. Acad. Sci. USA 83:5194, 1986.

69. Saglio, G., Camaschella, C., Serra, A., Bertero, T., Rege Cambrin, G., Guerrasiqo, A., Mazza, U., Izzo, P., Terragni, F., Giglioni, B., et al.: Italian type of deletional hereditary persistence of fetal hemoglobin. Blood 68:646, 1986.

70. Camaschella, C., Serra, A., Gottardi, E., Alfarano, A., Revello, D., Mazza, U., and Saglio, G.: A new hereditary persistence of fetal hemoglobin deletion has the breakpoint within the 3' β-globin gene enhancer. Blood 75:1000, 1990.

71. Baglioni, C.: A child homozygous for persistence of foetal haemoglobin. Nature 298:1177, 1963.

72. Huisman, T. H. J., Schroeder, W. A., Charache, S., Bethlen-Falvay, N. C., Bouver, N., Shelton, J. R., Shelton, J. B., and Apell, G.: Hereditary persistence of fetal hemoglobin: Heterogeneity of fetal hemoglobin in homozygotes and in conjunction with β-thalassemia. N. Engl. J. Med. 285:711, 1971.

73. Charache, S., Clegg, J. B., and Weatherall, D. J.: The Negro

variety of hereditary persistence of fetal hemoglobin is a mild form of thalassemia. Br. J. Haematol. 34:527, 1976.

74. Huisman, T. H. J., Wrightstone, R. N., Wilson, J. B., Schroeder, W. A., and Kendall, A. G.: Hemoglobin Kenya: The product of fusion of γ- and β-polypeptide chains. Arch. Biochem. Biophys. 152:850, 1972.

75. Kendall, A. G., Ojwang, P. J., Schroeder, W. A., and Huisman, T. H. J.: Hemoglobin Kenya, the product of a γβ fusion gene: Studies of the family. Am. J. Hum. Genet. 25:548, 1973.

76. Nute, P. E., Wood, W. G., Stamatoyannopoulos, G., Olweny, C., and Fialkow, P. J.: The Kenya form of hereditary persistence of fetal hemoglobin: Structural studies and evidence for homogeneous distribution of haemoglobin F using fluorescent anti-haemoglobin F antibodies. Br. J. Haematol. 32:55, 1976.

77. Ojwang, P. J., Nakatsuji, T., Gardiner, M. B., Reese, A. L., Gilman, J. G., and Huisman, T. H. J.: Gene deletion as the molecular basis for the Kenya-γ-HPFH condition. Hemoglobin 7:115, 1983.

78. Ottolenghi, S., and Giglioni, B.: γβ Thalassemia is due to a gene deletion. Cell 9:71, 1976.

79. Ramirez, F., O'Donnell, J. V., Marks, P. A., Bank, A., Musumeci, S., Schiliro, G., Pizzarelli, G., Russo, G., Luppis, B., and Gambino, R.: Abnormal or absent β mRNA in β Ferrara and gene deletion in δβ thalassemia. Nature 263:471, 1976.

80. Bernards, R., Kooter, J. M., and Flavell, R. A.: Physical mapping of the globin gene deletion in δβ thalassemia. Gene 6:265, 1979.

81. Ottolenghi, S., and Giglioni, B.: The deletion in a type of δβ thalassemia begins in an inverted Alu I repeat. Nature 300:770, 1982.

82. Ottolenghi, S., Giglioni, B., Taramelli, R., Comi, P., Mazza, U., Saglio, G., Camaschella, C., Izzo, P., Cao, A., Galanello, R., et al.: Molecular comparison of δβ thalassemia and hereditary persistence of fetal hemoglobin DNAs: Evidence of a regulatory area? Proc. Natl. Acad. Sci. USA 79:2347, 1982.

83. Anagnou, N. P., Papayannopoulou, Th., Stamatoyannopoulos, G., and Nienhuis, A. W.: Structurally diverse molecular deletions in the β-globin gene cluster exhibit an identical phenotype on interaction with the βˢ gene. Blood 65:1245, 1985.

84. Palena, A., Blau, A., Stamatoyannopoulos, G., and Anagnou, N. P.: Molecular characterization of a novel (δβ)-thalassemia deletion with increased expression of fetal hemoglobin in a family of Eastern European origin. Blood 79:6a, 1992.

85. Matsunaga, E., Kimura, A., Yamada, H., Fukumaki, Y., and Takagi, Y.: A novel deletion in δβ-thalassemia found in Japan. Biochem. Biophys. Res. Commun. 126:185, 1985.

86. Shiokawa, S., Yamada, H., Takihara, Y., Matsunaga, E., Ohba, Y., Yamamoto, K., and Fukumaki, Y.: Molecular analysis of Japanese δβ-thalassemia. Blood 72:1771, 1988.

87. Wainscoat, J. S., Thein, S. L., Wood, W. G., Weatherall, D. J., Metaxotou-Mavromati, A., Tzotzos, S., Kanavakis, E., and Kattamis, C.: A novel deletion in the β-globin gene complex. Ann. N.Y. Acad. Sci. 445:20, 1985.

88. Kulozik, A. E., Yarwood, N., and Jones, R. W.: The Corfu δβ-thalassemia. A small deletion acts at a distance to selectively abolish β-globin gene expression. Blood 71:457, 1988.

89. Traeger-Synodinos, J., Tzetis, M., Kanavakis, E., Metaxotou-Mavromati, A., and Kattamis, C.: The Corfu δβ-thalassemia mutation in Greece: Haematological phenotype and prevalence. Br. J. Haematol 79:302, 1991.

90. Galanello, R., Melis, M. A., Podda, A., Monne, M., Perseu, L., Loudianos, G., Cao, A., Pirastu, M., and Piga, A.: Deletion δ thalassemia: The 7.2 kb deletion of Corfu δβ-thalassemia in a non β-thalassemia chromosome. Blood 75:1747, 1990.

91. Zhang, J.-W., Stamatoyannopoulos, G., and Anagnou, N. P.: Laotian (δβ)⁰-thalassemia: Molecular characterization of a novel deletion associated with increased production of fetal hemoglobin. Blood 72:983, 1988.

92. Kulozik, A. E., Bellan-Koch, A., Kohne, E., and Kleihauer, E.: A deletion/inversion rearrangement of the β-globin gene

cluster in a Turkish family with δβ-thalassemia intermedia. Blood 79:2455, 1992.

93. Efremov, G. D., Nikolov, N., Hattori, Y., Bakioglu, I., and Huisman, T. H. J.: The 18- to 23-kb deletion of the Macedonian δβ-thalassemia includes the entire δ and β globin genes. Blood 68:971, 1986.

94. Trent, R. J., Svirklys, L., and Jones, P.: Thai (δβ)⁰-thalassemia and its interaction with γ-thalassemia. Hemoglobin 12:101, 1988.

95. Baglioni, C.: The fusion of two peptide chains in hemoglobin Lepore and its interpretation as a genetic deletion. Proc. Natl. Acad. Sci. USA 48:1880, 1962.

96. Flavell, R. A., Kooter, J. M., de Boer, E., Little, P. F., and Williamson, R.: Analysis of the βδ globin gene loci in normal and Hb Lepore DNA: Direct determination of gene linkage and intergene distance. Cell 15:25, 1978.

97. Baird, M., Schreiner, H., Driscoll, C., and Bank, A.: Localization of the site of recombination in formation of the Lepore Boston globin gene. J. Clin. Invest. 68:560, 1981.

98. Mavilio, F., Giampaolo, A., Care, A., Sposi, N. M., and Marinucci, M.: The δβ crossover region in Lepore Boston hemoglobinopathy is restricted to a 59 base pair region around the 5′ splice junction of the large globin gene intervening sequence. Blood 62:230, 1983.

99. Dobkin, C., Clyne, J., Metzenberg, A., and Bank, A.: Expression of a cloned Lepore globin gene. Blood 67:168, 1986.

100. Jones, R. W., Old, J. M., Trent, R. J., Clegg, J. B., and Weatherall, D. J.: Major rearrangement in the human β globin gene cluster. Nature 291:39, 1981.

101. Jennings, M. W., Jones, R. W., Wood, W. G., and Weatherall, D. J.: Analysis of an inversion with the human β globin gene cluster. Nucleic Acids Res. 13:2897, 1985.

102. Henthorn, P. S., Smithies, O., Nakatsuji, T., Felice, A. E., Gardiner, M. B., Reese, A. L., and Huisman, T. H. J.: (ᴬγδβ)⁰-Thalassemia in blacks is due to a deletion of 34 kbp of DNA. Br. J. Haematol. 59:343, 1985.

103. Orkin, S. H., Alter, B. P., and Altay, C.: Deletion of the ᴬγ gene in ᴳγδβ thalassemia. J. Clin. Invest. 64:866, 1979.

104. Trent, R. J., Jones, R. W., Clegg, J. B., Weatherall, D. J., Davidson, R., and Wood, W. G.: (ᴬγδβ) Thalassaemia: Similarity of phenotype in four different molecular defects, including one newly described. Br. J. Haematol. 57:279, 1984.

105. George, E., Faridah, K., Trent, R. J., Padanilam, B. J., Huang, H. J., and Huisman, T. H. J.: Homozygosity for a new type of ᴳγ (ᴬγδβ)⁰-thalassemia in a Malaysian male. Hemoglobin 10:353, 1986.

106. Jones, R. W., Old, J. M., Trent, R. J., Clegg, J. B., and Weatherall, D. J.: Restriction mapping of a new deletion responsible for ᴳγ (δβ)⁰ thalassemia. Nucleic Acids Res. 9:6813, 1981.

107. Mager, D. L., Henthorn, P. S., and Smithies, O.: A Chinese ᴳγ (ᴬγδβ)⁰ thalassemia deletion: Comparison to other deletions in the human β-globin gene cluster and sequence analysis of the breakpoints. Nucleic Acids Res. 13:6559, 1985.

108. Anagnou, N. P., Papayannopoulou, Th., Nienhuis, A. W., and Stamatoyannopoulos, G.: Molecular characterization of a novel form of (ᴬγδβ)⁰-thalassemia deletion with a 3′ breakpoint close to those of HPFH-3 and HPFH-4: Insights for a common regulatory mechanism. Nucleic Acids Res. 16:6057, 1988.

109. Zeng, Y. T., Huang, S. Z., Chen, B., Liang, Y. C., Chang, Z. M., Harano, T., and Huisman, T. H. J.: Hereditary persistence of fetal hemoglobin or (δβ)⁰-thalassemia: Three types observed in South-Chinese families. Blood 66:1430, 1985.

110. Zhang, J.-W., Song, W.-F., Zhao, Y.-J., Wu, G.-Y., Qiu, Z.-M., Wang, F.-N., Chen, S.-S., and Stamatoyannopoulos, G.: Molecular characterization of a novel form of (ᴬγδβ)⁰ thalassemia deletion in a Chinese family. Blood 81:1624, 1993.

111. Losekoot, M., Fodde, R., Gerritsen, E. J. A., van de Kuit, I., Schreuder, A., Giordina, P. C., Vossen, J. M., and Bernini, L. F.: Interaction of two different disorders in the β-globin gene cluster associated with an increased Hb F production:

A novel deletion type of ᴳγ + (ᴬγδβ)⁰-thalassemia and a hereditary persistence of fetal hemoglobin determinant. Blood 77:861, 1991.

112. Fucharoen, S., Winichagoon, P., Chaicharoen, S., and Wasi, P.: Different molecular defects of ᴳγ(ᴬγδβ)⁰-thalassemia in Thailand. Eur. J. Haematol. 39:154, 1987.

113. Winichagoon, P., Fucharoen, S., Thonglairoam, V., and Wasi, P.: Thai ᴳγ(Aγδβ)⁰-thalassemia and its interaction with a single γ-globin gene on a chromosome carrying β⁰-thalassemia. Hemoglobin 14:185, 1990.

114. Driscoll, M. C., Dobkin, C. S., and Alter, B. P.: γδβ-Thalassemia due to a de novo mutation deleting the 5′ β-globin gene activation–region hypersensitive sites. Proc. Natl. Acad. Sci. USA 86:7470, 1989.

115. Curtin, P., Pirastu, M., Kan, Y. W., Gobert-Jones, J. A., Stephens, A. D., and Lehmann, H.: A distant gene deletion affects β-globin gene function in an atypical γδβ-thalassemia. J. Clin. Invest. 76:1554, 1985.

116. Kioussis, D., Vanin, E., deLange, T., Flavell, R. A., and Grosveld, F. G.: β-Globin gene inactivation by DNA translocation in β-thalassemia. Nature 306:662, 1983.

117. Vanin, E. F., Henthorn, P. S., Kioussis, D., Grosveld, F., and Smithies, O.: Unexpected relationships between four large deletions in the human β-globin gene cluster. Cell 35:701, 1983.

118. Wright, S., Taramelli, R., Rosenthal, A., de Boer, E., Antoniou, M., Kioussis, D., Wilson, F., Hurst, J., Bartram, C., Athanassiadou, A., et al.: DNA sequences required for regulated expression of the human β-globin gene. Prog. Clin. Biol. Res. 191:251, 1985.

119. Orkin, S. H., Goff, S. C., and Nathan, D. G.: Heterogeneity of the DNA deletion in γδβ-thalassemia. J. Clin. Invest. 67:878, 1981.

120. Pirastu, M., Kan, Y. W., Lin, C. C., Baine, R. M., and Holbrook, C. T.: Hemolytic disease of the newborn caused by a new deletion of the entire β-globin cluster. J. Clin. Invest. 72:602, 1983.

121. Fearon, E. R., Kazazian, H. H., Jr., Waber, P. G., Lee, J. I., Antonarakis, S. E., Orkin, S. H., Vanin, E. F., Henthorn, P. S., Grosveld, F. G., Scott, A. F., et al.: The entire β-globin gene cluster is deleted in a form of γδβ-thalassemia. Blood 61:1269, 1983.

122. Diaz-Chico, J. C., Huang, H. J., Juri, D., Efremov, G. D., Wadsworth, L. D., and Huisman, T. H. J.: Two new large deletions resulting in εγδβ-thalassemia. Acta Haematol. (Basel) 80:79, 1988.

123. Flavell, R. A., Bernards, R., Kooter, J. M., de Boer, E., Little, P. F., Annison, G., and Williamson, R.: The structure of the human β-globin gene in β-thalassemia. Nucleic Acids Res. 6:2749, 1979.

124. Orkin, S. H., Old, J. M., Weatherall, D. J., and Nathan, D. G.: Partial deletion of β-globin gene DNA in certain patients with β⁰-thalassemia. Proc. Natl. Acad. Sci. USA 76:2400, 1979.

125. Orkin, S. H., Kolodner, R., Michelson, A., and Husson, R.: Cloning and direct examination of a structurally abnormal human β⁰ thalassemia globin gene. Proc. Natl. Acad. Sci. USA 77:3558, 1980.

126. Spritz, R. A., and Orkin, S. H.: Duplication followed by deletion accounts for the structure of an Indian deletion β thalassemia. Nucleic Acids Res. 10:8025, 1982.

127. Padanilam, B. J., Felice, A. E., and Huisman, T. H. J.: Partial deletion of the 5′ β-globin gene region causes β⁰-thalassemia in members of an American black family. Blood 64:941, 1984.

128. Anand, R., Boehm, C. D., Kazazian, H. H., Jr., and Vanin, E. F.: Molecular characterization of a β⁰-thalassemia resulting from a 1.4 kilobase deletion. Blood 72:636, 1988.

129. Gilman, J. G., Huisman, T. H. J., and Abels, J.: Dutch β⁰-thalassemia: A 10 kilobase DNA deletion associated with significant γ-chain production. Br. J. Haematol. 56:339, 1984.

130. Gilman, J. G.: The 12.6 kilobase DNA deletion in Dutch β⁰-thalassemia. Br. J. Haematol. 67:369, 1987.

131. Diaz-Chico, J. C., Yang, K. G., Kutlar, A., Reese, A. L., Aksoy, M., and Huisman, T. H. J.: An approximately 300 bp deletion involving part of the 5' β-globin gene region is observed in members of a Turkish family with β-thalassemia. Blood 70:583, 1987.

132. Spiegelberg, R., Aulehla-Scholz, C., Erlich, H., and Horst, J.: A β-thalassemia gene caused by a 290-base pair deletion: Analysis by direct sequencing of enzymatically amplified DNA. Blood 73:1695, 1989.

133. Aulehla-Scholz, C., Spiegelberg, R., and Horst, J.: A β-thalassemia mutant caused by a 300-bp deletion in the human β-globin gene. Hum. Genet. 81:298, 1989.

134. Popovich, B. W., Rosenblatt, D. S., Kendall, A. G., and Nishioka, Y.: Molecular characterization of an atypical β-thalassemia caused by a large deletion in the 5' β-globin gene region. Am. J. Hum. Genet. 39:797, 1986.

135. Waye, J. S., Cai, S.-P., Eng, B., Clark, C., Adams, J. G., III, Chui, D. H. K., and Steinberg, M. H.: High hemoglobin A_2 β^0-thalassemia due to a 532-basepair deletion of the 5' β-globin gene region. Blood 77:1100, 1991.

136. Fucharoen, S., Shimizu, K., and Fukumaki, Y.: A novel C-T transition within the distal CCAAT motif of the $^G\gamma$-globin gene in the Japanese HPFH: Implication of factor binding in elevated fetal globin expression. Nucleic Acids Res. 18:5245, 1990.

137. Surrey, S., Delgrosso, K., Malladi, P., and Schwartz, E.: A single base change at position −175 in the 5'-flanking region of the $^G\gamma$-globin gene from a black with $^G\gamma\beta^+$-HPFH. Blood 71:807, 1988.

138. Ottolenghi, S., Nicolis, S., Taramelli, R., Malgaretti, N., Mantovani, R., Comi, P., Giglioni, B., Longinotti, M., Dore, F., Oggiano, L., et al.: Sardinian $^G\gamma$-HPFH: A T→C substitution in a conserved "octamer" sequence in the $^G\gamma$-globin promoter. Blood 71:815, 1988.

139. Collins, F. S., Stoeckert, C. J., Jr., Serjeant, G. R., Forget, B. G., and Weissman, S. M.: $^G\gamma\beta^+$ Hereditary persistence of fetal hemoglobin: Cosmid cloning and identification of a specific mutation 5' to the $^G\gamma$ gene. Proc. Natl. Acad. Sci. USA 81:4894, 1984.

140. Oner, R., Kutlar, F., Gu, L.-H., and Huisman, T. H. J.: The Georgia type of nondeletional hereditary persistence of fetal hemoglobin has a C→T mutation at nucleotide −114 of the $^A\gamma$-globin gene. Blood 77:1124, 1991.

141. Gilman, J. G., Mishima, N., Wen, X. J., Stoming, T. A., Lobel, J., and Huisman, T. H. J.: Distal CCAAT box deletion in the $^A\gamma$ globin gene of two black adolescents with elevated fetal $^A\gamma$ globin. Nucleic Acids Res. 16:10635, 1988.

142. Gelinas, R., Endlich, B., Pfeiffer, C., Yagi, M., and Stamatoyannopoulos, G.: G to A substitution in the distal CCAAT box of the $^A\gamma$-globin gene in Greek hereditary persistence of fetal haemoglobin. Nature 313:323, 1985.

143. Collins, F. S., Metherall, J. E., Yamakawa, M., Pan, J., Weissman, S. M., and Forget, B. G.: A point mutation in the $^A\gamma$-globin gene promoter in Greek hereditary persistence of fetal haemoglobin. Nature 313:325, 1985.

144. Ottolenghi, S., Camaschella, C., Comi, P., Giglioni, B., Longinotti, M., Oggiano, L., Dore, F., Sciarratta, G., Ivaldi, G., Saglio, G., et al.: A frequent $^A\gamma$-hereditary persistence of fetal hemoglobin in Northern Sardinia: Its molecular basis and haematological phenotype in heterozygotes with β thalassemia. Hum. Genet. 79:13, 1988.

145. Huang, H. J., Stoming, T. A., Harris, H. F., Kutlar, F., and Huisman, T. H. J.: The Greek $^A\gamma\beta^+$-HPFH observed in a large black family. Am. J. Hematol. 25:401, 1987.

146. Stoming, T. A., Stoming, G. S., Lanclos, K. D., Fei, Y. I., Altay, C., Kutlar, F., and Huisman, T. H. J.: An $^A\gamma$ type of nondeletional hereditary persistence of fetal hemoglobin with a T→C mutation at position −175 to the cap site of the $^A\gamma$ globin gene. Blood 73:329, 1989.

147. Costa, F. F., Zago, M. A., Cheng, G., Nechtman, J. F., Stoming, T. A., and Huisman, T. H. J.: The Brazilian type of nondeletional $^A\gamma$-fetal hemoglobin has a C-G substitution at nucleotide −195 of the $^A\gamma$-globin gene. Blood 76:1896, 1990.

148. Giglioni, B., Casini, C., Mantovani, R., Merli, S., Comi, P., Ottolenghi, S., Saglio, G., Camaschella, C., and Mazza, U.: A molecular study of a family with Greek hereditary persistence of fetal hemoglobin and β-thalassemia. EMBO J 3:2641, 1984.

149. Farquhar, M., Gelinas, R., Tatsis, B., Murray, J., Yagi, M., Mueller, R., and Stamatoyannopoulos, G.: Restriction endonuclease mapping of γδβ globin region in $^G\gamma(\beta)^+$ HPFH and a Chinese $^A\gamma$ HPFH variant. Am. J. Hum. Genet. 35:611, 1983.

150. Gelinas, R., Bender, M., Lotshaw, C., Waber, P., Kazazian, H., Jr., and Stamatoyannopoulos, G.: Chinese $^A\gamma$ HPFH: C to T substitution at position −196 of the $^A\gamma$ gene promoter. Blood 67:1777, 1986.

151. Tate, V. E., Wood, W. G., and Weatherall, D. J.: The British form of hereditary persistence of fetal hemoglobin results from a single base pair mutation adjacent to an S1 hypersensitive site 5' to the $^A\gamma$ globin gene. Blood 68:1389, 1986.

152. Weatherall, D. J., Cartner, R., Clegg, J. B., Wood, W. G., Macrae, I. A., and Mackenzie, A.: A form of hereditary persistence of fetal haemoglobin characterized by uneven cellular distribution of haemoglobin F and the production of haemoglobins A and A_2 in homozygotes. Br. J. Haematol. 29:205, 1975.

153. Gilman, J. G., Mishima, N., Wen, X. J., Kutlar, F., and Huisman, T. H. J.: Upstream promoter mutation associated with modest elevation of fetal hemoglobin expression in human adults. Blood 72:78, 1988.

154. Marti, H. R.: Normale und anormale menschliche Hamoglobine. Berlin, Springer-Verlag, 1987, pp. 81–89.

155. Stamatoyannopoulos, G., Wood, W. G., Papayannopoulou, Th., and Nute, P. E.: A new form of hereditary persistence of fetal hemoglobin in Blacks and its association with sickle cell trait. Blood 46:683, 1975.

156. Wood, W. G., Weatherall, D. J., and Clegg, J. B.: Interaction of heterocellular hereditary persistence of foetal haemoglobin with β thalassemia and sickle cell anaemia. Nature 264:247, 1976.

157. Zago, M. A., Wood, W. G., Clegg, J. B., Weatherall, D. J., O'Sullivan, M., and Gunson, H.: Genetic control of F cells in human adults. Blood 53:977, 1979.

158. Milner, P. F., Leibfarth, J. D., Ford, J., Barton, B. P., Grenett, H. E., and Garver, F. A.: Increased Hb in sickle cell anemia is determined by a factor linked to the β^S gene from one parent. Blood 63:64, 1984.

159. Gianni, A. M., Bregni, M., Cappellini, M. D., Fiorelli, G., Taramelli, R., Giglioni, B., Comi, P., and Ottolenghi, S.: A gene controlling fetal hemoglobin expression in adults is not linked to the non−α globin cluster. EMBO J. 2:921, 1983.

160. Giampaolo, A., Mavilio, F., Sposi, N. M., Care, A., Massa, A., Cianetti, L., Petrini, M., Russo, R., Cappellini, M. D., and Marinucci, M.: Heterocellular hereditary persistence of fetal hemoglobin (HPFH). Molecular mechanisms of abnormal γ-gene expression in association with β thalassemia and linkage relationship with the β-globin gene cluster. Hum. Genet. 66:151, 1984.

161. Cappellini, M. D., Fiorellia, G., and Bernini, L. F.: Interaction between homozygous β^0 thalassemia and the Swiss type of hereditary persistence of fetal haemoglobin. Br. J. Haematol. 48:561, 1981.

162. Martinez, G., Novelletto, A., DiRienzo, A., Felicetti, L., and Colombo, B.: A case of hereditary persistence of fetal hemoglobin caused by a gene not linked to the β-globin cluster. Hum. Genet. 82:335, 1989.

163. Dover, G. J., Boyer, S. H., and Pembrey, M. E.: F-cell production in sickle cell anemia: Regulation by genes linked to β-hemoglobin locus. Science 211:1441, 1981.

164. Prchal, J., and Stamatoyannopoulos, G.: Two siblings with unusually mild homozygous β-thalassemia: A didactic example of the effect of a nonallelic modifier gene on the expressivity of a monogenic disorder. Am. J. Med. Genet. 10:291, 1981.

165. Boyer, S. H., Dover, G. J., Sergeant, G. R., Smith, K. D.,

Antonarakis, S. E., Embury, S. H., Margolet, L., Noyes, A. N., Boyer, M. L., and Bias, W. B.: Production of F cells in sickle cell anemia: Regulation by a genetic locus or loci separate from the β-globin gene cluster. Blood 64:1053, 1984.

166. Brittenham, G. B., Schechter, A. N., and Noguchi, C. T.: Hemoglobin S polymerization: Primary determinant of the hemolytic and clinical severity of the sickling syndromes. Blood 65:183, 1985.

167. Serjeant, G. R., Serjeant, B. E., and Mason, K.: Heterocellular hereditary persistence of fetal haemoglobin and homozygous sickle-cell disease. Lancet 1:795, 1977.

168. Perrine, R. P., Brown, M. J., Clegg, J. B., Weatherall, D. J., and May, A.: Benign sickle-cell anaemia. Lancet 2:1163, 1972.

169. Wood, W. G., Penbrey, M. E., Serjeant, G. R., Perrine, R. P., and Weatherall, D. J.: Hb F synthesis in sickle cell anaemia: A comparison of Saudi Arabian cases with those of African origin. Br. J. Haematol. 45:431, 1980.

170. Ali, S. A.: Milder variant of sickle-cell disease in Arabs in Kuwait associated with unusually high level of foetal haemoglobin. Br. J. Haematol. 19:613, 1970.

171. Nienhuis, A. W., and Maniatis, T.: Structure and expression of globin genes in erythroid cells. In Stamatoyannopoulos, G., Nienhuis, A. W., Leder, P., and Majerus, P. W. (eds.): The Molecular Basis of Blood Diseases. Philadelphia, W. B. Saunders Co., 1987, pp. 28–65.

172. Eaton, W. A.: The relationship between coding sequences and function in hemoglobin. Nature 284:183, 1980.

173. Go, M.: Correlation of DNA exonic regions with protein structural units in hemoglobin. Nature 291:90, 1981.

174. Orkin, S. H.: GATA-binding transcription factors in hematopoietic cells. Blood 80:575, 1992.

175. Evans, T., Reitman, M., and Felsenfeld, G.: An erythrocyte-specific DNA-binding factor recognizes a regulatory sequence common to all chicken globin genes. Proc. Natl. Acad. Sci. USA 85:5976, 1988.

176. Wall, L., de Boer, E., and Grosveld, F.: The human β-globin gene 3′ enhancer contains multiple binding sites for an erythroid-specific protein. Genes Dev. 2:1089, 1988.

177. Martin, D. I. K., Tsai, S.-F., and Orkin, S. H.: Increased γ-globin expression in a nondeletion HPFH mediated by an erythroid-specific DNA-binding factor. Nature 338:435, 1989.

178. Nicolis, S., Ronchi, A., Malgaretti, N., Mantovani, R., Giglioni, B., and Ottolenghi, S.: Increased erythroid-specific expression of a mutated HPFH γ-globin promoter requires the erythroid factor NFE-1. Nucl. Acids Res. 17:5509, 1989.

179. Tsai, S.-F., Martin, D. I. K., Zon, L. I., D'Andrea, A. D., Wong, G. G., and Orkin, S. H.: Cloning of cDNA for the major DNA-binding protein of the erythroid lineage through expression in mammalian cells. Nature 339:446, 1989.

180. Zon, L. I., Tsai, S.-F., Burgess, S., Matsudaira, P., Bruns, G. A. P., and Orkin, S. H.: The major human erythroid DNA-binding protein (GF-1): Primary sequence and localization of the gene to the X chromosome. Proc. Natl. Acad. Sci. USA 87:668, 1990.

181. Evans, T., and Felsenfeld, G.: The erythroid-specific transcription factor ERYF1: A new finger protein. Cell 58:877, 1989.

182. Trainor, C. D., Evans, T., Felsenfeld, G., and Boguski, M. S.: Structure and evolution of a human erythroid transcription factor. Nature 343:92, 1990.

183. Evans, T., and Felsenfeld, G.: Trans-activation of a globin promoter in nonerythroid cells. Mol. Cell. Biol. 11:843, 1991.

184. Martin, D. I. K., and Orkin, S. H.: Transcriptional activation and DNA binding by the erythroid factor GF-1/NF-E1/ERYF 1. Genes Dev. 4:1886, 1990.

185. Yang, H. Y., and Evans, T.: Distinct roles for the two cGATA-1 finger domains. Mol. Cell. Biol. 12:4562, 1992.

186. Yamamoto, M., Ko, L. J., Leonard, M. W., Beug, H., Orkin, S. H., and Engel, J. D.: Activity and tissue-specific expression of the transcription factor NF-E1 multigene family. Genes Dev. 4:1650, 1990.

187. Martin, D. I. K., Zon, L. I., Mutter, G., and Orkin, S. H.: Expression of an erythroid transcription factor in megakaryocytic and mast cell lineages. Nature 344:444, 1990.

188. Romeo, P.-H., Prandini, M.-H., Joulin, V., Mignotte, V., Prenant, M., Vainchenker, W., Marguerie, G., and Uzan, G.: Megakaryocytic and erythrocytic lineages share specific transcription factors. Nature 344:447, 1990.

189. Mouthon, M.-A., Bernard, O., Mitjavila, M.-T., Romeo, P.-H., Vainchenker, W., and Mathieu-Mahul, D.: Expression of tal-1 and GATA-binding proteins during human hematopoiesis. Blood 81:647, 1993.

190. Sposi, N. M., Zon, L. I., Care, A., Valtieri, M., Testa, U., Gabbianelli, M., Mariani, G., Bottero, L., Mather, C., Orkin, S. H., and Peschle, C.: Cell cycle–dependent initiation and lineage-dependent abrogation of GATA-1 expression in pure differentiating hematopoietic progenitors. Proc. Natl. Acad. Sci. USA 89:6353, 1992.

191. Crotta, S., Nicolis, S., Ronchi, A., Ottolenghi, S., Ruzzi, L., Shimada, Y., Migliaccio, A. R., and Migliaccio, G.: Progressive inactivation of the expression of an erythroid transcriptional factor in GM- and G-CSF–dependent myeloid cell lines. Nucleic Acids Res. 18:6863, 1990.

192. Ko, L. J., Yamamoto, M., Leonard, M. W., George, K. M., Ting, P., and Engel, J. D.: Murine and human T-lymphocyte GATA-3 factors mediate transcription through a cis-regulatory element within the human T-cell receptor δ gene enhancer. Mol. Cell. Biol. 11:2778, 1991.

193. Ho, I.-C., Vorhees, P., Marin, N., Oakley, B. K., Tsai, S.-F., Orkin, S. H., and Leiden, J. M.: Human GATA-3: A lineage-restricted transcription factor that regulates the expression of the T cell receptor α gene. EMBO J. 10:1187, 1991.

194. Zon, L. I., Mather, C., Burgess, S., Bolce, M. E., Harland, R. M., and Orkin, S. H.: Expression of GATA-binding proteins during embryonic development in Xenopus laevis. Proc. Natl. Acad. Sci. USA 88:10642, 1991.

195. Pevny, L., Simon, M. C., Robertson, E., Klein, W. H., Tsai, S.-F., D'Agati, V., Orkin, S. H., and Costantini, F.: Erythroid differentiation in chimaeric mice blocked by a targeted mutation in the gene for transcription factor GATA-1. Nature 349:257, 1991.

196. Mignotte, V., Eleouet, J. F., Raich, N., and Romeo, P. H.: Cis- and trans-acting elements involved in the regulation of the erythroid promoter of the human porpholbilinogen deaminase gene. Proc. Natl. Acad. Sci. USA 86:6548, 1989.

197. Mignotte, V., Wall, L., de Boer, E., Grosveld, F., and Romeo, P. H.: Two tissue-specific factors bind the erythroid promoter of the human porpholbilinogen deaminase gene. Nucleic Acids Res. 17:37, 1989.

198. Ney, P. A., Sorrentino, B. P., McDonagh, K. T., and Nienhuis, A. W.: Tandem AP-1–binding sites within the human β-globin dominant control region function as an inducible enhancer in erythroid cells. Genes Dev. 4:993, 1990.

199. Ney, P. A., Sorrentino, B. P., Lowrey, C. H., and Nienhuis, A. W.: Inducibility of the HS II enhancer depends on binding of an erythroid specific nuclear protein. Nucleic Acids Res. 18:6011, 1990.

200. Andrews, N. C., Erdjument-Bromage, H., Davidson, M. B., Tempst, P., and Orkin, S. H.: Globin locus control region enhancer binding factor (NF-E2): An hematopoietic-specific basic-leucine zipper protein. Nature 362:722, 1993.

201. Ney, P. A., Andrews, N. C., Jane, S. M., Safer, B., Purucker, M. E., Goff, S. C., Orkin, S. H., and Nienhuis, A. W.: Purification of the human NF-E2 complex: cDNA cloning of the hematopoietic-specific subunit and evidence for an associated partner. Mol. Cell Biol. (in press).

202. Stevens, P. W., Dodgson, J. B., and Engel, J. D.: Structure and expression of the chicken ferritin H-subunit gene. Mol. Cell. Biol. 7:1751, 1987.

203. Peters, L. L., Andrews, N. C., Eicher, E. M., Davidson, M. B., Orkin, S. H., and Lux, S. E.: The hematopoietic transcription factor NF-E2 is the site of the hypochromic microcytic

anemia mutation, mk, located on mouse chromosome 15. Blood 80:949, 1993.

204. Jarman, A. P., Wood, W. G., Sharpe, J. A., Gourdon, G., Ayyub, H., and Higgs, D. R.: Characterization of the major regulatory element upstream of the human α-globin gene cluster. Mol. Cell. Biol. 11:4679, 1991.

205. Strauss, E. C., Andrews, N. C., Higgs, D. R., and Orkin, S. H.: In vivo footprinting of the human α-globin locus upstream regulatory element by guanine and adenine ligation-mediated polymerase chain reaction. Mol. Cell. Biol. 12:2135, 1992.

206. Taketani, S., Inazawa, J., Nakahashi, Y., Abe, T., and Tokunaga, R.: Structure of the human ferrochelatase gene. Exon/intron gene organization and location of the gene to chromosome 18. Eur. J. Biochem. 205:217, 1992.

207. Walters, M., and Martin, D. I. K.: Functional erythroid promoters created by interaction of the transcription factor GATA-1 with CACCC and AP-1/NFE-2 elements. Proc. Natl. Acad. Sci. USA 89:10444, 1992.

208. Gong, Q., and Dean, A.: Enhancer-dependent transcription of the ε-globin promoter requires promoter-bound GATA-1 and enhancer-bound AP-1/NF-E2. Mol. Cell. Biol. 13:911, 1993.

209. Green, A. R., and Begley, C. G.: SCL and related hemopoietic helix-loop-helix transcription factors. Int. J. Cell Cloning 10:269, 1992.

210. Begley, C. G., Aplan, P. D., Davey, M. P., Nakahara, K., Tchorz, K., Kurtzberg, J., Hershfield, M. S., Haynes, B. F., Cohen, D. I., Waldmann, T. A., and Kirsch, I. R.: Chromosomal translocation in a human leukemic stem-cell line disrupts the T-cell antigen receptor δ-chain diversity region and results in a previously unreported fusion transcript. Proc. Natl. Acad. Sci. USA 86:2031, 1989.

211. Aplan, P. D., Lombardi, D. P., Reaman, G. H., Sather, H. N., Hammond, G. D., and Kirsch, I. R.: Involvement of the putative hematopoietic transcription factor SCL in T-cell acute lymphoblastic leukemia. Blood 79:1327, 1992.

212. Green, A. R., Lints, T., Visvader, J., Harvey, R., and Begley, C. G.: SCL is coexpressed with GATA-1 in hemopoietic cells but is also expressed in developing brain. Oncogene 7:653, 1992.

213. Begley, C. G., Aplan, P. D., Denning, S. M., Haynes, B. F., Waldmann, T. A., and Kirsch, I. R.: The gene SCL is expressed during early hematopoiesis and encodes a differentiation-related DNA-binding motif. Proc. Natl. Acad. Sci. USA 86:10128, 1989.

214. Aplan, P. D., Nakahara, K., Orkin, S. H., and Kirsch, I. R.: The SCL gene product: A positive regulator of erythroid differentiation. EMBO J. 11:4073, 1992.

215. Green, A. R., DeLuca, E., and Begley, C. G.: Antisense SCL suppresses self-renewal and enhances spontaneous erythroid differentiation of the human leukaemic cell line K562. EMBO J. 10:4153, 1991.

216. Mantovani, R., Superti-Furga, G., Gilman, J., and Ottolenghi, S.: The deletion of the distal CCAAT box region of the ᴬγ-globin gene in Black HPFH abolishes the binding of the erythroid specific protein NFE3 and of the CCAAT displacement protein. Nucl. Acids Res. 17:6681, 1989.

217. Jane, S. M., Ney, P. A., Vanin, E. F., Gumucio, D. L., and Nienhuis, A. W.: Identification of a stage selector element in the human γ-globin gene promoter that fosters preferential interaction with the 5' HS2 enhancer when in competition with the β-promoter. EMBO J. 11:2961, 1992.

218. Gong, Q.-H., Stern, J., and Dean, A.: Transcriptional role of a conserved GATA-1 site in the human ε-globin gene promoter. Mol. Cell. Biol. 11:2558, 1991.

219. Yu, C.-Y., Motamed, K., Chen, J., Bailey, A. D., and Shen, C.-K.J.: The CACC box upstream of human embryonic ε globin gene binds Sp1 and is a functional promoter element in vitro and in vivo. J. Biol. Chem. 266:8907, 1991.

220. Raich, N., Enver, T., Nakamoto, B., Josephson, B., Papayannopoulou, Th., and Stamatoyannopoulos, G.: Autonomous developmental control of human embryonic globin gene switching in transgenic mice. Science 250:1147, 1990.

221. Shih, D. M., Wall, R. J., and Shapiro, S. G.: Developmentally regulated and erythroid-specific expression of the human embryonic β-globin gene in transgenic mice. Nucleic Acids Res. 18:5465, 1990.

222. Raich, N., Papayannopoulou, Th., Stamatoyannopoulos, G., and Enver, T.: Demonstration of a human ε-globin gene silencer with studies in transgenic mice. Blood 79:861, 1992.

223. Cao, S. X., Gutman, P. D., Davie, H. P., and Schechter, A. N.: Identification of a transcriptional silencer in the 5'-flanking region of the human ε-globin gene. Proc. Natl. Acad. Sci. USA 86:5306, 1989.

224. Wada-Kiyama, Y., Peters, B., and Noguchi, C. T.: The ε-globin gene silencer. J. Biol. Chem. 267:11532, 1992.

225. Peters, B., Merezhinskaya, N., Diffley, J. F. X., and Noguchi, C. T.: Protein-DNA interactions in the ε-globin gene silencer. J. Biol. Chem. 268:3430, 1993.

226. Park, K., and Atchison, M. L.: Isolation of a candidate repressor/activator, NF-E1 (YY-1,δ), that binds to the immunoglobulin k3' enhancer and the immunoglobulin heavy-chain μE1 site. Proc. Natl. Acad. Sci. USA 88:9804, 1991.

227. Hariharan, N., Kelley, D. E., and Perry, R. P.: Delta, a transcription factor that binds to downstream elements in several polymerase II promoters, is a functionally versatile zinc finger protein. Proc. Natl. Acad. Sci. USA 88:9799, 1991.

228. Xiao, J. H., Davidson, I., Matthes, H., Garnier, J.-M., and Chambon, P.: Cloning, expression, and transcriptional properties of the human enhancer factor TEF-1. Cell 65:551, 1991.

229. Shi, Y., Seto, E., Chang, L.-S., and Shenk, T.: Transcriptional repression by YY1, a human GLI-kruppel-related protein, and relief of repression by adenovirus E1A protein. Cell 67:377, 1991.

230. Gumucio, D. L., Heilstedt-Williamson, H., Gray, T. A., Tarle, S. A., Shelton, D. A., Tagle, D. A., Slightom, J. L., Goodman, M., and Collins, F. S.: Phylogenetic footprinting reveals a nuclear protein which binds to silencer sequences in the human γ and ε globin genes. Mol. Cell. Biol. 12:4919, 1992.

231. Bodine, D. M., and Ley, T. J.: An enhancer element lies 3' to the human ᴬγ globin gene. EMBO J. 6:2997, 1987.

232. Jane, S. M., Gumucio, D. L., Ney, P. A., Cunningham, J. M., and Nienhuis, A. W.: Methylation enhanced binding of Sp1 to the stage selector element of the human γ-globin gene promoter may regulate developmental specificity of expression. Mol. Cell. Biol. 13:3272, 1993.

233. Choi, O. R., and Engel, J. D.: Developmental regulation of β-globin gene switching. Cell 55:17, 1988.

234. van der Ploeg, L. H., and Flavell, R. A.: DNA methylation in the human γδβ-globin locus in erythroid and nonerythroid tissues. Cell 19:947, 1980.

235. Mavilio, F., Giampaolo, A., Car, E. A., Migliaccio, G., Calandrini, M., Russo, G., Pagliardi, G. L., Mastroberardino, G., Marinucci, M., and Peschle, C.: Molecular mechanisms of human hemoglobin switching: Selective undermethylation and expression of globin genes in embryonic, fetal, and adult erythroblasts. Proc. Natl. Acad. Sci USA 80:6907, 1983.

236. Bird, A.: The essentials of DNA methylation. Cell 70:5, 1992.

237. Enver, T., Zhang, J.-W., Papayannopoulou, Th., and Stamatoyannopoulos, G.: DNA methylation: A secondary event in globin gene switching? Genes Dev. 2:698, 1988.

238. Gumucio, D. L., Rood, K. L., Gray, T. A., Riordan, M. F., Sartor, C. I., and Collins, F. S.: Nuclear proteins that bind the human γ-globin gene promoter: Alterations in binding produced by point mutations associated with hereditary persistence of fetal hemoglobin. Mol. Cell. Biol. 8:5310, 1988.

239. Mantovani, R., Malgaretti, N., Nicolis, S., Ronchi, A., Giglioni, B., and Ottolenghi, S.: The effects of HPFH mutations in the human γ-globin promoter on binding of ubiquitous and erythroid specific nuclear factors. Nucleic Acids Res. 16:7783, 1988.

240. McDonagh, K. T., and Nienhuis, A. W.: Induction of the human γ-globin gene promoter in K562 cells by sodium

butyrate: Reversal of repression by CCAAT displacement protein. Blood 78:255a, 1991.

241. Skalnik, D. G., Strauss, E. C., and Orkin, S. H.: CCAAT displacement protein as a repressor of the myelomonocytic-specific gp91-phox gene promoter. J. Biol. Chem. 266:16736, 1991.

242. McDonagh, K. T., Lin, H. J., Lowrey, C. H., Bodine, D. M., and Nienhuis, A. W.: The upstream region of the human γ-globin gene promoter. Identification and functional analysis of nuclear protein binding sites. J. Biol. Chem. 266:11965, 1991.

243. Ottolenghi, S., Mantovani, R., Nicolis, S., Ronchi, A., Malgaretti, N., Giglioni, B., and Gilman, J.: Altered binding to the γ-globin promoter of two erythroid specific nuclear proteins in different HPFH syndromes. Prog. Clin. Biol. 316A:229, 1989.

244. Nicolis, S., Ronchi, A., Malgaretti, N., Mantovani, R., Giglioni, B., and Ottolenghi, S.: Increased erythroid-specific expression of a mutated HPFH γ-globin promoter requires the erythroid factor NFE-1. Nucleic Acids Res. 17:5509, 1989.

245. Gumucio, D. L., Lockwood, W. K., Weber, J. L., Saulino, A. M., Delgrosso, K., Surrey, S., Schwartz, E., Goodman, M., and Collings F. S.: The −175 T—C mutation increases promoter strength in erythroid cells: Correlation with evolutionary conservation of binding sites for two *trans*-acting factors. Blood 75:756, 1990.

246. Ronchi, A., Nicholis, S., Santoro, C., and Ottolenghi, S.: Increased Sp1 binding mediates erythroid-specific overexpression of a mutated (HPFH) γ-globin promoter. Nucleic Acids Res. 17:10231, 1989.

247. Gumucio, D. L., Rook, K. L., Blanchard-McQuate, K. L., Gray, T. A., Saulino, A., and Collins, F. S.: Interaction of Sp1 with the human γ globin promoter: Binding and transactivation of normal and mutant promoters. Blood 78:1853, 1991.

248. Ulrich, M. J., Gray, W. J., and Ley, T. J.: An intramolecular DNA triplex is disrupted by point mutations associated with hereditary persistence of fetal hemoglobin. J. Biol. Chem. 267:18649, 1992.

249. Purucker, M., Bodine, D., Lin, H., McDonagh, K., and Nienhuis, A. W.: Structure and function of the enhancer 3′ to the human A γ globin gene. Nucleic Acids Res. 18:7407, 1990.

250. Ponce, E., Lloyd, J. A., Pierani, A., Roeder, R. G., and Lingrel, J. B.: Transcription factor OTF-1 interacts with two distinct DNA elements in the A γ-globin gene promoter. Biochemistry 30:2961, 1991.

251. Forrester, W. C., Thompson, C., Elder, J. T., and Groudine, M.: A developmentally stable chromatin structure in the human β-globin gene cluster. Proc. Natl. Acad. Sci. USA 83:1359, 1986.

252. Lumelsky, N. L., and Forget, B. G.: Negative regulation of globin gene expression during megakaryocytic differentiation of a human erythroleukemic cell line. Mol. Cell. Biol. 11:3528, 1991.

253. Dickinson, L. A., Joh, T., Kohwi, Y., and Kohwi-Shigematsu, T.: A tissue-specific MAR/SAR DNA-binding protein with unusual binding site recognition. Cell 70:631, 1992.

254. Eissenberg, J. C., and Elgin, S. C.: Boundary functions in the control of gene expression. Trends Genet. 7:335, 1991.

255. Antoniou, M., deBoer, E., Habets, G., and Grosveld, F.: The human β-globin gene contains multiple regulatory regions: Identification of one promoter and two downstream enhancers. EMBO J. 7:377, 1988.

256. deBoer, E., Antoniou, M., Mignotte, V., Wall, L., and Grosveld, F.: The human β-globin promoter; nuclear protein factors and erythroid specific induction of transcription. EMBO J. 7:4203, 1988.

257. Antoniou, M., and Grosveld, F.: β-Globin dominant control region interacts differently with distal and proximal promoter elements. Genes Dev. 4:1007, 1990.

258. Kollias, G., Wrighton, N., Hurst, J., and Grosveld, F.: Regulated expression of human A γ-, β-, and hybrid γ β-globin genes in transgenic mice: Manipulation of the developmental expression patterns. Cell 46:89, 1986.

259. Trudel, M., and Costantini, F.: A 3′ enhancer contributes to the stage-specific expression of the human β-globin gene. Genes Dev. 1:954, 1987.

260. Trudel, M., Magram, J., Bruckner, L., and Costantini, F.: Upstream G γ-globin and downstream β-globin sequences required for stage-specific expression in transgenic mice. Mol. Cell. Biol. 7:4024, 1987.

261. Behringer, R. R., Hammer, R. E., Brinster, R. L., Palmiter, R. D., and Townes, T. M.: Two 3′ sequences direct adult erythroid-specific expression of human β-globin genes in transgenic mice. Proc. Natl. Acad. Sci. USA 84:7056, 1987.

262. Magram, J., Niederreither, K., and Constantini, F.: β-Globin enhancers target expression of a heterologous gene to erythroid tissues of transgenic mice. Mol. Cell. Biol. 9:4581, 1989.

263. Myers, R. M., Tilly, K., and Maniatis, T.: Fine structure genetic analysis of a β-globin promoter. Science 232:613, 1986.

264. Cowie, A., and Myers, R. M.: DNA sequences involved in transcriptional regulation of the mouse β-globin promoter in murine erythroleukemia cells. Mol. Cell. Biol. 8:3122, 1988.

265. Hartzog, G. A., and Myers, R. M.: Discrimination among potential activators of the β-globin CACCC element by correlation of binding and transcriptional properties. Mol. Cell. Biol. 13:44, 1993.

266. Mantovani, R., Malgaretti, N., Nicolis, S., Giglioni, B., Comi, P., Cappellini, N., Bertero, M. T., Caligaris-Cappio, F., and Ottolenghi, S.: An erythroid specific nuclear factor binding to the proximal CACCC box of the β-globin gene promoter. Nucleic Acids Res. 16:4299, 1988.

267. Stuve, L. L., and Myers, R. M.: A directly repeated sequence in the β-globin promoter regulates transcription in murine erythroleukemia cells. Mol. Cell. Biol. 10:972, 1990.

268. Myers, R. M., Cowie, A., Stuve, L., Hartzog, G., and Gaensler, K.: Genetic and biochemical analysis of the mouse β-major globin promoter. Prog. Clin. Biol. Res. 316A:117, 1989.

269. Collis, P., Antoniou, M., and Grosveld, F.: Definition of the minimal requirements within the human β-globin gene and the dominant control region for high level expression. EMBO J. 9:233, 1990.

270. Watt, P., Lamb, P., Squire, L., and Proudfoot, N.: A factor binding GATAAG confers tissue specificity on the promoter of the human ζ-globin gene. Nucleic Acids Res. 18:1339, 1990.

271. Yu, C. Y., Chen, J., Lin, L. I., Tam, M., and Shen, C. K.: Cell type–specific protein-DNA interactions in the human ζ-globin upstream promoter region: Displacement of Sp1 by the erythroid cell–specific factor NF-E1. Mol. Cell. Biol. 10:282, 1990.

272. Humphries, R. K., Ley, T., Turner, P., Moulton, A. D., and Nienhuis, A. W.: Differences in human α-, β-, and δ-globin gene expression in monkey kidney cells. Cell 30:173, 1982.

273. Treisman, R., Green, M. R., and Maniatis, T.: *Cis* and *trans* activation of globin gene transcription in transient assays. Proc. Natl. Acad. Sci. USA 80:7428, 1983.

274. Brickner, H. E., Zhu, X. X., and Atweh, G. F.: A novel regulatory element of the human α-globin gene responsible for its constitutive expression. J. Biol. Chem. 266:15363, 1991.

275. Kim, C. G., Swendeman, S. L., Barnhart, K. M., and Sheffery, M.: Promoter elements and erythroid cell nuclear factors that regulate α-globin gene transcription in vitro. Mol. Cell. Biol. 10:5958, 1990.

276. Lim, L. C., Swendeman, S. L., and Sheffery, M.: Molecular cloning of the α-globin transcription factor CP2. Mol. Cell. Biol. 12:828, 1992.

277. Tuan, D., Solomon, W., Li, Q., and London, I. M.: The "β-like-globin" gene domain in human erythroid cells. Proc. Natl. Acad. Sci. USA 82:6384, 1985.

278. Van der Ploeg, L. H., Konings, A., Oort, M., Roos, D., Bernini, L., and Flavell, R. A.: γ-β-Thalassemia studies showing that

deletion of the γ- and δ-genes influences β-globin gene expression in man. Nature 283:637, 1980.

279. Kioussis, D., Vanin, E., deLange, T., Flavell, R. A., and Grosveld, F. G.: β-Globin gene inactivation by DNA translocation in γβ-thalassemia. Nature 306:662, 1983.

280. Curtin, P., Pirastu, M., Kan, Y. W., Gobert-Jones, J. A., Stephens, A. D., and Lehmann, H.: A distant gene deletion affects β-globin gene function in an atypical γδβ-thalassemia. J. Clin. Invest. 76:1554, 1985.

281. Driscoll, M. C., Dobkin, C. S., and Alter, B. P.: γδβ-Thalassemia due to a de novo mutation deleting the 5′ β globin gene activation-region hypersensitive sites. Proc. Natl. Acad. Sci. USA 86:7470, 1989.

282. Forrester, W. C., Epner, E., Driscoll, M. C., Enver, T., Brice, M., Papayannopoulou, Th., and Groudine, M.: A deletion of the human β-globin locus activation region causes a major alteration in chromatin structure and replication across the entire β-globin locus. Genes Dev. 4:1637, 1990.

283. Grosveld, F., van Assendelft, G. B., Greaves, D. R., and Kollias, G.: Position-independent, high-level expression of the human β-globin gene in transgenic mice. Cell 51:975, 1987.

284. Higgs, D. R., Wood, W. G., Jarman, A. P., Sharpe, J., Lida, J., Pretorius, I. M., and Ayyub, H.: A major positive regulatory region located far upstream of the human α-globin gene locus. Genes Dev. 4:1588, 1990.

285. Sharpe, J. A., Chan-Thomas, P. S., Lida, J., Ayyub, H., Wood, W. G., and Higgs, D. R.: Analysis of the human α globin upstream regulatory element (HS-40) in transgenic mice. EMBO J. 11:4565, 1992.

286. Greaves, D. R., Wilson, F. D., Lang, G., and Kioussis, D.: Human CD2 3′-flanking sequences confer high-level, T cell–specific, position-independent gene expression in transgenic mice. Cell 56:979, 1989.

287. Lang, G., Mamalaki, C., Greenberg, D., Yannoutsos, N., and Kioussis, D.: Deletion analysis of the human CD2 gene locus control region in transgenic mice. Nucleic Acids Res. 19:5851, 1991.

288. Aronow, B. J., Silbiger, R. N., Dusing, M. R., Stock, J. L., Yager, K. L., Potter, S. S., Hutton, J. J., and Wiginton, D. A.: Functional analysis of the human adenosine deaminase gene thymic regulatory region and its ability to generate position independent transgene expression. Mol. Cell. Biol. 12:4170, 1992.

289. Bonifer, C., Vidal, M., Grosveld, F., and Sippel, A. E.: Tissue specific and position independent expression of the complete gene domain for chicken lysozyme in transgenic mice. EMBO J. 9:2843, 1990.

290. Townes, T. M., Lingrel, J. B., Chen, H. Y., Brinster, R. L., and Palmiter, R. D.: Erythroid-specific expression of human β-globin genes in transgenic mice. EMBO J. 4:1715, 1985.

291. Blom van Assendelft, G., Hanscombe, O., Grosveld, F., and Greaves, D. R.: The β-globin dominant control region activates homologous and heterologous promoters in a tissue-specific manner. Cell 56:969, 1989.

292. Tuan, D., Solomon, W. B., London, I. M., and Lee, D. P.: An erythroid-specific, developmental-stage–independent enhancer far upstream of the human "β-like globin" genes. Proc. Natl. Acad. Sci. USA 86:2554, 1989.

293. Ren, S., Luo, X. N., and Atweh, G. F.: The major regulatory element upstream of the α-globin gene has classical and inducible enhancer activity. Blood 81:1058, 1993.

294. Pondel, M. D., George, M., and Proudfoot, N. J.: The LCR-like α-globin positive regulatory element functions as an enhancer in transiently transfected cells during erythroid differentiation. Nucleic Acids Res. 20:237, 1992.

295. Epner, E., Forrester, W. C., and Groudine, M.: Asynchronous DNA replication within the human β-globin gene locus. Proc. Natl. Acad. Sci. USA 85:8081, 1988.

296. Dhar, V., Mager, D., Iqbal, A., and Schildkraut, C. L.: The coordinate replication of the human β-globin gene domain reflects its transcriptional activity and nuclease hypersensitivity. Mol. Cell. Biol. 8:4958, 1988.

297. Philipsen, S., Talbot, D., Fraser, P., and Grosveld, F.: The β-globin dominant control region: Hypersensitive site 2. EMBO J. 9:2159, 1990.

298. Talbot, D., Philipsen, S., Fraser, P., and Grosveld, F.: Detailed analysis of the site 3 region of the human β-globin dominant control region. EMBO J. 9:2169, 1990.

299. Talbot, D., Grosveld, F.: The 5′ HS2 of the globin locus control region enhances transcription through the interaction of a multimeric complex binding at two functionally distinct NF-E2 binding sites. EMBO J. 10:1391, 1991.

300. Pruzina, S., Hanscombe, O., Whyatt, D., Grosveld, F., and Philipsen, S.: Hypersensitive site 4 of the human β globin locus control region. Nucleic Acids Res. 19:1413, 1991.

301. Ellis, J., Talbot, D., Dillon, N., and Grosveld, F.: Synthetic human β-globin 5′HS2 constructs function as locus control regions only in multicopy transgene concatemers. EMBO J. 12:127, 1993.

302. Lowrey, C. H., Bodine, D. M., and Nienhuis, A. W.: Mechanism of DNase I hypersensitive site formation within the human globin locus control region. Proc. Natl. Acad. Sci. USA 89:1143, 1992.

303. Sorrentino, B., Ney, P., Bodine, D., and Nienhuis, A. W.: A 46 base pair enhancer sequence within the locus activating region is required for induced expression of the γ-globin gene during erythroid differentiation. Nucleic Acids Res. 18:2721, 1990.

304. Caterina, J. J., Ryan, T. M., Pawlik, K. M., Palmiter, R. D., Brinster, R. L., Behringer, R. R., and Townes, T. M.: Human β-globin locus control region: Analysis of the 5′ DNase I hypersensitive site HS 2 in transgenic mice. Proc. Natl. Acad. Sci. USA 88:1626, 1991.

305. Curtin, P. T., Liu, D. P., Liu, W., Chang, J. C., and Kan, Y. W.: Human β-globin gene expression in transgenic mice is enhanced by a distant DNase I hypersensitive site. Proc. Natl. Acad. Sci. USA 86:7082, 1989.

306. Moi, P., and Kan, Y. W.: Synergistic enhancement of globin gene expression by activator protein-1–like proteins. Proc. Natl. Acad. Sci. USA 87:9000, 1990.

307. Forrester, W. C., Novak, U., Gelinas, R., and Groudine, M.: Molecular analysis of the human β-globin locus activation region. Proc. Natl. Acad. Sci. USA 86:5439, 1989.

308. Morley, B. J., Abbott, C. A., Sharpe, J. A., Lida, J., Chan Thomas, P. S., and Wood, W. G.: A single β-globin locus control region element (5′ hypersensitive site 2) is sufficient for developmental regulation of human globin genes in transgenic mice. Mol. Cell. Biol. 12:2057, 1992.

309. Fraser, P., Hurst, J., Collis, P., and Grosveld, F.: DNaseI hypersensitive sites 1, 2 and 3 of the human β-globin dominant control region direct position-independent expression. Nucleic Acids Res. 18:3503, 1990.

310. Walters, M., Kim, C., and Gelinas, R.: Characterization of a DNA binding activity in DNAse I hypersensitive site 4 of the human globin locus control region. Nucleic Acids Res. 19:5385, 1991.

311. Strauss, E. C., and Orkin, S. H.: In vivo protein-DNA interactions at hypersensitive site 3 of the human β-globin locus control region. Proc. Natl. Acad. Sci. USA 89:5809, 1992.

312. Ikuta, T., and Kan, Y. W.: In vivo protein-DNA interactions at the β-globin gene locus. Proc. Natl. Acad. Sci. USA 88:10188, 1991.

313. Reddy, P. M., and Shen, C. K.: Protein-DNA interactions in vivo of an erythroid-specific, human β-globin locus enhancer. Proc. Natl. Acad. Sci. USA 88:8676, 1991.

314. Liu, D., Chang, J. C., Moi, P., Liu, W., Kan, Y. W., and Curtin, P. T.: Dissection of the enhancer activity of β-globin 5′ DNAse I–hypersensitive site 2 in transgenic mice. Proc. Natl. Acad. Sci. USA 89:3899, 1992.

315. Philipsen, S., Pruzina, S., and Grosveld, F.: The minimal requirements for activity in transgenic mice of hypersensitive site 3 of the β globin locus control region. EMBO J. 12:1077, 1993.

316. Walsh, C. E., Liu, J. M., Xiao, X., Young, N. S., Nienhuis, A. W., and Samulski, R. J.: Regulated high level expression of a human γ-globin gene introduced into erythroid cells by

an adeno associated virus vector. Proc. Natl. Acad. Sci. USA 89:7257, 1992.

317. Miller, J. L., Walsh, C. E., Ney, P. A., Samulski, R. J., and Nienhuis, A. W.: Single copy transduction and expression of human γ-globin in K562 erythroleukemia cells using recombinant adeno-associated virus vectors: the effect of mutations in NF E2 and GATA-1 binding motifs within the HS2 enhancer. Blood (in press).

318. Felsenfeld, G.: Chromatin as an essential part of the transcriptional mechanisms. Nature 355:219, 1992.

319. Engel, J. D., Choi, O. R., Endean, D. J., Foley, K. P., Gallarda, J. L., and Yang, Z. Y.: Genetics and biochemistry of the embryonic to adult switch in the chicken ε- and β-globin genes. Prog. Clin. Biol. Res. 316A:89, 1989.

320. Jimenez, G., Griffiths, S. D., Ford, A. M., Greaves, M. F., and Enver, T.: Activation of the β-globin locus control region precedes commitment to the erythroid lineage. Proc. Natl. Acad. Sci. USA 89:10618, 1992.

321. Orlic, D., Anderson, S., Nishikawa, S.-I., Nienhuis, A. W., and Bodine, D. M.: Gene expression in purified murine hematopoietic stem cells. Blood 80:245a, 1992.

322. Taylor, I. C., Workman, J. L., Schuetz, T. J., and Kingston, R. E.: Facilitated binding of GAL4 and heat shock factor to nucleosomal templates: Differential function of DNA-binding domains. Genes Dev. 5:1285, 1991.

323. Workman, J. L., and Kingston, R. E.: Nucleosome core displacement in vitro via a metastable transcription factor–nucleosome complex. Science 258:1780, 1992.

324. Baron, M. H., and Maniatis, T.: Rapid reprogramming of globin gene expression in transient heterokaryons. Cell 46:591, 1986.

325. Elgin, S. C.: Chromatin structure and gene activity. Curr. Opin. Cell. Biol. 2:437, 1990.

326. Tazi, J., and Bird, A.: Alternative chromatin structure at CpG islands. Cell 60:909, 1990.

327. Fleenor, D. E., and Kaufman, R. E.: Characterization of the DNase I hypersensitive site 3′ of the human β globin gene domain. Blood (in press).

328. Feingold, E. A., and Forget, B. G.: The breakpoint of a large deletion causing hereditary persistence of fetal hemoglobin occurs within an erythroid DNA domain remote from the β-globin gene cluster. Blood 74:2178, 1989.

329. Forget, B. G.: Developmental control of human globin gene expression. Prog. Clin. Biol. Res. 352:313, 1990.

330. Li, Q., Zhou, B., Powers, P., Enver, T., and Stamatoyannopoulos, G: Primary structure of the goat β-globin locus control region. Genomics 9:488, 1991.

331. Li, Q. L., Zhou, B., Powers, P., Enver, T., and Stamatoyannopoulos, G.: β-Globin locus activation regions: Conservation of organization, structure, and function. Proc. Natl. Acad. Sci. USA 87:8207, 1990.

332. Moon, A. M., and Ley, T. J.: Conservation of the primary structure, organization, and function of the human and mouse β-globin locus-activating regions. Proc. Natl. Acad. Sci. USA 87:7693, 1990.

333. Hug, B. A., Moon, A. M., and Ley, T. J.: Structure and function of the murine β-globin locus control region 5′ HS-3. Nucleic Acids Res. 20:5771, 1992.

334. Jimenez, G., Gale, K. B., and Enver, T.: The mouse β-globin locus control region: Hypersensitive sites 3 and 4. Nucleic Acids Res. 20:5797, 1992.

335. Reitman, M., and Felsenfeld, G.: Developmental regulation of topoisomerase II sites and DNase I–hypersensitive sites in the chicken β-globin locus. Mol. Cell. Biol. 10:2774, 1990.

336. Reitman, M., Lee, E., Westphal, H., and Felsenfeld, G.: Site independent expression of the chicken β A-globin gene in transgenic mice. Nature 348:749, 1990.

337. Evans, T., Felsenfeld, G., and Reitman, M.: Control of globin gene transcription. Annu. Rev. Cell. Biol. 6:95, 1990.

338. Vyas, P., Vickers, M. A., Simmons, D. L., Ayyub, H., Craddock, C. F., and Higgs, D. R.: Cis-acting sequences regulating expression of the human α-globin cluster lie within constitutively open chromatin. Cell 69:781, 1992.

339. Higgs, D. R., Vickers, M. A., Wilkie, A. O., Pretorius, I. M.,

Jarman, A. P., and Weatherall, D. J.: A review of the molecular genetics of the human α-globin gene cluster. Blood 73:1081, 1989.

340. Romao, L., Osorio-Almeida, L., Higgs, D. R., Lavinha, J., and Liebhaber, S. A.: α-Thalassemia resulting from deletion of regulatory sequences far upstream of the α-globin structural genes. Blood 78:1589, 1991.

341. Hatton, C. S., Wilkie, A. O., Drysdale, H. C., Wood, W. G., Vickers, M. A., Sharpe, J., Ayyub, H., Pretorius, I. M., Buckle, V. J., and Higgs, D. R.: α-Thalassemia caused by a large (62 kb) deletion upstream of the human α globin gene cluster. Blood 76:221, 1990.

342. Hanscombe, O., Vidal, M., Kaeda, J., Luzzatto, L., Greaves, D. R., and Grosveld, F.: High-level, erythroid-specific expression of the human hemoglobin in murine erythrocytes. Genes Dev. 3:1572, 1989.

343. Ryan, T. M., Behringer, R. R., Townes, T. M., Palmiter, R. D., and Brinster, R. L.: High-level erythroid expression of human α-globin genes in transgenic mice. Proc. Natl. Acad. Sci. USA 86:37, 1989.

344. Jarman, A. P., Wood, W. G., Sharpe, J. A., Gourdon, G., Ayyub, H., and Higgs, D. R.: Characterization of the major regulatory element upstream of the human α-globin gene cluster. Mol. Cell. Biol. 11:4679, 1991.

345. Strauss, E. C., Andrews, N. C., Higgs, D. R., and Orkin, S. H.: In vivo footprinting of the human α-globin locus upstream regulatory element by guanine and adenine ligation-mediated polymerase chain reaction. Mol. Cell. Biol. 12:2135, 1992.

346. Kingsley, C., and Winoto, A.: Cloning of GT box-binding proteins: a novel Sp1 multigene family regulating T-cell receptor gene expression. Mol. Cell. Biol. 12:4251, 1992.

347. Costantini, F., Radice, G., Magram, J., Stamatoyannopoulos, G., Papayannopoulou, Th., and Chada, K.: Developmental regulation of human globin genes in transgenic mice. Cold Spring Harb. Symp. Quant. Biol. 50:361, 1985.

348. Spangler, E. A., Andrews, K. A., and Rubin, E. M.: Developmental regulation of the human ζ globin gene in transgenic mice. Nucleic Acids Res. 18:7093, 1990.

349. Pondel, M. D., Proudfoot, N. J., Whitelaw, C., and Whitelaw, E.: The developmental regulation of the human ζ-globin gene in transgenic mice employing β-galactosidase as a reporter gene. Nucleic Acids Res. 20:5655, 1992.

350. Sabath, D. E., Spangler, E. A., Rubin, E. M., and Stamatoyannopoulos, G.: Analysis of the human ζ globin promoter in transgenic mice. Blood (in press).

351. Albitar, M., Katsumata, M., and Liebhaber, S. A.: Human α-globin genes demonstrate autonomous developmental regulation in transgenic mice. Mol. Cell. Biol. 11:3786, 1991.

352. Enver, T., Raich, N., Ebens, A. J., Papayannopoulou, Th., Costantini, F., and Stamatoyannopoulos, G.: Developmental regulation of human fetal-to-adult globin gene switching in transgenic mice. Nature 344:309, 1990.

353. Behringer, R. R., Ryan, T. M., Palmiter, R. D., Brinster, R. L., and Townes, T. M.: Human γ- to β-globin gene switching in transgenic mice. Genes Dev. 4:380, 1990.

354. Dillon, N., and Grosveld, F.: Human γ-globin genes silenced independently of other genes in the β-globin locus. Nature 350:252, 1991.

355. Stamatoyannopoulos, G., Josephson, B., Zhang, J.-W., and Li, Q.: Developmental regulation of human γ globin genes in transgenic mice. Mol. Cell. Biol. (submitted for publication).

356. Stamatoyannopoulos, G.: Human hemoglobin switching. Science 252:383, 1991.

357. Hanscombe, O., Whyatt, D., Fraser, P., Yannoutsos, N., Greaves, D., Dillon, N., and Grosveld, F.: Importance of globin gene order for correct developmental expression. Genes Dev. 5:1387, 1991.

358. Kim, C. G., Epner, E. M., Forrester, W. C., and Groudine, M.: Inactivation of the human β-globin gene by targeted insertion into the β-globin locus control region. Genes Dev. 6:928, 1992.

359. Peterson, K. R., and Stamatoyannopoulos, G.: Developmental regulation of human γ and β globin genes is independent of their spatial order. Mol. Cell. Biol. (in press).

360. Peterson, K. R., Clegg, C. H., Huxley, C., Josephson, B. M., Haugen, H. S., Furukawa, T., and Stamatoyannopoulos, G.: Transgenic mice containing a 248 kb human β locus yeast artificial chromosome display proper developmental control of human globin genes. Proc. Natl. Acad. Sci. U.S.A. (in press).

361. Svedberg, T., and Hedenius, A.: The sedimentation constants of the respiratory proteins. Biol. Bull. 66:191, 1934.

362. McCutcheon, F. H.: Hemoglobin function during the life history of the bullfrog. J. Cell Comp. Physiol. 8:63, 1936.

363. Stamatoyannopoulos, G., Papayannopoulou, Th., Brice, M., Kurachi, S., Nakamoto, B., Lim, G., and Farquhar, M.: Cell biology of hemoglobin switching I. The switch from fetal to adult hemoglobin formation during ontogeny. In Stamatoyannopoulos, G., and Nienhuis, A. W. (eds.): Hemoglobins in Development and Differentiation. New York, Alan R. Liss, 1981, pp. 287–305.

364. Ingram, V. M.: Embryonic red cell formation. Nature 235:338, 1972.

365. Chapman, B. S., and Tobin, A. J.: Distribution of developmentally regulated hemoglobins in embryonic erythroid populations. Dev. Biol. 69:375, 1979.

366. Brotherton, T. W., Chui, D. H. K., Gauldie, J., and Patterson, M.: Hemoglobin ontogeny during normal mouse fetal development. Proc. Natl. Acad. Sci. USA 76:2853, 1979.

367. Le Douarin, N.: Ontogeny of hematopoietic organs studied in avian embryo interspecific chimeras. In Clarkson, B., Marks, P. A., and Till, J. (eds.): Differentiation in Normal and Neoplastic Hemopoietic Cells. New York, Cold Spring Harbor, 1978, pp. 5–31.

368. Beaupain, D., Martin, C., and Dieterlen-Lievre, F.: Origin and evolution of hemopoietic stem cells in the avian embryo. In Stamatoyannopoulos, G., and Nienhuis, A. W. (eds.): Hemoglobins in Development and Differentiation. New York, Alan R. Liss, 1981, pp. 161–169.

369. Chui, D. H. K., Mentzer, W. C., Patterson, M., Iarocci, T. A., Embury, S. H., Perrine, S. P., Mibashan, R. S., and Higgs, D. R.: Human embryonic ζ-globin chains in fetal and newborn blood. Blood 74:1409, 1989.

370. Peschle, C., Migliaccio, A. R., Migliaccio, G., Petrini, M., Calandrini, M., Russo, G., Mastroberardino, G., Presta, M., Gianni, A. M., Comi, P., Giglioni, B., and Ottolenghi, S.: Embryonic to fetal Hb switch in humans: Studies on erythroid bursts generated by embryonic progenitors from yolk sac and liver. Proc. Natl. Acad. Sci. USA 81:2416, 1984.

371. Stamatoyannopoulos, G., Constantoulakis, P., Brice, M., Kurachi, S., and Papayannopoulou, Th.: Coexpression of embryonic, fetal, and adult globins in erythroid cells of human embryos: Relevance to the cell-lineage models of globin switching. Dev. Biol. 123:191, 1987.

372. Weatherall, D. J., Clegg, J. B., and Wood, W. G.: A model for the persistence or reactivation of fetal haemoglobin production. Lancet 2:660, 1976.

373. Weatherall, D. J., Edwards, J. A., and Donohoe, W. T. A.: Haemoglobin and red cell enzyme changes in juvenile myeloid leukaemia. Br. Med. J. 1:679, 1968.

374. Alter, B. P., Jackson, B. T., Lipton, J. M., Piasecki, G. J., Jackson, P. L., Kudisch, M., and Nathan, D. G.: Control of simian fetal hemoglobin switch at the progenitor cell level. J. Clin. Invest. 67:458, 1981.

375. Alter, B. P., Jackson, B. T., Lipton, J. M., Piasecki, G. J., Jackson, P. L., Kudisch, M., and Nathan, D. G.: Three classes of erythroid progenitors that regulate hemoglobin synthesis during ontogeny in the primate. In Stamatoyannopoulos, G., and Nienhuis, A. W. (eds.): Hemoglobins in Development and Differentiation. New York, Alan R. Liss, 1981, pp. 331–340.

376. Kidoguchi, K., Ogawa, M., Karam, J. D., McNeil, J. S., and Fitch, M. S.: Hemoglobin biosynthesis in individual bursts in culture: Studies of human umbilical cord blood. Blood 53:519, 1979.

377. Weinberg, R. S., Goldberg, J. D., Schofield, M. J., Lenes, A. L., Styczynski, R., and Alter, B. P.: Switch from fetal to adult hemoglobin is associated with a change in progenitor cell population. J. Clin. Invest. 71:785, 1983.

378. Deisseroth, A., and Hendrick, D: Human α-globin gene expression following chromosomal dependent gene transfer into mouse erythroleukemia cells. Cell 15:55, 1978.

379. Papayannopoulou, Th., Brice, M., and Stamatoyannopoulos, G.: Analysis of human globin switching in MEL × human fetal erythroid cell hybrids. Cell 46:469, 1986.

380. Willing, M. C., Nienhuis, A. W., and Anderson, W. F.: Selective activation of human β- but not γ-globin gene in human fibroblast × mouse erythroleukaemia cell hybrids. Nature 277:534, 1979.

381. Pyati, J., Kucherlapati, R. S., and Skoultchi, A. I.: Activation of human β-globin genes from nonerythroid cells by fusion with murine erythroleukemia cells. Proc. Natl. Acad. Sci. USA 77:3435, 1980.

382. Ley, T. J., Chiang, Y. L., Haidaris, D., Anagnou, N. P., Wilson, V. L., and Anderson, W. F.: DNA methylation and regulation of the human β-globin–like genes in mouse erythroleukemia cells containing human chromosome. Proc. Natl. Acad. Sci. USA 81:6618, 1984.

383. Chiang, Y. L., Ley, T. J., Sanders-Haigh, L., and Anderson, W. F.: Human globin gene expression in hybrid 2S MEL × human fibroblast cells. Somatic Cell. Mol. Genet. 10:399, 1984.

384. Takegawa, S., Brice, M., Stamatoyannopoulos, G., and Papayannopoulou, Th.: Only adult hemoglobin is produced in fetal non-erythroid × MEL cell hybrids. Blood 68:1384, 1986.

385. Papayannopoulou, Th., Lindsley, D., Kurachi, S., Lewison, K., Hemenway, T., Melis, M., Anagnou, N. P., and Najfeld, V.: Adult and fetal human globin genes are expressed following chromosomal transfer into MEL cells. Proc. Natl. Acad. Sci. USA 82:780, 1985.

386. Papayannopoulou, Th., Enver, T., Takegawa, S., Anagnou, N. P., and Stamatoyannopoulos, G.: Activation of developmentally mutated human globin genes by cell fusion. Science 242:1056, 1988.

387. Melis, M., Demopulos, G., Najfeld, V., Zhang, J., Brice, M., Papayannopoulou, Th., and Stamatoyannopoulos, G.: A chromosome 11–linked determinant controls fetal globin expression and the fetal to adult globin switch. Proc. Natl. Acad. Sci. USA 84:8105, 1987

388. Oppe, T. E., and Fraser, I. D.: Foetal haemoglobin in haemolytic disease of the newborn. Arch. Dis. Child. 36:507, 1961.

389. Bard, H.: Postnatal synthesis of adult and fetal hemoglobin in infants with congenital cyanotic heart disease. Biol. Neonate 28:219, 1976.

390. Bard, H.: The effect of placental insufficiency on fetal and adult hemoglobin synthesis. Am. J. Obstet. Gynecol. 120:67, 1974.

391. Bromberg, Y. M., Abrahamov, A., and Salzberger, M.: The effect of maternal anoxaemia on the foetal haemoglobin of the newborn. J. Obstet. Gynecol. 63:875, 1956.

392. Bischoff, H.: Untersuchungen über die Resistenz des Hämoglobins des Menschenblutes mit besonderer Berücksichtigung des Sauglingsalters. Z. Gesamte Exp. Med. 48:472, 1925.

393. della Torre, L., and Meroni, P.: Studi sul sangue fetole nota I: Livelli di emoglobina fetale e adulta nella gravidanza fisiologica; relazione con la maturita fetal. Ann. Ostet. Ginecol. 91:148, 1969.

394. Bard, H., Makowski, E. L., Meschia, G., and Battaglia, F. C.: The relative rates of synthesis of hemoglobins A and F in immature red cells of newborn infants. Pediatrics 45:766, 1970.

395. Bard, H.: Postnatal fetal and adult hemoglobin synthesis in early preterm newborn infants. J. Clin. Invest. 52:1789, 1973.

396. Zanjani, E. D., Lim, G., McGlave, P. B., Clapp, J. F., Mann, L. I., Norwood, T. H., and Stamatoyannopoulos, G.: Adult haematopoietic cells transplanted to sheep fetuses continue to produce adult globins. Nature 295:244, 1982.

397. Zanjani, E. D., McGlave, P. B., Bhakthavathsalan, A., and Stamatoyannopoulos, G.: Sheep fetal haematopoietic cells

produce adult haemoglobin when transplanted in the adult animal. Nature 280:495, 1979.

398. Bunch, C., Wood, W. G., Weatherall, D. J., Robinson, J. S., and Corp, M. J.: Haemoglobin synthesis by fetal erythroid cells in an adult environment. Br. J. Haematol. 49:325, 1981.

399. Wood, W. G., Bunch, C., Kelly, S., Gunn, Y., and Breckon, G.: Control of haemoglobin switching by a developmental clock? Nature 313:320, 1985.

400. Papayannopoulou, Th., Nakamoto, B., Agostinelli, F., Manna, M., Lucarelli, G., and Stamatoyannopoulos, G.: Fetal to adult hemopoietic cell transplantation in man: Insights into hemoglobin switching. Blood 67:99, 1986.

401. Delfini, C., Saglio, G., Mazza, U., Muretto, P., Filippetti, A., and Lucarelli, G.: Fetal haemoglobin synthesis following fetal liver transplantation in man. Br. J. Haematol. 55:609, 1983.

402. Wood, W. G., Nash, J., Weatherall, D. J., Robinson, J. S., and Harrison, F. A.: The sheep as an animal model for the switch from fetal to adult hemoglobins. In Stamatoyannopoulos, G., and Nienhuis, A. W. (eds.): Cellular and Molecular Regulation of Hemoglobin Switching. New York, Grune & Stratton, 1979, pp. 153–167.

403. Wintour, E. M., Smith, M. B., Bell, R. J., McDougall, J. G., and Cauchi, M. N.: The role of fetal adrenal hormones in the switch from fetal to adult globin synthesis in the sheep. J. Endocrinol. 104:165, 1985.

404. Dover, G. J., Boyer, S. H., and Zinkham, W. H.: Production of erythrocytes that contain fetal hemoglobin in anemia. J. Clin. Invest. 63:173, 1979.

405. Alter, B. P.: Fetal erythropoiesis in stress hematopoiesis. Exp. Hematol. 7:200, 1979.

406. Papayannopoulou, Th., Vichinsky, E., and Stamatoyannopoulos, G.: Fetal Hb production during acute erythroid expansion. I. Observations in patients with transient erythroblastopenia and postphlebotomy. Br. J. Haematol. 44:535, 1980.

407. Alter, B. P., Rappeport, J. M., Huisman, T. H. J., Schroeder, W. A., and Nathan, D. G.: Fetal erythropoiesis following bone marrow transplantation. Blood 48:843, 1976.

408. Sheridan, B. L., Weatherall, D. J., Clegg, J. B., Pritchard, J., Wood, W. G., Callender, S. T., Durrant, I. J., McWhirter, W. R., Ali, M., Partridge, J. W., and Thompson, E. N.: The patterns of fetal haemoglobin production in leukaemia. Br. J. Haematol. 32:487, 1976.

409. DeSimone, J., Biel, S. I., and Heller, P.: Stimulation of fetal hemoglobin synthesis by hemolysis and hypoxia. Proc. Natl. Acad. Sci. USA 75:2937, 1978.

410. DeSimone, J., Biel, M., and Heller, P.: Maintenance of fetal hemoglobin (HbF) elevations in the baboon by prolonged erythropoietic stress. Blood 60:519, 1982.

411. Nute, P. E., Papayannopoulou, Th., Chen, P., and Stamatoyannopoulos, G.: Acceleration of F-cell production in response to experimentally induced anemia in adult baboons (Papio cynocephalus). Am. J. Hematol. 8:157, 1980.

412. DeSimone, J., Heller, P., Biel, M., and Zwiers, D.: Genetic relationship between fetal Hb levels in normal and erythropoietically stressed baboons. Br. J. Haematol. 49:175, 1981.

413. Stamatoyannopoulos, G., Veith, R., Galanello, R., and Papayannopoulou, Th.: Hb F production in stressed erythropoiesis: Observations and kinetic models. Ann. N.Y. Acad. Sci. 445:188, 1985.

414. Pembrey, M. E., Weatherall, D. J., and Clegg, J. B.: Maternal synthesis of haemoglobin F in pregnancy. Lancet:1350, 1973.

415. Popat, N., Wood, W. G., Weatherall, D. J., and Turnbull, A. C.: Pattern of maternal F-cell production during pregnancy. Lancet:377, 1977.

416. Al-Khatti, A., Veith, R. W., Papayannopoulou, Th., Fritsch, E. F., Goldwasser, E., and Stamatoyannoulos, G.: Stimulation of fetal hemoglobin synthesis by erythropoietin in baboons. N. Engl. J. Med. 317:415, 1987.

417. Umemura, T., Al-Khatti, A., Papayannopoulou, Th., and Stamatoyannopoulos, G.: Fetal hemoglobin synthesis in vivo: Direct evidence for control at the level of erythroid progenitors. Proc. Natl. Acad. Sci. USA 85:9278, 1988.

418. Ellis, M. J., and White, J. C.: Studies on human foetal haemoglobin. II. Foetal haemoglobin levels in healthy children and adults and in certain haematological disorders. J. Haematol. 6:201, 1960.

419. Salvati, F., Strippoli, P., Barchetti, M., and Scatizzi, A.: Effect on hemoglobin F synthesis by erythropoietin in patients with anemia of end-stage renal disease maintained by chronic hemodialysis. Nephron 60:371, 1992.

420. Nagel, R. L., Bookchin, R. M., Johnson, J., Labie, D., Wajcman, H., Isaac-Sodeye, W. A., Honig, G. R., Schiliro, G., Crookston, J. H., and Matsutomo, K.: Structural bases of the inhibitory effects of hemoglobin F and hemoglobin A2 on the polymerization of hemoglobin S. Proc. Natl. Acad. Sci. USA 76:670, 1979.

421. Goldberg, M. A., Husson, M. A., and Bunn, H. F.: Participation of hemoglobins A and F in polymerization of sickle hemoglobin. J. Biol. Chem. 252:3414, 1977.

422. Sunshine, H. R., Hofrichter, J., and Eaton, W. A.: Gelation of sickle cell hemoglobin in mixtures with normal adult and fetal hemoglobins. J. Mol. Biol. 133:435, 1979.

423. Cheetam, R. C., Heuhns, E. R., and Rosemeyer, M. A.: Participation of haemoglobins A, F, A2 and C in polymerisation of haemoglobin S. J. Mol. Biol. 129:45, 1979.

424. Benesch, R. E., Edalji, R., Benesch, R., and Kwong, S.: Solubilization of hemoglobin S by other hemoglobins. Proc. Natl. Acad. Sci. USA 77:5130, 1980.

425. Bertles, J. F., and Milner, P. F. A.: Irreversibly sickled erythrocytes: A consequence of the heterogeneous distribution of hemoglobin types in sickle-cell anemia. J. Clin. Invest. 47:1731, 1968.

426. Singer, K., and Fisher, B.: Studies of abnormal hemoglobins. V. The distribution of type S (sickle cell) hemoglobin and type F (alkali resistant) hemoglobin within the red cell population in sickle cell anemia. Blood 7:1216, 1952.

427. Dover, G. J., Boyer, S. H., Charache, S., and Heintzelman, H.: Individual variation in the production and survival of F-cells in sickle cell disease. N. Engl. J. Med. 299:1428, 1978.

428. Brittenham, G., Lozoff, B., Harris, J. W., Mayson, S. M., Miller, A., and Huisman, T. H. J.: Sickle cell anemia and trait in southern India: Further studies. Am. J. Hematol. 6:107, 1979.

429. Labie, D., Pagnier, J., Lapoumeroulie, C., Rouabhi, F., Dunda-Belkhodja, O., Chardin, P., Beldjord, C., Wajcman, H., Fabry, M. E., and Nagel, R. L.: Common haplotype dependency of high Gγ-globin gene expression and high Hb F levels in β-thalassemia and sickle cell anemia patients. Proc. Natl. Acad. Sci. USA 82:2111, 1985.

430. Nagel, R. L., Fabry, M. E., Pagnier, J., Zohoun, I., Wajcman, H., Baudin, V., and Labie, D.: Hematologically and genetically distinct forms of sickle cell anemia in Africa. N. Engl. J. Med. 312:880, 1985.

431. Nagel, R. L., and Ranney, H. M.: Genetic epidemiology of structural mutations of the β globin gene. Semin. Hematol. 37:342, 1990.

432. Miller, B. A., Salameh, M., Ahmed, M., Wainscoat, J., Antognetti, G., Orkin, S., Weatherall, D., and Nathan, D.: High fetal hemoglobin production in sickle cell anemia in the eastern province of Saudi Arabia is genetically determined. Blood 67:1404, 1986.

433. Pembrey, M. E., Wood, W. G., Weatherall, D. J., and Perrine, R. P.: Fetal haemoglobin production and the sickle gene in the oases of eastern Saudi Arabia. Br. J. Haematol. 40:415, 1978.

434. Fessas, P.: Thalassemia clinical and patho-physiological considerations. Trans. R. Soc. Trop. Med. Hyg. 61:164, 1967.

435. Alter, B. P., Rappeport, J. M., and Parkman, R.: The bone marrow failure syndromes. In Nathan, D. G., and Oski, F. A. (eds.): Hematology of Infancy and Childhood. Philadelphia, W. B. Saunders Co., 1981, pp. 168–249.

436. Shahidi, N. T., Gerald, P. S., Diamond, L. K.: Alkali-resistant hemoglobin in aplastic anemia of both acquired and congenital types. N. Engl. J. Med. 266:117, 1962.

437. Bloom, G. E., and Diamond, L. K.: Prognostic value of fetal hemoglobin levels in acquired aplastic anemia. N. Engl. J. Med. 278:304, 1968.

438. Lipton, J. M., Kudisch, M., Gross, R., and Nathan, D.: Defective erythroid progenitor differentiation system in congenital hypoplastic (Diamond-Blackfan) anemia. Blood 67:962, 1986.

439. Fanconi, G.: Familial constitutional panmyelopathy, Fanconi's anemia. I. Clinical aspects. Semin. Hematol. 4:233, 1967.

440. Bernard, J., Mathe, G., et al.: Contribution à l'étude clinique et physiopathologique de la maladie de Fanconi. Rev. Franc. Etudes Clin. Biol. III:599, 1958.

441. Jones, J. H.: Foetal haemoglobin in Fanconi type anaemia. Nature 192:982, 1961.

442. Beard, M. E. J., Young, D. E., Bateman, C. J., et al.: Fanconi's anemia. Qt. J. Med. 42:403, 1973.

443. Weatherall, D. J., Edwards, J. A., and Donohoe, W. T. A.: Haemoglobin and red cell enzyme changes in juvenile myeloid leukaemia. Br. Med. J. 1:679, 1968.

444. Maurer, H. S., Vida, L. N., and Honig, G. R.: Similarities of the erythrocytes in juvenile chronic myelogenous leukemia to fetal erythrocytes. Blood 39:778, 1972.

445. Dover, G. J., Boyer, S. H., Zinkham, W. H., Kazazian, H. H., Jr., Pinney, D. J., and Sigler, A.: Changing erythrocyte populations in juvenile chronic myelocytic leukemia: Evidence for disordered regulation. Blood 49:355, 1977.

446. Alter, B. P.: Fetal erythropoiesis in bone marrow failure syndromes. In Stamatoyannopoulos, G., and Nienhuis, A. W. (eds.): Cellular and Molecular Regulation of Hemoglobin Switching. New York, Alan R. Liss, 1979, pp. 87–105.

447. Papayannopoulou, Th., Halfpap, L., Chen, S. H., Fukuda, M., Hoffman, R., Dow, L., and Hill, S.: Fetal red cell markers and their relationships in patients with hematologic malignancies. In Stamatoyannopoulos, G., and Nienhuis, A. W. (eds.): Hemoglobins in Development and Differentiation. New York, Alan R. Liss, 1981 pp. 443–456.

448. Bagby, G. C., Jr., Richert-Boe, K., and Koler, R. D.: 32P and acute leukemia: Development of leukemia in a patient with hemoglobin Yakima. Blood 52:350, 1978.

449. Pagnier, J., Lopez, M., Mathiot, C., Habibi, B., Zamet, P., Varet, B., and Labie, D.: An unusual case of leukemia with high fetal hemoglobin: Demonstration of abnormal hemoglobin synthesis localized in a red cell clone. Blood 50:249, 1977.

450. Krauss, J. S., Rodriguez, A. R., and Milner, P. F.: Erythroleukemia with high fetal hemoglobin after therapy for ovarian carcinoma. Am. J. Clin. Pathol. 76:721, 1981.

451. Chudwin, D. S., Rucknagel, D. L., Scholnik, A. P., Waldmann, T. A., and McIntire, K. R.: Fetal hemoglobin and α-fetoprotein in various malignancies. Acta Haematol. 58:288, 1977.

452. Dainiak, N., and Hoffman, R.: Hemoglobin-F production in testicular malignancy. Cancer 45:2177, 1980.

453. Nyman, M., Skolling, R., and Steiner, H.: Acquired macrocytic anemia and hemoglobinopathy—a paraneoplastic manifestation? Am. J. Med. 41:815, 1966.

454. Stewart, T. C.: The occurrence of foetal haemoglobin in a patient with hepatoma. Med. J. Aust. 2:664, 1971.

455. Lozzio, C., and Lozzio, B.: Human chronic myelogenous leukemia cell line with a positive Philadelphia chromosome. Blood 45:321, 1975.

456. Rutherford, T., Clegg, J. B., Higgs, D. R., Jones, R. W., Thompson, J., and Weatherall, D. J.: Embryonic erythroid differentiation in the human cell line K562. Proc. Natl. Acad. Sci. USA 78:348, 1981.

457. Enver, T., Zhang, J., Anagnou, N. P., Stamatoyannopoulos, G., and Papayannopoulou, Th.: Developmental programs of human erythroleukemia cells: Globin gene expression and methylation. Mol. Cell. Biol. 8:4917, 1988.

458. Martin, P., and Papayannopoulou, Th.: HEL cells: A new human erythroleukemia cell line with spontaneous and induced globin expression. Science 216:1233, 1982.

459. Okano, H., Okamura, J., Yagawa, K., Tasaka, H., and Motomura, S.: Human erythroid cell lines derived from a patient with acute erythremia. Cancer Res. Clin. Oncol. 102:49, 1981.

460. Papayannopoulou, Th., Nakamoto, B., Kurachi, S., Tweeddale, M., and Messner, H.: Surface antigenic profile and globin phenotype of two new human erythroleukemia lines: Characterization and interpretations. Blood 72:1029, 1988.

461. Hirata, J., Sato, H., Takahira, H., Shiokawa, S., Endo, T., Nishimura, J., Katsuno, M., Masuda, S., Sasaki, R., Fukumaki, Y., Nawata, H., and Okano, H.: A novel CD10-positive erythroid cell line, RM10, established from a patient with chronic myelogenous leukemia. Leukemia 4:365, 1990.

462. Fukuda, T., Kishi, K., Ohnishi, Y., and Shibata, A.: Bipotential cell differentiation of KU-812: Evidence of a hybrid line that differentiates into basophils and macrophage-like cells. Blood 70:612, 1987.

463. Sato, T., Fuse, A., Eguchi, M., Hayashi, Y., Ryo, R., Adachi, M., Kishimoto, Y., Teramura, M., Mozoguchi, H., Shima, Y., Komori, I., Sunami, S., Okimoto, Y., and Nakajima, H.: Establishment of a human leukaemic cell line (CMK) with megakaryocytic characteristics from a Down's syndrome patient with acute megakaryoblastic leukaemia. Br. J. Hematol. 72:184, 1989.

464. Komatsu, N., Nakauchi, H., Miwa, A., Ishihara, T., Eguchi, M., Moroi, M., Okada, M., Sato, Y., Wada, H., Yawata, Y., Suda, T., and Miura, Y.: Establishment and characterization of a human leukemic cell line with megakaryocytic features; Dependency on granulocyte-macrophage colony-stimulating factor, interleukin 3, or erythropoietin for growth and survival. Cancer Res. 51:341, 1991.

465. Miura, Y., Komatsu, N., and Suda, T.: Growth and differentiation of two human megakaryoblastic cell lines: CMK and UT-7. Prog. Clin. Biol. Res. 356:259, 1990.

466. Hitomi, K., Fujita, K., Sasaki, R., Chiba, H., Okuno, Y., Ichiba, S., Takahashi, T., and Imura, H.: Erythropoietin receptor of a human leukemic cell line with erythroid characteristics. Biochem. Biophys. Res. Commun. 154:902, 1988.

467. Morgan, D., Gumucio, D. L., and Brodsky, I.: Granulocyte-macrophage colony-stimulating factor–dependent growth and erythropoietin-induced differentiation of a human cell line MB-02. Blood 78:2860, 1991.

468. Chiba, S., Takaku, F., Tange, T., Shibuya, K., Misawa, C., Sasaki, K., Miyagawa, K., Yazaki, Y., and Hirai, H.: Establishment and erythroid differentiation of a cytokine-dependent human leukemic cell line F-36: A parental line requiring granulocyte-macrophage colony-stimulating factor or interleukin-3, and a subline requiring erythropoietin. Blood 78:2261, 1991.

469. Seigneurin, D., Champelovier, P., Mouchiroud, G., Berthier, R., Leroux, D., Prenant, M., McGregor, J., Starck, J., Morle, F., Micouin, C., Pietrantuono, A., and Kolodie, L.: Human chronic myeloid leukemia cell line with positive Philadelphia chromosome exhibits megakaryocytic and erythroid characteristics. Exp. Hematol. 15:822, 1987.

470. Ogura, M., Morishima, Y., Ohno, R., Kato, Y., Hirabayashi, N., Nagura, H., and Saito, H.: Establishment of a novel human megakaryoblastic leukemia cell line, MEG-01, with positive Philadelphia chromosome. Blood 66:1384, 1985.

471. Morle, R., Laverriere, A. C., and Godet, J.: Globin genes are actively transcribed in the human megakaryoblastic leukemia cell line MEG-01. Blood 70:3094, 1992.

472. Kitamura, T., Tange, T., Terasawa, T., Chiba, T., Kuwaki, T., Miyagawa, K., Piao, Y-F., Miyazono, K., Urabe, A., and Takaku, F.: Establishment and characterization of a unique human cell line that proliferates dependently on GM-CSF, IL-3, or erythropoietin. J. Cell. Physiol. 140:323, 1989.

472a. Papayannopoulou, Th.: Unpublished data.

473. Papayannopoulou, Th., Brice, M., and Stamatoyannopoulos, G.: Stimulation of fetal hemoglobin synthesis in bone marrow cultures from adult individuals. Proc. Natl. Acad. Sci. USA 73:2033, 1976.

474. Stamatoyannopoulos, G., Kurnit, D. M., and Papayannopoulou, Th.: Stochastic expression of fetal hemoglobin in adult erythroid cells. Proc. Natl. Acad. Sci. USA 78:7005, 1981.

475. Constantoulakis, P., Walmsley, M., Patient, R., Papayannopoulou, Th., Enver, T., and Stamatoyannopoulos, G.: Cell lines

produce factors that induce fetal hemoglobin in human BFUe-derived colonies. Blood 80:2650, 1992.

476. Papayannopoulou, Th., Kurachi, S., Nakamoto, B., Zanjani, E. D., and Stamatoyannopoulos, G.: Hemoglobin switching in culture: Evidence for a humoral factor that induces switching in adult and neonatal but not fetal erythroid cells. Proc. Natl. Acad. Sci. USA 79:6579, 1982.

477. Stamatoyannopoulos, G., Nakamoto, B., Kurachi, S., and Papayannopoulou, Th.: Direct evidence for interaction between human erythroid progenitor cells and a hemoglobin switching activity present in fetal sheep serum. Proc. Natl. Acad. Sci. USA 80:5650, 1983.

478. Stamatoyannopoulos, G., Papayannopoulou, Th., Nakamoto, B., and Kurachi, S.: Hemoglobin switching activity. In Stamatoyannopoulos, G., and Nienhuis, A. W. (eds.): Globin Gene Expression and Hematopoietic Differentiation New York, Alan R. Liss, 1983, pp. 347–363.

479. Rosenblum, B. B., Strahler, J. R., Hanash, S. M., Whitten, C. F., Butkunas-Puskorius, R., and Roberts, A.: Peripheral blood erythroid progenitors from patients with sickle cell anemia: HPLC separation of hemoglobins and the effect of a Hb F switching factor. In Stamatoyannopoulos, G., and Nienhuis, A. W. (eds.).: Experimental Approaches for the Study of Hemoglobin Switching. New York, Alan R. Liss, 1985, pp. 397–410.

480. Constantoulakis, P., Nakamoto, B., Papayannopoulou, Th., and Stamatoyannopoulos, G.: Fetal calf serum contains activities which induce fetal hemoglobin in adult erythroid cell cultures. Blood 75:1862, 1990.

481. Migliaccio, A-R., Migliaccio, G., Brice, M., Constantoulakis, P., Stamatoyannopoulos, G., and Papayannopoulou, Th.: Influence of recombinant hemopoietins and of fetal calf serum on the globin synthetic pattern of human BFUe. Blood 76:1150, 1990.

482. Fujimori, Y., Ogawa, M., Clark, S. C., and Dover, G. J.: Serum-free culture of enriched hematopoietic progenitors reflects physiologic levels of fetal hemoglobin biosynthesis. Blood 745:1718, 1990.

483. Gabbianelli, M., Pelosi, E., Labbaye, C., Valtieri, M., Testa, U., and Peschle, C.: Reactivation of Hb F synthesis in normal adult erythroid bursts by IL-3. Br. J. Haematol. 74:114, 1986.

484. Miller, B. A., Perrine, S. P., Bernstein, A., Lyman, S. D., Williams, D. E., Bell, L. L., and Oliveri, N. F.: Influence of Steel factor on hemoglobin synthesis in sickle cell disease. Blood 79:1861, 1992.

485. Papayannopoulou, Th., Kalamantis, T., and Stamatoyannopoulos, G.: Cellular regulation of hemoglobin switching: Evidence for inverse relationship between fetal hemoglobin synthesis and degree of maturity of human erythroid cells. Proc. Natl. Acad. Sci. USA 76:6420, 1979.

486. Chui, D. H. K., Wong, S. C., Enkin, M. W., Patterson, M., and Ives, R. A.: Proportion of fetal hemoglobin synthesis decreases during erythroid cell maturation. Proc. Natl. Acad. Sci. USA 77:2757, 1980.

487. Dover, G. J., and Boyer, S. H.: Quantitation of hemoglobins within individual red cells: Asynchronous biosynthesis of fetal and adult hemoglobin during erythroid maturation in normal subjects. Blood 56:1082, 1980.

488. Wood, W. G., and Jones, R. W.: Erythropoiesis and hemoglobin production: A unifying model involving sequential gene activation. In Stamatoyannopoulos, G., and Nienhuis, A. W. (eds.): Hemoglobins in Development and Differentiation. New York, Alan R. Liss, 1981, pp. 243–261.

489. Farquhar, M. N., Turner, P. A., Papayannopoulou, Th., Brice, M., Nienhuis, A. W., and Stamatoyannopoulos, G.: The asynchrony of γ- and β-chain synthesis during human erythroid cell maturation. Dev. Biol. 85:403, 1981.

490. Papayannopoulou, Th., Brice, M., and Stamatoyannopoulos, G.: Hemoglobin F synthesis in vitro: Evidence for control at the level of primitive erythroid stem cells. Proc. Natl. Acad. Sci. USA 74:2923, 1977.

491. Papayannopoulou, Th., Bunn, H. F., and Stamatoyannopoulos, G.: Cellular distribution of hemoglobin F in a clonal hemopoietic stem-cell disorder. N. Engl. J. Med. 298:72, 1978.

492. Papayannopoulou, Th., Rosse, W., Stamatoyannopoulos, G., Chen, P., and Adams, J.: Fetal hemoglobin in paroxysmal nocturnal hemoglobinuria (PNH): Evidence for derivation of Hb F–containing erythrocytes (F cells) from the PNH clone as well as from normal hemopoietic stem cell lines. Blood 52:740, 1978.

493. Bunch, C., Wood, W. G., Weatherall, D. J., and Adamson, J. W.: Cellular origins of the fetal-haemoglobin–containing cells of normal adults. Lancet 1:1163, 1979.

494. Hoffman, R., Papayannopoulou, Th., Landaw, S., Wasserman, L. R., DeMarsh, Q. B., Chen, P., and Stamatoyannopoulos, G.: Fetal hemoglobin in polycythemia vera: Cellular distribution in 50 unselected patients. Blood 53:1148, 1979.

495. Stamatoyannopoulos, G., and Papayannopoulou, Th.: Fetal hemoglobin and the erythroid stem cell differentiation process. In Stamatoyannopoulos, G., and Nienhuis, A. W. (eds.): Cellular and Molecular Regulation of Hemoglobin Switching. New York, Grune & Stratton, 1979, pp. 323–349.

496. Macklis, R. M., Javid, J., Lipton, J. M., Kudisch, M., Pettis, P., and Nathan, D. G.: Synthesis of hemoglobin F in adult simian erythroid progenitor–derived colonies. J. Clin. Invest. 70:752, 1982.

497. Dover, G. J., and Ogawa, M.: Cellular mechanisms for increased fetal hemoglobin production in culture. J. Clin. Invest. 66:1175, 1980.

498. Kidoguchi, K., Ogawa, M., and Karam, J. D.: Hemoglobin biosynthesis in individual erythropoietic bursts in culture. J. Clin. Invest. 63:804, 1979.

499. Peschle, C., Migliaccio, G., Covelli, A., Lettieri, F., Migliaccio, A. R., Condorelli, M., Comi, P., Pozzoli, M. L., Giglioni, B., Ottolenghi, S., Cappellini, M. D., Polli, E., and Gianni, A. M.: Hemoglobin synthesis in individual bursts from normal adult blood: All bursts and subcolonies synthesize $^G\gamma$- and $^A\gamma$-globin chains. Blood 56:218, 1980.

500. Torrealba de Ron, A., Papayannopoulou, Th., and Stamatoyannopoulos, G.: Studies of Hb F in adult nonanemic baboons: Hb F expression in erythroid colonies decreases as the level of maturation of erythroid progenitors advances. Exp. Hematol. 13:919, 1985.

501. Boyer, S. H., Dover, G. J., Smith, K. D., and Scott, A.: Some interpretations of in vivo studies of globin gene switching in man and primates. In Stamatoyannopoulos, G., and Nienhuis, A. W. (eds.): Hemoglobin in Development and Differentiation. New York, Alan R. Liss, 1981, pp. 225–241.

502. Miyoshi, K., Kaneto, Y., Kawai, H., Ohchi, H., Niki, S., Hasegawa, K., Shirakami, A., and Yamano, T.: X-linked dominant control of F cells in normal adult life: Characterization of the Swiss type hereditary persistence of fetal hemoglobin regulated dominantly by gene(s) on X chromosome. Blood 72:1854, 1988.

503. Dover, G. J., Smith, K. D., Chang, Y. C., Purvis, S., Mays, A., Meyers, D. A., Chells, C., and Sergeant, G.: Fetal hemoglobin levels in sickle cell disease and normal individuals are partially controlled by an X-linked gene located at Xp22.2. Blood 80:816, 1992.

504. Stamatoyannopoulos, J. A., and Nienhuis, A. W.: Therapeutic approaches to hemoglobin switching in treatment of hemoglobinopathies. Annu. Rev. Med. 43:497, 1992.

505. Platt, O. S., Thorington, B. D., Brambilla, D. J., Milner, P. F., Rosse, W. F., Vichinsky, E., and Kinney, T. R.: Pain in sickle cell disease: Rates and risk factors. N. Engl. J. Med. 325:11, 1991.

506. Vesel, Y. J.: Mode of action and effects of 5-azacytidine and of its derivatives in eukaryotic cells. Pharmacol. Ther. 28:227, 1985.

507. Jones, P. A.: Effects of 5-azacytidine and its 2′-deoxyderivative on cell differentiation and DNA methylation. Pharmacol. Ther. 28:17, 1985.

508. DeSimone, J., Heller, P., Hall, L., and Zwiers, D.: 5-Azacytidine stimulates fetal hemoglobin synthesis in anemic baboons. Proc. Natl. Acad. Sci. USA 79:4428, 1982.

509. DeSimone, J., Heller, P., Schimenti, J. C., and Duncan, C. H.:

Fetal hemoglobin production in adult baboons by 5-azacytidine or by phenylhydrazine-induced hemolysis is associated with hypomethylation of globin gene DNA. *In* Stamatoyannopoulos, G., and Nienhuis, A. W. (eds.): Globin Gene Expression and Hematopoietic Differentiation. New York, Alan R. Liss, 1983, pp. 489–500.

510. Ley, T. J., DeSimone, J., Anagnou, N. P., Keller, G. H., Humphries, R. K., Turner, P. H., Young, N. S., Heller, P., and Nienhuis, A. W.: 5-Azacytidine selectively increases γ-globin synthesis in a patient with β+ thalassemia. N. Engl. J. Med. 307:1469, 1982.

511. Nienhuis, A. W., Ley, T. J., Humphries, R. K., Young, N. S., and Dover, G.: Pharmacological manipulation of fetal hemoglobin synthesis in patients with severe β-thalassemia. Ann. N. Y. Acad. Sci. 445:198, 1985.

512. Charache, S., Dover, G., Smith, K., Talbot, Jr., C. C., Moyer, M., and Boyer, S.: Treatment of sickle cell anemia with 5-azacytidine results in increased fetal hemoglobin production and is associated with nonrandom hypomethylation of DNA around the γ-δ-β-globin gene complex. Proc. Natl. Acad. Sci. USA 80:4842, 1983.

513. Dover, G. J., Charache, S., Boyer, S. H., Vogelsang, G., and Moyer, M.: 5-Azacytidine increases Hb F production and reduces anemia in sickle cell disease: Dose-response analysis of subcutaneous and oral dosage regimens. Blood 66:527, 1985.

514. Ley, T. J., and Nienhuis, A. W.: Induction of hemoglobin F synthesis in patients with β-thalassemia. Annu. Rev. Med. 36:485, 1985.

515. Editorial: 5-azacytidine for beta-thalassemia? Lancet 1:36, 1983.

516. Lowery, C. H., and Nienhuis, A. W.: Pharmacologic manipulation of globin gene expression with 5-azacytidine has produced long term therapeutic benefits in two patients with β-thalassemia. Blood 80:368a, 1992.

517. Torrealba de Ron, A., Papayannopoulou, Th., Knapp, M. S., Fu, M., Knitter, G., and Stamatoyannopoulos, G.: Perturbations in the erythroid marrow progenitor cell pools may play a role in the augmentation of Hb F by 5-azacytidine. Blood 63:201, 1984.

518. Humphries, R. K., Dover, G., Young, N. S., Moore, J. G., Charache, S., Ley, T., and Nienhuis, A. W.: 5-Azacytidine acts directly on both erythroid precursors and progenitors to increase production of fetal hemoglobin. J. Clin. Invest. 75:547, 1985.

519. Galanello, R., Stamatoyannopoulos, G., and Papayannopoulou, Th.: Mechanism of Hb F stimulation by S-stage compounds: in vitro studies with bone marrow cells exposed to 5-azacytidine, ara-C or hydroxyurea. J. Clin. Invest. 81:1209, 1988.

520. Miller, B. A., Platt, O., Hope, S., Dover, G., and Nathan, D. G.: Influence of hydroxyurea on fetal hemoglobin production in vitro. Blood 70:1824, 1987.

521. Papayannopoulou, Th., Torrealba de Ron, A., Veith, R., Knitter, G., and Stamatoyannopoulos, G.: Arabinosylcytosine induces fetal hemoglobin in baboons by perturbing erythroid cell differentiation kinetics. Science 224:617, 1984.

522. Letvin, N. L., Linch, D. C., Beardsley, G. P., McIntyre, K. W., and Nathan, D. G.: Augmentation of fetal-hemoglobin production in anemic monkeys by hydroxyurea. N. Engl. J. Med. 310:869, 1984.

523. Veith, R., Papayannopoulou, Th., Kurachi, S., and Stamatoyannopoulos, G.: Treatment of baboon with vinblastine: Insights into the mechanisms of pharmacologic stimulation of Hb F in the adult. Blood 66:456, 1985.

524. Platt, O. S., Orkin, S. H., Dover, G., Beardsley, G. P., Miller, B., and Nathan, D. G.: Hydroxyurea enhances fetal hemoglobin production in sickle cell anemia. J. Clin. Invest. 74:652, 1984.

525. Veith, R., Galanello, R., Papayannopoulou, Th., and Stamatoyannopoulos, G.: Stimulation of F-cell production in Hb S patients treated with Ara-C or hydroxyurea. N. Engl. J. Med. 313:1571, 1985.

526. Kaufman, R. E.: Hydroxyurea: Specific therapy for sickle cell anemia? Blood 79:2503, 1992.

527. Charache, S., Dover, G. J., Moyer, M. A., and Moore, J. W.: Hydroxyurea-induced augmentation of fetal hemoglobin production in patients with sickle cell anemia. Blood 69:109, 1987.

528. Dover, G. J., Humphries, R. K., Moore, J. G., Ley, T. J., Young, N. S., Charache, S., and Nienhuis, A. W.: Hydroxyurea induction of hemoglobin F production in sickle cell disease: Relationship between cytotoxicity and F cell production. Blood 67:735, 1986.

529. Rodgers, G. P.: Recent approaches to the treatment of sickle cell anemia. JAMA 265:2097, 1991.

530. Rodgers, G. P., Dover, G. J., Noguchi, C. T., Schechter, A. N., and Nienhuis, A. W.: Hematologic responses of patients with sickle cell disease to treatment with hydroxyurea. N. Engl. J. Med. 322:1037, 1990.

531. Charache, S., Dover, G. J., Moore, R. D., Eckert, S., Ballas, S. K., Koshy, M., Milner, P. F. A., Orringer, E. P., Phillips G., Jr., Platt, O. S., and Thomas, G. H.: Hydroxyurea: Effects on hemoglobin F production in patients with sickle cell anemia. Blood 79:2555, 1992.

532. Ballas, S. K., Dover, G. J., and Charache, S.: The effect of hydroxyurea on the rheological properties of sickle erythrocytes in vivo. Am. J. Hematol. 32:104, 1989.

533. Goldberg, M. A., Brugnara, C., Dover, G. J., Schapira, L., Carache, S., and Bunn, H. F.: Treatment of sickle cell anemia with hydroxyurea and erythropoietin. N. Engl. J. Med. 323:366, 1990.

534. Blau, C. A., Constantoulakis, P., Al-Khatti, A., Spadaccino, E., Goldwasser, E., Papayannopoulou, Th., and Stamatoyannopoulos, G.: Fetal hemoglobin in acute and chronic states of erythroid expansion. Blood 81:227, 1993.

535. Al-Khatti, A., Umemura, T., Clow, J., Abels, R. I., Vance, J., Papayannopoulou, Th., and Stamatoyannopoulos, G.: Erythropoietin stimulates F-reticulocyte formation in sickle cell anemia. Trans. Assoc. Am. Physicians 101:54, 1988.

536. Nagel, R. L., Vichinsky, E., Shah, M., Johnson, R., Spadaccino, E., Fabry, M. E., Mangahas, L., Abel, R., and Stamatoyannopoulos, G.: F reticulocyte response in sickle cell anemia treated with recombinant human erythropoietin: A double blind study. Blood 81:9, 1993.

537. Al-Khatti, A., Papayannopoulou, Th., Knitter, G., Fritsch, E. F., and Stamatoyannopoulos, G.: Cooperative enhancement of F-cell formation in baboons treated with erythropoietin and hydroxyurea. Blood 72:817, 1988.

538. McDonagh, K. T., Dover, G. J., Donahue, R. E., Nathan, D. G., Agricola, B., Byrne, E., and Nienhuis, A. W.: Hydroxyurea-induced Hb F production in anemic primates: Augmentation by erythropoietin, hematopoietic growth factors, and sodium butyrate. Exp. Hematol. 20:1156, 1992.

539. Rodgers, G. P., Dover, G. J., Uyesaka, N., Noguchi, C. T., Schechter, A. N., and Nienhuis, A. W.: Augmentation by erythropoietin of the fetal-hemoglobin response to hydroxyurea in sickle cell disease. N. Engl. J. Med. 328:73, 1993.

540. Umemura, T., Al-Khatti, A., Donahue, R. E., Papayannopoulou, Th., and Stamatoyannopoulos, G.: Effects of interleukin-3 and erythropoietin on in vivo erythropoiesis and F-cell formation in primates. Blood 74:1571, 1989.

541. Kruh, J.: Effects of sodium butyrate, a new pharmacologic agent, on cells in culture. Mol. Cell. Biochem. 42:65, 1982.

542. Leder, A., and Leder, P.: Butyric acid, a potent inducer of erythroid differentiation in cultured erythroleukemic cells. Cell 5:319, 1975.

543. Papayannopoulou, Th., Nakamoto, B., Kurachi, S., and Nelson, R.: Analysis of the erythroid phenotype of HEL cells: Clonal variation and the effect of inducers. Blood 70:1764, 1987.

544. Ginder, G. D., Whitters, M. J., and Pohlman, J. K.: Activation of a chicken embryonic globin gene in adult erythroid cells by 5-azacytidine and sodium butyrate. Proc. Natl. Acad. Sci. USA 81:3954, 1984.

545. Bard, H., and Prosmanne, J.: Relative rates of fetal hemoglobin and adult hemoglobin synthesis in cord blood of infants of insulin dependent diabetic mothers. Pediatrics 75:1143, 1985.

546. Perrine, S. P., Greene, M. F., and Faller, D. V.: Delay in the fetal globin switch in infants of diabetic mothers. N. Engl. J. Med. 312:334, 1985.

547. Perrine, S. P., Rudolph, A., Faller, D. V., et al.: Butyrate infusions in the ovine fetus delay the biologic clock for globin gene switching. Proc. Natl. Acad. Sci. USA 85:8540, 1988.

548. Constantoulakis, P., Papayannopoulou, Th., and Stamatoyannopoulos, G.: α-Amino-N-butyric acid stimulates fetal hemoglobin in the adult. Blood 72:1961, 1988.

549. Constantoulakis, P., Knitter, G., and Stamatoyannopoulos, G.: On the induction of fetal hemoglobin by butyrates: In vivo and in vitro studies with sodium butyrate and comparison of combination treatments with 5-AzaC and AraC. Blood 74:1963, 1989.

550. Perrine, S. P., Miller, B. A., Faller, D. V., Cohen, R. A., Vichinsky, E. P., Hurst, D., Lubin, B. H., and Papayannopoulou, Th.: Sodium butyrate enhances fetal globin gene expression in erythroid progenitors of patients with Hb SS and β thalassemia. Blood 74:454, 1989.

551. Blau, C. A., Constantoulakis, P., Shaw, C. M., and Stamatoyannopoulos, G.: Fetal hemoglobin induction with butyric acid: Efficacy and toxicity. Blood 81:529, 1993.

552. Perrine, S. P., Ginder, G. D., Faller, D. V., Dover, G. H., Ikuta, T., Witkowska, H. E., Cai, S.-P., Vichinsky, E. P., and Oliveri, N. F.: A short-term trial of butyrate to stimulate fetal-globin-gene expression in the β-globin disorders. N. Engl. J. Med. 328:81, 1993.

553. Dover, G. J., Charache, S. C., and Brusilow, S. W.: Sodium phenylbutyrate increases fetal hemoglobin production in patients with sickle cell disease. Blood 80:73a, 1992.

554. Riggs, M. G., Whittaker, R. G., Neumann, J. R., and Ingram, V. M.: N-butyrate causes histone modification in HeLa and friend erythroleukemia cells. Nature 268:462, 1977.

555. Thorne, A. W., Kmiciek, D., Mitchelson, K. Sautiere, P., and Crane-Robinson, C.: Patterns of histone acetylation. Eur. J. Biochem. 193:701, 1990.

556. McKnight, G. S., Hager, L., and Palmiter, R. D.: Butyrate and related inhibitors of histone deacetylation block the induction of egg white genes by steroid hormones. Cell 22:469, 1980.

557. Glauber, J. G., Wandersee, N. J., Little, J. A., and Ginder, G. D.: 5'-Flanking sequences mediate butyrate stimulation of embryonic globin gene expression in adult erythroid cells. Mol. Cell. Biol. 11:4690, 1991.

5

The Thalassemias

D. J. Weatherall

INTRODUCTION

The thalassemias are the most common single-gene disorders in the world population. They were among the first diseases to be studied by the methods of molecular biology and remain the prime model for understanding the relationship between molecular pathology and phenotypic diversity. Because of their particularly high frequency in many parts of the developing world, control of the thalassemias presents a major opportunity and challenge for applying the methods of molecular genetics to clinical practice.

Historical Perspective[1]

A form of severe anemia occurring early in life and associated with splenomegaly and characteristic bone changes was first described by Thomas Cooley and Pearl Lee in 1925.[2] The condition was later named thalassemia, from θαλασσα, "the sea," by George Whipple, since the first patients on whom he carried out autopsies were all of Mediterranean background.[3] It was only after 1940 that the true genetic nature of thalassemia was fully appreciated. It became clear that the disease described by Cooley and Lee is the homozygous state for a recessive autosomal gene. Subsequently, it was found that thalassemia is not restricted to the Mediterranean area but occurs widely throughout the Middle East, the Indian subcontinent, and Southeast Asia.

In the early 1950s, following the discovery of the molecular basis of sickle cell anemia by Linus Pauling and his colleagues,[4] the hemoglobin of patients with different clinical forms of thalassemia was studied in many parts of the world. It was soon realized that thalassemia is not a single disease but is extremely heterogeneous. Analyses of the hemoglobin patterns of patients with different types of thalassemia who had also inherited structural hemoglobin variants led to the suggestion by Vernon Ingram and Anthony Stretton that there might be two main types, α and β thalassemia.[5] The development of methods for studying hemoglobin synthesis in vitro led to the experimental validation of this hypothesis and to the further analysis of thalassemia,[6] so that by the early 1970s it was apparent that many different forms exist, all associated with defective synthesis of one or more of the globin chains of hemoglobin.

By the early 1970s, a great deal was known about the genetic control of human hemoglobin, many structural variants had been characterized, and the biosynthetic defects and remarkable heterogeneity of the thalassemias had been established.[7] The human hemoglobin field was, therefore, an ideal testing ground for application of the new techniques of recombinant DNA. First, with the use of soluble hybridization it was possible to demonstrate reduced amounts of globin messenger RNA (mRNA) and, then, deletions of the globin genes in some forms of thalassemia. Later, the advent of Southern blotting and cloning technology led to the definition of the molecular pathology of many forms of thalassemia, so paving the way for an understanding of the molecular basis of many human single-gene disorders.

Definition and Classification[7, 8]

The thalassemias are defined as a heterogeneous group of inherited disorders of hemoglobin synthesis, all characterized by the absence or reduced output of one or more of the globin chains of hemoglobin. They can be classified at several levels. First, there is a clinical classification that simply describes the degree of severity. Second, the thalassemias can be defined by the particular globin chain that is synthesized at a reduced rate. Finally, it is now often possible to subclassify them according to the particular mutation that is responsible for defective globin chain synthesis.

Clinical Classification

The descriptive classification of thalassemia, though it has no strict genetic basis, is still useful in clinical practice. The thalassemias are divided into the major forms of the illness, which are severe and transfusion dependent, and the symptomless minor forms, which usually represent the carrier state, or trait. Thalassemia major results either from the homozygous inheritance of a particular mutation or from the compound heterozygous state for two different mutations.

The term "thalassemia intermedia" describes conditions that, though not as severe as the major forms, are associated with a more severe degree of anemia than is the trait. In practice, this term encompasses a wide clinical spectrum ranging from disorders that are almost as serious as the major forms to asymptomatic conditions that are only slightly more severe than the trait.

Finally, some forms of thalassemia trait are clinically and hematologically completely silent; they are designated "silent" carrier states.

Genetic Classification

The thalassemias are classified according to their genetic basis by describing the globin chain that is synthesized at a reduced rate. A classification of the thalassemia syndromes is shown in Table 5–1.

The structure and genetic control of human hemoglobin are summarized in Figure 5–1. Human adult hemoglobin is a mixture of proteins consisting of a major component, hemoglobin A (Hb A), and a minor component, Hb A_2, which constitutes about 2.5 per cent of the total. During early development, several embryonic hemoglobins are present, after which the main hemoglobin during intrauterine life is Hb F.

The structures of these hemoglobins are similar. Each consists of two separate pairs of identical globin chains. Except for some of the embryonic hemoglobins, all the normal human hemoglobins have one pair

TABLE 5–1. THE THALASSEMIAS AND RELATED DISORDERS

α Thalassemia
  α^0
  α^+
    Deletion $(-\alpha)$
    Non-deletion (α^T)
β Thalassemia
  β^0
  β^+
  Normal Hb A_2
  "Silent"
δβ Thalassemia
  $(\delta\beta)^0$
  $(^A\gamma\,\delta\beta)^0$
  $(\delta\beta)^+$
γ Thalassemia
δ Thalassemia
  δ^0
  δ^+
εγδβ Thalassemia
Hereditary persistence of fetal hemoglobin
  Deletion
    $(\delta\beta)^0\,(^A\gamma\delta\beta)^0$
  Non-deletion
    Linked to β globin genes
      $^G\gamma\beta^+\,^A\gamma\beta^+$
    Unlinked to β globin genes

of α chains: In Hb A they are combined with β chains ($\alpha_2\beta_2$), in Hb A_2 with δ chains ($\alpha_2\delta_2$), and Hb F with γ chains ($\alpha_2\gamma_2$). Human hemoglobin shows further heterogeneity, particularly in fetal life, an observation that has important implications for understanding the thalassemias. Hb F is a mixture of two molecular forms, with the formulas $\alpha_2\gamma_2^{136Gly}$ and $\alpha_2\gamma_2^{136Ala}$. The γ chains containing glycine at position 136 are designated $^G\gamma$ chains, and those that contain alanine at this position are called $^A\gamma$ chains.

Before the eighth week of intrauterine life, there are three embryonic hemoglobins: Hb Gower 1 ($\zeta_2\epsilon_2$), Hb Gower 2 ($\alpha_2\epsilon_2$), and Hb Portland ($\zeta_2\gamma_2$). The ζ and ε chains are the embryonic counterparts of the adult α and β chains and γ and δ chains, respectively. Although thalassemia involving the embryonic globin genes has not been described, these genes are of importance in the thalassemia field because in some forms of α thalassemia ζ chain synthesis is persistent.

The classification of the thalassemias according to which chain is produced at a reduced rate reflects the structure of the globin gene clusters that are involved in their synthesis (Fig. 5–1). The β-like globin chains are controlled by a gene cluster on chromosome 11 in which the different genes are arranged in the order $5'$-ε-$^G\gamma$-$^A\gamma$-ψβ-δ-β-$3'$. The α-like gene cluster is on chromosome 16, p13.3, and the genes are arranged in the order $5'$-ζ-ψζ-φα-α2-α1-θ-$3'$.

As shown in Table 5–1, the thalassemias are classified into α, β, γ, δβ, δ, and εγδβ varieties, depending on which chain or chains are synthesized at a reduced rate.

α **THALASSEMIA.** Because there are two α globin genes per haploid genome, four in all, the α thalassemias are classified according to the relative output of both α genes. When both α globin genes on a chromosome are inactivated, the condition is called α^0 thalassemia. The heterozygous genotype can be written $--/\alpha\alpha$. When one of the linked α globin genes is inactivated, the condition is called α^+ thalassemia, and the genotype can be written $-\alpha/\alpha\alpha$ in cases in which one of the α globin genes is deleted, or $\alpha^T\alpha/\alpha\alpha$ if one of the linked α genes is inactivated by a mutation. In other words, the terms α^0 and α^+ thalassemia describe an α globin haplotype, that is, the state of the *two* linked α globin genes on a particular chromosome; in α^0 thalassemia, there is no output of α globin from the particular chromosome, and in α^+ thalassemia there is some output but usually only the product of a single α globin locus.

β **THALASSEMIA.** There are two main varieties of β-thalassemia: β^0 thalassemia, in which no β globin chains are produced, and β^+ thalassemia, in which some β chains are produced but at a reduced rate. Some forms of β thalassemia are designated β^{++} to indicate that the defect in β chain production is particularly mild.

The diagnostic feature of β thalassemia is an elevated level of Hb A_2 in heterozygotes, which is found in most forms of β^0 and β^+ thalassemia. There are, however, less common forms of β thalassemia in which the Hb A_2 level is normal in heterozygotes. These so-called "normal Hb A_2 β thalassemias" are also heterogeneous. They are classified into two varieties: type 1, in which there are no associated hematological changes, and type 2, in which the hematological find-

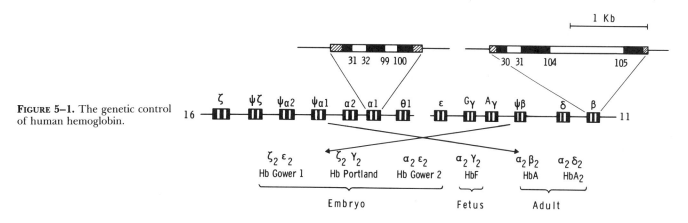

FIGURE 5–1. The genetic control of human hemoglobin.

ings are typical of β thalassemia trait with a raised Hb A$_2$. Type 1 normal Hb A$_2$ β thalassemia is also called "silent β thalassemia." Both these forms of β thalassemia with normal Hb A$_2$ levels are heterogeneous at the molecular level.

δβ THALASSEMIA. The δβ thalassemias are also heterogeneous. In some cases, no δ or β chains are synthesized. In the past, it was customary to classify these conditions according to the structure of the γ chains of the Hb F that is produced—$^G\gamma^A\gamma(\delta\beta)^0$ and $^G\gamma(\delta\beta)^0$ thalassemia, for example. This system was illogical and out of line with the classification of thalassemia according to the chain that is ineffectively synthesized. Thus, these conditions are best described as $(\delta\beta)^0$ and $(^A\gamma\delta\beta)^0$ thalassemias.

There are also $(\delta\beta)^+$ forms of δβ thalassemia. In many of these conditions, an abnormal hemoglobin is produced that has normal α chains combined with non-α chains that are constituted by the N-terminal residues of the δ chain fused to the C-terminal residues of the β chain. These δβ fusion variants, collectively called the Lepore hemoglobins, are synthesized inefficiently and produce the clinical phenotype of δβ thalassemia.

δ THALASSEMIA. Several different mutations give rise to a reduced output of δ chains and hence a reduced level of Hb A$_2$. These conditions are clinically silent and are of importance only insofar as when they are inherited together with β thalassemia they may prevent an elevation of the level of Hb A$_2$.

εγδβ THALASSEMIA. This is a rare form of thalassemia that results from loss of either the whole or part of the β-like globin gene cluster. Homozygotes have not been encountered, presumably because the condition would not be compatible with life; heterozygotes have the clinical phenotype of β thalassemia with a normal Hb A$_2$ level.

γ THALASSEMIA. There have been a few reports of deletions involving one or the other γ globin genes.[8] These deletions have been identified by determining the level of $^G\gamma$ and $^A\gamma$ chains in Hb F and do not appear to be of clinical significance. They are not considered further in this chapter.

HEREDITARY PERSISTENCE OF FETAL HEMOGLOBIN (HPFH) AS A FORM OF β OR δβ THALASSEMIA. This is another heterogeneous group of disorders of hemoglobin synthesis that are characterized by persistent fetal hemoglobin synthesis in adult life in the absence of major hematological abnormalities. They are described in detail in Chapter 4. By virtue of their interaction with the β thalassemias, and from other evidence, it is apparent that many of these conditions are extremely well compensated forms of β or δβ thalassemia. In addition, HPFH is important in the thalassemia field because of the way in which it can modify the clinical phenotype of the β thalassemias.

As shown in Table 5–1, HPFH is classified along similar lines to the thalassemias. First, there are those forms in which no δ or β globin chains are produced but in which there is almost complete compensation by a high output of γ chains; these conditions are

designated $(\delta\beta)^0$ HPFH. Second, there is a family of HPFH variants in which there is β and probably δ chain synthesis in *cis* to the HPFH determinant. These conditions are designated $^G\gamma(\delta\beta)^+$ or $^A\gamma(\delta\beta)^+$ HPFH, depending on the structure of the Hb F. Finally, there is a group of conditions, probably heterogeneous, in which much lower levels of Hb F are found in otherwise normal individuals. Evidence is increasing that the genetic determinant for at least some types of this form of HPFH may not be linked to the β globin gene cluster.

The first two types of HPFH are characterized by relatively high levels of Hb F production in heterozygotes, usually 15 to 25 per cent of the total hemoglobin, which is relatively homogeneously distributed among the red cells. In the latter group, levels of persistent Hb F production are much lower, in the 2 to 10 per cent range, usually heterogeneously distributed among the red cells. Thus, HPFH is also classified as either pancellular or heterocellular, although as knowledge of its molecular pathology increases, this subdivision is becoming less useful.

Molecular Classification

As their molecular pathology has been worked out, it has been possible to develop a more accurate approach to the designation of the different types of α and β thalassemia. For example, in many cases it is now possible to describe the genotype of a patient with the clinical picture of β thalassemia major according to the particular mutations at the homologous pairs of β globin chain loci. Homozygotes for a common Mediterranean nonsense mutation would have the following genotype: $\alpha\alpha/\beta^{39C\rightarrow T}\beta^{39C\rightarrow T}$. On the other hand, compound heterozygotes for this mutation and another common Mediterranean RNA-processing mutation would have the following genotype: $\alpha\alpha/\beta^{39C\rightarrow T}\beta^{IVS-1,1G\rightarrow A}$.

We shall consider the molecular classification of different forms of thalassemia in more detail as their molecular pathology is described in later sections.

The Complexity of the Thalassemias; The Thalassemia Syndromes

It is clear from the classifications of the thalassemias outlined in the previous section that all the common forms of thalassemia, particularly the α, β, and δβ thalassemias, are extremely heterogeneous. However, the complexity of these disorders does not end here. In many populations in which thalassemia is common, there is also a high frequency of structural hemoglobin variants, particularly Hb S, Hb C, or Hb E. Thus, it is quite common for an individual to inherit thalassemia from one parent and a structural hemoglobin variant from another. Similarly, both α and β thalassemias occur at a high frequency, and therefore individuals may inherit one or more different α thalassemia alleles and β thalassemia as well.

In countries like Thailand, where there is a high frequency of all forms of thalassemia and a particular structural hemoglobin variant—in this case, Hb E—the many different interactions of these different mutations produce a bewilderingly complex series of clinical phenotypes ranging from disorders that are lethal to those that are symptomless and are recognized only by mild anemia or morphological changes in the red cells.[7, 8]

In the sections that follow, I describe each of the different types of thalassemia separately and then attempt to define the clinical phenotypes that are produced by their interactions. As will become apparent, although we have a sophisticated understanding of the molecular pathology of many of these disorders, our knowledge about the clinical consequences of their interaction is, in many cases, still fragmentary.

α THALASSEMIA

Background and Classification

The evolution of our understanding of the α thalassemias[7-9] has taken longer than for β thalassemia, largely because for many years it was not appreciated that normal individuals have four α globin genes, two per haploid genome. The first intimation of the existence of α thalassemia came from the discovery of patients with thalassemia-like blood profiles and varying amounts of a hemoglobin variant that was later shown to be a homotetramer composed of four β chains (β_4). This abnormal hemoglobin was discovered in the mid-1950s, when new electrophoretic hemoglobin variants were designated by letters of the alphabet, and was called Hb H. A few years later, another variant of this type—in this case, a homotetramer of γ chains, γ_4—was discovered in an anemic baby at St. Bartholomew's Hospital in London. By then no letters of the alphabet were left for new hemoglobins, which had to be named by their place of discovery; the γ_4 variant was called Hb Bart's, the abbreviated form of "St. Bartholomew's Hospital"! Thus, it appeared that Hb Bart's and Hb H might reflect defective α chain production, α thalassemia, in fetal and adult life, respectively.

Subsequently, it became apparent that α thalassemia has two main clinical forms. First, there is the Hb Bart's hydrops fetalis syndrome, a disorder characterized by a severe deficiency of α chains and death late in uterine life. The second important variety of α thalassemia, Hb H disease, is characterized by a moderately severe anemia associated with variable amounts of Hb H in the blood. Analysis of the parents of patients with the Hb Bart's hydrops fetalis syndrome or hemoglobin H disease led to the idea that two types of α thalassemia trait exist: a severe form, called α thalassemia 1, and a much milder condition, α thalassemia 2, which may be hematologically silent.

When it was realized that two α globin genes are found on each of the homologous pairs of chromo-some 16, and when methods for their direct analysis became available, it was possible to clarify the genetics of α thalassemia. It became clear that two types exist: α^0 thalassemia, in which no normal α globin is produced from the α globin gene complex, and α^+ thalassemia, in which the output is reduced. Further work showed that α^+ thalassemia usually results from the deletion or inactivation by a mutation of one of the linked pairs of α globin gene. Thus, the terms α thalassemia 1 and 2 have now been replaced by α^0 and α^+ thalassemia, respectively.

A general model of the interaction of the α^0 and α^+ thalassemias is shown in Figure 5–2. The Hb Bart's hydrops syndrome results from the homozygous state for α^0 thalassemia, whereas Hb H disease usually reflects the compound heterozygous state for α^0 and α^+ thalassemia.

Now that the molecular pathology of the α globin genes is worked out, it is possible to classify the α thalassemias further.[9] The normal α globin haplotype may be written αα, representing the α2 and α1 genes, respectively. Therefore, a normal individual has the genotype αα/αα. A deletion involving one (−α) or both (− −) α genes may be further classified on the basis of its size, written as a superscript; thus $-\alpha^{3.7}$ indicates a deletion of 3.7 kilobases (kb) of DNA, including one α gene. In cases in which the size of a deletion has not yet been established, a superscript describing the geographical or individual origin of the

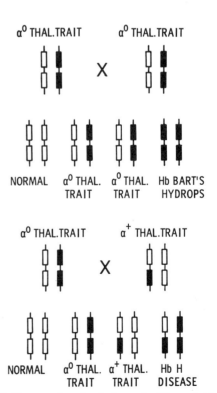

FIGURE 5–2. The genetics of α thalassemia. The α globin genes are represented as boxes. The black α genes represent gene deletions or otherwise inactivated α genes. The open boxes represent normal α genes. The terms α^0 thalassemia and α^+ thalassemia are defined in the text.

deletion is used; thus, $^{--\text{MED}}$ describes a deletion of both α genes first identified in individuals of Mediterranean origin. Finally, in those α thalassemic haplotypes in which both linked α globin genes are intact, the nomenclature $\alpha^T\alpha$ or $\alpha\alpha^T$ is used, indicating a thalassemia mutation at one or the other of the linked α genes. When the precise molecular defect is known, as for example, in the α globin chain termination mutant Hb Constant Spring, $\alpha^T\alpha$ can be replaced by the more precise $\alpha^{CS}\alpha$.

This nomenclature has provided a useful shorthand way of describing the complex interactions of the different forms of α thalassemia. For example, the genotype $^{--\text{SEA}}/\alpha^{CS}\alpha$ denotes the interaction of a chromosome containing the Hb Constant Spring mutation with a chromosome containing the common Southeast Asian form of α^0 thalassemia, a common finding in patients with Hb H disease.

The Structure of the α Globin Gene Complex

The molecular pathology of the α thalassemias is best understood against the background of recent work on the structure of the α globin gene cluster on chromosome 16.[9] It lies at the tip of chromosome 16 and has been assigned to 16p13.3.[10] It includes the duplicated α genes, α2 and α1; an embryonic α-like gene (ζ2); and three pseudogenes, ψζ1, ψα1, and ψα2, arranged in the order 5'-ζ2-ψζ1-ψα2-ψα1-α2-α1-θ-3' (Figs. 5–1 and 5–3). Analysis of the normal map of this region and that of a patient with a deletion of the terminal part of chromosome 16 has shown that the α complex is arranged with the ζ2 gene at the telomeric end of the array and the α1 gene at the centromeric end.[11]

The 26 kb segment of DNA that contains the α globin genes and an extended cloned segment flanking the cluster are part of a long G + C–rich isochore.[9] The α globin cluster and its boundaries have many of the characteristics of such regions; it is G + C rich, is early replicating, is within a Giemsa-negative band, and contains many *Alu* family repeats. Usually, such regions of the genome are thought to contain a high proportion of housekeeping genes; the α globin genes are an exception.

Structure and Expression of the α-like Globin Genes

The α globin gene family has evolved through a series of gene duplications and sequence divergences, so that now the functional α and ζ genes show only 58 per cent homology in their 141 amino acids.[9, 12] In contrast, the α1 and α2 genes are highly homologous, encode identical proteins, and differ in sequence only within IVS-2 and in their 3' non-coding regions. Like all globin genes, the α genes are divided into three exons by two non-coding intervening sequences. All the α-like globin genes and their flanking regions have been sequenced, and the entire region from the telomere of 16p to beyond the α globin gene complex has been cloned and partially mapped. From a provisional analysis of the long-range map of this region, it appears that the high GC content and the density of CpG-rich islands may extend as far as two megabases from the α genes.[9]

Both α and ζ genes are expressed in the primitive erythroblasts of the yolk sac up to 6 or 7 weeks of gestation, although ζ globin synthesis predominates during this period; definitive-line erythroblasts synthesize α globin almost exclusively. The expression of the

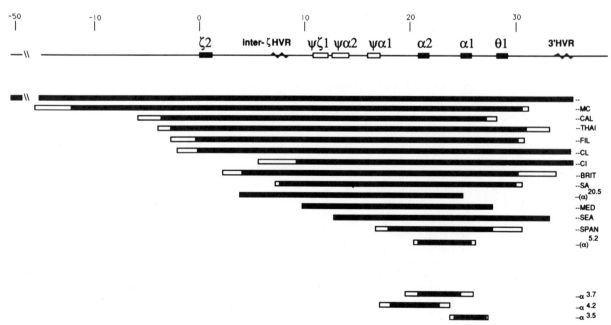

FIGURE 5–3. The arrangement of the α globin genes and the deletions that result in α^0 or α^+ thalassemia.

α2 gene predominates over that of the α1 gene by approximately 3:1 throughout all stages of development and in adult life. With sensitive assays, low levels of ζ globin expression can be detected throughout fetal life and in up to 80 per cent of cord blood samples. Although the function of the θ gene is unknown, θ mRNA can be detected at all stages of development.[9]

Each of the α genes contains typical promoter box structures at its 5′ terminal flanking region. Recent studies of α globin synthesis in mouse erythroleukemia cells and in transgenic mice, combined with an analysis of the position of DNase I–hypersensitive sites and naturally occurring deletions upstream from the α globin gene complex, have defined an element 40 kb upstream from the α globin gene cluster that has the properties of a locus control region (LCR) similar to that which has been identified upstream from the β globin gene cluster.[13] This element has been sequenced and shown to contain binding sites for NFE2/AP1, GATA-1, and CAC box proteins in an arrangement similar to that of the β globin LCR. As we shall see later, deletion of the α LCR sequences completely inactivates the α globin gene complex, suggesting that it is a major regulatory region involved in α globin gene expression in erythroid tissues.

Polymorphisms and Normal Variability at the α Globin Gene Complex

In interpreting the molecular pathology of α thalassemia, it is important to appreciate structural variability in the α globin gene cluster that is not associated with any hematological abnormalities. Its structure is highly polymorphic. There are numerous point mutations, rearrangements, and gene conversions that have no apparent effect on the expression of the α globin genes.[9] Analysis of the patterns of these polymorphisms in chromosomes derived from individuals representing 25 different populations has led to the definition of a number of specific α globin haplotypes that are extremely valuable for anthropological and population studies and, in particular, for tracing the origins and distribution of the α thalassemia mutations.[9, 14]

HYPERVARIABLE REGIONS. The α globin gene cluster contains several tandemly repeated segments of DNA, or minisatellites. They were first identified as polymorphic hypervariable regions (HVRs) located at the 3′ end of the complex (α globin 3′-HVR), between the ζ2 and ψζ1 genes (interζ HVR), and within the introns of the ζ-like genes (ζ intron HVRs).[9] More recently, HVRs have been located in the 5′ flanking region of the cluster; a particularly informative polymorphic locus lies 70 kb upstream of the ζ2 gene, a region that has been designated the 5′-HVR.[15] Together with other polymorphisms, these regions have been of great value in the genetic analysis of the α globin cluster.

VARIATION IN THE NUMBER OF α-LIKE GLOBIN GENES.[8, 9] As a result of unequal genetic exchange, phenotypically normal individuals may have four, five, or six α genes and three, four, five, or six ζ-like genes. The ααα chromosome arrangement occurs at a relatively high frequency, 0.01 to 0.08 in most populations. Even in the homozygous state for the triplicated α gene arrangement, no hematological abnormalities are present.

Chromosomes carrying a single ζ gene instead of the usual ζ2-ψζ1 arrangement are also quite common, with a gene frequency of about 0.05 in West Africa. The triplicated ζ gene arrangement usually has the structure ζ2-φζ1-φζ and occurs in parts of Southeast Asia at a frequency of 0.09 to 0.20; it is particularly common throughout Melanesia, Micronesia, and Polynesia, where phenotypically normal homozygotes (ζζζ/ζζζ) have been described. This arrangement is uncommon in other parts of the world.

The molecular basis of the generation of these novel arrangements of the ζ and α globin genes is considered in detail in a later section that describes the deletion forms of α+ thalassemia.

GENE CONVERSIONS.[9] Sequence analyses suggest that gene conversion events have taken place between the α1 and α2 and the ζ2 and ψζ1 genes during evolution.

Studies of the downstream ζ-like gene in several populations have shown that it exists in two distinct forms, one typically that of a pseudogene (ψζ1) and the other in which the ψζ1 gene has undergone a gene conversion by the ζ2 gene such that it becomes similar to the functional ζ gene. The frequency of the ζ2-ζ1 chromosome varies between populations, and normal individuals homozygous for either the ζ2-ψζ1 or the ζ2-ζ1 chromosome have been observed.

DELETIONS AND INSERTIONS IN THE α GLOBIN COMPLEX.[9] Several phenotypically silent deletions and insertions have been identified in the α globin complex. No hematological abnormalities are present. It is important to recognize that these changes can be found in normal individuals if they are not to be misinterpreted as the cause of unusual types of α thalassemia.

Molecular Pathology

In defining the molecular pathology of the α thalassemias, it is necessary to describe the molecular events that cause the loss of both α globin genes, and hence that produce the phenotype of α0 thalassemia, and those that lead to the inactivation of one of the linked pairs of α genes and underlie the phenotype of α+ thalassemia. It turns out that the α0 thalassemias are due to a heterogeneous series of deletions that involve either the α globin gene complex itself or the α globin LCR. On the other hand, the α+ thalassemias may result either from deletions of one or the other of the linked pairs of α globin genes or from mutations that, though they leave the genes intact, cause their partial or complete inactivation.

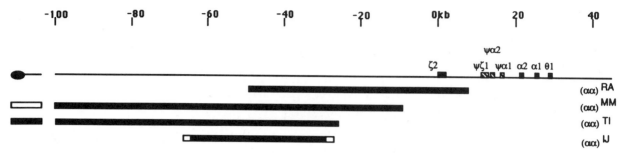

FIGURE 5–4. Deletions upstream from the α globin genes that inactivate the α globin gene complex by removing the locus control region (LCR).

α⁰ Thalassemia

DELETIONS THAT REMOVE ALL OR MOST OF THE α GLOBIN GENE CLUSTER. To date, 14 different lesions that remove both α globin genes have been described (Fig. 5–3).[9] The majority of these lesions remove both α genes, although in two cases they remove one gene and part of the other. It is clear, therefore, that chromosomes containing these deletions can produce no α globin chains, and hence molecular lesions of this type are all associated with the phenotype of α⁰ thalassemia.

In contrast to the α⁺ thalassemia deletions, which are described later, the α⁰ thalassemia deletions are limited in their geographical distribution. For example, the $--^{BRIT}$ mutation has been observed in 36 different families, all of which come from a small region in the north of England.[16] Analysis of polymorphic markers upstream of the common α⁰ thalassemias of Southeast Asia and the Mediterranean region, $--^{SEA}$ and $--^{MED}$, suggests that each of these mutations has arisen only once during evolution and reached its current high frequency by selection.[9]

Detailed analyses of the sequences across the breakpoints of these deletions have provided some evidence about the molecular events that have produced them.[9, 17] A number of mechanisms have been demonstrated, including illegitimate recombination, reciprocal translocation, and truncation of chromosome 16. Hence the study of these lesions has provided valuable information about the ways in which deletions of human chromosomes may occur.

It turns out that several of the 3′ breakpoints of the α⁰ thalassemia deletions fall within a 6 to 8 kb region at the 3′ end of the α globin complex, suggesting that this may represent a breakpoint cluster region *(bcr)*, similar to those observed in the chromosomal translocations associated with certain forms of leukemia. In some of the deletions, $--^{MED}$, $--^{SEA}$, $--^{20.5}$, $--^{SA}$, $--^{BRIT}$, the 5′ breakpoints also appear to cluster (Fig. 5–3). It seems, therefore, that the 5′ breakpoints are located approximately the same distance apart and in the same order along the chromosome as their respective 3′ breakpoints.[17] These observations are consistent with similar findings in a group of deletions of the β globin gene cluster. It has been suggested that such staggered deletions may result from illegitimate recombination events that lead to the deletion of an integral number of chromatin loops as they pass through their nuclear attachment points during replication.[18]

One of these deletions, $--^{MED}$, also involves a more complex rearrangement in which a new piece of DNA bridges the two breakpoints in the α globin gene cluster.[17] The inserted sequence originates upstream from the α globin gene cluster, where it normally exists in an inverted orientation to that found between the breakpoints of the deletion. Thus, it appears to have been incorporated into the junction in a way that reflects its close proximity to the deletion breakpoint regions during replication.

Further sequence analyses have shown that members of the dispersed family of *Alu* repeats are found frequently at or near the breakpoints of these deletions. One deletion, $--$RA, seems to have resulted from simple homologous recombination between two *Alu* repeats that are usually 62 kb apart.[17] *Alu* family repeats have been involved in similar recombinational events elsewhere in the genome.[19]

Recently, another mechanism for the generation of α⁰ thalassemia has been identified. In this case, there was a terminal truncation of the short arm of chromosome 16 to a site 50 kb distal to the α globin genes.[20] It is interesting that the telomeric consensus sequence (TTAGGG)n had been added directly to the site of the break. Since this mutation was shown to be stably inherited, it appears that telomeric DNA alone is sufficient to stabilize the broken chromosome end. This novel finding raises the possibility that other genetic diseases may result from chromosomal truncations.

DELETIONS INVOLVING THE α GLOBIN LCR. Several deletions that appear to downregulate the α globin genes by removal of the α globin LCR[21-23] have been identified (Fig. 5–4). In each case, the α globin genes have been left intact, although in one case, RA, the 3′ breakpoint is found between the ζ2 and ψζ1 genes, thus removing the ζ2 gene.[21] It appears that these deletions completely inactivate the α globin gene complex. They have not been observed in the homozygous state, presumably because it would be lethal.

α⁺ Thalassemia

So far, all the α⁺ thalassemias have been found to result either from deletions of one or the other of the duplicated α globin genes or from mutations that inactivate them.

α⁺ THALASSEMIA DUE TO DELETIONS. The most common types of α⁺ thalassemia involve the deletion of one or the other of the duplicated α globin genes, $-\alpha^{3.7}$ and $-\alpha^{4.2}$. These conditions are among the most common human genetic disorders and are found in all populations in which α thalassemia is common.

The mechanism that has led to the generation of the α⁺ thalassemia deletions reflects the underlying structure of the α globin complex.[12, 24] Each α gene lies within a boundary of homology approximately 4 kb long, interrupted by two small non-homologous regions. The homologous regions were probably generated by an ancient duplication and then subsequently were subdivided, presumably by insertions and deletions, to give three homologous subsegments, which are designated X, Y, and Z (Fig. 5–5). The duplicated Z boxes are 3.7 kb apart, and the X boxes are 4.2 kb apart. As shown in Figure 5–5, misalignment and reciprocal cross-over between these segments at meiosis produce a chromosome with either single ($-\alpha$) or triplicated ($\alpha\alpha\alpha$) α globin genes. If the cross-over occurs between homologous Z boxes, 3.7 kb of DNA is lost, an event that is described as a "rightward deletion," $-\alpha^{3.7}$. A similar process occurring between the two X boxes deletes 4.2 kb, the leftward deletion, $-\alpha^{4.2}$. The corresponding triplicated α gene arrangements are called $\alpha\alpha\alpha^{\text{anti-3.7}}$ and $\alpha\alpha\alpha^{\text{anti-4.2}}$.[25-28] Chromosomes with four α genes, $\alpha\alpha\alpha\alpha^{\text{anti-3.7}}$ or $\alpha\alpha\alpha\alpha^{\text{anti-4.2}}$, presumably arose from similar types of cross-overs involving the $\alpha\alpha\alpha^{\text{anti-3.7}}$ and $\alpha\alpha\alpha^{\text{anti-4.2}}$ chromosomes, respectively.[29]

Rearrangements involving the Z box are more frequent than those involving the X or Y region. The Z box rearrangements can be subdivided into three types, $-\alpha^{3.7I}$, $-\alpha^{3.7II}$, and $-\alpha^{3.7III}$, depending on the site of the cross-over with respect to three restriction enzyme sites that differ between the α2 and α1 Z boxes.[30] From population data, it appears that the frequency of each of these subtypes is related to the length of homology within each subsegment. The mechanism by which the fifth type of α⁺ thalassemia, which involves a deletion of 3.5 kb, $-\alpha^{3.5}$, arises is not yet clear.[31]

The five deletions involving single α globin genes, $-\alpha^{3.7I}$, $-\alpha^{3.7II}$, $-\alpha^{3.7III}$, $-\alpha^{4.2}$, and $-\alpha^{3.5}$, all lead to a reduced output of α chains from the affected chromosome (see Fig. 5–2). Since the output of the α2 gene is two to three times greater than that of the α1 gene, it would be expected that phenotypic differences between these conditions would exist. It is interesting that the phenotypes of homozygotes for the $-\alpha^{4.2}$ or $-\alpha^{3.7III}$ determinants are similar, suggesting that removal of the α2 gene results in a partial compensatory increase in the expression of the remaining α1 gene on the $-\alpha^{4.2}$ chromosome.[32] In fact, a compensatory increase in expression of the α1 gene when the α2 gene is deleted has been demonstrated at the RNA level.[33] Thus, the phenotypic effects of these deletions follow the pattern of all lesions of this type involving the globin gene clusters in that they exert an effect on the expression of nearby genes.

It appears, therefore, that homologous genetic recombination occurs relatively frequently within the human α globin gene cluster. It is not known whether such rearrangements occur between misaligned chromosomes or between chromatids during meiosis. The finding of a triplicated α globin gene arrangement, $\alpha\alpha\alpha$, at a low frequency in most populations suggests that the single α globin gene arrangement that forms the basis for the deletion form of α⁺ thalassemia has come under strong selection in those parts of the world where α⁺ thalassemia is common.[9] We return to this theme later in the chapter when we consider the population genetics of the α thalassemias.

NON-DELETION TYPES OF α⁺ THALASSEMIA. Non-deletion α⁺ thalassemias are conditions in which the output of α globin from one of the linked α globin genes is defective yet the affected gene is grossly intact. These disorders result from single or oligonucleotide mutations of the particular α globin gene. Most of them involve the α2 gene, but since the output from this locus is two to three times greater than that from the α1 gene, this may reflect ascertainment bias due to a greater effect on the phenotype and, possibly, a greater selective advantage. In contrast to the effects of deletions of the α2 gene, which underlie the $-\alpha^{4.2}$ form of α⁺ thalassemia, there appears to be no compensatory increase in expression of the α1 gene when the α2 gene is inactivated by a point mutation. It follows, therefore, that the non-deletion α⁺ thalasse-

(A)

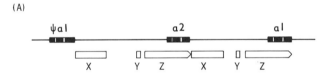

(B) RIGHTWARD CROSSOVER

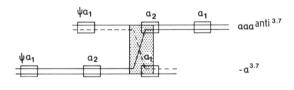

(C) LEFTWARD CROSSOVER

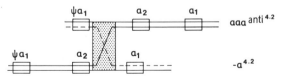

FIGURE 5–5. **The mechanisms of unequal cross-over that give rise to the $-\alpha^{3.7}$ and $-\alpha^{4.2}$ deletions.** *A,* The fine structure of the duplicated α globin genes with the positions of the homology boxes X, Y, and Z. *B,* The rightward cross-over occurs when genetic exchange takes place between misaligned homologous Z boxes, giving rise to a chromosome with either one ($-\alpha^{3.7}$) or three ($\alpha\alpha\alpha^{\text{anti-3.7}}$) α globin genes. *C,* The leftward cross-over occurs when genetic exchange takes place between the misaligned homologous X boxes, giving rise to a chromosome with either one ($-\alpha^{4.2}$) or three ($\alpha\alpha\alpha^{\text{anti-4.2}}$) α globin genes.

TABLE 5–2.   MUTATIONS THAT CAUSE NON-DELETION FORMS OF α^+ THALASSEMIA

MUTATION	RACE	REFERENCE
Non-functional mRNA		
Nonsense mutations		
Codon 116 (G → T)	Black	41
Frameshift mutations		
Codon 30/31 (−4 nt)	Black	9
Initiator codon mutations		
ATG → ACG	Mediterranean	34
CCCACCATG → CCCCATG	Mediterranean	35a
ATG → GTG	Mediterranean, black	35
Terminator codon mutations		
α^{CS} Hb Constant Spring (TAA → CAA)	Southeast Asian, Mediterranean	36, 37
α^{KD} Koya Dora (TAA → TCA)	Indian	39
α^{IC} Hb Icaria (TAA → AAA)	Mediterranean	38
α^{SR} Hb Seal Rock (TAA → GAA)	Black	40
RNA-processing mutants		
Splice junction changes		
IVS-1 donor site		
(GGTGAGGCT → GGCT)	Mediterranean	42
RNA cleavage; polyadenylation site		
AATAAA–AATAAG	Arab	44
	Mediterranean	45
Unstable globins		
$\alpha^{Quong\ Sze}$ (codon 125, Leu → Pro)	Southeast Asian	46
$\alpha^{Suan\ Dok}$ (codon 109, Leu → Arg)	Southeast Asian	46
$\alpha^{Petah\ Tikwah}$ (codon 110, Ala → Asp)	Middle East	46
$\alpha^{Evanston}$ (codon 14, Trp → Arg)	Black	46

mias have a greater phenotypic effect than do the deletion forms.

Some of the mutations that cause non-deletion α^+ thalassemia are summarized in Table 5–2. They are much less common than the deletion forms of α^+ thalassemia, and their geographical distribution is limited. Depending on the particular mutations involved, these lesions may exert their effect at the translational level or by interfering with processing of α globin mRNA.

Several types of mutations involving the α2 gene interfere with the translation of its mRNA. First are those that involve initiation. In two cases, the initiation codon is completely inactivated, ATG→ACG or GTG.[34, 35] In another, the efficiency of initiation is reduced by a dinucleotide deletion in the consensus sequence around the start signal (CCCAC-CATG→CCCCATG).[35a] Another family of mutations involves substitutions in the α2 globin termination codon, TAA.[36] Each replacement specifically changes this codon so that an amino acid is inserted instead of

the chain terminating. This is followed by readthrough of α globin mRNA, which is not normally translated until another in-phase stop codon is reached. The result is an elongated α globin chain with 31 additional residues at the C-terminal end. Four variants of this kind have been identified, Hb Constant Spring, Hb Icaria, Hb Koya Dora, and Hb Seal Rock.[36–40] They are all identical except for the residue at position 142, which reflects different substitutions in the chain termination codon (Fig. 5–6). Although it is not absolutely clear why the readthrough of normally untranslated mRNA leads to a reduced output from the α2 gene, considerable evidence exists that in some way it destabilizes the mRNA. Whatever the mechanism, the output from the α2 gene is markedly reduced; in homozygotes for Hb Constant Spring, the level of the variant hemoglobin, representing the output of both α2 genes, is only about 5 per cent of the total hemoglobin.[36] Finally, a mutation identified in a black patient from Mississippi causes premature termination of translation by changing codon 116 in exon 3 to an

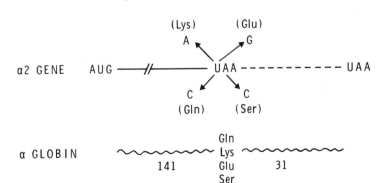

FIGURE 5–6. **The α globin chain termination mutations.** Above is shown the different mutations that have been described in the α globin termination codon UAA. Each results in insertion of an amino acid and readthrough of mRNA that is not normally translated, until another in-phase termination codon. The elongated α globin chains with different residues at position 142 are shown below.

in-phase termination codon (GAG→UAG),[41] and a 4 nucleotide (nt) deletion, also found in a black patient, leads to a shift in the α globin mRNA reading frame.[9]

Other mutations that produce non-deletion forms of α⁺ thalassemia involve the processing of the α globin mRNA transcript. One such mutation results from a pentanucleotide deletion, including the 5′ splice site of IVS-1 of the α2 gene. This deletion involves the invariant GT donor splicing sequence (G*G*TGAGGCT→GGCT) and abolishes the removal of IVS-1 during processing.[42, 43] The other mutations of this type involve substitutions in the poly (A) addition signal (AATAA*A*→AATAA*G*) and downregulate the α2 gene by interfering with the 3′ end processing of its mRNA and possibly with termination of transcription.[44, 45] It is interesting that this mutation seems to downregulate both the α2 and the α1 globin genes. Although it was originally reported that the linked α1 gene has an additional point mutation on the chromosome containing the poly(A) addition site substitution, this is not the case and the α1 gene appears to be completely normal.[45] But the function of *both* linked α globin genes is affected by this mutation, as is the case for other non-deletion forms of α thalassemia involving the dominant α2 locus. We shall return to the possible mechanisms for this observation in a later section.

Finally, the phenotype of non-deletion α⁺ thalassemia can be caused by mutations in the α2 gene that give rise to highly unstable α globin variants; these include Hb Quong Sze, Hb Suan Dok, Hb Petah Tikvah, and Hb Evanston.[9, 46]

Pathophysiology

The α thalassemia mutations, like all thalassemia mutations, lead to their phenotypic effects—in particular, anemia of varying severity—in two ways. First, and most important, is the deleterious effect of the globin chains that are produced in excess on red cell production and survival. Second, a reduced amount of hemoglobin production contributes to the anemia and causes the hypochromic blood profile that is characteristic of all the thalassemias. As in the case of β thalassemia, however, the critical factor in determining the severity of the phenotype in α thalassemia is the degree of imbalanced globin chain synthesis.

The pathophysiology of α thalassemia differs fundamentally from that of β thalassemia because of the properties of the globin chains that are produced in excess. Excess γ chains in fetal life or β chains in adults form homotetramers, Hb Bart's and Hb H. Although, particularly in the case of Hb H, they are unstable, unlike the excess α chains that are produced in β thalassemia they do not precipitate to any important degree in the red cell precursors in the bone marrow. Thus, in contrast to the β thalassemias, ineffective erythropoiesis resulting from destruction of developing red cells is not a major feature of α thalassemia. Rather, Hb H tends to precipitate and

form inclusion bodies in mature red cells as they age in the circulation. Cells containing inclusions of this type are trapped in the spleen and other parts of the reticuloendothelial system, resulting in a hemolytic anemia. Thus, the anemia of α thalassemia is due to a combination of shortened red cell survival and a reduced amount of hemoglobin production.

The other major pathophysiological mechanism that may have a profound phenotypic effect in α thalassemia is the functional properties of Hb Bart's and Hb H.[7] Because they are homotetramers, they show no heme-heme interaction and they have an extremely high oxygen affinity, which makes them physiologically useless as oxygen transporters. Thus, the clinical picture of α thalassemia reflects a complex combination of hypochromic anemia, hemolysis, and defective oxygen transport due to the properties of varying amounts of physiologically inefficient hemoglobin in the red cells. The resulting degree of tissue hypoxia may, therefore, be much greater than might be expected for the degree of anemia, a phenomenon that is well exemplified by the findings in the homozygous states for α⁰ thalassemia, the Hb Bart's hydrops syndrome.

Another factor adding to the complexity of the pathophysiology of the α thalassemias is that a critical level of reduction in α globin output is required for the production of homotetramers of γ or β chains. Furthermore, regardless of the type of α thalassemia mutation, the degree of globin chain imbalance seems to vary at different stages of development. For example, in many, but not all, infants who are heterozygous for deletion forms of α⁺ thalassemia (−α/αα), it is possible to demonstrate small amounts of Hb Bart's in the cord blood, and homozygotes for this condition have approximately 5 to 10 per cent Hb Bart's at birth. Yet in both cases the Hb Bart's disappears over the first few months of life and is not replaced by a similar amount of Hb H.[7-9] These observations suggest that during this phase of development any defect in α globin chain production may be exaggerated, possibly because some imbalance of α and non-α chain synthesis is present in many normal infants during the transition from γ to β chain production.

It is also clear that a critical level of reduction of α chain production is required before Hb H appears in a soluble form in the red cells. The most sensitive way of identifying trace amounts of Hb H is by finding inclusion bodies in the red cells after incubation with redox agents like the dye brilliant cresyl blue. Although inclusions of this type can be found in heterozygotes for α⁰ thalassemia, they are rarely present in α⁺ thalassemia heterozygotes or homozygotes.[47] The presence of sufficient Hb H to be demonstrated by electrophoresis usually requires the deletion of three of the four α globin genes (−α/− −) or the homozygous state for non-deletion mutations, which seem to downregulate both α2 and α1 genes (αᵀα/αᵀα). Thus, the production of soluble homotetramers depends both on the stage of development and on very subtle factors involving the precise level of excess β chain production in adults.

Another curious feature about the pathophysiology of Hb H disease is that many patients with this condition appear to produce Hb Bart's in adult life. This finding suggests that a modest increase in γ chain production may occur after the neonatal period. As is the case with Hb F production in β thalassemia (see a later section), γ chain production appears to be heterogeneously distributed among the red cells. It is possible that the presence of Hb Bart's in Hb H disease may reflect a very low level of γ chain production; also, because the γ_4 tetramer is more stable than the β_4 tetramer, there may be some selective survival of cells containing Hb Bart's.

It is against this complex background that the relationship between the molecular pathology and the phenotypic findings in the different clinical forms of α thalassemia has to be interpreted.

Interaction of the α Thalassemia Haplotypes and the Clinical Phenotypes of α Thalassemia

As mentioned earlier, it is convenient to describe α thalassemia mutations as haplotypes, that is the overall effect of a particular mutation on the output of both linked α globin genes. Although this is self-evident in the case of the deletions that remove both of them, it is equally valid for describing the effect of point mutations in one gene, particularly because many of them have an effect on the output of their normal partner in cis.

Currently, more than 30 different α thalassemia haplotypes have been described, and since these can interact with any other haplotype on the homologous chromosome 16, the potential exists for between 400 and 500 different phenotypes.[8, 9] In practice, these interactions produce a remarkable degree of phenotypic variability, ranging from complete normality to death during intrauterine life. Despite this complexity, for clinical purposes the α thalassemias can be divided into the Hb Bart's hydrops fetalis syndrome, Hb H disease, the homozygous state for Hb Constant Spring, α thalassemia minor, and the silent carrier states. These different clinical forms of α thalassemia, together with their underlying α globin haplotypes, are summarized in Table 5–3.

The Hemoglobin Bart's Hydrops Fetalis Syndrome

This condition occurs commonly in Southeast Asia and in the Mediterranean region.[7, 9, 48] It usually results from the homozygous inheritance of the two forms of α^0 thalassemia that are common in this region, $--^{SEA}/--^{SEA}$ or $--^{MED}/--^{MED}$. Hence fetuses with this disorder produce no α globin chains, and their hemoglobin consists of about 80 per cent Hb Bart's and about 20 per cent Hb Portland, the synthesis of which

TABLE 5–3. INTERACTIONS OF α THALASSEMIA HAPLOTYPES

		α^0	α^+				
			$\alpha\alpha$	$\alpha\alpha^T$	$-\alpha$	$\alpha^T\alpha$	$-\alpha^T$
α^0		Hy	T	H	H	H,Hy	—
α^+	$-\alpha^T$		T	—	H	T	H
	$\alpha^T\alpha$		T	—	T	H	—
	$-\alpha$		T	—	T		
	$\alpha\alpha^T$		T	—			
	$\alpha\alpha$		N				

Hy = Hb Bart's hydrops; H = Hb H disease; T = α thalassemia trait.

persists up to birth in this condition.[7] A few exceptions to this rule have been described, however. There have been reports of hydropic infants from Greece and Southeast Asia who have very low levels of α chain synthesis. Preliminary gene mapping analyses suggest that these infants have a common α^0 thalassemia determinant on one chromosome and a non-deletion mutation on the other; the nature of the latter has yet to be determined.[49, 50] It is possible that these non-deletion mutations are similar to the poly (A) addition site mutations in that they reduce the output of both linked α globin genes.

Babies with this syndrome die either in utero between 30 and 40 weeks' gestation or soon after birth. Several cases have been reported in which babies were delivered early, transfused, and nursed intensively; they have been maintained on regular blood transfusions and have survived to develop normally.[51, 52]

Clinically, the infant is pale and edematous, with signs of cardiac failure and severe intrauterine hypoxia.[7, 48, 53] Massive hypertrophy of the placenta is present. Hepatosplenomegaly is always found, and there is a significant increase in the occurrence of other congenital abnormalities. The hemoglobin level at birth ranges from 3 to 20 g/dl, and the blood film is characterized by variation in the shape and size of the red cells, which are grossly hypochromic; there are large numbers of nucleated red cells in the peripheral blood.

The other important feature of this syndrome is the high frequency of maternal complications, including hypertension, antepartum hemorrhage, malpresentation, difficult vaginal delivery (often necessitating cesarean section), retained placenta, and postpartum hemorrhage.[53]

It is clear, therefore, that the pathological changes in the Hb Bart's hydrops fetalis syndrome are the result of gross intrauterine hypoxia. These changes are not always seen in infants who are born with similar hemoglobin levels for other reasons and reflect the hemoglobin constitution of these babies. As mentioned earlier, Hb Bart's is physiologically useless, and hence the only way that oxygen can be transported is via Hb Portland, which usually makes up only about

20 per cent of the hemoglobin. Functionally, therefore, these babies are profoundly anemic, and it is surprising that so many of them survive to term.

Hemoglobin H Disease

Hemoglobin H disease usually results from the interaction of α^+ and α^0 thalassemia and is therefore found predominantly in Southeast Asia ($^{--SEA}/-\alpha^{3.7}$) and the Mediterranean region ($^{--MED}/-\alpha^{3.7}$).[9] In Southeast Asia, it also results from the inheritance of α^0 thalassemia and Hb Constant Spring ($--/\alpha^{CS}\alpha$). It may also result from the homozygous inheritance of mutations (non-deletion α^+ thalassemia) that affect the predominant $\alpha2$ gene, $\alpha^T\alpha/\alpha^T\alpha$.[34, 45, 54] In Algeria, homozygotes for chromosomes carrying the $-\alpha^{3.7II}$ deletion together with a non-deletion α thalassemia mutation on the remaining α gene ($-\alpha^T/-\alpha^T$) seem to have typical Hb H disease.[55]

As evidenced from the deletion forms of Hb H disease—$^{--SEA}/-\alpha$, for example—the loss of three of four α genes leads to a sufficient excess of β chains to generate viable β_4 tetramers. The same overall deficit of α chains must occur in the homozygous state for the non-deletion forms of α^+ thalassemia. On the other hand, homozygotes for the deletion forms of α^+ thalassemia, $-\alpha/-\alpha$, do not have Hb H disease. When the $\alpha2$ gene is inactivated by a mutation, the $\alpha1$ gene does not increase its output in the way that it does when the $\alpha2$ gene is deleted (Fig. 5–7). This finding may reflect the fact that competition exists between the α genes for activating factors that bind to their promoters, both of which are retained in the non-deletion α^+ thalassemias, or a more subtle effect reflecting the position of the $\alpha1$ gene relative to the αLCR on the deletion chromosomes. Whatever the

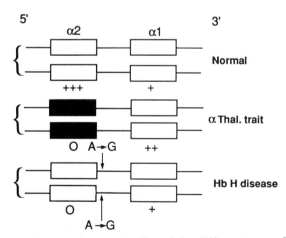

FIGURE 5–7. The phenotypic effect of the different types of α^+ thalassemia. Normally, the output from the $\alpha2$ gene exceeds that from the $\alpha1$ gene by 3:1. In the homozygous state for α^+ thalassemia due to a deletion of the $\alpha2$ gene, the output from the remaining $\alpha1$ genes is increased, and hence there is a mild phenotype similar to thalassemia trait. However, when both $\alpha2$ genes have a point mutation—in this case, in the poly (A) addition site—the output of the linked $\alpha1$ gene is not increased, and hence the phenotype is much more severe.

mechanism, the overall deficit of α chains in non-deletion α^+ thalassemia homozygotes is sufficient to lead to the phenotype of Hb H disease (Fig. 5–7).

Hemoglobin H disease is characterized by anemia and splenomegaly, together with typical thalassemic changes in the red cells, which contain variable amounts of Hb H. This clinical picture is extremely variable, however. Some patients with Hb H disease are asymptomatic, whereas others have severe anemia and require blood transfusions. Considering how much is known about the molecular pathology of this condition, it is disappointing to reflect on our lack of understanding about the reasons for this clinical heterogeneity. It appears that, overall, Hb H disease due to compound heterozygosity for α^0 and α^+ thalassemia is milder than if the disorder results from the interaction of α^0 thalassemia with a haplotype that carries a non-deletion form of α^+ thalassemia.[9, 56] For example, in Southeast Asia there is evidence that individuals with the former type of Hb H disease are less anemic and have, on average, lower levels of Hb H than do those who have the genotype $^{--SEA}/\alpha^{CS}\alpha$.[9, 57] This difference may reflect the milder defect in α chain production from the $-\alpha$ chromosome compared with the $\alpha^{CS}\alpha$ haplotype. But otherwise very little information exists about the reason for the clinical variability of Hb H disease, even between individuals who have the same molecular lesions.

The hematological findings in Hb H disease include a variable degree of anemia, hypochromic microcytic red cells, and levels of Hb H ranging from 2 to 40 per cent; when the cells are incubated with redox dyes, this is reflected in the number of them that contain typical Hb H inclusions. Overall, fetal hemoglobin levels appear to be normal in this condition, although in many patients, in addition to Hb H, small amounts of Hb Bart's have been observed, suggesting that γ chain production may be slightly increased after birth. For reasons that are not absolutely clear, there have been occasional reports of individuals with the phenotype of Hb H disease in whom the level of Bart's is higher than the level of Hb H.[7] The level of Hb A_2 is either normal or subnormal.

The most common complication of Hb H disease is the development of increasing splenomegaly and hypersplenism. Others include infection, leg ulcers, gallstones, and folic acid deficiency. Progressive iron loading, which is so common in β thalassemia, is not a major feature. Because of the sensitivity of Hb H to redox agents, there may be exacerbation of the hemolysis after the administration of drugs with redox potential.

The Homozygous State for Hemoglobin Constant Spring

We have already seen how the homozygous states for some non-deletion forms of α^+ thalassemia are associated with the clinical picture of Hb H disease. Presumably this is because they involve the dominant $\alpha2$ gene and because they also seem to downregulate the linked $\alpha 1$ gene, or at least prevent the compensatory increase in its output that occurs when the $\alpha 2$ gene is lost by a deletion. The homozygous state for the non-deletion form of α^+ thalassemia due to the Hb Constant Spring mutation on the $\alpha 2$ gene has a different phenotype, however. Because this α globin chain termination variant occurs at a high frequency in many parts of Southeast Asia, the homozygous state has been encountered often enough for its clinical phenotype to have been well established.[58, 59]

The clinical picture is characterized by a moderate degree of anemia, mild icterus, and splenomegaly.[58] The red cells are hypochromic and show variation in shape and size with marked basophilic stippling. The reticulocyte count is elevated, usually in the region of 10 per cent. The red cell survival is considerably reduced, but ferrokinetic studies indicate only a mild degree of ineffective erythropoiesis.

The hemoglobin consists of 5 to 8 per cent Hb Constant Spring, normal levels of Hb A_2 and Hb F, and the persistence of Hb Bart's into adult life at about 1 to 2 per cent of the total.

Hemoglobin biosynthetic studies demonstrate an overall defect in α globin chain synthesis, which becomes more marked during erythroid maturation, suggesting that α globin mRNA from the α^{CS} locus is unstable.[59] Hb Constant Spring is not itself unstable, and therefore the anemia seems to result mainly from defective α chain production consequent on the instability of α^{CS} mRNA. Presumably, this in turn results from the translation of $3'$ α globin mRNA sequence, which is not normally utilized. Biosynthetic studies clearly demonstrate a pool of free β chains in the cells of these patients, but it is not usually possible to demonstrate Hb H in the peripheral blood. Why they produce small amounts of Hb Bart's and not Hb H has not been satisfactorily explained. We shall encounter this problem again when we consider the interactions of α thalassemia with some of the β globin variants, such as Hb E. It appears that under certain conditions excess β chains do not form stable β_4 tetramers, but why this occurs is not clear.

Homozygous or Compound Heterozygous States for α^+ Thalassemia[60]

The clinical phenotype of the homozygous states for α^+ thalassemia varies, depending on the particular type of α thalassemia variant. Homozygotes for the deletion forms of α^+ thalassemia, $-\alpha^{3.7}/-\alpha^{3.7}$, for example, have a phenotype typical of thalassemia trait. Their red cells are hypochromic and microcytic, and they may be mildly anemic, but otherwise their adult hemoglobin pattern is normal. At birth, there is 5 to 10 per cent Hb Bart's, which disappears over the first few months of life, not to be replaced by Hb H.

As already mentioned, homozygotes for at least some non-deletion forms of α^+ thalassemia have a more severe deficit of α chains and may show the clinical phenotype of Hb H disease. It is clear, therefore, that if the $\alpha 2$ globin genes are inactivated by

mutations but are otherwise intact, the overall deficit of α chains is much greater than if the same genes are deleted.

The compound heterozygous states for deletion and non-deletion forms of α^+ thalassemia have been well described in the Saudi Arabian population.[54] The genotype $-\alpha/\alpha^{Saudi}\alpha$, where α^{Saudi} represents a poly (A) addition site mutation in the $\alpha 2$ gene, is characterized by findings typical of thalassemia trait.

α^0 Thalassemia Trait

The α^0 thalassemia trait is characterized by a very mild anemia and a reduction in the mean cell hemoglobin (MCH) and mean cell volume (MCV).[60] In adult life, there are no changes in the hemoglobin pattern, but at birth there is 5 to 10 per cent Hb Bart's. This Hb Bart's is not replaced by electrophoretically demonstrable amounts of Hb H in adult life, although on incubation of the red cells with redox dyes a few cells containing Hb H inclusion bodies can usually be found. In cases in which the embryonic ζ genes are spared, trace amounts of ζ chains can be demonstrated in the red cells.[9]

α^+ Thalassemia Trait

The α^+ thalassemia traits are all associated with extremely mild hematological changes, and the hemoglobin level and red cell indices may be normal.[60] Studies of newborn infants with this condition have shown that some of them have a slight elevation of Hb Bart's, in the 1 to 2 per cent range, but this is not always the case, and it is not possible to identify this condition with certainty in the neonatal period, or at any other time, other than by DNA analysis. The only exception to this rule is the heterozygous state for Hb Constant Spring or related chain termination variants in which it is possible to observe 0.1 to 1.5 per cent of the variant hemoglobin, using sensitive methods of hemoglobin electrophoresis.

Interaction of α Thalassemia with Structural Hemoglobin Variants

Because the inherited disorders of hemoglobin occur commonly in many parts of the world, individuals quite often inherit more than one condition of this type. We consider the results of the inheritance of both α and β thalassemia later in this chapter. Here we briefly review the various phenotypes that result from the inheritance of α thalassemia with either α or β globin structural variants. It is beyond the scope of this chapter to describe all these interactions in detail. Readers who wish to learn more about this subject are referred to several reviews and monographs.[7, 8, 9, 60] However, now that the molecular pathology of α thalassemia has been worked out by direct analysis of the structure of the α globin genes, it is possible to derive some general principles from the study of these interesting experiments of nature.

α Thalassemia with α Chain Variants [9, 60]

Some of the α globin chain variants that have been found in association with α thalassemia are summarized in Table 5–4. Unless the variants are unstable, the associated clinical phenotype is simply that of the particular form of α thalassemia. Because normal individuals have four α globin genes, if one of them carries a mutation for a structural hemoglobin variant, in heterozygotes the abnormal hemoglobin should make up approximately 25 per cent of the total. Although some variability exists, depending on whether the mutation involves the α2 or α1 gene, this expectation has been borne out in most of these interactions. If the variant occurs on a chromosome in which the linked α globin gene is deleted, that is on one with a deletion form of α^+ thalassemia, the relative level of the variant in heterozygotes will be higher, approximately 30 per cent of the total hemoglobin. Homozygotes for α globin variants—Hb J Tongariki, for example—on chromosomes of this type have no Hb A, since their genotype is $-\alpha^J/-\alpha^J$. Similarly, their inheritance, together with a chromosome carrying an α^0 thalassemia deletion, results in the clinical phenotype of Hb H disease in which the hemoglobin consists only of the variant form, and again there is no Hb A $(--/-\alpha^x)$.

As shown in Table 5–4, many of the α globin chain variants have been found on chromosomes with α thalassemia. Some occur on several different types of chromosomes, indicating that they represent independent mutations. For example, Hb G^{Philadelphia} ($\alpha^{68Asn\rightarrow Lys}$) has been found in at least four different racial groups and on both normal and α^+ thalassemia chromosomes.

α Thalassemia with β Chain Variants [8]

Because α thalassemia occurs so frequently in Africa and Southeast Asia, it is often encountered in individuals who also have the β chain hemoglobin variants that occur commonly in these populations. The clinical phenotypes resulting from the inheritance of α thalassemia with the sickle cell trait or sickle cell anemia have been well characterized in individuals of African

background. Similarly, the consequences of inheriting different types of α thalassemia with Hb E have been well documented in Thailand. The only phenotypic effects of these complex interactions on the sickle cell or Hb E trait are the hematological features of the particular form of α thalassemia and a lower level of the β globin variant than is usually found in heterozygotes. The reason for the latter finding lies in the differential affinity of α chains for normal and variant β chains. It appears that α chains have a higher affinity for normal β chains than for β^S or β^E chains. Thus, if there is an overall deficit of α chains, those that are synthesized bind preferentially to β^A chains, and therefore there is a relatively lower level of the abnormal hemoglobin than is usually found in heterozygotes.

This differential affinity of α chains for normal or variant β chains also explains the findings in individuals who have the genotype of Hb H disease but who also have the Hb S or Hb E traits. The hematological picture is very similar to that of Hb H disease, and the hemoglobin consists of Hb A, with a very low level (in the 10 per cent range) of Hb S or Hb E. Hb H is never seen in the red cells in these interactions, although it is usual to find small amounts of Hb Bart's. Presumably, with a severe degree of α chain deficiency, such α chains as are synthesized combine preferentially with normal β chains to produce Hb A. The β^S or β^E chains, an excess of which results, are unable to form stable tetramers and hence do not appear in the peripheral blood. Similarly, because α chains have a higher affinity for β than γ chains, if γ chain synthesis persists, excess γ chains produce Hb Bart's (γ_4).

Because of the very high frequency of Hb E together with α^0 and α^+ thalassemia in Thailand and other parts of Southeast Asia, a variety of different clinical phenotypes that result from the co-inheritance of the Hb E gene with different combinations of α thalassemia have been defined. It should be remembered that because the mutation that causes Hb E also produces a mild form of thalassemia, some of these conditions have quite severe clinical phenotypes. As mentioned above, the inheritance of the Hb E trait with the genotype of Hb H disease gives rise to a well-defined disorder that is clinically similar to Hb H disease but in which the hemoglobin pattern consists of Hb A + Hb E + Hb Bart's. The homozygous state for Hb E in combination with the genotype of Hb H disease is

TABLE 5–4.   THE INTERACTION OF α THALASSEMIA WITH α GLOBIN VARIANTS

VARIANT		GENOTYPE	POPULATION(s)
Hb Evanston	α^{14} Trp → Arg	$-\alpha^{3.7}$	Black
Hb Hasharon	α^{47} Asp → His	$-\alpha^{3.7}$ and αα	Mediterranean, Ashkenazi Jews
Hb G Philadelphia	α^{68} Asn → Lys	$-\alpha^{3.7}$ and αα	Algerian, Mediterranean, black, Melanesian
Hb Q (Mahidol)	α^{74} Asp → His	$-\alpha^{4.2}$	Southeast Asian
Hb Duan	α^{75} Asp → Ala	$-\alpha^{4.2}$	Chinese
Hb Nigeria	α^{81} Ser → Lys	Not determined	Black
Hb J Capetown	α^{92} Arg → Gln	$-\alpha^{3.7I}$	South African
Hb J Tongariki	α^{115} Ala → Asp	$-\alpha^{3.7III}$	Melanesian

From Higgs, D. R., Vickers, M. A., Wilkie, A. O. M., Pretorius, I.-M., Jarman, A. P., and Weatherall, D. J.: A review of the molecular genetics of the human α globin gene cluster. Blood 73:1081, 1989; with permission.

associated with a severe form of thalassemia intermedia in which the hemoglobin pattern consists of Hb E + Hb Bart's with an elevated level of Hb F.

The clinical effects of the inheritance of α thalassemia on sickle cell anemia have been characterized in several populations.[61] Comparisons of patients with sickle cell anemia who are homozygous for α+ thalassemia with those who do not have α thalassemia have shown that the group with α thalassemia has a higher hemoglobin level, typical thalassemic red cell indices, a greater likelihood of splenomegaly after early childhood, and, possibly, fewer episodes of the acute chest syndrome and chronic leg ulceration. They also have lower levels of Hb F. In vitro studies have shown that the deformability of sickle cells is enhanced if α thalassemia is also present, thus providing a cellular basis for these observations.[61a]

World Distribution and Population Genetics

Because of the difficulties of identifying the genotypes of α thalassemia from their hematological phenotypes, it is only following the advent of DNA analysis that it has been possible to start to determine the distribution and frequency of α thalassemia in different parts of the world.[7, 9, 60] The approximate frequency of α+ and α0 thalassemia among the world populations is illustrated in Figure 5–8. It is clear that α+ thalassemia occurs commonly across tropical Africa, the Middle East, and certain regions of India, as well as throughout Southeast Asia. The disorder reaches its highest frequency in some of the Pacific island populations. Although detailed population analyses of the varieties of α+ thalassemia have been

limited, it appears that the $-\alpha^{3.7}$ types predominate in Africa, whereas both $-\alpha^{3.7}$ and $-\alpha^{4.2}$ mutations occur frequently throughout Southeast Asia and the Pacific islands. The variant of the $-\alpha^{3.7}$ deletion, $-\alpha^{3.7III}$, is found commonly in Melanesia.

α^0 Thalassemia, on the other hand, is limited in its distribution to the Mediterranean region and parts of Southeast Asia, particularly southern China, Thailand, and Vietnam. This observation accounts for the uneven distribution of the Hb Bart's hydrops fetalis syndrome and Hb H disease in the world population. These conditions are found frequently only in regions where α^0 thalassemia occurs, that is in Southeast Asia and the Mediterranean area. In Saudi Arabia, Hb H disease occurs quite commonly, but this reflects a high frequency of the non-deletion form of α^+ thalassemia due to a mutation in the poly (A) addition site of the α2 gene, which, in the homozygous state, produces typical Hb H disease.[54] When there is a relatively high frequency of both deletion and non-deletion forms of α thalassemia, a number of complex genotypes are observed, including the heterozygous and homozygous states for the deletion forms of α^+ thalassemia, $-\alpha/\alpha\alpha$ and $-\alpha/-\alpha$, respectively; the compound heterozygous state for the deletion and non-deletion forms, $-\alpha/\alpha^T\alpha$; and the homozygous state for the non-deletion form of α^+ thalassemia, $\alpha^T\alpha/\alpha^T\alpha$.[54] Sporadic cases of Hb H due to the homozygous state for other non-deletion forms of α^+ thalassemia have been found in several racial groups.[9]

The occurrence of the different triplicated α globin gene arrangements ($\alpha\alpha\alpha^{anti-3.7}$; $\alpha\alpha\alpha^{anti-4.2}$) in most populations suggests that the cross-over events that lead to the deletion forms of α^+ thalassemia happen quite frequently.[9] Analysis of the α globin restriction frag-

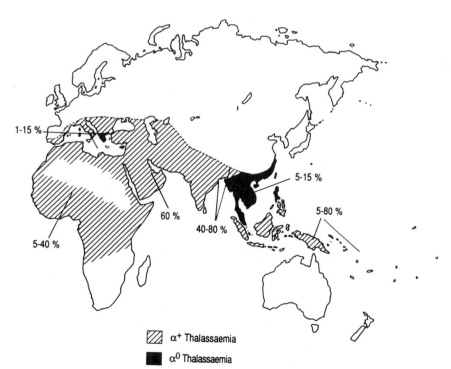

1-15 %

5-15 %

60 %

40-80 %

5-80 %

5-40 %

▨ α+ Thalassaemia

■ α0 Thalassaemia

FIGURE 5–8. The world distribution of α thalassemia.

ment length polymorphism (RFLP) haplotypes associated with these disorders also indicates that they have had multiple origins within both the same and different populations. The finding of extremely high frequencies of the deletion chromosomes in some populations suggests that they may have come under selection. In recent years, the application of DNA analysis to this problem has provided strong circumstantial evidence that a major factor responsible for the high frequency of α thalassemia is protection against *Plasmodium falciparum* malaria. Most of this evidence comes from work in the Pacific island populations.

It has been firmly established that a strong positive correlation exists throughout Melanesia between malarial endemicity and the frequency of α thalassemia.[62] In Papua New Guinea, where α thalassemia affects more than 80 per cent of the population in some regions, the relationship is altitude dependent. Throughout Melanesia a north to south, east to west decrease in malarial endemicity is closely paralelled by a decrease in the gene frequency of α thalassemia. A number of other loci, not linked to the α globin gene cluster, have been analyzed to see if any other polymorphisms have this particular distribution pattern, but none have been found. Furthermore, investigation of the molecular structure of α^+ thalassemia in this region shows that a few types, $-\alpha^{4.2}$, two haplotypes with $-\alpha^{3.71}$, and the $-\alpha^{3.7III}$ variant, predominate.[62] Furthermore, all these mutations are found on α globin gene haplotypes—that is, particular combinations of RFLPs—that are common to Melanesia and extremely rare elsewhere. These findings suggest that the α^+ thalassemia determinants found throughout this malaria cline originated in Melanesia and were amplified to a high frequency by a locally operating selective mechanism rather than being imported by population migrations from outside the region, from Southeast Asia, for example.

In a series of control studies, α thalassemia gene frequencies have been analyzed in areas where malaria has never been recorded.[63, 64] These include Iceland and Japan and many of the island archipeligos of Micronesia and Polynesia as Oceanic controls. There is virtually no α thalassemia in either Iceland or Japan, but, surprisingly, gene frequencies as high as 12 per cent are seen in parts of Polynesia. However, recent population studies suggest that the variant has been carried into the eastern Pacific during the migrations of proto-Polynesian colonizers.[64]

It appears, therefore, that a very strong correlation exists between the frequency of α thalassemia and present or past *P. falciparum* malaria. It is still not clear whether protection is afforded to heterozygotes or homozygotes for α^+ thalassemia, but this question should be settled by case control studies designed to examine the relative frequency of these different genotypes in patients with severe *P. falciparum* infections. If protection is mediated in this way, the question of how remains. Detailed in vitro studies in which the rates of invasion and growth of *P. falciparum* in α

thalassemic red cells were compared with these same factors normal red cells have shown no differences.[65] However, it has been found recently that infected α thalassemic cells bind significantly more antibody from the sera of patients with acute *P. falciparum* malaria than do normal red cells.[65] It is not clear whether this finding reflects more efficient exposure of malarial antigens by the thalassemic cells or whether these cells expose red cell neoantigens related to senescence more effectively than do normal cells when invaded by the parasite; changes of this kind have been well documented in parasitized red cells. If these observations are confirmed, they raise a completely new avenue of investigation for the protective effect of thalassemia against *P. falciparum* malaria and suggest that it may be immune mediated rather than due to the direct properties of the small thalassemic red cell.

α Thalassemia and Mental Retardation

In 1980, three patients who had varying degrees of mental retardation associated with the phenotype of Hb H disease were described.[66] Subsequently, there were several reports of a similar syndrome.[67, 68] Some unusual features were noted about this particular form of α thalassemia. First, the patients were all of Caucasian origin, which, as we have seen, is unusual for α thalassemia. Second, although one parent showed evidence of a mild form of α thalassemia in each family, the other parent was completely normal. Thus, it appeared that this condition was quite unlike the forms of Hb H disease described in other populations, both in its genetic transmission and in the associated mental retardation, which is not seen in the inherited types of Hb H disease. It was suggested that these patients might have received a de novo mutation, which had occurred in the germ cells of one of their parents and which was responsible for both α thalassemia and mental retardation. Because the condition had been identified only because of the chance inheritance of α thalassemia from the one parent, leading to the phenotype of Hb H disease, it was predicted that individuals would be found with mental retardation and the phenotype of α^0 thalassemia trait. Over the past few years, this prediction has been borne out, and more individuals or families with this syndrome have been identified.

It is now clear that two different varieties of the α thalassemia mental retardation syndrome exist.[69, 70] First, there is a group of patients who have relatively mild mental handicap and a variable constellation of facial and skeletal dysmorphisms. These individuals have long deletions involving the α globin gene cluster, removing at least 1 megabase (Mb). It appears that this condition can arise in several ways, including unbalanced translocation involving chromosome 16, truncation of the tip of chromosome 16, and the loss of the α globin gene cluster and parts of its flanking regions by other mechanisms. These findings localize a region of about 1.7 Mb in band 16p13.3, proximal to the α globin genes, as being involved in mental handicap.[71]

The second group is characterized by defective α globin synthesis associated with severe mental retardation and a strikingly homogeneous pattern of dysmorphism, including a similar facial appearance and genital abnormalities.[70] These patients have a relatively mild form of Hb H disease and so far have all had a male karyotype. Extensive structural studies have shown no abnormalities of the α globin genes, the activity of which appears to be reduced in both *cis* and *trans*. These chromosomes direct the synthesis of normal amounts of α globin in mouse erythroleukemia cells, suggesting that the α thalassemia is due to a deficiency of a *trans*-acting factor involved in the regulation of the α globin genes.

The finding of a typical facial appearance in the non-deletion form of this condition has led to the discovery of several more families. The retarded patients with α thalassemia are all males, and it is clear that the transmission is X linked.[70, 71] There seems to be extreme inactivation of the affected X chromosome in the female carriers. The availability of these families has allowed linkage analysis to be carried out, and the locus involved has been assigned to the short arm of the X chromosome. It seems likely, therefore, that an X chromosome–encoded *trans*-acting factor regulates α globin synthesis and is deficient in these children. Whether this factor is involved in development or, as seems more likely, this condition represents a contiguous gene syndrome that involves the locus for the α globin regulation factor, together with other genes, remains to be determined.

It appears, therefore, that a heterogeneous collection of conditions affect 16p13.3 and result in the clinical phenotype of α thalassemia associated with mental retardation. The further definition of the molecular defects that underlie these syndromes should throw light on normal developmental mechanisms, on the regulation of the α globin gene cluster, and on the pathogenesis of mental retardation in general.

α Thalassemia and Leukemia

The association of the phenotype of Hb H disease with myeloproliferative disorders is well established.[72, 73] In the cases described in the literature, there is a strong predominance of males and the condition occurs in older populations. It is usually seen in the setting of the myelodysplastic syndrome, although some patients have developed a more florid form of acute leukemia.

It appears that this is a clonal disorder that involves the neoplastic cell line. The peripheral blood profile is dimorphic, with both normal and hypochromic populations. In some patients, the hypochromic population expands, so that there is an almost complete absence of α chain synthesis in the red cell progenitors and reticulocytes.[72] Thus, it appears that the deficiency of α chains is mediated in both *cis* and *trans*. Cell fusion experiments have suggested that it can be corrected when the affected human chromosomes 16 are transferred into mouse erythroleukemia cells,[73] although these results must be interpreted with caution because of difficulties in defining the origin of the human cells. In all cases that have been studied in detail, the α globin genes have been intact and extensive mapping studies have shown no abnormalities. Thus, the findings are not unlike those observed in the non-deletion form of α thalassemia with mental retardation, but further work is required to determine whether the factor responsible for defective α chain synthesis is encoded by the X chromosome.

β THALASSEMIA

The β thalassemias are among the most intensively studied monogenic disorders in man. Close to 100 different mutations that give rise to the clinical phenotype of β thalassemia have been identified. Although the elucidation of the molecular pathology of the first few cases of β thalassemia that were studied involved sequencing random β thalassemia genes, the identification of new mutations was greatly facilitated by the observation that within any population each β thalassemia mutation is in strong linkage disequilibrium with specific arrangements of RFLPs in the β globin complex, called haplotypes.[74] Furthermore, as different populations were studied, it was found that in every case the bulk of β thalassemias resulted from a small number of common mutations, together with varying numbers of rare ones, and that each ethnic group has its own particular β thalassemia alleles. It has been inferred from these observations that the β thalassemias originated independently in these populations and were then subjected to positive selection, presumably because heterozygotes were protected against *P. falciparum* malaria. It turns out that about 20 different alleles account for more than 80 per cent of β thalassemia genes in the world population.

Because several different common β thalassemia mutations exist in all the populations in which there is a high frequency of the disorder, it follows that many patients with β thalassemia major, rather than being homozygous for a particular mutation, are compound heterozygotes for two different β thalassemia alleles. The only exception to this rule is in populations having a high frequency of consanguineous marriages. Because the mutations that underlie β+ thalassemia vary widely in their effect on β chain production, it follows that there is considerable possibility for phenotypic diversity based on different interactions of β thalassemia alleles in compound heterozygotes.

The β Globin Gene Cluster

The β globin gene cluster on chromosome 11 contains the non–α globin genes arranged in the following order: ε-^{G}γ-^{A}γ-ψβ-δ-β (see Fig. 5–1). Much of this region of DNA has been sequenced, and many of the major regulatory regions have been defined. It contains many RFLPs, although, in contrast to the α globin gene cluster, no minisatellite (hypervariable) sequences have been identified. The arrangement of RFLPs is not random between different populations. Rather, each population has a limited number of common arrangements of RFLPs, or β globin haplotypes, a finding that has been of considerable value in evolutionary studies of human populations and of the β globin genes.

The first indication of the existence of major regulatory sequences in this gene cluster came from studies that identified sites hypersensitive for DNase 1, five located far upstream and one far downstream from the cluster itself. These sites are erythroid specific but developmentally stable; that is, they represent regions of chromatin that are open at all stages of development. As described earlier for the α globin gene cluster, the region identified by DNase sensitivity 5' to the cluster has now been characterized in detail and designated the LCR.[75] It seems to be of major importance in regulating the expression of the entire β globin gene cluster in erythroid tissue and, in addition, appears to have classical enhancer-like function that is relatively specific for cells of erythroid origin. A number of other sequences with enhancer-like properties have been defined within the β globin gene cluster.

Molecular Pathology

The deficiency or absence of β globin chains that characterizes β thalassemia reflects the action of mutations that affect every level of β globin gene function, that is, transcription, mRNA processing, translation, and post-translational stability of the β globin chain product. Some of these mutations are illustrated in Figure 5–9 and listed in Table 5–5, grouped according to the mechanism by which they affect β globin gene expression. They have been the subject of several recent reviews,[76, 77] so only those of particular phenotypic importance are described here.

Nearly all the different β thalassemia mutations that have been identified so far behave like alleles of the β

globin gene and involve it directly. As we shall see in a later section, mutations many kilobases upstream from the β globin locus may cause its defective function, as occurs in some of the α thalassemias, but these lesions also involve γ and δ chain production and therefore do not give rise to the clinical phenotype of β thalassemia.

Gene Deletions

Unlike the α thalassemias, the β thalassemias are not commonly caused by gene deletion. Only a handful of different deletions affecting only the β globin gene have been described (Fig. 5–10). Of these, only a 619 bp deletion involving the 3' end of the β globin gene is common, and even this is restricted to the Sind populations of India and Pakistan, where it constitutes about 30 per cent of the β thalassemia alleles.[78] The other deletions that result in β thalassemia are extremely rare.[79–84] In each case, the 5' end of the β globin gene is lost and the δ gene remains intact. As we shall see later, these deletions are of particular phenotypic interest because they are all associated with an unusually high level of Hb A$_2$ production in heterozygotes.

Mutations in Promoter Regions of the β Globin Gene

Several mutations have been observed in or around the highly conserved sequences 5' to the β globin gene, which constitute the various promoter boxes.[77, 85–87] They involve single nucleotide substitutions in the TATA box, at around −30 nt from the transcription start site, or in the proximal or distal promoter elements, CACACCC at −90 nt and −105 nt. These mutations result in decreased β globin mRNA production in transient expression systems, ranging from 10 to 25 per cent of the output from a normal β globin gene, indicating that they are responsible for the associated β thalassemia phenotype. It is interesting that no mutations have yet been observed in the CCAAT box at −70 nt.

One mutation, C→T at position −101 nt to the β globin gene, appears to cause an extremely mild deficit

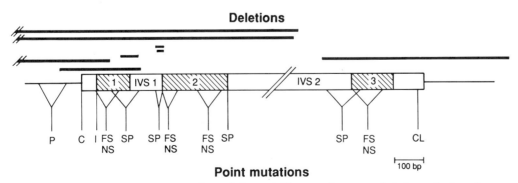

FIGURE 5–9. The major classes of mutations of the β globin gene that cause β thalassemia. P = Promoter boxes; C = CAP site; I = initiation codon; FS = frameshift; NS = nonsense; SP = splice junction, consensus sequence, or cryptic splice site; CL = RNA cleavage (poly [A]) site.

TABLE 5–5. MOLECULAR PATHOLOGY OF THE β THALASSEMIAS

MUTATION	β⁰ or β⁺ THALASSEMIA	RACIAL ORIGIN
1. Non-functional mRNA		
Nonsense mutants		
Codon 17 (A→T)	0	Chinese
Codon 39 (C→T)	0	Mediterranean, European
Codon 15 (G→A)	0	Asian Indian
Codon 121 (A→T)	0	Polish, Swiss
Codon 37 (G→A)	0	Saudi Arabian
Codon 43 (G→T)	0	Chinese
Codon 61 (A→T)	0	Black
Codon 35 (C→A)	0	Thai
Frameshift mutants		
−1 Codon 1 (−G)	0	Mediterranean
−2 Codon 5 (−CT)	0	Mediterranean
−1 Codon 6 (−A)	0	Mediterranean
−2 Codon 8 (−AA)	0	Turkish
+1 Codons 8/9 (+G)	0	Asian Indian
−1 Codon 11 (−T)	0	Mexican
+1 Codons 14/15 (+G)	0	Chinese
−1 Codon 16 (−C)	0	Asian Indian
+1 Codons 27–28 (+C)	0	Chinese
−1 Codon 35 (−C)	0	Indonesian
−1 Codons 36–37 (−T)	0	Iranian
−1 Codon 37 (−G)	0	Kurdish
−7 Codons 37–39	0	Turkish
−4 Codons 41/42 (−CTTT)	0	Asian Indian, Chinese
−1 Codon 44 (−C)	0	Kurdish
+1 Codon 47 (+A)	0	Surinamese black
−1 Codon 64 (−G)	0	Swiss
+1 Codon 71 (+T)	0	Chinese
+1 Codons 71/72 (+A)	0	Chinese
−1 Codon 76 (−C)	0	Italian
−1 Codons 82/83 (−G)	0	Azarbaijani
+2 Codon 94 (+TG)	0	Italian
+1 Codons 106/107 (+G)	0	American black
−1 Codon 109 (−G)	+	Lithuanian
−2, +1 Codon 114 (−CT, +G)	+	French
−1 Codon 126 (−T)	+	Italian
−4 Codons 128–129	0	
−11 Codons 132–135	0	Irish
+5 Codon 129	0	
Initiator codon mutants		
ATG → AGG	0	Chinese
ATG → ACG	0	Yugoslavian
2. RNA-processing mutants		
Splice junction changes		
IVS-1 position 1 (G→A)	0	Mediterranean
IVS-1 position 1 (G→T)	0	Asian Indian, Chinese
IVS-2 position 1 (G→A)	0	Mediterranean, Tunisian, American black
IVS-1 position 2 (T—G)	0	Tunisian
IVS-1 position 2 (T→C)	0	Black
IVA-1 3′ end—17 bp	0	Kuwaiti
IVS-1 3′ end—25 bp	0	Asian Indian
IVS-1 3′ end (G→C)	0	Italian
IVS-2 3′ end (A→G)	0	American black
IVS-2 3 end (A→C)	0	American black
IVS-1 5 end—44 bp	0	Mediterranean
IVS-1 3′ end (G→A)	0	Egyptian
Consensus changes		
IVS-1 position 5 (G→C)	+	Asian Indian, Chinese, Melanesian
IVS-1 position 5 (G→T)	+	Mediterranean, black
IVS-1 position 5 (G→A)	+	Algerian
IVS-1 position 6 (T→C)	+	Mediterranean
IVS-1 position −1 (G→C) (codon 30)	?	Tunisian, black
IVS-1 position −1 (G→A) (codon 30)	?	Bulgarian
IVS-1 position −3 (C→T) (codon 29)	?	Lebanese
IVS-2 3′ end CAG-AAG	+	Iranian, Egyptian, black
IVS-1 3′ end TAG-GAG	+	Saudi Arabian
IVS-2 3′ end −8 (T→G)	+	Algerian

TABLE 5–5. MOLECULAR PATHOLOGY OF THE β THALASSEMIAS *Continued*

MUTATION	β⁰ or β⁺ THALASSEMIA	RACIAL ORIGIN
Internal IVS changes		
IVS-2 position 110 (G→A)	+	Mediterranean
IVS-1 position 116 (T→G)	0	Mediterranean
IVS-1 position 705 (T→G)	+	Mediterranean
IVS-2 position 745 (C→G)	+	Mediterranean
IVS-2 position 654 (C→T)	0	Chinese
Coding region substitutions affecting processing		
Codon 26 (G→A)	E	Southeast Asian, European
Codon 24 (T→A)	+	American black
Codon 27 (G→T)	Knossos	Mediterranean
Codon 19 (A→G)	Malay	Malaysian
3. Transcriptional mutants		
−101 C→T	+	Turkish
−92 C→T	+	Mediterranean
−88 C→T	+	American black, Asian Indian
−88 C→A	+	Kurdish
−87 C→G	+	Mediterranean
−86 C→G	+	Lebanese
−31 A→G	+	Japanese
−30 T→A	+	Turkish
−30 T→C	+	Chinese
−29 A→G	+	American black, Chinese
−28 A→C	+	Kurdish
−28 A→G	+	Chinese
	+	
4. RNA cleavage + polyadenylation mutants		
AATAA A–rAACAAA	+	American black
AATAAA–AATAAG	+	Kurdish
AATAA–A)–AATAA)	+	Arab
AATAAA–AATGAA	+	Mediterranean
AATAAA–AATAGA	+	Malaysian
5. CAP site mutants		
+1 A–C	+	Asian Indian

Adapted from Kazazian, H. H., and Boehm, C. D.: Molecular basis and prenatal diagnosis of β-thalassemia. Blood 72:1107, 1988; and Kazazian, H. H.: The thalassemia syndromes: Molecular basis and prenatal diagnosis in 1990. Semin. Hematol. 27:209, 1990; with permission.

of β globin mRNA.[88] As we shall see later, this allele is so mild that it is completely silent in carriers, but it can be identified by its interaction with more severe β thalassemia alleles in compound heterozygotes.

Splice Site Mutations Involving Intron/Exon Boundaries

The boundaries between exons and introns are characterized by the invariant dinucleotides GT at the donor (5′) site and AG at the acceptor (3′) site. Mutations that affect either of these sites completely abolish normal splicing and give rise to the phenotype of β⁰ thalassemia.[74, 77, 85, 89] The transcription of genes carrying these mutations appears to be normal, but there is a complete inactivation of splicing at the altered junction. In every case, other donor-like sequences located elsewhere in the mRNA precursor are employed in splicing. Because these sites are not normally involved, they are referred to as cryptic splice sites. For this reason, abnormally processed products accumulate at low levels, in both in vivo erythroid precursors and in vitro expression systems, as a result of splicing to the cryptic sites in the surrounding exons or introns.

Mutations Involving Splice Site Consensus Sequences

Although only the GT dinucleotide is invariant at the donor splice site, there is conservation of adjacent

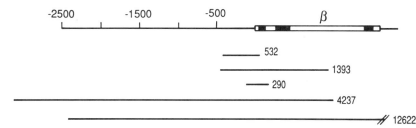

FIGURE 5–10. Deletions of the β globin gene that cause β⁰ thalassemia.

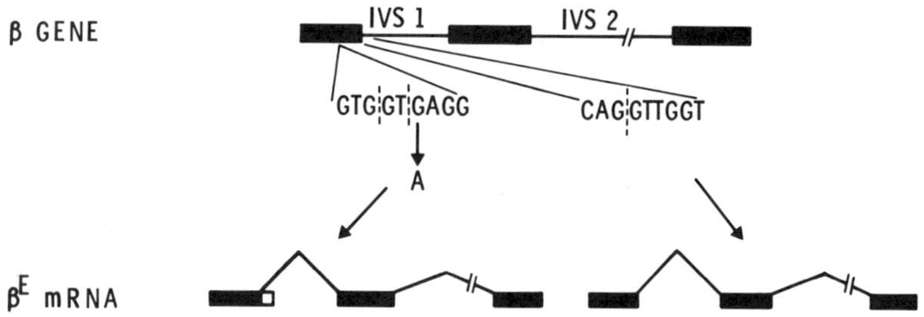

β GENE

IVS 1   IVS 2

GTG GT GAGG   CAG GTTGGT

A

βᴱ mRNA

FIGURE 5–11. Activation of a cryptic splice site in exon 1 of the β globin gene as the basis for the thalassemic phenotype associated with Hb E. Splicing occurs at both the normal splice junction and the cryptic splice site with the production of both normal and abnormal types of mRNA.

nucleotides, and a consensus sequence of these regions can be identified. Mutations within this sequence can reduce the efficiency of splicing to varying degrees and lead to alternate splicing at the surrounding cryptic sites.[74, 77, 89, 90–93] For example, mutations at position 5 of IVS-1, G to C or T, result in a moderately severe reduction of β chain production and in the phenotype of severe β⁺ thalassemia.[74] On the other hand, the substitution of C for T at position 6 in IVS-1 leads to a very mild reduction in the output of β chains.[74] This mutation, which is called the Portuguese form of β thalassemia, is particularly common in the Mediterranean population.[94] It is interesting that far more mutations have been found in the consensus donor sequence of IVS-1 than of IVS-2.

Mutations at Cryptic Sites in Exons

One of the cryptic splice sites involved in alternative splicing in mutations affecting the IVS-1 donor site spans codons 24 to 27 of exon 1 of the β globin gene. This site contains a GT dinucleotide, and adjacent substitutions that alter it so that it more closely resembles the consensus donor splice site result in its activation, even though the normal splice site is intact. For example, a mutation at codon 24, GGT→GGA, though it does not alter the amino acid normally found at this position in the β globin chain (glycine), allows some splicing to occur at this site instead of at the exon/intron boundary. This mutation results in the production of both normal and abnormally spliced β globin mRNA and in the clinical phenotype of severe β⁺ thalassemia.[95]

Mutations at codon 19 (A→G), 26 (G→A), and 27 (G→T) result both in a reduced production of mRNA caused by abnormal splicing and in an amino acid substitution when the mRNA that is spliced normally is translated into protein (Fig. 5–11). The abnormal hemoglobins produced are Hb Malay, Hb E, and Hb Knossos, respectively.[96–98] All these variants are associated with a mild β thalassemia–like phenotype.

Mutations that involve the cryptic donor splice site in exon 1 illustrate how sequence changes in coding rather than intervening sequences may influence RNA processing. Furthermore, they underline the importance of competition between potential splice site sequences in generating both normal and abnormal varieties of β globin mRNA.

Mutations at Cryptic Sites in Introns

Cryptic splice sites in introns may also carry mutations that activate them, even though the normal site remains intact. The first mutation of this type to be characterized involved a base substitution at position 110 in IVS-1.[99, 100] This region contains a sequence similar to a 3′ acceptor splice site, though it lacks the invariant AG dinucleotide (Fig. 5–12). The change of the G to A at position 110 creates this dinucleotide. The result is that about 90 per cent of the RNA transcript splices to this particular site and only 10 per cent to the normal site, producing the phenotype of severe β⁺ thalassemia. The product of the abnormal splicing is a non-functional β globin mRNA that contains an extra 19 nt derived from IVS-1. It can be detected in low amounts in reticulocyte or marrow RNA.

Several β thalassemia mutations that generate new donor sites within IVS-2 of the β globin gene have been described.[74, 90] Their effects are complex. In each case, a cryptic acceptor site within IVS-2 following nucleotide 580 is used for processing abnormal transcripts. No normal β globin mRNA appears to be processed from a gene with an A→G substitution at IVS-2 position 654, and hence the clinical phenotype is β⁰ thalassemia.[90] This is a curious observation because the IVS-2 donor and acceptor sites are entirely normal. It appears that all stable transcripts are spliced from the normal IVS-2 donor to the cryptic acceptor site and from the abnormal new donor site to the

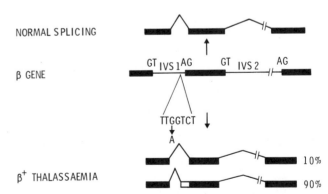

NORMAL SPLICING

β GENE

GT IVS 1 AG   GT IVS 2   AG

TTGGTCT

A

β⁺ THALASSAEMIA   10%   90%

FIGURE 5–12. The activation of a splice site in IVS-1 of the β globin gene due to a G→A change at position 110. Since the abnormal splice site is utilized to a greater extent than the normal site, and hence a large amount of abnormal β globin mRNA is generated, this mutation results in a severe β⁺ thalassemia phenotype.

normal IVS-2 acceptor. The processed β globin mRNA contains an insertion derived from IVS-2. It is not clear why splicing from the normal donor to acceptor sites does not occur.

Polyadenylation Signal Mutations

The sequence AAUAAA in the 3' untranslated region of β globin mRNA is the signal for cleavage and polyadenylation of the β gene transcript. Several different mutations of this region have been described.[77, 101–103] For example, a T→C substitution in the β globin gene in this sequence leads to only one tenth of the normal amount of β globin mRNA transcript and hence to a phenotype of severe β[+] thalassemia.[101] A small amount of an extended β globin mRNA molecule can be found in reticulocytes, presumably polyadenylated at a downstream site.

CAP Site Mutations

One example of a mutation involving the β globin mRNA CAP site has been described. This involves the substitution of the first A residue with C. It is not clear how this change leads to defective β globin chain production. It could be mediated by a reduction in the rate of transcription or by slowing down the 5' capping process, which, in turn, might reduce β globin mRNA stability.[104]

Mutations That Result in Abnormal Translation of β Globin mRNA

There are three main classes of mutations of this kind. First, base substitutions that change an amino acid codon to a chain termination codon prevent translation of β globin mRNA and result in the phenotype of β[0] thalassemia.[77, 105, 106] Several mutations of this kind have been described, the most common being a codon 17 mutation that occurs widely throughout Southeast Asia,[106] and a codon 39 mutation that is very common in Mediterranean populations.[105] Curiously, low levels of nuclear and cytoplasmic β globin mRNA have been found in red cell precursors in association with these mutations.[107, 108] It is not clear how the generation of a premature chain termination codon could reduce the overall amount of β globin mRNA that is synthesized.

Mutations in the second group of this class involve the insertion or deletion of 1, 2, or 4 nt in the coding region of the β globin gene.[74, 77, 103] These disrupt the normal reading frame, cause a frameshift, and therefore interfere with the translation of β globin mRNA. The end result is the insertion of anomalous amino acids after the frameshift until a termination codon is reached in the new reading frame. This type of mutation always leads to the phenotype of β[0] thalassemia.

Finally, two mutations involve the β globin initiation codon, ATG→AGG or ACG, and presumably reduce the efficacy of translation.[77, 102]

Unstable β Globin Chain Variants

As is the case in the unstable α globin variants, it might be expected that the synthesis of a highly unstable β globin variant that is incapable of forming a stable tetramer and that is rapidly degraded might produce the phenotype of β[0] thalassemia.[109–112] In many of these conditions, no abnormal globin chain product can be demonstrated by protein analysis or globin synthesis studies, and the molecular pathology has to be interpreted simply on the basis of a derived sequence of the variant β chain obtained from DNA analysis. In some cases, small quantities of abnormal globin chains have been identified by hemoglobin synthesis studies.

Recent studies have started to shed some light on the complex clinical phenotypes that may result from the synthesis of unstable β globin products. It turns out that there is a spectrum of disorders ranging from a family of exon 3 mutations that give rise to a moderately severe form of thalassemia in heterozygotes, through conditions that are characterized by a mild hypochromic anemia, to those in which the major feature is hemolysis due to precipitation of unstable β chain hemoglobin variants in the peripheral circulation. We return to this theme later in this chapter.

Pathophysiology

The pathophysiology of β thalassemia has been the subject of several extensive reviews.[7, 8, 12, 113] Only those aspects of the topic that are essential for an understanding of the relationship between the molecular pathology and the clinical phenotypes are summarized here.

The main cause of the anemia of β thalassemia is imbalanced globin chain synthesis and the deleterious effects of excess α chains on erythroid maturation and survival. It follows, therefore, that the major factor in determining the clinical phenotype is the magnitude of α chain excess in the red cell precursors. Although this reflects the degree of defective β chain production, other factors are involved, particularly the level of γ chain synthesis and, much less important, δ chain production. The degree of globin chain imbalance may also be modified by the level of α chain synthesis—in particular, the coexistence of α thalassemia. Although it has been suggested that other factors such as differences in the rate of proteolysis of excess α chains may also modify the phenotype of β thalassemia, it has been much more difficult to obtain solid evidence to this effect.

The Consequences of Imbalanced Globin Chain Synthesis

Measurements of in vitro globin chain synthesis in the blood or bone marrow of patients with different types of β thalassemia have shown either an absence or a reduction of β chains, together with the synthesis of a variable excess of α chains. Unpaired α chains are unable to form a viable hemoglobin tetramer and hence precipitate in red cell precursors.[114] The resulting inclusion bodies can be demonstrated by both light and electron microscopy.[115] In the bone marrow, α chain precipitation occurs in the earliest hemoglobinized precursors and throughout the erythroid maturation pathway.[116] These inclusions are responsible for the intramedullary destruction of red cell precursors and hence the ineffective erythropoiesis that characterizes all the β thalassemias. It has been calculated that a large proportion of the developing erythroblasts are destroyed in the bone marrow in severe forms of β thalassemia.[117] The precipitation of α chains can also be demonstrated in the red cell progenitors of β thalassemia heterozygotes, although the α chains are scanty. Presumably, the bulk of excess α chains are degraded by proteolytic enzymes; notwithstanding, a mild degree of ineffective erythropoiesis is present.[118]

The anemia of β thalassemia also has a hemolytic component. Such red cells that enter the circulation contain inclusions that result in their damage as they pass through the microcirculation, particularly the spleen. In addition to this physical mechanism for hemolysis, many abnormalities of red cell metabolism have been demonstrated in both severe and mild forms of β thalassemia.[119, 120] These include oxidant damage to the membrane as a consequence of lipid peroxidation, presumably resulting from the generation of superoxide and the formation of hemichrome by the precipitated globin chains.[120] These changes may be enhanced by excess iron in the red cells and by vitamin E deficiency. Damage to the red cell membranes is reflected by a variety of abnormalities of permeability—in particular, an increased rate of potassium loss.[119]

It appears therefore that the shortened red cell survival in β thalassemia is the consequence of both physical damage due to the presence of inclusion bodies and a complex series of secondary metabolic changes resulting from the effects of hemoglobin precipitation and damage to the red cell membranes. As we shall see, all these changes vary in severity between the heterogeneous cell populations that are found in the peripheral blood in severe forms of β thalassemia.

Persistent Fetal Hemoglobin Production and Cellular Heterogeneity

One of the earliest observations on the hemoglobin patterns of children with severe β thalassemia was that a variable amount of Hb F production persists into childhood and later life.[7] Indeed, in the β⁰ thalassemias, except for small amounts of Hb A$_2$, Hb F is the only hemoglobin produced. Examination of the peripheral blood, using staining methods that are specific for Hb F, shows that it is heterogeneously distributed among the red cells. There are still many unanswered questions about the mechanism of persistent γ chain synthesis in the β thalassemias. From such evidence as

is available, it is clear that both cell selection and genetic factors that modify γ chain production are involved.

CELL SELECTION. Normal adults produce small quantities of Hb F, which are also heterogeneously distributed among the red cells; cells with demonstrable Hb F are called F cells. It is clear that one important mechanism for the apparent persistence of Hb F production in β thalassemia is cell selection. As mentioned earlier, the major cause of ineffective erythropoiesis and shortened red cell survival in β thalassemia is the deleterious effect of excess α chains on erythroid maturation and survival of red cells in the blood. It follows, therefore, that any red cell precursors that produce significant numbers of γ chains will have an advantage in an environment where excess α chains are present; the latter will combine with γ chains to produce Hb F, and therefore the magnitude of α chain precipitation will be less. Differential centrifugation experiments and in vivo labeling studies have shown that populations of red cells with relatively large amounts of Hb F are more efficiently produced and survive longer in the blood than do those with low levels or no Hb F.[121, 122] This is one of the main reasons for the heterogeneity of cell populations in the peripheral blood of persons with severe β thalassemia. These cell populations show remarkable differences with respect to their survival; there are those that contain predominantly Hb A or virtually no hemoglobin that are very rapidly destroyed in the spleen and elsewhere, cells with a longer survival that contain relatively more Hb F, and cells of intermediate survival and hemoglobin constitution. These changes in hemoglobin content and constitution are mirrored by variability in the associated metabolic abnormalities.[123]

Whether cell selection of this type is the only mechanism for the presence of relatively large amounts of Hb F in the blood of transfusion-dependent patients with β thalassemia is not clear. Because of the gross destruction of red cell progenitors, the marked expansion of the erythron, and the cellular heterogeneity of distribution of Hb F, it is very difficult to calculate absolute amounts of Hb F production in this disease. Although it has been suggested that the marked increase in the turnover of red cell progenitors and the increased rate of red cell maturation may create an environment that favors γ chain production, it has not been possible to obtain any definite evidence that this is the case. Other dyserythropoietic and hemolytic anemias are not associated with very high levels of Hb F production, although of course in these disorders there is no reason for the selection of progenitors that are synthesizing γ chains. It remains a possibility, however, that there may be an absolute increase in Hb F production; this is certainly so in some milder forms of homozygous β thalassemia, but, as we shall see, other genetic factors may be responsible for the relatively high level of γ chain synthesis in these conditions.

GENETIC FACTORS THAT MODIFY γ CHAIN SYNTHESIS. Despite the fact that it has been evident for a long time that genetic factors play a major role in determining the level of Hb F production in β thalassemia, knowledge about their nature remains incomplete. However, from such information as is available it is clear that they fall into three major groups. First, there is growing evidence that the mutations involving the β globin genes or their flanking regions that give rise to β thalassemia may themselves have some effect on the output of Hb F. Second, it appears that polymorphisms involving the εγδβ globin gene cluster may modify the amount of Hb F produced in the face of defective β chain production. Finally, genetic determinants unlinked to the cluster seem to modify the level of Hb F production in adult life, in both normal and β thalassemic individuals. These different mechanisms for modifying Hb F production in β thalassemia are summarized in Figure 5–13.

One approach to determining the effect of individual β thalassemia mutations on γ chain synthesis is to analyze Hb F levels in homozygotes or compound heterozygotes for those mutations that produce a very mild deficit of β chains. Since imbalanced globin chain synthesis and cell selection play an important role in determining the level of Hb F in β thalassemia, it might be expected that the Hb F level would be relatively low in such individuals. This supposition is borne out by careful phenotypic analysis of homozygotes for the common IVS-1-6 (T→C) β$^+$ thalassemia mutation, the Portuguese mutation, which occurs widely in the Mediterranean. Persons with this mutation have a very mild phenotype, with levels of Hb F in the 10 to 20 per cent range.[94] On the other hand, it has been realized for many years that β thalassemia is particularly mild in black populations.[7] Many homozygotes with hemoglobin levels of 9 to 12 g/dl have been described. Yet nearly all these persons have Hb F levels between 40 and 60 per cent of the total hemoglobin.[7, 91] It is now clear that most of them are either homozygotes or compound heterozygotes for two common promoter mutations, −29 (A→G) and −88 (C→T).[85, 91] Homozygotes or compound heterozygotes for these mutations, whether they occur in blacks[91] or other populations,[124] usually have inappropriately high levels of Hb F for the degree of imbalanced globin chain synthesis. It is possible, therefore, that in conditions of relative hematopoietic stress in which γ chain synthesis is more likely to occur, the level of γ chain production may be modified by com-

petition for transcriptional regulatory sequences between the γ and β chain loci; mutations in or near these transcriptional boxes that cause β thalassemia may favor γ chain production. This hypothesis is strengthened by the observation that heterozygotes for the deletion forms of β thalassemia that remove the 5′ flanking regions of the β globin genes, in addition to unusually high levels of δ chain production, have, on average, higher levels of Hb F than is usual in β thalassemia heterozygotes.[125]

Analyses of this kind are complicated, however, by increasing evidence that polymorphisms or mutations of the γ globin genes *cis* to the β globin genes that contain β thalassemia mutations may have a considerable effect in modifying γ chain production. An extreme example of this kind is the finding of the common nonsense mutation at codon 39 in the β globin gene associated with a point mutation at position −196 upstream of the ^{A}γ gene on the same chromosome in Sardinian patients with a form of β^0 thalassemia associated with a very mild phenotype and high levels of γ chain production. We consider the way in which this type of chromosome has been generated in a later section that deals with the pathogenesis of δβ thalassemia.

One approach to asking whether *cis*-acting sequences may modify γ chain production is to determine whether any particular β globin RFLP haplotypes are associated with β thalassemia and unusually high levels of Hb F.[126] This approach is based on the idea that if this is the case, it is likely that the genetic determinant responsible for the increased level of Hb F production is within or close to the εγδβ globin gene cluster. There has been particular interest in the relationship between Hb F production and a C→T polymorphism at position 158 in the ^{G}γ globin gene. This substitution can be identified with the restriction enzyme *Xmn*-1, which makes it possible to analyze large populations for its presence or absence.[127] Studies in Asian, Mediterranean, and Middle Eastern populations have shown that this polymorphism is associated predominantly with one common β globin RFLP haplotype and is not found on chromosomes carrying the other common haplotypes in these regions.[128] Extensive analysis of β thalassemic persons of Afro-Asian, Mediterranean, and Turkish backgrounds has shown a strong, though not absolute, correlation between

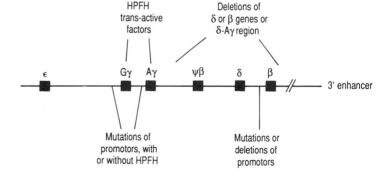

FIFURE 5–13. A summary of some of the genetic mechanisms that modify the level of Hb F production in β thalassemia.

increased γ chain production and the presence of the Xmn-1 polymorphism.[128-130]

Similar, though less consistent, observations have been made on Hb F production in sickle cell anemia in relation to this polymorphism.[131-133] The lack of an absolute association between haplotype and Hb F production and the clear demonstration in Indian[134, 135] and Saudi Arabian[136] populations that other genetic factors are involved in setting the fetal hemoglobin level in β thalassemia and sickle cell anemia suggest that the Hb F response to β chain disorders reflects the complex interactions of a number of different genetic determinants. One condition of particular importance in this respect is HPFH.

Strong evidence exists that there are forms of HPFH (see Chapter 4), the genetic determinants of which are not linked to the β globin gene cluster, that produce a slight elevation of the level of Hb F in the blood of normal individuals.[137] Extensive family data indicate that the co-inheritance of these types of HPFH with β thalassemia causes β thalassemia heterozygotes to have an unusually high level of Hb F; homozygotes have a mild phenotype, presumably because of the large amounts of Hb F that they produce.[138-140] It appears that this form of HPFH is also heterogeneous; there is some, though not unequivocal, evidence that at least one form is encoded by the X chromosome[141]; there is equally clear evidence that other forms are not.[140]

It is clear, therefore, that the genetic factors modifying Hb F production in β thalassemia are extremely complex and are still not fully worked out. As mentioned earlier, extensive data suggest that, by and large, the β globin promoter mutations that cause mild forms of thalassemia are associated with relatively high levels of γ chain production. Interpretation of these observations is complicated by the finding that nearly all the common promoter mutations that are found in black populations occur on a chromosome that carries the Xmn polymorphism. On the other hand, it seems unlikely that this is the only reason for the high level of Hb F production in these individuals, since homozygotes for the promoter mutations in other populations also produce unusually high levels of Hb F. Perhaps both mechanisms are involved. It is possible that the C→T change at position 158 acts as a more efficient promoter for γ chain production in conditions of increased red cell production and turnover.

In summary, the Hb F response to β thalassemia probably reflects a complex series of genetic variables, including the nature of the individual β thalassemic mutation, polymorphisms of the γ globin genes cis to the affected β globin gene, and the interaction of other genes unlinked to the β globin gene cluster, set against a background of cell selection and an increased likelihood of producing γ chains that results from the accelerated level of erythropoiesis consequent on the destruction of red cell precursors, which is due to the underlying β thalassemic mutation.

Variability in α Chain Production

It is clear that the major pathophysiological mechanism that leads to the anemia of β thalassemia is the deleterious effect of excess α chains on red cell maturation. It follows, therefore, that a relative deficit of α chain production should ameliorate the clinical phenotype of β thalassemia. As we shall see later in this chapter, many experiments of nature providing clear-cut evidence that the excess of α chains is the major factor in the pathogenesis of β thalassemia have been encountered. Individuals who inherit one or more α thalassemia determinants together with β thalassemia have a milder clinical phenotype than do those with β thalassemia who have four intact α genes.[142] Similarly, β thalassemia carriers who inherit chromosomes with three α genes (ααα) have an unusually severe phenotype.[142] We shall describe the phenotypic consequences of these interactions in a later section.

Acquired Factors [7]

In trying to assess the genotype/phenotype relationships in β thalassemia, it is very important to remember that several acquired factors may modify the clinical phenotype. Indeed, unless these are carefully controlled, it is almost impossible to compare patients with the same molecular defects in an attempt to relate molecular lesions to clinical phenotypes.

Constant bombardment of the spleen with abnormal red cells in persons with β thalassemia gives rise to the phenomenon of "work hypertrophy." Progressive splenomegaly may exacerbate the anemia. Enlarged spleens act as a sump for red cells and may sequestrate a considerable proportion of the peripheral red cell mass. Furthermore, splenomegaly may cause plasma volume expansion, a complication that may be exacerbated by massive hypertrophy of the erythroid bone marrow. The latter may also lead to folate deficiency. All these factors may combine to cause considerable worsening of the anemia in β thalassemia.

In β thalassemia homozygotes who are severely anemic, there is an increase in intestinal iron absorption that is related to the degree of expansion of the red cell precursor population.[7] Iron may also accumulate following regular blood transfusion. Iron accumulation occurs in the parenchymal cells of the liver, in endocrine glands, in the pancreas, and, most important, in the myocardium. The consequences of iron loading include diabetes, hyperparathyroidism, hypogonadism, and cardiac failure.[7, 8, 113]

Thus, in attempting to relate the genotype to the phenotype of β thalassemia, it is essential to take into consideration the widespread secondary complications of the disease, which may modify the phenotype.

Genotype/Phenotype Relationships

Given the considerable molecular heterogeneity of β thalassemia, and the many other genetic and acquired factors that have the potential to modify its phenotype, it is not surprising that the clinical spectrum produced by different β thalassemia mutations is so broad. Homozygotes or compound heterozygotes for different β thalassemia mutations may show a clinical picture ranging from a disease that is lethal in the first few months of life to a completely asymptomatic disorder that may be ascertained only by routine hematological analysis. Similarly, although the heterozygous states are usually asymptomatic, it is now apparent that a small subset of carriers have a moderately severe disease that is clearly inherited in a dominant fashion.

Severe Transfusion-Dependent Forms of β Thalassemia

Because most racial groups with a high frequency of β thalassemia have only a few common mutations, the severe phenotypes usually result from the homozygous or compound heterozygous states, which cause a severe deficit of β chain production. In the Mediterranean population, for example, severe disease is seen frequently in homozygotes for codon 39 (C→T) or IVS-1-110 (G→A) mutations or in compound heterozygotes who have received one of these mutations from each parent. In Melanesia, where there is only one common mutation—in this case, G→C at position IVS-1-5—all severely affected individuals are homozygous for this particular allele.

In populations such as those of the Mediterranean, in which the frequency of a mild β thalassemia allele is relatively high—in this case IVS-1-6 (T→C)—many compound heterozygotes who have received this mutation from one parent and a more severe β thalassemia allele from the other are encountered. As experience of these interactions is growing, it is becoming possible to define the resulting clinical phenotypes. For example, although the co-inheritance of the codon 39 (C→T) mutation with the IVS-1-6 (T→C) mutation produces a slightly milder phenotype, it is usually transfusion dependent. On the other hand, many patients who are compound heterozygotes for the IVS-1-6 (T→C) mutation and the IVS-1-110 (G→A) mutation have the phenotype of non–transfusion-dependent thalassemia intermedia (see below).

Intermediate Forms of β Thalassemia

These conditions are extremely heterogeneous,[7, 142] with respect both to their underlying genotype and to the spectrum of their clinical phenotypes, which range from a relatively severe degree of anemia requiring intermittent blood transfusion to an asymptomatic condition that is identified by chance hematological study. Some of the different genotypes associated with the phenotype of thalassemia intermedia are presented in Table 5–6, and the mechanisms modifying the severity of β thalassemia are summarized in Figure 5–14.

MILD β THALASSEMIA MUTATIONS. The homozygous state for particularly mild mutations, such as IVS-1-6 (T→C) and those involving the promoter regions, −88 (C→T) and −29 (A→G), are characterized by extremely mild clinical phenotypes.[91, 94] This

TABLE 5–6. β-THALASSEMIA INTERMEDIA

Mild forms of β thalassemia
  Homozygosity for mild β⁺ thalassemia alleles
  Compound heterozygosity for two mild β⁺ thalassemia alleles
  Compound heterozygosity for a mild and more severe β thalassemia allele
Inheritance of α and β thalassemia
  β⁺ Thalassemia with α⁰ thalassemia (−/αα) or α⁺ thalassemia (−α/αα or −α/−α)
  β⁺ Thalassemia with genotype of Hb H disease (−/−α)
β Thalassemia with elevated γ chain synthesis
  Homozygous β thalassemia with heterocellular HPFH
  Homozygous β thalassemia with ᴳγ or ᴬγ promotor mutations
  Compound heterozygosity for β thalassemia and deletion forms of HPFH
Compound heterozygosity for β thalassemia and β chain variants
  Hb E/β thalassemia
  Other interactions with rare β chain variants
Heterozygous β thalassemia with triplicated α chain genes (ααα)
Dominant forms of β thalassemia (see Table 5–7)
Interactions of β and (δβ)⁺ or (δβ)⁰ thalassemia

HPFH = Hereditary persistence of fetal hemoglobin.

mildness probably reflects the moderate reduction in the output of β globin chains, although in the case of the promoter box mutations may also depend to some degree on relatively high levels of γ chain production. When these particular forms of thalassemia are present with more severe β thalassemia mutations in compound heterozygotes, a greater degree of anemia and a more severe form of β thalassemia intermedia results. As mentioned earlier, the results of these interactions depend on whether the more severe β thalassemia mutation is of the β⁺ or β⁰ variety. For example, there are many compound heterozygotes for the IVS-1-6 (T→C) mutation and the IVS-1-110 (G→A) β⁺ thalassemia mutation who, although anemic, survive with only intermittent transfusions.

COEXISTENT α THALASSEMIA. Extensive data collected from the populations of the Mediterranean and Southeast Asia indicate that the coexistence of α thalassemia may modify the phenotype of homozygotes or compound heterozygotes for different β thalassemia mutations.[143–148] Again, the phenotypes are com-

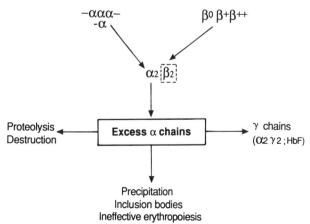

FIGURE 5–14. Major factors that modify the phenotype of β thalassemia.

plex and depend on the number of α globin genes that are inactivated, together with whether the β thalassemia is of the β^0 or β^+ variety. For example, it is clear that the coexistence of the heterozygous state for α^+ thalassemia and the homozygous state for β^0 thalassemia has very little effect on the phenotype. On the other hand, individuals who are either α^+ thalassemia homozygotes or α^0 thalassemia heterozygotes and who also are homozygous for β^+ thalassemia may have a mild form of β thalassemia intermedia that is not transfusion dependent. The same applies even to patients who have the genotype of Hb H disease together with homozygous β^+ or compound heterozygous β^+/β^0 thalassemia. These remarkable experiments of nature are the best evidence we have that the most important factor in determining the phenotype of β thalassemia is the degree of imbalanced globin chain synthesis.

β THALASSEMIA WITH UNUSUALLY HIGH LEVELS OF HB F PRODUCTION. As mentioned earlier, many genetic factors may modify the level of Hb F production in β thalassemia (see Fig. 5–13). Perhaps the most extreme examples are β^0 thalassemic persons of Afro-Asian or Middle Eastern origin who are asymptomatic, with hemoglobin values of 9 to 11 g/dl, and whose hemoglobin consists almost entirely of Hb F with a small amount of Hb A_2.[128–130] Family studies have shown no evidence of HPFH. Most, but not all, of these individuals seem to be homozygous or heterozygous for the β globin RFLP haplotype that carries the Xmn-1 polymorphism. It is likely, though by no means certain, that these mild phenotypes result from the fact that the β thalassemia mutation is on a chromosome carrying the C→T change at position 158 in the $^G\gamma$ globin gene. Studies of the Hb F have shown a predominance of $^G\gamma$ chains, in keeping with this hypothesis.

In addition to mild forms of β thalassemia of this type, there are many examples of the co-inheritance of definable forms of deletion or non-deletion types of HPFH together with β thalassemia that give rise to a phenotype of β thalassemia intermedia.[138–140] In the case of deletion forms of HPFH, such persons are compound heterozygotes for HPFH and β thalassemia. In the case of non-deletion forms of HPFH, notably those that are unlinked to the β globin gene cluster, β thalassemia homozygotes or compound heterozygotes seem to have an increased production of Hb F in both *cis* and *trans* that results from the action of the HPFH determinant.

COMPOUND HETEROZYGOUS STATES FOR β THALASSEMIA AND "SILENT" β THALASSEMIA. In a few patients with the phenotype of mild β thalassemia intermedia, genetic studies suggest that affected individuals have received a severe β thalassemia allele from one parent and a completely silent allele from the other. Sequence analysis of the silent allele has, in some cases, revealed no abnormality, although genetic studies indicate that β chain synthesis is defective. In one family, the silent allele was found to be associated with a C→T mutation at position −101 in the β globin

gene promoter.[88] Although there have been reports that the genetic determinant for the silent allele segregated independently of the β globin gene cluster,[149] these remain to be confirmed. The nature of the "silent β thalassemia" alleles, at least in some families, is unknown.

TRIPLICATED α GLOBIN GENES TOGETHER WITH β THALASSEMIA. As mentioned earlier in this chapter, triplicated α globin gene arrangements, ααα, occur in most populations at a low frequency. When they are inherited with β thalassemia trait, they may produce the picture of thalassemia intermedia.[150–154] The clinical phenotypes vary, depending on the nature of the β thalassemia allele. If it is a β^+ thalassemia, the condition is mild; the most severe interaction is with exon 3 mutations that produce dominantly inherited forms of β thalassemia,[155] as described in the following section.

DOMINANT FORMS OF β THALASSEMIA. In some families, particularly those of northern European and Japanese origin, a form of β thalassemia intermedia is inherited as a mendelian dominant. A disorder characterized by moderately severe anemia with jaundice and splenomegaly can be traced vertically and horizontally through different generations, indicating that the phenotype is due to the inheritance of a single gene and not to the co-inheritance of two different alleles.[155, 156] This condition is also characterized by the presence of inclusion bodies in the red cell precursors and has therefore also been called "inclusion body" β thalassemia. However, since all severe forms of β thalassemia have inclusions in the red cell precursors, the term "dominantly inherited β thalassemia" is preferred.

Recently, some insights into the molecular pathology of these conditions have been obtained. With β globin RFLP linkage analysis, it has been found that these disorders segregate with the β globin gene, indicating that they are due to mutations at or near this locus.[155] Sequence analysis has shown that they are heterogeneous at the molecular level but that the majority of them seem to involve mutations of exon 3 of the β globin gene (Table 5–7). These include frameshifts, premature chain termination (nonsense) mutations, and complex rearrangements that lead to the synthesis of truncated or elongated and highly unstable β globin gene products.[76, 109–112, 155–167] The most common mutation of this type is a GAA→TAA change at codon 121, which leads to the synthesis of a truncated β globin chain.[159] Although it is unusual to demonstrate an abnormal β chain product from loci affected by mutations of this type, many of these conditions have been designated "hemoglobin variants" (see Table 5–7).

A comparison of the lengths of abnormal gene products due to nonsense or frameshift mutations in the β globin gene (Fig. 5–15A) has suggested a mechanism to explain why most heterozygous forms of β thalassemia are mild, whereas those due to mutations that involve exon 3 are more severe.[155] Nonsense or frameshift mutations that produce truncated β chains

TABLE 5–7.   MOLECULAR FORMS OF DOMINANT β THALASSEMIA AND STRUCTURAL VARIANTS ASSOCIATED WITH A β THALASSEMIA PHENOTYPE

MUTATION	EXON	PHENOTYPE	DESIGNATION	RACE	REFERENCE
		Dominant β Thalassemia			
Codon 128 −4 bp, +5 bp, −11 bp; F/S terminates codon 154	III	Thalassemia intermedia Inclusion bodies	—	Irish	155
Codon 121 GAA → TAA*	III	Thalassemia intermedia Inclusion bodies	—	Swiss-French Greek-Polish	155 158 159 173
Codon 127 CAA → TAA	III	Thalassemia intermedia	—	English	111
Codon 114 −CT +G F/S terminates codon 157	III	Thalassemia intermedia	β^{Geneva}	Swiss-French	156
Codon 126 −T F/S terminates codon 157*	III	Thalassemia intermedia Inclusion bodies	β^{Vercelli}	Italian	161
Codon 94 +TG F/S terminates codon 157*	II	Severe thalassemia intermedia Inclusion bodies	β^{Agnana}	Italian	158 161
Codon 123 −A F/S terminates codon 157	III	Thalassemia intermedia Inclusion bodies	β^{Makabe}	Japanese	162
Codons 123–125 − 8 bp β chain 135 residues	III	Severe thalassemia intermedia with Hb E Inclusion bodies	β$^{Khon Kaen}$	Thai	163
Codon 127 Gin → Pro	III	Thalassemia intermedia	β^{Houston}	British	157
Codons 109–110 −G F/S terminates codon 157	III	Thalassemia intermedia	β^{Manhattan}	Ashkenazi Jew	157
Codons 32/34 −GGT*	II	Thalassemia intermedia	β^{Korea}	Korean	112
Codon 106 Leu → Arg†	III	Thalassemia intermedia	β$^{Terre Haute}$	European	164
Codon 28 Leu → Arg	I	Thalassemia intermedia Inclusion bodies	β^{Chesterfield}	English	165
Codon 60 Val → Glu	II	Thalassemia intermedia	β^{Cagliari}	Italian	166
		Thalassemia Trait			
Codon 110 Leu → Pro	III	β thalassemia trait	β$^{Showa-Yakushiji}$	Japanese	110
Codons 127/128 −3 bp β chain 145 residues	III	β thalassemia trait	β^{Gunma}	Japanese	167
β^{132} Lys → Gln	III	β thalassemia trait	β$^{K Woolwich}$	British	46
β^{134} Lys → Gln	III	Milk microcytosis S/β thalassemia interaction with Hb S	Hb North Shore–Caracas		46

*De novo mutations.
†Originally reported as Hb Indianapolis.
F/S = Frameshift.

up to about 72 residues in length are usually associated with a mild phenotype in heterozygotes. Presumably, these short β chain fragments are degraded, and the resulting small excess of α chains is removed in the same way. However, many exon 3 mutations produce longer truncated products. It is likely that the severe phenotypes associated with these products reflect their heme-binding properties and instability. Those with only 72 residues or fewer cannot bind heme, whereas those truncated to residue 120 or longer should bind heme, since only helix H is missing. Furthermore, such heme-containing products should have secondary structure and hence be less susceptible to proteolytic degradation. Furthermore, the lack of helix H, which would expose one of the hydrophobic patches of helix G and the hydrophobic patches of helix E and F, would also lead to aggregation. It is suggested, therefore, that the large inclusions in the red cell progenitors of these patients consist of aggregates of precipitated β chain products together with excess α chains (Fig. 5–15B). This theory would certainly explain the marked degree of dyserythropoiesis that is observed

in this interesting condition. The rarity of these dominant forms, as well as their occurrence mainly in Northern Europeans, suggests that they have had no selective value. Indeed, some of them represent de novo mutations (Table 5–7).

These conditions, unlike the unstable hemoglobin disorders, in which intact hemoglobin molecules precipitate in the red cells and cause a hemolytic anemia, are characterized by ineffective erythropoiesis due to the early precipitation of these unstable β globin products in the red cell precursors. Indeed, the pattern that is emerging from these studies is that there is a spectrum of disorders of β globin synthesis, which, in the heterozygous state, range from typical β thalassemia trait with hypochromic red cells, through the pattern of dominantly inherited β thalassemia with severe ineffective erythropoiesis, to a pure hemolytic anemia with effective erythropoiesis and destruction of the red cells in the peripheral blood due to instability of β globin chain variants. The main factors that determine the phenotype appear to be the length of the primary globin gene product, its ability to bind

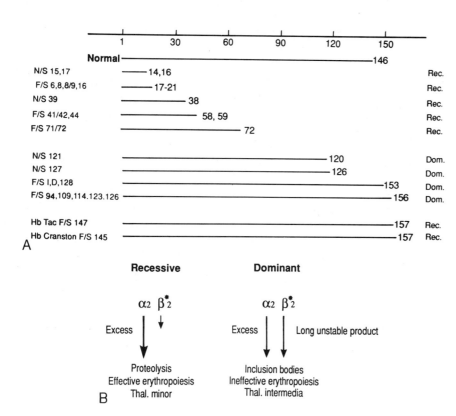

FIGURE 5–15. The molecular mechanisms for the dominant forms of β thalassemia. A, Mutations that result in truncated β globin gene products up to 70 residues are associated with the phenotype of β^0 thalassemia trait. The family of mutations that involve exon 3, many of which lead to elongated and highly unstable gene products, are associated with the genotype of dominant β thalassemia. B, The cellular basis for dominant β thalassemia.

heme and to form an α/β dimer and tetramer, and the stability of the tetramer in the developing red cell precursor and peripheral circulation.

Some unstable β globin variants, as exemplified by Hb Showa-Yakushigi, β^{110} Leu→Pro, produce a phenotype much more like that of β thalassemia trait.[110] There is a mild anemia with hypochromic red cells and no evidence of ineffective erythropoiesis. This variant introduces a proline residue into the middle of the G helix, which would disrupt all four $\alpha_1 \beta_1$ contact points in the helix and hence may lead to very rapid post-translational catabolism.

Although many questions remain, it seems likely that whether an unstable β globin chain variant produces hypochromic anemia similar to that seen with β thalassemia trait, or the more severe phenotype of dominantly inherited β thalassemia, depends on the properties of the unstable β globin chains. If they can be incorporated into a tetramer, or have enough tertiary structure to be relatively insensitive to proteases, the red cell precursors will contain both excess α chains and precipitates of the unstable β globin chain. This situation may be sufficient to damage the precursors and to lead to ineffective erythropoiesis. On the other hand, if the unstable product is rapidly degraded, the resulting phenotype may be a hypochromic anemia. Those variants that form a relatively stable tetramer and that precipitate only later in the life of the red cell give rise to the typical unstable hemoglobin disorders.

INTERACTION OF β THALASSEMIA WITH δβ THALASSEMIA.[7] The δβ thalassemias are described in a later section. The co-inheritance of β and δβ thalassemia is associated with a variable phenotype, depending on the particular type of δβ thalassemia mutation. For example, the co-inheritance of β thalassemia with $(\delta\beta)^+$ thalassemia of the Lepore variety, in which the output of γ chains from the Hb Lepore–containing chromosome is low, is often associated with a severe transfusion-dependent form of β thalassemia. In contrast, the co-inheritance of β thalassemia with a deletion form of $(\delta\beta)^0$ thalassemia leads to a milder phenotype because of the high output of γ chains generated by the chromosome containing the $(\delta\beta)^0$ thalassemia mutation.

β THALASSEMIA IN ASSOCIATION WITH STRUCTURAL VARIANTS OF β GLOBIN.[7] The consequences of the compound inheritance of β thalassemia with β globin chain variants depend on the nature of the particular structural variant. For example, since the action of the β thalassemia gene is to reduce the output of Hb A, the phenotypes of sickle cell β thalassemia and Hb C β thalassemia depend mainly on the properties of Hb S and Hb C. The most important interaction of this type is Hb E thalassemia, which is extremely common throughout the eastern part of the Indian subcontinent and Southeast Asia. This disorder varies in severity but usually has the phenotype of thalassemia major or severe thalassemia intermedia. As mentioned earlier, Hb E results from a mutation in exon 1 that activates a cryptic splice site. Hence this variant is associated with a phenotype of a mild form of β thalassemia. When this variant interacts with β^0 thalassemia or the severe form of β^+ thalassemia, there is a marked deficit of β globin chains, resulting in the phenotype of a severe form of β thalassemia. This may not be the whole story, however.

There are still considerable gaps in our understanding of the molecular pathophysiology of Hb E β thalassemia. Although both the phenotypic changes and the mutation that activates the cryptic splice site as the basis for Hb E suggest that this is a mild form of β thalassemia, the homozygous state for Hb E is an extremely mild disorder. The hemoglobin level is usually normal or only slightly reduced, there is no evidence of hemolysis or ineffective erythropoiesis (where measured), globin chain synthesis has been balanced, and the level of Hb F is not increased. These findings are quite different from those observed even in the mildest forms of homozygous β⁺ thalassemia. On the other hand, the inheritance of severe forms of β⁺ thalassemia, or β⁰ together with Hb E in the compound heterozygous state, can produce a disorder that is phenotypically indistinguishable from severe transfusion-dependent homozygous β thalassemia. Hb E is slightly unstable, but even in the homozygous state there is no evidence of hemolysis and no features similar to those observed in the unstable hemoglobin disorders. However, Hb E is unusually susceptible to oxidant damage, and it could be that this property, when combined with the oxidant stress associated with marked globin chain imbalance caused by the co-inheritance of a β thalassemia mutation, results in increased instability of Hb E. It is possible that under these conditions precipitation of both excess α chains and subunits of Hb E takes place.[7] However, this is pure speculation, and the reasons for the extraordinary clinical severity of the interaction of Hb E and β thalassemia remain to be determined.

The other feature of Hb E β thalassemia that is yet unexplained is the wide clinical diversity of the phenotype. Although some of this diversity is related to the particular variety of β thalassemia, this is by no means the entire picture. However, in Southeast Asia, where this condition is particularly common, α thalassemia occurs with high frequency. Unfortunately, there have been no studies in which variation in the phenotype of Hb E β thalassemia has been combined with a full analysis of the α globin genes. Nor have studies of this problem included a detailed family analysis for the presence of different forms of HPFH. Thus, the reasons for the remarkable clinical diversity of Hb E β thalassemia remain unclear.

β GLOBIN CHAIN VARIANT GENES THAT ALSO CONTAIN β THALASSEMIA MUTATIONS. Several examples have been discovered in which a β globin gene containing a sickle mutation has also been found to carry a β⁺ thalassemia mutation.[168] Affected individuals have the phenotype of β thalassemia trait with an elevated level of Hb A₂ and an unusually low level of Hb S, in the 10 per cent range. In one example of this type, the β⁺ thalassemia mutation was found to be the −88 C→T, which is a common form of β⁺ thalassemia in the black population. The same β⁺ thalassemia mutation has also been found in a β globin

gene carrying the mutation β$^{75Leu→0}$, which is responsible for the unstable variant, Hb Vicksburg.[169] The phenotype in this case is more severe and resembles thalassemia intermedia.

β Thalassemia Trait

The β thalassemia traits, whether β⁺ or β⁰, are usually characterized by mild anemia and small, poorly hemoglobinized red cells. The Hb A₂ is elevated to about twice the normal level. This increase is the result of both a relative deficiency of β chains and an absolute rise in the output of δ chains both in *cis* and *trans* to the β thalassemia mutation.[7] There is a slight elevation of Hb F in about 50 per cent of cases.

Rarer variant forms of β thalassemia trait exist, many of which have now been analyzed at the molecular level.

β THALASSEMIA TRAIT WITH UNUSUALLY HIGH LEVELS OF HB A₂. As mentioned earlier, this condition almost invariably results from deletions that remove part or all of the β globin gene, including its 5′ promoter sequences, but that leave the δ globin gene intact. It appears, therefore, that in the absence of the β globin gene promoter there is an absolute increase in δ chain synthesis above that seen in the usual forms of β thalassemia trait. This increase may reflect the availability of regulatory elements that normally compete for the promoters of the β and δ globin genes.

NORMAL HB A₂ β THALASSEMIA. In populations in which β thalassemia is common, individuals who have the features of β thalassemia trait but a normal Hb A₂ level are occasionally encountered. The molecular mechanisms for this form of β thalassemia are, again, quite heterogeneous. The bulk of cases seem to result from the co-inheritance of both β and δ thalassemia; we will consider the mutations that give rise to δ thalassemia in a later section.

Another relatively common cause of normal Hb A₂ β thalassemia in Middle Eastern and Mediterranean populations is the mutation at codon 26, GCC→TCC, which generates Hb Knossos, a variant that is not detectable by electrophoresis under standard conditions. As is the case for Hb E, this mutation results in both the insertion of a different amino acid and a reduced production of β globin mRNA.[98] However, although this mutation is associated with a β thalassemia–like disorder, the Hb A₂ level is not elevated. Recent studies suggest that the chromosome that carries the Hb Knossos mutation also has a mutation of the δ globin gene, the loss of an A in codon 59, which completely inactivates it.[170] Since most patients with Hb Knossos seem to share the same β globin RFLP haplotype, it appears that the δ⁰/β^{Knossos} allele has been disseminated throughout the Mediterranean region.

Finally, under the heading of "normal A₂ β thalassemia" should be included the silent β thalassemias, which were described earlier, and the carrier state for εγδβ thalassemia, a condition that is discussed later in this chapter.

As mentioned earlier, it has been customary to

define the normal Hb A$_2$ β thalassemias into type 1, or silent β thalassemia, and type 2, in which the hematological profile is typical of β thalassemia trait. As will have become apparent from this discussion, this classification, although still useful clinically, has little genetic meaning.

Clinical and Hematological Features

It is beyond the scope of this chapter to consider the clinical features of the β thalassemias in detail. They are the subject of several monographs,[7, 71, 113] and readers who wish to obtain a detailed account of this aspect of the thalassemia field are referred to these sources. Here I simply outline the major clinical features of the three main clinical groups of β thalassemia, the molecular basis and pathophysiology of which have been considered in the previous sections.

The Major Forms of β Thalassemia

These conditions often present during the first year of life as the level of Hb F declines. They usually declare themselves by failure to thrive, pallor, or anemia, which is discovered during an intercurrent illness such as an infection. Left untreated, affected infants are incapable of maintaining a hemoglobin level above 5 g/dl. Their subsequent clinical course and physical findings depend on whether they are placed on an adequate transfusion regimen at this stage or whether they are given insufficient blood to develop normally.

The standard textbook account of the major form of thalassemia, Cooley's anemia, describes the disease as it is seen in children who have been inadequately transfused. These children show early growth retardation, pallor, icterus, and, as they grow older, brown pigmentation of the skin. Progressive expansion of the bone marrow in response to anemia leads to characteristic skeletal changes, including bossing of the skull, overgrowth of the zygomas, and protrusion of the jaws. These changes may ultimately lead to the classic "thalassemic facies." These changes are associated with characteristic radiological abnormalities, including a "hair on end" appearance of the skull and thinning and trabeculation of the bones of the hands and the long bones. The bone changes may become so marked as to lead to repeated pathological fractures. Hepatosplenomegaly is progressive, and this may lead to a secondary dilutional anemia, with leukopenia and thrombocytopenia. These poorly developed children are particularly prone to infection, which, during the early years of life, is the most common cause of morbidity and mortality.[171]

In children who have been transfused regularly to maintain hemoglobin levels above 9 to 10 g/dl, growth and development are usually normal until early puberty. The splenomegaly that is common in inadequately transfused children is not so prominent, and hypersplenism rarely develops. However, by the age of 10 to 15 years, patients treated in this way, unless they have received regular chelation therapy to remove excess iron derived from transfusions, start to show signs of progressive hepatic, cardiac, and endocrine dysfunction, associated with a reduced pubertal growth spurt and failure of sexual maturation. On the other hand, children who have had adequate chelation therapy may have normal sexual maturation. Even they often have some growth retardation, however.

The hematological findings also depend on the type of transfusion regimen. In inadequately transfused children, the peripheral blood shows typical thalassemic red cell morphology with anisocytosis and poikilocytosis, target cells, and red cell fragments, all set against a background of marked hypochromia. Nucleated red cells are usually present and after splenectomy may become very frequent. The white cell and platelet count varies, depending on the degree of hypersplenism. In adequately transfused children, the peripheral blood count is often remarkably normal, simply reflecting the suppression of the patient's bone marrow.

The bone marrow shows intense erythroid hyperplasia. The red cell precursors show nuclear and cytoplasmic abnormalities and contain inclusions formed from precipitated α chains. Ferrokinetic and erythrokinetic studies demonstrate an extreme degree of ineffective erythropoiesis with a reduced survival of the red cells in the peripheral blood.

In untransfused or inadequately transfused patients, the hemoglobin consists of a variable amount of Hb F; in patients with no β chain production, there is no Hb A and the hemoglobin consists entirely of Hb F with a small proportion of Hb A$_2$. The level of Hb A$_2$ in homozygotes or compound heterozygotes for severe forms of β thalassemia is of no diagnostic value. It tends to be low in red cells that contain predominantly Hb F and relatively higher in those that contain Hb A; the level of Hb A$_2$ in the blood represents an average of its different distribution in these heterogeneous cell populations.[7]

β Thalassemia Intermedia

As might be expected from the heterogeneity of its molecular basis, β thalassemia intermedia is an ill-defined clinical entity with a very broad spectrum ranging from a condition little different from thalassemia major to a symptomless disorder that is discovered only by chance examination of the blood. One of the most useful indications that β thalassemia is going to follow a milder course is its time of presentation; babies with β thalassemia intermedia tend to present late in the first year and often well into the second year of life.[171] Otherwise, the clinical features are characterized by a varying degree of anemia and splenomegaly and, in the more severe forms, bone changes similar to those found in the major form of the illness.

At the severe end of the spectrum, the hemoglobin level settles down to 5 to 7 g/dl, and by the age of 2 and 3 years it is clear that development is not normal and there are already signs of the skeletal changes, particularly deformity of the skull and face, characteristic of untreated thalassemia major. If these children are transfused, which may not need to be as frequent as for those with thalassemia major, these changes can be arrested and future skeletal development is normal. However, at the other end of the spectrum, patients may not become symptomatic until they reach adult life, and they may remain transfusion free, with hemoglobin levels at 8 to 12 g/dl. However, they may develop complications as they get older, including increasing splenomegaly and hypersplenism, iron loading due to increased absorption, painful arthritis, gallstones, leg ulcers, and an increased proneness to infection.[7]

The hematological picture is similar to that of thalassemia major. The hemoglobin composition is extremely variable. Those who are homozygous for β^0 thalassemia have only Hb F and Hb A_2, whereas others who have inherited mild β^+ thalassemia mutations may have Hb F levels as low as 5 to 10 per cent. The relationship of the level of Hb F to particular mutations was considered earlier in this chapter.

Dominantly Inherited β Thalassemia

The phenotype of this condition is different from that of other forms of β thalassemia intermedia in several respects.[172, 173] Variable degrees of anemia, splenomegaly, and morphological changes of the red cells are present. The bone marrow shows marked erythroid hyperplasia with well-formed inclusion bodies in the red cell precursors. However, hemoglobin analysis reveals a raised level of Hb A_2 but normal or only slightly elevated levels of Hb F. These findings, together with the pattern of dominant inheritance, are diagnostic.

β Thalassemia Trait

The heterozygous states for β^0 and β^+ thalassemia are invariably asymptomatic and, despite their molecular heterogeneity, show a remarkably uniform hematological profile. There is microcytosis and hypochromia with low MCV and MCH values together with an increased level of Hb A_2. The level of Hb F is slightly increased in about 50 per cent of cases. The only exceptions are β thalassemia heterozygotes who also have α thalassemia trait in whom, for reasons that are not clear, the MCH and MCV are much closer to normal. The Hb A_2 level, however, is elevated.

The hematological findings in the subtypes of β thalassemia, such as those with unusually high levels of Hb A_2 or those with normal levels of Hb A_2, are similar; these conditions are defined by the Hb A_2 levels.

World Distribution and Population Genetics

The world distribution of the β thalassemias and the mutations that occur in different populations are summarized in Figure 5–16.

Gene frequency data for β thalassemia in different parts of the world are often based on small samples, and for many populations there are only sporadic reports of individual cases. It is clear, however, that with a few exceptions, such as Liberia, the condition occurs at a low frequency throughout tropical Africa, although higher frequencies have been observed in North Africa. It is particularly common throughout

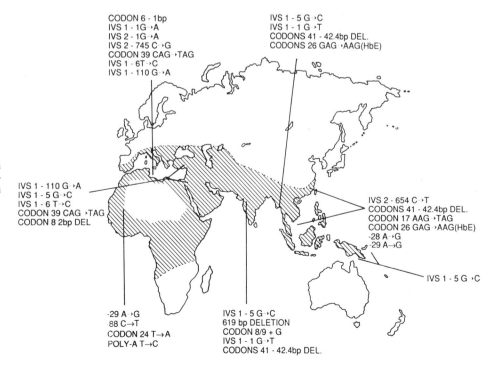

FIGURE 5–16. The world distribution of the different β thalassemia mutations. Nomenclature is described in the text.

CODON 6 - 1bp
IVS 1 - 1G ›A
IVS 2 - 1G ›A
IVS 2 - 745 C ›G
CODON 39 CAG ›TAG
IVS 1 - 6T ›C
IVS 1 - 110 G ›A

IVS 1 - 5 G ›C
IVS 1 - 1 G ›T
CODONS 41 - 42.4bp DEL.
CODONS 26 GAG ›AAG(HbE)

IVS 1 - 110 G ›A
IVS 1 - 5 G ›C
IVS 1 - 6 T ›C
CODON 39 CAG ›TAG
CODON 8 2bp DEL

IVS 2 - 654 C ›T
CODONS 41 - 42.4bp DEL.
CODON 17 AAG ›TAG
CODON 26 GAG ›AAG(HbE)
-28 A ›G
-29 A→G

IVS 1 - 5 G ›C

-29 A ›G
-88 C→T
CODON 24 T→A
POLY-A T→C

IVS 1 - 5 G ›C
619 bp DELETION
CODON 8/9 + G
IVS 1 - 1 G ›T
CODONS 41 - 42.4bp DEL.

the Mediterranean region, parts of the Middle East, and India and Burma.[7] It is also common throughout Southeast Asia in a line starting in southern China, stretching through Thailand, Cambodia, and Laos, and down the Malay peninsula into Indonesia. It is distributed sporadically in Melanesia.

In each of the high-frequency areas, there are a few common mutations with a varying number of rare ones (see Fig. 5–16). Furthermore, in each of these populations the pattern of mutations is different.[85, 89, 91, 130, 174–178] Even when the same mutation occurs in different populations, it is usually found together with a different β globin gene RFLP haplotype. It is likely, therefore, that the β thalassemia mutations have arisen independently in different populations and achieved their high frequency by selection. Although some movement of the β thalassemia genes may have occurred between populations, by drift and so on, little doubt exists that independent mutation and selection have been the major factors responsible for the world distribution of the β thalassemias.

Population studies suggest that a major factor that has maintained the β thalassemia polymorphism is protection of heterozygotes against *P. falciparum* malaria. Recent studies in Melanesia have shown that there is a frequency-dependent altitude correlation with malaria, as has been shown for α thalassemia.[178] It is still not absolutely clear how β thalassemia heterozygotes are protected against *P. falciparum* malaria. In vitro culture studies have shown that *P. falciparum* invades and develops in β thalassemic red cells in the same way as normal cells.[65] In an earlier section, we described how parasitized α thalassemic cells bind significantly greater amounts of antibody from the serum of patients with malaria than do control red cells. The same phenomenon has been demonstrated with red cells from β thalassemia heterozygotes.[65] These findings suggest that the protective effect of the thalassemias against malaria might be related, at least in part, to enhanced immune recognition and hence clearance of parasitized cells.

It appears, therefore, that the relative resistance of heterozygotes to *P. falciparum* malaria has been a major factor in maintaining the high frequency of β thalassemia in the world population. Whether other factors are involved remains to be determined.

δβ THALASSEMIAS

Globally, the δβ thalassemias are much less common than the β thalassemias.[7] But like the β thalassemias, they are extremely heterogeneous in their molecular pathology and clinical phenotype.

Classification

It is useful to divide the δβ thalassemias into the (δβ)+ and (δβ)0 thalassemias to indicate whether there is any output of δ and β chains from the affected chromosome.

The (δβ)+ thalassemias fall into two main classes. The first category comprises those that result from abnormal crossing over and the production of δβ fusion hemoglobin variants, of which Hb Lepore is the prototype. The second category consists of complex disorders that result from the presence of two different mutations in the εγδβ globin gene cluster such that either the δ or the β globin gene is partially or completely inactivated, and there is also a mutation involving the promoter region of the γ globin gene or another mutation that results in increased γ gene expression. As knowledge of the molecular pathology of these rare conditions has increased, it has become apparent that many of them are not true δβ thalassemias, but because they appear in the thalassemia literature under this heading, they are considered in this section. Depending on the nature of the mutations involved—in particular, whether they include the β or δ gene—the (δβ)+ thalassemias can be divided into δ+β0, δ0β+, and (δβ)+ varieties.

The (δβ)0 thalassemias usually result from long deletions involving the εγδβ globin gene cluster, which remove the β and δ genes but which leave either one or both of the γ genes intact. They produce a phenotype that is very similar to the phenotype of deletion forms of HPFH, which are described in detail in Chapter 4, and also are similar in that there is a high output of γ chains from the γ locus or loci *cis* to the mutation. Indeed, HPFH can be regarded as a form of (δβ)0 thalassemia in which there is almost, but not quite, complete compensation for defective β chain synthesis by persistent γ chain production.

Molecular Pathology

The molecular pathology of the δβ thalassemias, although of interest for its own sake, has been studied in particular detail because it was hoped that it might help to define the regions of the εγδβ globin gene cluster that are involved in the regulation of the transition from γ to β globin chain synthesis during development. This subject is of particular interest with respect to the lengths and sites of the deletions that underlie the deletion forms of δβ thalassemia compared with HPFH.

(δβ)+ Thalassemia

FUSION CHAIN VARIANTS. A family of hemoglobin variants has arisen by non-homologous crossing over within the εγδβ globin gene complex (Fig. 5–17). The first to be discovered, Hb Lepore, named after the family in which it was found, contains normal α chains and non-α chains that consist of the first 50 to 80 amino acid residues of the δ chain and the last 60 to 90 residues of the normal C-terminal sequence of the β chains.[179] Thus, the Hb Lepore non-α chain is a δβ fusion chain. Three different variants of Hb Lepore,

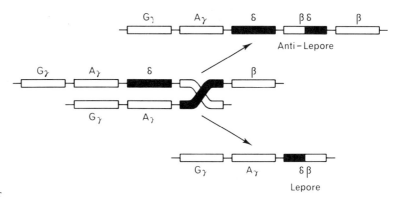

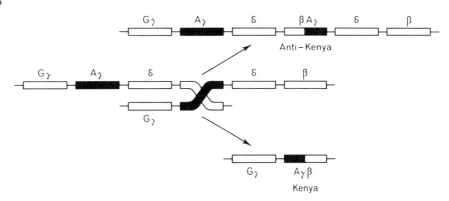

FIGURE 5–17. The abnormal crossing over mechanisms involved in the generation of the Lepore and anti-Lepore hemoglobins and Hb Kenya.

in which the transition from δ to β sequences occurs at different points, have been described.[180] Hemoglobin Kenya is analogous except that in this case the abnormal hybrid chain contains γ and β sequences; that is, it is a γβ fusion chain.[7]

These fusion globin chains have arisen by non-homologous crossing over between part of the δ locus on one chromosome and part of the β locus on the complementary chromosome (see Fig. 5–17). This event results from misalignment of chromosome pairs during meiosis, so that a δ chain gene pairs with a β chain gene instead of its homologous partner. As shown in Figure 5–17, this mechanism should give rise to two abnormal chromosomes. The Lepore chromosome has no normal δ or β loci and carries a δβ fusion gene. On the opposite of the homologous pairs of chromosomes, there is an anti-Lepore (βδ) fusion gene together with normal δ and β loci. Similarly, in the generation of the γβ fusion variant, Hb Kenya, an anti-Kenya chromosome with intact ^Aγ, δ, and β loci is produced. A variety of anti-Lepore–like hemoglobins have been discovered, including Hb Miwada, Hb E-Congo, Hb Lincoln Park, and Hb P-Nilotic.[180]

Another variant with δβ chains, Hb Parchman, is more complex in that the non-α chain has δ sequences at the N- *and* C-terminal ends and β sequences in the middle. It is likely that this arose by a double cross-over event.[180]

These δβ fusion chains are synthesized ineffectively and hence give rise to the clinical phenotype of severe δβ thalassemia. In contrast to the (δβ)⁰ thalassemias,

there is very little compensation by the γ globin genes on the same chromosome, and hence the homozygous state for Hb Lepore is associated with a severe clinical disorder. On the other hand, the chromosome carrying the ^Aγβ fusion product, Hb Kenya, is not associated with an abnormal phenotype because there is a high output of γ chains and hence the clinical picture of HPFH.

(δβ)⁺ Thalassemia-like Disorders Due to Two Mutations in the β Globin Gene Cluster

A heterogeneous family of non-deletion δβ thalassemias that result from two mutations in the εγδβ globin gene cluster has been described. Strictly speaking, they are not all δβ thalassemias, but because their phenotypes resemble the deletion forms of (δβ)⁰ thalassemia, which are described in the next section, they appear in the literature under this title.

In the Sardinian form of δβ thalassemia,[181] the β globin gene has the common Mediterranean codon 39 nonsense mutation, which leads to an absence of β globin synthesis. However, there is a relatively high expression of the ^Aγ gene in *cis*, which gives this condition the phenotype of δ⁺β⁰ thalassemia; this is because a point mutation occurs at position -196 upstream from the ^Aγ gene. Heterozygotes for this condition have thalassemic red cell changes, 15 to 20 per cent Hb F, and normal levels of Hb A₂. Thus, this disorder is a phenocopy of δβ thalassemia.

Another condition that has the phenotype of δβ

thalassemia, with more than 20 per cent Hb F in heterozygotes, has been described in a Chinese patient in whom defective β globin gene synthesis appears to be due to an A→G change in the ATA sequence in the promoter region of the β globin gene.[182] The increased γ chain synthesis, which appears to involve both $^G\gamma$ and $^A\gamma$ genes *cis* to this mutation, remains unexplained.

Another condition that was originally called δβ thalassemia has been described in the Corfu population.[183] Again, this condition results from two mutations in the β globin gene cluster.[184] First, a 7201 bp deletion starts in the δ globin gene, IVS-2, position 818 to 822, and extends upstream to a 5′ breakpoint located 1719 to 1722 bp 3′ to the ψβ gene termination codon. In addition, a G→A mutation is found at position 5 in the donor site consensus region of IVS-1 of the β globin gene. The output from this novel chromosome consists of relatively high levels of γ chains with very low levels of β chains. The $^A\gamma$ and $^G\gamma$ globin genes have been sequenced, including the upstream promoter regions from position −360 to the CAP sites, but no other mutations have been found. It is presumed, therefore, that the high level of γ chain production from this chromosome in adult life is related to the deletion.

Homozygotes for the Corfu form of thalassemia have almost 100 per cent Hb F with traces of Hb A but no Hb A_2. Curiously, heterozygotes have only slightly elevated levels of Hb F; the phenotype is similar to that of "normal Hb A_2 β thalassemia." Thus, strictly speaking, this condition is a $\delta^0\beta^+$ thalassemia with unusually high levels of Hb F in homozygotes.

(δβ)⁰ Thalassemia

These conditions result from deletions of various lengths that remove the δ and β globin genes. They can be classified into the (δβ)⁰ and ($^A\gamma$δβ)⁰ thalassemias, depending on the length of the deletion, that is, whether the $^A\gamma$ genes are involved or not. The extent of these deletions is illustrated in Figure 5–18. References to the original descriptions of these deletions are given in reference 185 and in the legend to Figure 5–18.

The (δβ)⁰ thalassemia deletions remove or inactivate only the δ and β globin genes. They are relatively small and are contained within the β gene cluster. One exception, however, is the Spanish type, in which the deletion extends much farther on the 3′ side, beyond the 3′ end of the (δβ)⁰ HPFH lesions.[186]

The deletions that underlie ($^A\gamma$δβ)⁰ thalassemias extend into or beyond the $^A\gamma$ gene on the 5′ side, as well as removing the δ and β genes. On the 3′ side, most of them terminate within 20 kb of the β gene, but again there is one exception, the Chinese type, that extends much farther.[187] The Indian form is not a simple deletion but reflects a complex rearrangement with two deletions, one affecting the $^A\gamma$ gene and the other the δ and β genes; the intervening region remains but is inverted.[188] This was the first example of

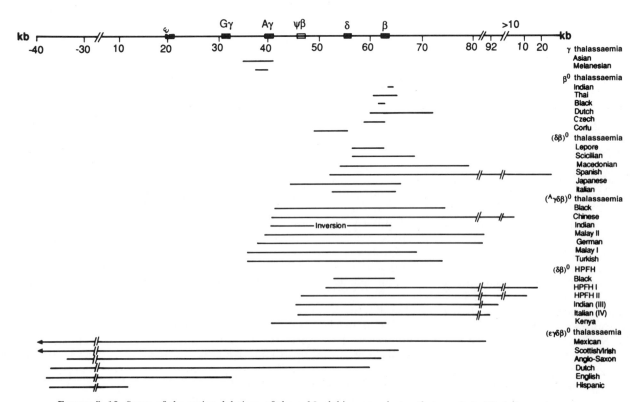

FIGURE 5–18. Some of the major deletions of the εγδβ globin gene cluster that result in δβ thalassemia and HPFH. (Data from references 8, 185, and 191 to 195.)

a major gene inversion underlying a genetic disease in man.

Genotype/Phenotype Relationships

The major phenotypic difference between the β and most of the δβ thalassemias reflects the relatively high output of γ globin chain production that occurs in δβ thalassemia and that leads to a milder disorder. The exception is the Hb Lepore disorders, in which there is a low output of γ chains and a severe deficit of non-α chain production leading to a clinical phenotype similar to that of β thalassemia. In all the other δβ thalassemias, there is a relatively high output either of $^G\gamma$ and $^A\gamma$ or of $^G\gamma$ chains. With the exception of the Sardinian[179] and Chinese[180] forms, in which upstream mutations involving the γ globin gene, similar to those observed in the non-deletion forms of HPFH (see Chapter 4) have been demonstrated, the reason for the high output of γ chains is not obvious, and it is assumed, therefore, that this must be due to the effect of the extensive deletions of the β-like globin gene cluster.

As described in Chapter 4, there is a family of deletion forms of HPFH that produce a very similar clinical phenotype to that of (δβ)⁰ thalassemia but in which the output of γ chains is higher and therefore the phenotype is even milder. The two African forms of (δβ)⁰ HPFH are both due to extensive deletions, of similar length but with staggered ends, differing phenotypically only in the proportions of γ chains produced. A third form of HPFH of this type, found in Indians, is associated with a more severe phenotype, particularly when co-inherited with β thalassemia (Fig. 5–18). It should be emphasized that the difference between the output of γ chains in HPFH and δβ thalassemia is only a matter of degree; homozygotes for the deletion forms of HPFH have small red cells and imbalanced globin chain synthesis.[189]

Because of the problems of cell selection due to imbalanced globin chain synthesis, which is found in δβ thalassemia homozygotes and even to some degree in HPFH homozygotes, the most valid comparisons of the phenotypic expression of these conditions are made in heterozygotes. With the exception of the Corfu form, heterozygotes for (δβ)⁰ thalassemia have levels of Hb F that greatly exceed those of β thalassemia heterozygotes, usually in the range of 5 to 15 per cent. On the other hand, heterozygotes for deletion forms of HPFH have Hb F values in the range of 15 to 25 per cent. Clearly, therefore, γ chain output is more effective in HPFH. However, detailed analyses of the underlying deletions have not provided a unifying hypothesis to explain these differences. In general, deletions that start within the β globin gene complex and extend 3′ to it appear to leave the surviving γ genes active in adult life. Although this observation could reflect the effects of newly opposed 3′ promoter sequences on γ chain synthesis, the number of different deletions of this type makes it difficult to imagine that each one mediates its effect in the same way. Furthermore, two of the deletions, those associated with Hb Kenya and the Indian form of $(^A\gamma\delta\beta)^0$ thalassemia, leave intact the 3′ end of the β gene and beyond (see Fig. 5–18). Comparison of (δβ)⁰ thalassemia and (δβ)⁰ HPFH does not identify any single region between the $^A\gamma$ and δ genes that remains intact in one condition but that is lost in the other, and it has not been possible to identify a sequence in the gene cluster that might be involved in modifying γ chain output in these different conditions.

One approach to this problem has been to compare the 5′ ends of the (δβ)⁰ HPFH and (δβ)⁰ thalassemia deletions that are closest together. For example, two deletions that cause these conditions end in a pair of Alu 1 repeats 5′ to the δ gene. The HPFH deletion ends in the 5′ Alu 1 repeat of the bipolar pair, the δβ thalassemia deletion in the 3′ Alu 1 repeat.[183] Thus, the two deletions have endpoints that are within 500 nt of each other; the larger deletion is associated with a significantly higher output of γ chains than is the smaller one. This observation suggested that there might exist a critical regulatory region involved with γ chain production within these Alu repeats. However, this whole region is deleted in the Corfu form of δβ thalassemia, yet heterozygotes do not have elevated levels of Hb F.[183, 184] Thus, all that can be concluded is that deletions starting within the complex and extending 3′ all appear to leave the remaining γ genes active to a variable extent in adult life. The reasons for the subtle phenotypic differences between δβ thalassemia and HPFH remain to be explained.

Clinical and Hematological Findings[7]

Homozygous δβ Thalassemia

The homozygous states for the (δβ)⁺ thalassemias, as typified by the Hb Lepore disorders, are characterized by a disorder very similar to β thalassemia major. Severe anemia, splenomegaly, and associated skeletal changes are present. The hemoglobin consists of F and Lepore only.

The homozygous states for the (δβ)⁰ thalassemias are quite different. In these, the clinical picture is a mild to moderate form of thalassemia intermedia. Typical thalassemic red cell changes are seen, and the hemoglobin is made up entirely of the fetal variety; Hb A and Hb A₂ are absent. Depending on the underlying molecular pathology, the Hb F consists of both $^G\gamma$ and $^A\gamma$ forms or only $^G\gamma$. The homozygous state for Corfu δβ thalassemia is very similar to (δβ)⁰ thalassemia, except that trace amounts of Hb A are present in the peripheral blood.

Globin chain synthesis in these disorders is imbalanced, with α/non-α synthesis ratios in the range of 2 to 3:1.

δβ Thalassemia Trait

All the carrier states for δβ thalassemia are characterized by hypochromic, microcytic red cells with a reduced MCH and MCV. In heterozygotes for $(\delta\beta)^+$ thalassemia of the Lepore variety, the hemoglobin consists of Hb A, Hb Lepore, and Hb A_2; the level of Hb Lepore constitues about 10 per cent of the total hemoglobin, and the mean level of Hb A_2 is approximately 2 per cent, significantly reduced.

$(\delta\beta)^0$ Thalassemia heterozygotes have 5 to 15 per cent Hb F with normal or just subnormal levels of Hb A_2. An exception to this rule is the heterozygote for the Corfu type of $\delta\beta$ thalassemia, who does not have elevated levels of Hb F.

δ THALASSEMIA

Thalassemia involving the δ globin locus is of no clinical significance except insofar as when inherited together with β thalassemia it may prevent the usual elevation of Hb A_2 that occurs in β thalassemia heterozygotes. As mentioned earlier, the co-inheritance of β and δ thalassemia is one of the most common causes of "normal A_2 β thalassemia."

Molecular Pathology

Like other forms of thalassemia, δ thalassemia can be classified into δ^0 and δ^+ thalassemia, depending on the particular molecular lesion. Some of the mutations that cause δ thalassemia are summarized in Figure 5–19, and their original descriptions are given in references 170 and 190.

One type of δ^0 thalassemia that is due to a partial deletion of the δ globin gene occurs in the Mediterranean population. This particular lesion was described in the previous section as part of the molecular pathology of the Corfu form of $\delta\beta$ thalassemia.[184] The deletion involves the loss of 7201 bp with a 5' breakpoint at a site 3' to the $\psi\beta$ globin gene and a 3' breakpoint in the middle of IVS-2 of the δ globin gene. This deletion has been observed on chromosomes with a normal β globin gene in patients in the Mediterranean population.[190] Presumably, the Corfu form of $\delta\beta$ thalassemia arose as a recombinational event with a chromosome containing a β gene with the IVS-1-5 G→A mutation. Several other molecular forms of δ^0 thalassemia have been described as shown

in Figure 5–19. Similarly, several mutations should give rise to the phenotype of δ^+ thalassemia, since they are similar to those in the β globin gene that cause its partial inactivation.

It is interesting that at least three of the mutations that have been found in δ thalassemia have their equivalents in the same position in the β globin chain in β thalassemia. These are δ^+27, δ^0 IVS-1-1, and G→C at codon 30.[190] It is presumed that identical nucleotide substitutions in the β and δ genes have arisen either as independent mutations or as the result of gene conversion events. Most of the δ thalassemias have been observed in *trans* to β thalassemia. However, the δ^+27 mutation has been observed in both *cis* and *trans*. As mentioned in an earlier section, the form of δ thalassemia that results from a loss of an A in codon 59 occurs on the same chromosome as the Hb Knossos mutation, thus explaining the normal level of Hb A_2 associated with this mild form of β thalassemia.[170]

Clinical and Hematological Implications

The δ thalassemias are not associated with any hematological changes. Because they prevent an elevation of Hb A_2 when inherited together with β thalassemia, they are of diagnostic importance for genetic counseling and screening. Although no population surveys have been done, it seems likely that these thalassemias occur at a low frequency, since there is no reason for them to have come under any form of selection.

εγδβ THALASSEMIA

This thalassemia is a rare form that results from several different long deletions that start approximately 50 to 100 kb upstream from the globin gene cluster and extend 3', where they remove all or part of the cluster. Since even if they spare the β globin gene it is inactivated, they are all considered $(\epsilon\gamma\delta\beta)^0$ thalassemias.

The approximate extent of these deletions is illustrated in Figure 5–18. In cases in which the deletion spares the β globin gene—the Dutch[191] and English[192] forms, for example—no β chain production occurs,

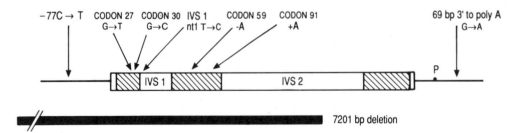

FIGURE 5–19. The mutations that cause δ thalassemia. (Data from Olds, R. J., et al.: A novel δ^0 mutation in *cis* with Hb Knossos: A study of different genetic interactions in three Egyptian families. Br. J. Haematol. 78:430, 1991; and Piratsu, M., et al.: Molecular analysis of atypical β-thalassemia heterozygotes. Ann. N. Y. Acad. Sci. 612:90, 1990.)

even though the gene is expressed in heterologous systems. Similarly, the Spanish deletion, which extends upstream 5' from the ε gene, is also associated with defective β chain production.[193]

The reason for the inactivation of the β globin gene *cis* to these deletions has been clarified recently by the discovery of the LCR about 50 kb upstream from the εγδβ globin gene cluster.[75] Just as occurs when the α globin LCR is inactivated by a deletion, as described earlier in this chapter, the removal of this critical regulatory region seems to inactivate completely the downstream globin gene complex. The Hispanic form of this condition[194] results from a deletion that includes most of the LCR, including four of the five sites hypersensitive to DNase 1. These lesions appear to close down the chromatin domain, which is usually open in erythroid tissues. They also delay the replication of the β genes in the cell cycle. Thus, although these are rare mutations, they have been of considerable importance, since it was analysis of the Dutch deletion that first pointed to the possibility of there being a major control region upstream from the β-like globin gene cluster and that ultimately led to the discovery of the β globin LCR.

The clinical and hematological phenotypes associated with (εγδβ)⁰ thalassemia vary, depending on the stage of development.[195] Presumably, the homozygous states would not be compatible with fetal survival. At birth, heterozygotes are anemic, with hypochromic red cells and a variable degree of hemolysis. In some cases, this condition has necessitated blood transfusion in the neonatal period. Three of nine infants with the Dutch variety of the disorder died. Five of the six living children with this condition required blood transfusions, whereas the remaining one survived with no treatment.

In adult life, the condition is characterized by the hematological picture of β thalassemia trait with a normal Hb A_2 level. Why this condition is so severe in some, but not all, heterozygotes in the neonatal period remains unexplained.

THALASSEMIAS FOR WHICH THE CAUSE HAS NOT BEEN DETERMINED

Despite intensive work in many laboratories over the past 15 years, there remain a significant number of thalassemia-like disorders for which the cause has not yet been determined. Most laboratories that study the disorder have encountered in the order of 5 per cent of cases in which the hematological findings and globin synthesis data suggest a thalassemic defect yet complete sequence analysis of the appropriate globin gene and its flanking regions has revealed no abnormality.

It seems quite likely that some of these disorders are due to mutations involving the LCR for the α or β globin genes. The strategy of studying these areas in unusual cases of α thalassemia has already disclosed five different deletions involving this region. It seems

likely that similar lesions will be found in the β globin LCR. In addition to the extensive deletions involving this region that have been found to date, more subtle deletions or even point mutations may be found. It is also possible, of course, that there are regulatory regions that control expression of the globin genes that are not close to the globin gene clusters or even on other chromosomes. The recent discovery that one form of α thalassemia associated with mental retardation is due to a lesion on the X chromosome suggests that such regulatory loci exist and that they may be involved in the genesis of some thalassemic disorders.

THE CONTROL AND TREATMENT OF THE THALASSEMIAS

The hemoglobin disorders are probably the most common single-gene diseases in the world population. Because they occur with a particularly high frequency in the developing world, where the rate of population increase is the greatest, it is likely that their prevalence will tend to increase, even if the major selective force that has maintained these polymorphisms in the past is removed. With the resurgence of malaria in many parts of the world, it may be a very long time before this occurs. Indeed, the World Health Organization has estimated that by the year 2000 approximately 7 per cent of the world's population will be carriers for important globin disorders.

It is beyond the scope of this chapter to deal with the population control and clinical management of the thalassemias in detail. Readers who wish to learn more about this topic are referred to two monographs that cover all aspects of the care of thalassemic patients.[7, 171] Here we concentrate on those aspects of the control of thalassemia that are based on an understanding of the molecular basis of these disorders.

Screening and Prenatal Diagnosis

In many ways, the thalassemias are ideal recessive disorders for developing population screening programs and prenatal diagnosis.[196, 197] The carrier states for the important α and β thalassemias can be identified hematologically and by hemoglobin analysis in the majority of cases. Occasionally, difficulty in distinguishing these traits from iron deficiency may be encountered, and complex interactions, particularly the co-inheritance of α and β thalassemia, may cause problems for screening, but overall the carrier states can be identified by any hematology laboratory with appropriately trained personnel.[196, 197]

Because the treatment of important forms of α and β thalassemia is still unsatisfactory, the best approach to their control is screening followed by prenatal diagnosis. Originally, this was accomplished by obtaining fetal blood from the placenta or umbilical cord, followed by analysis of globin chain synthesis.[197] In this way, it was possible to identify the important varieties of α thalassemia and the β⁰ and β⁺ thalassemias. Despite the technical difficulties involved, this technique was applied widely and very successfully in many populations.[196-200] Its main disadvantage is that fetal blood sampling cannot be carried out until well into the second trimester of pregnancy. Hence if the fetus is afflicted with a form of severe thalassemia, the pregnancy has to be terminated toward the end of the second trimester, which may be extremely distressing for the mother.

With the advent of DNA technology, prenatal diagnosis was carried out on fetal DNA, first obtained from amniotic fluid[201] and later by chorionic villus sampling (CVS) between 9 and 12 weeks of pregnancy.[202, 203] Although recent studies have suggested that the rate of fetal loss is slightly higher after CVS than after amniocentesis, many women are still willing to accept this rather than go through the trauma of a second trimester diagnosis. For this reason, many centers now use CVS as their first line and retain amniocentesis or fetal blood sampling for those pregnancies in which the mother presents too late for CVS.

The diagnostic techniques used for fetal DNA analysis have evolved over the past 10 years.[76, 77, 196] The earliest prenatal diagnoses were carried out by Southern blotting of fetal DNA, either using RFLP linkage analysis[203] or, in those cases in which a mutation could be identified directly, using a specific restriction enzyme. The use of RFLP analysis for prenatal detection of genetic disease entails three steps. First, an appropriate RFLP marker is chosen, one that is either within or closely linked to the disease locus and for which an individual at risk of transmitting the disease is heterozygous. Second, it is necessary to determine which of the marker alleles is on the chromosome carrying the disease allele; this step involves the study of family members, ideally a previously affected or normal child. Finally, with use of the markers, fetal DNA is examined to see whether the fetus has inherited the chromosome (or chromosomes) carrying the gene (or genes) for the particular form of thalassemia, or its normal allele. The disadvantage of this method is that it is necessary to establish, by a family study, that appropriate markers are available. Although it has been largely superseded by more direct approaches of identifying thalassemia mutations in fetal DNA, it is still a valuable method to fall back on in families at risk for having children with rare forms of thalassemia. α⁰ Thalassemia and the few forms of β⁰ thalassemia that result from gene deletions can be identified directly by Southern blotting.[197] In addition, approximately 20 different β thalassemia mutations alter a particular restriction enzyme site and can therefore be identified in the same way.[197]

More recently, following the development of the polymerase chain reaction (PCR), the identification of thalassemia mutations in fetal DNA has been greatly facilitated.[204-207] For example, it can be used for the very rapid detection of mutations that alter the cutting sites of restriction enzymes. The appropriate fragment of the β globin gene is amplified approximately 30 times, after which the DNA fragments are digested with the appropriate enzyme and separated by electrophoresis. Because PCR produces so much DNA, these fragments can be detected by either ethidium bromide or silver staining of DNA bands on gels; no radioactive probes are required.

Now that the mutations have been determined in so many different forms of α and β thalassemia, most centers that have prenatal diagnosis programs are using the direct detection of these mutations as their first-line approach. Since most racial groups have only a few common β thalassemia mutations, it is possible in many cases to determine the mutations in the parents and then to analyze fetal DNA for their presence. The development of PCR, combined with the use of oligonucleotide probes to detect individual mutations, has offered a variety of new approaches for facilitating the speed and accuracy of carrier detection and prenatal diagnosis. For example, diagnoses can be made using hybridization of specific ³²P-end-labeled oligonucleotides to an amplified region of the β globin gene dotted onto a nylon membrane.[76, 77] Because the β globin gene sequence of interest is amplified more than 10⁶-fold, hybridization time can be limited to 1 hour, and the entire procedure can be carried out in 2 hours.

A number of variations on this theme have been developed. For example, another approach to the identification of mutations that uses PCR, called the amplification refractory mutation system (ARMS), also allows the diagnosis to be made in 1 to 2 hours.[208] This method is based on the observation that in many cases oligonucleotides for the 3′ mismatched residue will, under appropriate conditions, not function as primers in the PCR. This method makes use of two primers. The normal one is refractory to PCR on mutant template DNA; the mutant sequence is refractory to PCR on normal DNA. The difference between normal DNA and that carrying a particular mutation is identified by size differences of the amplified fragments (Fig. 5–20). Other modifications of the PCR involve the use of non–radioactively labeled probes.[207, 209, 210] For example, it is feasible to use horseradish peroxidase labeling of the 5′ end of oligonucleotides designed to detect mutations.

In establishing a prenatal diagnosis program, it is first necessary to determine the common α or β thalassemia mutations in the population. It is then possible to identify the majority of them by dot blotting, using PCR and radioactively labeled probes. There will be a few rare β thalassemias in each population that can be analyzed by rapid sequencing methods or, if they are not available, by RFLP linkage analysis or by fetal blood sampling and globin chain synthesis.

The error rate with these different approaches varies, depending on a number of factors, particularly the experience of the laboratory. Fetal blood sampling with globin synthesis analysis is usually associated with an error rate of 2 to 3 per cent, although in very experienced hands this may be reduced to less than 1

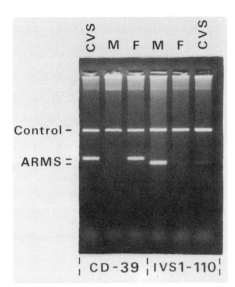

FIGURE 5–20. The rapid prenatal diagnosis of β thalassemia by the ARMS (*a*mplification *r*efractory *m*utation *s*ystem), a development for the rapid identification of mutations based on the polymerase chain reaction. One parent has the common Mediterranean codon 39 (CD) mutation, the other the IVS-1-110-G→A mutation. The fetus is heterozygous for the codon 39 mutation. M = Mother; F = father; CVS = fetal DNA from chorionic villus sampling.

the birth of babies with β thalassemia is a remarkable testament to their effectiveness (Fig. 5–21). The majority of centers that are carrying out this work have switched successfully from fetal blood sampling to DNA diagnostic techniques. Even in less developed parts of the world, provided one center can develop simple dot blot technology, it is possible to establish a prenatal diagnosis program that will cover 80 or 90 per cent of cases. Centers in Greece, Cyprus, and Italy have succeeded in lowering the birth rate of β thalassemic babies to 10 per cent or less of the prescreening levels (see Fig. 5–21).

Major prevention programs have started recently in Israel, China, and Thailand. However, it should be remembered that in many countries, particularly those with large Islamic populations, this approach to the control of genetic disease is incompatible with religious beliefs. This problem is highlighted in the United Kingdom, where there are large Cypriot and Afro-Asian populations; new cases of thalassemia have become very rare in the Cypriot population, but there has been virtually no reduction in the birth of β thalassemic infants in Afro-Asians.

per cent. Low error rates, of less than 1 per cent, have been reported from most laboratories using fetal DNA analysis. Potential sources of error include maternal contamination of fetal DNA, non-paternity, and genetic recombination in cases in which RFLP linkage analysis is used.

Despite the apparent "high technology" of some of these approaches, they have been established successfully in many countries, and the overall reduction in

Treatment

Since the α thalassemias cause either intrauterine death or a relatively mild disorder in adult life, they do not pose a major health burden in countries where they are common. The major public health problem for countries where the thalassemias are common is the management of severe forms of β thalassemia.

FIGURE 5–21. The effects of the development of prenatal diagnosis programs in different countries on the births of homozygous β thalassemic persons. (Reproduced, by permission, from Modell, B., and Bulyzhenkov, V.: Distribution and control of some genetic disorders. World Health Stat. Q. 41:209–218, 1988, Fig. 4, p. 217.)

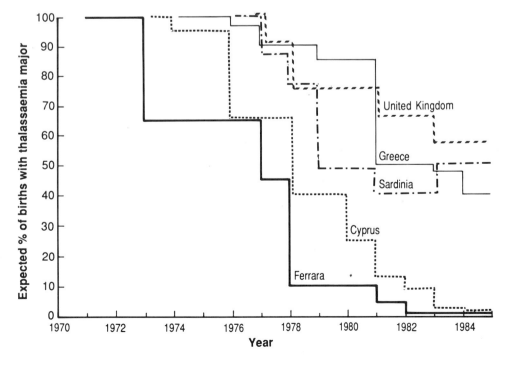

Symptomatic

For many years, the standard approach to managing severe β thalassemia has been regular blood transfusion, chelation therapy to remove excess iron, and the judicious use of splenectomy.[7] Children who are treated in this way survive into adult life, have a normal puberty, and may have children.[211] However, all this is at a great price to both the patients and their families. The only useful form of chelation therapy is desferrioxamine given as an overnight infusion.[212] Many children cannot cope with this regimen and, particularly as they grow older, a high level of noncompliance results.[213] For children who are not able to manage regular chelation therapy, the prognosis is poor and few of them survive after the age of 20 years; death usually results from iron loading of the myocardium and either acute or chronic cardiac failure, often precipitated by infection. The recent development of new families of oral chelating agents may improve the situation,[214] although the safety of these drugs for long-term administration has yet to be determined. For these reasons, the symptomatic treatment of β thalassemia is far from satisfactory.

Marrow Transplantation

In recent years, interest in the use of bone marrow transplantation for β thalassemia has been increasing. Good results have been obtained, provided that the procedure is carried out early in life.[215, 216] Unfortunately, however, successful engraftment requires the availability of a sibling or relative with a complete human leukocyte antigen (HLA) match; therefore, this form of treatment is available only to a limited number of children with thalassemia.

Experimental Approaches

A number of experimental approaches to the management of thalassemia are under evaluation. Since it is clear that the production of high levels of fetal hemoglobin can protect those with β thalassemia, much interest has been generated in finding ways to stimulate Hb F production. The methods being explored are based on earlier observations that there is a transient reversal to fetal hemoglobin synthesis during recovery from marrow suppression after the use of cytotoxic drugs for the treatment of leukemia[217] or after bone marrow transplantation.[218] It is assumed, therefore, that cytotoxic drugs alter the pattern of erythropoiesis in such a way that it favors the expression of the γ globin genes. Several cytotoxic agents have been used, including hydroxyurea and the demethylating agent 5-azacytidine. The current status of these studies has been the subject of a recent review.[219] Although there is no doubt that the use of cytotoxic agents or, under certain circumstances, erythropoietin can produce a significant rise in the number of Hb F–containing reticulocytes and in the level of Hb F, it is still not certain whether this approach will be of value in the management of thalassemia.

The other major area of investigation for the management of the thalassemias and other single-gene disorders is somatic gene therapy. The idea of this therapy is to try to replace or correct defective globin genes in the patient's hematopoietic stem cells. For gene replacement therapy, one or more copies of a normal globin gene would be inserted into the hematopoietic stem cell to produce sufficient amounts of the missing gene product to correct the disorder or at least convert it into a heterozygous phenotype. On the other hand, correction therapy involves lining up a normal globin gene with the defective gene under conditions that would favor a recombination event between the two genes and hence correct the thalassemic defect.

The present status of somatic gene therapy has been the subject of several recent reviews.[220-222] Currently, retroviruses seem to be the most promising vectors for gene transfer. It turns out that the genes for viral proteins, which constitute nearly 80 per cent of the retroviral genome, can be deleted and replaced by DNA sequences encoding the gene to be transferred. Cells containing such a recombinant retrovirus are not able to produce infectious particles unless the structural viral proteins are supplied from elsewhere. This problem has been overcome by the development of specific packaging lines. Bone marrow cells from mice, primates, and humans have been transfected with a variety of retroviral vectors containing different human genes. The results of these experiments have been encouraging. However, the selection of retroviral producer clones on the basis of expression in murine fibroblast cell lines has not always correlated with what happens in primary hematopoietic cells. For example, it has been found that although excellent expression can be obtained in fibroblasts or hematopoietic cell lines, there may be only a low level of expression in primary murine hematopoietic cells.

Further problems have been encountered in obtaining long-term expression of genes introduced into hematopoietic stem cells. Expression has usually been at a low level and in a minority of cell populations, and it is often short lived. A "waxing and waning" phenomenon has been observed, suggesting that only a small number of stem cells have been transfected and that hematopoiesis, at least in the mouse, may reflect the sequential activation of different stem cell clones. It is not yet known whether this phenomenon is relevant to human stem cells. The pluripotent stem cell makes up only a small proportion of bone marrow cells. Furthermore, for successful retroviral transfection these cells must be in cycle; it appears that the bulk of hematopoietic stem cells are out of cycle at any particular time. This finding suggests that the short-lived expression of transfected genes may reflect the fact that the bulk of cells that are transfected are more mature and hence have a limited life span. Some improvements have resulted from the addition of hematopoietic growth factors during infection, and a variety of approaches to select for transfected cells are being explored.

Efforts to insert globin gene sequences into the human β globin locus by site-directed homologous recombination have met with some success, although currently the major difficulty with this approach is its extremely low efficiency.[223]

Although formidable obstacles are still to be overcome in the cell biology of gene therapy, recent successes in defining the major regulatory loci for the α and β globin genes, together with the gradual improvement in the efficiency of gene transfer systems, suggest that it may ultimately be possible to correct some forms of thalassemia. But before this is achieved, it may be necessary to develop better methods for purifying human stem cell populations. Furthermore, the safety of the retroviral approach is still uncertain; although the development of ingenious packaging systems seems to have largely overcome the danger of generating infectious virus particles, some concern about the oncogenic properties of the retrovirus vectors still remains. Perhaps long-term site-directed recombination offers the most attractive approach to gene replacement therapy. It is also possible that with increasing expertise in developing minichromosomes—using the technology of yeast genetics, for example—it may be possible to develop safer and more effective gene transfer systems. But whatever method is successful in the long term, it seems unlikely that gene replacement therapy for β thalassemia will be a major therapeutic option in the immediate future.

REFERENCES

1. Weatherall, D. J.: Toward an understanding of the molecular biology of some common inherited anemias: The story of thalassemia. *In* Wintrobe, M. M. (ed.): Blood, Pure and Eloquent. New York, McGraw-Hill Book Co., 1980, pp. 373–414.
2. Cooley, T. B., and Lee P.: A series of cases of splenomegaly in children with anemia and peculiar bone changes. Trans. Am. Pediatr. Soc. 37:29, 1925.
3. Whipple, G. H., and Bradford, W. L.: Mediterranean disease–thalassemia (erythroblastic anemia of Cooley); associated pigment abnormalities simulating hemochromatosis. J. Pediatr. 9:279, 1933.
4. Pauling, L., Itano, H. A., Singer, S. J., and Wells, I. C.: Sickle-cell anemia, a molecular disease. Science 10:543, 1949.
5. Ingram, V. M., and Stretton, A. O. W.: Genetic basis of the thalassaemia diseases. Nature 184:1903, 1959.
6. Weatherall, D. J., Clegg, J. B., and Naughton, M. A.: Globin synthesis in thalassaemia: An *in vitro* study. Nature 208:1061, 1965.
7. Weatherall, D. J., and Clegg, J. B.: The Thalassaemia Syndromes. 3rd ed. Oxford, England, Blackwell Scientific Publications, 1981.
8. Weatherall, D. J., Clegg, J. B., Higgs, D. R., and Wood, W. G.: The hemoglobinopathies. *In* Scriver, C. R., Beaudet, A. L., Sly, W. S., and Valle, D. (eds.): The Metabolic Basis of Inherited Disease. 6th ed. New York, McGraw-Hill Book Co., 1989, pp. 2281–2366.
9. Higgs, D. R., Vickers, M. A., Wilkie, A. O. M., Pretorius, I.-M., Jarman, A. P., and Weatherall, D. J.: A review of the molecular genetics of the human α globin gene cluster. Blood 73:1081, 1989.
10. Buckle, V. J., Higgs, D. R., Wilkie, A. O. M., Super, M., and Weatherall, D. J.: Localisation of human α globin to 16p 13.3-pter. J. Med. Genet. 25:847, 1988.
11. Wilkie, A. O. M., Higgs, D. R., Rack, K. A., Buckle, V. J., Spurr, N., Fischel-Ghodsian, N., Ceccherini, I., Brown, W. R. A., and Harris, P. C.: Stable length polymorphism of up to 260 kb at the tip of the short arm of chromosome 16. Cell 64:595, 1991.
12. Lauer, J., Shen, C.-K. J., and Maniatis, T.: The chromosomal arrangement of human α-like globin genes: Sequence homology and α-globin gene deletions. Cell 20:119, 1980.
13. Higgs, D. R., Wood, W. G., Jarman, A. P., Sharpe, J., Lida, J., Pretorius, I.-M., and Ayyub, H.: A major positive regulatory region located far upstream of the human α-globin gene locus. Genes Dev. 4:1588, 1990.
14. Higgs, D. R., Wainscoat, J. S., Flint, J., Hill, A. V. S., Thein, S. L., Nicholls, R. D., Teal, H., Ayyub, H., Peto, T. E. A., Jarman, A., Clegg, J. B., and Weatherall D. J.: Analysis of the human α globin gene cluster reveals a highly informative genetic locus. Proc. Natl. Acad. Sci. USA 83:5165, 1986.
15. Jarman, A. P., and Higgs, D. R.: A new hypervariable marker for the human α-globin gene cluster. Am. J. Hum. Genet. 42:2490, 1988.
16. Higgs, D. R., Ayyub, H., Clegg, J. B., Hill, A. V. S., Nicholls, R. D., Teal, H., Wainscoat, J. S., and Weatherall, D. J.: α-Thalassaemia in British people. Br. Med. J. 290:1303, 1985.
17. Nicholls, R. D., Fischel-Ghodsian, N., and Higgs, D. R.: Recombination at the human α-globin gene cluster: Sequence features and topological constraints. Cell 49:369, 1987.
18. Vanin, E. F., Henthorn, P. S., Kioussis, G., Grosveld, F., and Smithies, O.: Unexpected relationships between four large deletions in the human β-globin gene cluster. Cell 35:701, 1983.
19. Meuth, M.: Illegitimate recombination in mammalian cells. *In* Berg, D., Howe, M. (eds.): Mobile DNA. Washington, D.C., American Society of Microbiology, 1988.
20. Wilkie, A. O. M., Lamb, J., Harris, P. C., Finney, R. D., and Higgs, D. R.: A truncated human chromosome 16 associated with α thalassaemia is stabilized by addition of telomeric repeat $(TTAGGG)_n$. Nature 346:868, 1990.
21. Hatton, C. S. R., Wilkie, A. O. M., Drysdale, H. C., Wood, W. G., Vickers, M. A., Sharpe, J., Ayyub, H., Pretorius, I.-M., Buckle, V. J., and Higgs, D. R.: α-Thalassaemia caused by a large (62 kb) deletion upstream of the human α globin gene cluster. Blood 76:221, 1990.
22. Liebhaber, S. A., Griese, E.-U., Weiss, I., Cash, F. E., Ayyub, H., Higgs, D. R., and Horst, J.: Inactivation of human α-globin gene expression by a *de novo* deletion located upstream of the α-globin gene cluster. Proc. Natl. Acad. Sci. USA 87:9431, 1990.
23. Romao, L., Osorio-Almeida, L., Higgs, D. R., Lavinha, J., and Liebhaber, S. A.: α-Thalassaemia resulting from deletion of regulatory sequences far upstream of the α-globin structural gene. Blood 78:1589, 1991.
24. Embury, S. H., Miller, J. A., Dozy, A. M., Kan, Y. W., Chan, V., and Todd, D.: Two different molecular organizations account for the single α-globin gene of the α-thalassemia-2 genotype. J. Clin. Invest. 66:1319, 1980.
25. Higgs, D. R., Old, J. M., Pressley, L., Clegg, J. B., and Weatherall, D. J.: A novel α-globin gene arrangement in man. Nature 284:632, 1980.
26. Goossens, M., Dozy, A. M., Embury, S. H., Zachariades, Z., Hadjiminas, M. G., Stamatoyannopoulos, G., and Kan, Y. W.: Triplicated α-globin loci in humans. Proc. Natl. Acad. Sci. USA 77:518, 1980.
27. Trent, R. J., Higgs, D. R., Clegg, J. B., and Weatherall, D. J.: A new triplicated α-globin gene arrangement in man. Br. J. Haematol. 49:149, 1981.
28. Lie-Injo, L. E., Herrera, A. R., and Kan, Y. W.: Two types of triplicated α globin loci in humans. Nucleic Acids Res. 9:3707, 1981.
29. Gu, Y. C., Landman, H., and Huisman, T. H. J.: Two different quadruplicated α globin gene arrangements. Br. J. Haematol. 66:245, 1987.
30. Higgs, D. R., Hill, A. V. S., Bowden, D. K., Weatherall, D. J., and Clegg, J. B.: Independent recombination events be-

tween duplicated human α globin genes: Implications for their concerted evolution. Nucleic Acids Res. 12:6965, 1984.

31. Kulozik, A., Kar, B. C., Serjeant, B. E., Serjeant, G. R., and Weatherall, D. J.: The molecular basis of α-thalassemia in India: Its interaction with sickle cell disease. Blood 71:467, 1988.

32. Bowden, D. K., Hill, A. V. S., Higgs, D. R., Oppenheimer, S. J., Weatherall, D. J., and Clegg J. B.: Different hematologic phenotypes are associated with leftward ($-\alpha^{4.2}$) and rightward ($-\alpha^{3.7}$) α^+-thalassemia deletions. J. Clin. Invest. 79:39, 1987.

33. Liebhaber, S. A., Cash, F. E., and Main, D. M.: Compensatory increase in α1-globin gene expression in individuals heterozygous for the α-thalassemia-2 deletion. J. Clin. Invest. 76:1057, 1985.

34. Pirastu, M., Saglio, G., Chang, J. C., Cao, A., and Kan Y. W.: Initiation codon mutation as a cause of α thalassemia. J. Biol. Chem. 259:12315, 1984.

35. Moi, P., Cash, F. E., Liebhaber, S. A., Cao, A., and Pirastu, M.: An initiation codon mutation (AUG→GUG) of the human α1-globin gene: Structural characterisation and evidence for a mild thalassemic phenotype. J. Clin. Invest. 80:1416, 1987.

35a. Morle, F., Lopez, B., Henni, T., and Godet, J.: α-Thalassaemia associated with the deletion of two nucleotides at position -2 and -3 preceding the AUG codon. EMBO J. 4:1245, 1985.

36. Weatherall, D. J., and Clegg, J. B.: The α-chain termination mutants and their relationship to the α-thalassaemias. Philos. Trans. R. Soc. Lond. [Biol.] 271:411, 1975.

37. Milner, P. F., Clegg, J. B., and Weatherall, D. J.: Haemoglobin H disease due to a unique haemoglobin variant with an elongated α chain. Lancet 1:729, 1971.

38. Clegg, J. B., Weatherall, D. J., Contopoulos-Griva, I., Caroutsos, K., Poungouras, P., and Tsevrenis, H.: Haemoglobin Icaria, a new chain termination mutant which causes α-thalassaemia. Nature 251:245, 1974.

39. De Jong, W. W., Khan, P. M., and Bernini, L. F.: Hemoglobin Koya Dora; high frequency of a chain termination mutant. Am. J. Hum. Genet. 27:81, 1975.

40. Bradley, T. B., Wohl, R. C., and Smith, G. J.: Elongation of the α-globin chain in a black family: Interaction with Hb G Philadelphia. Clin. Res. 23:131, 1975.

41. Liebhaber, S. A., Coleman, M. B., Adams, J. G., III, Cash, F. E., and Steinberg, M. H.: Molecular basis for non-deletion α-thalassemia in American blacks α2$^{116GAG→UAG}$. J. Clin. Invest. 80:154, 1987.

42. Orkin, S. H., Goff, S. C., and Hechtman, R. L.: Mutation in an intervening sequence splice junction in man. Proc. Natl. Acad. Sci. USA 78:5041, 1981.

43. Felber, B. K., Orkin, S. H., and Hamer, D. H.: Abnormal RNA splicing causes one form of α thalassemia. Cell 29:895, 1982.

44. Higgs, D. R., Goodbourn, S. E. Y., Lamb, J., Clegg, J. B., Weatherall, D. J., and Proudfoot, N. J.: α-Thalassaemia caused by a polyadenylation signal mutation. Nature 306:398, 1983.

45. Thein, S. L., Wallace, R. B., Pressley, L., Clegg, J. B., Weatherall, D. J., and Higgs, D. R.: The polyadenylation site mutation in the α-globin gene cluster. Blood 71:313, 1988.

46. Adams, J. G., III, and Coleman, M. B.: Structural hemoglobin variants that produce the phenotype of thalassemia. Semin. Hematol. 27:229, 1990.

47. Galanello, R., Paglietti, E., Melis, M. A., Giagu, L., and Cao, A.: Hemoglobin inclusions in heterozygous α-thalassemia according to their α-globin genotype. Acta Haematol. 72:34, 1984.

48. Pootrakul, S., Wasi, P., and Na-Nakorn, S.: Haemoglobin Bart's hydrops foetalis in Thailand. Ann. Hum. Genet. 30:283, 1967.

49. Sharma, R. S., Yu, V., and Walters, W. A. W.: Haemoglobin Bart's hydrops fetalis syndrome in an infant of Greek origin and prenatal diagnosis of alpha-thalassaemia. Med. J. Aust. 2:404, 1979.

50. Todd D.: Personal communication, 1987.

51. Beaudry, M. A., Ferguson, D. J., Pearse, K., Yanofsky, R. A., Rubin, E. M., and Kan, Y. W.: Survival of a hydropic infant with homozygous α-thalassemia-1. J. Pediatr. 108:713, 1986.

52. Bianchi, D. W., Beyer, E. C., Start, A. R., Saffan, D., Sachs, B. P., and Wolfe L.: Normal long-term survival with α-thalassemia. J. Pediatr. 108:716, 1986.

53. Liang, S. T., Wong, V. C. W., So, W. W. K., Ma, H. K., Chan, V., and Todd, D.: Homozygous α-thalassaemia: Clinical presentation, diagnosis and management. A review of 46 cases. Br. J. Obstet. Gynaecol. 92:680, 1985.

54. Pressley, L., Higgs, D. R., Clegg, J. B., Perrine, R. P., Pembrey, M. E., and Weatherall D. J.: A new genetic basis for hemoglobin-H disease. N. Engl. J. Med. 303:1383, 1980.

55. Henni, T., Morle, F., Lopez, B., Colonna, P., and Godet, J.: α-Thalassemia haplotypes in the Algerian population. Hum. Genet. 75:272, 1987.

56. Galanello, R., Pirastu, M., Melis, M. A., Paglietti, E., Moi, P., and Cao, A.: Phenotype-genotype correlation in haemoglobin H disease in childhood. J. Med. Genet. 20:425, 1983.

57. Winichagoon, P., Adirojnanon, P., and Wasi, P.: Levels of haemoglobin H and proportions of red cells with inclusion bodies in the two types of haemoglobin H disease. Br. J. Haematol. 46:507, 1980.

58. Pootrakul, P., Winichagoon, P., Fucharoen, S., Pravatmuang, P., Piankijagum, A., and Wasi, P.: Homozygous haemoglobin Constant Spring: A need for revision of concept. Hum. Genet. 59:250, 1981.

59. Derry, S., Wood, W. G., Pippard, M., Clegg, J. B., Weatherall, D. J., Wickramasinghe, S., Darley, J., Winichagoon, P., and Wasi, P.: Hematologic and biosynthetic studies in homozygous hemoglobin Constant Spring. J. Clin. Invest. 73:1673, 1984.

60. Higgs, D. R., and Weatherall, D. J.: α-Thalassemia. In Piomelli, S, and Yachnin, S (eds.): Current Topics in Hematology. 4th ed. New York, Alan R. Liss, 1983, pp. 37–97.

61. Higgs, D. R., Aldridge, B. E., Lamb, J., Clegg, J. B., Weatherall, D. J., Hayes, R. J., Grandison, Y., Lowrie, Y., Mason, K. P., Serjeant, B. E., and Serjeant, G. R.: The interaction of alpha-thalassemia and homozygous sickle-cell disease. N. Engl. J. Med. 306:1441, 1982.

61a. Noguchi, C. T., Dover, G. J., Rodgers, G. P., Serjeant, G. R., Antonarakis, S. E., Anagnou, N. P., Higgs D. R., Weatherall, D. J., and Schechter A. N.: α Thalassemia changes erythrocyte heterogeneity in sickle cell disease. J. Clin. Invest. 75:1632, 1985.

62. Flint, J., Hill, A. V. S., Bowden, D. K., Oppenheimer, S. J., Sill, P. R., Serjeantson, S. W., Bana-Koiri, J., Bhatia, K., Alpers, M. P., Boyce, A. J., Weatherall, D. J., and Clegg, J. B.: High frequencies of α thalassemia are the result of natural selection by malaria. Nature 321:744, 1986.

63. Flint, J., Hill, A. V. S., Weatherall, D. J., Clegg, J. B., and Higgs, D. R.: Alpha globin genotypes in two North European populations. Br. J. Haematol. 63:796, 1986.

64. O'Shaughnessy, D. F., Hill, A. V. S., Bowden, D. K., Weatherall, D. J., and Clegg, J. B.: Globin genes in Micronesia: Origin and affinities of Pacific island peoples. Am. J. Hum. Genet. 46:144, 1990.

65. Luzzi, G. A., Merry, A. H., Newbold, C. I., Marsh, K., Pasvol, G., and Weatherall, D. J.: Surface antigen expression on Plasmodium falciparum–infected erythrocytes is modified in α- and β-thalassaemia. J. Exp. Med. 173:785, 1991.

66. Weatherall, D. J., Higgs, D. R., Bunch, C., Old, J. B., Hunt, D. M., Pressley, L., Clegg, J. B., Bethlenfalvay, N. C., Sjolin, S., Koler, R. D., Magenic, E., Francis, J. L., and Bebbington, D.: Hemoglobin H disease and mental retardation. A new syndrome or a remarkable coincidence? N. Engl. J. Med. 305:607, 1981.

67. Hutz, M. H., Marmitt, C. R., Schuler, L., and Salzano, F. M.: Hereditary anemias in Brazil—new case of Hb H disease with mental retardation (abstract). Seventh International Congress of Human Genetics, Berlin, 1986, p. 458.

68. Bowcock, A. M., Tonder, S. V., and Jenkins, T.: The hemoglobin H disease mental retardation syndrome: Molecular

studies on the South African case. Br. J. Haematol. 56:69, 1984.

69. Wilkie, A. O. M., Buckle, V. J., Harris, P. C., Lamb, J., Bartin, N. J., Reeders, S. T., Lindenbaum, R. H., Nicholls, R. D., Barrow, M., Bethlenfalvay, N. C., Hutz, M. H., Tolmie, J. L., Weatherall, D. J., and Higgs D. R.: Clinical features and molecular analysis of the α thalassemia/mental retardation syndromes. I. Cases due to deletions involving chromosome band 16p13.3. Am. J. Hum. Genet. 46:1112, 1990.

70. Wilkie, A. O. M., Zeitlin, H. C., Lindenbaum, R. H., Buckle, V. J., Fischel-Ghodsian, N., Chui, D. H. K., Gardner-Medwin, D., MacGillivray, M. H., Weatherall, D. J., and Higgs, D. R.: Clinical features and molecular analysis of the α thalassemia/mental retardation syndromes. II. Cases without detectable abnormality of the α globin complex. Am. J. Hum. Genet. 46:1127, 1990.

71. Gibbons, R. J., Wilkie, A. O. M., Weatherall, D. J., and Higgs, D. R.: A newly defined X-linked mental retardation syndrome associated with α thalassaemia. J. Med. Genet. 28:729, 1991.

72. Higgs, D. R., Wood, W. G., Barton, C., and Weatherall, D. J.: Clinical features and molecular analysis of acquired Hb H disease. Am. J. Med. 75:181, 1983.

73. Anagnou, N. P., Ley, T. J., Chesbro, B., Wright, G., Kitchens, C., Liebhaber, S., Nienhuis, A. W., and Deisseroth, A. B.: Acquired α-thalassemia in preleukemia is due to decreased expression of all four α-globin genes. Proc. Natl. Acad. Sci. USA 80:6051, 1983.

74. Orkin, S. H., Kazazian, H. H., Jr., Antonarakis, S. E., Goff, S. C., Boehm, C. D., Sexton, J. P., Waber, P. G., and Giardina, P. J. V.: Linkage of β-thalassemic mutations and β-globin gene polymorphisms with DNA polymorphisms in the human β-globin gene cluster. Nature 296:727, 1982.

75. Grosveld, F., van Assendelft, G. B., Greaves, D. R., and Kollias, G.: Position-independent, high-level expression of the human β-globin gene in transgenic mice. Cell 51:975, 1987.

76. Kazazian, H. H., and Boehm, C. D.: Molecular basis and prenatal diagnosis of β-thalassemia. Blood 72:1107, 1988.

77. Kazazian, H. H.: The thalassemia syndromes: Molecular basis and prenatal diagnosis in 1990. Semin. Hematol. 27:209, 1990.

78. Thein, S. L., Old, J. M., Wainscoat, J. S., and Weatherall D. J.: Population and genetic studies suggest a single origin for the Indian deletion β⁰ thalassemia. Br. J. Haematol. 57:271, 1984.

79. Anand, R., Boehm, C. D., Kazazian, H. H., Jr., and Vanin, E. F.: Molecular characterization of a β⁰-thalassemia resulting from a 1.4 kb deletion. Blood 72:636, 1988.

80. Aulehla-Scholtz, C., Spielberg, R., and Horst, J.: A β-thalassemia mutant caused by a 300 bp deletion in the human β-globin gene. Hum. Genet. 81:298, 1989.

81. Diaz-Chico, J. C., Yang, K. G., Kutlar, A., Reese, A. L., Aksoy, M., and Huisman, T. H. J.: A 300 bp deletion involving part of the 5′ β-globin gene region is observed in members of a Turkish family with β-thalassemia. Blood 70:583, 1987.

82. Gilman, J. G.: The 12.6 kilobase deletion in Dutch β⁰-thalassemia. Br. J. Haematol. 67:369, 1987.

83. Padanilam, B. J., Felice, A. E., and Huisman, T. H. J.: Partial deletion of the 5′ β-globin gene region causes β⁰-thalassemia in members of an American black family. Blood 64:941, 1984.

84. Popovich, B. W., Rosenblatt, D. S., Kendall, A. G., and Nishioka, Y.: Molecular characterization of an atypical β-thalassemia caused by a large deletion in the 5′ β-globin gene region. Am. J. Hum. Genet. 39:797, 1986.

85. Antonarakis, S. E., Orkin, S. H., Cheng, T.-C., Scott, A. F., Sexton, J. P., Trusco, S. P., Charache, S., and Kazazian, H. H.: β-Thalassemia in American blacks: Novel mutations in the TATA box and IVS-2 acceptor splice site. Proc. Natl. Acad. Sci. USA 81:1154, 1984.

86. Orkin, S. H., Antonarakis, S. E., and Kazazian, H. H., Jr.: Base substitution at position −88 in a β-thalassemic globin gene: Further evidence for the role of distal promoter element ACACCC. J. Biol. Chem. 259:8679, 1984.

87. Orkin, S. H., Sexton, J. P., Cheng, T.-C., Goff, S., Giardina, P. J. V., Lee, J. I., and Kazazian, H. H.: ATA box transcription mutation in β-thalassemia. Nucleic Acids Res. 11:4727, 1983.

88. Gonzalez-Redondo, J. H., Stoming, T. A., Kutlar, F., Lanclos, K. D., Howard, E. F., Fei, Y. J., Aksoy, M., Altay, C., Gurgey, A., Basak, A. N., Efremov, G. D., Petkov, G., and Huisman, T. H. J.: A C→T substitution at nt −101 in a conserved DNA sequence of the promoter region of the β-globin gene is associated with "silent" β-thalassemia. Blood 73:1705, 1989.

89. Kazazian, H. H., Jr., Orkin, S. H., Antonarakis, S. E., Sexton, J. P., Boehm, C. D., Goff, S. C., and Waber, P. G.: Molecular characterization of seven β-thalassemia mutations in Asian Indians. EMBO J. 3:593, 1984.

90. Cheng, T., Orkin, S. H., Antonarakis, S. E., Potter, M. J., Sexton, J. P., Markham, A. F., Giardina, P. J. V., Lia, A., and Kazazian, H. H.: β-Thalassemia in Chinese: Use of in vivo RNA analysis and oligonucleotide hybridization in systematic characterization of molecular defects. Proc. Natl. Acad. Sci. USA 81:2821, 1984.

91. Gonzalez-Redondo, J. H., Stoming, T. A., Lanclos, K. D., Gu, Y. C., Kutlar, A., Kutlar, F., Nakasuji, T., Deng, B., Han, I. S., McKie, V. C., and Huisman, T. H. J.: Clinical and genetic heterogeneity in Black patients with homozygous β-thalassemia from the Southeastern United States. Blood 72:1007, 1988.

92. Hill, A. V. S., Bowden, D. K., O'Shaughnessy, D. F., Weatherall, D. J., and Clegg, J. B.: β-Thalassemia in Melanesia: Association with malaria and characterization of a common variant. Blood 72:9, 1988.

93. Lapoumeroulie, C., Pagnier, J., Bank, A., Labie, D., and Krishnamoorthy, R.: β-Thalassemia due to a novel mutation in IVS-1 sequence donor site consensus sequence creating a restriction site. Biochem. Biophys. Res. Commun. 139:709, 1986.

94. Tamagnini, G. P., Lopes, M. C., Castanheira, M. E., Wainscoat, J. S., and Wood, W. G.: β⁺ Thalassaemia—Portuguese type: Clinical, haematological and molecular studies of a newly defined form of β thalassaemia. Br. J. Haematol. 54:189, 1983.

95. Goldsmith, M. E., Humphries, R. K., Ley, T., Cline, A., Kantor, J. A., and Nienhuis, A. W.: Silent substitution in β⁺-thalassemia gene activating a cryptic splice site in β-globin RNA coding sequence. Proc. Natl. Acad. Sci. USA 80:2318, 1983.

96. Yang, K. G., Kutlar, F., George, E., Wilson, J. B., Kutlar, A., Stoming, T. A., Gonzalez-Redondo, J. M., and Huisman, T. H. J.: Molecular characterization of β-globin gene mutations in Malay patients with Hb E-β-thalassaemia and thalassaemia major. Br. J. Haematol. 72:73, 1989.

97. Orkin, S. H., Kazazian, H. H., Jr., Antonarakis, S. E., Oster, H., Goff, S. C., and Sexton, J. P.: Abnormal RNA processing due to the exon mutation of the βᴱ-globin gene. Nature 300:768, 1982.

98. Orkin, S. H., Antonarakis, S. E., and Loukopoulos, D.: Abnormal processing of βᴷⁿᵒˢˢᵒˢ RNA. Blood 64:311, 1984.

99. Spritz, R. A., Jagadeeswaran, P., Choudary, P. V., Biro, P. A., Elder, J. D., de Riel, J. K., Manley, J. L., Gefter, M. L., Forget, B. G., and Weissman, S. M.: Base substitution in an intervening sequence of a β⁺-thalassemic human globin gene. Proc. Natl. Acad. Sci. USA 78:2455, 1981.

100. Westaway, D., and Williamson, R.: An intron nucleotide sequence variant in a cloned β⁺-thalassemia globin gene. Nucleic Acids Res. 9:1777, 1981.

101. Orkin, S. H., Cheng, T.-C., Antonarakis, S. E., and Kazazian, H. H.: Thalassemia due to a mutation in the cleavage-polyadenylation signal of the human β-globin gene. EMBO J. 4:4543, 1985.

102. Jankovic, L., Efremov, G. D., Petkov, G., Kattamis, C., George, E., Yang, K.-G., Stoming, T. A., and Huisman, T. H. J.: Three novel mutations leading to β-thalassemia. Blood 24:226A, 1989.

103. Rund, D., Filon, D., Rachmilewitz, E. A., Cohan, T., Dowling,

C., Kazazian, H. H., and Oppenheim, A.: Molecular analysis of β-thalassemia in Kurdish Jews: Novel mutations and expression studies. Blood 74:821A, 1989.

104. Wong, C., Antonarakis, S. E., Goff, S. C., Orkin, S. H., Boehm, C. D., and Kazazian, H. H.: On the origin and spread of β-thalassemia: Recurrent observation of four mutations in different ethnic groups. Proc. Natl. Acad. Sci. USA 83:6529, 1986.

105. Trecartin, R. F., Liebhaber, S. A., Chang, J. C., Lee, K. Y., Kan, Y. W., Furbetta, A., Angius, A., and Cao, A.: β⁰-Thalassemia in Sardinia is caused by a nonsense mutation. J. Clin. Invest. 68:1012, 1981.

106. Chang, J. C., and Kan, Y. W.: β⁰-Thalassemia, a nonsense mutation in man. Proc. Natl. Acad. Sci. USA 76:2886, 1979.

107. Takeshita, K., Forget, B. G., Scarpa, A., and Benz, E. J.: Intranuclear defect in β globin mRNA accumulation to a premature termination codon. Blood 64:13, 1984.

108. Humphries, R. K., Ley, T. J., Anagnou, N. P., Baur, A. W., and Nienhuis A. W.: β⁰-39-thalassemia gene: A premature termination codon causes β mRNA deficiency without changing cytoplasmic β mRNA stability. Blood 64:23, 1984.

109. Adams, J. G., Steinberg, M. H., Boxer, L. A., Baehner, R. L., Forget, B. G., and Tsistrakis, G. A.: The structure of hemoglobin Indianapolis [beta 112(G14) arginine]. An unstable variant detectable only by isotopic labeling. J. Biol. Chem. 254:3479, 1979.

110. Kobayashi, Y., Fukumaki, Y., Komatsu, N., Ohba, Y., Miyaji, T., and Miura, Y.: A novel globin structural mutant, Showa-Yakushiki (β¹¹⁰ Leu→Pro) causing a β-thalassemia phenotype. Blood 70:1688, 1987.

111. Hall, G. W., Franklin, I. M., Sura, T., and Thein, S. L.: A novel mutation (nonsense β127) in exon 3 of the β globin gene produces a variable thalassaemia phenotype. Br. J. Haematol. 79:342, 1991.

112. Park, S. S., Barnetson, R., Kim, S. W., Weatherall, D. J., and Thein, S. L.: A spontaneous deletion of β33/34 val in exon 2 of the β globin gene (Hb Korea) produces the phenotype of dominant β thalassaemia. Br. J. Haematol. 78:581, 1991.

113. Bunn, H., and Forget, B. G.: Hemoglobin: Molecular, Genetic and Clinical Aspects. Philadelphia, W. B. Saunders Co., 1986.

114. Fessas, P.: Inclusions of hemoglobin in erythroblasts and erythrocytes of thalassemia. Blood 21:21, 1963.

115. Wickramasinghe, S. N., and Hughes, M.: Some features of bone marrow macrophages in patients with homozygous β-thalassaemia. Br. J. Haematol. 38:23, 1978.

116. Yataganas, X., and Fessas, P.: The pattern of hemoglobin precipitation in thalassemia and its significance. Ann. N. Y. Acad. Sci. 165:270, 1969.

117. Finch, C. A., Deubelbeiss, K., Cook, J. D., Eschbach, J. W., Harker, L. A., Funk, D. D., Marsaglia, G., Hillman, R. S., Slichter, S., Adamson, J. W., Ganzoni, A., and Giblett, E. R.: Ferrokinetics in man. Medicine (Balt) 49:17, 1970.

118. Chalevelakis, G., Clegg, J. B., and Weatherall, D. J.: Imbalanced globin chain synthesis in heterozygous β-thalassemic bone marrow. Proc. Natl. Acad. Sci. USA 72:3853, 1975.

119. Nathan, D. G., Stossel, T. B., Gunn, R. B., Zarkowsky, H. S., and Laforet, M. T.: Influence of hemoglobin precipitation in alpha and beta thalassemia J. Clin. Invest. 48:33, 1969.

120. Shinar, E., and Rachmilewitz, E. A.: Differences in the pathophysiology of hemolysis of α- and β-thalassemic red blood cells. Ann. N. Y. Acad. Sci. 612:106, 1990.

121. Gabuzda, T. G., Nathan, D. G., and Gardner, F. H.: The turnover of hemoglobins A, F and A₂ in the peripheral blood of three patients with thalassemia. J. Clin. Invest. 42:1678, 1963.

122. Loukopoulos, D., and Fessas, P.: The distribution of hemoglobin types in thalassemic erythrocyte. J. Clin. Invest. 44:231, 1965.

123. Nathan, D. G., and Gunn, R. B.: Thalassemia: The consequences of unbalanced hemoglobin synthesis. Am. J. Med. 41:815, 1966.

124. Camaschella, C., Alfarano, A., Gottardi, E., Serra, A., Revello,

D., and Saglio, G.: The homozygous state for the −87 C→G β⁺ thalassemia. Br. J. Haematol. 75:132, 1990.

125. Thein, S. L., Hesketh, C., Brown, J. M., Anstey, A. V., and Weatherall, D. J.: Molecular characterisation of a high A₂ β thalassemia by direct sequencing of single strand enriched amplified genomic DNA. Blood 73:924, 1989.

126. Wainscoat, J. S., Thein, S. L., Higgs, D. R., Bell, J. I., Weatherall, D. J., Al-Awamy, B., and Serjeant, G.: A genetic marker for elevated levels of haemoglobin F in homozygous sickle cell disease. Br. J. Haematol. 60:261, 1985.

127. Gilman, J. G., and Huisman, T. H. J.: DNA sequence variation associated with elevated fetal ᴳγ globin production. Blood 66:783, 1985.

128. Thein, S. L., Sampietro, M., Old, J. M., Cappellini, M. D., Fiorelli, G., Modell, B., and Weatherall, D. J.: Association of thalassaemia intermedia with a beta-globin gene halpotype. Br. J. Haematol. 65:3670, 1987.

129. Thein, S. L., Hesketh, C., Wallace, R. B., and Weatherall, D. J.: The molecular basis of thalassaemia major and thalassaemia intermedia in Asian Indians: Application to prenatal diagnosis. Br. J. Haematol. 70:225, 1988.

130. Diaz-Chico, J. C., Yang, K. G., Stoming, T. A., Efremov, D. G., Kutlar, A., Kutlar, F., Aksoy, N., Altay, C., Gurgey, A., Kining, Y., and Huisman, T. H. J.: Mild and severe β-thalassemia among homozygotes from Turkey: Identification of the types by hybridization of amplified DNA with synthetic probes. Blood 71:248, 1988.

131. Kulozik, A. E., Wainscoat, J. S., Serjeant, G. R., Al-Awamy, B., Essan, F., Falusi, Y., Haque, S. K., Hilali, A. M., Kate, S., Sanasinghe, W. A. E. P., and Weatherall, D. J.: Geographical survey of βˢ-globin gene haplotypes: Evidence for an independent Asian origin of the sickle-cell mutation. Am. J. Hum. Genet. 39:239, 1986.

132. Nagel, R. L., Fabry, M. E., Pagnier, J., Zohoun, I., Wajcman, H., Baudin, V., and Labie, D.: Hematologically and genetically distinct forms of sickle cell anemia in Africa. N. Engl. J. Med. 312:880, 1985.

133. Labie, D., Dunda-Belkhodja, O., Rouabhi, F., Pagnier, J., Ragusa, A., and Nagel, R. L.: The −158 site 5' to the ᴳγ gene and ᴳγ expression. Blood 66:1463, 1985.

134. Kulozik, A. E., Kar, B. C., Satapathy, R. K., Serjeant, B. E., Serjeant, G. R., and Weatherall, D. J.: Fetal hemoglobin levels and βˢ globin haplotypes in an Indian population with sickle cell disease. Blood 69:1742, 1987.

135. Kulozik, A. E., Thein, S. L., Kar, B. C., Wainscoat, J. S., Serjeant, G. R., and Weatherall, D. J.: Raised Hb F levels in sickle cell disease are caused by a determinant linked to the β globin gene cluster. In Stamatoyannopoulos, G. (ed.): Hemoglobin Switching. 5th ed. New York, Alan R. Liss, 1987, pp. 427–439.

136. Miller, B. A., Salameh, M., Ahmen, M., Wainscoat, J. S., Antognetti, G., Orkin, S., Weatherall, D. J., and Nathan, D. G.: High fetal hemoglobin production in sickle cell anemia in the eastern province of Saudi Arabia is genetically determined. Blood 67:1404, 1986.

137. Zago, M. A., Wood, W. G., Clegg, J. B., Weatherall, D. J., O'Sullivan, M., and Gunson, H. H.: Genetic control of F-cells in human adults. Blood 53:977, 1979.

138. Wood, W. G., Weatherall, D. J., and Clegg, J. B.: Interaction of heterocellular hereditary persistence of foetal haemoglobin with β thalassaemia and sickle cell anaemia. Nature 264:247, 1976.

139. Cappellini, M. D., Fiorelli, G., and Bernini, L. F.: Interaction between homozygous β⁰ thalassaemia and the Swiss type of hereditary persistence of fetal haemoglobin. Br. J. Haematol. 48:561, 1981.

140. Jeffreys, A. J., Wilson, V., Thein, S. L., Weatherall, D. J., and Ponder, B. A. J.: DNA "fingerprints" and segregation analysis of multiple markers in human pedigrees. Am. J. Hum. Genet. 39:11, 1986.

141. Miyoshi, K., Kaneto, Y., Kawai, H., Ohchi, H., Niki, S., Haseqawa, K., Shirakami, A., and Yamano, T.: X-linked dominant control of F cells in normal adult life: Characterization of the Swiss type as hereditary persistence of fetal

hemoglobin regulated dominantly by gene(s) on X-chromosome. Blood 72:1854, 1988.

142. Wainscoat, J. S., Thein, S. L., and Weatherall, D. J.: Thalassaemia intermedia. Blood Rev. 1:273, 1987.

143. Weatherall, D. J., Pressley, L., Wood, W. G., Higgs, D. R., and Clegg, J. B.: The molecular basis for mild forms of homozygous β thalassaemia. Lancet 1:527, 1981.

144. Wainscoat, J. S., Old, J. M., Weatherall, D. J., and Orkin, S. H.: The molecular basis for the clinical diversity of β thalassaemia in Cypriots. Lancet 1:1235, 1983.

145. Kanavakis E., Wainscoat, J. S., Wood, W. G., Weatherall, D. J., Cao, A., Furbeta, M., Galanello, R., Georgiou, D., and Sophocleous, T.: The interaction of α thalassaemia with heterozygous β thalassaemia. Br. J. Haematol. 52:465, 1982.

146. Rosatelli, C., Falchi, A. M., Scalas, M. T., Tuveri, T., Furbetta, M., and Cao, A.: Hematological phenotype of double heterozygous state for alpha and beta thalassemia. Hemoglobin 8:25, 1984.

147. Wainscoat, J. S., Bell, J. I., Old, J. M., Weatherall, D. J., Furbetta, M., Galanello, R., and Cao, A.: Globin gene mapping studies in Sardinian patients homozygous for β⁰ thalassaemia. Mol. Biol. Med. 1:1, 1983.

148. Wainscoat, J. S., Kanavakis, E., Wood, W. G., Letsky, E. A., Huehns, E. R., Marsh, G. W., Higgs, D. R., Clegg, J. B., and Weatherall, D. J.: Thalassaemia intermedia in Cyprus—the interaction of α- and β-thalassaemia. Br. J. Haematol. 53:411, 1983.

149. Semenza, G. L., Delgrosso, K., Poncz, M., Malladi, P., Schwartz, E., and Surrey, S.: The silent carrier allele: β-Thalassaemia without a mutation in the β-globin gene or its immediate flanking regions. Cell 39:123, 1984.

150. Kanavakis, E., Metaxatou-Mavromati, A., Kattamis, C., Wainscoat, J. S., and Wood, W. G.: The triplicated α gene locus and β thalassaemia. Br. J. Haematol. 54:201, 1983.

151. Sampietro, M., Cazzola, M., Cappellini, M. D., and Fiorelli, G.: The triplicated alpha-gene locus and heterozygous beta thalassaemia: A case of thalassaemia intermedia. Br. J. Haematol. 55:709, 1983.

152. Kulozik, A. E., Thein, S. L., Wainscoat, J. S., Gale, R., Kay, L., Weatherall, D. J., Wood, J. K., and Huehns, E. R.: Thalassaemia intermedia: Interaction of the triple α-globin gene arrangement and heterozygous β-thalassaemia. Br. J. Haematol. 66:109, 1987.

153. Camaschella, C., Bertero, M. T., Serra, A., Dall'Acqua, M., Gasparini, P., Trento, M., Vettore, L., Perona, G., Saglio, G., and Mazza, U.: A benign form of thalassemia intermedia may be determined by the interaction of triplicated α locus and heterozygous β thalassemia. Br. J. Haematol. 66:103, 1987.

154. Galanello, R., Ruggeri, R., Paglietti, E., Addis, M., Melis, A., and Cao, A.: A family with segregating triplicated alpha globin loci and beta thalassemia. Blood 62:1035, 1983.

155. Thein, S. L., Hesketh, C., Taylor, P., Temperley, P., Hutchison, R. M., Old, J. M., Wood, W. G., Clegg, J. B., and Weatherall, D. J.: Molecular basis for dominantly inherited inclusion body β thalassemia. Proc. Natl. Acad. Sci. USA 87:3924, 1990.

156. Beris, R. P., Miescher, P. A., Diaz-Chico, J. C., Han, I.-S., Kutlar, A., Hu, H., Wilson, J. B., and Huisman, T. H. J.: Inclusion body β-thalassemia trait in a Swiss family is caused by an abnormal hemoglobin (Geneva) with an altered and extended β chain carboxy-terminus due to a modification in codon β114. Blood 72:801, 1988.

157. Kazazian, H. H., Jr., Dowling, C. E., Hurwitz, R. L., Coleman, M., and Adams, J. G., III: Thalassemia mutations in exon 3 of the β-globin gene often cause a dominant form of thalassemia and show no predilection for malarial-endemic regions of the world. Am. J. Hum. Genet. 45:A242, 1989.

158. Fei, Y. J., Stoming, T. A., Kutlar, A., Huisman, T. H. J., and Stamatoyannopoulos, G.: One form of inclusion body β-thalassemia is due to a GAA→TAA mutation at codon 121 of the β chain. Blood 73:1075, 1989.

159. Kazazian, H. H., Jr., Orkin, S. H., Boehm, C. D., Goff, S. C., Wong, C., Dowling, C. E., Newberger, P. E., Knowlton, R.

G., Brown, V., and Donis-Keller, H.: Characterization of a spontaneous mutation to a β-thalassemia allele. Am. J. Hum. Genet. 38:860, 867, 1986.

160. Murru, S., Loudianos, G., Deiana, M., Camaschella, C., Sciarratta, G. V., Agosti, S., Parodi, M. I., Cerruti, P., Cao, A., and Pirastu, M.: Molecular characterization of β-thalassemia intermedia in patients of Italian descent and identification of three novel β-thalassemia mutations. Blood 77:1342, 1991.

161. Ristaldi, M. S., Pirastu, M., Murru, S., Casula, L., Loudianos, G., Cao, A., Sciarratta, G. V., Agosti, S., Parodi, M. I., Leone, D., and Melesendi, C.: A spontaneous mutation produced a novel elongated β⁰ globin chain structural variant (Hb Agnana) with a thalassemia-like phenotype. Blood 75:1378, 1990.

162. Fucharoen, S., Kobayashi, Y., Fucharoen, G., Ohba, Y., Miyazono, K., Fukumaki, Y., and Takaku, F.: A single nucleotide deletion in codon 123 of the β-globin gene causes an inclusion body β-thalassemia trait: A novel elongated globin chain βMakabe. Br. J. Haematol. 75:393, 1990.

163. Fucharoen, G., Fucharoen, S., Jetsrisuparb, A., and Fukumaki, Y.: Eight-base deletion of the β-globin gene produced a novel variant (β Khon Kaen) with an inclusion body β-thalassemia trait. Blood 78: 537, 1991.

164. Coleman, M. B., Steinberg, M. H., and Adams, J. G., III: Hemoglobin Terre Haute [β106 (G8) Arginine]: A posthumous correction to the original structure of Hb Indianapolis. Blood 76:57A, 1990.

165. Thein, S. L., Best, S., Sharpe, J., Paul, B., Clark, D. J., and Brown, M. J.: Hemoglobin Chesterfield (β28 Leu→Arg) produces the phenotype of inclusion body β thalassemia. Blood 77:2791, 1991.

166. Podda, A., Galanello, R., Maccioni, L., Melis, M. A., Rosatelli, C., Perseu, L., and Cao, A.: Hemoglobin Cagliari (β69 [E4] VAL→GLU): A novel unstable thalassemic hemoglobinopathy. Blood 77:371, 1991.

167. Fucharoen, S., Fucharoen, G., Fukumaki, Y., Nakamaya, Y., Hattori, Y., Yamamoto, K., and Ohba, Y.: Three-base deletion in exon 3 of the β-globin gene produced a novel variant (βGunma) with a thalassemia-like phenotype. Blood 76:1894, 1990.

168. Baklouti, F., Ouazana, R., Gonnet, C., Lapillonne, A., Delaunay, J., and Godet, J.: β⁺-thalassemia in cis of a sickle cell gene: Occurrence of a promoter mutation on a βˢ chromosome. Blood 74:1817, 1989.

169. Adams, J. G., III, Steinberg, M. H., Newman, M. V., Morrison, W. T., Benz, E. J., and Iyer, R.: β-Thalassemia present in cis to a new β-chain structural variant: Hb Vicksburg [β75 (E19) leu→0]. Proc. Natl. Acad. Sci. USA 78:469, 1981.

170. Olds, R. J., Sura, T., Jackson, B., Wonke, B., Hoffbrand, A. V., and Thein, S. L.: A novel δ⁰ mutation in cis with Hb Knossos: A study of different genetic interactions in three Egyptian families. Br. J. Haematol. 78:430, 1991.

171. Modell, C. B., and Berdoukas, V. A.: The Clinical Approach to Thalassemia. New York, Grune and Stratton, 1981.

172. Weatherall, D. J., Clegg, J. B., Knox-Macaulay, H. H. M., Bunch, C., Hopkins, C. R., and Temperley, I. J.: A genetically determined disorder with features both of thalassaemia and congenital dyserythropoietic anaemia. Br. J. Haematol. 24:681, 1973.

173. Stamatoyannopoulos, G., Woodson, R., Papayannopoulou, T., Heywood, D., and Kurachi, M. S.: Inclusion-body β-thalassemia trait. A form of β thalassemia producing clinical manifestations in simple heterozygotes. N. Engl. J. Med. 290:939, 1974.

174. Chehab, F. F., Der Kaloustian, V., Khouri, F. P., Deeb, S. S., and Kan, Y. W.: The molecular basis of β-thalassemia in Lebanon: Application to prenatal diagnosis. Blood 69:1141, 1987.

175. Kazazian, H. H., Jr., Orkin, S. H., Markham, A. F., Chapman, C. R., Youssoufian, H., and Waber, P. G.: Quantification of the close association between DNA haplotypes and specific β-thalassemia mutations in Mediterraneans. Nature 310:152, 1984.

176. Thein, S. L., Hesketh, C., and Weatherall, D. J.: The molecular basis of β-thalassemia in UK Asian Indians: Applications to prenatal diagnosis. Br. J. Haematol. 70:225, 1988.

177. Thein, S. L., Winichagoon, P., Hesketh, C., Fucharoen, S., Wasi, P., and Weatherall, D. J.: The molecular basis of β thalassemia in Thailand: Application to prenatal diagnosis. Am. J. Hum. Genet. 47:369, 1990.

178. Hill, A. V. S., Bowden, D. K., O'Shaughnessy, D. F., Weatherall, D. J., and Clegg, J. B.: β-Thalassemia in Melanesia: Association with malaria and characterization of a common variant (IVS-1 nt 5G-C). Blood 72:9, 1988.

179. Baglioni, C.: The fusion of two peptide chains in hemoglobin Lepore and its interpretation as a genetic deletion. Proc. Natl. Acad. Sci. USA 48:1880, 1962.

180. Efremov, G. D.: Hemoglobins Lepore and anti-Lepore. Hemoglobin 2:197, 1978.

181. Ottolenghi, S., Giglioni, B., Pulazzini, A., Comi, P., Camaschella, C., Serra, A., Guerrasio, A., and Saglio, G.: Sardinian δβ⁰-thalassemia: A further example of a C to T substitution at position −196 of the ᴬγ globin gene promoter. Blood 69:1058, 1061, 1987.

182. Atweh, G. F., Zhu, X.-X., Brickner, H. W., Dowling, C. H., Kazazian, H. H., Jr., and Forget, B. G.: The β-globin gene on the Chinese δβ-thalassemia chromosome carries a promoter mutation. Blood 70:1470, 1987.

183. Wainscoat, J. S., Thein, S. L., Wood, W. G., Weatherall, D. J., Tzotos, S., Kanavakis, E., Metaxatou-Mavromati, A., and Kattamis, C.: A novel deletion in the β globin gene complex. Ann. N. Y. Acad. Sci. 445:20, 1985.

184. Kulozik, A., Yarwood, N., and Jones, R. W.: The Corfu δβ⁰ thalassemia: A small deletion acts at a distance to selectively abolish β globin gene expression. Blood 71:457, 1988.

185. Poncz, M., Henthorn, P., Stoeckert, C., and Surrey, S.: Globin gene expression in hereditary persistence of fetal haemoglobin and (δβ)⁰-thalassaemia. In Maclean, N. (ed.): Oxford Surveys on Euykaryotic Genes. Vol. 5. Oxford, England, Oxford University Press, 1988, pp. 163–203.

186. Ottolenghi, S., Giglioni, B., Taramelli, R., Comi, P., Mazza, U., Saglio, G., Camaschella, C., Izzo, P., Cao, A., Galenello, R., Gimgerra, E., Baiget, M., and Gianni, A.: Molecular comparison of δβ-thalassemia and hereditary persistence of fetal hemoglobin DNAs: Evidence of a regulatory area. Proc. Natl. Acad. Sci. USA 79:2347, 1982.

187. Jones, R. W., Old, J. M., Trent, R. J., Clegg, J. B., and Weatherall D. J.: Restriction mapping of a new deletion responsible for ᴳγ(δβ)⁰ thalassaemia. Nucleic Acids Res. 9:6813, 1981.

188. Jones, R. W., Old, J. M., Trent, R. J., Clegg, J. B., and Weatherall, D. J.: Major rearrangement in the human β-globin gene cluster. Nature 291:39, 1981.

189. Charache, S., Clegg, J. B., and Weatherall, D. J.: The Negro variety of hereditary persistence of fetal haemoglobin is a mild form of thalassemia. Br. J. Haematol. 34:527, 1976.

190. Pirastu, M., Ristaldi, M. S., Loudianos, G., Murru, S., Sciarratta, G. V., Parodi, M. I., Leone, D., Agosti, S., and Cao, A.: Molecular analysis of atypical β-thalassemia heterozygotes. Ann. N. Y. Acad. Sci. 612:90, 1990.

191. Fearon, E. F., Kazazian, H. H., Waber, P. G., Lee, J. I., Antonarakis, E., Orkin, S. H., Vanin, E. F., Henthron, P. A., Grosveld, F. G., Scott, F., and Buchanan, G. R.: The entire β-globin gene cluster is deleted in a form of γδβ-thalassemia. Blood 61:1269, 1983.

192. Pirastu, M., Kan, Y. W., Lin, C. C., Baine, R., and Holbrook, C. T.: Hemolytic disease of the newborn caused by a new deletion of the entire β-globin gene cluster. J. Clin. Invest. 72:602, 1983.

193. Orkin, S. H., Goff, S. C., and Nathan, D. G.: Heterogeneity of DNA deletion in γδβ-thalassemia. J. Clin. Invest. 67:878, 1981.

194. Driscoll, M. C., Dobkin, C. S., and Alter, B. P.: γδβ-Thalassemia due to a de novo mutation deleting the 5′ β-globin gene activation-region hypersensitive sites. Proc. Natl. Acad. Sci. USA 86:7470, 1989.

195. Trent, R. J., Williams, B. G., Kearney, A., Wilkinson, T., and

Harris, P.: Molecular and hematological characterisation of Scottish-Irish type (εγδβ)⁰ thalassemia. Blood 76:2132, 1990.

196. Weatherall, D. J.: Prenatal diagnosis of haematological disease. In Hann, I. M., Gibson, B. E. S., and Letsky, E. A. (eds.): Fetal and Neonatal Haematology. London, Bailliere Tindall, 1991, pp. 285–314.

197. Weatherall, D. J.: Prenatal diagnosis of inherited blood diseases. Clin. Haematol. 14:747, 1985.

198. Cao, A., Rosatelli, M. C., Battista, G., Tuveri, T., Scalas, M. T., Monni, G., Olla, G., and Galanello, R.: Antenatal diagnosis of β-thalassemia in Sardinia. Ann. N.Y. Acad. Sci. 612:215, 1990.

199. Loukopoulos, D., Hadji, A., Papadakis, M., Karababa, P., Sinopoulou, K., Boussiou, M., Kollia, P., Xenakis, M., Antsaklis, A., Mesoghitis, S., Loutradi, A., and Fessas, P.: Prenatal diagnosis of thalassemia and of the sickle cell syndromes in Greece. Ann. N. Y. Acad. Sci. 612:226, 1990.

200. Alter, B. P.: Antenatal diagnosis: Summary of results. Ann. N. Y. Acad. Sci. 612:237, 1990.

201. Kazazian, H. H., Jr., Phillips, J. A., III, Boehm, C. D., Vik, T., Mahoney, M. J., and Ritchey, A. K.: Prenatal diagnosis of β-thalassemia by amniocentesis: Linkage analysis of multiple polymorphic restriction endonuclease sites. Blood 56:926, 1980.

202. Old, J. M., Ward, R. H. T., Petrou, M., Karagozlu, F., Modell, B., and Weatherall, D. J.: First trimester diagnosis for haemoglobinopathies: A report of 3 cases. Lancet 2:1413, 1982.

203. Old, J. M., Fitches, A., Heath, C., Thein, S. L., Weatherall, D. J., Warren, R., McKenzie, C., Rodeck, C. H., Modell, B., Petrou, M., and Ward, R. H. T.: First trimester fetal diagnosis for haemoglobinopathies: Report on 200 cases. Lancet 2:763, 1986.

204. Pirastu, M., Kan, Y. W., Cao, A., Conner, B. J., Teplitz, R. L., and Wallace, R. B.: Prenatal diagnosis of β-thalassemia: Detection of a single nucleotide mutation in DNA. N. Engl. J. Med. 309:284, 1983.

205. Kogan, S. C., Doherty, M., and Gitschier J.: An improved method for prenatal diagnosis of genetic diseases by analysis of amplified DNA sequences: Application to hemophilia A. N. Engl. J. Med. 317:985, 1987.

206. Chehab, F., Doherty, M., Cai, S., Cooper, S., and Rubin, E.: Detection of sickle cell anemia and thalassaemia. Nature 329:293, 1987.

207. Saiki, R. K., Chang, C.-A., Levenson, C. H., Warren, T. C., Boehm, C. D., Kazazian, H. H., Jr., and Erlich, H. A.: Diagnosis of sickle cell anemia and β-thalassemia with enzymatically amplified DNA and non-radioactive allele-specific oligonucleotide probes. N. Engl. J. Med. 319:537, 1988.

208. Old, J. M., Varawalla, N. Y., and Weatherall, D. J.: The rapid detection and prenatal diagnosis of β-thalassaemia in the Asian Indian and Cypriot populations in the UK. Lancet 336:834, 1990.

209. Cai, S. P., Chang, C. A., Zhang, J. Z., Saiki, R. K., Erlich, H. A., and Kan, Y. W.: Rapid prenatal diagnosis of β-thalassemia using DNA amplification and nonradioactive probes. Blood 73:372, 1989.

210. Saiki, R. K., Walsh, P. S., Levenson, C. H., and Erlich, H. A.: Genetic analysis of amplified DNA with immobilized sequence-specific oligonucleotide probes. Proc. Natl. Acad. Sci. USA 86:6230, 1989.

211. Piomelli, S.: Cooley's anemia management: 25 years of progress. In Buckner, C. D., Gale, R. P., and Lucarelli, G. (eds.): Progress in Clinical and Biological Research. Vol. 309: Advances and Controversies in Thalassemia Therapy. New York, Alan R. Liss, 1989, pp. 23–26.

212. Weatherall, D. J., Pippard, M. J., and Callender, S. T.: Iron loading in thalassaemia—five years with the pump. N. Engl. J. Med. 308:456, 1983.

213. Vullo, C., and Di Palma, A.: Compliance with therapy in Cooley's anemia. In Buckner, C. D., Gale, R. P., and Lucarelli, G. (eds.): Progress in Clinical and Biological Research. Vol. 309: Advances and Controversies in Thalassemia Therapy. New York, Alan R. Liss, 1989, pp. 43–49.

214. Hershko, C., and Weatherall, D. J.: Iron chelating therapy. Clin. Lab. Sci. 26:303, 1988.
215. Thomas, E. D., Buckner, C. D., Sanders, J. E., Papayannopoulou, T., Borgna-Pignatti, C., de Stafano, P., Sullivan, K. M., Clift, R. A., and Storb, R.: Marrow transplantation for thalassaemia. Lancet 2:227, 1982.
216. Lucarelli, G., Galimberti, M., Polchi, P., Angelucci, E., Baronciani, D., Giardini, C., Politi, P., Durazzi, S. M. T., Muretto, P., and Albertini, F.: Bone marrow transplantation in patients with thalassemia. N. Engl. J. Med. 322:417, 1990.
217. Sheridan, B. L., Weatherall, D. J., Clegg, J. B., Pritchard, J., Wood, W. G., Callender, S. T., Durrant, I. J., McWhirter, W. R., Ali, M., Partridge, J. W., and Thompson, E. N.: The patterns of fetal haemoglobin production in leukaemia. Br. J. Haematol. 32:487, 1976.
218. Alter, B. P., Rappeport, J. M., Huisman, T. H. J., Schroeder, W. A., and Nathan, D. G.: Fetal erythropoiesis following bone marrow transplantation. Blood 48:843, 1976.
219. Ley, T. J.: The pharmacology of hemoglobin switching: Of mice and men. Blood 77:1146, 1991.
220. Weatherall, D. J.: Gene therapy in perspective. Nature 349:275, 1991.
221. Apperley, J. F., and Williams, D. A.: Gene therapy: Current status and future directions. Br. J. Haematol. 75:148, 1990.
222. Friedman, T.: Gene therapy. In Friedman, T. (ed.): Therapy for Genetic Disease. Oxford, England, Oxford University Press, 1991, pp. 107–121.
223. Smithies, P., Gregg, R. G., Boggs, S. S., Koralewski, M. A., and Kucherlapati, R. S.: Insertion of DNA sequences into the human chromosomal β-globin locus by homologous recombination. Nature 317:230, 1985.

Sickle Hemoglobin and Other Hemoglobin Mutants

H. Franklin Bunn

INTRODUCTION

The study of hemoglobins, both normal and mutant, has provided fundamental and continued insights into structure-function relationships of proteins in general and, in particular, the molecular basis of oxygen transport. The discovery by Pauling and Itano[1] that sickle hemoglobin has an abnormal electrophoretic mobility ushered us into the era of molecular medicine. With the advent of recombinant DNA technology, research on hemoglobin provided early and important information about the organization and regulation of genes as well as insights into how ontogeny affects gene expression. The switch from fetal to adult hemoglobin production, a topic of vital importance in developmen-

tal biology, is discussed in Chapter 4, whereas Chapter 5 covers the thalassemias, inherited defects in globin biosynthesis.

This chapter begins with a description of normal human hemoglobin, its structure and physiologic function. In the first edition of this book, Perutz[2] reviewed this topic in a considerably more detailed and authoritative manner. The minor hemoglobin components are also discussed in this chapter, since measurement of these species can offer valuable clues to the diagnosis of both congenital and acquired disorders. The human hemoglobin mutants are discussed both in the context of underlying mutations in globin gene structure and in terms of their phenotypic expression. A major portion of the chapter is devoted to sickle

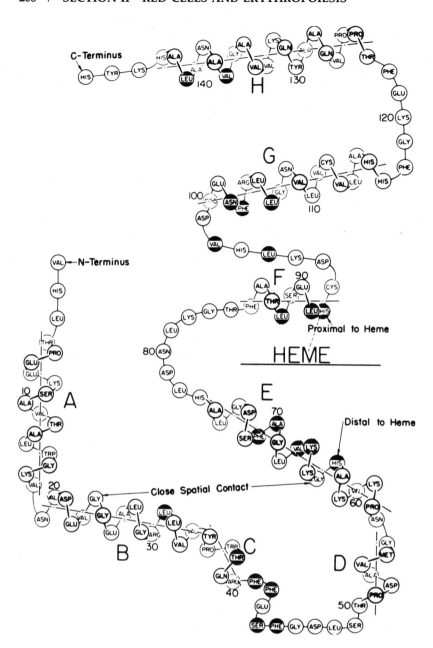

FIGURE 6–1. Primary and secondary structure of the β chain of human hemoglobin. The eight helices are shown, designated A through H. The iron atom of the heme group is covalently attached to the "proximal histidine," residue 92, with the helical location F8. (Reprinted with permission from Huisman, T. H. J., and Schroeder, W. A.: New Aspects of the Structure, Function and Synthesis of Hemoglobins. Boca Raton, Fla., CRC Press, 1971. Copyright CRC Press, Inc., Boca Raton, FL.)

hemoglobin and sickle cell disease, since contemporary molecular biology has had a major and growing impact on our understanding of the pathogenesis of this important disease and the development of rational approaches to therapy.

NORMAL HUMAN HEMOGLOBIN

Structure

Hemoglobin is a 64.4 kDa tetramer composed of two pairs of unlike globin polypeptide chains designated by Greek letters (e.g., $\alpha_2\beta_2$). A heme group, ferroprotoporphyrin IX, is linked covalently at a specific site to each chain. In the reduced (ferrous) state, it can bind reversibly with gaseous ligands, such as

oxygen or carbon monoxide. Approximately 75 per cent of hemoglobin in its native state is in the form of an α helix (Fig. 6–1). Individual residues can be assigned to one of eight helices or to adjacent nonhelical stretches. This has greatly facilitated establishment of homology between globin subunits. Thus, in all hemoglobins whose primary structure is known, the heme iron is linked covalently to a histidine at the eighth residue of the F helix. In human hemoglobins, His F8 is residue 87 of the α chain and 92 of the β chain (Fig. 6–1). Residues that have charged side groups, such as lysine, arginine, and glutamic acid, lie on the surface of the molecule in contact with the surrounding water solvent. Uncharged residues are generally oriented toward the hydrophobic interior of the molecule. Unlike most proteins, hemoglobin contains no disulfide bonds.

From X-ray analyses of crystals of hemoglobins, Max Perutz at the Medical Research Council Laboratory in Cambridge, England, determined the three-dimensional structure of human hemoglobin.[2] This remarkable achievement, which earned Perutz the Nobel Prize, has enabled a thorough understanding of the relationship between structure and function. The hemoglobin tetramer is a globular molecule (5.0 × 5.4 × 6.4 nm) with a single (dyad) axis of symmetry. The polypeptide chains are themselves folded in such a way that the four heme groups lie in clefts on the surface of the molecule equidistant from one another. Recent X-ray analyses are of sufficiently high resolution that the coordinates of all atoms in the molecule are known to within 0.2 nm.[3, 4] As shown in Figure 6–2, the molecule undergoes a marked change in conformation upon deoxygenation. The β chains rotate apart by about 0.7 nm. In contrast, liganded forms, including oxyhemoglobin, carboxyhemoglobin, and cyanmethemoglobin, all appear to be isomorphous. The conformational change that occurs upon removal and addition of ligand accounts for the many known differences in physical and chemical properties of oxyhemoglobin and deoxyhemoglobin. Perutz[2] has shown that deoxyhemoglobin is stabilized in a constrained or taut (T) configuration by the presence of intersubunit and intrasubunit salt bonds (Fig. 6–3A). These include residues responsible for the Bohr effect (Fig. 6–3B) and for the binding of 2,3-diphosphoglycerate (2,3-DPG) (discussed below). Upon the addition of ligand, such as oxygen, these salt bonds are sequentially broken. The fully liganded hemoglobin is in the so-called relaxed (R) configuration. In this state, considerably less bonding energy is present between subunits, and the liganded molecule is able to dissociate reversibly according to the following reaction: $\alpha_2\beta_2 \rightleftharpoons 2\alpha\beta$. The formation of αβ dimers is required for hemoglobin to bind to haptoglobin and to traverse renal glomeruli.[5] As shown in Figure 6–2, each subunit in the tetramer is oriented toward the two unlike subunits in different ways (i.e., $\alpha^1\beta^1$ and $\alpha^1\beta^2$). The dissociation of the liganded tetramer into dimers occurs at the $\alpha^1\beta^2$ interface. Thus, binding is stronger between α^1 and β^1 subunits than between α^1 and β^2 subunits. Furthermore, during oxygenation and deoxygenation (T⇌R), there is considerable movement along the $\alpha^1\beta^2$ interface. As will be discussed, hemoglobin mutants having an amino acid substitution in this interface are likely to have markedly abnormal functional properties.

Functional Properties

The oxygenation of hemoglobin, as depicted by the classical sigmoid oxyhemoglobin dissociation curve shown in Figure 6–4, can be characterized by two important properties: oxygen affinity and cooperativity.

A convenient index of oxygen affinity is P_{50}, or the partial pressure of oxygen at which hemoglobin is half-saturated. If the oxyhemoglobin dissociation curve is shifted to the right, P_{50} is increased and oxygen affinity is decreased. Thus, P_{50} varies inversely with oxygen affinity. As discussed in detail in this section, P_{50} depends on temperature, pH, organic phosphates, and P_{CO_2}. Under physiologic conditions (37°C, pH of 7.40, 2,3-DPG = 5 mM, P_{CO_2} = 40 mm Hg), the P_{50} of normal adult blood is 26 mm Hg.

The sigmoid shape of the oxyhemoglobin-binding curve indicates that hemoglobin binds oxygen in a cooperative fashion. Cooperativity means that when hemoglobin is partially saturated with oxygen, the affinity of the remaining hemes on the tetramer for oxygen increases markedly. This phenomenon can be considered in terms of two hemoglobin conformations: deoxy (or T) and oxy (or R). The T form has a lower affinity for ligands such as oxygen and carbon monoxide than the R form has. At some point during the sequential addition of oxygen to the four hemes of the molecule, a transition from the T to the R conformation occurs. At this point, the oxygen affinity of the partially liganded molecule increases markedly. In this way, hemoglobin can be considered a prototype of a more general class of allosteric enzymes, in which the binding of a ligand to a protein alters the affinity for the ligand at a different site on the same macromolecule.[6]

During the past 25 years, a generation of biochemists and biophysicists have focused intently on the question of whether the oxygenation of hemoglobin faithfully adheres to the two-state model of Monod, Wyman, and Changeux (MWC).[6] Because of the concerted transition implicit in a highly cooperative molecule, only the unligated (deoxy) and the fully ligated hemoglobins are present in sufficient amounts for structural and functional analyses. Since the partially oxygenated intermediates are present in such low quantities, investigators have gone to great lengths to prepare and study hybrid molecules in which heme groups have been partially replaced by substitutes that stably impose upon the subunit either the deoxy or the liganded tertiary structure. In general, the properties of these hybrid hemoglobins are in reasonable agreement with the MWC two-state model, although some deviations have been noted.*

When two or three molecules of oxygen are bound, the $\alpha^1\beta^2$ interface is sufficiently destabilized to flip the quaternary structure from T to R, thereby increasing the affinity of the remaining heme (or hemes) for oxygen. How can the seemingly small structural perturbation resulting from the oxygenation of two or three heme groups cause sufficient alteration in the

---

*Ackers and his colleagues[7] have coupled the preparation of hybrid hemoglobins with meticulous measurements of dimer-tetramer equilibria, which, through thermodynamic linkage considerations, provide a valid measurement of the free energy of subunit cooperativity. They find that certain partially ligated species depart significantly from the pure T (deoxy) and R (oxy) quaternary states. They present evidence for a third allosteric state (and quaternary structure) consisting of either singly ligated species or the tetramer in which one αβ dimer is fully oxygenated and the other is unligated.

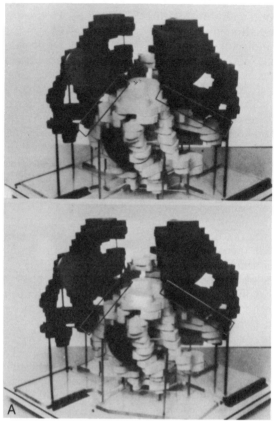

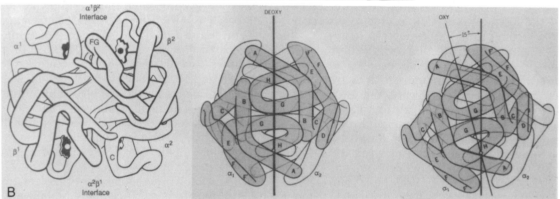

FIGURE 6–2. *A,* A three-dimensional model of hemoglobin, based on early X-ray crystallographic analysis. The α chains are shown in white, the β chains in black; the boxed areas are the αβ contact areas. The heme groups are depicted as disks inserted into each subunit. There is an axis of symmetry that is parallel to the plane of the paper. Note the difference in conformation between oxyhemoglobin and deoxyhemoglobin. (From Muirhead, H., Cox, J. M., Mazzarella, L.: Structure and function of haemoglobin. 3. A three-dimensional fourier synthesis of human deoxyhaemoglobin at 5.5 Angstrom resolution. J. Mol. Biol. 28:117, 1967; with permission.) *B,* Diagram showing the folding of the subunits in deoxyhemoglobin and oxyhemoglobin. The α helices (A through H) are also shown. In the left-hand panel, the dyad axis of symmetry is perpendicular to the plane of the paper. The middle and right-hand panels are oriented the same way as the solid model shown in *A.* These panels depict the change in quaternary structure upon oxygenation. (From Ackers, G. K., Doyle, M. L., Myers, D. M., and Daugherty, M. A.: Molecular code for cooperativity in hemoglobin. Science 255:54, 1992; with permission. Copyright 1992 by the AAAS.)

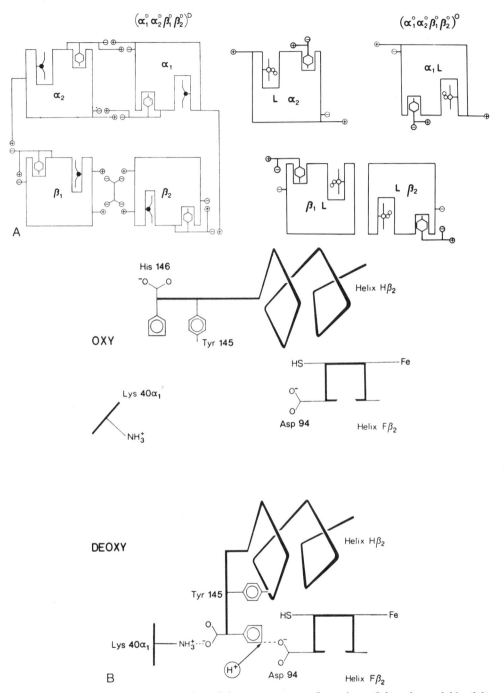

FIGURE 6–3. *A,* Diagrammatic representation of the quaternary configurations of deoxyhemoglobin *(left)* and oxyhemoglobin *(right).* A molecule of 2,3-DPG is depicted between the β subunits. Its negatively charged groups interact with positively charged residues on the β subunits. Intrasubunit and intersubunit salt bonds are broken upon oxygenation. *B,* Effect of oxygenation on the contacts of C-terminal residues of the β chain. The salt bridges of β146 His break when the quaternary structure changes from T to R or when the β chain hemes take up oxygen, whichever comes first. The proton shown in this figure, as explained in the text, is a major contributor to the Bohr effect. (*A* modified and *B* reprinted by permission from *Nature,* Vol. 228, p. 734; copyright © 1970 Macmillan Magazines Limited.)

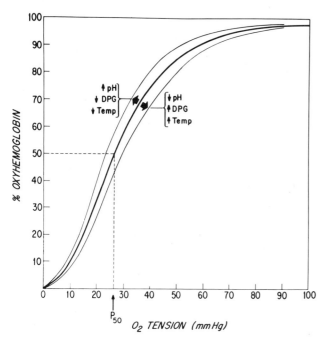

FIGURE 6–4. The principal factors that influence the position of the oxyhemoglobin dissociation curve in red cells: temperature, pH, and the intracellular concentration of 2,3-DPG.

protein conformation to have impact on subunit interactions? This question has persistently occupied Perutz's attention during the 25 years that have elapsed since he solved the structures of oxyhemoglobin and deoxyhemoglobin. In the latter, the iron atoms lie outside the plane of the porphyrin ring by about 0.038 nm.[8] The trigger that effects this allosteric transition appears to be the decrease in the atomic radius of heme iron upon the addition of ligand. The smaller iron atom is now able to snap into the plane of the porphyrin ring. The resulting alteration in heme configuration is amplified by an intramolecular path that transduces this chemical signal across the $\alpha^1\beta^2$ interface, resulting in increased ligand affinity. Under physiologic conditions (i.e., in the presence of organic phosphates), when deoxyhemoglobin binds oxygen, the α chain hemes are favored.

During the past several years, a considerable amount has been learned about the environment within the heme pocket, thanks to a combination of (1) high-resolution structural analyses of hemoglobin and model ("picket fence") heme compounds; (2) studies on site-directed mutants of hemoglobin, which can be produced in high quantities in *Escherichia coli*[9–11]; and (3) ultrafast measurements of the kinetics of ligand binding and conformational transitions.[12, 13] This collective body of information has provided fresh and penetrating insights about physiologically important properties of hemoglobin, such as the relative affinity of hemoglobin for oxygen versus carbon monoxide and the rate of auto-oxidation of hemoglobin. In free heme, the affinity for oxygen is several thousand–fold lower than that for carbon monoxide. Such a molecule could not serve as a physiologic oxygen transporter,

since it would remain saturated by the carbon monoxide that is continually produced by heme catabolism. Accordingly, one of the challenges in the evolutionary engineering of hemoglobin was to increase oxygen affinity relative to carbon monoxide.* In the α chains of hemoglobin, a nitrogen atom on the imidazole of the distal (E7) histidine forms a hydrogen bond with the bound oxygen, thereby significantly increasing oxygen affinity. When α E7 His is replaced with a glycine residue by means of site-directed mutagenesis, the affinity for carbon monoxide increases fourfold.[9] Mutagenesis at E7 His has also provided insights into hemoglobin's remarkable ability to resist spontaneous oxidation of its heme iron atoms, resulting in the conversion to non-functional methemoglobin. Auto-oxidation is considerably facilitated by protons. Perutz[14] has suggested that the distal histidine acts as proton trap and shuttle, protecting the ferrous heme iron from auto-oxidation. No other amino acid side chain could function in this way: "Evolution is a brilliant chemist."[14]

Cooperativity (or heme-heme interaction) depends on interaction between unlike globin subunits. This phenomenon has considerable physiological importance. The familiar sigmoid shape of the oxyhemoglobin dissociation curve (see Fig. 6–4) allows a considerable amount of oxygen to be released over a relatively small drop in oxygen tension. In contrast, heme proteins, such as myoglobin and hemoglobin (Hb) H (β_4) and Hb Bart's (γ_4), which lack cooperativity, have a hyperbolic curve, which allows much less oxygen unloading.

Effectors of Hemoglobin Function

Inside the red cell, the oxygen affinity of hemoglobin is modulated by protons, carbon dioxide, and 2,3-DPG. As will be explained, these allosteric effectors bind preferentially to deoxyhemoglobin and alter the equilibrium between T and R quaternary structures.

PROTONS. In 1904, Bohr and colleagues[15] discovered that the oxygen affinity of hemoglobin decreased with increasing carbon dioxide tension. It was later shown that this phenomenon depends primarily on pH. Thus, over a pH range of 6 to 8.5, oxygen affinity varies directly with pH. A thermodynamic corollary of this statement is that deoxyhemoglobin binds protons more strongly than does oxyhemoglobin. Under physiologic conditions, a molecule of hemoglobin releases about 2.8 protons upon oxygenation:

$$HbH + 4O_2 \rightleftharpoons Hb(O_2)_4 + 2.8H^+$$

High-resolution X-ray data in conjunction with experiments on chemically modified hemoglobins[16] have permitted the identification of specific acid groups on hemoglobin that yield Bohr protons. After nearly a

---

*The Haldane coefficient (K_{CO}/K_{O_2}) for the hemoglobins of man and other mammals is about 210, at least 10-fold lower than that of free heme.

decade of controversy, recent high-resolution proton nuclear magnetic resonance (NMR) analyses[17] have confirmed one of Perutz's earliest and boldest predictions: A substantial portion of the Bohr effect is due to an intrasubunit salt bond between the positively charged imidazole of β146 histidine and the negatively charged carboxyl of β94 aspartate. This salt bridge is one of the important bonds that stabilize the deoxy conformation (see Fig. 6–3B). When hemoglobin is oxygenated, these bonds are broken and protons are released.

The Bohr effect offers a physiological advantage in facilitating oxygen unloading. At the tissue level, the drop in pH due to carbon dioxide influx lowers oxygen affinity, thereby enhancing oxygen release. In contrast, at the pulmonary level, the increase in pH due to the efflux of carbon dioxide increases oxygen affinity and uptake.

CARBAMINO ADDUCTS. Carbon dioxide can bind free amino groups on hemoglobin to form carbamino complexes according to the following reaction:

$$RNH_2 + CO_2 \rightleftharpoons RNHCOO^- + H^+$$

Only non-protonated amino groups can react with carbon dioxide. The only amino groups in globin whose pKs are low enough to be partially non-protonated at physiologic pH are at the N-termini of the α and β chains. Deoxyhemoglobin forms carbamino complexes more readily than does oxyhemoglobin. From this, it follows that at a given pH, carbon dioxide lowers oxygen affinity. Under physiologic conditions, only about 10 per cent of the carbon dioxide produced by tissue metabolism is transported to the lungs in the form of carbamino hemoglobin.[5]

2,3-DPG. The red cell contains an unusually high concentration of 2,3-DPG (about 5 mmol/l). This compound is a potent modifier of hemoglobin function.[18] The addition of increasing amounts of 2,3-DPG to a solution of purified Hb A results in a progressive lowering of oxygen affinity. This helps explain the long-known fact that whole blood has a lower oxygen affinity than does a solution of dialyzed hemoglobin, studied under comparable conditions. The mechanism by which 2,3-DPG lowers oxygen affinity can be explained by the fact that it binds to human deoxyhemoglobin rather avidly ($K_d = 2 \times 10^{-5}$ M) in a 1:1 molar ratio but only weakly to oxyhemoglobin. Model fitting and X-ray diffraction measurements[19] have established the sites on hemoglobin involved in 2,3-DPG binding. 2,3-DPG is situated in the central cavity between the two β chains. Its negative charges are neutralized by positively charged groups: β NH$_2$-terminus, β2 histidine, β82 lysine, and β143 histidine. This information on the binding of 2,3-DPG to hemoglobin suggests the following simple reaction:

$$HbDPG + 4O_2 \rightleftharpoons Hb(O_2)_4 + DPG$$

(Note the similarity of this equation and that for the Bohr effect previously given.) This equilibrium expresses both the preferential binding of 2,3-DPG for deoxyhemoglobin and the 1:1 stoichiometry. Furthermore, changing concentrations of 2,3-DPG shift the oxygen-binding equilibrium in accord with the experimental results cited above.

The position of the oxyhemoglobin dissociation curve is influenced by a number of factors. As depicted in Figure 6–4, the three most important are temperature, pH, and red cell 2,3-DPG. Oxygen affinity varies inversely with temperature. This phenomenon is physiologically appropriate because, during a period of relative hyperthermia, oxygen requirement is likely to be increased. The decrease in oxygen affinity at elevated body temperature would facilitate the unloading of oxygen to tissues. The effects of pH and 2,3-DPG on hemoglobin function have already been discussed. Conventionally, whole blood oxygen saturation curves are corrected to pH 7.4, 37°C. Thus, the main variable leading to fluctuation in the position of the standardized oxygen dissociation curve is red cell 2,3-DPG.

How does the oxygen affinity of the blood affect the delivery of oxygen to tissues? This subject has been reviewed in detail.[5, 20] At a given blood flow and hemoglobin concentration, the amount of oxygen that is unloaded depends on the position of the oxyhemoglobin dissociation curve. As shown in Figure 6–4, red cells that are right shifted have enhanced oxygen release when going from a normal arterial Po$_2$ (95 mm Hg) to a normal mixed venous Po$_2$ (40 mm Hg). With this decrease in Po$_2$, a steeper portion of the oxygen dissociation curve is encompassed, and therefore more oxygen is unloaded. In contrast, if the oxyhemoglobin dissociation curve is shifted to the left, less oxygen is unloaded. This phenomenon bears on several clinical states, including hemoglobin mutants associated with polycythemia, discussed at the end of this chapter.

Other Hemoglobin Components

In red cells of adults and children over 6 months of age, Hb A ($\alpha_2\beta_2$) accounts for more than 90 per cent of the total hemoglobin. However, other globin genes are preferentially expressed during embryonic and fetal development. The ontogeny and regulation of globin gene expression are discussed in Chapter 4. Several of these hemoglobins provide useful information on the diagnosis of a variety of congenital and acquired hematological disorders. Furthermore, post-translational modifications of hemoglobin have been exploited in the monitoring of certain non-hematological disorders.

HEMOGLOBIN F. After the eighth week of gestation, Hb F ($\alpha_2\gamma_2$) becomes the predominant hemoglobin. Other primates and ruminants also have structurally different γ chains. In humans, the γ chain differs from the β chain in 39 of 146 residues. Unlike the other human globin subunits, the γ chain has structural heterogeneity.[21] In newborns, about two thirds of the γ chains have glycine at position 136, whereas the remaining γ chains have alanine. This ratio falls during the switch from γ to β chain production. The two

F hemoglobins ($\alpha_2{}^G\gamma_2$ and $\alpha_2{}^A\gamma_2$) have very similar properties.[22] The $^G\gamma$ and $^A\gamma$ chains are products of adjacent genes located between the ϵ and δ genes. In addition, there is structural heterogeneity at position 75, whereas in certain populations, the γ chain contains threonine instead of isoleucine.[23] The incidence of this substitution ranges from 0 to 40 per cent. Only the $^A\gamma$ gene carries this polymorphism. The determination of these differences in primary sequences has provided new insights into the thalassemias and hereditary persistence of fetal hemoglobin. (See Chapters 4 and 5.)

About 20 per cent of Hb F in the developing fetus has a post-translational modification: The N-terminus of the γ chain is acetylated (Hb F).[24] In contrast, no other human globin subunits are acetylated, except for mutants that have substitutions of the N-terminal residue.[5]

Fetal red cells have a considerably higher oxygen affinity than do adult red cells. This phenomenon, which has been observed in a number of mammalian species,[5] may facilitate the transport of oxygen across the placenta. In the human, this discrepancy in relative oxygen affinities is due to the diminished interaction of Hb F with red cell organic phosphates.[25, 26] Hb F has the special property of being remarkably resistant to denaturation at extremes of pH. The measurement of alkali-resistant hemoglobin has proved a very useful, although indirect, way of estimating the content of Hb F within a hemolysate.

The red cells of the newborn contain about 80 per cent Hb F and 20 per cent Hb A (Fig. 6–5A). By the time individuals are older than 6 months, Hb F constitutes less than 1 per cent of the total hemoglobin and is distributed unevenly among red cells.[27, 28] Normally, only 0.1 to 7 per cent of red cells contain detectable amounts of fetal hemoglobin. These "F cells" contain about 5 pg of Hb F, approximately 20 per cent of the total hemoglobin in the cell. As explained in more detail in Chapter 4, F cell production is genetically controlled.

Hemoglobin F is increased to a variable extent in several hereditary disorders, including β thalassemia, hereditary persistence of fetal hemoglobin (Chapter 5), and sickle cell anemia (discussed below).

HEMOGLOBIN A$_2$. About 2.5 per cent of the hemoglobin in normal red cells is Hb A$_2$ ($\alpha_2\delta_2$). It can be readily separated from Hb A by electrophoresis or ion-exchange chromatography (see Fig. 6–5). This minor component is evenly distributed among red cells, and its functional behavior is very similar to that of Hb A.[5] The amino acid sequence of δ and β chains is identical in all but 10 of 146 residues. The level of Hb A$_2$ is altered in a variety of congenital and acquired diseases.[29] The increased percentage of Hb A$_2$ in β thalassemia is a useful diagnostic aid. (See Chapter 5.) By contrast, Hb A$_2$ is decreased in α thalassemia, as well as in iron deficiency and sideroblastic anemias. The relative rate of synthesis of this minor component is markedly curtailed in the final stages of erythroid development.[30, 31] The level of Hb A$_2$ appears to

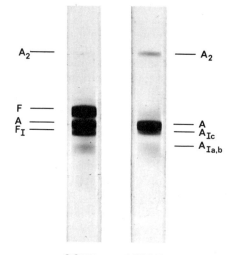

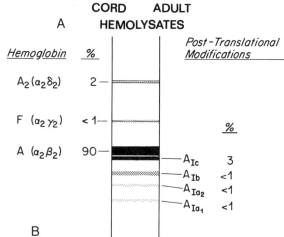

FIGURE 6–5. *A,* Analysis of human umbilical cord and adult blood hemolysates by gel electrofocusing. The gels have been overloaded in order to demonstrate Hb A$_2$. *B,* Separation of hemoglobin components in a normal hemolysate by means of gel electrofocusing. Glycated hemoglobins are shown on the right, along with the percentage of components in normal individuals. (*A* from Bunn, H. F., and Forget, B. G.: Hemoglobin: Molecular, Genetic and Clinical Aspects. Philadelphia, W. B. Saunders Company, 1986, p. 62.)

depend on the rate of assembly of hemoglobin subunits, as discussed later in this chapter.

GLYCATED HEMOGLOBINS. When the hemoglobin from normal adult red cells is carefully analyzed by column chromatography,[32, 33] several minor components that have lower isoelectric points than the main Hb A can be detected (Fig. 6–5B). These are designated A$_{Ia1}$, A$_{Ia2}$, A$_{Ib}$, and A$_{Ic}$. Hb A$_{Ic}$ accounts for approximately 3 per cent of the hemoglobin in normal adult red cells.[34] This minor component differs from Hb A only at the N-terminal amino group of each β chain, where glucose is attached non-enzymatically by a ketoamine linkage.[35, 36] In addition, approximately 5 per cent of hemoglobin molecules have glucose linked to certain lysine residues. These adducts cannot be separated from unmodified hemoglobins by ordinary chromatography or electrophoresis, but they can be isolated by means of an affinity resin containing phenylboronate, which binds to sugar hydroxyl groups. In like manner, sugar phosphates and other red cell metabolites combine with hemoglobin at the β N-terminus to form less abundant adducts. Hb A_{Ib} is an adduct of pyruvate with the β N-terminus.[37]

Glycated hemoglobins are formed slowly and continuously throughout the 120-day life span of the red cell. Consequently, individuals who have increased red cell turnover (hemolysis) have decreased levels of these minor hemoglobin components.[38]

Patients with diabetes mellitus have levels of Hb A_{Ic} that are two to three times higher than normal (see reference 39 for a review). The measurement of Hb A_{Ic} has proved a useful independent assessment of the degree of diabetic control, as it is not subject to fluctuations of the blood glucose level. Furthermore, Hb A_{Ic} is a prototype of glycosylation of other proteins, which could contribute to the long-term complications of the disease.

OTHER POST-TRANSLATIONAL MODIFICATIONS. Although glucose adducts are by far the most common and abundant type of chemical modification of hemoglobin, other small molecules also are capable of forming covalent linkages and thereby may reflect significant metabolic perturbations. Examples include cyanate adducts in uremic patients,[40] acetaldehyde adducts in alcoholics,[41, 42] and porphyrin-substituted hemoglobin in patients with lead poisoning.[43, 44]

HUMAN HEMOGLOBIN MUTANTS

To date, more than 500 structurally different human hemoglobin mutants have been discovered.[45] They are classified in Table 6–1 according to type of mutation and affected subunit.

In heterozygotes, the β globin mutant hemoglobin

generally constitutes about half of the total hemoglobin in the red cell, in keeping with the presence of two β globin genes. In contrast, normal individuals have four α globin genes. Accordingly, α globin mutants usually constitute about 25 per cent of the hemolysate. This fraction increases with concurrent α thalassemia. The two tandem α globin genes differ significantly in transcriptional efficiency: α-2 > α-1. Therefore, stable mutants expressed by the α-2 gene tend to be relatively more abundant than those expressed by the α-1 gene.[46]

There are nearly twice as many known β chain mutants as α chain mutants. This observation may seem surprising because there are two α globin genes. However, α mutants, because of their relatively low abundance, often escape clinical detection. Occasionally, δ chain and γ chain mutants have been encountered and characterized, but again the frequency of detection is limited by their low abundance.

The majority of these hemoglobin mutants are not associated with any clinical manifestations. Many were discovered during the course of large population surveys. The simplest and most practical diagnostic tool for the detection of new hemoglobin mutants is zone electrophoresis, which separates proteins that differ in charge. However, in recent years a number of more sophisticated techniques have been applied to the detection of mutant hemoglobins, including high-performance liquid chromatography,[47, 48] mass spectrometry,[48] and sequencing of DNA fragments generated by the polymerase chain reaction.[49, 50]

ASSEMBLY OF MUTANT HEMOGLOBINS. The proportion of normal and mutant hemoglobins in red cells of heterozygotes provides insight into the assembly of human hemoglobins.[51, 52] The great majority of β chain mutants are synthesized at the same rate as $β^A$ (see reference 53) and have normal stability. Therefore, heterozygotes would be expected to have equal amounts of normal and mutant hemoglobin. However, measurements of the proportion of normal and abnormal hemoglobins in heterozygotes have revealed unexpected variability. Figure 6–6A shows a comparison of stable β chain mutants. The positively charged mutants, such as Hb S, Hb C, Hb D-Los Angeles, Hb C, and Hb E constitute significantly less than half of the total hemoglobin in heterozygotes and are reduced further in the presence of α thalassemia (Fig. 6–6B)[51, 52, 54] In contrast, many of the negatively charged mutants are present in amounts exceeding that of Hb A. In two heterozygotes who had a negatively charged mutant (Hb J-Baltimore or Hb J-Iran) in conjunction with α thalassemia, the proportion of the mutant hemoglobin was found to be further increased. This analysis of the proportion of β chain mutant in heterozygotes suggests that alterations in surface charge contribute to different rates of assembly of the hemoglobin tetramer. This hypothesis is supported by in vitro mixing experiments on normal and mutant β subunits showing that when α chains are present in limiting amounts (mimicking α thalassemia), negatively

TABLE 6–1. MOLECULAR MECHANISMS UNDERLYING GLOBIN MUTATIONS

MECHANISM	α	β	γ	δ
Single base substitution → amino acid replacement (S, C, E, etc.)	162	288	62	20
Two replacements in same subunit (C-Harlem, etc.)	2	16		
Fusion hemoglobins: δβ—3 (Lepore variants) βδ—4 (Miyada, P-Congo, etc.) δβδ—1 (Parchman) γβ—1 (Kenya)				
Deletion (Gun Hill, etc.)	2	12		
Insertion (Grady, Koriyama, Catonsville)	2	1		
Deletion/insertion (Montreal, Galacia, Birmingham)		3		
Extended subunit:				
Termination codon mutation (Constant Spring, etc.)	3			
Frameshift (Wayne, Tak, Cranston, Saverne)	1	3		
N-terminal mutation → retention of initiator methionine (Long Island–Marseille, etc.)	1	3		

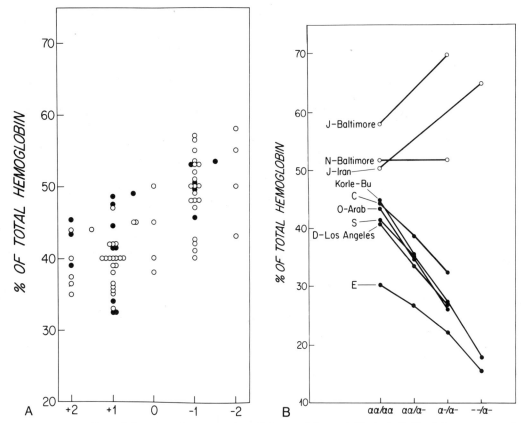

FIGURE 6–6. *A,* Effect of charge on the proportion of abnormal hemoglobin in individuals heterozygous for 72 stable β globin variants. Each data point represents a mean value for a given variant. The solid circles denote measurements of Huisman (Am. J. Hematol. 14:393, 1983), utilizing high-resolution chromatography. Substitutions involving a histidine residue were scored as a change of one-half charge. The "−1" group differs significantly from the "+1" group ($p < .001$) and from the "0" group ($p \leq .05$). (From Bunn, H. F., and Forget, B. G.: Hemoglobin: Molecular, Genetic and Clinical Aspects. Philadelphia, W. B. Saunders Company, 1986, p. 420.) *B,* Effect of α thalassemia on the proportion of six positively charged β chain variants *(solid circles)* and of three negatively charged variants *(open circles).* (Modified and updated by permission from *Nature,* Vol. 306, p. 498; Copyright © 1983 Macmillan Magazines Limited.)

charged mutants are formed much more readily than positively charged mutants.[55]

This electrostatic model of hemoglobin assembly has clinical implications. Differences in rates of assembly explain not only the low proportion of Hb S in sickle trait (AS) but also the higher proportion of Hb S in sickle C (SC) disease. The prominent clinical manifestations of SC disease and their absence in sickle trait can be attributed in part to differences in the intracellular content of Hb S.[52] This model also provides an explanation for differences in the levels of Hb A$_2$[52] and Hb F[56, 57] that accompany certain hematological disorders.

CLINICAL PHENOTYPES. Individuals with hemoglobin mutants come to the attention of physicians because the mutation affects hemoglobin solubility, oxygenation, or synthesis (Table 6–2). In this clinical classification of the hemoglobinopathies, by far the most important are the sickle syndromes, either homozygous (SS) disease or the compound heterozygous states SC and S/β thalassemia. Hb S causes morbidity

by its propensity, when deoxygenated, to aggregate into rigid polymers, thereby occluding flow in the microcirculation. Hb C is also less soluble than Hb A, forming crystals rather than long polymers (see reference 58 and references therein). More important, Hb C, either in the homozygous state (CC) or in the heterozygous states (SC, AC), induces red cell dehydration.[59–61] The sickle syndromes and Hb C are discussed in detail below. The unstable mutants are also relatively insoluble. Rather than forming ordered polymers or crystals, these mutant molecules aggregate into amorphous precipitates (Heinz bodies) that cause hemolysis because they impair red cell pliability and damage the erythrocyte membrane. Hemoglobin mutants with abnormally high oxygen affinity are associated with secondary erythrocytosis owing to impaired oxygen delivery to tissues, whereas the much less common low-affinity mutants are sometimes so undersaturated with oxygen that they may cause cyanosis. Cyanosis may also be due to mutants (the M hemoglobins) in which the heme iron is locked in the ferric or

TABLE 6–2. CLINICALLY IMPORTANT HEMOGLOBIN MUTANTS

I. The sickle syndromes
   A. Sickle cell trait
   B. Sickle cell disease
      1. SS
      2. SC
      3. S/β thalassemia
II. Structural mutants that result in a thalassemic phenotype (approximately 15 mutants)
III. The unstable hemoglobins (congenital Heinz body anemia) (approximately 80 mutants)
IV. Mutants with abnormal oxygen affinity
   A. High affinity (familial erythrocytosis) (approximately 35 mutants)
   B. Low affinity (Hb Kansas, Hb Beth Israel → familial cyanosis)
V. The M hemoglobins → familial cyanosis (7 mutants)

methemoglobin form. Finally, if the synthesis of a mutant hemoglobin is sufficiently impaired, it may be associated with a thalassemic phenotype. These clinical phenotypes are discussed in the remainder of this chapter.

SICKLE HEMOGLOBIN AND SICKLE CELL DISEASE

Molecular Pathogenesis

The packaging of a very high concentration (32 to 34 g/dl) of hemoglobin into red cells requires that the protein be extraordinarily soluble. The substitution of valine for glutamic acid at β6 results in a marked decrease in the solubility of Hb S when it is deoxygenated. The aggregation of deoxy Hb S into polymers is the primary event in the molecular pathogenesis of sickle cell disease. Under physiologic conditions of pH, ionic strength, and temperature extant in the circulating red blood cell, the polymer assumes the form of an elongated rope-like fiber that usually aligns with other fibers, resulting in distortion into the classic crescent or sickle shape and a marked decrease in cell deformability. These rigid cells are responsible for the vaso-occlusive phenomena that are the hallmark of sickle cell disease.

Structure of the Sickle Fiber

Following deoxygenation, Hb S–containing cells assume a variety of interesting shapes readily appreciated by light microscopy and even more clearly by scanning electron microscopy, as shown in Figure 6–7. To understand the molecular events responsible for these morphological changes, much higher resolution is necessary. Transmission electron microscopy provides structural information at roughly 3 nm resolution. Analyses of deoxygenated sickle cells reveal the presence of parallel bundles of long fibers that are oriented along the axis of sickling.[62–65] In cells that

assume a holly leaf shape, bundles of Hb S fibers point in the direction of each projection. Higher resolution electron micrographs with negative staining showed that the sickle fiber is a solid structure.[66] The high quality of these electron micrographs enabled Edelstein and his colleagues[67] to utilize optical diffraction and image reconstruction to obtain a three-dimensional structure of the fiber. This analysis showed that individual fibers have an elliptical cross-section with a maximum diameter of about 23 nm and a minimum diameter of about 18 nm. Since hemoglobin tetramers are globular molecules with a diameter of about 5.5 nm, one can calculate that up to about 15 molecules could be packed into a cross-sectional area. Longitudinal views, as shown in Figure 6–8A, reveal a subtle but regular undulating pattern, in keeping with the elliptical cross-section and suggestive of a helical structure.[67] The helix has a high pitch with a periodicity of about 300 nm. The twisted rope-like structure, shown in Figure 6–8B, is composed of 14 strands, an inner core of 4 surrounded by a sheath of 10 (Fig. 6–8C). Each strand is a string of deoxy Hb S beads aligned in head-to-tail (or axial) array. Even higher resolution views revealed additional structural features: a hexagonal cross-section composed of seven pairs of molecules[68, 69] (Fig. 6–9A). Analyses of longitudinal views indicated that the components of each double strand are staggered by half a molecule. Verification of the double strand as the primary structural unit in the sickle fiber was provided by the finding of occasional fibers that lack one pair of strands (or even two) but no fibers that lack only a single strand.[66] These elegant electron micrographs provided sufficient detail to establish the directionality or polarity of the double strands as shown in Figure 6–9B.[68, 69] Such information on polarity is essential in determining intermolecular contacts in the fiber, compared with those in the crystal, described below.

Although these electron microscopy and optical diffraction studies have provided critical information on the packing of the sickle fiber, they lack sufficient resolution to address two important issues: the orientation of the hemoglobin tetramer in the polymer and the contacts with neighboring tetramers. Earlier optical measurements indicated that the long molecular x-axis (6.5 nm dimension) was within 20° of the fiber axis.[70, 71]* To address these questions in detail, it was necessary to employ X-ray diffraction. X-ray analyses of sickle fibers in gels of deoxy Hb S provided independent evidence for the presence of double strands but lacked sufficient resolution to convey information on molecular orientation or contacts.[72] Love and his associates[73] prepared crystals of deoxy Hb S in 10 to 15 per cent polyethylene glycol and performed X-ray diffraction analysis, initially at 0.5 nm resolution. Subsequently, the structure was solved at 0.3 nm resolution and then extensively refined.[74, 75] The primary

---

*Accordingly, the dyad axis of symmetry would be nearly perpendicular to the fiber axis.

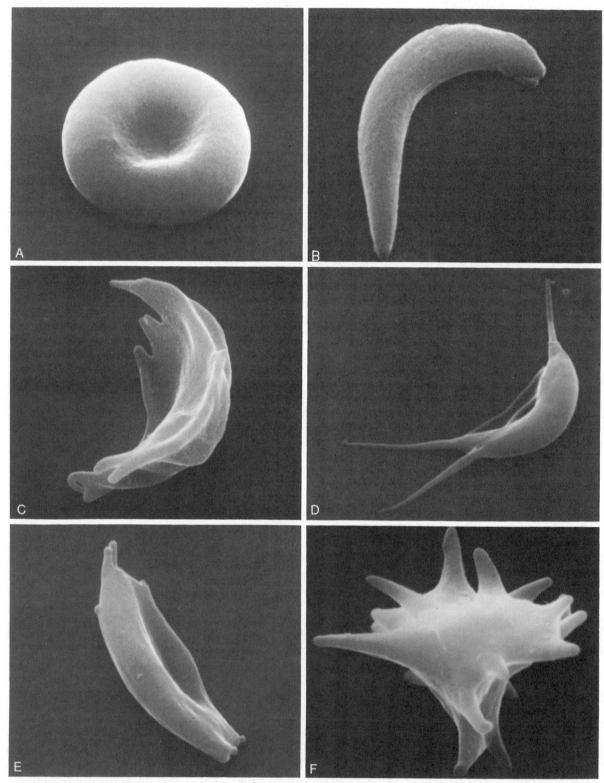

FIGURE 6–7. **Scanning electron micrographs of SS erythrocytes.** *A,* Oxygenated discocyte. *B,* Irreversibly sickled cell (ISC). Note the elongated shape and smooth contour. *C–F,* Deoxygenated discocytes (reversibly sickled cells). Cell D has a few elongated spiculated projections, giving rise to an elongated sickle shape, whereas cell F has multiple projections, giving rise to a holly leaf shape. (Prepared by Dr. James White. For further information, see Arch Intern. Med. 133:545, 1974.)

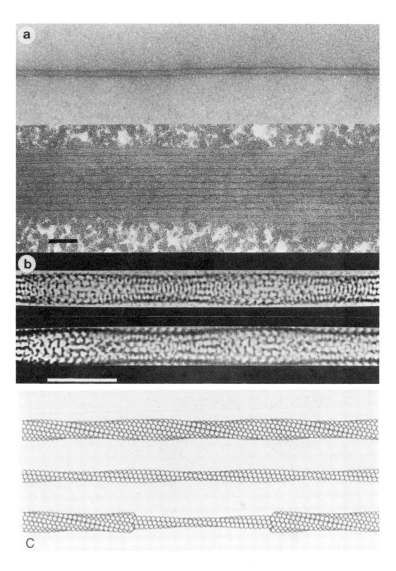

FIGURE 6–8. *A,* Electron micrographs of negatively stained sickle fibers. A single fiber and multiple aligned fibers are shown. *B,* Fiber images showing the twist of the strands within each fiber (*A* and *B* from Rodgers, D. W., Crepeau, R. H., and Edelstein, S. J.: Pairings and polarities of the 14 strands in sickle cell hemoglobin fibers. Proc. Natl. Acad. Sci. USA 84:6157, 1987; with permission.) *C,* Three-dimensional image reconstruction of the fiber. Each sphere represents a Hb S tetramer. The inner core of 4 strands and the outer sheath of 10 strands are shown. (Prepared by Dr. S. Edelstein.)

structural unit in the crystal is a double strand in which hemoglobin molecules are half-staggered. Adjacent molecules in the unit cell are related to one another by a 180° (twofold) screw symmetry. This finding motivated the search for and identification of comparable double strands in the fiber. The crystal contains alternate layers of double strands of opposite polarity. The structure of individual tetramers of deoxy Hb S is indistinguishable from that of deoxy Hb A except for a shift in the A helix of one of the β subunits, which enables contact with the β E and F helices of the neighboring molecule in the other strand (Fig. 6–10). The hemoglobin tetramer $\alpha^1\beta^1\alpha^2\beta^2$ is oriented in such a way that the 6(A3) Val of one of the two β subunits (β^2) forms a hydrophobic contact with a complementary or acceptor site at 70(E14) Ala, 85(F1) Phe, and 88(F4) Leu on the β^1 subunit of the partner strand.* It is noteworthy that the 6 Val of the β^1 subunit makes no contacts in the crystal structure

or in the fiber structure. As discussed below, this observation bears directly on the participation of non-S hemoglobins in the polymerization process. Moreover, the contact between β6 Val and an acceptor site on the partner strand is possible only when Hb S is in the T or deoxy conformation. R or oxygenated molecules cannot fit into the polymeric structure.

There is rather convincing evidence that the structure of the double strand in the crystal, including intermolecular contacts, is nearly identical with that in the fiber. Accordingly, the high-resolution information available from the crystal structure can be applied directly to the fiber, which, as stated previously, is the physiologically relevant structure. The double strands that are stacked in an antiparallel linear array in the crystal are slightly twisted in the fiber (Fig. 6–11). Stretching of the outer strands in the fiber limits its size to seven pairs.

Prior to these direct structural analyses, a considerable body of important information on the contacts between molecules in the polymer was generated by Bookchin and Nagel,[76–78] who studied the gelation of mixtures of Hb S with Hb A, Hb A_2, Hb F, and a

---

*Similar, but not identical, contacts are made with 6 Val of β_2 in the other strand: 70(E14) Ala, 73(E17) Asp, and 88(F4) Leu.

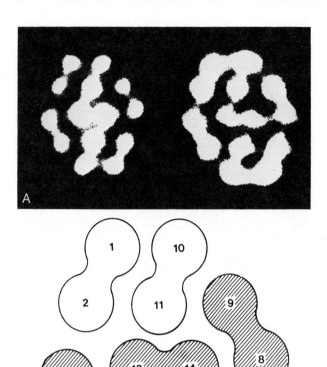

FIGURE 6–9. *A*, Cross-sectional views calculated from correlated images of fibers. *B*, Relationship between the above cross-sectional views and strand pairing and the polarity of the pairs. (*B* from Rodgers D. W., Crepeau, R. H., and Edelstein, S. J.: Pairings and polarities of the 14 strands in sickle cell hemoglobin fibers. Proc. Natl. Acad. Sci. USA 84:6157, 1987; with permission.)

large number of β globin mutants. Subsequently, Benesch and Benesch[79, 80] performed similar experiments with α globin mutants. When Hb S ($\alpha_2\beta^S_2$) and a β globin mutant ($\alpha_2\beta^X_2$) are mixed, the tetramers readily dissociate into αβ dimers, which then can reassociate to form hybrid tetramers $(\alpha_2\beta^S\beta^X)$[81] as well as the parent tetramers. Since only one β6 Val is required for polymerization at position β_2, the participation of the hybrid tetramer in the gel provides unambiguous information about contacts in the β_1 *(trans)* subunit. Taken together, the results of these gelation experiments are in remarkably good agreement with the X-ray analyses. The mutants that are indistinguishable from Hb A when mixed with Hb S generally have amino acid substitutions at sites not involved in contacts. The β globin mutants that do affect gelation tend to be on the β_1 or *trans* subunit and involve either lateral contacts between partners of the double strand or axial contacts between members of a single strand. In contrast, α contacts tend to be either axial or

between double strands.[82, 83]* Preparation and testing of genetically engineered site-directed globin mutants are providing further information about the contacts in the polymer. For example, the double mutant β6 Val, β121 Gln polymerizes much more readily than does Hb S.[84] This result fully supports the earlier finding of enhanced polymerization in a mixture of Hb S and Hb O-Arab (β121 Gln), confirming this site as a contact in the fiber. Another mutagenesis experiment has shown that β6 Val is not required for polymerization. Replacement of β6 Glu (in Hb A) by another hydrophobic residue, isoleucine, results in a hemoglobin ($\alpha_2\beta^{6Ile}_2$) that polymerizes even more readily than Hb S.[85]

Sickle Hemoglobin Polymerization

The polymerization of sickle hemoglobin involves the self-association of identical molecules. The detailed information on the structure of the polymer summarized in the previous section indicates that no accessory molecules are involved. Accordingly, the assembly process should and does obey simple chemical rules. During the past 15 years, a rigorous body of thermodynamic and kinetic measurements, primarily from the laboratory of Eaton and Hofrichter,† has provided a thorough understanding of the mechanistic pathway for Hb S polymerization both in pure solution and in the intact red cell. This information is critical to an understanding of the pathogenesis of the vaso-occlusive events in sickle cell disease.

EQUILIBRIUM MEASUREMENTS. When a gelled solution of deoxygenated Hb S is carefully examined by various physicochemical probes, large polymers (fibers) and free tetramers can be readily demonstrated, but species of intermediate size cannot be detected. This finding indicates that the polymerization of Hb S is a highly concerted process and therefore can be regarded as a simple phase change. Accordingly, the equilibrium between sol and gel can be studied by a measurement of the concentration of free hemoglobin in solution after segregating the polymer, such as by high-speed centrifugation[86–88] (Fig. 6–12). As in any bona fide solubility measurement, the result is independent of the total hemoglobin concentration.‡ For pure deoxy Hb S at pH 7 and 20°C, the solubility is 20 g/dl, considerably lower than the concentration of hemoglobin inside the red cell. Such solubility measurements have provided highly reliable information on the effect of a number of physiologically relevant parameters, such as fractional oxygenation, pH, tem-

---

*For a complete compilation of the experimental data on mixtures of Hb S with naturally occurring hemoglobin mutants, see references 83 and 86.

†These investigators have recently written a definitive review of this topic (reference 86). See References 89 and 90 for recent reviews that are less detailed and comprehensive.

‡This statement does not hold for partially oxygenated solutions or mixtures of S and non-S hemoglobins, owing to considerations of non-ideality and differences in the composition of the polymer and solution phases.

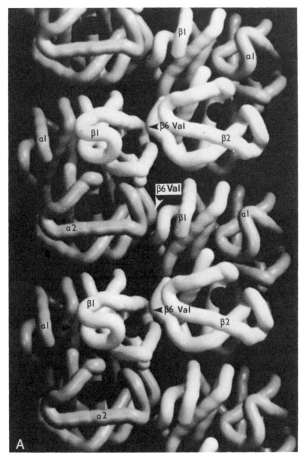

FIGURE 6–10. *A,* Intermolecular contacts in the sickle double strand. The α subunits are dark shaded, and the β subunits are light shaded. The β6 valine on the β$_2$ subunit forms a hydrophobic contact with a complementary site on the β$_1$ subunit of the adjacent strand. (Prepared by Drs. S. Watowich, L. Grass, and Robert Josephs.) *B,* Detail of the contacts between β6 Val and the complementary site located on the adjacent strand. Note that normal Hb A with β6 Glu cannot make this hydrophobic contact with the complementary site. (Prepared by I. Geis.)

FIGURE 6–11. Comparison between the linear double strand in the deoxy Hb S crystal and the twisted double strand in the deoxy Hb S fiber. (Prepared by Drs. S. Watowich, L. Grass, and Robert Josephs.)

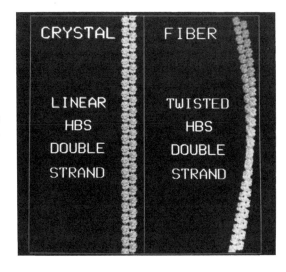

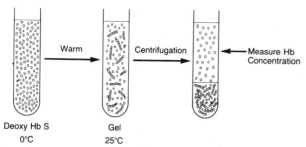

FIGURE 6–12. Measurement of the solubility of deoxy Hb S. A concentrated hemoglobin solution is warmed from 0°C to 25°C, allowing gelation to occur. After high-speed centrifugation, Hb S polymer forms a pellet at the bottom of the tube. The concentration of hemoglobin in the supernatant provides an accurate measurement of the solubility.

perature, ionic strength, organic phosphates, and the presence of non-S hemoglobins.

Fractional Oxygenation. Since, as mentioned above, the crystal structure of Hb S is nearly identical with that of Hb A, it is not surprising that in dilute solution the two hemoglobins have identical oxygen-binding curves under a variety of solvent conditions. However, at concentrations above the solubility of deoxy Hb S, the oxygen-binding curve is progressively right shifted.[91–93] Since Hb S polymerizes only when it is in the T quaternary conformation, it is not surprising that the polymer binds oxygen non-cooperatively and with low affinity.[94] The principles of thermodynamic linkage dictate that oxygen affinity is lowered in direct proportion to the amount of polymer formed. Moreover, because of the reciprocal relationship between oxygen binding and polymerization, it follows that the solubility of Hb S increases directly with oxygen saturation. Fully oxygenated molecules of Hb S or partially oxygenated molecules that assume the R conformation cannot be incorporated into the polymer but indirectly lower the solubility because their large excluded volume greatly increases the chemical activity of the coexisting T-state molecules,[95] thereby favoring their aggregation. This non-ideality consideration[95, 101] applies equally well to the solubility of mixtures of S and non-S hemoglobins and is a particularly important determinant of polymer formation at very high hemoglobin concentrations, such as those found in red blood cells.

pH. The solubility of deoxy Hb S is lowest between pH 6.0 and 7.2 and rises quite sharply at higher and lower pH values.[96, 97] Accordingly, in the pH range 6.5 to 7.5, the alkaline Bohr effect is enhanced in concentrated solutions of Hb S as well as in SS red cells.[98]

Temperature. The polymerization of Hb S is an endothermic process,[99–101] consistent with the importance of hydrophobic interactions. Therefore, polymer formation is entropically driven, resulting from the release of ordered water molecules from the surface of free hemoglobin. Sickle polymers are melted by cooling. Accordingly, a temperature jump is a simple and effective way of initiating polymerization and thereby enabling kinetic measurements.

Ionic Strength. The solubility of deoxy Hb S depends on salt and buffer conditions. At salt concentrations spanning the physiologic range, solubility increases with ionic strength,[102] but it decreases markedly at high ionic strength.[102, 103] This salting out effect allows experiments to be performed with relatively small amounts of hemoglobin. In general, the solubility data obtained in high phosphate buffers agree well, but not perfectly,[104] with measurements made under physiologic conditions.

Organic Phosphates. As mentioned at the beginning of this chapter, the primary modulator of oxygen affinity in the red cell is 2,3-DPG. An increase in red cell 2,3-DPG favors Hb S polymerization in three ways: lowered oxygen affinity, increasing deoxygenation; a reduction in intracellular pH; and a direct effect on the conformation of deoxy Hb S, the latter two ways directly enhancing aggregation.[105, 106]

Non-S Hemoglobins. As mentioned above, in the description of the structure of the sickle fiber, a considerable amount has been learned about intermolecular contacts from measurements of the gelation or solubility of mixtures of S and non-S hemoglobins. Of particular and practical importance is the effect of Hb F, Hb A, and Hb, C which commonly coexist in high concentration in the red cells of patients with various sickle genotypes. Information on the copolymerization of Hb S with these hemoglobins has provided important insights into the pathogenesis and clinical severity of the various sickle syndromes, including SS with increased levels of Hb F, S/β⁰ thalassemia, S/β⁺ thalassemia, SC disease, and AS (sickle trait). Moreover, as mentioned above, these studies have provided early and reliable information on intermolecular contacts in the sickle fiber. The solubility of a mixture of equal amounts of Hb S and Hb A (and that of Hb S + Hb C) is only about 40 per cent higher than that of Hb S alone. In this mixture, half of the hemoglobin is asymmetrical hybrid tetramers ($\alpha_2\beta^S\beta^A$). Since only one of the two β6 Val residues is engaged in an intermolecular contact, there is a 50 per cent chance that the hybrid tetramer will enter the polymer in such a way that all the proper contacts are made. Indeed, incorporation of αβ dimers of Hb A into the sickle polymer has been experimentally documented.[55, 96] In contrast, the Hb A tetramers ($\alpha_2\beta_2$), which constitute 25 per cent of the mixture, fail to be incorporated into the polymer. Nevertheless, by virtue of their excluded volume,[95] the solubility is further lowered.

In contrast to Hb A and Hb C, Hb F and Hb A_2 inhibit polymerization. Accordingly, the hybrid tetramers $\alpha_2\beta\gamma$ and $\alpha_2\beta\delta$ fail to be incorporated into the sickle polymer. Hb F ($\alpha_2\gamma_2$) affects polymerization by means of the asymmetrical hybrid $\alpha_2\beta^S\gamma$.[96, 107] Thus, the inhibition is *trans* to the β6 Val contact. Nagel and his colleagues[77] have presented evidence that γ87 is one of the important inhibitory sites. This residue constitutes one of the lateral contacts in the double strand of the sickle fiber.

KINETICS OF POLYMERIZATION. The information presented thus far on the structure of the sickle fiber

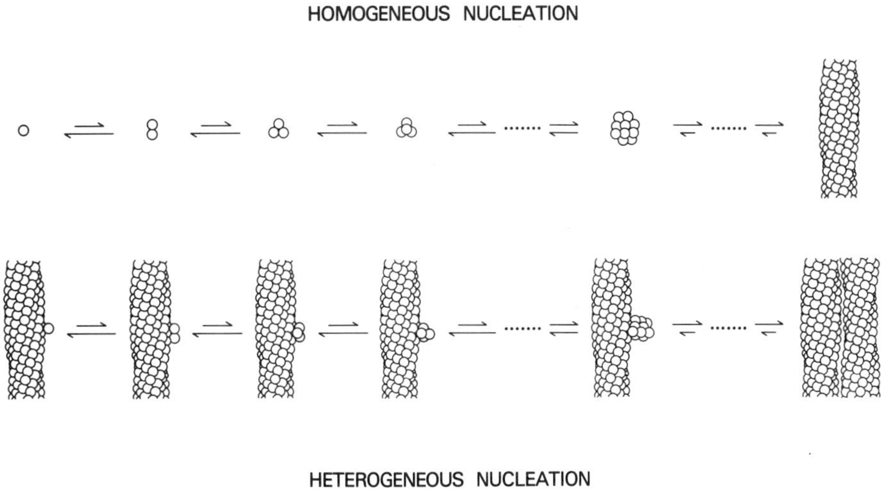

HOMOGENEOUS NUCLEATION

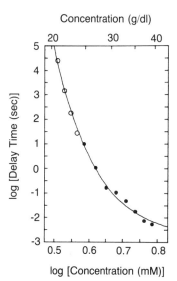

HETEROGENEOUS NUCLEATION

FIGURE 6–13. Schematic representation of homogeneous and heterogeneous nucleation. In the homogeneous pathway, nuclei form in solution, whereas in the heterogeneous pathway, nuclei form on the surface of existing fibers. Initially, the formation of small aggregates is thermodynamically unfavorable. As the aggregate increases in size, each participating hemoglobin molecule has relatively more contacts, providing enhanced stability, which overcomes the unfavorable entropic forces. Once this critical nucleus is formed, propagation of the polymer is very rapid. (Prepared by Dr. William A. Eaton. From Bunn, H. F., and Forget B. G.: Hemoglobin: Molecular, Genetic and Clinical Aspects. Philadelphia, W. B. Saunders Company, 1986, p. 472.)

as well as on the thermodynamics of gelation may lead to the false impression of a rather static process. In fact, the polymerization of sickle hemoglobin is a remarkably dynamic event. Rigorous measurements, primarily made by Eaton and Hofrichter and their colleagues,[108, 109] of the kinetics of polymer formation, both in pure Hb S solutions and in sickle erythrocytes, have provided critical insights into the pathogenesis of vaso-occlusive crises, which play such a dominant role in sickle cell disease. Their studies led directly to information on the nucleation mechanism responsible for fiber formation. Their experiments on intact red cells have provided an explanation at the molecular level of the morphological changes that are observed following the deoxygenation of cells, both in vitro and in vivo. Finally, understanding the kinetics of polymerization has enabled them to propose a novel and workable approach to the assessment of new antisickling therapy.

Solution Studies. The time course for polymerization of a concentrated solution of Hb S can be monitored after either rapid removal of ligand such as by photolysis or (as mentioned above) by rapidly increasing the temperature of deoxy Hb S, taking advantage of the markedly endothermic nature of the process. The formation of sickle fibers can be documented by a variety of physicochemical techniques, including turbidity, light scattering, calorimetry, and NMR spectroscopy. The subsequent alignment of fibers is best monitored by measurement of birefringence. Following ligand removal or temperature jump, there is a clearly measurable time lag before occurrence of a signal reflecting the presence of detectable polymer. Simultaneous calorimetry and birefringence measurements document the formation of fibers and their subsequent alignment. The progress of polymer formation is exponential. During the delay time, the amount of polymer is insufficient to provide a signal, owing to limitations of sensitivity of the above-mentioned methods for monitoring. Fiber formation begins with a nucleation process, shown in Figure 6–13, in which a relatively small number of hemoglobin molecules assemble to form a lattice upon which fiber

growth can take place. The approximate number of molecules in the nucleus can be estimated from the slope of the concentration dependence of the delay time (Fig. 6–14). At high concentrations of hemoglobin, the slope is about 15, whereas at lower concentrations, it increases to about 30. As shown in Figure 6–13, aggregates smaller than the critical nucleus are thermodynamically unfavored. In contrast, once the nucleus is formed, subsequent addition of molecules is highly favored, and fiber growth becomes very rapid (approximately 250 hemoglobin tetramers per second).[110] Ferrone, Eaton, and Hofrichter[111] observed that delay times on relatively concentrated solutions, although short, were highly reproducible; to their surprise, when measurements were made on small volumes of more dilute solutions, the longer delay

FIGURE 6–14. Concentration dependence of the delay time of polymerization of deoxy Hb S from laser photolysis of very concentrated solutions *(solid circles)* and temperature jump measurements of less concentrated solutions *(open circles)*. The slope of this curve provides an approximation of the "order" of the polymerization reaction and therefore of the size of the critical nucleus. (From Eaton, W. A., and Hofrichter, J.: Hemoglobin S gelation and sickle cell disease. Blood 70:1245, 1987; with permission.)

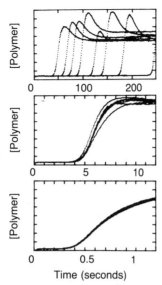

FIGURE 6–15. Kinetic plots of the progress curves for the polymerization of deoxy Hb S. In a concentrated solution (*bottom panel*), where the delay time is short (approximately 0.4 second), replicate experiments are highly reproducible. In contrast, in a more dilute solution (*top panel*), replicate experiments are highly variable, with delay times ranging from 40 to 175 seconds. This stochastic behavior reflects the formation and propagation of a single polymer domain. (From Eaton, W. A., and Hofrichter, J.: Hemoglobin S gelation and sickle cell disease. Blood 70:1245, 1987; with permission.)

times varied markedly. This stochastic behavior, shown in Figure 6–15, suggested to them that each signal had been amplified from a single nucleation event. Statistical thermodynamic modeling of their results[111, 112] led these investigators to propose two pathways for the nucleation of sickle hemoglobin fibers. In one, nucleation of individual fibers occurs in the bulk solution phase and is called homogeneous nucleation. In the second, nucleation occurs on the surface of existing polymers, which leads to autocatalytic formation of fibers and hence the delay period. This second pathway is called heterogeneous nucleation. As shown in Figure 6–13, in highly concentrated solutions of deoxy Hb S, homogeneous nucleation is favored. Polarizing microscopy reveals multiple domains of polymers giving rise to birefringent spherulites. These are probably the tactoids that Harris first observed in solutions of deoxy Hb S.[113] In less concentrated solutions of deoxy Hb S, heterogeneous nucleation predominates, leading to fewer domains of aligned sickle fibers. Recently, the kinetics of formation of individual fibers has been observed directly by means of video-enhanced differential interference contrast microscopy.[110] The growth of new fibers from branch points provides direct support for a heterogeneous nucleation mechanism.

Cellular Studies. The extension of the equilibrium and kinetic studies of polymerization to erythrocytes is greatly complicated by the marked heterogeneity of SS cells, owing to a wide range of oxygen affinity, an even wider distribution of intracellular hemoglobin concentration (20 to 50 g/dl), and the heterogeneous

distribution of Hb F. However, when these variables are taken into account, the delay times of SS red cells and the amount of polymer per cell at equilibrium are remarkably close to what is encountered in hemoglobin solutions.[114] This conclusion is consistent with the finding that the cytosolic surface of the red cell membrane has no effect on the delay time.[115]

The kinetics of polymerization plays a critical role in the rheology and morphology of circulating red cells.[116] Equilibrium measurements of the polymer content of red cells, whether by oxygen-binding curves,[117] by NMR spectroscopy,[118, 119] or by differential polarization microscopy,[120] grossly overestimate the amount of intracellular polymer that is formed in vivo as SS red cells are deoxygenated in the arterioles and capillaries. Because the range of transit times in the microcirculation is short, relative to the range of delay times of SS red cells, the great majority (perhaps 95 per cent) of cells fail to form polymer during their flow through arterioles and capillaries.[116] In contrast, if these cells were equilibrated at the oxygen tensions in the microcirculation, virtually all of them would contain polymer and as a result would have markedly decreased deformability.

As shown in Figure 6–16, kinetics is the critical determinant of cell shape and morphology. A number of early experiments clearly demonstrated that when SS red cells are deoxygenated slowly, they form the classical elongated (sickle) shapes. This observation is a vivid demonstration of homogeneous nucleation, wherein one domain propagates by fiber growth and alignment to distort the cell into a classical sickle shape. With somewhat more rapid deoxygenation, a few independent domains will induce a more irregular

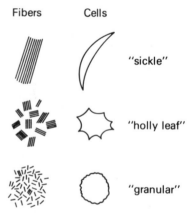

FIGURE 6–16. Relationship between the number of polymer domains and the shape of the sickled cell. *Top,* When cells sickle slowly, there is likely to be a single polymer domain, which propagates into very long fibers with further alignment of fibers along a single long axis, giving rise to the classic banana or sickle shape. *Middle,* With intermediate rates of polymerization, there will be several polymer domains composed of shortened aligned fibers, resulting in multiple spiculated projections and a holly leaf shape (see Fig. 6–7F). When polymerization is very rapid, there will be multiple domains with randomly oriented fibers, resulting in a granular appearance with no projections from the cell surface. (From Eaton, W. A., and Hofrichter, J.: Hemoglobin S gelation and sickle cell disease. Blood 70:1245, 1987; with permission.)

shape.[121] In contrast, when deoxygenation is rapid, multiple spherulitic domains result in a granular or cobblestone texture with no gross distortion of cell shape. Because the shape of the sickled cell is so dependent on the number of independent polymer domains, it is possible to convert a holly leaf cell into an elongated sickle shape by partial reoxygenation![122] As discussed in detail below, the distortion of cell shape by projections of aligned Hb S fibers plays a critical role in the pathogenesis of the membrane lesion.

The Erythrocyte Membrane in Sickle Cell Disease

Although information on the kinetics and thermodynamics of Hb S polymerization has provided remarkably penetrating insights into the pathogenesis of sickle cell disease, a fuller understanding depends on reckoning with the complexities of the flow of sickle erythrocytes in the microcirculation. The red cell membrane is the fulcrum that links primary intracellular events (polymer formation, growth, and orientation) with secondary changes that have impact on red cell deformability as well as interactions with the vascular endothelium. Several hundred papers have been written on this subject during the past decade. For more detailed coverage than is possible in this chapter, the recent review by Hebbel[123] is recommended.

Membrane Proteins

LIPID BILAYER–SKELETON UNCOUPLING. The red cell skeleton is composed of a two-dimensional hexagonal lattice of interacting spectrin tetramers, stabilized by actin and protein 4.1. This flexible yet sturdy "geodesic dome" is covered snugly by a lipid bilayer, in which is embedded a variety of proteins such as erythroid-specific glycophorins and transport proteins, including the anion channel (protein 3) and Na-K-ATPase and other cation channels. Ankyrin provides a bridge between spectrin and protein 3, whereas protein 4.1 is linked to glycophorins A and C and to aminophospholipids on the cytoplasmic side of the lipid bilayer. The spicules that are observed following slow deoxygenation of SS erythrocytes contain protein 3 but not spectrin.[124] These spicules represent the penetration of bundles of aligned sickle fibers through the skeleton, thereby dissociating it from the lipid bilayer.[124]* When the red cell is reoxygenated, the sickle polymers melt and the bilayer lipids at the tip of the spicule are released from the cells in the form of hemoglobin-rich lipid vesicles. A large proportion of the additional perturbations in the structure and function of red cell membrane proteins and lipids that

are discussed in this section are a direct consequence of the rather draconian distortions imposed by projections of sickle polymer.

Irreversibly Sickled Cells. The earliest evidence of the impaired structure and function of SS erythrocyte membranes came with the recognition of irreversibly sickled cells (ISCs), which remain locked in an elongated shape despite full oxygenation and absence of polymer. Unlike reversibly sickled cells, which usually contain multiple sharp projections (see Fig. 6–7), ISCs have a relatively smooth contour. The persistence of the elongated (sickled) shape, even after removal of the membrane lipid by a detergent, provided convincing evidence that the architecture of the skeleton was irreversibly perturbed.[126] This shape change is a consequence of plastic deformation of membrane skeletal proteins induced by rearrangement of spectrin heterodimers.[127]

Anywhere between 1 and 50 per cent of the red cells in blood films from patients with SS disease have an elongated shape. However, about half of these cells are reversibly sickled, having such low oxygen affinity that polymerized Hb S persists during the preparation of the specimen.[128] Truly *irreversibly* sickled cells are those that retain an elongated shape after all of the intracellular polymer has been melted by equilibrating the blood specimen with carbon monoxide prior to preparing the microscope slide.[128]

ISCs are generally very dense cells, with mean corpuscular hemoglobin concentrations (MCHCs) as high as 50 g/dl. In a given patient, ISCs have lower levels of Hb F than do less dense cells.[129] Moreover, among a large group of patients with SS disease in the absence of concurrent α thalassemia, the percentage of ISCs correlates inversely with the percentage of Hb F.[130, 131] SS red cells lacking Hb F have a much higher potential for forming polymer than do SS F cells, for reasons discussed above. Therefore, it is very likely that the ISC is the consequence of repeated cycles of in vivo sickling. In vitro experiments provide support for this claim. ISCs can be formed in vitro by repetitive cycles of deoxygenation (see references 132 and 133 and the references therein) and, importantly, by a single deoxygenation step if the oxygen removal is slow enough to allow the SS cell to assume an elongated, sickle shape.[134] Under these conditions, K leak exceeds Na gain, and the cell becomes dehydrated, contributing further to deoxy Hb S polymerization. Earlier reports notwithstanding, ATP depletion is not necessary for in vitro ISC formation, whereas external Ca is required.[134] The latter finding suggests that the Gardos channel may contribute to the K loss that accompanies ISC formation. (See Disordered Volume Control, later).

ISCs tend to be young red cells.[135] Moreover, because of their very high MCHC and stiff membrane, they are inordinately rigid cells that understandably have a markedly shortened life span. Thus, these cells are morphological reminders of the autocatalytic processes that are such a fundamental feature of sickle cell disease.

---

*In like manner, the vesicles that are shed following repeated cycles of in vitro sickling are free of spectrin.[125]

DISORDERED MEMBRANE PROTEIN INTERACTIONS. The structure and function of a number of membrane proteins are perturbed in SS red cells. The demonstration that inside-out vesicles from SS red cells show decreased binding to normal spectrin implies an abnormality in ankyrin.[136] Similarly, protein 4.1 from SS red cells has a decreased capability for binding to normal inside-out vesicles that have been depleted of endogenous protein 4.1. Moreover, SS vesicles have a decreased content of protein 4.1.[137] It is not clear whether these findings reflect impaired binding of protein 4.1 to aminophospholipids or to glycophorin. The altered function of protein 4.1 from SS red cells may be due to oxidative damage (see below).[137] The interaction of Hb S with the cytosolic surface may also contribute to disordered membrane function. Hb S binds more readily than Hb A to normal inside-out vesicles (see references 138 and 139 and the references therein). Nevertheless, this interaction does not appear to alter the kinetics of intracellular polymerization of Hb S.[115] A small amount of globin appears to be covalently linked to spectrin in SS red cells as well as in other types of dehydrated cells.[140] The adherence of Hb S to the red cell membrane contributes significantly to the static rigidity of SS red cells.[141]

These abnormalities in the organization of proteins on the cytoplasmic surface of SS membranes are matched by equally striking alterations on the cell surface. In particular, glycophorin[142, 143] and protein 3[143] are abnormally clustered. The aggregates of protein 3 may lead to the enhanced binding of immunoglobulin that has been observed on the surface of circulating SS red cells. It has been suggested, but not yet proved, that clustering of glycophorin and protein 3 may be provoked by the formation of Heinz bodies (aggregates of denatured Hb S).[123] The abnormal distribution of these highly charged surface proteins in SS red cells may contribute significantly to the pathogenesis of vaso-occlusion either because of adhesion to endothelial cells or, less likely, as a source of procoagulant. The enhanced binding of immunoglobulin to SS red cells may trigger accelerated clearance by the mononuclear phagocyte system.

OXIDATION OF SS MEMBRANE PROTEINS. Considerable effort has been expended seeking and documenting oxidant damage to membranes of SS red cells.[123] There is a significant, although modest, reduction in free sulfhydryl groups of SS membrane proteins.[144, 145] The formation of interprotein disulfide bonds cannot be extensive, since protein-sizing gels fail to reveal high molecular weight aggregates that are commonly associated with oxidant-type hemolytic anemia. Oxidant damage can impose other structural alterations on specific proteins in SS membranes. For example, in protein 4.1, decreased free sulfhydryl content is accompanied by large protein aggregates, half of which appeared to be disulfide cross-links, and also by oxidized amino acids.[137]

Why should SS red cells be unduly susceptible to oxidant damage? In an attempt to answer this question, Hebbel and his colleagues have amassed experimental data indicating that oxidized Hb S is the culprit.[123] They found that purified Hb S auto-oxidized 1.7 times faster than Hb A purified from the same AS donor[146] and that Hb S had a comparably increased rate of dissociation of heme. These investigators propose that these abnormalities are responsible for the twofold increased deposition of heme and heme proteins, such as hemichromes, that has been documented on the membranes of SS red cells.[147, 148] Because these heme moieties can serve as a biological Fenton reagent, they may be responsible for the enhanced rate of hydroxyl radical generated from superoxide and peroxide in SS red cells.[149, 150]

Two issues remain controversial: (1) the mechanisms responsible for the formation of hemichrome and activated oxygen compounds in SS red cells and (2) the contribution of these phenomena to the damage of SS membranes.

It is not at all clear that the above-mentioned modest increase in the rate of auto-oxidation of Hb S[146] is the cause of the twofold increase in the generation of superoxide and hydroxyl radical. Current understanding of the three-dimensional structure of hemoglobin and the molecular events responsible for auto-oxidation and hemichrome formation does not predict that the $\beta6$ Glu$\rightarrow$Val replacement would have any impact. Moreover, there are stable mutants such as Hb Kansas that have markedly higher rates of hemoglobin auto-oxidation than that reported for Hb S and yet are not associated with any evidence of red cell membrane damage or hemolysis. Moreover, like individuals with SS disease, Hb Kansas heterozygotes have no detectable methemoglobinemia. Rather than auto-oxidation, another more striking abnormality of SS red cells may be responsible for hemichrome formation: Upon mechanical shaking in room air, Hb S denatures more readily than Hb A and other common mutants,[151, 152] with a twofold increase in the release of hemin.[153] This enhanced denaturation at the liquid-gas interface may have a parallel at the cytosol-membrane interface within the red cell.

There is general agreement that hemichromes (irreversibly oxidized hemoglobin) are modestly increased (twofold to threefold) in SS red cells. How much do these products contribute to the multiplicity of structural and functional perturbations in SS membranes? Much higher levels of hemichromes are encountered in red cells of individuals having unstable hemoglobin mutants, yet the clinical and laboratory phenotype in this disorder bears only superficial similarity to sickle cell disease. In vitro loading of hemin onto normal red cell skeletons does induce membrane defects similar to what has been reported in SS red cells.[154, 155] However, differences in the dose of hemin and its presentation in the membrane raise concern about the relevance of these in vitro experiments to the pathophysiology of sickle cell disease. A similar concern may be raised about the pathophysiological significance of the comparably modest (twofold) increase in the production of superoxide and hydroxyl radical by SS red cells. However, it may be that in SS red cells the enhanced production of activated oxygen compounds synergizes with the increased levels of heme and non-heme iron in the membrane, resulting in significant oxidant damage.[123]

Membrane Lipids

INSTABILITY OF THE LIPID BILAYER. In a variety of biological membranes, the distribution of phospholipids is asymmetrical. In the lipid bilayer of the human red cell, more than 75 per cent of the choline-containing phospholipids (phosphatidylcholine [PC] and sphingomyelin) are on the outer leaflet, whereas more than 80 per cent of phosphatidylethanolamine (PE) and all of phosphatidylserine (PS) are on the inner leaflet. This asymmetry is maintained by two independent mechanisms: (1) an ATP-dependent aminophospholipid translocase, which catalyzes the transfer of PE and PS from the plasma across the outer leaflet to the inner leaflet[156]; and (2) the binding of the aminophospholipids (PE and PS) to proteins of the skeleton (spectrin and protein 4.1). The importance of the second mechanism is controversial (see reference 157 and the references therein).

In a variety of hemolytic disorders, including SS disease, reduction of membrane stability has been documented by a decrease in phospholipid asymmetry and by increased rates of transit of choline phospholipids across the bilayer. In SS red cells, aminophospholipids have been noted in the outer leaflet of ISCs, as well as in the outer leaflet of discoid SS cells that have been induced to sickle.[158] The precise extent of the flip-flop is unclear, since the methods used to monitor phospholipid asymmetry are likely to perturb the equilibrium between phospholipids in the inner and outer leaflets. In both ISCs and in deoxygenated discoid SS cells, reduction of phospholipid asymmetry is accompanied by an increase in PC translocation.[159–161] These phenomena appear to be a direct result of the marked upheaval in the organization of the skeleton, as discussed in detail above. Polymerization-induced deformation of red cell shape is necessary to induce both enhanced PC translocation and loss of phospholipid asymmetry. When discoid SS cells are deoxygenated under conditions that produce multiple domains of polymer but no spicules or gross membrane distortion, the stability of the lipid bilayer is maintained.[160, 161] Moreover, when SS cells have been stressed by multiple cycles of deoxygenation and reoxygenation, the vesicles that are formed from the shed spicules have markedly decreased phospholipid asymmetry, whereas the remnant despiculated cell appears to have normal membrane stability.[159] These findings again underscore the primacy of polymerization-induced distortion of cell shape in the pathogenesis of the membrane lesions in sickle cell disease.

The loss of phospholipid asymmetry in SS red cells may contribute to the vaso-occlusive manifestations of the disease. ISCs, sickled discocytes, and the vesicles shed from sickled cells, like PE-enriched liposomes, are potent procoagulants.[156, 162, 163] The literature on abnormalities in hemostasis in sickle cell disease is large and confusing. The aggregate of clinical and laboratory data suggests that thrombosis may play a significant, albeit secondary, role (see reference 164 and the references therein).

LIPID PEROXIDATION. Oxidant stress affects the structure not only of proteins, as discussed previously, but also of lipids. Membranes of SS red cells have about twofold higher levels of lipid peroxidation than do normal red cells.[165, 166] Moreover, ISCs have a novel phospholipid composed of PE and PS cross-linked by malondialdehyde,[167] a product of lipid peroxidation. It is likely that increased amounts of both denatured hemoglobin[168] and non-heme iron[169] in SS membranes generate activated oxygen compounds responsible for increased lipid peroxidation.

The pathophysiological significance of a twofold increase in lipid peroxidation is not clear. Considering the fact that such a tiny mole fraction of membrane lipid is modified, it seems plausible that this phenomenon is overshadowed by the impact of oxidant stress on the structure and function of SS membrane proteins. However, lipid peroxidation may induce enhanced recognition of SS red cells by macrophages,[170] thereby contributing to the shortened in vivo survival of SS red cells.

Disordered Volume Control*

The rate and extent of polymer formation in a circulating SS red cell depend on three primary variables: the cell's hemoglobin composition,† its degree of deoxygenation, and its intracellular hemoglobin concentration (MCHC). During their 120-day survival, circulating normal AA red cells lose a small amount of solute and water with a concomitant increase in MCHC. Therefore, normal red cells have a significant but narrow distribution of MCHC and density that depends in part on in vivo aging. Although the MCHC and mean cell density of the overall population of SS red cells are close to what is found in normal red cells, the density distribution of SS red cells is unusually broad. The substantial population of low density SS cells reflects a high number of reticulocytes that have a relatively low MCHC. The marked increase in dense cells is a result of enhanced dehydration of a comparably substantial proportion of circulating cells. The ISC, discussed in the beginning of this section, is the final stage of this process. Since the polymerization of deoxy Hb S is so markedly dependent on hemoglobin concentration, dense SS cells are much more prone to sickle and thus contribute disproportionately to the vaso-occlusive and hemolytic aspects of the disease. Arguably, this accelerated in vivo dehydration is the most relevant pathophysiological consequence of the

---

*For more detailed coverage of this topic, see the recent review by Bookchin et al.[171]

†In particular, whether Hb F is present in the SS red cell and, if so, what is its concentration?

above-described perturbations in the structure of the membrane in SS red cells.

There is convincing evidence that four independent phenomena contribute to the dehydration of SS red cells: (1) KCl cotransport, (2) Ca-activated K efflux, (3) passive K and Na leak, and (4) decrease in osmotic pressure. All but the first of these are triggered by intracellular polymerization of Hb S.

KCL COTRANSPORT. Sheep erythrocytes that are genetically low in K have a ouabain- and bumetanide-resistant transport system that is a major pathway for the flux of K and Cl.[172, 173] KCl cotransport was first demonstrated in human red cells by Brugnara and his colleagues.[61, 174] In normal AA red cells, this channel is active only in reticulocytes[175, 176] and may contribute to the above-mentioned decrease in MCHC that accompanies normal in vivo red cell aging. Much higher levels of KCl cotransport are observed in CC[61, 177] and SS[174, 177] red cells. This finding cannot be due merely to hemolysis with an increase in young red cells, since KCl cotransport is also elevated in AC and AS red cells,[178] which have normal life spans. Thus, it is likely that the function of this transporter is affected by these mutants, which are known to have enhanced binding to the cytosolic surface of the red cell membrane.[138] KCl cotransport is induced by hypo-osmolarity and also by a modest decrease in pH (to 7.0). As discussed in more detail below, the latter stimulus likely pertains in vivo, particularly at sites of stagnant circulation. Conversely, the pathway is markedly (90 per cent) inhibited by DIOA ([[(dihydroindenyl) oxy]alkanoic acid).[179] This agent is not fully specific, since it also inhibits the anion channel.

KCl cotransport probably plays a major role in the marked dehydration that is a hallmark of CC[61] and SC[180] red cells. In SS cells, this pathway is particularly active in those cells lacking Hb F and thus could contribute to progressive dehydration of these cells.[181] Nevertheless, Hb F per se does not directly inhibit this pathway.[135] KCl cotransport is significantly inhibited by deoxygenation, probably because of the accompanying rise in free cytosolic Mg.[182, 183] The overall contribution of KCl cotransport to the dehydration of SS red cells must be weighed against sickling-induced mechanisms, discussed below.

CALCIUM-DEPENDENT K CHANNEL. SS red cells have increased amounts of Ca.[184, 185] Because Ca is compartmentalized within intracellular vesicles,[186, 187] the steady-state levels of free ionized Ca are normal.[171] However, when cells undergo sickling, there is an increase in the permeability of a number of cations, including not only Ca[171] but also K, Na,[188] and Mg.[189] This leak appears to be limited to cations, since sickling fails to affect the permeability of sulfate anion, erythritol, mannitol, or arabinose.[190] Similar to other perturbations in SS membrane structure and function, which are discussed above, this non-specific leak in cations requires not only the formation of sickle polymer but also the distortion of the membrane by elongated spicules. ATP is maintained at normal levels in SS red cells, and therefore the Ca ATPase, which

efficiently pumps Ca out of the cell or into vesicles, remains fully active. However, when the cell membrane is stretched by sickling, the transient increase in free cytosolic Ca is sufficient to trigger the Ca-dependent (Gardos) K channel, thereby providing a pathway for sickling-induced loss of K and water, leading to cell dehydration. This process could be accentuated by inhibition of Ca ATPase. Although Ca ATPase levels are probably normal in SS red cells (reviewed in reference 171), enzyme activity could be low in vulnerable SS cells, since the enzyme is susceptible to both reversible and permanent damage by oxidants known to be produced by SS cells.[191]

PASSIVE K AND NA LEAK. Forty years ago, Tosteson showed that when SS cells were deoxygenated they became leaky to Na and K.[192] These ion movements are unaffected by furosemide or by anion replacement and do not involve a Na-K exchange mechanism. The Na and K leak can be inhibited by stilbene disulfonates, such as DIDS (4,4′-diisothiocyano-2,2′-disulfostilbene), but in a manner independent of inhibition of the anion channel (protein 3).[193] As mentioned above, this increase in cation permeability requires true sickling with gross deformation and stretching of the cell membrane.[188, 193a] Subsequent measurements confirmed that sickling-induced passive influx of K and efflux of Na are almost precisely balanced.[194] However, because the red cell sodium pump (Na-K-ATPase) has a stoichiometry of 3 K out for 2 Na in, repeated cycles of sickling should result in a net loss of total cation and water. Recent modeling studies[171, 195] suggest that the dehydration caused by sickling-induced K and Na leak is likely to be slow and modest and probably does not account for the rapid transition from young reticulocyte to dense ISC that has been noted in vivo.[135] However, simulation experiments suggest that oxidant damage to SS membranes may act synergistically with mechanical distortion to magnify cation leaks.[196, 197]

DECREASE IN OSMOTIC PRESSURE. A fourth mechanism for sickling-induced cell dehydration evolves directly from thermodynamic principles. As sickle hemoglobin polymerizes inside the red cell, osmolarity may change significantly, with an accompanying shift in water across the cell membrane. The solute concentration in the water that is trapped within sickle polymers does not appear to differ significantly from that in the free cytosol.[198] Accordingly, intracellular polymerization of Hb S should be associated with a fall in osmolarity and therefore with prompt cell shrinkage. Previous measurements of this phenomenon have given conflicting results owing to pH changes and difficulties in accurately measuring red cell volumes. However, recent and carefully obtained measurements verify that deoxygenation of SS red cells is associated with a small but significant degree of cell shrinkage. Since the kinetics of deoxy Hb S polymerization depend so exquisitely on hemoglobin concentration, this phenomenon could be an amplification factor, increasing the rate and extent of polymerization during flow in the microcirculation. It should be noted that this process depends on polymer formation but, unlike

Ca-induced K efflux or passive Na and K leaks, does not depend on sickling-induced distortion of the cell membrane. Moreover, unlike the other three means for dehydration of SS cells, discussed above, the polymerization-induced change in osmolarity is instantaneous and fully reversible.

Bookchin and Lew[135, 195] have presented an integrated model that places in perspective the four independent mechanisms, discussed above, that can induce rapid dehydration of young SS red cells. In contrast to mature red cells, reticulocytes do not return to their original steady state following transient perturbations. Brief spurts of either acidosis or sickling-induced Ca influx can trigger K and water efflux. As shown in Figure 6–17, positive cooperativity exists between these two processes. K efflux is accompanied by an equivalent Cl efflux, which is compensated by co-influx of Cl and protons via the Jacobs-Stewart mechanism. This secondary acidosis would trigger further K and water loss via KCl cotransport. In essence, red cells in general and reticulocytes in particular do not have an effective way of dealing with K loss. A transient period of sickling can set in motion K and water loss through cooperation of the Gardos and KCl cotransport channels, resulting in hysteresis and drift, setting the young SS cell on a downhill trajectory that leads eventually to the ISC.

The rapid conversion of SS reticulocytes to ISCs has been documented in vivo by the clinical observations of Embury and colleagues.[199] They observed that oxygen therapy during pain crisis acutely suppressed erythropoiesis. Cessation of oxygen administration was associated with a sequential increase in plasma erythropoietin levels, reticulocytes, and ISCs.

In Vivo Sickling

The two salient clinical manifestations of sickle cell disease are severe hemolysis and vaso-occlusive episodes. Just as an understanding of the molecular basis of sickle hemoglobin polymerization helps to explain many of the complex perturbations of SS membranes described above, these membrane abnormalities provide insights into how sickle red cells might interact with other cells in ways that contribute to the pathophysiology of the disease. Specifically, enhanced binding of SS erythrocytes to monocytes or macrophages may contribute importantly to hemolysis; similarly, the adherence of SS red cells to vascular endothelial cells could play a critical role in vaso-occlusive crises. The most mysterious and challenging aspect of the disease is the episodic and unpredictable nature of these events, both temporally and spatially. Although the unique kinetic features of Hb S polymerization are the primary determinant of the stochastic nature of these vaso-occlusive events, complex secondary phenomena such as membrane changes, cell-cell interactions, and vicissitudes in the microcirculation are likely to be important contributors.

Adherence of SS Erythrocytes to Macrophages

Red cell destruction in sickle cell disease is primarily extravascular, in keeping with only modest elevation of plasma hemoglobin levels. The enhanced rigidity of ISCs and sickled discocytes would lead to extravascular destruction, akin to that of rigid cells encountered in a host of other hemolytic disorders, such as hereditary spherocytosis and congenital Heinz body

FIGURE 6–17. Scheme depicting the mechanism proposed by Lew and Bookchin[135, 195] for the conversion of SS reticulocytes directly into ISCs. K and Cl efflux is triggered by either sickling-induced Ca influx, which activates the Gardos channel (*lower left*), or by transient acidosis, which triggers the KCl cotransport pathway (*lower right*). The latter is particularly active in reticulocytes. In compensating for Cl efflux, the Jacobs-Stewart mechanism is activated (*upper right*), leading to further acidification and a positive feedback cycle. (From Lew, V. L., Freeman, C. J., Ortiz, O. E., and Bookchin, R. M.: A mathematical model on the volume, pH and ion content regulation in reticulocytes: Application to the pathophysiology of sickle cell dehydration. Reproduced from the *Journal of Clinical Investigation*, 1991, Vol. 87, pp. 100–112, by copyright permission of the American Society for Clinical Investigation.)

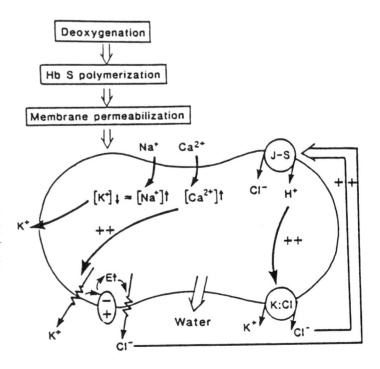

hemolytic anemia (see later). In addition, hemolysis in SS disease may be amplified by immune recognition and clearance. SS red cells have enhanced adherence to monocytes and macrophages[200, 201] and more readily undergo erythrophagocytosis.[200, 202] Two mechanisms have been offered to explain these phenomena. As mentioned previously, the external surface of a subpopulation of SS red cells has increased deposits of immunoglobulin G (IgG),[200, 203, 204] which appear to be abnormally clumped[205] and thereby more susceptible to recognition by Fc receptors on macrophages. Adherence and phagocytosis can be inhibited either by Fc blockade[200] or by elution of IgG.[206] Alternatively, monocytes and macrophages may recognize the abnormal display of PE and PS in the outer membrane leaflet of sickled cells.[201] (See Membrane Lipids, earlier.) This may explain why the adherence of monocytes to deoxygenated SS cells is reversed upon oxygenation. In general, a strong correlation exists between monocyte adherence and maneuvers that increase the display of surface PS on SS as well as on normal red cells. Moreover, this process can be partially blocked by preincubation of monocytes with PS liposomes.

Adherence of SS Erythrocytes to Endothelial Cells

The potential for the initiation of a vaso-occlusive event by a sickled cell depends primarily on whether the delay time for sickling is within the range of the capillary transit time.[89] Therefore, any secondary phenomena that retard the transit of SS red cells in the microcirculation could have a critical impact on the pathogenesis of vaso-occlusion in sickle cell disease. Accordingly, considerable interest has been shown in studies demonstrating enhanced adherence of SS red cells to endothelial cells.[206-208] Most of the experiments described below have utilized human umbilical vein endothelial cells (HUVEC)[207-211] or endothelium from bovine aorta.[206, 212]* Initially, Hebbel and his colleagues measured adherence by incubating radiolabeled sickle and normal red cells with a HUVEC monolayer, followed by successive washings. Subsequently, the development of flow chambers has provided a more physiological way to study the adherence of red cells to endothelial cells.[209-211] Mohandas and Evans[212, 214, 215] have devised a micropipette technique that enables them to make direct measurements on individual red cells, including the quantitation of strength of adherence at shear forces that would be anticipated in the microcirculation. Irregularly shaped discocytes are more adherent than regularly shaped discocytes. These micropipette experiments confirmed that ISCs are the least adherent,[207, 214] probably because their rigidity precludes their forming extensive surface contact with the endothelial cell. This consideration may

explain why deoxygenated sickled discocytes also have relatively weak adherence.[207]

In a flow chamber, shear stresses that simulate in vivo flow in the microcirculation can be applied. At low shear rates, simulating flow in capillaries and venules, high-density SS red cells adhered to HUVEC less readily than did low-density cells,[210] probably owing in part to the poor binding of ISCs (mentioned previously). All populations of SS red cells were markedly more adherent than AA or AS cells. However, AA red cells with a high proportion of reticulocytes behaved similarly to SS red cells. Thus, there appear to be surface determinants on young red cells per se, independent of hemoglobin composition, that facilitate adherence to endothelium. The fact that patients with other types of hemolytic anemia do not have sickle-type crises argues that adherence of SS cells to vascular endothelium is not sufficient for the development of vaso-occlusive events.

In addition to red cell age, other intrinsic properties more specific to SS erythrocytes have been implicated as contributors to endothelial cell adherence. These include glycophorin clustering, oxidation of membrane proteins or lipids, aminophospholipid externalization, and dehydration.[123]

Plasma appears to be required for optimal adherence,[214, 216] even though in an albumin-buffer medium SS red cells are more adherent than normal cells. SS plasma, particularly samples obtained during crises, supports adherence more than normal plasma.[209, 216] These results implicate the participation of acute phase reactants in the plasma. Fibrinogen has been suggested as an important plasma contributor, since adherence is strengthened by addition and weakened by depletion of this abundant plasma protein.[216] Experiments showing that adherence is inhibited by EDTA (ethylenediaminetetra-acetic acid) and restored by excess Ca[214] suggest that adhesive molecules such as the integrins are involved in this phenomenon. The demonstration that adherence can be partially blocked by the removal of collagen-binding proteins[214] or by the addition of RGDS peptide (Arg-Gly-Asp-Ser) lends further support to this conclusion.[211, 215] There is a growing body of evidence that high molecular weight multimers of von Willebrand protein (vWF) play a critical role. Specific depletion of this protein markedly inhibits adhesion,[209, 211] as does the addition of antibodies to GpIb or GpIIbIIIa,[217] platelet plasma membrane molecules that bind to vWF. Ex vivo adherence of SS red cells to the endothelium of rat mesentery is enhanced by pretreating the animal with DDAVP (D-amino-8-D-arginine-vasopressin),[218] an agent that enhances the secretion of vWF multimers from endothelial cells. Von Willebrand multimer is a particularly appealing mediator of adherence because its huge size would permit bridging between red cells and endothelial cells over a distance sufficient to minimize repulsion owing to the negative charge on the surfaces of the two cells. To further delineate the precise role of integrins in this phenomenon, it will be necessary to search for receptors on sickle red cells,

---

*As discussed later, SS erythrocytes have also been shown to have increased adherence ex vivo to vascular endothelium of rat mesentery.[213]

akin to platelet GpIb, that bind specifically and with high affinity to vWF multimers.

The pathophysiological importance of the adherence of SS red cells to endothelium is underscored by the finding that unlike a host of other laboratory parameters that have been examined, the degree of adherence correlates strongly with clinical severity in a large number of patients with SS disease and other sickle genotypes.[208] About 20 per cent of pain crises occur in the setting of infections, both viral and bacterial. It is tempting to speculate that this association is due to enhanced adherence as a result of increases in acute phase proteins such as vWF and fibrinogen. Moreover, infectious agents may directly condition endothelial cells. HUVEC cells infected with herpes simplex virus type 1 had enhanced adherence to SS red cells, mediated through an increase in the expression of receptors for the Fc portion of IgG.[219]

Sickling in the Microcirculation

The neural and humoral control of blood flow in the microcirculation, coupled with temporal and spatial variability in oxygen consumption, adds greatly to the complexity of ex vivo sickling.* Recently, significant advances have been made in the development of in vivo or ex vivo models of sickle vaso-occlusion. Kaul and his colleagues[213, 221] have studied the behavior of SS and AA red cells infused into the vascular bed of rat mesocecum. This preparation permits both direct microscopic visualization of the transit of individual red cells in the microcirculation and measurements of pressure, flow, and vascular resistance. These experiments have shown convincingly that the enhanced adherence of SS red cells, described previously, pertains to in vivo blood flow. The extent of adherence of oxygenated cells varied inversely with blood flow. Consistent with in vitro results in a flow chamber,[210] adherence varied inversely with red cell density, with reticulocytes and young discocytes being the most adherent, particularly in immediate postcapillary venules and at vessel bends and near vessel junctions. Shear rates would be expected to be significantly lower here than in the arterioles or capillaries, thereby reducing the chance for red cell detachment. Adherence was associated with an increase in peripheral resistance, particularly when the infusate included the most dense cells, which are, per se, the least adherent. Thus, it is likely that the adherence of low-density discocytes results in secondary trapping of rigid, dense SS cells, including the ISCs (Fig. 6–18). Preferential trapping of dense SS cells has been observed during perfusion of the femoral artery in the rat.[221] ^{31}P magnetic resonance measurements showed that the vaso-occlusion was associated with acidosis and edema, both indicators of tissue ischemia. In contrast, low density, deformable SS red cells adhered to the vascular endothelium but did not cause obstruction to flow.[221a]

Rodgers and his colleagues have utilized a number of non-invasive methods to investigate in vivo blood flow in patients having SS disease and other sickle syndromes in comparison to normal individuals.[222–224] Cutaneous microvascular flow can be monitored by laser-Doppler velocimetry.[222, 223, 225] About 50 per cent of patients with SS disease, 12 per cent of patients with SC disease, and an occasional AA individual[226] have oscillations in blood flow, termed periodic microcirculatory flow. This phenomenon is thought to represent a compensatory response to impaired blood flow caused by sickle vaso-occlusion. When patients with SS disease are subjected to progressive periods of partial occlusion of forearm blood flow, the postocclusive hyperemia was associated with proportional increases in blood flow and in the magnitude of the flow oscillations, as well as with a significant delay in the peak level of blood flow.[223] It is of interest that a similar pattern was observed in two patients with homozygous Hb C disease,[223, 225] in whom red cells are dehydrated but not subject to sickling. In one SS patient, the abnormal flow pattern was reversed by exchange transfusion.[223]

Studies of in vivo blood flow can be complemented by non-invasive assessment of tissue function and metabolism. For example, positron emission tomography has demonstrated focal abnormalities in cerebral metabolic rate in sites not identified by conventional computed tomographic scans.[227]

The application of these accurate non-invasive techniques to studies of vaso-occlusion in sickle cell disease provides a special opportunity to make objective assessments of both conventional and new therapeutic modalities. For example, the administration of an arteriolar vasodilator, nifedipine, was shown to result in significant improvement in microvascular flow in the retina and conjunctiva.[224] The development of transgenic animal models for sickle cell disease (discussed later) will also be useful in assessing whether therapeutic maneuvers result in improvement of blood flow in the microcirculation and in prevention of vaso-occlusive events.

PATHOGENESIS OF SICKLE CRISES. Among the protean manifestations of sickle cell disease, the feature most enigmatic to clinicians is the acute pain crisis. In a given patient, none of the many readily available laboratory or diagnostic parameters currently in use correlate with the frequency of crises or serve as predictors for their onset. Recent analyses of large numbers of patients with SS disease indicate that the frequency of crises varies directly with hemoglobin level[228–230] and inversely with the level of Hb F.[229] Surprisingly, the potential for a patient's red cells to form sickle polymer is sometimes *not* a good predictor of pain crises.[231] For example, the frequency of acute crises in S/β^0 thalassemia appears to be greater than that in SS disease,[229, 231] even though the degree of polymer formation would be less, owing to the lower intracellular hemoglobin concentration. For this reason, it is doubtful whether sophisticated (yet greatly oversimplified) numerical calculations of intracellular

---

*For more detailed information, see reviews by Eaton and Hofrichter[89] and by Francis and Johnson.[220]

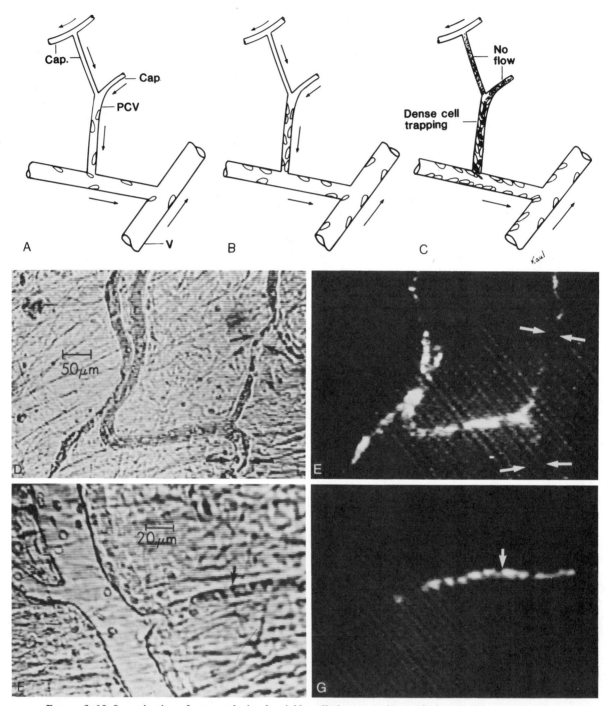

FIGURE 6–18. Investigation of vaso-occlusion by sickle cells in an ex vivo perfusion model. *A–C,* Diagrammatic representation of adhesion of deformable SS cells (reticulocytes and discocytes) *(A and B)* followed by secondary trapping of dense SS cells and subsequent occlusion of the post-capillary venule *(C).* (From Kaul D. K., Fabry, M. E., Nagel, R. L.: Erythrocytic and vascular factors influencing the microcirculatory behavior of blood in sickle cell anemia. Ann. N. Y. Acad. Sci. 565:316, 1989; with permission.) *D–G,* Demonstration of selective trapping of dense cells. A mixture of unlabeled low-density SS discocytes and fluorescently labeled high-density SS cells were infused into the rat mesoappendix. The epifluorescence illumination in the figures on the right shows high concentration of dense cells that obstruct postcapillary venules. (From Kaul, D. K., Fabry, M. E., and Nagel, R. L.: Microvascular sites and characteristics of sickle cell adhesion to vascular endothelium in shear flow conditions: Pathophysiological implications. Proc. Natl. Acad. Sci. USA 86:3356, 1989; with permission.)

polymer fraction[232-234] offer additional insight into the pathophysiology of the vaso-occlusive complications of sickle cell disease.

It is likely that the development of acute pain crises reflects perturbations in the macrocirculation and microcirculation sufficiently complex and multifactorial to elude current understanding. From decades of careful clinical observations, Serjeant[231] has proposed that pain crises are sometimes triggered by circulatory reflexes. The acute onset of pain in an extremity following cold exposure may result in the diversion of blood flow away from the skin and bone marrow to shunts in the muscle with subsequent vaso-occlusion in the marrow. This mechanism would explain the remarkable symmetry of the distribution of pain, swelling, and osteonecrosis in the hand-foot syndrome as well as a significant proportion of pain crises in older patients. This interesting hypothesis begs for rigorous investigation in the whole organism.

Confusion exists in the literature about the relationship between acute pain crises and the properties of SS red cells. There appears to be no consistent change in the percentage of circulating ISCs with the development of pain crises, although some of the ISCs have been noted to acquire a spiculated (echinocytic) shape during crisis.[235] The filterability of partially and fully oxygenated SS red cells is significantly decreased for several days following the onset of crises.[236-238a] Since MCHC is the main determinant of red cell deformability, these observations are consistent with the recent report of a 54 per cent increase in the fraction of dense cells 3 to 4 days after the crisis.[239] These density distribution measurements are difficult to reconcile with reports from another institution of a 51 per cent *decrease* in the fraction of dense cells 3 to 4 days following the onset of acute pain crisis (see reference 240 and the references therein).

TRANSGENIC MOUSE MODEL. The large chasm between our thorough knowledge of the molecular basis of polymerization of Hb S and our rudimentary understanding of the temporal, regional, humoral, and neural factors that affect in vivo sickling is unlikely to be bridged by continuation of "traditional" investigations either at the laboratory bench or at the bedside. There is a critical need for an animal model that faithfully duplicates the hematological and vaso-occlusive manifestations of the disease. The recent development of transgenic mice bearing the β^S gene is a major advance toward achieving this end. It appears increasingly likely that this model will provide not only a deeper understanding of the pathogenesis of sickle cell disease but also an efficient and rigorous way of testing new and innovative therapies, prior to clinical trials in patients.

The animal is prepared by the injection of DNA bearing the transgene into the pronucleus of fertilized ova, which are then allowed to develop in the uterus of a foster mother. Of the full-term fetuses, a substantial fraction will have the transgene incorporated randomly and with variable copy number into the genome. Subsequent generations can be bred to produce homozygotes. In the application of this technology to the study of globin gene regulation, considerable effort has been devoted to the identification and characterization of the important tissue and developmental specific *cis*-acting elements of the human α and β genes that are responsible for their high level of expression in erythroid cells.*

A number of independent research groups have made transgenic mice that express the β^S gene. In an initial report,[241] only a small amount of β^S was expressed in the homozygote because the transgene lacked the above-mentioned control elements. The red cells failed to sickle in part because β^S/total β was only 10 per cent and in part because the hybrid tetramer $\alpha^M_2\beta^S_2$ lacks the appropriate α subunit contacts,[242] owing to differences in primary sequence between mouse and man. These early experiments showed that it is necessary for the mouse red cells to contain high levels of human Hb S. Increased expression of Hb S has been achieved by injecting both α and β^S transgenes, each of which contains the appropriate globin gene control elements.[243, 244] These animals have 30 per cent to as much as 80 per cent Hb S in their red cells. Although they are not anemic or hemolytic, their red cells form polymer and assume classical sickle shapes when deoxygenated. The relative amount of Hb S in these transgenic animals can be further improved by breeding them into a background of mouse β thalassemia[241, 244, 245] and α thalassemia.[245a] Indeed, the β thalassemic mice that express the β^S transgene enjoy a partial correction of their anemia and red cell abnormalities, owing to an improvement in chain imbalance.[245]

Additional strategies are available to increase sickling further in order to make the transgenic animal mimic the patient with SS disease. One approach is to breed the Hb S–bearing transgene into mice that have left-shifted oxygen-binding curves resulting from mutant hemoglobins (R. Popp, personal communication, 1992). This method would enhance the proportion of oxygen released from Hb S and therefore promote sickling. Another option is to add mutations other than $\beta6$ Val that would further promote polymerization. (See Structure of the Sickle Fiber, previously.) The naturally occurring mutant $\beta^{S-Antilles}$ sickles more readily than β^S because the $\beta6$ Val substitution is combined with $\beta23$ Ile, which further stabilizes the sickle polymer.[246] Transgenic mice having 50 per cent $\beta^{S-Antilles}$ (in a β thalassemic background) had readily demonstrable in vitro sickling and a widening of their red cell volume profile when they were exposed to 10 days of hypoxia.[247] Recently, mice have been prepared with a transgene containing $\beta6$ Val, $\beta23$ Ile, and a third mutation, $\beta121$ Gln (D-Los Angeles), which also promotes polymerization.[248] When bred into a homozygous β thalassemia background and a heterozygous α thalassemia background, the resulting SAD (S-Antilles, D-Los Angeles) transgenic mice have a severe

---

*For further information on this topic, see Chapters 4 and 5.

hemolytic disease having several features in common with SS disease, including hemolytic anemia and splenomegaly.[248, 249]

Epidemology of Sickle Cell Disease

Origin of the β^S Gene

In 1978, Kan and Dozy[250] discovered that in African-Americans with SS disease the β^S gene is linked to a polymorphic restriction site (*Hpa* I) in the 5' flanking region. This finding led to the use of additional restriction enzymes, which identified other β globin polymorphisms in populations with common hemoglobin disorders, particularly the thalassemias* and sickle cell disease. Populations in which large-scale migrations have been absent or limited have only a small number of specific polymorphism patterns, called haplotypes. These can be regarded as ancestral sequences of DNA. Study of the haplotypes of the β globin gene complex has provided valuable information on important and diverse issues such as the antenatal diagnosis of β thalassemia, the origin of the β^S and other β globin mutations, the migration of affected populations, and the phenotypic contribution of other genes or regulatory elements in *cis* to the β globin gene.

Labie, Nagel, and their colleagues[251-253] have conducted extensive field trips in Africa to explore the genetic background of β^S genes and its impact on phenotype.† They have identified regions in central Africa, shown in Figure 6–19A, designated (from west to east) Senegal, Benin, and Bantu (or Central African Republic), in which the β^S gene is nearly exclusively associated with a single and specific haplotype (Fig. 6–19B).‡ In each region, individuals with β^A genes have not only this haplotype but also a few others. Therefore, it can be assumed that in each of these regions the β^S gene arose as a spontaneous mutation in a chromosome bearing this haplotype. Because the gene confers fitness to malaria (see further on), it became fixed in this region with a high frequency. Haplotypes identified by restriction site polymorphisms have been verified and refined by the association of specific variable tandem repeat polymorphisms.[253] These collective data strongly suggest that the β^S gene arose independently in at least three different times and locations in central Africa.

Further detailed analyses of these haplotypes have revealed subtle variations within each of these three population groups. In the Senegal, Benin, and Bantu areas fewer than 10 per cent of the β^S chromosomes have atypical restriction polymorphism patterns. About 80 per cent of the β^S Bantu chromosomes have

undergone a conversion event between the ^Gγ and ^Aγ genes.[255] Of these, about half have a 6 base pair (bp) deletion 5' to the ^Gγ gene.[256] Heterogeneity at the 5' end of the Bantu haplotype can be explained by recombination in a hot spot in the ψβ pseudogene 5' to the β gene.[257]

POPULATION MIGRATIONS. The study of β^S haplotypes has provided valuable insights into the history and route of movement of populations. For example, the geographical distribution of the Bantu haplotype supports earlier linguistic evidence for the eastward and southward spread of the blacks originally located in West Africa.[254] In contrast, populations sharing the Benin β^S haplotype migrated northward to Morocco, Algeria, and Egypt as well as across the Mediterranean to Sicily,[258] Greece,[259] and Turkey.* The fact that in Sicily 100 per cent of the β^S chromosomes have the Benin haplotype, whereas none of the β^A chromosomes do, provides compelling evidence for this northward migration.[258] The β^S chromosomes in the western Arabian peninsula also have the Benin haplotype, indicating that the above-mentioned migration also extended northeastward across the Red Sea (see Fig. 6–19A).

In contrast, in the eastern Arabian peninsula, individuals who have the β^S gene share a common and unique haplotype with those in the subcontinent of India. The frequency of the β^S gene is very high among the scheduled tribes that are distributed throughout central and southern India. These tribal peoples live apart, outside the mainstream of the Indian caste system.[254] The finding that these widely dispersed tribes share a common β^S haplotype provides evidence not only for a unicentric origin of the β^S gene in India but also for a common ancestry among the tribes.[260] The fact that all β^S chromosomes in eastern Arabia also share this haplotype begs the question of the actual origin of this mutation and the direction of the subsequent migration.

Investigation of β^S haplotypes also provides independent information about the slave trade to the New World. Analyses of β^S haplotypes in Jamaica, Cuba, and the United States are in remarkably good agreement with historical records from the seventeenth to nineteenth centuries of the place of origin of the slaves.[254]

MALARIA AND THE SICKLE GENE. Both the high frequency of the β^S gene in Central Africa and the fact that it has originated in at least three different locations can be explained by the finding that in heterozygotes the gene confers increased fitness, almost certainly by enhancing resistance against malaria.[261, 262] In evolutionary terms, high morbidity and mortality in the SS homozygote are small prices to pay for improved survival of the much more common heterozygote. This phenomenon is probably the best studied and best understood example in human

---

*For discussion of globin polymorphisms in the thalassemias, see Chapter 5.

†See the recent review by Nagel and Ranney[254] for more detailed coverage of this topic.

‡Recently, a fourth African haplotype, differing from the other three in both 5' and 3' regions, has been found in a specific and restricted ethnic group designated Eton, originating in Cameroon.[254]

---

*In Portugal, all three haplotypes are found in association with the β^S gene, in keeping with the impact of frequent and extensive maritime voyages on the gene pool.[254]

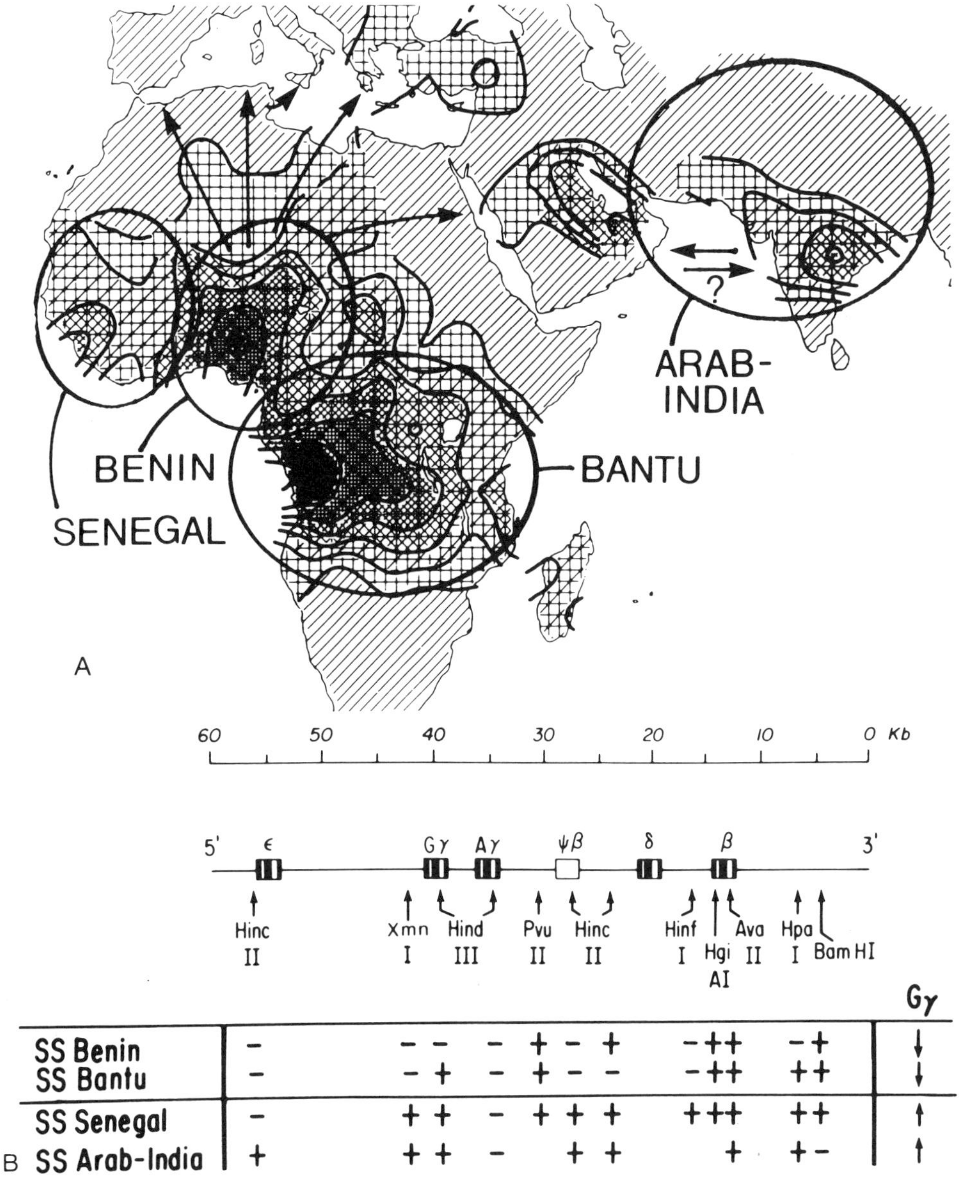

FIGURE 6–19. *A,* Map of Africa and Asia Minor and the Indian subcontinent. Regions of high frequency of the β^S gene are depicted by the dark-hatched textures. The four major β^S haplotypes are labeled according to their respective locales. The arrows depict flow of the β^S gene to North Africa, the Mediterranean, and the Arabian Peninsula. *B,* The β globin gene cluster and the major restriction fragment length polymorphisms (RFLPs) that determine the four major β^S-linked haplotypes. (*A* and *B* from Nagel, R. L., and Ranney, H. M.: Genetic epidemiology of structural mutations of the β-globin gene. Semin. Hematol. 27:342, 1990; with permission.)

biology of "balanced polymorphism." AS heterozygotes become infected with *Plasmodium falciparum* at about the same rate as AA individuals, but fewer die of the infection.[263] The molecular basis for this enhanced resistance is still not fully understood. In 1970, Luzzatto and his colleagues[264] reported that parasitization of AS red cells greatly accelerated their rate of sickling. The enhanced clearance of these rigid cells thus facilitated the host's destruction of the parasite. The sickling of parasitized AS red cells may be further enhanced by the adherence of trophozoite-induced knobs to the venular endothelium.[265] The decreased rate of growth of *P. falciparum* in AS red cells compared with AA red cells has been attributed to a lower level of intracellular K induced by sickling. However, it is likely that intracellular polymerization, rather than cation content, is the primary deterrent to parasite growth.[261] Sickle polymers are a poor substrate for malarial proteases.

Genetic Modulators of Sickle Cell Disease

RELATION OF β^S HAPLOTYPE TO PHENOTYPE. The demonstration of multiple origins of the β^S gene, as discussed above, raises questions about whether, among these genes, there are differences in *cis* that impact significantly on disease phenotype. To answer this question, Nagel and his colleagues, as well as others, have collected a considerable amount of genetic and clinical information both in the United States and all over the world. There is solid agreement that the β^S haplotype has a significant bearing on the ratio of $^G\gamma$ to $^A\gamma$ production, which is normally about 60:40 at birth but after about 4 months of life changes to about 40:60. (See Chapter 4.) The Senegal and the Arab-Indian haplotypes are associated with maintenance of the newborn ratio, whereas the Benin and Bantu haplotypes are associated with a ratio similar to that of the adult.[131, 266]

SS individuals homozygous for the Senegal β^S haplotype also appear to have higher levels of Hb F than do Benin and Bantu homozygotes, although the data are considerably spread.[131, 254, 266] This relationship may be stronger for African patients[131, 266] than for patients with SS disease in the United States, where conflicting results have been obtained.[267–269] An even more complex issue is whether the β^S haplotype affects the degree of anemia and the clinical course of SS homozygotes. Again, conflicting results have been reported.[267–269] In interpreting these reports, two separate issues are relevant. First, there may be additional genetic modulators, not linked to the β^S gene, that are fixed in African populations and have independent impact on the severity of SS disease among the Senegals, Benins, and Bantus. Second, despite the large number of American and Jamaican patients studied (60 in reference 267; 113 in reference 268), the results are confounded by genetic admixture. The Benin haplotype is strongly favored. Therefore, access to Benin homozygotes is ample, whereas there exists a relative paucity of Americans and Jamaicans homozygous for the Senegal and Bantu haplotypes. Results on the remaining heterozygotes are difficult to interpret.

SS homozygotes from eastern Arabia and India, who, as mentioned above, share a common and distinct β globin haplotype, have unusually mild disease, owing primarily to high levels of Hb F and perhaps also to a very high gene frequency for α thalassemia (see below). The high Hb F level appears to be linked to the β^S gene.[270] Thus, the Arab-Indian haplotype can be considered a marker for increased expression of Hb F.* Hemolytic stress is apparently required for this effect, since it is seen only in SS homozygotes. AS heterozygotes bearing this haplotype have normal levels of Hb F. In addition, other genetic modulators may have an impact on γ gene expression in these populations.

X-LINKED DETERMINANT OF HB F PRODUCTION. A survey of a large number of people in Japan revealed that the distribution of Hb F and F cells was affected by gender.[271] Relatively high levels (>0.7 per cent Hb F and >4.4 per cent F cells) were encountered in about 10 per cent of men and 20 per cent of women. Family studies on these individuals with high Hb F levels strongly suggested an X-linked determinant of Hb F production. Dover and his colleagues have confirmed these findings in African-Americans. From analysis of polymorphic restriction sites on sib pairs of SS homozygotes, they have shown that this Hb F production gene is controlled by a locus on Xp22.2.[272]

CONCURRENT α THALASSEMIA. As explained in detail in Chapter 5, deletion of one of the two tandem α globin genes is commonly encountered among all populations in which the β^S gene is fixed at high frequency. About 30 per cent of African-Americans are heterozygotes ($-\alpha/\alpha\alpha$), and about 3 per cent are homozygotes ($-\alpha/-\alpha$).[273, 274] The frequency of α thalassemia is even higher among Arabs and Asian Indians who have the β^S gene. Among Africans, the vast majority have the "rightward deletion" $-\alpha$ haplotype[275] (see also Chapter 5), although the "leftward deletion" has been reported.[276] Deletion of both α globin genes ($--$) occurs rarely in Africans.[277] Accordingly, α thalassemia per se is of little clinical significance among Africans. However, the coexistence of $-\alpha/\alpha\alpha$ or $-\alpha/-\alpha$ in Africans with the β^S gene is of considerable importance, since it affects the phenotype of both sickle trait (AS) and homozygous (SS) disease.

A trimodal distribution of Hb S and Hb A in the red cells of AS heterozygotes correlates precisely with the number of α globin genes. Non-thalassemic AS individuals have about 40 per cent Hb S, whereas those with $-\alpha/\alpha\alpha$ have about 35 per cent and those

---

*This contention is supported by the observation that although the Arab-Indian haplotype is encountered only rarely in Jamaican patients with SS disease, it is invariably associated with high levels of Hb F.[270] Non-linked genes for enhanced γ globin expression in the Arab-Indian populations would be diluted in these Jamaican patients.

with $-\alpha/-\alpha$ have about 28 per cent[54] (see Fig. 6–6B). The most reliable and uniform manifestation of in vivo sickling in AS individuals is a defect in the ability of the renal medulla to produce concentrated urine. This defect varies directly with the percentage of Hb S in the AS red cells and therefore with the number of α globin genes.[278]

The impact of α thalassemia on SS disease is more complex and of greater clinical significance.* As expected, the mean corpuscular volume (MCV) decreases in proportion to the number of α globin genes deleted. Of note is a parallel reduction in the severity of anemia. SS patients with the $-\alpha/-\alpha$ genotype have a mean hemoglobin of 9.0 g/dl, compared with 7.9 g/dl in those without α thalassemia.[281–283] α Thalassemia ameliorates the degree of hemolysis[284] primarily by a reduction in dense cells, in ISCs, and in intracellular hemoglobin concentration, phenomena that greatly inhibit intracellular polymerization. The combination of fewer reticulocytes (light cells) and fewer dense cells results in a more narrow red cell density distribution profile.[285] Cation leak in deoxygenated SS cells is significantly reduced in the presence of α thalassemia,[286] in keeping with a decreased potential for intracellular polymerization. In like manner, the deformability of SS red cells is increased in proportion to the number of α globin genes deleted.[287] However, at a given density fraction, deformability is unaffected by α thalassemia.[287] Thus, α thalassemia affects the properties of the SS red cell primarily through its impact on cell density and intracellular hemoglobin concentration. The coexistence of α thalassemia is associated with a slight decrease in the percentage of Hb F and F cells, in keeping with a comparatively slight reduction in the preferential survival of F cells.[285, 288] Because of their lower MCHC, the non-F cells do not undergo such a rapid transition to dense cells[285] and therefore have improved survival.

Even though α thalassemia has significant impact on hematological values in SS disease and on the properties of SS red cells, it has little impact on the clinical manifestations of the disease. Specifically, three studies[269, 282, 283] agree that the incidence of acute pain crises is not affected by the α globin gene number. Concurrent α thalassemia may be associated with a lower incidence of leg ulcers[269, 282] but with an increased risk of developing avascular bone necrosis[289, 290] and perhaps retinopathy.[291] It is of interest that these latter two complications also occur often in SC disease and S/β thalassemia. The development of bone necrosis and retinopathy may be fostered by a relatively high hemoglobin level, a feature that is shared by all three of these forms of sickle cell disease. Since α thalassemia has such little impact on the clinical manifestations of SS disease, it is surprising that it has been associated with improved survival.[292] This report

needs to be verified by the study of a larger, well-characterized population.

It may be overly simplistic to assume that the effects of α thalassemia on SS disease all stem from a reduction in cell density and intracellular hemoglobin concentration. The low MCV or the more redundant red cell membrane in SS patients with α thalassemia might have independent impact on the hematological or clinical phenotype.[280]

GLUCOSE-6-PHOSPHATE DEHYDROGENASE DEFICIENCY. The most common genetic abnormality among populations with a high frequency of the β^S gene is deficiency of erythrocyte glucose-6-phosphate dehydrogenase (G6PD). About 10 per cent of African-American males are deficient in this enzyme, which is encoded by a gene on the X chromosome. About the same proportion of American males with SS disease are G6PD deficient. Past reports (cited in reference 293) have been conflicting, claiming that the deficiency state has a beneficial, harmful, or nonexistent influence on the hematological or clinical manifestations of SS disease. Recently, the Cooperative Study of Sickle Cell Disease has settled this issue by a definitive analysis of a large number (801) of male patients with SS disease.[293] G6PD deficiency had no effect on the hematological values, morbidity (pain crises, episodes of sepsis, anemic crises), or mortality of these patients with SS disease.

Compound Heterozygous States

SC Disease

HEMOGLOBIN C. To understand the molecular pathogenesis of SC disease, it is necessary first to discuss the properties and phenotypic features of Hb C (β6 Glu→Lys), the third most commonly encountered mutant worldwide, next to Hb S and Hb E. The frequency of the β^C gene in areas of West Africa, particularly Ghana and Upper Volta, approaches 0.15.[5] Among American blacks, the gene frequency is 0.010 to 0.012. AC heterozygotes have no clinical manifestations and normal hematological values except for slightly dehydrated and dense red cells, which appear as target cells on stained blood films. CC homozygotes have a mild hemolytic anemia and moderate splenic enlargement. CC red cells are markedly dehydrated with increased MCHC. The primary morphological feature is the presence of plump target cells.

The clinical and hematological phenotype of AC and CC individuals can be explained by two relevant properties of Hb C. The replacement of β6 glutamic acid by lysine results in a significant decrease in the solubility of both oxygenated and deoxy forms, resulting in the formation of crystals. In CC patients who have undergone splenectomy, occasional red cells will contain elongated rectangular crystals of oxyhemoglobin.[58] Larger and more frequent crystals can be induced by incubating CC red cells in a hypertonic

---

*For more information on this topic, see reviews by Steinberg and Embury[279] and by Embury.[280]

medium. The crystallization of oxy Hb C is inhibited by the presence of Hb F, primarily at γ87 Gln.[294] Accordingly, no Hb F is incorporated into the crystal. In contrast, the presence of Hb S increases the rate at which Hb C forms crystals.[295] Moreover, such crystals contain Hb S in addition to Hb C. The other relevant property of Hb C is its ability to stimulate KCl cotransport to an even greater extent than Hb S[61] (see Disordered Volume Control, discussed earlier). As a result of K efflux and accompanying water loss, CC red cells rapidly become dehydrated, dense, and targeted. It is not known why CC and even AC red cells have enhanced KCl cotransport. It is noteworthy that Hb C binds more avidly than does Hb A to protein 3 in the inner surface of the red cell membrane.[296]

CLINICAL FEATURES OF SC DISEASE. Among American blacks, the β^S gene occurs about three times as frequently as the β^C gene. However, the prevalence of SC disease is comparable to that of SS disease, owing to the higher mortality of the homozygous state. Patients with SC disease have a mild hemolytic anemia. The peripheral blood smear reveals plump target cells. Some are pointed at opposite ends, resembling broad-beamed canoes. Classic ISCs are not seen. Occasional cells contain crystals, and others may have round hemoglobin aggregates (billiard ball cells).[181, 297] Patients with SC disease may develop any of the vaso-occlusive complications seen in SS homozygotes, although such events are generally less frequent and severe. However, a few exceptions are noteworthy. Proliferative retinopathy is more common in patients with SC disease than in SS homozygotes. Aseptic necrosis of the femoral head and hematuria from renal medullary infarction occur almost as frequently in SC disease as in SS disease.

PATHOGENESIS OF SC DISEASE. Why do SC individuals have significantly more morbidity than do AS individuals? When incubated at decreased oxygen tensions, SC cells sickle much more readily than AS cells. The increased tendency to form polymer cannot be explained by enhanced copolymerization of Hb S with Hb C.[60, 298] The enhanced sickling of SC cells can be attributed to two independent phenomena.[60] First, SC cells contain about 25 per cent more Hb S than do AS cells, owing to a slower rate of assembly of Hb C compared with Hb A.[52] Second, SC red cells have a higher MCHC and a significantly higher proportion of dense cells than do AS cells,[59, 60] owing to the contribution of Hb C to increased KCl cotransport, which, as explained above (see Disordered Volume Control), leads to K and water loss.[61, 297] In view of the importance of intracellular hemoglobin concentration to the kinetics of polymerization of Hb S, it is not surprising that a patient with both SC disease and concurrent hereditary spherocytosis* had unusually severe clinical and laboratory evidence of sickling.[299]

S/β Thalassemia

Individuals who inherit the β^S gene from one parent and a β thalassemia gene from the other have a disorder that is highly variable in severity and laboratory manifestations. If the β thalassemia allele is incapable of producing any normal subunit, the patient will have S/β^0 thalassemia and red cells containing Hb S (80 to 95 per cent), Hb F (2 to 20 per cent), and Hb A_2 (2 to 4 per cent). In contrast, if the β thalassemia allele is capable of some synthesis of β^A, the patient will have S/β^+ thalassemia and red cells containing Hb S (55 to 75 per cent), Hb A (10 to 30 per cent), Hb F (1 to 13 per cent), and Hb A_2 (3 to 6 per cent). Large-scale clinical studies both in the United States and in Jamaica have demonstrated that the clinical and hematological severity of S/β^0 thalassemia is on a par with that of SS disease, although milder in certain features and perhaps more severe in others. As mentioned above, patients with S/β^0 thalassemia apparently have more frequent pain crises than do those with SS disease.[229, 231] In contrast, patients with S/β^+ thalassemia have relatively mild clinical manifestations. Like patients with SC disease, those with S/β^+ thalassemia have a high incidence of proliferative retinopathy.

The marked clinical severity of S/β^0 thalassemia is puzzling. Measurements of red cell indices consistently show a reduction in MCHC. Accordingly, the rate and extent of polymer formation should be correspondingly reduced. Careful measurements of cell density distributions in S/β^0 thalassemia blood specimens are needed. The fact that ISCs are commonly encountered must mean that accelerated cell dehydration is taking place. It may be that the α subunits, present in excess because of the imbalance in hemoglobin synthesis, trigger KCl cotransport, leading to increased K and water loss.

Advances in the Management of Sickle Cell Disease

Antenatal Diagnosis*

A family at risk for having a baby with SS disease might decide to interrupt the pregnancy if the diagnosis were established safely, accurately, and early in gestation. Clearly, this is a highly sensitive issue that requires skilled and empathetic counseling coupled with access to up-to-date diagnostic facilities.

Considerable advances have been made in the technology for antenatal diagnoses of the hemoglobinopathies. Initially, it was necessary to obtain a sample of fetal blood to establish in utero diagnoses of sickle cell disease or one of the clinically significant thalassemias. In the former case, this approach has been supplanted by analysis of β globin DNA.[301] Adaptation of the polymerase chain reaction[302, 303] has enabled accurate

---

*This congenital disorder of the red cell skeleton is associated with increased intracellular hemoglobin concentration.

*For more information on this topic, see the recent review by Old et al.[300]

diagnoses of the SS, AS, and AA genotypes to be made simply and rapidly on very small amounts of DNA, thus eliminating the time and expense involved in culturing fetal cells. The development of chorionic villus biopsy[304] permits samples to be obtained safely during weeks 6 to 10 of gestation, whereas amniocentesis cannot be performed prior to week 15.

In a recent worldwide survey of all antenatal diagnoses done for hemoglobinopathies from 1974 through 1989, 2800, or 14 per cent, were on fetuses at risk for sickle cell disease.[305] Nearly all of these cases were from the United States and Canada. In recent years, almost 90 per cent of cases of sickle cell disease utilized analyses of DNA rather than fetal blood. The accuracy of diagnosis has increased to greater than 99.5 per cent, and the incidence of fetal loss has fallen to less than 2 per cent. Considering the safety, accuracy, and relative ease of diagnosis early in pregnancy, it is disappointing that the procedure has thus far had little impact on the prevention of SS disease. The figures cited above show that only a small fraction of the families in the United States at risk for having a baby with SS disease have taken advantage of antenatal diagnosis. Moreover, even when the diagnosis of SS disease is established in a fetus, approximately one third of families surveyed[305] have elected to continue the pregnancy. Recently, this percentage has dropped significantly, reflecting perhaps increased effectiveness of the diagnostic and counseling services that are now being provided to the families at risk.

Newborn Screening and Prophylaxis

During the past decade, considerable advances have been made in reducing the morbidity and mortality of SS disease, particularly during the first 10 years of life. Because the Hb F to Hb S switch does not occur until about 6 months after birth, SS newborns are clinically and phenotypically normal. Nevertheless, the diagnosis of SS disease and the clinically significant compound heterozygous states can be readily made on a small sample of umbilical cord blood either by routine electrophoretic methods or by analysis of DNA.[306] There is ample evidence that early diagnosis as a result of screening newborns has greatly improved the care of children with sickle cell disease.[307, 308] Parents benefit from an orderly and comprehensive education about the disease, including relevant preventive measures (see below) and advice on when and how to seek medical help. The child has a greater chance of enrolling in a health care system that is experienced and knowledgeable about sickle cell disease. Newborn screening and follow-up appear to be cost effective in regions that have a relatively high incidence of the β^S gene,[308] but probably not in regions where sickle cell disease is infrequently encountered.[309]

During infancy and early childhood, infections, especially those due to *Streptococcus pneumoniae*, are the major cause of morbidity and mortality. The incidence and severity of pneumococcal sepsis are retarded but not eliminated by polyvalent vaccination. Large-scale clinical trials[310, 311] have provided conclusive evidence for the efficacy of prophylactic penicillin. In comparison to a placebo group, those receiving oral penicillin G had an 84 per cent reduction in the incidence of pneumococcal sepsis.[311]

Rational Approaches to Antisickling Therapy

The preceding portion of this chapter presents a synopsis of biochemical, genetic, and clinical studies that have greatly advanced our understanding of the molecular and cellular pathogenesis of sickle cell disease. From the current body of information, three independent rational approaches to therapy have been proposed and developed:

1. Chemical inhibition of Hb S polymerization.
2. Reduction of intracellular hemoglobin concentration (MCHC).
3. Pharmacological induction of fetal hemoglobin (Hb F).

INHIBITORS OF HB S POLYMERIZATION. Detailed information on the three-dimensional structure of the Hb S polymer (see Figs. 6–8, 6–9, and 6–10) has facilitated the design and development of compounds that inhibit polymerization.[312–315] Although a review of the large literature on this topic is beyond the scope of this chapter, a few underlying principles merit discussion. Inhibitors of sickling can be classified as covalent or non-covalent and also according to their mechanism of action. Compounds that bind covalently to hemoglobin are more likely to have therapeutic potential. None of the non-covalent inhibitors described to date would be effective drugs because they bind relatively weakly to Hb S and therefore a high plasma concentration would be required in order for a significant fraction of the hemoglobin to be modified. However, it is possible that a non-covalent inhibitor could be designed that binds to Hb S with such high affinity that the plasma concentration would be relatively low and non-toxic. Inhibitors of sickling could work either by binding to contact sites on the Hb S fiber, thereby inhibiting polymer assembly or growth or both, or by increasing oxygen affinity, thereby decreasing the relative amount of deoxy Hb S in the red cell. The former strategy is preferable, since any compound that significantly increases oxygen affinity is very likely to induce an increase in red cell production. As discussed elsewhere in this chapter, there is growing clinical evidence that an increase in red cell mass has a significant negative impact on the clinical course of sickle cell disease.

The design of a safe and effective inhibitor of Hb S polymerization is a formidable challenge. The ideal agent should (1) be readily absorbed through the gastrointestinal tract, (2) circulate in the plasma without strong binding to plasma proteins, (3) readily penetrate the erythrocyte membrane, (4) bind strongly and specifically to Hb S in a way that will inhibit polymerization but will not affect physiologic oxygen transport, and (5) bind minimally to other biologically important molecules. Unfortunately, an Ehrlichian "magic bullet" for sickle cell disease still eludes us. No antisickling agents tested thus far can be regarded as safe and effective therapy.

REDUCTION OF MCHC. Because the rate of polymerization of sickle hemoglobin is so exquisitely dependent on Hb S concentration (see Fig. 6–14), any treatment that lowers mean MCHC has a sound rationale. The simplest approach and the only one to have undergone clinical trials is induction of hyponatremia, thereby causing osmotic swelling of red cells.[316] Although with careful monitoring this treatment appears to be effective, it is too cumbersome and risky to be adapted to chronic outpatient care.[317] There is current interest in the development of pharmacological agents that inhibit K and water loss from SS red cells, thereby resulting in a reduction in MCHC.

INDUCTION OF Hb F. In 1948, Watson reported that the red cells of newborns with sickle cell anemia did not sickle as readily as those of older children with the disease.[318] She attributed this to the high percentage of fetal hemoglobin (Hb F) that is still present at the time of birth. Subsequent studies (see discussion of non-S hemoglobins under Sickle Hemoglobin Polymerization, discussed earlier) confirmed that Hb F is indeed a very potent inhibitor of polymerization of deoxy Hb S. In certain populations such as Bedouin Arabs and Veddoid Indians, SS homozygotes produce relatively high amounts of Hb F (see Genetic Modulators of Sickle Cell Disease, discussed earlier). In view of the marked effect of Hb F in impeding Hb S polymerization, it is not surprising that these patients have relatively mild clinical manifestations. The inhibitory effect of Hb F extends to all homozygotes. A recent study of the natural history of patients with SS disease in the United States showed that the frequency of pain crises correlated inversely with the level of Hb F.[229]

Because of the compelling biochemical and clinical evidence that Hb F inhibits sickling, therapeutic agents that increase Hb F production would be expected to benefit patients with sickle cell disease. The first drug to be tested was 5-azacytidine, an antineoplastic drug known to inhibit maintenance methylation of DNA. DeSimone and his colleagues[319] knew that actively expressed genes are generally hypomethylated and that in erythroid cells, with the developmental switch from γ globin to β globin production, the inactive γ gene becomes methylated. Therefore, they reasoned that the administration of 5-azacytidine might turn on dormant γ globin production. They showed that anemic baboons developed a marked increase in Hb F a few weeks after receiving the drug. These results prompted limited clinical trials demonstrating significant, albeit somewhat less dramatic, induction of Hb F production in patients with homozygous β thalassemia and sickle cell disease.[320–322]

Hydroxyurea. Subsequently, other antitumor agents, including cytosine arabinoside[323, 324] and hydroxyurea,[325, 326] have also been shown to induce increased production of fetal hemoglobin in primates[323, 325] as well as in man.[324, 326–334] Since these agents are not known to induce hypomethylation, the molecular mechanism through which they induce Hb F production remains enigmatic.

Despite the considerable interest, discussed below, in alternate means of inducing Hb F in patients with sickle cell disease, hydroxyurea is currently the agent that holds the most promise for safe and effective therapy. It is relatively non-toxic, its myelosuppressive effects are readily reversible, and it is not known to induce secondary malignancies. Currently, the major use of hydroxyurea is in myeloproliferative diseases, in which it has been noted to induce modest increases in Hb F levels.[335] Much more impressive increases in Hb F have been noted in sickle cell disease.[326–334] In a recent analysis of 32 patients with SS disease who were treated with hydroxyurea, the mean Hb F level was 14.9 per cent, compared with a mean value of 3.7 per cent prior to treatment.[334] The great majority of patients with SS disease who are given sufficient doses to cause mild myelosuppression develop a marked increase in F cells and in the percentage of Hb F[327–333] as well as an increase in Hb F per F cell.[330, 332] This effect is accompanied by an increase in hemoglobin coupled with a decreased reticulocyte count indicative of a decrease in hemolytic rate. Prolonged survival of ^{51}Cr-labeled autologous red cells and reduction in serum non-conjugated bilirubin and lactate dehydrogenase document the decrease in hemolysis.[331, 332]

These improvements in hematological parameters during hydroxyurea therapy are accompanied by objective evidence of the inhibition of intracellular polymerization of Hb S. The proportion of ISCs[332, 333] and dense cells,[331–333] as well as in vitro measurements of sickling, is significantly decreased. There are conflicting reports on whether hydroxyurea therapy affects the cation content of SS red cells.[331–333] Preliminary data on a small number of SS patients indicate that treatment results in amelioration of pain crises.[329, 332] A large multicenter prospective study is now in progress to document the safety of hydroxyurea in patients with SS disease and to assess its efficacy in preventing vaso-occlusive events.

A comprehensive body of objective measurements is required to document the effect of hydroxyurea therapy on the properties and survival of sickle red cells. It is generally assumed that the beneficial effects of treatment of sickle cell disease with hydroxyurea are due to the induction of Hb F. However, it is possible that other effects of the drug also contribute. Treatment is invariably associated with macrocytosis. There is no reason, a priori, why an increase in red cell size should have a beneficial effect. A more relevant and critical question is whether hydroxyurea treatment lowers intracellular hemoglobin concentration, which would greatly inhibit polymerization of sickle hemoglobin. In one recent report on six patients with myeloproliferative diseases and Hb A, hydroxyurea-induced macrocytosis was accompanied by decreased MCHC and red cell density, indicative of enhanced red cell hydration.[336] However, this study did not measure red cell indices and density prior to initiation of therapy. A similar result has been noted in dogs treated with hydroxyurea.[333] The benefit of hydroxyurea therapy may be due in part to a marked reduction in reticulocytes and young (hypodense) (SS) red cells, since these cells have a particularly high adherence to vascular endothelium. Since treatment also partially suppresses erythropoiesis, this reduction of young, adherent cells imposes a limitation on the patient's steady-state red cell mass. A full compensatory response to the reduction in hemolysis would have adverse rheological consequences.

As experience with long-term treatment of sickle cell disease patients with hydroxyurea expands, there is appropriate concern about the possible induction of malignant transformation. The risk appears to be very small in patients with myeloproliferative disorders who have taken the drug for up to 10 years. In a recent study of 32 patients with sickle cell disease, Charache and associates[334] found that chromosomal abnormalities after 2 years of treatment were no greater than those prior to treatment. However, they concluded that the period of observation was too short to evaluate the risk of tumorigenesis.

Erythropoietin. Even though hydroxyurea is relatively non-toxic, there are legitimate concerns, mentioned above, about long-term administration of any antitumor drug to patients with a congenital non-malignant disorder. Accordingly, there is considerable interest in identifying safe alternatives for inducing Hb F production. Recombinant human erythropoietin (rhEpo) has proved to be both extremely effective and remarkably non-toxic therapy for the anemia of chronic renal disease.[337, 338] Preliminary studies indicated that rhEpo stimulated Hb F production not only in primates[339] but also in patients with sickle cell anemia.[340] When 6 patients with SS disease were treated with weekly high-dose rhEpo, however, no induction of F reticulocytes or F cells or increase in the percentage of Hb F occurred.[332] Subsequently, the same dosage schedule of rhEpo was given to nine patients with SS disease.[341] Five had no significant response. In four patients who also received supplemental iron therapy, rhEpo treatment was associated with a significant increase in F reticulocytes but no significant increase in F cells.

There has been recent interest in whether patients with SS disease might derive benefit from a combination of hydroxyurea and rhEpo. Three patients who had achieved maximal induction of Hb F from daily treatment with hydroxyurea had no significant increment from the addition of weekly high-dose rhEpo.[332] However, high-dose rhEpo, in combination with iron supplementation, induces further Hb F production in patients on pulse hydroxyurea therapy (4 consecutive days per week).[342] It is likely that this dose of hydroxyurea was suboptimal, because of both intermittent administration and the possibility that iron therapy partially offset the drug's inhibition of ribonucleotide reductase.[343] Further treatment trials with different dose schedules are needed to assess whether the addition of rhEpo will provide an effective and sustained increment in Hb F production, thereby permitting the use of lower and less toxic doses of hydroxyurea.

Butyrates. Considerable interest has recently been focused on the physiological and pharmacological roles of butyric acid and analogues thereof in the regulation of Hb F production. Ginder and his colleagues[344, 345] found that when adult anemic chickens were treated with a combination of 5-azacytidine and sodium butyrate, selective hypomethylation and reactivation of embryonic globin gene expression resulted. Perrine and coworkers[346] showed that the switch from Hb F to Hb A is delayed in infants of diabetic mothers in association with increased levels of α-amino-N-butyric acid. They found that the addition of this metabolite enhanced γ globin and suppressed β globin expression in cultured neonatal human cells.[347] Moreover, this metabolite as well as sodium butyrate enhanced γ globin gene expression in erythroid progenitors of patients with SS disease and β thalassemia.[348] These exciting results led to in vivo experiments. Infusions of butyrate into fetuses of sheep,[349] normal baboons,[350] and recently three patients with SS disease[351] have in all cases resulted in increases of Hb F production. Clearly, enthusiasm is considerable for further investigation of this potentially non-teratogenic and non-mutagenic means of inducing Hb F production in man.

HEMOGLOBIN MUTANTS WITH A THALASSEMIA PHENOTYPE

Thus far, about 30 human hemoglobin mutants have been found to be associated with a thalassemia-like red cell morphology, including microcytosis, hypochromia, and stippling.[352, 353]* These include 14 α globin mutants, 13 β globin mutants, and 3 $\delta\beta$ fusion mutants (the Lepore hemoglobins). Clinical severity in heterozygotes varies considerably, from normal hemoglobin levels and reticulocyte counts to marked hemolysis and/or ineffective erythropoiesis.

Some of these thalassemia-like mutants have arisen because of interesting molecular mechanisms, summarized at the beginning of this chapter. (See Human Hemoglobin Mutants.) These include elongated subunits, such as Hb Constant Spring, caused by mutations in the termination codon; the $\delta\beta$ fusion products due to non-homologous cross-over; and mutations such as Hb E that cause abnormal splicing.

Hb E is the second most commonly encountered hemoglobin mutant. The frequency of the Hb E gene approaches 0.5 in regions of Laos and Thailand.[254] As discussed in detail in Chapter 5, the production of Hb E, both at the mRNA level and at the protein level, is impaired because the base substitution giving rise to β26 Glu→Lys also created a surrogate splice junction leading to a reduction in the level of correctly spliced

---

*These mutants are discussed in more detail in Chapter 5. In addition, Adams and Coleman[352] have recently reviewed this topic.

mRNA. Hb EE homozygotes have microcytic red cells but no significant anemia, hemolysis, or clinical problems. Hb E poses a problem only when it coexists in the compound heterozygous state with β thalassemia.

Several of the α globin mutants have a thalassemia phenotype because they are invariably linked to a tandem α globin gene deletion. The most common of these are Hb G-Philadelphia and Hb Hasharon.

Some mutants consist of single amino acid replacements that confer such instability that the mutant subunit can be detected only by special techniques such as radioactive labeling of newly synthesized transient subunits. The first and best known example of this is Hb Terre Haute (β112 Leu→Arg), originally called Hb Indianapolis.* As information accumulates on well-characterized mutant hemoglobins, it is becoming apparent that there is a continuum that blurs the boundaries between those inducing a thalassemia phenotype and those that give rise to congenital Heinz body hemolysis. The former mutants (described above) have such extreme instability that they are readily degraded in bone marrow precursor cells, resulting in a thalassemia phenotype with ineffective erythropoiesis. The latter mutants, described in the next section, have intermediate stability and form Heinz bodies in circulating red blood cells, resulting in hemolysis.

THE UNSTABLE HEMOGLOBIN MUTANTS (CONGENITAL HEINZ BODY HEMOLYTIC ANEMIA)

In 1952, Cathie[355] described a patient with congenital non-spherocytic hemolytic anemia associated with jaundice, splenomegaly, and pigmenturia. Subsequently, other patients with similar clinical findings were suspected of having a structurally abnormal hemoglobin because their hemolysates formed a precipitate readily upon heating. In most cases, structural analyses have demonstrated mutant hemoglobins. So-called congenital Heinz body hemolytic anemia (CHBA) constitutes an important type of congenital hemolytic disease. Although the term is widely used, CHBA is a misnomer. Because of its variable severity, clinical manifestations may not appear until later in childhood or in adulthood, and Heinz bodies are not always present.

Unstable hemoglobinopathy has an autosomal dominant pattern of inheritance. Thus, affected individuals are heterozygotes. The unstable hemoglobin con-

stitutes only a minority (10 to 30 per cent) of the total. As expected in the heterozygous state, the remaining hemoglobin is predominantly normal Hb A. A sizeable minority of cases of unstable hemoglobinopathy appear to have arisen because of a spontaneous mutation, with both parents being unaffected.[356] Viewed another way, of the instances of apparent spontaneous mutations among hemoglobin mutants reported to date, approximately two thirds involve patients with unstable hemoglobins. This is not surprising because many cases are sufficiently severe that medical attention and evaluation are sought. In contrast, the chances are very remote of finding an asymptomatic individual with a hemoglobin mutant due to a spontaneous mutation. Furthermore, the potential of patients with severe unstable hemoglobinopathy to have healthy offspring may be slightly decreased.

Pathogenesis

Thus far, more than 100 structurally different unstable hemoglobin mutants have been documented. Many of these show only mild instability in vitro and are not associated with any significant clinical manifestations. About three fourths of these are β chain mutants. Many of them are amino acid replacements in the vicinity of the heme pocket (Fig. 6–20). The majority are neutral replacements, such as Hb Köln (β98 Val→Met). Such an alteration in primary structure may cause considerable perturbations in the hydrophobic interior of the molecule. Considering the nature of such amino acid replacements, it is not surprising that many of these mutants have electrophoretic mobility identical to that of Hb A. Others may appear as single or multiple bands having isoelectric points higher than those of Hb A. If these bands are no longer visible following the addition of hemin to the hemolysate, it is likely that the abnormal electrophoretic mobility was due to heme loss (or heme displacement) rather than to an alteration in the charge of a globin subunit. About one fifth of the unstable mutants involve a replacement by proline. Proline residues can prevent the formation of an α helix. Thus, instability may result from disruption of the secondary structure of the subunit. Some unstable mutants contain deletions of one to five amino acids in sequence (see Table 6–1) and probably arose because of frameshift mutagenesis in the region of the reiterated nucleotide sequence.[5] This mechanism is supported by the finding of "mirror image" mutants: Hb Gun Hill, which has a five residue deletion at position 93 to 97, and Hb Koriyama, which has a tandem insertion of the same five residues.[50] A few unstable mutants have insertions within deletions (see Table 6–1).

The mechanism by which red cells hemolyze is still uncertain. Much of the red cell destruction occurs in the bone marrow.[357] There is convincing evidence that normally placed hemes confer considerable stability on their respective globin subunits. In many of the

---

*By means of elegant high-resolution analyses of radiolabeled peptides, Adams and his colleagues initially concluded that this mutant was β112 Cys→Arg. However, a second report of a mutant with this replacement but without a thalassemic phenotype prompted these investigators to re-examine their case. The patient was deceased, and the only available specimen was some old bone marrow slides. Analysis of minute amounts of DNA from cells scraped off these slides by means of the polymerase chain reaction showed conclusively that the correct replacement was β106 Leu→Arg.[354]

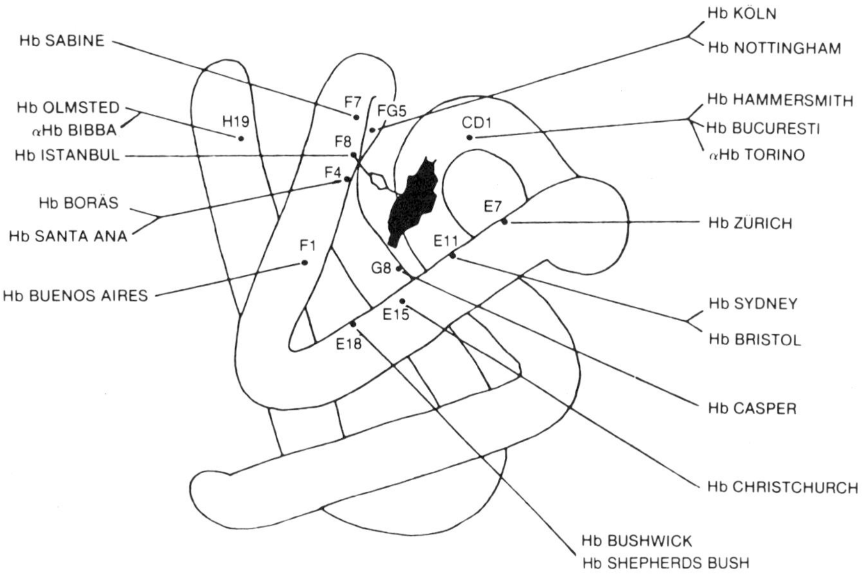

FIGURE 6–20. Three-dimensional representation of β chain showing sites of amino acid substitutions at the heme pocket that make the mutant hemoglobins unstable. (From Milner, P. F., and Wrightstone, R. N.: *In* Wallach, D. [ed.]: The Function of Red Blood Cells. New York, Alan R. Liss, Inc. 1981. Copyright © 1981 by John Wiley & Sons, Inc. Reprinted by permission of John Wiley & Sons, Inc.)

unstable hemoglobin mutants, the amino acid substitution prevents a normal heme-globin linkage. Once the heme becomes detached from its normal position in the cleft on the surface of the involved subunit, it probably binds non-specifically to another site on the globin. Both spectrophotometric and electron spin resonance measurements indicate that the formation of hemichrome may be an intermediate step in the denaturation of unstable hemoglobins.[358] Following heme displacement, the globin subunits aggregate to form a coccoid precipitate having the morphological characteristics of a Heinz body. The Heinz bodies and the heat-induced precipitate contain equal amounts of α and β chains and probably a normal complement of heme.[359] Red cells containing Heinz bodies have reduced deformability[360] and are likely to be entrapped in the microcirculation. There is convincing morphological evidence that these Heinz bodies become selectively removed, or "pitted," during circulation through the sinusoids of the spleen.[361] Therefore, it is not surprising that patients who have undergone splenectomy have an increased number of Heinz bodies and, in most cases, a greater percentage of the hemoglobin mutant relative to normal Hb A.

The intracellular release of heme from these unstable mutants may contribute to decreased deformability of CHBA red cells and therefore to the rate of hemolysis. The release of reactive oxidants such as hydrogen peroxide, superoxide, and hydroxyl radical may damage the red cell membrane by both lipid peroxidation and cross-linking of membrane proteins.[362, 363]

Because the degree of instability of these hemoglobin mutants spans a wide range, the extent of hemolysis varies considerably. In some, such as Hb Zürich, an additional oxidant stress, such as the ingestion of certain drugs, is required for significant hemolysis. Fever may also increase the hemolytic rate.[364] Many patients, however, have continuous and marked red cell breakdown. The degree of anemia is influenced

not only by the severity of the hemolysis but also by the ability of the blood to unload oxygen.[5] Thus, patients having unstable mutants of high oxygen affinity, such as Hb Köln, may have a near-normal hemoglobin level (i.e., compensated hemolysis). In contrast, the hemoglobin level is likely to be much lower in patients having mutants with decreased oxygen affinity, such as Hb Hammersmith.

The structural alteration in Hb Zürich leads to particularly interesting functional and clinical consequences.[365, 366] The replacement of the distal histidine by arginine at βE7 causes a larger space in the heme pocket where gas ligands bind. Accordingly, carbon monoxide is able to bind in a non-constrained fashion and with much higher affinity. Carbon monoxide protects this mutant from oxidative denaturation. Individuals with Hb Zürich who smoke tend to accumulate high levels of carboxyhemoglobin and have less hemolysis than do affected family members who do not smoke.

As discussed in the beginning of this section, a few hemoglobin mutants are so unstable that virtually no mutant gene product can be detected in the hemolysate. Examples include Hb Terre Haute,[354] Hb Showa-Yakushiji,[367] and Hb Geneva.[368] Heterozygotes have a phenotype of thalassemia intermedia with moderate anemia, splenomegaly, microcytic red cells, Heinz bodies, and elevated levels of Hb A_2.

Clinical Features

These pathophysiological considerations explain a number of the clinical features of this disorder. Patients usually present in early childhood with a hemolytic anemia accompanied by jaundice and splenomegaly. In some cases, hemolysis is markedly aggravated by fever or the ingestion of an oxidant-type drug. The red cell morphology is somewhat variable. Often, patients with a functioning spleen have normal-looking red cells. Slight hypochromia and prominent basophilic stippling are common features. Indeed, the intensity of the basophilic stippling may equal or even exceed that noted in pyrimidine 5'-nucleotidase deficiency. In both conditions, the stippling may be due to excessive clumping of ribosomes. The blood may have to be incubated in order to demonstrate Heinz bodies. In some cases, routine blood films reveal occasional red cells that appear as if a bite had been taken from a margin, and it is tempting to speculate that a Heinz body had been pitted at this site. After splenectomy, red cells appear much more abnormal. Heinz bodies are larger and more numerous. The extent of symptoms varies markedly with the degree of anemia. As mentioned earlier, one of the two parents is affected in about two thirds of cases. Some patients give a history of passing dark urine. Although this pigment has not been completely characterized, it appears to be a dipyrrole (mesobilifuscin) and may be the consequence of aberrant (perhaps non-enzymatic) heme catabolism. Dipyrroles have also been detected in CHBA red cells by means of fluorescence microscopy.[369]

HEMOGLOBIN MUTANTS WITH ABNORMAL OXYGEN BINDING

In 1966, Charache and coworkers[370] described a family with erythrocytosis due to the presence of a hemoglobin mutant, Hb Chesapeake (α92 Arg→Leu). Oxygen equilibria done on both whole blood and the isolated abnormal hemoglobin revealed a marked increase in oxygen affinity and a reduction in subunit cooperativity. Because of the "shift to the left" and consequent reduction in oxygen unloading, individuals with a high-affinity hemoglobin mutant have compensatory erythrocytosis via increased production of erythropoietin.[371] To date, more than 50 other mutants with very high oxygen affinity have been discovered. In each case, affected family members have erythrocytosis. Unlike the unstable hemoglobins, which may also have abnormal oxygen affinity, these mutants are not associated with any hemolysis or abnormal red cell morphology. The high-affinity mutants have provided an unusual bounty of information on both physiologic oxygen transport in man and structure-function relationships of hemoglobin.

The location and nature of the amino acid substitutions in these mutants have been useful in establishing specific sites on the hemoglobin molecule that are critical to its function. A number of these mutants, including Hb Kempsey, have substitutions at the $\alpha^1\beta^2$ interface. As Figure 6–21 shows, in normal Hb A the interaction of β99 Asp with α42 Tyr at this subunit interface contributes to the stability of the T structure. In Hb Kempsey, the substitution β99 Asp→Asn prevents this interaction. There is good experimental evidence that the high oxygen affinity of Hb Kempsey is due to destabilization of the T (deoxy) conformation. In contrast, the oxy or R conformation of Hb A is

stabilized by an interaction at the $\alpha^1\beta^2$ interface between β102 Asn and α94 Asp (Fig. 6–21). The *low* oxygen affinity of Hb Kansas can be attributed to decreased stability of the R form, owing to the replacement of β102 asparagine by threonine.[5] A second group of high oxygen affinity mutants has substitutions at the C-terminus of the abnormal subunit. As explained at the beginning of this chapter and depicted in Figure 6–3*B*, electrostatic interactions at the C-terminus of the β subunit are important contributors to the stability of the T quaternary conformation and to the Bohr effect. Hb Hiroshima (β146 His→Asp) is one of several variants in which replacement of the C-terminal histidine gives rise to increased oxygen affinity and diminished Bohr effect (Fig. 6–22). A third group of mutants with high oxygen affinity has substitutions at the 2,3-DPG–binding site, which results in impaired binding to 2,3-DPG and increased intracellular oxygen affinity.[5]

Other than demonstrating erythrocytosis, affected individuals have minimal clinical manifestations. In most cases, the increase in red cell mass is probably appropriate to ensure tissue oxygenation. Hemodynamic studies on these individuals have produced somewhat variable results. Some patients have had increased cardiac output or low mixed venous PO_2 or both when subjected to graded exercise or bled down to a normal red cell mass.[5] Packed cell volumes seldom reach levels high enough to necessitate therapeutic phlebotomy for increased blood viscosity. There are many reports of affected mothers carrying unaffected offspring to term. In these cases, the oxygen affinity of the maternal blood was probably greater than that of the fetus. The lack of any untoward complications[372] argues against the physiological importance of increased oxygen affinity of fetal blood.

The possibility of a functionally abnormal hemoglobin should be considered in any case of unexplained erythrocytosis. A positive family history and an abnormal hemoglobin electrophoresis are very helpful. However, I have seen one child in whom neither of these findings was present. She was found to have Hb Bethesda, which apparently arose as a spontaneous mutation. In such cases, a measurement of oxygen affinity is required to establish the diagnosis. Not all familial erythrocytosis is due to a functionally abnormal hemoglobin mutant; in some families, there may be either an enhanced production of erythropoietin or enhanced sensitivity to normal levels of erythropoietin.[373]

M HEMOGLOBINS

The appearance of blue or dusky skin and mucous membranes is a common and informative finding on physical examination. In the vast majority of cases, cyanosis is due to an excess of deoxyhemoglobin in the blood, owing to cardiac or pulmonary dysfunction or both and rarely to a stable mutant hemoglobin

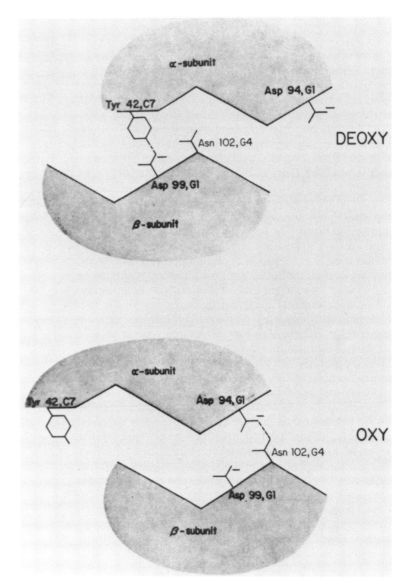

FIGURE 6–21. Mechanism by which substitutions at the α¹β² interface affect oxygen affinity. Upon oxygenation, the area of contact between subunits shifts in a dovetail fashion. Deoxyhemoglobin is normally stabilized by a hydrogen bond between α42 Tyr and β99 Asp. This bond cannot form in a set of high oxygen mutants, including Hb Kempsey (β99 Asp→Asn). Conversely, oxyhemoglobin is stabilized by a bond between α94 Asp and β102 Asn. This bond cannot form in Hb Kansas (β102 Asn→Thr), Hb Beth Israel (β102 Asn→Thr), and Hb Titusville (α94 Asp→Asn). (From Perutz, M. F.: New Scient. Sci. J., June 1971; with permission.)

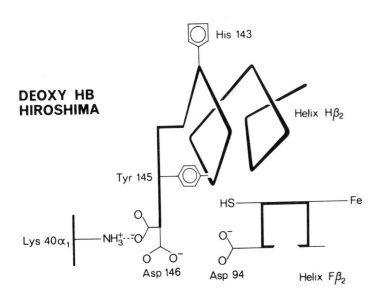

FIGURE 6–22. Diagram of the contacts of β^Hiroshima in which the C-terminal 146 histidine is replaced by aspartic acid. Compare with Figure 6–3B. The substitution prevents the salt bond with βAsp 94 and explains why Hb Hiroshima has high oxygen affinity and half-normal Bohr effect. (From Perutz, M. F.: Molecular anatomy, physiology, and pathology of hemoglobin. *In* Stamatoyannopoulos, G., Nienhuis, A. W., Leder, P., and Majerus, P. W.: The Molecular Basis of Blood Diseases. Philadelphia, W. B. Saunders Company, 1981; p. 127.)

(such as Hb Kansas) that has unusually low oxygen affinity.

Much less often, cyanosis is due to oxidized hemoglobin (methemoglobin or sulfhemoglobin or both) in circulating red cells. Congenital methemoglobinemia is usually caused by a deficiency of the enzyme cytochrome b_5 reductase (also called diaphorase I or NADH-dependent methemoglobin reductase), which enables red cell hemoglobin to be maintained in the reduced form. A more uncommon cause of congenital methemoglobinemia is the presence of one of the M hemoglobins. Like the other types of functionally abnormal hemoglobins discussed in detail in this chapter, the M hemoglobins are inherited according to an autosomal dominant pattern. Affected individuals present with cyanosis but are otherwise asymptomatic. Generally, no evidence of anemia is present. The blood has a peculiar mahogany color "like that of Japanese soy sauce."[374] Spectral examination of the hemoglobin shows an abnormal pattern that is similar to, but not identical with, that of methemoglobin. Hemoglobin electrophoresis reveals an abnormal band with a slightly anodal mobility. The normal A and abnormal M hemoglobins may be separated more readily if the entire hemolysate is converted to methemoglobin prior to electrophoresis.

Seven M hemoglobins have been described (Table 6–3). The α and β chain mutants have been detected in unrelated families all over the world. Six of the seven M hemoglobins represent substitution of either the proximal (F8) or the distal (E7) histidine by tyrosine. It is likely that the side group of the substituted tyrosine can serve as an internal ligand, stabilizing the heme iron in the ferric form (Fig. 6–23). As anticipated, the M hemoglobins are functionally abnormal. Both α chain mutants have decreased oxygen affinity and decreased Bohr effect.[5] The whole blood oxygen affinity of individuals with Hb M may be markedly decreased, owing in part to the intrinsic functional abnormality of the hemoglobin mutant and in part to increased 2,3-DPG in the red cell.[5] Furthermore, individuals who have one of the M hemoglobins may have mild hemolysis. However, the M hemoglobins should not be confused with some of the unstable mutants, such as Hb Freiburg and Hb St. Louis, in which a high proportion of the abnormal subunit oxidizes to methemoglobin. Hbs FM-Osaka (γ63 His→Tyr)[375] and FM-Fort Ripley (γ92 His→Tyr)[376] were discovered in cyanotic newborns. The cyanosis

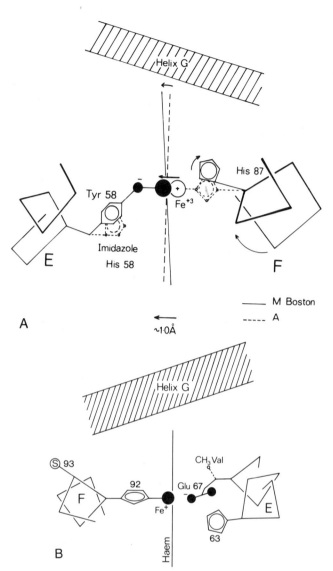

FIGURE 6–23. *A*, Diagram of the heme pocket of $\beta^{M\text{-Boston}}$ showing that the oxidized (Fe^{3+}) iron atom forms a bond with the substituted tyrosine at α58 (E7) on the distal side of the heme rather than with the proximal F8 histidine. (From Pulsinelli, P. D., Perutz, M. F., and Nagel, R. L.: Structure of hemoglobin M Boston, a variant with a five-coordinated ferric heme. Proc. Natl. Acad. Sci. USA: 70:3870, 1973; with permission.) *B*, Comparable diagram of $\beta^{M\text{-Milwaukee-1}}$ showing the binding of the carboxyl group of the substituted β67 glutamic acid with the oxidized heme iron. (Reprinted by permission from *Nature* [New Biol], Vol. 237, p. 259; copyright © 1972 Macmillan Magazines Limited.)

disappeared during the first few months of life as β chains replaced γ chains.

In this disorder, treatment is neither indicated nor possible. The M hemoglobins are perhaps of more interest and concern to molecular biologists than to the individuals affected.

TABLE 6–3. PROPERTIES OF THE M HEMOGLOBINS

HEMO-GLOBIN	STRUCTURE	HELICAL RESIDUE	O_2 AFFINITY AT P_{50}	BOHR EFFECT
M-Boston	α58 His → Tyr	E7	Decreased	Decreased
M-Iwate	α86 His → Tyr	F8	Decreased	Decreased
M-Saskatoon	β63 His → Tyr	E7	Normal	Present
M-Hyde Park	β92 His → Tyr	F8	Normal	Present
M-Milwaukee-1	β67 Val → Glu	E11	Decreased	Present
FM-Osaka	γ63 His → Tyr	E7		
FM-Fort Ripley	γ92 His → Tyr	F8		

REFERENCES

1. Pauling, L., Itano, H., Singer, S. J., and Wells, I. C.: Sickle cell anemia: A molecular disease. Science 110:543, 1949.
2. Perutz, M. F.: Molecular anatomy, physiology, and pathology

of hemoglobin. *In* Stamatoyannopoulos, G., Nienhuis, A. W., et al. (eds.): The Molecular Basis of Blood Diseases. Philadelphia, W. B. Saunders Co., 1987, p. 127.

3. Shaanan, B.: The structure of human oxyhaemoglobin at 2.1: A resolution. J. Mol. Biol. 171:31, 1983.

4. Fermi, G., Perutz, M. F., and Shaanan, B.: The crystal structure of human deoxyhemoglobin at 1,74: A resolution. J. Mol. Biol. 175:159, 1984.

5. Bunn, H. F., and Forget, B. G.: Hemoglobin: Molecular, Genetic and Clinical Aspects. Philadelphia, W. B. Saunders Co., 1986.

6. Monod, J., Wyman, J., and Changeux, J. P.: On the nature of allosteric transitions: A plausible model. J. Mol. Biol. 12:88, 1965.

7. Ackers, G. K., Doyle, M. L., Myers, D. M., and Daugherty, M. A.: Molecular code for cooperativity in hemoglobin. Science 255:54, 1992.

8. Fermi, G., Perutz, M. F., and Shulman, R. G.: Iron distances in hemoglobin: Comparison of x-ray crystallographic and extended x-ray absorption fine structure studies. Proc. Natl. Acad. Sci. USA 84:6167, 1987.

9. Nagai, K., Perutz, M. F., and Poyart, C.: Studies of haemoglobin functions by site-directed mutagenesis. Philos. Trans. R. Soc. Lond. [A] 317:443, 1986.

10. Nagai, K., Luisi, B., Shih, D., Miyazaki, G., Imai, K., Poyart, C., De Young, A., Kwiatkowsky, L., Noble, R. W., Lin, S.-H., and Yu, N.-T.: Distal residues in the oxygen binding site of haemoglobin studied by protein engineering. Nature 329:858, 1987.

11. Hoffman, S. J., Looker, D. L., Roehrich, J. M., Cozart, P. E., Durfee, S. L., Tedesco, J. L., and Stetler, G. L.: Expression of fully functional tetrameric human hemoglobin in *Escherichia coli.* Proc. Natl. Acad. Sci. USA 87:8521, 1990.

12. Murray, L. P., Hofrichter, J., Henry, E. R., Ikeda-Saito, M., Kitagishi, K., Yonetani, T., and Eaton, W. A.: The effect of quaternary structure on the kinetics of conformational changes and nanosecond geminate rebinding of carbon monoxide to hemoglobin. Proc. Natl. Acad. Sci. USA 85:2151, 1988.

13. Murray, L. P., Hofrichter, J., Henry, E. R., and Eaton, W. A.: Time-resolved optical spectroscopy and structural dynamics following photodissociation of carbonmonoxyhemoglobin. Biophys. Chem. 29:63, 1988.

14. Perutz, M. F.: Mechanisms regulating the reactions of human hemoglobin with oxygen and carbon monoxide. Annu. Rev. Physiol. 52:1, 1990.

15. Bohr, C., Hasselbalch, K., and Krogh, A.: Ueber einen in biologischer Beziehung wichtigen Einfluss. den die Kohlensauerespannung des Blutes auf dessen Sauerstoffbinding ubt. Skand. Arch. Physiol. 16:402, 1904.

16. Riggs, A. F.: The Bohr effect. Annu. Rev. Physiol. 50:181, 1988.

17. Busch, M. R., Mace, J. E., Ho, N. T., and Ho, C.: Roles of the β146 histidyl residue in the molecular basis of the Bohr effect of hemoglobin: A proton nuclear magnetic resonance study. Biochemistry 30:1865, 1991.

18. Benesch, R., and Benesch, R. E.: Intracellular organic phosphates as regulators of oxygen release by haemoglobin. Nature 221:618, 1969.

19. Arnone, A.: X-ray diffraction study of binding of 2,3-diphosphoglycerate to human deoxyhaemoglobin. Nature 237:146, 1972.

20. Adamson, J. W., and Finch, C. A.: Hemoglobin function, oxygen affinity and erythropoietin. Annu. Rev. Physiol. 38:351, 1975.

21. Huisman, T. H. J., Schroeder, W. A., Bannister, W. H., and Grech, J. L.: Evidence for four nonallelic structural genes for the γ chain of human fetal hemoglobin. Biochem. Genet. 7:131, 1972.

22. Adachi, K., Kim, J., Asakura, T., and Schwartz, E.: Characterization of two types of fetal hemoglobin: α2Gγ2 and α2Aγ2. Blood 75:2070, 1990.

23. Ricco, G., Mazza, U., Turi, R. M., Pich, P. G., Camaschella, C., Saglio, G., and Bernini, L. F.: Significance of a new type

24. of human fetal hemoglobin carrying a replacement isoleucine-threonine at position 75 (E 19) of the γ chain. Hum. Genet. 32:305, 1976.

24. Schroeder, W. A., Cua, J. T., Matsuda, G., and Fenninger, W. D.: Hemoglobin F₁, an acetyl-containing hemoglobin. Biochem. Biophys. Acta 63:532, 1962.

25. Bauer, C., Ludwig, I., and Ludwig, M.: Different effects of 2,3-diphosphoglycerate and adenosine triphosphate on the oxygen affinity of adult and fetal human hemoglobin. Life Sci. 7:1339, 1968.

26. Tyuma, I., and Shimizu, K.: Different response to organic phosphates of human fetal and adult hemoglobins. Arch. Biochem. Biophys. 129:404, 1969.

27. Boyer, S. H., Belding, T. K., Margolet, L., and Noyes, A. N.: Fetal hemoglobin restriction to few erythrocytes (F cells) in normal human adults. Science 188:361, 1975.

28. Wood, W. G., Stamatoyannopoulos, G., Lim, G., and Nute, P. E.: F-cells in the adult: Normal values and levels in individuals with hereditary and acquired elevation of Hb F. Blood 46:671, 1975.

29. Steinberg, M. H., and Adams, J. G. III: Hemoglobin A₂: Origin, evolution, and aftermath. Blood 78:2165, 1991.

30. Rieder, R. F., and Weatherall, D. J.: Studies on hemoglobin biosynthesis: Asynchronous synthesis of hemoglobin A and hemoglobin A₂ by erythrocyte precursors. J. Clin. Invest. 44:42, 1965.

31. Roberts, A. V., Weatherall, D. J., and Clegg, J. B.: The synthesis of human hemoglobin A₂ during erythroid maturation. Biochem. Biophys. Res. Commun. 47:81, 1972.

32. Allen, D. W., Schroeder, W. A., and Balog, J.: Observations on the chromatographic heterogeneity of normal adult and fetal human hemoglobins. J. Am. Chem. Soc. 80:1628, 1958.

33. McDonald, M. J., Shapiro, R., Bleichman, M., Solway, J., and Bunn, H. F.: Glycosylated minor components of human adult hemoglobin. J. Biol. Chem. 253:2327, 1978.

34. Garlick, R. L., Mazer, J. S., Higgins, P. J., and Bunn, H. F.: Characterization of glycosylated hemoglobins. Relevance to monitoring of diabetic control and analysis of other proteins. J. Clin. Invest. 71:1062, 1983.

35. Bookchin, R. M., and Gallop, P. M.: Structure of hemoglobin A₁c: Nature of the N-terminal β chain blocking group. Biochem. Biophys. Res. Commun. 32:86, 1968.

36. Bunn, H. F., Haney, D. N., Gabbay, K. H., and Gallop, P. M.: Further identification of the nature and linkage of the carbohydrate in hemoglobin A₁c. Biochem. Biophys. Res. Commun. 67:103, 1975.

37. Prome, D., Blouquit, Y., Ponthus, C., Prome, J. C., and Rosa, J.: Structure of the human adult hemoglobin minor fraction A1b by electrospray and secondary ion mass spectrometry. Pyruvic acid as amino-terminal blocking group. J. Biol. Chem. 266:13050, 1991.

38. Bunn, H. F., Haney, D. N., Kamin, S., Gabbay, K. H., and Gallop, P. M.: Biosynthesis of human hemoglobin A₁c. Slow glycosylation of hemoglobin in vivo. J. Clin. Invest. 57:1652, 1976.

39. Bunn, H. F., Gabbay, K. H., and Gallop, P. M.: The glycosylation of hemoglobin: Relevance to diabetes mellitus. Science 220:21, 1978.

40. Fluckiger, R., Harmon, W., Meier, W., Loo, S., and Gabbay, K. H.: Hemoglobin carbamylation in uremia. N. Engl. J. Med. 304:823, 1981.

41. Stevens, V. J., Fantl, W. J., Newman, C. B., Sims, R. V., Cerami, A., and Peterson, C. M.: Acetaldehyde adducts with hemoglobin. J. Clin. Invest. 67:361, 1981.

42. Hoberman, H. D.: Post-translational modification of hemoglobin in alcoholism. Biochem. Biophys. Res. Commun. 113:1004, 1983.

43. Charache, S., and Weatherall, D. J.: Fast hemoglobin in lead poisoning. Blood 28:377, 1966.

44. Lamola, A. A., Piomelli, S., Poh-Fitzpatrick, M. G., Yamane, T., and Harber, L. C.: Erythropoietic protoporphyria and lead intoxication: The molecular basis for difference in cutaneous photosensitivity. II. Different binding of eryth-

rocyte protoporphyrin to hemoglobin. J. Clin. Invest. 56:1528, 1975.

45. International Hemoglobin Information Center: List of hemoglobin variants. Hemoglobin 15:139, 1991.

46. Cash, F. E., Monplaisir, N., Goossens, M., and Liebhaber, S. A.: Locus assignment of two α-globin structural mutants from the Caribbean basin: α Fort de France (α$^{45\ Arg}$) and Spanish Town (α$^{27\ Val}$). Blood 74:833, 1989.

47. Wilson, J. B., Chen, S. S., Webber, B. B., Kutlar, A., Kutlar, F., Villegas, A., and Huisman, T. H. J.: The identification of five rare β-chain abnormal hemoglobins by high performance liquid chromatographic procedures. Hemoglobin 10:49, 1986.

48. Lubin, B. H., Witkowska, E., and Kleman, K.: Laboratory diagnosis of hemoglobinopathies. Clin. Biochem. 24:363, 1991.

49. Schnee, J., Aulehla-Scholz, C., Eigel, A., and Horst, J.: Hb D Los Angeles (D-Punjab) and Hb Presbyterian: Analysis of the defect at the DNA level. Hum. Genet. 84:365, 1990.

50. Codrington, J. F., Kutlar, F., Harris, H. F., Wilson, J. B., Stoming, T. A., Huisman, T. H. J.: Hb A$_2$− Wrens or α$_2$δ$_2$98 (FG5) Val → Met, an unstable δ chain variant identified by sequence analysis of amplified DNA. Biochim. Biophys. Acta 1009:87, 1989.

51. Bunn, H. F., and McDonald, M. J.: Electrostatic interactions in the assembly of haemoglobin. Nature 306:498, 1983.

52. Bunn, H. F.: Subunit assembly of hemoglobin: An important determinant of hematologic phenotype. Blood 69:1, 1987.

53. Liebhaber, S. A., Cash, F. E., and Cornfield, D. B.: Evidence for posttranslational control of Hb C synthesis in an individual with Hb C trait and α-thalassemia. Blood 71:502, 1988.

54. Huisman, T. H. J.: Percentages of abnormal hemoglobins in adults with a heterozygosity for an α-chain and/or β-chain variant. Am. J. Hematol. 14:393, 1983.

55. Mrabet, N. T., McDonald, M. J., Turci, S., Sarkar, R., Szabo, A., and Bunn, H. F.: Electrostatic attraction governs the dimer assembly of dimers of human hemoglobin. J. Biol. Chem. 261:5222, 1986.

56. Adams, J. G. III, Coleman, M. B., Hayes, J., Morrison, W. T., and Steinberg, M. H.: Modulation of fetal hemoglobin synthesis by iron deficiency. N. Engl. J. Med. 313:1402, 1985.

57. Chui, D. H. K., Patterson, M., Dowling, C. E., Kazazian, H. H., Jr., and Kendall, A. G.: Hemoglobin Bart's disease in an Italian boy. An interaction between α-thalassemia and hereditary persistence of fetal hemoglobin. N. Engl. J. Med. 323:179, 1990.

58. Hirsch, R. E., Raventos-Suarez, C., Olsen, J. A., and Nagel, R. L.: Ligand state of intraerythrocytic circulating Hb C crystals in homozygous CC patients. Blood 66:775, 1985.

59. Fabry, M. E., Kaul, D. K., Raventos-Suarez, C., Chang, H., and Nagel, R. L.: SC red cells have an abnormally high intracellular hemoglobin concentration: Pathophysiologic consequences. J. Clin. Invest. 70:1315, 1982.

60. Bunn, H. F., Noguchi, C. T., Hofrichter, J., Schechter, G. P., Schechter, A. N., and Eaton, W. A.: The molecular and cellular pathogenesis of hemoglobin SC disease. Proc. Natl. Acad. Sci. USA 79:7527, 1982.

61. Brugnara, C., Kopin, A. S., Bunn, H. F., and Tosteson, D. C.: Regulation of cation content and cell volume in hemoglobin erythrocytes from patients with homozygous hemoglobin C disease. J. Clin. Invest. 75:1608, 1985.

62. White, J. G.: The fine structure of sickled hemoglobin in situ. Blood 31:561, 1968.

63. Bertles, J. F., and Dobler, J.: Reversible and irreversible sickling: A distinction by electron microscopy. Blood 33:884, 1969.

64. Edelstein, S. J., Telford, J. N., and Crepeau, R. H.: Structure of fibers of sickle cell hemoglobin. Proc. Natl. Acad. Sci. USA 70:1104, 1973.

65. Dykes, G. W., Crepeau, R. H., and Edelstein, S. J.: Three-dimensional reconstruction of the fibers of sickle cell haemoglobin. Nature 272:506, 1978.

66. Garrell, R. L., Crepeau, R. H., and Edelstein, S. J.: Cross-

sectional views of hemoglobin S fibers by electron microscopy and computer modeling. Proc. Natl. Acad. Sci. USA 76:1140, 1979.

67. Dykes, G., Crepeau, R. H., and Edelstein, S. J.: Three-dimensional reconstruction of the 14-filament fibers of hemoglobin S. J. Mol. Biol. 130:451, 1979.

68. Rodgers, D. W., Crepeau, R. H., and Edelstein, S. J.: Pairings and polarities of the 14 strands in sickle cell hemoglobin fibers. Proc. Natl. Acad. Sci. USA 84:6157, 1987.

69. Carragher, B., Bluemke, D. A., Gabriel, B., Potel, M. J., and Josephs, R.: Structural analysis of polymers of sickle cell hemoglobin. I. Sickle hemoglobin fibers. J. Mol. Biol. 199:315, 1988.

70. Perutz, M. F., and Mitchison, J. M.: State of haemoglobin in sickle-cell anaemia. Nature 166:677, 1950.

71. Hofrichter, J., Hendricker, D., and Eaton, W. A.: Structure of hemoglobin S fibers: Optical determination of the molecular orientation in sickled erythrocytes. Proc. Natl. Acad. Sci. USA 70:3604, 1973.

72. Magdoff-Fairchild, B., and Chiu, C. C.: X-ray diffraction studies of fibers and crystals of deoxygenated sickle cell hemoglobin. Proc. Natl. Acad. Sci. USA 76:223, 1979.

73. Wishner, B. C., Ward, K. B., Lattman, E. E., and Love, W. E.: Crystal structure of sickle-cell deoxyhemoglobin at 5 Å resolution. J. Mol. Biol. 98:179, 1975.

74. Padlan, E. A., and Love, W. E.: Refined crystal structure of deoxyhemoglobin S. I. Restrained least squares refinement at 3.0-Å resolution. J. Biol. Chem. 260:8272, 1985.

75. Padlan, E. A., and Love, W. E.: Refined crystal structure of deoxyhemoglobin S. II. Molecular interactions in the crystal. J. Biol. Chem. 260:8280, 1985.

76. Bookchin, R. M., Nagel, R. L., and Ranney, H. M.: Structure and properties of hemoglobin C-Harlem, a human hemoglobin variant with amino acid substitutions in 2 residues on the β-polypeptide chain. J. Biol. Chem. 242:248, 1967.

77. Nagel, R. L., Bookchin, R. M., Johnson, J., Labie, D., Wajcman, H., Isaac-Sodeye, W. A., Honig, G. R., Schiliro, G., Crookston, J. H., and Matsutomo, K.: Structural bases of the inhibitory effects of hemoglobin F and hemoglobin A$_2$ on the polymerization of hemoglobin S. Proc. Natl. Acad. Sci. USA 76:670, 1979.

78. Nagel, R. L., Johnson, J., Bookchin, R. M., Garel, M. C., Rosa, J., Schiliro, G., Wajcman, H., Labie, D., Moo-Penn, W., and Castro, O.: β-Chain contact sites in the haemoglobin S polymer. Nature 283:832, 1980.

79. Benesch, R. E., Yung, S., Benesch, R., Mack, J., and Schneider, R. G.: α-Chain contacts in the polymerization of sickle haemoglobin. Nature 260:219, 1976.

80. Benesch, R. E., Kwong, S., and Benesch, R.: The effect of α chain mutations cis and trans to the β6 mutation on the polymerization of sickle cell haemoglobin. Nature 299:231, 1982.

81. Bunn, H. F., and McDonough, M.: Asymmetrical hemoglobin hybrids. An approach to the study of subunit interactions. Biochemistry 13:988, 1974.

82. Edelstein, S. J.: Molecular topology in crystals and fibers of hemoglobin S. J. Mol. Biol. 150:557, 1981.

83. Watowich, S. J., Gross, L. J., and Josephs, R.: Intermolecular contacts within sickle hemoglobin fibers. J. Mol. Biol. 209:821, 1989.

84. Adachi, K., Kim, J., Ballas, S., Surrey, S., and Asakura T.: Facilitation of Hb S polymerization by the substitution of Glu for Gln at β121. J. Biol. Chem. 263:5607, 1988.

85. Baudin-Chich, V., Pagnier, J., Marden, M., Bohn, B., Lacaze, N., Kister, J., Schaad, O., Edelstein, S. J., and Poyart, C.: Enhanced polymerization of recombinant human deoxyhemoglobin β6 Glu-Ile. Proc. Natl. Acad. Sci. USA 87:1845, 1990.

86. Eaton, W. A., and Hofrichter, J.: Sickle cell hemoglobin polymerization. Adv. Protein Chem. 40:63, 1990.

87. Bertles, J. F., Rabinowitz, R., and Dobler, J.: Hemoglobin interaction: Modification of solid phase composition in the sickling phenomenon. Science 169:375, 1970.

88. Briehl, R. W., and Ewert, S.: Effects of pH, 2,3,-diphospho-

glycerate and salts on gelation of sickle cell deoxyhemoglobin. J. Mol. Biol. 80:445, 1973.

89. Eaton, W. A., and Hofrichter, J.: Hemoglobin S gelation and sickle cell disease. Blood 70:1245, 1987.

90. Briehl, R. W.: Sickle-cell hemoglobin. Encyclopedia of Human Biology 7:1, 1991.

91. Gill, S. J., Skold, R., Fall, L., Shaeffer, T., Spokane, R., and Wyman, J.: Aggregation effects on oxygen binding of sickle cell hemoglobin. Science 201:362, 1978.

92. Benesch, R. E., Edalji, R., Kwong, S., and Benesch, R.: Oxygen affinity as an index of hemoglobin S polymerization: A new micromethod. Anal. Biochem. 89:162, 1978.

93. Gill, S. J., Benedict, R. C., Fall, L., Spokane, R., and Wyman, J.: Oxygen binding to sickle cell hemoglobin. J. Mol. Biol. 130:175, 1979.

94. Sunshine, H. R., Hofrichter, J., Ferrone, F. A., and Eaton, W. A.: Oxygen binding by sickle cell hemoglobin polymers. J. Mol. Biol. 158:251, 1982.

95. Minton, A. P.: Non-ideality and the thermodynamics of sickle-cell hemoglobin gelation. J. Mol. Biol. 110:89, 1977.

96. Goldberg, M. A., Husson, M. A., and Bunn, H. F.: The participation of hemoglobins A and F in the polymerization of sickle hemoglobin. J. Biol. Chem. 252:3414, 1977.

97. Briehl, R. W.: Gelation of sickle cell hemoglobin IV. Phase transitions in hemoglobin S gels: Separate measures of aggregation and solution-gel equilibrium. J. Mol. Biol. 123:521, 1978.

98. Ueda, Y., and Bookchin, R. M.: Effects of carbon dioxide and pH variations in vitro on blood respiratory function, red cell volume, transmembrane pH gradients and sickling in sickle cell anemia. J. Lab. Clin. Med. 104:146, 1984.

99. Ross, P. D., Hofrichter, J., and Eaton, W. A.: Calorimetric and optical characterization of sickle cell hemoglobin gelation. J. Mol. Biol. 96:239, 1975.

100. Magdoff-Fairchild, B., Poillon, W. N., Li, T.-I., and Bertles, J. F.: Thermodynamic studies of polymerization of deoxygenated sickle cell hemoglobin. Proc. Natl. Acad. Sci. USA 73:990, 1976.

101. Ross, P. D., Hofrichter, J., and Eaton, W. A.: Thermodynamics of gelation of sickle cell deoxyhemoglobin. J. Mol. Biol. 115:111, 1977.

102. Poillon, W. N., and Bertles, J. F.: Deoxygenated sickle hemoglobin. Effects of lyotropic salts on its solubility. J. Biol. Chem. 254:3462, 1979.

103. Adachi, K., Ozguc, M., and Asakura, T.: Nucleation-controlled aggregation of deoxyhemoglobin S. Participation of hemoglobin A in the aggregation of deoxyhemoglobin S in concentrated buffer. J. Biol. Chem. 255:3092, 1980.

104. Roth, E. F., Jr., Bookchin, R. M., and Nagel, R. L.: Deoxyhemoglobin S gelation and insolubility at high ionic strength are distinct phenomena. J. Lab. Clin. Med. 93:867, 1979.

105. Swerdlow, P. H., Bryan, R. A., Bertles, J. F., Poillon, W. N., Magdoff-Fairchild, B., and Milner, P. F.: Effect of 2,3-diphosphoglycerate on the solubility of deoxy sickle hemoglobin. Hemoglobin 1:527, 1977.

106. Poillon, W. N., and Kim, B. C.: 2,3-Diphosphoglycerate and intracellular pH as interdependent determinants of the physiologic solubility of deoxyhemoglobin S. Blood 76:1028, 1990.

107. Bookchin, R. M., Nagel, R. L., and Balazs, T.: Role of hybrid tetramer formation in gelation of hemoglobin S. Nature 256:667, 1975.

108. Hofrichter, J., Ross, P. D., and Eaton, W. A.: Kinetics and mechanism of deoxyhemoglobin S gelation: A new approach to understanding sickle cell disease. Proc. Natl. Acad. Sci. USA 71:4864, 1974.

109. Hofrichter, J., Ross, P. D., Eaton, W. A.: Supersaturation in sickle cell hemoglobin solutions. Proc. Natl. Acad. Sci. USA 73:3034, 1976.

110. Samuel, R. E., Salmon, E. D., and Briehl, R. W.: Nucleation and growth of fibres and gel formation in sickle cell haemoglobin. Nature 345:833, 1990.

111. Ferrone, F. A., Hofrichter, J., Sunshine, H. R., and Eaton, W. A.: Kinetic studies on photolysis-induced gelation of sickle

112. Hofrichter, J.: Kinetics of sickle hemoglobin polymerization. III. Nucleation rates determined from stochastic fluctuations in polymerization progress curves. J. Mol. Biol. 189:553, 1986.

113. Harris, J. W.: Studies on the destruction of red blood cells. VII. Molecular orientation in sickle cell hemoglobin solutions. Proc. Soc. Exp. Biol. Med. 75:197, 1950.

114. Coletta, M., Hofrichter, J., Ferrone, F. A., and Eaton, W. A.: Kinetics of sickle haemoglobin polymerization in single red cells. Nature 300:194, 1982.

115. Goldberg, M. A., Lalos, A. T., and Bunn, H. F.: The effect of erythrocyte membrane preparations on the polymerization of sickle hemoglobin. J. Biol. Chem. 256:193, 1981.

116. Mozzarelli, A., Hofrichter, J., and Eaton, W. A.: Delay time of hemoglobin S polymerization prevents most cells from sickling in vivo. Science 237:500, 1987.

117. Winslow, R. M.: Hemoglobin interactions and whole blood oxygen equilibrium curves in sickling disorders. In Caughey, W. S. (ed.): Clinical and Biochemical Aspects of Hemoglobin Abnormalities. New York, Academic Press, 1978, p. 369.

118. Noguchi, C. T., Torchia, D. A., and Schechter, A. N.: Determination of deoxyhemoglobin S polymer in sickle erythrocytes upon deoxygenation. Proc. Natl. Acad. Sci. USA 77:5487, 1980.

119. Noguchi, C. T., Torchia, D. A., and Schechter, A. N.: Intracellular polymerization of sickle cell hemoglobin. Effects of cell heterogeneity. J. Clin. Invest. 72:846, 1983.

120. Mickols, W. E., Corbett, J. D., Maestre, M. F., Tinoco, I., Jr., Kropp, J., and Embury, S. H.: The effect of speed of deoxygenation on the percentage of aligned hemoglobin in sickle cells. J. Biol. Chem. 263:4338, 1988.

121. Horiuchi, K., Ballas, S. K., and Asakura, T.: The effect of deoxygenation rate on the formation of irreversibly sickled cells. Blood 71:46, 1988.

122. Horiuchi, K., and Asakura, T.: Oxygen promotes sickling of SS cells. Ann. N. Y. Acad. Sci. (Sickle Cell Disease) 565:395, 1989.

123. Hebbel, R. P.: Beyond hemoglobin polymerization: The red blood cell membrane and sickle disease pathophysiology. Blood 77:214, 1991.

124. Liu, S.-C., Derick, L. H., Zhai, S., and Palek, J.: Uncoupling of the spectrin-based skeleton from the lipid bilayer in sickled red cells. Science 252:574, 1991.

125. Allan, D., Limbrick, A. R., Thomas, P., and Westerman, M. P.: Release of spectrin free spicules on reoxygenation of sickled erythrocytes. Nature 295:612, 1982.

126. Lux, S. E., John, K. M., and Karnovsky, M. J.: Irreversible deformation of the spectrin-actin lattice in irreversibly sickled cells. J. Clin. Invest. 58:955, 1976.

127. Liu, S. C., Derick, L. H., Zhai, S., and Palek, J.: Ultrastructural anatomy of the red cell membrane lesion in sickle cells: Penetration of the hemoglobin S polymers through the membrane skeleton and the reorganization of the skeletal lattice. Blood (Suppl 1.) 74:44a, 1989.

128. Rodgers, G. P., Noguchi, C. T., and Schechter, A. M.: Irreversibly sickled erythrocytes in sickle cell anemia: A quantitative reappraisal. Am. J. Hematol. 20:17, 1985.

129. Bertles, J. F., and Milner, P. F. A.: Irreversibly sickled erythrocytes: A consequence of the heterogeneous distribution of hemoglobin types in sickle-cell anemia. J. Clin. Invest. 47:1731, 1968.

130. Fabry, M. E., Mears, J. G., Patel, P., Schaefer-Rego, K., Carmichael, L. D., Martinez, G., and Nagel, R. L.: Dense cells in sickle cell anemia: The effects of gene interaction. Blood 64:1042, 1984.

131. Nagel, R. L., Fabry, M. E., Pagnier, J., Zohoun, I., Wajcman, J., Baudin, V., and Labie, D.: Hematologically and genetically distinct forms of sickle cell anemia in Africa: The Senegal type and the Benin type. N. Engl. J. Med. 312:880, 1985.

132. Horiuchi, K., and Asakura, T.: Formation of light irreversibly

sickled cells during deoxygenation-oxygenation cycles. J. Lab. Clin. Med. 110:653, 1987.

133. Horiuchi, K., Ohata, J., Hirano, Y., and Asakura, T.: Morphologic studies of sickle erythrocytes by image analysis. J. Lab. Clin. Med. 115:613, 1990.

134. Horiuchi, K., Ballas, S. K., and Asakura, T.: The effect of deoxygenation rate on the formation of irreversibly sickled cells. Blood 71:46, 1988.

135. Bookchin, R. M., Ortiz, O. E., and Lew, V. L.: Evidence for a direct reticulocyte origin of dense red cells in sickle cell anemia. J. Clin. Invest. 87:113, 1991.

136. Platt, O. S., Falcone, J. F., and Lux, S. E.: Molecular defect in the sickle erythrocyte skeleton: Abnormal spectrin binding to sickle inside-out vesicles. J. Clin. Invest. 75:266, 1985.

137. Schwartz, R. S., Rybicki, A. C., Heath, R. H., and Lubin, B. H.: Protein 4.1 in sickle erythrocytes. Evidence for oxidative damage. J. Biol. Chem. 262:15666, 1987.

138. Klipstein, F. A., and Ranney, H. M. Electrophoretic components of the hemoglobin of red cell membranes. J. Clin. Invest. 39:1894, 1960.

139. Fung, L. W.-M., Litvin, S. D., and Reid, T. M.: Spin-label detection of sickle hemoglobin-membrane interaction at physiological pH. Biochemistry 22:864, 1983.

140. Fortier, N., Snyder, L. M., Garver, F., Kiefer, C., McKenney, J., and Mohandas, N.: The relationship between in vivo generated hemoglobin skeletal protein complex and increased red cell membrane rigidity. Blood 71:1427, 1988.

141. Evans, E. A., and Mohandas, N.: Membrane-associated sickle hemoglobin: A major determinant of sickle erythrocyte rigidity. Blood 70:1443, 1987.

142. Hebbel, R. P., Yamada, O., Moldow, C. F., Jacob, H. S., White, J. G., and Eaton, J. W.: Abnormal adherence of sickle erythrocytes to cultured vascular endothelium: A possible mechanism for microvascular occlusion in sickle cell disease. J. Clin. Invest. 65:154, 1980.

143. Waugh, S. M., Willardson, B. M., Kannan, R., Labotka, R. J., and Low, P. S.: Heinz bodies induce clustering of band 3, glycophorin, and ankyrin in sickle cell erythrocytes. J. Clin. Invest. 78:1155, 1986.

144. Rank, B. H., Carlsson, J., and Hebbel, R. P.: Abnormal redox status of membrane-protein thiols in sickle erythrocytes. J. Clin. Invest. 75:1531, 1985.

145. Rice-Evans, C., Omorphos, S. C., and Baysal, E.: Sickle cell membranes and oxidative damage. Biochem. J. 237:265, 1986.

146. Hebbel, R. P., Morgan, W. T., Eaton, J. W., and Hedlund, B. E.: Accelerated autooxidation and heme loss due to instability of sickle hemoglobin. Proc. Natl. Acad. Sci. USA 85:237, 1988.

147. Asakura, T., Minakata, K., Adachi, K., Russell, M. O., and Schwartz, E.: Denatured hemoglobin in sickle erythrocytes. J. Clin. Invest. 59:633, 1977.

148. Kuross, S. A., Rank, B. H., and Hebbel, R. P.: Excess heme in sickle erythrocyte inside-out membranes: Possible role in thiol oxidation. Blood 71:876, 1988.

149. Hebbel, R. P., Eaton, J. W., Balasingam, M., and Steinberg, M. H.: Spontaneous oxygen radical generation by sickle erythrocytes. J. Clin. Invest. 70:1253, 1982.

150. Repka, T., and Hebbel, R. P.: Hydroxyl radical formation by sickle erythrocyte membranes: Role of pathologic iron deposits and cytoplasmic reducing agents. Blood 78:2753, 1991.

151. Asakura, T.: Mechanical instability of the oxy-form of sickle hemoglobin. Nature 244:437, 1973.

152. Asakura, T.: Abnormal precipitation of oxyHb S by mechanical shaking. Proc. Natl. Acad. Sci. USA 71:1594, 1974.

153. Liu, S.-C., Zhai, S., and Palek, J.: Detection of hemin release during hemoglobin S denaturation. Blood 71:1755, 1988.

154. Liu, S.-C., Zhai, S., Lawler, J., and Palek, J.: Hemin-mediated dissociation of erythrocyte membrane skeletal proteins. J. Biol. Chem. 260:12234, 1985.

155. Jarolim, P., Lahav, M., Liu, S.-C., and Palek, J.: Effect of hemoglobin oxidation products on the stability of red cell membrane skeletons and the associations of skeletal proteins: Correlation with a release of hemin. Blood 76:2125, 1990.

156. Middelkoop, E., Lubin, B. H., Bevers, E. M., Op den Kamp, J. A. F., Comfurius, P., Chiu, D. T.-Y., Zwaal, R. F. A., van Deenen, L. L. M., and Roelofsen, B.: Studies on sickled erythrocytes provide evidence that the asymmetric distribution of phosphatidlyserine in the red cell membrane is maintained by both ATP-dependent translocation and interaction with membrane skeletal proteins. Biochim. Biophys. Acta 937:281, 1988.

157. Devaux, P. F.: Static and dynamic lipid asymmetry in cell membranes. Biochemistry 30:1163, 1991.

158. Lubin, B., Chiu, D., Bastacky, J., Roelofsen, B., and van Deenen, L. L. M.: Abnormalities in membrane phospholipid organization in sickled erythrocytes. J. Clin. Invest. 67:1643, 1981.

159. Franck, P. F. H., Bevers, E. M., Lubin, B. H., Comfurius, P., Chiu, D. T.-Y., Op den Kamp, J. A. F., Zwaal, R. F. A., van Deenen, L. L. M., and Roelofsen, B.: Uncoupling of the membrane skeleton from the lipid bilayer. The cause of accelerated phospholipid flip-flop leading to an enhanced procoagulant activity of sickled cells. J. Clin. Invest. 75:183, 1985.

160. Mohandas, N., Rossi, M., Bernstein, S., Ballas, S., Ravindranath, Y., Wyatt, J., and Mentzer, W.: The structural organization of skeletal proteins influences lipid translocation across erythrocyte membrane. J. Biol. Chem. 260:14264, 1985.

161. Blumenfeld, N., Zachowski, A., Galacteros, F., Beuzard, Y., and Devaux, P. F.: Transmembrane mobility of phospholipids in sickle erythrocytes: Effect of deoxygenation on diffusion and asymmetry. Blood 77:849, 1991.

162. Chiu, D., Lubin, B., Roelofsen, B., van Deenen, L. L. M.: Sickled erythrocytes accelerate clotting in vitro: An effect of abnormal membrane lipid asymmetry. Blood 58:398, 1981.

163. Westerman, M. P., Cole, E. R., Wu, K.: The effect of spicules obtained from sickle red cells on clotting activity. Br. J. Haematol. 56:557, 1984.

164. Richardson, S. G. N., Matthews, K. B., Stuart, J., Geddes, A. M., and Wilcox, R. M.: Serial changes in coagulation and viscosity during sickle-cell crisis. Br. J. Haematol. 41:95, 1979.

165. Das, S. K., and Nair, R. C.: Superoxide dismutase, glutathione peroxidase, catalase and lipid peroxidation of normal and sickled erythrocytes. Br. J. Haematol. 44:87, 1980.

166. Hebbel, R. P., and Miller, W. J.: Phagocytosis of sickle erythrocytes: Immunologic and oxidative determinants of hemolytic anemia. Blood 64:733, 1984.

167. Jain, S. K., and Shohet, S. B.: A novel phospholipid in irreversibly sickled cells: Evidence for in vivo peroxidative membrane damage in sickle cell disease. Blood 63:362, 1984.

168. Van den Berg, J. J. M., Kuypers, F. A., Qju, J. H., Chiu, D., Lubin, B., Roelofsen, B., and Op den Kamp, J. A. F.: The use of cis-parinaric acid to determine lipid peroxidation in human erythrocyte membranes. Comparison of normal and sickle erythrocyte membranes. Biochim. Biophys. Acta 944:29, 1988.

169. Kuross, S. A., and Hebbel, R. P.: Nonheme iron in sickle erythrocyte membranes: Association with phospholipids and potential role in lipid peroxidation. Blood 72:1278, 1988.

170. Hebbel, R. P., and Miller, W. J.: Unique promotion of erythrophagocytosis by malondialdehyde. Am. J. Hematol. 29:222, 1988.

171. Bookchin, R. M., Ortiz, O. E., and Lew, V. L.: Mechanisms of red cell dehydration in sickle cell anemia. Application of an integrated red cell model. In Raess, B. U., and Tunnicliff, G. (eds.): The Red Cell Membrane: A Model for Solute Transport. Clifton, N. J., Humana Press, 1989.

172. Lauf, P. K., and Theg, B. E.: A chloride dependent K$^+$ flux induced by N-ethylmaleimide in genetically low K$^+$ sheep and goat erythrocytes. Biochem. Biophys. Res. Commun. 92:1422, 1980.

173. Dunham, P. B., and Ellory, J. C.: Passive potassium transport

in low potassium sheep red cells: Dependence upon cell volume and chloride. J. Physiol. 318:511, 1981.

174. Brugnara, C., Bunn, H. F., and Tosteson, D. C.: Regulation of erythrocyte cation and water content in sickle cell anemia. Science 232:388, 1986.

175. Hall, A. C., and Ellory, J. C.: Evidence for the presence of volume-sensitive K:Cl transport in "young" human red cells. Biochim. Biophys. Acta 858:317, 1986.

176. Brugnara, C., and Tosteson, D. C.: Cell volume, K$^+$ transport and cell density. Am. J. Physiol. 21:C269, 1987.

177. Canessa, M., Spalvins, A., and Nagel, R. L.: Volume-dependent and NEM-stimulated K$^+$:Cl$^-$ transport is elevated in oxygenated SS, SC and CC human red cells. FEBS Lett. 200:197, 1986.

178. Olivieri, O., Vitoux, D., Galacteros, F., Bachir, D., Blouquit, Y., Beuzard, Y., and Brugnara, C.: Hemoglobin variants and activity of the (K$^+$Cl$^-$) cotransport system in human erythrocytes. Blood 79:793, 1992.

179. Vitoux, D., Olivieri, O., Garay, R. P., Cragoe, E. J., Galacteros, F., and Beuzard, Y.: Inhibition of K$^+$ loss and dehydration of sickle cells by DIOA: An inhibitor of the [K$^+$CL$^-$] cotransport system. Proc. Natl. Acad. Sci. USA 86:4273, 1989.

180. Lawrence, C., Fabry, M. E., and Nagel, R. L.: The unique red cell heterogeneity of SC disease: Crystal formation, dense reticulocytes, and unusual morphology. Blood 78:2104, 1991.

181. Fabry, M. E., Romero, J. R., Buchanan, I. D., Suzuka, S. M., Stamatoyannopoulos, G., Nagel, R. L., and Canessa, M.: Rapid increase in red blood cell density driven by K:Cl cotransport in a subset of sickle cell anemia reticulocytes and discocytes. Blood 78:217, 1991.

182. Brugnara, C., and Tosteson, D. C.: Inhibition of K transport by divalent cations in sickle erythrocytes. Blood 70:1810, 1987.

183. Canessa, M., Fabry, M. E., and Nagel, R. L.: Deoxygenation inhibits the volume-stimulated Cl$^-$-dependent K$^+$ efflux in SS and young AA cells: A cytosolic Mg^{2+} modulation. Blood 70:1861, 1987.

184. Eaton, J. W., Skelton, T. D., Swofford, H. S., Koplin, C. E., and Jacob, H. S.: Elevated erythrocyte calcium in sickle cell disease. Nature 246:105, 1973.

185. Palek, J.: Red cell calcium content and transmembrane calcium movements in sickle cell anemia. J. Lab. Clin. Med. 89:1365, 1977.

186. Lew, V. L., Hockaday, A., Sepulveda, M. I., Somlyo, A. P., Somlyo, A. V., Ortiz, O. E., and Bookchin, R. M.: Compartmentalization of sickle cell calcium in endocytic inside-out vesicles. Nature 315:586, 1985.

187. Williamson, P., Puchulu, E., Westerman, M., and Schlegel, R. A.: Erythrocyte membrane abnormalities in sickle cell disease. Biotechnol. Appl. Biochem. 12:523, 1990.

188. Mohandas, N., Rossi, M. E., and Clark, M. R.: Association between morphologic distortion of sickle cells and deoxygenation-induced cation permeability increase. Blood 68:450, 1986.

189. Ortiz, O. E., Lew, V. L., and Bookchin, R. M.: Deoxygenation permeabilizes sickle cell anaemia red cells to magnesium and reverses its gradient in the dense cells. J. Physiol. 427:211, 1990.

190. Clark, M. R., and Rossi, M. E.: Permeability characteristics of deoxygenated sickle cells. Blood 76:2139, 1990.

191. Hebbel, R. P., Shalev. O., Foker, W., and Rank, B. H.: Inhibition of erythrocyte Ca^{2+}-ATPase by activated oxygen through thiol- and lipid-dependent mechanisms. Biochim. Biophys. Acta 862:8, 1986.

192. Tosteson, D. C., Shea, E., and Darling, R. C.: Potassium and sodium of red blood cells in sickle cell anemia. J. Clin. Invest. 31:406, 1952.

193. Joiner, C. H.: Deoxygenation-induced cation fluxes in sickle cells: II. Inhibition by stilbene disulfonates. Blood 76:212, 1990.

193a. Sugihara, T., and Hebbel, R. P.: Exaggerated cation leak from oxygenated sickle red blood cells during deformation: Evidence for a unique leak pathway. Blood 80:2374, 1992.

194. Joiner, C. H., Platt, O. S., and Lux, S. E.: Cation depletion by the sodium pump in red cells with pathological cation leaks. Sickle cells and xerocytes. J. Clin. Invest. 78:1487, 1986.

195. Lew, V. L., Freeman, C. J., Ortiz, O. E., and Bookchin, R. M.: A mathematical model of the volume, pH, and ion content regulation in reticulocytes. Application to the pathophysiology of sickle cell dehydration. J. Clin. Invest. 87:100, 1991.

196. Ney, P. A., Christopher, M. M., and Hebbel, R. P.: Synergistic effects of oxidation and deformation on erythrocyte monovalent cation leak. Blood 75:1192, 1990.

197. Sugihara, T., Rawicz, W., Evans, E. A., and Hebbel, R. P.: Lipid hydroperoxides permit deformation-dependent leak of monovalent cation from erythrocytes. Blood 77:2757, 1991.

198. Lew, V. L., and Bookchin, R. M.: Osmotic effects of protein polymerization: Analysis of volume changes in sickle cell anemia red cells following deoxy-hemoglobin S polymerization. J. Membrane Biol. 122:55, 1991.

199. Embury, S. H., Garcia, J. F., Mohandas, N., Pennathur-Das, R., and Clark, M. R.: Oxygen inhalation by subjects with sickle cell anemia. Effects on endogenous erythropoietin kinetics, erythropoiesis, and pathophysiologic properties of sickle blood. N. Engl. J. Med. 311:291, 1984.

200. Hebbel, R. P., and Miller, W. J.: Phagocytosis of sickle erythrocytes: Immunologic and oxidative determinants of hemolytic anemia. Blood 64:733, 1984.

201. Schwartz, R. S., Tanaka, Y., Fidler, I. J., Chiu, D. T.-Y., Lubin, B., and Schroit, A. J.: Increased adherence of sickled and phosphatidylserine-enriched human erythrocytes to cultured human peripheral blood monocytes. J. Clin. Invest. 75:1965, 1985.

202. Solanki, D. L.: Erythrophagocytosis in vivo in sickle cell anemia. Am. J. Hematol. 20:353, 1985.

203. Petz, L. D., Yam, P., Wilkinson, L., Garratty, G., Lubin, B., and Mentzer, W.: Increased IgG molecules bound to the surface of red blood cells of patients with sickle cell anemia. Blood 64:301, 1984.

204. Galili, U., Clark, M. R., and Shohet, S. B.: Excessive binding of natural anti-alpha-galactosyl immunoglobulin G to sickle erythrocytes may contribute to extravascular cell destruction. J. Clin. Invest. 77:27, 1986.

205. Schluter, K., and Drenckhahn, D.: Co-clustering of denatured hemoglobin with band 3: Its role in binding of autoantibodies against band 3 to abnormal and aged erythrocytes. Proc. Natl. Acad. Sci. USA 83:6137, 1986.

206. Hoover, R., Rubin, R., Wise, G., and Warren, R.: Adhesion of normal and sickle erythrocytes to endothelial monolayer cultures. Blood 54:872, 1979.

207. Hebbel, R. P., Yamada, O., Moldow, C. F., Jacob, H. S., White, J. G., and Eaton, J. W.: Abnormal adherence of sickle erythrocytes to cultured vascular endothelium: A possible mechanism for microvascular occlusion in sickle cell disease. J. Clin. Invest. 65:154, 1980.

208. Hebbel, R. P., Boogaerts, M. A. B., Eaton, J. W., and Steinberg, M. H.: Erythrocyte adherence to endothelium in sickle cell anemia: Possible determinant of disease severity. N. Engl. J. Med. 302:992, 1980.

209. Smith, B. D., and La Celle, P. L.: Erythrocyte-endothelial cell adherence in sickle cell disorders. Blood 68:1050, 1986.

210. Barabino, G. A., McIntire, L. V., Eskin, S. G., Sears, D. A., and Udden, M.: Endothelial cell interactions with sickle cell, sickle trait, mechanically injured, and normal erythrocytes under controlled flow. Blood 70:152, 1987.

211. Wick, T. M., Moake, J. L., Udden, M. M., Eskin, S. G., Sears, D. A., and McIntire, L. V.: Unusually large von Willebrand factor multimers increase adhesion of sickle erythrocytes to human endothelial cells under controlled flow. J. Clin. Invest. 80:905, 1987.

212. Mohandas, N., and Evans, E.: Adherence of sickle erythrocytes to vascular endothelial cells: Requirement for both cell membrane changes and plasma factors. Blood 64:282, 1984.

213. Kaul, D. K., Fabry, M. E., and Nagel, R. L.: Microvascular

sites and characteristics of sickle cell adhesion to vascular endothelium in shear flow conditions: Pathophysiological implications. Proc. Natl. Acad. Sci. USA 86:3356, 1989.

214. Mohandas, N., and Evans, E.: Sickle erythrocyte adherence to vascular endothelium. Morphologic correlates and the requirement for divalent cations and collagen-binding plasma proteins. J. Clin. Invest. 76:1605, 1985.

215. Mohandas, N., and Evans, E.: Rheological and adherence properties of sickle cells. Potential contribution to hematologic manifestations of the disease. Ann. N. Y. Acad. Sci. (Sickle Cell Disease) 565:327, 1989.

216. Hebbel, R. P., Moldow, C. F., and Steinberg, M. H.: Modulation of erythrocyte-endothelial interactions and the vasoocclusive severity of sickling disorders. Blood 58:947, 1981.

217. Wick, T. M., Moake, J. I., Udden, M. M., and McIntire, L. V.: Unusually large vWF multimers preferentially promote young sickle and non-sickle erythrocyte adhesion to endothelial cells. Am. J. Hematol (in press).

218. Kaul, B. K., Nagel, R. L., Chen, D., and Tsai, H.-M.: Sickle erythrocyte–endothelial interactions in microcirculation: The role of von Willebrand factor and implications for vasoocclusion. Blood (in press).

219. Hebbel, R. P., Visser, M. R., Goodman, J. L., Jacob, H. S., and Vercellotti, G. M.: Potentiated adherence of sickle erythrocytes to endothelium infected by virus. J. Clin. Invest. 80:1503, 1987.

220. Francis, R. B., Jr., and Johnson, C. S.: Vascular occlusion in sickle cell disease: Evolving concepts and unanswered questions. Blood 77:1405, 1991.

221. Fabry, M. E., Rajanayagam, V., Fine, E., Holland, S., Gore, J. C., Nagel, R. L., and Kaul, D. K.: Modeling sickle cell vasoocclusion in the rat leg: Quantification of trapped sickle cells and correlation with ^{31}P metabolic and ^{1}H magnetic resonance imaging changes. Proc. Natl. Acad. Sci. USA 86:3808, 1989.

221a. Fabry, M. E., Fine, E., Rajanayagam, V., Factor, S. M., Gore, J., Sylla, M., and Nagel, R. L.: Demonstration of endothelial adhesion of sickle cells in vivo: A distinct role for deformable sickle cell discocytes. Blood 79:1602, 1992.

222. Rodgers, G. P., Schechter, A. N., Noguchi, C. T., Klein, H. G., Neinhuis, A. W, and Bonner, R. F.: Periodic microcirculatory flow in patients with sickle cell disease. N Engl. J. Med. 311:1534, 1984.

223. Rodgers, G. P., Schechter, A. N., Noguchi, C. T., Klein, H. G., Nienhuis, A. W., and Bonner, R. F.: Microcirculatory adaptations in sickle cell anemia: reactive hyperemia response. Am. J. Physiol. 258:H113, 1990.

224. Rodgers, G. P., Roy, M. S., Noguchi, C. T., and Schechter, A. N.: Is there a role for selective vasodilation in the management of sickle cell disease? Blood 71:597, 1988.

225. Kennedy, A. P., Williams, B., Meydrech, E. F., and Steinberg, M. H.: Regional and temporal variation in oscillatory blood flow in sickle cell disease. Am. J. Hematol. 28:92, 1988.

226. Brody, A. S., Embury, S. H., Mentzer, W. C., Winkler, M. L., and Gooding, C. A.: Preservation of sickle cell blood-flow patterns during MR imaging: An in vivo study. Am. J. Radiol. 151:139, 1988.

227. Rodgers, G. P., Clark, C. M., Larson, S. M., Rapoport, S. I., Nienhuis, A. W., and Schechter, A. N.: Brain glucose metabolism in neurologically normal patients with sickle cell disease. Arch. Neurol. 45:78, 1988.

228. Baum, K. F., Dunn, D. T., Maude, G. H., and Serjeant, G. R.: The painful crisis of homozygous sickle cell disase. Arch. Intern. Med. 147:1231, 1987.

229. Platt, O. S., Thorington, B. D., Brambilla, D. J., Milner, P. F., Rosse, W. F., Vichinsky, E., and Kinney, T. R.: Pain in sickle cell disease: Rates and risk factors. N. Engl. J. Med. 325:11, 1991.

230. Lande, W. M., Andrews, D. L., Clark, M. R., Braham, N. V., Black, D. M., Embury, S. H., and Mentzer, W. C.: The incidence of painful crisis in homozygous sickle cell disease: Correlation with red cell deformability. Blood 72:2056, 1988.

231. Serjeant, G. R., and Chalmers, R. M.: Current concerns in

haematology 1. Is the painful crisis of sickle cell disease a "steal" syndrome? Clin. Pathol. 43:789, 1990.

232. Brittenham, G. M., Schechter, A. N., and Noguchi, C. T.: Hemoglobin S polymerization: Primary determinant of the hemolytic and clinical severity of the sickling syndromes. Blood 65:183, 1985.

233. Noguchi, C. T., Rodgers, G. P., Serjeant, G., and Schechter, A. N.: Levels of fetal hemoglobin necessary for treatment of sickle cell disease. N. Engl. J. Med. 318:96, 1988.

234. Keidan, A. J., Sowter, M. C., Johnson, C. S., Noguchi, C. T., Stevens, S. M. E., and Stuart, J.: Effect of polymerization tendency on haematological, rheological and clinical parameters in sickle cell anaemia. Br. J. Haematol. 71:551, 1989.

235. Warth, J. A., and Rucknagel, D. L.: Density ultracentrifugation of sickle cells during and after pain crisis: Increased dense echinocytes in crisis. Blood 64:507, 1984.

236. Rieber, E. E., Veliz, G., and Pollack, S.: Red cells in sickle cell crisis: Observations on the pathophysiology of crisis. Blood 49:967, 1977.

237. Kenney, M. W., Meaken, M., Worthington, D. J., and Stuart, J.: Erythrocyte deformability in sickle crisis. Br. J. Haematol. 49:103, 1981.

238. Lucas, G. S., Caldwell, N. M., and Stuart, J.: Fluctuating deformability of oxygenated sickle erythrocytes in the asymptomatic state and in painful crisis. Br. J. Haematol. 59:363, 1985.

238a. Akinola, N. O., Stevens, S. M. E., Franklin, I. M., Nash, G. B., and Stuart, J.: Rheological changes in the prodromal and established phases of sickle cell vasoocclusive crisis. Br. J. Haematol. 81:598, 1992.

239. Ballas, S. K., and Smith, E. D.: Red cell changes during the evolution of the sickle cell painful crisis. Blood 79:2154, 1992.

240. Billett, H. H., Nagel, R. L., and Fabry, M. E.: Evolution of laboratory parameters during sickle cell painful crisis: Evidence compatible with dense red cell sequestration without thrombosis. Am. J. Med. Sci. 296:293, 1988.

241. Rubin, E. M., Lu, R., Cooper, S., Mohandas, N., and Kan, Y. W.: Introduction and expression of the human β^S-globin gene in transgenic mice. Am. J. Hum. Genet. 42:585, 1988.

242. Rhoda, M. D., Domenget, C., Vidaud, M., Bardakdjian-Michau, J., Rouyer-Fessard, P., Rosa, J., and Beuzard, Y.: Mouse α chains inhibit polymerization of hemoglobin induced by human β^S or β$^{S\ Antilles}$ chains. Biochim. Biophys. Acta 952:208, 1989.

243. Greaves, D. R., Fraser, P., Vidal, M. A., Hedges, M. J., Ropers, D., Luzzatto, L., and Grosveld, F.: A transgenic mouse model of sickle cell disorder. Nature 343:183, 1990.

244. Ryan, T. M., Townes, T. M., Reilly, M. P., Asakura, T., Palmiter, R. D., Brinster, R. L., and Behringer, R. R.: Human sickle hemoglobin in transgenic mice. Science 247:566, 1990.

245. Rubin, E. M., Kan, Y. W., and Mohandas, N.: Effect of human β^S-globin chains on cellular properties of red cells from β-thalassemic mice. J. Clin. Invest. 82:1129, 1988.

245a. Fabry, M. E., Nagel, R. L., Pachnis, A., Suzuka, S. M., and Costantini, F.: High expression of human β^S and α-globins in transgenic mice: I. Hemoglobin composition and hematological consequences. Proc. Natl. Acad. Sci. USA (in press).

246. Monplaisir, N., Merault, G., Poyart, C., Rhoda, M. D., Craescu, C., Vidaud, M., Galacteros, F., Blouquit, Y., and Rosa, J.: Hemoglobin S Antilles: A variant with lower solubility than hemoglobin S and producing sickle cell disease in heterozygotes. Proc. Natl. Acad. Sci. USA 83:9363, 1986.

247. Rubin, E. M., Witkowska, H. E., Spangler, E., Curtin, P., Lubin, B. H., Mohandas, N., and Clift, S. M.: Hypoxia-induced in vivo sickling of transgenic mouse red cells. J. Clin. Invest. 87:639, 1991.

248. Trudel, M., Saadane, N., Garel, M.-C., Bardakdjian-Michau, J., Blouquit, Y., Guerquin-Kern, J.-L., Rouyer-Fessard, P., Vidaud, D., Pachnis, A., Romeo, P.-H., Beuzard, Y., and Costantini, F.: Towards a transgenic mouse model of sickle cell disease: Hemoglobin SAD. EMBO J. 10:3157, 1991.

249. Saadane, N., Trudel, M., Garel, M.-C., Bardakdjian-Michau,

J., Blouquit, Y., Guerquin-Kern, J.-L., Rouyer-Fessard, P., Vidaud, D., Pachnis, A., Romeo, P.-H., Costantini, F., and Beuzard, Y.: Sickle cell anemia in transgenic SAD mice. Blood 78:369a, 1991.

250. Kan, Y. W., and Dozy, A. M.: Polymorphism of DNA sequence adjacent to the human beta-globin structural gene: Relationship to sickle mutation. Proc. Natl. Acad. Sci. USA 75:5631, 1978.

251. Pagnier, J., Mears, J. G., Dunda-Belkodja, O., Schaefer-Rego, K. E., Beldjord, C., Nagel, R. L., and Labie, D.: Evidence of the multicentric origin of the hemoglobin S gene in Africa. Proc. Natl. Acad. Sci. USA 81:1771, 1984.

252. Labie, D., Pagnier, J., Lapoumeroulie, C., Rouabhi, F., Dunda-Belkhodja, O., Chardin, P., Beldjord, C., Wajcman, H., Fabry, M. E., and Nagel, R. L.: Common haplotype dependency on high $^G\gamma$-globin gene expression and high Hb F levels in β-thalassemia and sickle cell anemia patients. Proc. Natl. Acad. Sci. USA 82:2111, 1985.

253. Chebloune, Y., Pagnier, J., Trabuchet, G., Faure, C., Verdier, G., Labie, D., and Nigon, V.: Structural analysis of the 5' flanking region of the β-globin gene in African sickle cell anemia patients: Further evidence of three origins of the sickle cell mutation in Africa. Proc. Natl. Acad. Sci. USA 85:4431, 1988.

254. Nagel, R. L., and Ranney, H. M.: Genetic epidemiology of structural mutations of the β-globin gene. Semin. Hematol. 27:342, 1990.

255. Bouhassira, E. E., Lachman, H., Krishnamoorthy, R., Labie, D., and Nagel, R. L.: A gene conversion located 5' to the $^A\gamma$ gene in linkage disequilibrium with the Bantu haplotype in sickle cell anemia. J. Clin. Invest. 83:2070, 1989.

256. Bouhassira, E. E., and Nagel, R. L.: A 6-bp deletion 5' to the $^G\gamma$ globin gene in β^S chromosomes bearing the Bantu haplotype. Am. J. Hum. Genet. 47:161, 1990.

257. Srinivas, R., Dunda, O., Krishnamoorthy, R., Fabry, M. E., Georges, A., Labie, D., and Nagel, R. L.: Atypical haplotypes linked to the β^S gene in Africa are likely to be the product of recombination. Am. J. Hematol. 29:60, 1988.

258. Ragusa, A., Lombardo, M., Sortino, G., Lombardo, T., Nagel, R. L., and Labie, D.: β^S Gene in Sicily is in linkage disequilibrium with the Benin haplotype: Implications for gene flow. Am. J. Hematol. 27:139, 1988.

259. Boussiou, M., Loukopoulos, D., Christakis, J., and Fessas, P.: The origin of sickle mutation in Greece: Evidence from β^S globin gene cluster polymorphisms. Hemoglobin 15:459, 1991.

260. Labie, D., Srinivas, R., Dunda, O., Dode, C., LaPoumeroulie, C., Devi, V., Devi, S., Ramasami, K., Elion, J., Ducrocq, R., Krishnamoorthy, R., and Nagel, R. L.: Haplotypes in tribal Indians bearing the sickle gene: Evidence for unicentric origin of the β^S mutation and the unicentric origin of the tribal populations of India. Hum. Biol. 61:479, 1989.

261. Nagel, R. L., and Roth, E. F.: Malaria and red cell genetic defects. Blood 74:1213, 1989.

262. Nagel, R. L.: Innate resistance to malaria: The intraerythrocytic cycle. Blood Cells 16:321, 1990.

263. Allison, A. C.: Protection afforded by sickle-cell trait against subtertian malarial infection. Br. Med. J. 1:190, 1954.

264. Luzzatto, L., Nwachukes-Jarrett, E. S., and Reddy, S.: Increased sickling of parasitized erythrocytes as mechanisms of resistance against malaria in sickle cell trait. Lancet 1:319, 1970.

265. Raventos-Suarez, C., Kaul, D. K., Macaluso, F., and Nagel, R. L.: Membrane knobs are required for themicrocirculatory obstruction induced by *Plasmodium falciparum*–infected erythrocytes. Proc. Natl. Acad. Sci. USA 82:3829, 1985.

266. Nagel, R. L., Rao, S. K., Dunda-Belkhodja, O., Connolly, M. M., Fabry, M. E., Georges, A., Krishnamoorthy, R., and Labie, D.: The hematologic characteristics of sickle cell anemia bearing the Bantu haplotype: The relationship between $^G\gamma$ and HbF level. Blood 69:1026, 1987.

267. Nagel, R. L., Erlingsson, S., Fabry, M. E., Croizat, H., Sushuka, S. M., Lachman, H., Sutton, M., Driscoll, C., Bouhassira, E., and Billett, H. H.: The Senegal DNA haplotype is associated

with the amelioration of anemia in Afro-American sickle cell anemia patients. Blood 77:1371, 1991.

268. Rieder, R. F., Safaya, S., Gilette, P., Fryd, S., Hsu, H., Adams, J. G., and Steinberg, M. H.: Effect of β-globin gene cluster haplotype on the hematological and clinical features of sickle cell anemia. Am. J. Hematol. 36:184, 1991.

269. Powars, D., Chan, L. S., and Schroeder, W. A.: The variable expression of sickle cell disease is genetically determined. Semin. Hematol. 27:360, 1990.

270. Wainscoat, J. S., Thein, S. L., Higgs, D. R., Bell, J. I., Weatherall, D. J., Al-Awamy, B. H., and Serjeant, G. R.: A genetic marker for elevated levels of haemoglobin F in homozygous sickle cell disease? Br. J. Haematol. 60:261, 1985.

271. Miyoshi, K., Kaneto, Y., Kawai, H., Ohchi, H., Niki, S., Hasegawa, K., Shirakami, A., and Yamano, T.: X-linked dominant control of the F cells in normal adult life: Characterization of the Swiss type as hereditary persistence of fetal hemoglobin regulated dominantly by gene(s) on X chromosome. Blood 72:1854, 1988.

272. Dover, G. J., Smith, K. D., Chang, Y. C., Purvis, S., Mays, A., Meyers, D. A., Sheils, C., and Sergeant, G.: Hb F production in sickle cell disease and normal individuals is controlled by an X-linked gene located at Xp 22.2. Blood 80:816, 1992.

273. Davis, J. R., Dozy, A. M., Lubin, B., Koenig, H. M., Peirce, H. I., Stamatoyannopoulos, G., and Kan, Y. W.: Alpha thalassemia in blacks is due to gene deletion. Am. J. Hum. Genet. 31:569, 1979.

274. Dozy, A. M., Kan, Y. W., Embury, S. H., Mentzer, W. C., Wang, W. C., Lubin, B., Davis, J. R., Jr., and Koenig, H. M.: Alpha globin gene organization in blacks precludes the severe form of alpha thalassemia. Nature 280:605, 1979.

275. Embury, S. H., Miller, J., Dozy, A. M., Kan, Y. W., Chan, V., and Todd, D.: Two different molecular organizations account for the single α-globin gene of the α-thalassemia-2 genotype. J. Clin. Invest. 66:1319, 1980.

276. Embury, S. H., Gholson, M. A., Gillette, P., Rieder, R. F., and the National Cooperative Study of Sickle Cell Disease: The leftward deletion of α-Thal-2 haplotype in a black subject with hemoglobin SS. Blood 65:769, 1985.

277. Steinberg, M. H., Coleman, M. B., Adams, J. G., III, Hartmann, R. C., Saba, H., and Anagnou, N. P.: A new gene deletion in the α-like globin gene cluster as the molecular basis for the rare α-thalassemia-1 (− − /αα) in blacks: HbH disease in sickle cell trait. Blood 67:469, 1986.

278. Gupta, A. K., Kirchner, K. A., Nicholson, R., Adams, J. G., III, Schechter, A. N., Noguchi, C. T., and Steinberg, M. H.: Effects of α-thalassemia and sickle polymerization tendency on the urine-concentrating defect of individuals in sickle cell trait. J. Clin. Invest. 88:1963, 1991.

279. Steinberg, M. H., and Embury, S. H.: α-Thalassemia in blacks: Genetic and clinical aspects and interactions with the sickle hemoglobin gene. Blood 68:985, 1986.

280. Embury, S. H.: Alpha thalassemia, a modifier of sickle cell disease. Ann. N. Y. Acad. Sci. (Sickle Cell Disease) 565:213, 1989.

281. Embury, S. H., Dozy, A. M., Miller, J., Davis, J. R., Jr., Kleman, K. M., Preisler, H., Vichinsky, E., Lande, W. N., Lubin, B. H., Kan, Y. W., and Mentzer, W. C.: Concurrent sickle-cell anemia and α-thalassemia: Effect on severity of anemia. N. Engl. J. Med. 306:270, 1982.

282. Higgs, D. R., Aldridge, B. E., Lamb, J., Clegg, J. B., Weatherall, D. J., Hayes, R. J., Grandison, Y., Lowrie, Y., Mason, K. P., Serjeant, B. E., and Serjeant, G. R.: The interaction of alpha-thalassemia and homozygous sickle-cell disease. N. Engl. J. Med. 306:1441, 1982.

283. Steinberg, M. H., Rosenstock, W., Coleman, M. B., Adams, J. G., Platica, O., Cedeno, M., Rieder, R. F., Wilson, J. T., Milner, P., West, S., and the Cooperative Study of Sickle Cell Disease: Effects of thalassemia and microcytosis on the hematologic and vasoocclusive severity of sickle cell anemia. Blood 63:1353, 1984.

284. DeCeulear, K., Higgs, D. R., Weatherall, D. J., Hayes, R. J., Serjeant, B. E., and Serjeant, G. R.: α-Thalassemia reduces

the hemolytic rate in homozygous sickle cell disease. N. Engl. J. Med. 309:189, 1984.

285. Noguchi, C. T., Dover, G. J., Rodgers, G. P., Serjeant, G. R., Antonarakis, S. E., Anagnou, N. P., Higgs, D. R., Weatherall, D. J., and Schechter, A. N.: α-Thalassemia changes erythrocyte heterogeneity in sickle cell disease. J. Clin. Invest. 75:1632, 1985.

286. Embury, S. H., Backer, K., and Glader, B. E.: Monovalent cation changes in sickle erythrocytes: A direct reflection of α-globin gene number. J. Lab. Clin. Med. 106:75, 1985.

287. Embury, S. H., Clark, M. R., Monroy, G. M., and Mohandas, N.: Concurrent sickle cell anemia and α-thalassemia: Effect on pathological properties of sickle red cells. J. Clin. Invest. 73:116, 1984.

288. Dover, G. J., Chang, V. T., Boyer, S. H., Serjeant, G. R., Antonarakis, S., and Higgs, D. R.: The cellular basis for different fetal hemoglobin levels among sickle cell individuals with two, three, and four alpha-globin genes. Blood 69:341, 1987.

289. Hawker, H. R., Neilson, R., Hayes, R. J., and Serjeant, G. R.: Haematological factors associated with avascular necrosis of the femoral head in homozygous sickle cell disease. Br. J. Haematol. 50:29, 1982.

290. Milner, P. F., Kraus, A. P., Sebes, J. I., Sleeper, L. A., Dukes, K. A., Embury, S. H., Bellevue, R., Koshy, M., Moohr, J. W., and Smith, J.: Sickle cell disease as a cause of osteonecrosis of the femoral head. N. Engl. J. Med. 325:1476, 1991.

291. Hayes, R. J., Condon, P. I., and Serjeant, G. R.: Haematologic factors associated with proliferative retinopathy in homozygous sickle cell disease. Br. J. Ophthalmol. 65:29, 1981.

292. Mears, J. G., Lachman, H. M., Labie, D., Nagel, R. L.: Alpha-thalassemia as related to prolonged survival in sickle cell anemia. Blood 62:286, 1983.

293. Steinberg, M. H., West, M. W., Gallagher, D., Mentzer, W., and The Cooperative Study of Sickle Cell Disease: Effects of glucose-6-phosphate dehydrogenase deficiency upon sickle cell anemia. Blood 71:748, 1988.

294. Hirsch, R. E., Lin, M. J., and Nagel, R. L.: The inhibition of hemoglobin C crystallization by hemoglobin F. J. Biol. Chem. 263:5936, 1988.

295. Lin, M. J., Nagel, R. L., and Hirsch, R. E.: Acceleration of hemoglobin C crystallization by hemoglobin S. Blood 74:1823, 1989.

296. Reiss, G., Ranney, H. M., and Shaklai, N.: The association of hemoglobin C with red cell ghosts. J. Clin. Invest. 70:946, 1982.

297. Diggs, L. W., and Bell, A.: Intraerythrocytic hemoglobin crystals in sickle cell hemoglobin C disease. Blood 25:218, 1965.

298. Bookchin, R. M., and Balazs, T.: Ionic strength dependence of the polymer solubilities of deoxyhemoglobins S + C and S + A mixtures. Blood 67:887, 1986.

299. Warkentin, T. E., Barr, R. D., Ali, M. A. M., and Mohandas, N.: Recurrent acute splenic sequestration crisis due to interacting genetic defects: Hemoglobin SC disease and hereditary spherocytosis. Blood 75:266, 1990.

300. Old, J. M., Thein, S. L., Weatherall, D. J., Cao, A., and Loukopoulos, D.: Prenatal diagnosis of the major haemoglobin disorders. Mol. Biol. Med. 6:55, 1989.

301. Chang, J. C., and Kan, Y. W.: A sensitive new prenatal test for sickle-cell anemia. N. Engl. J. Med. 307:30, 1982.

302. Embury, S. H., Scharf, S. J., Saiki, R. K., Gholson, M. A., Golbus, M., Arnheim, N., and Erlich, H. A.: Rapid prenatal diagnosis of sickle cell anemia by a new method of DNA analysis. N. Engl. J. Med. 316:656, 1987.

303. Chehab, F. F., Doherty, M., Cai, S., Kan, Y. W., Cooper, S., and Rubin, E. M.: Detection of sickle cell anaemia and thalassaemias. Nature 329:293, 1987.

304. Rhoads, G. G., Jackson, L. G., Schlesselman, S. E., de la Cruz, F. F., Desnick, R. J., Golbus, M. S., Ledbetter, D. H., Lubs, H. A., Mahoney, M. J., Pergament, E., Simpson, J. L., Carpenter, R. J., Elias, S., Ginsberg, N. A., Goldberg, J. D., Hobbins, J. C., Lynch, L., Shiono, P. H., Wapner, R. J., and Zachary, J. M.: The safety and efficacy of chorionic villus

305. Alter, B. P.: Antenatal diagnosis: Summary of results. Ann. N. Y. Acad. Sci. 612:237, 1990.

306. Rubin, E. M., Andrews, K. A., and Kan, Y. W.: Newborn screening by DNA analysis of dried blood spots. Hum. Genet. 82:134, 1989.

307. Pearson, H.: A neonatal program for sickle cell anemia. Adv. Pediatr. 33:381, 1986.

308. Vichinsky, E., Hurst, D., Earles, A., Kleman, K., and Lubin, B.: Newborn screening for sickle cell disease: Effect on mortality. Pediatrics 81:749, 1988.

309. Tsevat, J., Wong, J. B., Pauker, S. G., and Steinberg, M. H.: Neonatal screening for sickle cell disease: A cost-effectiveness analysis. J. Pediatr. 118:546, 1991.

310. John, A. B., Ramlal, A., Jackson, H., Maude, G. H., Waight Sharma, A., and Serjeant, G. R.: Prevention of pneumococcal infection in children with homozygous sickle cell disease. Br. Med. J. 288:1567, 1984.

311. Gaston, M. H., Verter, J. I., Woods, G., Peglow, C., Kelleher, J., Presbury, G., Zarkowsky, H., Vichinsky, E., Iyer, R., Lobel, J. S., Diamond, S., Gill, S., Falletta, J. M.: Prophylaxis with oral penicillin in children with sickle cell anemia: A randomized trial. N. Engl. J. Med. 314:1593, 1986.

312. Cerami, A., and Manning, J. M.: Potassium cyanate as an inhibitor of the sickling of erythrocytes in vitro. Proc. Natl. Acad. Sci. USA 68:1180, 1971.

313. Walder, J. A., Zaugg, R. H., Walder, R. Y., Steele, J. M., and Klotz, I. M.: Diaspirins that cross-link β chains of hemoglobin: Bis(3.5-dibromosalicyl) succinate and bis(3.5-dibromosalicyl) fumarate. Biochemistry 18:4265, 1979.

314. Abraham, D. J., Perutz, M. F., and Phillips, S. E.: Physiological and x-ray studies of potential antisickling agents. Proc. Natl. Acad. Sci. USA 80:324, 1983.

315. Manning, J. M.: Covalent inhibitors of the gelation of sickle cell hemoglobin and their effects on function. Adv. Enzymol. Rel. Areas Mol. Biol. 64:55, 1991.

316. Rosa, R. M., Bierer, B. E., Thomas, R., Stoff, J. S., Kruskall, M., Robinson, S., Bunn, H. F., and Epstein, F. H.: A study of induced hyponatremia in the prevention and treatment of sickle cell crises. N. Engl. J. Med. 303:1138, 1980.

317. Charache, S., and Walker, W. G.: Failure of desmopressin to lower serum sodium or prevent crisis in patients with sickle cell anemia. Blood 58:892, 1981.

318. Watson, J., Stahman, A. W., and Bilello, F. P.: The significance of the paucity of sickle cells in newborn Negro infants. Am. J. Med. Sci. 215:419, 1948.

319. DeSimone, J. P., Heller, P., Hall, L., and Zweirs, D.: 5-Azacytidine stimulates fetal hemoglobin (Hb F) synthesis in anemic baboons. Proc. Natl. Acad. Sci. USA 79:4428, 1982.

320. Ley, T. J., DeSimone, J., Anagnou, N. P., Keller, G. H., Humphries, R. K., Turner, P. H., Young, N. S., Heller, P., and Nienhuis, A. W.: 5-Azacytidine selectively increases χ-globin synthesis in a patient with β+ thalassemia. N. Engl. J. Med. 307:1469, 1982.

321. Ley, T. J., DeSimone, J., Noguchi, C. T., Turner, P. H., Schechter, A. N., Heller, P., and Nienhuis, A. W.: 5-Azacytidine increases gamma-globin synthesis and reduces the proportion of dense cells in patients with sickle cell anemia. Blood 62:370, 1983.

322. Dover, G. J., Charache, S., Boyer, S. H., Vogelsang, G., and Moyer, M.: 5-Azacytidine increases HbF production and reduces anemia in sickle cell disease: Dose-response analysis of subcutaneous and oral dosage regimens. Blood 66:527, 1985.

323. Papayannopoulou, T., Torrealba De Ron, A., Veith, R., Knitter, G., and Stamatoyannopoulos, G.: Arabinosylcytosine induces fetal hemoglobin in baboons by perturbing erythroid cell differentiation kinetics. Science 224:617, 1984.

324. Veith, R., Galanello, R., Papayannopoulou, T., and Stamatoyannopoulos, G.: Stimulation of F-cell production in patients with sickle cell anemia treated with cytarabine or hydroxyurea. N. Engl. J. Med. 313:1571, 1985.

325. Letvin, N. L., Linch, D. C., Beardsley, G. P., McIntyre, K. W.,

and Nathan, D. G.: Augmentation of fetal hemoglobin production in anemic monkeys by hydroxyurea. N. Engl. J. Med. 310:869, 1984.

326. Platt, O. S., Orkin, S. H., Dover, G., Beardsley, G. P., Miller, B., and Nathan, D. G.: Hydroxyurea enhances fetal hemoglobin production in sickle cell anemia. J. Clin. Invest. 74:652, 1984.

327. Sumoza, A., and Bisotti, R. S.: Treatment of sickle cell anemia with hydroxyurea: Results in 26 patients. Blood 68:67A, 1986.

328. Dover, G. J., Humphries, R. K., Moore, J. G., Ley, T. J., Young, N. S., Charache, S., and Nienhuis, A. W.: Hydroxyurea induction of hemoglobin F production in sickle cell disease: Relationship between cytotoxicity and F cell production. Blood 67:735, 1986.

329. Charache, S., Dover, G. J., Moyer, M. A., and Moore, J. W.: Hydroxyurea-induced augmentation of fetal hemoglobin production in patients with sickle cell anemia. Blood 69:109, 1987.

330. Rodgers, G. P., Dover, G. J., Noguchi, C. T., Schechter, A. N., and Nienhuis, A. W.: Hematological responses of sickle cell patients treated with hydroxyurea. N. Engl. J. Med. 322:1037, 1990.

331. Ballas, S. K., Dover, G. J., and Charache, S.: Effect of hydroxyurea on the rheological properties of sickle erythrocytes in vitro. Am. J. Hematol. 32:104, 1989.

332. Goldberg, M. A., Brugnara, C., Dover, G. J., Schapira, L., Charache, S., and Bunn, H. F.: Evaluation of hydroxyurea and erythropoietin therapy in sickle cell anemia. N. Engl. J. Med. 323:366, 1990.

333. Orringer, E., Blythe, D., Phillips, G., Dover, G., and Parker, J. C.: Effects of hydroxyurea on hemoglobin F and water content in the red blood cells of dogs and of patients with sickle cell anemia. Blood 78:212, 1991.

334. Charache, S., Dover, G. J., Moore, R. D., Eckert, S., Ballas, S. K., Koshy, M., Milner, P. F. A., Orringer, E. P., Phillips, G., Jr., Platt, O. S., and Thomas, G. H.: Hydroxyurea: Effects on hemoglobin F production in patients with sickle cell anemia. Blood 79:2555, 1992.

335. Alter, B. P., and Gilbert, H. S.: The effect of hydroxyurea on hemoglobin F in patients with myeloproliferative syndromes. Blood 66:373, 1985.

336. Burns, E. R., Reed, L. J., and Wenz, B.: Volumetric erythrocyte macrocytosis induced by hydroxyurea. Am. J. Clin. Pathol. 85:337, 1986.

337. Eschbach, J. W., Egrie, J. C., Downing, M. R., Browne, J. K., and Adamson, J. W.: Correction of the anemia of end-stage renal disease with recombinant human erythropoietin. N. Engl. J. Med. 316:73, 1987.

338. Winearls, C. G., Pippard, M. J., Downing, M. R., Oliver, D. O., Reid, C., and Cotes, P. M.: Effect of human erythropoietin derived from recombinant DNA on the anaemia of patients maintained by chronic haemodialysis. Lancet 2:1175, 1986.

339. Al-Khatti, A., Veith, R. W., Papayannopoulou, T., Fritsch, E. F., Goldwasser, E., and Stamatoyannopoulos, G.: Stimulation of fetal hemoglobin synthesis by erythropoietin in baboons. N. Engl. J. Med. 317:415, 1987.

340. Al-Khatti, A., Umemura, T., Clow, J., Abels, R. I., Vance, J., Papayannopoulou, T., and Stamatoyannopoulos, G.: Erythropoietin stimulates F-reticulocyte formation in sickle cell anemia. Trans. Assoc. Am. Physicians 101:54, 1988.

341. Vichinsky, E., Nagel, R. L., Shah, M., Johnson, R., Spadacino, E., Fabry, M. F., Mangahas, L., and Stamatoyannopoulos, G.: The stimulation of fetal hemoglobin by rhErythropoietin in sickle cell anemia: A double blind study. In Stamatoyannopoulos, G., and Nienhuis, A. (eds.).: The Regulation of Hemoglobin Switching (Proceedings of the Seventh Conference on Hemoglobin Switching). Baltimore, Johns Hopkins University Press, 1991, p. 394.

342. Rodgers, G. P., Dover, G. J., Uyesaka, N., Noguchi, C. T., Schechter, A. N., and Nienhuis, A. W.: Augmentation by erythropoietin of fetal hemoglobin response to hydroxyurea in sickle cell patients. N. Engl. J. Med. 328:73, 1993.

343. Oblender, M., and Carpentieri, U.: Effects of iron, copper and zinc on the activity of ribonucleotide reductase in normal and leukemic human lymphocytes. Anticancer Res. 10:123, 1990.

344. Ginder, D. G., Whitters, J. M., and Pohlman, K. J.: Activation of a chicken embryonic globin gene in adult erythroid cells by 5-azacytidine and sodium butyrate. Proc. Natl. Acad. Sci. USA 81:3954, 1984.

345. Burns, J. L., Glauber, G. J., and Ginder, D. G.: Butyrate induces selective transcriptional activation of a hypomethylated embryonic globin gene in adult erythroid cells. Blood 72:1536, 1988.

346. Perrine, S. P., Greene, M. F., and Faller, D. V.: Delay in the fetal globin switch in infants of diabetic mothers. N. Engl. J. Med. 312:334, 1985.

347. Perrine, S. P., Miller, B. A., Greene, M. F., Cohen, R. A., Cook, N., Shackleton, C., and Faller, D. V.: Butyric acid analogs augment γ globin gene expression in neonatal erythroid progenitors. Biochem. Biophys. Res. Commun. 148:694, 1987.

348. Perrine, S. P., Miller, B. A., Faller, D. V., Cohen, R. A., Vichinsky, E. P., Hurst, D., Lubin, B. H., and Papayannopoulou, T.: Sodium butyrate enhances fetal globin gene expression in erythroid progenitors of patients with Hb SS and β thalassemia. Blood 74:454, 1989.

349. Perrine, S. P., Rudolph, A., Faller, D. V., Roman, C., Cohen, R. A., Chen, S.-J., and Kan, Y. W.: Butyrate infusions in the ovine fetus delay the biologic clock for globin gene switching. Proc. Natl. Acad. Sci. USA 85:8540, 1988.

350. Constantoulakis, P., and Stamatoyannopoulos, G.: On the induction of fetal hemoglobin by butyrates: In vivo and in vitro studies with sodium butyrate and comparison of combination treatments with 5-AzaC and AraC. Blood 74:1963, 1989.

351. Perrine, S. P., Ginder, G., Faller, D. V., Dover, G., Ikuta, T., Witkowska, H. E., Cai, S., Vichinsky, E., and Olivieri, N.: A short-term trial of butyrate to stimulate fetal globin gene expression in the β globin gene disorders. N. Engl. J. Med. 328:81, 1993.

352. Adams, J. G., and Coleman, M. B.: Structural hemoglobin variants that produce the phenotype of thalassemia. Semin. Hematol. 27:229, 1990.

353. Kazazian, H. H., Jr., and Adams, J. G., III: Two distinct dominantly inherited phenotypes associated with exon 3 mutations in the β-globin gene (submitted for publication).

354. Coleman, M. B., Steinberg, M. H., and Adams, J. G., III: Hemoglobin Terre Haute arginine β106: A posthumous correction to the original structure of hemoglobin Indianapolis. J. Biol. Chem. 266:5798, 1991.

355. Cathie, I. A. B.: Apparent idiopathic Heinz body anemia. Great Ormond St. J. 3:43, 1952.

356. Stamatoyannopoulos, G., Nute, P. E., and Miller, M.: De novo mutations producing unstable hemoglobins or hemoglobins M. Hum. Genet. 58:396, 1981.

357. Vissers, M. C., Winterbourn, C. C., and Carrell, R. W.: Rapid proteolysis of unstable globins in human bone marrow. Br. J. Haematol. 53:417, 1983.

358. Rachmilewitz, E. A.: Denaturation of the normal and abnormal hemoglobin molecule. Semin. Hematol. 11:441, 1974.

359. Winterbourn, C. C., and Carrell, R. W.: Characterization of Heinz bodies in unstable hemoglobin. Nature 240:150, 1972.

360. Jandl, J. H., Simmons, R. L., and Castle, W. B.: Red cell filtration and the pathogenesis of certain hemolytic anemias. Blood 18:133, 1961.

361. Rivkind, R. A.: Heinz body anemia: An ultrastructural study. II. Red cell sequestration and destruction. Blood 26:433, 1965.

362. Flynn, T. P., Allen, D. W., Johnson, G. J., and White, J. G.: Oxidant damage of the lipids and proteins. J. Clin. Invest. 71:1215, 1983.

363. Allen, D. W., Burgoyne, C. F., Groat, J. D., Smith, C. M., II, and White, J. G.: Comparison of hemoglobin Koln erythrocyte membranes with malondialdehyde-reacted normal erythrocyte membranes. Blood 64:1263, 1984.

364. Winterbourn, C. C., Williamson, D., Vissers, M. C., and Carrell, R. W.: Unstable haemoglobin haemolytic crises: Contributions of pyrexia and neutrophil oxidants. Br. J. Haematol. 49:111, 1981.

365. Tucker, P. W., Phillips, S. E., Perutz, M. F., Houtchens, R., and Caughey, W. S., et al.: Structure of hemoglobins Zurich [His E7(63) β-Arg] and Sydney [Val E11(67) β-Ala] and role of the distal residues in ligand binding. Proc. Natl. Acad. Sci. USA 75:1076, 1978.

366. Zinkham, W. H., Houtchens, R. A., and Caughey, W. S.: Carboxyhemoglobin levels in an unstable hemoglobin disorder (Hb Zurich): Effect on phenotypic expression. Science 209:406, 1980.

367. Kobayashi, Y., Fukumaki, Y., Komatsu, N., Ohba, Y., Miyaji, T., and Miura, Y.: A novel globin structural mutant. Showa-Yakushiji (β$^{110Leu-Pro}$) causing a β-thalassemia phenotype. Blood 70:1688, 1987.

368. Beris, P., Miescher, P. A., Diaz-Chico, J. C., Han, I. S., Kutlar, A., Hu, H., Wilson, J. B., and Huisman, T. H.: Inclusion body β-thalassemia trait in a Swiss family is caused by an abnormal hemoglobin (Geneva) with an altered and extended β chain carboxy-terminus due to a modification in codon β114. Blood 72:801, 1988.

369. Eisinger, J., Flores, J., Tyson, J. A., and Shohet, S. B.: Fluorescent cytoplasm and Heinz bodies of hemoglobin Koln erythrocytes: Evidence for intracellular heme catabolism. Blood 65:886, 1985.

370. Charache, S., Weatherall, D. J., and Clegg, J. B.: Polycythemia associated with a hemoglobinopathy. J. Clin. Invest. 45:813, 1966.

371. Adamson, J. W., Parer, J. T., and Stamatoyannopoulos, G.: Erythrocytosis associated with hemoglobin Rainier: Oxygen equilibria and marrow regulation. J. Clin. Invest. 48:1376, 1969.

372. Charache, S., Catalano, P., Burns, S., Jones, R. T., Koler, R. D., Rutstein, R., Williams, R. R.: Pregnancy in carriers of high-affinity hemoglobins. Blood 65:713, 1985.

373. Adamson, J. W.: Familial polycythemia. Semin. Hematol. 12:383, 1975.

374. Shibata, S., Miyaji, T., Iuchi, I., Ohba, Y., and Yamamoto, K.: Hemoglobins M of the Japanese. Bull. Yamaguchi Med. School 14:141, 1967.

375. Priest, J. R., Watterson, J., Jones, R. T., Faassen, A. E., and Hedlund, B. E.: Mutant fetal hemoglobin causing cyanosis in a newborn. Pediatrics 83:734, 1989.

376. Hayashi, A., Fujita, T., Fujimura, M., and Titani, K.: A new abnormal fetal hemoglobin, Hb FM Osaka (α$_2$γ$_2$$^{63His-Tyr}$). Hemoglobin 4:447, 1980.

ACKNOWLEDGMENTS: The preparation of this chapter was greatly facilitated by the cooperation of 25 colleagues who generously supplied reprints and preprints. Drs. Stuart Edelstein, Robert Josephs, Dhananjaya Kaul, and James White kindly prepared figures for this chapter. Drs. Carlo Brugnara, William Eaton, Robert Hebbel, and Jiri Palek provided critical comments on portions of the chapter.

The Erythrocyte Membrane and Cytoskeleton: Structure, Function, and Disorders

Edward J. Benz, Jr.

INTRODUCTION

The plasma membrane (plasmalemma) is the integument of the cell. It demarcates the boundary between the cell's interior milieu and the external environment in which it must survive and function. Membranes are fluid, semipermeable lipid-protein mosaics whose bio-chemical properties allow them to act both as a barrier to diffusion and as the surface through which regulated entry and egress of nutrients, macromolecules, hormones, ions, and information can occur. These features place the plasma membrane at the center of many life-sustaining processes. Selective permeability provides for retention of essential intracellular components, exclusion of unwanted toxins, uptake of nutrients, and excretion of metabolic by-products. Channels and pumps embedded in membranes modulate intracellular ion content, which in turn determines each cell's osmotic pressure and electrical potential. The plasma membrane also functions as the primary site for interaction and communication with the external environment. For example, the ability of hematopoietic cells of a given lineage to respond to hormones or growth factors depends on the presence and density of appropriate receptor proteins embedded in the lipid bilayer. Cell-cell and cell-matrix interactions essential for stem cell homing phenomena, hematopoiesis, or contact-dependent cellular activation depend on the topological array of membrane-bound cell adhesion molecules and their receptors. Immune recognition by antibodies or effector cells requires presentation of antigens and cofactor proteins on the exterior face of the membrane. An intact and functioning plasmalemma is, therefore, indispensable for cellular life.

The classical notion of membranes as static, semipermeable "sacs" surrounding cells and organelles is incomplete. The plasma membrane is a dynamic entity utilized as a major locus for organizing, localizing, and regulating metabolic processes. Membranes have the capacity to compartmentalize and sequester key molecules involved in metabolic regulation. In some cases, enzymes or cofactors attach to membranes to form topological arrays that modulate the efficiency of a particular metabolic process—for example, electron transport along the inner leaflet mitochondrial cristae. Conversely, reversible attachment to membranes can sequester proteins until their activity is appropriate to cellular function.

Membranes are highly ordered yet fluid structures that spontaneously form thin hydrophobic sheets or layers when suspended in aqueous fluids. (To conserve space, references for some aspects of the material in these introductory sections, those that summarize general well-established principles and facts, are limited to several excellent reviews of the relevant topics.[1-7] These should be utilized as resource material to gain access to the primary literature.) They are non-covalent, self-assembling, and self-sealing mosaics composed of several types of lipids and many types of proteins. Lipid-protein complexes do not themselves possess sufficient tensile strength or rigidity to confer stability of shape, physical tolerance to shear stress, or topological order on the membrane. These properties are attained by attachment to underlying protein complexes that form a firm, elastic network called the cytoskeleton (Fig. 7–1). The *cortical cytoskeleton* is that portion that forms the interior lining of the plasma membrane. Analogous skeletal networks also penetrate further into the interior of cells and form the structural underpinnings of organelles such as mitochondria and nuclei. The protein-lipid bilayer complex thus provides a hydrophobic barrier and membrane fluidity, whereas the cytoskeleton plays the major role in defining the size and shape and compartmentalization of the encased space. Tensile strength, elasticity, and exterior topology of the entire cell are determined by the interaction between the bilayer and cytoskeleton.

Any attempt to understand the physiology of hematopoietic cells or the pathophysiology of their diseases must include a thorough examination of the biology of hematopoietic cell membranes. This chapter summarizes current knowledge about the structure and function of a particular membrane, the erythrocyte membrane, its cytoskeleton, and disorders attributable to their derangement. At the present time, erythrocytes are the only cells about which detailed information is available concerning the normal structure and function of their cytoskeleton and about the molecular pathology of disorders due primarily to abnormal membrane or cytoskeletal structure. The erythrocyte membrane remains the paradigm for ongoing studies of other cell types.

We first consider the basic elements of membranes and cytoskeletal structures. We then discuss unique features that adapt the red cell to withstand the prolonged physical and metabolic stresses associated with extended life in the circulation. Finally, we survey current understanding of the pathophysiology and molecular basis of representative disorders of the red cell membrane and cytoskeleton.

STRUCTURE AND FUNCTION OF CELL MEMBRANES

To a first approximation, the membrane lipids sustain barrier function, whereas the protein components provide the receptors, channels, and pumps by which the barrier can be breached for purposes of solute transport and exterior-to-interior communication. The hydrophobicity of the lipid bilayer is the essential property that provides for the diffusion barrier.[4] Most cells live in an aqueous external environment; intracellular metabolic reactions also occur largely in the aqueous phase. Most substances that are soluble in water cannot traverse the highly hydrophobic environment of the lipid bilayer. The bilayer thus prevents dispersion of vital intracellular components and precludes their random admixture with molecules on the outside.

Proteins embedded in, or attached to, the bilayer provide the means by which both substances and information can traverse the bilayer.[1-3] Substances enter via transmembrane pumps or channels. Membrane-spanning proteins also convey information to the interior of the cell by undergoing allosteric conformational changes of their cytoplasmic domains upon binding to substances on the exterior face. These changes signal the occurrence of external events to signal transduction elements on the inside, without the need for the provoking molecule to enter the cell.

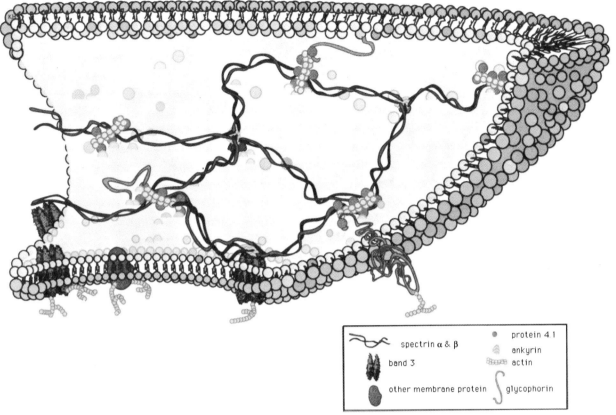

spectrin α & β

protein 4.1

ankyrin

band 3

actin

other membrane protein

glycophorin

FIGURE 7–1. A three-dimensional view of the cell membrane from the interior and exterior of the cell. The lipid bilayer is shown as hydrophilic head groups *(shaded circles)* attached to hydrophobic tails, forming the lipid bilayer. The underlying cytoskeletal meshwork, consisting of spectrin fibers arranged in a hexagonal, anastomosing lattice, is attached to the bilayer by means of band 3, actin, protein 4.1, and ankyrin. The principal transmembrane proteins at which the cytoskeleton is attached, band 3 and glycophorin, are shown spanning the lipid bilayer. The lipid components of the membrane are presented in more detail in Figure 7–2, and the arrangements of proteins, in Figures 7–3 and 7–4. (From Morrow, J.: Plasma membrane dynamics and organization. *In* Hoffman, R., Benz, E. J., Jr., Shattil, S., Furie, B., and Cohen, H. [eds.]: Hematology: Basic Principles and Practice. New York, Churchill Livingstone, 1991, pp. 36–50; with permission.)

Lipid Components of Membranes

Membrane lipids consist of cholesterol and two types of amphipathic lipids: phospholipids and glycolipids (cf. references 1, 3, and 4). The term "amphipathic" refers to the possession of both hydrophobic and hydrophilic tendencies. Most amphipathic lipids contain aliphatic carbon chains at one end of the molecule attached to "polar headgroups," consisting of more highly charged moieties, such as acidic, phosphate, or sugar residues. The hydrophobic tails of these molecules tend to associate with one another to exclude water and form a non-aqueous interior, whereas the polar headgroups remain in contact with the aqueous solution. This arrangement leads to the formation of "micelles" or globules (Fig. 7–2). Free fatty acids, the simplest amphipathic lipids, are not usually found in cell membranes because they form spherical globules lacking the flexibility and linearity essential for a viable membrane. Membrane lipids generally have highly polar headgroups and bulky hydrophobic tails; they can satisfy their need to exist in a hydrophobic environment only by aligning in linear micelles (cf. reference 1) (Fig. 7–2A).

Two types of phospholipids account for most of the amphipathic lipid membranes: phosphoglycerides, derived from glycerol, and sphingomyelin, derived from ceramide, a derivative of sphingosine[1, 3] (Fig. 7–2B). The most abundant phospholipid is phosphatidylcholine. Other major components include phosphatidylethanolamine, phosphatidylserine, and phosphatidylinositol. The long hydrocarbon tails of these lipids are modified to varying degrees by the formation of double bonds between carbon moieties, creating unsaturated phospholipids. As the degree of desaturation increases, the packing of hydrophobic tails in the core of the bilayer is increasingly disrupted, thereby enhancing the "fluidity" of the membrane.

The glycolipids present in eukaryotic membranes are largely based on sphingosine and therefore are called glycosphingolipids.[2, 4] Glucocerebroside and galactocerebroside are the simplest examples; more complex arrangements of sugar residues or the lipid core result in the formation of substances called gangliosides. Glycolipids tend to be located almost exclusively on the extracellular face of the plasma membrane, with the result that the sugar residues protrude into the extracellular space. The precise biological impor-

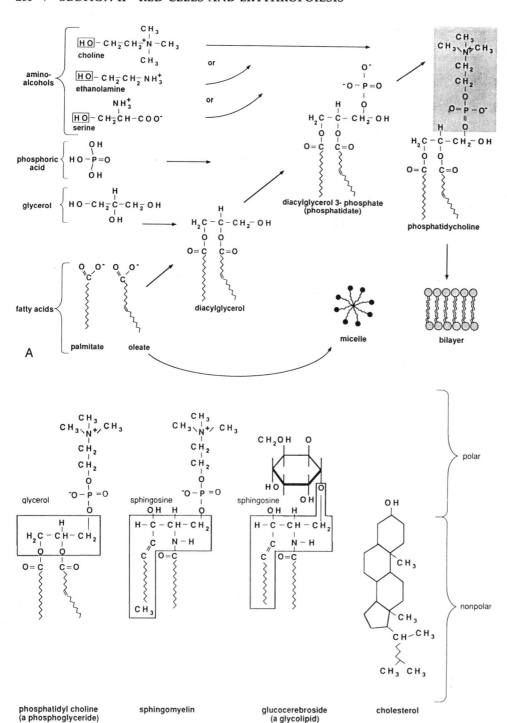

FIGURE 7–2. Lipid components of membranes. A shows the basic chemical structures of lipids found in membranes. The bulky polar head groups of lipids actually found in membranes (cf. text) favor exclusion of water in such a way as to form a lipid bilayer, rather than the spherical micelle formed by simple fatty acids. B shows the structures of the major phospholipid, sphingomyelin, glycolipid, and cholesterol moieties found in naturally occurring membranes. (Adapted from Morrow, J.: Plasma membrane dynamics and organization. In Hoffman, R., Benz, E. J., Jr., Shattil, S., Furie, B., and Cohen, H. [eds.]: Hematology: Basic Principles and Practice. New York, Churchill Livingstone, 1991, pp. 36–50; with permission.)

tance of this asymmetry is unknown. Asymmetry of and in itself may permit biochemical discrimination between the interior and exterior faces of the membrane.

Cholesterol, the third lipid component, is unique among membrane lipids because it is almost entirely hydrophobic. Its primary role appears to be to control membrane fluidity. Interspersion of cholesterol among the phospholipids and glycolipids interferes with packing of their hydrophobic tails into highly ordered arrays. Cholesterol contributes to maintenance of membrane fluidity, even under conditions, such as low temperature, that might lead to phospholipid crystallization and rigidification of the bilayer.

Lipids account for 50 to 60 per cent of membrane mass. The remainder is protein. Although lipids are clearly critical for the membrane organization, disease states due primarily to derangements in membrane lipids are uncommon. A few illustrative examples are discussed later. The remainder of this chapter focuses primarily on *proteins* associated with the membrane. Proteins play the predominant role in conferring tensile strength and specialized functional properties on membranes of individual cell types. Most "membrane diseases" that have been well characterized are due to abnormal membrane proteins.

Membrane Proteins

Membrane proteins are classified according to the ease with which they can be removed from membranes.[1, 5, 6] "Peripheral" proteins are more loosely associated; they are extractable by high- or low-salt or high-pH extraction (Fig. 7–3A). "Integral" proteins are firmly embedded into or through the lipid bilayer by hydrophobic domains within their amino acid sequences. They can be extracted only by harsh reagents such as chaotropic solvents or detergents.[5, 6] Peripheral proteins are typically associated with only one face of the membrane (i.e., exterior or extracellular versus interior or cytoplasmic), whereas many integral proteins often protrude into both spaces.

The intimacy with which proteins associate with the

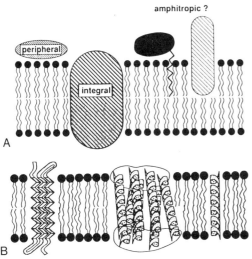

FIGURE 7–3. Types of membrane proteins and their interactions with membranes. The schematic (A) illustrates the different types of membrane proteins, based on the intimacy of their relationship to the lipid bilayer. Peripheral proteins, shown at the far left, are reversibly attached by non-covalent weak forces or by non-covalent binding to more firmly embedded proteins. At the other extreme, integral proteins are firmly embedded in the membrane by virtue of their extensive regions of hydrophobic α helices or β-pleated sheets. Amphitropic proteins, shown at the right, are partially or more reversibly embedded in the membrane by virtue of less extensive hydrophobic domains (illustrated on the far right) or reversible attachments to fatty acid moieties (proteins shown second from the right). These interactions are discussed in more detail in the text. B illustrates the helical and β-pleated sheet motifs characteristic of firmly embedded proteins. On the far left is shown a protein with a single bilayer spanning the α helix (e.g., glycophorin); in the center is shown a globular protein with multiple membrane-spanning helices (e.g., band 3); and on the right is shown a β-pleated sheet (e.g., porin). (See text for details.) (Adapted from Morrow, J.: Plasma membrane dynamics and organization. *In* Hoffman, R., Benz, E. J., Jr., Shattil, S., Furie, B., and Cohen, H. [eds.]: Hematology: Basic Principles and Practice. New York, Churchill Livingstone, 1991, pp. 36–50; with permission.)

membrane is not a static property. Rather, proteins can become more or less tightly bound according to their state of phosphorylation, methylation, glycosylation, or lipid modification (myristylation, palmitylation, or farnesylation).[1] The term "amphitropic" (Fig. 7–3) is used to describe the changeable affinity of these proteins for the hydrophobic environment of the lipid bilayer.[6]

Integral proteins may be embedded in the membrane or anchored to it.[1, 5–7] *Embedded* proteins are intimately, and usually permanently, associated with the lipid bilayer by virtue of extensive amphipathic α helices or β-pleated sheet structures within their amino acid sequences (Fig. 7–3B). Examples include transmembrane proteins such as growth factor receptors, transport ATPases, and bacterial rhodopsin. *Anchored* proteins associate by means of covalent reversible attachments to the bilayer. Examples include the phosphoinositide linkages that attach complement decay-accelerating factor (DAF) or the CD4 antigen to the exterior surface of the membrane, or certain metabolic enzymes that become reversibly anchored in the lipid bilayer by farnesylation or myristylation.[2, 8] Peripheral proteins are *attached* indirectly to the lipid bilayer by means of covalent or non-covalent binding to the (usually) cytoplasmic domains of embedded or anchored proteins.

Embedded proteins generally contain large domains of hydrophobic residues. Some, like the prototype glycophorin A, form α helices approximately 20 amino acids long, spanning a distance just sufficient to traverse the lipid bilayer.[9, 10] Others, such as the bacterial membrane protein porin, utilize β-pleated sheet structures for the same purpose.[11] One or both ends of the protein are typically hydrophilic. The generic structure of an embedded protein is thus one in which hydrophobic domains are insinuated in the lipid bilayer, whereas the hydrophilic extremities of the molecule protrude either into the extracellular or the cytoplasmic space or into both.

Anchored proteins, on the other hand, tend to possess short consensus sequences at their amino- or carboxy-termini that serve as recognition sites for myristylation, farnesylation, or attachment of phosphoinositides. They fall into two general classes: those attached by direct covalent bonding between the lipid bilayer and amino acid residues on the protein and those insinuated into the bilayer by covalent linkage to a lipid moiety. The former are exemplified by proteins, such as CD4,[2] that bind to phosphoinositide. The latter possess conserved structural motifs at the amino- or carboxy-terminus that promote covalent modification by lipid moieties such as palmitate or myristate.[8] These moieties confer hydrophobic tendencies that favor partial insertion into the lipid bilayer. This association can be reversed by cleavage of the bond between the protein and its lipid modifier. Myristylation and farnesylation are being increasingly recognized as mechanisms whereby proteins can be anchored or sequestered in order to enhance, compartmentalize, or diminish their availability for metabolic impact on cells.

Attached proteins bind reversibly to the membrane by covalent or non-covalent linkage to the cytoplasmic domains of embedded or anchored proteins.[12, 13] Attached proteins are often multivalent, permitting reversible assembly of complex multimolecular aggregates. Assembly is a dynamic process because binding affinities can be readily modulated by modifications such as methylation, phosphorylation, attachment of phosphoinositide groups, and/or conformational changes induced by interaction of the attached proteins with other proteins, cofactors, metabolites, or ions.

Structural motifs originally discovered in cytoskeletal proteins are increasingly being encountered as fundamental structures in many cytoplasmic and nuclear proteins. The importance of these motifs remains to be established. Some proteins, including certain homeotic gene products, such as the *Drosophila notch* gene product, possess structural repeats homologous to the mammalian cytoskeletal protein ankyrin.[14] It is tempting to speculate that the ability of these factors to enter the nucleus and exert effects on gene expression could be modulated by the tendency of the ankyrin-like repeats to attach to cytoskeletal structures, thereby sequestering the factor from the site of its biological activity.

Maintenance of Asymmetry and Topological Organization of the Membrane

Lipids and embedded membrane proteins are freely diffusible in *lateral* directions *along* the plane of the lipid bilayer. Phospholipids or proteins embedded in the bilayer could, based on a typical diffusion constant, circumnavigate the red cell membrane in a matter of seconds.[15] In contrast, *transverse* mobility is highly constrained because of the bulkiness of polar head groups, amino acid side chains, or end modifications, such as sugar residues.[16] The free energy expenditure required to drag these bulky hydrophilic groups *through* the hydrophobic membrane prohibits "flip flopping" across the bilayer. These chemical constraints maintain asymmetry of the interior and exterior faces of the membrane; this is critical for communication and regulatory functions. Even though many integral membrane proteins should be freely diffusible in the lateral plane, their actual mobilities are usually far more restricted (e.g., by binding to the cytoskeleton) than their potential.[17] Restricted mobility begets non-random aggregation and clustering of proteins in specific parts of the membrane, thus allowing development of localized functions, cell polarity, formation of pseudopods for cell motility, pinocytosis, and other organized behaviors.[18-21]

Membrane organization arises from interactions between integral membrane proteins and other molecules contacting the hydrophilic faces of the membrane, and by protein-protein or protein-lipid interactions within the bilayer itself.[21-25] The best studied examples of *exterior organization* are those that occur when multivalent extracellular ligands or antibodies bind to their receptors or epitopes, forming clusters or patches of receptor multimers, or antigen-antibody complexes.[21] Antigen "capping" and the formation of receptor dimers or oligomers that activate signal transduction events are widely known examples.[26, 27]

Integral membrane proteins can interact with one another or with lipids *within the lipid bilayer*. Stable associations between the subunits of multicomponent channels and pumps are often maintained by interaction of the transmembrane segments with one another, whereas other proteins maintain association with one another by interacting with lipids such as phosphatidylinositol 4,5-bisphosphate (PIP_2). An important membrane cytoskeletal protein, protein 4.1, regulates one of its affinities for membranes via this type of lipid interaction.

Interactions on the *cytoplasmic* face of the protein are usually mediated by the cortical cytoskeleton. This structure consists of a submembranous scaffold of spectrin-actin fibers connected to the membrane at multiple points by the multivalent linking proteins ankyrin and protein 4.1. Ankyrin and protein 4.1 attach by binding to spectrin or complexes of spectrin and actin, on the one hand, and to the cytoplasmic domains of integral membrane proteins, such as band 3, glycophorin, the Na^+K^+ATPase, and the Na channel, on the other. The avidity of these attachments is modulated by post-translational modifications of the participating proteins, such as phosphorylation.[1, 12, 13, 23-28]

By utilizing the cytoplasmic domains of embedded proteins as attachment points, the cytoskeleton not only affixes itself to the lipid bilayer but also provides a means to order the topological arrangement of the transmembrane proteins; the act of attachment constrains motion along the transverse plane. For example, the localization of the Na^+K^+ATPase to the basolateral, but not the apical, surface of renal epithelial cells is achieved in part by fixing the enzyme to recognition domains on ankyrin and thereby to the spectrin-actin cytoskeleton.[24, 25]

THE ERYTHROCYTE MEMBRANE AND ITS CYTOSKELETON

Red cells circulate for 120 days, devoid of a nucleus, mitochondria, polyribosomes, or nucleic acids.[29-31] They have no capacity to synthesize new proteins to replace those lost or damaged by life in the blood stream. During this odyssey, they traverse the circulation more than 100,000 times, facing enormous mechanical and metabolic challenges during each passage. For example, many capillary beds have interior diameters smaller than the 7.5 μm diameter of the red cell. The red cell must deform to "squeeze" through these capillaries and then resume its normal shape upon emergence into more capacious venules at the distal end of the capillaries. The enormous burden of intracellular protein (hemoglobin) creates a large oncotic pressure gradient. Erythrocytes thus tend to swell in isotonic solutions and to shrivel in hypertonic solutions. In the distal tubules and collecting system of the kidney, red cells pass through zones having molarities ranging from isotonic to nearly six times isotonic and back again in a matter of milliseconds. Iron and hemichromes released from damaged hemoglobin molecules add further redox stresses, intensified by marked changes in the pH and pO_2 that must be endured in the kidney, spleen, and muscle.[32–34] These challenges demand that red cells possess several properties to remain structurally sound. The membrane must be highly pliable yet sufficiently resilient to resist fragmentation in the face of substantial shear stresses. It must be distensible enough to accommodate rapid changes in osmotic pressure. In addition, the bilayer and its underpinnings (the cortical cytoskeleton) must be resistant to damage resulting from oxidation, proteolysis, or other noxious stimuli in the circulation, since no replacement of damaged proteins is possible. The erythrocyte membrane is highly adapted to meet these demands.

Physical and Mechanical Properties of Erythrocytes

From a physiological and clinical perspective, the single most important property that must be possessed by red cells for normal survival is *cellular deformability*.[35, 36] This term refers to the ability of the erythrocyte to undergo distortions and deformations and then to resume its normal shape without fragmentation or loss of integrity. Red cells normally have a biconcave discoid shape. Under the hydrostatic pressure of the circulation, the erythrocyte is distorted to an ellipsoidal shape when it must pass through narrow vascular conduits in the capillary beds; upon entering more capacious vessels on the venous side of the circulation, normal red cells resume their discoid shape. Normal red cells must also be able to swell and shrink in response to changes in osmolality without bursting or imploding. The *cellular* deformability of erythrocytes is now known to depend predominantly on three variables: geometry (biconcave disc shape), cytoplasmic viscosity, and *membrane* deformability.[37]

The *biconcave disc shape* of red cells is critical for their survival. Objects with this surface geometry have a high ratio of surface area to enclosed volume. In the red cell, for example, the normal volume is 90 μm³; the minimum surface area that could encase this volume would be a sphere of 98 μm³ (cf. reference 30). The surface area of a biconcave disc enclosing this volume is 140 μm³. Thus, shape alone provides the red cell with a considerable amount of redundant membrane and cytoskeleton. This feature provides for the extra membrane area needed when red cells swell. More importantly, the geometrical arrangement allows red cells to be stretched as they undergo deformation and distortion in response to mechanical stress. Loss of membrane, by partial phagocytosis in immune he-

molytic anemias or by fragmentation of bits of membrane from the cell in patients with cytoskeletal defects, leads to elliptocytic or spherocytic shapes having greatly reduced surface area and, therefore, much less deformability.[30, 37–39] The consequent reduction in tolerance of these cells to osmotic stress explains why anemias due to membrane defects are often accompanied by osmotic fragility, the basis for a useful clinical laboratory test. Conversely, if erythrocytes are engorged with water, they become macrospherocytic and less deformable.

Red cell viscosity is largely determined by hemoglobin content.[30, 37] At normal intracellular concentrations (27 to 35 g/dl), viscosity contributes very little to cellular deformability. When erythrocytes become dehydrated, the effective intracellular hemoglobin concentration rises, and viscosity increases exponentially. Membrane pumps and channels normally maintain intracellular volumes that hold hemoglobin concentrations below the level at which cytoplasmic viscosity has an impact on deformability. Inherited anomalies of pumps or channels (e.g., hereditary xerocytosis)[39] or derangements of them by polymerized or crystallized hemoglobin (e.g., sickle cell anemia or HbCC disease)[37, 38] lead to cellular dehydration and greatly increased red cell viscosity.

Red cells experience mechanical stress when forced through the narrow conduits of small capillaries and venules under hydrostatic pressure. This force, which can be mimicked by laboratory devices such as the ektacytometer,[39] deforms the discoid erythrocyte to an elliptocytic shape, which reverts to the normal disc when the force is removed.[40, 41] Excessive or prolonged application of force exceeds deformability, resulting in permanent deformation; application of even higher levels of force begins to produce red cell fragmentation. *Membrane deformability*[40–42] is the material property of the membrane-cytoskeletal unit that determines the extent to which the membrane is distorted by application of a defined level of force. The *stability* of the membrane, in contrast, is defined as the maximum extent of deformation that is reversible[39, 40]; in other words, membrane stability reflects the maximum force that can be tolerated before the membrane becomes irreversibly deformed by application of force. Decreased deformability results in rigid red cells, whereas decreased membrane stability results in increased susceptibility to fragmentation under normal circulating stresses.[40] Defects of membrane and cytoskeletal proteins have been shown to cause temporary deformation, permanent (plastic) deformation, and/or fragmentation at lower than normal forces.[37, 40]

The Red Cell Cytoskeleton—The Molecular Basis for Red Cell Deformability and Stability

The deformability and stability of red cells depend on the topology of the cytoskeleton and the means by which it is attached to the fragile lipid bilayer. The

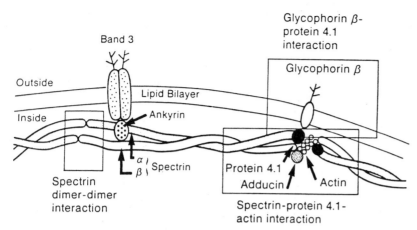

FIGURE 7–4. Arrangement of the major membrane and cytoskeletal proteins within and attached to the erythrocyte membrane. This diagram is best appreciated by comparison to Figure 7–1. The transmembrane proteins band 3 and glycophorin are shown traversing the lipid bilayer. The spectrin latticework illustrated in Figure 7–1 is represented here by the shaded intertwined α and β subunits, shown with the spectrin-spectrin association between the amino-terminus of the α subunit and the carboxy-terminus of the β subunit. Attachment of the latticework to the membrane is mediated by the formation of spectrin/actin/protein 4.1 junctional complexes that in turn attach to the cytoplasmic domain of glycophorin, and the binding of ankyrin to both spectrin and the cytoplasmic domain of band 3, an interaction thought to be facilitated by protein 4.2.

basic structure of the cytoskeleton is a hexagonal latticework[43] composed of spectrin and actin filaments onto which are attached additional proteins that fasten the lattice to the lipid bilayer[1, 13, 29, 40] (Figs. 7–1 and 7–4). Additional proteins intersect at the attachment points to stabilize or weaken the attachment. Attachment occurs at regular intervals by means of multivalent proteins (ankyrin, protein 4.1) that bind both to the lattice and to the cytoplasmic domains for the integral proteins glycophorin and band 3.[5, 13, 29, 44]

The spectrin and actin filaments can be regarded as firm but spring-like rods. In the resting state, the folded helical segments of spectrin (described later) are in a relatively highly coiled state.[30, 37] Deformation is accompanied by a rearrangement of the network. Some spectrin molecules become uncoiled and extended, whereas others become more compressed and folded, resulting in no net change in surface area. Thus, shape changes but surface area does not. The extent to which this stretching and compression are possible determines the extent of deformability. Further distortion of shape requires an increase in membrane surface area, which can occur only if the attachments to the cytoskeleton are broken at the protein 4.1/glycophorin/spectrin/actin junction points (described later).[40, 44] At this point, the membrane fails, becoming permanently deformed or fragmented.

Clearly, deformability will be increased or decreased by increasing or decreasing the chemical associations of the spectrin-actin hexagonal network with molecules influencing their ability to coil or uncoil. Membrane stability will be decreased by any state or event that weakens the junctional complexes. Mutations or acquired alterations of membrane and cytoskeletal proteins could exert either or both effects. Thus, a single mutation might simultaneously exert adverse effects on deformability and stability.

Components of the Erythrocyte Membrane and Underlying Cytoskeleton

Lipid Components

The red cell membrane consists of 52 per cent protein, 40 per cent lipid, and 8 per cent carbohydrate,

proportions typical of most mammalian membranes (cf. references 45 and 46). The lipid component consists of roughly equimolar quantities of phospholipids and unesterified cholesterol and minimal amounts of free fatty acids and glycolipids (see Fig. 7–2). The four major phospholipids are phosphatidylcholine (PC, 30 per cent), sphingomyelin (SM, 25 per cent), phosophatidylethanolamine (PE, 28 per cent), and phosphatidylserine (PS, 14 per cent). Other phospholipids, such as phophatidylinositol 4,5-bisphosphate (PIP$_2$), constitute to 2 to 3 per cent. These lipids are highly asymmetrical with respect to the interior and exterior faces of the membrane. The relatively uncharged phospholipids, PC and SM, exist largely in the outer monolayer (leaflet); 80 per cent of the highly charged phospholipids, PE and PS, are localized to the inner leaflet. Cholesterol freely diffuses into and through the bilayer.

Red cells have no capacity to synthesize new lipids, but lipids in the circulation exchange relatively freely with the membrane, resulting in considerable turnover, usually without significant changes in overall lipid composition. This mechanism provides for rejuvenation and renewal of the lipid components. In certain pathological situations, such as advanced cirrhosis and abetalipoproteinemia, abnormal circulating lipid profiles and/or abnormal mechanisms of exchange can generate morphological abnormalities (e.g., acanthocytosis) or actual hemolytic anemia (cf. references 30 and 31).

Protein Components

Mild detergent extraction of red cell membranes removes lipids, leaving behind the hexagonal protein latticework of the cortical cytoskeleton.[43] The individual proteins composing this structure were first named according to their mobility in a sodium dodecyl sulfate (SDS)–acrylamide gel system described by Fairbanks.[5, 6] The slowest migrating band was band 1 (or protein 1), the next slowest band, band 2 (or protein 2), and so on (cf. Fig. 7–5). Subbands were designated with decimals. Thus, for example, the terms protein 4.1 and 4.2 designated two subbands constituting a zone at the position of the fourth most slowly migrat-

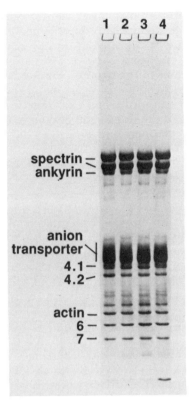

FIGURE 7–5. Proteins of the red cell membrane and cytoskeleton. The figure shows a Coomassie blue–stained sodium dodecyl sulfate (SDS)–acrylamide gel. All four lanes were loaded with protein extracted from normal red cell membranes. The individual α and β chains of spectrin (band 1 and band 2) are not resolved on this particular electrophoretogram. Band 3, the anion transporter, migrates as a diffuse band because of its extensive glycosylation. The same region of diffuse staining also contains the heavily glycosylated isoforms of glycophorin. Band 5 was subsequently proved to be red cell actin, as indicated by the label. The function of band 6 remains unknown. The example shown does not resolve subbands, such as band 7.2 and 4.1A. (Adapted, by permission, from the New England Journal of Medicine, Vol. 323, p. 1046, 1990.)

ing band (see Fig. 7–5). Some of these proteins were later renamed when they were better characterized. For example, proteins 1 and 2 are the α and β chains of spectrin, protein 3 is the anion transport channel, and protein 5 is actin. Other proteins critical to red cell function, such as proteins 4.1 and 4.2, have never been renamed.

The original Fairbanks gels resolved about a dozen major cytoskeletal proteins.[5, 6] Many more proteins have subsequently been found, but only about 15 merit detailed consideration, because of their quantity, function, or role in hereditary anemias. The most notable of these at the present time are the two spectrin subunits (α and β), ankyrin, protein 4.1, actin, the glycophorins, band 3, protein 4.2, adducin, and protein 4.9. Other potentially important proteins, such as the Rh D antigen core protein, a recently described 28 kDa water channel, or the Na^+K^+ATPase, are either insufficiently understood or insufficiently abundant to warrant detailed discussion at this time.

The major embedded red cell proteins are band 3 and the glycophorins (cf. references 29 and 30). The other cytoskeletal proteins are attached to and arrayed along the inner (cytoplasmic) leaflet of the lipid bilayer (cf. Figs. 7–1 and 7–4). They associate to form a cytoskeletal lattice that is composed largely of tetrameric spectrin filaments, connected to one another at nodes that also contain F-actin filaments and protein 4.1. The nodes attach to the overlying lipid bilayer by the binding of protein 4.1 to glycophorin and of the multivalent linking protein ankyrin to both spectrin and the cytoplasmic tail of band 3. The attachments are dynamic, subject to modification by phosphorylation or direct interaction with lipids such as PIP_2. Adducin, protein 4.2, and protein 4.9 appear to stabilize the interaction of spectrin and actin as well as the bundling of actin.

Major Integral Membrane Proteins

Band 3

Band 3, a transmembrane glycoprotein with a molecular mass of 100 kDa,[29, 47, 48] is the major anion transport protein in erythrocytes. It is also being increasingly appreciated as a critical regulator of red cell deformability, membrane assembly, intermediary metabolism, and red cell senescence.[49–51] It is highly abundant (10^6 copies per erythrocyte).[52] The 43 kDa (400 amino acids) cytoplasmic domain is located at the amino-terminal end of the protein.[48, 50] The remainder of the amino acid sequence folds into helices and β sheets to form 12 to 14 membrane-spanning segments containing the anion transport channels. The boundary between the cytoplasmic tail and the first membrane-spanning segment (amino acids 400 to 404) is highly conserved in erythrocytes of diverse species.[53, 54] In particular, the proline at position 403 is thought to be critical for creating either a β bend or a random coil at the membrane junction, thereby giving the tail freedom of movement (interdomain hinge).[53, 55] This feature is essential for red cell flexibility; mutations in this region produce rigid erythrocytes.[56] (Fig. 7–6). The physiologically functional form in which interactions with cytoplasmic molecules occur most efficiently appears to be a tetramer.[50, 57]

Recent findings suggest that protein 3 is of central importance for several basic aspects of red cell homeostasis.[51, 53] First, it is the major anion (Cl^-, HCO_3^-) transport channel. Second, the cytoplasmic tail interacts with the cytoskeleton, by binding to ankyrin, protein 4.1, protein 4.2, and possibly spectrin. Third, the cytoplasmic tail is the target for binding by hemichromes, which are generated by denaturation or oxidation of hemoglobin. Fourth, band 3 may regulate metabolic pathways by sequestering key pathway enzymes, such as glucose-3-phosphate dehydrogenase. Fifth, protein 3 may be a key organizing element during membrane biogenesis in erythroblasts.[58]

Binding of the 43 kDa cytoplasmic domain to ankyrin is a critical attachment mechanism. The inter-

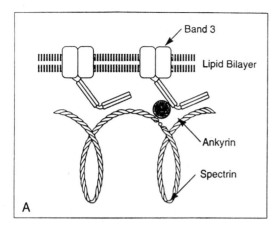

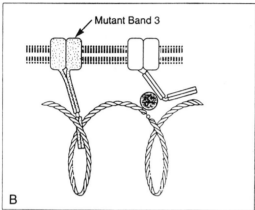

FIGURE 7–6. Diagrammatic representation of the functional configuration of band 3 in association with the membrane and cytoskeletal lattice. *A* shows how the "interdomain hinge" in the cytoplasmic domain of band 3 permits it to interact flexibly and non-obstructively with ankyrin and spectrin. Mutations in band 3 that abolish the hinge, shown in *B*, cause the cytoplasmic domain to interfere with and become entangled in the latticework. The importance of this arrangement is discussed in more detail in the section on hereditary ovalocytosis. (Adapted from the Journal of Clinical Investigation, 1992, Vol. 89, pp. 686–692, by copyright permission of the American Society for Clinical Investigation.)

domain hinge at the attachment point may be a crucial determinant of the flexibility or rigidity of erythrocytes.[56, 57] Binding of band 3 by hemichromes appears to stimulate aggregation into "patches," which are uniquely recognized by a red cell senescence isoantibody, leading to opsonization of the cell and its removal from the circulation by the reticuloendothelial (RE) system.[29–31] Increasing evidence supports the notion that this is a major mechanism by which aging red cells are sequestered. Biogenesis of the red cell membrane in erythroblasts depends on the use of the cytoplasmic domain of band 3 as the nidus for stable assembly of the multimolecular complexes forming the spectrin latticework (cf. reference 58). Band 3 is thus crucial for biogenesis of the membrane, modulation of elasticity or rigidity, anion transport, and immune marking of aging red cells for removal.

The locus on chromosome 17 encoding erythrocyte band 3 is a member of a gene family encoding numerous isoforms expressed in many tissues.[59] The non-erythroid isoforms that have been characterized are transporters of anions or organic acids. These family members share significant but localized regional homology with erythroid band 3.[58, 59] The hydrophobic channel domains of the proteins tend to be conserved, but the cytoplasmic domains are more divergent, implying conservation of anion exchange properties but specialization of the domains that bind to the cytoskeleton. These binding functions may be adapted to particular cell types.

The Glycophorins

Glycophorins A, B, C, and D were originally identified as the most abundant integral membrane glycoproteins in erythrocytes.[55, 60, 61] Because of their high sialic acid content, they account for more than 95 per cent of the periodic acid–Schiff (PAS)–staining capacity of erythrocytes. In the aggregate, these proteins are highly abundant; glycophorin A is the major component (5 to 9 × 10^5 copies per cell) (cf. references 29 and 55). Glycophorins B, C, and D account for 0.8 to 3 × 10^5, 0.5 to 1 × 10^5, and 0.1 to 0.2 × 10^5 copies, respectively.[29, 52] Characterization of complementary DNA (cDNA) and genomic clones encoding the glycophorins has revealed that they fall into two distinct subgroups.[62–68] Glycophorins A and B are homologous to each other and are encoded by two closely linked genes. Glycophorins C and D arise from a single locus bearing no particular homology to the genes for glycophorins A and B. Glycophorin D differs from glycophorin C by use of a different translation start site created by alternative messenger RNA (mRNA) splicing. Recently, another gene linked in tandem with those for glycophorins A and B has been isolated; it would encode a putative fifth glycophorin, glycophorin E, which seems to have evolved from glycophorin A by homologous recombination at *Alu* repeats.[69, 70] No protein product of this gene has been identified.

The glycophorins are *O*-glycosylated (cf. references 60 and 61). Glycophorin A is 131 amino acids long; glycophorin B is 72 amino acids long; glycophorin E (also called *invariant [inv]*), if expressed, would be 78 amino acids long; glycophorin C is 128 amino acids long; and glycophorin D is 107 amino acids long. All have a single extracellular hydrophilic amino-terminal domain, a single membrane-spanning domain, and a carboxy-terminal cytoplasmic tail.

Glycophorins A and B are nearly identical, save for their cytoplasmic tails. The first 70 amino acids are exoplasmic, after post-translation cleavage of a leader peptide. A 22 amino acid membrane-spanning domain is next, and the C-terminal 39 residues form the cytoplasmic domain. Amino acids 90 to 93 appear to be particularly important for the formation of glycophorin A dimers, the predominant form encountered in the membrane; they may serve as an interdomain hinge.[71] Glycophorin B is quite similar, except that exon 3, which encodes residues 27 to 55 in the glycophorin A gene, is not retained in fully processed mRNA arising from the glycophorin B gene.[63, 65, 71, 72] The cytoplasmic domain is also foreshortened, containing only three amino acids in addition to the three amino acid hinge region.[63, 65]

The genes for glycophorins A, B, and E are located on chromosome 4q28–q31, in the order A → B → E.[73–76] Each contains seven exons. The promoters of all three genes are highly conserved and contain potential binding sites for important erythroid transcription factors, including NF-E$_1$ and NF-E$_2$.[76] Exons 1 and 2 encode cleavable leader peptides. The major differences between the three isoforms occur in exon 3, resulting in foreshortening of the exoplasmic domains of glycophorins B and E, and in the carboxy-terminal exons, causing premature termination of the cytoplasmic domains of glycophorins B and E. The three genes are so closely linked and homologous that unequal crossover events occur, yielding fused gene products, analogous to hemoglobin Lepore.[75]

The precise biological functions of the glycophorins are incompletely characterized. Because of their high sialic acid content, the glycophorins constitute more than 60 per cent of the net negative surface charge of red cells, suggesting that they are important for modulating red cell–red cell and red cell–endothelial interactions (cf. reference 59). For example, removal of sialic acids causes red cell clumping.[77] Glycophorins A and B are also relevant to clinical immunohematology[78, 79] (see also Chapter 8); blood groups M and N reside on glycophorin A. Group M differs from group N by polymorphic changes in amino acid residues 1 and 5.[55, 78, 79] Similarly, the Ss phenotype results from a polymorphism at amino acid 29 (methionine and threonine, respectively).[80] Certain rare variant blood groups, such as Miltenberger V, En(a−), and M^{k}M^k are glycophorin variants.[78–81] Miltenberger V[75] arises by a gene fusion event, whereas some forms of En(a−) result from deletion of the glycophorin A gene. Some "glycophorin-deficient" states, defined by lack of immunochemical reactivity, are actually due to unequal crossing over events that yield fusion genes giving rise to novel glycophorin immunotypes unreactive with established antisera.

No biological function has been assigned to glycophorin B other than its association with the Ss blood group. It, like glycophorin A, is found only in erythroid cells. Both are expressed only during terminal erythroid maturation, appearing for the first time at the proerythroblast stage.[55]

Most information about the function of glycophorins A and B has come from studies of glycophorin A. Glycophorin A–deficient red cells exhibit increased glycosylation of band 3, owing to the addition of extra sialic acid.[82] The quantitative increase almost exactly counterbalances the normal contribution expected from glycophorin A. This suggests that maintenance of total surface charge density is important for red cell survival. Glycophorin A–deficient red cells exhibit no abnormalities of shape or deformability, suggesting that these glycophorins are not critical for maintaining mechanical stability, deformability, or shape of the

membrane.[83, 84] Binding of immunologically "non-specific" ligands to red cells, such as wheat germ agglutinin, causes aggregation of glycophorin and decreased red cell deformability, but the clinical relevance of this alteration is not known (cf. reference 55). Also poorly understood is the observation that glycophorin-deficient red cells are considerably more resistant to invasion by malaria parasites than are normal cells.[55]

Glycophorins C and D are encoded by a single gene located on chromosome 2q14–q21.[67–68, 85] They differ in their use of alternative translation start sites; when translation is initiated at the first AUG, glycophorin C is produced. When initiation occurs at the AUG encoding methionine at position 20, a truncated protein, glycophorin D, is generated. Residues 21 to 128 of the two proteins are identical. The gene spans 13.5 kb and contains 4 exons.

Glycophorin C does not express a cleavable signal peptide.[86–88] The extracellular amino-terminal domain is 57 amino acids long, containing 1 N-glycosylation and 12 O-glycosylation sites, a 24 amino acid membrane-spanning segment, and a 47 residue C-terminal cytoplasmic domain. Residues 41 to 50 encode the Gerbich (Ge:3) blood group antigens.[89] Variants of glycophorin C give rise to unusual immunohematological phenotypes (cf. references 55 and 89), including Gerbich YUS and WEPB. These appear to arise by intragenic crossing over between the highly homologous exons 2 and 3, resulting in the deletion of exons or the generation of hybrid exons encoding novel epitopes.

Glycophorin C is expressed in multiple non-erythroid tissues, but the level of expression is far higher during erythropoiesis.[90, 91] This feature may result from the use of different transcription start sites. Post-translational modification of glycophorin C may change during erythropoiesis, as evidenced by the differential reactivity of early and later progenitors with different monoclonal antibodies raised against the protein.

Glycophorin C plays a critical role in regulating the stability, deformability, and shape of the membrane. Deficiency is associated with elliptocytic red cells without hemolytic anemia; these cells are less stable and less deformable than are normal red cells.[92–95] Naturally occurring mutations in the exoplasmic domain appear to have no effect on these properties, suggesting that the abnormalities of deficient cells arise from absence of the cytoplasmic domain. The cytoplasmic tail probably interacts with protein 4.1, since protein 4.1 deficiency leads to glycophorin C deficiency in vivo and increased detergent extractibility in vitro.[93–95] Reconstitution of these membranes with protein 4.1 restores the resistance of glycophorin C to detergent extraction. Thus, the cytoplasmic tail of glycophorin C, like that of band 3, appears to serve as an important anchoring site for attachment to the cytoskeleton.

Other Embedded Membrane Proteins

The red cell membrane contains small amounts (fewer than 10,000 copies per cell) of numerous ion pumps and channels, including the Na$^+$K$^+$ATPase and the calcium-dependent potassium channel (Gardos shunt) (cf. references 29 and 55). The activities of these proteins are often altered in response to primary abnormalities of membrane or cytoskeleton, but disease states originating with mutations in these proteins have not yet been described. Therefore, they will not be considered further. Similarly, knowledge is rapidly emerging about the structure and about the structure-function and structure-epitope relationships within the protein constituting the core determinant of the Rh antigen blood system, the Rh D peptide. The gene encoding this protein has recently been cloned and is rapidly being characterized (cf. reference 96). It appears that at least some Rh immunotypes arise as the result of the alternative splicing of Rh gene products. The molecular basis for the so-called Rh (null phenotype), a state associated with absence of Rh antigen activity and a chronic moderate-grade hemolytic diathesis, remains undefined but should emerge within the next few years.

An integral membrane protein of emerging interest is the so-called water channel (CHiP 28), whose encoding gene was recently isolated by Agre and coworkers.[97] This protein has already been shown to facilitate water exchange across the membrane, possibly contributing to the ability of the red cell to adjust rapidly to changes in osmolality. CHiP 28 appears to be a member of a large family of proteins involved in cell volume regulation via water transport in plants and other animals.

Cytoskeletal Proteins That Attach to the Membrane

The major proteins of the erythrocyte cortical cytoskeleton are spectrin; short filaments of F-actin; proteins 4.1, 4.2, and 4.9; ankyrin; and adducin. As noted earlier, these form an interlocking network or lattice that attaches to the membrane largely by binding to the cytoplasmic domains of the glycophorins and band 3.

The Spectrin Protein Family

Spectrin is the major constituent of the erythrocyte cortical skeleton, constituting 75 per cent of its mass; it is present at a concentration of 200,000 molecules per cell.[98] Non-erythroid isoforms of spectrin constitute the principal structural element of the cytoskeletons of other cell types. The fundamental structure of the spectrin molecule is that of a heterodimer, consisting of two highly homologous chains, the α and β chains. The α chain has a molecular mass of 280,000, and the β chain, 240,000[98] (Fig. 7–7A). The chains align and intertwine with each other in antiparallel fashion with respect to their amino-termini, to form flexible, rod-like heterodimers (Fig. 7–7B). These dimers further self-associate to form tetramers and higher order oligomers. From a physiological perspective, the critical functional unit is probably the tetramer, resulting from head-to-head linkages of the heterodimers (cf. references 13 and 44). Tetramers have a contour length of approximately 200 nm.

The α and β subunits of spectrin are highly homologous. Each consists of a series (21 in α spectrin, 17 in β spectrin) of tandem repeats, 106 amino acids long, "marked" by an invariant tryptophan residue surrounded by a short consensus sequence.[13, 99, 100] At some points along the subunit chains, some of the repeats exhibit more divergence from the canonical structure than others. In particular, repeat 10 and the amino- and carboxy-termini are somewhat more divergent.[101–107] The essential structural feature of each repeat is the formation of three amphipathic α helices, linked to one another by short sequences exhibiting less highly ordered structure; the linkage between adjacent repeats is also by relatively short random coil sequences. For this reason, the spectrin molecule is often portrayed as "links of sausage on a chain," as depicted in Figure 7–7. Each "link" is composed of three helical segments. The somewhat more open structures present at the termini give the rod-like structure a barbell appearance.

The amino- and carboxy-termini appear to be the key regions accessible for dimer-dimer associations and for interaction with actin, ankyrin, and protein 4.1.[108–111] The amino-terminus of β spectrin contains the binding site for protein 4.1; ankyrin binding occurs in repeats β15 and β16[112] near the C-terminus. More moderately divergent repeats along the chain appear to be utilized as recognition sites for binding to other modifiers, perhaps kinases, calmodulin, and so forth.[113–115] The overall effect of this repeating structure is to provide for a strong, elastic, rod-like filament that can associate into complex multimolecular assemblies capable of lending shape and resiliency to the overlying plasma membrane via formation of a meshwork linkable to integral membrane proteins. Direct interactions of a weaker nature might also occur between the spectrin filament and the lipid bilayer itself.

The genes encoding erythroid α and β spectrins have been cloned and characterized at both the cDNA and the genomic levels.[98, 101–109] Analysis of genomic DNA, RNA expression, and immunologically cross-reactive molecules from a variety of tissues and organisms has revealed that the erythroid spectrin chains are prototypical members of a multigene family that includes fodrin ("brain spectrin"), dystrophin, the fibrillar protein in muscle that is absent in Duchenne muscular dystrophy, and α actinin (cf. references 98 and 99). Each of these proteins contains multiple helical repeats separated by short regions of random coil, forming rod-like filaments capped at each end by looser "barbell-like" structures that interact with other molecules. For example, the C-terminus of α spectrin forms a potential calcium-binding EF hand structure. The spectrin family might well represent the fundamental motif utilized by cells for the formation of intracellular scaffolds and matrices.

Heterodimer formation between α and β chains

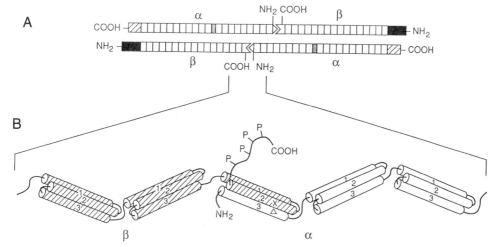

FIGURE 7–7. Subunit structure and self-association of spectrin chains. *A* diagrams the regular array of internal repeating subunits in the α and β chains of spectrin. The shaded area at approximately repeat 11 of the α chain shows a region in which the repeating structure is interrupted. This region appears to be a target for spectrin modification and binding to other proteins. The head-to-head association between two dimers is diagrammed in both *A* and *B*. *B* demonstrates how the association of the amino-terminus of the α chain with the carboxy-terminus of the β chain "fills in" the missing helical segments needed to maintain the stable trihelical structure. (See text for details.) (Adapted from Winkelmann, J. C., and Forget, B. G.: Spectrin and nonerythroid Spectrins. Blood [in press]; and from the Journal of Clinical Investigation, 1990, Vol. 86, p. 909, by copyright permission of the American Society for Clinical Investigation.)

appears to depend on appropriate alignment and intercalation of helical coils from one chain, with "grooves" provided by gaps in the helical array on the other chains.[98, 99] In other words, there appears to be helix-helix interaction along most of the chains. Tetramer formation may well depend on the fact that the usual three-coil helix motif is not well preserved near the ends of the α and β chains. Rather, one chain has a two-coil repeat, whereas the other has a one-coil repeat.[116] It is postulated that these combine to form the apparently more stable three-helix structure, thereby linking two heterodimers together (see Fig. 7–7B). The exact physical description of these interactions is still being established; their importance is illustrated by the fact that, as discussed later, that some hereditary hemolytic anemias arise as a result of defective heterodimer or tetramer formation.

The gene for erythrocyte α spectrin is located on chromosome 1,[117] and that for erythroid β spectrin is found on chromosome 14[110]; the major non-erythroid α isoform, fodrin, is encoded on chromosome 9,[118] and the major non-erythroid β isoform is encoded on chromosome 2.[119] Each of these genes exhibits similar intron/exon structure, but the exons do not correspond exactly to 106 amino acid repeats. The promoters and regulatory sequences responsible for tissue-specific expression of the mRNAs are in the process of being characterized. Of particular note is the fact that spectrin, like several other cytoskeletal proteins, appears to utilize alternative mRNA splicing as a favored mechanism for the establishment of unique tissue-specific isoforms. For example, a muscle isoform of β spectrin appears to result from alternative mRNA splicing of the mRNA transcript of the erythroid β spectrin gene.[120, 121] The splice alters transla-

tion termination near the C-terminus, leading to elongation of the C-terminus of the muscle form.

Mild proteolytic cleavage of spectrin subdivides the protein into a reproducible pattern of domains of the α (αI through αV, in order of decreasing size) and β (βI through βV) chains, 20 to 80 kDa in size. (See Spectrin Defects, below.) These patterns provide useful "fingerprints" of the normal molecule that are changed by many mutations altering spectrin function. Mild tryptic or chymotryptic digestion is thus used to localize and partially characterize mutations of these very large proteins.[122]

Proteins That Bind to Spectrin

PROTEIN 4.1. In erythrocytes, protein 4.1 is an 80 kDa phosphoprotein present in about 80,000 copies per cell.[29, 123] It can be subdivided by mild chymotryptic digestion into four domains, of apparent molecular weight of 30 kDa, 16 kDa, 10 kDa, and 22 to 24 kDa, proceeding from amino-terminus to carboxy-terminus[124] (Fig. 7–8). It is variably but highly phosphorylated; other distinctive features are clustering of cysteine residues near the N-terminus, glycosylation in the 10 kDa domain, a markedly acidic carboxy-terminus, and a markedly basic amino-terminus.[124–127] Phosphorylation sites are located near the carboxy-terminal extremity of the 30 kDa domain and in the middle of the 10 kDa domain.[126, 127] The latter appears to be cyclic AMP (cAMP) dependent, whereas the others may be modulated by protein kinase C. Protein 4.1 is the prototype of non-membrane proteins that are glycosylated by an *O*-linked *N*-acetylglucosamine mechanism, a feature that contributes to its higher apparent molecular weight on acrylamide gels than

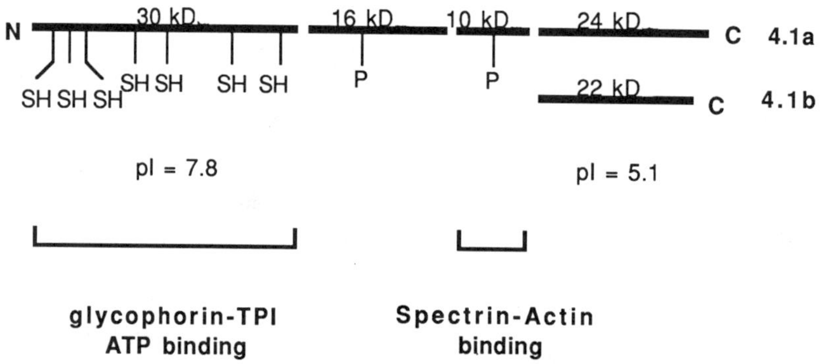

FIGURE 7–8. Molecular model of human protein 4.1. The diagram indicates the five chymotryptic digestion fragments described in the text. The amino-terminal 30 kDa domain is thought to be necessary for binding to the cytoplasmic domain of glycophorin in the presence of phospholipids. The central domain, 10 kDa in length, has been shown to be necessary and sufficient for binding to spectrin-actin. The 24 kDa domain, present in protein 4.1a, and the 22 kDa present in its place in protein 4.1b are now known to differ only by deamidation of asparagine residues at positions 478 and 502. The "SH" designations mark positions of sulfhydryl groups, and the "P" designations mark prominent sites of phosphorylation. The black boxes indicate insertions into erythroid protein 4.1 sequence.

predicted on the basis of known amino acid sequence.[125] In red cells, two molecular weight forms, protein 4.1a and protein 4.1b, are consistently seen.[128] Protein 4.1a, which is of *higher* molecular weight, increases as red cells age. It is barely apparent in young red cells. Recent studies have shown that 4.1a results from the deamidation of two asparagine residues (478 and 502) in a non-enzymatic, age-dependent fashion.[128] These lower the mobility of the protein in gels, producing a band of higher apparent molecular weight. The functional significance of glycosylation and deamidation, if any, is unknown, but the latter provides a useful marker of red cell age.

Protein 4.1 links the spectrin-actin framework to the lipid bilayer (see Fig. 7–4) by facilitating complex formation between spectrin-actin itself, the cytoplasmic domain of band 3, and glycophorin C.[29, 111] Protein 4.1 is thus critical for the strength of the membrane. Abnormalities and deficiencies produce hereditary elliptocytosis.[29, 55]

Protein 4.1 was originally thought to be expressed only in red cells. It is now known to be widely expressed in a variety of tissues, identifiable as immunologically cross-reactive forms that are heterogeneous with respect to molecular weight, abundance, and intracellular localization (cf. references 29, 129, and 130). These isoforms arise from a single genomic locus, positioned near the Rh locus at chromosome 1q32–9ter.[131] The gene is 100 to 150 kDa long; its primary mRNA transcript is subjected to extensive alternative splicing, giving rise to a family of mRNAs 6.5 to 7.0 kb long.[132–136] There are at least 10 alternately spliced exons, as well as an important cryptic acceptor site, that lead to the production of a diverse protein family from a single gene (Fig. 7–9). Mature mRNA transcripts representing many of the 10^3 possible mRNA spliceoforms have been identified by cDNA cloning or polymerase chain reaction (PCR) analysis, but splicing events in only two regions have

functional relevance in red cells: that encoding the spectrin-actin–binding domain and that encoding the 5′ untranslated region.

Three alternatively spliced exons are located in the region encoding the amino-terminal end of the 10 kDa domain.[135, 136] This domain is known to encompass the spectrin-actin–binding activity of the protein.[137] In particular, the amino-terminal end of the 10 kDa fragment was tentatively implicated as the binding site on the basis of competition assays and analysis with peptide-specific antibodies. One of the three exons, exon 15, is 63 bases long and codes for 21 amino acids found at the amino-terminus of the red cell form (see Fig. 7–9). This sequence is present in mature erythroid mRNA and protein but absent from most non-erythroid forms. The erythroid mRNA splicing pattern depends on tissue-specific and differentiation stage–specific alternative splicing that is induced late in the course of terminal erythroid maturation.[132, 133, 136] Recombinant isoforms containing these 21 amino acids bind to spectrin-actin complexes efficiently.[138] Otherwise identical recombinant proteins lacking the sequence fail to bind. Thus, alternative splicing of this exon during late erythropoiesis is essential to generate a functioning protein isoform.

Muscle and testes (and, to a lesser degree, brain) are the only non-erythroid tissues that express exon 15 in significant amounts.[134, 136] The relevance of the "erythroid" splicing pattern to testicular and muscle cell function remains unknown; however, it is intriguing that a major isoform of β spectrin expressed in muscle is the erythroid form. The erythroid isoform of β spectrin, whose amino-terminus is the binding site for protein 4.1, is also abundant in brain, in which small to moderate amounts of protein 4.1 mRNA containing exon 15 can be found.[111, 120, 121]

Two additional exons are adjacent to the one responsible for binding to erythroid spectrin-actin. There are thus eight possible variants of the 10 kDa

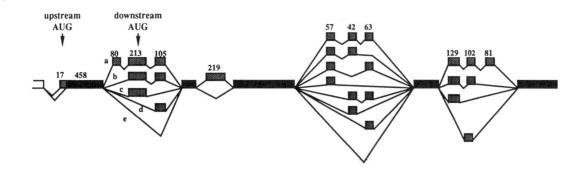

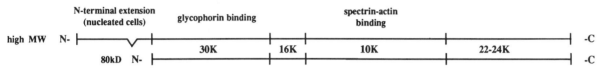

FIGURE 7–9. **Alternative splicing of protein 4.1 mRNAs.** Portions of the protein 4.1 mRNA transcribed into mRNA in all tissues are shown in black. Exons expressed selectively in certain tissues are shown as stippled regions, with length in nucleotides indicated. One exon, 80 bases in length, does not code for a protein because it contains translation termination codons in all three reading frames. For simplicity, some exons expressed at extremely low levels in many tissues have been omitted from the diagram. The key exons described in the text are the 17 base and 213 base exons containing AUG translation start codons and the 63 base exon important for spectrin-actin binding. The latter is expressed in large amounts predominantly in red cells and to a lesser extent in muscle and testes. The 17 base "exon," which inserts an upstream AUG, permitting synthesis of a high molecular weight isoform with an N-terminal extension, is called exon 2 in the text. The 213 base exon containing the downstream AUG must be expressed for synthesis of the 80 kDa isoform in red cells, which do not express the 17 base exon 2. The 63 base exon, described as exon 15 in the text, is essential for spectrin-actin binding.

spectrin-actin–binding domain arising from combinatorial splicing of three consecutive exons.[134, 136] In lymphocytes, none of the exons are retained in the majority of the mRNA transcripts; in brain, multiple isoforms containing various combinations of the exons are encountered, whereas in erythrocytes, all of the protein 4.1 contains only exon 15.[134] This multiplicity of isoforms may be important for interaction with spectrin isoforms in different cell types.

The biochemical role of protein 4.1 in linking spectrin to the membrane is complex (see references 29, 58, and 137 for reviews). Spectrin binds actin weakly, as does protein 4.1. Protein 4.1 greatly facilitates and stabilizes spectrin-actin interaction and the formation of a ternary complex that can bind to glycophorin or protein 3. This binding is weakened by phosphorylation of protein 4.1. Much less is known about the structural requirements for binding of protein 4.1 to the cytoplasmic domains of transmembrane proteins or to lipids. Lipid binding may facilitate binding to the proteins. Two alternatively spliced exons located near the C-terminus of the 30 kDa domain are expressed differentially to significant degrees in some tissues, but no functional significance has been attached to these splicing patterns.[133–137]

As illustrated in Figure 7–9, two splicing events that modify the structure of the 5′ untranslated region of erythroid protein 4.1 can generate, in non-erythroid tissues, a high molecular weight isoform resulting from initiation of mRNA translation at an upstream initia-

tion codon inserted by use of a cryptic acceptor splice site in exon 2.[133–135] The high molecular weight isoform (apparent molecular weight of 120 kDa) has been identified immunochemically in cells by the use of antibodies generated against the novel upstream peptides.

In most non-erythroid tissues, the higher molecular weight isoforms (120 to 150 kDa) and low molecular weight isoforms (60 to 90 kDa) coexist in varying ratios. These presumably represent two different families of protein spliceoforms translated from the upstream (high molecular weight) or downstream (low molecular weight) translation start site. The relative amounts of each family produced could depend on the relative amounts of alternative mRNA splicing or the preferential use of one or the other translation start sites. Recent work has shown that the upstream translation start site, when present, is used almost exclusively, thus greatly reducing the likelihood of translational regulation.[139] These studies indirectly, but strongly, implicate the regulated use of a cryptic splice site in exon 2 as the determinant of high and low molecular weight isoform distribution.

The functional importance of the high molecular weight isoforms remains unknown. The C-terminal 80 kDa of these isoforms is identical to their low molecular weight analogues. It is possible that the additional amino acid residues form a "headpiece" that alters the behavior of the 30 kDa membrane-binding domain or causes localization of the protein to other regions of the cell. Preliminary data suggest that the spectrin-actin binding is not affected, provided that exon is expressed.[137] Multiple alternative mRNA splicing events might generate isoforms with different affinities for membrane and intracellular structures. The diverse array of spliceoforms would then account for the fact that in non-erythroid tissues protein 4.1 is found in several locations (perinuclear regions, stress fibers, cytoplasmic filaments of unknown significance, and centrioles), in addition to its erythroid localization underneath the plasma membrane (cf. references 29 and 58).

The alternate splicing events leading to the production of high molecular weight isoforms of protein 4.1 are highly relevant to the pathophysiology of certain protein 4.1 deficiency states, even though the normal functional significance of adding a headpiece to protein 4.1 remains unknown. The high molecular weight isoforms are completely absent from mature red cells.[134] Indeed, mRNA containing the 17 amino acid extension of exon 2 needed for the synthesis of high molecular weight forms is essentially absent from erythroid cells, at least from the proerythroblast stage forward.[133–136] Thus, only the downstream translation initiation site is available for protein 4.1 biosynthesis during erythropoiesis. Mutations abolishing this site will lead to protein 4.1 deficiency in red cells, but deficiency of only the low molecular weight family of isoforms in non-erythroid cells (since the upstream methionine will be available for synthesis of high molecular weight forms).[140, 141] Erythropoiesis is marked by the induction of splicing events leading to retention of the spectrin-actin–binding sequence motif in the 10 kDa domain, but exclusion of the sequences containing the upstream translation initiator codon needed for production of high molecular weight isoforms. Mutations altering either of these events can thus cause selective deficiencies or abnormalities in red cells.

ANKYRIN. Ankyrin, previously designated protein 2.1, is a 210 kDa sulfhydryl-rich molecule containing three defined domains: an amino-terminal 89 kDa domain that contains sites for binding to the anion exchanger (protein 3), a 62 kDa domain containing spectrin-binding sites, and a 55 kDa regulatory domain at the C-terminus.[29, 30, 142] It is present in about 100,000 copies per cell. Ankyrin is globular but, like protein 4.1, highly asymmetrical.[143–145] The band 3–binding domain is basic; the central spectrin-binding domain is neutral, but heavily phosphorylated; and the regulatory domain is highly acidic, at least in the predominant erythroid form.[145] Phosphorylation occurs by casein kinase and cAMP-independent protein kinase.[146, 147] Phosphorylation markedly weakens the binding of ankyrin to spectrin tetramers, but not to dimers, and reduces affinity for the anion transporter.

The amino-terminal domain contains tandem repeats marked by fascinating short sequence motifs that are found throughout nature in protein implicated in the control of tissue differentiation and cell cycle regulation.[148, 149] These repeats have been called "CYC2" repeats because of their presence in cell cycle control genes. The amino-terminal 90 kDa domain contains a complex repeated internal structure that gives rise to multiple binding sites for the cytoplasmic tail of band 3. There are 23 highly conserved 33 amino acid sequence repeats. Repeat numbers 12 to 23 have been shown to be important for ankyrin and perhaps tubulin binding. Each repeat is relatively hydrophobic, predicting a high order of secondary structure that may favor packing into a highly globular domain with charged residues presented on the outside. The amino-terminal repeats are probably far more ordered than is the spectrin-binding domain.

The locus encoding ankyrin is on chromosome 8p11.2.[148, 149] Multiple erythroid-specific isoforms arise from this locus by alternative mRNA splicing events that generate diversity of the carboxy-terminal regulatory domain.[149] The most important of these quantitatively is protein 2.2, which has been truncated by removal of the 162 amino acids that render the regulatory domain of protein 2.1 highly acidic. The alternatively spliced isoform, protein 2.2, has a higher affinity for both the cytoplasmic domain of band 3 and spectrin, suggesting that the acidic portion of the regulatory domain exerts an inhibitory effect on ankyrin binding.[150]

Erythrocyte ankyrin is expressed primarily in red cells, but to some degree in other tissues as well.[150–152] Multiple non-erythroid ankyrin isoforms have been defined, and their cDNAs cloned. The genomic locus for these isoforms, some of which probably arise by alternative splicing, is on chromosome 4.[151, 152]

Ankyrin is multivalent, binding to the carboxy-terminal region of the spectrin β chain with its 55 kDa central domain and to the cytoplasmic tail of the anion exchanger via repeated sequences in the amino-terminal 90 kDa domain.[150] Binding creates a tight association between spectrin and protein 3, but the strength of binding can be modified by phosphorylation. The stoichiometry of the abundance of spectrin and ankyrin suggests strongly that one ankyrin molecule is available to link each spectrin tetramer to the membrane. Moreover, the binding interactions are cooperative. Attachment of ankyrin to band 3 greatly facilitates the ability of the molecule to organize the spectrin to which it is attached into tetramers.[150] Conversely, spectrin binding enhances the affinity for protein 3. Ankyrin thus functions both as an attachment point for the spectrin-actin latticework and, with band 3, as a nidus for organization of the lattice itself.

PROTEIN 4.2. Protein 4.2, 72,000 kDa, is present at about 200,000 copies per erythrocyte.[153] It is encoded by a gene located on chromosome 15q15–q21 and gives rise to a principal isoform, protein 4.2 "long" (p4.2L), and a minor short isoform (p4.2S) by alternative mRNA splicing.[154–156] Its amino acid sequence places it, surprisingly, in a protein family including factor XIII and guinea pig transglutaminase. Indeed, the protein shows strong conservation with many transglutaminase genes. However, protein 4.2 cannot catalyze cross-linking of proteins like other transglutaminase because it possesses alanine, instead of the essential cysteine, in its potential active site.[157]

Protein 4.2 binds to several proteins, including band 3, protein 4.1, ankyrin, and ankyrin–protein 3 complexes.[153, 158] The major function of protein 4.2 is probably to stabilize the spectrin-actin-ankyrin association with protein 3. It has also been proposed that protein 4.2 protects the cytoskeleton from premature aging by binding calcium and other cofactors that normally activate red cell transglutaminases.[156] Since these transglutaminases would otherwise cross-link proteins, possibly leading to their inactivation in an age-dependent manner, protein 4.2 has been postulated to act as a "false agonist." As discussed later, the importance of protein 4.2 to cytoskeletal integrity is supported by the existence of hereditary hemolytic anemias due to deficiency states.

OTHER PROTEINS THAT ASSOCIATE WITH SPECTRIN-ANKYRIN COMPLEXES. Adducin, dematin (protein 4.9), tropomyosin, myosin, proteins related to troponin, and other proteins known to be associated with actin in non-erythroid cells are found in variable amounts in red cells (see references 29, 58, and 142 for reviews). The functional role of these proteins has not been defined. There is reason to doubt that several of them are important for the behavior of mature red cells. Protein 4.9, for example, declines in amount during erythroid maturation. It may be more important for red cell development than for life in the circulation. Similarly, adducin is present in only 30,000 copies per cell. It appears to compete with protein 4.1 for binding to spectrin-actin complexes, but its presence in such small amounts suggests that it is unlikely to be quantitatively significant as a modulator of junctional complex formation. No deficiency states associated with red cell abnormalities have been defined for these proteins. Therefore, they shall not be considered further.

BIOGENESIS AND ASSEMBLY OF THE MEMBRANE DURING RED CELL DEVELOPMENT

A great deal of information has been gathered about red cell membrane biogenesis, but no clear picture of the sequence of steps involved has emerged. Several issues have confounded mechanistic analysis (see references 58 and 142 for reviews). First, it has been difficult to obtain synchronized erythroid precursors representing each stage of erythropoiesis from BFUE/CFUE through reticulocytes in sufficient amounts and purity. Second, knowledge of the diversity of protein isoforms and isoform switching occurring during erythropoiesis is still emerging. Nucleic acid and antibody probes for specific subregions of these proteins and their mRNAs have become available only recently. Recent discovery of these multiple alternatively spliced or translated isoforms complicates interpretation of earlier studies of the erythrocyte membrane biogenesis; these studies detected only entire proteins, or mRNA transcripts, which are actually composites of several isoforms increasing or decreasing in amount during various stages of erythropoiesis. Third, reliance on inducible transformed cell lines, such as the mouse erythroleukemia cell (MELC), as an alternative source of pure synchronized cells has been compromised by the fact that these lines appear to support an imperfect and incomplete mode of membrane development during erythroblast maturation. Despite these limitations, some features of red cell membrane biogenesis are beginning to emerge. Most of this information has been gathered by use of murine or avian cells obtained during early embryonic or fetal life, when partial synchronization can be achieved by purifying cells from yolk sac or fetal liver as a function of time after gestation or by the use of cells undergoing stress erythropoiesis in response to a pharmacological or hormonal (erythropoietin) manipulation.

Only a few studies have attempted to provide point-by-point temporal correlations of mRNA levels, protein biosynthetic rates, steady-state accumulation of protein in the cell, and stable quantitative incorporation of the protein products into the membrane. When those correlative measurements have been made, mRNA and protein biosynthetic levels have correlated well (cf. reference 142). Therefore, the discussion that follows refers to mRNA and protein biosynthetic levels interchangeably. In contrast, the primary rates of protein biosynthesis often do *not* correlate well with stable incorporation into the membrane.[142] One consistent principle of membrane protein biosynthesis appears to be that some proteins are synthesized in excess of the others. The proteins synthesized in lesser amounts thus become rate limiting for the assembly of macromolecular complexes. The unused excess amounts of the proteins synthesized in higher initial abundance tend to be catabolized. Only small pools of unincorporated membrane proteins exist, particularly during the later stages of erythropoiesis.

Membrane protein biosynthesis occurs asynchronously during erythropoiesis. There is no evidence to support the idea of a coordinate simultaneous induction of the genes encoding the red cell membrane proteins.[159–165] Rather, biosynthesis of different components peaks at different stages of erythropoiesis. Those components expressed in the earlier stages could direct assembly of the cytoskeleton as additional components are produced in the later stages. In some cases, modification of the multiple mRNA products of a single gene proceeds in temporally separated stages. In the case of protein 4.1 gene expression, the mRNA splicing event that *excludes* the upstream translation start codon (used for biosynthesis of high molecular weight forms in non-erythroid cells) occurs at very early stages, probably well before the proerythroblast stage. In contrast, the splicing event that leads to *inclusion* of the 63 base exon 15 encoding the erythroid spectrin-actin–binding domain does not occur until the mid to late stages of erythroblast maturation.[129–133]

Careful studies in avian erythroblasts, corroborated in part by studies of murine and human cells, provide convincing evidence for the notion that the early stages of red cell membrane assembly are directed by production of the erythroid form of protein 3.[160, 162] Protein 3, once inserted into the membrane, directs the assembly of stable macromolecular complexes as the other protein components appear. There are complicated switches in the predominance of the 9.0 kb and 7.0 kb mRNA transcripts arising from the ankyrin gene in mice and humans.[160] Although both transcripts are found at all stages of erythropoiesis, the 9.0 kb transcript tends to predominate in early cells, whereas the 7.5 kb transcript is far more abundant in later cells.[166] Ankyrin also appears to be synthesized at relatively high levels during early stages of erythropoiesis, suggesting that it, too, is an important element for assembly by virtue of its direct interaction with band 3.[160, 162]

The biosynthesis and assembly of spectrin subunits is complex. β Spectrin biosynthesis exceeds that of α spectrin in the early erythroblasts derived from both embryonic (yolk sac) and fetal/adult (liver/spleen) origins (cf. references 166 to 168). This ratio is preserved during later stages of erythropoiesis in embryonic cells, but not in fetal/adult-derived late erythroblasts and reticulocytes. In these latter cells, α spectrin gene expression increases, whereas β spectrin gene expression remains constant, resulting in a predominance of α mRNA protein during the late stages, when active assembly of the actual membrane is occurring most rapidly. To some degree, these changing ratios may reflect differential sensitivity to erythropoietin or other stimulants of "stress erythropoiesis"; β spectrin gene expression has been shown to increase selectively in erythropoietin-stimulated Friend leukemia virus–infected spleen cells, induced MELC, and human ankyrin-deficient erythroblasts. α Spectrin gene expression predominates in late human erythroid precursors.

The feature of spectrin biosynthesis relevant to the analysis of hereditary hemolytic anemias is that spectrin subunits are incorporated into the membrane in a 1:1 α/β stoichiometric ratio, regardless of their primary rates of biosynthesis on polyribosomes.[165–168] Chains not incorporated must be unstable, since large pools do not accumulate. Human α spectrin synthesis exceeds that of β-spectrin by a factor of nearly 2:1 during the later stages of erythropoiesis, when, presumably, membrane assembly is proceeding rapidly. The availability of β spectrin subunits thus determines the maximum rate and amount of stable spectrin assembly. Therefore, mutations reducing steady-state levels of newly synthesized β spectrin should have a far greater phenotypic impact than do mutations causing comparable decreases in α spectrin biosynthesis. Preliminary analyses of some patients with hereditary hemolytic anemias support this prediction.[169]

Considerable remodeling and maturation of the red cell membrane occur after enucleation of late erythroblasts (see reference 30 for a review). Some biosynthesis of protein 4.1 and glycophorin C continues in the newly enucleated reticulocyte, but most membrane remodeling occurs post-translationally. The reticulocyte is multilobular and motile; it possesses mitochondria, polyribosomes, and numerous membrane proteins that are either absent or much less abundant in mature red cells. In addition, phospholipid composition and inside-outside lipid distribution are different. Reticulocytes are far less deformable and considerably more unstable mechanically than are mature erythrocytes. Maturation begins in the bone marrow and lasts for 2 or 3 days. It is completed in the circulation and perhaps in the spleen (splenic polishing). Reticulocytes first become cup shaped before acquiring their final biconcave disc shape. This process involves major reorganization of both membrane phospholipids and cytoskeletal and embedded proteins, as well as the loss of lipids and numerous proteins, including transferrin receptors, insulin receptors, and fibronectin receptors. At the end of this process, deformability is close to that of the mature red cell.

Understanding of membrane protein gene regulation during erythropoiesis will require re-examination in the light of new knowledge concerning tissue- and differentiation-specific isoforms, as well as the role of alternative mRNA splicing in generating these isoforms. The primary rates of production of these proteins are probably not major determinants. Rather, post-translational events, including stabilization of newly synthesized proteins by assembly processes, may be the key regulatory foci. These considerations greatly complicate attempts to relate mutations of membrane proteins to particular clinical syndromes. A single mutation can have pleiotropic effects on synthesis, assembly, remodeling, and/or biochemical function in the mature cell. The fact that particular morphological abnormalities, degrees of clinical severity, and patterns of inheritance in particular kindreds do not always correlate in a straightforward way with the nature or location of a particular mutation is more understandable in view of these complexities.

DISORDERS OF THE RED CELL MEMBRANE LIPIDS

Inherited and acquired abnormalities of the red cell membrane manifest as morphological abnormalities accompanied by shortened red cell life spans and hemolytic anemias of varying degree. Only a few are severe enough to require therapeutic intervention. Most of the acquired abnormalities are in fact important primarily as stigmata of particular diseases or of disease progression in other organ systems. We first focus on a very brief survey of disorders attributable to abnormal membrane lipids and then devote more detailed attention to disorders of the membrane proteins, about which far more molecular information is available. (*Note:* The material in this section has been reviewed in references 58, 142, and 170; the reader is referred to these excellent summaries for access to the primary literature.)

Target Cells

Target cells result from an increase in surface-to-volume ratio, due either to increased membrane surface area or to decreased intracellular volume. The latter occurs when cells are poorly hemoglobinized, in part because the negative charge of hemoglobin tends to draw sodium and, thereby, water into cells. Thus, microcytic target cells are encountered with variable frequency in iron deficiency and the thalassemia syndromes. Hemoglobin C, which crystallizes in red cells and thus lowers its effective intracellular concentration, is also characterized by the presence of target cells.

The most commonly encountered occurrences of target cells are the result of increased red cell membrane lipids in liver disease associated with intrahepatic cholestasis. Net uptake of free plasma cholesterol and phospholipids by the membrane is increased because the cholesterol/phospholipid/protein ratios of low density lipoproteins are abnormal in these conditions, resulting in redistribution. Target cells have an increased surface area with normal or only slightly increased cell volumes. They exhibit normal survival, although they are osmotically fragile.

Target cells are also encountered in a rare autosomal dominant condition called lecithin cholesterol acyltransferase (LCAT) deficiency. The normal function of LCAT is to transfer fatty acids from phosphatidylcholine to cholesterol. LCAT is normally complexed to high density lipoproteins in the plasma. Deficient patients have increased cholesterol and phospholipid content in their membranes and large numbers of target cells on the peripheral smear. These cells have a mildly shortened survival. LCAT deficiency is marked by the presence of so-called "sea blue histiocytes" because of storage cells in the bone marrow; compensatory erythropoiesis by the bone marrow appears to be impaired for unknown reasons. The most severe consequence of LCAT deficiency is premature atherosclerosis. Target cells and the mild anemia are useful diagnostic manifestations.

Acanthocytosis and Spur Cell Anemia

Acanthocytes, so named because of the "thorn"-like projections of the membrane protruding from the body of the red cell, arise from several conditions, many of which are associated with abnormal membrane lipid composition and altered distribution of lipids between the outer and inner leaflets of the bilayer. These include severe liver disease, abetalipoproteinemia, and chorea-acanthocytosis syndrome. Acanthocytes also appear to be associated with the inheritance of certain polymorphisms of red cell antigens, such as the McLeod blood group. The molecular pathophysiology of acanthocytosis has been most thoroughly examined in the acquired condition of severe end-stage liver disease. Only a small percentage of patients with liver disease acquire the syndrome of "spur cell hemolytic anemia," but the prevalence of liver disease is so high that these individuals account for the majority of cases of acanthocytosis encountered clinically.

Acanthocytes, like target cells, result from increased acquisition of free cholesterol from the plasma due to abnormal cholesterol/lipoprotein ratios. In severe liver disease, an extraordinarily high ratio of free cholesterol to phospholipids is found in lipoproteins; the free cholesterol readily partitions into the membrane, where it preferentially associates with the outer leaflet. The outer leaflet becomes less fluid; attempts to remodel the membrane are made by the spleen, producing rigid spherical cells possessing the characteristic spiculated projections. On subsequent passes through the spleen, these poorly deformable cells have difficulty in negotiating the narrow sinusoids of the splenic circulation and are hemolyzed. Spur cell anemia is an ominous clinical marker of the terminal stages of liver disease. It is primarily important as a sign of worsening liver function; the anemia itself is rarely a major clinical problem. Prior to the availability of liver transplantation, patients reaching this stage rarely lived for more than a few weeks.

Spur cell anemia is sometimes confused with "Zieve's syndrome," a transient, relatively mild spherocytic hemolytic anemia that occurs during acute fatty metamorphosis accompanied by hyperglycemia. The molecular basis of this membrane abnormality remains unknown. Numerous conditions are also associated with cells having *regular* projections from the red cell membrane, called echinocytes, or burr cells. These include malnutrition and renal disease. Essentially nothing is known about the molecular basis of burr cell formation. ATP depletion, abnormal calcium loading, and the binding of certain drugs have all been implicated. Like acanthocytes, burr cells seem to result from asymmetry in the lipid content of the outer and inner leaflets of the membrane. In experimental models, overloading of the outer leaflet results in spiculated cells, whereas overloading of the inner leaflet results in stomatocytic (mouth-like) cells.

Abetalipoproteinemia

Abetalipoproteinemia is an autosomal recessive disorder characterized by the complete absence of apolipoprotein B (cf. reference 170). Affected patients are unable to secrete the newly synthesized apoprotein into the plasma. They have a mild anemia, dramatic acanthocytosis, retinitis pigmentosa, neuromuscular abnormalities, and other multisystem defects.

Acanthocytes in abetalipoproteinemia are characterized by overloading of the outer leaflet with sphingomyelin. Indeed, the discoid shape can be restored by mild extraction of lipids from the outer leaflet or by incubation of red cells with chlorpromazine, which binds to the inner leaflet, thus restoring the balance of inner and outer leaflet mass. These acanthocytes are not as rigid as in liver disease; consequently, the hemolytic diathesis is not as severe. Less impressive degrees of acanthocytosis are seen in a related syndrome of hypobetalipoproteinemia, chorea-acanthocytosis syndrome, an autosomal recessive disorder characterized primarily by neurological movement disorders and high levels of unsaturated fatty acids in the red cell membrane, but no anemia (cf. references 142 and 170).

DISORDERS OF RED CELL CYTOSKELETAL PROTEINS

Clinically relevant derangements of the red cell membrane proteins include the following: (1) hereditary hemolytic anemias due to genetic defects of these proteins; (2) acquired abnormalities of membrane proteins due to derangement of other red cell components, especially abnormal hemoglobins or hemoglobin-derived products; (3) alterations in membrane proteins, notably band 3, that occur with advancing red cell age and lead to eventual sequestration and destruction; and (4) incompletely understood hemolytic states associated with abnormal membrane antigens. The final common pathway characterizing these disorders appears to be loss of the amount or function, or both, of cytoskeletal proteins, leading to reduced deformability or reduced mechanical stability, or both. The focus of this discussion is on the genetic defects and the molecular basis of the pathophysiology of the disorders. For detailed discussion of natural history, clinical diagnosis, management, and genetic counseling, the reader is referred to several excellent recent reviews.[57, 142, 170-172] To conserve space, individual literature citations are not provided for the well-established clinical principles outlined in this section. The reader is referred to the aforementioned references for access to this vast literature.

Inherited Defects of the Red Cell Cytoskeleton

Inherited red cell abnormalities attributable to primary genetic defects in red cell membrane proteins were originally classified by their morphological presentation. They include hereditary spherocytosis (HS), hereditary elliptocytosis (HE), hereditary pyropoikilocytosis (HPP), and hereditary ovalocytosis/stomatocytosis (HO). Less common conditions, such as hereditary xerocytosis and hereditary stomatocytosis, are also thought to arise from red cell membrane protein abnormalities, but their etiology is less clear. We shall focus on the better characterized disorders: HS, HE, HPP, and HO.

Each of the inherited disorders of red cell membrane proteins is extremely heterogeneous, both clinically and in terms of the primary molecular defect. There is also considerable overlap, both morphologically and genetically. For example, in some patients with HPP, elliptocytes are common. In some kindreds only HE is encountered, whereas in others both HE and HPP are found in different family members. These facts, coupled with rapidly expanding knowledge of the structure, function, biogenesis, and molecular pathology of the membrane proteins, make a simple classification of these disorders difficult. One cannot correlate a particular abnormality, such as HS, strictly with a particular pattern of inheritance or membrane protein defect. For example, spectrin mutations can participate in the pathogenesis of HE, HPP, and HS. Conversely, HS can arise from defects in spectrin, protein 4.2, ankyrin, or protein 3. Therefore, the discussion that follows attempts to organize knowledge about these disorders in two tiers. First, we consider the traditional nosology of HS, HE, HPP, and HO. Second, molecular defects of the individual membrane proteins and the diverse disorders produced by these mutations are surveyed.

Hereditary Spherocytosis (HS)

Hereditary spherocytosis is characterized by the predominance of spherocytic erythrocytes on the peripheral smear. The most common form is an autosomal dominant hemolytic anemia of variable severity. Autosomal recessive forms, which are usually quite severe in their clinical presentation, and very mild forms that present late in life are also common. HS occurs sporadically in all ethnic groups but tends to be somewhat more frequent in the Western world, notably in northern Europeans. However, this apparent preponderance may reflect observer bias because the disease can go unnoticed without sophisticated testing.

PATHOGENESIS. The common feature of HS red cells is a marked decrease in surface area due to reduced amounts of all lipid components of the membrane (Fig. 7–10). Loss of redundant surface area makes these cells less capable of distention in hypo-osmolar solutions, leading to increased susceptibility to rupture (osmotic fragility). This phenomenon is the basis for a clinical test in which the ability of normal red cells and the ability of test red cells to resist lysis under conditions of progressively decreasing tonicity are compared (osmotic fragility test). The osmotic fragility test is thus regarded as a standard maneuver during the diagnostic workup of hereditary hemolytic anemias (cf. references 170 and 171).

Red cells in HS are also less deformable, because of the loss of the redundant surface area needed for the flexible disc shape. They tend to become entrapped in the fenestrations in the wall of splenic sinuses. This leads to engorgement of the spleen and an increased time of residency in contact with splenic macrophages. Further damage and loss of membrane and increased osmotic fragility occur. Damage occurs cumulatively, resulting in eventual premature sequestration and destruction by macrophages in the spleen, liver, or perhaps other tissues; hemolytic anemia results.

Most red cells exhibit quantitative reductions of 25 to 50 per cent in spectrin content. Spectrin deficiency is a hallmark of HS cells; this defect probably accounts

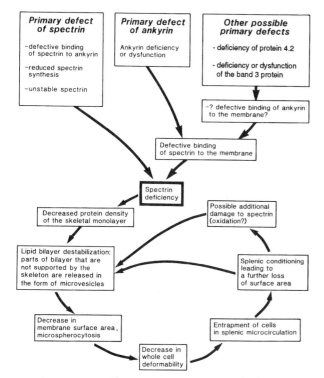

FIGURE 7–10. Diverse biochemical etiologies producing a common pathophysiology of hereditary spherocytosis (HS). The schematic illustrates the development of spectrin deficiency by multiple mechanisms as a common pathway leading to membrane destabilization and loss of red cell surface area. As indicated by the upper part of the schematic, spectrin deficiency can result from primary defects in the production, stability, or function of spectrin or from secondary loss of spectrin from stable membrane-bound cytoskeletal structures, due to deficiencies or functional defects of proteins necessary for interaction with spectrin during formation of these stable complexes. Because of the inadequate amounts of spectrin, greater proportions of the lipid bilayer are left unattached to the stabilizing cytoskeleton, resulting in progressive vesiculation of the unsupported lipid, loss of membrane surface area, loss of deformability, entrapment in the spleen, possible further damage by splenic macrophages, and aggravation of the membrane instability, leading to the vicious circle and ultimate red cell destruction indicated in the diagram. (See text for further discussion.) (Adapted from Palek, J.: Red cell membrane disorders. *In* Hoffman, R., Benz, E. J., Jr., Furie, B., Shattil, S., and Cohen, H. [eds.]: Hematology: Basic Principles and Practice. New York, Churchill Livingstone, 1990, pp. 472–504; with permission.)

for the reduced surface area of the overlying membrane (see Fig. 7–10). Normally, the lipid bilayer fragments or sheds microvesicles when subjected to severe shear stress, leading to loss of surface area. This tendency is counteracted by the dense hexagonal network of spectrin filaments attached to the membrane (cf. references 30, 58, and 142). Spectrin deficiency leads to an increase in the amount of lipids that are not stabilized by this anchoring mechanism. Microvesiculation and fragmentation thus occur in response to the normal mechanical and biochemical stresses of the circulation. Mechanical fragility can be demonstrated by ektacytometry[30]; susceptibility to biochemically induced fragmentation can be induced by allowing red cells to incubate in the absence of glucose, which leads to ATP depletion, membrane fragmenta-

tion, and, ultimately, hemolysis.[170] HS cells are far more susceptible to hemolysis under these conditions than are normal cells. This phenomenon forms the basis for the "autohemolysis" test. Microvesicles released as the result of these stresses contain integral membrane proteins, but no cytoskeletal proteins, suggesting that they do indeed result from a failure to be anchored to the cytoskeleton.

Many secondary abnormalities of red cell membrane function have been described, including increased sodium influx, associated with a paradoxical *dehydration*, possibly due to secondary overactivity of the Na^+K^+ATPase. Since the sodium pump extrudes three sodiums for every two potassiums entering the cell, the net effect of uncompensated overactivity is loss of cations and cellular dehydration.

CLINICAL MANIFESTATIONS. The clinical manifestations of HS are extremely variable. The most common form is inherited as an autosomal dominant disorder associated with minimal, mild, or moderate hemolysis. Anemia is rarely severe; the blood count is often normal. In the mildest cases, spherocytes are seen on the peripheral smear, but hemolytic stigmata (anemia reticulocytosis, hepatosplenomegaly, jaundice to hyperbilirubinemia, bilirubin gallstones leading to premature gallbladder disease, or leg ulcers) are present. Some patients have reticulocytosis or mild anemia or both. Occasionally, these patients present in adult life with secondary complications of chronic hemolysis, such as premature biliary tract disease, acute onset of anemia due to decompensation of compensatory erythropoiesis ("aplastic" or "hypoplastic" crises caused by suppression of erythropoiesis by viral infections, cytotoxic drugs, and so on), or superimposition of a second hemolytic diathesis, such as conditions predisposing to hypersplenism. It is the exceptional patient, usually one with the rare autosomal recessive forms of the disease, who exhibits severe chronic hemolytic anemia with all of the associated stigmata.

INHERITANCE. The patterns of inheritance of HS are complex.[142, 171, 172] Spontaneous mutations are common. Mildly symptomatic patients can coexist in kindreds with asymptomatic or more severely symptomatic individuals in the same kindred. This is due to heterozygosity for silent, mild, or more severe alleles; homozygosity for alleles that may be clinically silent in the simple heterozygous state; or double heterozygosity for mild ("silent carrier") and more severe alleles.

As discussed later in more detail, HS can arise from mutations in the genes for ankyrin, α spectrin, β spectrin, protein 4.2, and possibly protein 3.[170, 171] In all cases, the biochemical abnormalities arising from these mutations lead, as a final common pathway, to instability of the spectrin-actin association with the lipid bilayer. Membrane cytoskeletal proteins, including spectrin, that are not stabilized by this association tend to be catabolized. Instability of membrane association thus leads to a net spectrin deficiency. Quantitative measurements of membrane-associated spectrin can, when performed by properly qualified laboratories, be a useful adjunct to diagnosis.[142, 171]

Although spectrin deficiency is a hallmark of HS, it is not a finding exclusively associated with HS. Spectrin deficiency can also occur as part of the pathogenesis of acquired membrane defects resulting from oxidation of the cytoskeleton by hemichromes or binding to certain structurally abnormal hemoglobins or free globin chains.

DIAGNOSIS AND THERAPY. Clinical diagnosis of HS is usually based on the characteristic appearance of the red cells. In contrast to many other conditions accompanied by the presence of spherocytes, such as immune hemolytic anemia and hypersplenism, the peripheral blood smear of most patients with HS shows a relatively *uniform* population of spherocytes. Moreover, the mean corpuscular hemoglobin concentration (MCHC) value tends to be rather high in HS patients, reflecting the secondary defects that generate dehydrated red cells. These changes are far less dramatic in other conditions associated with spherocytosis. Subtle but useful and reproducible differences in measurements of osmotic fragility and autohemolysis are also helpful in diagnosis.

Most patients with HS require no therapeutic intervention. Individuals who inherit severe forms, notably the autosomal recessive form, require transfusion support until they are old enough to tolerate splenectomy. In general, the response to splenectomy is good, leading to amelioration or elimination of the anemia. Hemolysis may persist, however, particularly in the autosomal recessive form.

Hereditary Elliptocytosis and Hereditary Pyropoikilocytosis

Hereditary elliptocytosis and hereditary pyropoikilocytosis are distinct but interrelated disorders sometimes found within a single kindred (cf. reference 58). The morphological hallmark of HE is the predominance of elliptical red cells on the peripheral blood smear. In HPP, red cell morphology is extremely bizarre, consisting of fragmented red cells, spiculated cells, and elliptocytes. HPP erythrocytes are thermally unstable, acquiring bizarre morphology and undergoing fragmentation at lower temperatures than normal cells.[172] HPP is rare, tends to be inherited in a complex but recessive fashion, often in kindreds with HE, and is usually associated with significant clinical hemolytic anemia. In contrast, HE is extremely variable in terms of clinical severity (usually mild) and inheritance.

PATHOGENESIS. The molecular basis of HE is heterogeneous (cf. references 58 and 170 to 172). Five major categories have been identified: first, spectrin defects involving abnormal cell association of heterodimers to tetramers; second, defects of spectrin resulting in abnormal binding to protein 4.1 or ankyrin; third, deficiencies or abnormal functions of protein 4.1; fourth, deficiencies of glycophorin C; and fifth, abnormalities of protein 4.2.

The common feature uniting these diverse defects

is that each weakens the formation of the junctional complexes important for structural integrity of the spectrin latticework (Fig. 7–11). Thus, the spectrin abnormalities underlying HE tend to be those disrupting dimer-dimer association to form tetramers, or β spectrin mutations affecting binding to protein 4.1. Glycophorin C deficiency leads to secondary protein 4.1 deficiency, which, like defects of protein 4.1 itself, removes the essential component necessary for forming the spectrin/actin/protein 4.1/protein 4.2 junctional complex. Protein 4.2 defects have the same impact. Thus, spectrin self-association or spectrin association with other components of the junctional complex is the molecular hallmark of these disorders.

These abnormalities have been characterized in the literature as "horizontal" defects, as opposed to the "vertical" defects in HS that affect the stability of direct attachment to the overlying membrane (cf. references 58 and 173). The latter result in deficiencies of spectrin, producing fragile, non-deformable, physically unstable membranes (see Fig. 7–11). In HE, the *quantity* of spectrin in the latticework appears to be nearly normal. Qualitative defects disrupt the junctional complexes. The net effect is a membrane that is less tolerant of shear stress. These membranes are more susceptible to permanent "plastic" deformation in the circulation because of the loss of resiliency. This may be the reason that they acquire the elliptocytic shape, although the molecular basis for acquisition of this shape remains unknown.

Hereditary pyropoikilocytosis appears, in those cases that have been studied, to represent a compound heterozygous state in which clinical manifestations are more severe because there is co-inheritance of spectrin deficiency—for example, a biosynthetic defect—and a mutation that results in qualitative deficiency of normal spectrin.[171] Cells from these patients might be expected to exhibit features of both decreased deformability and resiliency and increased membrane fragmentation, resulting in a syndrome with morphology different from that of either HE or HS. In this regard, it is interesting to note that some of the more severe forms of HE are associated with poikilocytosis and that the thermal instability that is highly characteristic of HPP can also be encountered in some HE patients carrying a similar spectrin mutation.

The exact pathophysiology responsible for the formation of elliptocytes and poikilocytes in HE and HPP is not yet clear (cf. references 58 and 170). Bone marrow precursor cells have normal morphology, suggesting that the shapes are acquired in the circulation. The elliptical shapes of HE cells are retained by the membrane skeleton and membrane ghosts after detergent extraction in vitro, a situation similar to that observed when normal red cells are subjected to enough mechanical stress to induce plastic deformation. The weakened complexes thought to arise from mutations producing HE may lead to this plastic deformation under normal shear stress.

Poikilocytes occur in patients with severely defective self-association of spectrin dimers into tetramers. The

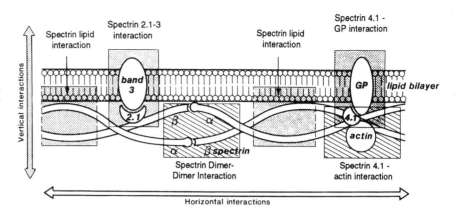

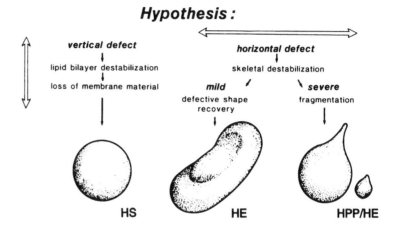

FIGURE 7–11. Different molecular origins of HS and HE/HPP based on the hypothesis of "vertical" and "horizontal" defects. As discussed in more detail in the text, vertical interactions are those needed to stabilize the attachment of the spectrin lattice to the lipid bilayer. Failures of this attachment or reduction in the number of attachment sites results in destabilization of the lipid bilayer, membrane loss, and HS, by mechanisms outlined in Figure 7–10. Horizontal interactions are those by which spectrin dimers and tetramers are held together in a firm but elastic manner, permitting reversible stretching and distortion of the red cell membrane. Weakening or derangement of these interactions results in fragility or loss of elasticity. (See text for details.) (Adapted from Palek, J.: Red cell membrane disorders. *In* Hoffman, R., Benz, E. J., Jr., Furie, B., Shattil, S., and Cohen, H. [eds.]: Hematology: Basic Principles and Practice. New York, Churchill Livingstone, 1990, pp. 472–504; with permission.)

spectrin latticework in these patients is disrupted by fixation into an "extended" state by mild to moderate shear stress. Indeed, HPP might represent the biochemically extreme form of defective self-association present in moderately severe forms of HE. The disruption of the latticework adds the element of mechanical instability to that of lost resiliency.

CLINICAL MANIFESTATIONS. HE is usually either asymptomatic or associated with mild hemolytic anemia. Superimposition of other hemolytic diatheses, such as disseminated intravascular coagulation (DIC), can result in sporadic periods of more severe hemolytic anemia. Occasionally, neonates with HE due to an α spectrin mutation have been found to exhibit worsened hemolysis during fetal life; poikilocytosis or hemolysis or both disappear during the first postnatal year as fetal hemoglobin in the circulation is replaced by adult hemoglobin.[174] This phenotypic "switch" results from the fact that fetal hemoglobin binds 2,3-diphosphoglycerate (2,3-DPG) much more poorly than adult hemoglobin. 2,3-DPG, like other phosphorylated compounds, tends to weaken the formation of junctional complexes. The higher "free" 2,3-DPG levels in cells with high hemoglobin F content accentuate the defective behavior of the mutant spectrin.

INHERITANCE. HE is usually inherited as an autosomal dominant trait. Homozygosity for particular spectrin or protein 4.1 mutations and compound heterozygosity for two mutations produce variable de-

grees of more severe hemolysis, depending on the severity of the functional defect encoded by the mutation. At the extreme end, these patients resemble those with HPP as much as those with severe HE, because of the appearance of substantial numbers of poikilocytes in the peripheral blood.

Hereditary pyropoikilocytosis results from co-inheritance of a mutant spectrin that impairs self-association with a mutation causing quantitative deficiency of spectrin. Parents of the propositus have HE or are asymptomatic (cf. references 58 and 171). In some families, the self-association mutant is co-inherited with an apparent "thalassemia"-like allele that results in quantitative spectrin deficiency. In others, the second allele carries a mutation that results in spectrin instability. The net effect is to combine quantitative deficiency of spectrin with dysfunction of the small amount of spectrin that is incorporated. The characteristic poikilocytosis and thermal instability of cells at 49°C are observed.

DIAGNOSIS AND THERAPY. Diagnosis is usually appreciated by the presence of abnormal morphology on the blood film, anemia, or, in severe cases, stigmata of both anemia and chronic hemolysis. Because of the fact that elliptocytes and poikilocytes, like spherocytes, tend to be sequestered in the spleen, splenectomy can cure symptoms in severe cases. Rare forms of HE in which there are also defects in erythropoiesis (ineffective erythropoiesis) and mild to moderate defects in platelet function have been reported. Otherwise, no involvement of non-erythroid tissues has been reported in patients with these red cell disorders.

Hereditary Ovalocytosis

Two major subtypes of hereditary ovalocytosis have been defined (cf. references 54, 58, and 142). The first, also called *spherocytic HE,* is characterized by clear evidence of hemolytic anemia accompanied by a blood film showing somewhat rounded elliptical cells, but no poikilocytes or fragmented forms. Osmotic fragility is increased into the range found in patients with HS. In one case, complete protein 4.1 deficiency was detected. As noted above, patients with partial deficiency usually have relatively mild HE with normal osmotic fragilities.

Southeast Asian ovalocytosis (ovalocytosis/stomatocytosis) is extraordinarily common in some South Asian populations. Nearly 30 per cent of the population in some regions of Malaysia and Papua New Guinea have HO. The red cells have a characteristic oval cup shape, reminiscent of, but not identical to, stomatocytes. Heterozygotes are virtually asymptomatic; mild hemolysis occurs in homozygous cases.

Ovalocytes are remarkably rigid because of mutations of protein 3 that *enhance* the tightness of association between protein 3 (cf. Fig. 7–6), ankyrin, and the spectrin lattice.[54] It is interesting that the treatment of normal red cells with cross-linking agents also generates rigid ovalocytes with tightened associations among cytoskeletal components.[58, 142] The mutations causing HO occur either in the interdomain hinge or in the domain involved in ankyrin binding.

The remarkably high incidence of HO in South Asian populations could be due to the marked resistance of HO red cells to invasion by malaria parasites.[175] HE cells also are somewhat resistant to invasion, a fact that may account for the somewhat higher frequency of HE in equatorial African populations.

Hereditary Stomatocytosis (Hydrocytosis)

Stomatocytes, like ovalocytes, have a cup or bowl shape with a transverse slit or stoma.[170] Hereditary stomatocytoses are a heterogeneous group of autosomal dominant disorders characterized by moderate to severe hemolytic anemia and a predominance of stomatocytes on peripheral smear. In contrast to patients with HO, the osmotic fragility is markedly increased in patients with hereditary stomatocytosis; the cells look and behave like "swollen" red cells. Membrane lipids and surface area are increased.

Cells from patients with stomatocytosis exhibit a marked increase in intracellular sodium and water due to a vastly increased sodium "leak." $Na^+K^+ATPase$ pump activity is much higher than normal but inadequate to compensate for the leak, resulting in engorged, distended cells. The precise molecular defect is unknown. Various abnormalities in membrane proteins have been reported but have been found to be unrelated to the primary defect upon follow-up study (cf. reference 70).

Hereditary Xerocytosis

Hereditary xerocytosis, also called desiccocytosis, is a rare autosomal hemolytic anemia in which the red cells are *dehydrated* but have *reduced* osmotic fragility.[170] MCHC is increased. Dehydration appears to result from a loss of potassium that is uncompensated by sodium intake. The molecular basis of xerocytosis is not understood. Some patients exhibit features of both stomatocytosis and xerocytosis. These patients have been described as having "intermediate syndromes." Their exact biochemical abnormalities and molecular basis are under investigation. Stomatocytes are also encountered in a variety of acquired conditions, such as hepatobiliary disease and alcoholism. The molecular basis of these findings is unclear; the condition rarely causes significant hematological abnormalities.

Rh Deficiency Syndrome

Rh deficiency syndrome, also called the Rh null phenotype, is a mild to moderate hemolytic anemia associated with stomatocytes, spherocytes, and complete or near absence of the Rh blood group antigen.[96, 176] This clinically heterogeneous disorder is inherited as an autosomal recessive allele. Many defects in osmotic fragility, membrane surface area, potassium transport, and $Na^+K^+ATPase$ activity have been reported. Membrane phospholipid distribution may also be abnormal, but the molecular pathophysiology remains incompletely understood. The recent isolation of the gene encoding the Rh antigen core protein should facilitate molecular analysis.

The McLeod Antigen

The McLeod syndrome is characterized by decreased expression of the Kell antigen on the red cell surface and by acanthocytosis (see reference 170 for review). Chronic granulomatous disease, retinitis pigmentosa, and Duchenne muscular dystrophy have been associated with the McLeod syndrome, because of the close proximity of the genes responsible for the above disorders to the genes for the Kell antigen system on chromosome Xp21. Early reports that attempted to associate red cell morphological abnormalities with Duchenne muscular dystrophy may in fact simply have reflected simultaneous loss of the Kell and Duchenne loci from the X chromosome. The Kell antigen consists of two components. A 37 kDa protein carries the Kx antigen and serves as a precursor necessary for expression of the other protein, a 93 kDa protein that carries the Kell blood group antigen. McLeod red cells lack Kx and have a partial deficiency of the 93 kDa protein. It is not clear why acanthocytes form under these circumstances: Lipid composition, overall protein composition, membrane fluidity, and red cell enzyme and ATP levels have all been found to be normal; phosphorylation of some proteins and lipids, water permeability, and the density of intramembrane particles are abnormal. The acanthocytosis is corrected by exposure of McLeod cells to agents expanding the inner leaflet. Therefore, the reduced amounts of the 93 kDa protein or loss of the Kx protein or both must lead to either expansion of the outer leaflet or contraction of the inner leaflet, thereby producing acanthocytes.

Red Cell Cytoskeletal Proteins and Normal Red Cell Aging

The survival of normal red cells in the circulation is both remarkably long (120 days) and remarkably uniform. They experience progressive loss of vital constituents as they age in the circulation, yet their morphology and biochemistry remain remarkably normal until they are abruptly sequestered from the circulation. Many theories have been advanced to explain this abrupt senescence and destruction.[7, 31] The "geometric" theory is based on the supposition that red cells progressively lose small amounts of membrane as they pass through the spleen, resulting eventually in the formation of rigid spherocytes that are sequestered. The "metabolic" theory states that progressive loss of red cell enzymes causes diminished glycolysis, decreased membrane pump function, and loss of reducing capacity, with consequent oxidation of hemoglobin and membrane protein damage. Neither of these theories satisfactorily explains the uniform appearance and biochemical behavior of erythrocytes that are heterogeneous with respect to age.

Recently, Low and coworkers[32, 33, 177–179] have suggested that immune clearance of senescent red cells accounts for normal red cell destruction. Acceleration of the conditions leading to immune clearance may also explain premature destruction of red cells bearing abnormal hemoglobins, enzyme defects, and/or dysfunctional membrane components.[132, 177] The hypothesis states that metabolic aging results first in oxidation of intracellular hemoglobin, followed by the generation of hemichromes from the denatured hemoglobin. Hemichromes have a high affinity for the cytoplasmic domain of protein 3; upon binding, they promote the aggregation of protein 3 into localized membrane clusters or patches.[34, 177, 178] Thus, hemoglobin denaturation due to any cause results in alteration of the external topology of the red cell. Humans possess an autologous immunoglobulin G (IgG) antibody that recognizes band 3 clusters, but not normally configured protein 3.[178, 179] This polyvalent IgG binds to the erythrocyte, and the immune complex is cleared by macrophages.

From a clinical perspective, delineation of this clearance mechanism is of fundamental importance for understanding the hemolytic component of many inherited and acquired red cell abnormalities, including the hemoglobinopathies and enzymopathies. A final common pathway in these conditions is hemoglobin denaturation with release of hemichromes. Thus, hemoglobin sickling, denaturation of unstable hemoglobins, or hemoglobins oxidized because of red cell enzyme deficiencies could result in sufficient hemichrome formation to accelerate protein 3 clustering and lead to premature clearance (i.e., hemolysis) of the affected red cells. Evidence for the acceleration of this type of immune clearance in sickle cell anemia and thalassemia has recently been published.[173, 180–182]

Red Cell Membrane Proteins in Patients with Hemoglobinopathies

Changes in the membrane cytoskeleton have been implicated in the hemolytic diathesis accompanying sickle cell anemia and the thalassemia syndromes. Spectrin deficiency reminiscent of that encountered in HS has been documented in these patients (cf. reference 172). Controversy exists regarding the exact mechanism by which spectrin deficiencies develop. Binding of denatured hemoglobin, hemichromes, or free globin chains to the cytoskeleton, probably directly to spectrin, has been reported.[183] However, the relevance of the binding phenomena as a cause of spectrin deficiency is unknown. Spectrin deficiency may contribute to the shape changes seen in these diseases as well as to the hemolytic diathesis.

MOLECULAR DEFECTS UNDERLYING RED CELL MEMBRANE PROTEIN DISORDERS

The foregoing discussion has emphasized the fact that different defects in the same cytoskeletal protein can give rise to different forms of hereditary hemolytic anemia; conversely, a single clinical syndrome can arise from defects in many different proteins. Thus, HS, which results from "vertical" abnormalities in the band 3/spectrin/ankyrin association, could conceivably arise from abnormalities of any of those proteins (see Fig. 7–11). HE, which seems to involve abnormal spectrin self-association and weakened "horizontal" junctions, could arise from defects in spectrin, protein 4.1, protein 4.2, or glycophorin C (cf. references 142 and 170). These predictions have been verified by direct analysis of the genes and mRNAs encoding abnormal proteins in patients with HS, HE, HPP, and HO. In general, the characterization of these mutations has utilized a common approach. Membrane abnormalities were first correlated with biochemical deficiencies or abnormalities of individual proteins in a given patient or kindred. The abnormality was then characterized at the genetic level, usually by use of the PCR reaction to amplify segments of the genes or mRNAs predicted to be abnormal by protein analyses. Mutations in the genes encoding α spectrin, β spectrin, ankyrin, protein 4.1, glycophorin C, protein 4.2, and band 3 have all been implicated as the cause of HE, HS, HPP, and/or HO. In this section, we examine the defects in each gene, noting the syndromes associated with particular defects.

Spectrin Defects

Spectrin defects constitute the most complex and thoroughly analyzed group of mutations. Because of the large size of the spectrin α and β chains, their mRNAs, and their genomic loci, it was important to have preliminary methods for "scanning" the spectrin chains for the likely location of the mutation. This scanning would then allow analysis of a limited region along the mRNA sequence by the use of PCR technology. Fortunately, spectrin can be subdivided into reproducible domains by limited proteolytic digestion at 0°C.[184] A fingerprint of normal spectrin domains (Fig. 7–12A) can be obtained by one-dimensional or two-dimensional electrophoresis and can be compared with comparable fingerprints from patients. The fragments are named according to their chain of origin, size order (I = largest, II = next largest, and so on), and apparent molecular weight (Fig. 7–12B). Thus, $\alpha^{I/80}$ refers to the largest peptide domain of the spectrin α chain, having a molecular weight of approximately 80 kDa; $\alpha^{I/74}$ refers to an abnormal peptide of 74 kDa, rather than 80 kDa, found in some patients with spectrin mutations.[185–187] Domains of interest in which spectrin mutations have been identified are αI, αII, and βIV; mutations have also been identified at the extreme C-terminus of the spectrin β chain.[58, 142, 170]

α Spectrin Mutations

The most common α spectrin mutations affect the αI domain, which is located at the amino-terminal end of spectrin (Fig. 7–13); this region is critical for interaction with β spectrin to form dimers and for dimer-dimer association to form tetramers (cf. references 142, 170, and 171). Mutations alter the size of the α domain by deranging folding, thereby exposing normally inaccessible recognition sequences to the protease and altering the digestion pattern. Mutations have been subclassified by the size of the abnormal peptide. The most common, important, and interesting mutations at the present time are those producing the $\alpha^{I/74}$ peptide; these expose arginine 45 or lysine 48 for cleavage, thereby truncating the normal αI domain.[188–191]

In competition experiments, purified normal αI domains compete well with intact α spectrin in the oligomerization reaction, implying that $\alpha^{I/80}$ possesses the essential information necessary for dimer and tetramer formation.[189] Since $\alpha^{I/74}$ does not compete, the key information must reside in the first 45 to 48 amino acids that form the first helix of α spectrin. Since this helix interacts with two helices at the C-terminus of β spectrin to form dimers (see Fig. 7–7), it is not surprising that mutations in these regions of the α and β chains are the most common and most widespread cause of defective self-association. Amino acid 28 is a particularly common site at which mutations causing HE generate the $\alpha^{I/74}$ fragment.[188, 189, 191, 193] Less common mutations foreshorten the αI domain to 65, 50, or 78 kDa (cf. references 192, 194–202). All of these mutations share certain features: They are base substitutions producing single amino acid changes that affect the ability of spectrin dimers to form tetramers. The positions of these mutations localize specific amino acids that are critical for self-associations, such as amino acids 41 to 49, amino acid

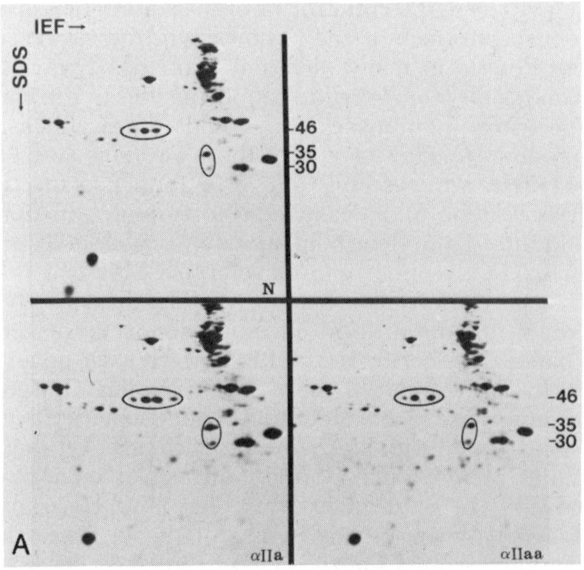

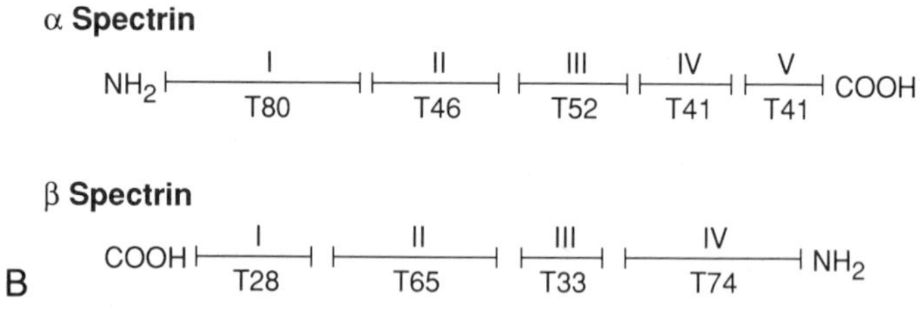

α Spectrin

β Spectrin

B

FIGURE 7–12. Analyses of normal and abnormal spectrins by two-dimensional fingerprint analysis of partial tryptic digest. *A* shows fingerprints of a normal (N) and two abnormal spectrin preparations from patients with HE (αIIa, αIIaa). After mild digestion at 0°C with limiting amounts of trypsin, the digested proteins are separated by SDS gel electrophoresis in one dimension and by isoelectric focusing (IEF) in the other, as indicated above the panel labeled N. The approximate molecular weights, based on gel markers not shown in this figure, are shown for the fragments relative to this analysis at 46, 35, and 30 kDa. On the basis of the large body of work obtained with normal spectrin α and β chains, the tryptic digestion map shown in *B* has been obtained. The panel labeled αIIa in *A* shows that the 46 kDa family of spots is different by the addition of a spot in this patient with HE, and the panel labeled αIIaa shows a change in charge of a prominent spot at approximately 30 kDa. As discussed in the text, further analysis of these abnormal spots reveals their derivation from a particular tryptic domain, in this case the αII domain, and guides the use of polymerase chain reaction analyses of mRNA for precise identification of the mutation. In *B*, the letter T indicates that the fragments (domains) are obtained by digestion with trypsin, and the numbers indicate the approximate molecular weight of the normal fragments. (Adapted, with permission, from the Annual Reviews in Cell Biology, Vol. 1, © 1985 by Annual Reviews, Inc.; and from the Journal of Clinical Investigation, 1987, Vol. 80, p. 191, by copyright permission of the American Society for Clinical Investigation.)

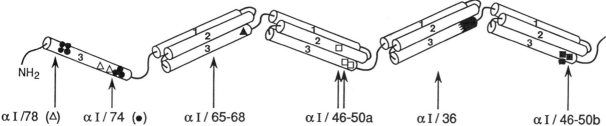

FIGURE 7–13. **Representative location of mutations at the amino-terminus of the α spectrin chain that produce HE or HPP.** The diagram shows only the first 80 kDa at the amino-terminus of the α spectrin chain. The three helical segments within each repeating subunit that form the basic three-dimensional structure of spectrin are indicated. Note that helices 1 and 2 at the extreme amino-terminus of α spectrin are provided by the extreme carboxy-terminus of β spectrin (see Fig. 7–14). Shown underneath the diagram are positions of mutations that alter the tryptic digestion patterns, producing abnormal fragments of indicated sizes. (Adapted and updated from Gallagher, P. G., Tse, W. T., and Forget, B. G.: Clinical and Molecular aspects of disorders of the erythrocyte membrane skeleton. Semin. Perinatol. 14:351–367, 1990; with permission.)

28, or region around amino acid 260, and amino acid 470. Most of these changes cause mild to moderately severe HE. The $\alpha^{I/74}$ and $\alpha^{I/50a}$ mutation can produce HPP in the doubly heterozygous or homozygous state. $\alpha^{I/65}$ Homozygotes have moderately severe HE.

A single mutation in the αII domain of spectrin, alanine to arginine in the αIX helix, is asymptomatic in the heterozygous state but produces autosomal recessive HS in the homozygous state.[203, 204] The biochemical defect caused by this mutation is not defined, but spectrin association does not appear to be involved. It is tempting to speculate that this mutation might influence interaction with ankyrin. A second mutation, spectrin Jendouba, does disrupt dimer-dimer contact.[205] It is located in repeat 7. Like the αI mutations, it produces mild HE.

β Spectrin Mutations

Several mutations of β spectrin have now been characterized[206–213] (Fig. 7–14). One amino-terminal mutation that produces dominantly inherited HS results from a TRP → ARG substitution at position 202 and disrupts contact and complex formations between spectrin and protein 4.1.[213] For unknown reasons, this mutation results in a secondary spectrin deficiency, possibly due to the weakened formation of junctional complexes. The reciprocal mutation of protein 4.1 that weakens the junctions does not, interestingly, cause HS; rather, mild to moderate HE results (cf. reference 170).

Most of the β spectrin mutations have been found near the extreme C-terminus.[206–212, 214] This is the site on β spectrin that interacts with α spectrin to initiate chain-to-chain contact and dimer-dimer association into tetramers.[142, 170] Mutations in this region of β spectrin should and do produce effects similar to those of the amino-terminus of α spectrin. The genetic mechanism underlying most of these mutations, however, is different. In contrast to a predominance of amino acid substitutions occurring in the αI domain, these abnormal β spectrins tend to be truncated at the C-terminal end as a result of mutations that disrupt

splicing or lead to frameshifts, or both.[208–212] Two exons, called X and Y, near the 3' end of the spectrin gene, are involved in most of these mutations. In one case, exon Y is skipped entirely; the abnormal splice results in a frameshift and premature chain termination within exon X. In other cases, mutations altering the reading frame or splicing of exon X result in the creation of premature chain terminations, usually owing to frameshifts. For example, one mutation is an interstitial 7 bp deletion that alters the reading frame.

Some β spectrin mutations, such as ALA → PRO at position 2053 in exon X, are particularly instructive. The β spectrin mutation at residue 2053 was originally detected and characterized as an $\alpha^{I/74}$ mutation.[190, 193, 194] Analysis of these patients revealed no abnormalities of the α spectrin sequence. The generation of the $\alpha^{I/74}$ peptide results from the disruptive effects of the abnormal β spectrin on the folding of the amino-terminus of α spectrin. Thus, mutations in one spectrin chain can clearly alter the configuration and, presumably, the function or stability of the other chain.

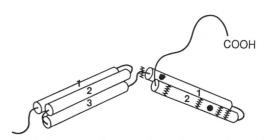

FIGURE 7–14. **Representative mutations of β spectrin producing hereditary elliptocytosis (HE) and hereditary pyropoikilocytosis (HPP).** Only the extreme C-terminus of the molecule is shown. Note that β spectrin supplies only helices 1 and 2 near the C-terminus. Helix 3, as noted in Figure 7–13, is supplied by the amino-terminus of α spectrin. As noted in the text, some of these mutations actually cause abnormalities in the digestion pattern of α spectrin. (Adapted and updated from Gallagher, P. G., Tse, W. T., and Forget, B. G.: Clinical and Molecular aspects of disorders of the erythrocyte membrane skeleton. Semin. Perinatol. 14:351–367, 1990; with permission.)

Ankyrin Mutations

Ankyrin deficiency has been documented to be the primary defect in a mouse model of HS, the *nb* mutation.[168] Ankyrin deficiency, analyzed at the level of protein biochemistry, has been documented in some cases of HS.[142, 170, 215, 216] Complete deletion of the ankyrin gene from chromosome 8 in patients with HS associated with mental retardation has been identified.[217–219] It does seem likely that ankyrin mutations produce some forms of HS. Co-inheritance of HS in a large kindred and a restriction fragment length polymorphism (RFLP) of the ankyrin gene has been reported.[219] As of this writing, unfortunately, direct association of ankyrin mutations with common forms of HS has not yet been demonstrated. An exception is ankyrin Prague,[220] which is dominantly co-inherited with mild HS and is associated with a fast-migrating ankyrin variant exhibiting deranged function of the regulatory domain.

Protein 4.1 Defects

Two major classes of molecular abnormality of protein 4.1 have been reported: those producing selective deficiency of protein 4.1 from red cells and those disrupting the erythroid-specific spectrin-actin–binding domain (exon 15).[140, 141, 221–227] Both categories are associated with mild HE in the simple heterozygous state. Homozygous protein 4.1 deficiency, the only homozygous state described thus far, is associated with severe HE and is common in North Africa.[140, 141]

Two abnormalities of the spectrin-actin–binding domain of protein 4.1 have been identified.[221, 222] One produces an elongated protein, 95 kDa long, resulting from duplication of three exons encoding the spectrin-actin domain, with consequent duplication of amino acids 407 to 529. Duplication causes mild abnormality of junctional complex formation. A truncated form of protein 4.1, protein 4.1[68/65], lacks the spectrin-actin–binding domain because of deletion of the exons encoding the spectrin-actin–binding site and amino acids 407 to 486, with consequent weakened interaction with spectrin and actin.

In the forms of protein 4.1 deficiency studied thus far, the deficiency occurs selectively in red cells, because of the complex regulation of tissue-specific alternative mRNA splicing that occurs during erythropoiesis.[133, 138–141] As shown in Figure 7–9, and discussed in an earlier section, non-erythroid cells synthesize considerable amounts of a high molecular weight isoform of protein 4.1, owing to splicing events at the 5' end of the gene that convert a portion of the 5' untranslated region into translatable sequence. The high molecular weight isoform thus contains the entire 80 kDa segment found in erythroid protein 4.1, plus a 209 amino acid "headpiece" added to the amino-terminus.[133] These splicing events are totally suppressed at an early stage of erythropoiesis, so that virtually no high molecular weight isoform is present in mature red cells. Rather, the translation of the protein is initiated at an internal methionine codon. One form of selective erythroid protein 4.1 deficiency has been shown to arise by deletion and/or gene rearrangement that removes the exon containing this internal translation initiation site.[140] Thus, erythroid cells, lacking the ability to translate from the upstream start site, cannot produce protein 4.1 from the mutant allele. Non-erythroid cells, possessing the upstream start site, synthesize the high molecular weight form. A form of protein 4.1 deficiency encountered in Spaniards has been shown to result from an analogous mechanism, a point mutation that abolishes the downstream initiator methionine.[141]

Glycophorin Defects

As noted earlier, multiple mutations resulting in the production of abnormal or deficient glycophorin A and B have been documented (cf. reference 55). None of these result in phenotypic abnormalities of red cells, other than alteration of blood group phenotypes and increased resistance to malarial invasion. Two mutations have been associated with mild HE and complete absence of glycophorin C in homozygotes.[228] These rare mutations are asymptomatic in the heterozygous state. One results in deletion of exons 3 and 4, whereas the other is a frameshift in codons 44 and 45. In both cases, frameshifting and premature translation termination result. An interesting aspect of these mutations is the fact that protein 4.1 deficiency occurs concomitantly in these cells, suggesting once again that protein stability after translation depends on successful incorporation into the cytoskeleton (cf. reference 55).

Protein 4.2 Defects

Even though the function of protein 4.2 is incompletely understood, its role in stabilizing the formation of the spectrin/actin/protein 4.1 junctional complex appears to be physiologically important, because of the fact that deficiencies or defects in this protein are being increasingly appreciated as causes of varying forms of HE and HS. Most of the mutations are point mutations that presumably alter function.[158, 229]

Band 3 Defects

As previously noted, some defects of protein 3, characterized at the level of protein function, have been correlated with acanthocytosis and, possibly, the chorea-acanthocytosis syndrome. Protein 3 defects have also been associated by RFLP linkage with cases of HS marked by selective deficiency of band 3 and by functional studies with some cases of dominantly inherited HS.[142, 170] Band 3 mutations may be a common source of the more prevalent forms of HS; DNA analysis of the band 3 gene in HS is under way in several laboratories.[230, 231]

The most thoroughly studied and understood band 3 defects are those associated with Southeast Asian hereditary ovalocytosis (cf. references 50 to 54, 56, and 57). Molecular analysis of the common form has identified an intron/exon deletion that results in loss of amino acids 400 to 408; this is the "interdomain" hinge region that may be important for the flexibility of the cytoskeleton at the point of the protein 3/ankyrin/spectrin association.[54] A tightly linked polymorphism at codon 56 is co-inherited with the most common of these defects.[56] Mutations that alter the hinge region produce marked reductions in lateral mobility, increased phosphorylation, tightening and rigidification of the vertical association of band 3 with the cytoskeleton, and rigid red cells. The anion transport function of band 3 may also be abnormal, since binding to the specific inhibitor of the protein, DIDS, and actual anion transport have both been shown to be altered.[57]

Impact of the Cytoskeletal Protein Mutations on Non-erythroid Tissues

For the most part, hereditary hemolytic anemias due to abnormal cytoskeletal proteins exhibit clinical abnormalities confined to the red cells, despite the fact that many of these cytoskeletal proteins are widely expressed. In some cases, the selectivity of clinical abnormalities can be attributed to the fact that the defects occur only in erythroid-specific genes or isoforms. Most non-erythroid tissues rely, for example, on a different gene for production of the α spectrin isoform, fodrin; similarly, abnormal or deficient protein 4.1 in some forms of hereditary elliptocytosis is due to abnormalities that affect only the erythroid-specific spliceoforms. This explanation alone is not completely satisfying, however, because "erythroid-specific" forms of some of these proteins are in fact expressed selectively in some other tissues. For instance, the erythroid form of β spectrin and the exon associated with the erythroid spectrin-actin–binding domain of protein 4.1 both appear to be expressed abundantly in muscle. Erythroid ankyrin may be expressed in muscle, kidney, and some parts of the central nervous system, even though a brain-specific isoform of ankyrin clearly exists. Indeed, ankyrin deficiency in mice and in some forms of HS has been associated with mental retardation and spinal cord abnormalities, although none of these have been directly attributed to the cytoskeletal protein deficiency. Nonetheless, the vast majority of patients with cytoskeletal protein defects are phenotypically normal except for their red cells.[55, 58, 142, 170, 171] These findings demand explanation of the ability of quantitative or qualitative defects of cytoskeletal proteins to disrupt erythroid homeostasis without deranging function in at least some other tissues.

A mutation producing an abnormal cytoskeletal protein could impair red cell function without causing significant abnormalities in non-erythroid cells because of the unique mechanical and biochemical demands placed on the membrane and cytoskeleton of erythrocytes. For the most part, the mutations that cause hereditary hemolytic anemia are those that alter the ability of the membrane to withstand shear stress. Indeed, in the most commonly encountered forms of these diseases, these abnormalities are relatively mild. They are detected more often by a distinctive morphology than by any clinical symptomatology. It is doubtful that comparably mild defects in other organ systems would come to clinical attention. Indeed, mutations that primarily affect mechanical stability under conditions of shear stress may not produce any deleterious effects on the cytoskeletons of non-circulating cells.

Red cells are unique in that they must survive for long periods, even though they cannot repair or replenish their proteins. A final pathway common to forms of hereditary spherocytosis and elliptocytosis is quantitative deficiency of the protein, resulting in mild to moderate shortening of red cell survival. In other tissues, it is possible, even likely, that these deficiencies can be overcome by the continual biosynthesis of new proteins. As noted in an earlier section, actual assembly of most cytoskeletal components appears to be limited more by post-translational incorporations of these proteins into the cytoskeleton than by the rates of de novo biosynthesis. Deficiencies in red cells result largely because the erythrocyte is released into the circulation with only the amount of protein that is already incorporated into the cytoskeleton. Once lost from the cytoskeleton, these proteins cannot be replaced. This is probably not the case for nucleated cells. Red cell membrane protein defects are instructive for understanding the complex relationships that can exist between a mutation and its ultimate phenotypic expression in different tissues.

SUMMARY AND CONCLUSIONS

Membranes form the boundaries of cells, defining their interface with the external environment and protecting them from noxious materials in that environment, while at the same time permitting communication and selective molecular exchange with it. Membranes also provide hydrophobic sites for sequestration, compartmentalization, and regulation of intracellular metabolic events. The ability of membranes to serve these fundamental biological functions is, as outlined in this chapter, dependent on the precise assembly and non-covalent interaction of a complex array of lipids, integral proteins, and the attached proteins that form the cytoskeleton. In particular, membranes can survive and function only because of their interaction with cytoskeletal protein frameworks that confer shape and mechanical stability on the lipid bilayer.

Abnormalities of the membrane-cytoskeletal unit that lead to human disease have been best exemplified by defects of the red cell membrane that produce morphological abnormalities or frank hemolytic anemias. These conditions have stimulated successful attempts to isolate and characterize the major lipid and protein components of both the membrane and the underlying cytoskeleton, to isolate and characterize their genes, and to identify mutations that derange function. As noted in the preceding section, the structure-function relationships, as well as the abnormalities created by the mutations studied thus far, may represent special cases largely applicable only to the unique membrane and cytoskeleton of red cells. However, these investigations have provided the core biochemical knowledge needed to pursue the study of cell membranes in general.

It is clear from the analysis of erythrocytes that the cytoskeleton is a vital element of the cell necessary for membrane function, motility, response to metabolic demands altering shape, and extracellular-intracellular signaling. The characterization of erythroid and non-erythroid forms of the key cytoskeletal proteins is now largely complete, an advance that should pave the way for application of the experimental paradigm used for red cell membranes to the studies of normal and disease functions of non-erythroid cells. The mutations producing red cell membrane defects also appear to offer the most promising, well-defined system available at the present time to study the pleiotropic effects of mutations upon formation of complex multimolecular assemblies.

REFERENCES

1. Morrow, J.: Plasma membrane dynamics and organization. *In* Hoffman, R., Benz, E. J., Jr., Shattil, S., Furie, B., and Cohen, H. (eds.): Hematology: Basic Principles and Practice. New York, Churchill Livingstone, 1991, pp. 36–50.
2. Stryer, L.: Biochemistry. 3rd ed. New York, W. H. Freeman, 1988.
3. Alberts, B., Bray, D., Lewis, J., Raff, M., Roberts, K., and Watson, J. D.: Molecular Biology of the Cell. 2nd ed. New York, Garland, 1989.
4. Tanford, C.: The Hydrophobic Effect: Formation of Micelles and Biological Membranes. 2nd ed. New York, Wiley-Interscience, 1980.
5. Fairbanks, G., Steck, T. L., and Wallach, D. F. H.: Electrophoretic analysis of the major polypeptides of the human erythrocyte membrane. Biochemistry 10:2606, 1971.
6. Steck, T. L., Fairbanks, G., and Wallach, D. F. H.: Disposition of the major proteins in the isolated erythrocyte membrane. Proteolytic dissection. Biochemistry 10:2617, 1971.
7. Agre, P., and Parker, J. C. (eds.): Red Blood Cell Membranes. New York, Marcel Dekker, 1989.
8. Skene, J. H., and Virag, I.: Posttranslational membrane attachment and dynamic fatty acylation of a neuronal growth cone protein, GAP-43. J. Cell Biol. 108:613, 1989.
9. Tomita, M., Furthmayr, H., and Marchesi, V. T.: Primary structure of human erythrocyte glycophorin A: Isolation and characterization of peptides and complete amino acid sequence. Biochemistry 17:4756, 1978.
10. Marchesi, V. T.: Functional adaptations of transbilayer proteins. *In* Dhindsu, D. S., and Bahl, O. P. (eds.): Molecular and Cellular Aspects of Reproduction. New York, Plenum, 1986, p. 107.
11. Kleffel, B., Garavito, R. M., Baumeister, W., and Rosenbusch, J. P.: Secondary structure of a channel-forming protein: Porin from *E. coli* outer membranes. EMBO J. 4:1589, 1985.
12. Bennett, V.: The spectrin actin junction of erythrocyte membrane skeletons. Biochim. Biophys. Acta. 988:107, 1989.
13. Marchesi, V. T.: The stabilizing infrastructure of cell membranes. Annu. Rev. Cell Biol. 1:531, 1985.
14. Lux, S. C., John, K. M., and Bennett, V.: Analysis of cDNA for human erythrocyte ankyrin indicates a repeated structure with homology to tissue-differentiation and cell-cycle control proteins. Nature 344:36, 1990.
15. Vaz, W. L. C., Derzko, Z. I., and Jacobson, K. A.: Photobleaching measurements of the lateral diffusion of lipids and proteins in artificial phospholipid bilayer membranes. Cell Surf. Rev. 8:83, 1982.
16. Kornberg, R. D., and McConnell, H. M.: Inside-outside transitions of phospholipids in vesicle membranes. Biochemistry 10:1111, 1971.
17. Golan, D. E.: Red blood cell membrane protein and lipid diffusion: *In* Agre P., and Parker, J. C. (eds.): Red Blood Cell Membranes: Structure, Function, Clinical Implications. New York, Marcel Dekker, 1989, p. 367.
18. Yechiel, E., and Edidin M.: Micrometer-scale domains in fibroblast plasma membranes. J. Cell Biol. 105:755, 1987.
19. Bloch, R., and Morrow J. S.: An unusual β-spectrin associated with clustered acetylcholine receptors. J. Cell Biol. 108:481, 1989.
20. Mahaffey, D. T., Moore M. S., Brodsky F. M., and Anderson, R. G.: Coat proteins isolated from clathrin coated vesicles can assemble into coated pits. J. Cell Biol. 108:1615, 1989.
21. Buck, C. A., and Horwitz, A. F.: Cell surface receptors for extracellular matrix molecules. Annu. Rev. Cell Biol. 3:179, 1987.
22. Gumbiner, B., and Louvard D.: Localized barriers in the plasma membrane: A common way to form domains. Trends Biochem. Sci. 10:435, 1985.
23. Elgsaeter, A., and Branton, D.: Intramembrane particle aggregation in erythrocyte ghosts. I. The effects of protein removal. J. Cell Biol. 63:1018, 1974.
24. Nelson, W. J., and Veshnock, P. J.: Ankyrin binding to (Na$^+$K)ATPase and implications for the organization of membrane domains in polarized cells. Nature 328:533, 1987.
25. Srinivasan, Y., Elmer, L., Davis, J., Bennett, V., and Angelides, K.: Ankyrin and spectrin associate with voltage-dependent sodium channels in brain. Nature 333:177, 1988.
26. Anderson, R. A., and Marchesi, V. T.: Regulation of the association of membrane skeletal protein 4.1 with glycophorin by a polyphosphoinositide. Nature 318:295, 1985.
27. Sato, S. B., and Ohnishi, S.: Interaction of a peripheral protein of the erythrocyte membrane, band 4.1, with phosphatidylserine-containing liposomes and erythrocyte inside-out vesicles. Eur. J. Biochem. 130:19, 1983.
28. Morrow, J. S., and Marchesi, V. T.: Self-assembly of spectrin oligomers in vitro: A basis for a dynamic cytoskeleton. J. Cell Biol. 88:463, 1981.
29. Becker, P. S., and Benz, E. J., Jr.: Molecular biology of the red cell membrane proteins. *In* Chien, S. (ed.): Molecular Biology of the Cardiovascular System. Philadelphia, Lea and Febiger, 1990, pp. 155–182.
30. Mohandas, N.: The red cell membrane. *In* Hoffman, R., Benz, E. J., Jr., Shattil, S., Furie, B., and Cohen, H. (eds.): Hematology: Basic Principles and Practice. New York, Churchill Livingstone, 1991, pp. 264–269.
31. Brewer, G. (ed.): The Red Cell: Seventh Ann Arbor Conference. New York, Alan R. Liss, 1989.
32. Kannan, R., Yuan J., and Low P. S.: Isolation and partial characterization of antibody and globin-enriched complexes from membranes of dense human erythrocytes. Biochem. J. 278:57, 1991.
33. Waugh, S. M., and Low, P. S.: Hemochrome binding to band 3: Nucleation of Heinz bodies on the erythrocyte membrane. Biochemistry 24:34, 1985.
34. Low, P. S.: Interaction of native and denatured hemoglobins with band 3: Consequences for erythrocyte structure and function. *In* Agre P., and Parker, J. C. (eds.): Red Blood Cell Membranes. New York, Marcel Dekker, 1989, pp. 237–260.
35. Weed, R. I.: The importance of erythrocyte deformability. Am. J. Med. 49:147, 1970.

36. Chien, S.: Red cell deformability and its relevance to blood flow. Annu. Rev. Physiol. 49:177, 1987.

37. Mohandas, N., Chasis, J. A., and Shohet, S. B.: The influence of membrane skeleton on red cell deformability, membrane material properties, and shape. Semin. Hematol. 20:225, 1983.

38. Mohandas, N., Phillips, W. M., and Bessis, M.: Red blood cell deformability and hemolytic anemias. Semin. Hematol. 16:95, 1979.

39. Palek, J.: Hereditary elliptocytosis, spherocytosis and related disorders: Consequences of a deficiency or a mutation of membrane skeletal proteins. Blood Rev. 1:147, 1987.

40. Chasis, J. A., Agre, P., and Mohandas, N.: Decreased membrane mechanical stability and in vivo loss of surface area reflect spectrin deficiencies in hereditary spherocytosis. J. Clin. Invest. 82:617, 1988.

41. Evans, E. A., and La Celle, P. L.: Intrinsic material properties of erythrocyte membrane indicated by mechanical analysis of deformation. Blood 45:29, 1975.

42. Hochmuth, R. M., and Waugh, R. E.: Erythrocyte membrane elasticity and viscosity. Annu. Rev. Physiol. 49:209, 1987.

43. Liu, S. C., Derick, L. H., and Palek, J.: Visualization of the hexagonal lattice in the erythrocyte membrane skeleton. J. Cell Biol. 104:527, 1987.

44. Fowler, V., and Taylor, D. L.: Spectrin plus band 4.1 cross-link actin: Regulation by micromolar calcium. J. Cell Biol. 85:361, 1980.

45. Ways, P., and Hanahan, D. J.: Characterization and quantitation of red cell lipids in normal man. J. Lipid Res. 5:318, 1964.

46. Verkleij, A. J., Zwaal, R. F. A., Roelofsen, B., et al.: The asymmetric distribution of phospholipids in the human red cell membrane. A combined study using phospholipases and freeze-etch electron microscopy. Biochim. Biophys. Acta 323:178, 1973.

47. Bennet, V., and Stenbuck, P. J.: Association between ankyrin and the cytoplasmic domain of ban 3 isolated from the human erythrocyte membrane. J. Biol. Chem. 225:6426, 1980.

48. Hargreaves, W. R., Giedd, K. N., Verkleij, A., and Branton, D.: Reassociation of ankyrin with band 3 in erythrocyte membranes and lipid vesicles. J. Biol. Chem. 225:11965, 1980.

49. Drickamer, L. K.: Fragmentation of the band 3 polypeptide from human erythrocyte membranes. J. Biol. Chem. 252:6909, 1977.

50. Liu, S. C., Zhai, S., Palek, J., Golan, D. E., Amato, D., Hassan, K., Nurse, G. T., Babona, T., Koetzer, T., Jarolim, P., Zaik, M., and Borwein, S.: Molecular defect of the band 3 protein in Southeast Asian ovalocytosis, N. Engl. J. Med. 323:1530, 1990.

51. Low, P. S., Willardson, B. M., Thevenin, B., Kannan, R., Mahler, E., Geahlen, R. L., and Harrison, M.: The other functions of erythrocyte membrane band 3. In Hamasaki, N., and Jennings, M. J. (eds.): Anion Transport Proteins of the Red Cell Membrane. Amsterdam, Elsevier, 1989, pp. 103–118.

52. Lux, S. E., John, K. M., Kopito, R. R., and Lodish, H. F.: Cloning and characterization of band 3, the human erythrocyte anion exchange protein (AE1). Proc. Natl. Acad. Sci. USA 86:9089, 1989.

53. Low, P. S.: Structure and function of the cytoplasmic domain of band 3: Center of erythrocyte membrane–peripheral protein interactions. Biochim. Biophys. Acta 864:145, 1986.

54. Mohandas, N., Winardi, R., Knowles, D., Leung, A., Parra, M., George, E., Conboy, J., and Chasis, J.: Molecular basis for membrane rigidity of hereditary ovalocytosis: A novel mechanism involving the cytoplasmic domain of band 3. J. Clin. Invest. 89:686, 1992.

55. Chasis, J. A., and Mohandas, N.: Red cell glycophorins. Blood 80:1869, 1992.

56. Golan, D. E., and Veatch, W.: Lateral mobility of band 3 in the human erythrocyte membrane studied by fluorescence photobleaching recovery: Evidence for control by cytoskeletal interactions. Proc. Natl. Acad. Sci. USA 77:2537, 1980.

57. Tanner, M. J. A., Wainwright, S. D., and Martin, P. G.: The structure and molecular genetics of the human erythrocyte anion transport protein. In Hamasaki, N., and Jennings, M. J. (eds.): Anion Transport Proteins of the Red Cell Membrane. Amsterdam, Elsevier, 1989, pp. 121–132.

58. Palek, J., and Sahr, K. E.: Mutations of the red cell membrane proteins: From clinical evaluation to detection of the underlying genetic defect. Blood 80:308, 1992.

59. Kopito, R. R., Andersson, M., and Lodish, H. F.: Structure and organization of the murine band 3 gene. J. Biol. Chem. 262:8035, 1987.

60. Tomita, M., and Marchesis, V. T.: Amino-acid sequence and oligosaccharide attachment sites of human erythrocyte glycophorin. Proc. Natl. Acad. Sci. USA 72:2964, 1975.

61. Tomita, M., Furthmayr, H., and Marchesi, V. T.: Primary structure of human erythrocyte glycophorin-A. Isolation and characterization of peptides and complete amino acid sequence. Biochemistry 17:4756, 1978.

62. Siebert, P. D., and Fukuda, M.: Isolation and characterization of human glycophorin A cDNA clones by a synthetic oligonucleotide approach: Nucleotide sequence and mRNA structure. Proc. Natl. Acad. Sci. USA 83:1665, 1986.

63. Siebert, P. D., and Fukuda, M.: Molecular cloning of human glycophorin-B cDNA: Nucleotide sequence and relationship to glycophorin-A. Proc. Natl. Acad. Sci. USA 85:421, 1987.

64. Colin, Y., Rahuel, C., London, J., Romeo, P. H., d'Auriol, L., Galibert, F., and Cartron, J. P.: Isolation of cDNA clones for human erythrocyte glycophorin C. J. Biol. Chem. 261:229, 1986.

65. Blanchard, D., Dahr, W., Hummel, M., Latron, F., Beyreuther, K., and Cartron, J. P.: Glycophorin-B and C from human erythrocyte membranes: Purification and sequence analysis. J. Biol. Chem. 262:5808, 1987.

66. Blanchard, D., El-Maliki, B., Hermand, P., Dahr, W., and Cartron, J. P.: Structural homology between glycophorins C and D, two minor glycoproteins of the human erythrocyte membrane carrying blood group Gerbich antigen. In Proceedings of the IXth International Symposium on Glycoconjugates, Lille, France, 1987, p. F54.

67. Mattei, M. G., Colin, Y., LeVan Kim, C., Mattei, J. F., and Cartron, J. P.: Localization of the gene for human erythrocyte-C to chromosome 2, q14–q21. Hum. Genet. 74:420, 1986.

68. Tate, C. G., and Tanner, M. J. A.: Isolation of cDNA clones for human erythrocyte membrane sialoglycoproteins α and δ. Biochem. J. 254:743, 1988.

69. Kudo, S., and Fukuda, M.: Identification of a novel human glycophorin, glycophorin E, by isolation of genomic clones and complementary DNA clones utilizing polymerase chain reaction. J. Biol. Chem. 265:1102, 1990.

70. Vignal, A., Rahuel, C., London, J., Cherif-Zahar, B., Schaff, S., Hattab, C., Okubo, Y., and Cartron, J. P.: A novel member of the glycophorin A and B family. Molecular cloning and expression. Eur. J. Biochem. 191:619, 1990.

71. Welsh, E. J., and Thom, D.: Molecular organization of glycophorin A: Implications for molecular interactions. Biopolymers 24:2301, 1985.

72. Furthmayr, H.: Glycophorins A, B, C: A family of sialoglycoproteins. Isolation and preliminary characterization of trypsin-derived peptides. J. Supramol. Struct. 9:79, 1978.

73. Rahuel, C., London, J., d'Auriol, L., Mattei, M. G., Tournamille, C., Skrzynia, C., Lebouc, Y., Galibert, F., and Cartron, J. P.: Characterization of cDNA clones for human glycophorin A. Use for gene localization and for analysis of normal and glycophorin A deficient (Finnish type) genomic DNA. Eur. J. Biochem. 172:147, 1988.

74. Kudo, S., and Fukuda, M.: Structural organization of glycophorin A and B genes: Glycophorin B gene evolved by homologous recombination at Alu repeat sequences. Proc. Natl. Acad. Sci. USA 86:4619, 1989.

75. Vignal, A., Rahuel, C., El Maliki, B., LeVan, Kim, C., London, J., Blanchard, D., d'Auriol, L., Galibert, F., Blajchman, M.

A., and Cartron, J. P.: Molecular analysis of glycophorin A and B gene structure and expression in homozygotes Milterberger class V (Mi^V) human erythrocytes. Eur. J. Biochem. 184:337, 1989.

76. Vignal, A., London, J., Rahuel, C., and Cartron, J. P.: Promoter sequence and chromosomal organization of the genes encoding glycophorins A, B and E. Gene 95:289, 1990.

77. Chien, S., and Sung, L. A.: Physiochemical basis and clinical implications of red cell aggregation. Clin. Hemorheology 7:71, 1987.

78. Dahr, W.: Immunochemistry of sialoglycoproteins in human red blood cell membranes. *In* Vengelen-Tyler, V., and Judd, W. J. (eds.): Recent Advances in Blood Group Biochemistry. Arlington, Va, American Association of Blood Banks, 1986, p. 23.

79. Anstee, D. J.: The blood group MNSs-active sialoglycoproteins. Semin. Hematol. 18:13, 1981.

80. Dahr, W., Beyreuther, K., Steinbach, H., Gielen, W., and Kruger, J.: Structure of the Ss blood group antigens. II. A methionine/threonine polymorphism within the N-terminal sequence of the Ss glycoprotein. Hoppe-Seyler's Z Physiol. Chem. 361:895, 1980.

81. Cook, P. J. L., Lindenbaum, R. H., Salonen, R., De La Chapelle, A., Daker, M. G., Buckton, K. E., Noades, J. E., and Tippett, P.: The MNSs blood group of families with chromosome 4 rearrangements. Ann. Hum. Genet. 45:39, 1981.

82. Reid, M. E., Anstee, D. J., Jensen, R. H., and Mohandas, N.: Normal membrane function of abnormal β-related erythrocyte sialoglycoproteins. Br. J. Haematol. 67:467, 1987.

83. Tanner, M. J. A., and Anstee, D. J.: The membrane change in En(A−) human erythrocytes. Absence of the major erythrocyte sialoglycoprotein. Biochem. J. 153:271, 1976.

84. Tokunaga, E., Sasakawa, S., Tamaka, K., Kawamata, H., Giles, C. M., Ikin, E. W., Poole, J., Anstee, D. J., Mawby, W., and Tanner, M. J. A.: Two apparently healthy Japanese individuals to type M^kM^k have erythrocytes which lack both the blood group MN and Ss-active sialoglycoproteins. J. Immunogenet. 6:383, 1979.

85. Cartron, J. P., Colin, Y., Kudo, S., and Fukuda, M.: Molecular genetics of human erythrocyte sialoglycoproteins Glycophorins A, B, C and D. *In* Harris, J. R. (ed.): Blood Cell Biochemistry. Vol. 1, New York, Plenum, 1990, p. 322.

86. El-Maliki, B., Blanchard, D., Dahr, W., Beyreuther, K., and Cartron, J. P.: Structural homology between glycophorins C and D of human erythrocytes. Eur. J. Biochem. 183:639, 1989.

87. Colin, Y., Le Van Kim, C., Tsapis, A., Clerget, M., d'Auriol, L., London, J., and Cartron, J. P.: Human erythrocyte glycophorin-C. Gene structure and rearrangement in genetic variants. J. Biol. Chem. 264:3773, 1989.

88. High, S., and Tanner, M. J. A.: Human erythrocyte membrane sialoglycoprotein-β. The cDNA sequence suggests the absence of a cleaved N-terminal signal sequence. Biochem. J. 243:277, 1987.

89. Dahr, W., Kiedrowski, S., Blanchard, D., Hermand, P., Moulds, J. J., and Cartron, J. P.: High frequency of human erythrocyte membrane sialoglycoproteins. V. Characterization of the Gerbich blood group antigens. Ge2 and Ge3. Biol. Chem. Hoppe-Seyler, 368:1375, 1987.

90. LeVan Kim, C., Colin, Y., Mitjavila, M. T., Clerget, M., Dubart, A., Nakazawa, M., Vainchenker, W., and Cartron, J. P.: Structure of the promoter region and tissue specificity of the human glycophorin C. J. Biol. Chem. 264:20407, 1989.

91. Villeval, J. L., LeVan Kim, C., Bettaieb, A., Debili, N., Colin, Y., El Maliki, B., Blanchard, D., Vainchenker, W., and Cartron, J. P.: Early expression of glycophorin-C during normal and leukemic human erythroid differentiation. Cancer Res. 49:2626, 1989.

92. Telen, M. J., LeVan Kim, C., Chung, A., Cartron, J. P., and Colin, Y.: Molecular basis for elliptocytosis associated with glycophorin C and D deficiency in Leach phenotype. Blood 78:1603, 1991.

93. Alloisio, N., Morle, L., Bachir, D., Guetarni, D., Colonna, D., and Delaunay, J.: Red cell membrane sialoglycoprotein in homozygous and heterozygous 4.1(−) hereditary elliptocytosis. Biochem. Biophys. Acta 816:57, 1985.

94. Reid, M. E., Takakuwa, Y., Conboy, J., Tchernia, G., and Mohandas, N.: Glycophorin-C content of human erythrocyte membrane is regulated by protein 4.1. Blood 75:2229, 1990.

95. Sondag, D., Alloisio, N. N., Blanchard, D., Ducluzeau, M. T., Colonna, P., Bachir, D., Bloy, C., Cartron, J. P., and Delaunay, J.: Gerbich reactivity in 4.1(−) hereditary elliptocytosis and protein 4.1 level in blood group Gerbich deficiency. Br. J. Haematol. 65:43, 1987.

96. Agre, P., and Cartron, J.-P.: Molecular biology of the Rh antigens. Blood 78:551, 1991.

97. Preston, G. M., Carroll, T. P., Guggino, W. B., and Agre, P.: Appearance of water channels in *Xenopus* oocytes expressing red cell CHIP28 protein. Science 256:385, 1992.

98. Winkelmann, J. C., and Forget, B. G.: Erythroid and nonerythroid spectrins. Blood 81:373, 1993.

99. Bennett, V., and Lambert, S.: The spectrin skeleton: From red cells to brain. J. Clin. Invest. 87:1483, 1991.

100. Speicher, D. W., and Marchesi, V. T.: Erythrocyte spectrin is comprised of many homologous triple helical segments. Nature 311:177, 1984.

101. Sahr, K. E., Laurila, P., Kotula, L., Scarpa, A. L., Coupal, E., Leto, T. L., Linnenbach, A. J., Winkelmann, J. C., Speicher, D. W., Marchesi, V. T., Curtis, P. J., and Forget, B. G.: The complete cDNA and polypeptide sequences of human erythroid α-spectrin. J. Biol. Chem. 265:4434, 1990.

102. Sahr, K. E., Tobe, T., Scarpa, A., Laughinghouse, K., Marchesi, S. L., Agre, P., Linnenbach, A. J., Marchesi, V. T., and Forget, B. G.: Sequence and exon-intron organization of the DNA encoding to αI domain of human spectrin. Applications to the study of mutations causing hereditary elliptocytosis. J. Clin. Invest. 84:1243, 1989.

103. Kotula, L., Laury-Kleintop, L. D., Showe, L., Shar, K., Linnenbach, A. J., Forget, B. G., and Curtis, P. J.: The exon-intron organization of the human erythrocyte α spectrin gene. Genomics 9:131, 1991.

104. Cioe, L., Laurila, P., Meo, P., Krebs, K., Goodman, S., and Curtis, P. J.: Cloning and nucleotide sequence of a mouse erythrocyte β-spectrin cDNA. Blood 70:915, 1987.

105. Byers, T. J., Husain-Chishti, A., Dubreuil, R., Branton, D., and Goldstein L. S. B.: Sequence similarity of the amino-terminal domain of Drosophila beta spectrin to alpha actinin and dystrophin. J. Cell Biol. 109:1160, 1989.

106. Prchal, J. T., Morley, B. J., Yoon, S.-H., Coetzer, T. L., Palek, J., Conboy, J. G., and Kan, Y. W.: Isolation and characterization of cDNA clones for human erythrocyte β-spectrin. Proc. Natl. Acad. Sci. USA 84:7468, 1987.

107. Winkelmann, J. C., Leto, T. L., Watkins, P. C., Eddy, R., Shows, T. B., Linnenbach, A. J., Sahr, K. E., Kathuria, N., Marchesi, V. T., and Forget, B. G.: Molecular cloning of the cDNA for human erythrocyte beta-spectrin. Blood 72:328, 1988.

108. Tanaka, T., Kadowaki, K., Lazarides, E., and Sobue, K.: Ca^{2+}-dependent regulation of the spectrin/actin interaction by calmodulin and protein 4.1. J. Biol. Chem. 266:1134, 1991.

109. Cohen, C. M., and Langley, R. C., Jr.: Functional characterization of human erythrocyte spectrin alpha and beta chains: Association with actin and erythrocyte protein 4.1. Biochemistry 23:4488, 1984.

110. Fukushima, Y., Byers, M. G., Watkins, P. C., Winkelmann, J. C., Forget, B. G., and Shows, T. B.: Assignment of the gene for β-spectrin (SPTB) to chromosome 14q23 → q24.2 by *in situ* hybridization. Cytogenet. Cell Genet. 53:232, 1990.

111. Becker, P. S., Schwartz, M. A., Morrow, J. S., and Lux, S. E.: Radiolabel-transfer cross-linking demonstrates that protein 4.1 binds to the N-terminal region of beta spectrin and to actin in binary interactions. Eur. J. Biochem. 193:827, 1990.

112. Kennedy, S. P., Warren S. L., Forget, B. G., and Morrow, J. S.: Ankyrin binds to the 15th repetitive unit of erythroid and nonerythroid β-spectrin. J. Cell Biol. 115:267, 1991.

113. Harris, H. W., Jr., and Lux, S. E.: Structural characterization

of the phosphorylation sites of human erythrocyte spectrin. J. Biol. Chem. 225:11512, 1980.

114. Mische, S. M., and Morrow, J. S.: Multiple kinases phosphorylate spectrin. In Cohen, C. M., and Palek, J. (eds.): Molecular and Cellular Biology of Normal and Abnormal Erythrocyte Membranes. New York, Alan R. Liss, 1990, p. 113.

115. Mische, S. M., and Morrow, J. S.: Spectrin phosphorylation regulates spectrin subunit interactions (abstract). J. Cell Biol. 107:469a, 1989.

116. Tse, W. T., Lecomte, M.-C., Costa, F. F., Garbarz, M., Feo, C., Boivin, P., Dhermy, D., and Forget, B. G.: Point mutation in β-spectrin gene associated with αI/74 hereditary elliptocytosis. J. Clin. Invest. 86:909, 1990.

117. Huebner, K., Palumbo, A. P., Isobe, M., Kozak, C. A., Monaco, S., Rovera, G., Croce, C. M., and Curtis, P. J.: The α-spectrin gene is on chromosome 1 in mouse and man. Proc. Natl. Acad. Sci. USA 82:3790, 1985.

118. Leto, T. L., Fortugno-Erikson, D., Barton, B. E., Yang-Feng, T. L., Francke, U., Morrow, J. S., Marchesi, V. T., and Benz, E. J., Jr.: Comparison of nonerythroid α spectrin genes reveals strict homology among diverse species. Mol. Cell Biol. 8:1, 1988.

119. Watkins, P. C., Eddy, R. L., Forget, B. G., Chang, J. G., Byers, M. G., Rochelle, R., and Shows, T. B.: Assignment of the gene for non-erythroid β spectrin (SPTBN1) human chromosome 2p21 (abstract). Cytogenet. Cell Genet. 51:1103, 1989.

120. Winkelmann, J. C., Costa, F. F., Linzie, B. L., and Forget, B. G.: β Spectrin in human skeletal muscle: Tissue-specific differential processing of 3′ β spectrin pre-mRNA generates a β spectrin isoform with a unique carboxyl terminus. J. Biol. Chem. 265:20449, 1990.

121. Chu, Z.-L., and Winkelmann, J. C.: Murine erythroleukemia cells are able to splice human β spectrin pre-mRNA in a tissue-specific manner (abstract). Clin. Res. 39:317A, 1991.

122. Marchesi, S. L., Letsinger, J. T., Speicher, D. W., Marchesi, V. T., Agre, P., Hyun, B., and Gulati, G.: Mutant forms of spectrin α-subunits in hereditary elliptocytosis. J. Clin. Invest. 80:191, 1987.

123. Leto, T. L., and Marchesi, V. T.: A structural model of human erythrocyte protein 4.1. J. Biol. Chem. 259:4603, 1984.

124. Cohen, C. M.: The molecular organization of the red cell membrane skeleton. Semin. Hematol. 20:141, 1983.

125. Miller, J. A., Gravallese, E., and Bunn, H. F.: Nonenzymatic glycosylation of erythrocyte membrane proteins. J. Clin. Invest. 65:896, 1980.

126. Wolfe, L. C., Luz, S. E., and Ohanian, V.: Regulation of spectrin-actin binding by protein 4.1 and polyphosphates. J. Cell Biol. 87:203a, 1980.

127. Cohen, C. M., Liu, S. C., Lawler, J., and Palek, J.: Identification of the protein 4.1 binding site to phosphatidylserine vesicles. Biochemistry 27:614, 1988.

128. Inaba, M., Gupta, K. C., Kuwabara, M., Takahashi, T., Benz, E. J., Jr., and Maeda, Y.: Deamidation of human erythrocyte protein 4.1: Possible role in aging. Blood 79:3355, 1992.

129. Tang, K. T., Leto, T. L., Marchesi, V. T., and Benz, E. J., Jr.: Expression of specific isoforms of protein 4.1 in erythroid and non-erythroid tissues. In Tavassoli, M., Zanjani, E. D., Ascensao, J. L., Abraham, N. G., and Levin, A. S. (eds.): Molecular Biology of Hemopoiesis: Advances in Experimental Medicine and Biology. New York, Plenum, 1989, Vol. 241, pp. 81–95.

130. Tang, T. K., Qin, Z., Leto, T., Marchesi, V. T., and Benz, E. J., Jr.: Membrane skeletal protein 4.1 of human erythroid and non-erythroid cells is composed of multiple isoforms with novel sizes, functions and tissue specific expression. In Cohen, C. M., and Palek, J. (eds.): Cellular and Molecular Biology of Normal and Abnormal Erythroid Membranes. New York, Alan R. Liss, 1990, pp. 43–59.

131. Conboy, J., Kan, Y. W., Shobet, S. B., and Mohandas, N.: Molecular cloning of protein 4.1: A major structural element of the human erythrocyte membrane cytoskeleton. Proc. Natl. Acad. Sci. USA 83:9512, 1986.

132. Tang, T. K., Leto, T. L., Correas, I., Alonso, M., Marchesi, V.

133. T., and Benz, E. J., Jr.: Selective expression of an erythroid-specific isoform of protein 4.1. Proc. Natl. Acad. Sci. USA 85:3713, 1988.

133. Tang, T. K., Qin, Z., Leto, T. L., Marchesi, V. T., and Benz, E. J., Jr.: Heterogeneity of mRNA and protein products arising from the protein 4.1 gene in erythroid and nonerythroid tissues. J. Cell Biol. 110:617, 1990.

134. Huang, J. P., Tang, C. J., Kou, G. H., Marchesi, V. T., Benz, E. J., Jr., Tang, T. K.: Genomic structure of the locus encoding protein 4.1. Structural basis for complex combinational patterns of tissue-specific alternative RNA splicing. J. Biol. Chem. 268:3758, 1993.

135. Ngai, J., Stack, J. W., Moon, R. T., and Lazerides, E.: Regulated expression of multiple chicken erythroid membrane skeleton protein 4.1 variants is governed by differential RNA processing and translation control. Proc. Natl. Acad. Sci. USA 84:4432, 1987.

136. Conboy, J. G., Chan, J. Y., Chasis, J. A., Kan, Y. W., and Mohandas, N.: Tissue- and development-specific alternative RNA splicing regulates expression of multiple isoforms of erythroid membrane protein 4.1. J. Biol. Chem. 266:8273, 1991.

137. Correas, I., Leto, T. L., Speicher, D. W., and Marchesi, V. T.: Identification of the functional site of erythrocyte protein 4.1 involved in spectrin actin binding. J. Biol. Chem. 261:3310, 1986.

138. Horne, W., Tang, T. K., Marchesi, V. T., and Benz, E. J., Jr.: Tissue specific alternative splicing of protein 4.1 inserts, an exon necessary for erythrocyte spectrin-actin binding. Blood (in press).

139. Huang, S., Tang, T. K., Baklouti, F., and Benz, E. J., Jr.: Differential utilization of translation initiation sites in alternatively spliced mRNAs arising from the protein 4.1 gene (abstract). Clin. Res. 40(2):212A, 1992.

140. Conboy, J. G., Chasis, J. A., Winardi, R., Tchernia, G., Kan, Y. W., and Mohandas, N: Tissue-specific deficiency of protein 4.1 as a consequence of usage of an alternative translation initiation site. Blood 78 (Suppl.):365a, 1991.

141. Venezia, N. D., Gilsanz, F., Alloisio, N., Ducluzeau, M. T., Benz, E. J., Jr., and Delaunay, J.: Homozygous 4.1(−) hereditary elliptocytosis associated with point mutation in downstream initiation codon of protein 4.1 gene. J. Clin. Invest. 90:1713, 1992.

142. Palek, J., and Lambert, S.: Genetics of the red cell membrane skeleton. Semin. Hematol. 27:290, 1990.

143. Davis, J. Q., and Bennet, V.: Brain ankyrin purification of a 72,000 M_r spectrin binding domain. J. Biol. Chem. 259:1874, 1984.

144. Wallin, R., Culp, E. N., and Coleman, D. B.: A structural model of human erythrocyte band 2.1: Alignment of chemical and functional domains. Proc. Natl. Acad. Sci. USA 81:4095, 1984.

145. Weaver, D. C., and Marchesi, V. T.: The structural basis of ankyrin function, Parts I and II. J. Biol. Chem. 259:6165; 6170, 1984.

146. Cianci, C. D., Giorgi, M., and Morrow, J. S.: Phosphorylation of ankyrin downregulates its cooperative interaction with spectrin and protein 3. J. Cell Biochem. 37:301, 1988.

147. Lu, P.-W., Soong, C. F., and Tao, M.: Phosphorylation of ankyrin decreases its affinity for spectrin tetramer. J. Biol. Chem. 262:14958, 1985.

148. Lambert, S., Yu, H., Prchal, J. T., and Palek, J.: The cDNA sequence for human erythrocyte ankyrin. Proc. Natl. Acad. Sci. USA 87:1730, 1990.

149. Lambert, S., Lawler, J., Yu, H., and Palek, J.: A conserved repeating unit within the structure of human erythrocyte ankyrin. J. Cell Biol. 107:469a, 1989.

150. Hall, T. G., and Bennett, V.: Regulatory domains of erythrocyte ankyrin. J. Biol. Chem. 262:10537, 1987.

151. Tse, W. T., Zhong, W., Yang-Feng, T. L., and Forget, B. G.: Cloning of a novel gene related to the erythroid ankyrin gene. Blood 74:61a, 1989.

152. Otto, E., McLaughlin, F., Lux, S. E., and Bennet, V.: Isolation and sequence of a human brain ankyrin cDNA: Evidence for a multigene family. J. Cell Biol. 109:264a, 1989.

153. Korsgren, C., and Cohen, C. M.: Association of human eryth-

rocyte band 4.2 binding to ankyrin and to the cytoplasmic domain of band 3. J. Biol. Chem. 263:10212, 1988.

154. Sung, L. A., Chien, S., Chang, L. S., Lambert, K., Bliss, S. A., Bouhassira, E. E., Nagel, R. L., Schwartz, R. S., and Rybicki, A. C.: Molecular cloning of human protein 4.2: A major component of the erythrocyte membrane. Proc. Natl. Acad. Sci. USA 87:955, 1990.

155. Korsgren, C., Lawler, J., Lambert, S., Speicher, P., and Cohen, C. M.: Complete amino acid sequence and homologies of human erythrocyte membrane protein band 4.2. Proc. Natl. Acad. Sci. USA 87:613, 1990.

156. Chang, L. S., Fan, Y. S., Lambert, K., Zhu, L., Lam, J. S., Lin, C. C., Chien, S., and Sung, L. A.: Human erythrocyte protein 4.2: Differential splicing, isoform expression, and chromosomal assignment. Blood (in press).

157. Folk J. G.: Transglutaminases. Annu. Rev. Biochem. 49:517, 1980.

158. Rybicki, A. C., Heath, R., Wolf, J. S., Lubin, B., and Schwartz, R. S.: Deficiency of protein 4.2 in erythrocytes from a patient with a Coombs negative hemolytic anemia: Evidence for a role of protein 4.2 in stabilizing ankyrin on the membrane. J. Clin. Invest. 81:898, 1988.

158a. Rix, M., Bjerrum, P. J., Wieth, J. O., and Fradsen, B.: Congenital stomatocytosis with hemolytic anemia—with abnormal cation permeability and defective membrane proteins. Ugeskr. Laeger 153:724, 1991.

158b. Eber, S. W., Lande, W. M., Iarocci, T. A., Mentzer, W. C., Hohn, P., Wiley, J. S., and Schroter, W.: Hereditary stomatocytosis: Consistent association with an integral membrane protein deficiency. Br. J. Haematol. 72:452, 1989.

158c. Morle, L., Pothier, B., Alloisio, N., Feo, C., Garay, R., Bost, M., and Delaunay, J.: Reduction of membrane band 7 and activation of volume stimulated (K+, Cl−)− cotransport in a case of congenital stomatocytosis. Br. J. Haematol. 71:141, 1989.

158d. Stewart, G. W., Hepworth-Jones, B. E., Keen, J. N., Dash, B. C. J., Argent, A. C., and Casimir, C. M.: Isolation of cDNA coding for an ubiquitous membrane protein deficient in high Na+, low K+ stomatocytic erythrocytes. Blood 79:1593, 1992.

158e. Wang, D., Mentzer, W. C., Cameron, T., and Johnson, R. M.: Purification of band 7.2b, a 31-kDa integral phosphoprotein absent in hereditary stomatocytosis. J. Biol. Chem. 266:17826, 1991.

158f. Moore, R. B., Plishker, G. A., and Shriver, S. K.: Purification and measurement of calpromotin, the cytoplasmic protein which activates calcium-dependent potassium transport. Biochem. Biophys. Res. Commun. 166:146, 1990.

158g. Moore, R. B., Mankad, M. V., Shriver, S. K., Mankad, V. N., and Plishker, G. A.: Reconstitution of Ca-dependent K transport in erythrocyte membrane vesicles requires a cytoplasmic protein. J. Biol. Chem. 266:17833, 1991.

159. Koury, M. J., Bondurant, M. C., and Rana, S. S.: Changes in erythroid membrane proteins during erythropoietin-mediated terminal differentiation. J. Cell. Physiol. 133:438, 1987.

160. Lazarides, E.: From genes to structural morphogenesis: The genesis and epigenesis of a red blood cell. Cell 51:345, 1987.

161. Cox, J. V., Stack, J. H., and Lazarides, E.: Erythroid anion transporter assembly is mediated by a developmentally regulated recruitment onto a preassembled membrane cytoskeleton. J. Cell Biol. 105:1405, 1987.

162. Woods, C. M., Boyer, B., Vogt, P. K., and Lazarides E.: Control of erythroid differentiation: Asynchronous expression of the anion transporter and the peripheral components of the membrane skeleton in AEV- and S13-transformed cells. J. Cell Biol. 103:1789, 1986.

163. Moon, R. T., and Lazarides, E.: Biogenesis of the avian erythroid membrane skeleton: Receptor-mediated assembly and stabilization of ankyrin (globin) and spectrin. J. Cell Biol. 98:1899, 1984.

164. Blikstad, I., Nelson, W. J., Moon, R. T., and Lazarides, E.: Synthesis and assembly of spectrin during avian erythropoi-esis: Stoichiometric assembly, but unequal synthesis of α and β spectrin. Cell 32:1081, 1983.

165. Hanspal, M., and Palek, J.: Synthesis and assembly of membrane skeletal proteins in mammalian red cell precursors. J. Cell. Biol. 105:147, 1987.

166. Peters, L. L., Turtzo, L. C., Birkenmeier, C., and Barker, J. E.: Distinct fetal ANK-1 and ANK-2 related proteins and mRNA's in normal and nb/nb mice. Blood 81:2144, 1993.

167. Peters, L. L., White, R. A., Birkenmeier, C., Bloom, M. L., Lux, S. E., and Barker, J. E.: Changing in cytoskeletal mRNA expression and protein synthesis patterns during murine erythropoiesis in vivo. Proc. Natl. Acad. Sci. USA (in press).

168. Bodine, D. M., Birkenmeier, C. S., and Barker, J. E.: Spectrin deficient inherited hemolytic anemias in the mouse: Characterization by spectrin synthesis and mRNA activity in reticulocytes. Cell 37:721, 1984.

169. Marchesi, S. L., Agre, P. A., Speicher, D. W., Tse, W. T., and Forget, B. G.: Mutant spectrin αII domain in recessively inherited spherocytosis. Blood 74:213a, 1989.

170. Palek, J.: Red cell membrane disorders. In Hoffman, K., Benz, E. J., Jr., Furie, B., Shattil, S., and Cohen, H. (eds.): Hematology: Basic Principles and Practice. New York, Churchill Livingstone, 1990, pp. 472–504.

171. Gallagher, P. G., Tse, W. T., and Forget, B. G.: Clinical and molecular aspects of disorders of the erythrocyte membrane skeleton. Semin. Perinatol. 14:351, 1990.

172. Lux, S. E.: Disorders of the red cell membrane skeleton: Hereditary spherocytosis and hereditary elliptocytosis. In Stanbury, J. B., Wyngaarden, J. B., and Fredrickson, D. S. (eds.): The Metabolic Basis of Inherited Disease. 5th ed., New York, McGraw-Hill, 1983.

173. Lutz, H., Bussolino, F., Flapp, R., Fasier, S., Kazatchkine, M. D., and Arese, P.: Naturally-occurring anti-band-3 antibodies and complement together mediate phagocytosis of oxidatively stressed human erythrocytes. Proc. Natl. Acad. Sci. USA 84:7368, 1987.

174. Mentzer, W. C., Jr., Iarocci, T. A., and Mohandas, N.: Modulation of erythrocyte membrane mechanical fragility by 2,3 diphosphoglycerate in neonatal poikilocytosis/elliptocytosis syndrome. J. Clin. Invest. 79:943, 1987.

175. Nagel, R.: Red cell cytoskeletal abnormalities: Implications for malaria. N. Engl. J. Med. 323:1558, 1990; and Malaria and red cell genetic defects. Blood 74:1213, 1989.

176. Nash, R., and Shojania, A. M.: Hematological aspects of Rh deficiency syndrome: A case report and a review of the literature. Am. J. Hematol. 24:267, 1987.

177. Low, P. S., Waugh, S. M., Zinke, K., and Drenckhahn, D.: The role of hemoglobin denaturation and band 3 clustering in red blood cell aging. Science 227:531, 1985.

178. Turrini, F., Arese, P., Yuan, J., and Low, P. S.: Clustering of integral membrane proteins of the human erythrocyte membrane stimulates autologous IgG binding, complement deposition and phagocytosis. J. Biol. Chem. 266:23611, 1991.

179. Low, P. S., and Kannan, R.: Effect of hemoglobin denaturation on membrane structure and IgG binding: Role in red cell aging. In Brewer, G. (ed.): The Red Cell. Seventh Ann Arbor Conference. New York, Alan R. Liss, 1989, pp. 525–552.

180. Kannan, R., Labotka, R., and Low, P. S.: Isolation and characterization of the hemochrome-stabilized membrane protein aggregates from sickle erythrocytes: Major site of autologous antibody binding. J. Biol. Chem. 263:13766, 1988.

181. Yuan, J., Kannan, R., Shinar, E., Rachmilewitz, E. A., and Low, P. S.: Isolation characterization and immunoprecipitation studies of immune complexes from membranes of β-thalassemic erythrocytes. Blood 79:3007, 1992.

182. Waugh, S. M., Willardson, B. M., Kannan, R., Labotka, R. J., and Low, P. S.: Heinz bodies induce clustering of band 3, Clycophorin and ankyrin in sickle cell erythrocytes. J. Clin. Invest. 78:1155, 1986.

183. Shinar, E., Shaley, O., Rachmilewitz, E. A., and Schreier, S. L.: Erythrocyte membrane skeleton abnormalities in severe beta thalassemia. Blood 70:158, 1987.

184. Marchesi, S. L.: The erythrocyte cytoskeleton in hereditary elliptocytosis and spherocytosis. *In* Agre, P., and Parker, J. C. (eds.): Red Blood Cell Membranes: Structure, Function, Clinical Implications, New York, Marcel Dekker, 1989, pp. 77–110.

185. Speicher, D. W., Morrow, J. S., Knowles, W. J., and Marchesi, V. T.: A structural model of human erythrocyte spectrin. Alignment of chemical and functional domains. J. Biol. Chem. 257:9093, 1982.

186. Speicher, D. W., Morrow, J. S., Knowles, W. J., and Marchesi, V. T.: Identification of proteolytically resistant domains of human erythrocyte spectrin. Proc. Natl. Acad. Sci. USA 77:5673, 1980.

187. Morrow, J. S., Speicher, D. W., Knowles, W. J., Hsu, J., and Marchesi, V. T.: Identification of functional domains of human erythrocyte spectrin. Proc. Natl. Acad. Sci. USA 77:6592, 1980.

188. Garbarz, M., Lecomte, M. D., Feo, C., Devaux, I., Picat, C., Lefebvre, C., Galibert, F., Gautero, H., Bournier, O., Galand, C., Forget, B. G., Boivin, P., and Dhermy, D.: Hereditary pyropoikilocytosis and elliptocytosis in a white French family with the spectrin $\alpha^{1/74}$ variant related to CGT to CAT codon change (Arg to His) at position 22 of the spectrin αI domain. Blood 75:1691, 1990.

189. Morle, L., Roux, A.-F., Alloisio, N., Pothier, B., Starck, J., Denroy, J., Morle, F., Rudigoz, R.-C., Forget, B. G., Delaunay, J., and Godet, J.: Two elliptocytogenic $\alpha^{1/74}$ variants of the spectrin αI domain spectrin Culoz (GGT → GTT; αI 40 GLY → Val) and spectrin Lyon (CTT → TTT; α I43 Leu → Phe). J. Clin. Invest. 86:548, 1990.

190. Tse, W. T., Lecomte, M. C., Costa, F. F., Garbarz, M., Feo, C., Boivin, P., Dhermy, D., and Forget, B.: Point mutation in the β-spectrin gene associated with $\alpha^{1/74}$ hereditary elliptocytosis. J. Clin. Invest. 86:909, 1990.

191. Speicher, D. W., Davis, G., and Marchesi, V. T.: Structure of human erythrocyte spectrin. II. The sequence of the α-I domain. J. Biol. Chem. 258:14938, 1983.

192. Coetzer, T., Sahr, K., Prchal, J., Blacklock, H., Peterson, L., Koler, R., Doyle, J., Manaster, J., and Palek, J.: Four different mutations in codon 28 of α spectrin are associated with structurally and functionally abnormal spectrin $\alpha^{1/74}$ in hereditary elliptocytosis. J. Clin. Invest. 88:743, 1991.

193. Floyd, P. B., Gallagher, P. G., Valentino, L. A., Davis, M., Marchesi, S. L., and Forget, B. G.: Heterogeneity of the molecular basis of hereditary pyropoikilocytosis and hereditary elliptocytosis associated with increased levels of the spectrin $\alpha^{1/74}$-kilodalton tryptic peptide. Blood 78:1364, 1991.

194. Coetzer, T., Palek, J., Lawler, J., Liu, S. C., Jarolim, P., Lahav, M., Prchal, J. T., Wang, W., Alter, B. P., Schewitz, G., Mankad, V., Gallanello, R., and Cao, A.: Structural and functional heterogeneity of α spectrin mutations involving the spectrin heterodimer self-association site: Relationships to hematologic expression of homozygous hereditary elliptocytosis and hereditary pyropoikilocytosis. Blood 75:2235, 1990.

195. Marchesi, S. L., Letsinger, J. T., Speicher, D. W., Marchesi, V. T., Agre, P., Hyun, B., and Gulati, G.: Mutant forms of spectrin α-subunits in hereditary elliptocytosis. J. Clin. Invest. 80:191, 1987.

196. Morle, L., Roux, A.-F., Morle, R., Alloisio, N., Pothier, B., Sahr, K. E., Forget, B. G., Godet, J., and Delaunay, J.: The diversity of hereditary elliptocytosis in North Africa: Protein aspects and molecular genetics. *In* Cohen, C. M., and Palek, J. (eds.): Cellular and Molecular Biology of Normal and Abnormal Erythroid Membranes. UCLA Syposium on Molecular and Cellular Biology, New Series 118:223, 1990.

197. Roux, A. F., Morle, F., Guetarni, D., Colonna, P., Sahr, K., Forget, B. G., Delaunay, J., and Godet, J.: Molecular basis of Sp $\alpha^{1/65}$ hereditary elliptocytosis in North Africa: Insertion of a TTG triplet between codons 147 and 149 in the α-spectrin gene from five unrelated families. Blood 73:2196, 1989.

198. Sahr, K. E., Tobe, T., Scarpa, A., Laughinghouse, K., Mar-

chesi, S. L., Agre, P., Linnenbach, A. J., Marchesi, V. T., and Forget, B. G.: Sequence and exon-intron organization of the DNA encoding the αI domain of human spectrin: Application to the study of mutations causing hereditary elliptocytosis. J. Clin. Invest. 84:1243, 1989.

199. Gallagher, P. G., Tse, W. T., Coetzer, T., Zarkowsky, H. S., Lecomte, M. C., Garbarz, M., Baruchel, A., Ballas, S. K., Dhermy, D., Palek, J., and Forget, B. G.: A common type of the spectrin αI 46–50a kDa peptide abnormality in hereditary elliptocytosis and pyropoikilocytosis is associated with a mutation distant from the proteolytic cleavage site. J. Clin. Invest. 89:892, 1992.

200. Gallagher, P. G., Marchesi, S. L., and Forget, B. G.: A new point mutation associated with αI/50b kDa hereditary elliptocytosis (HE) and hereditary pyropoikilocytosis (HPP). Clin. Res. 39:313a, 1991.

201. Lecomte, M. C., Garbarz, M., Grandchamp, B., Feo, C., Gautero, H., Devaux, I., Bournier, O., Galand, C., d'Auriol, L., Galibert, F., Sahr, K. E., Forget, B. G., Boivin, P., and Dhermy, D: Sp $\alpha^{1/78}$. A mutation of the αI spectrin domain in a white kindred with HE and HPP phenotypes. Blood 74:1126, 1989.

202. Morle, L., Morle, F., Roux, A. F., Godet, J., Forget, B. G., Denoroy, L., Garbarz, M., Dhermy, D., Kastally, R., and Delaunay, J.: Spectrin Tunis (Sp $\alpha^{1/78}$), an elliptocytogenic variant, is due to the CGG → TGG codon change (Arg → Trp); at position 35 of the αI domain. Blood 74:828, 1989.

203. Marchesi, S. L., Agre, P. A., Speicher, D. W., Tse, W. T., and Forget, B. G.: Mutant spectrin αII domain in recessively inherited spherocytosis. Blood 74 (Suppl. 13B):213, 1989.

204. Marchesi, S. L., Agre, P. A., and Speicher, D. W.: Abnormal spectrin αII domain in recessive spherocytosis. J. Cell. Biochem. (Suppl. 13B):213, 1989.

205. Alloisio, N., Baklouti, F., Morle, L., Wilmott, R., Marechal, J., Ducluzeau, M.-T., Denoroy, L., Forget, B. G., Kastally, R., and Delaunay, J.: $\alpha^{II/31}$ Spectrin Jendouba: An elliptocytogenic αII domain variant associated with the αII 112 ASP → GLU (GAC → GAA) mutation. Blood 76 (Suppl.):23a, 1990.

206. Lecomte, M. C., Gautero, H., Garbarz, M., Boivin, P., and Dhermy, D.: Abnormal tryptic peptide from the spectrin α- or β-chain mutations: two genetically distinct forms of the Sp $\alpha^{1/74}$ variant. Br. J. Haematol. 76:406, 1990.

207. Pothier, B., Alloisio, N., Morle, L., Marechal, J., Barthelemy, H., Ducluzeau, M. T., Dorier, A., and Delaunay, J.: Two distinct variants of erythrocyte β IV domain. Hum. Genet. 83:373, 1989.

208. Gallagher, P. G., Tse, W. T., Costa, F., Scarpa, A., Boivin, P., Delaunay, J., and Forget, B. G.: A splice site mutation of the β-spectrin gene causing exon skipping in hereditary elliptocytosis associated with a truncated β-spectrin chain. J. Biol. Chem. 266:23, 1991.

209. Garbarz, M., Tse, W. T., Gallagher, P. G., Picat, C., Lecomte, M. C., Galibert, F., Dhermy, D., and Forget, B. G.: Spectrin Rouen ($\beta^{220/218}$), a novel shortened β-chain variant in a kindred with hereditary elliptocytosis. J. Clin. Invest. 88:76, 1991.

210. Yoon, S. H., Ut, H., Eber, S., and Prchal, J. T.: Molecular defect of truncated β-spectrin Gottingen. J. Biol. Chem. 266:8490, 1991.

211. Tse, W. T., Gallagher, P. G., Pothier, B., Costa, F. F., Scarpa, A., Delaunay, J., and Forget, B. G.: An insertional frameshift mutation of the β-spectrin gene associated with elliptocytosis in spectrin Nice ($\beta^{220/216}$). Blood 78:517, 1991.

212. Garbarz, M., Feldman, L., Boulanger, L., Lecomte, M. C., Gautero, H., Galand, C., Boivin, P., and Dhermy, D.: Molecular basis of spectrin Tandil, a shortened β spectrin variant associated with hereditary elliptocytosis. Blood 78:84a, 1991.

213. Becker, P. S., Morrow, J. S., and Lux, S. E.: Abnormal oxidant sensitivity and β-chain structure of spectrin in hereditary spherocytosis associated with defective spectrin-protein 4.1 binding. J. Clin. Invest. 80:557, 1987.

214. Alloisio, N., Morlé, L., Maréchal, J., Roux, A. F., Ducluzeau,

M. T., Guetarni, D., Pothier, B., Baklouti, F., Ghanem, A., Kastally, R., and Delaunay, J.: Sp α$^{V/41}$: A common spectrin polymorphism at the α^{IV}-α^{V} domain junction. Relevance to the expression level of hereditary elliptocytosis due to α-spectrin variants located in trans. J Clin Invest 87:2169, 1991.

215. Agre, P., Casella, J. F., Zinkham, W. H., McMillan, C., and Bennett, V.: Partial deficiency of erythrocyte spectrin in hereditary spherocytosis. Nature 314:380, 1985.

216. Hanspal, M., Yoon, S. H., Yu, H., Hanspal, J. S., Palek, J., and Prchal, J. T.: Molecular basis of spectrin and ankyrin deficiencies in severe hereditary spherocytosis: Evidence implicating a primary defect of ankyrin. Blood 77:165, 1991.

217. Lux, S. E., Tse, W. T., Menninger, J. C., John, K. M., Harris, P., Shalev, O., Chilcote, R. R., Marchesi, S. L., Watkins, P. C., Bennett, V., McIntosh, S., Collins, F. S., Francke, U., Ward, D. C., and Forget, B. G.: Hereditary spherocytosis associated with deletion of human erythrocyte ankyrin gene on chromosome 8. Nature 345:736, 1990.

218. Cohen, H., Walker, H., Delhanty, J. D. A., Lucus, S. B., and Huehns, E. R.: Congenital spherocytosis, B19 parvovirus infection and inherited interstitial deletion of the short arm of chromosome 8. Br. J. Haematol. 78:251, 1991.

219. Costa, F. F., Agre, P., Watkins, P. C., Winkelmann, J. C., Tang, T. K., John K. M., Lux, S. E., and Forget, B. G.: Linkage of dominant hereditary spherocytosis to the gene for the erythrocyte membrane skeleton protein ankyrin. N. Engl. J. Med. 323:1046, 1990.

220. Jarolim, P., Brabec, V., Lambert, S., Liu, S. C., Zhou, Z., and Palek, J.: Ankyrin Prague: A dominantly inherited mutation of the regulatory domain of ankyrin associated with hereditary spherocytosis. Blood 76 (Suppl.):37a, 1990.

221. Marchesi, S. L., Conboy, J., Agre, P., Letsinger, J. T., Marchesi, V. T., Speicher, D. W., and Mohandas, N.: Molecular analysis of insertion/deletion mutations in protein 4.1 elliptocytosis. I. Biochemical identification of rearrangements in the spectrin/actin binding and functional characterizations. J. Clin. Invest. 86:516, 1990.

222. Conboy, J., Marchesi, S., Kim, R., Agre, P., Kan, Y. W., and Mohandas, N.: Molecular analysis of insertion/deletion mutations in protein 4.1 in elliptocytosis. II. Determination of molecular genetic origins of rearrangements. J. Clin. Invest. 86:524, 1990.

223. Conboy, J., Mohandas, N., Tchernia, G., and Kan, Y. W.: Molecular basis of hereditary elliptocytosis due to protein 4.1 deficiency. N. Engl. J. Med. 315:680, 1986.

224. Feddal, S., Brunet, G., Roda, L., Chabanis, S., Alloisio, N., Morle, L., Ducluzeau, M.-T., Marechal, J., Robert, J.-M., Benz, E. J., Delaunay, J., and Baklouti, F.: Molecular analysis of a variety of 4.1(−) hereditary elliptocytosis with reduced protein 4.1 in the French Northern Alps. Blood 78:2113, 1991.

225. Feddal, S., Hayette, S., Baklouti, F., Rimokh, R., Wilmotte, R., Magaud, J. P., Marechal, J., Benz, E. J., Jr., Girot, R., Delaunay, J., and Morle, L.: Prevalent skipping of an individual exon accounts for shortened protein 4.1 Presles. Blood 80:2925, 1992.

226. Alloisio, N., Morle, L., Dorleac, E., Gentilhomme, O., Bachir, D., Guetarni, D., Colonna, P., Bost, M., Zouaoui, Z., and Roda, L.: The heterozygous form of 4.1(−) hereditary elliptocytosis (the 4.1[−] train). Blood 65:46, 1985.

227. Dhermy, D., Garbarz, M., Lecomte, M. C., Feo, C., Bournier, O., Chaveroche, I., Gautero, H., Galand, C., and Boivin, P.: Hereditary elliptocytosis: Clinical, morphological and biochemical studies of 38 cases. Nouv. Rev. Fr. Hematol. 28:129, 1986.

228. Telen, M. J., Le Van Kim, C., Chung, A., Cartron, J.-P., and Colin, Y.: Varying molecular basis of elliptocytosis due to glycophorin C. deficiency. Blood 76 (Suppl.):18a, 1990.

229. Schwartz, R. S., Yawata, Y., Ata, K., Nagel, R. L., and Rybicki, A. C.: An alanine threonine substitution in protein 4.2 cDNA is associated with a Japanese form of hereditary hemolytic anemia. Clin. Res. 39:313a, 1991.

230. Rybicki, A. C., Musto, S., Nagel, R. L., and Schwartz, R. S.: Red cell protein 4.2 deficiency associated with a defect in the cytoplasmic domain of band 3. Blood 78 (Suppl.):81a, 1991.

231. Jarolim, P., Palek, J., Rubin, H. L., Prchal, J. T., Korsgren, C., and Cohen, C. M.: Band 3 Tuscalossa: PRO^{327} → ARG^{327} substitution in the cytoplasmic domain of erythrocyte band 3 protein associated with spherocytic hemolytic anemia and partial deficiency of protein 4.2. Blood 78 (Suppl.):252a, 1991.

ACKNOWLEDGMENTS: The author is indebted to Ms. Julia Fallon, Ms. Carol Doria, and Ms. Dawne Newcombe for expert preparation of the manuscript and to Drs. Bernard Forget, Patrick Gallagher, William Tse, John Morrow, and Jiri Palek for permission to utilize their outstanding illustrations as the basis for some of the figures in this chapter.

Red Cell Membrane Antigens

John B. Lowe

INTRODUCTION

The human erythrocyte represents a therapeutic entity when used to replenish oxygen-carrying capacity lost through hemorrhage. In many ways, the red cell transfusion represents an organ transplantation procedure. As in other transplantation procedures, it is to be expected that the recipient's immune system may identify non-self molecules on the transfused red cells and will thus mount an immune response. It was appreciated early on that infusion of red cells obtained from one individual could provoke either immediate or delayed untoward reactions in the recipient.[1, 2] Laboratory and clinical investigation of red cell "incompatibility" in the context of transfusion has led to the identification of "blood groups" whose expression is genetically determined. Subsequent studies have assigned distinct erythrocyte surface molecules to many of these blood group antigens. As discussed below, inherited structural polymorphisms in these molecules or interindividual (genetic) differences in the ability to express them, or both, are in many instances responsible for red cell incompatibility. It will also be clear that the expression of many of these molecules is in fact not restricted to erythrocytes; many are also elaborated and displayed by other tissues.

A relatively recent compilation of blood group antigens lists more than 243 different determinants, which in turn belong to 1 of 19 distinct blood group systems or else to "collections" of antigenic determinants that exhibit allelism.[3] This chapter focuses on a major subset of these antigen systems whose biochemical, genetic, and molecular properties are best understood (Table 8–1). Polypeptide antigen systems are discussed first, followed by the polymorphic systems whose component antigens are composed of complex carbohydrate molecules. The clinical significance of these molecules is discussed only briefly; readers desiring additional detailed diagnostic and therapeutic information related to blood group determinants are urged to consult a recent text on transfusion medicine.[4, 5]

THE Rh BLOOD GROUP SYSTEM

The Rh blood group system was discovered in the context of a case of erythroblastosis fetalis, or hemolytic disease of the newborn.[6–8] It is now understood that the pathogenesis of this disorder involves maternal alloimmunization by Rh antigens encoded by paternal genes and displayed on the surface of the fetal red cells. Alloimmunization generates antibodies that can cross the placenta and destroy fetal red cells.

The term Rh, from rhesus, derives from studies performed simultaneously by Landsteiner and Wiener[9] involving the generation of heteroantisera. In these studies, guinea pigs and rabbits were immunized with red cells taken from *Macaca mulatta* (rhesus) monkeys. Antisera taken from these immunized animals, after appropriate absorption and dilution, were found to detect one or more antigens present on the red cells of roughly 85 per cent of humans. This new antigen was termed Rhesus or Rh.

At the time, it was proposed that the specificities of the human alloantibody and the heteroantibody were similar or identical.[7, 9] Some 20 years later, it was demonstrated that these antibodies detect different molecules.[10, 11] The heteroantibody was renamed LW after the investigators (Landsteiner and Wiener) who discovered that antigenic system. The human alloantibody continued to be called Rh. It is now known that RH and LW are antigenic systems determined by distinct gene complexes found, respectively, on chromosome 1 and chromosome 19. There is, however, a relationship between the expression of antigens determined by the *RH* and *LW* loci, in that rare persons

TABLE 8–1. MAJOR HUMAN BLOOD GROUP SYSTEMS

BLOOD GROUP	ANTIGEN TYPE	ANTIGEN COPY NUMBER PER RED CELL	NUMBER OF ALLELES	GENE ISOLATED	CHROMOSOME
Rh	Protein complex		~48 Haplotypes includes minor C/c and E/e alleles	Yes	1p34.3–p36.1
	D	~2×10^4	2 Major (D "+" or D "−")		
	C/c	~2×10^4	2 Major (C or c)		
	E/e	~2×10^4	2 Major (E or e)		
MN (glycophorin A)	Glycoprotein	~1×10^6	2 Major (M or N); multiple minor	Yes	4q28–q31
Ss (glycophorin B)	Glycoprotein	~1.5×10^5	2 Major (S or s); multiple minor	Yes	4q28–q31
Gerbich (Ge) (glycophorins C and D)	Glycoproteins	~1×10^5 (glycophorin C) ~2×10^4 (glycophorin D)	1 Major (Ge:1, 2, 3, 4); multiple minor	Yes	2q14–q21
Kell	Glycoprotein	~5×10^3	2 Major (KEL1, KEL2); several minor	Yes	Unknown
Kidd	Glycoprotein	~14,000	2 Major (Jk^a, Jk^b); several minor	No	18
Fy (Duffy)	Glycoprotein	~12,000–17,000	2 Major (Fy^a and Fy^b)	No	1
Lutheran	Glycoprotein	~1,600–4,100	3 Major (Lu^a, Lu^b, recessive null)	No	19
Ch/Rg (Chido/Rodgers)	Glycoprotein; 4th component of complement (C4A and C4B)	~10^3	Ch (1 major, several minor) Rg (1 major, several minor)	Yes	6
Cromer glycoprotein (Decay-accelerating factor)	Glycoprotein	~10^3	2 Major (Cr^a, Cr^b); several minor	Yes	1q32
ABO	Oligosaccharide	8×10^5–2×10^6	3 Major; several minor (*cis*-AB, subgroups)	Yes	9
H	Oligosaccharide	See ABO	1 Major; several minor (Bombay, para-Bombay)	Yes	19
Secretor	Oligosaccharide	See Lewis	2 Major (secretor, non-secretor)	No	19
Lewis	Oligosaccharide	4,500–7,300	2 Major (Lewis "+" and Lewis "−")	Yes	19
Ii	Oligosaccharide	See ABO	1 Major (I); at least 1 minor (i)	Yes	Unknown
P	Oligosaccharide	~10^3	Complex	No	Unknown

whose red cells do not express Rh antigens (Rh$_{null}$) are also deficient in LW antigen expression (reviewed in reference 12). As discussed later in this section, it is likely that the LW and Rh antigens associate in the membrane and that LW expression requires Rh polypeptide expression.

Serology

In Caucasians, approximately 85 per cent of persons are termed Rh "positive," whereas roughly 15 per cent are classified as Rh "negative." These terms refer, respectively, to whether or not the red cells display the Rh D antigen (Rh "positive") or do not display that determinant (Rh "negative"). The RH blood group system is made complex by the fact that there are other antigens (the Cc and Ee antigens) in this system, whose expression is determined by a second locus distinct from but extraordinarily tightly linked to the locus that determines D antigen expression. Alleles at these two loci are inherited together in a group termed a haplotype (Table 8–2).[13] Numerous antigens in the C/c and E/e groups have been defined, whereas it has been found that virtually all red cells either are D positive or lack D expression (Rh negative) (reviewed in reference 13). Three distinct nomenclatures have evolved to describe the various antigens (Table 8–3). It should be noted that in contrast to the C/c and E/e groups, there is no product of the hypothetical d allele of the D gene—hence the absence of the d antigen in this system.

In Caucasians, there are eight relatively common Rh gene complexes (see Table 8–2) if one considers D, C, c, E, and e alleles only. Wiener[14] suggested that these three groups of Rh antigens (D, C/c, E/e) are displayed by a single protein encoded by a single gene. By contrast, Fisher proposed that these three Rh antigens correspond to three distinct polypeptides encoded by three closely linked genes (cited in reference 15). As discussed below, however, emerging information about the genes encoding these antigens is consistent with a genetic model in which the C/c and E/e antigens are displayed on two polypeptides encoded by a single locus, whereas the D antigen is expressed on a structurally similar protein encoded by a second distinct locus that is tightly linked to the C/c-E/e locus and that

is partially or completely deleted in Rh-negative individuals.

Clinical Relevance

The Rh antigens are among the most antigenic of the polymorphic red cell surface polypeptide molecules (reviewed in references 4 and 13). Consequently, these antigens have been implicated in immune hemolytic transfusion reactions and figure prominently in hemolytic disease of the newborn. The D determinant is a highly immunogenic alloantigen. Nearly 80 per cent of Rh-"negative" persons will generate anti-D reactivity following immunization with D-positive red cells (reviewed in reference 4). Formation of anti-C and anti-E antibodies in conjunction with immunization against D determinants has been described, but formation of these antibodies in subjects who are D positive and do not form anti-D antibodies is an uncommon circumstance.[4] Antibodies directed against Rh determinants are typically of the immunoglobulin (Ig) G class and consequently may lead to extravascular hemolysis, and a delayed hemolytic transfusion reaction, if antigen-positive red cells are subsequently transfused. Similarly, Rh antigen–negative mothers sensitized to Rh antigens as a consequence of pregnancy or transfusion may generate IgG anti-D antibodies that can cross the placenta, bind to Rh antigen–positive fetal red cells, and mediate destruction of fetal erythrocytes. This disorder now occurs relatively infrequently, since Rh immune globulin, routinely given to RhD-negative mothers giving birth to D-positive infants, eliminates circulating and potentially immunogenic fetal red cells before they are recognized by the maternal immune system.[5]

Biochemical Characteristics and Molecular Genetics

The C/c and E/e antigens are displayed by distinct but structurally similar proteins with sizes approximating 33,100 daltons. The D antigen is expressed on a 31,900 dalton protein[16–18] that is also structurally similar to the C/c and E/e polypeptides.[19, 20] Amino acid sequence information indicates that the NH$_2$-termini of the D, C/c, and E/e proteins are identical through at least the first 41 residues.[21–23]

Cloned cDNAs corresponding to purified Rh

TABLE 8–3. NOMENCLATURE OF Rh ANTIGENS

FISHER-RACE	WIENER	ROSENFIELD (numerical)
D	Rho	RH1
C	rh'	RH2
E	rh''	RH3
c	hr'	RH4
e	hr''	RH5

TABLE 8–2. COMMON Rh GENE COMPLEXES IN CAUCASIANS

HAPLOTYPE	FREQUENCY	ANTIGENS PRODUCED
CDe	0.41	C, D, e
cde	0.39	c, e
cDE	0.14	c, D, E
cDe	0.026	c, D, e
cdE	0.012	c, E
Cde	0.010	C, e
CDE	Rare	C, D, E
CdE	Very rare	C, E

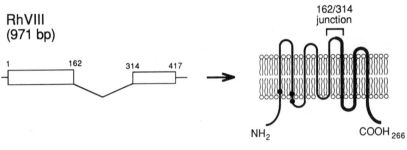

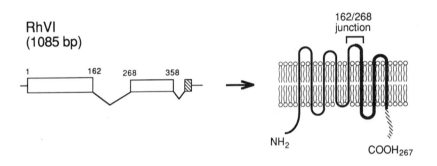

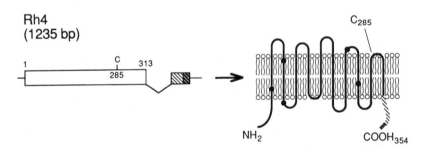

FIGURE 8–1. Structures of Rh polypeptide cDNAs and predicted transmembrane topologies of their polypeptide products.[29] The cDNA structures are depicted at the left; open boxes correspond to coding sequence. Numbers above the coding segments refer to amino acid sequence positions, numbered according to the predicted product of the RhIX b cDNA. Splicing patterns that delete polypeptide sequence in RhVIII, RhVI, and Rh4 are indicated by the thin, angled lines connecting portions of the coding segments. The amino acid sequence positions of the deletion endpoints are indicated by the numbers above the splice junctions. Protein sequence generated by frameshifting is indicated by the patterns filling the COOH-terminal portions of RhVI and Rh4. The proteins encoded by the cDNAs are predicted to maintain multiple membrane-spanning segments. The orientations of the COOH-terminal portions of the RhVIII and RhVI proteins are predicted to be inverted (indicated by the *bolder line*) relative to the RhIX b protein. The extracellular cysteine at position 285 in RhIX b and Rh4 is believed to correspond to the free sulfhydryl group whose oxidation destroys Rh antigenic reactivity. Amino acid sequence polymorphisms are denoted by the small solid circles.

proteins[23, 24] localize the cognate gene to chromosome 1p34.3–p36.1.[25] This position corresponds to the location of the Rh blood group locus determined by genetic mapping studies.[26] DNA sequence analysis of the open reading frame in the initially described cDNAs predicts a 417 amino acid long polypeptide without sequence similarity to known proteins. No potential asparagine-linked glycosylation sites are present, consistent with earlier work indicating that the Rh proteins are not glycosylated.[18, 27] The predicted amino acid sequence corresponds perfectly to the NH_2-termini of the purified Rh proteins. Southern blot analysis of genomic DNA suggests a model in which D-positive persons maintain two tightly linked and very homologous genes.[28] One of these (the *D* gene) en-

codes the RhD protein, and the second (the *Cc/Ee* gene) encodes both C/c- and E/e-reactive polypeptides. RhD-negative individuals are homozygous for complete deletions of the *D* gene, but the gene encoding the C/c- and E/e-reactive proteins remains intact. The Southern blot data[28] also suggest that in most individuals who do not display antigens of the C/c and/or E/e complex, the *Cc/Ee* gene remains largely intact but has suffered mutations that render it unable to generate its polypeptide products. The generation of C and E determinants by the *Cc/Ee* gene has been suggested by results of sequencing of Rh complementary DNAs (cDNAs)[23, 24, 29] (Fig. 8–1). The *Cc/Ee* gene can potentially generate at least four distinct membrane-spanning polypeptide products, by utilizing alternative splicing mechanisms. The large protein encoded by the RhIXb cDNA (see Fig. 8–1) corresponds to the E or e protein, whereas one or more of the other cDNAs yield a protein with C or c activity. This model is consistent with one proposed recently in which one gene encodes the D polypeptide and the other encodes both the C/c and the E/e polypeptides.[30]

The Rh cDNA sequences predict polypeptides with identical NH_2-termini (see Fig. 8–1), consistent with protein-sequencing studies. Hydropathy analysis and other considerations suggest that these proteins maintain multiple membrane-spanning segments, connected by short segments displayed at the surface of the cell or within the cytosol, with topologies as shown in Figure 8–1. These topologies are supported by other biochemical analyses.[22, 24, 31–33] In some instances, the membrane-spanning domains may in fact cross the membrane twice without hydrophilic extramembrane connections. It is noteworthy that four of the five NH_2-terminal domains of each protein contain acidic amino acid residues, whereas the third and fifth transmembrane segments are predicted to maintain an amphipathic helical configuration (reviewed in reference 34). These observations suggest the possibility that the putative transmembrane segments might function as part of a transmembrane channel. There is no cleavable signal sequence in these proteins, implying that their NH_2-termini are displayed on the cytosolic face of the membrane.[35]

The Rh polypeptides are post-translationally modified by fatty acylation[36] and are palmitylated via a thioester linkage to free sulfhydryls on cysteine residues, by analogy with other palmitylated polypeptides. The position (or positions) of palmitylation has yet to be defined, and the functional significance of this modification remains to be determined.

Rh antigenic reactivity is influenced by the lipid composition of the membrane environment, including alterations in red cell membrane cholesterol/phospholipid ratios.[37, 38] These observations are consistent with the predicted transmembrane orientation of the Rh proteins and indicate that alterations of the plasma membrane lipid concentration can modulate the display or conformation, or both, of the Rh determinants. There is also evidence that the Rh polypeptides interact with the red cell membrane skeleton. Under conditions in which the major protein components of the membrane skeleton (spectrin, actin, and other associated proteins) remain insoluble (low concentrations of non-ionic detergents), the Rh polypeptides may be found associated with these proteins.[39–41] Several pieces of evidence indicate that the Rh proteins maintain a physical association with other membrane polypeptides.[16, 42, 43] Some of these share substantial amounts of NH_2-terminal amino acid sequence identity with the RhD and RhC/c-E/e proteins[42, 43] and are thus termed "Rh-related" proteins, but the nature of these associated molecules remains unclear. One of the polypeptides that physically associate with the Rh proteins is the LW antigen, a glycoprotein with a deglycosylated molecular mass of 25,000 Da.[20, 33, 44] The COOH-terminal portion of the LW glycoprotein is displayed at the surface of the red cell and contributes to epitope (or epitopes) recognized by anti-LW antibodies. Two-dimensional peptide mapping studies demonstrate conclusively that the RhD polypeptide and the LW glycoprotein are distinct molecules.[20]

Rh_{null} and Rh_{mod} Phenotypes

Rh_{null} cells are completely deficient in Rh antigens and exhibit stomatocytosis, spherocytosis, and increased in vitro osmotic fragility. The rare individuals with the Rh_{null} phenotype typically suffer from a chronic, mild to moderate, non-immune hemolytic anemia (reviewed in reference 45). These cells also exhibit abnormalities in ion transport, ATPase activity, and water content[46, 47]; their membranes are relatively deficient in cholesterol content[47]; and they maintain an abnormal membrane phospholipid distribution.[48] A similar phenotype, known as Rh_{mod}, has also been described.[49] Rh_{mod} red cells have very low levels of Rh antigens, and like individuals with the Rh_{null} phenotype, persons with the Rh_{mod} phenotype also suffer from a mild compensated hemolytic anemia.

Rh_{null} (and Rh_{mod}) red cells also have diminished or absent expression of other blood group determinants,[30] including glycophorin B (the Ss antigens; see reference 50) and Duffy determinants (reviewed in reference 12). These cells are also deficient in other membrane-associated molecules, including the Rh-related glycoproteins and the LW glycoprotein,[20, 22, 33, 43, 44, 51] as well as others defined by monoclonal antibodies.[52, 53]

Genetic considerations reviewed in reference 45 indicate that the Rh_{null} phenotype may be accounted for either by homozygosity for silent alleles at the RH locus (the less common "amorph type" Rh_{null}) or by homozygosity for an allele (termed X^0r) at an autosomal locus that is genetically independent of the RH locus (the more common "regulator type" of Rh_{null}). The Rh_{mod} phenotype is believed to be a consequence of homozygosity for an allele (termed X^Q) at an autosomal locus distinct from the RH locus.[49] It is not known if the X^0r and X^Q correspond to alleles at the same locus.

Function

The abnormalities in the Rh_{null} and Rh_{mod} cells and the biochemical data summarized above are consistent with the notion that the Rh polypeptides play an essential role in facilitating normal surface display of the Rh-related glycoproteins and the other molecules whose expression is diminished or absent in Rh_{null} and Rh_{mod} red cells. By physically associating with these molecules, the Rh peptides may operate to fix them within the membrane or otherwise stabilize their conformations, possibly via their presumed association with proteins of the membrane skeleton.

The proposed multimembrane-spanning topology of the Rh proteins suggests that they may represent components of a membrane transporter complex, but this function, or any other, remains to be demonstrated. Several groups have proposed that the Rh polypeptides may participate in a process that maintains the asymmetrical distribution of phospholipids in red cell membranes (reviewed in reference 54). This process requires an enzyme termed ATP-dependent phosphatidylserine translocase, or PS flippase. It seems unlikely, however, that the Rh polypeptides participate in these events, since recent studies have shown that the PS flippase activities in Rh_{null} cells and in normal red cells are virtually identical and demonstrate that the PS flippase activity is unperturbed by Rh antibodies.[55]

Remaining questions for this area include those centered on understanding the physical and functional organization of the Rh locus and the molecular basis for antigenic polymorphisms in the Rh system, on understanding the topological relationships between the Rh polypeptides and the Rh-related polypeptides, and on determining the function (or functions) of the Rh complex.

GLYCOPHORINS A, B, AND E, AND THE MNSs BLOOD GROUP LOCUS

The red cell antigens M and N were first discovered by Landsteiner and Levine,[56] using antisera prepared from rabbits immunized with human red cells. The S and s antigens were later defined with human antisera.[57–59] Detailed discussions of the MNSs blood group system may be found in references 12 and 13.

Early genetic and immunological studies indicated that the M and N determinants represent allelic products of a single gene closely linked to another gene that gives rise to the allelic S and s determinants. Four common haplotypes at these two loci exist, with frequencies that depend on the population examined. Northern European populations, for example, maintain haplotype frequencies of approximately 0.38 for Ns, 0.30 for Ms, 0.24 for MS, and 0.07 for NS. Other phenotypes within the MNSs system also deserve mention. The U antigen, first described in 1953 by Wiener and colleagues,[60] is expressed by most Caucasian red cells but is absent from the red cells of approximately 1 per cent of black individuals. Among S-negative and s-negative blacks, approximately 84 per cent also have red cells that are deficient in the U determinant, whereas the remainder express low levels of the U determinant.

Two other high-frequency antigens have been described in Caucasians. The En^a antigen is absent from red cells taken from individuals with the En(a−) phenotype. As discussed later in this section, En(a−) red cells are deficient in part or all of the glycophorin A (GpA) protein. Another high-frequency antigen, known as the Wr^b determinant, is also absent from some individuals whose red cells are deficient in GpA

and glycophorin B (GpB). The molecular basis for its absence in rare individuals is poorly understood.

In addition to these high-frequency determinants, a large number of MN and Ss variants are encoded by alleles at the corresponding loci. These have typically been identified by investigating alloantibodies generated during transfusion or in pregnancy. These variants include those of the Miltenberger (Mi) class, Henshaw (He), and St^a, for example.

The clinical significance of the MNSs blood group system is relatively minor.[4, 5, 12] Many anti-M and anti-N antibodies are found as "naturally occurring" antibodies. These antibodies may often be heterogeneous mixtures of IgM and IgG molecules that display enhanced binding at low temperatures (i.e., cold-reactive antibodies). They are generally of little clinical significance. Examples of alloantibodies directed against the M and N determinants are rare. Anti-S and anti-s antibodies may be generated after exposure to antigen-positive red cells, via transfusion or pregnancy, although this is also a relatively infrequent occurrence. These antibodies are typically of the IgG class and have been known to be responsible for transfusion reactions and hemolytic disease of the newborn.[4, 5, 12]

Glycophorins

Biochemical and immunological methods have assigned the MN antigens to the glycophorin A (GpA) red cell surface sialoglycoprotein and the Ss antigens to glycophorin B (GpB) (reviewed in references 61 and 62).

The GpA gene (Fig. 8–2) gives rise to three transcripts of 2.8, 1.7, and 1.0 kb.[63–66] The 5' ends of these transcripts are virtually identical; transcript length heterogeneity is dictated by the use of alternate polyadenylation sites.[66, 67] GpA is synthesized with a cleavable leader peptide that ultimately yields a type I transmembrane protein 131 amino acids long. The protein is heavily glycosylated, carrying a single asparagine-linked glycan and 15 serine/threonine-linked oligosaccharide units. Carbohydrate constitutes approximately 60 per cent of the mass of GpA. The M and N antigens on GpA are determined by amino acid polymorphism at positions 1 and 5 of the mature polypeptide. The M antigen is defined by a serine at amino acid position 1 and a glycine at position 5, whereas the N antigen is defined by a leucine at position 1 and a glutamine at position 5. Anti-M and anti-N antibodies can recognize these peptide determinants exclusively but may also exhibit carbohydrate-dependent recognition properties.[68, 69]

Glycophorin B is a structurally similar type I transmembrane protein derived from a gene consisting of five exons (see Fig. 8–2). This gene yields a single 0.6 kb transcript.[63–66, 70] GpB is synthesized with a cleavable signal sequence, to yield a type I transmembrane protein 72 amino acids in length. There are no asparagine-linked carbohydrate chains on this molecule, whereas there are about 11 serine/threonine-linked

FIGURE 8–2. Glycophorins A, B, and E gene and protein structures. The glycophorin A (GpA) gene comprises seven exons. Exon 1 yields a leader peptide, whereas the extracellular domain is encoded by exons 2, 3, and 4. Exon 5 encodes the transmembrane domain. Exons 6 and 7 generate the cytosolic domain and 3′ untranslated region. Positions of amino acid residues corresponding to domain boundaries are indicated below the GpA protein. Amino acid sequence polymorphisms encoded by exon 2 yield either an M-specific glycophorin A molecule (serine at position 1 and glycine at residue 5) or an N-specific molecule (leucine at residue 1 and glutamine at residue 5).

The glycophorin B (GpB) gene comprises five functional exons (Nos. 1, 2, 4, 5, and 6); sequences corresponding to exon 3 are designated a pseudoexon, as they are not present in GpB transcripts as a consequence of a non-functional splice acceptor sequence at its 3′ border. Exon 1 yields a leader peptide. The extracellular domain is encoded by exons 2 and 4, and exon 5 encodes a short cytosolic segment and the transmembrane domain. Exon 6 generates the 3′ untranslated region. Positions of amino acid residues corresponding to domain boundaries are indicated below the GpB protein. Amino acid sequence polymorphisms encoded by exon 4 yield either an S-specific glycophorin B molecule (methionine at position 29) or an s-specific molecule (threonine at residue 29). The amino acid sequence encoded by exon 2 yields the "N" antigen, with leucine at position 1 and glutamine at position 5.

The glycophorin E (GpE) gene is predicted to comprise four functional exons (Nos. 1, 2, 5, and 6) and two non-utilized pseudoexons (Nos. 3 and 4). Exon 1 yields a leader peptide, exon 2 encodes the putative extracellular domain, and exon 5 encodes the predicted transmembrane segment. Exon 6 generates the 3′ untranslated region. Positions of amino acid residues corresponding to domain boundaries are indicated below the GpE protein. The extracellular domain is predicted to display M antigenic specificity. Thick lines correspond to segments of the GpE gene most similar to corresponding segments in the GpB gene, whereas thin lines denote regions most similar to corresponding locations in the GpA gene.

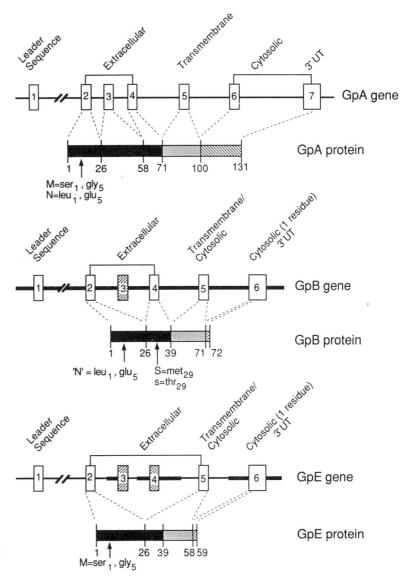

oligosaccharide chains. Approximately 50 per cent of the mass of GpB consists of oligosaccharide. The peptide sequence that determines N antigen reactivity on GpA is also found on GpB. This antigen, termed "N," is relatively weakly expressed, probably because substantially fewer copies of the GpB molecule are expressed at the surface of the red cell (0.15×10^6 copies per cell), relative to GpA copy number (approximately 1×10^6 copies per cell). The blood group Ss antigens are specified by amino acid polymorphism at position 29. The S antigen maintains a methionine at this position, whereas the s antigen displays a threonine here.[71]

Molecular cloning studies have been used to identify a gene homologous to the *GpA* and *GpB* genes, termed the *GpE* gene.[72, 73] Its sequence predicts a mature GpE protein 59 amino acids long, with residues 1 and 5 occupied by serine and glycine, respectively (i.e., corresponding to the blood group M determinant). The *GpE* gene lacks DNA sequences corresponding to amino acid residues 27 to 39 of GpB, encompassing the position of the Ss amino acid sequence polymorphism in GpB. The *GpE* also contains a DNA sequence insertion, relative to the *GpB* and *GpA* genes, at a position corresponding to exon 5 of the *GpA* gene. This insertion is predicted to encode eight amino acids not present in GpA or GpB. Efforts to identify a polypeptide product corresponding to the *GpE* gene have been largely unsuccessful, although recent immunoblotting studies using a murine anti-M monoclonal antibody suggest the *GpE* gene product can be identified as a 20,000 dalton molecule (reviewed in reference 74). The *GpA*, *GpB*, and *GpE* genes are tandemly oriented in a gene cluster (Fig. 8–3).

Molecular Basis of Antigenic Variation

The molecular basis has been determined for a variety of variant phenotypes of the MNSs blood group system (reviewed in references 62 and 75) (Fig. 8–4). These variants may be grouped into sets, accord-

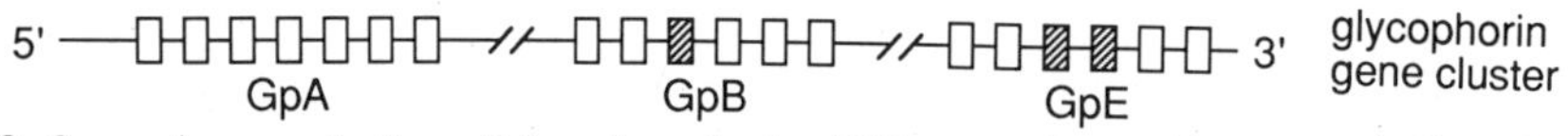

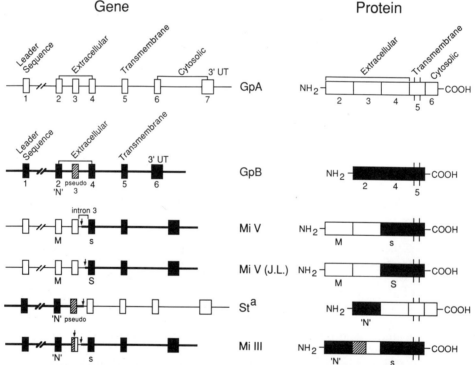

FIGURE 8–3. Genomic organization of the glycophorin ABE gene cluster. Exons are indicated by the open boxes. Pseudoexons in the GpB and GpE genes are denoted by the hatched boxes.

ing to the apparent mechanisms that generated them. Members of one of these sets appear to have been derived as a consequence of genetic cross-over events between intron 3 of the *GpA* gene and intron 3 of the *GpB* gene (Fig. 8–5). Members of a second group of variants appear to have been generated via gene replacement events (either double cross-over events or gene conversion) that have substituted a portion of the *GpB* gene pseudoexon 3 and intron 3 with a corresponding segment of the *GpA* gene derived from exon 3 and intron 3. A third group consists of members derived by structurally significant deletions of the *GpA* or *GpB* gene or both. Last, variants have been described whose antigenic properties are different from the wild-type versions by virtue of alterations in the serine/threonine-linked glycans attached to otherwise normal GpA and GpB polypeptides.

Examples of variants produced by unequal crossover include the MiV, MiV (J.L.), and St[a] phenotypes

(see Figs. 8–4 and 8–5) (reviewed in reference 76). The cross-over events that have engendered these phenotypes yield chimeric glycophorin protein products derived from the donor genes. In the case of the MiV and MiV (J.L.) phenotypes, this yields hybrid glycophorin molecules derived from the first three exons of the *GpA* gene and the last three exons of the *GpB* gene. These two phenotypes differ by virtue of the particular *Ss* allele derived from the donor *GpB* gene (see Fig. 8–4). By contrast, the St[a] phenotype is derived from a hybrid glycophorin molecule encoded by a chimeric gene constructed from the first two exons of the *GpB* gene and the last three exons of the *GpA* gene (see Figs. 8–4 and 8–5).

Examples of variants produced by sequence replacement mechanisms include the MiIII, MiX, and MiVI variants.[76] Molecular analysis of these variants has shown that a segment of the *GpB* gene between the 3′ portion of pseudoexon 3 and a position within intron

FIGURE 8–4. Genomic structures and polypeptides of representative variant glycophorins A and B. The structures of the wild-type GpA (*open boxes* and *thin lines*) and GpB (*solid black boxes* and *thick lines*) genes (*left*) and their corresponding proteins (*right*) are displayed at the top. Variant glycophorin genes, and their corresponding products, are displayed below the wild-type sequences. The MiV and MiV (J.L.) variant glycophorins arise as a consequence of recombination events (see Fig. 8–5) that have juxtaposed 5′ segments of the GpA gene with 3′ segments of the GpB gene, with the cross-overs (denoted by an *arrow*) occurring within the intron 3′ to GpA exon 3 and the intron 5′ to GpB exon 4. These hybrid molecules display M and S, or M and s, determinants, depending on the Ss genotype of the donor GpB segment. A reciprocal cross-over event is apparently responsible for generating the St[a] variant glycophorin. Double cross-over events, or gene conversion events, are apparently responsible for replacing a segment of the GpB gene with a corresponding portion of the GpA gene (denoted by paired vertical arrows), to generate the Mi III glycophorin variant.

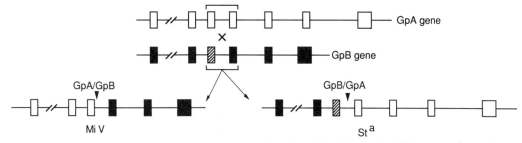

FIGURE 8–5. Recombination events predicted to yield variant glycophorin A and B genes and proteins.

3 has been replaced by a corresponding segment of the *GpA* gene (see Fig. 8–4). In each instance, the replacement events have occurred at different positions and are of different sizes. Nonetheless, in each case the GpA insert constitutes the 3′ end of exon 3 from the *GpA* gene, as well as sequences corresponding to the 5′ end of intron 3 of the *GpA* gene. This segment incorporates a functional 5′ splice junction derived from *GpA* intron 3 and therefore replaces the non-functional corresponding splice site at the distal end of *GpB* pseudoexon 3. Consequently, the chimeric molecules contain a peptide sequence encoded by portions of *GpB* pseudoexon 3, as well as a peptide sequence derived from the distal end of *GpA* exon 3.

Variants derived from partial or complete deletion of the *GpA* and/or *GpB* genes naturally are detected as red cells with deficiencies of the GpA or GpB proteins or both. Red cells with no detectable MN antigens fall into the En(a−) class of such variants. Two types of En(a−) variant are known. In an extensively studied Finnish pedigree, Southern blot analyses indicate that substantial portions of the *GpA* gene are absent, whereas the *GpB* sequences are virtually intact.[77] These observations, as well as biochemical studies, indicate that absence of GpA in En(a−) individuals in this pedigree is due to a homozygous deletion in the *GpA* gene. By contrast, in an En(a−) pedigree studied in the United Kingdom, genomic studies indicate that this *En(UK)* gene is a hybrid consisting of the 5′ end of the *GpA* gene linked to the 3′ portion of the *GpB* gene.[78] This chimeric gene presumably gives rise to a hybrid glycophorin molecule composed of the NH_2-terminal portion of an M-specific GpA linked to the COOH-terminal portion of a GpB molecule with S specificity.[77–79]

Red cells deficient for the Ss and U determinants are found rarely among North American populations but are present at low to moderate levels in populations of certain regions of Africa.[80] Biochemical analyses indicate that S− s− U− red cells are deficient in GpB or express a non-glycosylated, defective form of this protein.[81, 82] Southern blot hybridization analyses on DNA from S− s− U− persons indicate that in most instances absence of red cell GpB expression correlates with large deletions of the *GpB* gene.[83, 84] Rare individuals of the S− s− U− phenotype who maintain partial deletions of the *GpB* gene[83] or an apparently normal gross *GpB* gene structure[84] have been identified. In these instances, it is probable that

expression of the GpB polypeptide is deficient as a consequence of the partial deletions observed on Southern blots or as a result of point mutations or small deletions not detectable by Southern blot analyses.

Finally, phenotypes that are apparently due to deletion of the *GpA* and *GpB* genes have been described.[73, 85] In heterozygotes of the Mk variant,[86] red cell MN and Ss antigens are present at 50 per cent of the wild-type levels. In homozygotes,[87] red cells lack detectable GpA and GpB proteins, as well as all MN and Ss antigens, Wr^b determinants, and the En^a antigen.[12, 13, 88] Southern blot analyses have confirmed that the *GpA* and *GpB* loci are deleted in one such homozygous Mk individual.[73, 85] It is interesting that homozygous individuals exhibit no obvious detrimental phenotype associated with complete deficiency of the GpA and GpB proteins. There are no red cell morphological abnormalities, and red cell function and survival are essentially normal. These observations suggest that the GpA and GpB polypeptides have no essential function (reviewed in references 61, 62, and 89). Thus, the function or functions of the human glycophorins A, B, and E, if any, remain to be defined.

GLYCOPHORINS C AND D AND THE GERBICH BLOOD GROUP LOCUS

Antigens of the Gerbich (Ge) blood group were first described by Rosenfield and colleagues in 1960.[90] Except for rare variants, these antigens are found on the red cells from nearly all individuals. Consequently, generation of alloantibodies directed against Gerbich blood group determinants in the context of transfusion or pregnancy is an exceedingly rare event.[4] Four high-frequency antigens within the Gerbich blood group have been defined by human antisera and Gerbich variant red cells.[91, 92] These are denoted Ge:1, Ge:2, Ge:3, and Ge:4. These determinants define four phenotypes, including the most common phenotype, Ge:1, 2, 3, 4, and three variants that lack one or more of these determinants. These variants are known as the Melanesian type, which lacks the Ge:1 determinant (Ge:−1, 2, 3, 4); the Yussef type (Ge:−1, −2, 3, 4); and the Gerbich type (Ge:−1, −2, −3, 4). There is, in addition, a rare variant known as the "Leach" phenotype (Ge:−1, −2, −3, −4).[92–97]

Red cells taken from individuals with the Leach

phenotype are elliptocytotic and are deficient in red cell membrane proteins glycophorin C (GpC) and glycophorin D (GpD).[96, 97] This observation demonstrated that the Gerbich antigens correspond to determinants on GpC and/or GpD. Biochemical and immunological analyses indicate that the Ge:3 determinant may be destroyed by neuraminidase treatment or trypsin digestion and that it is expressed on GpC and GpD.[98–100] By contrast, the Ge:2 determinant, although neuraminidase and trypsin sensitive, is found only on GpD.[99, 100] The positions of the Ge:1 and Ge:2 determinants remain to be defined.

Cloned cDNAs encoding GpC have been obtained from a human reticulocyte cDNA library using peptide sequence information.[101, 102–104] The cDNA sequence predicts a 128 amino acid protein with a molecular weight of 14,000 daltons (Fig. 8–6A). This size predicted for the primary translation product is substantially smaller than the size of the GpC protein observed on sodium dodecyl sulfate (SDS) polyacrylamide gel (32,000 daltons; see references 102 and 105). This discrepancy can be accounted for by extensive post-translational modification by glycosylation, at the single predicted asparagine-linked glycosylation site and the multiple potential serine/threonine-linked glycosylation sites. These positions are located within a 57 amino acid long domain at NH_2-terminus that is predicted to be displayed at the surface of the red cell. A 24 amino acid long hydrophobic segment is appended to this extracellular domain and is predicted to constitute a membrane-spanning segment, whereas the COOH-terminal portion presumably resides in the cytosolic compartment.

Protein-sequencing studies indicate that GpD represents a molecular variant of the GpC molecule, corresponding to residues 22 to 128 of GpC.[106] This hypothesis is supported by immunochemical studies indicating that the COOH-terminal domain of GpD

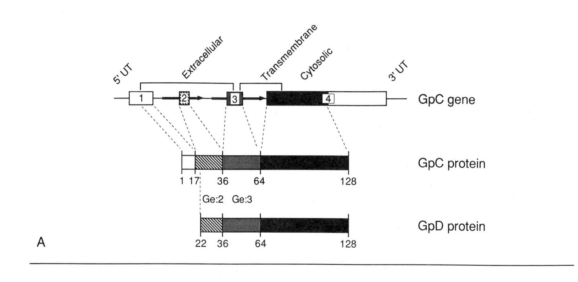

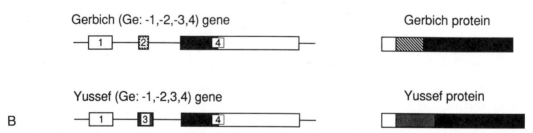

FIGURE 8–6. Glycophorin C (GpC) gene and variants. *A*, Wild-type GpC gene and derived protein products. The glycophorin C (GpC) gene comprises four exons. The extracellular domain of GpC is encoded by exons 1 and 2. Its transmembrane segment is encoded by exons 3 and 4, and the cytosolic portion by exon 4. Arrows encompassing exons 2 and 3 represent repeat sequences believed to be involved in recombination events that have deleted exon 2 or 3 in some glycophorin C variants (see *B*). Glycophorin D (GpD) is believed to be derived from the same transcript that yields GpC, via translation initiation at an internal methionine residue corresponding to residue 22 of GpC. Positions of amino acid residues corresponding to exon boundaries are indicated below the GpC and GpD proteins. The Ge:2 and Ge:3 determinants have been localized to positions corresponding to exons 2 and 3, respectively. *B*, Variant GpC proteins. The Gerbich-type variant GpC gene lacks sequences corresponding to exon 3, via a postulated recombination event occurring between repeated sequences depicted in *A*. This variant gene encodes a shortened GpC molecule deficient in amino acid residues corresponding to exon 3. The Yussef-type variant GpC gene lacks sequences corresponding to exon 2, via a similar mechanism, and is predicted to express a shortened protein deficient in amino acid residues corresponding to exon 2.

cross-reacts immunologically with GpC, whereas monoclonal antibodies specific for an NH_2-terminal segment of GpC do not react with GpD.[107] These considerations are also consistent with the observation that GpC (32,000 daltons) is approximately 9000 daltons larger than GpC (23,000 daltons). Inspection of the cDNA sequence encoding GpC suggests that the same transcript yields both GpC and GpD via a mechanism involving translation initiation at an internal ATG codon corresponding to the methionine residue at amino acid 22 in the GpD protein sequence.

GpC is encoded by a gene comprising four exons[62, 108, 109] (see Fig. 8–6A). The extracellular portion of GpC is encoded by exons 1 and 2, and a large part of exon 3, whereas the transmembrane segment and COOH-terminal cytosolic domains are encoded by exon 4. This gene represents a single copy sequence located on chromosome 2q14–q21.[110, 111] The fact that this represents a single copy sequence that yields a single 1.1 kb transcript in the erythroid lineage provides additional support for the idea that a single transcript yields both GpC and GpD proteins.

The molecular basis for several of the variants of the Gerbich blood group antigens has been determined. As noted previously, Leach variant red cells exhibit elliptocytosis and are deficient in the GpC and GpD cell surface sialoglycoproteins. Four unrelated individuals with the Leach phenotype have been examined by Southern blot analyses using segments of the GpC gene.[109, 112, 113] These studies indicate that three of these individuals are homozygous for a deletion of the GpC gene encompassing exons 3 and 4, whereas exons 1 and 2 are grossly intact. These reports did not provide information on whether or not these aberrant genes were transcribed, although it would be predicted that this would yield aberrant GpC and GpD molecules deficient in the membrane-spanning and cytoplasmic segments. Molecular analyses of a fourth individual of the Leach phenotype identified, by Southern blotting, a grossly normal GpC gene that also generated an apparently normal transcript. Nonetheless, sequence analysis of this transcript identified DNA sequence alterations at a position corresponding to codons 44 and 45.[113] These alterations change the tryptophan codon at position 44 to a leucine codon and also delete a single nucleotide in the adjacent codon. The frameshift mutation yields a termination codon at a position corresponding to residue 56 of the native protein, and the resulting predicted protein would thus consist of 43 residues derived from the native sequence followed by 12 new amino acids. This aberrant polypeptide, if expressed, would presumably not be displayed at the cell surface, since it would not contain a transmembrane segment.

Red cells of the Yussef type and Gerbich type variants lack membrane GpC and GpD molecules but display instead a single structurally related glycoprotein with a molecular weight intermediate between that displayed by GpC and GpD. Structural analysis of the GpC gene in Yussef-type individuals indicates that it has suffered a deletion of exon 2[110, 112] (Fig. 8–

6B). Similarly, the gene in Gerbich-type individuals has suffered a deletion of sequences corresponding to exon 3[110, 112] (Fig. 8–6B). It has been hypothesized that these deletions occur as a consequence of recombination between direct repeats within the GpC gene[108, 109] (Fig. 8–6A and B).

The deletion in the Yussef-type variant yields a transcript derived from exons 1 and 3 that is in turn translated into a 109 amino acid long protein deficient in the 19 residues encoded by exon 2. By contrast, a deletion in Gerbich-type individuals yields a transcript that is translated into a 100 amino acid long protein deficient in the 28 amino acids encoded by exon 3. These aberrant GpC molecules thus retain a transmembrane and COOH-terminal, cytosolic domain but display truncated forms of the extracellular domain. It is of interest that recent work indicates that alternative splicing of exon 2 of the wild-type GpC gene may occur normally in some tissues, to yield a truncated polypeptide identical to that expressed by the Yussef-type variant.[114] It is predicated that variant GpD molecules will also be synthesized by these molecular variants, via the internal initiation mechanism outlined above, although these molecules have yet to be described.

Other variants of the Gerbich blood group have been described, including the Ls^a phenotype, in which the red cells display larger GpC and GpD variant molecules as a consequence of duplicated exon 3.[115] The Webb (Wb) variant is a trypsin-sensitive antigen displayed by an aberrant GpC molecule.[116–118] Sequence analysis of a Wb allele identified a single base pair sequence difference within the codon corresponding to the asparagine residue at amino acid 8. This alteration changes the asparagine codon to a serine codon and thus removes the single asparagine-linked glycosylation site found on wild-type GpC. Thus, absence of the asparagine-linked glycan chain at this position accounts for the smaller size observed for Wb GpC.[118]

The elliptocytotic morphology exhibited by Leach erythrocytes (deficient in GpC and GpD molecules) suggests that these proteins function to maintain the normal shape of the red cell, via interactions with the erythrocytes of skeletal proteins.[93, 94, 119–123] Biochemical analyses indicate that GpC and GpD remain associated with red cell membrane skeleton proteins following extraction with non-ionic detergent.[94, 120] Similarly, patients who are genetically deficient in red cell protein 4.1 are concomitantly deficient in GpC and GpD molecules and Gerbich blood group determinants.[124, 125] These observations imply that the surface display of GpC and GpD depends on an interaction with protein 4.1, as has been shown in a recent study.[126]

THE KELL BLOOD GROUP SYSTEM

The Kell blood group system was first discovered in 1945[127] and named for the individual who made antibodies leading to its discovery. A total of 24 alloanti-

TABLE 8–4. NOMENCLATURE AND FREQUENCIES OF SOME KELL BLOOD GROUP ANTIGENS

Number	Letter	Antigen frequency (percentage)	Name
Kel1 (K1)	K	9.0	Kell
Kel2 (K2)	k	99.8	Cellano
Kel3 (K3)	Kp^a	2.0	Penny
Kel4 (K4)	Kp^b	>99.9	Rautenberg
Kel5 (K5)	Ku	>99.9	Peltz (K$_0$)
Kel6 (K6)	Js^a	<1.0 in whites; 19.5 in blacks	Sutter
Kel7 (K7)	Js^b	>99.9 in whites; 99.9 in blacks	Matthews
Kel15 (K15)	Kx	>99.9	

From Parsons, S. F., Mallinson, G., Judson, P. A., Anstee, D. J., Tanner, M. J. A., and Daniels, G. L.: Evidence that the Lu^b blood group antigen is located on red cell membrane glycoproteins of 85 and 78 kd. Transfusion 27:61, 1987; with permission.

gens have been described (reviewed in reference 128). Historically, these alloantigens have been referred to by a rather complex nomenclature that has been substantially simplified to one based on a simple numbering system (Table 8–4).[128]

The K1 antigen is highly immunogenic, relative to other human blood group alloantigens; it is second only to the RhD determinant in its immunogenicity. Approximately 5 per cent of K1-deficient recipients will mount an alloantibody response to the K1 determinant following transfusion with a single unit of K1-positive red cells.[129] Thus, anti-K1 antibodies are relatively frequently represented among the alloantibodies found in association with both immediate and delayed hemolytic transfusion reactions, as well as in hemolytic disease of the newborn (reviewed in reference 4). Indeed, anti-K1 accounts for approximately two thirds of non-Rh immune red cell alloantibodies.[4] Alloantibodies directed against other Kell determinants have been implicated in transfusion reactions and hemolytic disease of the newborn. These antibodies are substantially less common, largely because most represent high-frequency antigens. In most instances, anti-K1 antibodies are IgG; it has been estimated that approximately 17 per cent of these antibodies are competent to activate complement when bound to K1-positive red cells.[130]

Red cells display approximately 5000 Kell determinants.[131, 132] Immunoprecipitation studies using monospecific anti-Kell antibodies identify a single 93,000 dalton red cell membrane protein that displays two different Kell epitopes.[133] This molecule may exist as part of a larger complex under non-reducing conditions, migrating with sizes ranging from 115,000 daltons to more than 200,000 daltons. Immunoblotting experiments suggest that the Kell glycoprotein may exist as a homodimer in the membrane.[134, 135] The 93,000 dalton Kell reactive polypeptide was not detectable on red cells taken from individuals of the K$_0$ (K$_{null}$) type, which are known to be deficient in all Kell determinants.[133–135]

Sequence of a cDNA encoding the Kell protein[136] predicts an 83,000 dalton polypeptide 732 amino acids long. This protein is predicted to maintain a topology consisting of a cytosolic NH$_2$-terminal segment, a single hydrophobic membrane-spanning segment, and a large COOH-terminal extracellular domain (Fig. 8–7). Six potential asparagine-linked glycosylation sites and 15 cysteine residues are located in the extracellular domain. The Kell protein displays two heptad arrays of leucine residues, with clustered cysteine residues, in a motif known as a leucine zipper, that may be involved in protein-protein interactions.[137] By sequence homology, the Kell glycoprotein appears to be a member of the family of zinc-binding neutral endopeptidases.[136]

Two unusual Kell phenotypes have been described. The first, known as K$_0$ or K$_{null}$ phenotype, refers to the absence of the Kell glycoprotein from red cells[138] (reviewed in reference 128). Red cells of persons

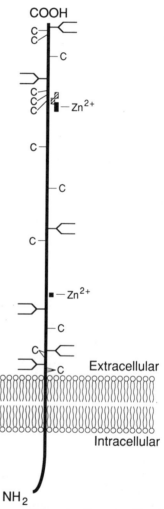

FIGURE 8–7. Transmembrane topology predicted for the Kell protein. Molecular cloning and biochemical studies outlined in the text predict that the Kell protein maintains a single transmembrane segment, with a large COOH-terminal extracellular domain. Positions of potential asparagine-linked glycosylation sites are indicated by the small branched structure. Locations of extracellular cysteine residues are indicated by C. Putative leucine zipper motifs are depicted by the small patterned boxes. Potential zinc coordination sites are shown by the small solid boxes.

homozygous for the K° allele are deficient in all known Kell antigens. K_{mod} is a rare, genetically heterogeneous phenotype in which the red cells display extraordinarily weak Kell antigen reactivity (reviewed in reference 130). Kell$_{null}$ and Kell$_{mod}$ red cells display a normal morphology and survive normally in vivo.

The McLeod syndrome is an X-linked disorder wherein affected males have acanthocytic red cells with a shortened in vivo survival. The common Kell antigens on these red cells are substantially depressed or not detectable. The locus responsible for the McLeod syndrome[139] has been termed Xk and is closely linked to the loci of chronic granulomatous disease and Duchenne muscular dystrophy.[140, 141] The product of this locus is a 37,000 dalton polypeptide that carries the Kx or Kell 5 determinant.[142] It is hypothesized that the product of the Xk gene directly facilitates red cell membrane expression of the Kell determinants. Red cells of patients with the McLeod syndrome display markedly decreased levels of Kell antigen activity because of a reduced amount of the 93,000 dalton Kell glycoprotein[142] and of the Kx determinant. These abnormalities yield an acanthocytic red cell morphology, as well as reduced in vivo survival.[143] Female carriers of a defective Xk locus display two populations of red cells, as a consequence of X-chromosome lyonization. One red cell population maintains a normal shape and displays a quantitatively normal amount of Kell determinants. The second population displays acanthocytosis and is presumably derived from an erythroid progenitor clone wherein the wild-type Xk allele has been inactivated.

THE KIDD BLOOD GROUP SYSTEM

The Kidd blood group system was first described in 1951, in the context of a case of hemolytic disease of the newborn.[144] The pathological IgG antibody here was directed against an antigen termed Jk^a. An antibody against a distinct Kidd allele, termed Jk^b, was described in 1953.[145] These two antigenic determinants (Jk^a and Jk^b) represent the only common alleles in most populations. The gene frequency for the Jk^a allele in Caucasians is 0.514 and is 0.486 for the Jk^b allele. Thus, approximately 26 per cent of such individuals have red cells with the phenotype Jk(a+ b−), corresponding to the genotype $Jk^a Jk^a$. Roughly 50 per cent of individuals have red cells with the phenotype Jk(a+b+), corresponding to the genotype $Jk^a Jk^b$, whereas 24 per cent of such individuals are of the genotype $Jk^b Jk^b$, with red cells of the phenotype Jk(a−b+). Rare individuals with a red cell phenotype of Jk(a−b−) have been described.[146–148] Anti-Jk^a and anti-Jk^b antibodies are typically generated in the context of pregnancy or transfusion and are most often IgG class antibodies, although IgM antibodies have also been described. Anti-Jk^a and anti-Jk^b antibodies have been implicated in hemolytic transfusion reactions and are among the more common types of antibodies implicated in delayed hemolytic transfusion reactions.[4]

Some Jk(a−b−) individuals generate antibodies capable of reacting with both Jk^a and Jk^b determinants.[146] Transfused or multiparous Jk(a−b−) individuals may generate an antibody termed Jk3, which recognizes Kidd blood group determinants distinct from the Jk^a and Jk^b determinants.[147, 148] By analogy to null phenotypes in other blood group systems (i.e., K$_{null}$, Rh negative), these observations point to the possibility that some Jk(a−b−) individuals may be genetically deficient in the ability to express meaningful amounts of the Kidd molecule.

Approximately 14,000 Kidd molecules are expressed at the surface of the red cell.[149] The Kidd determinant (or determinants) reside on a 45,000 dalton protein,[150] which most probably functions in transporting urea or other solutes.[151–153] This molecule has not yet been fully structurally characterized. Jk(a−b−) individuals exhibit a defective ability to concentrate their urine,[154] suggesting the possibility that the Kidd blood group determinants reside on a urea transporter molecule that is also expressed in the kidney (reviewed in references 155 and 156). Anti-Jk^a and anti-Jk^b antibodies have been used to screen λ gt11 cDNA expression libraries prepared from human reticulocytes.[157, 158] Preliminary sequence analyses of such clones suggest that they encode a polypeptide containing hydrophobic segments that may participate in generating a transmembrane topology. Functional analyses have not yet been done to confirm that this cDNA indeed encodes the Kidd blood group antigen or that it functions as the red cell urea transporter.

THE DUFFY (Fy) BLOOD GROUP SYSTEM

In Caucasians, there are two major alleles in the Duffy blood group system, Fy^a and Fy^b, with roughly equivalent frequencies (0.425 and 0.557, respectively) (reviewed in reference 159). Two other alleles also exist; Fy^x determines the expression of a weakly reactive version of Fy^b, whereas a null allele termed Fy generates neither Fy^a or Fy^b determinants. In most populations, the Fy^x and Fy alleles are found with frequencies substantially less than 0.02. By contrast, the Fy allele is common in blacks with African ancestry, and in certain regions in Africa all endogenous inhabitants are homozygous for this null allele.

Anti-Fy^a typically represents an IgG-type immune antibody; it has been implicated in hemolytic transfusion reactions and in hemolytic disease of the newborn. Anti-Fy^b is typically an anti-IgG antibody, although it is detected much less frequently than is anti-Fy^a.

The Fy^a and Fy^b determinants are found on one or more glycoproteins that migrate as a broad band with a molecular weight of between 38,000 daltons and 90,000 daltons.[160, 161] A significant amount of the mass of the immunoreactive molecule corresponds to asparagine-linked oligosaccharides, which probably accounts for its heterogeneous migration properties in its native state.[162] The antigenic determinant (or determinants) recognized by anti-Fy[a] antibodies is most likely a peptide sequence and is not created by post-translational glycosylation.

A protein termed Pd showing immunoreactivity with anti-Duffy antibody has also been isolated,[163] but its relationship to the Fy[a]- and Fy[b]-reactive molecules[160–162] remains to be determined.

Duffy antigens are essential for invasion of human red cells by *Plasmodium vivax,* an agent of human malaria, and also by *Plasmodium knowlesi,* a parasite that affects Old World monkeys but that is also capable of invading human red cells (reviewed in reference 164). Merozoites derived from these parasites are competent to attach to both Duffy-positive and Duffy-negative (Fy[a−b−]) human erythrocytes. After binding, the merozoite reorients (on both types of red cells) so that its apical end contacts the erythrocyte surface. Successful entry of the merozoite into the red cell requires the subsequent formation of a junction between the apex of the merozoite and the red cell.[165] Formation of this junction and penetration of the merozoite into the erythrocyte occur only on Duffy-positive red cells. Consequently, humans who lack Duffy blood group antigens are resistant to infection by *P. vivax,* accounting for the observation that infection with this parasite is rarely seen in West Africa, where the frequency of the Duffy locus null allele (*Fy*) is nearly 1.0.

THE LUTHERAN BLOOD GROUP SYSTEM

The Lutheran blood group system[12, 166] was first described during an investigation of an antibody formed in a patient who had received two blood transfusions.[167] Four major phenotypes are observed in this system. Approximately 90 per cent of individuals maintain the phenotype Lu(a−b+), and nearly all have the genotype *Lu[b]Lu[b]*. Most other individuals exhibit the phenotype Lu(a+b+), with the genotype *Lu[a]Lu[b]*. The phenotype Lu(a+b−) is relatively infrequent, owing to the low frequency of the *Lu[a]* allele in most populations. Rare individuals display no detectable Lutheran determinants (phenotype Lu[a−b−]). This Lutheran null phenotype is a consequence of three known genetic backgrounds. One represents homozygosity for null alleles at the *Lutheran* locus.[12, 166] A second corresponds to inheritance of a rare, autosomal dominant inhibitor gene termed (*In[Lu]*), which is not linked to the Lutheran locus.[168, 169] *In(Lu)* also suppresses expression of antigens from other blood group systems, including the P[1] and i antigens[170] and the CD44 epitope.[171, 172] Since two of these antigens are composed of oligosaccharide determinants (P[1], i) and the others represent glycoproteins (Lu and CD44), it is possible that the *In(Lu)* gene encodes a glycosyltransferase that masks or otherwise alters these determinants by glycosylation. The third, an X-linked dominantly acting inhibitor gene termed "*XS2*," can also suppress Lutheran antigen expression.[173] In homozy-

gotes for the null alleles, Lutheran antigens are not detectable, whereas in persons who have inherited an inhibitor gene, Lutheran antigens are expressed at low levels.

Anti-Lu[a] or anti-Lu[b] antibodies are rarely encountered, and virtually always in the context of transfusion or prior pregnancy. Immune anti-Lu[a] or anti-Lu[b] antibodies have typically not been associated with transfusion reactions or hemolytic disease of the newborn.[12, 166]

The Lutheran determinants are displayed by a pair of membrane glycoproteins with molecular weights of 78,000 daltons and 83,000 daltons.[174] Other antithetical antigens encoded by the *Lutheran* locus (Lu[6] and Lu[9]; Lu[8] and Lu[14]) and the so-called para-Lutheran antigens (Lu[4], Lu[12], and Lu[17], for example) also appear to be displayed by these two polypeptides.[175] The Auberger blood group determinants Au[a] and Au[b] are also located on the Lutheran glycoproteins.[176, 177]

In blood, the Lutheran blood group proteins are apparently restricted in their expression to erythrocytes. Lutheran blood group proteins, or antigenically related ones, are expressed by kidney endothelial cells and by hepatocytes.[178] The structures of Lutheran blood group proteins have not yet been determined, their genes remain to be isolated, and their functions are as yet unknown.

COMPLEMENT SYSTEM PROTEINS AS BLOOD GROUP DETERMINANTS—THE CHIDO/RODGERS ANTIGENS AND CROMER-RELATED ANTIGENS

The Chido (Ch) and Rodgers (Rg) blood group determinants were identified by corresponding alloantibodies that were generated in transfused patients.[179, 180] Ch or Rg determinants also circulate in plasma.[179–181] Antibodies directed against these determinants are typically of the IgG class and are generated only in transfused patients who lack Ch or Rg determinants. Ch or Rg alloantibodies are encountered relatively infrequently, since more than 95 per cent of random donors are Ch positive[181, 182] and more than 95 per cent are Rg positive.[180] Except in rare circumstances,[183] these antibodies are not clinically significant,[184, 185] most probably because the circulating forms of the corresponding antigens neutralize the antibody reactivities in vivo. Nonetheless, these antibodies can present difficulties during cross-matching procedures.

The Chido and Rodgers determinants are displayed by the two isotypes of the fourth component of complement, C4A and C4B (reviewed in reference 186). The human C4 molecules are glycoproteins with a molecular weight of approximately 210,000 daltons.[186] They are synthesized as single-chain precursors (pro-C4A and pro-C4B), which are converted to mature forms consisting of three disulfide bond–linked polypeptide chains. Complement activation cleaves the C4 molecules into specific fragments. The α chain of the mature form ultimately yields a fragment, termed C4d, that remains stably associated with the red cell membrane. Biochemical studies have demonstrated that the Ch and Rg determinants localize to the C4d fragment.[187] These molecules thus represent antigens that are acquired from plasma. It is believed that in vivo, the C4 proteins are subject to a constant, low-level fluid-phase activation that ultimately yields red cell–associated C4d molecules (reviewed in reference 188). Genetic, biochemical, and serological studies indicate that in most instances the Rodgers determinant corresponds to rare amino acid sequence polymorphisms within a region of the C4d fragment derived from the C4A isotype, within a region between amino acid residues 1054 and 1191 (summarized in reference 186). Similarly, Chido antigenic determinants generally correlate with rare amino acid sequence polymorphisms within the same region of the C4d fragment derived from the C4B isotype.[186] Rare exceptions to these assignments have been described in which variants of the C4A and C4B molecules (i.e., C4A1 and C4B5) express the Chido and Rodgers determinants typically assigned to the other C4 isotype.[189, 190]

The complement regulatory protein decay-accelerating factor, or DAF, also displays polymorphic antigens that may associate with the red cell membrane (reviewed in reference 191). These molecules have been termed "Cromer-related antigens," after the patient who made the alloantibody used to discover the Cromer-related system. Antibodies against these determinants have been described independently numerous times. In addition to being termed *Cromer (Cr^a)*, the locus that determines the expression of these antigens has been independently termed *Tc, Dr, WES, Es,* and *UMC*.[191] The rare Inab phenotype corresponds to a complete deficiency in Cromer-related antigens.[192]

Antibodies directed against Cromer-related antigens normally are not clinically significant,[193] although exceptions have been described in which these antibodies diminish red cell survival.[194] Biochemical and immunochemical approaches have been used to demonstrate that the Cromer-related antigens are carried on DAF.[195, 196] This assignment is further supported by the observation that Inab phenotype cells are deficient in DAF expression[197] and by identifying a specific amino acid sequence polymorphism in DAF (Ser 165 → Leu) that defines the *Dr^b* allele within the Cromer system.[198] The molecular basis for other polymorphisms within the DAF molecule that are identified as Cromer-related antigens remains to be defined.

THE *ABO* BLOOD GROUP LOCUS

At the beginning of this century, Landsteiner and associates, as well as other investigators, discovered a system of genetically polymorphic erythrocyte surface molecules that came to be known as the ABO blood group system.[199, 200] Humans could be grouped into distinct classes, depending on the presence or absence of substances in the serum that would agglutinate red cells from humans of other classes. These early results quickly found practical use in the field of blood transfusion.[4, 5, 201] The antigens of the ABO system, known as A, B, and H determinants, are expressed by the erythrocyte and by many other tissues, including the epithelium that lines glands and internal organs, and the vascular endothelium.[202] The cells of some human tissues can elaborate water-soluble forms of these molecules, as components of the glycans on secreted and soluble glycoproteins, on glycosphingolipids, and on free oligosaccharides. The ability to elaborate soluble ABH-active blood group molecules is a genetically inherited trait determined by the *Secretor* or *Se* locus.

Oligosaccharide Structure

The immunoreactive portions of the ABO blood group determinant are displayed at the termini of structurally heterogeneous oligosaccharides (Fig. 8–8). The membrane-associated A, B, and H determinants are components of integral membrane proteins and membrane-associated glycolipids (reviewed in references 203 and 204). A, B, and H blood group molecules are constructed by sequential action of distinct glycosyltransferases that are in turn each encoded by a distinct genetic locus (Fig. 8–9). These enzymes operate on one of four structurally distinct oligosaccharide precursor types known to be synthesized in human cells (see Fig. 8–8). Type 1 and type 2 precursors are found at the termini of linear and branched chain oligosaccharides that are themselves linked to proteins (see Fig. 8–8) via some asparagine residues (asparagine-linked oligosaccharides, Fig. 8–10A) or via some serine or threonine residues (serine/threonine-linked oligosaccharides, Fig. 8–10B). Type 1 and type 2 chains may also be displayed as components of lipid-linked oligosaccharides (Fig. 8–8 and Fig. 8–10C). Type 3 chains are found exclusively as components of serine/threonine-linked oligosaccharides (see Fig. 8–8), whereas type 4 chains are restricted to lipids (see Fig. 8–8). Type 1 oligosaccharide precursors are in general synthesized only by the epithelia lining the digestive, respiratory, urinary, and reproductive tracts, as well as by some exocrine glandular epithelium.[202] ABH determinants displayed by proteins and lipids in body fluids and secretions generally derive from these sources and thus are largely represented by type 1 molecules. By contrast, the ABH determinants displayed by erythrocytes and the epidermis are based largely on type 2 precursor chains.[202, 203, 205] Type 3 A, B, and H antigens are relatively abundant components of mucins that are elaborated by the gastric mucosa or by the cells that line ovarian cysts (reviewed in references 205 and 206). Type 3 ABH determinants are not found on human erythrocytes.[207] A variant of type 3 ABH-active chains, however, known as the "A associated" type 3 chain (Fig. 8–11), has been shown to be present in the glycolipids isolated from blood group A red cells.[207, 208] Human red cell glycolipids also contain A, B, and H determinants based on type 4 chains.[209, 210]

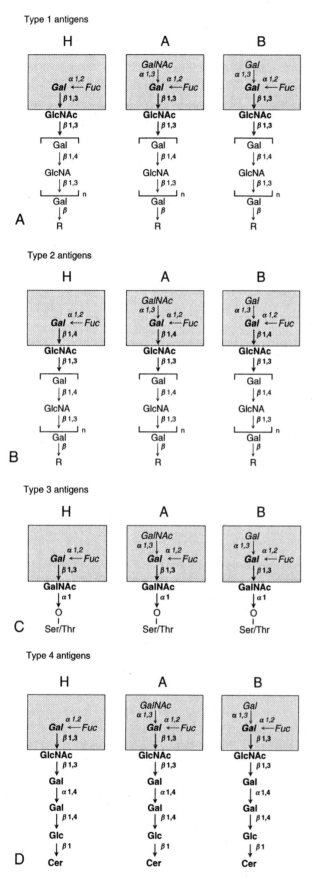

FIGURE 8–8. Oligosaccharide structures that display red cell ABH blood group determinants. The immunodominant part of each antigen is enclosed within a shaded box, and its monosaccharide components are italicized. Component monosaccharides displayed in bold type determine whether the oligosaccharide may be classified as type 1, 2, 3, or 4.

A and *B* display type 1 and type 2 determinants, respectively. R represents the asparagine-linked, serine/threonine-linked, or lipid-linked glycoconjugate backbone (see Fig. 8–10). Single lactosamine units are bracketed; this unit may be represented many times as a component of a linear polymer, where n may be 1 to more than 5, or it may not be found at all (n = 0). Not shown are β1,6-linked G1cNAc residues that yield I antigenic determinants (see Figs. 8–10 and 8–19) and multiple A, B, and H determinants on a branched oligosaccharide.

C displays type 3 A, B, and H determinants. These oligosaccharides are attached to some serines (Ser) or threonines (Thr) via an α-linked *N*-acetylgalactosamine moiety.

D displays type 4 A, B, and H determinants. Monosaccharide components of the globo-series backbone shown here are indicated by bold type. These molecules associate with the erythrocyte membrane via their ceramide (Cer) moiety. Similar oligosaccharides based on ganglio-series glycolipid precursors (Galβ1, 3GalNAcβ1, 3Galβ1, 4G1cβ1-Cer) also exist in human tissues (reviewed in reference 205).

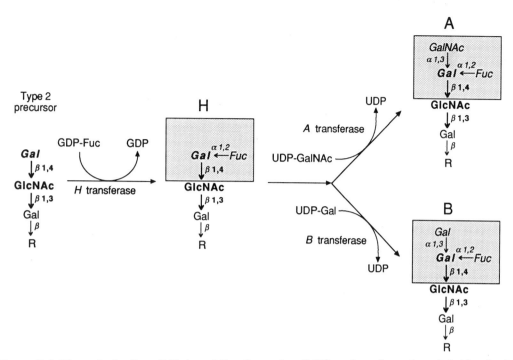

FIGURE 8–9. Biosynthesis of type2 H, A, and B antigens. An α(1,2)fucosyltransferase (encoded either by the *H* locus or by the *Secretor* locus) operates on the type 2 precursor oligosaccharide to form an H determinant. The H determinant may in turn be utilized by the α(1,3)*N*-acetylgalactosaminyltransferase activity encoded by the *A* blood group locus and/or by the α(1,3)galactosyltransferase encoded by the *B* blood group locus, to form, respectively, the A or B blood group antigen. The *A* transferase requires UDP-*N*-acetylgalactosamine (UDP-GalNAc) as its sugar nucleotide donor, whereas the *B* transferase utilizes UDP-galactose (UDP-Gal). Types 1, 3, and 4 A, B, and H determinants are constructed in a manner virtually identical to the reactions shown here. R represents the asparagine-linked, serine/threonine-linked, or lipid-linked glycoconjugate backbone.

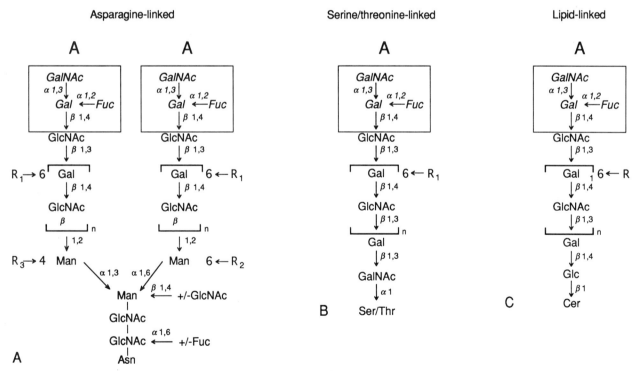

FIGURE 8–10. Glycoconjugate substructures that display the ABH blood group determinants. An A-active asparagine-linked oligosaccharide is shown in *A*, a serine/threonine-linked A determinant is displayed in *B*, and *C* shows a lipid-linked A-active oligosaccharide molecule. R_1 denotes branching oligosaccharide chains linked via β1 → 6–linked GlcNAc residues that form portions of I determinants (see Fig. 8–19). R_2 and R_3 indicate positions where other GlcNAc residues may be added to form tri- and tetra-antennary oligosaccharides.[242] Lactosamine units that may be polymerized (n = 0 to 5 or more) are enclosed in brackets.

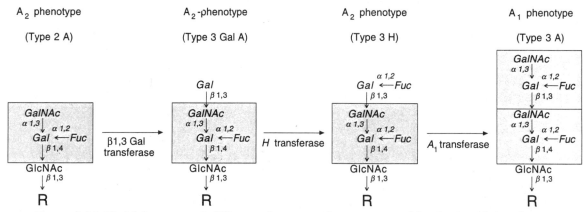

FIGURE 8–11. Model for structural differences between antigens constructed by the A₁ and A₂ subgroup transferases.[205] Type 2 A determinants representative of the A₂ phenotype (*far left*) are constructed by both A₁ and A₂ subgroup transferases. These determinants are then modified by a β1,3galactosyltransferase (β1,3Gal transferase) to form a type 3 precursor (type 3 Gal A, or "A-associated" determinant) also typical of the A₂ phenotype. This precursor is then fucosylated by the *H* locus–encoded α(1,2)fucosyltransferase to yield a type 3 H determinant. Type 3 H determinants are efficiently utilized by the A₁ transferase to form a repetitive A-reactive unit that terminates with a type 3 A structure. These moieties are proposed to be responsible for the A₁ phenotype.[205] By contrast, the A₂ transferase is unable to complete this reaction efficiently.[213] R represents the underlying glycosphingolipid substructure, as shown in Figure 8–10C. A-reactive portions of the molecule are boxed, and the component monosaccharides of these moieties are italicized.

Glycosyltransferases

During the formation of the ABO blood group determinants, oligosaccharide precursors are first modified in a transglycosylation reaction catalyzed by α(1,2)fucosyltransferases (see Fig. 8–9). These enzymes utilize the nucleotide sugar substrate GDP-fucose and transfer the fucose moiety to carbon 2 of the galactose molecule at the oligosaccharide precursor's non-reducing terminus. The fucose is attached in α anomeric linkage and forms the blood group H determinant, represented by the disaccharide unit Fucα(1,2)Galβ – (reviewed in reference 203). As discussed in detail below, genetic and biochemical evidence is consistent with the notion that the human genome encodes at least two different α(1,2)fucosyltransferases. These are thought to correspond to the products of the *H* and the *Se* blood group loci. The α(1,2)fucosyltransferases encoded by the two loci exhibit characteristic tissue-specific expression patterns (reviewed in reference 211) and display different affinities for the various ABH blood group precursor types. For example, the *H*-encoded enzyme, expressed in erythrocyte precursors, utilizes type 2[212] and type 4[213] precursors to form type 2 (see Figs. 8–8 and 8–9) and type 4 H determinants (see Fig. 8–8). By contrast, the *Se* α(1,2)fucosyltransferase, expressed in endodermally derived epithelia,[211] operates on type 1[212] and type 3[208] precursors to form the corresponding type 1 and 3 H determinants (see Fig. 8–8).

Codominant glycosyltransferases encoded by the *ABO* blood group locus in turn utilize type 1, 2, 3, or 4 H determinants to form A or B blood group determinants (reviewed in reference 203). The *A* allele at the *ABO* locus encodes an α1,3N-acetylgalactosaminyltransferase that utilizes H molecules to form the blood group A molecule (see Fig. 8–9). The blood group *B* allele, by contrast, encodes an α1,3galactosyltransferase that operates on H-active oligosaccharide precursors to form the blood group B determinant (see Fig. 8–9). The *O* allele represents a null allele incapable of encoding a functional glycosyltransferase that will further modify H-active precursors. Thus, an individual's complement of alleles at his or her *ABO* locus will determine whether that individual is capable of constructing the A molecule exclusively (genotype *AA* or *AO*), only B determinants (genotype *BB* or *BO*), or both A and B determinants (genotype *AB*). Individuals who maintain two null alleles at the *ABO* locus (genotype *OO*) do not modify their H-active precursors, and their red cells and tissues thus do not construct A or B determinants.

Expression in the Red Blood Cell

Most of the ABH determinants expressed on human erythrocytes are found as components of membrane-associated glycoproteins. Roughly 80 per cent of the red cell ABH determinants (1 to 2 million molecules per red cell; see reference 214) are displayed by the anion transport protein, also known as band 3.[215] The red cell glucose transport protein (band 4.5) also displays a significant number of ABH determinants (roughly 5 × 10⁵ molecules; see references 216 and 217). These two polypeptides are integral membrane proteins, and each displays ABH determinants on a single asparagine-linked oligosaccharide molecule.[217, 218] This asparagine-linked oligosaccharide is a branched poly N-acetylgalactosaminoglycan, whose terminal branches may display several ABH determinants (see Fig. 8–10).[219] Other red cell glycoproteins, including the Rh-related proteins discussed above, also display ABH determinants, albeit in smaller numbers.[220] The structural nature of the A-, B-, and H-active glycans attached to these proteins is not yet defined. Red cell membrane–associated glycolipids account for the rest of the red cell ABH molecules (approximately 5×10^5 determinants per red cell). These molecules are also poly N-acetylactosaminoglycan based and have been termed polyglycosylceramides, or macroglycolipids[221, 222] (see Fig. 8–10).

Anti-A and Anti-B Antibodies

The structural polymorphisms in these erythrocyte surface-localized oligosaccharides, determined by the *ABO* locus, are very clinically important entities under some circumstances.[4, 5] During infancy, the human immune system elaborates IgM antibodies specific for ABO oligosaccharide determinants that are *not* displayed by that person's erythrocytes or by other cells or tissues. It is believed that this immune response is a consequence of exposure to microbial oligosaccharide antigens that are structurally similar to, or identical to, the A and B blood group molecules. For example, type O persons lack A and B determinants and consequently maintain substantial titers of naturally occurring IgM antibodies, or isoagglutinins, reactive with A and B blood group molecules. Similarly, blood group B individuals maintain anti-A IgM-type isoagglutinins, but not anti-B isoagglutinins. In addition, sera taken from blood group A individuals contain IgM-type anti-B antibodies, but not anti-A antibodies. Finally, blood group AB persons make neither anti-A nor anti-B IgM-type isoagglutinins. In most individuals, antibodies directed against H determinants are not formed, because a substantial number of the blood group H precursors are not enzymatically converted to A or B determinants, or both, even in persons with a functional *A* or *B* allele. However, as noted below in more detail, individuals exist whose cells and tissues are relatively or completely deficient in H determinants. These persons, with the Bombay or para-Bombay phenotype, do typically generate anti-H antibodies, as well as anti-A and anti-B antibodies, since these persons cannot construct A or B determinants, regardless of their genotype at the *ABO* locus (see Fig. 8–9).

The naturally occurring IgM isoagglutinins efficiently fix complement and are present in sufficiently high titer to allow them to rapidly lyse transfused erythrocytes that display the corresponding antigen. This event typically is accompanied by the other clinical manifestations of an immediate or acute transfusion reaction and is normally avoided by the now routine ABO blood group typing and cross-matching procedures that were implemented earlier in this century.[4, 5] These procedures ensure compatibility between the ABO phenotype of transfused red cells and recipient plasma, or, conversely, compatibility between transfused plasma and a recipient's red cells.

A and B Subgroups

Routine ABO blood group typing and cross-matching procedures identify variants of blood group A determinants, termed A subgroups.[4, 223, 224] For example, blood group A individuals may be subgrouped according to whether or not their red cells will be agglutinated with an appropriately diluted solution of a carbohydrate-binding protein, or lectin, termed *Dolichos biflorus*.[225] Red cells that are agglutinated with this procedure are termed A_1 cells, whereas the red cells that are not agglutinated are termed A_2 cells. Antibody specific for A_1 cells may be prepared from group O or group B sera by prior adsorption with A_2 cells. In contrast, antibody specific for A_2 cells cannot be prepared by the converse procedure, via adsorption with A_1 cells.[4] The A_1 and the A_2 traits correspond to different alleles at the *ABO* locus.[203] Their frequency varies among different ethnic groups.[226] The A_1 trait is substantially more frequent than the A_2 trait. The A_1 and A_2 enzymes differ in their isoelectric points, metal ion requirements, pH activity profiles, and nucleotide sugar substrate affinities (reviewed in reference 203). The absolute number of immunodominant molecules is greater on A_1 cells than on A_2 cells[227, 228] (see Fig. 8–11). The antigens of the A_1 and A_2 subgroups also differ in their molecular structure.[227, 229–231] Other, relatively rare, subgroups of A also exist (reviewed in references 223 and 224) and represent biochemically distinct α 1,3N-acetylgalactosaminyltransferase activities and relatively unique antigenic properties. Unusual, weakly reactive blood group B antigens also exist[4, 223, 224] and most certainly also correspond to variant *B* transferase alleles.

The *cis*-AB phenotype has been described in rare pedigrees in which the ability to express both A and B determinants is inherited on a single chromosome transmitted from one parent.[232–234] In most such pedigrees, the *cis*-AB phenotype is characterized by a weakly reactive A antigen, similar in reactivity to A_2 cell reactivity. Red cells taken from *cis*-AB individuals also display only weak B antigen reactivity.

Two genetic models, supported by family studies,[235–237] account for this phenotype. In one model, the *cis*-AB phenotype is determined by two closely linked loci each of which encodes separate transferases, one with A-like activity and one with B-like activity. Such duplicated alleles could have arisen via an intrachromosomal duplication of an *A* or *B* allele to first yield a pair of tandemly repeated but otherwise identical transferase loci. In the second model, a wild-type *A* or *B* transferase allele has evolved to yield a single polypeptide capable of utilizing both UDP-N-acetylgalactosamine and UDP-galactose and thus also capable of synthesizing both A and B determinants.

Molecular Genetics

The human *A* transferase cDNA has been cloned and sequenced.[238, 239] The sequence predicts a 353

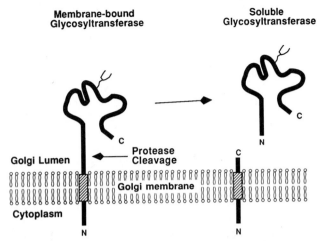

Membrane-bound Glycosyltransferase

Soluble Glycosyltransferase

Golgi Lumen

Protease Cleavage

Golgi membrane

Cytoplasm

FIGURE 8–12. Topology and biosynthesis of type II transmembrane-oriented mammalian glycosyltransferases. The enzyme's NH_2-terminus (N) of the full-length enzyme orients to the cytosolic face of the Golgi membrane, whereas its larger COOH-terminal catalytic domain (C) resides within the lumen of the Golgi apparatus. A short hydrophobic transmembrane segment (*hatched boxes*) anchors the enzyme within the Golgi membrane. The A, B, H, and Lewis blood group transferases are each predicted to contain one or more asparagine-linked glycosylation sites (oligosaccharide is represented by the branched structure attached to the protein backbone). Soluble, catalytically active forms of mammalian glycosyltransferases (*right*) derive from their membrane-bound precursors by one or more proteolytic events that release the catalytic domain from its membrane-associated NH_2-terminus.

amino acid long protein with a 15 residue NH_2-terminal segment, a 24 residue hydrophobic segment, and a 314 residue COOH-terminal domain. The hydrophobic segment most likely functions as a signal anchor sequence, to yield a protein with a type II transmembrane orientation (Fig. 8–12). This topology will position the protein's short NH_2-terminus within the cytosol and will place the longer COOH-terminal

segment "outside" the cell or, in this case, within the lumen of the Golgi apparatus. This is a topology that has been described for several other mammalian glycosyltransferases (reviewed in reference 240) and places the enzyme's COOH-terminal catalytic domain within the membrane-delimited compartments of the Golgi apparatus and the trans-Golgi network,[241] where terminal glycosylation reactions occur.[242] The peptide sequence predicts a single potential site for asparagine-linked glycosylation, suggesting the possibility that this enzyme is itself synthesized as a glycoprotein, as are other mammalian glycosyltransferases.[240] The enzyme exhibits a substantial amount of primary amino acid sequence similarity with murine and bovine $\alpha(1,3)$galactosyltransferases[243, 244] and a human $\alpha(1,3)$galactosyltransferase pseudogene,[245] but not to any other previously described proteins.

Although the cDNA sequence predicts a transmembrane enzyme, the A transferase was purified as a soluble, catalytically active polypeptide from human lung.[238] The NH_2-terminus of the soluble enzyme corresponds to the alanine residue encoded by codon 54 of the cDNA sequence, indicating that the soluble, catalytically active form of the A transferase is derived from its transmembrane precursor by one or more specific proteolytic events (see Fig. 8–12). Similar processes have been described for other mammalian glycosyltransferases, which exist both in membrane-associated forms and as soluble catalytically active forms.[240] It is presumed that such proteolytic events also generate the soluble A and B transferase activities found in human serum (reviewed in reference 203).

The molecular basis for polymorphism at the *ABO* locus has been delineated (Fig. 8–13).[246] The blood group O phenotype is due to a single base pair deletion of one nucleotide in the codon for amino acid 87 of the A transferase. This frameshift mutation generates

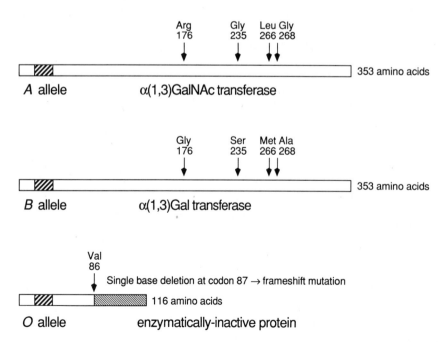

Arg 176   Gly 235   Leu Gly 266 268

353 amino acids

A allele $\alpha(1,3)$GalNAc transferase

Gly 176   Ser 235   Met Ala 266 268

353 amino acids

B allele $\alpha(1,3)$Gal transferase

Val 86

Single base deletion at codon 87 → frameshift mutation

116 amino acids

O allele   enzymatically-inactive protein

FIGURE 8–13. Molecular basis for polymorphism at the *ABO* locus. The ABO polypeptides are displayed as boxes. NH_2-terminal transmembrane segments are denoted by the hatched portion within each box. The *A* locus encodes an $\alpha(1,3)N$-acetylgalactosaminyltransferase 354 amino acids long (*top*). The $\alpha(1,3)$galactosyltransferase encoded by the *B* locus is of an identical length. The A and B transferases differ at the four amino acid positions indicated by the numbered arrows above the boxes. The sequence of the *O* allele–encoded protein (*bottom*) is identical to the sequences of A and B transferases up to a valine residue at amino acid position 86. It is different at the 30 subsequent positions (indicated by the *fine hatched lines* at the COOH-terminus of the box depicting the *O*-encoded protein) because of a frameshifting single base deletion within codon 87 of the *A* and *B* alleles. A termination codon within the altered reading frame truncates the resulting protein at 116 residues, to yield a non-functional protein.

a protein whose amino acid sequence differs completely from that of the A transferase at residues distal to amino acid residue 86 (see Fig. 8–13). The frameshifted reading frame stops at a termination codon that corresponds to amino acid 117 of the A transferase. This single base pair deletion in the O allele thus predicts the synthesis of an altered and shortened polypeptide that lacks a functional catalytic domain and that is consequently catalytically inactive. These results explain why no detectable A or B transferase activity is found in the sera taken from blood group O individuals (genotype OO) and why the erythrocytes of these individuals are devoid of A or B determinants.

Comparisons of the sequences of the cDNAs isolated from A and/or B phenotype cell lines identified seven nucleotide sequence differences within their protein-coding segments.[246] Three of these represent functionally neutral polymorphisms. The other four generate amino acid sequence differences between the A and B transferases (see Fig. 8–13). The four amino acid sequence polymorphisms are located at residues 176 (arginine, A; glycine, B), 235 (glycine, A; serine, B), 266 (leucine, A; methionine, B), and 268 (glycine, A; alanine, B). The polymorphisms at positions 266 and 268 exert a strong influence on the enzyme's ability to discriminate between UDP-GalNAc and UDP-Gal.[247] Thus, leucine at 266 and glycine at 268 generate an A phenotype, independent of the polypeptide sequence at the other two polymorphic positions; similarly, a B transferase phenotype is observed whenever B transferase residues are placed at these positions (methionine at 266, alanine at 268), irrespective of the residues at positions 176 and 235. The polymorphism at position 176 has virtually no detectable influence on substrate discrimination.

Function

The functions of the ABO blood group oligosaccharides remain unknown. Numerous associations between ABO blood group phenotype and relative risk for a number of maladies have been reported (reviewed in references 248 and 249). These associations are, without exception, substantially imperfect, and without an identifiable causal relationship. Examples include the association between group A phenotype and slight increase in the relative risk for stomach cancer (relative risk of approximately 1.2; see reference 250) and the association between blood group O phenotype and a mildly increased propensity to develop peptic ulcers (relative risk of roughly 1.3; see reference 251). Selective advantage, such as protection from various infectious agents, has been invoked to explain the establishment of ABO blood group frequencies in human populations (reviewed in reference 252), but no evidence from population or other studies has been provided in support of this idea. It is possible that environmental pressures once selected for, or perhaps against, expression of A or B determinants or both, but that such pressures are no longer widely operative (discussed in reference 252). The nature of such pressures remains a subject for speculation.

THE H AND Se BLOOD GROUP LOCI

H blood group oligosaccharide precursors represent essential substrates for the transferases encoded by the ABO locus (see Fig. 8–9). H-active precursors maintain terminal Fucα1,2Galβ linkages, which are also an integral part of the A and B antigenic determinants (see Figs. 8–8 and 8–9). H-active Fucα1,2Galβ linkages are synthesized by α(1,2)fucosyltransferases (GDP-fucose:Galβ 2-α-L-fucosyltransferase, E.C.2.4.1.69) (see Fig. 8–9). These transferases can utilize types 1, 2, 3, or 4 glycoprotein or glycolipid substrates (reviewed in reference 203), as well as low molecular weight β-D-galactosides.[253]

In humans, the ability to synthesize H-active blood group substances, and thus also A- or B-active substances (depending on the ABO locus genotype), is determined by at least two discrete genetic loci. These loci are termed the H locus and the Secretor (Se) locus (reviewed in references 202 and 203). The Se locus determines expression of an α(1,2)fucosyltransferase activity, as well as membrane-associated and soluble H-active blood group substances, in epithelial cells that line the digestive, respiratory, and urinary tracts, for example, and in the acinar cells of the salivary glands. In secretor-positive individuals, it is possible to detect such soluble group-active substances by testing saliva for their presence, using hemagglutination-inhibition methods.[4] Nearly all of this soluble blood group–active substance is constructed from type 1 precursors[202] and is elaborated largely by the sublingual and submaxillary glands, and to a lesser extent by the parotid gland.[254, 255] If the tested individual also maintains a functional A or B allele or both, the saliva will contain soluble A- or B-active blood group molecules or both, in addition to H-active blood group substance, since the ABO locus is also expressed in these tissues. By contrast, the saliva taken from non-secretor individuals does not contain H-active blood group substance or significant levels of α(1,2)fucosyltransferase activity. Moreover, because H determinants represent essential precursors for the synthesis of A and B determinants, their absence precludes synthesis of A- and B-active molecules, regardless of the non-secretor's ABO locus genotype.

It is generally true that erythrocytes taken from both secretors and non-secretors maintain an essentially identical complement of H determinants and of A or B determinants, depending on the ABO locus genotype. This is because the synthesis of α(1,2)fucosyltransferase activity, and thus H determinants, in erythrocyte precursors is directed by the H locus.[202] Rare individuals have been described, however, whose red cells are deficient in H (and also A and B) determinants. These individuals maintain two null alleles at the H locus. The first description of such individuals termed this the Bombay (O_h) blood group phenotype,[256] based on the city of origin of the pedigree. The saliva and other secretions taken from individuals with the Bombay phenotype in this pedigree, and from similar such individuals in other subsequently described Bombay pedigrees, are also deficient in H determinants, as well as A and B determinants. Consequently, individuals with the Bombay phenotype maintain high titers of naturally occurring isoagglutinins that react with H determinants (and with A and B antigens as well). As with A and B isoagglutinins in O phenotype individuals, it is again presumed that these IgM-type anti-H antibodies develop in response to H antigens elaborated by microbes. These anti-H isoagglutinins render these individuals cross-match incompatible with all blood group donors, except other Bombay donors whose red cells do not display H determinants.[4, 5]

Subsequent studies have identified a related phenotype, termed the para-Bombay phenotype.[257] Red cells taken from these individuals are relatively deficient in H, A, and B determinants, but their saliva contains an essentially normal amount of H blood group substance.

Genetic Models

A model accounting for each of the four possible phenotypes described to date (Fig. 8–14) proposes that the *H* and *Se* loci correspond to distinct genes encoding different α(1,2)fucosyltransferases with disparate tissue-specific expression patterns.[258] This model proposes that the *H* locus is expressed predominantly by cells of the erythroid lineage, by keratinocytes in the epidermis, and by primary sensory neurons within the peripheral nervous system.[202, 205, 259] By contrast, the *Se* locus is proposed to encode an α(1,2)fucosyltransferase whose expression is generally restricted to the epithelia lining the respiratory, digestive, biliary, and urinary tracts and to the acinar cells of salivary glands.[260, 261] Individuals with the common

secretor phenotype (roughly 80 per cent of most populations; see reference 262) are thus believed to maintain at least one functional allele at both the *H* locus and the *Se* locus. Individuals with the nonsecretor phenotype (nearly all of the remaining 20 per cent of individuals) maintain two null alleles at the *Se* locus, but at least one wild-type *H* allele. The model proposes that the rare Bombay phenotype is the consequence of homozygosity for null alleles at the *H* locus, and at the *Se* locus, whereas the equally rare para-Bombay phenotype results from a state of homozygosity for null alleles at the *H* locus, in the context of at least one functional *Se* allele (see Fig. 8–14).

Molecular Genetics

The two-locus model is supported by a number of biochemical and genetic observations. Careful analysis of the catalytic activities of the α(1,2)fucosyltransferase determined by the *H* locus, and the corresponding enzyme determined by the *Se* locus, indicates that the *Se*-determined α(1,2)fucosyltransferase maintains a significantly higher affinity for type 1 precursors than does the *H*-determined enzyme.[263–265] These observations are additionally consistent with the finding that blood group–active substances elaborated by secretory epithelia (where the *Se* locus is expressed) are constructed mainly from type 1 precursors, whereas erythrocyte H determinants, synthesized by the *H*-encoded α(1,2)fucosyltransferase, are based largely on type 2 precursors (reviewed in references 202 and 211). These observations also support a hypothesis that optimal utilization of the stereochemically distinct type 1 and type 2 precursors should require structurally and enzymatically distinct α(1,2)fucosyltransferases (reviewed in reference 266). Furthermore, genetic and biochemical studies of several H-deficient pedigrees indicate that although the *H* and *Se* loci are closely linked on chromosome 19 (lod score of 12.9 at 1 per cent recombination; see reference 258), they nonethe-

Phenotype	Phenotype (trivial name)	Genotype
H (A&B) on red cells		*HH* or *Hh*
	Secretor	
H (A&B) in secretions		*Sese* or *SeSe*
H (A&B) on red cells		*HH* or *Hh*
	Non-Secretor	
H (A&B) absent from secretions		*sese*
weak or absent H (A&B) on red cells (antigens adsorbed from plasma)		*hh*
	para-Bombay	
H (A&B) in secretions		*Sese* or *SeSe*
H (A&B) absent from red cells		*hh*
	Bombay, or O$_h$	
H (A&B) absent from secretions		*sese*

FIGURE 8–14. The two-locus model for H and Se phenotypes. The two-locus model proposes that the *H* and *Se* loci correspond to distinct, chromosome 19–localized α(1,2)fucosyltransferase genes with different tissue-specific expression patterns. The figure displays the red cell and secretion antigenic phenotypes predicted by this model for various genotypes at the two loci. A and B antigens are included in parentheses to indicate that they will be displayed also only if the individual maintains a functional *A* or *B* transferase allele. Red cells of para-Bombay individuals display H (and A or B) antigens weakly, or not at all, because they are acquired in low amounts from glycosphingolipid-based antigens circulating in the plasma.

less determine expression of α(1,2)fucosyltransferases with distinctly different catalytic properties.

A human α(1,2)focusyltransferase gene that is a candidate for the human *H* blood group locus has been isolated recently (Fig. 8–15).[264, 267] The sequence of a corresponding cloned cDNA[268] predicts a 365 amino acid long polypeptide with the type II transmembrane topology characteristic of mammalian glycosyltransferases.[240] The amino acid sequence predicts an 8 amino acid long NH₂-terminal cytosolic domain, a 17 residue hydrophobic domain that presumably spans the Golgi membrane, and a 340 amino acid long COOH-terminal domain corresponding to a Golgi-localized catalytic domain (see Figs. 8–12 and 8–15). Two potential asparagine-linked glycosylation sites are located within the COOH-terminal domain, suggesting that the fucosyltransferase is synthesized as a glycoprotein. The enzyme does not exhibit significant primary sequence similarity to any known polypeptide, including other mammalian glycosyltransferases. Gene fusion experiments have demonstrated that catalytic activity may be generated by the enzyme's COOH-terminal domain and have directly confirmed that the cDNA encodes an α(1,2)fucosyltransferase.[268]

The α(1,2)fucosyltransferase encoded by this cDNA exhibits affinities for acceptor and donor substrates that are essentially identical to those previously ascribed to the human *H* α(1,2)fucosyltransferase.[263, 269] The properties of this enzyme are significantly different, however, from those attributed to the *Se* α(1,2)fucosyltransferase activity.[265] This gene has been localized to human chromosome 19,[268] where the human *H* locus is found,[270] further suggesting that this cDNA corresponds to the human *H* blood group locus.

The structure and function of this gene have been examined in Bombay and para-Bombay pedigrees.[271] Analysis of this gene (see Fig. 8–15) in a Bombay pedigree identified a termination codon corresponding to a tyrosine at amino acid residue 316 (Tyr 316 → ter, Fig. 8–15). Gene transfer experiments have confirmed that the mutation inactivates this allele. The Bombay propositus is homozygous for this mutation, whereas the parents are heterozygous.

In a para-Bombay pedigree (secretor positive, erythroid H deficient; see reference 257), the propositus is a compound heterozygote for two functionally significant mutations that segregate separately in the family. One represents a missense mutation in the

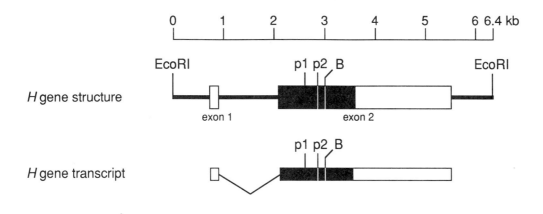

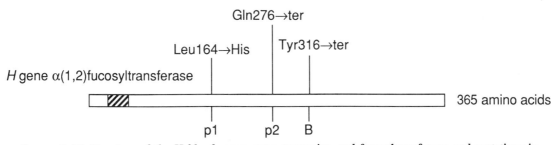

FIGURE 8–15. **Structure of the H blood group gene, transcript, and fucosyltransferase, and mutations in Bombay and para-Bombay alleles.** The gene and its transcript are drawn to the scale indicated at the top of the figure. The two exons of the human *H* gene are encompassed within a 6.4 kb *EcoRI* DNA restriction fragment. Exon 2 contains the entire coding region (*solid region*). The gene yields a 3.6 kb mRNA transcript (*middle*). The positions of inactivating mutations in Bombay (B) and para-Bombay (p1 and p2) pedigrees are indicated on the gene structure and its transcript. The transcript yields a 365 amino acid type 2 transmembrane protein (*bottom,* not to scale; transmembrane segment indicated by the *hatched segment*). The positions and identities of the amino acids corresponding to inactivating mutations in the Bombay and para-Bombay alleles are displayed above and below the schematic of the α(1,2)fucosyltransferase.

DNA sequence corresponding to amino acid residue 164; the other creates a termination codon corresponding to amino acid residue 276 (Glu 276 → ter) (see Fig. 8–15). Gene transfer experiments indicate that both the nonsense mutation and the missense mutation yield an inactive α(1,2)fucosyltransferase gene. These findings demonstrate that the cloned α(1,2)fucosyltransferase gene determines expression of H blood group antigen on red cells, and thus corresponds to the *H* locus. They also imply that the human genome must contain a second functional α(1,2)fucosyltransferase gene distinct from the *H* locus, since the para-Bombay individual who contains the two inactivated α(1,2)fucosyltransferase alleles is still capable of expressing wild-type, *Se* locus–determined α(1,2)fucosyltransferase activity. Final confirmation of this hypothesis, as well as a definition of the molecular basis for the non-secretor phenotype, will await isolation of the human *Se* blood group locus.

Function

As is the case with the *ABO* locus, no clear functions have been assigned to the oligosaccharides whose synthesis is determined by the *H* and *Se* loci. Many associations between secretor status and predilection for various illnesses have been reported.[248, 249, 252] These include an increased relative risk for peptic ulceration exhibited by non-secretors[272] and an increased relative risk for recurrent urinary tract infection in non-secretor females.[273] These latter observations may reflect influences exerted by soluble blood group substances on the binding of bacterial pathogens to oligosaccharide receptors displayed by urothelial surfaces.[274, 275] Most other such reported associations have had no obvious causal relationship demonstrated, however. The apparently normal phenotype of Bombay subjects suggests that oligosaccharides containing terminal, H-active Fucα(1,2)Galβ moieties determined by the *H* and *Se* α(1,2)fucosyltransferases are not essential molecules, unless one invokes the existence of still other α(1,2)fucosyltransferase genes (proposed in reference 276) with essential (if as yet unidentified) functions during embryogenesis (discussed in references 252 and 277).

THE *LEWIS* BLOOD GROUP LOCUS

The first description of the human Lewis blood group system was reported as part of an investigation into two cases of hemolytic disease of the newborn.[278] The term "Lewis" is derived from the last name of one of the women with anti-Lewis antibodies. The antigenic portions of the Lewis blood group–active molecules are composed of carbohydrates[279–281] (Fig. 8–16).

Expression of Lewis a (Le^a) or Lewis b (Le^b) antigens, or of no Lewis antigens at all, by human red cells, is a function of an individual's *Se* and Lewis (*Le*) genotypes.

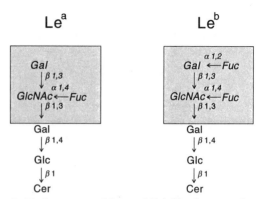

FIGURE 8–16. Structures of Le^a and Le^b blood group glycosphingolipids. The immunodominant portion of each molecule is highlighted by a shaded rectangle. Component monosaccharides are italicized. The molecule associates with the erythrocyte membrane via the ceramide moiety (Cer).

Le^a and Le^b antigens displayed by red cells are not themselves synthesized by red cell precursors. They are instead adsorbed by the erythrocyte membrane via an apparently passive process that utilizes Lewis-active glycosphingolipid molecules (see Fig. 8–16) circulating in plasma.[282] These Le^a- and Le^b-active glycosphingolipid molecules[280, 281] (see Fig. 8–16) are found in the plasma as complexes with low- and high-density lipoproteins and as aqueous dispersions.[282] It has been estimated that there are between approximately 4500 and 7300 Le^a molecules per red cell.[283]

Antibodies directed against Lewis determinants are relatively common entities and in most cases are naturally occurring (reviewed in reference 4). High-titer anti-Le^a antibodies have in some cases played causative roles in clinically significant hemolytic transfusion reactions, whereas anti-Le^b antibodies typically are not associated with clinical problems.[4] Circulating anti-Lewis antibodies are effectively neutralized in most cases by transfused plasma,[4, 5] which contains soluble Le^a or Le^b substances.[284] In addition, transfused Lewis antigen–positive erythrocytes can rapidly become Lewis antigen negative after transfusion, via reversal of the passive absorptive process by which they acquire these antigens in the donor.[4, 5] Red cells taken from newborns are typically deficient in Lewis antigens. These determinants appear at approximately 10 days after birth and are displayed first as Le^a activity in Lewis-positive infants.[285] The full complement of red cell Lewis antigens is realized at approximately 24 months of age.[286]

Synthesis of the Le^a and Le^b antigens is catalyzed by two distinct fucosyltransferases whose expression is independently controlled by the *Le* blood group locus and the *Se* blood group locus (reviewed in references 202 and 203) (Figs. 8–16 and 8–17). Strong biochemical and genetic evidence indicates that the *Le* locus corresponds to an α(1,3/1,4)fucosyltransferase gene.[287–290] The enzyme encoded by this gene is capable of operating on a structurally diverse group of oligosaccharide precursors. This enzyme can utilize unsubstituted type 1 oligosaccharide precursors to

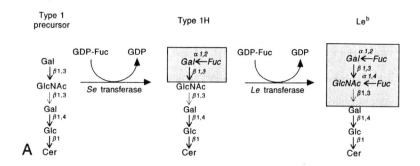

Lewis-positive, Secretor-positive

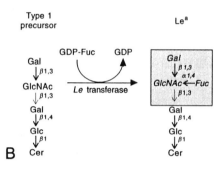

Lewis-positive, Non-secretor

FIGURE 8–17. Biosynthesis of the Le^a and Le^b determinants. The α(1,3/1,4)fucosyltransferase encoded by the *Lewis* locus (*Le* fucosyltransferase) and the α(1,2)fucosyltransferase determined by the *Secretor* locus (*Se* transferase) operate singly, or sequentially, on type 1 glycosphingolipid precursors. The final product depends on the genotype at both loci (see text for details). The oligosaccharide products of each of the four possible phenotypes are indicated in *A* through *D*. The immunodominant portion of each antigen is highlighted by a shaded rectangle. Component monosaccharides are italicized.

Lewis-negative, Secretor-positive

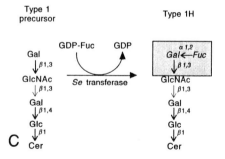

Lewis-negative, Non-secretor

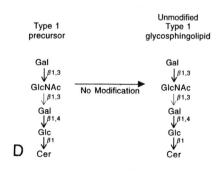

form the Le[a] determinant, for example, and can also efficiently utilize type 1 H determinants to construct Le[b] determinants.[287–289] Histochemical and biochemical procedures identify *Le* locus–dependent expression of Le[a] and Le[b] molecules by epithelia lining the respiratory, urinary, and digestive tracts, salivary glands, and bile ducts, for example (reviewed in references 202, 203, and 211). These tissues correspond almost perfectly to the tissue types capable of expression of type 1 H molecules, whose synthesis is determined by the *Se* locus.

Since the *Lewis* $\alpha(1,3/1,4)$fucosyltransferase can utilize the oligosaccharide products formed by the *Se*-determined $\alpha(1,2)$fucosyltransferase, and because the *Se* and *Le* fucosyltransferases are expressed in many of the same tissues, it follows that the genotype at these two loci will determine which, if any, of the Lewis-active oligosaccharide molecules will be constructed (see Fig. 8–17). In secretor-positive individuals, type 1 oligosaccharide precursors initially are converted to type 1 H molecules.[203] These in turn represent substrates for the action of the *Lewis* locus–encoded $\alpha(1,3/1,4)$fucosyltransferase, which converts these to Le[b]-active molecules (Le[a−b+] phenotype, Fig. 8–17*A*). By contrast, non-secretors are incapable of constructing type 1 H determinants in secretory epithelia, and these unsubstituted type 1 molecules are thus converted into Le[a]-active oligosaccharides by the action of the *Le*-encoded $\alpha(1,3/1,4)$fucosyltransferase (Le[a+b−] phenotype, Fig. 8–17*B*). In individuals homozygous for null alleles at the *Le* locus, two possible outcomes are observed. In secretor-positive, Lewis-negative individuals, type 1 H determinants are constructed but remain unconverted to Le[b] determinants (Fig. 8–17*C*). Alternatively, in Lewis-negative, secretor-negative persons, the type 1 precursors remain unsubstituted by the action of either blood group fucosyltransferase (Fig. 8–17*D*). In either of the latter two circumstances, the individual's phenotype is denoted Le(a−b−).

Molecular Genetics

A cloned cDNA tentatively assigned to the human *Lewis* blood group locus has been isolated, using a gene transfer approach.[289] Sequence analysis of this cDNA predicts a 361 amino acid long type II transmembrane protein that maintains a 15 amino acid long NH_2-terminal cytosolic segment, a 19 residue transmembrane segment, and a 327 amino acid long COOH-terminal, Golgi-localized catalytic domain. The enzyme encoded by this cDNA is capable of efficiently constructing several types of $\alpha(1,3)$fucosylated and $\alpha(1,4)$fucosylated oligosaccharides. These include Le[a], Le[b], Le[x] (SSEA-1), and Le[y] molecules and sialylated forms of the Le[a] and Le[x] determinants[289, 290] (Figs. 8–17 and 8–18).

The gene corresponding to this cDNA maps to chromosome 19 and is a member of an $\alpha(1,3)$fucosyltransferase gene family, whose members

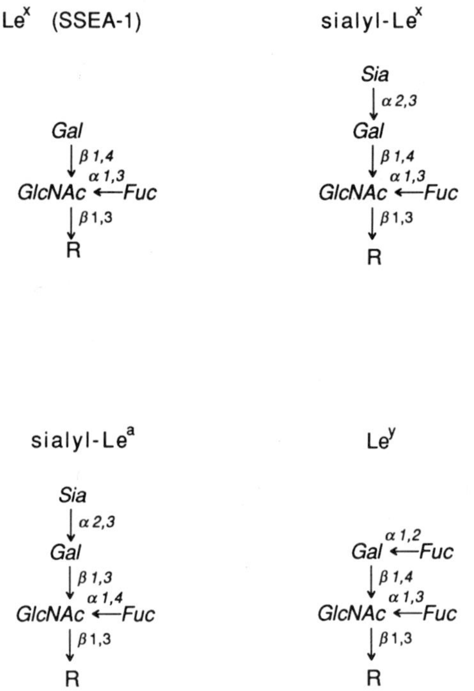

FIGURE 8–18. Le[x], sialyl-Le[x], sialyl-Le[a], and Le[y] structures. The Lewis x determinant (CD15) has also been described as a murine stage-specific embryonic antigen, termed SSEA-1.[277] R denotes the underlying glycoconjugate, which may be represented by a protein- or lipid-linked oligosaccharide or by free oligosaccharide. Monosaccharide components of each epitope are italicized.

maintain substantial primary sequence similarity and overlapping catalytic activities.[291, 292–295] Two other human $\alpha(1,3)$fucosyltransferase genes are also found on chromosome 19, whereas the fourth is localized to human chromosome 11.[292, 295] Southern blot analyses indicate that the human genome may contain still other structurally related $\alpha(1,3)$fucosyltransferase genes.[295]

Function

These $\alpha(1,3)$fucosyltransferase genes and two members of the Lewis family of oligosaccharide determinants have been implicated in important functions in the human inflammatory response and in a new class of oligosaccharide-dependent cell adhesion mechanisms (reviewed in reference 296). Essential early events in the inflammatory process involve the binding of neutrophils and monocytes to vascular endothelium, followed by the transmigration of these cells through the endothelial barrier to arrive at inflammatory loci in the extravascular space. Binding of myeloid lineage cells to the interior of the vessel wall is mediated by endothelial leukocyte adhesion molecule-1 (ELAM-1)[297] or E-selectin,[298] an adhesion receptor expressed by activated vascular endothelial cells. E-selectin exhibits structural similarity[297] to members of the family of C-type carbohydrate-binding proteins (lectins).[299] It has been shown to mediate myeloid cell adhesion via binding interactions with the sialyl Le[x] determinants that are abundantly expressed at the surface of the myeloid cells[290, 300-302] (see Fig. 8–18). More recently, the sialyl Le[a] determinant (see Fig. 8–18) has been shown also to bind with high affinity to E-selectin.[302-304] Although these sialylated forms of the Lewis blood group determinants are not found on erythrocytes, they are not infrequently "aberrantly" expressed by a variety of malignancies.[305] Aberrant expression of these determinants may occur as a consequence of aberrant expression of the Lewis blood group α(1,3/1,4)fucosyltransferase gene, or other α(1,3)fucosyltransferase genes and may function to facilitate E-selectin–dependent spread of malignant cells.[290, 303, 304] Moreover, the sialyl Le[a] and sialyl Le[x] oligosaccharides can function as counterreceptors for P-selectin[306, 307] and possibly also L-selectin,[308] two other members of the selectin family of cell adhesion molecules.[298] These two oligosaccharides may therefore play important roles in the acute inflammatory response (via P-selectin[306, 307]; reviewed in reference 296) and in lymphocyte recirculation (via L-selectin; see reference 308).

The importance of the sialyl Le[x] determinant in the normal human inflammatory response is well illustrated by the phenotype of individuals with the recently described leukocyte adhesion deficiency type II.[309] These patients exhibit a life-threatening susceptibility to bacterial infections, in addition to displaying a variety of other functional and morphological abnormalities. The immunodeficiency in these patients is believed to occur because their neutrophils and monocytes lack the normal complement of cell surface sialyl Le[x] determinants and are therefore incapable of completing normal, E-selectin–dependent endothelial binding and transmigration in response to bacterial invasion. The cells of these patients are incapable of synthesizing fucosylated oligosaccharides under normal circumstances, despite having a normal complement of fucosyltransferase activities (J. C. Paulson, K. Ketchum, B. W. Weston, and J. B. Lowe, unpublished data). As might be expected, these patients also exhibit a Lewis-negative, Bombay phenotype, since they are incapable of constructing the H or Lewis blood group molecules.[309] These patients most likely inherit a defect in the ability to synthesize normal amounts of intracellular GDP-fucose,[310] the substrate for all known human fucosyltransferases.

It remains to be demonstrated if members of the Lewis family of oligosaccharide molecules possess other functions, since other associations between Lewis phenotype and disease susceptibility remain weak and without demonstrated mechanistic relationship (reviewed in references 249 and 311).

THE Ii BLOOD GROUP SYSTEM

The Ii blood group system was discovered during an investigation of a cold hemagglutinating antibody in a patient with acquired hemolytic anemia.[312] In order to find unreactive cells for transfusion into this patient, several thousand blood donors were screened for cross-match compatibility. The antigen identified by the cold agglutinin antibody was found to be absent from the red cells of just 5 of some 22,000 tested individuals. The commonly expressed antigen was called I, and its absence was denoted i. Subsequent studies identified cold agglutinins with relative specificity for i-type cells.[313] Later studies demonstrated that expression of these antigens on red cells is developmentally regulated.[314] Red cells taken from the embryo or from umbilical cord blood are relatively deficient in I determinants but are strongly reactive with anti-i antibodies. During the first 18 months of life, this relationship is reversed, to yield red cells with robust anti-I reactivity and diminished i reactivity, as is observed in most adults.

The Ii antigens are carbohydrate molecules and correspond to portions of the oligosaccharide chains that function as precursors to the ABO and H blood group determinants (reviewed in references 315 and 316). Molecules with i reactivity correspond to oligosaccharide chains containing at least two repeating N-acetyl-lactosamine units (Fig. 8–19). By contrast, I activity corresponds to branched oligosaccharide structures formed by an N-acetyl-lactosamine unit attached in β1,6 linkage to a galactose residue within linear lactosamine polymers (see Fig. 8–19).[317, 318] These structural results are consistent with studies demonstrating that neonatal erythrocyte oligosaccharide chains are largely unbranched, whereas those in adult red cells are highly branched[319, 320] and suggest that the increase in I reactivity, with a corresponding decrease in i reactivity, that occurs during early infancy corresponds to the elaboration and display of increasing numbers of β1,6-linked lactosamine units. These observations are also consistent with the idea that I reactivity is determined by a locus encoding an N-acetylglucosaminyltransferase that is expressed in a developmentally regulated fashion in most individuals, except rare individuals (i phenotype) who are homozygous for null alleles at this locus.[321] This particular β1,6N-acetylglucosaminyltransferase activity and a chain-elongating β1,3N-acetylglucosaminyltransferase activity (see Fig. 8–19) have been described in human serum[322, 323] and in animal cells and tissues.[324, 325] A candidate cDNA for the I transferase has recently been isolated (M. Fukuda and M. Buirhuizen, personal communication). Ii-reactive oligosaccharide chains are ubiquitous entities displayed at the surfaces of many human cell lines and tissues,[325, 326-329] including those of the erythroid lineage.[330, 331] Ii determinants are also displayed as developmentally regulated cell surface molecules during murine embryogenesis.[332] Nonetheless, the functions of these molecules remain to be defined.

THE P BLOOD GROUP SYSTEM

The P blood group system was discovered during experiments designed to uncover new human red cell

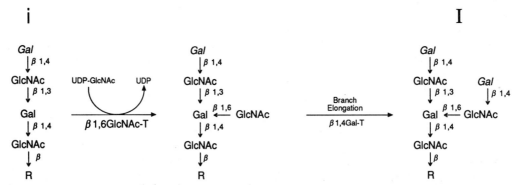

FIGURE 8–19. Antigens and biosynthesis of the I/i blood group system. Linear polymers of lactosamine units (Galβ1,4GlcNAcβ1,3) represent i-reactive oligosaccharide antigens. These molecules are utilized by a β(1,6)GlcNAc transferase (whose expression is determined by the *I* locus), which attaches *N*-acetylglucosamine in β(1,6) linkage to internal galactose residues. These β(1,6)-linked *N*-acetylglucosamine moieties are then modified, forming branched oligosaccharide determinants with I reactivity. (These positions are also indicated in Fig. 8–10.) R denotes the underlying glycoconjugate, which may be represented by a protein- or lipid-linked oligosaccharide or by free oligosaccharide.

alloantigens by immunizing rabbits with human red cells.[333] The nomenclature, biochemistry, and genetics of this system are complex, largely because the nature of the corresponding genes is not well established (reviewed in references 315 and 334). The system is perhaps best understood by first considering the chemical structures and biosynthesis of its antigens. The P antigens are displayed for the most part by red cell membrane–associated glycosphingolipids, although glycoprotein-based P group antigens may also exist (Fig. 8–20; reviewed in reference 315). Like the antigens of the *ABO, H,* and *Lewis* blood group loci, P molecules are constructed by the sequential action of a series of distinct glycosyltransferases.

Biosynthesis of the P system molecules[334] may be divided into two distinct pathways; lactosylceramide serves as a common precursor for both (Fig. 8–20A). P antigen biosynthesis is initiated by the action of an α(1,4)galactosyltransferase (*P^k* transferase) that creates the P^k antigen. The P^k antigen in turn serves as a precursor for the action of a β(1,3)GalNAc transferase, termed the *P* transferase, which forms the P antigen. Polymorphisms are observed in the ability to express each of these two glycosyltransferase activities, as discussed below, which in turn can lead to polymorphism in P and P^k antigen expression.

In the parallel pathway that directs the synthesis of the P_1 antigen, lactosylceramide serves as a precursor for the synthesis of paragloboside, via two of the enzymatic glycosylations that are apparently not polymorphic (Fig. 8–20B). Paragloboside in turn serves as a substrate for the action of *P_1* transferase, which forms the P_1 molecule. Polymorphisms are often observed in the ability to express *P_1* transferase activity, and thus in P_1 antigen expression.

Phenotypes and Genotypes

A consideration of these pathways and antigens, and of the functional polymorphisms in the three enzyme activities that determine their synthesis, can account for the observed red cell phenotypes in virtually all individuals. The most common phenotype, termed P_1, is the result of full activity of each of the polymorphic enzyme activities (Table 8–5). Consequently, P_1 red cells display normal amounts of both P and P_1 antigens. Small amounts of P^k determinants are also detectable because the *P* transferase is apparently incapable of completely converting all P^k precursor determinants into P determinants.

The P_2 phenotype represents the other most common phenotype (see Table 8–5). These persons presumably maintain two null alleles at the *P_1* transferase locus. Their red cells consequently do not display a normal complement of P_1 determinants but do express levels of the P and P^k antigens similar to those found on P_1 cells.

Three rare phenotypes have also been described. Individuals with the P_1^k phenotype are deficient in *P* transferase activity and thus presumably maintain two null alleles at this locus.[335–337] These persons therefore do not convert their P^k molecules into P determinants and thus express supranormal amounts of P^k determinants. The parallel pathway for P_1 synthesis is intact and yields normal amounts of P_1 determinants.

Persons with the rare P_2^k phenotype are presumably homozygous for null alleles at the *P* transferase and the *P_1* transferase loci.[335, 336] Neither pathway is completed, leading to deficiencies in both P and P_1 antigen expression, but with increased expression of P^k molecules.

Finally, red cells of the p phenotype are deficient in all three P antigens (P, P_1, and P^k).[13, 335, 338] Homozygosity for null alleles at the *P^k* transferase and *P_1* transferase loci can account for this phenotype.[338–340] Normal levels of P antigen are not synthesized, regardless of *P* transferase activity, because the P precursor (P^k) is not available. Nonetheless, red cells of the p phenotype typically display low levels of P reactivity because the *P* transferase can utilize attach

P antigen biosynthesis

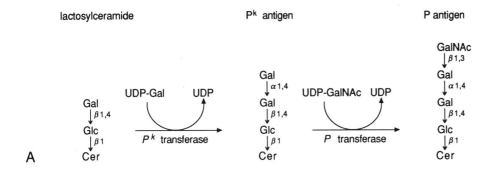

P₁ antigen biosynthesis

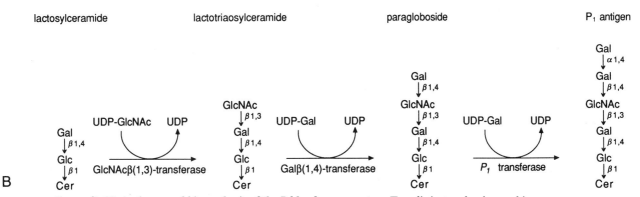

FIGURE 8–20. Antigens and biosynthesis of the P blood group system. Two distinct and polymorphic enzymes operate to construct the P^k and P antigens (*A*). The P₁ antigen is constructed (*B*) from lactosylceramide via the action of two apparently non-polymorphic enzymes (yielding the precursor paragloboside), followed by the action of the polymorphic P₁ transferase.

a galactose moiety in α(1,4) linkage to paragloboside, formed in the other pathway, which yields a molecule with P antigen reactivity (see Fig. 8–20).

The discussion above assumes that the *P*, *P₁*, and *P^k* transferases represent distinct enzymes, encoded by three different loci. However, at least two alternative, biochemically and genetically consistent models may be proposed to explain the p phenotype and the others

(discussed in reference 334). One such model[341] proposes that the *P₁* transferase and the *P^k* transferase "activities" in fact correspond to a single tranferase locus that in most instances encodes one enzyme capable of constructing both P^k and P₁ determinants (P₁ phenotype). A second model proposes that the *P₁* locus encodes a regulatory molecule capable of modulating the substrate specificity of an α(1,4)galacto-

TABLE 8–5. COMMON AND RARE P BLOOD GROUP SYSTEM PHENOTYPES*

PHENOTYPE	FREQUENCY	RED CELL ANTIGENS	POSSIBLE GENOTYPES			SERUM ANTIBODIES
P₁	75%	P, P₁, (weak P^k)	$P^k/-$	$P/-$	$P_1/-$	None
P₂	25%	P, (weak P^k)	$P^k/-$	$P/-$	p_1/p_1	Anti-P₁
P₁^k	Rare	P₁, p^k	$P^k/-$	p/p	$P_1/-$	Anti-P
P₂^k	Rare	p^k	$P^k/-$	p/p	p_1/p_1	Anti-P
P	Rare	(Weak P)	p^k/p^k	$-/-$	p_1/p_1	Anti-PP₁P^k (or anti-Tj^a)

Phenotype frequencies are those observed in Caucasian populations. Predicted genotypes are based on the three–glycosyltransferase locus model discussed in the text. Dashed lines indicate that a functional or a null allele will yield the same phenotype. Antigens expressed at low levels are preceded by the term "weak" and are enclosed within parentheses.

syltransferase encoded by the p^k locus.[334] Which, if any, of these three models is correct remains to be determined, as their cognate genes have not yet been isolated.

Function

Similarly, functions for these oligosaccharides remain unknown, and few significant associations have been made between pathological states and P blood group phenotype. Perhaps the most compelling one centers on the observation that some uropathogenic strains of *Escherichia coli* express pili that recognize the Galα(1,4)Gal moiety of the P^k and P_1 antigens (see references 274, 342, and 343, for example). The latter determinant is relatively more abundant on the urothelium of P_1 persons and might conceivably function to mediate bacterial attachment and invasion to the urinary tract lining. This possibility is consistent with reports that individuals with the P_1 blood group are at a slightly increased relative risk for urinary tract infection and for pyelonephritis[275, 344, 345] compared with persons having the P_2 phenotype. Roles for P determinants in other circumstances remain to be discovered.

Antibodies directed against the P_1 antigen are often found in persons of the P_2 phenotype.[4, 13] These are typically naturally occurring, cold-agglutinating IgM molecules and have only rarely been associated with red cell destruction. Antibodies against P, P_1, and P^k determinants (anti-PP$_1$P^k or anti-Tj^a; see reference 4) are found in individuals with the p phenotype. These antibodies have been implicated in hemolytic transfusion reactions and in hemolytic disease of the newborn, and they may play causative roles in some women who experience spontaneous abortion early in pregnancy.[346] Anti-P antibodies with similar characteristics have also been described in P_1^k and P_2^k individuals. Cold, complement-fixing "Donath-Landsteiner" antibodies responsible for intravascular hemolysis in paroxysmal cold hemoglobinuria display anti-P specificity.[4]

REFERENCES

1. Landsteiner, K., Levine, P., and Janes, M. L.: On the development of isoagglutinins following transfusions. Proc. Soc. Exp. Biol. 25:672, 1928.
2. Landsteiner, K.: Individual differences in human blood. Science 73:405, 1931.
3. Lewis, M., Anstee, D. J., and Bird, G. W. G, et al.: Blood group terminology 1990. Vox Sang. 58:152, 1990.
4. Mollison, P. L., Engelfriet, C. P., and Contreras, M.: Blood Transfusion in Clinical Medicine. 8th ed. Oxford, England, Blackwell, 1987.
5. Rossie, E. C., Simon, T. L., and Moss, G. S. (eds.): Principles of Transfusion Medicine. Baltimore, The Williams and Wilkins Co., 1991.
6. Levine, P., and Stetson, R. E.: An unusual case of intragroup agglutination. J.A.M.A. 113:126, 1939.
7. Levine, P., Burnham, L., Katzin, E. M., and Vogel, P.: The role of isoimmunization in the pathogenesis of erythroblastosis fetalis. Am. J. Obstet. Gynecol. 42:925, 1941.
8. Levine, P., Katzin, E. M., and Burnham, L.: Isoimmunization in pregnancy, its possible bearing on etiology of erythroblastosis fetalis. J.A.M.A. 116:825, 1941.
9. Landsteiner, K., and Wiener, A. S.: An agglutinable factor in human blood recognized by immune sera for rhesus blood. Proc. Soc. Exp. Biol. Med. 43:223, 1940.
10. Levine, P., Cellano, M., and Fenichel, R.: A "D-like" antigen in rhesus monkey, human Rh positive and human Rh negative red blood cells. J. Immunol. 87:747, 1961.
11. Levine, P., Cellano, M. J., Wallace, J., and Sanger, R.: A human "D-like" antibody. Nature 198:596, 1963.
12. Issitt, P. D.: Applied Blood Group Serology. 3rd ed. Miami, Montgomery Scientific Publications, 1985.
13. Race, R. R., and Sanger, R.: Blood Groups in Man. 6th ed. Oxford, England, Blackwell, 1975.
14. Wiener, A. S.: The Rh series of allelic genes. Science 100:595, 1944.
15. Race, R. R.: An "incomplete" antibody in human serum. Nature 153:771, 1944.
16. Moore, S., and Green, C.: The identification of specific Rhesus polypeptide blood group ABH active glycoprotein complexes in the human red cell membrane. Biochem. J. 244:735, 1987.
17. Agre, P., Saboori, A. M., Asimos, A., and Smith, B. L.: Purification and partial characterization of the Mr 30,000 integral membrane protein associated with the erythrocyte Rh(D) antigen. J. Biol. Chem. 262:17497, 1987.
18. Bloy, C., Blanchard, D., Lambin, P., Goossens, D., Rouger, P., Salmon, C., and Cartron, J. P.: Human monoclonal antibody against Rh(D) antigen: Partial characterization of rh Rh(D) polypeptide from human erythrocytes. Blood 69:1491, 1987.
19. Blanchard, D., Bloy, C., Hermand, P., Cartron, J. P., Saboori, A. M., Smith, B. L., and Agre, P.: Two-dimensional iodopeptide mapping demonstrates erythrocyte RhD, c, and E polypeptides are structurally homologous but nonidentical. Blood 72:1424, 1988.
20. Bloy, C., Hermand, P., Cherif-Zahar, B., Sonneborn, H. H., Cartron, J. P.: Comparative analysis by two-dimensional iodopeptide mapping of the RhD protein and LW glycoprotein. Blood 75:2245, 1990.
21. Saboori, A. M., Smith, B. L., and Agre, P.: Polymorphism in the Mr 32,000 Rh protein purified from Rh(D) positive and negative erythrocytes. Proc. Natl. Acad. Sci. USA 85:4042, 1988.
22. Avent, N. D., Ridgwell, K., Mawby, W. J., Tanner, M. J., Anstee, D. J., and Kumpel, B.: Protein-sequence studies of Rh-related polypeptides suggest the presence of at least two groups of proteins which associated in the human red-cell membrane. Biochem. J. 256:1043, 1988.
23. Avent, N. D., Ridgwell, K., Tanner, M. J. A., and Anstee, D. J.: cDNA cloning of a 30 kDa erythrocyte membrane protein associated with Rh (Rhesus)-blood-group-antigen expression. Biochem. J. 271:821, 1990.
24. Cherif-Zahar, B., Bloy, C., Le Van Kim, C., Blanchard, D., Bailly, P., Hermand, P., Salmon, C., Cartron, J. P., and Colin, Y.: Molecular cloning and protein structure of a human blood group Rh polypeptide. Proc. Natl. Acad. Sci. USA 87:6243, 1990.
25. Cherif-Zahar, B., Mattei, M. G., Le Van Kim, C., Bailly, P., Cartron, J. P., and Colin, Y.: Localization of the human Rh blood group gene structure to chromosome 1p34.3–1p36.1 region by in situ hybridization. Hum. Genet. 86:398, 1991.
26. Bruns, G. A. P., and Sherman, S. L.: Report of the committee on genetic constitution of chromosome I. Cytogenet. Cell Genet. 51:67, 1989.
27. Gahmberg, C. G.: Molecular characterization of the human red-cell Rho(D) antigen. EMBO J. 2:223, 1983.
28. Colin, Y., Cherif-Zahar, B., Le Van Kim, C., Raynal, V., Van Huffel, V., and Cartron, J. P.: Genetic basis of the RhD-positive and RhD-negative blood group polymorphism as determined by Southern analysis. Blood 78:2747, 1991.
29. Le Van Kim, C., Cherif-Zahar, B., Raynal, V., Mouro, I., Lopez, M., Cartron, J.-P., and Colin, Y.: Multiple Rh mes-

senger RNA isoforms are produced by alternative splicing. Blood 80:1074, 1078, 1992.

30. Tippett, P.: Regulator genes affecting red cell antigens. Transf. Med. Rev. 4:56, 1990.

31. Avent, N. D., Butcher, S. K., Liu, W., Mawby, W. J., Mallison, G., Parsons, S. F., Anstee, D. J., and Tanner, M. J. A.: Localization of the C termini of the Rh (Rhesus) polypeptides to the cytosolic face of the human erythrocyte membrane. J. Biol. Chem. 267:15134, 1992.

32. Suyama, K., and Goldstein, J.: Membrane orientation of Rh(D) polypeptide and partial localization of its epitope-containing domain. Blood 79:808, 1992.

33. Bloy, C., Hermand, P., Blanchard, D., Cherif-Zahar, B., Goossens, D., and Cartron, J.-P.: Surface orientation and antigen properties of Rh and LW polypeptides of the human erythrocyte. J. Biol. Chem. 265:21482, 1990.

34. Agre, P., and Cartron, J.-P.: Molecular biology of the Rh antigens. Blood 78:551, 1991.

35. Hartmann, E., Rapoport, T. A., and Lodish, H. F.: Predicting the orientation of eukaryotic membrane-spanning proteins. Proc. Natl. Acad. Sci. USA 86:5786, 1989.

36. DeVetten, M. P., and Agre, P.: The Rh polypeptide is a major fatty acid acylated erythrocyte membrane protein. J. Biol. Chem. 263:18193, 1988.

37. Shinitzky, M., and Souroujon, M.: Passive modulation of blood group antigens. Proc. Natl. Acad. Sci. USA 76:4438, 1979.

38. Basu, M. K., Flamm, M., Schacter, D., Bertles, J. F., and Maniatis, A.: Effects of modulating erythrocyte membrane cholesterol on Rho(D) antigen expression. Biochem. Biophys. Res. Commun. 95:887, 1980.

39. Gahmberg, C. G., and Karhi, K. K.: Association of Rho(D) polypeptides with the membrane skeleton in Rho(D)-positive human red cells. J. Immunol. 133:334, 1984.

40. Ridgwell, K., Tanner, M. J. A., and Anstee, D. J.: The Rhesus(D) polypeptide is linked to the human erythrocyte cytoskeleton. FEBS Lett. 174:7, 1984.

41. Moore, S., Woodrow, C. F., and McClelland, D. B.: Isolation of membrane components associated with human red cell antigens Rh₀(D), (c), (E), and Fyª. Nature 295:529, 1982.

42. Von dem Borne, A. E., Bos, M. J., Lomas, C., Tippett, P., Bloy, C., Hermand, P., Cartron, J. P., Admiraal, L. G., van de Graaf, J., and Overbeeke, M. A.: Murine monoclonal antibodies against a unique determinant of erythrocytes related to Rh and U antigens. Br. J. Haematol. 75:254, 1990.

43. Avent, N. D., Judson, P. A., Parsons, S. F., Mollison, G., Anstee, D. J., Tanner, M. J., Evans, P. R., Hodges, E., Maciver, A. G., and Holmes, C.: Monoclonal antibodies that recognize different membrane proteins that are deficient in Rh-RH_null human erythrocytes. Biochem. J. 251:499, 1988.

44. Bloy, C., Blanchard, D., Hermand, P., Kardowicz, M., Sonneborn, H. H., and Cartron, J. P.: Properties of the blood group LW glycoprotein and preliminary comparison with Rh proteins. Mol. Immunol. 26:1013, 1989.

45. Nash, R., and Shojania, A. M.: Hematological aspect of Rh deficiency syndrome: A case report and review of the literature. Am. J. Hematol. 24:267, 1987.

46. Lauf, P. K., and Joiner, C. H.: Increased potassium transport and ouabain binding in human Rh null red blood cells. Blood 48:457, 1976.

47. Ballas, S., Clark, M. R., Mohandas, N., Colfer, H. F., Caswell, M. S., Bergren, M. O., Perkins, H. A., and Shohet, S. B.: Red cell membranes and cation deficiency in Rh null syndrome. Blood 63:1046, 1984.

48. Kuypers, F., van Linde-Sibenius-Trip, M., Roelofsen, B., Tanner, M. J., Anstee, D. J., Op den Kamp, J. A.: Rh-RH_null human erythrocytes have an abnormal membrane phospholipid organization. Biochem. J. 221:931, 1984.

49. Chown, B., Lewis, M., Kaita, H., and Lowen, B.: An unlinked modifier of Rh blood groups: Effect when heterozygous and homozygous. Am. J. Hum. Genet. 24:623, 1972.

50. Dahr, W., Kordowicz, M., Moulds, J., Gielen, W., Lebeck, L., and Kruger, J.: Characterization of the Ss sialoglycoprotein and its antigens in Rh-RH_null erythrocytes. Blut 54:13, 1987.

51. Mallinson, G., Martin, P. G., Anstee, D. J., Tanner, M. J., Merry, A. H., Tills, D., and Sonneborn, H. H.: Identification and partial characterization of the human erythrocyte membrane component(s) which express the antigens of the LW blood group system. Biochem. J. 234:649, 1986.

52. Miller, Y. E., Daniels, G. L., Jones, C., and Palmer, D. K.: Identification of a cell-surface antigen produced by a gene on human chromosome 3 (cenq22) and not expressed by Rh-RH_null cells. Am. J. Hum. Genet. 41:1061, 1987.

53. Sonneborn, H. H., Ernst, M., Tills, D., Lomas, C. G., Gorick, B. D., and Hughes-Jones, N. C.: Comparison of the reactions of the Rh-related murine monoclonal antibodies BS58 and R6A. Vox Sang. 58:219, 1990.

54. Zachowski, A., and Devaux, P. F.: Transmembrane movements of lipids. Experientia 46:644, 1990.

55. Smith, R. E., and Daleke, D. L.: Phosphatidylserine transport in Rh_null erythrocytes. Blood 76:1021, 1990.

56. Landsteiner, K., and Levine, P.: A new agglutinable factor differentiating individual human bloods. Proc. Soc. Exp. Biol. 24:600, 1927.

57. Sanger, R., and Race, R. R.: Subdivisions of the MN blood groups in man. Nature 160:505, 1947.

58. Sanger, R., Race, R. R., Walsh, R. J., and Montgomery, C.: An antibody which subdivides the human MN blood groups. Heredity 2:131, 1948.

59. Levine, P., Kuhmichel, A. B., Wigod, M., and Koch, E.: A new blood factor, s allelic to S. Proc. Soc. Exp. Biol. 78:218, 1951.

60. Wiener, A. S., Unger, L. J., and Gordon, E. B.: Fatal hemolytic transfusion reaction caused by sensitization to a new blood factor U. J.A.M.A. 153:1444, 1953.

61. Blanchard, D.: Human red cell glycophorins: Biochemical and antigenic properties. Transf. Med. Rev. 4:170, 1990.

62. Cartron, J. P., Colin, Y., Kudo, S., and Fukuda, M.: Molecular genetics of human erythrocyte sialoglycoproteins, glycophorins A, B, C, and D. In Harris, J.R. (ed.): Blood Cell Biochemistry. Vol. 1. New York, Plenum Press, 1990, pp 299–335.

63. Siebert, P. D., and Fukuda, M.: Molecular cloning of human glycophorin B cDNA: Nucleotide sequence and genomic relationship to glycoprotein A. Proc. Natl. Acad. Sci. USA 84:6735, 1987.

64. Tate, C. G., and Tanner, M. J. A.: Isolation of cDNA clones for human erythrocyte membrane sialoglycoproteins α and δ. Biochem. J. 254:743, 1988.

65. Siebert, P. D., and Fukuda, M.: Isolation and characterization of human glycophorin A cDNA clones by a synthetic oligonucleotide approach: Nucleotide sequence and mRNA structure. Proc. Natl. Acad. Sci. USA 83:1665, 1986.

66. Rahuel, C., Vignal, A., London, J., Hamel, S., Romeo, P. H., Colin, Y., and Cartron, J. P.: Structure of the 5′ flanking region of the glycophorin A gene and analysis of its multiple transcripts. Gene 85:471, 1989.

67. Hamid, J., and Burness, A. T. H.: The mechanism of production of multiple mRNAs for human glycophorin A. Nucleic Acids Res. 18:5829, 1990.

68. Judd, W. J., Issitt, P. D., Pavone, B. G., Anderson, J., and Aminoff, D.: Antibodies that define NANA-independent MN-system antigens. Transfusion 19:12, 1979.

69. Lisowska, E.: Antigenic properties of human erythrocyte glycophorins. In Wu, A. M. (ed.): Molecular Immunology of Complex Carbohydrates. New York, Plenum Press, 1989.

70. Le Van Kim, C., Colin, Y., Mitjavila, M. T., Clerget, M., Dubart, A., Nakazawa, M., Vainchenker, W., and Cartron, J. P.: Structure of the promoter region and tissue specificity of the human glycophorin C. J. Biol. Chem. 264:20407, 1989.

71. Dahr, W., Beyreuther, K., Steinbach, H., Gielen, W., and Kruger, J.: Structure of the Ss blood group antigens. II. A methionine/threonine polymorphism within the N-terminal sequence of Ss glycoprotein. Hoppe-Seyler's Z. Physiol. Chem. 361:895, 1980.

72. Kudo, S., and Fukuda, M.: Identification of a novel human glycophorin, glycophorin E, by isolation of genomic clones

and complementary DNA clones utilizing polymerase chain reaction. J. Biol. Chem. 265:1102, 1990.

73. Vignal, A., Rahuel, C., London, J., Cherif-Zahar, B., Schaff, S., Hattab, C., Okubo, Y. and Cartron, J. P.: A novel gene member of the human glycophorin A and B gene family. Molecular cloning and expression. Eur. J. Biochem. 191:619, 1990.

74. Anstee, D. J.: The nature and abundance of human red cell surface glycoproteins. J. Immunogenet. 17:219, 1990.

75. Huang, C.-H., Johe, K. K., Seifter, S., and Blumenfeld, O. O.: Biochemistry and molecular biology of MNSs blood group antigens. Baillieres Clin. Haematol. 4:821, 1991.

76. Huang, C. H., and Blumenfeld, O. O.: Molecular genetics of human erythrocyte MiIII and MiVI glycophorins. J. Biol. Chem. 266:7248, 1991.

77. Dahr, W., Uhlenbruck, G., Leikola, J., and Wagstaff, W.: Studies on the membrane glycoprotein defect of En(a−) erythrocytes. III. N-terminal amino acids of sialoglycoproteins from normal and En(a−) red cells. J. Immunogenet. 5:117, 1978.

78. Rahuel, C., London, J., Vignal, A., Cherif-Zahar, B., Colin, Y., Siebert, P., Fukuda, M., and Cartron, J. P.: Alteration of the genes for glycophorin A and B in glycophorin A deficient individuals. Eur. J. Biochem. 177:605, 1988.

79. Bigbee, W. L., Langlois, R. G., Vanderlaan, M., and Jensen, R. H.: Binding specificities of eight monoclonal antibodies to human glycophorin A. Studies with MᶜM and MᵏEn(UK) variant erythrocytes and M- and MNᵛ-type chimpanzee erythrocytes. J. Immunol. 133:3149, 1984.

80. Lowe, R. F., and Moores, P. P.: Red cell factor in Africans of Rhodhesia, Malawi, Mozambique and Natal. Hum. Hered. 22:344, 1972.

81. Dahr, W., Uhlenbruck, G., Issitt, P., and Allen, F. H.: SDS-polyacrylamide gel electrophoretic analysis of the membrane glycoproteins from S− s− U− erythrocytes. J. Immunogenet. 2:249, 1975.

82. Tanner, M. J. A., Anstee, D., and Judon, P. A.: A carbohydrate-deficient membrane glycoprotein in human erythrocytes of phenotype S− s−. Biochem. J. 165:157, 1977.

83. Huang, C. H., Lu, W. M., Boots, M. E., Guizzo, M. L., and Blumenfeld, O. O.: Two types of δglycophorin gene alterations in S− s− U− individuals. Transfusion 29:35S, 1989.

84. Rahuel, C., London, J., Vignal, A., Ballas, S. K., and Cartron, J. P.: Erythrocyte glycophorin B deficiency may occur by two distinct gene alterations. Am. J. Hematol. 37:57, 1991.

85. Tate, C. G., Tanner, M. J. A., Judson, P. A., and Anstee, D. J.: Studies on human red-cell membrane glycophorin A and glycophorin B genes in glycophorin-deficient individuals. Biochem. J. 263:993, 1989.

86. Metaxas, N. N., and Metaxas-Buhler, M.: An apparently silent allele at the MN locus. Nature 202:1123, 1964.

87. Tokunaga, E., Sasakama, S., Tamaka, K., Kawamata, H., Giles, C. M., Ikin, E. W., Poole, J., Anstee, D. J., Mawby, W., and Tanner, M. J. A.: Two apparently healthy Japanese individuals of type Mk/Mk have erythrocytes which lack both the blood group MN and Ss active sialoglycoproteins. J. Immunogenet. 6:383, 1979.

88. Issitt, P. D.: The MN Blood Group System. Miami, Montgomery Scientific Publications, 1981.

89. Furthmayr, H.: Structural comparison of glycophorins and immunochemical analysis of genetic variants. Nature 271:519, 524, 1978.

90. Rosenfield, R. E., Haber, G. V., Kissmeyer-Nielson, J. A., Jack, J. A., Sanger, R., and Race, R. R.: Ge, a very common red cell antigen. Br. J. Haematol. 6:344, 1960.

91. Booth, P. B., and McLoughlin, K.: The Gerbich blood group system especially in Melanesians. Vox Sang. 22:73, 1972.

92. McShane, K., and Chung, A.: A novel human allo antibody in the Gerbich system. Vox Sang. 57:205, 1989.

93. Anstee, D. J., Parsons, S. F., Ridgwell, K., Tanner, M. J. A., Merry, A. H., Thomson, E. E., Judson, P. A., Johnson, P., Bates, S., and Fraser, I. D.: Two individuals with elliptocytic red cells lack three minor erythrocyte membrane sialoglycoproteins. Biochem. J. 218:615, 1984.

94. Anstee, D. J., Ridgwell, K., Tanner, M. J. A., Daniels, G. L., and Parsons, S. F.: Individuals lacking the Gerbich blood-group antigen have alterations in the human erythrocyte membrane sialoglycoproteins β and γ. Biochem. J. 221:97, 1984.

95. Daniels, G. L., Reid, M. E., Anstee, D. J., Beattie, K. M., and Judd, W. J.: Transient reduction in erythrocyte membrane sialoglycoprotein β associated with the presence of elliptocytes. Br. J. Haematol. 70:477, 1988.

96. Rountree, J., Chen, J., Moulds, M. K., Moulds, J. J., Green, A. M., and Telen, M. J.: A second family demonstrating inheritance of the Leach phenotype. Tranfusion 29 (Suppl):15S, 1989.

97. Daniels, G. L., Reid, M. E., Anstee, D. J., Beattie, K. M., and Judd, W. J.: Transient reduction in erythrocyte membrane sialoglycoprotein β associated with the presence of elliptocytes. Br. J. Haematol. 70:477, 1988.

98. Dahr, W., Moulds, J., Baumeister, G., Moulds, M., Kiedrowski, S., and Hummel, M.: Altered membrane sialoglycoproteins in human erythrocytes lacking the Gerbich blood group antigens. Biol. Chem. Hoppe-Seyler 366:201, 1985.

99. Dahr, W., Kiedrowski, S., Blanchard, D., Hermand, P., Moulds, J. J., and Cartron, J. P.: High frequency of human erythrocyte membrane sialoglycoproteins. V. Characterization of the Gerbich blood group antigens: Ge2 and Ge3. Biol. Chem. Hoppe-Seyler 368:1375, 1987.

100. Reid, E. M., Anstee, D. J., Tanner, M. J. A., Ridgwell, K., and Nurse, C. T.: Structural relationships between human erythrocyte sialoglycoproteins β and γ and abnormal sialoglycoproteins found in certain rare human erythrocyte variants lacking the Gerbich blood-group antigen(s). Biochem. J. 244:123, 1987.

101. Furthmayr, H.: Glycophorins A, B, C: A family of sialoglycoproteins. Isolation and preliminary characterization of trypsin-derived peptides. J. Supramol. Struct. 9:79, 1978.

102. Colin, Y., Rahuel, C., London, J., Romeo, P. H., d'Auriol., L., Galibert, F., and Cartron, J. P.: Isolation of cDNA clones for human erythrocyte glycophorin C. J. Biol. Chem. 261:229, 1986.

103. Dahr, W., Beyreuther, K., Kordowicz, M., and Kruger, J.: N-terminal amino acid sequence of sialoglycoprotein D (glycophorin C) from human erythrocyte membranes. Eur. J. Biochem. 125:57, 1982.

104. Blanchard, D., Dahr, W., Hummal, M., Latron, F., Beyreuther, K., and Cartron, J. P.: Glycophorins B and C from human erythrocyte membranes: Purification and sequence analysis. J. Biol. Chem. 262:5808, 1987.

105. High, S., and Tanner, M. J. A.: Human erythrocyte membrane sialoglycoprotein β. The cDNA sequence suggests the absence of a cleaved N-terminal signal sequence. Biochem. J. 243:277, 1987.

106. El-Maliki, B., Blanchard, D., Dahr, W., Beyreuther, K., and Cartron, J. P.: Structural homology between glycophorins C and D of human erythrocytes. Eur. J. Biochem. 183:639, 1989.

107. Dahr, W., Blanchard, D., Kiedrowski, S., Poschmann, A., Cartron, J. P., and Moulds, J.: High frequency antigens of human erythrocyte membrane sialoglycoproteins. VI. Monoclonal antibodies reacting with the N-terminal domain of glycophorin C. Biol. Chem. Hoppe-Seyler 370:849, 1989.

108. Colin, Y., Le Van Kim, C., Tsapis, A., Clerget, M., d'Auriol., L., London, J., Galibert, F., and Cartron, J. P.: Human erythrocyte glycophorin C gene structure and rearrangement in genetic variants. J. Biol. Chem. 264:3773, 1989.

109. High, S., Tanner, M. J. A., Macdonald, E. B., and Anstee, D. J.: Rearrangements of the red cell membrane glycophorin C (sialoglycoprotein β) gene. Biochem. J. 262:47, 1989.

110. Le Van Kim, C., Colin, Y., Blanchard, D., Dahr, W., London, J., and Cartron, J. P.: Gerbich group deficiency of the Ge: 1, −2, −3 and Ge: −1, −2, 3 types. Eur. J. Biochem. 165:571, 1987.

111. Mattei, M. G., Colin, Y., Le Van Kim, C., Mattei, J. F., and Cartron, J. P.: Localization of the gene for human erythro-

cyte glycophorin C to chromosome 2q14–q21. Hum. Genet. 74:420, 1986.

112. Tanner, M. J. A., High, S., Martin, P. G., Anstee, D. J., Judson, P. A., and Jones, T. J.: Genetic variants of human red cell membrane sialoglycoprotein β. Study of the alterations occurring in the sialoglycoprotein β gene. Biochem. J. 250:407, 1988.

113. Telen, M. J., Le Van Kim, C., Chung, A., Cartron, J. P., and Colin, Y.: Molecular basis for elliptocytosis associated with glycophorin C deficiency in the Leach phenotype. Blood 78:1603, 1991.

114. Le Van Kim, C., Mitjavila, M.-T., Clerget, M., Cartron, J. P., and Colin, Y.: An ubiquitous isoform of glycophorin C is produced by alternative splicing. Nucleic Acids Res. 18:3076, 1990.

115. Macdonald, E. B., Condon, J., Ford, D., Fisher, B., and Gerns, L. M.: Abnormal beta and gamma sialoglycoprotein associated with the low-frequency antigen Lsᵃ. Vox Sang. 58:300, 1990.

116. Macdonald, E. B., and Gerns, L. M.: An unusual sialoglycoprotein associated with the Webb-positive phenotype. Vox Sang. 50:112, 1986.

117. Reid, M. E., Shaw, M. A., Rowe, G., Anstee, D. J., and Tanner, M. J. A.: Abnormal minor human erythrocyte membrane sialoglycoprotein β in association with the rare blood-group antigen Webb (Wb). Biochem. J. 232:289, 1985.

118. Telen, M. J., Le Van Kim, C., Guizzo, M. L., Cartron, J. P., and Colin, Y.: Erythrocyte Webb-type glycophorin C variant lacks N-glycosylation due to an asparagine to serine substitution. Am. J. Hematol. 37:51, 1991.

119. Nash, G. B., Parmar, J., and Reid, M. E.: Effects of deficiencies of glycophorins C and D on the physical properties of the red cell. Br. J. Haematol. 76:282, 1990.

120. Mueller, T. J., and Morrison, M.: Glycoconnection (PAS 2), a membrane attachment site for the human erythrocyte cytoskeleton. In Kruckenberg, W. C., Eaton, J. W., and Brewer, G. J. (eds.): Erythrocyte Membrane 2: Recent Clinical and Experimental Advances. New York, Alan R. Liss, 1981, pp. 95–112.

121. Bennett, V.: Spectrin-based membrane skeleton: A multipotential adaptor between plasma membrane and cytoplasm. Physiol. Rev. 70:1029, 1990.

122. Chasis, J. A., and Mohandas, N.: Erythrocyte membrane deformability and stability: Two distinct membrane properties that are independently regulated by skeletal protein associations. J. Cell Biol. 103:343, 1986.

123. Reid, E. M., Chasis, J. A., and Mohandas, N.: Identification of a functional role for human erythrocyte sialoglycoproteins β and γ. Blood 69:1068, 1987.

124. Alloisio, N., Morle, L., Bachir, D., Guetarni, D., Colonna, P., and Dulaunay, J.: Red cell membrane sialoglycoprotein in homozygous and heterozygous 4.1(−) hereditary elliptocytosis. Biochem. Biophys. Acta 816:57, 1985.

125. Sondag, D., Alloisio, N., Blanchard, D., Ducluzeau, M. T., Colonna, P., Bachir, D., Bloy, C., Cartron, J. P., and Delaunay, J.: Gerbich reactivity in 4.1(−) hereditary elliptocytosis and protein 4.1 level in blood group Gerbich deficiency. Br. J. Haematol. 65:43, 1987.

126. Reid, M. E., Takakuwa, Y., Conboy, J., Tchernia, G., and Mohandas, N.: Glycophorin C content of human erythrocyte membrane is regulated by protein 4.1. Blood 75:2229, 1990.

127. Coombs, R. R. A., Mourant, A. E., and Race, R. R.: New test for the detection of weak and "incomplete" Rh agglutinins. Br. J. Exp. Pathol. 26:255, 1945.

128. Marsh, W. L., and Redman, C. M.: The Kell blood group system: A review. Transfusion 30:158, 1990.

129. Giblett, E. R.: A critique of the theoretical hazard of inter- vs. intraracial transfusion. Transfusion 1:233, 1961.

130. Marsh, W. L., and Redman, C. M.: Recent developments in the Kell blood group system. Trans. Med. Rev. 1:4, 1987.

131. Masouredis, S. P., Sudora, E., Mahan, L. C., and Victoria, E. J.: Immunoelectron microscopy of Kell and Cellano antigens on red cell ghosts. Haematologia (Budap) 13:59, 1980.

132. Hughes-Jones, N. L., and Gardner, B.: The Kell system

133. Redman, C. M., Avellino, G., and Pfeffer, S. R.: Kell blood group antigens are part of a 93,000-dalton red cell membrane protein. J. Biol. Chem. 261:9521, 1987.

134. Jaber, A., Blanchard, D., Goossens, D., Bloy, C., Lambin, P., Rouger, P., Salmon, C., and Cartron, J-P.: Characterization of the blood group Kell (K1) antigen with a human monoclonal antibody. Blood 73:1597, 1989.

135. Wallas, C., Simon, R., Sharpe, M. A., and Byler, C.: Isolation of a Kell-reactive protein from red cell membranes. Transfusion 26:173, 1986.

136. Lee, S., Zambas, E. D., Marsh, W. L., and Redman, C. M.: Molecular cloning and primary structure of Kell blood group protein. Proc. Natl. Acad. Sci. USA 88:6353, 1991.

137. Johnson, P. F., and McKnight, S. L.: Eukaryotic transcriptional regulatory proteins. Annu. Rev. Biochem. 58:799, 1989.

138. Chown, B., Lewis, M., and Kaita, K.: A "new" Kell bloodgroup phenotype (letter). Nature 180:7111, 1957.

139. Allen, F. H., Crabbe, S. M. R., and Corcoran, P. A.: A new phenotype (McLeod) in the Kell blood-group system. Vox Sang. 6:555, 1961.

140. Bertelson, C. J., Pogo, A. O., and Chaudhuri, A.: Localization of the McLeod locus (Xk) within Xp21 by deletion analysis. Am. J. Hum. Genet. 42:703, 1988.

141. Franke, U., Ochs, H. D., and de Martinville, B.: Minor Xp21 chromosome deletion in a male associated with expression of Duchenne muscular dystrophy, chronic granulomatous disease, retinitis pigmentosa, and the McLeod syndrome. Am. J. Hum. Genet. 37:250, 1985.

142. Redman, C. M., Marsh, W. L., Scarborough, A., Johnson, C. L., Rabin, B. I., and Overbeeke, M.: Biochemical studies on McLeod phenotype red cells and isolation of Kx antigen. Br. J. Haematol. 68:131, 1988.

143. Wimer, B., Marsh, W. L., Taswell, H. F., and Galey, W. R.: Haematological changes associated with the McLeod phenotype of the Kell blood group system. Br. J. Haematol. 36:219, 1977.

144. Allen, F. H., Jr., Diamond, L. K., and Niedziela, B.: A new blood group antigen. Nature 167:482, 1951.

145. Plaut, G., Ikin, E. W., Mourant, A. E., Sanger, R., and Race, R. R.: A new blood-group antibody, anti Jkᵇ. Nature 171:431, 1953.

146. Pinkerton, F. J., Mermod, L. E., Liles, B. A., Jack, J. A., Jr., and Noades, J.: The phenotype of Jk(a−b−) in the Kidd blood group system. Vox Sang. 4:155, 1959.

147. Woodfield, D. G., Douglas, R., Smith, J., Simpson, A., Pinder, L., and Staveley, J. M.: The Jk(a−b−) phenotype in New Zealand Polynesians. Transfusion 22:276, 1982.

148. Okubo, Y. H., Yamaguchi, H., Nagao, N., Tomita, T., Seno, T., and Tanaka, M.: Heterogeneity of the phenotype Jk(a−b−) found in Japanese. Transfusion 26:237, 1986.

149. Masouredis, S. P., Sudora, E., Mahan, L., and Victoria, E. J.: Quantitative immunoferritin microassay of Fyᵃ, Fyᵇ, Jkᵃ, U and Diᵇ antigen site numbers on human red cells. Blood 56:969, 1980.

150. Sinor, L. T., Eastwood, K. L., and Plapp, F. V.: Dot blot purification of the Kidd blood group antigen. Med. Lab. Sci. 44:294, 1987.

151. Heaton, D. C., and McLaughlin, K.: Jk(a−b−) red blood cells resist urea lysis. Transfusion 22:70, 1982.

152. Edwards-Moulds, J., and Kasschau, M.: The effect of 2M urea on Jk(a−b−) red cells. Vox Sang. 55:181, 1988.

153. Froelich, O., Macy, R. I., Edwards-Moulds, J., Gargas, J. J., and Gunn, R. B.: Urea transport deficiency in Jk(a−b−) erythrocytes. Am. J. Physiol. 260 (Cell Physiol. 29): C778, 1991.

154. Sands, J. M., Gargus, J. J., Froehlich, O., Gunn, R. B., and Kokko, J. P.: Importance of carrier-mediated urea transport to urine concentrating ability in patients with the Jk(a−b−) blood type. J. Am. Soc. Nephrol. 1:678, 1990.

155. Gargus, J. J., and Mitas, M.: Physiological processes revealed through analysis of inborn errors. J. Am. Physiol. Soc. 255:F1047, 1988.

156. Gunn, R. B., Gargus, J. J., and Froehlich, O.: The Kidd antigens and urea transport. *In* Agre, P., and Cartron, J. P. (eds.): Protein Blood Group Antigens of the Human Red Cell. Baltimore, Johns Hopkins University Press, 1992, pp. 88–100.

157. Allen, J. R., Mitas, M., Malone, L., Brunner-Jackson, B., Wimalasena, D. S., and Gargus, J. J.: Inborn error in human urea transport: Analysis of the cDNA encoding the putative transporter. Am. J. Hum. Genet. 43:A1, 1988.

158. Gargus, J. J., Steele, E., Feng, Y., Whaley, W. L., and Malone, L.: Expression studies of human urea transporter cDNA. Biophys. J. 59:330a, 1991.

159. Issitt, P. D., and Issitt, C. H.: The Duffy blood group system. *In* Applied Blood Group Serology. 3rd ed. Miami, Montgomery Scientific Publications, 1985, pp. 278–288.

160. Moore, S., Woodrow, C. F., and McClelland, D. B. L.: Isolation of membrane components associated with human red cell antigens Rh (D), (c), (E) and Fyª. Nature 295:429, 1982.

161. Hadley, T. J., David, P. H., and McGinniss, M. H.: Identification of an erythrocyte component carrying the Duffy blood group Fyª antigen. Science 223:597, 1984.

162. Tanner, M. J. A., Anstee, D. J., and Mallinson, G.: Effect of endoglycosidase F preparations on the surface components of the human erythrocyte Carbohydr. Res. 178:203, 1988.

163. Chaudhuri, A., Zbrzezna, V., Johnson, C., Nichols, M., Rubinstein, P., Marsh, W. L., and Pogo, A. O.: Purification and characterization of an erythrocyte membrane protein complex carrying Duffy blood group antigenicity. Possible receptor for *Plasmodium vivax* and *Plasmodium knowlesi* malaria parasite. J. Biol. Chem. 264:13770, 1989.

164. Barnwell, J. W., and Wertheimer, S. P.: *Plasmodium vivax*: Merozoite antigens, the Duffy blood group, and erythrocyte invasion. Prog. Clin. Biol. Res. 313:1, 1989.

165. Miller, L. H., Alkawa, M., Johnson, J. G., and Shiroishi, T.: Interaction between cytochalasin B–treated malarial parasites and erythrocytes. Attachment and junction formation. J. Exp. Med. 149:172, 1979.

166. Crawford, M. N.: The Lutheran blood group systems: Serology and genetics: *In* Pierce, S. R., and MacPherson, C. R. (eds.): Blood Group Systems: Duffy, Kidd, and Lutheran. Arlington, Va., American Association of Blood Banks, 1988.

167. Callendar, S., Race, R. R., and Paykoc, Z. V.: Hypersensitivity to transfused blood. Br. Med. J. 2:83, 1945.

168. Shaw, M.-A., Leak, M. R., Daniels, G. L., and Tippett, P.: The rare Lutheran blood group phenotype Lu(a−b−): A genetic study. Ann. Hum. Genet. 48:229, 1984.

169. Marsh, W. L., Brown, P. J., and DiNapoli, J.: Anti-Wj: An autoantibody that defines a high-incidence antigen modified by the *In(Lu)* gene. Transfusion: 23:128, 1983.

170. Norman, P. C., Tippett, P., and Beal, R. W.: An Lu(a−b−) phenotype caused by an X-linked recessive gene. Vox Sang. 51:49, 1986.

171. Spring, F. A., Dalchau, R., Daniels, G. L., Mallinson, G., Judson, P. A., Parson, S. F., Fabre, J. W., and Anstee, D. J.: The Inª and Inᵇ blood group antigens are located on a glycoprotein of 80,000 MW (the CD44 glycoprotein) whose expression is influenced by the *In(Lu)* gene. Immunology 64:37, 1988.

172. Picker, L. J., de los Toyos, J., Telen, M. J., Haynes, B. F., and Butcher, E. C.: Identity of CD44 [In(Lu)-related p80], Pgp-1, and the Hermes class of lymphocyte homing receptors. J. Immunol. 142:2046, 1989.

173. Norman, P. C., Tippett, P., and Beal, R. W.: An Lu(a−b−) phenotype caused by an X-linked recessive gene. Vox Sang. 51:49, 1986.

174. Parsons, S. F., Mallinson, G., Judson, P. A., Anstee, D. J., Tanner, M. J. A., and Daniels, G. L.: Evidence that the Luᵇ blood group antigen is located on red cell membrane glycoproteins of 85 and 78 kd. Transfusion 27:61, 1987.

175. Daniels, G., and Khalid, G.: Identification, by immunoblotting, of the structures carrying Lutheran and para-Lutheran blood group antigens. Vox Sang. 57:137, 1989.

176. Daniels, G.: Evidence that the Auberger blood group antigens

177. Daniels, G. L., Le Pennec, P. Y., Rouger, P., Salmon, C., and Tippett, P.: The red cell antigens Auª and Auᵇ belong to the Lutheran system. Vox Sang. 60:191, 1991.

178. Anstee, D. J., Mallinson, G., and Yendle, J. E.: Evidence for the occurrence of Luᵇ-active glycoproteins in human erythrocytes, kidney and liver (abstract). Proceedings of the XXth Congress of the International Society of Blood Transfusions. Manchester, England, British Blood Transfusion Society, 1988, p. 263.

179. Harris, J. P., Tegoli, J., Swanson, J., Fisher, N., Gavin, J., and Noades, J.: A nebulous antibody responsible for cross-matching difficulties (Chido). Vox Sang. 12:140, 1967.

180. Longster, G., and Giles, C. M.: A new antibody specificity, anti-Rgª, reacting with a red cell and serum antigen. Vox Sang. 30:175, 1976.

181. Middleton, J., and Crookston, M. C.: Chido-substance in plasma. Vox Sang. 23:256, 1972.

182. Humphreys, J., Stout, T. D., Middleton, J., and Crookston, M. C.: The identification of Chido-negative donors by a plasma-inhibition test. Washington D. C., Communications of the International Congress of Blood Transfusion (abstract), 1972, p. 57.

183. Westhoff, C. M., Sipherd, B. D., Wylie, D. E., and Toalson, L. D.: Severe anaphylactic reactions following transfusions of platelets to a patient with anti-Ch. Transfusion 32:576, 1992.

184. Moore, H. C., Issitt, P. D., and Pavone, B. G.: Successful transfusion of Chido-positive blood to two patients with anti-Chido. Transfusion 15:266, 1975.

185. Tilley, C. A., Crookston, M. C., Haddad, S. A., and Shumak, K. H.: Red blood cell survival studies in patients with anti-Chª, and anti-Ykª, anti-Ge, and anti-Vel. Transfusion 17:171, 1977.

186. Yu, C. Y., Campbell, R. D., and Porter, R. R.: A structural model for the location of the Rodgers and the Chido antigenic determinants and their correlation with the human complement component C4A/C4B isotypes. Immunogenetics 27:399, 1988.

187. Tilley, C. A., Romans, D. G., and Crookston, M. C.: Localisation of Chido and Rodgers determinants to the C4d fragment of human C4. Nature 276:713, 1978.

188. Atkinson, J. P., Chan, A. C., Karp, D. R., Killion, C. C., Brown, R., Spinella, D., Schreffler, D. C., and Levine, R. P.: Origin of the fourth component of complement related Chido and Rodgers blood group antigens. Complement 5:65, 1988.

189. Rittner, C., Giles, C. M., Roos, M. H., Demant, P., and Mollenhauer, E.: Genetics of human C4 polymorphism: Detection and segregation of rare and duplicated haplotypes. Immunogenetics 19:321, 1984.

190. Roos, M. H., Giles, C. M., Demant, P., Mollenhauer, E., and Rittner, C.: Rodgers (Rg) and Chido (Ch) determinants on human C4; characterisation of two C4B 5 subtypes, one of which contains Rg and Ch determinants. J. Immunol. 133:2634, 1984.

191. Daniels, G. L.: Cromer-related antigens—blood group determinants on decay-accelerating factor. Vox Sang. 56:205, 1989.

192. Daniels, G. L., Tohyama, H., and Uchikawa, M.: A possible null phenotype in the Cromer blood group complex. Transfusion 22:362, 1982.

193. Smith, K. J., Coonce, L. S., and South, S. F.: Anti-Crª: Family study and survival of chromium-labeled incompatible red cells in a Spanish-American patient. Transfusion 23:167, 1983.

194. McSwain, B., and Robins, C.: A clinically significant anti-Crª. Transfusion 28:289, 1988.

195. Telen, M. J., Hall, S. E., and Green, A. M.: Identification of human erythrocyte blood group antigens on decay accelerating factor (DAF) and an erythrocyte phenotype negative for DAF. J. Exp. Med. 167:93, 1988.

196. Parsons, S. F., Spring, F. A., and Merry, A. H.: Evidence that Cromer-related blood group antigens are carried on decay accelerating factor (DAF) suggests that the Inab phenotype is a novel form of DAF deficiency (abstract). Manchester,

England, XXth Congress of the International Society of Blood Transfusion, 1988, p. 116.

197. Telen, M. J., and Green, A. M.: The Inab phenotype: Characterization of the membrane protein and complement regulatory defect. Blood 74:437, 1989.

198. Lublin, D. M., Thompson, E. S., Green, A. M., Levene, C., and Telen, M. J.: Dr(a−) polymorphism of decay accelerating factor. Biochemical, functional, and molecular characterization and production of allele-specific transfectants. J. Clin. Invest. 87:1945, 1991.

199. Landsteiner, K.: Zur Kenntnis der antifermentativen, lytischen und agglutinierenden Wirkungen des Blutserums und der Lymphe. Zbl. Batk. 27:357, 1900.

200. Landsteiner, K.: Uber agglutinationserscheinungen normalen menschlichen Blutes. Wien. Klin. Wochenschr. 14:1132, 1901.

201. Walker, R. H. (ed.): American Association of Blood Banks Technical Manual. Arlington, Va., American Association of Blood Banks, 1990.

202. Oriol, R., Le Pendu, J., and Mollicone, R.: Genetics of ABO, H, Lewis, X and Related Antigens. Vox Sang. 51:161, 1986.

203. Watkins, W. M.: Biochemistry and Genetics of the ABO, Lewis, and P blood group systems. Adv. Hum. Genet. 10:1, 1980.

204. Hakomori, S.: Blood group ABH and Ii antigens of human erythrocytes: Chemistry, polymorphism, and their developmental change. Semin. Hematol. 18:39, 1981.

205. Clausen, H., and Hakomori, S.: ABH and related histo-blood group antigens: Immunochemical differences in carrier isotypes and their distribution. Vox Sang. 46:1, 1989.

206. Sadler, J. E.: Biosynthesis of glycoproteins: Formation of O-linked oligosaccharides. In Ginsburg, V., and Robbins, P. (eds.): Biology of Carbohydrates. Vol. 2. New York, Wiley, 1984, pp. 199–288.

207. Clausen, H., Levery, S. B., Nudelman, E., Tsuchiya, S., and Hakomori, S.: Repetitive A epitope (type 3 chain A) defined by blood group A_1–specific monoclonal antibody TH-1: Chemical basis of qualitative A_1 and A_2 distinction. Proc. Natl. Acad. Sci. USA 82:1199, 1985.

208. Le Pendu, J., Lambert, F., Samuelsson, B. E., Breimer, M. E., Seitz, R. C., Urdaniz, M. P., Suesa, N., Ratcliffe, M., Francoise, A., Poschmann, A., Vinas, J., and Oriol, R.: Monoclonal antibodies specific for type 3 and type 4 chain–based blood group determinants: Relationship to the A1 and A2 subgroups. Glycoconjugate J. 3:255, 1986.

209. Clausen, H., Levery, S. B., Nudelman, E., Baldwin, M., and Hakomori, S.: Further characterization of type 2 and type 3 chain blood group A glycosphingolipids from human erythrocyte membranes. Biochemistry 25:7075, 1986.

210. Kannagi, R., Levery, S. B., and Hakomori, S.: Blood group H antigen with globo-series structure: Isolation and characterization from human blood group O erythrocytes. FEBS Lett. 175:397, 1984.

211. Oriol, R.: Genetic control of the fucosylation of ABH precursor chains. Evidence for new epistatic interactions in different cells and tissues. J. Immunogenet. 17:235, 1990.

212. Betteridge, A., and Watkins, W. M.: Acceptor substrate specificities of human α-2-L-fucosyltransferases from different tissues. Biochem. Soc. Trans. 13:1126, 1986.

213. Clausen, H., Holmes, E., and Hakomori, S.: Novel blood group H glycolipid antigens exclusively expressed in blood group A and AB erythrocytes (type 3 chain H). II. Differential conversion of different H substrates by A_1 and A_2 enzymes, and type 3 chain H expression in relation to secretor status. J. Biol. Chem. 261:1388, 1986.

214. Laine, R. A., and Rush, J. S.: Chemistry of human erythrocyte polylactosamine glycopeptides (erythroglycans) as related to ABH blood group antigenic determinants. Adv. Exp. Med. Biol. 228:331, 1988.

215. Steck, T. L.: The organisation of proteins in the human red blood cell membrane. J. Cell Biol. 62:1, 1974.

216. Allard, W. J., and Lienhard, G. E.: Monoclonal antibodies to the glucose transporter from human erythrocytes. J. Biol. Chem. 160:8668, 1985.

217. Tanner, M. J. A., Martin, P. G., and High, S.: The complete amino acid sequence of the human erythrocyte membrane anion-transport protein deduced from the cDNA sequence. Biochem. J. 256:703, 1988.

218. Mueckler, M., Caruso, C., and Baldwin, S. A.: Sequence and structure of a human glucose transporter. Science 229:941, 1985.

219. Fukuda, M., and Fukuda, M. N.: Changes in cell surface glycoproteins and carbohydrate structures during the development and differentiation of human erythroid cells. J. Supramol. Struct. 17:313, 1974.

220. Moore, S. J., and Green, C.: The identification of Rhesus polypeptide-blood group ABH-active glycoprotein complex in the human red cell membrane. Biochem. J. 244:735, 1987.

221. Dejter-Juszynski, M., Harpaz, N., Flowers, H. M., and Sharon, N.: Blood-group ABH-specific macroglycolipids of human erythrocytes: Isolation in high yield from a crude membrane glycoprotein fraction. Eur. J. Biochem. 83:363, 1978.

222. Koscielak, J., Miller-Podraza, H., Krauze, R., and Piasek, A.: Isolation and characterization of poly(glycosyl)ceramides (megaloglycolipids) with A, H, and I blood-group activities. Eur. J. Biochem. 71:9, 1976.

223. Salmon, C. H., and Cartron, J. P.: ABO phenotypes. In Greenwalt, T. J., and Steane, E. A. (eds.): CRC Handbook Series in Clinical Laboratory Science. Section D: Blood Banking. Vol. 1. Cleveland, CRC Press, 1977, p. 71.

224. Salmon, C., Cartron, J.-P., and Rouger, P.: The Human Blood Groups. New York, Masson Publishers USA, 1984.

225. Bird, G. W. G.: Haemagglutinins in seeds. Br. Med. Bull. 15:165, 1959.

226. Mourant, A. E., Kopèc, A. C., and Domaniewska-Sobczak, K.: The Distribution of the Human Blood Groups and Other Biochemical Polymorphisms. 2nd ed. Oxford, England, Oxford University Press, 1976.

227. Economidou, J., Hughes-Jones, N. C., and Gardner, B.: Quantitative measurements concerning A and B antigen sites. Vox Sang. 12:321, 1967.

228. Mäkela, O., Ruoslahti, E., and Ehnholm, C.: Subtypes of human ABO blood groups and subtype-specific antibodies. J. Immunol. 10:763, 1969.

229. Kisailus, E. C., and Kabat, E. A.: Immunochemical studies on blood groups. LXVI. Competitive binding assays of A_1 and A_2 blood group substances with insolubilized anti-A serum and insolubilized A agglutinine from Dolichos biflorus. J. Exp. Med. 147:830, 1978.

230. Mohn, J. F., Cunningham, R. K., and Bates, J. F.: Qualitative distinctions between subgroups A_1 and A_2. In Mohn, J., Plunkett, R., Cunningham, R., and Lambert, R. (eds.): Human Blood Groups. New York, Karger, 1977, pp. 316–325.

231. Moreno, C., Lundblad, A., and Kabat, E. A.: Immunochemical studies on blood groups. LI. A comparative study of the reaction of A_1 and A_2 blood group glycoproteins with human anti-A. J. Exp. Med. 134:439, 1971.

232. Yamaguchi, H., Okubo, Y., and Hazama, F.: Another Japanese A_2B_3 blood-group family with the propositus having O-group father. Proc. Jpn. Acad. 42:417, 1966.

233. Seyfried, H., Walewska, I., and Verblinska, B.: Unusual inheritance of ABO group in a family with weak B antigens. Vox Sang. 9:268, 1964.

234. Lopez, M., Liberge, G., Gerbal, A., Brocteur, J., and Salmon, C.: Cis AB blood groups. Immunologic, thermodynamic and quantitative studies of ABH antigens. Biomedicine 24:265, 1976.

235. Yoshida, A., Yamaguchi, H., and Okubo, Y.: Genetic mechanism of cis-AB inheritance. I. A case associated with unequal chromosomal crossing over. Am. J. Hum. Genet. 32:332, 1980.

236. Yoshida, A., Yamaguchi, H., and Okubo, Y.: Genetic mechanism of Cis-AB inheritance. II. Cases associated with structural mutation of blood group glycosyltransferases. Am. J. Hum. Genet. 32:645, 1980.

237. Watkins, W. M., Greenwell, P., and Yates, A. D.: The genetic and enzymatic regulation of the synthesis of the A and B

determinants in the ABO blood group system. Immunol. Commun. 10:83, 1981.

238. Clausen, H., White, T., Takio, K., Titani, K., Stroud, M., Holmes, E., Karkov, J., Thim, L., and Hakomori, S.: Isolation to homogeneity and partial characterization of a histo-blood group A defined Fuc $\alpha 1 \rightarrow 2$Gal $\alpha 1 \rightarrow 3$-N-acetylgalactosaminyltransferase from human lung tissue. J. Biol. Chem. 265:1139, 1990.

239. Yamamoto, F.-I., Marken, J., Tsuji, T., White, T., Clausen, H., and Hakomori, S.-I.: Cloning and characterization of DNA complementary to human UDP-GalNAc:Fuc$\alpha 1 \rightarrow 2$Gal $\alpha 1 \rightarrow 3$GalNAc transferase (histo-blood group A transferase) mRNA. J. Biol. Chem. 264:1146, 1990.

240. Lowe, J. B.: Molecular cloning, expression, and uses of mammalian glycosyltransferases. Semin. Cell Biol. 2:289, 1991.

241. Griffiths, G., and Simons, K.: The trans Golgi network: Sorting at the exit site of the Golgi complex. Science 234:438, 1986.

242. Kornfeld, R., and Kornfeld, S.: Assembly of asparagine-linked oligosaccharides. Annu. Rev. Biochem. 54:631, 1985.

243. Larsen, R. D., Rajan, V. P., Ruff, M. M., Kukowska-Latallo, J., Cummings, R. D., and Lowe, J. B.: Isolation of a cDNA encoding a murine UDPgalactose:b-D-galactosyl-1,4-N-acetyl-D-glucosaminide α-1,3-galactosyltransferase: Expression cloning by gene transfer. Proc. Natl. Acad. Sci. USA 86: 8227, 1989.

244. Joziasse, D. H., Shaper, J. H., van den Eijnden, D. H., Van Tunen, A. J., and Shaper, N. L.: Bovine $\alpha 1 \rightarrow 3$-galactosyltransferase: Isolation and characterization of a cDNA clone. Identification of homologous sequences in human genomic DNA. J. Biol. Chem. 264:14290, 1989.

245. Larsen, R. D., Rivera-Marrero, C. A., Ernst, L. K., Cummings, R. D., and Lowe, J. B.: Frameshift and nonsense mutations in a human genomic sequence homologous to a murine UDP-Gal:β D-Gal(1,4)-D-GlcNAc α(1,3)-galactosyltransferase cDNA. J. Biol. Chem. 265:7055, 1990.

246. Yamamoto, F.-I., Clausen, H., White, T., Marken, J., and Hakomori, S.-I.: Molecular genetic basis of the histo-blood group ABO system. Nature 345:229, 1990.

247. Yamamoto, F.-I., and Hakomori, S.-I.: Sugar-nucleotide donor specificity of histo-blood group A and B transferases is based on amino acid substitutions. J. Biol. Chem. 265:19257, 1990.

248. Roberts, J. A. Fraser: Blood groups and susceptibility to disease. Br. J. Prev. Soc. Med. 11:107, 1957.

249. Mourant, A. E.: Blood Groups and Diseases: A Study of Associations of Diseases with Blood Groups and Other Polymorphisms. Oxford, England, Oxford University Press, 1978.

250. Aird, I., and Bentall, H. H.: A relationship between cancer of the stomach and the ABO blood groups. Br. Med. J. 1:799, 1953.

251. Aird, I., Bentall, H. H., Mehigan, J. A., and Roberts, J. A. Fraser: The blood groups in relation to peptic ulceration and carcinoma of colon, rectum, breast, and bronchus: An association between the ABO groups and peptic ulceration. Br. Med. J. 2:315, 1954.

252. Le Pendu, J.: A hypothesis on the dual significance of the ABH, Lewis, and related antigens. J. Immunogenet. 16:53, 1989.

253. Chester, M. A., Yates, A. D., and Watkins, W. M.: Phenyl-β-D-galactopyranoside as an acceptor substrate for the blood-group H gene associated guanosine diphosphate L-fucose:β-D-galactosyl α-2-L-fucosyltransferase. Eur. J. Biochem. 69:583, 1976.

254. Wolf, R. O., and Taylor, L. L.: The concentration of blood-group substances in the parotid, sublingual and submaxillary salivas. J. Dent. Res. 43:272, 1964.

255. Milne, R. W., and Dawes, C.: The relative contributions of different salivary glands to the blood group activity of whole saliva in humans. Vox Sang. 25:298, 1973.

256. Levine, P., Robinson, E., Celano, M., Briggs, O., and Falkinburg, L.: Gene interaction resulting in suppression of blood group substance B. Blood 10:1100, 1955.

257. Solomon, J., Waggoner, R., and Leyshon, W. C.: A quantitative immunogenetic study of gene suppression evoking A_1 and

258. Oriol, R., Danilovs, J., and Hawkins, B. R.: A new genetic model proposing that the Se gene is a structural gene closely linked to the H gene. Am. J. Hum. Genet. 33:421, 1981.

259. Mollicone, R., Davies, D. R., Evans, B., Dalix, A. M., and Oriol, R.: Cellular expression and genetic control of ABH antigens in primary sensory neurons of marmoset, baboon and man. J. Neuroimmunol. 10:255, 1986.

260. Szulman, A. E.: The ABH and Lewis antigens of human tissues during prenatal and postnatal life. *In* Mohn, J. Plunkett, R., Cunningham, R., and Lambert, R. (eds.): Human Blood Groups. Basel, Karger, 1977, pp. 426–436.

261. Rouger, P., Poupon, R., Gane, P., Mallissen, B., Darnis, F., and Salmon, C.: Expression of blood group antigens including HLA markers in human adult liver. Tissue Antigens 27:78, 1986.

262. Gaensslen, R. E., Bell, S. C., and Lee, H. C.: Distribution of genetic markers in United States populations: I. Blood group and secretor systems. J. Forensic Sci. 32:1016, 1987.

263. Le Pendu, J., Cartron, J. P., Lemieux, R. U., and Oriol, R.: The presence of at least two different H-blood-group–related $\beta DGal$ α-2-L-fucosyltransferases in human serum and the genetics of blood group H substances. Am. J. Hum. Genet. 37:749, 1985.

264. Rajan, V. P., Larsen, R. D., Ajmera, S., Ernst, L. K., and Lowe, J. B.: A cloned human DNA restriction fragment determines expression of a GDP-L-fucose:β-D-galactoside 2-α-L-fucosyltransferase in transfected cells, J. Biol. Chem. 24:11158, 1991.

265. Sarnesto, A., Kohlin, T., Hindsgaul, O., Thurin, J., and Blaszczyk-Thurin, M.: Purification of the secretor-type beta-galactoside alpha 1 $\rightarrow$ 2-fucosyltransferase from human serum. J. Biol. Chem. 267:2737, 1992.

266. Lemieux, R. U.: Human blood groups and carbohydrate chemistry. Chem. Soc. Rev. 7:423, 1978.

267. Ernst, L. K., Rajan, V. P., Larsen, R. D., Ruff, M. M., and Lowe, J. B.: Stable expression of blood group H determinants and GDP-L-fucose:β-D-galactoside 2-α-L-fucosyltransferase in mouse cells after transfection with human DNA. J. Biol. Chem. 264:3436, 1989.

268. Larsen, R. D., Ernst, L. K., Nair, R. P., and Lowe, J. B.: Molecular cloning, sequence, and expression of human GDP-L-fucose:β-D-galactoside 2-α-L-fucosyltransferase cDNA that can form the H blood group antigen. Proc. Natl. Acad. Sci. USA 87:6674, 1990.

269. Sarnesto, A., Kohlin, T., Thurin, J., and Blaszczyk-Thurin, M.: Purification of H gene–encoded β-galactoside α 1-2 fucosyltransferase from human serum. J. Biol. Chem. 265:15067, 1990.

270. Ball, S. P., Tongue, N., Gibaud, A., Le Pendu, J., Mollicone, R., Gerard, G., and Oriol, R.: The human chromosome 19 linkage group FUT1 (H), FUT2 (SE), LE, LU, PEPD, C3, APOC2, D19S7, and D19S9. Ann. Hum. Genet. 55 (pt. 3):225, 1991.

271. Kelly, R. J., Ernst, L. K., Larsen, R. D., Bryant, J. G., Robinson, J. S., and Lowe, J. B.: Molecular basis for H blood group deficiency in Bombay (O_h) and para-Bombay individuals (submitted for publication).

272. Clarke, C. A., Edwards, J. Wyn, Haddock, D. R. W., Howel-Evans, A. W., McConnell, R. B., and Sheppard, P. M.: ABO blood groups and secretor character in duodenal ulcer. Br. Med. J. 2:725, 1956.

273. Sheinfeld, J., Schaeffer A. J., Cordon-Cardo, C., Rogatko, A., and Fair, W. R.: Association of the Lewis blood group phenotype with recurrent urinary tract infections in women. N. Engl. J. Med. 320:773, 1989.

274. Lund, B., Lindberg, F. P., Baga, M., and Normark, S.: Globoside-specific adhesions of uropathogenic *Escherichia coli* are encoded by similar trans-complementable gene clusters. J. Bacteriol. 162:1293, 1985.

275. Lomberg, H., and Eden, C. S.: Influence of P blood group phenotype on susceptibility to urinary tract infection. FEMS Microbiol. Immunol. 1:363, 1989.

276. Blaszczyk-Thurin, M., Sarnesto, A., Thurin, J., Hindsgaul, O., and Koprowski, H.: Biosynthetic pathways for the Leb and Y glycolipids in the gastric carcinoma cell line KATO III as analyzed by a novel assay. Biochem. Biophys. Res. Commun. 151:100, 1988.

277. Feizi, T.: Demonstration by monoclonal antibodies that carbohydrate structures of glycoproteins and glycolipids are onco-developmental antigens. Nature 314:53, 1985.

278. Mourant, A. E.: A "new" human blood group antigen of frequent occurrence. Nature 158:237, 1946.

279. Rege, V. P., Painter, T. J., Watkins, W. M., and Morgan, W. T. J.: Isolation of a serologically active fucose containing trisaccharide from human blood group Le^a substrate. Nature 240:740, 1964.

280. Hanfland, P., and Graham, H.: Immunochemistry of the Lewis blood group system: Partial characterization of Le^a, Le^b, and H type 1 (Le^{dh}) blood group active glycosphingolipids from human plasma. Arch. Biochem. Biophys. 220:383, 1981.

281. Hanfland, P., Kardowicz, M., Peter-Katalinic, J., Pfannschmidt, G., Crawford, R. J., Graham, H. A., and Egge, H.: Immunochemistry of the Lewis blood group system: Isolation and structures of the Lewis c active and related glycosphingolipids from the plasma of blood-group OLe(a−b−) nonsecretors. Arch. Biochem. Biophys. 246:655, 1986.

282. Marcus, D. M., and Cass, L. E.: Glycosphingolipids with Lewis blood group activity: Uptake by human erythrocytes. Science 164:553, 1969.

283. Holburn, A. M.: Quantitative studies with [^{125}I]IgM anti-Le^a Immunology 24:1019, 1973.

284. Mollison, P. L., and Polley, M. J.: Temporary suppression of the Lewis blood-group antibodies to permit incompatible transfusion. Lancet 1:909, 1963.

285. Cutbush, M., Giblett, E. R., and Mollison, P. L.: Demonstration of the phenotype Le(a+b+) in infants and adults. Br. J. Haematol. 2:210, 1956.

286. Grubb, R., and Morgan, W. T. J.: The "Lewis" blood group characters of erythrocytes and body fluids. Br. J. Exp. Pathol. 30:198, 1949.

287. Johnson, P. H., Yates, A. D., and Watkins, W. M.: Human salivary fucosyltransferases: Evidence for two distinct α-3-L-fucosyltransferase activities one of which is associated with the Lewis blood group Le gene. Biochem. Biophys. Res. Commun. 100:1611, 1981.

288. Prieels, J. P., Monnom, D., Dolmans, M., Beyer, T. A., and Hill, R. L.: Copurification of the Lewis blood group N-acetylglucosaminide α1 → 4 fucosyltransferase and an N-acetylglucosaminide α1 → 3 fucosyltransferase from human milk. J. Biol. Chem. 256:10456, 1981.

289. Kukowska-Latallo, J. F., Larsen, R. D., Nair, R. P., and Lowe, J. B.: A cloned human cDNA determines expression of a mouse stage-specific embryonic antigen and the Lewis blood group α(1,3/1,4)fucosyltransferase. Genes Devel. 4:1288, 1990.

290. Lowe, J. B., Stoolman, L. M., Nair, R. P., Larsen, R. D., Berhend, T. L., and Marks, R. M.: ELAM-1–dependent cell adhesion to vascular endothelium determined by a transfected human fucosyltransferase cDNA. Cell 63:475, 1990.

291. Lowe, J. B., Kukowska-Latallo, J. F., Nair, R. P., Larsen, R. D., Marks, R. M., Macher, B. A., Kelly, R. J., and Ernst, L. K.: Molecular cloning of a human fucosyltransferase gene that determines expression of the Lewis x and VIM-2 epitopes but not ELAM-1–dependent cell adhesion. J. Biol. Chem. 266:17467, 1991.

292. Weston, B. W., Nair, R. P., Larsen, R. D., and Lowe, J. B.: Isolation of a novel human α(1,3)fucosyltransferase gene and molecular comparison to the human Lewis blood group α(1,3/1,4)fucosyltransferase gene. J. Biol. Chem. 267:4152, 1992.

293. Goelz, S. E., Hession, C., Goff, D., Griffiths, B., Tizard, R., Newman, B., Chi-Rosso, G., and Lobb, R.: ELFT: A gene that directs the expression of an ELAM-1 ligand. Cell 63:1349, 1990.

294. Kumar, R., Potvin, B., Muller, W. A., and Stanley, P.: Cloning of a human α(1,3)fucosyltransferase gene that encodes ELFT but does not confer ELAM-1 recognition on CHO transfections. J. Biol. Chem. 266:21777, 1991.

295. Weston, B. W., Smith, P. L., Kelly, R. J., and Lowe, J. B.: Molecular cloning of a fourth member of a human α(1,3)fucosyltransferase gene family: Multiple homologous sequences that determine expression of the Lewis x, sialyl Lewis x, and difucosyl sialyl Lewis x epitopes. J. Biol. Chem. 267:24575, 1992.

296. Lowe, J. B.: Specificity and expression of carbohydrate ligands. In Wegner, C. D. (ed.): The Handbook of Immunopharmacology. Orlando, Fla., Academic Press (in press).

297. Bevilacqua, M. P., Stengelin, S., Gimbrone, M. A., and Seed, B.: Endothelial leukocyte adhesion molecule 1: An inducible receptor for neutrophils related to complement regulatory proteins and lectins. Science 243:1160, 1989.

298. Bevilacqua, M., Butcher, E., Furie, B., Furie, B., Gallatin, M., Gimbrone, M., Harlan, J., Kishimoto, K., Lasky, L., and McEver, R.: Selectins: A family of adhesion receptors. Cell 67:233, 1991.

299. Drickamer, K.: Two distinct classes of carbohydrate-recognition domains in animal lectins. J. Biol. Chem. 263:9557, 1988.

300. Phillips, M. L., Nudelman, E., Gaeta, F. C., Perez, M., Singhal, A. K., Hakomori, S., and Paulson, J. C.: ELAM-1 mediates cell adhesion by recognition of a carbohydrate ligand, sialyl-Lex. Science 250:1130, 1990.

301. Walz, G., Aruffo, A., Kolanus, W., Bevilacqua, M., and Seed, B.: Recognition by ELAM-1 of the sialyl-Lex determinant on myeloid and tumor cells. Science 250:1132, 1990.

302. Tyrrel, D., Pames, P., Rao, N., Foxall, C., Abbas, S., Dasgupta, F., Nashed, M., Hasegawa, A., Kiso, M., Asa, D., Kidd, J., and Brandley, B. K.: Structural requirements for the carbohydrate ligand of E-selectin. Proc. Natl. Acad. Sci. USA 88:10372, 1991.

303. Berg, E. L., Robinson, M. K., Mansson, O., Butcher, E. C., and Magnani, J. L.: A carbohydrate domain common to both sialyl Lea and sialyl Lex is recognized by the endothelial cell leukocyte adhesion molecule ELAM-1. J. Biol. Chem. 266:14869, 1991.

304. Takada, A., Ohmori, K., Takahashi, N., Tsuyuoka, K., Yago, A., Zenita, K., Hasegawa, A., and Kannagi, R.: Adhesion of human cancer cells to vascular endothelium mediated by a carbohydrate antigen, sialyl Lewis A. Biochem. Biophys. Res. Commun. 179:713, 1991.

305. Kim, Y. S., and Itzkowitz, S.: Carbohydrate antigen expression in the adenoma-carcinoma sequence. Prog. Clin. Biol. Res. 279:241, 1988.

306. Zhou, Q., Moore, K. L., Smith, D. F., Varki, A., McEver, R. P., and Cummings, R. D.: The selectin GMP-140 binds to sialylated, fucosylated lactosaminoglycans on both myeloid and nonmyeloid cells. J. Cell Biol. 115:557, 1991.

307. Polley, M. J., Phillips, M. L., Wayner, E., Nudelman, E., Singhal, A. K., Hakomori, S.-I., and Paulson, J. C.: CD62 and endothelial cell–leukocyte adhesion molecule 1 (ELAM-1) recognize the same carbohydrate ligand, sialyl-Lewis x. Proc. Natl. Acad. Sci. USA 88:6224, 1991.

308. Brandley, B. K., Watson, S. R., Dowbenko, D., Fennie, C., Lasky, L. A., Hasegawa, A., Kiso, M., and Foxall, C.: The sialyl Lewis x oligosaccharide is a ligand for L-selectin. FASEB J. A1890, 1992.

309. Etzioni, A., Frydman, M., Pollack, S., Avidor, I., Phillips, M. L., Paulson, J. C., and Gershoni-Baruch, R.: Brief report: Recurrent severe infections caused by a novel leukocyte adhesion deficiency. N. Engl. J. Med. 327:1789, 1992.

310. Reitman, M. L., Trowbridge, I. S., and Kornfeld, S.: Mouse lymphoma cell lines resistant to pea lectin are defective in fucose metabolism. J. Biol. Chem. 255:9900, 1980.

311. Marcus, D. M.: The ABO and Lewis blood-group system. Immunochemistry, genetics and relationship to human disease. N. Engl. J. Med. 280:994, 1969.

312. Wiener, A. S., Unger, L. T., and Cohen, L.: Type-specific cold autoantibodies as a cause of acquired hemolytic anemia and hemolytic transfusion reactions: Biologic test with bovine red cells. Ann. Intern. Med. 44:221, 1956.

313. Marsh, W. L., and Jenkins, W. J.: Anti-i: A new cold antibody. Nature 188:753, 1960.

314. Marsh, W. L.: Anti-i: A cold antibody defining the Ii relationship in human red cells. Br. J. Haematol. 7:200, 1961.

315. Hakomori, S.-I.: Blood group ABH and Ii antigens of human erythrocytes: Chemistry, polymorphism, and their developmental change. Semin. Hematol. 18:39, 1981.

316. Feizi, T.: The blood group Ii system: A carbohydrate antigen system defined by naturally monoclonal or oligoclonal autoantibodies of man. Immunol. Commun. 10:127, 1981.

317. Niemann, H., Watanabe, K., Hakomori, S., Childs, R. A., and Feizi, T.: Blood group i and I activities of "lacto-N-norhexaosyl-ceramide" and its analogues: The structural requirements for i-specificities. Biochem. Biophys. Res. Commun. 81:1286, 1978.

318. Watanabe, K., Hakomori, S., Childs, R. A., and Feizi, T.: Characterization of a blood group I–active ganglioside: structural requirements for I and i specificities. J. Biol. Chem. 254:3221, 1979.

319. Koscielak, J., Zdebska, E., Wileznska, Z., Miller-Podraza, H., and Dzierzkowa-Borodej, W.: Immunochemistry of Ii-active glycosphingolipids of erythrocytes. Eur. J. Biochem. 96:331, 1979.

320. Watanabe, K., and Hakomori, S.: Status of blood group carbohydrate chains in ontogenesis and oncogenesis. J. Exp. Med. 144:644, 1976.

321. Koscielak, J., Zdebska, E., Wilczynska, Z., Miller-Podraza, H., and Dzierzkowa-Borodej, W.: Immunochemistry of Ii-active glycosphingolipids of erythrocytes. Eur. J. Biochem. 96:331, 1979.

322. Yates, A. D., and Watkins, W. M.: Enzymes involved in the biosynthesis of glycoconjugates. A UDP-2-acetamido-2-deoxy-D-glucose: beta-D-galactopyranosyl-(1 → 4)-saccharide (1 → 3)-2-acetamido-2-deoxy-beta-D-glucopyranosyltransferase in human serum. Carbohydr. Res. 120:251, 1983.

323. Piller, F., and Cartron, J. P.: UDP-GlcNAc:Galβ1 → 4Glc(NAc)β1 → 3N-acetylglucosaminyltransferase. Identification and characterization in human serum. J. Biol. Chem. 258:12293, 1983.

324. Van den Eijnden, D. H., Winterwerp, H., Smeeman, P., and Schiphorst, W. E.: Novikoff ascites tumor cells contain N-acetyllactosaminide β1 → 3 and β1 → 6 N-acetylglucosaminyltransferase activity. J. Biol. Chem. 258:3435, 1983.

325. Gu, J., Nishikawa, A., Fujii, S., Gasa, S., and Taniguchi, N.: Biosynthesis of blood group I and i antigens in rat tissues. Identification of a novel β1-6-N-acetylglucosaminyltransferase. J. Biol. Chem. 267:2994, 1992.

326. Childs, R. A., Kapadia, A., and Feizi, T.: Blood group I and i antigens as common surface antigens on a variety of human and animal cell lines. In Schauer, R., Boer, P., Buddecke, E., Karamer, M. F., Vliegenthart, J. F. G., and Wiegandt, H. (eds.): Glycoconjugates. Stuttgart, Georg Thieme, pp. 518–519, 1979.

327. Childs, R. A., Kapadia, A., and Feizi, T.: Expression of blood group I and i active carbohydrate sequences on cultured human and animal cell lines assessed by radioimmunoassays with monoclonal cold agglutinins. Eur. J. Immunol. 10:379, 1980.

328. Shumak, K. H., Rachkewich, R. A., Crookston, M. C., and Crookston, J. H.: Antigens of the Ii system on lymphocytes. Nature New Biol. 231:148, 1971.

329. Thomas, D. B.: The i antigen complex: A new specificity unique to dividing human cells. Eur. J. Immunol. 4:819, 1974.

330. Fukuda, M.: K562 human leukaemic cells express fetal type (i) antigen on different glycoproteins from circulating erythrocytes. Nature 285:405, 1980.

331. Papayannopoulou, T., Chen, P., Maniatis, A., and Stamatoyannopoulos, G.: Simultaneous assessment of i-antigenic expression and fetal hemoglobin in single red cells by immuno-fluorescence. Blood 55:221, 1980.

332. Kapadia, A., Feizi, T., and Evans, M. J.: Changes in expression and polarization of blood group I and i antigens in post-implantation embryos and teratocarcinomas of mouse associated with cell differentiation. Exp. Cell. Res. 131:185, 1981.

333. Landsteiner, K., and Levine, P.: Further observations on individual differences of human blood. Proc. Soc. Exp. Biol. Med. 24:941, 1927.

334. Marcus, D. M., Kundu, S. K., and Suzuki, A.: The P blood group system: Recent progress in immunochemistry and genetics. Semin. Hematol. 18:63, 1981.

335. Kortekangas, A. E., Kaarsalo, E., and Melartin, L.: The red cell antigen P^k and its relationship to the P system. The evidence of three more Pk families. Vox Sang. 10:385, 1965.

336. Matson, G. A., Swandon, J., and Noades, J.: A "new" antigen and antibody belonging to the P blood group system. Am. J. Hum. Genet. 11:26, 1959.

337. Kijimoto-Ochiai, S., Naiki, M., and Makita, A.: Defects of glycosyltransferase activities in human fibroblast of P^k and p blood group phenotypes. Proc. Natl. Acad. Sci. USA 74:5407, 1973.

338. Marcus, D. M., Naiki, M., and Kundu, S. K.: Abnormalities in the glycosphingolipid content of human P^k and p erythrocytes. Proc. Natl. Acad. Sci. USA 73:3262, 1976.

339. Fellous, M., Gerbal, A., and Tessier, C.: Studies on the biosynthetic pathway of human P erythrocyte antigens using somatic cells in culture. Vox Sang. 26:518, 1974.

340. Fellous, M., Gerbal, A., and Nobillot, G.: Studies on the biosynthetic pathway of human P erythrocyte antigens using genetic complementation tests between fibroblasts from rare p and P^k phenotype donors. Vox Sang. 32:262, 1977.

341. Graham, H. A., and Williams, A. N.: A genetic model for the inheritance of the P_1P_1 and P^k antigens. Transfusion 18:638, 1978.

342. Leffler, H., and Svanborg, E. C.: Chemical identification of a glycosphingolipid receptor for Escherichia coli attaching to human urinary epithelial cells and agglutinating human erythrocytes. FEMS Microbiol. Lett. 8:127, 1980.

343. Wold, A. E., Thorssen, M., Hull, S., and Svanborg, E. C.: Attachment of Escherichia coli to mannose or Galα1-4Galβ containing receptors in human colonic epithelial cells. Infect. Immunol. 56:2531, 1988.

344. Lomberg, H., Hanson, L. A., Jacobsson, B., Jodal, U., Leffler, H., and Svanborg, E. C.: Correlation of P blood group, vesicoureteral reflux, and bacterial attachment in patients with recurrent pyelonephritis. N. Engl. J. Med. 308:1189, 1983.

345. Tomisawa, S., Kogure, T., Kuroume, T., Leffler, H., Lomberg, H., Shimabukoro, N., Terao, K., and Svanborg Eden, C.: P blood group and proneness to urinary tract infection in Japanese children. Scand. J. Infect. Dis. 21:403, 1989.

346. Levine, P., and Koch, E. A.: The rare human isoagglutinin and anti-Tjᵃ and habitual abortion. Science 120:239, 1954.

The Molecular Biology of Enzymes of Erythrocyte Metabolism

Ernest Beutler

INTRODUCTION

Of all the mutations of man, the most common are probably those that affect the erythrocyte. This is so because considerable compromise in the function of the red cell is quite compatible with extrauterine existence. Such mutations may affect the structure or quantity of hemoglobin or of the membrane proteins. They may also impair the enzymatic machinery that allows the red cell to maintain ionic gradients, its shape, its flexibility, and the functional state of the hemoglobin within the cell.

Abnormalities of red cell metabolism were among the first to be defined at the biochemical level. Our understanding of this field began in the 1940s and 1950s with the recognition that hereditary enzyme deficiencies existed and that some were relatively common. Acatalasemia, the absence of red cell catalase, was discovered in 1948[1]; deficiencies of glucose-6-phosphate dehydrogenase (G6PD)[2] and of galactose-1-phosphate uridyl transferase were discovered in 1956,[3] and deficiency of pyruvate kinase in 1961.[4] It is notable that only two of these four mutations cause a hematological disease. In the case of acatalasemia

331

and galactose-1-phosphate uridyl transferase, the red cell served as a convenient biopsy tissue to allow investigators to discover the cause of a disorder that was manifested clinically elsewhere in the body.

It was only in the 1960s and 1970s, through more detailed biochemical characterization, that it became evident that within any given deficiency a great deal of heterogeneity existed. In the 1980s and 1990s, understanding of the red cell enzyme defects has been transformed by the powerful tools of molecular biology. Thus far, only in the case of G6PD does a large body of information exist regarding the mutations and their population distribution. There are so many other red cell enzyme defects and some are so rare that most of the genes concerned have not yet been cloned.

This chapter reviews the normal metabolism of the erythrocyte, the genetic defects of red cell metabolism that are known, and, particularly in the case of G6PD, the emerging insights that the tools of molecular biology have made possible.

METABOLISM OF THE NORMAL ERYTHROCYTE

The human erythrocyte, like all other body cells, is the product of a nucleated cell with the capacity to synthesize DNA, RNA, and protein and to divide. By the time that it leaves the marrow as a reticulocyte, the erythrocyte has been endowed with virtually all of the proteins that it requires for its 120 day life span. The reticulocyte contains mere vestiges of ribosomes and messenger RNA (mRNA), of mitochondria, and of lysosomes, and these, too, disappear within a few days.[5] Although bereft of most synthetic functions, the mature erythrocyte retains the capacity to metabolize glucose. This capacity provides the energy needed for it to actively reduce methemoglobin to hemoglobin; to pump Na^+, K^+, and Ca^{2+} against concentration gradients; and to carry out synthesis of a few small molecules, including adenine, guanine, and pyrimidine nucleotides, glutathione, and lipids.

The Metabolism of Glucose

Glycolysis

Glucose is the main source of energy for the circulating erythrocyte of man. The erythrocytes of some mammals lose their permeability to glucose after infancy[6] and may use purine nucleosides as substrates instead.[7] The glycolytic pathway (Fig. 9–1) serves to phosphorylate glucose, transferring the phosphate to ADP to yield ATP, and ultimately to form two molecules of lactic acid from each molecule of glucose.[8, 9] This pathway also provides NADH to reduce methemoglobin to hemoglobin, and 2,3-diphosphoglycerate, an allosteric effector of the hemoglobin molecule, is formed in the Rapoport-Luebering cycle.[10] The enzymes that catalyze the steps of the glycolytic pathway are listed in Table 9–1.

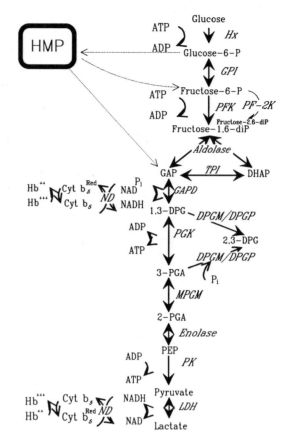

FIGURE 9–1. The glycolytic and related pathways of red cell metabolism. The names of enzymes or their abbreviations (see Table 9–1) are shown in italics.

The Hexose Monophosphate (HMP) Shunt

The second major pathway of glucose metabolism is the HMP shunt (Fig. 9–2).[48, 49] In this pathway, the first product of glucose phosphorylation, glucose-6-phosphate, undergoes oxidation, followed by a series of rearrangements eventuating in the formation of fructose-6-phosphate and glyceraldehyde-3-phosphate, both intermediates in the glycolytic pathway. The HMP shunt is the only source of NADPH in the erythrocytes, and it also produces the ribose needed for synthesis of nucleotides in the salvage pathways. Because NADPH is required for the reduction of oxidized glutathione, and possibly of protein sulfhydryl groups,[50] the HMP shunt plays a vital role in red cell metabolism: When the pathway is prevented from functioning normally by a deficiency of the enzyme that catalyzes its first step, G6PD, red cell life span may be markedly shortened.[51] Red cells are a particularly rich source of catalase. Like glutathione peroxidase, this enzyme removes peroxide from the erythrocyte[52] but is relatively inefficient at low peroxide levels. Catalase has the ability to bind NADPH tightly,[53, 54] and the inactive form, compound II, is reactivated by NADPH. Thus, the activity of the HMP shunt removes peroxidase not only through the action of glutathione peroxidase but also by activating catalase.[54] Despite the important role that catalase may

TABLE 9–1. GLYCOLYTIC ENZYMES AND ENZYMES OF RELATED PATHWAYS IN THE ERYTHROCYTE

ENZYME (ABBREVIATION)	INHERITANCE*	EFFECT OF DEFICIENCY	MOLECULAR BIOLOGY	SELECTED REFERENCES†
Hexokinase (HK)	A	NSHA‡	Unique reticulocyte enzyme; number of loci controversial; not cloned	11–15
Glucosephosphate isomerase (GPI)	A	NSHA	Cloned and partly sequenced	16–19
Phosphofructokinase (PFK)	A	Compensated hemolysis, ± erythrocytosis and myopathy identified	Both subunits M and L have been cloned and sequenced; An M subunit mutation has been discovered	20–22 23–25
Fructose-6-phosphate 2-kinase (PF 2-K)		Deficiency unknown	Rat muscle enzyme cloned	26–28
Aldolase	A	NSHA; ?mental retardation and glycogen storage disease	Cloned; mutation identified in one case	29–31
Triosephosphate isomerase (TPI)	A	NSHA and severe neuromuscular disease	Cloned; mutations identified in several cases	32–34 35, 36
Diphosphoglycerate mutase/ diphosphoglycerate phosphatase (DPGM/DPGP)	A	Erythrocytosis	Cloned; mutations detected	37–39, 39a
Phosphoglycerate kinase (PGK)	X	NSHA; mental retardation sequencing	Cloned; several mutations detected by DNA and protein analysis	40–43 43a
Monophosphoglycerate mutase (MPGM)	A	Deficiency unknown	—	
Enolase	A	?NSHA	—	
Pyruvate kinase (PK)	A	NSHA	Cloned; some mutations detected	44, 45, 45a
Lactate dehydrogenase (LDH)	A	None	—	
NADH-diaphorase (ND)	A	Methemoglobinemia with or without mental retardation	Some mutations identified	46, 47, 47a

*A = Autosomal; X = X-linked.
†Selected to emphasize recent advances in molecular biology.
‡Hereditary non-spherocytic hemolytic anemia.

play in erythrocyte metabolism, the erythrocyte is able to compensate very well for its absence, presumably by utilizing glutathione peroxidase. Cu^{2+}/Zn^{2+} superoxide dismutase is found in the red cells, where it presumably functions to remove free radicals.[55] Since a deficiency of this enzyme has never been described, its precise role in the erythrocyte remains to be defined. The enzymes that catalyze the steps of the HMP shunt and the enzymes associated with this pathway are summarized in Table 9–2.

The Metabolism of Purines and Pyrimidines

Although the erythrocyte lacks the capacity for de novo synthesis of purine and pyrimidine nucleotides, it is able to form some of these compounds by "salvage" of the preformed bases. For example, adenine moiety is continually lost from the circulating red cell by deamination of adenosine to inosine by adenosine deaminase and by deamination of AMP to IMP by AMP deaminase. Yet the adenine nucleotide pool of cells that are near the end of their life span is actually larger than that of young cells.[74–76] This pool is replenished from preformed adenine, which reacts with phosphoribosyl pyrophosphate (PRPP) to synthesize AMP in the adenine phosphoribosyl transferase

(APRT) reaction (Fig. 9–3). An analogous reaction, the hypoxanthine-guanine phosphoribosyl transferase (HGPRT) reaction, may be utilized to replenish the supply of guanine nucleotides (Fig. 9–3). Erythrocytes also have the capacity to synthesize NAD from nicotinamide and from nicotinic acid[11] and flavine adenine dinucleotide from riboflavin and ATP.[77]

The red cell has numerous enzymes that interconvert different nucleotides. Among the most active of these is adenylate kinase, which catalyzes the equilibrium between the three adenine nucleotides, ATP, ADP, and AMP. In addition, there are enzymes that transfer phosphate from ATP to GMP[78] and that deaminate GTP to ITP[79] and AMP to IMP.[79]

The utilization of the bond energy in nucleotides results in their hydrolysis. Thus, ATP-powered ion pumps have ATPase activity. These activities are usually largely present in the membrane. Red cells have Na^+-K^+-ATPase,[80] Mg^{2+}-ATPase,[81] Ca^{2+}-ATPase,[82] oxidized glutathione-(GSSG)-activated ATPase,[83] glutathione synthetase conjugate–activated ATPase,[84] Mg^{2+}-GTPase,[85] and ITPase.[86, 87] The transport functions of some of these enzymes are implicit in the substance that stimulates their activity; in the case of others, the function is unknown. Red cells also contain other nucleotidases that may play a role in reticulocyte maturation, such as pyrimidine 5′-nucleotidase[88–91] and thymidine nucleotidase.[88, 92]

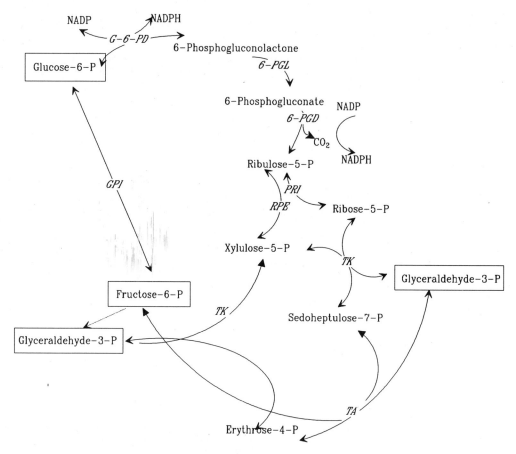

FIGURE 9–2. The hexosemonophosphate (HMP) shunt of erythrocytes. Intermediates of the glycolytic pathway are enclosed in rectangles. Abbreviations of the enzymes of the HMP are italicized and are defined in Table 9–2.

TABLE 9–2. HEXOSE MONOPHOSPHATE (HMP) AND RELATED ENZYMES IN HUMAN ERYTHROCYTES

ENZYME (ABBREVIATION)	INHERITANCE*	EFFECT OF DEFICIENCY	MOLECULAR BIOLOGY	SELECTED REFERENCES†
Glucose-6-phosphate dehydrogenase (G6PD)	X	Drug-induced hemolytic anemia and NSHA‡	Many variants sequenced on DNA level (see Table 9–3)	56, 57
6-Phosphogluconolactonase (6-PGL)	A	None known	—	58
6-Phosphogluconate dehydrogenase (6-PGD)	A	None known	—	59
Transketolase (TK)	?	None known	—	60, 61
				62, 63
Transaldolase (TA)	?	—	—	60, 64
Phosphoribose isomerase (PRI)	?	—	—	64, 65
Ribulose-phosphate 4-epimerase (RPE)	?	—	—	66
Glutathione peroxidase (GSH-Px)	A	?NSHA	Cloned	67
Glutathione reductase (GR)	A	Favism	cDNA cloned	68, 69
NADPH diaphorase	A	None	—	70
Catalase	A	Oral	Cloned; mutation identified in one case	71
Superoxide dismutase	?	—		72, 73

*X = X-linked; A = autosomal.
†Selected to emphasize recent advances in molecular biology.
‡Hereditary non-spherocytic hemolytic anemia.

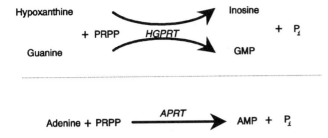

FIGURE 9–3. The hypoxanthine guanine phosphoribosyl transferase (HGPRT) and adenine phosphoribosyl transferase (APRT) reactions. These reactions serve to convert the preformed purine bases hypoxanthine, guanine, and adenine into the mononucleotides inosine, guanosine monophosphate (GMP), and adenine monophosphate (AMP). The ribose and phosphate are donated by phosphoribosyl pyrophosphate (PRPP), and inorganic phosphate (P_i) is a reaction product.

CLINICAL CONSEQUENCES OF RED CELL ENZYME ABNORMALITIES

Glycolytic Enzymes and Associated Abnormalities

Hereditary deficiencies of many of the enzymes that catalyze the sequential breakdown of glucose to lactic acid have been documented. As summarized in Table 9–1, many of these deficiencies are characterized clinically by hemolytic anemia.

Designated hereditary non-spherocytic hemolytic anemia, this disorder is distinguished from hereditary spherocytosis by the fact that the red cells are morphologically normal and manifest a normal osmotic fragility. Although a few abnormal cells may appear on the blood film, this is of no assistance in establishing a diagnosis,[93] except in pyrimidine 5'-nucleotidase deficiency, in which erythrocyte morphology is characteristic. In this case, prominent basophilic stippling provides the clue that may lead to the diagnosis.[94]

In some instances, hemolysis is the only consistently observed clinical consequence of the abnormality. A deficiency of type R (red cell) and L (liver) pyruvate kinase, the most common of these defects, is such a disorder. It is likely that the type M enzyme, which is under separate genetic control, serves to protect other tissues from the metabolic effects of the deficiency.[95–97] The clinical effects of glucosephosphate isomerase deficiency and hexokinase deficiency also appear to be limited to the erythrocyte.

Because 2,3-diphosphoglycerate (2,3-DPG) regulates the oxygen affinity of hemoglobin, enzyme defects that lower the levels of this intermediate may cause polycythemia. Deficiencies of the bifunctional diphosphoglycerate mutase/diphosphoglycerate phosphatase (DPGM/DPGP) enzyme[37, 98] and of phosphofructokinase[99, 100] have this effect. Similarly, increased activity of red cell phosphoglycerate kinase, presumably occurring as a result of inappropriate expression of the M_2-type enzyme in erythrocytes,[101] results in elevated red cell ATP and decreased 2,3-DPG levels,[102–104] also leading to polycythemia.

In the case of some of the other defects of glycolytic enzymes, clinical manifestations secondary to involvement of tissues other than red cells also occur. Among the most devastating of these disorders is triosephosphate isomerase deficiency. In this disorder, the enzyme is absent from all tissues that have been examined,[36] and the clinical course is characterized by neuromuscular degeneration that usually terminates fatally during the first decade of life.[105] Deficiency of the M subunit of phosphofructokinase causes muscle glycogen storage disease[22]; and although hemolysis may be present,[106] as noted above, mild polycythemia may also occur as a result of the lowered 2,3-DPG levels that result from the metabolic block.[99, 100] Phosphoglycerate kinase deficiency appears to be associated with emotional disturbances[107] and with muscle abnormalities.[108, 109] Usually, but not always,[110] hemolytic anemia is also present.

Deficiency of the NADH diaphorase that transfers electrons from NADH to cytochrome b_5 in the methemoglobin-reducing pathway produces methemoglobinemia. When the deficiency is limited to red cells, methemoglobinemia is the only consequence, but a more generalized form of the defect has also been described, and this disorder is associated with mental retardation.[111]

Some glycolytic enzyme deficiencies in the red cell seem to be without any consequences. Almost total lack of the principal (H) subunit of lactate dehydrogenase does not seem to cause any abnormality.[112] Mild deficiencies of glyceraldehyde phosphate dehydrogenase also do not seem to be associated with any functional deficit.[113]

Hexose Monophosphate Enzymes and Associated Pathways

Glucose-6-Phosphate Dehydrogenase (G6PD) Deficiency

The principal clinical consequence of G6PD deficiency is hemolytic anemia. The common (polymorphic) forms of the deficiency are associated with little or no shortening of the red cell life span in the absence of stress,[114–118] but brisk hemolysis may occur during febrile illnesses[119–126] and on exposure to certain drugs[127, 128] and to fava beans. Neonatal icterus may also occur in patients with some of the more severely deficient variants,[129–135] but this may be due more to impairment of liver function than to hemolysis.[129] In some of the functionally more severe, sporadic forms of the deficiency, chronic hemolysis occurs, and this may be punctuated by hemolytic crises during febrile illnesses and sometimes on exposure to hemolytic drugs. A variety of non-hematological manifestations have been attributed to G6PD deficiency, including a lower incidence of cancer,[136–138] certain types of mental disease,[139] diabetes,[140] and cataracts,[141] but none of these associations have stood the test of time.[142–146]

6-Phosphogluconate Dehydrogenase Deficiency

6-Phosphogluconate dehydrogenase is very polymorphic electrophoretically,[147] but severe deficiency has been reported only once.[148] The deficiency did not appear to cause any clinical manifestations.

6-Phosphogluconolactonase Deficiency

A partial (heterozygous) deficiency state for 6-phosphogluconolactonase has been reported[58] and appears not to cause any clinical manifestations; severe deficiency has never been reported.

Glutathione Synthetase (GSH-S) Deficiency

GSH-S deficiency was originally described as a cause of hereditary non-spherocytic hemolytic anemia.[149] Subsequently, it was recognized that a totally different disorder, 5-oxoprolinuria, was also characterized by a deficiency of red cell GSH-S.[150–152] It now appears that when the enzyme deficiency is limited to the erythrocyte, the clinical presentation is limited to hemolytic anemia. A generalized form of the disorder apparently generally leads to the neurological form of the disease.[153]

γ-Glutamyl Cysteine Synthetase (GC-S) Deficiency

γ-Glutamyl cysteine synthetase (GC-S) deficiency is very rare; only two families have been described. In both, affected patients had chronic hemolytic anemia. In one family, spinocerebellar degeneration was present in the patients[154]; in the other, the single affected individual was neurologically normal.[155]

Glutathione Reductase Deficiency

Glutathione reductase deficiency is commonly the result of suboptimal riboflavin intake.[156–158] In one family, severe glutathione reductase deficiency was associated with sensitivity to the hemolytic effect of the fava bean.[68]

Glutathione S-Transferase Deficiency

Only one patient with glutathione S-transferase deficiency has been described, and this patient had mild hemolytic anemia.[159] However, the patient was an adopted orphan, and in the absence of family studies it is not at all certain that a cause-and-effect relationship existed.

Glutathione Peroxidase (GSH-Px) Deficiency

It has frequently been suggested that reduction of GSH-Px activity to about one half of normal causes hemolytic anemia.[160–165] However, the fact that more severe deficiencies of the red cell enzyme may be observed in patients with a benign polymorphism that in the homozygous state reduces the enzyme to one half of normal[166, 167] and in those with selenium deficiency[168, 169] casts doubt on this interpretation. Recently, we have examined the blood of a child with hemolytic anemia and only about 10 per cent of normal GSH-Px activity.

Abnormalities of Enzymes of Purine Metabolism

Increased Adenosine Deaminase (ADA) Activity

Deficiencies of ADA and purine nucleoside phosphorylase are well-known causes of immunodeficiency. Another abnormality of ADA is of special interest with regard to its role in the cause of hereditary nonspherocytic hemolytic anemia. In this disorder, the ADA in red cells is greatly increased to levels as high as 100 times normal. In other tissues, however, the level of ADA seems to be normal. The high ADA presumably depletes the erythrocytes of vital adenine nucleotides, impairing their metabolism.[170–172] The residual enzyme in this disorder seems to be normal, and complete sequencing of the gene, including its promotor, has revealed no abnormality.[173, 174] Attaching the promotor to a reported gene produced a modest increase above normal levels of enzyme activity in the K562 cell line,[170] but the differences observed did not approach those observed in vivo.

AMP Deaminase Deficiency

AMP deaminase deficiency has been documented in several families.[175–177] Lack of this enzyme does not appear to cause any disease state but is associated with increased red cell ATP levels, indicating that this enzyme plays a role in the homeostasis of the adenine nucleotide pool in erythrocytes.

Pyrimidine 5'-Nucleotidase (P-5'-N) Deficiency

A deficiency of P-5'-N is a cause of hemolytic anemia characterized by red cells with marked basophilic stippling.[94, 178, 179] The enzyme is exquisitely sensitive to inhibition by lead, and the levels of erythrocyte P-5'-N are markedly reduced in lead intoxication.[180, 181] The enzyme deficiency results in accumulation of large amounts of pyrimidine nucleotides in the erythrocyte. These inhibit the outward transport of GSSG from the red cells,[182, 183] a finding that probably accounts for the high GSH level that has been documented in the red cells of patients with this defect.[184, 185]

Accumulation of another type of pyrimidine nucleotide, namely, cytidine diphosphate (CDP)–choline, has been documented in a patient with chronic hemolytic anemia.[186] The enzymatic defect that causes this abnormality is not known.

ITPase Deficiency

Hereditary deficiency of ITPase results in the accumulation of ITP in red cells.[187, 188] This autosomal recessive enzyme deficiency has no known clinical consequences.

ATPase Deficiency

A single case of putative ATPase deficiency has been reported,[189] but the evidence that this is actually an entity is not clear. There are, however, ethnic differences in ATPase activity that apparently have a genetic basis.[190]

Adenylate Kinase (AK) Deficiency

A deficiency of AK has been associated with hemolytic anemia in several kindreds, but in one family virtually total absence of this enzymatic activity was documented in one hematologically normal sib,[191] casting doubt on the capacity of this enzyme deficiency to produce anemia. In several reported families, AK deficiency was inherited together with G6PD deficiency,[192–194] and it is conceivable that the combined deficiencies were responsible for the shortening of the red cell life span that occurred.

Other Erythrocyte Enzyme Deficiencies and Enzyme Deficiencies in Non-hematological Disease

Non-hematological disease states are beyond the scope of this chapter, but it is useful to point out that a number of hereditary non-hematological diseases are best diagnosed by examination of red blood cells, which share the enzyme deficiency, although they themselves are not involved directly in the pathological process. The three types of galactosemia,[195] the porphyrias,[196] hypoxanthine-guanine phosphoribosyl transferase deficiency[197–199] and prolidase deficiency[200–202] are such disorders. Among the immunodeficiencies, adenosine deaminase deficiency[203] and purine nucleoside phosphorylate deficiency[204, 205] are diagnosed by measuring the enzyme activity of erythrocytes. Adenine phosphoribosyl transferase deficiency[206–208] and PRPP synthetase deficiency[209] are causes of gout that are detected by studying the erythrocytes. Acatalasemia was the first red cell enzyme deficiency to have been described.[1] It was serendipitously discovered in Japan when Takahara treated the oral mucosa of a dental patient with hydrogen peroxide and noted that the peroxide did not foam and that tissues and blood turned black.[210] In the Japanese form of the deficiency, oral gangrene is the only clinical manifestation, while in the Swiss form of the disease[211] no clinical manifestations have been found. Recently, the basis of the Japanese mutation has been found to be a splicing mutation.[71]

Hereditary absence of red cell cholinesterase was reported in an asymptomatic individual in 1962,[212] and another case with moderate deficiency has been detected subsequently.[213] The lack of this enzyme appears to be entirely asymptomatic. AMP deaminase deficiency[176] is another red cell enzyme abnormality that does not appear to cause any clinical consequences. The fact that ATP levels are increased in deficient erythrocytes confirms that this enzyme is rate limiting in the catabolism of ATP.

MOLECULAR BIOLOGY AND BIOCHEMISTRY OF RED CELL ENZYMES

The molecular biology of G6PD has been studied extensively, and some information has emerged about the molecular biology of pyruvate kinase, phosphofructokinase, and adenosine deaminase. However, as indicated in Table 9–1, little is as yet known of the molecular biology of many of the red cell enzymes.

Glucose-6-Phosphate Dehydrogenase

G6PD is composed of 515 amino acid subunits with a calculated molecular weight of 59,256 daltons. Aggregation of the inactive monomers into catalytically active dimers and higher forms requires the presence of NADP.[214] Thus, NADP appears to be bound to the enzyme both as a structural component and as one of the substrates of the reaction.[215–217] The binding site or sites for this coenzyme have not been identified at the biochemical level, but examination of mutants has established that amino acids 386 and 387 seem to bind one of the phosphates of NADP[218] (see below). It has also been suggested, on the basis of the deduced conformation of the peptide chain of the yeast enzyme, that the NADP-binding site may be elsewhere,[219] but data on the human enzyme seem much more compelling. The glucose-6-phosphate binding site has been identified at amino acid 205 by locating a lysine at this position that is reactive in competition with glucose-6-phosphate.[220–223]

G6PD was cloned and sequenced by Persico and colleagues[224–227] and subsequently independently by Takizawa and Yoshida and associates.[228] The gene itself is over 20 kb in length, containing 13 exons. The first exon contains no coding sequence, which begins in exon 2. The intron between exons 2 and 3 is extraordinarily long, extending for 9857 base pairs (bp). The entire gene has recently been sequenced.[229] In 1989, Kanno and coworkers[230] suggested that G6PD was, in reality, a translation product made from two separate mRNAs. Protein sequence data were interpreted as showing that the enzyme was a fusion protein, with an amino-terminus that was coded by a gene on chromosome 6 and a carboxyl-terminus derived from the gene on the X chromosome. However, study of the reactivity of red cell G6PD with antibodies made against peptides in these two portions of the molecule[231] indicated that only the X chromosome–encoded sequence was present. Antibody made against the chromosome 6–derived sequence reacted with GMP reductase[231]; it had been pointed out that the sequence of this part of the molecule was homologous to that enzyme.[232] Characterization of enzymes made from the X chromosome–encoded and the putative fusion sequence also led to the unequivocal conclusion that the enzyme was actually made only from the X chromosome sequence.[233] The original claim was retracted, with the suggestion that the fusion protein was an artifact of purification.[234]

Some heterogeneity in the mRNA of G6PD has been found, but its functional significance is doubtful. The existence of an alternatively spliced form has been documented,[235, 236] but the amount of this mRNA, which contains 138 nucleotides (nt) of what is usually the 3' end of intron 7 without losing frame, is always very small.

At the 5' end of the gene is a CpG-rich island. Differential demethylation of some of the CpG's is associated with expression of the gene on the active X chromosome,[237] and these CpG's appear to be preserved between man and the mouse.[238] A 2850 bp segment of the 5' end has been fused to a reporter, and deletional analysis showed that a 436 bp region was sufficient for full expression.[239]

Because most mutants of G6PD have abnormal properties, either electrophoretically or kinetically, or both, it was to be expected that the mutations affecting this enzyme would be found in the coding region. This has, indeed, proved to be the case. Facile polymerase chain reaction (PCR)–based methods for the detection of mutations have been developed,[240, 241] and these have made it possible to define the mutations in many individuals with mutant G6PD[241a] (Table 9–3).

Understanding of the structure-function relationships of G6PD is still somewhat rudimentary because it has not been possible to solve the crystal structure of the mammalian enzyme, although extensive efforts have been made to obtain this information. Thus, we currently depend on the analysis of mutants and site-specific inhibitor studies for our understanding of the location of functional domains in the G6PD molecule.

Pyruvate Kinase

The molecular biology of pyruvate kinase is more complex than that of G6PD in that two different genetic loci make two different forms of the enzyme, and further heterogeneity is introduced by the existence of tissue-specific promoters and alternative splicing. The type L (liver) and type R (red cell) enzymes are products of the same gene: Genetically determined deficiency of the red cell enzyme is accompanied by a deficiency of the liver enzyme.[261–263] Apparently, a different promoter is utilized in the liver and in the red cell precursor,[264] and splicing of the two enzymes occurs in a different fashion, so that the first exon is utilized for the amino-terminal of the R enzyme and the second exon for the L enzyme. The type M (muscle) enzyme is encoded by a separate gene.[179] This isozyme has kinetic properties that are quite different from those of the erythrocyte and liver enzymes,[265]

and it is the product of this gene that is present in normal leukocytes.

POPULATION GENETICS OF RED CELL ENZYME DEFICIENCIES

Prevalence of Red Cell Enzyme Deficiencies

Mild red cell enzyme deficiencies are relatively common. These may be due to inheritance of genes that cause partial deficiency or to heterozygosity for genes that produce severe deficiency. Deficiencies of GSH-Px,[166, 167] pyridoxal kinase,[266, 267] galactokinase,[268] galactose-1-phosphate uridyl transferase,[269, 270] and Na+-K+-ATPase[190] are in the first category. In the case of each of these enzymes, polymorphisms that lower the level found in red cells have been discovered; homozygotes have about one-half normal activity. No advantage has been demonstrated to accrue to the individuals who are deficient, nor has any disadvantage been found.

Mutations that result in the loss of most or all of the activity of a red cell enzyme are considerably rarer in the population, with the exception of those that result in a deficiency of G6PD. The most common of such enzyme deficiencies may be those of pyruvate kinase and of APRT. The gene frequency for pyruvate kinase–deficient genes is probably on the order of .005, so that about 1 per cent of the population is heterozygous.[271–273] The incidence may be higher in the Asian population[273, 274] and in the Middle East.[275] One may speculate that lowered pyruvate kinase activity might have a selective advantage, since this may be accompanied by a slightly right-shifted oxygen dissociation curve,[262, 276] possibly an advantage under certain circumstances. The incidence of heterozygosity for APRT deficiency is also about 1 per cent,[277] and no obvious advantage of the partially deficient state presents itself. Systematic study of the red cells of a large number of newborns has suggested that certain other enzyme deficiencies may also be relatively common.[271, 278, 279] Lowered triosephosphate isomerase activity was found in almost 1 per cent of black infants, and enolase activity was diminished in 1 per cent of black and 0.5 per cent of white newborns.

The exception to the rarity of red cell enzyme deficiencies is that of G6PD. Mutations of this enzyme are common; indeed, it has been suggested that 100 million persons worldwide are deficient in this enzyme.[280] Consequently, much has been learned about the mutations that affect this enzyme and the distribution of these mutations.

Malaria and Glucose-6-Phosphate Dehydrogenase Deficiency

The high gene frequency of G6PD deficiency in some ethnic groups implies that this gene confers or in the past conferred a selective advantage to those who inherited it. The distribution of the gene in

TABLE 9–3.   MUTATIONS OF GLUCOSE-6-PHOSPHATE DEHYDROGENASE (G6PD)

VARIANT	NUCLEOTIDE SUBSTITUTION	WHO CLASS*	AMINO ACID SUBSTITUTION	REFERENCES
Gaohe[a]	95 A→G	2	32 His→Arg	242
Sunderland	103–105 deletion	1	Ile deletion	243
Metaponto	172 G→A	3	58 Asp→Asn	244
A−[b]	202 G→A / 376 A→G	3	68 Val→Met / 126 Asn→Asp	235
Ube Konan	241 C→T	3	81 Arg→Cys	244a
A(+)	376 A→G	4	126 Asn→Asp	245
Ilesha	466 G→A	3	156 Glu→Lys	244
Mahidol	487 G→A	3	163 Gly→Ser	246
Santamaria	542 A→T / 376 A→G	2	181 Asp→Val / 126 Asn→Asp	247
Mediterranean[c]	563 C→T	2	188 Ser→Phe	244
Santiago	593 G→C	1	198 Arg→Pro	248
Minnesota[d]	637 G→T	1	213 Val→Leu	240
Harilaou	648 T→G	1	216 Phe→Leu	241, 247
Mexico City	689 G→A		227 Arg→Gly	248
A−	680 G→T / 376 A→G	3	227 Arg→Leu / 126 Asn→Asp	235
Wayne	769 G→C	1	257 Arg→Gly	249
"Chinese-3"	835 A→T	2	279 Thr→Ser	250
Seattle[e]	844 G→C	2	282 Asp→His	251
Montalbano	854 G→A	3	285 Arg→His	252
Viangchan[f]	871 G→A	2	291 Val→Met	249
A−[g]	968 T→C / 376 A→G	3	323 Leu→Pro / 126 Asn→Asp	235
Chatham	1003 G→A	3	335 Ala→Thr	244
Greece	1057 C→T	2	353 Pro→Ser	248
Loma Linda	1089 C→A	1	363 Asn→Lys	240
Tomah	1153 T→C	1	385 Cys→Arg	244
Iowa[h]	1156 A→G	1	386 Lys→Glu	218
Guadalajara	1159 C→T		387 Arg→Cys	248
Beverly Hills[i]	1160 G→A	1	387 Arg→His	218
Nashville[j]	1178 G→A	1	393 Arg→His	240
Alhambra	1180 G→C	1	394 Val→Leu	248
Puerto Limon	1192 G→A	1	398 Glu→Lys	247
Riverside	1228 G→T	1	410 Gly→Cys	218
"Japan"	1229 G→A	1	410 Gly→Asp	248
Tokyo	1246 G→A	1	416 Glu→Lys	249a
Pawnee	1316 G→C		439 Arg→Pro	248
Santiago de Cuba	1339 G→A	1	447 Gly→Arg	244
"Chinese-2"	1360 C→T	2	454 Arg→Cys	250
Andalus	1361 G→A	1	454 Arg→His	253
Taiwan-Hakka[k]	1376 G→T	2	459 Arg→Leu	254
Kaiping[l]	1388 G→A	2	463 Arg→His	254

*Class 1 = Non-spherocytic hemolytic anemia; Class 2 = severe deficiency; Class 3 = moderate deficiency; Class 4 = not deficient.
[a-l]Other variants with the same mutation(s): (a) A−[242], Gaozhou[242]; (b) Distrito Federal,[255] Matera,[244] Castilla,[255] Alabama (E. Beutler, unpublished data), Betica,[256] Tepic,[255] Ferrara[257]; (c) Dallas,[258] Birmingham,[258] Sassari,[251] Cagliari,[251] Panama (E. Beutler, unpublished data); (d) Marion,[240] Gastonia[240]; (e) Modena,[257] Lodi[259]; (f) Jammu[249]; (g) Betica,[235] Selma[235]; (h) Walter Reed,[218] Iowa City,[218] Springfield[218]; (i) Genova (A. Argusti et al., personal communication), Worcester (E. Beutler, unpublished data); (j) Anaheim,[240] Calgary[240]; (k) Gifu-like,[254] Agrigento-like,[254] Canton[260]; (l) Anant,[254] Dhon,[254] Petrich-like,[254] Sapporo-like.[254]

tropical areas in which *Plasmodium falciparum* malaria was common led to the suggestion that the advantage of G6PD deficiency might be that it provided resistance to infection with malaria,[281–283] although direct inoculation of volunteers did not provide support for this concept[284] and population studies gave ambiguous results.[285–287] Some of the difficulties in demonstrating a possible beneficial effect of G6PD deficiency on the course of malaria may be the relatively small advantage that is required to maintain relatively high equilibrium levels of the gene and the suggestion that there is no advantage to hemizygous males or homozygous females, with only heterozygous females showing any

level of protection.[288] The elegant studies of Luzzatto and colleagues[289] in heterozygotes for G6PD A− clearly demonstrated that parasites preferred cells with normal enzyme activity to those that were deficient. Using an indirect histochemical method, these investigators counted the number of parasites in the blood cells of women with malaria who were also heterozygotes for G6PD deficiency. Since G6PD is X linked, the red cells of such women are a mosaic of normal and deficient cells.[290] The number of parasites in normal cells greatly exceeded the number in enzyme-deficient cells, indicating either that the parasites were unable to grow normally in deficient cells or that the enzyme-deficient parasitized cells were destroyed prematurely.

With the development of methods for culturing malaria parasites, this question was able to be addressed more directly in the 1980s. Red blood cells from hemizygotes and heterozygotes for G6PD deficiency were found to support growth of *Plasmodium falciparum* less effectively than were normal red cells.[291] Moreover, it was demonstrated that plasmodia were able to adapt to G6PD-deficient cells after several growth cycles.[292, 293] Although it was initially proposed that this adaptation was due to induction of the parasite's own G6PD,[292, 294] the development of more sensitive methods for the measurement of parasite G6PD has indicated that this is not the case[295]: Malarial G6PD appears to be produced constitutively in normal or G6PD-deficient red cells.

The Glucose-6-Phosphate Dehydrogenase Polymorphism

Over the past 25 years, G6PD variants have been studied extensively, using biochemical techniques standardized in 1967 by an expert committee of the WHO.[296] More than 400 variants believed to be distinct from one another were described, and these have been summarized in recently published tabulations.[57, 297] However, it has been clear that biochemical characterization was not entirely satisfactory for a number of reasons. Mutant enzymes are often unstable and change their properties during storage purification. In spite of efforts to standardize techniques, differences in commercial reagents and minor differences in technique can produce qualitative differences that are difficult to interpret. An impressive illustration of the limitations inherent in biochemical characterization was provided by the finding that G6PD Cornell and G6PD Chicago, variants that appeared to be quite distinct, were from members of the same extended family.[298] Accurate definition of the mutations affecting G6PD had to await sequencing of the genetic material itself.

African Variants

Electrophoretic and kinetic studies suggested that two variants were common in Africa: G6PD A(+), an electrophoretically rapid variant that has normal activity, and G6PD A−, also electrophoretically fast but moderately deficient. It had been suggested that these variants were related, one representing a mutation that produced a change in charge and the other a superimposed regulatory mutation.[299] It had also been proposed that G6PD A(+) was heterogeneous[300] and that there was an amino acid substitution in G6PD A(+).[301] However, none of the questions dealing with its possible heterogeneity or its relationship to G6PD A(+) could be investigated until it become possible to sequence the G6PD gene.

With the application of this technology, G6PD A(+) has been found to be characterized by a G→A mutation at nt 376. The same mutation is found in G6PD A−, but in addition there is a mutation at nt 202 in most cases. In a few patients, however, the second mutation is not at nt 202 but rather at nt 680 or nt 968.[256, 301] Thus, where there was thought to be a single variant designated G6PD A−, we now recognize the existence of three variants. A fourth mutation at nt 542, that of G6PD Santamaria, is also found together with the mutation at nt 376.[247] This mutation eliminates a negatively charged aspartic acid, changing it to valine, while the mutation at nt 376 produces a negatively charged aspartic acid from asparagine. Therefore, G6PD Santamaria has a normal electrophoretic mobility and was not recognized as a form of G6PD A−. Many G6PD variants that were thought to be unique merely turn out to be examples of G6PDA−. These include G6PDs Ferrara,[257] Betica,[256] Tepic,[255] Distrito Federal,[255] Castilla,[255] Alabama,[302] and Matera.[244]

The fact that at least four G6PD mutations have occurred on the background of the nt 376 mutation suggests that the latter is of relatively ancient origin, a conclusion that is also borne out by determining the G6PD haplotype in which the G6PD A(+) and the common G6PD A− mutations are found.[303–305] But studies of the nucleotide sequence of the chimpanzee G6PD indicate that the primordial human G6PD was, in reality, G6PD B.[256]

The fact that the deficiency mutations were all associated with the nt 376 mutations was initially believed to indicate that the nt 376 mutation was the most common genotype in Africa at the time that deficiency mutations arose.[256, 306] However, recent studies of recombinant G6PD suggested that the nt 202 mutation alone does not produce enzyme deficiency, but that deficiency is observed when it is found in combination with the nt 376 mutation.[307] Thus, it may be that the incidence of the nt 376 mutation was not very high in the population, but that second mutations had a special advantage.

Mediterranean Variants

G6PD in the Mediterranean region was thought to be very heterogeneous. This turns out not to be the case. It has been found that most cases of G6PD deficiency are due to a C→T transition at nt 563 of the G6PD-coding region, a mutation characteristic of the common G6PD Mediterranean. This mutation includes variants as diverse as Cagliari,[251] Sassari,[251] Dallas,[258] and Birmingham.[258] It is interesting that when this mutation is found in southern Europe and in the Middle East, it is almost always associated with a T at nt 1311, a polymorphism that is present in about 20 per cent of the European population. In contrast, when the G6PD 563T mutation is found in the Indian subcontinent, it has been associated with a C at nt 1311 in all three patients we have studied thus far. This finding implies that the common G6PD Mediterranean 563T mutation arose independently in

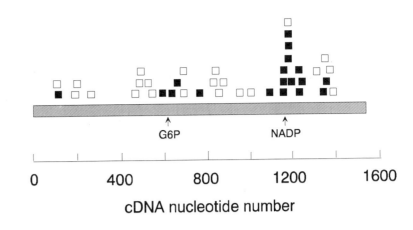

FIGURE 9–4. The locations of mutations that have been detected in glucose-6-phosphate dehydrogenase (G6PD), shown in terms of their position along the linear sequence of the mRNA. The putative binding sites for glucose-6-phosphate (G6P) and NADP are indicated by arrows. The mutations that cause chronic hemolytic anemia are shown in solid boxes. They cluster around the NADP- and G6P-binding sites. The exact location of the mutation shown on this figure is presented in Table 9–3.

these two parts of the world. Less commonly, a mutation at nt 844 causes G6PD deficiency in southern Europe. This mutation, designated G6PD Seattle (or Seattle-like),[251] has been variously known as G6PD Lodi[259] and G6PD Modena.[257]

Sporadic Variants

Some G6PD variants are functionally so severely deficient that a chronic hemolytic anemia results (Fig. 9–4). Any slight advantage that such variants may confer with respect to resistance to malaria is obviously more than counterbalanced by the effect of chronic anemia on fitness. Thus, they do not reach polymorphic frequencies but rather occur sporadically in people of all ethnic origins.

The results of analyzing the DNA of such patients have been surprising: The same mutations are encountered repeatedly in unrelated patients with hereditary non-spherocytic hemolytic anemia. Study of such variants has made it possible for us to identify the NADP-binding site.[218] Moreover, most of the variants studied so far have been limited either to the region of this newly identified NADP-binding site or to the region of the previously identified putative binding site for glucose-6-phosphate.

FUTURE PROSPECTS

The relative ease with which genes can now be cloned and the rapid methods of sequence analysis that are becoming available promise to increase greatly our knowledge of the molecular biology of red cell enzymes over the next few years. As more mutations are found, not only in G6PD but in other enzymes as well, and as the crystal structure of some of the enzymes is resolved, new insights regarding structure-function relationships are sure to emerge.

Until now, treatment of hereditary red cell enzyme deficiencies has been purely symptomatic. The clinical manifestations of many of these defects are quite mild, and in those cases little more is needed than is now available. On the other hand, some enzyme defects have catastrophic defects. In such circumstances, gene transfer therapy may be expected ultimately to play an important role in management. In the case of deficiencies of enzymes such as pyruvate kinase, in which the disease phenotype appears to be purely a function of the red cell enzyme deficiency, transfer of genes into hematopoietic stem cells should be curative. In disorders such as triosephosphate deficiency and some forms of methemoglobin reductase and glutathione synthetase deficiency, it will be necessary to correct the defect in other tissues as well, and the challenge will be correspondingly greater.

REFERENCES

1. Takahara, S., and Miyamoto, H.: Three cases of progressive oral gangrene due to lack of catalase in the blood. Nippon Jibiinkoka Gakkai Kaiho 51:163, 1948.
2. Carson P. E., Flanagan C. L., Ickes C. E., and Alving A. S.: Enzymatic deficiency in primaquine-sensitive erythrocytes. Science 124:484, 1956.
3. Isselbacher, K. J., Anderson, E. P., Kurahashi, E., and Kalckar, H. M.: Congenital galactosemia, a single enzymatic block in galactose metabolism. Science 123:635, 1956.
4. Valentine, W. N., Tanaka, K. R., and Miwa, S.: A specific erythrocyte glycolytic enzyme defect (pyruvate kinase) in three subjects with congenital non-spherocytic hemolytic anemia. Trans. Assoc. Am. Physicians 74:100, 1961.
5. Bull, B. S., Breton-Gorius, J., and Beutler, E.: Morphology of the erythron. In Williams, W. J., Beutler, E., Erslev, A. J., and Lichtman M. A. (eds.): Hematology. 4th ed. New York, McGraw-Hill Book Co., 1990, pp. 297–316.
6. Kim, H. D., and McManus, T. J.: Studies on the energy metabolism of pig red cells. I. The limiting role of membrane permeability in glycolysis. Biochim. Biophys. Acta 230:1, 1971.
7. Kim, H. D.: Is adenosine a second metabolic substrate for human red blood cells. Biochim. Biophys. Acta 1036:113, 1990.
8. Beutler, E.: Red cell metabolism. In Rossi, E. C., Simon, T. L., and Moss, G. S. (eds.): Principles of Transfusion Medicine. Baltimore, The Williams & Wilkins Co., 1990, pp. 35–40.

9. Beutler, E.: Red cell enzyme defects. Hematol. Pathol. 4:103, 1990.
10. Sasaki, R., Ikura, K., Narita, H., Yanagawa, S., and Chiba, H.: 2,3-Bisphosphoglycerate in erythroid cells. TIBS Rev. 7:140, 1982.
11. Micheli, V., Simmonds, H. A., Sestini, S., and Ricci, C.: Importance of nicotinamide as an NAD precursor in the human erythrocyte. Arch. Biochem. Biophys. 283:40, 1990.
12. Rijksen, G., and Staal, G. E. J.: Purification and some properties of human erythrocyte hexokinase. Biochim. Biophys. Acta 445:330, 1976.
13. Haritos, A. A., and Rosemeyer, M. A.: Purification and physical properties of hexokinase from human erythrocytes. Biochim. Biophys. Acta 873:335, 1986.
14. Magnani, M., and Stocchi, V.: Hexokinase: One gene or two. Blood 76:854, 1990.
15. Murakami, K., Blei, F., Tilton, W., Seaman, C., and Piomelli, S.: An isozyme of hexokinase specific for the human red blood cell (HK$_R$). Blood 75:770, 1990.
16. Baughan, M. A., Valentine, W. N., Paglia, D. E., Ways, P. O., Simon, E. R., and De Marsh, Q. B.: Hereditary hemolytic anemia associated with glucosephosphate isomerase (GPI) deficiency—a new enzyme defect of human erythrocytes. Blood 32:236, 1968.
17. Detter, J. C., Ways, P. O., Giblett, E. R., Baughan, M. A., Hopkinson, D. A., Povey, S., and Harris, H.: Inherited variations in human phosphohexose isomerase. Ann. Hum. Genet. 31:329, 1968.
18. Walker, J. I., Faik, P., and Morgan, M. J.: Characterization of the 5′ end of the gene for human glucose phosphate isomerase (GPI). Genomics 7:638, 1990.
19. Carter, N. D., and Yoshida, A.: Purification and characterization of human phosphoglucose isomerase. Biochim. Biophys. Acta 181:12, 1969.
20. Vora, S.: Isozymes of human phosphofructokinase: Biochemical and genetic aspects. *In* Rattazzi, M. C., Scandalios, J. G., and Whitt, G. S. (eds.): Isozymes: Current Topics in Biological and Medical Research. New York, Alan R. Liss, 1983, pp. 3–23.
21. Nakajima, H., Noguchi, T., Yamasaki, T., Kono, N., Tanaka, T., and Tarui, S.: Cloning of human muscle phosphofructokinase cDNA. FEBS Lett. 223:113, 1987.
22. Tarui, S., Okuno, G., Ikura, Y., Tanaka, T., Suda, M., and Nishikawa, M.: Phosphofructokinase deficiency in skeletal muscle. A new type of glycogenosis. Biochem. Biophys. Res. Commun. 19:517, 1965.
23. Levanon, D., Danciger, E., Dafni, N., and Groner, Y.: Construction of a cDNA clone containing the entire coding region of the human liver–type phosphofructokinase. Biochem. Biophys. Res. Commun. 147:1182, 1987.
24. Sharma, P. M., Reddy, G. R., Babior, B. M., and McLachlan, A.: Alternative splicing of the transcript encoding the human muscle isoenzyme of phosphofructokinase. J. Biol. Chem. 265:9006, 1990.
25. Nakajima, H., Kono, N., Yamasaki, T., Hotta, K., Kawachi, M., Kuwajima, M., Noguchi, T., Tanaka, T., and Tarui, S.: Genetic defect in muscle phosphofructokinase deficiency. Abnormal splicing of the muscle phosphofructokinase gene due to a point mutation at the 5′-splice site. J. Biol. Chem. 265:9392, 1990.
26. Fujii, S., Matsuda, M., Okuya, S., Yoshizaki, Y., Miura-Kora, Y., and Kaneko, T.: Fructose-6-phosphate, 2-kinase activity in human erythrocytes. Blood 70:1211, 1987.
27. Colomer, D., Gallego, C., Corrons, J. L. V., Carreras, J., and Bartrons, R.: Fructose 2,6-biphosphate and 6-phosphofructo 2-kinase in density-fractionated human red blood cells. Med. Sci. Res. 17:405, 1989.
28. Sharma, P. M., Reddy, G. R., Vora, S., Babior, B. M., and McLachlan, A.: Cloning and expression of a human muscle phosphofructokinase cDNA. Gene 77:177, 1989.
29. Kishi, H., Mukai, T., Hirono, A., Fujii, H., Miwa, S., and Hori, K.: Human aldolase A deficiency associated with a hemolytic anemia: Thermolabile aldolase due to a single base mutation. Proc. Natl. Acad. Sci. USA 84:8623, 1987.
30. Beutler, E., Scott, S., Bishop, A., Margolis, N., Matsumoto, F., and Kuhl, W.: Red cell aldolase deficiency and hemolytic anemia: A new syndrome. Trans. Assoc. Am. Physicians 86:154, 1974.
31. Beutler, E.: Comment on " 'aldolase A' deficiency with syndrome of growth and developmental retardation, midfacial hypoplasia, hepatomegaly, and consanguineous parents" by R. B. Lowry and J. W. Hanson. Birth Defects 13:227, 1977.
32. Marquat, L. E., Chilcote, R., and Ryan, P. M.: Human triosephosphate isomerase cDNA and protein structure. J. Biol. Chem. 260:3748, 1989.
33. Schneider, A. S., Valentine, W. N., Hattori, M., and Heins, H. L., Jr.: Hereditary hemolytic anemia with triosephosphate isomerase deficiency. N. Engl. J. Med. 272:229, 1965.
34. Kahn, A., Kaplan, J.-C., and Dreyfus, J. C.: Advances in hereditary red cell enzyme anomalies. Hum. Genet. 50:1, 1979.
35. Valentine, W. N., Schneider, A. S., Baughan, M. A., Paglia, D. E., and Heins, H. L., Jr.: Hereditary hemolytic anemia with triosephosphate isomerase deficiency. Am. J. Med. 41:27, 1966.
36. Skala, H., Dreyfus, J. C., Vives-Corrons, J. L., Matsumoto, F., and Beutler, E.: Triose phosphate isomerase deficiency. Biochem. Med. 18:226, 1977.
37. Rosa, R., Prehu, M.-O., and Beuzard, Y.: The first case of a complete deficiency of diphosphoglycerate mutase in human erythrocytes. J. Clin. Invest. 62:907, 1976.
38. Garel, M. C., Lemarchandel, V., Prehu, M. O., Calvin, M. C., Arous, N., Rosa, R., Rosa, J., and Cohen-Solal, M.: Natural and artificial mutants of the human 2,3-biphosphoglycerate as a tool for the evaluation of structure-function relationships. Biomed. Biochim. Acta 49:166, 1990.
39. Joulin, V., Garel, M. C., Le Boulch, P., Valentin, C., Rosa, R., Rosa, J., and Cohen-Solal, M.: Isolation and characterization of the human 2,3-biphosphoglycerate mutase gene. J. Biol. Chem. 263:15785, 1988.
39a. Lemarchandel, V., Joulin, V., Valentin, C., Rosa, R., Galactros, F., Rosa, J., and Cohen-Solal, M.: Compound heterozygosity in a complete erythrocyte bisphosphoglycerate mutase deficiency. Blood 80:2643, 1992.
40. Michelson, A. M., Markham, A. F., and Orkin, S. H.: Isolation and DNA sequence of a full-length cDNA clone for human X chromosome–encoded phosphoglycerate kinase. Proc. Natl. Acad. Sci. USA 80:472, 1983.
41. Fujii, H., and Yoshida, A.: Molecular abnormality of phosphoglycerate kinase–Uppsala associated with chronic nonspherocytic hemolytic anemia. Proc. Natl. Acad. Sci. USA 77:5461, 1980.
42. Maeda, M., and Yoshida, A.: Molecular defect of a phosphoglycerate kinase variant (PGK-Matsue) associated with hemolytic anemia: Leu→Pro substitution caused by T/A→C/G transition in exon 3. Blood 77:1348, 1991.
43. Maeda, M., Bawle, E., Kulkarni, R., Beutler, E., and Yoshida, A.: Molecular abnormalities of a phosphoglycerate kinase variant generated by spontaneous mutation. Blood 79:2759, 1992.
43a. Fujii, H., Kanno, H., Hirono, A., Shiomura, T., and Miwa, S.: A single amino acid substitution (157 Gly → Val) in a phosphoglycerate kinase variant (PGK Shizuoka) associated with chronic hemolysis and myoglobinuria. Blood 79:1582, 1992.
44. Neubauer, B., Lakomek, M., Winkler, H., Parke, M., Hofferbert, S., and Schröter W.: Point mutations in the L-type pyruvate kinase gene of two children with hemolytic anemia caused by pyruvate kinase deficiency. Blood 77:1871, 1991.
45. Kanno, H., Fujii, H., Hirono, A., and Miwa, S.: cDNA cloning of human R-type pyruvate kinase and identification of a single amino acid substitution (Thr^{384}→Met) affecting enzymatic stability in a pyruvate kinase variant (PK Tokyo) associated with hereditary hemolytic anemia. Proc. Natl. Acad. Sci. USA 88:8218, 1991.
45a. Kanno, H., Fujii, H., Hirono, A., Omine, M., and Miwa, S.: Identical point mutations of the R-type pyruvate kinase (PK)

cDNA found in unrelated PK variants associated with hereditary hemolytic anemia. Blood 79:1347, 1992.

46. Tomatsu, S., Kobayashi, Y., Fukumaki, Y., Yubisui, T., Orii, T., and Sakaki, Y.: The organization and the complete nucleotide sequence of the human NADH–cytochrome $b5$ reductase gene. Gene 80:353, 1989.

47. Kobayashi, Y., Fukumaki, Y., Yubisui, T., Inoue, J., and Sakaki, Y.: Serine-proline replacement at residue 127 of NADH–cytochrome $b5$ reductase causes hereditary methemoglobinemia, generalized type. Blood 75:1408, 1990.

47a. Shirabe, K., Yubisui, T., Borgese, N., Tang, C., Hultquist, D. E., and Takeshita, M.: Enzymatic instability of NADH–cytochrome $b5$ reductase as a cause of hereditary methemoglobinemia type I (red cell type). J. Biol. Chem. 267:20416, 1992.

48. Eggleston, L. V., and Krebs, H. A.: Regulation of the pentose phosphate cycle. Biochem. J. 138:423, 1974.

49. Beutler, E.: Abnormalities of the hexose monophosphate shunt. Semin. Hematol. 8:311, 1971.

50. Srivastava, S. K., and Beutler, E.: Glutathione metabolism of the erythrocyte. The enzymic cleavage of glutathione-haemoglobin preparations by glutathione reductase. Biochem. J. 119:353, 1970.

51. Beutler, E.: Drug induced hemolytic anemia and non-spherocytic hemolytic anemia. In Yoshida, A., and Beutler, E. (eds.): Glucose-6-Phosphate Dehydrogenase. Orlando, Fla., Academic Press, 1986, pp. 3–12.

52. Gaetani, G. F., Galiano, S., Canepa, L., Ferraris, A. M., and Kirkman, H. N.: Catalase and glutathione peroxidase are equally active in detoxification of hydrogen peroxide in human erythrocytes. Blood 73:334, 1989.

53. Kirkman, H. N., and Gaetani, G. F.: Catalase: A tetrameric enzyme with four tightly bound molecules of NADPH. Proc. Natl. Acad. Sci. USA 81:4343, 1984.

54. Kirkman, H. N., Galiano, S., and Gaetani, G. F.: The function of catalase-bound NADPH. J. Biol. Chem. 262:660, 1987.

55. Winterbourn, C. C., and Stern, A.: Human red cells scavenge extracellular hydrogen peroxide and inhibit formation of hypochlorous acid and hydroxyl radical. J. Clin. Invest. 80:1486, 1987.

56. Luzzatto, L., and Mehta, A.: Glucose 6-phosphate dehydrogenase deficiency. In Scriver, C. R., Beaudet, A. L., Sly, W. S., and Valle D. (eds.): The Metabolic Basis of Inherited Disease. 6th ed. New York, McGraw-Hill Information Services Co., 1990, pp. 2237–2265.

57. Beutler, E.: Genetics of glucose-6-phosphate dehydrogenase deficiency. Semin. Hematol. 27:137, 1990.

58. Beutler, E., Kuhl, W., and Gelbart, T.: 6-Phosphogluconolactonase deficiency, a hereditary erythrocyte enzyme deficiency: Possible interaction with glucose-6-phosphate dehydrogenase deficiency. Proc. Natl. Acad. Sci. USA 82:3876, 1985.

59. Parr, C. W., and Fitch, L. I.: Hereditary partial deficiency of human-erythrocyte phosphogluconate dehydrogenase. Biochem. J. 93:28C, 1964.

60. Brownstone, Y. S., and Denstedt, O. F.: The pentose phosphate metabolic pathway in the human erythrocyte. II. The transketolase and transaldolase activity of the human erythrocyte. Can. J. Biochem. 39:533, 1961.

61. Kaufmann, A., Uhlhaas, S., Friedl, W., and Propping, P.: Human erythrocyte transketolase: No evidence for variants. Clin. Chim. Acta 162:215, 1987.

62. Kaczmarek, M. J., and Nixon, P. F.: Variants of transketolase from human erythrocytes. Clin. Chim. Acta 130:349, 1983.

63. Wolfe, S. J., Brin, M., and Davidson, C. S.: The effect of thiamine deficiency on human erythrocyte metabolism. J. Clin. Invest. 37:1476, 1958.

64. Dische, Z., and Sigeura, H.: Interconversion of ribose-5-phosphate and hexose-6-phosphate in human blood. Biochim. Biophys. Acta 24:87, 1957.

65. Bruns, F. H., Noltmann, E., and Vahlhaus, E.: Über den Stoffwechsel von Ribose-5-phosphat in Hämolysaten. I. Aktivitaets-messung und Eigenschaften der Phosphoribose-iso-

merase. II. Der Pentosephosphate-Cyclus in roten Blutzellen. Biochem. Z. 330:483, 1958.

66. Karmali, A., Drake, A. F., and Spencer, N.: Purification, properties and assay of D-ribulose 5-phosphate 3-epimerase from human erythrocytes. Biochem. J. 211:617, 1983.

67. McBride, O. W., Mitchell, A., Lee, B. J., Mullenbach, G., and Hatfield, D.: Gene for selenium-dependent glutathione peroxidase maps to human chromosomes 3, 21 and X. BioFactors 1:285, 1989.

68. Loos, H., Roos, D., Weening, R., and Houwerzijl, J.: Familial deficiency of glutathione reductase in human blood cells. Blood 48:53, 1976.

69. Tutic, M., Lu, X., Schirmer, R. H., and Werner, D.: Cloning and sequencing of mammalian glutathione reductase cDNA. Eur. J. Biochem. 188:523, 1990.

70. Sass, M. D., Caruso, C. J., and Farhangi, M.: TPNH-methemoglobin reductase deficiency: A new red-cell enzyme defect. J. Lab. Clin. Med. 70:760, 1967.

71. Wen, J.-K., Osumi, T., Hashimoto, T., and Ogata, M.: Molecular analysis of human acatalasemia. Identification of a splicing mutation. J. Mol. Biol. 211:383, 1990.

72. Touati, D.: Molecular genetics of superoxide dismutases. Free Radic. Biol. Med. 5:393, 1988.

73. Guemouri, L., Artur, Y., Herbeth, B., Jeandel, C., Cuny, G., and Siest, G.: Biological variability of superoxide dismutase, glutathione peroxidase, and catalase in blood. Clin. Chem. 37:1932, 1991.

74. Dale, G. L., and Norenberg, S. L.: Time-dependent loss of adenosine 5′-monophosphate deaminase activity may explain elevated adenosine 5′-triphosphate levels in senescent erythrocytes. Blood 74:2157, 1989.

75. Suzuki, T., and Dale, G. L.: Senescent erythrocytes: Isolation of in vivo aged cells and their biochemical characteristics. Proc. Natl. Acad. Sci. USA 85:1647, 1988.

76. Paglia, D. E., Valentine, W. N., Nakatani, M., and Brockway, R. A.: AMP deaminase as a cell-age marker in transient erythroblastopenia of childhood and its role in the adenylate economy of erythrocytes. Blood 74:2161, 1989.

77. Mandula, B., and Beutler, E.: Synthesis of riboflavin nucleotides by mature human erythrocytes. Blood 36:491, 1970.

78. Agarwal, K. C., and Parks, R. E., Jr.: Adenosine triphosphate–guanosine 5′–phosphate phosphotransferase. Mol. Pharmacol. 8:128, 1972.

79. Henderson, J. F., Zombor, G., and Burridge, P. W.: Guanosine triphosphate catabolism in human and rabbit erythrocytes: Role of reductive deamination of guanylate to inosinate. Can. J. Biochem. 56:474, 1978.

80. Schmalzing, G., Pfaff, E., and Breyer-Pfaff, U.: Red cell ouabain binding sites, Na$^+$K$^+$-ATPase, and intracellular Na$^+$ as individual characteristics. Life Sci. 29:371, 1981.

81. Morrot, G., Zachowski, A., and Devaux, P. F.: Partial purification and characterization of the human erythrocyte Mg^{2+}-ATPase. FEBS Lett. 266:29, 1990.

82. Niggli, V., Penniston, J. T., and Carafoli, E.: Purification of the Ca-Mg-ATPase from human erythrocyte membranes using a calmodulin affinity column. J. Biol. Chem. 254:9955, 1979.

83. Kondo, T., Kawakami, Y., Taniguchi, N., and Beutler, E.: Glutathione disulfide–stimulated Mg^{2+}-ATPase of human erythrocyte membranes. Proc. Natl. Acad. Sci. USA 84:7373, 1987.

84. Sharma, R., Gupta, S., Ahmad, H., Ansari, G. A. S., and Awasthi, Y. C.: Stimulation of a human erythrocyte membrane ATPase by glutathione conjugates. Toxicol. Appl. Pharmacol. 104:421, 1990.

85. Beutler, E., and Kuhl, W.: Guanosine triphosphatase activity in human erythrocyte membranes. Biochim. Biophys. Acta 601:372, 1980.

86. Parks, R. E., Jr., Brown, P. R., and Kong, C. M.: Incorporation of purine analogs into the nucleotide pools of human erythrocytes. In Sperling, O., De Vries, A., and Wyngaarden, J. B. (eds.): Purine Metabolism in Man. New York, Plenum Publishing Corp., 1973, pp. 117–127.

87. Ericson, A., Niklasson, F., and de Verdier, C.-H.: Metabolism of guanosine in human erythrocytes. Vox Sang. 48:72, 1985.

88. Paglia, D. E., Valentine, W. N., and Brockway, R. A.: Identification of thymidine nucleotidase and deoxyribonucleotidase activities among normal isozymes of 5'-nucleotidase in human erythrocytes. Proc. Natl. Acad. Sci. USA 81:588, 1984.

89. Paglia, D. E., and Valentine, W. N.: Characteristics of a pyrimidine-specific 5'-nucleotidase in human erythrocytes. J. Biol. Chem. 250:7973, 1975.

90. Torrance, J. D., Whittaker, D., and Beutler, E.: Purification and properties of human erythrocyte pyrimidine 5'-nucleotidase. Proc. Natl. Acad. Sci. USA 74:3701, 1977.

91. Beutler, E., and West, C.: Tissue distribution of pyrimidine-5'-nucleotidase. Biochem. Med. 27:334, 1982.

92. Paglia, D. E., Valentine, W. N., Keitt, A. S., Brockway, R. A., and Nakatani, M.: Pyrimidine nucleotidase deficiency with active dephosphorylation of dTMP: Evidence for existence of thymidine nucleotidase in human erythrocyte. Blood 62:1147, 1983.

93. Valentine, W. N., Tanaka, K. R., and Paglia, D. E.: Hemolytic anemias and erythrocyte enzymopathies. Ann. Intern. Med. 103:245, 1985.

94. Valentine, W. N., Fink, K., Paglia, D. E., Harris, S. R., and Adams, W. S.: Hereditary hemolytic anemia with human erythrocyte pyrimidine 5'-nucleotidase deficiency. J. Clin. Invest. 54:866, 1974.

95. Marie, J., Kahn, A., and Boivin, P.: Pyruvate kinase isozymes in man. I. M. type isozymes in adult and foetal tissues, electrofocusing and immunological studies. Hum. Genet. 31:35, 1976.

96. Kahn, A., Marie, J., and Boivin, P.: Pyruvate kinase isozymes in man. II. L type and erythrocyte-type isozymes. Electrofocusing and immunologic studies. Hum. Genet. 33:35, 1976.

97. Ibsen, K. H.: Interrelationships and functions of the pyruvate kinase isozymes and their variant forms: A review. Cancer Res. 37:341, 1977.

98. Galacteros, F., Rosa, R., Prehu, M.-O., Najean, Y., and Calvin, M.-C.: Deficit en diphosphoglycerate mutase: Nouveaux cas associes a une polyglobulie. Nouv. Rev. Fr. Hematol. 26:69, 1984.

99. Vora, S., Corash, L., Engel, W. K., Durham, S., Seaman, C., and Piomelli, S.: The molecular mechanism of the inherited phosphofructokinase deficiency associated with hemolysis and myopathy. Blood 55:629, 1980.

100. Vora, S., Davidson, M., Seaman, C., Miranda, A. F., Noble, N. A., Tanaka, K., Frenkel, E. P., and DiMauro, S.: Heterogeneity of the molecular lesions in inherited phosphofructokinase deficiency. J. Clin. Invest. 72:1995, 1983.

101. Max-Audit, I., Rosa, R., and Marie, J.: Pyruvate kinase hyperactivity genetically determined: Metabolic consequences and molecular characterization. Blood 56:902, 1980.

102. Zürcher, C., Loos, J. A., and Prins, H. K.: Hereditary high ATP content of human erythrocytes. Bibl. Haematol. 23:549, 1965.

103. Staal, G. E. J., Jansen, G., and Roos, D.: Pyruvate kinase and the "high ATP syndrome." J. Clin. Invest. 74:231, 1984.

104. Ouwerkerk, R., Van Echteld, C. J. A., Staal, G. E. J., and Rijksen, G.: Distribution of phosphorylated metabolites and magnesium in the red cells of a patient with hyperactive pyruvate kinase. Blood 72:1224, 1988.

105. Schneider, A. S., Valentine, W. N., Baughan, M. A., Paglia, D. E., Shore, N. A., and Heins, H. L., Jr.: Triosephosphate isomerase deficiency. A multi-system inherited enzyme disorder: Clinical and genetic aspects. In Beutler, E. (ed.): Hereditary Disorders of Erythrocyte Metabolism. New York, Grune & Stratton, 1968, pp. 265–272.

106. Waterbury, L., and Frenkel, E. P.: Hereditary nonspherocytic hemolysis with erythrocyte phosphofructokinase deficiency. Blood 39:415, 1972.

107. Konrad, P. N., McCarthy, D. J., Mauer, A. M., Valentine, W. N., and Paglia, D. E.: Erythrocyte and leukocyte phospho-

108. DiMauro, S., Dalakas, M., and Miranda, A. F.: Phosphoglycerate kinase deficiency: Another cause of recurrent myoglobinuria. Ann. Neurol. 13:11, 1983.

109. Rosa, R., George, C., Fardeau, M., Calvin, M. C., Rapin, M., and Rosa, J.: A new case of phosphoglycerate kinase deficiency: PGK Creteil associated with rhabdomyolysis and lacking hemolytic anemia. Blood 60:84, 1982.

110. Krietsch, W. K. G., Krietsch, H., Kaiser, W., Duennwald, M., Kuntz, G. W. K., Duhm, J., and Buecher, T.: Hereditary deficiency of phosphoglycerate kinase: A new variant in erythrocytes and leucocytes, not associated with haemolytic anaemia. Eur. J. Clin. Invest. 7:427, 1977.

111. Leroux, A., Junien, C., and Kaplan J.-C.: Generalised deficiency of cytochrome b5 reductase in congenital methaemoglobinaemia with mental retardation. Nature 258:619, 1975.

112. Miwa, S., Nishina, T., Kakehashi, Y., Kitamura, M., Hiratsuka, A., and Shizume, K.: Studies on erythrocyte metabolism in a case with hereditary deficiency of H-subunit of lactate dehydrogenase. Acta Haematol. Jpn. 34:2, 1971.

113. McCann, S. R., Finkel, B., Cadman, S., and Allen, D. W.: Study of a kindred with hereditary spherocytosis and glyceraldehyde-3-phosphate dehydrogenase deficiency. Blood 47:171, 1976.

114. Bernini, L., Latte, B., Siniscalco, M., Piomelli, S., Spada, U., Adinolfi, M., and Mollison, P. L.: Survival of 51 Cr-labelled red cells in subjects with thalassemia-trait or G6PD deficiency or both abnormalities. Br. J. Haematol. 10:171, 1964.

115. Chan, T. K., Chesterman, C. N., McFadzean, A. J. S., and Todd D.: The survival of glucose-6-phosphate dehydrogenase–deficient erythrocytes in patients with typhoid fever on chloramphenicol therapy. J. Lab. Clin. Med. 77:177, 1971.

116. Dern, R. J., Weinstein, I. M., Le Roy, G. V., Talmage, D. W., and Alving, A. S.: The hemolytic effect of primaquine. I. The localization of the drug-induced hemolytic defect in primaquine-sensitive individuals. J. Lab. Clin. Med. 43:303, 1954.

117. Zail, S. S., Charlton, R. W., and Bothwell, T. H.: The haemolytic effect of certain drugs in Bantu subjects with a deficiency of glucose-6-phosphate dehydrogenase. S. Afr. J. Med. Sci. 27:95, 1962.

118. McCurdy, P. R., and Morse, E. E.: Glucose-6-phosphate dehydrogenase deficiency and blood transfusion. Vox Sang. 28:230, 1975.

119. Raoult, D., Lena, D., Perrimont, H., Gallais, H., Walker, D. H., and Casanova, P.: Haemolysis with Mediterranean spotted fever and glucose-6-phosphate dehydrogenase deficiency. Trans. R. Soc. Trop. Med. Hyg. 80:961, 1986.

120. Tugwell, P.: Glucose-6-phosphate-dehydrogenase deficiency in Nigerians with jaundice associated with lobar pneumonia. Lancet 1:968, 1973.

121. Rosenbloom, B. E., Weingarten, S., Rosenfelt, F. P., and Weinstein, I. M.: Severe hemolytic anemia due to glucose-6-phosphate dehydrogenase deficiency and Epstein-Barr virus infection. Mt. Sinai J. Med. 55:404, 1988.

122. Hersko, C., and Vardy, P. A.: Haemolysis in typhoid fever in children with G-6-PD deficiency. Br. Med. J. 1:214, 1967.

123. Lampe, R. M., Kirdpon, S., Mansuwan, P., and Benenson, M. W.: Glucose-6-phosphate dehydrogenase deficiency in Thai children with typhoid fever. J. Pediatr. 87:576, 1975.

124. Whelton, A., Donadio, J. V., Jr., and Elisberg, B. L.: Acute renal failure complicating rickettsial infections in glucose-6-phosphate dehydrogenase–deficient individuals. Ann. Intern. Med. 69:323, 1968.

125. Walker, D. H., Hawkins, H. K., and Hudson, P.: Fulminant Rocky Mountain spotted fever. Arch. Pathol. Lab. Med. 107:121, 1983.

126. Burka, E. R., Weaver, Z., III, and Marks, P. A.: Clinical spectrum of hemolytic anemia associated with G 6 PD deficiency. Ann. Intern. Med. 64:817, 1966.

127. Beutler, E.: Hemolytic Anemia in Disorders of Red Cell Metabolism. New York, Plenum Press, Inc., 1978.

glycerate kinase deficiency with neurologic disease. J. Pediatr. 82:456, 1973.

128. Beutler, E.: Glucose-6-phosphate dehydrogenase deficiency. *In* Williams, W. J., Beutler, E., Erslev, A. J., and Lichtman, M. A. (eds.): Hematology. 4th ed. New York, McGraw-Hill Book Co., 1990, pp. 591–606.

129. Piomelli, S.: G6PD deficiency and hemolytic anemia: G6PD-related neonatal jaundice. *In* Yoshida, A., and Beutler, E. (eds.): Glucose-6-Phosphate Dehydrogenase. Orlando, Fla., Academic Press, 1986, pp. 95–108.

130. Wolf, B. H. M., Schutgens, R. B. H., Nagelkerke, N. J. D., and Weening, R. S.: Glucose-6-phosphate dehydrogenase deficiency in ethnic minorities in the Netherlands. Trop. Geogr. Med. 40:322, 1988.

131. Szeinberg, A., Oliver, M., Schmidt, R., Adam, A., and Sheba, C.: Glucose-6-phosphate dehydrogenase deficiency and haemolytic disease. Arch. Dis. Child. 38:23, 1963.

132. Panizon, F.: L'ictere grave du nouveau-ne associé à une déficience en glucose-6-phosphate dehydrogenase. Biol. Neonate 2:167, 1960.

133. Panizon, F.: Erythrocyte enzyme deficiency in unexplained kernicterus. Lancet 2:1093, 1960.

134. Flatz, G., Thanangkul, O., Simarak, S., and Manmontri, M.: Glucose-6-phosphate dehydrogenase deficiency and jaundice in newborn infants in Northern Thailand. Ann. Pediatr. 203:39, 1964.

135. Doxiadis, S. A., and Valaes, T.: The clinical picture of glucose 6-phosphate dehydrogenase deficiency in early infancy. Arch. Dis. Child. 39:545, 1964.

136. Naik, S. N., and Anderson, D. E.: G-6-PD deficiency and cancer. Lancet 1:1060, 1970.

137. Naik, S. N., and Anderson, D. E.: The association between glucose-6-phosphate dehydrogenase deficiency and cancer in American Negroes. Oncology 25:356, 1971.

138. Beaconsfield, P., Rainsbury, R., and Kalton, G.: Glucose-6-phosphate dehydrogenase deficiency and the incidence of cancer. Oncology 19:11, 1965.

139. Dern, R. J., Glynn, M. F., and Brewer, G. J.: Studies on the correlation of the genetically determined trait, glucose-6-phosphate dehydrogenase deficiency, with behavioral manifestations in schizophrenia. J. Lab. Clin. Med. 62:319, 1963.

140. Chanmugam, D., and Frumin, A. M.: Abnormal oral glucose tolerance response in erythrocyte glucose-6-phosphate dehydrogenase deficiency. N. Engl. J. Med. 271:1202, 1964.

141. Orzalesi, N., Sorcinelli, R., and Guiso, G.: Increased incidence of cataract in male subjects deficient in glucose-6-phosphate dehydrogenase. Arch. Ophthalmol. 99:69, 1981.

142. Panich, V., and Na-Nakorn, S.: G 6 PD deficiency in senile cataracts. Hum. Genet. 55:123, 1980.

143. Eppes, R., Brewer, G., De Gowin, R., McNamara, J., Flanagan, C., Schrier, S., Tarlov, A., Powell, R., and Carson, P.: Oral glucose tolerance in Negro men deficient in G-6-PD. N. Engl. J. Med. 275:855, 1966.

144. Meloni, T., Carta, F., Forteleoni, G., Carta, A., Ena, F., and Meloni, G. F.: Glucose-6-phosphate dehydrogenase deficiency and cataract of patients in Northern Sardinia. Am. J. Ophthalmol. 110:661, 1990.

145. Ferraris, A. M., Broccia, G., Meloni, T., Forteleoni, G., and Gaetani, G. F.: Glucose-6-phosphate dehydrogenase deficiency and incidence of hematologic malignancy. Am. J. Hum. Genet. 42:516, 1988.

146. Cocco, P., Dessi, S., Avataneo, G., Picchiri, G., and Heinemann, E.: Glucose-6-phosphate dehydrogenase deficiency and cancer in a Sardinian male population: A case-control study. Carcinogenesis 10:813, 1989.

147. Giblett, E. R.: Genetic Markers in Human Blood. Philadelphia, F. A. Davis Co., 1969.

148. Parr, C. W., and Fitch, L. I.: Inherited quantitative variations of human phosphogluconate dehydrogenase. Ann. Hum. Genet. 30:339, 1967.

149. Mohler, D. N., Majerus, P. W., Minnich, V., Hess, C. E., and Garrick, M. D.: Glutathione synthetase deficiency as a cause of hereditary hemolytic disease. N. Engl. J. Med. 283:1253, 1970.

150. Boivin, P., Galand, C., and Schaison, G.: Déficit en glutathion-synthetase avec 5-oxoprolinurie. Deux nouveaux cas et revue de la littérature. Presse Med. 7:1531, 1978.

151. Jellum, E., Kluge, T., Boerresen, H. C., Stokke, O., and Eldjarn, L.: Pyroglutamic aciduria—a new inborn error of metabolism. Scand. J. Clin. Lab. Invest. 26:327, 1970.

152. Eldjarn, L., Jellum, E., and Stokke, O.: Pyroglutamic aciduria: Studies on the enzymic block and on the metabolic origin of pyroglutamic acid. Clin. Chim. Acta 40:461, 1972.

153. Beutler, E.: Glutathione deficiency, pyroglutamic acidemia and amino acid transport. N. Engl. J. Med. 295:441, 1976.

154. Richards, F., II, Cooper, M. R., Pearce, L. A., Cowan, R. J., and Spurr, C. L.: Familial spinocerebellar degeneration, hemolytic anemia, and glutathione deficiency. Arch. Intern. Med. 134:534, 1974.

155. Beutler, E., Moroose, R., Kramer, L., Gelbart, T., and Forman, L.: Gamma-glutamylcysteine synthetase deficiency and hemolytic anemia. Blood 75:271, 1990.

156. Beutler, E.: Glutathione reductase: Stimulation in normal subjects by riboflavin supplementation. Science 165:613, 1969.

157. Beutler, E.: Effect of flavin compounds on glutathione reductase activity: In vivo and in vitro studies. J. Clin. Invest. 48:1957, 1969.

158. Glatzle, D., Weber, F., and Wiss, O.: Enzymatic test for the detection of a riboflavin deficiency. NADPH-dependent glutathione reductase of red blood cells and its activation by FAD in vitro. Experientia 24:1122, 1968.

159. Beutler, E., Dunning, D., Dabe, I. B., and Forman, L.: Erythrocyte glutathione S-transferase deficiency and hemolytic anemia. Blood 72:73, 1988.

160. Whaun, J. M., and Oski, F. A.: Relation of red blood cell glutathione peroxidase to neonatal jaundice. J. Pediatr. 76:555, 1970.

161. Steinberg, M., Brauer, M. J., and Necheles, T. F.: Acute hemolytic anemia associated with erythrocyte glutathione-peroxidase deficiency. Arch. Intern. Med. 125:302, 1970.

162. Boivin, P., Galand, C., Hakim, J., and Blery, M.: Déficit en glutathion-peroxydase érythrocytaire et anémie hémolytique médicamenteuse. Une nouvelle observation. Presse Med. 78:171, 1970.

163. Necheles, T. F., Steinberg, M. H., and Cameron, D.: Erythrocyte glutathione-peroxidase deficiency. Br. J. Haematol. 19:605, 1970.

164. Boivin, P., Galand, C., Hakim, J., Roge, J., and Gueroult, N.: Anémie hémolytique avec déficit en glutathion-peroxydase chez un adulte. Enzyme 10:68, 1969.

165. Necheles, T. F., Maldonado, N., Barquet-Chediak, A., and Allen, D. M.: Homozygous erythrocyte glutathione-peroxidase deficiency: Clinical and biochemical studies. Blood 33:164, 1969.

166. Beutler, E., and Matsumoto, F.: Ethnic variation in red cell glutathione peroxidase activity. Blood 46:103, 1975.

167. Golan, R., Ezzer, J. B., and Szeinberg, A.: Red cell glutathione peroxidase in various Jewish ethnic groups in Israel. Hum. Hered. 30:136, 1980.

168. Kien, C. L., and Ganther, H. E.: Manifestations of chronic selenium deficiency in a child receiving total parenteral nutrition. Am. J. Clin. Nutr. 37:319, 1983.

169. Thomson, C. D., Rea, H. M., Doesburg, V. M., and Robinson M. F.: Selenium concentrations and glutathione peroxidase activities in whole blood of New Zealand residents. Br. J. Nutr. 37:457, 1977.

170. Kanno, H., Tani, K., Fujii, H., Iguchi-Ariga, S. M. M., Ariga, H., Kozaki, T., and Miwa, S.: Adenosine deaminase (ADA) overproduction associated with congenital hemolytic anemia: Case report and molecular analysis. Jpn. J. Exp. Med. 58:1, 1988.

171. Miwa, S., Fujii, H., Matsumoto, N., Nakatsuji, T., Oda, S., Asano, H., and Asano, S.: A case of red-cell adenosine deaminase overproduction associated with hereditary hemolytic anemia found in Japan. Am. J. Hematol. 5:107, 1978.

172. Valentine, W. N., Paglia, D. E., Tartaglia, A. P., and Gilsanz, F.: Hereditary hemolytic anemia with increased red cell

adenosine deaminase (45- to 70-fold) and decreased adenosine triphosphate. Science 195:783, 1977.

173. Chottiner, E. G., Gribbin, T. E., Ginsburg, D., and Mitchell, B. S.: Erythrocyte-specific overproduction of adenosine deaminase: Molecular genetic studies. In Brewer, G. J. (ed.): The Red Cell: Seventh Ann Arbor Conference. New York, Alan R. Liss, 1989, pp. 55–68.

174. Chottiner, E. G., Cloft, H. J., Tartaglia, A. P., and Mitchell, B. S.: Elevated adenosine deaminase activity and hereditary hemolytic anemia: Evidence for abnormal translational control of protein synthesis. J. Clin. Invest. 79:1001, 1987.

175. Ogasawara, N., Goto, H., Yamada, Y., and Hasegawa, I.: Deficiency of erythrocyte type isozyme of AMP deaminase in human. Adv. Exp. Med. Biol. 195:123, 1986.

176. Ogasawara, N., Goto, H., Yamada, Y., Nishigaki, I., Itoh, T., Hasegawa, I., and Park, K. S.: Deficiency of AMP deaminase in erythrocytes. Hum. Genet. 75:15, 1987.

177. Ogasawara, N., Goto, H., Yamada, Y., Nishigaki, I., Itoh, T., and Hasegawa, I.: Complete deficiency of AMP deaminase in human erythrocytes. Biochem. Biophys. Res. Commun. 122:1344, 1984.

178. Beutler, E., Baranko, P. V., Feagler, J., Matsumoto, F., Miro-Quesada, M., Selby, G., and Singh, P.: Hemolytic anemia due to pyrimidine-5′-nucleotidase deficiency: Report of eight cases in six families. Blood 56:251, 1980.

179. Paglia, D. E., and Valentine, W. N.: Haemolytic anaemia associated with disorders of the purine and pyrimidine salvage pathways. Clin. Haematol. 10:81, 1981.

180. Paglia, D. E., Valentine, W. N., and Dahlgren, J. G.: Effects of low-level lead exposure on pyrimidine 5′-nucleotidase and other erythrocyte enzymes. J. Clin. Invest. 56:1164, 1975.

181. Valentine, W. N., Paglia, D. E., Fink, K., and Madokoro, G.: Lead poisoning. Association with hemolytic anemia, basophilic stippling, erythrocyte pyrimidine 5′-nucleotidase deficiency, and intraerythrocytic accumulation of pyrimidines. J. Clin. Invest. 58:926, 1976.

182. Kondo, T., Dale, G. L., and Beutler, E.: Glutathione transport by inside-out vesicles from human erythrocytes. Proc. Natl. Acad. Sci. USA 77:6359, 1980.

183. Kondo, T., Ohtsuka, Y., Shimada, M., Kawakami, Y., Hiyoshi, Y., Tsuji, Y., Fujii, H., and Miwa, S.: Erythrocyte-oxidized glutathione transport in pyrimidine 5′-nucleotidase deficiency. Am. J. Hematol. 26:37, 1987.

184. Valentine, W. N., and Paglia, D. E.: Syndromes with increased red cell glutathione. Hemoglobin 4:799, 1980.

185. Valentine, W. N., Bennett, J. M., Krivit, W., Konrad, P. N., Lowman, J. T., Paglia, D. E., and Wakem, C. J.: Nonspherocytic haemolytic anaemia with increased red cell adenine nucleotides, glutathione and basophilic stippling and ribosephosphate pyrophosphokinase (RPK) deficiency: Studies on two new kindreds. Br. J. Haematol. 24:157, 1973.

186. Paglia, D. E., Valentine, W. N., Nakatani, M., and Rauth, B. J.: Selective accumulation of cytosol CDP-choline as an isolated erythrocyte defect in chronic hemolysis. Proc. Natl. Acad. Sci. USA 80:3081, 1983.

187. Vanderheiden, B. S.: Human erythrocyte "ITPase": An ITP pyrophosphohydrolase. Biochim. Biophys. Acta 215:555, 1970.

188. Vanderheiden, B. S.: Genetic studies of human erythrocyte inosine triphosphatase. Biochem. Genet. 3:289, 1969.

189. Hanel, H. K., Cohn, J., and Harvald, B.: Adenosine-triphosphatase deficiency in a family with nonspherocytic haemolytic anemia. Hum. Hered. 21:313, 1971.

190. Beutler, E., Kuhl, W., and Sacks, P.: Sodium-potassium-ATPase activity is influenced by ethnic origin and not by obesity. N. Engl. J. Med. 309:756, 1983.

191. Beutler, E., Carson, D., Dannawi, H., Forman, L., Kuhl, W., West, C., and Westwood, B.: Metabolic compensation for profound erythrocyte adenylate kinase deficiency. J. Clin. Invest. 72:648, 1983.

192. Szeinberg, A., Gavendo, S., and Cahane, D.: Erythrocyte adenylate-kinase deficiency. Lancet 1:315, 1969.

193. Szeinberg, A., Kahana, D., Gavendo, S., Zaidman, J., and Ben-

194. Kende, G., Ben-Bassat, I., Brok-Simoni, F., Holtzman, F., and Ramot, B.: Adenylate kinase deficiency associated with congenital non-spherocytic hemolytic anemia. Abstr. XIX Int. Soc. Haematol. 19:224, 1982.

195. Beutler, E.: Galactosemia: Screening and diagnosis. Clin. Biochem. 24:293, 1991.

196. Rimington, C.: A review of the enzymic errors in the various porphyrias. Scand. J. Clin. Lab. Invest. 45:291, 1985.

197. Fairbanks, L. D., Simmonds, H. A., and Webster, D. R.: Use of intact erythrocytes in the diagnosis of inherited purine and pyrimidine disorders. J. Inherited Metab. Dis. 10:174, 1987.

198. Kelley, W. N., and Wyngaarden, J. B.: Clinical syndromes associated with hypoxanthine-guanine phosphoribosyltransferase deficiency. In Stanbury, J. B., Wyngaarden, J. B., Fredrickson, D. S., Goldstein, J. L., and Brown, M. S. (eds.): The Metabolic Basis of Inherited Disease. 5th ed. New York, McGraw-Hill Book Co., 1983, pp. 1115–1143.

199. Seegmiller, J. E., Rosenbloom, F. M., and Kelley, W. N.: Enzyme defect associated with a sex-linked human neurological disorder and excessive purine synthesis. Science 155:1682, 1967.

200. Wysocki, S. J., Hahnel, R., Mahoney, T., Wilson, R. G., and Panegyres P. K.: Prolidase deficiency: A patient without hydroxyproline-containing iminodipeptides in urine. J. Inherited Metab. Dis. 11:161, 1988.

201. Kodama, H., Mikasa, H., Ohhashi, T., Ohno, T., and Arata, J.: Biochemical investigations on prolidase and prolinase in erythrocytes from patients with prolidase deficiency. Clin. Chim. Acta 173:317, 1988.

202. Endo, F., Matsuda, I., Ogata, A., and Tanaka, S.: Human erythrocyte prolidase and prolidase deficiency. Pediatr. Res. 16:227, 1982.

203. Agarwal, R. P., Crabtree, G. W., Parks, R. E., Jr., Nelson, J. A., Keightley, R., Parkman, R., Rosen, F. S., Stern, R. C., and Polmar, S. H.: Purine nucleoside metabolism in the erythrocytes of patients with adenosine deaminase deficiency and severe combined immunodeficiency. J. Clin. Invest. 57:1025, 1976.

204. Rich, K. C., Arnold, W. J., Palella, T., and Fox, I. H.: Cellular immune deficiency with autoimmune hemolytic anemia in purine nucleoside phosphorylase deficiency. Am. J. Med. 67:172, 1979.

205. Staal, G. E., Stoop, J. W., Zegers, B. J., Siegenbeek van Heukelom, L. H., van der Vlist, M. J., Wadman, S. K., and Martin, D. W.: Erythrocyte metabolism in purine nucleoside phosphorylase deficiency after enzyme replacement therapy by infusion of erythrocytes. J. Clin. Invest. 65:103, 1980.

206. Delbarre, F., Auscher, C., Amor, B., De Gery, A., Cartier, P., and Hamet, M.: Gout with adenine phosphoribosyl transferase deficiency. Biomedicine 21:82, 1974.

207. Cartier, P., and Hamet, M.: Une nouvelle maladie métabolique: Le déficit complet en adenine-phosphoribosyltransferase avec lithiase de 2,8-dihydroxyadenine. C. R. Acad. Sci. (Paris) 279:883, 1974.

208. Van Acker, K. J., Simmonds, A., Potter, C., and Cameron, J. S.: Complete deficiency of adenine phosphoribosyltransferase. Report of a family. N. Engl. J. Med. 297:127, 1977.

209. Johnson, M. G., Rosenzweig, S., and Switzer, R. L.: Evaluation of the role of 5-phosphoribosyl-alpha-1-pyrophosphate synthetase in congenital hyperuricemia and gout: A simple isotopic assay and an activity stain for the enzyme. Biochem. Med. 10:266, 1974.

210. Takahara, S.: Acatalasemia in Japan. In Beutler, E. (ed.): Hereditary Disorders of Erythrocyte Metabolism. New York, Grune & Stratton, 1968, pp. 21–48.

211. Aebi, H., Bossi, E., Cantz, M., Matsubara, S., and Suter, H.: Acatalas(em)ia in Switzerland. In Beutler, E. (ed.): Hereditary Disorders of Erythrocyte Metabolism. New York, Grune & Stratton, 1968, pp. 41–65.

212. Johns, R. J.: Familial reduction in red-cell cholinesterase. N. Engl. J. Med. 267:1344, 1962.

Ezzer, J.: Hereditary deficiency of adenylate kinase in red blood cells. Acta Haematol. (Basel) 42:111, 1969.

213. Shinohara, K., and Tanaka, K. R.: Hereditary deficiency of erythrocyte acetylcholinesterase. Am. J. Hematol. 7:313, 1979.
214. Kirkman, H. N., and Hendrickson, E. M.: Glucose-6-phosphate dehydrogenase from human erythrocytes. II. Subactive states of the enzyme from normal persons. J. Biol. Chem. 237:2371, 1962.
215. De Flora, A., Morelli, A., and Giuliano, F.: Human erythrocyte glucose 6-phosphate dehydrogenase. Content of bound coenzyme. Biochem. Biophys. Res. Commun. 59:406, 1974.
216. De Flora, A., Morelli, A., Benatti, U., Giuliano, F., and Molinari, M. P.: Human erythrocyte glucose 6-phosphate dehydrogenase. Interaction with oxidized and reduced coenzyme. Biochem. Biophys. Res. Commun. 60:999, 1974.
217. Canepa, L., Ferraris, A. M., Miglino, M., and Gaetani, G. F.: Bound and unbound pyridine dinucleotides in normal and glucose-6-phosphate dehydrogenase-deficient erythrocytes. Biochim. Biophys. Acta 1074:101, 1991.
218. Hirono, A., Kuhl, W., Gelbart, T., Forman, L., Fairbanks, V. F., and Beutler, E.: Identification of the binding domain for NADP⁺ of human glucose-6-phosphate dehydrogenase by sequence analysis of mutants. Proc. Natl. Acad. Sci. USA 86:10015, 1989.
219. Persson, B., Jörnvall, H., Wood, I., and Jeffery, J.: Functionally important regions of glucose-6-phosphate dehydrogenase defined by the Saccharomyces cerevisiae enzyme and its differences from the mammalian and insect forms. Eur. J. Biochem. 198:485, 1991.
220. Camardella, L., Caruso, C., Rutigliano, B., Romano, M., Di Prisco, G., and Descalzi-Cancedda, F.: Human erythrocyte glucose-6-phosphate dehydrogenase: Identification of a reactive lysyl residue labelled with pyridoxal 5'-phosphate. Eur. J. Biochem. 171:485, 1988.
221. Jeffery, J., Wood, I., Macleod, A., Jeffery, R., and Jörnvall, H.: Glucose-6-phosphate dehydrogenase. Characterization of a reactive lysine residue in the Pichia jadinii enzyme reveals a limited structural variation in a functionally significant segment. Biochem. Biophys. Res. Commun. 160:1290, 1989.
222. Jeffery, J., Hobbs, L., and Jörnvall, H.: Glucose-6-phosphate dehydrogenase from Saccharomyces cerevisiae: Characterization of a reactive lysine residue labeled with acetylsalicyclic acid. Biochemistry 24:666, 1985.
223. Bhadbhade, M. M., Adams, M. J., Flynn, T. G., and Levy, H. R.: Sequence identity between a lysine-containing peptide from Leuconostoc mesenteroides glucose-6-phosphate dehydrogenase and an active site peptide from human erythrocyte glucose-6-phosphate dehydrogenase. FEBS Lett. 211:243, 1987.
224. Persico, M. G., Viglietto, G., Martini, G., Dono, R., D'Urso, M., Toniolo, D., Vulliamy, T., and Luzzatto, L.: Analysis of the primary structure of human G 6 PD deduced from the cDNA sequence. In Yoshida, A., and Beutler, E., (eds.): Glucose-6-Phosphate Dehydrogenase. Orlando, Fla., Academic Press, 1986, pp. 503–516.
225. Persico, M. G., Viglietto, G., Martino, G., Toniolo, D., Paonessa, G., Moscatelli, C., Dono, R., Vulliamy, T., Luzzatto, L., and D'Urso, M.: Isolation of human glucose-6-phosphate dehydrogenase (G6PD) cDNA clones: Primary structure of the protein and unusual 5'-non-coding region. Nucleic Acids Res. 14:2511, 7822, 1986.
226. Martini, G., Toniolo, D., Vulliamy, T., Luzzatto, L., Dono, R., Viglietto, G., Paonessa, G., D'Urso, M., and Persico, M. G.: Structural analysis of the X-linked gene encoding human glucose-6-phosphate dehydrogenase. EMBO J. 5:1849, 1986.
227. Toniolo, D., Persico, M. G., Battistuzzi, G., and Luzzatto, L.: Partial purification and characterization of the messenger RNA for human glucose-6-phosphate dehydrogenase. Mol. Biol. Med. 2:89, 1984.
228. Takizawa, T., Huang, I. Y., Ikuta, T., and Yoshida, A.: Human glucose-6-phosphate dehydrogenase: Primary structure and cDNA cloning. Proc. Natl. Acad. Sci. USA 83:4157, 1986.
229. Chen, E. Y., Cheng, A., Lee, A., Kuang, W.-J., Hillier, L.,

Green, P., Schlessinger, D., Ciccodicola, A., and D'Urso, M.: Sequence of human glucose-6-phosphate dehydrogenase cloned in plasmids and a yeast artificial chromosome (YAC). Genomics 10:792, 1991.
230. Kanno, H., Huang, I.-Y., Kan, Y. W., and Yoshida, A.: Two structural genes on different chromosomes are required for encoding a single chain human red cell glucose-6-phosphate dehydrogenase subunit. Cell 58:595, 1989.
231. Beutler, E., Gelbart, T., and Kuhl, W.: Human red cell glucose-6-phosphate dehydrogenase: All active enzyme has sequence predicted by the X-chromosome encoded cDNA. Cell 62:7, 1990.
232. Henikoff, S., and Smith, J. M.: The human mRNA that provides the N-terminus of chimeric G6PD encodes GMP reductase. Cell 58:1021, 1989.
233. Mason, P. J., Bautista, J. M., Vulliamy, T. J., Turner, N., and Luzzatto, L.: Human red cell glucose-6-phosphate dehydrogenase is encoded only on the X chromosome. Cell 62:9, 1990.
234. Yoshida, A., and Kan, Y. W.: Origin of "fused" glucose-6-phosphate dehydrogenase. Cell 62:11, 1990.
235. Hirono, A., and Beutler, E.: Molecular cloning and nucleotide sequence of cDNA for human glucose-6-phosphate dehydrogenase variant A(−). Proc. Natl. Acad. Sci. USA 85:3951, 1988.
236. Hirono, A., and Beutler, E.: Alternative splicing of human glucose-6-phosphate dehydrogenase mRNA in different tissues. J. Clin. Invest. 83:343, 1989.
237. Toniolo, D., Martini, G., Migeon, B. R., and Dono, R.: Expression of the G6PD locus on the human X chromosome is associated with demethylation of three CpG islands within 100 kb of DNA. EMBO J. 7:401, 1988.
238. Toniolo, D., Filippi, M., Dono, R., Lettieri, T., and Martini, G.: The CpG island in the 5' region of the G6PD gene of man and mouse. Gene 102:197, 1991.
239. Ursini, M. V., Scalera, L., and Martini, G.: High levels of transcription driven by a 400 bp segment of the human G6PD promoter. Biochem. Biophys. Res. Commun. 170:1203, 1990.
240. Beutler, E., Kuhl, W., Gelbart, T., and Forman, L.: DNA sequence abnormalities of human glucose-6-phosphate dehydrogenase variants. J. Biol. Chem. 266:4145, 1991.
241. Poggi, V., Town, M., Foulkes, N. S., and Luzzatto, L.: Identification of a single base change in a new human mutant glucose-6-phosphate dehydrogenase gene by polymerase-chain-reaction amplification of the entire coding region from genomic DNA. Biochem. J. 271:157, 1990.
241a. Vulliamy, T., Beutler, E., and Luzzatto, L.: Variants of glucose-6-phosphate dehydrogenase are due to missense mutations spread throughout the coding region of the gene. Hum. Mut. (in press).
242. Chao, L., Du, C.-S., Louie, E., Zuo, L., Chen, E., Lubin, B., and Chiu, D. T. Y.: A to G substitution identified in exon 2 of the G6PD gene among G6PD deficient Chinese. Nucleic Acids Res. 19:6056, 1991.
243. MacDonald, D., Town, M., Mason, P., Vulliamy, T., Luzzatto, L., and Goff, D. K.: Deficiency in red blood cells. Nature 350:115, 1991.
244. Vulliamy, T. J., D'Urso, M., Battistuzzi, G., Estrada, M., Foulkes, N. S., Martini, G., Calabro, V., Poggi, V., Giordano, R., Town, M., Luzzatto, L., and Persico, M. G.: Diverse point mutations in the human glucose-6-phosphate dehydrogenase gene cause enzyme deficiency and mild or severe hemolytic anemia. Proc. Natl. Acad. Sci. USA 85:5171, 1988.
244a. Hirono, A., Fujii, H., and Miwa, S.: Molecular abnormality of G6PD Konan and G6PD Ube. Hum. Genet. (in press).
245. Takizawa, T., Yoneyama, Y., Miwa, S., and Yoshida, A.: A single nucleotide base transition is the basis of the common human glucose-6-phosphate dehydrogenase variant A(+). Genomics 1:228, 1987.
246. Vulliamy, T. J., Wanachiwanawin, W., Mason, P. J., and Luzzatto, L.: G6PD Mahidol, a common deficient variant in South East Asia is caused by a (163)glycine→serine mutation. Nucleic Acids Res. 17:5868, 1989.

247. Beutler, E., Kuhl, W., Sáenz, G. F., and Rodriguez, W.: Mutation analysis of G6PD variants in Costa Rica. Hum. Genet. 87:462, 1991.
248. Beutler, E., Westwood, B., Prchal, J., Vaca, G., Bartsocas, C. S., and Baronciani, L.: New G6PD mutations from various ethnic groups. Blood 80:255, 1992.
249. Beutler, E., Prchal, J. T., Westwood, B., and Kuhl W.: Definition of the mutations of G6PD Wayne, G6PD Viangchan, G6PD Jammu and G6PD "LeJeune." Acta Haematol. (Basel) 86:179, 1991.
249a. Hirono, A., Fujii, H., Hirono, K., Kanno, H., and Miwa, S.: Molecular abnormality of a Japanese glucose-6-phosphate dehydrogenase variant (G6PD Tokyo) associated with hereditary non-spherocytic hemolytic anemia. Hum. Genet. 88:347, 1992.
250. Beutler, E., Westwood, B., Kuhl, W., and Hsia, Y. E.: G6PD variants in Hawaii. Hum. Hered. 42:327, 1992.
251. De Vita, G., Alcalay, M., Sampietro, M., Cappellini, M. D., Fiorelli, G., and Toniolo, D.: Two point mutations are responsible for G6PD polymorphism in Sardinia. Am. J. Hum. Genet. 44:233, 1989.
252. Viglietto, G., Montanaro, V., Calabrò, V., Vallone, D., D'Urso, M., Persico, M. G., and Battistuzzi, G.: Common glucose-6-phosphate dehydrogenase (G6PD) variants from the Italian population: Biochemical and molecular characterization. Ann. Hum. Genet. 54:1, 1990.
253. Vives-Corrons, J.-L., Kuhl, W., Pujades, M. A., and Beutler, E.: Molecular genetics of G6PD Mediterranean variant and description of a new G6PD mutant, G6PD Andalus[1361A]. Am. J. Hum. Genet. 47:575, 1990.
254. Zuo, L., Chen, E., Du, C. S., Chang, C. N., and Chiu, D. T. Y.: Genetic study of Chinese G6PD variants by direct PCR sequencing. Blood (Suppl.)76:51a, 1990.
255. Beutler, E., Kuhl, W., Ramirez, E., and Lisker, R.: Some Mexican glucose-6-phosphate dehydrogenase (G-6-PD) variants revisited. Hum. Genet. 86:371, 1991.
256. Beutler, E., Kuhl, W., Vives-Corrons, J.-L., and Prchal, J. T.: Molecular heterogeneity of G6PD A−. Blood 74:2550, 1989.
257. Fiorelli, G., Anghinelli, L., Carandina, G., Toniolo, D., Sempietro, M., Cappellini, M. D., and Pareti, F. I.: Point mutations in two G6PD variants previously described in Italy. Blood (Suppl.)76:7a, 1990.
258. Beutler, E., and Kuhl, W.: The NT 1311 polymorphism of G6PD: G6PD Mediterranean mutation may have originated independently in Europe and Asia. Am. J. Hum. Genet. 47:1008, 1990.
259. Ninfali, P., Bresolin, N., Baronciani, L., Fortunato, F., Comi, G., Magnani, M., and Scarlato, G.: Glucose-6-phosphate dehydrogenase Lodi[844C]: A study on its expression in blood cells and muscle. Enzyme 45:180, 1991.
260. Stevens, D. J., Wanachiwanawin, W., Mason, P. J., Vulliamy, T. J., and Luzzatto, L.: G6PD Canton, a common deficient variant in South East Asia caused by a 459 Arg→Leu mutation. Nucleic Acids Res. 18:7190, 1990.
261. Nakashima, K., Miwa, S., Oda, S., Tanaka, T., Imamura, K., and Nishina T.: Electrophoretic and kinetic studies of mutant erythrocyte pyruvate kinases. Blood 43:537, 1974.
262. Kahn, A., Marie, J., Galand, C., and Boivin, P.: Chronic haemolytic anaemia in two patients heterozygous for erythrocyte pyruvate kinase deficiency. Scand. J. Haematol. 16:250, 1976.
263. Imamura, K., Tanaka, T., Nishina, T., Nakashima, K., and Miwa, S.: Studies on pyruvate kinase (PK) deficiency II. Electrophoretic, kinetic, and immunological studies on pyruvate kinase of erythrocytes and other tissues. J. Biochem. (Tokyo) 74:1165, 1973.
264. Noguchi, T., Yamada, K., Inoue, H., Matsuda, T., and Tanaka, T.: The L- and R-type isozymes of rat pyruvate kinase are produced from a single gene by use of different promoters. J. Biol. Chem. 262:14366, 1987.
265. Kechemir, D., Max-Audit, I., and Rosa, R.: Comparative study of human M_2-type pyruvate kinases isolated from human leukocytes and erythrocytes of a patient with red cell pyruvate kinase hyperactivity. Enzyme 41:121, 1989.

266. Chern, C. J., and Beutler, E.: Pyridoxal kinase: Decreased activity in red blood cells of Afro-Americans. Science 187:1084, 1975.
267. Martin, S. K., Miller, L. H., Kark, J. A., Hicks, C. U., Okoye, V. C., and Esan, G. J. F.: Low erythrocyte pyridoxal-kinase activity in blacks: Its possible relation to falciparum malaria. Lancet 1:466, 1978.
268. Tedesco, T. A., Bonow, R., Miller, K., and Mellman, W. J.: Galactokinase: Evidence for a new racial polymorphism. Science 178:176, 1972.
269. Beutler, E., Baluda, M. C., Sturgeon, P., and Day, R. W.: The genetics of galactose-1-phosphate uridyl transferase deficiency. J. Lab. Clin. Med. 68:646, 1966.
270. Beutler, E., Baluda, M. C., Sturgeon, P., and Day, R.: A new genetic abnormality resulting in galactose-1-phosphate uridyltransferase deficiency. Lancet 1:353, 1965.
271. Mohrenweiser, H. W.: Functional hemizygosity in the human genome: Direct estimate from twelve erythrocyte enzyme loci. Hum. Genet. 77:241, 1987.
272. Blume, K. G., Löhr, G. W., Praetsch, O., and Rüdiger, H. W.: Beitrag zur Populationsgenetik der Pyruvatkinase menschlisher Erythrocyten. Humangenetik 6:261, 1968.
273. Wu, Z.-L., Yu, W.-D., and Chen, S.-C.: Frequency of erythrocyte pyruvate kinase deficiency in Chinese infants. Am. J. Hematol. 20:139, 1985.
274. Fung, R. H. P., Keung, Y. K., and Chung, G. S. H.: Screening of pyruvate kinase deficiency and G6PD deficiency in Chinese newborn in Hong Kong. Arch. Dis. Child. 44:373, 1969.
275. Karadsheh, N. S.: Pyruvate kinase and glucose-6-phosphate dehydrogenase deficiencies in Jordan. Dirasat 12:75, 1985.
276. Tanaka, K. R., and Paglia, D. E.: Pyruvate kinase deficiency. Semin. Hematol. 8:367, 1971.
277. Srivastava, S. K., Villacorte, D., and Beutler, E.: Correlation between adenylate metabolizing enzymes and adenine nucleotide levels of erythrocytes during blood storage in various media. Transfusion 12:190, 1972.
278. Mohrenweiser, H. W., and Neel, J. V.: Frequency of thermostability variants: Estimation of total "rare" variant frequency in human populations. Proc. Natl. Acad. Sci. USA 78:5729, 1981.
279. Mohrenweiser, H. W.: Frequency of enzyme deficiency variants in erythrocytes of newborn infants. Proc. Natl. Acad. Sci. USA 78:5046, 1981.
280. Carson, P. E.: Glucose-6-phosphate dehydrogenase deficiency in hemolytic anemia. Fed. Proc. 19:995, 1960.
281. Allison, A. C.: Glucose-6-phosphate dehydrogenase deficiency in red blood cells of East Africans. Nature 186:531, 1960.
282. Allison, A. C., and Clyde, D. F.: Malaria and glucose-6-phosphate dehydrogenase. Br. Med. J. 2:521, 1961.
283. Motulsky, A. G.: Glucose-6-phosphate dehydrogenase deficiency haemolytic disease of the newborn, and malaria. Lancet 1:1168, 1961.
284. Powell, R., Brewer, G. J., De Gowin, R., and Carson, P.: Effects of glucose-6-phosphate dehydrogenase deficiency upon the host and upon host-drug-malaria parasite interactions. Milit. Med. 131:1039, 1966.
285. Livingstone, F. B.: Malaria and human polymorphisms. Annu. Rev. Genet. 5:33, 1971.
286. Martin, S. K., Miller, L. H., Alling, D., Okoye, V. C., Esan, G. J. F., Osunkoya, B. O., and Deane, M.: Severe malaria and glucose-6-phosphate-dehydrogenase deficiency: A reappraisal of the malaria/G-6-PD hypothesis. Lancet 1:524, 1979.
287. Bernstein, S. C., Bowman, J. E., and Noche, L. K.: Population studies in Cameroon. Hum. Hered. 30:251, 1980.
288. Bienzle, U., Lucas, A. O., Ayeni, O., and Luzzatto, L.: Glucose-6-phosphate dehydrogenase and malaria. Greater resistance of females heterozygous for enzyme deficiency and of males with non-deficient variant. Lancet 1:107, 1972.
289. Luzzatto, L., Usanga, E. A., and Reddy, S.: Glucose 6-phosphate dehydrogenase deficient red cells: Resistance to infection by malarial parasites. Science 164:839, 1969.
290. Beutler, E., Yeh, M., and Fairbanks, V. F.: The normal human

female as a mosaic of X-chromosome activity: Studies using the gene for G-6-PD deficiency as a marker. Proc. Natl. Acad. Sci. USA 48:9, 1962.

291. Roth, E. F., Jr., Raventos-Suarez, C., Rinaldi, A., and Nagel, R. L.: Glucose-6-phosphate dehydrogenase deficiency inhibits in vitro growth of *Plasmodium falciparum*. Proc. Natl. Acad. Sci. USA 80:298, 1983.

292. Usanga, E. A., and Luzzatto, L.: Adaptation of *Plasmodium falciparum* to glucose 6-phosphate dehydrogenase–deficient host red cells by production of parasite-encoded enzyme. Nature 313:793, 1985.

293. Roth, E., Jr., and Schulman, S.: The adaptation of *Plasmodium falciparum* to oxidative stress in G6PD deficient human erythrocytes. Br. J. Haematol. 70:363, 1988.

294. Luzzatto, L., O'Brien, S., Usanga, E., and Wanachiwanawin, W.: Origin of G6PD polymorphism: Malaria and G6PD deficiency. *In* Yoshida, A., and Beutler, E. (eds.): Glucose-6-Phosphate Dehydrogenase. Orlando, Fla., Academic Press, 1986, pp. 181–193.

295. Kurdi-Haidar, B., and Luzzatto, L.: Expression and characterization of glucose-6-phosphate dehydrogenase of *Plasmodium falciparum*. Mol. Biochem. Parasitol. 41:83, 1990.

296. Betke, K., Beutler, E., Brewer, G. J., Kirkman, H. N., Luzzatto, L., Motulsky, A. G., Ramot, B., and Siniscalco, M.: Standardization of procedures for the study of glucose-6-phosphate dehydrogenase. Report of a WHO scientific group. WHO Tech. Rep. Ser. No. 366, 1967.

297. Beutler, E., and Yoshida, A.: Genetic variation of glucose-6-phosphate dehydrogenase: A catalog and future prospects. Medicine (Baltimore) 67:311, 1988.

298. Fairbanks, V. F., Nepo, A. G., Beutler, E., Dickson, E. R., and Honig, G.: Glucose-6-phosphate dehydrogenase variants: Reexamination of G6PD Chicago and Cornell and a new variant (G6PD Pea Ridge) resembling G6PD Chicago. Blood 55:216, 1980.

299. Porter, I. H., Boyer, S. H., Watson-Williams, E. J., Adam, A., Szeinberg, A., and Siniscalco, M.: Variation of glucose-6-phosphate dehydrogenase in different populations. Lancet 1:895, 1964.

300. Luzzatto, L., and Allan, N. C.: Different properties of glucose-6-phosphate dehydrogenase from human erythrocytes with normal and abnormal enzyme levels. Biochem. Biophys. Res. Commun. 21:547, 1965.

301. Yoshida, A.: A single amino acid substitution (asparagine to aspartic acid) between normal (B+) and the common negro variant (A+) of human glucose-6-phosphate dehydrogenase. Proc. Natl. Acad. Sci. USA 57:835, 1967.

302. Beutler, E., Lisker, R., and Kuhl, W.: Molecular biology of G6PD variants. Biomed. Biochim. Acta 49:236, 1990.

303. Beutler, E., and Kuhl, W.: Linkage between a PvuII restriction fragment length polymorphism and G6PD A$-^{202A/376G}$: Evidence for a single origin of the common G6PD A− mutation. Hum. Genet. 85:9, 1990.

304. Vulliamy, T. J., Othman, A., Town, M., Nathwani, A., Falusi, A. G., Mason, P. J., and Luzzatto, L.: Polymorphic sites in the African population detected by sequence analysis of the glucose-6-phosphate dehydrogenase gene outline the evolution of the variants A and A−. Proc. Natl. Acad. Sci. USA 88:8568, 1991.

305. Kay, A. C., Kuhl, W., Prchal, J. T., and Beutler, E.: The origin of G6PD polymorphisms in Afro-Americans. Am. J. Hum. Genet. 50:394, 1992.

306. Beutler, E.: Glucose-6-phosphate dehydrogenase: New perspectives. Blood 73:1397, 1989.

307. Town, M., Bautista, J. M., Mason, P. J., and Luzzatto, L.: Both mutations in G6PD A− are necessary to produce the G6PD deficient phenotype. Hum. Mol. Genet. 1:171, 1992.

Molecular Mechanisms of Iron Metabolism

Joe B. Harford, Tracey A. Rouault, Helmut A. Huebers, and Richard D. Klausner

INTRODUCTION

Iron is essential to virtually all life forms but is highly toxic when present in excess. Consequently, a variety of mechanisms exist to allow diverse organisms to obtain iron from the environment, to regulate their content of iron, and to maintain iron intracellularly in a non-toxic state.[1-5] Iron is utilized in a large number of critical enzymatic reactions, especially those in which electron transfer occurs. Enzymes contain iron either in the porphyrin ring structure of heme or as a variety of non-heme forms, such as iron-sulfur clusters. Heme (iron protoporphyrin) is the prosthetic group found on enzymes required for oxidative phosphorylation, on enzymes involved in splitting hydrogen peroxide, and on other enzymes associated with detoxification of chemical agents or drugs. Heme also serves as a functional group for the binding of oxygen by hemoglobin and myoglobin, which together represent the repository for most of the body's total iron. Iron-sulfur clusters are contained in a number of critical cellular enzymes. Representative of these is the Krebs cycle enzyme aconitase. In addition, there exist a number of cellular enzymes that contain neither heme nor an iron-sulfur cluster but that nonetheless either contain bound iron or require iron for activity. Notable in this group is the enzyme ribonucleotide reductase, which catalyzes the rate-limiting step in DNA replication needed for cell division.

IRON ACQUISITION BY MICROORGANISMS

Because of the myriad of important reactions in which iron participates, living organisms require a mechanism for assimilation to avoid the ill effects of iron deficiency. Although iron is the fourth most abundant element and the second most abundant metal in the earth's crust, it exists virtually entirely in the highly insoluble, oxidized ferric form rather than in the more soluble, reduced ferrous form. Organisms from archaebacteria to man possess means of acquiring iron from their environment despite its insolubility. For example, many plants actively acidify the soil around their roots. This acidification has the effect of increasing the bioavailability of iron, since ferric iron is considerably more soluble at lower pH. Many plants and certain unicellular organisms secrete iron-binding proteins called siderophores (Fig. 10–1). These relatively complex organic molecules that chelate iron are chemically derived from either phenol catechols or hydroxamic acid.[4–6] Siderophores are synthesized by enzymatic mechanisms and secreted. Their very high affinity for ferric iron facilitates formation of iron-chelate complexes despite the very low concentration of soluble ferric iron in the extracellular milieu. The iron-siderophore complexes are generally taken up by the microorganism via a specific membrane receptor. In organisms employing this strategy, the proteins involved in iron acquisition are the enzymes required for synthesis of the siderophore and the membrane receptor for the iron-siderophore complex. Once inside the cell, the complex is broken down, with release of iron for metabolic uses. In *Escherichia coli* the genes for these proteins are part of a single operon, present on a virulence plasmid (Fig. 10–1). Expression of operon genes is under the control of a regulatory molecule called "fur" that represses transcription when iron is bound to the fur molecule.[7, 8] Under conditions of low intracellular iron, the repressor is relatively inactive, and expression of the operon leads to synthesis of both the siderophore (known as aerobactin) and the siderophore receptor. As the iron level is increased, active repressor accumulates, and the operon is turned off.

An alternative strategy for iron solubilization and acquisition is used by yeast, including *Saccharomyces cerevisiae*. Yeast lack siderophores, but they absorb iron without difficulty. *S. cerevisiae* accomplish this absorption by expressing a membrane ferric reductase.[9, 10] This activity utilizes electron donors (e.g., NADH or NADPH) in the cytoplasm to reduce extracellular ferric iron. Once reduced, the iron is transported into cells via a ferrous transport system (Fig. 10–2). The gene encoding the membrane-associated ferric reductase of *S. cerevisiae* has been molecularly cloned and sequenced, and this activity has been shown to be involved in the intracellular uptake of iron.[9] The yeast reductase has limited sequence similarity to a subunit of the respiratory burst oxidase of mammalian neutrophils.[10] It is interesting that the respiratory burst oxidase catalyzes single-electron transport across a lipid bilayer from cytoplasmic reducing equivalents, with molecular oxygen being the electron acceptor.

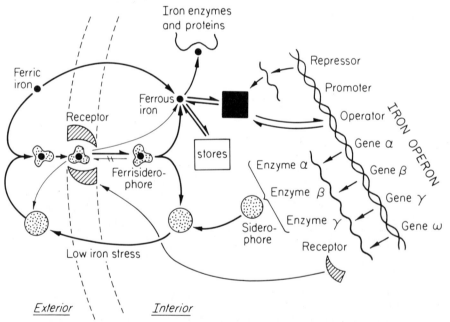

FIGURE 10–1. Iron metabolism in bacteria. *Escherichia coli* organisms synthesize and secrete a siderophore (termed aerobactin). Siderophores are low molecular weight chelators that bind extracellular iron. The siderophore-iron complex is recognized by a specific receptor that mediates passage through the plasma membrane. Once inside the cell, the complex is degraded and iron is released for utilization. A single operon encodes the siderophore receptor and enzymes involved in siderophore synthesis (here denoted m). The operon may be either on a plasmid or integrated into the bacterial genome. Binding of iron to the repressor protein (termed "fur" and depicted as the black square) increases its affinity for the operator, leading to decreased transcription of the genes of the operon. In conditions of iron deficiency, the repressor is released, and transcription of the operon gene products is increased, with the end result being greater iron uptake via the siderophore-receptor system. (Adapted with permission from Lewin, R.: How microorganisms transport iron. Science 225:401; 1984. Copyright 1984 by the American Association for the Advancement of Science.)

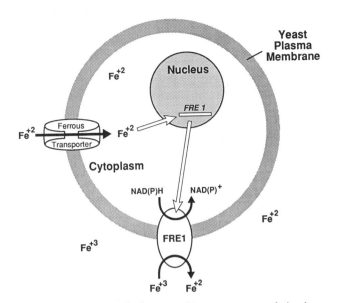

FIGURE 10–2. Iron uptake by yeast. Yeast express on their plasma membranes a ferric iron reductase termed FRE1 and a transport system for ferrous iron. Yeast lacking the FRE1 gene product do not grow well in iron-deficient media. Iron availability controls the expression of the FRE1 gene at the level of transcription with much less FRE1 mRNA expression when iron is abundant. FRE1 achieves electron transport from a cytoplasmic electron donor (probably NADPH or NADH). FRE1 has sequence similarity to the mammalian electron transporter involved in the oxidative burst of neutrophils. (Adapted from Dancis, A., et al.: Genetic evidence that ferric reductase is required for iron uptake in *Saccharomyces cerevisiae*. Mol. Cell. Biol. 10: 29, 1990; and Dancis, A., et al.: Ferric reductase of *Saccharomyces cerevisiae*: Molecular characterization, role in iron uptake, and transcriptional control by iron. Proc. Natl. Acad. Sci. 89:3869, 1992; with permission.)

The ferric reductase of yeast is envisioned as being a related activity, with ferric iron as the electron acceptor. The transporter of ferrous iron in yeast awaits molecular characterization.

As will become evident, higher eukaryotes utilize mechanisms for iron acquisition that are variations on the two strategies for iron acquisition by microorganisms outlined above. Plasma transferrin (Tf) serves as the functional equivalent of a siderophore in that it binds and solubilizes extracellular ferric iron. It differs, of course, in that it is a large protein rather than a small organic compound. But like the siderophores, Tf is recognized by a specific cell surface receptor and internalized. Once inside the cell, iron is released for utilization. Higher eukaryotes also appear to utilize the ferric reduction/ferrous transport strategy. This is thought to be at least one of the means by which dietary iron is moved across the gut mucosal cells and into the plasma. It may also be the way in which iron taken into cells via the transferrin receptor (TfR) is moved from the endocytic compartment into the cytoplasm.

THE BODY'S IRON ECONOMY

To date, four major proteins with roles in the iron homeostasis of higher eukaryotes have been charac-

terized. Human iron metabolism is discussed in this chapter in the context of the functions of these four proteins. As mentioned above, vertebrates absorb iron and utilize the protein carrier Tf for transport of iron in the circulation in a soluble state. The TfR, a specific membrane protein with high affinity for ferric Tf, is used to get iron into most cells. The cytoplasmic protein ferritin is used for intracellular sequestration of iron in a non-toxic form, thus providing both protection from the propensity of free iron to engage in oxidative damage to components of the cell and a source of usable intracellular iron. Controlling the expression of ferritin and the TfR is an RNA-binding protein, the iron-responsive element–binding protein (IRE-BP) which is itself an iron-sulfur protein. The IRE-BP appears to serve as the means by which eukaryotic cells sense changes in the availability of iron.

In humans, the amount of iron in the body is regulated by control of iron absorption.[11] Factors that determine the level of iron absorption include the amount of iron in the diet, the content of the diet, and the dietary form of iron (heme versus non-heme).[12] The average American diet contains 15 mg of iron per day, of which approximately 3 mg is taken into cells of the duodenum and proximal jejunum, with about 1 mg finding its way into the plasma (Fig. 10–3). The daily requirement for iron increases dramatically during pregnancy, with approximately 5 mg/day being transferred to the fetus via the placenta.[13] Regulation of the intestinal transfer of iron to the plasma depends on the existing level of iron stores and the rate of erythropoiesis (iron absorption is enhanced in certain disease states characterized by ineffective erythropoiesis).[14–16] Iron excretion is limited to obligatory losses occurring as a consequence of the shedding of epithelial cells from the intestinal and urinary tracts and from the skin and small amounts of intestinal bleeding. No regulatory mechanism seems to exist for the excretion of iron. Essential to the economy of iron is the recycling process whereby erythrocyte iron is reutilized for synthesis of new hemoglobin[16] (Fig. 10–3). Tf, a serum protein to which iron is bound in the ferric form, has a central role in this cycling process. Although only 3 to 5 mg of iron is associated with Tf in the plasma of a normal adult individual, the flux through this pool is 30 to 35 mg/day, of which approximately 1 mg is derived by absorption and the remainder by reutilization.

Approximately 80 to 90 per cent of the iron traffic borne by Tf is destined for hemoglobin synthesis.[1, 16] Although this movement of iron from erythroid precursors to the circulation within red cells and later to reticuloendothelial (RE) cells constitutes the major portion of erythroid iron turnover, some red cell iron short-circuits the circulating red cell mass.[1, 17] In the process of hemoglobin formation, some erythrocyte iron is deposited as ferritin and subsequently is removed from the red cell and processed by the RE cells of the marrow or spleen. A small fraction of hemoglobin combines with haptoglobin in the plasma and is cleared by hepatocytes.[18, 19] These various red cell

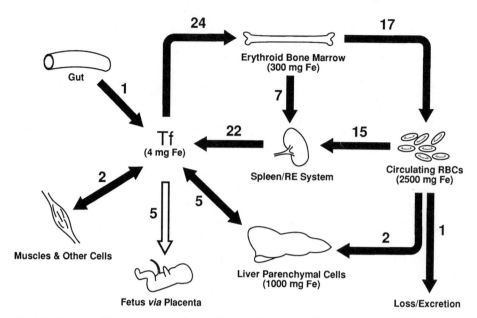

FIGURE 10–3. Pathways of human iron exchange. Dietary iron enters from the gut and is incorporated into plasma transferrin (Tf). Tf iron is the source of iron for the erythroid bone marrow and other dividing cells (and is delivered to the fetus via the placenta). Effete red blood cells (RBCs) are catabolized by the reticuloendothelial (RE) system. Some RBC iron is processed as free hemoglobin by the liver, and the liver is the primary source of Tf synthesis. Iron is lost from the body by incidental bleeding as well as through loss of skin cells and hair. Numbers on the arrows of the figure represent amounts of iron, in milligrams per day, involved in the traffic in iron. Numbers in parentheses are the approximate total iron stores of the indicated tissues. Iron that is taken into gut mucosal cells but lost via sloughing of these cells without making it into the plasma is not considered absorbed iron. (Adapted from Bothwell, T. H., Charlton, R. W., Cook, J. D., and Finch, C. A.: Iron Metabolism in Man. Oxford, England, Blackwell Scientific Publications, 1979; with permission.)

pathways are subject to change with expansion or contraction of the red cell marrow and particularly with ineffective erythropoiesis of hemolysis or both.

Cellular uptake of iron in dividing cells of higher eukaryotes is mediated largely or exclusively by the interaction of Tf with a membrane receptor protein, the TfR. The ligand-receptor complex is endocytosed, and iron is released into the cell. Iron enters a soluble "chelatable" pool where it is partitioned between utilization for synthesis of essential cellular iron-containing constituents and deposition in ferritin as a nontoxic form (Fig. 10–4). Another form of intracellular iron is hemosiderin, an amorphous, insoluble aggregate of iron oxide and organic constituents that is thought to be a partially degraded form of ferritin.

Some insight into the physiology and pathophysiology of iron exchange is provided by the distribution of iron stores. In the normal adult, about two thirds of reserve iron is in RE cells and about one third is in hepatocytes. RE cells occupy the most prominent position, supplying perhaps two thirds of iron passing through the plasma. Within the RE cell, there is a constantly changing distribution of iron processed from effete red cells between storage and return of iron to Tf.[20, 21] When more iron is required for red cell production, an increased amount of iron is returned to Tf, and in addition, storage iron is mobilized. The liver represents a major repository of body iron. Hepatocytes appear to be capable of iron uptake

by several distinct mechanisms, including the TfR, receptors for ferritin and for hemoglobin-haptoglobin, and uptake of lower molecular weight non–Tf-bound iron (NTBI). The interplay between these mechanisms in liver iron metabolism remains the subject of much debate. Historically, consideration of human iron metabolism has focused on the critical roles of Tf, the TfR, and ferritin. Much is known about the genes and structure of these proteins and how they interact to make iron available to the cell while protecting the cell from the inherent toxicity of ferric iron.

TRANSFERRIN

Our discussion focuses on serum Tf, but it is worth noting that this protein is part of a larger family. In addition to serum Tf, this family includes ovotransferrin, which is found in bird and reptile egg white[22]; lactoferrin, which is present in extracellular secretions (predominantly milk) and in neutrophils[23–26]; p97, a membrane protein discovered on human melanoma cells[27]; and B-lym, a transforming protein found in chicken B-cell lymphoma.[28] Although these proteins are related in sequence, their functions appear to be quite diverse. Human serum Tf is a single polypeptide chain glycoprotein with a molecular weight of 75,000 to 80,000.[29–32] One reason for having a macromolecular binder of iron rather than a low molecular weight

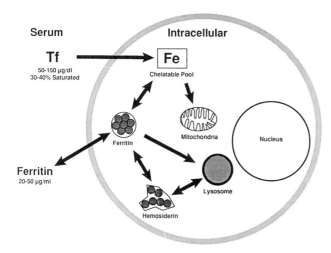

FIGURE 10–4. Cellular iron pools in normal individuals. From serum, transferrin (Tf) iron enters the cell via the transferrin receptor (see Fig. 10–11) and is transferred to a chelatable intracellular pool. Iron in the intracellular pool is utilized for the metabolic needs of cells (e.g., mitochondrial cytochromes) or incorporated into ferritin. Iron can be remobilized from ferritin, or the ferritin can be partially degraded to form hemosiderin, some of which may be seen in lysosomes. Small amounts of ferritin reach the serum by unknown means. Serum ferritin has a low iron content, but nonetheless the level of serum ferritin protein serves as an index of total body iron stores.

siderophore is that the larger size of Tf contributes to whole body iron retention, preventing loss in urine via kidney glomerular filtration. Tf consists of N-terminal and C-terminal domains, each of which has an iron-binding site. The two domains are partially homologous at the amino acid sequence level. Analysis of protein structure led to the suggestion that the two domains reflect a gene duplication event.

The Transferrin Gene

Complementary DNAs (cDNAs) for human Tf have been identified and sequenced,[33, 34] verifying the protein's structure as determined by biochemical techniques.[30] These cDNA clones have been used to iden-

tify genomic clones containing the human Tf gene.[35, 36] Fifteen exons have been characterized; two additional exons are thought to exist based on protein structure and analogy to the ovotransferrin gene (Fig. 10–5). The 15 exons are distributed over 30 kilobases (kb) of genomic DNA.

Analysis of gene structure has provided strong support for a gene duplication event in the evolution of Tf. Seven pairs of homologous exons can be identified from the N-terminal and C-terminal domains. These exons resemble each other by a 50 to 56 per cent sequence identity at both the amino acid and the nucleotide levels and by virtue of very similar size and preservation of splicing junctions. The gene is thought to have arisen by duplication, as depicted in Figure 10–6, with subsequent mutations resulting in diversity of exon structure and intron length characteristic of the two halves of the human Tf gene. The Tf gene has been mapped to the distal portion of the long arm of chromosome 3 (3q21→3qter).[37]

Transferrin Structure and Function

The Tf polypeptide has 679 amino acids.[31, 33, 34, 38] By weight it consists of 6 per cent carbohydrate[29, 30] present as branched structures joined by N-glycosidic linkages to asparagine residues 415 and 608, both of which are in the C-terminal domain of the protein.[30] X-ray crystallographic studies have verified that the protein folds into two domains, each of which contains an iron-binding site. There are 19 disulfide bridges in human Tf, 8 in the N-terminal domain and 11 in the C-terminal domain. Several of the disulfide bridges are positioned identically in the two domains of the protein and are also phylogenetically invariant.[39] A model of the three-dimensional structure showing the disulfide bridges and the two domains of the protein is given in Figure 10–7. A number of genetic variants of human Tf have been characterized: The most common is TfD1, in which there is a single amino acid substitution (Asp→Gly) at position 277.[29, 40] No functional significance of this or other substitutions has been established.

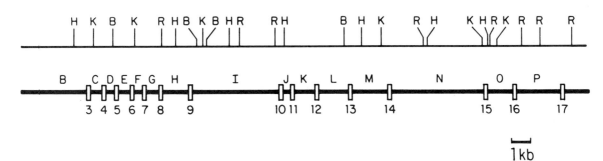

FIGURE 10–5. Structure of the Tf gene. The human Tf gene is located on chromosome 3. Exons are numbered, and introns are designated by a capital letter. The most 5′ exons shown here are inferred from the structure of the Tf protein and by comparison with the ovotransferrin gene. (Adapted from Schaeffer, E., Park, I., Cohen, G. N., and Zakin, M. M.: Organization of the human serum transferrin gene. *In* Spik, G., Montreuil, J., Crichton, R. R., and Mazurier, J. [eds.]: Structure and Function of Transferrins. New York, Elsevier, 1985, p. 361; with permission.)

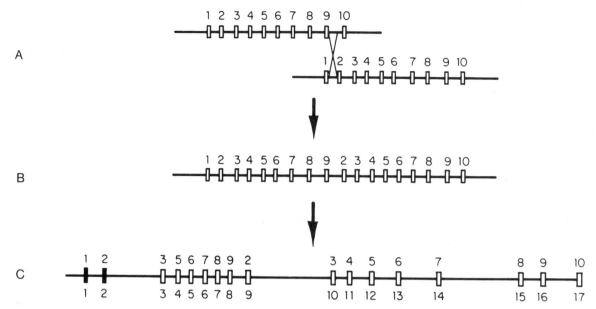

FIGURE 10–6. Possible gene duplication that produced the Tf gene in higher organisms. *A*, Unequal crossover between two primordial Tf genes by which several of the exons and introns are duplicated. *B*, The initial product of the cross-over event. *C*, Structure of the human Tf gene. Note that although the exon lengths and general arrangement of exons and introns are similar in the two halves of the human Tf gene, the lengths of introns are more variable. (Adapted from Schaeffer, E., Park, I., Cohen, G. N., and Zakin, M. M.: Organization of the human serum transferrin gene. *In* Spik, G., Montreuil, J., Crichton, R. R., and Mazurier, J. [eds.]: Structure and Function of Transferrins. New York, Elsevier, 1985, p. 361; with permission.)

The sites of interaction of iron with the protein have been deduced from spectroscopic, chemical modification, and sequence data.[41] Binding of iron to Tf is accompanied by binding of an anion, physiologically

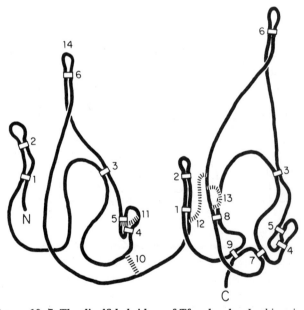

FIGURE 10–7. The disulfide bridges of Tf molecules. In this string model of the Tf protein, the positions of disulfide bonds that are common to human and chicken Tf molecules are shown as open boxes. The four disulfide bridges found in human Tf that are not in the chicken molecule are indicated by the hatched lines. (Adapted from Williams, J.: The evolution of transferrin. Trends Biol. Sci. 2:394, 1982; with permission.)

carbonate or bicarbonate. The protein's three-dimensional folding provides a pocket in which the metal- and anion-binding residues reside (Fig. 10–8). The anion is thought to interact at arginine 124. Initial binding of the iron may occur through tyrosine residues 185 and 188, with subsequent metal interaction with histidines 207 and 249. Conformational changes in the protein may be induced as a consequence of iron binding and formation of these interactions. Binding of iron is associated with the release of several protons.

Although Tf has a very high affinity for ferric iron ($K_a \sim 10^{-20}$ M), its affinity for ferrous iron is much less.[42] Release of ferric iron from Tf occurs predominantly, if not exclusively, in the intracellular environment. At least five mechanisms have been proposed as participating in the release of ferric iron from the protein: (1) protonation of the protein's iron-binding ligands, (2) reduction of bound ferric iron to ferrous iron, (3) a primary attack on the anion, (4) competition between Tf and a strong chelator, and (5) an influence on iron binding by the binding of ferric Tf to the TfR.

The presence of two iron-binding sites on Tf has led to the hypothesis that the two might function differently. Evidence of non-homogeneous behavior has been presented that indicates that one Tf metal-binding site transfers iron preferentially to reticulocytes, whereas the other site was thought to be specific for non-erythroid tissues.[43] Other evidence has indicated that the two monoferric Tf molecules with iron bound to either the N-terminal or the C-terminal

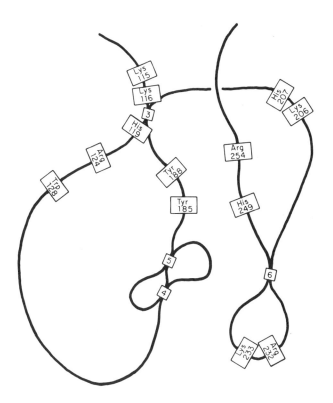

FIGURE 10–8. **Proposed iron- and anion-binding sites in the N-terminal domain of human Tf.** Iron is thought to bind to tyrosines 185 and 188 and to two of the three histidines found at 119, 206, and 207. Arginine 124 represents the probable site of anion binding. Four disulfide bonds (boxes 3 to 6) are similarly indicated in Figure 10–7. (Adapted from Chasteen, N. D.: The identification of the probable locus of iron and anion binding in the transferrins. Trends Biol. Sci. 2:272, 1983; with permission.)

domain are similar, if not identical, in their rate of iron delivery to cells, although there is a strong preference in binding for diferric Tf.[44, 45] Recently, it has been demonstrated that association with the TfR influences differentially the affinities of the two Tf iron sites within the acidic environment of the endosomal compartment.[46, 47]

Synthesis and Degradation of Transferrin

Most or all of serum Tf is synthesized in the liver.[48] Lymphocytes, Sertoli cells, and cells in the muscle, brain, and mammary gland also have the capacity for Tf synthesis.[49–51] Whether Tf synthesized in these sites functions locally or is secreted is unknown. The rate of Tf synthesis may be modulated by iron level.[52, 53] Although variations in Tf concentration are observed in disease states such as iron deficiency or various inflammatory conditions, the molecular basis of these variations has not been elucidated. The Tf protein has a half-life of 7 to 10 days,[54] in contrast to the half-life of Tf-bound iron, which is only 2 hours, indicating that Tf may be used to deliver iron about 100 times in its life time. Clearance and degradation of desialiated Tf molecules can occur via the asialoglycopro-

tein receptor of hepatocytes,[55, 56] although it is not known whether this is the physiologically relevant degradative pathway.

THE TRANSFERRIN RECEPTOR

The polypeptide that forms the TfR is a 760 amino acid glycoprotein of molecular weight approximately 90,000.[57–64] Carbohydrate represents 5 per cent by weight and is distributed in three N-linked oligosaccharide chains. The functional TfR is composed of two identical, disulfide-linked polypeptides (Fig. 10–9). Each chain has an N-terminal cytoplasmic domain of 61 amino acids and an extracellular segment of 671 residues. The transmembrane domain of the TfR is 28 amino acids located at residues 62 to 89. The TfR polypeptide lacks an N-terminal leader sequence.[59–61] It resembles the asialoglycoprotein receptor in having the majority of its C-terminal segment as an external domain. Integration into the membrane is thought to occur via the hydrophobic transmembrane segment that functions as an internal signal peptide.[65] The mature receptor contains covalently bound fatty acid,[66] which might also have a role in its integration into the membrane. Serine residues within the N-terminal segment may be phosphorylated.[57] It is not yet clear what functional significance, if any, is associated with posttranslational modification of the TfR.[64] Analysis of the cDNA sequence has indicated that the TfR lacks similarity to other proteins involved in iron metabolism, including Tf.[59, 61] Limited sequence similarity exists between the TfR and the mouse epidermal growth factor (EGF) precursor. The region of relatedness

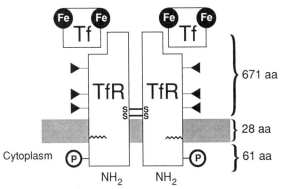

FIGURE 10–9. **Structure and orientation in the plasma membrane of the transferrin receptor (TfR).** The TfR is depicted as a disulfide-linked homodimer with two molecules of diferric Tf bound. The amino-terminus of each polypeptide is oriented toward the cytoplasm. The intracellular domain contains a site for phosphorylation by protein kinase C. There is also a site for covalently bound fatty acid (depicted as a squiggle in the membrane-spanning domain). In addition to the ligand-binding domain, the extracellular portion of each polypeptide contains sites for the addition of three N-linked carbohydrate chains (depicted as triangles). (Adapted from Harford, J. B., Casey, J. L., Koeller, D. M., and Klausner, R. D.: Structure, function, and regulation of the transferrin receptor: Insights from molecular biology. *In* Steer, C. J., and Hanover, J. A. [eds.]: Intracellular Trafficking of Proteins. Cambridge, England, Cambridge University Press, 1991, p. 302; with permission.)

within the EGF precursor overlaps with a region of similarity to the low density lipoprotein (LDL) receptor.[67] The respective regions of similarity to the EGF precursor within the TfR and the LDL receptor lie just outside their membrane-spanning domains.

The gene for the TfR is found in 19 exons distributed over 31 kb of genomic DNA (Fig. 10–10). It has been mapped to the distal portion of the long arm of chromosome 3 (3q26→3qter)[68, 69] in the same region where the genes for Tf[37] and the p97 antigen[70] that has homology to Tf have been mapped. Transcriptional control sequences for the TfR gene have been localized in the immediate 5' flanking region.[71] These sequences may be involved in induction of gene expression in response to iron deprivation or in response to various growth factors. Two nuclear proteins (termed TREF-1 and TREF-2) have been identified as binding to the transcriptional control region of the TfR gene.[72]

Cellular Uptake of Iron: The Transferrin Cycle

The existence of a specific receptor for Tf was proposed in 1963,[54] but the purification and detailed characterization of the TfR did not begin until more than a decade later.[62, 63] It was initially observed more than 20 years ago by electron microscopy that Tf entered reticulocytes in endocytic vesicles.[73, 74] These fundamental observations that Tf first interacts with its specific high-affinity receptor and is subsequently internalized by the cell provided the basis for understanding the iron delivery process. The TfR is thus placed in that large group of receptors that mediate internalization of their specific ligands, and the Tf cycle can be understood in terms of the general pathway of receptor-mediated endocytosis.[75, 76]

Most cells possess, on their surface, numerous different receptors, each having a high affinity for a specific ligand. These receptors mediate the action of hormones, neurotransmitters, growth factors, differentiation factors, and chemotactic factors. They also provide for the specific recognition of serum transport proteins, such as Tf, LDL, and transcobalamin, and other important molecules, such as IgG, IgE, IgA, and lysosomal enzymes. Microscopy and, in particular, electron microscopy allowed the visualization of the interaction of both specific and non-specific proteins within the cell. In the late 1950s, Bessis and coworkers observed the uptake of single molecules of ferritin

into pinocytotic vesicles.[77] Their striking observation was that the sites of entry into the cell were definable as small indentations in the plasma membrane. By the early 1960s, these indentations were identified as coated pits because of the appearance in electron micrographs of a fuzzy electron-dense coat beneath the invagination.[78] Coated pits have been observed in virtually all cells (except mature enucleated erythrocytes) and serve as the site of entry of receptors and their ligands.

Although many of the molecular events underlying the endocytic pathway remain obscure, studies using a wide variety of receptors and ligands in many cell types have elucidated a general process. The first event in the endocytosis of a ligand is the binding to the surface receptor. Dissociation constants for a wide array of ligand-receptor interactions range from 10^{-7} M to 10^{-10} M. Most receptors, in the absence of ligand, are found randomly distributed in the plane of the plasma membrane. Some, including the TfR, are preferentially clustered into coated pits even in the apparent absence of ligand.[79] The coat itself is composed of a polygonal structure reminiscent of geodesic domes formed by a mixture of hexagons and pentagons that are made up of the 180,000 dalton protein called clathrin and several smaller proteins.[80, 81]

The coated pit regions of cells are constantly invaginating, with the coat most likely closing into a completed polygonal cage around a cytoplasmic vesicle referred to as a coated vesicle. Receptor-ligand complexes contained within the invaginating pit are thus internalized. These coated vesicles are short lived, and the newly formed vesicle most likely loses its coat. This smooth-walled vesicle containing newly internalized material is referred to as an endocytic vesicle, or endosome.[82] The endosome compartment comprises a highly polymorphic set of vesicles and tubules found in the cell periphery. After 15 to 45 minutes, the evolving endosome (or some vesicular structure derived from the endosome) fuses with a lysosome, thereby delivering the internalized contents for hydrolytic degradation. It is important to note that endocytosis defines a pathway of vesicular transfer of external molecules to lysosomes. This pathway per se does not provide a route for the transfer of molecules from outside the cell (or from inside the endosome) into the cytoplasm.

The one-way pathway from the cell surface to the lysosome is taken by the vast majority of ligands. The fate of most receptors is quite different from that of

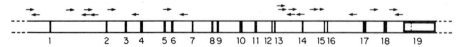

FIGURE 10–10. Organization of the human TfR gene. The gene encoding the human TfR is distributed over more than 33 kb of genomic DNA on human chromosome 3. The exons are numbered, and positions of repetitive DNA sequences within the introns are indicated by horizontal arrows. (Adapted with permission from McClellar, A., Kuhn, L. C., and Ruddle, F. H.: The human transferrin receptor gene: Genomic organization and the complete primary structure of the receptor deduced for a cDNA sequence. Cell 39:267, 1984. Copyright by Cell Press.)

their ligands, and one of the most striking aspects of this general pathway is the recycling of receptors.[83] Thus, many receptors mediate the internalization and degradation of scores of ligand molecules without their being degraded. These receptors can be recycled to the plasma membrane and reutilized again and again for the internalization of new ligand molecules. At some point subsequent to internalization, the ligand and receptor take different physical paths, the former going to lysosomes and the latter avoiding lysosomes and returning to the plasma membrane. The prerequisite for this divergence is a physicochemical mechanism for the intravesicular dissociation of the ligand from the receptor. The observation that the interior of endosomes is acidic provided this mechanism, and this observation was followed by the demonstration that ligands actually dissociate from their receptors within the endosome and that this dissociation was due to the acidification of that organelle.[84, 85] The acidification of the endosome is the result of an ATP-dependent proton pump present in the membrane of these organelles, similar, if not identical, to that found in lysosomal membranes.[86] The majority of endocytic receptor-ligand interactions are highly pH dependent, with the ligand rapidly dissociating at pHs below 5.5. Once the ligand is released into the fluid phase of the lumen of the endocytic vesicle, a still mysterious sorting process occurs whereby the freed ligand enters a vesicular pathway leading to fusion with lysosomes while the membrane receptor is recycled to the cell surface.

Studies over a number of years have clarified the somewhat unusual endocytic pathway taken by Tf[87–91] and referred to as the Tf cycle (Fig. 10–11). Monoferric or diferric Tf binds to the cell surface TfR and is rapidly internalized via coated pits. Shortly after internalization, the transferrin is detected in acidified endocytic vesicles.[92] Up to this point, Tf endocytosis is indistinguishable from the generalized pathway taken by other ligands. However, in contrast to these other ligands, the Tf is not delivered to lysosomes and is therefore not degraded. Rather, the Tf is rapidly released from the cell. In a single cycle through the cell, the vast majority of diferric Tf is released as apotransferrin after about a 5 to 15 minute transit. The efficiency of this recycling is greater than 95 per cent. As with many other receptor systems, the TfR recycles and is reutilized. The rates of cycling of the TfR and its ligand Tf are the same.

How does Tf avoid delivery to and degradation in the lysosome? The answer lies in the interesting details of the pH dependence of the ligand-receptor interaction.[92–94] Soon after internalization, the Tf-receptor complex finds itself in an acidic vesicle. It is here that the iron is released, and the acidity of the environment is an absolute requirement for this iron release.[95–97] This leaves apotransferrin bound to its receptor. At neutral pH, this would result in a rapid dissociation because of the extremely low affinity of apotransferrin for the TfR. However, the dissociation constant of the apotransferrin-receptor interaction is much lower at acidic pH, so that the apotransferrin, in contrast to other ligands, remains bound to its receptor in the acidic endosome. The normally recycling receptor carries the apotransferrin back to the cell surface, where, upon encountering the neutral pH of the outside environment, the apotransferrin rapidly dissociates and is released from the membrane. This cycle allows for the reutilization of both ligand and receptor, the former to be reloaded with ferric iron and the latter to engage in additional rounds of endocytosis. The acidic endosome in this and other systems provides the mechanism for sorting components of endocytic systems. During the uptake of ligands such as LDL and asialoglycoproteins, the pH-dependent dissociation allows the ligand to be delivered without its receptor to lysosomes. During iron uptake, the iron is released from Tf in the acidic milieu. The acidic environment of the endosome, while necessary, is likely insufficient to account for iron unloading of Tf, since even at pH 5, release of Tf-bound iron is much slower than the endocytic cycle. The interaction of Tf with the TfR also appears to facilitate release of iron from Tf,[46, 47] and an intraendosomal chelator may also participate. The molecular details of the transfer of iron from the endosome to the cytoplasm remain obscure but likely involve a reductase and transporter,[9] analogous to the system described above for yeast iron uptake (compare Figs. 10–2 and 10–12).

Control of Transferrin Receptor Synthesis

Iron has several roles in cellular metabolic processes. Iron is required for the synthesis of ribonucleotide reductase, which is in turn required for DNA synthesis and cell division.[98, 99] Hence, the availability of iron may influence the rate of cell proliferation, and conversely, the number of receptors is highest on proliferating cells. Iron is also required for the synthesis of many other cellular proteins, such as the cytochromes involved in oxidative metabolism. Iron is also needed for certain specialized functions, such as hemoglobin synthesis in erythroid cells. Clearly, control of iron acquisition and utilization must be modulated to meet these varied and diverse demands.

Rapidly dividing cells require more iron than do quiescent cells. Moreover, growth arrest occurs upon removal of Tf from cell culture medium. This growth arrest can be explained by the requirement for iron to synthesize essential enzymes such as ribonucleotide reductase.[99] The fact that the growth requirement for Tf is related to the iron it carries is evidenced by the fact that the addition of iron in a chelated form that passes through the cell membrane results in reinitiation of cell proliferation independent of the presence of Tf.[100, 101] Conversely, the addition of strong chelators such as desferrioxamine produces an arrest in cell growth independent of the presence of Tf.[102, 103] The level of TfR expression is related to the proliferative state of the cells[104–106] as well as to the induction of differentiation.[107–109] Resting lymphocytes express few,

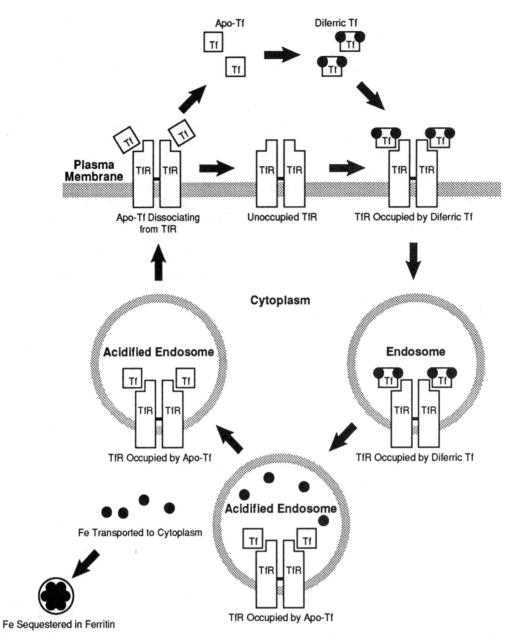

FIGURE 10–11. The Tf cycle for iron uptake. Tf and the TfR are depicted as in Figure 10–9. The Tf cycle involves binding of diferric Tf by the TfR, internalization of the TfR-Tf complex, endosome acidification, transfer of iron to the cytoplasm, externalization of the TfR-apotransferrin complex, and release of apotransferrin upon encounter with the neutral pH of the extracellular milieu. Details of the transfer of iron from the endosome are given in Figure 10–12. Cytoplasmic iron is either utilized or incorporated into ferritin (see Fig. 10–4). (Adapted from Harford, J. B., and Klausner, R. D.: Coordinate post-transcriptional regulation of ferritin and transferrin receptor expression: The role of regulated RNA-protein interaction. Enzyme 44:28, 1991; with permission of S. Karger AG, Basel.)

if any, TfR on their surface, but a rapid and dramatic increase in TfR expression occurs following lymphocyte activation.[110–112] The transcription rate of the TfR gene has also been assessed by nuclear run-off experiments in activated T cells[108] and in HL60 cells induced to differentiate toward monocytes with dibutyryl cyclic AMP (cAMP).[109] Activation of T cells leads to increased TfR expression, whereas cAMP treatment of HL60 results in decreased TfR expression. The corresponding changes in nuclear run-offs that were

observed in both instances are consistent with a transcriptional component to these regulations of TfR gene expression.

Receptor number may also be modulated by the redistribution of receptor molecules between the surface and internal membranes.[113–116] Fluctuations that occur during the cell cycle may reflect such partitioning. Many more receptors are found on the surface during the S phase of the cell cycle than during the G_1 phase.[106, 117, 118] Treatment of human fibroblasts

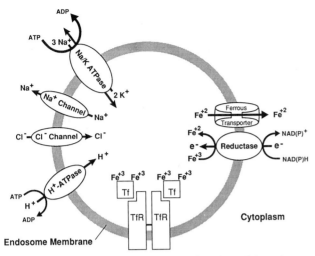

FIGURE 10–12. Iron release within the endocytic vesicle and transfer to the cytoplasm. Iron release from Tf depends on the acidic pH of the endosome. Vesicle acidification is envisioned here as being dependent on a proton-pumping ATPase. Chloride influx and sodium efflux may be involved in neutralization of the electrical gradient produced by the proton pumping. A sodium-potassium ATPase would maintain a sodium gradient across the endosome membrane. In addition to the lowered pH, other factors may participate in the release of iron from Tf, including the interaction of the Tf with the TfR. Once released, ferric iron would be reduced to ferrous iron, using an electron-transporting reductase with electrons coming from cytoplasmic reducing equivalents (NADH or NADPH). The resultant ferrous iron would be moved to the cytoplasm by a ferrous transporter. The endosome reductase-transporter for transmembrane movement of iron bears at least functional resemblance to the iron uptake system of yeast depicted in Figure 10–2. (Adapted from Nunez, M. T., Gaete, V., Watkins, J. A., and Glass, J.: Mobilization of iron from endocytic vesicles: The effects of acidification and reduction. J. Biol. Chem. 265:6688, 1990; with permission.)

with EGF results in a rapid increase in the ability of the cell membrane to bind Tf by accelerating the return of internalized receptors retarding their internalization or both.[113] Exposure of human erythroleukemia cells to a monoclonal antibody with specificity for the TfR results in internalization of the antibody-receptor complex.[114] An increased fraction of the receptor is directed to lysosomes for degradation compared with internalization initiated by Tf binding, leading to a decrease in surface receptor number. Furthermore, rapid, short-term changes in receptor number that accompany activation of erythroleukemia cells by phorbol esters have been shown to reflect receptor redistribution from an intracellular pool.[115, 116] The TfR persists on maturing erythroblasts even beyond nuclear extrusion, as reflected by its presence in large numbers on reticulocytes. This feature ensures availability of iron for hemoglobin synthesis. After maturation of reticulocytes to red cells, the receptors appear to be shed.[119, 120] The mechanisms by which specialized cells control receptor number during maturation are largely unknown.

Within populations of proliferating cells, the expression of TfR is modulated by iron availability in a manner that resembles feedback regulation, such that fewer receptors are expressed when iron is abundant and more receptors are expressed when iron is scarce.[121–125] The predominant locus of iron regulation of TfR expression lies not in the promoter but in sequences corresponding to the 3'UTR of the TfR messenger RNA (mRNA). The portion of the TfR cDNA corresponding to the 3'UTR of the TfR mRNA has been shown to be sufficient to confer iron regulation on the expression of a chimeric transcript encoding heterologous genes.[126, 127] The region within the 3'UTR of the TfR mRNA that is the predominant locus of iron regulation has been defined as being within a fragment of 678 nucleotides (nt).[127] A very similar secondary structure can be formed from a corresponding sequence within the 3'UTR of the chicken TfR mRNA.[128, 129] One of the most exciting observations made upon inspection of the possible secondary structure of the regulatory region of the TfR mRNA was the discovery of five stem-loop structures within the TfR 3'UTR that bore striking similarity to the RNA motif termed IRE found within the 5'UTR of mRNAs encoding ferritin[127] (see below).

FERRITIN

Protection from the harmful effects of iron plus oxygen is in large measure accomplished by the process of iron sequestration. The best characterized protein that serves this function is ferritin, a highly conserved protein found in all vertebrates.[130, 131] Ferritin-like sequestration compounds have been reported in bacteria as well as in simple eukaryotes. Vertebrate ferritin subunits assemble into a well-characterized structure containing a total of 24 subunits that form a spherical shell into which as many as 4500 atoms of iron can be sequestered and detoxified as a ferric oxyhydroxide micelle. How iron that has entered ferritin can be remobilized for metabolic uses is still unclear. Ferritin, a ubiquitous protein found in all cells, is composed of 24 apoferritin subunits arranged to form a hollow sphere that may contain a large amount of iron.[38, 131–136] Two types of apoferritin subunits have been identified. The human L chain contains 174 residues and has a molecular weight of 19,700, whereas the human H chain has 182 residues with a molecular weight of 21,100. The H chain is four amino acids longer on either end than the L chain. Despite only 55 per cent identity at the protein sequence level, the secondary and tertiary conformations of the H and L chains are quite similar.

Ferritin Genes

Both the H and the L genes are part of relatively large multigene families.[134–144] There are at least 10 genes in the H chain gene family and more than a dozen in the L chain gene family. Most or all of these are on separate chromosomes. A functional gene for the H chain has been molecularly cloned and mapped

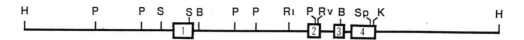

1 kb

FIGURE 10–13. Organization of the human ferritin H chain gene. The gene encoding expressed ferritin H chain is located on human chromosome 11. The gene covers approximately 3 kb of genomic DNA and is composed of four exons (numbered boxes). The letters at the top of the figure represent restriction enzyme cleavage sites, some of which were used to determine the gene organization. (Adapted from Hentze, M. W., Kein, S., Papadopoulos, P., O'Brien, S., Modi, W., Drysdale, J., Leonard, W. J., Harford, J. B., and Klausner, R. D.: Cloning, characterization, expression and chromosomal localization of a human ferritin heavy chain gene. Proc. Natl. Acad. Sci. 83:7226, 1986; with permission.)

to chromosome 11.[144] It is a relatively compact gene, having four exons and three introns, with a total size of only 3 kb (Fig. 10–13). An L chain gene with similar organization has also been cloned.[142] A functional L chain gene was mapped to chromosome 19 by immunological analyses using somatic cell hybrids.[145] Several of the H chain–related genes have been shown to be processed by intronless pseudogenes both by heteroduplex mapping of cloned DNA fragments, which revealed the absence of introns, and by DNA sequence analysis, which revealed inactivating mutations.[134, 135, 143] Such genes lack transcriptional control sequences and therefore are unlikely to function. Potentially interesting H chain–related sequences have been mapped to chromosomes 3 and 6.[135] The ferritin-related sequence on chromosome 3 is located close to the loci for the Tf gene,[37, 146] the TfR gene,[68, 69] and the gene encoding p97 antigen, a protein structurally related to Tf.[70] The gene for primary hemochroma-

tosis (see below) has been linked to the human leukocyte antigen (HLA) locus on chromosome 6 near the mapped H chain gene.[135] Ferritin has long been hypothesized to be involved in the hemochromatosis defect, so ferritin-related sequences on chromosome 6 have been the focus of some attention.

Ferritin Structure

Each ferritin subunit is folded into a roughly cylindrical molecule containing four long and nearly parallel right-handed helices (A, B, C, D), a shorter helix (E), a helical turn (P), a long extended chain (L), and some irregular regions (Fig. 10–14A).[132, 133] The relative orientation of the various subunits to one another in the assembly of the 24 subunit shell is illustrated in Figure 10–14B. An interesting feature of this quaternary structure is the presence of six channels with a

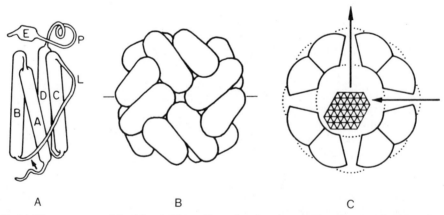

A   B   C

FIGURE 10–14. The structure of ferritin. A, Three-dimensional representation of an apoferritin subunit. The segments labeled A to E and P are helical in nature, whereas L is a non-helical loop. The numbers of amino acids in each helical segment are as follows: A, 27; B, 25; C, 28; D, 20; P, 7; and E, 10, with this being the order of the helical segments, starting with the amino-terminus. B, Quaternary structure of the apoferritin shell viewed down one axis of its fourfold axis of symmetry. The central opening represents a channel through which iron enters the ferritin core. C, A cross-sectional view of the ferritin shell following oxidation of ferrous iron to ferric iron as it enters. As many as 4500 atoms of iron may be sequestered within the ferritin shell, although typically the number is less. (Adapted with permission from Clegg, G. A., Fitton, J. E., Harrison, P. M., and Treffry, A.: Ferritin: Molecular structure and iron-storage mechanisms. Prog. Biophys. Mol. Biol. 36:56, 1980, Pergamon Press, Ltd.)

fourfold axis of symmetry that passes through the shell (Fig. 10–14C.) These channels may function to enable iron and other molecules necessary for its storage and mobilization to enter or to leave the central cavity.

Isoelectric focusing of ferritin molecules extracted from a variety of tissues revealed a very complex pattern with multiple bands.[132, 133, 147–150] This heterogeneity reflects, at least in part, the assembly of ferritin shells having variable numbers of H and L subunits. Indeed, variable expression of H and L chain genes occurs in different tissues. For example, the human liver contains predominantly L chains, whereas the heart contains predominantly H chains.[148, 149] The multiplicity of isoferritins detected could also reflect expression of more than the ferritin genes of the H and L types. Three distinct ferritin cDNAs have been characterized for frog red cells.[151] Post-translational modification of the ferritin polypeptides may also introduce heterogeneity into ferritin subunits[152–154] and contribute to the multiplicity of isoferritins demonstrable in various tissues.

Uptake and Release of Iron from Ferritin

Incorporation of iron is thought to follow assembly of the apoferritin subunit shell, although the possibility that the shell develops around preformed crystals has not been totally excluded. Relatively soluble ferrous iron is incorporated into the shell much more readily than is ferric iron.[132, 133, 147] Once ferrous ions traverse the channels, they are thought to associate with residues on the inner surface of the subunits, thereby facilitating oxidation to the ferric form, with subsequent deposition. Ultimately, as many as 4500 iron atoms may be accommodated within each protein shell, although ferritin molecules having many fewer iron atoms are common.

Release of iron from ferritin shells may be readily demonstrated in vitro. Various flavins or other reducing agents, such as cysteine, glutathione, or ascorbic acid or chelators, may facilitate such release.[132, 155–157] These substances are thought to be able to pass through the channels in the ferritin shell. Iron may be released within cells by similar mechanisms. Alternatively, ferritin shells may undergo degradation, either within lysosomes to form hemosiderin or within cytoplasm.[158] Iron exposed to cytoplasmic constituents following degradation of the ferritin subunit shell may be more readily mobilized.

Ferritin and hemosiderin iron are storage forms that are ultimately available for hemoglobin synthesis. The absence of storage iron in iron deficiency states and the mobilization of excess iron stores during phlebotomy of patients with hemochromatosis document the gradual flux from these storage forms into a metabolically active pool.[16] However, rapidly proliferating cells may depend exclusively on external Tf as a source of iron. Indeed, cells deprived of Tf or treated with chelators such as desferrioxamine experience growth arrest and alter expression of the TfR and ferritin despite having intracellular stores in the form of ferritin.[100, 103, 159]

Ferritin Synthesis

Ferritin genes are expressed in all cells, but the differential expression of the H and L chain genes in different tissues suggests tight regulation of ferritin gene expression. In addition to the cell type–specific expression of ferritins, cells possess the ability to respond quickly to increased exposure to iron by modulation of ferritin biosynthesis. Accelerated biosynthesis and assembly of apoferritin shells can be demonstrated within minutes of increasing intracellular iron concentration.[160–163] This increase in ferritin biosynthesis occurs by a post-transcriptional mechanism, as first evidenced by the observation that the increase occurred in response to iron even in the presence of actinomycin D, an inhibitor of RNA synthesis. Moreover, elevated rates of synthesis of ferritin occur independently of corresponding changes in the levels of apoferritin mRNA.[164, 165] This iron-dependent modulation of ferritin biosynthesis is now known to occur at the level of mRNA translation (see below).

CELLULAR IRON HOMEOSTASIS

There is evidence to indicate that three (Tf, TfR, and ferritin) of the four proteins now known to be involved in the acquisition of iron and in the regulation of its intracellular distribution are modulated in the rates of their biosynthesis by available iron. The fourth protein (the IRE-BP) is also regulated by iron, but at a post-translational level (see below). Although expression of both Tf and its receptor may be induced by iron deprivation and both genes have been localized to a single chromosomal region (3:q3→qter), the mechanism of regulation differs. Regulation of Tf synthesis appears to be primarily transcriptional. When cells are iron depleted, Tf levels increase, and conversely, under conditions of iron overload, Tf levels decrease.[53] Regulation of the TfR occurs through regulation of the stability of the mRNA. Regulation of ferritin synthesis occurs primarily at the translational level and is directly, rather than inversely, related to iron supply. The activity of the IRE-BP appears to be modulated by iron through its own reversible binding of iron. The role of the IRE-BP in the coordinate regulation of biosynthesis of ferritin and the TfR is discussed below.

The hepatocyte possesses additional mechanisms for iron uptake. Heme bound to hemopexin appears to be internalized via a specific receptor, and hemopexin is recycled to the circulation.[166–169] Similarly, uptake of a hemoglobin-haptoglobin complex has been reported to result in release of heme iron and degradation of both globin and haptoglobin.[170–172] There also appears to be a receptor for ferritin on hepatocytes,[173] although

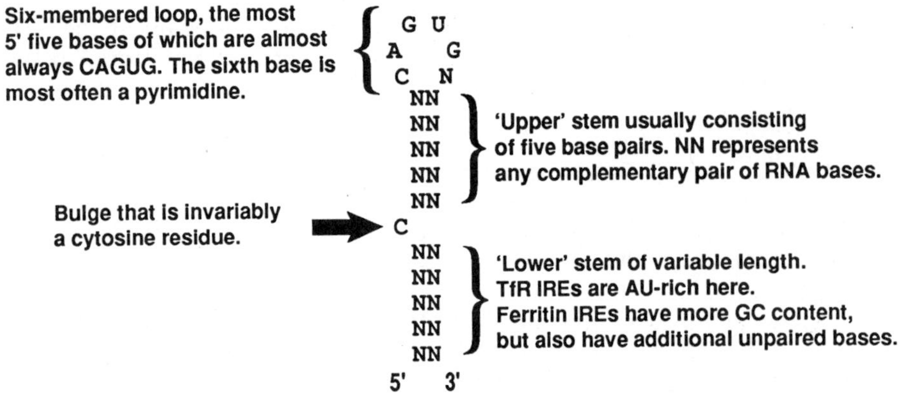

Six-membered loop, the most 5' five bases of which are almost always CAGUG. The sixth base is most often a pyrimidine.

```
        G  U
      A      G
    C          N
        NN
        NN      } 'Upper' stem usually consisting
        NN          of five base pairs. NN represents
        NN          any complementary pair of RNA bases.
        NN
```

Bulge that is invariably a cytosine residue. ➡ C

```
        NN
        NN      } 'Lower' stem of variable length.
        NN          TfR IREs are AU-rich here.
        NN          Ferritin IREs have more GC content,
        NN          but also have additional unpaired bases.
     5'    3'
```

FIGURE 10–15. The structure of an iron-responsive element (IRE). All known ferritin mRNAs contain a single IRE within their 5' untranslated region. All known TfR mRNAs contain five IREs within their 3' untranslated region. The consensus IRE shown is derived from the sequences and possible secondary structures of IREs from ferritin and TfR mRNAs. (Adapted from Harford, J. B., and Klausner, R. D.: Coordinate post-transcriptional regulation of ferritin and transferrin receptor expression: The role of regulated RNA-protein interaction. Enzyme 44:28, 1991; with permission of S. Karger AG, Basel.)

under normal circumstances very little iron reaches the liver by this mechanism. Both hepatocytes and macrophages can donate iron to plasma Tf. If plasma iron levels fall owing to iron depletion, the hepatocyte releases iron, whereas with an increase in plasma Tf saturation, there is an increased net flow into hepatocyte ferritin and hemosiderin stores.[174–176] One other aspect of hepatocyte-iron exchange that is unique among body cells is the ability to take up non-Tf iron from the plasma. Iron citrate or ascorbate that is injected intravenously in an organism that already has fully saturated Tf is nevertheless rapidly removed from circulation by the hepatocytes.[177, 178] Thus, by virtue of its large number of TfRs and additional mechanisms of iron uptake, the hepatocyte is often the immediate reservoir for excess iron from various sources.

Once iron enters eukaryotic cells, it may be used for enzyme synthesis or deposited in ferritin after brief passage through a chelatable pool (see Fig. 10–2). The size and physical nature of this chelatable pool remain obscure. The percentage of newly acquired iron incorporated into ferritin is directly proportional to the amount of ferritin available for iron deposition; iron partitions between ferritin and non-ferritin pools depend on ferritin levels.[179, 180] The mechanisms controlling this partitioning are obscure. The rates of synthesis of the TfR and ferritin are coordinately regulated but in opposite directions.[181] A decrease in iron availability to cells results in a minor increase in the transcription of the gene coding for the TfR and a major increase in total amounts of TfR mRNA because of decreased degradation of the transcript. Depletion of the "regulatory" iron pool leads to a rapid drop in the synthesis of ferritin because of a decrease in the rate of translation. The increased numbers of TfRs would be expected to result in an increase in iron uptake, whereas lowered ferritin synthesis would lead to decreased sequestration of intracellular iron. The decrease in ferritin levels would mean that a greater percentage of the iron entering via the Tf cycle would be available for metabolic and synthetic needs. As the iron supply rises, the "regulatory" pool fills, leading to an increase in ferritin synthesis and a concomitant increase in the rate of degradation of the TfR mRNA. Thus, the opposite synthetic rate responses to iron

changes for the receptor and ferritin produce a homeostatic response by reversible coordinate effects on iron uptake and intracellular iron sequestration. When iron is scarce, this homeostatic system serves to enhance the immediate availability of iron needed for synthesis of enzymes required for cell division and metabolism through up-modulation of the Tf cycle and down-modulation of iron sequestration. When iron is abundant, the system affords protection of organelles from iron toxicity by decreasing iron uptake and increasing iron sequestration.

Insight has been gained into the mechanism by which cells achieve simultaneous translational regulation of ferritin and regulation of the mRNA half-life of the TfR. The 5'UTR of ferritin mRNA and the 3'UTR of the TfR contain stem-loop sequences known as iron-responsive elements (IREs) (Fig. 10–15), which form a potential binding site for an intracellular regulatory protein known as IRE-BP. The IRE-BP binds to IREs when intracellular iron is depleted. Binding of the IRE-BP reduces translation of ferritin mRNA by interfering with the function of the translation apparatus; binding to some of the 3' IREs in the TfR mRNA interferes with degradation of the transcript, thereby increasing mRNA levels and TfR biosynthesis (Fig. 10–16).

The IRE-BP appears to be the master regulatory protein in iron homeostasis. Cloning of the protein has revealed an interesting homology to the mitochondrial enzyme aconitase.[182, 183] Aconitase has an iron-sulfur cluster that has an interesting feature in that the fourth iron of the iron-sulfur cluster is labile on purification. Thus, it may be that in vivo changes in the iron-sulfur cluster of the protein are directly transduced into changes in the binding affinity of the protein for IREs; when the fourth iron is absent because of relative intracellular iron depletion, the protein binds IREs tightly, but when the fourth iron is present, the protein binds IREs poorly. Thus, the IRE-BP would represent both the direct sensor of iron levels and the direct regulator of expression of proteins important in the maintenance of iron homeostasis. Recent evidence indicates that IREs are also present in the 5'UTR of porcine mitochondrial aconitase[184] and in the 5'UTR of erythrocyte δ-aminolevulinic acid (ALA) synthase,[184, 185] the rate-limiting

Ferritin mRNA

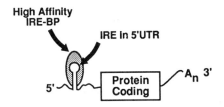

**IRE-BP Bound When Fe Is Scarce:
mRNA Translation Repressed**

TfR mRNA

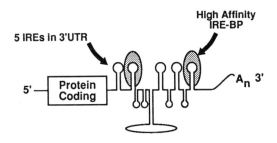

**IRE-BP Bound When Fe Is Scarce:
mRNA Degradation Repressed**

FIGURE 10–16. **Coordinate regulation of the expression of ferritin and the TfR.** The 5′ untranslated region of ferritin mRNA contains a single iron-responsive element (IRE). The 3′ untranslated region of the TfR mRNA contains five similar elements (see Fig. 10–15). When iron is scarce, a cytoplasmic, high-affinity IRE-binding protein (IRE-BP) interacts with the IREs of both mRNAs. In the case of the ferritin mRNA, this interaction serves to reduce the translation of the mRNA and results in reduced ferritin synthesis with no alteration in the level of ferritin mRNA. In the case of the TfR, the interaction of the high-affinity IRE-BP with the IREs results in protection of the mRNA from degradation. This in turn leads to more TfR synthesis owing to the elevated level of its mRNA. (Adapted from Harford, J. B., and Klausner, R. D.: Coordinate post-transcriptional regulation of ferritin and transferrin receptor expression: The role of regulated RNA-protein interaction. Enzyme 44:28; 1991; with permission of S. Karger AG, Basel.)

step in heme biosynthesis. Expression of these genes may also be subject to regulation by the IRE-BP.

DIETARY IRON ABSORPTION

The above discussion of iron uptake, utilization, storage, and regulation relates primarily to these functions within individual cells of higher eukaryotes. In complex, multicellular organisms (like humans), there exists another level on which iron metabolism must be understood. It is one thing to discuss how cells acquire

iron from diferric Tf in tissue culture or even from plasma Tf, but we must also understand how iron gets to plasma Tf from the environment outside the organism. Dietary iron absorption in humans is extremely complex, in part because our diets are complex and varied.[186–193] Dietary iron absorption is influenced by many factors, including existing total body iron stores, interactions between free iron and food components, the availability of gastric acid during digestion, gastric and small intestinal mobility, mucosal processing of iron, and movement of iron from the mucosal cell to the blood stream. Dietary iron is closely linked to caloric intake; about 6 to 7 mg of iron is taken in with each 1000 calories.[187] There are two types of absorbable iron in food.[154, 189–192] Heme iron is absorbed directly and catabolized inside the mucosal cell, whereas non-heme iron is taken up as free iron or in a protein-bound form or both. Humans absorb heme with great facility, an advantage when the human diet was rich in heme derived from the blood and meat of animals. Beginning with the cultivation of grain about 10,000 years ago, highly available heme iron in meat was replaced by less available non-heme iron in the cereal diet. Heme constitutes only 1 to 3 mg/day of iron in the average Western diet and even less in the diet of the world's poor population.[187, 193]

Dietary composition has a major effect on the absorption of non-heme iron. Facilitating substances such as ascorbic acid or meat are required for appreciable absorption, whereas non-heme iron uptake may be blocked by increasing amounts of tannins and phosphates.[194–197] Neither the chemical form nor the quantity of non-heme iron in food is as important as dietary factors that operate within the lumen to determine the availability of iron.

Gastric acid maintains the solubility of iron, especially that in the ferric form. Although the gastric mucosa cannot absorb iron, acid creates a low pH in the upper duodenum that is conducive to iron solubility. Each unit drop in pH results in a 1000-fold increase in the solubility of ferric iron.[5] The stomach also acts as a reservoir for releasing iron into the intestine; large doses of iron may be held there for many hours. Mucoproteins of gastric secretion have been thought to facilitate absorption,[198] and products of protein digestion, such as the amino acids, cysteine, and histidine, may also affect absorption.[199] Pancreatic juice with its high pH reduces solubility, particularly of ferric iron salts, although this may be counterbalanced by the action of pancreatic enzymes in liberating polypeptides and amino acids. Bile contains Tf that may facilitate absorption.[53] No other specific intraluminal regulators of iron absorption have been identified.

The primary mechanism by which the enterocyte absorbs iron from the gut is poorly understood. Iron salts are best absorbed in the duodenum and most actively by the epithelial cells at the tips of the villi.[200] Cellular uptake has been characterized by autoradiographs, by sensitive methods of iron staining, and by chemical fractionation of the mucosa.[201–206] There appears to be an initial interaction between iron salts and the intestinal brush border, with subsequent passage into the cell. Some ionized iron may diffuse between mucosal cells; this fraction may increase when large amounts of iron are present in the lumen. Iron absorbed from heme appears in the plasma later than does non-heme iron, suggesting that more time is required for the release of iron within the mucosal cell by heme oxidase. Newly acquired iron appears to enter a common pool within the mucosal cell. Some of the mucosal iron is temporarily stored as ferritin, to be released and absorbed over the next few hours. Other iron is held by ferritin until the cell is exfoliated.[190, 200] Evidence linking the absorptive process to mucosal cellular metabolism is suggested by the enhancing effect of phenobarbital and by the effect of inhibitors of protein synthesis in decreasing absorption.[207–209]

Absorbed radioactive tracer iron appears in the plasma within seconds in experimental animals, regardless of the state of iron balance, suggesting a relatively small intracellular iron pool in the mucosal epithelial cells (Fig. 10–17). Iron crossing the mucosal cell layer passes into the extravascular space of the lamina propria, where it can bind to plasma Tf, from which it can be utilized by individual cells having TfRs on their plasma membranes.

Several proteins that have iron-binding properties have been isolated from gut mucosa.[210–212] The precise role of these proteins in mucosal iron transport remains to be established, although some role is sug-

gested, since an antibody to a 54 kDa membrane glycoprotein isolated from human gut has been reported to block ^{59}Fe uptake by human microvillous membrane vesicles.[212]

Regulation of Dietary Iron Absorption

Normal individuals absorb approximately 1 mg of iron per day into the plasma. This may be increased to as much as 3.5 mg/day under conditions of iron deficiency or accelerated erythropoiesis and may be decreased to 0.5 mg/day in the presence of iron overload. The content and bioavailability of iron in the diet have major influences on iron absorption independent of the physiological state of the individual. For more than 40 years, it has been recognized that iron balance in humans is maintained by regulation of iron absorption.[213] In addition, more than 40 years ago, Granick proposed his "mucosal block" theory that envisioned the passage of iron through the enterocyte of the duodenum and into the plasma as being regulated by ferritin of the mucosa.[214] All iron entering the mucosal cell was envisioned as adding to the ferritin pool, from which it would be released to the plasma as needed. Later the mucosal block theory was modified to one that envisioned rapid transfer of iron from gut lumen to plasma as being the default pathway. Mucosal ferritin would compete with transfer from the enterocyte to the plasma, with the efficacy of this competition depending on ferritin content. With

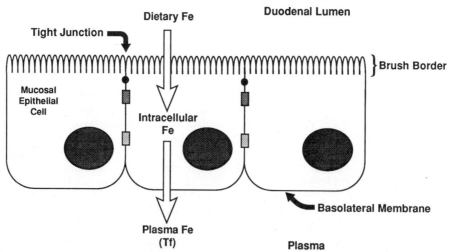

FIGURE 10–17. Absorption of dietary iron. The enterocyte of the duodenum is the primary site of iron absorption. Iron is transferred across the brush border plasma membrane. Once inside the mucosal epithelial cell, the intracellular iron is utilized for metabolic needs of the enterocyte, sequestered into mucosal ferritin, or transferred across the basolateral membrane, where it associates with plasma Tf. Only a fraction of the iron entering the epithelial cell is transported across the basolateral membrane and thus absorbed into the plasma. The means for transfer across the brush border membrane and the basolateral membrane remain obscure. This transport of iron across the lipid bilayers of the gut cells may be at least functionally similar to transmembrane transport of iron into yeast (see Fig. 10–2) or endosomal membrane transport of iron into the cytoplasm (see Fig. 10–12). Iron that crosses the brush border membrane but does not cross the basolateral membrane is removed from the body as the epithelial cells of the gut are sloughed. The fraction of dietary iron that is absorbed is in part governed by the total body iron stores. In patients with human leukocyte antigen (HLA)–linked hemochromatosis, this feedback loop is deranged, resulting in higher absorption than would be appropriate for the iron-overloaded individual.

relative iron sufficiency, ferritin synthesis would be induced, and a greater proportion of absorbed iron would partition to the ferritin pool within enterocytes. Enterocytes are routinely sloughed and excreted through the gastrointestinal tract. Thus, iron that has been taken into the enterocyte and sequestered in ferritin within the cytoplasm would be excreted when the cell was exfoliated. Conversely, during periods of iron deficiency, ferritin synthesis would be depressed, and more iron would pass through to the circulation. Loss of dietary iron by sloughing of gut enterocytes can be viewed as a type of excretory mechanism for iron, but this form of excreted iron was never really absorbed (i.e., it never reached the plasma). Once the duodenal mucosal barrier is passed, there are no other known effective excretory systems. Iron that has entered the plasma leaves the body only by loss of blood (an important consideration in menstruating individuals) and by such minor incidental means as loss of skin cells or hair.

The mucosal block theory was no doubt an oversimplified model to explain regulation of dietary iron absorption. Nonetheless, it provided a working hypothesis by which the influence of total body iron stores on dietary iron absorption was explained through iron's regulation of ferritin synthesis and ferritin's known ability to sequester iron. Although much concerning iron metabolism has been learned in the past half century, the underlying mechanism by which absorption is regulated remains to be established. It is clear that apotransferrin is not required for mucosal release of iron, as similar absorption occurs when circulating Tf is saturated[215, 216] and when individuals are afflicted with the genetic disorder atransferrinemia[217] (see the following section). Increased amounts of apotransferrin appear to be unable to enhance absorption.[218, 219] The iron-binding capacity of Tf in the extravascular fluid of the lamina propria is quite limited,[219] and, in all probability, this capacity is frequently exceeded, whereupon iron may enter the portal system either unbound to protein or non-specifically bound to albumin. NTBI is rapidly removed by the hepatocyte.[216, 220] Small amounts of iron pass directly into the lymphatics. Insoluble aggregates of iron may be taken up by macrophages in the intestinal wall. These cells may act as another barrier to plasma iron absorption.[221]

A very important determinant of iron absorption appears to be erythropoietic activity; phlebotomy increases absorption in humans and experimental animals.[15, 154, 210, 222–224] Animals with hemolytic anemia exhibit increased iron absorption. In humans, hemolytic anemia is usually not associated with a significant increase in absorption, but at very high rates of erythropoiesis—particularly with ineffective erythropoiesis—absorption is markedly increased.[16] Animals subjected to exchange transfusion with blood high in reticulocyte content experience an extremely rapid increase in iron absorption.[225] Thus, a regulatory mechanism exists that is able to convey the needs of the erythron to the intestinal mucosa. Increased retic-uloendothelial release of iron is also observed under these circumstances. The role of Tf in these adjustments has been a matter of debate.[32, 225]

Another determinant of intestinal iron absorption is the amount of iron held in ferritin and hemosiderin. Any increase in body iron stores is followed by a reduction in iron absorption and any depletion by increased absorption.[226] Such regulation can occur without any demonstrable change in plasma iron or Tf saturation.[32, 225] In the absence of apotransferrin, iron appears to bind to albumin and is removed from the portal blood by hepatocytes. Some modulation of iron absorption may occur by this mechanism.

DISORDERS OF IRON HOMEOSTASIS: IRON DEFICIENCY

There are two major causes of iron deficiency: blood loss and low iron absorption from the diet. The latter may occasionally be the consequence of sprue or gastric surgery but is usually related to inadequacy of the diet. In many geographical settings, iron deficiency is due to a combination of poor absorption and increased loss. For example, in tropical countries, iron deficiency is often due to the combination of poor nutrition and hookworm infection.[227, 228] In iron deficiency, the sequence of depletion of iron stores and the development of anemia is relatively well understood.[229] Three phases may be recognized: iron store depletion, associated with increased relative iron absorption, increased concentration of circulating Tf, and decreased serum ferritin; iron deficient erythropoiesis, associated with a Tf saturation of less than 16 per cent, a red cell protoporphyrin level less than 100 $\mu g/ml$ of red cells, and a serum ferritin level less than 12 $\mu g/l$, but no recognizable anemia; and iron deficiency anemia. The clinical and laboratory manifestations and differential diagnosis of iron deficiency anemia are described in standard textbooks of hematology.

Considerations of the consequences of iron deficiency have traditionally focused on effects of the anemia in reducing maximum oxygen consumption and maximum work performance in proportion to the severity of the anemia.[230, 231] Non-hematological effects related to iron deficiency have generally been regarded as late and unusual complications of severe iron deficiency. In the past, recognized tissue effects of iron deficiency were largely anatomical (spoon nails, cheilosis, glossitis, and esophageal webs). Achlorhydria was observed, but it was unclear whether this was the cause or the effect of iron deficiency. Enzyme depletion of cytochrome P-450 and cytochrome oxidase has been demonstrated in the intestinal mucosa without clear evidence that these deficiencies were causing symptoms or dysfunction.[230, 232]

Several studies have shown that amounts of other iron-containing proteins may decrease along with hemoglobin during iron depletion.[233] Fetal development in pregnant rats is retarded in the presence of maternal iron deficiency.[154, 230] Muscle dysfunction has been found in iron-deficient adult animals after the anemia has been corrected by exchange transfusion.[234] On exertion, these rats develop lactic acidosis, which prevents further activity. Decreased levels of the mitochondrial enzyme α-glycerophosphate oxidase appear to be responsible for the impaired cellular metabolism. Increased catecholamine levels have been described in iron-deficient children, and behavioral abnormalities have been associated with this deficiency.[230, 235] Other possible sequelae of iron deficiency relate to the common pathway of metal absorption. Several metals apparently compete with iron for absorption. A person with iron deficiency who is exposed to toxic metals such as lead, cadmium, and plutonium may absorb more than an individual with an adequate iron intake.[222, 236]

A rarity of the expected symptoms of iron deficiency has been noted in patients with polycythemia vera who were treated exclusively with venesections for periods up to 15 years.[237] Apparently, persons of middle age or older tolerate a degree of chronic iron deficiency sufficient to produce microcytosis of red cells without serious untoward effects.[231, 233] A similar degree of iron deficiency in infants and children may have quite different effects. Decreased motivation, decreased attention span, and an overall impairment in intellectual performance have been described, as well as a reduction in involuntary activity. These features disappear promptly with iron treatment, prior to any significant rise in hemoglobin level. The physiological mechanisms involved are largely speculative. Several areas of the brain contain large quantities of iron.[230, 238, 239] Iron is required for the activity of enzymes such as thyroxine hydroxylase, tryptophan hydroxylase, and monoamine oxidase that are important to amine neurotransmitter metabolism. Dopamine receptor function may be impaired in iron deficiency and lead to some of the observed neurophysiological changes.[240]

DISORDERS OF IRON HOMEOSTASIS: IRON OVERLOAD

Iron overload may result from increased dietary iron absorption or from the need for regular blood transfusions secondary to severe genetic or acquired anemia. Blood transfusions contain approximately 250 mg of iron per unit, and direct infusion of blood into the patient bypasses the mucosal uptake regulatory mechanisms. Increased dietary absorption is most often due to the genetic defect present in patients with primary (idiopathic) hemochromatosis. In South African Bantus, a syndrome of iron overload has been observed that has been previously attributed solely to markedly increased dietary intake of iron from alcohol that is brewed in iron pots. However, recently, careful analysis of this population suggests that a non–HLA-linked genetic defect is involved.[241]

Primary hemochromatosis is one of the more common genetic diseases, with a heterozygote frequency of about 10 per cent in the European and American populations.[242–249] The finding of a tight linkage between the gene responsible for this disease and the HLA-A locus has allowed the definition of the mode of inheritance and the discovery of the high incidence of the abnormal gene. The locus for the hemochromatosis gene is very close to the A locus of the HLA complex on human chromosome 6, with few, if any, cases of recombination between HLA-A and the disease locus having been documented. There is a particularly high association of one particular A locus allele, A3, with the disease; 75 to 80 per cent of patients possess this HLA-A3 allele. However, the frequency of HLA-A3 (30 per cent) in the general population militates against the value of screening for hemochromatosis by HLA typing, although the linkage disequilibrium involving the A3 and hemochromatosis alleles is useful for family studies and genetic counseling.[250, 251]

Primary hemochromatosis is transmitted as an autosomal recessive trait and is thought to result from excess intestinal absorption of dietary iron.[242–249] As stated earlier, there is no normal mechanism whereby the body can excrete iron once absorption from the enterocyte into the plasma has taken place. The excess iron absorbed by these patients, which may represent an excess of only 1 or 2 mg/day, inexorably accumulates in parenchymal tissue. Although the absorption defect is present from birth, it is the accumulation of 5 to 30 g of excess iron in hepatocytes, cardiac muscle, and other cells that eventually results in cellular toxicity and organ damage. Clinical manifestations are unusual before the mid-20s, and often initial clinical problems are first observed in the fourth to fifth decade of life. Symptoms, when present, are generally a combination of non-specific complaints of fatigue, malaise, weakness, arthralgia, and decreased libido, along with specific evidence of organ damage, such as arthritis, liver disease, and cardiomyopathy. Increased skin pigmentation is common but often subtle. Endocrine abnormalities due to iron overload are most commonly either primary gonadal failure or hypogonadotropic hypogonadism due to pituitary iron deposition. Diabetes, long considered a classic manifestation of the disease, is probably caused by deposition of iron in pancreatic islet cells. Adult-onset diabetes, when observed in families with primary hemochromatosis, segregates independently of the hemochromatosis gene.[252]

The severity of clinical manifestations is generally thought to correlate with the extent of iron overload. Thus, the probability of tissue damage in homozygotes may be modified by blood loss (especially menstruation) and the nature and amount of dietary iron. Phlebotomy remains the most effective treatment for patients with primary hemochromatosis. Significant clinical variability has been observed among patients in terms of both the severity and the spectrum of disease manifestations. Heterozygotes rarely, if ever, develop clinical problems. However, careful study of these patients demonstrates evidence for increased iron absorption, when compared with populations of patients entirely lacking the abnormal gene.[248] The heterozygous condition may be particularly deleterious in alcoholic gene carriers, who may experience alcoholic liver disease of earlier onset and greater severity. Thus, the primary defect is likely to be codominant, even though the mild elevation in iron absorption in heterozygotes does not generally lead to clinically significant iron overload; therefore, the clinical disease appears recessive.

Normal iron absorption is regulated at the level of the intestinal enterocyte. The feedback information from iron stores is somehow deranged in primary hemochromatosis. It is clear that the gene responsible for this disease plays either a structural or a regulatory role in this process. Homozygotes can regulate intestinal iron absorption, but the rate of absorption is chronically too high to prevent systemic iron accumulation. We do not completely understand all of the elements involved in iron absorption and do not know the nature of the gene affected by the hemochromatosis mutation (or mutations). Localization of the gene to chromosome 6, however, rules out certain candidates. Both Tf and the TfR are located on chromosome 3. Currently, the only known functional genes for the ferritins are on chromosomes 11 and 19. The gene for the IRE-BP has been localized to chromosome 9.[253] Thus, the major known proteins of iron metabolism cannot currently be directly implicated in the disease. Efforts to detect abnormalities in the handling of iron enterocytes have been inconclusive,[254] although apparent in vitro abnormalities of monocyte function[255–257] have been reported. One striking histological finding that characterizes the iron overload of primary hemochromatosis is that iron deposition is most marked in parenchymal cells, with a sparing of RE cells, early in the course of iron loading.[258–260] This sparing may reflect a defect in the ability of RE cells to retain iron.[261, 262] Whether the genetic defect is manifested in all cells or only in the enterocyte and perhaps RE cells is not known. This pattern of tissue iron distribution differs from the iron distribution of Bantu siderosis, in which iron deposition is pronounced in the RE system as well as in liver parenchymal cells.[241, 260]

In contrast to HLA-linked hemochromatosis, which, as indicated above, is a rather common genetic defect, there exists a much rarer condition known as neonatal hemochromatosis.[263] This disorder manifests itself in severe iron overload in the first few weeks and months after birth. Most patients die within a few months. As in HLA-linked, adult-onset hemochromatosis, patients manifest iron loading of parenchymal cells with relatively little iron accumulation in RE cells. Owing to the rarity of the disorder, it is difficult to establish whether the defect is genetic, although a few instances of affected siblings have been reported. No linkage to the HLA locus is found in patients with neonatal hemochromatosis or their families, and it is assumed that this disorder, while sharing the name and certain clinical manifestations with HLA-linked hemochromatosis, is in fact a distinct entity.

A common reason for iron overload is the multiple blood transfusions given to patients with a genetic defect in erythropoiesis.[264] The majority of such patients have severe β thalassemia, although other congenital anemias and acquired anemias that demand regular transfusion also lead inevitably to iron overload. The marked ineffective erythropoiesis, characteristic of B thalassemia, enhances iron absorption, so that such patients may accumulate iron by two routes.[265, 266] The clinical manifestations of iron overload reflect damage to the liver, endocrine glands, and—most importantly—the heart. The clinical course of patients with secondary hemochromatosis has been well described in several reviews.[264, 267, 268] Death from cardiac dysfunction by the mid-20s is inevitable in those patients with congenital transfusion-dependent anemias. Adults with acquired anemias exhibit cardiac dysfunction after receiving 100 to 200 units of blood. The clinical course of transfusion-dependent anemia has been modified by regular use of the iron chelator desferrioxamine.[267–271] Current clinical experience documents that regular use of this compound can delay the onset of cardiac dysfunction, although all of the manifestations of iron overload may not be prevented. Specifically, children with thalassemia often exhibit abnormalities of growth and sexual maturation. Secondary hemochromatosis due to excessive dietary absorption is rare, and even Bantu siderosis now appears to involve expression of a genetic abnormality in addition to excessive dietary intake (see above).

The importance of Tf for whole body iron homeostasis is highlighted in the very rare recessive genetic disorder known as atransferrinemia.[217, 272–274] The name atransferrinemia is probably a misnomer, since in most cases some immunoreactive Tf is measured and in all cases the serum contains a small but measurable amount of unsaturated iron-binding capacity. To date, modern molecular techniques have not been used to elucidate the molecular defect of this interesting condition. Paradoxically, greatly reduced Tf levels result in generalized iron overload of the liver but a profound refractory hypochromic, microcytic anemia caused by an inadequate iron supply to the erythron.[217, 272] Thus, whereas the lack of Tf results in inadequate transport of iron into erythroblasts, the liver accumulates even more iron than when Tf is present. In addition to its role in carrying iron to the erythron, Tf apparently serves as a plasma buffer for iron, and the liver is apparently very efficient at accumulating iron not bound to Tf. The absence of the additional capacity of Tf to bind iron, whether due to Tf saturation (in the case of hemochromatosis) or a generalized Tf deficiency (in the case of atransferrinemia), leads to iron overload in the liver.

MECHANISMS OF TISSUE DAMAGE BY IRON

Many hypotheses have been advanced to explain tissue iron toxicity (Fig. 10–18). Currently, the two

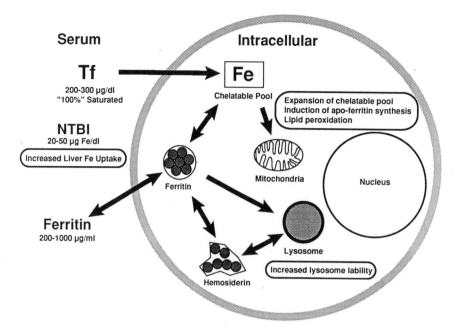

FIGURE 10–18. Cellular iron pools in an individual with HLA-linked hemochromatosis. Because of increased gut absorption of dietary iron, the serum Tf of the patient with hemochromatosis becomes saturated. With no unoccupied Tf to bind incoming iron, the level of non–Tf-bound iron (NTBI) is elevated. Although the molecular nature of this NTBI is unknown, it is taken up by the parenchymal cells (primarily of liver and heart), which become severely iron overloaded. Increased intracellular iron acquired through elevated uptake either via the TfR or via NTBI will lead to increased ferritin synthesis. In iron-overloaded individuals with hemochromatosis, serum ferritin levels are elevated. Increased Tf saturation, increased serum ferritin levels, and increased iron deposition in liver parenchymal cells are the most common indices of hemochromatosis. Excess intracellular iron can engage in oxidative reactions leading to lipid peroxidation, which in turn might be responsible for increased lysosome lability. In liver, the oxidative damage induced by excess iron is thought to cause fibrosis and to lead to an increased incidence of hepatocellular carcinoma in individuals with hemochromatosis.

favored hypotheses for the mechanism of hepatocellular injury in chronic iron overload are (1) peroxidative damage to the lipid membranes of cellular organelles, resulting in structural and functional alteration in cell integrity,[275–280] and (2) lysosomal fragility, resulting in the release of cell-damaging hydrolytic enzymes.[281, 282] These are not mutually exclusive theories, as lipid peroxidation may mediate the loss of lysosomal membrane integrity. Peroxidative damage to the membranes of myocardial cells has been shown to adversely affect their function in a cell culture system.[283] Addition of desferrioxamine inhibits peroxidation and restores normal contractility. An increase in the amount of "free iron" both within and outside cells may be responsible for peroxidative damage.[284, 285] Oxidation of membrane lipids may be influenced by various compounds, such as ascorbic acid[286, 287] and vitamin E.[288]

ADDITIONAL FUNCTIONS OF IRON AND IRON-BINDING PROTEINS

The requirement for iron in normal cell proliferation results in pleiotropic effects on hematological and immunological function. A direct role for iron-binding proteins in these processes has been proposed. Indeed, both ferritin and lactoferritin influence myelopoiesis, as assayed by in vitro culture methodologies.[289–291] Local release of these substances in vivo might modulate hematopoietic function, although such a role has not yet been defined. In addition, iron-binding proteins may have a role in immunoregulation by acting on cells of the lymphoid system.[292, 293] One physiological function of lactoferrin appears to be to inhibit bacterial growth in breast milk.[24, 25] By binding available iron, microbial growth is prevented because of lack of iron for essential cellular functions. This may also be a function of plasma Tf. There have been reports of increased systemic infections in hemochromatosis patients with high NTBI due to high Tf saturation.[24, 25] Low levels of ferritin are present in normal sera, and much higher levels are present with iron overload.[294, 295] Serum ferritin has a low iron content and therefore is unlikely to serve a transport function; rather, it serves as a convenient clinical measure of iron stores.

PERSPECTIVES FOR FUTURE RESEARCH

Humans, like all organisms, have critical metabolic needs for iron and must acquire it from the environment. In humans, this process involves consuming iron-containing foods, absorbing iron from them in a usable form, and moving that iron to sites of need around the body where systems for cellular uptake and intracellular utilization exist. Also in common with other organisms, we must deal with the possible toxicity that is the other side of the iron coin. The balance between the essentiality of iron and its possible toxicity underlies all aspects of human iron metabolism. Much has been learned about iron metabolism both at the cellular level and at the level of the whole organism; we have attempted to summarize this work here. Nonetheless, there remains much to be elucidated concerning iron metabolism.

Perhaps of foremost interest are the identity and function of the gene responsible for the very common human disorder known as hemochromatosis. To date, the most significant step forward has been the linkage of this disease to a gene near the HLA locus on chromosome 6.[244] Efforts attempting to localize this gene more precisely and to identify it by positional cloning are ongoing at several major research centers around the world. These and other research teams are also striving to identify new candidate genes by increasing our understanding of the components involved in cellular and whole body iron metabolism. Modern techniques of molecular biology have allowed scientists to gain much insight into the structure and function of Tf, the TfR, ferritin, and, more recently, the IRE-BP. However, chromosomal localizations of the genes encoding these proteins have indicated that none of them is at the hemochromatosis locus. A major player in iron metabolism remains to be identified. Candidates that come to mind include components of the reductase/transporter system responsible for the transmembrane movement of iron. The defect, however, may be not in these genes per se but in a yet undefined gene whose product regulates their expression or function. Similarly, given that the in vivo loading and unloading of the iron sequestration protein ferritin are poorly understood, components or regulators of these processes remain candidates for the hemochromatosis defect as well. The factors that account for the variations in age of onset and severity of HLA-linked hemochromatosis remain obscure, as does the connection between this disorder and neonatal hemochromatosis.

In addition to considerations related to hemochromatosis, there remains much to be discovered concerning human iron metabolism. The lives of patients suffering from transfusion iron overload (e.g., thalassemics) have been significantly improved through the development and widespread use of the iron-chelating drug desferrioxamine.[271] More research in this area is ongoing because desferrioxamine is not orally active and requires lengthy infusions several times a week to be effective.[296] The development of safe and effective oral iron-chelating drugs remains a great challenge. In addition to removal of excess iron, another possible avenue of clinical intervention in iron overload would be to negate its toxic effects within cells. This approach would require a significant increase in our understanding of the biochemical basis of the pathology of iron overload.

Far and away the most common worldwide health problem related to iron metabolism is iron deficiency. A minor portion of this chapter is devoted to this issue, since it lies outside the scope of this text. Although more nutritional research might reveal ways in which dietary iron might be made more available, the fundamental problem is dietary insufficiency. Basic biomedical research has already shown that iron is required for normal childhood development and that iron deficiency at critical points in the process can result in irreparable damage, including learning deficiencies.[228] It remains to be seen what will be done with this information.

REFERENCES

1. Bothwell, T. H., Charlton, R. W., Cook, J. D., and Finch, C. A.: Iron Metabolism in Man. Oxford, England, Blackwell Scientific Publications, 1979.
2. Emmery, T.: Iron metabolism in humans and plants. Am. Sci. 70:626, 1982.
3. London, I.: Iron and heme: Crucial carriers and catalysts. In Wintrobe, M. M. (ed.): Blood, Pure and Eloquent. New York, McGraw-Hill Book Co., 1980.
4. Lewin, R.: How micro-organisms transport iron. Science 225:401, 1984.
5. Crichton, R. R.: Inorganic Biochemistry of Iron Metabolism. New York, Ellis Horwood, 1991.
6. Neilands, J. B., and Nakamura, K.: Regulation of iron assimilation in microorganisms. Nutr. Rev. 43:193, 1985.
7. De Lorenzo, V., Bindereif, A., Paw, B. H., and Neilands, J. B.: Aerobactin biosynthesis and transport genes of plasmid ColV-K30 in Escherichia coli K-12. J. Bacteriol. 165:570, 1986.
8. Neilands, J. B., Bindereif, A., and Montgomerie, J. Z.: Genetic basis of iron assimilation in pathogenic Escherichia coli. Curr. Top. Microbiol. Immunol. 118:179, 1985.
9. Dancis, A., Klausner, R. D., Hinnebusch, A. G., and Barriocanal, J. G.: Genetic evidence that ferric reductase is required for iron uptake in Saccharomyces cerevisiae. Mol. Cell. Biol. 10:29, 1990.
10. Dancis, A., Roman, D. G., Anderson, G. J., Hinnebusch, A. G., and Klausner, R. D.: Ferric reductase of Saccharomyces cerevisiae: Molecular characterization, role in iron uptake, and transcriptional control by iron. Proc. Natl. Acad. Sci. USA 89:3869, 1992.
11. Finch, C. A., and Huebers, H. A.: Iron metabolism. Clin. Physiol. Biochem. 4:5, 1986.
12. Hallberg, L.: Bioavailability of dietary iron in man. Annu. Rev. Nutr. 1:123, 1981.
13. Van Dijk, J. P.: Regulatory aspects of placental iron transfer: A comparative study. Placenta 9:315, 1988.
14. Finch, C. A., and Huebers, H.: Perspectives in iron metabolism. N. Engl. J. Med. 306:1520, 1982.
15. Weintraub, L. R., Conrad, M. E., and Crosby, W. H.: Regulation of the intestinal absorption of iron by the rate of erythropoiesis. Br. J. Haematol. 11:432, 1965.
16. Finch, C. A., Deubelbeiss, K., Cook, J. D., Eachbach, J. W., Harker, L. A., Funk, D. D., Marsaglia, G., Hilman, R. S., Slichter, S., Adamson, J. W., Ganzoni, A., and Biblett, E. R.: Ferrokinetics in man. Medicine 49:17, 1970.
17. Morgan, E. H.: Transferrin: Biochemistry, physiology and clinical significance. Mol. Aspects Med. 4:1, 1981.
18. Garby, L., and Noyes, W. D.: Studies on hemoglobin metabolism. II. Pathways of hemoglobin iron metabolism in normal man. J. Clin. Invest. 38:1484, 1959.
19. Hershko, C., Cook, J. D., and Fiinch, C. A.: Storage iron kinetics. II. The uptake of hemoglobin iron by hepatic parenchymal cells. J. Lab. Clin. Med. 80:624, 1972.

20. Deiss, A.: Iron metabolism in reticuloendothelial cells. Semin. Hematol. 20:81, 1983.
21. Uchida, T., Akitsuki, T., Kimura, H., Tanaka, T., Matsuda, S., and Kariyone, S.: Relationship among plasma iron, plasma iron turnover, and reticuloendothelial iron release. Blood 61:799, 1983.
22. Williams, J., Ellerman, T. C., Kingston, I. B., Wilkins, A. C., and Kuhn, K. A.: The primary structure of hen ovotransferrin. Eur. J. Biochem. 122:297, 1982.
23. Mazurier, J., Metz-Boutique, M., Jolies, J., Spik, G., Montreuil, J., and Jolles, P.: Human lactotransferrin: Molecular, functional, and evolutionary comparisons with human serum transferrin and hen ovotransferrin. Experientia 39:135, 1983.
24. Weinberg, E. D.: Roles of iron in infection and neoplasia. J. Pharmacol. 16:358, 1985.
25. Weinberg, E. D.: Iron withholding: A defense against infection in neoplasia. Physiol. Rev. 64:65, 1984.
26. Metz-Boutique, M. H., Jolies, J., Mazurier, J., Schoentgen, F., Legrand, D., Spik, G., Montreuil, J., and Jolles, P.: Human lactotransferrin: Amino acid sequence and structural comparison with other transferrins. Eur. J. Biochem. 145:659, 1984.
27. Brown, J. P., Henwick, R. M., Hellstrom, L., Hellstrom, K. E., Doolittle, R. F., and Dreyer, W. J.: Human melanoma-associated antigen p97 is structurally and functionally related to transferrin. Nature 296:171, 1982.
28. Goubin, G., Goldman, D. S., Luce, J., Neiman, P. E., and Cooper, G. M.: Molecular cloning and nucleotide sequence of a transforming gene detected by transfection of chicken B-cell lymphoma DNA. Nature 302:114, 1983.
29. Aisen, P., and Brown, E. B.: Structure and function of transferrin. In Brown, E. B. (ed.): Progress in Hematology. New York, Grune and Stratton, 1975, p. 25.
30. MacGillivroy, R. T. A., Mendez, E., Shewale, J. G., Sinha S., Lineback-Zins, J., and Brew, K.: The primary structure of human serum transferrin. The structures of seven cyanogen bromide fragments and the assembly of the complete structure. J. Biol. Chem. 258:3543, 1983.
31. Williams, J.: The structure of transferrins. In Spik, G., Montreuil, J., Crichton, R. R., and Mazurier, J. (eds.): Proteins of Iron Storage and Transport. New York, Elsevier, 1985, p. 13.
32. Huebers, H. A., and Finch, D. A.: Transferrin: Physiologic behavior and clinical implications. Blood 64:763, 1984.
33. Uzan, G., Frain, M., Park, I., Besmond, C., Maessen, G., Triepat, J. S., Zakin, M. M., and Kahn, A.: Molecular cloning and sequence analysis of cDNA for human transferrin. Biochem. Biophys. Res. Commun. 119:273, 1984.
34. Yang, F., Lum, J. B., McGill, J. R., Moore, C. M., Naylor, S. L., van Bragt, P. H., Baldwin, W. D., and Bowman, B. H.: Human transferrin: cDNA characterization and chromosomal localization. Proc. Natl. Acad. Sci. USA 81:2752, 1984.
35. Park, I., Schaeffer, E., Sidoli, A., Baralle, F. E., Cohen, G. N., and Zakin, M. M.: Organization of the human transferrin gene: Direct evidence that it originated by gene duplication. Proc. Natl. Acad. Sci. USA 82:3149, 1985.
36. Schaeffer, E., Park, I., Cohen, G. N., and Zakin, M. M.: Organization of the human serum transferrin gene. In Spik, G., Montreuil, J., Crichton, R. R., and Mazurier, J. (eds.): Structure and Function of Transferrins. New York, Elsevier, 1985, p. 361.
37. Huerre, C., Uzan, G., Grzeschik, K. H., Weil, D., Levin, M., Hors-Cayla, M. C., Boue, J., Kahn, A., and Junien, C.: The structural gene for transferrin (TF) maps to 3q21 m3qter. Ann. Genet. (Paris) 27:5, 1984.
38. Aisen, P., and Listowski, I.: Iron transport and storage proteins. Ann. Rev. Biochem. 49:357, 1980.
39. Williams, J.: The evolution of transferrin. Trends Biol. Sci. 2:394, 1982.
40. Wang, A. C., and Sutton, H. E.: Human transferrins C and D1: Chemical differences in a peptide. Science 149:435, 1965.
41. Chasteen, N. D.: The identification of the probable locus of iron and anion binding in the transferrins. Trends Biol. Sci. 2:272, 1983.
42. Aisen, P., Leibman, A., and Zweier, J.: Stoichiometric and site characteristics of the binding of iron to human transferrin. J. Biol. Chem. 253:1930, 1978.
43. Fletcher, J., and Huehns, E. R.: Function of transferrin. Nature 218:1211, 1968.
44. Huebers, H. A., Huebers, E., Csiba, E., and Finch, C. A.: Heteogeneity of the plasma iron pool: Explanation of the Fletcher-Huehns phenomenon. Am. J. Physiol. 247:R280, 1984.
45. Huebers, H., Csiba, E., Huebers, E., and Finch, C. A.: Molecular advantage of diferric transferrin in delivering iron to reticulocytes: A comparative study. Proc. Soc. Exp. Biol. Med. 179:222, 1985.
46. Bali, P. K., Zak, O., and Aisen, P.: A new role for the transferrin receptor in release of iron from transferrin. Biochemistry 30:324, 1991.
47. Bali, P. K., and Aisen, P.: Receptor-modulated iron release from transferrin: Differential effects on the N- and C-terminal sites. Biochemistry 30:9947, 1991.
48. Morgan, E. H., and Peters, T., Jr.: The biosynthesis of rat transferrin. Evidence for rapid glycosylation, disulfide bond formation, and tertiary folding. J. Biol. Chem. 260:14793, 1985.
49. Bloch, B., Popovici, T., Levin, M. J., Tuil, D., and Kahn, A.: Transferrin gene expression visualized in oligodendrocytes of the rat brain by using in situ hybridization and immunohistochemistry. Proc. Natl. Acad. Sci. USA 82:6706, 1985.
50. Levin, M. J., Tuil, D., Uzan, G., Dreyfus, J. C., and Kahn, A.: Expression of the transferrin gene during development of non-hepatic tissues: High level of transferrin mRNA in fetal muscle and adult brain. Biochem. Biophys. Res. Commun. 122:212, 1984.
51. Skinner, M. K., Cosand, W. L., and Griswold, M. D.: Purification and characterization of testicular transferrin secreted by rat Sertoli cells. Biochem. J. 218:313, 1984.
52. McKnight, G. S., Lee, D. C., Hemmaplardh, D., Finch, C. A., and Palmiter, R. D.: Transferrin gene expression. Effects of nutritional iron deficiency. J. Biol. Chem. 255:144, 1980.
53. Idzerda, R. L., Huebers, H., Finch, C. A., and McKnight, G. S.: Rat transferrin gene expression: Tissue-specific regulation by iron deficiency. Proc. Natl. Acad. Sci. USA 83:3723, 1986.
54. Jandl, J. H., and Katz, J. H.: The plasma to cell cycle of transferrin. J. Clin. Invest. 42:314, 1963.
55. Debanne, M. T., Chindemi, P. A., and Regoeczi, E.: Binding of asialotransferrins by purified rat liver plasma membranes. J. Biol. Chem. 256:4929, 1981.
56. Young, S. P., Bomford, A., and Williams, R.: Dual pathways for the uptake of rat asialotransferrin by rat hepatocytes. J. Biol. Chem. 258:4972, 1983.
57. Schneider, C., Sutherland, R., Newman, R., and Greaves, M.: Structural features of the cell surface receptor for transferrin that is recognized by the monoclonal antibody OKT9. J. Biol. Chem. 257:8516, 1982.
58. Omary, M. B., and Trowbridge, I. S.: Biosynthesis of the human transferrin receptor in cultured cells. J. Biol. Chem. 256:12888, 1981.
59. Schneider, C., Owen, M. J., Banville, D., and Williams, J. G.: Primary structure of human transferrin receptor deduced from the mRNA sequence. Nature 311:675, 1984.
60. Kuhn, L. C., McClelland, A., and Ruddle, F. H.: Gene transfer, expression, and molecular cloning of the human transferrin receptor gene. Cell 37:95, 1984.
61. McClelland, A., Kuhn, L. C., and Ruddle, F. H.: The human transferrin receptor gene: Genomic organization, and the complete primary structure of the receptor deduced for a cDNA sequence. Cell 39:267, 1984.
62. Seligman, P. A., Schleicher, R. B., and Allen, R. H.: Isolation and characterization of the transferrin receptor from human placenta. J. Biol. Chem. 254:9943, 1979.
63. Enns, C. A., and Sussman, H. H.: Physical characterization of

the transferrin receptor in human placentae. J. Biol. Chem. 256:9820, 1980.

64. Harford, J. B., Casey, J. L., Koeller, D. M., and Klausner, R. D.: Structure, function and regulation of the transferrin receptor: Insights from molecular biology. *In* Steer, C. J., and Hanover, J. A. (eds.): Intracellular Trafficking of Proteins. Cambridge, England, Cambridge University Press, 1991, p. 302.

65. Zerial, M., Melancon, P. M., Schneider, C., and Garoff, H.: The transmembrane sequence of the transferrin receptor functions as a signal peptide. EMBO J. 5:1543, 1986.

66. Omary, M. B., and Trowbridge, I. S.: Covalent binding of fatty acid to the transferrin receptor in cultured human cells. J. Biol. Chem. 256:4715, 1981.

67. Gray, A., Dull, T. J., and Ullrich, A.: Nucleotide sequence of epidermal growth factor cDNA predicts a 128,000-molecular weight protein precursor. Nature 303:722, 1983.

68. Miller, Y. E., Jones, C., Scoggin, C., Morse, H., and Seligman, P.: Chromosome 3q (22-ter) encodes the human transferrin receptor. Am. J. Hum. Genet. 35:573, 1983.

69. Rabin, M., McClelland, A., Kuhn, L., and Ruddle, F. H.: Regional localization of the human transferrin receptor gene to 3q26 mqter. Am. J. Hum. Genet. 37:1112, 1985.

70. Plowman, G. D., Brown, J. P., Enns, C. A., Schroder, J., Nikinmaa, B., Sussman, H. H., and Hellstrom, K. E.: Assignment of the gene for human melanoma-associated antigen to chromosome 3. Nature 303:70, 1983.

71. Casey, J. L., Di Jeso, B., Rao, K., Klausner, R. D., and Harford, J. B.: Deletional analysis of the promotor region of the transferrin receptor. Nucleic Acids Res. 16:629, 1988.

72. Roberts, M. R., Miskimins, W. K., and Ruddle, F. H.: Nuclear proteins TREF-1 and TREF-2 bind to the transcriptional control element of the transferrin receptor gene and appear to be associated as a heterodimer. Cell Regul. 1:151, 1989.

73. Morgan, E. H., and Appleton, T. C.: Autoradiographic location of ^{125}I-labeled transferrin in rabbit reticulocytes. Nature 223:1371, 1969.

74. Sullivan, A. L., Grasso, J. A., and Weintraub, L. R.: Micropinocytosis of transferrin by developing red cells: An electron microscopic study utilizing ferritin-conjugates antibodies to transferrin. Blood 47:133, 1976.

75. Pastan, I. H., and Willingham, M. C.: Receptor-mediated endocytosis: Coated pits, receptosomes and the Golgi. Trends Biochem. Sci. 8:250, 1983.

76. Steinman, R. M., Mellman, I. S., Muller, W. A., and Cohn, Z. A.: Endocytosis and the recycling of plasma membrane. J. Cell Biol. 96:1, 1983.

77. Bessis, M.: Cytologic aspects of hemoglobin production. Harvey Lec. 58:125, 1963.

78. Roth, T. F., and Porter, K. R.: Yolk protein uptake in the oocyte of the mosquito *Aedes aegypti*. L. J. Cell Biol. 20:313, 1964.

79. Pastan, I., and Willingham, M. C.: The pathway of endocytosis. *In* Pastan, I., and Willingham, M. D. (eds.): Endocytosis. New York, Plenum Press, 1985, p. 1.

80. Pearse, B. M. F.: On the structural and functional components of coated vesicles. J. Mol. Biol. 126:803, 1978.

81. Steer, C. J., and Heuser, J.: Clathrin and coated vesicles: Critical determinants of intracellular trafficking. *In* Steer, C. J., and Hanover, J. A. (eds.): Intracellular Trafficking of Proteins. Cambridge, England, Cambridge University Press, 1991, p. 47.

82. Helenius, A., Mellman, I. L., Wall, D., and Hubbard, A.: Endosomes. Trends Biochem. Sci. 8:245, 1983.

83. Brown, M. S., Anderson, R. G. W., and Goldstein, J. L.: Recycling receptors: The round-trip itinerary of migrant membrane proteins. Cell 32:663, 1983.

84. Tycko, B., and Maxfield, F. R.: Rapid acidification of endocytic vesicles containing alpha-macroglobulin. Cell 28:643, 1982.

85. Harford, J., Wolkoff, A., Ashwell, G., and Klausner, R. D.: Intracellular dissociation of receptor-bound asialoglycoproteins in cultured hepatocytes. J. Cell Biol. 258:3191, 1983.

86. Galloway, C. J., Dean, G. E., Marsh, M., Rudnick, G., and Mellman, I.: Acidification of macrophage and fibroblast endocytic vesicles in vitro. Proc. Natl. Acad. Sci. USA 80:3343, 1983.

87. Karin, M., and Minz, B.: Receptor-mediated endocytosis of transferrin developmentally totipotent mouse teratocarcinoma cells. J. Biol. Chem. 256:3245, 1981.

88. Bleil, J. D., and Bretscher, M. S.: Transferrin receptor and its recycling in HeLa cells. EMBO J. 1:351, 1982.

89. Klausner, R. D., van Renswoude, J., Ashwell, G., Kempf, C., Schreichter, A. N., Dean, A., and Bridges, K. R.: Receptor-mediated endocytosis of transferrin K562 cells. J. Biol. Chem. 258:4715, 1983.

90. Lacopetta, B. J., Morgan, E. H., and Yeoh, G. C. T.: Receptor-mediated endocytosis of transferrin by developing erythroid cells from the fetal rat liver. J. Histochem. Cytochem. 31:336, 1983.

91. Ciechanover, A., Schwartz, A. L., Dautry-Varsat, A., and Lodish, H. F.: Kinetics of internalization and recycling of transferrin and the transferrin receptor in a human hepatoma cell line. J. Biol. Chem. 258:9681, 1983.

92. Van Renswoude, J. K., Bridges, K. R., Harford, J. B., and Klausner, R. D.: Receptor-mediated endocytosis of transferrin and the uptake of Fe in K562 cells: Identification of a non-lysosomal acidic compartment. Proc. Natl. Acad. Sci. USA 79:6186, 1982.

93. Klausner, R. D., Ashwell, G., van Renswoude, J., Harford, J. B., and Bridges, K. R.: Binding of apotransferrin to K562 cells: Explanation of the transferrin cycle. Proc. Natl. Acad. Sci. USA 80:2263, 1983.

94. Duatry-Varsat, A., Ciechanover, A., and Lodish, H. F.: pH and the recycling of transferrin during receptor-mediated endocytosis. Proc. Natl. Acad. Sci. USA 80:2258, 1983.

95. Morgan, E. H.: Inhibition of reticulocyte iron uptake by NH_4Cl and CH_3NH_2. Biochim. Biophys. Acta 642:119, 1981.

96. Rao, K., van Renswoude, J., Kempf, C., and Klausner, R. D.: Separation of Fe^{+3} from transferrin in endocytosis: Role of the acidic endosome. FEBS Lett. 160:213, 1983.

97. Klausner, R. D., van Renswoude, J., Kempf, C., Rao, K., Bateman, J. L., and Robbins, A. R.: Failure to release iron from transferrin in a Chinese hamster ovary cell mutant pleiotropically defective in endocytosis. J. Cell Biol. 98:1098, 1984.

98. Hoffbrand, A. V., Ganehaguru, K., Hooton, J. W. L., and Tattersall, M. H. N.: Effect of iron deficiency and desferrioxamine on DNA synthesis in human cells. Br. J. Haematol. 33:517, 1976.

99. Graslund, A., Ehrenberg, A., and Thelander, L.: Characterization of the free radical mammalian ribonucleotide reductase. J. Biol. Chem. 257:5711, 1982.

100. Robbins, E., and Pederson, T.: Iron: Its intracellular localization and possible role in cell division. Proc. Natl. Acad. Sci. USA 66:1244, 1970.

101. Stragand, J. J., and Hagemann, R. F.: An iron requirement for the synchronous progression of colonic cells following fasting and refeeding. Cell Tissue Kinet. 11:513, 1978.

102. Soyano, A., Chinea, M., and Romano, E. L.: The effect of desferrioxamine on the proliferative response of rat lymphocytes stimulated with various mitogens in vitro. Immunopharmacology 8:163, 1984.

103. Lederman, H. M., Cohen, A., Lee, J. W., Freedman, M. H., and Gelfand, E. W.: Deferoxamine: A reversible S-phase inhibitor of human lymphocyte proliferation. Blood 64:748, 1984.

104. Larrick, J. W., and Creswell, P.: Modulation of cell surface iron transferrin receptors by cellular density and state of activation. J. Supramol. Struct. 11:579, 1979.

105. Trowbridge, I. S., and Omary, M. B.: Human cell surface glycoprotein related to cell proliferation is the receptor for transferrin. Proc. Natl. Acad. Sci. USA 78:3039, 1981.

106. Chitambar, C. R., Massey, E. J., and Seligman, P. A.: Regulation of transferrin receptor expression on human leukemic cells during proliferation and induction of differentiation. Effects of gallium and dimethylsulfoxide. J. Clin. Invest. 72:1314, 1983.

107. Hu, H. Y., Gardner, J., and Aisen, P.: Inducibility of transfer-

rin receptors on friend leukemia cells. Science 197:559, 1977.

108. Kronke, M., Leonard, W. J., Depper, J. M., and Greene, W. C.: Sequential expression of genes involved in human T lymphocyte growth and differentiation. J. Exp. Med. 161:1593, 1985.

109. Trepel, J. B., Colamonici, O. R., Kelly, K., Schwab, G., Watt, R. A., Sausville, E. A., Jaffe, E. S., and Neckers, L. M.: Transcriptional inactivation of c-myc and the transferrin receptor in dibutyryl cyclic-AMP–treated HL60 cells. Mol. Cell. Biol. 7:2644, 1987.

110. Sutherland, R., Delia, D., Schneider, C., Newman, R., Keurhead, J., and Greaves, M.: Ubiquitous cell-surface glycoprotein on tumor cells is proliferation associated receptor for transferrin. Proc. Natl. Acad. Sci. USA 78:4515, 1981.

111. Galbraith, R. M., and Galbraith, G. M.: Expression of transferrin receptors on mitogen-stimulated human peripheral blood lymphocytes: Relation to cellular activation and related metabolic events. Immunology 44:703, 1981.

112. Hamilton, T. A.: Regulation of transferrin receptor expression in concanavalin A stimulated and gross virus transformed rat lymphoblasts. J. Cell. Physiol. 113:40, 1982.

113. Wiley, H. S., and Kaplan, J.: Epidermal growth factor rapidly induces a redistribution of transferrin receptor pools in human fibroblasts. Proc. Natl. Acad. Sci. USA 81:7456, 1984.

114. Weissman, A., Rao, K., Klausner, R. D., and Harford, J. B.: Exposure of K562 cells to anti-receptor monoclonal antibody OKT9 results in rapid redistribution and enhanced degradation of the transferrin receptor. J. Cell Biol. 102:951, 1986.

115. May, W. S., Jacobs, S., and Cuatrecasas, P.: Association of phorbol ester–induced hyperphosphorylation and reversible regulation of transferrin membrane receptors in HL60 cells. Proc. Natl. Acad. Sci. USA 81:2016, 1984.

116. Klausner, R. D., Harford, J., and van Renswoude, J.: Rapid internalization of the transferrin receptor in K562 cells is triggered by ligand binding or treatment with a phorbol ester. Proc. Natl. Acad. Sci. USA 81:3005, 1984.

117. Musgrove, E., Rugg, C., Taylor, I., and Hedley, D.: Transferrin receptor expression during exponential and plateau phase growth of human tumor cells in culture. J. Cell. Physiol. 118:6, 1984.

118. Sager, P. R., Brown, P. A., and Berlin, R. D.: Analysis of transferrin recycling in mitotic and interphase HeLa cells by quantitative fluorescence microscopy. 39:275, 1984.

119. Pan, B. T., Teng, K., Wu, C., Adam, M., and Johnstone, R. M.: Electron microscopic evidence for externalization of the transferrin receptor in vesicular form in sheep reticulocytes. J. Cell Biol. 101:942, 1985.

120. Harding, C., Heuser, J., and Stahl, P.: Endocytosis and intracellular processing of transferrin and colloidal gold–transferrin in rat reticulocytes: Demonstration of a pathway for receptor shedding. Eur. J. Cell Biol. 35:256, 1984.

121. Ward, J. H., Kushner, J. P., and Kaplan, J.: Regulation of HeLa cell transferrin receptors. J. Biol. Chem. 257:10317, 1982.

122. Pelicci, P. G., Tabillio, A., Thomopoulos, P., Titieux, M., Vainchenker, W., Rochant, H., and Testa, U.: Hemin regulates the expression of transferrin receptors in human hematopoietic cell lines. FEBS Lett. 145:350, 1982.

123. Mattia, E., Rao, K., Shapiro, D. S., Sussman, H. H., and Klausner, R. D.: Biosynthetic regulation of the human transferrin receptor by desferrioxamine in K562 cells. J. Biol. Chem. 529:2689, 1984.

124. Rao, D., Harford, J. B., Rouault, T., McClelland, A., Ruddle, F. H., and Klausner, R. D.: Transcriptional regulation by iron of the gene for the transferrin receptor. Mol. Cell. Biol. 6:236, 1986.

125. Rouault, T., Rao, K., Harford, J., Mattia, E., and Klausner, R. D.: Hemin, chelatable iron and the regulation of transferrin receptor biosynthesis. J. Biol. Chem. 260:14862, 1985.

126. Owen, D., and Kühn, L. C.: Noncoding 3′ sequences of the transferrin receptor gene are required for mRNA regulation by iron. EMBO J. 6:1287, 1987.

127. Casey, J. L., Hentze, M. W., Koeller, D. M., Caughman, S. W., Rouault, T. A., Klausner, R. D., and Harford, J. B.: Iron-responsive elements: Regulatory RNA sequences that control mRNA levels and translation. Science 240:924, 1988.

128. Koeller, D. M., Casey, J. L., Hentze, E. M., Chan, L.-N. L., Klausner, R. D., and Harford, J. B.: A cytosolic protein binds to structural elements within the iron regulatory region of the transferrin receptor mRNA. Proc. Natl. Acad. Sci. USA 86:3574, 1989.

129. Chan, L.-N. L., Grammatikakis, N., Banks, J. M., and Gerhardt, E. M.: Chicken transferrin receptor gene: Conservation of the 3′ noncoding sequences and expression in erythroid cells. Nucleic Acids Res. 17:3763, 1989.

130. Munro, H. N., and Linder, M. C.: Ferritin: Structure, biosynthesis, and role in iron metabolism. Physiol. Rev. 58:317, 1978.

131. Theil, E. C.: Ferritin: Structure, gene regulation, and cellular function in animals, plants, and microorganisms. Annu. Rev. Biochem. 56:289, 1987.

132. Clegg, G. A., Fitton, J. E., Harrison, P. M., and Treffry, A.: Ferritin: Molecular structure and iron-storage mechanisms. Prog. Biophys. Mol. Biol. 36:56, 1980.

133. Ford, G. C., Harrison, P. M., Rice, D. W., Smith, J. M., Treffry, A., White, J. L., and Yariv, J.: Ferritin: Design and formation of an iron-storage molecule. Philos. Trans. R. Soc. Lond. [Biol.] 304:551, 1984.

134. Munro, H. N., Leibold, E. A., Vass, J. K., Aziz, N., Roges, J., Murray, M., and White, K.: Ferritin gene structure and expression. In Spik, G., Montreuil, J., Crichton, R. R., and Mazurier, J. (eds.): Proteins of Iron Storage and Transport. New York, Elsevier, 1985, p. 331.

135. Drysdale, J., Jain, S. K., Boyd, D., Barrett, K. J., Vecoli, C., Belcher, D. M., Beaumont, C., Worwood, M., Lebo, R., McGill, J., and Crampton, J.: Human ferritins: Genes and proteins. In Spik, G., Montreuil, J., Crichton, R. R., and Mazurier, J. (eds.): Proteins of Iron Storage and Transport. New York, Elsevier, 1985, p. 343.

136. Lebo, R. V., Kan, Y. W., Cheung, M. C., Jain, S. K., and Drysdale, J. H.: Human ferritin light chain gene sequences mapped to several sorted chromosomes. Hum. Genet. 71:325, 1985.

137. Jain, S. K., Barrett, K. J., Boyd, D., Favreau, M. F., Crampton, J., and Drysdale, J. W.: Ferritin H and L chains are derived from different multigene families. J. Biol. Chem. 260:11762, 1985.

138. Boyd, D., Vecoli, C., Belcher, D. M., Jain, S. K., and Drysdale, J. W.: Structural and functional relationships of human ferritin H and L chains deduced from cDNA clones. J. Biol. Chem. 260:11755, 1985.

139. Boyd, D., Jain, S. K., Crampton, J., Barrett, K. J., and Drysdale, J.: Isolation and characterization of a cDNA clone for human ferritin heavy chain. Proc. Natl. Acad. Sci. USA 81:4751, 1984.

140. Dorner, M. H., Salfeld, J., Will, H., Leibold, E. W., Vass, J. K., and Munro, H. N.: Structure of human ferritin light subunit messenger RNA: Comparison with heavy subunit message and functional implications. Proc. Natl. Acad. Sci. USA 82:3139, 1985.

141. Leibold, E. A., Azia, N., Brown, A. J., and Munro, H. N.: Conservation in rat liver of light and heavy subunit sequences of mammalian ferritin. Presence of unique octopeptide in the light subunit. J. Biol. Chem. 259:4327, 1984.

142. Santoro, C., Marone, M., Ferrone, M., Costanzo, F., Colombo, M., Mingvanti, C., Cortese, R., and Silengo, L.: Cloning of the gene coding for human L apoferritin. Nucleic Acids Res. 11:2863, 1986.

143. Costanzo, F., Columbo, M., Staempfli, S., Santoro, C., Marone, M., Mingvanti, C., Cortese, R., and Silengo, L.: Structure of gene and pseudogenes of human apoferritin H. Nucleic Acids Res. 11:2863, 1986.

144. Hentze, M. W., Keim, S., Papadopoulos, P., O'Brien, S., Modi, W., Drysdale, J., Leonard, W. J., Harford, J. B., and Klausner, R. D.: Cloning, characterization, expression and chro-

mosomal localization of a human ferritin heavy chain gene. Proc. Natl. Acad. Sci. USA 83:7226, 1986.

145. Caskey, J. H., Jones, C., Miller, Y. E., and Seligman, P. A.: Human ferritin gene is assigned to chromosome 19. Proc. Natl. Acad. Sci. USA 80:482, 1983.

146. Yang, F., Lum, J. B., McGil, J. R., Moore, C. M., Naylor, S. L., van Bragt, P. H., Baldwin, W. D., and Bowman, B. H.: Human transferrin: cDNA characterization and chromosomal localization. Proc. Natl. Acad. Sci. USA 81:2752, 1984.

147. Harrison, P. M., White, J. L., Smith, J. M. A., Farrants, G. W., Ford, G. C., Rice, D. W., Addison, J. M., and Treffry, A.: Comparative aspects of ferritin structure, metal-binding and immunochemistry. In Spik, G., Montreuil, J., Crichton, R. R., and Mazurier, J. (eds.): Proteins of Iron Storage and Transport. New York, Elsevier, 1985, p. 67.

148. Arosio, P., Adelman, T. G., and Drysdale, J. W.: On ferritin heterogeneity. Further evidence for heteropolymers. J. Biol. Chem. 253:4451, 1978.

149. Drysdale, J. W., Adelman, T. G., Arosio, P., Casareale, D., Fitzpatrick, P., Hazard, J. T., and Yokota, M.: Human isoferritins in normal and disease states. Semin. Hematol. 14:71, 1977.

150. Hazard, J. T., Yokota, M., Arosio, P., and Drysdale, J. W.: Immunologic differences in human isoferritins: Implications for immunologic quantitation of serum ferritin. Blood 49:139, 1977.

151. Didsbury, J. R., Theil, E. C., Kaufman, R. E., and Dickey, L. F.: Multiple red cell ferritin mRNAs, which code for an abundant protein in the embryonic cell type, analyzed by cDNA sequence and by primer extension of the 5'-untranslated regions. J. Biol. Chem. 261:949, 1986.

152. Bomford, A., Conlon-Hollingshead, C., and Munro, H. M.: Adaptive responses of rat tissue isoferritins to iron administration. Changes in subunit synthesis, isoferritin abundance, and capacity for iron storage. J. Biol. Chem. 256:948, 1981.

153. Mertz, J. R., and Theil, E. C.: Subunit dimers in sheep spleen apoferritin. The effect on iron storage. J. Biol. Chem. 258:11719, 1983.

154. Treffry, A., Lee, P. J., and Harrison, P. M.: Iron-induced changes in rat liver isoferritins. Biochem. J. 220:717, 1984.

155. Funk, F., Lenders, J. P., Crichton, R. R., and Schneider, W.: Reductive mobilization of ferritin iron. Eur. J. Biochem. 152:167, 1985.

156. Pape, L., Multani, J. S., Stitt, C., and Saltman, P.: The mobilization of iron from ferritin by chelating agents. Biochemistry 7:613, 1968.

157. Sirivech, S., Freiden, E., and Osaki, S.: The release of iron from horse spleen ferritin by reduced flavins. Biochem. J. 143:311, 1974.

158. Weir, M. P., Gibson, J. F., and Peters, T. J.: Biochemical studies on the isolation and characterization of human spleen haemosiderin. Biochem. J. 223:31, 1984.

159. Ganeshaguru, K., Hoffbrand, A. V., Grady, R. W., and Cerami, A.: Effect of various iron chelating agents on DNA synthesis in human cells. Biochem. Pharmacol. 29:1275, 1980.

160. Aziz, N., and Munro, H. N.: Both subunits of rat liver ferritin are regulated at a translational level by iron induction. Nucleic Acids Res. 14:915, 1986.

161. Zahringer, J., Baliga, B. S., and Munro, H. N.: Novel mechanism for translational control in regulation of ferritin synthesis by iron. Proc. Natl. Acad. Sci. USA 73:857, 1976.

162. Shull, G. E., and Theil, E. C.: Translational control of ferritin synthesis by iron in embryonic reticulocytes of the bullfrog. J. Biol. Chem. 257:14187, 1982.

163. Schaefer, F. V., and Theil, E. C.: The effect of iron on the synthesis and amount of ferritin in red blood cells during ontogeny. J. Biol. Chem. 256:1711, 1981.

164. Rouault, T. A., Hentze, M. W., Dancis, A., Caughman, S. W., Harford, J. B., and Klausner, R. D.: Influence of altered transcription on the translational control of human ferritin expression. Proc. Natl. Acad. Sci. USA 84:6335, 1987.

165. Jain, S. K., Crampton, J., Gonzalez, I. L., Schmickel, R. D.,

and Drysdale, J. W.: Complementarity between ferritin H mRNA and 28S ribosomal RNA. Biochem. Biophys. Res. Commun. 131:863, 1985.

166. Smith, A., and Morgan, W. T.: Haem transport to the liver by haemopexin. Receptor-mediated uptake with recycling of the protein. Biochem. J. 182:47, 1979.

167. Majuri, R., and Grasbeck, R.: Isolation of the haemopexin-haem receptor from pig liver cells. FEBS Lett. 199:80, 1986.

168. Smith, A.: Intracellular distribution of haem after uptake by different receptors. Haem-haemopexin and haemasialo-haemopexin. Biochem. J. 231:663, 1985.

169. Smith, A., and Morgan, W. T.: Hemopexin-mediated heme transport to the liver. Evidence for a heme-binding protein in liver plasma membranes. J. Biol. Chem. 260:8325, 1985.

170. Kino, K., Tsunoo, H., Higa, Y., Takami, M., Hamaguchi, H., and Nakajima, H.: Hemoglobin receptor in rat liver plasma membrane. J. Biol. Chem. 255:9161, 1980.

171. Kino, K., Tsunoo, H., Higa, Y., Takami, H., and Nakajima, H.: Kinetic aspects of hemoglobin: Haptoglobin-receptor interaction in rat liver plasma membranes, isolated liver cells, and liver cells in primary culture. J. Biol. Chem. 257:4828, 1982.

172. Lowe, M. E., and Ashwell, G.: Solubilization and assay of an hepatic receptor for the haptoglobin-hemoglobin complex. Arch. Biochem. Biophys. 216:704, 1982.

173. Mack, U., Powell, L. W., and Halliday, J. W.: Detection and isolation of a hepatic membrane receptor for ferritin. J. Biol. Chem. 258:4672, 1983.

174. Bacon, B. R., and Tavill, A. S.: Role of the liver in normal iron metabolism. Semin. Liver Dis. 4:181, 1984.

175. Aisen, P.: Transferrin metabolism and the liver. Semin. Liver Dis. 4:193, 1984.

176. Aisen, P.: Transferrin and the alcoholic liver. Hepatology 5:902, 1985.

177. Fawwaz, R. A., Winchell, H. S., Pollycove, M., and Sargent, T.: Hepatic iron deposition in humans. I. First-pass hepatic deposition of intestinally absorbed iron in patients with low plasma latent iron-binding capacity. Blood 30:417, 1967.

178. Wheby, M. S., and Umpierre, G.: Effect of transferrin saturation on iron absorption in man. N. Engl. J. Med. 271:1391, 1964.

179. Klausner, R. D., Harford, J. B., Rao, K., Mattia, R., Weissman, A. M., Rouault, T., Ashwell, G., and van Renswoude, J.: Molecular aspects of the regulation of cellular iron metabolism. In Spik, G., Montreuil, J., Crichton, R. R., and Mazurier, J. (eds.): Proteins of Iron Storage and Transport. New York, Elsevier, 1985, p. 111.

180. Mattia, E., Josic, D., Ashwell, G., Klausner, R., and van Renswoude, J.: Regulation of intracellular iron distribution in K562 human erythroleukemia cells. J. Biol. Chem. 261:4587, 1986.

181. Harford, J. B., and Klausner, R. D.: Coordinate post-transcriptional regulation of ferritin and transferrin receptor expression: The role of regulated RNA-protein interaction. Enzyme 44:28, 1991.

182. Rouault, T. A., Stout, C. D., Kaptain, S., Harford, J. B., and Klausner, R. D.: Structural relationship between an iron-regulated RNA-binding protein (IRE-BP) and aconitase: Functional implications. Cell 64:881, 1991.

183. Kaptain, S., Downey, W. E., Tang, C., Philpott, C., Haile, D., Orloff, D. G., Harford, J. B., Rouault, T. A., and Klausner, R. D.: A regulated RNA binding protein also possesses aconitase activity. Proc. Natl. Acad. Sci. USA 88:10109, 1991.

184. Dandedar, T., Stripecke, R., Gray, N. K., Goosen, B., Constable, A., Johansson, H. E., and Hentze, M. W.: Identification of a novel iron-responsive element in murine and human erythroid δ-aminolevulinic acid synthase mRNA. EMBO J. 10:1903, 1991.

185. Cox, T. C., Bawden, M. J., Martin, A., and May, B. K.: Human erythroid 5-aminolevulinate synthase: Promoter analysis and identification of an iron-responsive element in the mRNA. EMBO J. 10:1891, 1991.

186. Savin, M. A., and Cook, J. D.: Mucosal iron transport by rat intestine. Blood 56:1029, 1980.

187. Cook, J. D., and Finch, C. A.: Iron nutrition. West. J. Med. 122:474, 1975.
188. Hallberg, L., and Rossander, L.: Bioavailability of iron from Western-type whole meals. Scand. J. Gastroenterol. 17:151, 1982.
189. Finch, C. A., and Cook, J. D.: Iron deficiency. Am. J. Clin. Nutr. 39:471, 1984.
190. Huebers, H., and Rummel, W.: Protein mediated epithelial iron transfer. In Csaky, T. Z. (ed.): Pharmacology of Intestinal Permeation. Berlin, Springer-Verlag, 1984, p. 513.
191. Callender, S. T., Mallett, B. J., and Smith, M. D.: Absorption of hemoglobin iron. Br. J. Haematol. 3:186, 1957.
192. Conrad, M. E., Weintraub, L. R., Sears, D. A., and Crosby, W. H.: Absorption of hemoglobin iron. Am. J. Physiol. 211:1123, 1966.
193. Hallber, L.: Iron nutrition and food fortification. Semin. Hematol. 19:31, 1982.
194. Cook, J. D., Morck, T. A., and Lynch, S. R.: The inhibitory effect of soy products on nonheme iron absorption in man. Am. J. Clin. Nutr. 34:2622, 1981.
195. Hunter, J. E.: Iron availability and absorption in rats fed sodium phytate. J. Nutr. 111:841, 1981.
196. Morck, T. A., Lynch, S. R., and Cook, J. D.: Inhibition of food iron absorption by coffee. Am. J. Clin. Nutr. 37:416, 1983.
197. Sorenson, E. W.: Studies on iron absorption. V. The effect of ascorbic acid and ethyl alcohol on the absorption of iron in iron-deficient subjects. Acta Med. Scand. 180:240, 1966.
198. Jacobs, A., Rhodes, J., Peters, D. K., Campbell, H., and Eakins, J. D.: Gastric acidity and iron absorption. Br. J. Haematol. 12:728, 1966.
199. Martinez-Torres, C., Romano, E., and Layrisse, M.: Effect of cysteine of iron absorption in man. Am. J. Clin. Nutr. 34:332, 1981.
200. Crosby, W. H.: Iron absorption. In Handbook of Physiology. Washington, D.C., American Physiological Society, 1968, p. 1553.
201. Bedard, Y. C., Pinkerton, P. H., and Simon, G. T.: Radioautographic observations on iron absorption by the duodenum of mice with iron overload, iron deficiency, and X-linked anemia. Blood 42:131, 1973.
202. Crosby, W. H.: The control of iron balance by the intestinal mucosa. Blood 22:441, 1963.
203. Parmley, R. T., Barton, J. C., and Conrad, M. E.: Ultrastructural cytochemical identification of the siderophilic enterocyte. J. Histochem. Cytochem. 32:724, 1984.
204. Huebers, H., Huebers, E., Rummel, W., and Crichton, R. R.: Isolation and characterization of iron-binding proteins from rat intestinal mucosa. Eur. J. Biochem. 66:447, 1976.
205. Humphrys, J., Walpole, B., and Worwood, M.: Intracellular iron transport in rat intestinal epithelium: Biochemical and ultrastructural observations. Br. J. Haematol. 36:209, 1977.
206. Kaufman, N., Wyllie, J. C., and Newkirk, M.: Two microsomal-associated iron-binding proteins observed in rat small intestine cells during iron absorption. Biochim. Biophys. Acta 497:719, 1977.
207. Thomas, F. B., Baba, N., Greenberger, N. J., and Salsburey, D.: Effect of phenobarbital on small intestinal structure and function in the rat. J. Lab. Clin. Med. 80:548, 1972.
208. Thomas, F. B., McCullough, F. S., and Greenberger, N. J.: Effect of phenobarbital on the absorption of inorganic and hemoglobin iron in the rat. Gastroenterology 62:590, 1972.
209. Bedard, Y. C., Clarke, S., Pinkerton, P. H., and Simon, G. T.: Effect of cycloheximide on iron absorption. Toxicity of iron. Lab. Invest. 30:155, 1974.
210. Conrad, M. E., Umbreit, J. N., Moore, E. G., Peterson, R. D. A., and Jones, M. B.: A newly identified iron binding protein in duodenal mucosa of rats: Purification and characterization of mobilferrin. J. Biol. Chem. 265:5273, 1990.
211. Stremmel, W., Lotz, G., Niederau, C., Teschke, R., and Strohmeyer, G.: Iron uptake by rat duodenal microvillous membrane vesicles: Evidence for a carrier mediated transport system. Eur. J. Clin. Invest. 17:136, 1987.
212. Teichmann, R., and Stremmel, W.: Iron uptake by human upper small intestine microvillous membrane vesicles. Indication for a facilitated transport mechanism mediated by a membrane iron-binding protein. J. Clin. Invest. 86:2145, 1990.
213. Winrobe, M. M.: Clinical Hematology. 3rd ed. Philadelphia, Lea & Febiger, 1951, p. 117.
214. Granick, S.: Ferritin: Its properties and significance for iron metabolism. Chem. Rev. 38:379, 1946.
215. Bergamaschi, G., Eng, M. J., Huebers, H. A., and Finch, C. A.: The effect of transferrin saturation on internal iron exchange. Proc. Soc. Exp. Biol. Med. 183:66, 1986.
216. Wheby, M. S., and Umpierre, G.: Effect of transferrin saturation on iron absorption in man. N. Engl. J. Med. 271:1391, 1964.
217. Goya, N., Mlyazakl, S., Kodate, S., and Ushlo, B.: A family of congenital atransferrinemia. Blood 14:239, 1972.
218. Schade, S. G., Bernier, G. M., and Conrad, M. E.: Normal iron absorption in hypertransferrinemic rats. Br. J. Haematol. 17:187, 1969.
219. Morgan, E. H.: The role of plasma transferrin in iron absorption in the rat. Q. J. Exp. Physiol. 65:239, 1980.
220. Fawwaz, R. A., Winchell, H. S., Pollycove, M., and Sargent, T.: Hepatic iron deposition in humans. I. First-pass hepatic deposition of intestinally absorbed iron in patients with low plasma latent iron-binding capacity. Blood 30:417, 1967.
221. Refsum, S. B., and Schreiner, B. B. J.: Regulation of iron balance by absorption and excretion. Scand. J. Gastroenterol. 19:867, 1984.
222. Bothwell, T. H., Charlton, R., and Motulsky, A. G.: Hemochromatosis. In Scriver, C. R., Beaudet, A. L., Sly, W. S., and Valle, D. (eds.): The Metabolic Basis of Inherited Disease. 6th ed. New York, McGraw Information Sciences Co., 1989, p. 1433.
223. Bothwell, T. H., Pirzio-Biroli, G., and Finch, C. A.: Iron absorption: I. Factors influencing absorption. J. Lab. Clin. Med. 51:24, 1958.
224. Weiden, P. L., Hackman, R. C., Deeg, H. J., Graham, T. C., Thomas, E. D., and Storb, R.: Long-term survival and reversal of iron overload after marrow transplantation in dogs with congenital hemolytic anemia. Blood 57:66, 1981.
225. Finch, C. A., Huebers, H., Eng, M., and Miller, L.: Effect of transfused reticulocytes on iron exchange. Blood 59:364, 1982.
226. Cook, J. D., and Monsen, E. R.: Food iron absorption: Use of a semisynthetic diet to study absorption of nonheme iron. Am. J. Clin. Nutr. 28:1289, 1975.
227. Charlton, R. W., and Bothwell, T. H.: Definition, prevalence and prevention of iron deficiency. Clin. Haematol. 11:309, 1982.
228. Scrimshaw, N. S.: Iron deficiency. Sci. Am. 265:46, 1991.
229. Bainton, D. F., and Finch, C. A.: The diagnosis of iron deficiency anemia. Am. J. Med. 37:62, 1964.
230. Finch, C. A., and Cook, J. D.: Iron deficiency. Am. J. Clin. Nutr. 39:471, 1984.
231. Pollitt, E., and Leibel, R. L.: Iron deficiency and behavior. J. Pediatr. 88:372, 1976.
232. Dallman, P. R., and Slimes, M. A.: Iron deficiency in infancy and childhood. INACG Report, 1979, p. 1.
233. Dallman, P. R., Beutler, E., and Finch, C. A.: Annotation: Effects of iron deficiency exclusive of anemia. Br. J. Haematol. 40:179, 1983.
234. Finch, C. A., Miller, L. R., Inamdar, A. R., Person, R., Seiler, K., and Mackler, B.: Iron deficiency in the rat: Physiological and biochemical studies of muscle dysfunction. J. Clin. Invest. 58:447, 1976.
235. Dillmann, E., Johnson, D. G., Martin, J., Mackler, B., and Finch, C. A.: Catecholamine elevation in iron deficiency. Am. J. Physiol. 237:R297, 1979.
236. Forth, W., and Rummel, W.: Gastrointestinal absorption of heavy metals. In IEPT—Pharmacology of Intestinal Absorption: Gastrointestinal Absorption of Drugs. Sect. 39B. Oxford, England, Pergamon Press, 1975, p. 599.
237. Rector, W. G., Jr., Fortuin, N. J., and Conley, C. L.: Nonhematologic effects of chronic iron deficiency. A study of

patients with polycythemia vera treated solely with venesections. Medicine 61:382, 1982.
238. Hill, J. M., Ruff, M. R., Weber, R. J., and Pert, C. B.: Transferrin receptors in rat brain: Neuropeptide-like pattern and relationship to iron distribution. Proc. Natl. Acad. Sci. USA 82:4552, 1985.
239. Cook, J. D., and Skikne, B. S.: Iron deficiency: Definition and diagnosis. J. Intern. Med. 226:349, 1989.
240. Youdim, M. B. H., Yehuda, S., Ben-Shachar, D., and Askenazi, R.: Behavioral and brain biochemical changes in iron-deficient rats. The involvement of iron in dopamine receptor function. In Pollitt, E., and Leibel, R. L. (eds.): Iron Deficiency: Brain Biochemistry and Behavior. New York, Raven Press, 1982, p. 39.
241. Gordeuk, V., Mukiibi, J., Hasstedt, S. J., Samowitz, W., Edwards, C. Q., West, G., Ndambire, S., Emmanual, J., Nkanza, N., Chapanduka, Z., Randall, M., Boone, P., Romano, P., Martell, R. W., Yamashita, T., Effler, P., and Brittenham, G.: Iron overload in Africa. Interaction between a gene and dietary iron content. N. Engl. J. Med. 326:95, 1992.
242. Bomford, A. B., Dymock, I. W., and Hamilton, E. B.: Genetic haemochromatosis. Gut (Suppl.):S111, 1991.
243. McLaren, G. D., Muir, W. A., and Kellermeyer, R. W.: Iron overload disorders: Natural history, pathogenesis, diagnosis, and therapy. CRC Crit. Rev. Lab. Sci. 19:205, 1983.
244. Simon, M., Bourel, M., and Genetet, B.: Idiopathic hemochromatosis: Demonstration of recessive transmission and early detection by family HLA typing. N. Engl. J. Med. 297:1017, 1977.
245. Cartwright, G. E., Edwards, C. Q., Kravitz, K., Skolnick, M., Amos, D. B., Johnson, A., and Buskjaer, L.: Hereditary hemochromatosis: Phenotypic expression of the disease. N. Engl. J. Med. 301:175, 1979.
246. Edwards, C. Q., Skolnick, M. H., and Kushner, J. P.: Hereditary hemochromatosis: Contributions of genetic analysis. Prog. Haematol. 12:43, 1981.
247. Kravitz, K., Skolnick, M., Cannings, C., Carmelli, D., Baty, B., Amos, B., Johnson, A., Mendell, N., Edwards, C., and Cartwright, G.: Genetic linkage between hereditary hemochromatosis and HLA. Am. J. Hum. Genet. 31:601, 1979.
248. Valberg, L. S., and Ghent, C. N.: Diagnosis and management of hereditary hemochromatosis. Annu. Rev. Med. 36:601, 1979.
249. Halliday, J. W.: Inherited iron overload. Acta Paediatr. Scand. (Suppl.) 361:86, 1989.
250. Milman, N., Graudal, N., Nielsen, L. S., and Srensen, S. A.: HLA determinants in idiopathic hemochromatosis. Dan. Med. Bull. 32:262, 1985.
251. Lin, H. J., Conte, W. J., and Rotter, J. I.: Disease risk estimates from marker association data. Application to individuals at risk for hemochromatosis. Clin. Genet. 27:127, 1985.
252. Niederau, C., Fischer, R., Sonnenberg, A., Stremmel, W., Trampisch, H. J., and Strohmeyer, G.: Survival and causes of death in cirrhotic and in noncirrhotic patients with primary hemochromatosis. N. Engl. J. Med. 313:1256, 1985.
253. Rouault, T. A., Tang, C. K., Kaptain, S., Burgess, W. H., Haile, D. J., Samaniego, F., McBride, O. W., Harford, J. B., and Klausner, R. D.: Cloning of the cDNA encoding an RNA regulatory protein: The human iron responsive element binding protein. Proc. Natl. Acad. Sci. USA 87:7958, 1990.
254. Cox, T. M., and Peters, T. J.: Uptake of iron by duodenal biopsy specimens from patients with iron-deficiency anemia and primary hemochromatosis. Lancet 1:123, 1978.
255. Jacobs, A., and Summers, M. R.: Iron uptake and ferritin synthesis by peripheral blood leukocytes in patients with primary idiopathic hemochromatosis. Br. J. Haematol. 49:649, 1981.
256. Bassett, M. L., Halliday, J. W., and Powell, L. W.: Monocyte ferritin synthesis in idiopathic hemochromatosis. J. Lab. Clin. Med. 100:137, 1982.
257. Bjorn-Rasmussen, E., Hagman, J., van Den Dungen, P., Prowit-Ksiazek, A., and Biberfeld, P.: Transferrin receptors

258. on circulating monocytes in hereditary hemochromatosis. Scand. J. Haematol. 34:308, 1985.
258. Halliday, C. E., Halliday, J. W., and Powell, L. W.: The clinical manifestations of chronic iron overload. Baillieres Clin. Haematol. 2:403, 1989.
259. Valberg, L. S., Simon, J. B., Manley, P. N., Corbett, W. E., and Ludwig, J.: Distribution of storage iron as body iron stores expand in patients with hemochromatosis. J. Lab. Clin. Med. 86:479, 1975.
260. Brink, B., Disler, P., Lynch, S., Jacobs, P., Charlton, R., and Bothwell, T.: Patterns of iron storage in dietary iron overload and idiopathic hemochromatosis. J. Lab. Clin. Med. 88:725, 1976.
261. Fillet, G., and Margaglia, G.: Idiopathic hemochromatosis: Abnormality in RBC transport of iron by the reticuloendothelial system. Blood 46:1007, 1975.
262. Stefanelli, M., Bentley, D. P., Cavill, I., and Roeser, J. P.: Quantitation of iron release from the RES in man. Am. J. Physiol. 247:R842, 1984.
263. Knisely, A. S., Magid, M. S., Dische, M. R., and Cutz, E.: Neonatal hemochromatosis. Birth Defects 23:75, 1987.
264. Ley, T. J., Griffth, P., and Nienhuis, A. W.: Transfusional hemosiderosis and chelation therapy. Clin. Haematol. 11:4376, 1982.
265. De Alarcon, P. A., Donovan, M., Forbes, G. B., Landaw, S. A., and Stockman, J. A.: Iron absorption in the thalassemia syndromes and its inhibition by tea. N. Engl. J. Med. 300:5, 1979.
266. Pippard, M. J., and Weatherall, D. J.: Iron absorption in nontransfused iron loading anemias: Prediction of risk for iron loading in response to iron chelation treatment in beta thalassemia intermedia and congenital sideroblastic anemias. Haematologica 17:17, 1984.
267. Nienhuis, A. W., and Wolfe, L.: The thalassemias: Disorders of hemoglobin synthesis. In Nathan, D. G., and Oski, F. A. (eds.): Hematology in Infancy and Childhood. Philadelphia, W. B. Saunders Co., 1987.
268. Modell, B., and Berdoukas, V.: The Clinical Approach to Thalassemia. New York, Grune and Stratton, 1984.
269. Modell, B., Letsky, E., Flynn, D. M., Peto, R., and Weatherall, D. J.: Survival and desferrioxamine in thalassemia major. Br. Med. J. 284:1081, 1982.
270. Wolfe, L., Olivieri, N., Sallan, D., Clan, S., Rose, V., Propper, R., Freedman, M. H., and Nathan, D. C.: Prevention of cardiac disease by subcutaneous deferoxamine in patients with thalassemia major. N. Engl. J. Med. 312:1600, 1985.
271. Barry, M., Flynn, D. M., Letsky, E. A., and Risdon, R. A.: Long term chelation therapy in thalassaemia major: Effect on liver iron concentration, liver histology and clinical progress. Br. Med. J. 2:16, 1974.
272. Heilmeyer, L., Keller, W., and Vivell, O.: Congenital transferrin deficiency in a seven-year-old girl. German Med. Meth. 6:385, 1961.
273. Sakata, T.: Atransferrinemia. J. Pediatr. Pract. 32:1523, 1969.
274. Fairbanks, V. F., and Beutler, E.: Congenital atransferrinemia and idiopathic pulmonary hemosiderosis. In Williams, W. J., Beutler, E., Erslev, A. J., and Lichtman, M. G. (eds.): Hematology. New York, McGraw-Hill Book Co., 1983, p. 489.
275. Gutteridge, J. M. C.: Iron and oxygen: A biologically damaging mixture. Acta Pediatr. Scand. (Suppl.) 361:78, 1989.
276. Bacon, B. R., and Britton, R. S.: The pathology of hepatic iron overload: A free radical–mediated process? Hepatology 11:127, 1990.
277. Jacobs, A.: The pathology of iron overload. In Jacobs, A., and Worwood, M. (eds.): Iron and Biochemistry in Medicine. London, Academic Press, 1980, p. 427.
278. Bassett, M. L., Halliday, J. W., and Powell, L. W.: Genetic hemochromatosis. Semin. Liver Dis. 4:217, 1984.
279. O'Connell, M. J., Ward, R. J., Baum, H., and Peters, T. J.: The role of iron in ferritin- and haemosiderin-mediated lipid peroxidation in liposomes. Biochem. J. 229:135, 1985.
280. Thomas, C. D., Morehouse, L. A., and Aust, S. D.: Ferritin

and superoxide-dependent lipid peroxidation. J. Biol. Chem. 260:3275, 1985.

281. Selden, C., Owen, M., Hopkins, J. N. P., and Peters, T. J.: Studies on the concentration and intracellular localization of iron proteins in liver biopsy specimens from patients with iron overload with special reference to their role in lysosomal disruption. Br. J. Haematol. 44:593, 1980.

282. Weir, M. P., Gibson, J. F., and Peters, T. J.: Hemosiderin and tissue damage. Cell Biochem. Funct. 2:186, 1984.

283. Link, G., Pinson, A., and Hershko, C.: Heart cells in culture: A model of myocardial iron overload in chelation. J. Lab. Clin. Med. 106:147, 1985.

284. Hershko, C., Graham, G., Bates, G. W., and Rachmilewitz, E. A.: Non-specific serum iron in thalassemia: An abnormal serum iron fraction of potential toxicity. Br. J. Haematol. 40:255, 1978.

285. Brissot, P., Wright, T. L., Ma, W. L., and Weiseger, R. A.: Efficient clearance of non–transferrin-bound iron by rat liver. Implications for hepatic iron loading in iron overload states. J. Clin. Invest. 76:1463, 1985.

286. Mak, I. T., and Weglicki, W. B.: Characterization of iron-mediated peroxidative injury in isolated hepatic lysosomes. J. Clin. Invest. 75:58, 1985.

287. Terao, J., Sugino, K., and Matsushita, S.: Fe2+ and ascorbic acid induced oxidation of cholesterol in phosphatidylcholine liposomes and its inhibition by alphatocopherol. J. Nutr. Sci. Vitaminol. (Tokyo) 31:499, 1985.

288. Dillard, C. J., Downey, J. E., and Tappel, A. L.: Effect of antioxidants on lipid peroxidation in iron-loaded rats. Lipids 19:127, 1984.

289. Broxmeyer, H. E., Juliano, L., Waheed, A., and Shadduck, R. K.: Release from mouse macrophages of acidic isoferritins that suppress hematopoietic progenitor cells is induced by purified L cell colony stimulating factor and suppressed by human lactoferrin. J. Immunol. 135:3224, 1985.

290. Sala, G., Worwood, M., and Jacobs, A.: The effect of isoferritins on granulopoiesis. Blood 67:436, 1986.

291. Dezza, L., Cazzola, M., Piacibello, W., Arosio, P., Levi, S., and Aglietta, M.: Effect of acidic and basic isoferritins on in vitro growth of human granulocyte-monocyte progenitors. Blood 67:789, 1986.

292. Akbar, A. N., Fitzgerald-Bocarsly, P. A., Desousa, M., Hilgartner, M. W., and Grady, R. W.: Decreased natural killer activity in thalassemia major: A possible consequence of iron overload. J. Immunol. 136:1635, 1986.

293. Akbar, A. N., Giardina, P. J., Hilgartner, M. W., and Grady, R. W.: Immunological abnormalities in thalassaemia major. I. A transfusion-related increase in circulating cytoplasmic immunoglobin-positive cells. Clin. Exp. Immunol. 62:397, 1985.

294. Worwood, M.: Serum ferritin. Clin. Sci. 70:215, 1986.

295. Worwood, M.: Ferritin in human tissues and serum. Clin. Haematol. 11:275, 1982.

296. Porter, J. B., Huehns, E. R., and Hider, R. C.: The development of iron chelating drugs. Baillieres Clin. Haematol. 2:257, 1989.

297. Nunez, M. T., Gaete, V., Watkins, J. A., and Glass, J.: Mobilization of iron from endocytic vesicles: The effects of acidification and reduction. J. Biol. Chem. 265:6688, 1990.

SECTION III

LYMPHOPOIESIS

Gene Rearrangements in Lymphoid Cells

Ilan R. Kirsch and W. Michael Kuehl

INTRODUCTION

The elucidation of the structure and organization of the genetic loci that encode the immunoglobulin and T-cell antigen receptor genes is one of the earliest and currently most important successes of the use of recombinant DNA technology. In terms of our understanding of cell growth, development, and differentiation, there are critical lessons to be learned from a molecular genetic analysis of the necessary and sufficient factors required for the generation of a humoral or cell-mediated immune response. Over the past 15 years, this work has not only solved the riddle of immune diversity but has also demonstrated a particularly profound example of the fundamental principle of genomic instability (see below). In terms of societal impact, the cloning and characterization of the immunoglobulin and T-cell antigen receptor genes have provided a set of extremely diverse, powerful, and specific reagents that can be applied to a variety of biomedical concerns, from the diagnosis, staging, and treatment of cancer[1, 2] to the synthesis of new kinds of "designer" catalytic enzymes.[3, 4]

Immunoglobulins became an early target of recombinant DNA research for two basic reasons. The mystery of how a higher organism was capable of responding specifically to a myriad of "foreign" antigenic stimuli, with which it might or might not come into contact during its lifetime, was an obviously important question that had been explored and debated for the previous century. What was required, however, to approach this problem at the outset of DNA cloning technology was a model system in which abundant immunoglobulin messenger RNA (mRNA) could be obtained for cloning studies. Today, essentially any gene or piece of DNA can be cloned, but initially an abundance of mRNA was a prerequisite to practical consideration of gene cloning. Such a model system existed for the immunoglobulin genes through the in vivo propagation and in vitro expansion in cell culture of murine plasmacytomas,[5] plasma cell tumors in which as much as 10 per cent of the total mRNA encoded a particular immunoglobulin molecule. With this resource at hand, the full force of a new technology could be brought to bear on the problem. The rest is history, and the result can now be delineated in textbook form.

THE QUESTION OF IMMUNE DIVERSITY

A species becomes a species because, over time, it can safeguard the integrity of its genetic material. Bacteria maintain this ability in part through the restriction-modification system exploited in recombinant DNA technology.[6] In higher organisms, it is not just the integrity of the DNA of the population, but also the protection (at least until reproductive age is achieved) of the viability of the cells that constitute the individual organism that provides a selective advantage for a particular species. Thus, higher organisms have developed a variety of mechanisms—for example, the mechanical barrier of the skin, the neuromuscular capacity of fight or flight, and the immune response—that protect them from discernible or invisible (e.g., microbial) threats within their environment. Inherent in the ability to perceive a threat is the ability to distinguish between oneself and the rest of the world. Our neurological system provides this function for the discernible world. Our immunological system provides this function with regard to the viruses, bacteria, fungi, and protozoa (or transformed cells) that we cannot see, but that can invade the sanctity of our bodies.

The immune system serves two defensive functions: (1) the recognition of a microbial agent or cell as "foreign" and (2) the processing and elimination of this foreign entity (the "effector" function). We are situated in the midst of a sea of foreign substances many of which are capable of invading and infecting us. We are capable of responding with great specificity to the majority of these substances via the recognition of specific "antigenic" determinants that these foreign molecules carry. This recognition is accomplished by the immune receptors (immunoglobulins and T-cell antigen receptors) expressed by our lymphocytes. We have the ability to respond to a myriad of antigens, only some of which can we count on being exposed to in our lifetime. What gives us this ability of being able to respond to this diversity of "foreignness"? How is this capability encoded in our DNA? This was a question that challenged immunologists for most of this century, stimulated by the work of Landsteiner, which established that the repertoire of the immune response was essentially infinite.[7]

This issue became the focus for the elucidation of immune diversity, an issue summarized by the following question: How can an essentially infinite repertoire of immune responsiveness be encoded in a finite amount of DNA? One possible solution to this question envisioned an expansive array of potentially functional immune receptor genes spread across and occupying a large proportion of germline DNA, one gene for each possible antigen with which the organism might come in contact. A diametrically opposed view suggested the existence of a single "platonic" immune receptor gene, which, upon antigenic stimulation, would mutate until it developed the capacity to recognize and interact with the antigen. The answer to this question was partially predicted by Dreyer and Bennett[8] and exists between the two extreme possibilities just described. These investigators suggested that the key to immune receptor diversity might reside in a structural reconfiguration of primary genetic material so as to associate one of multiple segments of variable sequence with a single segment of constant sequence. The implication of their suggestion was that the DNA of a functional, mature lymphocyte would, therefore, structurally no longer be the same as that of other cells. This was a novel and radical concept at the time of its suggestion and has been proved to be absolutely true.

THE BASIS OF IMMUNE DIVERSITY—A GENERIC OVERVIEW

Immune Receptor Proteins—Structure and Terminology

The proteins that combine to form the immunoglobulin and T-cell antigen receptors share common amino acid motifs (Figs. 11–1 and 11–2). Each of these proteins has domains that are more or less constant among all members of a particular immune receptor class. This "constancy" in fact defines a protein as a member of a particular class. In some cases, variations in these domains divide members of a particular class into subclasses. The immunoglobulin kappa (Igκ) and lambda (Igλ) and the T-cell antigen receptor alpha (TCRα), beta (TCRβ), gamma (TCRγ), and delta (TCRδ) classes all have a single such domain. The immunoglobulin heavy chain genes mu (Igμ), delta (Igδ), gamma (Igγ), epsilon (Igε), and alpha (Igα) are composed of three or four constant domains and a "hinge" sequence found between the first two constant domains.[9] Additional "constant" domains are associated with these immunoglobulin proteins when they are membrane bound (see below). Constant domains define the "effector" functions of these molecules, functions that are described more fully in Chapter 13.

The antigen recognition function of immune receptors is primarily handled by the amino-terminal domain of the molecule, which shows marked amino acid variability among all members of a particular class or subclass. Within this variable domain are regions that are "hypervariable," the complementarity determining regions (CDR), some of which have been shown by X-ray crystallography (at least for immunoglobulins) to be the parts of the protein that directly interact with antigen.[10–12]

Immunoglobulins have a basic four-chain structure consisting of two identical heavy chain peptides of the μ, δ, γ, ε, or α class (corresponding to IgM, IgD, IgG, IgE, and IgA antibodies, respectively) and two identical light chain peptides of the κ or λ class. For some classes of immunoglobulin, this basic structure undergoes oligomerization to form pentameric (e.g., IgM) or dimeric (e.g., IgA) proteins. T-cell antigen receptors form a basic two-chain structure consisting of an α/β or γ/δ heterodimer, although many other membrane proteins become associated with this primary structure.

The Germline Structure of Immune Receptor Genes[13–16]

The genes that will eventually encode the peptide chains of functional immune receptor proteins initially reside in germline DNA as a number of discrete, discontinuous segments (Fig. 11–3). For a given immune receptor, these segments can be found spread out across hundreds of thousands of nucleotides at a particular chromosomal location. Variations exist among these receptors in terms of the actual number and configurations of the segments (see below for a detailed description of each immune receptor locus), but a general structural theme is shared by all these genes. There are multiple (sometimes hundreds) of variable or "V" segments, each with its own leader sequence and promoter region. For some of the loci (IgH, TCRδ, TCRβ) there are diversity or "D" segments. For all the loci, one finds joining or "J" segments a few thousand nucleotides upstream from constant or "C" segments. These constant segments are the nucleic acid counterpart of the constant portion of the immune receptor polypeptide. The constant segment thus "defines" the locus. Sequences that are capable of enhancing the transcription of the locus are often found in proximity to these C regions.

As a prerequisite to the formation of a functional immunoglobulin or T-cell antigen receptor, one of the V segments undergoes a site-specific recombination event with a D, J, or previously site-specifically rearranged D-D or D-J segment. This forms a now contiguous VJ or VDJ continuous coding region still a few thousand nucleotides upstream of the constant segment. This contiguous VJ or VDJ region of DNA corresponds to the variable domain of the immune receptor polypeptide described above. The rearranged gene is transcribed into RNA and, after appropriate splicing out of intervening sequences, translated into protein. The recombination event is mediated by a set of enzymes that cause a DNA breakage and rejoining event that appears to commence with the recognition of specific "signal" sequences 3' of V segments, 5' of J segments, and flanking the interposed D segments. The signal sequences are shown schematically as triangles in Figure 11–3. (For a more complete description of this recombination event, see The Mechanism of V(D)J Recombination further on in this chapter.) The end result of this recombination is the irreversible structural reconfiguration of the DNA in the lymphocyte that has undergone the recombination event. Depending on the orientation of the various recombining segments, the recombination event can occur either via deletion or inversion of the DNA between the segments to be joined. Both deletions and inversions have been demonstrated as part of V(D)J recombination.[17, 18] As classically envisioned, V(D)J recombination occurs within a given immunoglobulin or T-cell antigen receptor locus, but it can occur between loci as well, via either sister chromatid exchange[19] or frank interchromosomal translocation or inversion.[20, 21]

Immune receptor diversity is achieved by the summation of five features of the structure and activation of these loci: (1) germline diversity, (2) combinatorial joining, (3) junctional diversity, (4) combinatorial association, and (5) somatic mutation.

Germline Diversity

This element of diversity arises from the proliferation over evolutionary time of V, D, and J segments

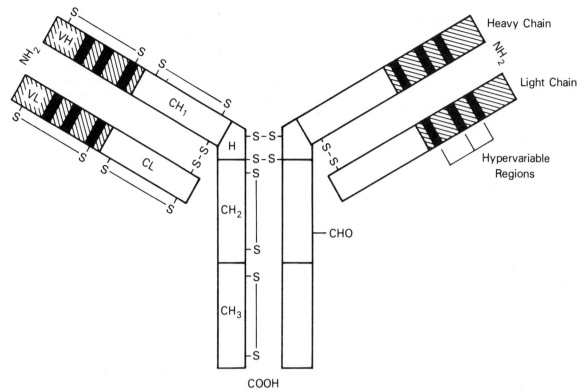

FIGURE 11–1. A schematic representation of an antibody molecule. The basic immunoglobulin consists of two identical "heavy" chains and two identical "light" chains. Each chain is divided into an amino (NH_2) terminal region, which is variable (V), and a carboxy (COOH) terminal region, which is constant (C) among all members of that heavy or light chain subclass. Within the variable regions are regions that show hypervariability from one chain to another. The hypervariable regions are predominantly responsible for the antigen-binding function of the molecule, and the constant regions mediate the molecule's "effector" function(s). The chains are glycosylated (CHO) and contain intrachain and interchain disulfide bonds (-S-S-). Heavy chain constant regions are composed of three or four constant domains (e.g., CH_1); light chains have a single constant segment. Some heavy chain classes have a separate "hinge" domain (H) between CH_1 and CH_2.

within immune receptor loci. Some loci contain hundreds of potential V segments. Most contain at least a handful of J segments (the TCRα locus contains dozens; see below). A few of the loci contain D segments as well.

Combinatorial Joining

Theoretically, any V segment can combine with any D and any J. Thus, diversity arises in this case simply from the number of distinctive segments that are available to participate in the process. For example, if any one of 100 V segments can recombine with any of 10 D and 5 J segments, 5000 distinct variable regions can be formed from these 115 discrete segments.

Junctional Diversity

Variation at the Point of Recombination/Nucleotide Deletion

Although site specific, the V(D)J recombination event is not absolutely precise to a specific nucleotide.

In fact, flexibility exists at the point of alignment between V, D, and J segments. The simplest example of this can be seen in studies of VJ rearrangement in the immunoglobulin light chain genes. The germline κ V segment can potentially encode amino acids 1 to 95 of the mature κ polypeptide. The amino acid sequence continues with amino acid 96 at the start of the J segment. This sequence is indeed formed if recombination occurs precisely between the end of codon 95 of the V segment and the beginning of codon 96 of the J segment, but that is not always the case. The rearrangement can occur within codon 95 or 96 to create a composite codon with nucleotides provided by each segment. This can alter the amino acid encoded by that codon and thus generate additional diversity as a result of the joining event itself. In Figure 11–4, this feature is illustrated for the TCRγ locus using one particular V_γ and one particular J_γ segment for the demonstration. The figure raises several issues for consideration. It should be noted that the heptamer signal sequences are not always exactly flush or in-frame with the known V or J coding segments. Next, the point needs to be made that the "flexibility" of point of joining is actually a reflection of variable deletion of nucleotides from one, the other,

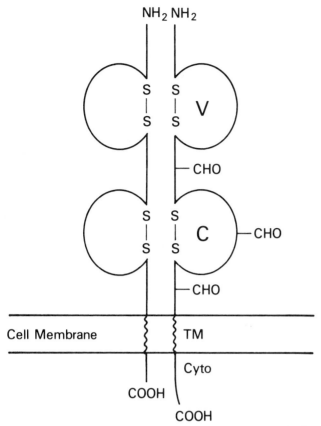

FIGURE 11–2. The T-cell antigen receptor heterodimer. The fundamental antigen recognition component of the T-cell antigen receptor consists of a heterodimeric molecule formed from an α and β chain or a γ and δ chain. Like immunoglobulins, these chains are divided into portions that are variable (V) and constant (C) among all members of the particular class. The amino (NH₂) portion of the molecule is extracellular, and the carboxy-terminus is within the cellular cytoplasm (cyto), with the two segments connected by a transmembrane (TM) domain. Like the membrane-associated immunoglobulin molecules, the T-cell antigen receptors are part of a macromolecular complex of proteins that confer stability and coordinate effector function (see text). The α/β heterodimer is interchain disulfide linked; one type of γ/δ heterodimer seems not to be.

or both partners in the rearrangement event. Initially, this flexibility was viewed as variability in the crossover point of recombination, but now it is recognized as being instead an example of the more general theme of exonucleolytic "nibbling" of the coding ends involved in V(D)J recombination. This realization has arisen because of the finding that the signal sequences from the two opposing segments are almost always joined in a precise and flush fashion without any loss of nucleotides.[22] The implication of this finding is that first a cut is made at the signal sequence/coding sequence border. The signal sequences are then joined together directly. The coding sequences, however, can be subjected to loss of nucleotides before ligation to each other. It should also be noted at this point that this "flexibility" of VJ joining need not always result in a recombination event that maintains a continuous reading frame from V segment through J segment. Indeed, in the characterization of these rearrangements, such "out-of-frame" non-functional recombi-

nants are frequently noted.[23, 24] The system is built so that absolute precision (and indeed guaranteed functionality) is sacrificed to enhance diversity. In one model system that has been studied extensively, one or the other of the rearranged coding ends (V, D, or J) shows nucleotide loss about 75 per cent of the time when compared with its germline sequence. The loss is usually less than 5 nucleotides (nt) from either end.[22]

Insertion

Nucleotide addition also occurs at the coding segment junctions in about 75 per cent of rearrangements (Fig. 11–5). The addition of these nucleotides appears to be of at least two types. The first type of nucleotide addition is related to the specific sequences found at the end of the coding segments that are joined and involves the creation of a 1 to 3 base pair (bp) inverted repeat of one and/or the other coding segment end. These inverted repeats are called "P" nucleotides and are postulated to occur through a sequence of cleavage, hairpin formation, endonucleolytic activity, and ligation.[25] "P" nucleotides are found only when no nucleotides have been lost from the coding strands, suggesting that the generation of these additional nucleotides occurs early in the process of V(D)J recombination and can be "erased" by subsequent exonucleolytic "nibbling" of the coding ends. The second type of nucleotide addition seen at the boundary of V, D, or J coding segment rearrangements appears to be DNA template independent. Usually fewer than five non-templated nucleotides are found at these junctions. The non-templated nucleotides often show a predisposition toward the addition of G and C residues. This is consistent with the preference for G and C residues by the enzyme terminal deoxynucleotidyl transferase (TdT), and indeed the presence of these non-templated nucleotides, "N" regions, correlates with the presence and level of TdT activity.[26–28] Rearrangements of the immunoglobulin heavy chain locus are almost invariably accompanied by N sequence addition, in contrast to immunoglobulin light chain rearrangements, in which N sequences are a rarity. This supports the observation that TdT is much more active at the time of IgH than IgL V(D)J recombination. Putative N sequences can be found with regularity in TCR gene rearrangements. There may be an additional requirement for complementary bases to exist at the ends of the two coding ends in order for a successful resolution and ligation of the ends to be achieved.[25]

Depending on (1) the relationship of the signal sequences to the V, D, and J coding segments, (2) the ability of the ends of the segments to form complementary base pairs with each other, (3) the stringency and universality of postulated "hairpin" (see Fig. 11–5) formation and reopening, and (4) the presence or absence of "nibbling" exonucleases and N sequences added by TdT, certain combinations of V's, D's, and J's may be favored at different times of development. For example (although there is no evidence that this

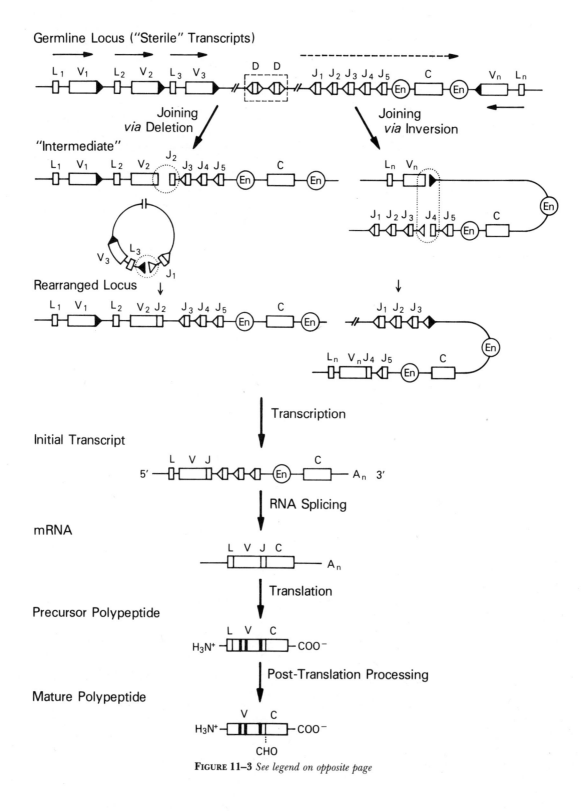

FIGURE 11–3 *See legend on opposite page*

example is true), if a rearrangement were to occur at a time when the exonuclease was not active, then only those V and J segments whose distance from the heptamer signals resulted in in-frame recombination would be functional. Thus, there would be a selection for certain V's to recombine with certain J's, D's, and so on. This example is complicated and possibly made irrelevant if the formation of 1 to 3 "P" nucleotides at the ends of the coding segments is a random process, since that would alter the reading frame randomly. Whether these or other factors do exert a selective effect on immune receptor expression is not yet established, but it does appear that in embryonic development, there may be a more restricted repertoire of immune receptors than during later development (see reference 28a and Table 11–1).

Combinatorial Association

There is no evidence that the particular rearrangement of one receptor biases the choice of V or J utilized by its dimerizing partner. Thus, additional diversity is generated by the possibility that (at least theoretically) any immunoglobulin heavy chain can dimerize with any immunoglobulin light chain, any TCRα with any TCRβ, or any TCRγ with any TCRδ. Once a functional immune receptor has been formed via V(D)J recombination, there appears to be a shutdown of any further recombinational activity on the other allele of that immune receptor. This results in the production of only a single functional immune receptor chain of any given type by a single cell (this is called "allelic exclusion" and will be dealt with more extensively later on in this chapter).

Somatic Mutation

Earlier in this chapter we contrasted two extreme views of the generation of immune receptor diversity, one in which all potential antigen-binding possibilities were encoded in place in germline DNA, the other in which a single gene became subject to a mechanism of hypermutation upon antigenic stimulation. We have seen that germline diversity does indeed exist, although it is not as extensive as in the extreme example. Similarly, at least for the immunoglobulin heavy and light chain loci, a mechanism of somatic hypermutation of the V(D)J regions formed by site-specific recombination has been amply demonstrated. Numerous cases have been described in which the V region sequence in a functionally rearranged immunoglobulin produced by a B lymphocyte differs from the germline V segment from which it arose, not just in junctional sequences but in the body of the segment as well. Most of these examples are found in B cells that have "switched" (see below) from a "primary" IgM response to an IgG or IgA "secondary" response. The conceptual framework in which somatic mutation is viewed postulates that such mutation acts to increase the binding affinity of antibody for antigen, and that those cells that have mutated their initial immunoglobulins to those of higher affinity for a particular antigen are more selectively stimulated by antigenic challenge.

The rate of somatic mutation within the V segments of immunoglobulin genes has been estimated to be remarkably high; by some investigators the estimate is as high as 10^{-3} per base pair per cell generation.[29] This process can continue during several cycles of cell division.[30] Remarkably, this mutational mechanism appears to be restricted to the variable regions of rearranged immunoglobulins in B cells; the rest of the genomic DNA is not affected. In fact, the rest of the immunoglobulin locus appears to be unaffected, with the 5' boundary of mutational activity being found near the promoter of the rearranged V segment and the 3' boundary about 1000 nt distal to the rearranged J segment.[31] Thus, there appears to be a mutational system activated in B lymphocytes that because of a

FIGURE 11–3. V(D)J recombination. A generalized schematic illustrating the structural reconfigurations of immune receptor loci that are a prerequisite to the formation of a functional polypeptide and therefore to the generation of immune diversity. The gene that will eventually constitute the immune receptor exists initially in germline DNA as a set of discrete, non-contiguous segments. There are multiple variable (V) segments with their upstream leader (L) exons that mediate transport of the polypeptide into or through a membrane. For certain of the immune receptor loci (IgH, TCRβ, TCRδ) there are diversity (D) segments. For all the loci, one finds joining (J) segments upstream from constant (C) segments. Prior to gene rearrangement, "sterile" transcription (*solid* and *dashed arrows* over the first line of the schematic) of the loci about to be rearranged occurs, probably indicative of a change in the status and "accessibility" of the chromatin at these sites (see text). Structural and irreversible rearrangement of the DNA occurs either by deletion of the DNA between the rearranging segments or by inversion. The reaction is essentially site specific, mediated by a recombinase enzyme complex that recognizes heterologous signal sequences (*solid* and *open triangles*) that flank the rearranging segments. Following recombination, a now contiguous V(D)J region is formed and still can begin from the promoter located 5' of the rearranged V segment, with transcriptional activity "enhanced" by enhancer elements (En) that are found around the DNA flanking the C segment. A precursor RNA is transcribed up to the point where addition of a run of adenosine residues (A_n) is sited. RNA intervening between coding segments is spliced out, yielding the mature messenger RNA (mRNA). The mRNA is translated into protein and transported to its position in the membrane. The mature polypeptide is finished after additional processing, which includes cleavage of the leader peptide and possible glycosylation (CHO) of certain sites within the peptide. (From Kirsch, I. R.: Genetics of pediatric tumors: The causes and consequences of chromosomal aberrations. *In* Pizzo, P., and Poplack, D. [eds.]: Principles and Practice of Pediatric Oncology. 2nd ed. Philadelphia, J. B. Lippincott, 1993; with permission.)

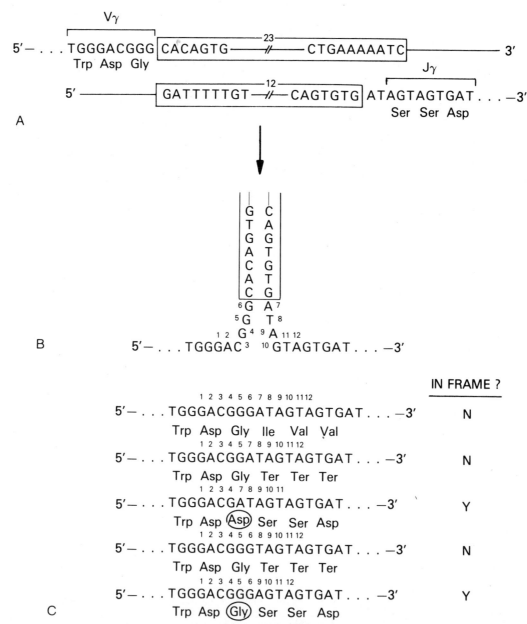

FIGURE 11–4. V(D)J recombination, signal sequences, "nibbling" of coding ends. *A*, The nucleotide sequence at the 3' border of a V segment and 5' border of a J segment is shown, using segments from the TCRγ locus in this example. The signal heptamer and nonamer sequences are boxed. There is a "spacer" of 23 nucleotides (nt) separating heptamer from nonamer 3' of a Vγ coding segment. A 12 nt spacer is found 5' of a Jγ segment. A signal sequence abuts the V coding segment but is separated from the J coding segment by 2 nt. The amino acids encoded at the border of these segments in their germline state are shown. *B*, the coding segments are approximated by the V(D)J recombinase complex, possibly aided by potential hydrogen bonding between complementary nucleotides of the opposing signal sequences. A DNA break occurs at the border of the signal sequences, which are then ligated to one another (see Fig. 11–3). *C*, Variable nucleotide deletion occurs at the ends of the coding segments prior to ligation. Depending on the extent of deletion, the resolved contiguous V-J region can maintain a single reading frame and be translatable into a functional TCRγ polypeptide, or it can become contiguous but out of frame and non-functional (see examples). For in-frame structures, additional variability can occur at the amino acid encoded at the V-J junction (in the example shown, Asp or Gly), depending on the deletion.

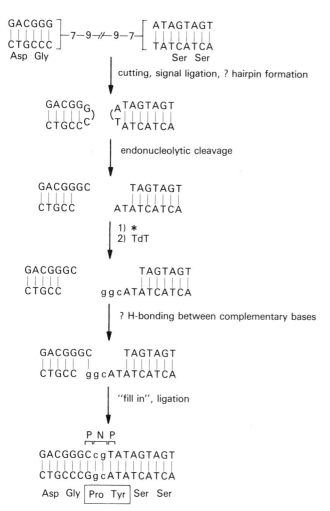

FIGURE 11–5. **V(D)J recombination, nucleotide insertion, "P" and "N" nucleotides.** An abbreviated and still speculative model is shown again, using (as in Fig. 11–4) a Vγ-Jγ juxtaposition. Following approximation of the signal ends, endonucleolytic cleavage occurs, generating short single strands at the ends of the coding segments (via a postulated hairpin intermediate). (*It is at this point where exonucleolytic nibbling might, but need not, occur. The consequent occurrence of nucleotide deletions is shown in Fig. 11–4.) Terminal deoxynucleotidyl transferase (TdT) adds non-templated nucleotides to the junctional coding ends. Complementarity of terminal nucleotides aids in aligning the two coding ends, and after double-stranded repair mechanisms and ligation a contiguous V-J segment is formed. The "P" nucleotides are the short, single-nucleotide, inverted repeats resulting from the endonucleolytic cleavage and repair. (They can be longer than single nucleotides, depending on the point of endonucleolytic cleavage.) The "N" sequences, shown in lower case, are the result of TdT activity. In this example, these two processes have combined to create additional diversity at the V-J junction. Two additional amino acids, proline and tyrosine, will now be part of the TCRγ polypeptide. (A more refined and extensive discussion of models like this one is available in reference 25 and particularly in reference 173.)

combination of structural information and transcriptional activity targets the rearranged V(D)J region in antigen-selected cells. This process does not appear to be active in T cells. Perhaps the different "recognition" requirements (see Chapter 13) of T cells make a hypermutation mechanism a disadvantage in this lineage.

The five mechanisms of generation of immune receptor diversity just described are responsible for the almost infinite variety of binding sites that allow a response to essentially any antigenic challenge (see Table 11–1).

THE MECHANISM OF V(D)J RECOMBINATION

The Recombinase Complex

In the above section, we have provided an overview of the process of the generation of immune receptor diversity, a process that relies largely, though not totally, on a structural, irreversible reconfiguration of the DNA encoding the immune receptor genes. In this section, we describe in greater detail some of the components and the mechanism of action of the "recombinase complex" that mediates V(D)J rearrangement. At present, there is no cell-free system for analysis of V(D)J recombination that can be readily utilized to dissect out and study the various components in the process. It seems that there are probably a number of enzymes whose concerted action leads to the recognition and juxtaposition of V, D, and J segments. Included among these are likely to be RAG-1 and RAG-2, the *scid* gene product, TdT, and recombination signal sequence–binding proteins.

RAG-1 and RAG-2

The *r*ecombination *a*ctivating *g*enes, RAG-1 and RAG-2, were discovered because of their ability to synergistically induce measurable V(D)J recombination activity (on an exogenously introduced substrate) when transfected into fibroblasts, cells that normally have no "recombinase" activity.[32, 33] These genes are tightly linked on human chromosome 11. Although it is formally possible that the protein products of these genes regulate the expression of the actual recombinase, circumstantial evidence suggests that they themselves are part of the recombinase complex. The genes are conserved in those species that are known to carry out V(D)J recombination. Their protein motifs are not consistent with other known classes of transcription activating factors. When transfected into fibroblasts, they initiate V(D)J recombination activity without initiating any other evidence of a lymphoid developmental program. Their dual expression is closely correlated with those lymphoid cells and cell lines that have demonstrated V(D)J recombinational activity and not with those that do not.

The *scid* Gene Product

In the mouse, there is a mutation, *scid*, which, when present in the homozygous form, abrogates normal B- and T-cell–mediated immunity.[34] It was demonstrated[35] that these mice were incapable of generating functionally V(D)J rearranged immune receptor genes. More refined molecular analysis revealed that

TABLE 11–1. POTENTIAL DIVERSITY OF HUMAN IMMUNOGLOBULIN (IG) AND TCR VARIABLE REGION DOMAINS*

	Ig			TCRαβ		TCRγδ	
	H	κ	λ	α	β	γ	δ
V segments	100	100	100	60	80	8	6
D segments	15	0	0	0	2	0	3
J segments	6	5	4	50	13	5	3
V(D)J combinations	10^4	500	400	3000	2000	40	18
N regions	2	0	0	1	2	1	4
V domains	10^{10}	10^4	10^4	10^6	10^9	10^4	10^{13}
V domain pairs	10^{14}			10^{15}		10^{17}	

*The approximate number of V, D, and J segments is indicated for each locus. The number of N regions corresponds to the number of joining events, except for Ig light chains (κ and λ), which rarely have N sequences. The approximate number of potential V domains for each locus is calculated as the number of V, (D), and J segment combinations multiplied by the potential extent of junctional diversity as a result of one or more joining events. As a rough estimate, joints lacking N sequences are assumed to have 10 possible amino acid sequences as a result of exonuclease nibbling and P sequences, whereas joints containing N sequences are assumed to have 1000 possible template-independent amino acid sequences. Additional variability of Ig V domains results from antigen-driven somatic hypermutation. Potential variability is decreased early in ontogeny owing to lack of N regions or preferential joining of specific V, D, and J segments, as indicated in the text. A more complete discussion of the potential variability at sites of joining can be found elsewhere (see reference 173).

recognition of signal sequences and DNA breakage was taking place in these animals but that the ends of the V, D, or J coding segments were not being ligated back together. The signal ends, however, were ligated without apparent problem.[36–38] Without this reaction, no functional immunoglobulins or T-cell antigen receptors could be formed and no antigen-driven stimulation and proliferation of lymphocytes achieved. Thus the product of this *scid* locus appears to be an integral part of the complex that mediates the site-specific V(D)J recombinational mechanism. The category of severe combined immunodeficiency in humans covers a broad range of genetic defects, including adenosine deaminase deficiency,[39] purine nucleoside phosphorylase deficiency,[40] and X-linked immunodeficiency,[41] among others.[42] Among those SCID patients whose defect has not yet been characterized, there may be individuals who manifest a syndrome analogous to that seen in the *scid* mice.

Terminal Deoxynucleotidyl Transferase

As noted above, the appearance of N sequences at the junction of V(D)J rearrangements is consistent with the known pattern of expression and demonstrated activity of this enzyme. Terminal transferase is a DNA polymerase that does not require a DNA template but does require a DNA primer, preferably a protruding 3′ hydroxyl-terminus.[43] TdT is capable of adding any of the four nucleoside triphosphates to this 3′ end of the molecule.

Recombination Signal Sequence–Binding Proteins

A number of investigators have used oligonucleotides based on the signal sequences that flank the recombining segments (see below) as a tool for dissecting out protein elements that may play a role in the process of recombination. So far, no gene identified in this way has been shown to be either necessary or sufficient for V(D)J recombination, nor has an

immunologically distinctive phenotype yet been associated with its loss or mutation. Nevertheless, one or more of these genes may indeed be components of the recombinase complex mediating one or another aspect of the recognition or breakage and rejoining reaction. One gene isolated in this manner shares an approximately 40 amino acid motif with other genes of known function in recombinational systems, namely, the bacteriophage λ "integrase" and certain recombinases of bacteria and yeasts.[44]

Signal Sequence Recognition

The activity of the recombinase complex is focused on certain sites in the genome where a specific nucleotide signal sequence occurs. This signal sequence is conserved in all species known to rearrange immune receptors via a recombinase complex. It consists of a heptamer with a consensus sequence "CACA/TGTG" separated by 12 or 23 random nt from a consensus nonamer sequence "ACAAAAACC" (or GGTTTTTGT, depending on the orientation). These sequences are found 3′ of the V segments, 5′ of the J segments, and flanking the D segments. The heptamer is always flush to the coding segments, and the nonamer is upstream or downstream of the heptamer, in the direction of the segment with which potential rearrangement can occur (see Fig. 11–4). For the recombinase complex to be able to join any two coding segments, it appears that one heptamer/nonamer must enclose a random spacer of 12 bp and the other heptamer/nonamer a spacer of 23 bp. This spacing corresponds roughly to one or two turns of a DNA double helix, suggesting a potential three-dimensional structure recognized by the recombinase complex.

A refined analysis of these signal sequences[45] has suggested that the heptamer sequence is more crucial for recombination than is the nonamer. Indeed V(D)J recombination can occur (though with less efficiency) even in the absence of the nonamer from one or the other side of the rearranging segments. The four bases of the heptamer closest to the coding segments are the most crucial nucleotides for signal recognition. Alterations of the sequence in this area can lower by more than 100-fold the efficiency of recombination of experimentally designed constructs introduced into cells in which the recombinase complex is known to be active. The efficiency of recombination is also markedly lowered if more than 2 bp are added or deleted from the spacer between the heptamer and nonamer.

Accessibility

The presence of appropriate signal sequences and active recombinase enzymes is probably not sufficient to cause structural reconfiguration of a particular immune receptor locus. Introduction of RAG-1 and RAG-2 into fibroblasts was sufficient to cause V(D)J-like rearrangement of exogenously introduced (and actively transcribed) substrates, but not of the immune receptor genes in the endogenous DNA of the fibroblast.[32, 33] This finding supported the concept that in addition to the enzymes and signal sequences, a locus must be "accessible" to the recombinase complex in order for recombination to occur. In a fibroblast, the immune receptor genes are inactive and transcriptionally silent. Thus, there is no evidence that a recombinase enzyme complex could gain access to them. Earlier work[46] had demonstrated that transcriptional activity can be detected from V segments prior to their rearrangement (see Fig. 11–3). Although it is possible that the "sterile" (not coding for a functional protein) transcript itself might play a role in the recombinational mechanism, it is perhaps equally likely that it is simply a marker of a change in the status of the chromatin in which the V segments reside. This latter argument would suggest that if a segment of DNA was accessible to an RNA polymerase, it might be similarly accessible to the recombinase complex. In lymphocytes in which IgH but not the endogenous immunoglobulin light chains or TCR loci are transcribed or subject to rearrangement, exogenously introduced substrates carrying immunoglobulin light chain genes or TCR genes are ready targets for V(D)J recombination as long as they are provided on a transcriptionally active vector.[47, 48] These experiments also supplied evidence that the same recombinase system was capable of rearranging immunoglobulin and T-cell antigen receptor loci. In other words, the regulation of rearrangement of these loci does not occur at the level of V(D)J recombinase recognition but more likely is decided by which loci are accessible to the recombinase complex at a point in lymphocyte development and lineage determination. If signal sequences are present within two given loci, and if the recombinase complex is active, those two loci are at risk of being rearranged if they are transcriptionally active, even if neither encodes an immune receptor.[49] Thus, the V(D)J recombinase complex can be an important factor in increasing genomic instability in

lymphocytes, instability that can cause chromosomal aberrations and, in so doing, contribute to malignant transformation by disrupting or dysregulating genes that control cell growth or development (this topic is discussed in greater detail later in this chapter). The concept that chromatin must be in an accessible conformation in order for breakage and rejoining events to occur may, indeed, transcend a discussion of V(D)J recombination and be generally relevant to the generation of most chromosomal aberrations.[50, 51]

REGULATION OF TRANSCRIPTION[16, 52–54]

At least four kinds of *cis* elements regulate transcription in mammalian cells: promoters, enhancers, silencers, and locus control regions (LCR). (See Chapters 2 and 4.) Promoters, which are the minimal element necessary for RNA polymerase to initiate transcription, are located immediately upstream from transcription initiation sites and function best (and in many cases only) in one orientation. Enhancers can increase transcription when present in either orientation and can be located either upstream or downstream of the transcription initiation site; in addition, they can be active over relatively long distances, more than 10 kilobases (kb) in many cases. Silencers repress transcription independent of the orientation or distance from a promoter or enhancer and can also be located either upstream or downstream of the promoter or enhancer.[53] LCRs, which have been best studied in the β globin locus, are defined as elements that confer site of integration independent tissue-specific expression of a heterologous gene, and can act in either orientation over very long distances, perhaps 100 kb or more. It is thought that the function of an LCR is mediated, at least in part, by establishing open chromatin domains over long distances.[54]

In fact, the four kinds of elements described above often occur in combinations. For example, promoters or LCRs can contain enhancer elements, and enhancers can contain silencers. Each kind of element is often associated with multiple DNA binding motifs, with several motifs contributing to generate a particular effect on transcription in a given cell type. Redundancy of function often occurs, so that removal of several DNA binding motifs from a regulatory element, or even removal of the entire regulatory element, may have no effect on transcription in a particular setting. For example, removal of an immunoglobulin heavy chain intronic enhancer has little effect on the transcription of heavy chain in a myeloma cell. Each DNA binding motif might bind a variety of *trans*-acting transcription factors, and the presence of these factors, or an active form of these factors, may depend on the cell type or the physiological state of the cell. For example, all immunoglobulin promoters and many immunoglobulin enhancers contain an octamer motif, which can interact with transcription factors called Oct-1 and Oct-2; most cells express Oct-1, whereas Oct-2 is restricted primarily to all stages of

B-cell development but only a limited number of other cell types. Other factors that are expressed in most tissues contribute to increased immunoglobulin transcription by binding to additional (non-octamer) motifs present in immunoglobulin promoters or enhancers. Another well-studied example of a B-cell tissue-specific transcriptional activator is NF-κB, which binds a 10 bp motif in the J-C$_\kappa$ intronic enhancer and is present in an active form in virtually all cells in the B-cell lineage except pre-B cells. In fact, NF-κB is present in an inactive form in most kinds of cells (including pre-B cells) and can be converted to an active form, even in the presence of protein synthesis inhibitors, by stimulating the cells through a variety of signaling pathways. In some cases, transcription factors interact with other proteins or each other, and thereby alter their DNA binding specificity or the effect of DNA binding.

As a result of the complex interplay of distinct DNA binding motifs and multiple transcription factors, any of the four regulatory elements described above may be active in one kind of cell but inactive in another kind of cell. For example, there is a silencer element that is located near an enhancer element downstream of the TCRα constant region.[53] The silencer element per se is active in non-T cells or γ/δ T cells but is inactive in α/β T cells. By contrast, the downstream enhancer per se is active in both kinds of T cells but is not active in non-T cells even if the silencer element is not present.

Despite progress in the past few years, we have only a fragmentary knowledge of how transcription of the immunoglobulin and T-cell antigen receptor loci is regulated in B and T lymphoid cells. Nonetheless, it is worthwhile summarizing a few general features of transcriptional regulation of the these loci. A strong association exists between transcriptional activity and "accessibility" of sequences for the unique recombinational processes that occur in lymphoid cells. In addition, it should be noted that transcriptional regulation of the immunoglobulin and T-cell antigen receptor loci is unique in that gene rearrangements lead to important changes in the distances over which transcriptional regulatory elements are separated from one another at different times in the maturation of lymphocytes. We will focus on the regulation of the immunoglobulin loci as more information is available in this system.

Depending on the state of B-cell maturation, there are a variety of transcripts that can be expressed from rearranged or unrearranged loci.[46, 47, 52, 55, 56] For example, early pre-B cells can express germline V$_H$ segment transcripts, germline Cμ transcripts initiating about 1 kb upstream from a germline μ constant region gene, DJC transcripts initiating upstream of DJ rearranged genes, and VDJC (heavy chain) transcripts after completion of rearrangements. Late pre-B cells can express germline V$_\kappa$ and germline JC$_\kappa$ transcripts, as well as VJC$_\kappa$ (κ light chain) transcripts after completion of rearrangements, but probably not germline V$_H$ transcripts. Beyond the pre-B cell stage, germline

V$_\kappa$ transcripts are not expressed. In fact, the B-cell developmental stage at which these germline or partially rearranged (i.e., DJ) loci are transcribed coincides with the time that these loci are involved in VDJ rearrangements (see below).[55, 56] Many of the transcripts from unrearranged loci appear to be "sterile" transcripts (i.e., transcripts that do not seem to encode a protein). However, in some cases, it appears that transcripts from an unrearranged locus do encode a protein; for example, a protein of uncertain significance is translated from the incompletely rearranged DJC$_H$ sequence.[57] Highly differentiated B cells continue to express rearranged H and L genes but prior to switching can express transcripts that initiate upstream of switch regions associated with constant regions that are programmed to be involved in the heavy chain switch recombination process (see below). Plasma cells transcribe heavy and light chain genes at significantly higher rates and have higher steady-state levels of the corresponding mRNAs than less mature B or pre-B cells (it should be noted that the higher levels of immunoglobulin heavy and light chain mRNAs in plasma cells are a consequence of both transcriptional and post-transcriptional mechanisms).[58]

A substantial amount of information is available for the promoters upstream of V segments, but not for the promoters upstream of most of the other transcripts described above.[16, 52] Similarly, intronic enhancers located between the J segments and the constant regions have been well defined for the IgH (see Fig. 11–13 below) and Igκ (compare with Fig. 11–3) loci. More recently, 3′ enhancers have been defined downstream of the κ and λ constant regions (compare with Fig. 11–3), as well as downstream of the 3′-most heavy chain constant region exon (i.e., the α constant region) (see Fig. 11–13). The IgH intronic enhancer functions reasonably well in all B cells, but the 3′ enhancer may be more active in plasma cells.[59] The light chain intronic (κ) and 3′ (κ and λ) enhancers are active in B cells and plasma cells but have little or no activity in pre-B cells. Although these and other data provide some insights, many questions remain to be answered regarding the *cis* elements and *trans* factors that regulate transcription and rearrangement of immunoglobulin loci:

1. What turns germline V$_H$ or V$_L$ transcripts on and then off as B lymphoid cells progress along a developmental pathway?

2. What accounts for the increased transcription of immunoglobulin genes in plasma cells compared with earlier B cells?

3. Are there LCR regions in the immunoglobulin loci, and if so, are the 3′ enhancers part of an LCR region?

4. Are the 3′ enhancers responsible for the dysregulation of translocated c-*myc* genes that is the sine qua non of Burkitt's lymphoma? (The translocations that invariably link immunoglobulin loci and the *myc* gene in Burkitt's lymphoma [see reference 141] are discussed in more detail below.)

5. What mechanisms determine transcription of constant regions that are selected for switch recombination?

6. Is transcription necessary for, or merely associated with, recombination?

T-CELL ANTIGEN RECEPTORS (TCR)

Structure and Function[60-68]

There are two basic kinds of TCRs, each composed of a pair of disulfide-linked heterodimeric glycoproteins (i.e., α/β or γ/δ) with a composite molecular weight of about 90 kDa (see Fig. 11–2). All four types of TCR chains (α, β, γ, and δ) have a similar size (30 to 40 kDa of amino acids) and structural organization, with a large extracellular region, a transmembrane domain of about 20 amino acids that includes a conserved lysine (as well as an arginine for α and δ chains), and a very small cytoplasmic domain containing fewer than 20 amino acids. Starting at the amino-terminus, the extracellular region is divided into three domains: a variable region with an intradomain disulfide bond, a constant region with an intradomain disulfide bond as well as several N-linked oligosaccharides, and a hinge or connecting domain containing a cysteine residue that can form an interchain disulfide bond with the other member of the heterodimer.[61-63]

Both kinds of TCR are non-covalently associated with a number of non-polymorphic glycopeptides that collectively are designated the CD3 complex.[64] The CD3 complex includes five polypeptides, that is, one copy each of CD3-γ, CD3-δ, and CD3-ε chains, as well as a disulfide linked dimer of CD3-ζ chains. All four kinds of CD3 polypeptides have similar structural features. Each chain includes an extracellular domain, a transmembrane domain containing a negatively charged amino acid, and an intracellular domain that contains conserved serine and tyrosine residues. It is thought that the negative charges in the transmembrane domains of CD3 chains interact with the positive charges in the transmembrane domains of the TCR chains, thus ensuring cell surface expression of a functional TCR-CD3 membrane complex. Moreover, the CD3 complex is thought to transduce the antigen/TCR binding signal to the interior of the cell by a process involving a change in the phosphorylation status of the serine or tyrosine residues, or both, on the cytoplasmic portions of the CD3 chains.

Although α/β TCRs appear later in ontogeny than γ/δ TCRs, the former represent 95 per cent or more of T cells in peripheral blood and secondary lymphoid tissues.[60] An α/β TCR cannot recognize free antigen but instead recognizes antigen expressed on a cell surface. More specifically, the α/β TCR is thought to recognize an antigenic determinant primarily as a breakdown product (derived from either an intracellular or an extracellular antigen) that is non-covalently complexed either to a major histocompatibility complex (MHC) class I (i.e., HLA-A, -B, or -C antigens) molecule or to an MHC class II (i.e., HLA-DR, -DS, or -SB) molecule on the surface of an appropriate cell. In fact, it appears that a functional TCR response requires simultaneous corecognition of the antigenic determinant and the MHC product by the TCR. The ability of T lymphocytes to recognize a complex composed of an antigenic determinant and an MHC class I or MHC class II molecule is enhanced by the additional interaction of T-cell receptors (CD4 and CD8) for the two respective MHC products. CD4 and CD8 receptors are composed of CD4 and CD8 glycopeptides, each of which is a member of the immunoglobulin supergene family that also includes immunoglobulin, TCR, MHC class I, and MHC class II genes. Thus, the functional interaction of antigen with an α/β TCR receptor includes not only an association of an antigen/MHC complex and the CD3 complex with TCR but also an interaction of CD8 with MHC class I molecules or CD4 with MHC class II molecules on the antigen-presenting cell. In general, cytotoxic T cells express CD8 so that they can recognize antigen/MHC class I complexes on essentially any cell. In contrast, helper T cells generally express CD4 so that they can efficiently recognize antigen/MHC class II complexes on macrophages or B lymphocytes.[60, 62-64]

Although it is not as well worked out, it appears that γ/δ TCRs also do not recognize free antigen but only antigen expressed on a cell surface, perhaps in association with the same or other MHC class I or MHC class II molecules. The functional distinction between a TCR composed of α/β and that composed of γ/δ heterodimers is not entirely clear, although a consistent difference in pattern of expression has been well established. T cells expressing γ/δ TCR heterodimers occur earlier in ontogeny, as supported by expression on CD4−8− cells, and also appear to be relatively more abundant in the epidermis and intestinal epithelium. Most T cells with γ/δ TCR receptors are CD4−8−, with a small fraction being CD4−8+ and an even smaller fraction being CD4+8−.[60-63, 65-66]

Chromosomal Localization and Genetic Organization

A knowledge of the chromosomal localization and genetic organization of the four TCR loci is critical for understanding the pattern and significance of normal and abnormal (e.g., chromosomal translocations) TCR gene rearrangements in normal and malignant cells. It should be noted that the overall organization of the four TCR loci is highly conserved for the extensively studied human and murine systems.[61, 62, 67, 68]

TCRβ Locus

The TCRβ locus has been localized to the long arm of human chromosome 7, at chromosome band 7q35, and includes more than 700 kb of DNA (Fig. 11–6). At the centromeric end of the locus, there are approx-

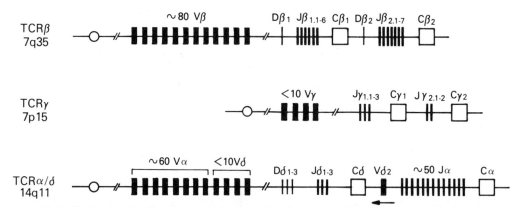

FIGURE 11-6. The human T-cell antigen receptor loci. The chromosomal localization and genetic organization of the three TCR loci are shown in schematic form, although not to scale. The positions of centromeres are depicted by open circles. V segments, each containing two exons, are indicated by dark boxes. D segments and J segments are indicated by thin and thick lines, respectively. Constant region genes, each of which contains a number of exons, are indicated by open boxes. The arrow indicates that the Vδ2 segment is transcribed toward the centromere, whereas all other segments are transcribed away from the centromere. See text for further details.

imately 80 known V segments. Each V segment contains 2 exons: a short exon encoding most of the leader or signal sequence (compare with Fig. 11–3) and a longer exon encoding the C-terminal end of the signal sequence and the bulk of the variable domain, including the two cysteines that form the intradomain disulfide bond in the variable region domain. The V segments can be divided into 21 subfamilies, with 15 subfamilies containing only one member (in general, members of a subfamily are defined either by sharing a protein sequence homology of 50 per cent or more, or by cross-hybridization at moderate to high stringency as detected on Southern blots; the close homology of subfamily members to one another suggests that they are more closely related, by evolution, to one another than to other V segments). Most, if not all, V segments have the same transcriptional orientation as the C genes, so that intrachromosomal joining of V to DJ results in deletion of intervening sequences (compare with Fig. 11–3). In an approximately 20 kb region at the telomeric end of the locus, there is a single D segment (D1) followed by one non-functional pseudo J and 6 functional (J1.1–1.6) J segments and a C gene (C1); then there is another D segment (D2) followed by 7 J segments (J2.1–2.7) and another C gene (C2). The two C genes, each of which includes four exons, are highly homologous, with only six amino acid substitutions distinguishing them. Not surprisingly, there is no known functional difference for these two β isotypes. Although the number and organization of C gene exons are not identical for all TCR C genes, collectively the C gene exons, including the Cβ gene exons, encode the constant region domain, a short connecting region containing the cysteine involved in the disulfide bond to the TCR heterodimeric partner, the transmembrane domain, the cytoplasmic domain, and the 3' untranslated region. The Cβ genes are unique among TCR genes in that there is a fourth cysteine of unknown significance located between the cysteines that form the intradomain disulfide bridge

in the constant region. The initial rearrangement event in this locus is D to J, and at a later time, V to DJ. Position and orientation dictate that D1 can join to any of the 13 J segments but that D2 can join only to J2.1–2.7 (see Fig. 11–6).

TCRγ Locus

The TCRγ locus, which has been localized to human chromosome 7 at band 7p15, includes 160 kb of DNA (see Fig. 11–6). At the centromeric end of the locus, there are 14 V segments, each containing two exons in the same orientation as the C genes, as described above for Vβ. By sequence homology, there are six subfamilies, with five subfamilies containing one sequence. Five of the V segments are pseudogenes, three of which are members of the large subfamily. There are no known D regions. In an approximately 30 kb region at the telomeric end of the locus, there are 3 J segments (J1.1–1.3) followed by a C gene (C1) and then 2 more J segments (J2.1–2.2) followed by another C gene (C2). The C1 gene has three exons, whereas the highly homologous C2 gene is represented by alleles with four or five exons, resulting from a duplication or triplication, respectively, of the second exon. In addition, the C2 gene lacks the cysteine residue that forms an interchain disulfide bridge for all other TCR heterodimeric pairs. Thus γ chains of subtype 2 (i.e., γ2 chains) are larger than γ chains of subtype 1 and other TCR chains and provide the only example of human or mouse TCR that cannot be disulfide linked to its heterodimeric partner. It should be noted that Cβ and Cγ are structurally more similar to each other than to either Cα or Cδ genes.

TCRα Locus

The TCRα locus, which has been localized to human chromosome 14 at band 14q11, includes more than 1 Mb of DNA (see Fig. 11–6). At the centromeric end of the locus, there are approximately 60 known V segments, each containing two exons and apparently in the same orientation as the C genes, as described above for Vβ. By sequence homology there are 22 V segment subfamilies, with 15 subfamilies containing only one member. Members of the same Vα segment subfamily can be adjacent or widely dispersed over more than 600 kb. There are no known D segments, but there are 47 known J segments covering an 80 kb region separated by about 100 kb from the 3'-most V segment. This pattern of numerous and broadly distributed J segments diverges markedly from the J clusters associated with other immune receptors. Approximately 5 kb from the 3'-most J segment is a single C gene, which contains four exons.

TCRδ Locus

The TCRδ locus is localized within the TCRα locus and has the same transcriptional orientation as the TCRα locus. All D, J, and Cδ sequences, and perhaps all Vδ sequences as well, are localized between the 3'-most Vα and 5'-most Jα gene segments (see Fig. 11–6). The interspersion of these two structurally and functionally related loci is consistent with the notion that one locus evolved from the other by gene duplication. Moreover, this unusual organization of these two loci results in deletion of the δ locus upon rearrangement of Vα and Jα segments. The single Cδ constant region gene, which contains four exons, is located about 80 kb upstream from the Cα constant region gene. There are three Jδ segments within a 10 kb sequence, with the most 3' J about 3 kb from the 5' end of the first Cδ exon. There are also three Dδ segments within a 10 kb sequence, with the most 3' D about 1 kb from the 5' J segment. Thus far, approximately half a dozen Vδ gene segments have been found, all of which are localized downstream of the Vα gene segments. There is at least one example demonstrating that the same V segment can be rearranged to either a Jα or a Dδ gene segment, with the possibility that the same V segment can be used in either TCRα or TCRδ chains in other instances as well. A single Vδ gene segment is localized about 3 kb 3' of the 3' exon of the Cδ gene, thus providing the first example in humans of a TCR V gene segment that is oriented in an opposite transcriptional orientation from the corresponding C gene; hence an inversion rather than a deletion will occur when this V gene segment is rearranged to a D segment. Finally, the TCRδ locus provides the only example of a TCR locus in which D-D joining occurs in addition to V-D or D-J joining. In fact, it appears that a functionally rearranged human δ gene includes three D segments and four sets of N sequences corresponding to the four joining events. In contrast to the rearrangement of TCRβ genes, which first join a D segment to a J segment and then a V segment to a DJ segment, there does not seem to be a consistent temporal sequence of joining the V, J, and multiple D segments in this locus.

T-Cell Receptor Gene Rearrangement and Diversity[61–63, 65, 66]

The structural organization of TCR genes and signal sequences for joining dictates how these genes can be rearranged to generate the vast number of different V regions to recognize the diverse antigenic determinants that are encountered by an individual. As described above, the heptamer/nonamer signals for joining are located so that the nonamer is adjacent to the structural sequence that is to be joined. In addition, the two structural gene segments (i.e., V, D, and J) to be joined are constrained in that the signal sequence adjacent to one segment must have a separation of 11 or 12 bp (about one turn of the DNA helix) between the heptamer and nonamer sequences, whereas the other segment must have a separation of 22 or 23 bp (about two turns of the DNA helix) between the heptamer and nonamer sequences (i.e., 12/23 bp rule). On the basis of the organization of signal sequences for joining as shown in Figure 11–7, one can predict which segments (V, D, and J) can be joined for each of the TCR genes, although not all possibilities occur at a detectable frequency. For all TCR loci, the heptamer/nonamer separation is 23 bp downstream of the V gene segment and 12 bp upstream of the J gene segment. Yet a V segment is directly joined to a J segment only in the α and γ loci. Similarly, since the heptamer and nonamer sequences are separated by 12 and 23 bp, respectively, for the joining signals upstream and downstream of D segments, it should be possible to join two D segments in either the β or the δ loci. Although the joining of three D segments occurs in the δ locus, the two D segments in the β locus have not been observed to join to each other. In both of the cases cited above, it is not understood why some apparently possible joining events do not occur at a detectable frequency.

For all four TCR loci, the various mechanisms described above (with the exception of somatic hypermutation) can be used to generate an incredible diversity of V regions.[61–63, 173] The relative contribution of different mechanisms is not identical for each locus, and there is also a striking difference in how a similar extent of potential diversity can be achieved for the α/β receptor compared with the γ/δ receptor. As summarized in Table 11–1, there are many more potential combinations of V segments or V and J segments for receptors composed of TCRα and TCRβ chains than for receptors composed of TCRγ and TCRδ chains. For each type of receptor, however, the relative contribution of junctional mechanisms would seem to outweigh greatly the contribution of the remainder of the V and J segments in generating TCR diversity. As a rationale for this finding, it has been hypothesized that the junctional region is critically involved in recognizing the vast number of antigenic determinants, whereas the remainder of the V region is important for recognizing the more limited number of MHC molecules. For each kind of receptor, one (i.e., β or δ) of the two chains has D segments, which mostly can

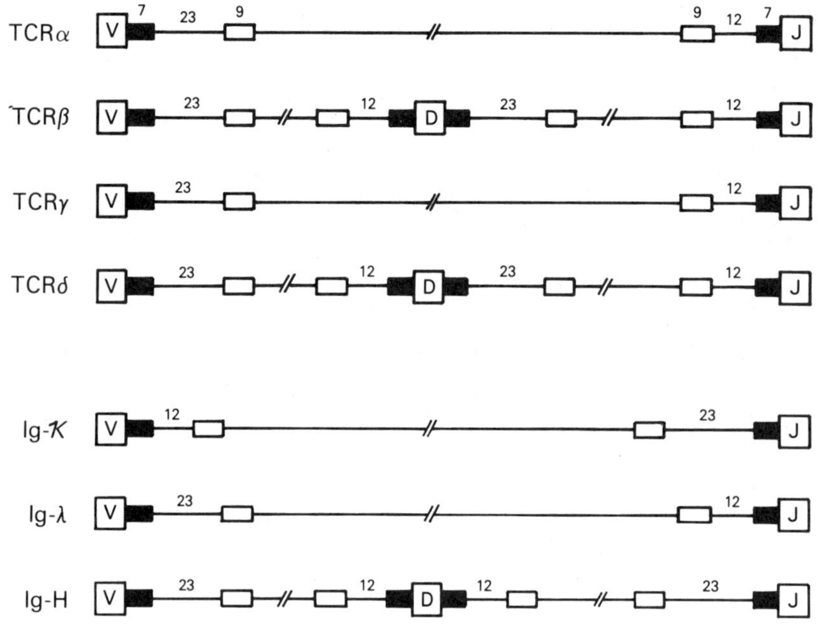

FIGURE 11–7. Organization of heptamer/nonamer sequences for V, D, and J segments located in the four TCR and three Ig loci. The V, D, and J segments are indicated by large open boxes, the heptamer by closed boxes, and the nonamers by small open boxes. The heptamer and nonamer sequences are separated by 12 or 23 base pairs (bp), creating two kinds of joining signals. Intralocus or, rarely, interlocus joining can occur between segments that have different joining signals, such as V_H to D or D to J_H but not V_H to J_H or D to D in the Ig-H locus. See text for details.

be read in three frames. Among all TCR and immunoglobulin loci, the powerful diversity mechanism of D-D joining apparently occurs only in the δ locus. For all loci and kinds of joints (VD, DD, DJ, VJ), there is a marked degree of flexibility (i.e., exonuclease nibbling, as described above) in the precise nucleotides that are used to join two segments. Similarly, for each of these instances as many as five or more N nucleotides can be added. Thus, one can predict the possibility of 10^{15} or more heterodimeric combinations for either α/β or γ/δ TCR (see Table 11–1).

Despite the incredible potential diversity of heterodimers, the actual diversity achieved may be considerably less, depending, for example, on the type of receptor and the age of the individual. For example, whereas δ chains in adult mice demonstrate D-D joining and the addition of N regions at all joints, the δ chains in fetal mice contain only one D and have few, if any, N regions.[61, 62] In addition, there seems to be a preferential rearrangement of Vγ genes, so that Vγ genes located most 3′ are rearranged first, with 5′ Vγ genes being rearranged at a latter time in murine development. In addition, for γ/δ TCR bearing T cells, a different predominant V region is expressed in fetal murine thymocytes compared with peripheral T cells; T cells associated with various kinds of epithelium express different but a highly restricted set of TCRγδ variable regions.[65, 66] Not enough evidence exists, particularly in humans, to assess whether these and other constraints limit the actual extent of heterodimeric TCR diversity.

Ontogeny of TCR Expression

The pattern and anatomical locations of T-lymphocyte development are similar in mouse and man.[60, 63, 72, 73] (See also Chapter 12.) A simplified version of the developmental pathways thought to be involved in this process is shown in Figure 11–8. Depending on the age of the individual, pluripotent hematopoietic stem cells in the yolk sac, fetal liver, or bone marrow give rise to pro-T cells that express CD7, as well as cytoplasmic TdT and possibly some components of the CD3 complex also localized in the cytoplasm. The pro-T cells migrate to the thymus, where they continue the developmental process as pre-T cells in the cortex of the thymus. In addition to CD7 and TdT, the earliest pre-T cells in the thymic cortex express CD1, CD2, and IL-2R but do not express surface CD3, CD4, or CD8. It is thought that a small fraction of these CD3−4−8− pre-T cells rearrange and express γ and δ genes, generating a population of CD3+4−8− cells that express low levels of a γ/δ TCR; the surface expression of CD3 and TCR apparently requires the expression of both complexes. A much larger fraction of the CD3−4−8− pre-T cells begin to express CD8 and then CD4. The CD3−4+8+ pre-T cells rearrange and express α and β TCR genes, generating a population of CD3+4+8+ cells that express very low levels of an α/β TCR. Late in ontogeny, the vast majority of cells in the thymus are CD4+8+, with a significant portion also expressing CD3 and low levels of α/β TCR but a substantial portion expressing neither CD3 nor any kind of TCR. This latter CD3−4+8+TCR− population includes cells that have not completed α and β TCR rearrangements, as well as cells that have made incorrect rearrangements and thus are no longer capable of generating a functional α/β TCR receptor. A small fraction of cells in the thymic cortex are CD3+4+8−TCRα/β or CD3+4−8+TCRα/β, although most of the cells with these two phenotypes are found in the thymic medulla.

On the basis of a variety of evidence, it appears that CD3+4+8+TCRα/β cells (as well as

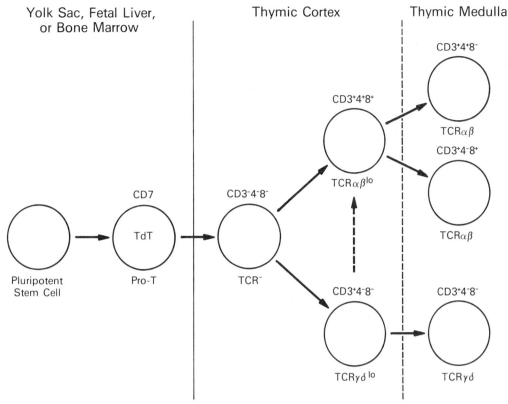

FIGURE 11–8. T-cell developmental pathway. This simplified scheme shows a limited number of intermediates in the developmental process and only a few of the known markers. It should be noted that TdT (terminal deoxynucleotidyl transferase), which is first expressed in pro-T cells, continues to be expressed in pre-T cells in the thymic cortex. The early pre-T cells generate more mature pre-T cells that express either TCRαβ or TCRγδ. The dashed arrow indicates that TCRγδ cells can turn off expression of TCRγδ and proceed to express TCRαβ as well as CD4 and CD8. The TCR receptor is subjected to a combination of positive and negative selection, resulting in a limited fraction of T cells that upregulate TCR expression as they progress to the thymic medulla. See text for additional details.

CD3−4+8+TCR− negative cells that have been unable to generate a functional TCR receptor by functionally rearranging both α and β TCR genes) pass through a selection process involving the thymic epithelium in which greater than 98 per cent of thymocytes die within the thymus. A negative selection process apparently eliminates cells expressing a functional TCR receptor that is reactive against self-antigen/MHC complexes. A positive selection process selects a subset of cells with functionally useful receptors, which results in the elimination of cells that do not express a functionally useful receptor, including cells that express no receptor owing to aberrant rearrangements. In any case, after these positive and negative selection processes, the selected cells present in the thymic medulla are presumably functional CD3+4+8−TCRαβ or CD3+4−8+TCRαβ thymocytes, which express much higher levels of the α/β TCR and also generate the various kinds of cytotoxic and helper T cells, respectively, that are found in the peripheral blood and secondary lymphoid organs. Although less well worked out, it appears that CD3+4−8− thymocytes with γ/δ TCR go through a similar selection process that presumably does not involve CD4 or CD8.[69–71]

Regulation of TCR Gene Formation

In general, it appears that individual T cells express a single species of functional TCR receptor.[63, 72, 74] Presumably this is necessary because of the stringent positive and negative selection processes involved in generating functional T cells and because of the need to produce a T cell having a TCR that recognizes only one kind of antigen/MHC interaction. Since the formation of variable regions by gene rearrangements, as described above, is not a precise process, the rearrangement and expression of TCR genes must be tightly regulated to achieve this goal of expressing only one kind of TCR receptor per cell. What are the results of this regulatory process? First, only one of the two kinds of TCR receptors (α/β TCR or γ/δ TCR) is expressed on a particular cell. Second, for each kind of chain expressed in a functional receptor, only one parental allele is used to encode that chain, and the other parental allele is excluded from encoding a chain that contributes to a functional receptor (i.e., the allelic exclusion phenomenon). Finally, it is important to take into account the apparent inefficiency of the rearrangement process in creating functionally rearranged genes. Since V and J segments can be read in only one reading frame, the flexible joining process probably results in an in-frame V(D)J one of three times (the efficiency would be even lower if TdT did not show a bias of adding G's or C's in N regions, or if D regions could be read in only one or two frames). The actual efficiency of forming an in-frame V(D)J sequence at a given locus might be somewhat higher than 33 per cent, since secondary rearrangements involving, for example, an upstream V and a downstream J are possible.

Although we do not have a thorough understanding of how and when these regulatory processes occur, there is information from studies of humans as well as normal and transgenic mice that sheds some light on how these goals are achieved. It is thought that the enzymes involved in V(D)J rearrangements are expressed prior to the onset of rearrangements (e.g., TdT is present before pro-T cells enter the thymic cortex and begin gene rearrangements) and that the timing of rearrangements is likely determined by the accessibility of the various loci. However, little is known about accessibility beyond what is known about the timing of TCR gene rearrangements and the tightly coupled transcription and translation of the rearranged genes.

In any case, the earliest rearrangements in ontogeny apparently occur in the δ locus, although V-J joining in the γ locus and D-J joining in the β locus also occur at a relatively early time.[60, 63, 72] A variety of evidence, including results with γ/δ transgenic mice, indicates that most thymocytes are destined to become cells that express α/β receptors and that this decision process involves the turning off of expression at the γ and perhaps δ loci through the occurrence of *cis* silencer sequences associated with these loci.[75] Since many, although not all, extrachromosomal circular DNA generated by Vα-Jα joinings retain the δ gene segments in the germline configuration, the decision to follow the α/β TCR pathway is often made before δ rearrangements.[76, 77] If this silencer mechanism is not used, expression of a functional γ/δ receptor is thought to block further rearrangements at many, if not all, of the four loci (perhaps by the mechanism described below).[74, 75]

Thymocytes in the α/β receptor pathway go on to rearrange a Vβ gene segment to a previously rearranged and transcribed DβJβ gene segment, forming a VDJ sequence that is transcribed and translated as a β chain. There is evidence, mainly from studies with transgenic mice,[74] that a functional β chain polypeptide somehow inhibits additional Vβ to DβJβ joining events as well as rearrangements in the δ and γ loci. In addition, a functional Vβ chain may provide a signal to promote rearrangements in the TCRα locus (perhaps by alleviating the effect of a silencer located 3' of the Cα gene) and also to enhance expression of CD4 and CD8. The expression of a functional α/β TCR in a transgenic mouse does not appear to prevent additional rearrangements in the TCRα locus. Thus, it is unclear why few clones of T cells express receptors with different α chains and a single β chain (a few

examples have been described). A possible explanation is that rearrangement and expression of a functional α/β TCR receptor occur at a later time in a normal compared with a transgenic animal; and expression of a functional α/β receptor at this later time results in a prompt inhibition of further rearrangements at all loci (see below).

It is of interest that a recent study[78] using human thymocytes demonstrated that RAG-1 and RAG-2 are expressed in TCR − CD3 − thymocytes and also in TCR + CD3 + 4 + 8 + thymocytes but not in TCR + CD3 + 4 + 8 − or TCR + CD3 + 4 − 8 + thymocytes, regardless of whether the latter were present in the cortex or medulla of the thymus. They also found that cross-linking of the CD3-TCR complex caused a rapid loss of expression of RAG-1 and RAG-2. Thus, it appears that the positive and or negative selection processes that act on the CD3-TCR complex may serve to shut down the enzymatic machinery required for TCR gene rearrangements. Perhaps this shutdown of recombinase activity occurs as a consequence of the selection of cells that express either kind of TCR receptor.

Finally, it is important to note that approximately 10 per cent of peripheral T cells have undergone DJ rearrangements in the IgH locus but rarely, if ever, have undergone VDJ rearrangements or rearrangements in the immunoglobulin light chain loci (see reference 123). Usually, however, the rearranged IgH genes are not transcribed in T cells. Since the TCR and immunoglobulin loci are thought to share identical enzymatic machinery for rearrangements,[48] the rearrangements of IgH loci in T cells suggest that there is a significant chance that the IgH locus becomes transiently accessible for rearrangement during the period when recombinase activity is occurring in T cells.

IMMUNOGLOBULINS

Structure and Function[10, 12–16, 56, 79–83]

Immunoglobulins are quite similar in structure and function to T-cell antigen receptors, but they pose some specialized problems and have unique solutions to these problems. First, although immunoglobulin can function as a B-cell surface receptor for antigen, most immunoglobulin is secreted from the cells to circulate in extracellular fluids. This problem is solved by generating distinct membrane and secreted forms of heavy chain mRNA by alternative processing of RNA generated from a single transcription unit. Second, different classes and subclasses of secreted immunoglobulin are able to mediate different effector functions, depending on the carboxy-terminal constant region domains present in the heavy chains. To preserve the same antigen-binding site but different classes of immunoglobulin in the progeny of a B-cell clone, B cells are able to alternatively process RNA (IgD) or rearrange DNA (all other isotypes) so that the heavy chain variable region (VDJ) is juxtaposed immediately upstream from the appropriate heavy chain constant region. Finally, immunoglobulins are able to somatically hypermutate both heavy and light chain variable regions to generate sites with higher affinity for antigen. The somatic hypermutation process occurs at a restricted time and in a particular site (germinal centers) after antigenic stimulation, with mutation rates as high as 10^{-3} per nucleotide per generation (see below).

As indicated above, immunoglobulins have a basic four-chain monomeric structure consisting of two identical heavy chains and two identical light chains, which are held together by interchain disulfide bonds (see Fig. 11–1). There are two light chain isotypes, κ and λ. The light chains contain an amino-terminal variable region domain (V_L) and a carboxy-terminal constant region domain (C_L), with each domain having a single intradomain disulfide bond. There are five heavy chain classes (μ, δ, γ, ε, and α), 4 γ subclasses (γ1–4), and 2 α subclasses (α1–2). Starting at the amino-terminal end of the heavy chain, there is a variable region domain (V_H), followed by the CH1, hinge region (in most cases), CH2, CH3, and, for some classes, CH4 domains. The V domain and the four CH domains contain intradomain disulfide bonds. The paired V_H/V_L domains constitute an antigen recognition site, so that each immunoglobulin monomer has two identical antigen recognition sites. Both the V_L and the V_H domains can be divided into alternating framework (FR1, FR2, FR3, and FR4) and complementarity (to antigen)–determining (CDR1, CDR2, CDR3) regions. The CDR regions are more variable in structure than are framework regions, particularly the CDR3 region, which is encoded by the VJ junctional region (light chain) or the D region plus the VD and DJ junctional regions (heavy chain). The paired C_L/CH1 domains are called the immunoglobulin CH1 domain. The paired CH2, CH3, and CH4 domains are responsible for the unique biological effector functions (e.g., complement fixation, histamine release by mast cells, binding to Fc receptors on monocytes) of different classes of subclasses of immunoglobulin. The secreted forms of IgM and IgA contain, respectively, five and two monomeric units that are disulfide bonded to each other and to a single J chain (J chain is a 15.5 kDa cysteine-rich protein that is expressed in activated B cells and all plasma cells but not at earlier stages of B-cell development).[84]

The membrane form of immunoglobulin differs only in that each class of heavy chain contains two additional carboxy-terminal domains, a transmembrane domain, and a short cytoplasmic domain, but otherwise the same light chain and the same basic structure. For most classes of immunoglobulin, expression of the membrane form of immunoglobulin on the cell surface requires that the immunoglobulin interact with a disulfide complex of two glycoproteins called Igα and Igβ.[82, 85] The Igα and Igβ heterodimer is analogous to the proteins composing the CD3 complex on T cells. It is thought that these two proteins

not only are required to anchor the immunoglobulin on the cell surface but also are involved in transduction of an antigenic signal from the outside to the inside of a B cell. Despite the similarities of the immunoglobulin receptor and the TCR, it should be noted that the former exists as a tetramer with two identical antigen-binding sites, whereas the latter exists as a dimer with a single antigen-binding site; however, in each case two chains have transmembrane domains.

Chromosomal Localization and Genetic Organization

Similar to the situation for TCR, a knowledge of the chromosomal localization and genetic organization of the three immunoglobulin loci is critical for understanding the pattern and significance of normal and abnormal Ig gene rearrangements in normal and malignant cells. Although the overall organization of these three loci is similar to that of the four TCR loci, there are important differences, particularly for the IgH locus. In general, the overall organization of the three immunoglobulin loci is highly conserved for the human and murine systems.[9, 56, 68, 80, 83, 83a]

Igκ Locus

The Igκ locus has been localized to the short arm of chromosome 2, at chromosome band 2p11, and covers more than 2.5 Mb (Fig. 11–9).

At the centromeric end of the locus, there are at least 70 known V segments. Like the V segments in each of the TCR and immunoglobulin loci, each of the κ V segments contains two exons, a short exon encoding most of the signal sequence and a longer exon encoding the C-terminal end of the signal sequence and the remainder of the variable domain. By sequence homology, the V segments are divided into six subgroups, with each member of a subgroup showing 75 per cent or more nucleic acid homology with other members of the same subgroup. In contrast to the situation in the mouse, the subgroups are not clustered but are interspersed among other V segments. The V segments may have the same or opposite transcriptional orientation as the J and C segments, although V segments with the same orientation tend to be clustered near one another. Approximately 25 per cent of known V segments are pseudogenes, which seem to be interspersed in the locus. In addition to the V segments in this locus, there are 5 Vk-like gene segments (at least three of which are pseudogenes) dispersed to chromosomes 1, 15, and 22, with the three on chromosome 22 being localized at band 22q11, centromeric to the λ V segments.

In a 5 kb region at the telomeric end of the locus, there are five functional J segments, separated from one another by about 300 bp, and a single C gene, which contains a single exon that encodes the entire constant region domain and the 3′ untranslated region. The J1 segment is about 25 kb from the 3′-most

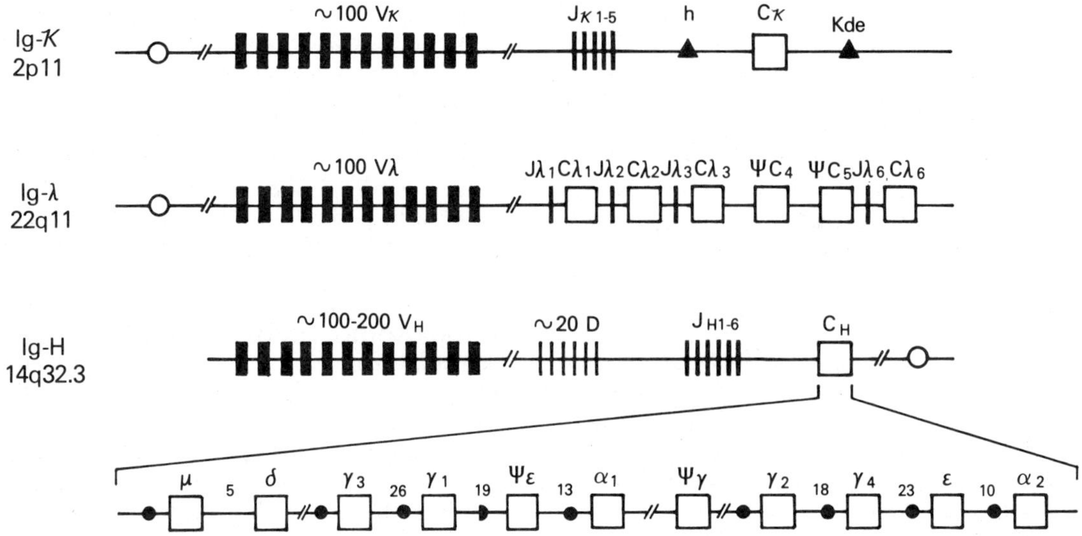

FIGURE 11–9. The human immunoglobulin loci. The chromosomal localization and genetic organization of the three Ig loci are shown in schematic form, although not to scale. The positions of centromeres are depicted by open circles, V segments by dark boxes, D segments by thin lines, J segments by thick lines, and constant (C) region genes by open boxes. Each V segment contains two exons, and each C gene contains multiple exons, as described in the text. With the exception of the δ C gene and the ψε and ψγ C genes, each Ig H chain constant region is preceded by a functional switch region, which is depicted by a dark circle. The distance (in kilobases) between each pair of Ig H chain constant regions is shown. The triangles in the Ig-κ locus represent an isolated intronic heptamer (h) and a nonamer/heptamer pair (Kde), which can be involved in developmentally regulated rearrangement events that specifically delete the Cκ constant region. See text for additional details.

V, and the J5 segment is separated by 2.5 kb from the C gene. Approximately 30 kb telomeric to the C gene is a conserved region called κde (κ deleting element), with a joining signal composed of a heptamer separated by 23 bp from the more centromeric nonamer. In addition, there is an isolated heptamer (h in Fig. 11–9) located in the JCκ intron between J5 and the intronic enhancer. The significance of h and κde is discussed below.[86]

Igλ Locus

The Igλ locus has been localized to the long arm of human chromosome 22, at chromosome band 22q11 (see Fig. 11–9). The size of the locus is unknown.

The V segments are located at the centromeric end of the locus. Sequence homology of genes and proteins that have been isolated has shown that there are 7 V segment subgroups. By Southern blot analysis, there appears to be an average of 10 V segments per subgroup, indicating that there must be a total of 70 or more V segments. It is not known if the transcriptional orientation of all V segments is the same as that of the C genes. Covering an approximately 40 kb region at the telomeric end of the locus, there are 6 C genes (C1–6), each composed of a single exon, which are spaced about 5 kb from one another. There are four highly homologous functional C genes (C1, C2, C3, and C6), each associated with its own upstream J segment. There are two pseudo C genes (C4 and C5), neither of which is associated with a clearly defined J segment. There are individuals with dupli-

cations of the C2/C3 genes, so that chromosomal loci from different individuals can contain a total of six to nine C genes. The V segments and C segments have not been physically linked.

In addition to conventional λ V or J gene segments and C genes, there are four related genes that are present on chromosome 22. One gene, which is called V-pre-B, is homologous to a V segment.[82, 87, 88] However, it is expressed uniquely in pre-B cells without gene rearrangement and encodes an approximately 16 kDa protein (see below). The V-pre-B gene is localized at the centromeric end of the V segments, perhaps centromeric to all of the V segments. The precise chromosomal location of the other three genes, each of which is homologous to λ C genes, is unclear, although they are probably not located between the V segments and the C genes.[82, 89] One of these genes, which is called 14.1, is expressed uniquely in pre-B cells without gene rearrangement and encodes an approximately 22 kDa protein that contains sequences homologous to J as well as C sequences (see below).[90] Parenthetically, the V-pre-B and 14.1 homologues in the mouse are separated by approximately 5 kb, suggesting that the human genes may not be that far apart.[82] A second gene, called 16.1, is similar to 14.1, although its expression pattern and full coding sequence have not been clearly established. The third gene, called 18.1, is a pseudogene that contains sequences homologous to C genes but not to J segments. Finally, there is a processed pseudogene (i.e., a pseudogene lacking intronic sequences, suggesting that it is derived from a processed RNA transcript) that is not present on chromosome 22.

IgH Locus

The immunoglobulin heavy chain locus is located on human chromosome 14, at band 14q32.3, and includes at least 2 Mb of DNA (see Fig. 11–9).

In contrast to all of the other TCR and immunoglobulin loci, the V segments are localized at the telomeric end of the locus. More than 60 V segments have been cloned, of which approximately one third are pseudogenes. By sequence homology, there are 6 V segment subgroups, which are interspersed throughout the locus. Unlike the Igκ V segments, all immunoglobulin heavy V segments are thought to have the same transcriptional orientation as the C genes.

Toward the centromeric end of the locus, there is an approximately 50 kb region containing at least 1 pseudo D segment and 12 functional D segments. Immediately adjacent to the 3′-most D segment, there are six functional J segments (J1–6), with three pseudo J segments interspersed among the functional J segments. Approximately 6 kb downstream from the J6 segment is the first C gene.

Unlike any of the other TCR or immunoglobulin loci, the IgH locus contains multiple C genes, with only the 5′-most C gene being associated with an immediately upstream J segment. There are 11 IgH C genes, including 2 pseudogenes, that occur in a region covering more than 100 kb. Evidence exists of a prior duplication at the 3′ end of this region (i.e., γ2-γ4-ε-α2 corresponding to γ3-γ1-ψε-α1). Each C gene contains multiple exons that generally correspond to functional domains in the corresponding H chain: CH1, hinge, CH2, CH3, and CH4. In addition, for each C gene there are two exons (M1 and M2) that together encode the transmembrane domain, the short cytoplasmic tail, and the 3′ untranslated portion of the membrane form of the corresponding mRNA (see below). Each functional C gene (except the δ and two pseudo C genes) has a switch region sequence (see below) located immediately upstream of the CH1 exon. The unique organization of the IgH C genes reflects the need for expression of different heavy chain constant region sequences with the same VDJ sequence (see below for heavy chain switching) at different times in the lifetime of a B cell and its progeny.

Immunoglobulin Gene Rearrangement and Diversity[12–16, 56, 173]

Depending on the transcriptional orientation of the V segment relative to the C gene, intrachromosomal gene rearrangement results in release of an extrachromosomal circle or a chromosomal inversion (see Fig. 11–3), with rearrangements between sister chromatids or homologous chromosomes occurring rarely.[16, 56, 91] The structural relationship of the V, D, and J segments to their corresponding signal sequence (or sequences) is shown in Figure 11–7. It is significant that the separation of heptamer/nonamer joining signals from

one another is the same on either side of the IgH D segments. Thus, in contrast to the situation with TCR receptors, D segments cannot be joined to one another, so that all functional IgH rearrangements result in a VDJ sequence. In addition, in contrast to the TCR loci, IgH D segments usually can be read in only one frame. Immunoglobulin loci are similar to TCR loci in that secondary rearrangements involving an upstream segment (e.g., V or D) and a downstream segment (e.g., D or J) are possible if appropriate joining signals remain available. For example, this is true for primary IgL VJ or IgH DJ joints but not primary IgH VDJ joints (in this latter case, all D segments have been deleted and the joining signals are not appropriate for the direct joining of an IgH V segment to a J segment). However, in contrast to the TCR and other immunoglobulin loci, another kind of secondary rearrangement (V region replacement) can result in replacement of the V segment portion of a rearranged IgH VDJ sequence with an upstream V segment.[56, 93] This IgH V segment replacement is possible, since there is a heptamer signal (but no nonamer signal) within the coding region at the 3′ end of many IgH V segments. The mechanisms that distinguish and regulate VDJ joining events, which are mediated by heptamer/nonamer signal sequences, and IgH V segment replacements, which apparently are mediated solely by a heptamer signal sequence, remain unclear. Although one can imagine the replacement of V segments with an upstream V segment by a gene conversion type of recombination, there is no evidence that this occurs at a significant rate at any of the TCR or immunoglobulin loci in humans or mice, although it is clearly an important mechanism in generating diversity of avian immunoglobulin genes.[94]

The potential diversity of immunoglobulin variable regions involves all of the mechanisms described above (including somatic hypermutation of immunoglobulin heavy and light chain variable regions), although it should be noted that immunoglobulin light chains rarely have N sequences.[28, 56] Table 11–1 summarizes the extent of potential diversity of immunoglobulin variable regions prior to somatic hypermutation. Since somatic hypermutation can occur within any portion of the heavy or light chain variable regions after antigenic stimulation, the potential diversity of immunoglobulin variable regions is seemingly infinite.[29–31]

As is true for TCR, the actual diversity achieved may be much more restricted, depending on the age of the animal, the type and situation of antigen exposure, and so forth. For example, IgH VDJ sequences from fetal or young individuals show few N regions. In addition, early in ontogeny, there may be a preferential rearrangement of certain V, D, and J segments (e.g., 3′-most V segments with 5′-most J segments or V segments and J segments that share a few nucleotides of homology at their joining ends).[29, 82, 173] Currently, however, we have limited evidence in humans to assess the constraints that bias or limit immunoglobulin variable region diversity.

Ontogeny of Immunoglobulin Rearrangements[56, 82, 95, 96]

The anatomical locations and patterns of B-lymphocyte development are similar in mice and humans.[82, 95, 96] (See also Chapter 12.) Depending on the age of the individual, pluripotent hematopoietic stem cells in the yolk sac, fetal liver, and finally the spleen and bone marrow give rise to progenitor B cells that progress through an ordered process of immunoglobulin gene rearrangements. These various stages of B-cell differentiation have been determined in humans and/or mice by analysis of normal tissues, hybridomas involving normal B-cell precursors, and various B-cell tumors (Fig. 11–10). It is thought that a lymphoid progenitor cell gives rise to a pro-B cell that is committed to the B-cell lineage. The pro-B cell expresses certain B-cell markers, including MHC class II antigens, CD19, TdT (and possibly RAG-1, RAG-2, V-pre-B, and 14.1), but has all Ig loci in an unrearranged germline state.[32, 33, 56, 82]

Pro-B cells progress to a stage (pre-B 1) in which there is joining of D segments to J segments at both IgH loci; secondary D to J rearrangements can also occur at this stage of development. Subsequently, the cells begin to express germline V gene transcripts, which correlates with cells at a developmental stage (pre-B 2) that join V segments to DJ segments generated at the pre-B 1 stage. The cells then progress to a stage (pre-B 3) in which TdT levels are low or absent, there are germline transcripts from Igκ V and J/C regions, and V segments are joined to J segments in the Igκ locus. The joining of V segments to J segments in the Igλ locus is thought to occur after rearrangements in the Igκ locus (see below).

If this sequence of gene rearrangements generates both functional immunoglobulin heavy chains and immunoglobulin light chains, the B cell has progressed through an antigen-independent pathway to a stage (immature B cell) in which a membrane IgM receptor is expressed. By analogy to the T-cell developmental pathway (see above), cells that express membrane IgM are selected to migrate into the blood and peripheral lymphoid tissues, and this selection process may provide the signal to turn off the recombinase (e.g., RAG-1 and RAG-2). Cells that express no membrane IgM or a membrane IgM directed against a self-component die for lack of a positive signal or because of a negative signal.

Regulation of Immunoglobulin Gene Formation: Allelic and IgL Isotype Exclusion

With rare exceptions, individual B cells express a single species of functional immunoglobulin.[16, 24, 56, 82, 98, 99] The immunoglobulin expressed by a cell contains *either* Igκ or Igλ light chains and thus requires *isotypic exclusion* of one of the isotypes (κ or λ) of immunoglobulin light chain. In addition, individual B cells express a single functional immunoglobulin heavy chain encoded by a functionally rearranged gene located in *either* the maternal or the paternal IgH locus, plus a single functional immunoglobulin light chain encoded by a functionally rearranged gene located in *either* the maternal or the paternal Igκ (or Igλ) locus. Thus, there is *allelic exclusion* involving both immunoglobulin loci that encode a functional immunoglobulin. Another reason why this process of immunoglobulin gene formation must be tightly regulated is that rearrangement is an inefficient process, succeeding perhaps in 1 of 3 and 1 of 9 primary attempts to generate in-frame VJ light chain and VDJ heavy chain genes, respectively. (It should be noted that in-frame joining may not be sufficient to ensure functionality; e.g., there may be mutations in one of the coding regions, such as a pseudo V.) If all primary rearrangements to generate a functional immunoglobulin heavy or light chain are unsuccessful, the cell either must proceed to attempt secondary rearrangements or replacements or must be eliminated, since B cells that do not express immunoglobulin are found only rarely in peripheral lymphoid tissues. On the basis of limited information regarding the coexistence of functional and non-functional Ig rearrangements in single B cells, it was initially proposed that allelic and isotype exclusion is actively regulated and is mediated by the products of the rearrangement process.[98, 99] Although non-regulated, stochastic models have also been proposed, most available evidence supports the hypothesis that allelic and isotypic exclusion is indeed mediated by the protein products that are encoded by the rearranged immunoglobulin or TCR genes.[56, 82]

Overall, there is a much better understanding of the regulation of immunoglobulin gene formation in B cells than of TCR gene formation in T cells. A possible model that suggests how immunoglobulin gene formation is regulated in B cells is shown in Figure 11–11 and described more fully below. The data for this model come from studies on normal and malignant B cells from humans and mice, as well as from studies of transgenic mice that contain a rearranged and functional immunoglobulin heavy and/or immunoglobulin light chain gene.[56, 82, 97, 119]

A fundamental assumption underlying this model is that the formation of VJ or VDJ sequences by gene rearrangement is immediately followed by transcription and translation of the newly rearranged gene.[56] If a rearranged immunoglobulin heavy chain (see Fig. 11–10, stage pre-B cell 2) is "functional," the cell stops additional V to DJ joining events. Correspondingly, if a rearranged immunoglobulin light chain (see Fig. 11–10, stage pre-B cell 3) is "functional," the cell stops additional V to J joining events at both immunoglobulin light chain loci. In fact, a similar hypothesis may apply to β, and possibly γ or δ, TCR gene rearrangements (see above). The key question is as follows: "How does a cell determine whether an individual chain is functional?" Since heavy chain gene rearrangements occur before light chain gene rearrangements, it was possible to propose that the "functionality" of a light chain is determined by the ability of

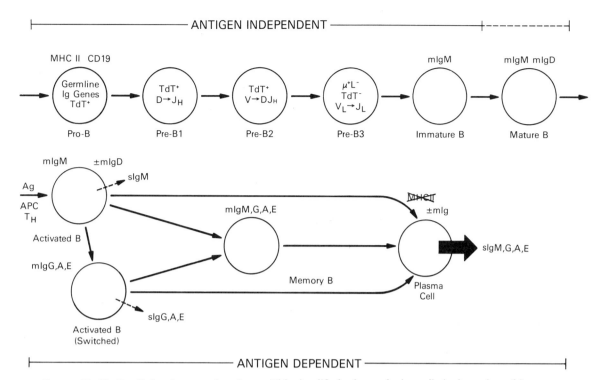

FIGURE 11–10. B-cell developmental pathway. This simplified scheme depicts a limited number of interme-diates in the developmental process and only a few of the known markers. This scheme focuses principally on cell intermediates that are involved either in V(D)J rearrangements to generate Ig H or L chain genes or in H chain switch recombination. The antigen-independent maturation events, at least through the immature B-cell stage, occur in the yolk sac, fetal liver, spleen, or bone marrow, depending on the age of the individual. Mature B cells, which coexpress mIgM and mIgD on the cell surface, are the major resting B cells in secondary lymphoid organs. Antigen-dependent maturation, which occurs principally in secondary lymphoid organs, usually requires both antigen-presenting cells (APC) and helper T cells (T_H) in addition to antigen (Ag). Some antigen-stimulated cells enter germinal centers in which Ig H and L chain variable regions are specifically subjected to a somatic hypermutation process for a limited number of divisions before progressing to either the memory B or the plasma cell stages. For additional details, see text and Chapter 12.

the light chain to form a functional complex with a functional heavy chain that was generated at an earlier stage.[56, 99] From studies of transgenic mice that received a rearranged and functional heavy chain, it was shown that the membrane form of the heavy chain can mediate this kind of regulation, whereas the secreted form of the heavy chain cannot.[97] Thus, the functionality of the IgH-IgL complex requires cell surface expression of this complex.

A tougher problem was to explain how the functionality of a newly rearranged immunoglobulin heavy chain can be determined, since the cells express no immunoglobulin light chain at the pre-B 2 stage of differentiation. If no light chain is available, the CH1 domain of the heavy chain binds to heavy chain–binding protein (BiP), which prevents secretion or surface expression of the heavy chain.[100] Parenthetically, the heavy chain in "heavy chain disease" (see below) usually has deleted the CH1 domain so that it does not bind to BiP and can then be expressed on the membrane or secreted. The apparent answer to the functionality problem is that pre-B cells express a surrogate light chain that is composed of two polypeptides that are encoded by the V-pre-B and λ 14.1 genes (see above).[87, 90, 101–105] A variety of evidence

indicates that V-pre-B encodes a 16,000 dalton poly-peptide called iota (ι) that is homologous to a λ V region but contains about 20 additional amino acids, having a significant net negative charge, at its carboxy-terminal end. Correspondingly, the λ 14.1 gene en-codes a 22,000 dalton polypeptide called omega (ω) that is homologous to a λ constant region at its car-boxy-terminal end but contains approximately 100 additional amino acids, with a substantial net positive charge, at its amino-terminus. In addition, the follow-ing have been shown: (1) ι and ω form a non-covalent complex, perhaps involving the non–immunoglobulin-like sequences at the carboxy-terminal and amino-terminal ends, respectively; (2) a ternary complex composed of a disulfide-linked heterodimer of μ heavy chain and ω plus a non-covalently associated ι chain has been identified in pre-B cells; and (3) the expres-sion of ι plus ω can substitute for a light chain in enabling a heavy chain to be secreted or expressed on the cell surface.

The model in Figure 11–11 summarizes this hy-pothesis. Following D to J joining events at both IgH loci, the cells progress from stage pre-B 1 to stage pre-B 2, in which they begin to make V to DJ rearrange-ments. It is not clear whether there is a positive signal

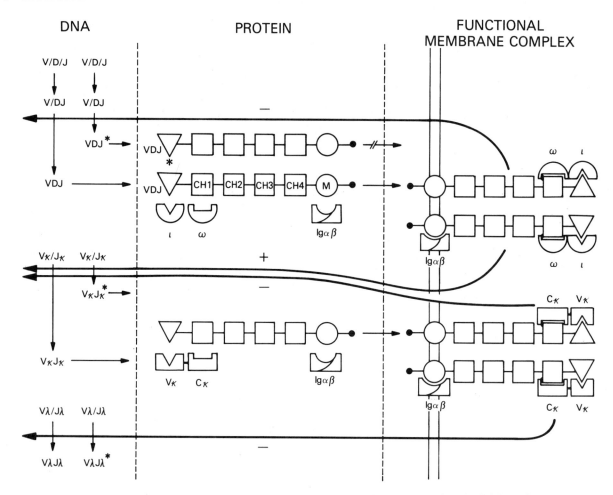

FIGURE 11–11. A possible model of allelic exclusion of Ig H and L chains. After the joining of D to J segments to form DJ segments on both chromosomes, V_H segments are joined to DJ segments, resulting in a functional VDJ or a non-functional VDJ*. A functional VDJ is immediately transcribed and translated to generate the membrane form of μ H chain. It is thought that the variable region domain (VDJ) interacts non-covalently with ι protein, while the CH1 domain interacts non-covalently and covalently (by formation of a disulfide bond) with the ω protein. This ternary complex interacts with the Igα and Igβ glycopeptides via the membrane (M) domain to form a functional membrane complex that is localized on the surface of the cell (the *closed circle* represents the cytoplasmic domain). Formation of this functional membrane complex signals the cell to stop V_H to DJ rearrangements (depicted as a negative signal), turn off TdT expression (not shown), and begin joining of Vκ segments to Jκ segments (depicted as a positive signal). A non-functional VDJ* is unable to form a functional membrane complex, thus permitting the cell to remain in the same state so that additional V_H to DJ rearrangements can be made. Rearrangements resulting in the formation of a functional VκJκ sequence produce a functional κ L chain gene that is immediately transcribed and translated. The functional κ L chain can associate with μ H chain, Igα, and Igβ to form a functional membrane complex that is localized on the cell surface. Formation of this second kind of functional membrane complex signals the cells to stop V_L to J_L rearrangements (depicted as a negative signal) at both κ and λ loci, thus leading to isotypic and allelic exclusion of L chains. Formation of a functional λ light chain would generate the same kind of functional membrane complex and signal the cell to stop V_L to J_L rearrangements. A non-functional V_LJ_L* is unable to form a functional membrane complex, so that the cell continues to make L chain gene rearrangements. See text for additional details.

to move from stage pre-B 1 to stage pre-B 2. When an in-frame VDJ rearrangement results in expression of a functional H chain, the H chain associates with Igα, Igβ, ι, and ω polypeptides to generate a complex that is expressed on the cell surface (see Fig. 11–11). It is presumed that the surface expression of this functional complex somehow generates a signal that results in differentiation to stage pre-B 3, which must then include the following: (1) an inhibition of further V to DJ joining events (perhaps by decreasing acces-

sibility of unrearranged V genes for transcription and rearrangements); (2) a turn-off of TdT expression; and (3) a turn-on of V to J joining in the Igκ locus. When an in-frame joining of V to J generates a functional light chain, it is hypothesized that the functional light chain associates with a functional immunoglobulin heavy chain so that a functional IgH/IgL receptor is expressed on the cell surface. It is presumed that the surface expression of this functional complex (see Fig. 11–11) generates a signal that prevents additional joining events. It remains to be determined how a surrogate light chain (ι plus ω chains)/heavy chain complex or a light chain (κ or λ)/heavy chain complex generates differential signals. In any case, signals generated by the presence of a functional light chain/heavy chain complex might decrease the accessibility of unrearranged V segments in both immunoglobulin light chain loci or might result in a shut-off of recombinase activity. Cells that do not express a functional IgH/IgL receptor might continue to make additional gene rearrangements but, if unable to do so, would eventually die.

It is unclear how and when a decision is made to rearrange and express λ light chain genes. It is well established that B cells expressing a κ light chain almost always possess germline λ genes, whereas B cells expressing a λ light chain have deleted or nonfunctionally rearranged both κ constant regions.[56, 119] Immunoglobulin λ light chain transgenic mice show a marked inhibition of rearrangement of endogenous κ and λ light chain genes.[106] Deletion of a κ constant region occurs by joining either a V segment or a JC_κ intronic heptamer element (h), which is not associated with a nonamer sequence, to the κde (see Fig. 11–9 and above).[86] Mainly on the basis of these data, it has been argued that rearrangements occur in the Igλ locus only when rearrangements in the Igκ locus have failed. Alternatively, it is possible that a cell becomes committed to rearrange either κ or λ genes and that the decision to rearrange Igλ genes somehow activates the deleting mechanism for the κ constant region.[56]

Expression of Alternative Forms of Heavy Chain by RNA Processing

As indicated above, all classes and subclasses of immunoglobulin can be expressed as a membrane-associated receptor or in a secreted form.[16, 80, 81] In each case, the membrane form of immunoglobulin heavy chain contains additional carboxy-terminal sequences that encode a transmembrane domain and a short cytoplasmic tail. The membrane and secreted forms of heavy chain are encoded by membrane and secreted forms of heavy chain mRNA that are generated by alternative polyadenylation and then joining of all adjacent splice donor/splice acceptor pairs.[81, 107] An example of how this works is shown for μ heavy chain in Figure 11–12A. Essentially the same alternative RNA-processing mechanism is used for all classes and subclasses of heavy chain. The differential expression of the membrane and secreted forms of heavy chain mRNA is developmentally regulated. For example, pre-B cells and resting B cells (e.g., immature, mature, and memory B cells, as shown in Fig. 11–10) express similar levels of the membrane and secreted forms of heavy chain mRNA. In contrast, activated B cells and terminally differentiated plasma cells express much higher levels of the secreted form than of the membrane form of heavy chain mRNA.

It is important to note that the presence of the membrane or secreted form of heavy chain mRNA does not ensure that the corresponding protein will be expressed, respectively, on the cell surface or in extracellular secretions. The site of expression of the membrane or secreted form of heavy chain (or immunoglobulin) is determined by developmentally regulated post-translational mechanisms. For example, expression of the membrane form of heavy chain on the cell surface generally does not occur in plasma cells, since plasma cells usually do not express a protein (Igα) that is necessary for cell surface expression (see above).[82, 85] Similarly, the secreted form of heavy chain is not secreted from immature or mature B cells. The lack of secretion of the secreted form of immunoglobulin from these early B cells is poorly understood but is not likely due to the absence of J chain expression at this time in B-cell development.[81]

Up to the immature B-cell stage of development (see Fig. 11–10), B cells express μ heavy chain and ultimately a cell surface IgM receptor when there is a functional pair of heavy and light chains. As the cells progress to the mature B-cell stage (i.e., the major kind of B cell in peripheral lymphoid tissues), they coexpress cell surface IgM and IgD receptors (but at a later developmental stage express only IgM again).[82, 95, 96] Parenthetically, the function of IgD in B cells remains enigmatic. In any case, IgM and IgD share the same light chain and the same VDJ sequence but differ in the heavy chain constant region associated with the VDJ sequence. As indicated above, the μ constant region gene is immediately downstream from the J segments, and the δ constant region gene is immediately downstream of the μ constant region (see Fig. 11–9). Since cells that coexpress μ and δ heavy chains have no DNA rearrangement involving the μ or δ heavy chain constant region genes, and can progress to a developmental stage in which they express only IgM again, it is hypothesized that a single transcription unit can generate μ and δ mRNAs by alternative RNA processing (see Fig. 11–12B). The developmentally regulated mechanism for this process is unclear. However, it differs from the mechanism for generating the membrane and secreted forms of heavy chain mRNA, since the decision to generate a δ mRNA requires that the VDJ splice donor site bypass all splice acceptor sites on μ exons to use the splice acceptor site on the CH1 δ exon.[81, 107]

Expression of Other Heavy Chain Classes by Switch Recombination

The stable expression of all classes of immunoglobulin except μ and δ requires a switch recombination event that juxtaposes the VDJ DNA segment and the appropriate constant region gene.[56, 108, 109] This developmentally regulated recombination event generally occurs within isotype-specific switch sequences that are located upstream of all heavy chain constant regions except δ (see Fig. 11–9). There are two clear structural consequences of the switch recombination event (Fig.

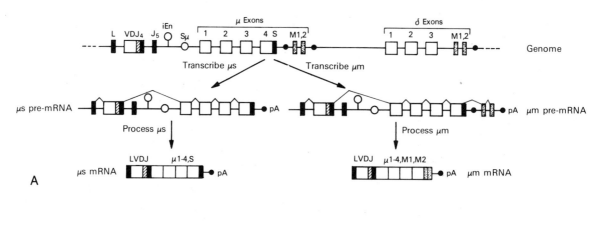

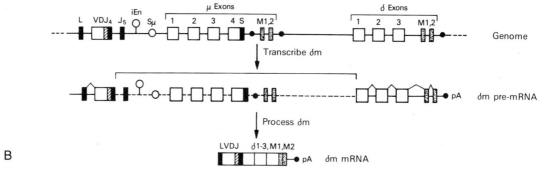

FIGURE 11–12. Generation of different Ig H chains by alternative RNA processing. *A,* Production of the secreted and membrane forms of μ H chain mRNAs by using two different polyadenylation signals. *B,* production of δ H chain mRNA by RNA processing to remove μ exons. The primary transcription unit, which includes a rearranged VDJ₄ variable region (L represents the first exon of the V segment), a μ constant region gene, and a δ constant region gene, is the same for *A* and *B*. The exons are shown as boxes. The open circle on the line is a switch sequence, the open circle above the line represents the intronic enhancer, and the closed circles represent polyadenylation sites. In *A,* the secreted form of μ H chain is derived from a $μ_s$ pre-mRNA primary transcript that uses the proximal polyadenylation site located between exon 4 and the first membrane exon (M1). The membrane form of μ H chain is derived from a $μ_m$ pre-mRNA primary transcript that uses the polyadenylation site downstream of the second membrane exon (M2). With the exception of the J5 splice site, all available splice donor and acceptor splice sites are used to generate the mature form of each kind of μ mRNA. Note that a splice donor site that occurs within μ exon 4 is used together with the acceptor splice site upstream of the μ M1 exon, so that the 3' end of exon 4 (i.e., S) is present in $μ_s$ but not in $μ_m$ mRNA. In *B,* the membrane form of δ mRNA is generated from a primary transcript that uses the polyadenylation site downstream of δ exon M2. The VDJ segment supplies a splice donor site that is used with a splice acceptor site on the 5' end of δ exon 1. The dashed line between VDJ and δ exon 1 in the primary transcript indicates the uncertainty of whether or not the primary transcript remains intact prior to the joining of VDJ and δ exon 1 sequences by splicing. It should also be noted that this figure does not include $δ_s$ exons.

11–13). First, the VDJ segment and the heavy chain intronic enhancer are positioned immediately upstream of the appropriate constant region gene. Second, there is formation of a hybrid switch region (e.g., Sμγ₁ in Fig. 11–13).

Switch sequences, which can be 1 to 10 kb in length, are composed of tandem repeats of unique nucleotide sequences containing about 10 to 100 nt per repeat, depending on the particular switch region. The switch regions associated with different constant region genes share limited homology to one another, including the presence of GAGCT and GGGGT or TGGGG pentanucleotide sequences in each kind of repeat. However, they differ substantially in the lengths, sequences, and organization of the repeats. The human and mouse switch sequences are highly homologous. The precise point at which heterologous switch sequences join is highly variable and can occur essentially anywhere within (and in some cases near) the switch sequences. There may be insertion, deletion, or substitutions of a limited number of nucleotides at or near the site of joining. The nature of the switch sequences and the hybrid switch joint indicates that recombination is a pseudo-homologous type of rearrangement,[109a] although it does not target a particular nucleotide in each switch region.[108–111] In contrast to VDJ recombination, the imprecision of the switch recombination process does not seem to have a functional consequence, since the process occurs within an intervening sequence and therefore has no effect on coding segments.

Switch recombination is similar to VDJ recombination in that most recombination events appear to be intrachromosomal.[108–111] The intervening sequences are eliminated from the cell as a switch recombination circle (see Fig. 11–13A). Rarely, it is possible for the

FIGURE 11–13. Mechanism of immunoglobulin heavy (Ig H) chain switch recombination. *A,* Intrachromosomal H chain switch recombination with formation of deletion circle. *B,* Interchromosomal H chain switch recombination with formation of unequal chromosomes. In each case, the chromosomes are shown with the same LVDJ and constant region segments. The various boxes represent the various gene or gene segments but do not reflect the organization of exons. The circles on the line depict switch regions, and the circles above the line represent the intronic enhancer (iEn) and the 3' enhancer (3'En) that is downstream of the most 3' constant region (Cα_2). The arrows represent the regions in which transcription is occurring, with the dashed portion indicating that transcription occurs only at certain stages of B-cell development. In *A,* intrachromosomal H chain switch results in the formation of a deletion circle that generally is lost during subsequent cell divisions. In *B,* interchromosomal (involving either sister chromatids or homologous chromosomes) H chain switch between duplex A (*solid line*) and duplex A' (*wavy line*) results in recombined chromosomes that have lost (A/A') or gained (A'/A) sequences, although there is no net loss or gain of sequences in a cell until the recombined chromosomes segregate at a subsequent cell division. However, unlike intrachromosomal recombination, both rearranged segments would contain a centromere and thus each rearranged chromosome would be retained in separate daughter cells. As indicated in the text, interchromosomal H chain switch recombination occurs, but at a much lower frequency than intrachromosomal H chain switch recombination.

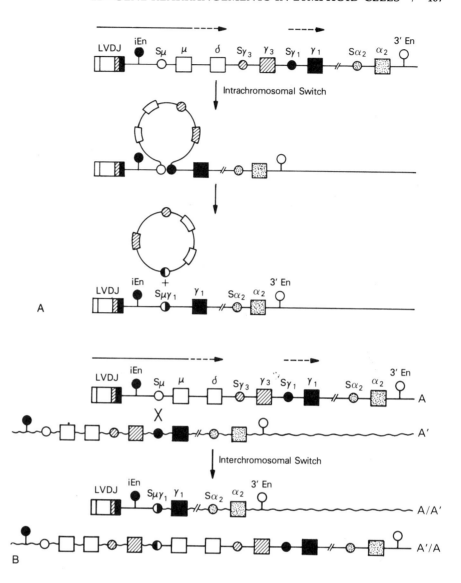

intervening sequences to invert, which probably would result in a non-functional transcription unit.[110] Interchromosomal switching events as a result of sister chromatid exchange or switch recombination involving IgH loci on homologous chromosomes occurs at a low but significant frequency (see Fig. 11–13*B*). It is of interest that a transgenic μ gene can undergo switch recombination with an endogenous IgH locus, which provides a situation analogous to chromosomal translocations mediated by class switch.[112] During interchromosomal switching, one chromosome loses sequences and the other chromosome gains the same sequences, with the chromosomal partners being segregated at the next cell division.

The mechanism and regulation of switch recombination are poorly understood. In general, it appears that switch recombination generally occurs from μ to another heavy chain constant region, although sequential switching has been observed. Back-switching (e.g., α to γ or μ) is unusual but can be explained by interchromosomal switch recombination. It is now thought that switch recombination is not a random process but can be regulated so that switching is targeted to specific constant region genes. Some evidence supporting this concept includes the following: (1) Switching often occurs to the same isotype of constant region at both IgH loci, even though only one IgH locus can express a functional heavy chain; (2) tumor cell lines can reproducibly switch from μ to one or a limited number of heavy chain constant regions; and (3) addition of helper T-cell cytokines can promote or inhibit switch recombination to specific IgH constant region genes. Many of these cytokines are elaborated by different types of helper T cells, supporting the concept that the context in which antigen, T cells, and B cells interact directs switching to specific heavy chain constant regions. The mechanism by which switch recombination is directed to specific heavy chain constant regions is thought to be mediated by accessibility of the target region. The increased accessibility of a particular constant region has been associated with some of the following events: (1) decreased DNA methylation or increased DNase I hypersensitivity or both; (2) deletions within the recipient switch region due to homologous recombination; and (3) sterile RNA transcripts, which can be initiated upstream of each switch region. It remains to be determined how the accessibility of the switch regions is controlled, although it is clear that different cytokines can cause an increased or decreased accessibility of specific constant region genes and their associated switch regions.[56, 108, 109, 113] Little is known about switch recombinase except that transfection experiments with model switch recombination substrates demonstrate that switch recombination can occur in an appropriate B-cell line but not in a fibroblast line.[92] Switch recombination is generally thought to require interaction of B cells with antigen and helper T cells. Moreover, it occurs at a time in development (see Fig. 11–10) when VDJ recombinase, as well as TdT, RAG-1, and RAG-2, do not seem to be expressed.[32, 33] Thus, it seems unlikely, though unproven, that VDJ and switch recombinases are closely related.

Timing of Gene Rearrangement and Somatic Hypermutation in Lymphoid Cells (a Summary)

As indicated above, there is a sequential pattern of VDJ rearrangements to generate functional TCR or immunoglobulin variable regions in lymphoid cells. This process is occurring in pre-T or pre-B cells (see above discussion and Figs. 11–6 and 11–10). TCR α genes and immunoglobulin light chain genes rearrange later than their respective counterparts. In addition, immunoglobulin light chain genes rarely contain N sequences, since TdT is not expressed at the pre-B cell stage in which light chain gene rearrangements are occurring. A normal or malignant lymphoid tumor can be classified as having progressed to a certain stage of differentiation based on the genotype as defined by the nature of these gene rearrangements. Similarly, lymphocyte-associated translocations can be classified with regard to the time of occurrence by the nature of the breakpoint. For example, a translocation to one of the light chain loci probably occurred at a later time in development than a translocation to the heavy chain locus. Switch recombination in the IgH locus generally occurs after antigen stimulation (see Fig. 11–10), which provides another genotypic marker for the stage of differentiation through which a B cell has passed or for the developmental stage at which a translocation into a switch region occurred. For example, the most common kind of translocation in endemic Burkitt's lymphoma, t(8;14), shows features characteristic of VDJ rearrangements (targeting near heptamer-nonamer signals), whereas the most common kind of translocation in sporadic Burkitt's lymphoma, also t(8;14), shows features suggesting an association with switch recombination (targeting an Ig switch region) (see reference 141). Thus, the translocation event in endemic Burkitt's lymphoma is presumed to have occurred in a cell at an early stage of B-cell maturation, whereas the translocation event in sporadic Burkitt's lymphoma is thought to have occurred at a late stage of B-cell maturation. Finally, somatic hypermutation occurs after antigen and helper T-cell stimulation and during a limited time period in germinal centers, with the selected progeny of this process generating memory cells or plasma cells or both (see Fig. 11–10).[114, 115] The presence or absence of somatic hypermutation of rearranged immunoglobulin heavy and/or light chains also provides a genotypic marker of whether or not a cell (e.g., plasmacytoma or B-cell lymphoma or B cells from a patient with combined variable immunodeficiency) has progressed through the stage of B-cell development in which somatic hypermutation occurs.

IMMUNE RECEPTOR GENE REARRANGEMENTS AS MARKERS OF CLONAL PROLIFERATION

In a previous section of this chapter, we described the foundation for immune receptor diversity. In that section it was emphasized that fundamental and irreversible structural reconfigurations of DNA accompany the formation of functional immune receptor genes. These gene rearrangements are not abstractions of strictly academic interest. They are real changes in the DNA of a lymphocyte that can be visualized and applied to answer questions posed in basic research and clinical patient care. At the basis of studies that utilize the study of gene rearrangements (genotyping) is the realization that these rearrangements distinguish one lymphocyte from any other not derived from it or a common parent. The structural diversity inherent and necessary to immune responsiveness creates a situation in which each rearranged lymphocyte carries within its DNA a unique "molecular fingerprint" based on its utilization of a particular V, D, and J segment with or without P and N region addition and somatic mutation.

The Recognition of Immune Receptor Gene Rearrangements

Southern Blot Analyses

Southern blot analysis (see Chapter 1) of DNA extracted from peripheral blood lymphocytes of normal individuals reveals only the germline pattern of immune receptor loci. The complete diversity of rearrangements present in the population cannot be appreciated by Southern blot analysis because the level of sensitivity is at best 1 per cent. That is, a particular pattern of gene rearrangement must be present in at least 1 of every 100 cells in order to be appreciated with this technique. If, however, one particular lymphocyte or clone of lymphocytes begins to proliferate selectively so that it constitutes 1 per cent or more of the population, its unique pattern of gene rearrangement begins to emerge through the background "haze" of all the other rearrangements present in the population (Figs. 11–14 and 11–15). Thus, this assay has found general use as a means of character-

POLYCLONAL

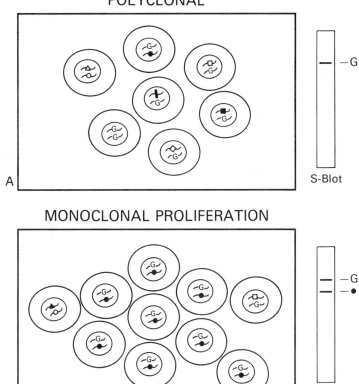

FIGURE 11–14. *A*, Polyclonal immune receptor gene rearrangements. In the schematic, "G" represents a germline, unrearranged allele of a particular immune receptor. The various other shapes represent different rearrangements of the same locus. Some cells have no rearrangements (they could be stem cells or granulocytes or the majority of T cells if one were considering Ig gene rearrangements). Other cells have one or both alleles rearranged. If a Southern blot analysis is performed (see Chapter 1 and Fig. 11–15), the sensitivity of the technique is such that only the germline band is recognizable. *B*, Monoclonal proliferation. If, however, one particular cell begins to predominate in the population (e.g., through transformation, growth stimulation, or abrogation of programmed cell death), its unique pattern of gene rearrangement starts to emerge through the background of all the other rearrangements present in the sample. In most laboratories, the sensitivity of detection of this predominant clone occurs at the 1 to 5 per cent level.

MONOCLONAL PROLIFERATION

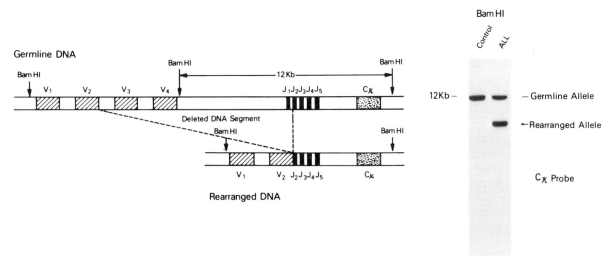

FIGURE 11–15. **Recognition of an Igκ V-J rearrangement in a leukemia by Southern blot analysis.** If germline DNA is digested with the restriction endonuclease *Bam*HI, size fractionated on an agarose gel, denatured and transferred to a solid matrix (like nitrocellulose), and hybridized to a probe homologous to the Cκ segment and autoradiographed, a single band of 12,000 base pairs is identified. In this example, the same analysis is performed on DNA extracted from the malignant cells of a patient with B-cell precursor acute lymphoblastic leukemia (ALL). Presumably as part of its normal development, the transformed cell had undergone a V-J rearrangement in which a Vκ segment had recombined in a site-specific fashion with a Jκ segment. This resulted in a deletion of DNA between the V and J and therefore, by definition, the introduction of a different 5' *Bam*HI site vis-à-vis the Cκ probe. This can be appreciated as a novel hybridizing band on the Southern blot lane to the right of the control (germline) DNA. The germline fragment is also present in the leukemic cells because only one of the two κ encoding alleles has rearranged. Despite the fact that the rearrangement of the κ gene most likely had nothing directly to do with the leukemic transformation, it provides a "molecular fingerprint" of the leukemic clone.

izing and establishing a tumor-specific marker for lymphoid malignancies. It is also valuable in the assessment of whether a proliferation of lymphocytes represents a polyclonal reaction, as might occur in a variety of inflammatory situations, or a monoclonal proliferation, most often associated with malignant transformation (see references 116 and 117). For example, a study of patients with mycosis fungoides at the plaque stage of the disease was able to demonstrate clonal TCR gene rearrangement even in circumstances in which histological and immunological assays were non-diagnostic.[118]

The identification of immunoglobulin and TCR gene rearrangments has provided tumor-specific markers despite the fact that in most cases the particular gene rearrangements themselves had nothing to do with the event (or events) that led to malignant transformation. Although this is generally assumed to be the case, it need not be universally true. For example, a particular immune receptor might provide a target for the binding of a particular transforming virus. A particular prolonged or substantial antigenic challenge may cause cells bearing a particular immune receptor to receive such a stimulus to further growth and expansion that this particular clone becomes a more likely mutational target for additional random growth-affecting events that contribute incrementally to malignant transformation. Despite these possible exceptions, most immune receptor gene rearrangements are probably incidental to the transforming etiology of the malignant clone in which they are found. The cell was engaged in its normal differentiated activity, which involved the structural rearrangement and elaboration of an immune receptor, at the time it was transformed.

In many cases, a study of immune receptor gene rearrangements offers a glimpse into the status of cellular development at the time transformation occurred.[119, 120] Classification of lymphoid neoplasms on the basis of immune receptor genotypic analyses should be viewed as an addition to and not a replacement of immunophenotypic analyses. Each technique has its limitations, ambiguities, and instructive insights.[121, 122] A telling example of this comes from a retrospective study of the malignant lymphocytes from 70 patients with immunophenotypic "B-cell precursor" acute lymphoblastic leukemia (ALL) of childhood.[123] These lymphoblasts were analyzed for rearrangements of all their immune receptor genes. All but three cases had rearranged their IgH locus, certainly consistent with their phenotypic lineage. However, 80 per cent had a rearrangement of TCRδ. In addition, rearrangements of TCRγ and TCRβ were seen in about 50 per cent of cases (Fig. 11–16). One question that arises from such a study is the issue of what it means to call something a B-cell when it has a germline IgH locus but a rearranged TCRδ gene. The safest answer to such a question is to not become constrained by forcing a cell into one or another lineage if it does not quite fit. Instead, the cell should be considered simply as a composite of its phenotypic, genotypic, and functional

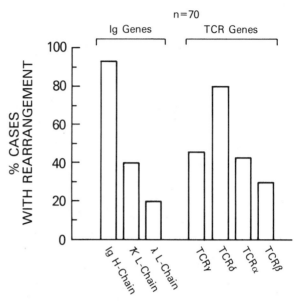

FIGURE 11–16. Ig and TCR gene rearrangements in a retrospective study of 70 patients with immunophenotypically defined "B-cell precursor" ALL of childhood. Percentages reflect cases with recombinational or deletional rearrangements or both. (From Felix, C. A., Poplack, D. G., Reaman, G. H., et al.: Characterization of immunoglobulin and T-cell receptor gene patterns in B-cell precursor acute lymphoblastic leukemia of childhood. J. Clin. Oncol. 8:431, 1990.)

attributes. The second issue raised by studies such as this one deals with the designation of these cells as B-cell precursors. More "mature" B-cell or T-cell malignancies or Epstein-Barr virus transformed–B-lymphoblastoid cell lines do not show nearly this level of simultaneous immunoglobulin and TCR locus rearrangement.[124–128] So one is left to ponder what these cells are the precursors of, since their more mature successors are not readily apparent. This question leads to the speculation that the target cell population in B-cell precursor ALL of childhood may represent a temporally or physiologically distinct entity. For example, it could be that the increased incidence of multiple immune receptor gene rearrangements could reflect a clone that, as a population of cells, spends more time at a stage at which the V(D)J recombinase complex is active.

The Use of Immune Receptor Gene Rearrangements for the Determination of Minimal Residual Disease

The sensitivity of Southern blot analysis for the detection of clonal proliferation is not distinctly greater than that offered by morphological diagnosis (e.g., bone marrow examination) for following the course of treatment and response of a patient with a lymphoid malignancy. Recently, however, molecular genetic techniques have been developed that greatly increase the sensitivity with which a particular leukemic cell can be identified. These techniques have provided the opportunity to determine minimal residual disease at the level of 1 cell per 10^5 to 10^6, as opposed to the 1 in 100 offered by Southern blot analysis.

The kinds of assays described in this section all make use of the polymerase chain reaction (PCR)[129] (see Chapter 1) to amplify the unique rearrangements that form a molecular "fingerprint" of a particular leukemic cell. The amplification proceeds to the point that evidence of the presence of the leukemic cell is unequivocal and easily visualized. The specificity of this technique can be made essentially absolute.

PCR analysis should be seen as part of the continuum of remarkable advances in recombinant DNA technology that have occurred over the past 20 years and that have brought a new era in biomedical endeavors. The underlying principle of PCR technology is beautifully simple. It is controlled and focused DNA replication. DNA polymerase requires a primer that starts it off on its synthesis of a complementary strand. In PCR, a specific segment of DNA is repeatedly replicated through the judicious choice of opposing primers, one specific for each complementary strand and oriented so that the direction of replication will be such as to replicate the region between the two primers. Repeated rounds of primer annealing, replication, denaturation, reannealing to the index and newly synthesized DNA, replication, and so on are accomplished via a thermal cycling machine and a heat-resistant DNA polymerase. Thirty-five such cycles could theoretically amplify a single segment of DNA 2^{35} times. It is also possible to amplify a specific mRNA by this process after an initial step in which the RNA is converted into complementary DNA (cDNA). This assay is fast, relatively inexpensive, automated, and amenable to the development of quality control standards in the hands of experienced personnel.[130] With appropriate resource allocation, the use of molecular genetics in the determination of minimal residual disease could be incorporated into protocols covering the care of almost every patient with ALL.

We have noted that malignant lymphocytes often have rearrangements of their immune receptor genes, which can be used to specifically identify the leukemic clone. In addition to these rearrangements, malignant lymphocytes—and hematopoietic malignancies in general—often carry a variety of disease-specific chromosomal rearrangements (see below, as well as Chapters 23 and 24) whose structure and unique configurations also make them available as tumor-specific markers. Either of these markers can theoretically provide the basis of minimal residual disease determination. The use of immunoglobulin or TCR gene rearrangements offers an advantage with regard to their being the most universally applicable to lymphoid malignancies, since more than 95 per cent of lymphoid leukemias or lymphomas involve lymphocytes that have rearranged either one or more immunoglobulin or TCR locus. The disadvantages of this approach include the following: (1) the need to individualize the assay for each patient (see below); (2) the fact that the assay itself is slightly more complicated than just screening

for a chromosomal aberration; (3) the fact that, in some cases, the focus of the assay (the specific immunoglobulin or TCR) may somatically mutate so as to become invisible, and therefore lead to a false-negative result; and finally (4) the fact that the genetic sequence being assayed is not causally related (in most cases) to the etiology of the transformation; as discussed earlier, it is an epiphenomenon. Assaying specific chromosomal breaks avoids these four disadvantages but at present is not as universally applicable because the majority of leukemia- or lymphoma-associated chromosomal aberrations have not been identified or characterized to the point where they are amenable to PCR-based assay. Furthermore, certain characterized chromosomal aberrations (e.g., *myc*-Ig) may have breakpoints too diverse and scattered for different patients to be amenable to PCR analysis using a single panel of primers.

The key to the use of immunoglobulin and TCR rearrangements for determination of minimal residual disease is the junctional diversity described earlier in this chapter. There are four basic steps to the use of Ig and TCR gene rearrangements in this assay:

1. Identification (of locus rearrangement).
2. Characterization (of the unique junctional sequence).
3. Determination (of the presence of leukemic cells in "remission" samples).
4. Quantitation (of the number of leukemic cells present).

Identification

On presentation of a patient with the clinical and morphological diagnosis of lymphoid malignancy, a determination must be made of whether there is a clonal immune receptor rearrangement carried by the malignant cells. Classically, this is accomplished by Southern blot analysis.

Denaturing Gradient Gel Electrophoresis

One way to speed up the identification process may be through the use of denaturing gradient gel electrophoresis (DGGE).[131] DGGE technology in this particular application begins with the fundamental PCR assay for junctional diversity. In this assay, one PCR primer (or group of primers) is synthesized so that it will be complementary to part of the variable segment of the immune receptor being studied. The part of the variable segment that is chosen for this primer is ideally the *least* variable part of the segment—for example, the 5' end of the V segment or, in some cases, framework region (FR) 3. This allows for the construction of a "consensus" V primer that can be utilized successfully to prime DNA replication from every or practically every V segment in that particular immune receptor locus. The downstream primer is related to the J segments, either a consensus J sequence or, if the structure of the locus is suitable, a primer from just 3' of the most 3' J segment. It is possible to use this exact 3′ sequence as a primer in those cases in which the J segments are few in number and not spread out over greater than 1000 nt of DNA. If this is the case, the amplified product of a V(D)J rearrangement will be less than 2000 bp. Products larger than 2000 bp cannot be amplified with an efficiency that makes them reasonable substrates for this analysis.

Once the appropriate primer pairs have been developed, they are then used to amplify V(D)J rearranged DNA in the sample to be analyzed. The vastly predominant clone in a sample population (as would be the case in a newly diagnosed lymphoid malignancy) will be the predominant amplified product. A consensus primer will work in most cases because (1) it need only bind to a particular sequence well enough and long enough to initiate replication, and (2) after the first cycle of replication, it will be identical to one end of all the newly synthesized DNA fragments. When placed on a denaturing gradient gel, the amplified fragment migrates until it begins to undergo regional denaturation[132] (the point at which this occurs is sequence specific), at which time migration is markedly slowed. After gel staining, the fragment (or fragments) associated with the clone appears as a notable band that emerges from the background haze caused by the migratory patterns of the other polyclonal rearrangements, which are below the level of detection in this particular kind of gel visualization. Without the use of DGGE, one could not distinguish a monoclonal proliferation from a polyclonal one because the size of the amplified fragments would be the same in either case. DGGE is sensitive to DNA sequence.

Which immune receptor should be studied for which disease? Depending on the type of lymphoid malignancy, it is more or less likely that a particular immune receptor gene will be rearranged. With regard to minimal residual disease determination, rather than screen every malignancy for rearrangement of every immune receptor, it is possible to play the percentages and screen only for those rearrangements that are the most likely and most usable in a PCR-based assay. Table 11–2 provides a general sense of the frequency of immune receptor gene rearrangements in acute leukemia. Clearly, studying immune receptor rearrangements is more or less applicable, depending on the leukemic type. For example, for B-cell precursor ALL, rearrangement of the IgH locus is most applicable and has indeed been used in preliminary studies.[133, 134] However, the use of IgH PCR amplification can be a problem because the great diversity of V segments in the IgH locus complicates the preparation of a "consensus" V_H segment. Furthermore, as noted above, the IgH locus is subject to continued somatic mutation, which can occasionally (although usually not in ALL; see above) change the unique molecular "fingerprint" and thus defeat the characterization and determination steps, to be described next. The TCRγ and δ loci are almost always rearranged in T-cell ALL, and each is rearranged in

TABLE 11–2. IG AND TCR GENE REARRANGEMENTS IN ACUTE LEUKEMIAS

	B-CELL PRECURSOR ALL (%)	T-CELL ALL (%)	AML (%)	ALL OF INFANCY (%)
IgH				
R	98	14	14	64
Igκ				
R	28	0	2	18
D	17	0	0	0
	45			
Igλ				
R	20	0	0	0
TCRβ				
R	33	89	7	9
TCRγ				
R	55	91	5	0
TCRδ				
R	54	68	8	NA
D	26	28	1	NA
	80	96	9	

ALL = Acute lymphoblastic leukemia; AML = acute myeloblastic leukemia; R = rearranged; D = deleted.
Data are derived from references 123, 137, and 174.

more than 50 per cent of B-cell precursor ALLs. The repertoire of V segments for these loci is much more restricted than for the IgH locus, and these loci are not subject to somatic hypermutation. Thus, in situations in which such TCR rearrangements can be identified, they may be logistically simpler to work with and interpret.[135, 136] For example, identifying both a TCRδ and an IgH rearrangement in the ALL cells of a patient with B-cell precursor ALL may be advantageous in terms of the more homologous (less "degenerate" in order to achieve consensus) primers that can be used for TCRδ. Having both of these loci available for the analysis of this patient would also provide a comforting and useful "backup" for pinpointing the minimal residual disease clone.

Characterization

This next step requires PCR amplification of the hypervariable, junctional part of the V(D)J rearranged region. Once amplified, the unique molecular fingerprint, which is the precise DNA sequence of this junction, must be determined. The most straightforward way to do this is by sequencing this region, which can be accomplished either by cloning and sequencing the PCR product or by newer sequencing techniques that may not give quite as much resolution but that are accomplished directly at the time of PCR amplification. "Nested" PCR analysis is an alternative to actually sequencing the junction. In nested analysis, PCR primers from inside the originally amplified fragment are used to amplify a shorter stretch of DNA that is almost pure hypervariable region. This fragment is then used as a probe of subsequent amplifications of the same patient's "remission" DNAs. The premise is that at very high stringency of hybridization, only the absolutely identical sequence will hybridize (here one is not asking merely for an oligonucleotide to transiently prime a polymerization reaction but rather for it to bind with high affinity and stay bound). Thus, a hybridization signal from a study performed using a "clonospecific" probe (derived at the patient's presentation) on a DNA sample from that patient would be indicative of residual leukemic cells even if morphological and clinical remission had been achieved. Actual sequencing of the junction provides a more controlled way of generating a smaller and completely specific oligonucleotide probe that can be utilized for such hybridization studies.

Determination

As just described, this step involves the preparation of DNA (or cDNA) from the patient's samples obtained at various times during a course of treatment. The appropriate consensus primers are used to amplify the V(D)J rearrangements present in the sample. A probe, prepared either from known sequence of the leukemic clone or by nested PCR, is then applied to the products of the amplification reaction. Positive hybridization indicates the presence of DNA that carries a molecular fingerprint identical to that of the probe and (the presumption is) therefore of residual leukemic cells. Obviously, crucial attention must be paid to making the conditions of the hybridization reaction high enough to be absolutely specific but such that the formation of double-stranded DNA is still allowed (in this case, one strand is the probe and the other the target DNA).

Quantitation

It may not be sufficient to know simply whether residual leukemic cells exist in a sample. It may be important to be able to at least roughly quantitate how many such cells remain. A variety of strategies exist for this quantitation. One strategy involves the cloning of products of a PCR amplification into bacteriophage and plating out the phage on a bacterial lawn. Duplicate lifts of phage DNA are then made, one lift hybridized to a clonospecific probe and the other to a probe that will recognize every V(D)J rearrangement of the particular immune receptor being analyzed in the sample. The ratio of clonospecific phage to total hybridizing phage provides one kind of quantitation when combined with morphological and immunophenotypic data concerning the proportion of lymphoid, erythroid, and myeloid cells in the sample.[133] Another means of quantitation involves making a standard titration curve by diluting known amounts of clonospecific cells in a background of miscellaneous cells. The signal generated from the sample containing an unknown amount of clonospecific DNA is then plotted on a standard curve (prepared as an internal control by mixing known quantities of clonal and polyclonal DNAs together) to provide a rough estimate of the number of leukemic cells in the sample.[134]

Preliminary Results

Enough pilot studies[133–137] have been performed using these methods to begin to have a rough picture of the dynamics of leukemic cell kill during current accepted therapy for ALL. Different studies yield varying results, but a consensus pattern seems to be emerging at present. Induction therapy results in a threefold to fourfold log reduction in the number of leukemic cells (down to about 0.01 per cent of cells in a given sample). This level of cells then seems to plateau for a while (usually measured in many months) often corresponding to the maintenance therapy phase of treatment. Whether these cells are viable and capable of cell division and "rekindling" of the leukemia is not known at this time. However, it is clear that the majority of children who complete a full 2- to 3-year course of therapy for ALL test negative for residual leukemic cells on these pilot assays. In at least one study,[136] differences in the duration of minimal residual disease were not associated with any particular clinical or hematological parameter of the underlying disease. Reappearance of the leukemic clone either during or following therapy is a bad prognostic sign and can precede clinical evidence of relapse by several months. Whether such information obtained a few months before clinical relapse would help rescue certain patients if acted upon by a physician is an issue that needs to be tested in prospective protocols.

IMMUNE RECEPTORS AS PARTICIPANTS IN THE GENERATION OF CHROMOSOMAL ABERRATIONS (Table 11–3)

The Burkitt's Lymphoma Precedent

It could be said that the study of gene rearrangements in lymphoid cells gave birth to the entire field of molecular genetic analysis of cancer-associated chromosomal aberrations. In 1982, the chromosomal localization of the murine and human immunoglobulin genes was established. It was striking that the chromosomal bands to which these genes had been localized were precisely those bands disrupted by the consistent translocations associated with the development of Burkitt's lymphoma in humans and plasmacytoma in BALB/c mice. One group of investigators studying the c-*myc* gene in plasmacytomas came across its structural juxtaposition to the IgH locus.[138] Two other groups approached the translocation breakpoint in Burkitt's lymphoma and murine plasmacytomas by the cloning and characterization of "peculiar," uncharacteristic rearrangements of the immunoglobulin genes in these malignant cells and similarly found that the IgH locus had rearranged with the c-*myc* proto-oncogene.[139, 140] This was the first time the genes that precisely flanked a cancer-associated chromosomal aberration had been identified. It was not only the simple fact of their identification but the fact of precisely what genes they were that made the finding so com-

TABLE 11–3. IMMUNE RECEPTORS IN THE GENERATION OF CHROMOSOMAL ABERRATIONS

TRANSLOCATION	CANCER	LOCI
Involvement of Ig Genes in Human B-Cell Malignancy		
t(5;14) (q31;q32)	ALL with hypereosinophilia	Il-3-IgH
t(8;14) (q24;q32.3)	Burkitt's lymphoma	c-Myc-IgH
t(2;8) (p12;q24)		Igκ-c-Myc
t(8;22) (q24;q11)		c-Myc-Igλ
t(10;14) (q24;q32)	High and low-grade lymphoma	Lyt10-Igα
t(11;14) (q13;q32.3)	Diffuse lymphoma, CLL, multiple myeloma	Bc11-IgH
t(14;18) (q32.3;q21)	Follicular lymphoma	IgH-Bc12
t(14;19) (q32;q11.3)	B-CLL	IgH-Bc13
Involvement of TCR Genes in Human T-Cell Malignancy		
t(1;7) (p34;q35)	T-ALL	Lck-TCRβ
t(1;14) (p33;q11.2)	Stem cell leukemia, T-ALL	Scl(Ta11,Tc15)-TCRδ
t(6;14) (q21;q11)	T-ALL	?-TCRα/δ
t(7;9) (q35;q34.2)	T-ALL	TCRβ-Ta12
t(7;9) (q35;q34)	T-ALL	TCRβ-Tan1
t(7;10) (q35;q24)	T-ALL	TCRβ-?
t(7;19) (q35;p13)	T-ALL	TCRβ-Ly1-1
t(8;14) (q24;q11)	T-ALL T-CLL	c-Myc-TCRα/δ
t(10;14) (q23;q11)	T-ALL	Hox11-TCRδ
t(11;14) (q13;q11)	T-ALL	Ttg2 (Rhom2)-TCRδ
t(11;14) (p15;q11)	T-ALL	Ttg1 (Rhom1)-TCRδ
t(12;14) (q24;q11)*	ATL	?-TCRα/δ
inv(14) (q11.2;q32.1)	T-PLL	TCRα/δ-?
t(14;14) (q11.2;q32.1)	T-CLL	TCRα-?
Involvement of TCR Genes in Clonal Proliferation/Malignancy in Ataxia-Telangiectasia		
t(7;14) (q35;q32.1)		TCRβ-?
inv(14) (q11.2;q32.1)		TCRα-?
t(14;14) (q11.2;q32.1)		TCRα-?
t(X;14) (q28;q11.2)		?-TCRα
Involvement of the Ig and TCR Loci in Chromosomal Aberration in Normal Individuals		
t(2;14) (p12;q32.3)†		Igκ-IgH
inv(7) (p13;q35)		TCRγ-TCRβ
t(7;7) (p13;p35)*		TCRγ-TCRβ
t(7;14) (p13;q11.2)		TCRγ-TCRα/δ
t(7;14) (q35;q11.2)*		TCRβ-TCRα/δ
inv(14) (q11.2;q32.3)†		TCRα-IgH
t(14;14) (q11.2;q32.3)*		TCRα-IgH
V(D)J Recombinase-Mediated Rearrangement of Other Genes		
del(1p33)‡	T-ALL	Sil-Scl
Involvement of Other Immune-Related Genes		
t(1;19) (q23;p13)	pre-B-ALL	E2A-Pbx1
t(2;8) (q34;q24)	T-ALL	?-c-Myc

*No cloning data available.
†Also seen in rare malignancies.
‡Not visible by routine cytogenetic analysis.
ALL = Acute lymphoblastic leukemia; CLL = chronic lymphocytic leukemia; B-CLL = B-cell CLL; T-ALL = T-cell ALL; ATL = adult T-cell leukemia; PLL = prolymphocytic leukemia.

pelling. In Burkitt's lymphoma, a B-cell tumor, the characteristic translocation carried by the malignant cells juxtaposed the primary differentiated product of those cells, immunoglobulins, with a gene, c-*myc*, whose dysregulation was associated with malignant transformation. It was impossible not to speculate that the translocated c-*myc* gene might now be inappropriately controlled by those factors that promoted transcription of the immunoglobulin genes, and that the net effect of this dysregulation would be a qualitatively and possibly quantitatively inappropriate expression of a gene with known growth-effecting properties. Although complete elucidation of the mechanism by which this translocation contributes to malignant transformation has not yet been achieved, the basic speculative premise just described is firmly established. Studies of many examples of sporadically occurring Burkitt's lymphoma suggested that in the approximately 80 per cent that involved the IgH locus (as opposed to the Igκ and Igλ loci) the heavy chain "switch" region had been targeted in the breakage and rejoining event.[141] Thus, not only was the immunoglobulin locus involved in the translocation but also its involvement seemed to be selected by one of its cell type–specific recombinational processes. The switch region of the Igα locus is similarly involved by the

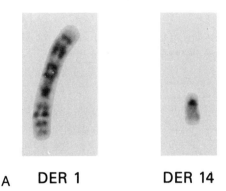

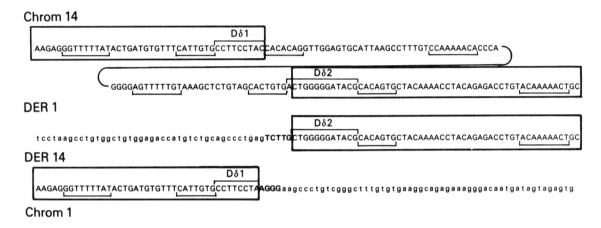

FIGURE 11–17. Analysis of the breakpoint in a t(1;14) translocation associated with the development of a stem cell leukemia. *A,* The reciprocal chromosome partners of the translocation, the derivative chromosome 1 (DER 1) (which maintains the chromosome 1 centromere) and the derivative chromosome 14 (DER 14) (maintaining the chromosome 14 centromere), are shown in a G-banded partial karyotype. *B,* Sequence analysis of a reciprocal t(1;14) translocation. The uppermost sequence is the germline chromosome 14 sequence (uppercase letters). Note the two Dδ segments flanked by heptamer and nonamer signal sequences (*underlined*) and the intervening DNA (*interrupted line*) between these segments. DER 1 shows the germline chromosome 14 sequence at the 3′ end and the germline chromosome 1 sequence (lowercase letters) at the 5′ end. Five nucleotides attributed to N-region diversity are shown in boldface letters. DER 14 shows 3′ germline chromosome 1 sequence, N nucleotides, and 5′ chromosome 14 sequence. Note that the intervening DNA between the Dδ segments has been deleted from the translocated chromosomes, suggesting that the translocation may have taken place during physiologic D-D rearrangement, which would have normally deleted this intervening DNA (see Fig. 11–18). The bottom line shows the germline chromosome 1 sequence with two possible heptamer signal sequences (*dashed underline*). A gap that corresponds to the area involved in N-region addition has been introduced into the germline chromosome 1 sequence to allow alignment of nucleotides on DER 1 and DER 14. (Modified from Begley, G. B., Aplan, P. A., Davey, M. P., et al.: Chromosomal translocation in a human leukemic stem cell line disrupts the TCRD δ region and results in a previously unreported fusion transcript. Proc. Natl. Acad. Sci. USA 86: 2031, 1989; with permission.)

t(14;19)(q32;q13.1) translocation associated with the development of some cases of B-cell chronic lymphocytic leukemia (CLL). The translocation juxtaposes the IgH locus with a putative cell cycle control–related gene, BCL3.[142] It is not known what enzymes and structural signals and conformations are necessary for the chromosomal breakage and rejoining events that involve these IgH switch regions.

V(D)J Recombinase–Mediated Chromosomal Aberrations

An even larger and more diverse number of chromosomal aberrations that occur within the immune receptor loci seem to implicate the V(D)J recombinase complex as playing some role in their occurrence. Characterization of the chromosomal regions involved in these aberrations often suggests that the deletion, inversion, or translocation occurred at the time that the immune receptor locus was undergoing its normal, physiologic segment rearrangements (Fig. 11–17*A* and *B*). Instead of completing the process within the locus, material from a different part of the genome becomes interposed. In many cases, the results of the aberration are essentially balanced. For example, a V segment for an immune receptor locus becomes contiguous with nucleotide X from another chromosome, and the J segment to which that V might have rearranged becomes contiguous with nucleotide X + 1 on the other chromosome. The material between that V and J is deleted as it might have been in normal intralocus VJ rearrangement. The structure of such chromosomal aberrations has strong implications for their mechanism of occurrence. Such balanced structures are not consistent with temporally unrelated times of breakage of the two involved regions. One cannot easily imagine a V and J segment becoming dislodged from each other and floating around in the nucleus of the cell until they encounter two new chromosomal regions to which they can ligate; and why should those two new chromosomal regions have any relationship to each other? It is conceptually simpler to visualize (Fig. 11–18) all of the participants in the generation of a chromosomal aberration being present at the same time. If chromosomal aberrations do indeed occur at a point in time (as seems most consistent with the data), then they almost certainly occur at a point in space, a point where relevant recombinase enzyme complexes can function and interact. The likely temporal and spatial localization for the occurrence of chromosomal aberrations in which the V(D)J recombinase plays a role suggests an inherent organization of the interphase nucleus and may provide as well a key to understanding the requirement of chromatin accessibility discussed in an earlier section of this chapter.

A Model

The speculative model depicted in Figure 11–18 attempts to suggest a temporal and spatial focus for one kind of V(D)J recombinase–mediated translocation. In this example, based on the cloning and characterization of a t(1;14) translocation associated with the development of a stem cell leukemia,[143] breaks occur at precise signal sequences flanking two diversity segments from the TCRδ locus (see Fig. 11–17A and B). The chromosomal breaks within the 3' SCL gene on chromosome 1 do not clearly focus on immune receptor–like signal sequences. (This 3' SCL breakpoint should be contrasted with the 5' SCL breakpoints seen in the interstitial deletion of part of chromosome 1, to be described below. The 5' breakpoints are proximate to clear heptamer/nonamer signal sequences.) This raises the question of whether the V(D)J recombinase is necessary but not sufficient for the occurrence of such translocations. The answer to this question will most likely not be settled until a cell-free system exists for studying the formation of chromosomal aberrations. Other structures that have been suggested as facilitating recombinase-mediated translocations (or, for that matter, chromosomal aberrations in general) include alternating stretches of purine and pyrimidine residues forming "Z" DNA configurations[144] and sequences with homology to the prokaryotic recombinogenic signal, "chi."[145, 146]

Hybrid Immune Receptor Genes

Invoking more complex mechanisms is not a problem when both partners in reciprocal chromosomal exchanges have reasonable heptamer sequences at their site of recombination. Such is the case in many aberrations associated with lymphoid malignancies. One common type would be a chromosomal aberration involving V(D)J recombination that occurs between two immune receptor loci instead of within one or the other locus. All humans carry within a subset of their peripheral blood lymphocytes chromosomal translocations or inversions that are formed by site-specific V(D)J recombination between two immune receptor loci. The result of these aberrations is to form hybrid genes with a V segment from one receptor and a J and C segment from another. The most common such abnormality appears to be a hybrid IgH variable–TCRα constant segment that occurs at a frequency as high as 0.1 per cent of a normal individual's peripheral blood T-cell population.[147, 148] Other such hybrids that have been extensively characterized include TCRγ-TCRδ hybrids caused by V(D)J-mediated t(7;14)(p13;q11.2) translocation[20] and TCRγ-TCRβ hybrids caused by V(D)J-mediated inv (7)(p13q35).[21] In general, these hybrid genes are found at low frequency, although their structures and expression suggest that they may make some contribution of their own to immune receptor diversity or stimulation of cellular proliferation. Although approximately 50 per cent of such hybrid junctions are in-frame at the DNA level, there is a selection for the expression of in-frame recombinants such that more than 90 per cent of such hybrid mRNAs are in-frame,[21] a phenomenon that could be related to antigenic selection or mRNA stability.[149] The same phenomenon has been observed for normal intralocus V(D)J recombinants and suggests that hybrid immune receptors can be expressed, translated, placed in the membrane of a host lymphocyte, and selected by antigenic stimulation. Given the apparent diversity of effector functions and lineage determination based on what immune receptor is expressed on a cell, the implications of having a TCRγ V segment expressed on a TCRβ constant segment could be significant, although, as yet, no particular function or phenotype has been associated with this or any other hybrid.

What has been observed with these hybrids is that their frequency is increased about 100-fold in patients suffering from the disease ataxia-telangiectasia (AT).[21] Ataxia-telangiectasia is a disease of protean manifestations, including progressive cerebellar degeneration, oculocutaneous telangiectasia, radiosensitivity, immunodeficiency, a predisposition to the development of certain malignancies (particularly lymphoid), and, as noted, an increase in cell type–specific chromosomal aberrations. This increase of hybrid gene formation reflects multiple independent events. Although as much as 10 per cent of an AT patient's peripheral T-cell population may carry an inversion of chromosome 7, this population, when analyzed at the level of the

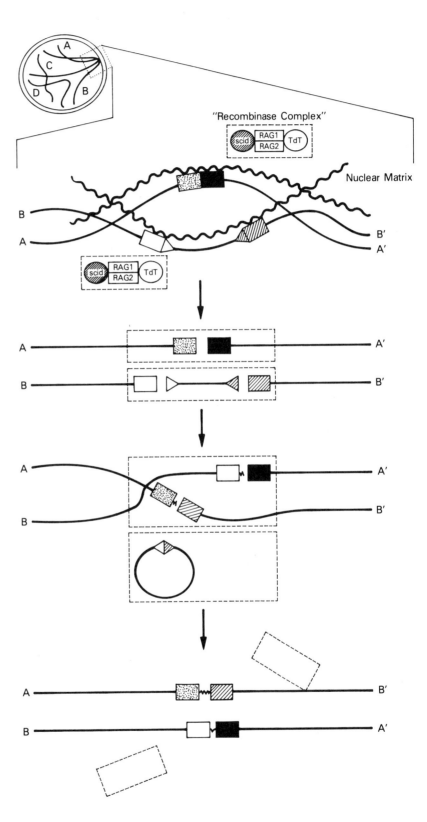

FIGURE 11–18. Postulated nuclear localization of the recombinase complex and targets of recombinase-mediated translocation. The circle at the very top of the figure represents a cell—for example, a lymphocyte—in which a part of chromosome A and a part of chromosome B are sequestered in a part of the nucleus, perhaps attached to the nuclear matrix (*wavy line*) because of their particular structure, function, chromatin status, or accessibility, or by chance. The recombinase complexes are operative in this part of the nucleus and act on the two chromosomes to cause breakage and rejoining events. The complex (*dashed line box*) consists of targeting, nucleolytic, and repair enzymes, including RAG-1, RAG-2, the *scid* gene product, and TdT. The hatched and open boxes delineate "coding" segments, the triangle "signal" sequences. The structure shown on chromosome B in the upper part of the figure is consistent with an immune receptor locus, such as the TCRDδ locus shown in Figure 11–17. Part of the recombination reaction proceeds normally; the ends of the intervening sequence carrying the signal segments are joined together in an extrachromosomal circle. However, the topography and topology of chromosomes A and B cause an interchromosomal rather than an intrachromosomal rearrangement, which results in a chromosomal translocation. (From Kirsch, I. R.: Genetics of pediatric tumors: The causes and consequences of chromosomal aberrations. *In* Pizzo, P., and Poplack, D. [eds.]: Principles and Practice of Pediatric Oncology. 2nd ed. Philadelphia, J. B. Lippincott, 1993; with permission.)

DNA, demonstrates an array of distinct Vγ recombined with any one of a number of Jβ segments. So the picture in the peripheral blood of a patient with AT represents an exaggeration of the normal polyclonal population of hybrid genes found in everyone's normal peripheral blood T-cell population.

What is the relationship of this finding in AT to other aspects of the phenotype of this complex disease? There is no evidence at present that the increase in hybrid gene formation is caused by an overexpression or overactivity of the V(D)J recombinase complex. One possibility might be that part of the AT phenotype is caused by an inappropriate "accessibility" of the genome to the activity of DNA interactive factors, such as the recombinase complex. This feature might explain why loci that are only rarely simultaneously accessible in normal lymphocytes (such as the TCRβ and TCRγ loci) are more frequently capable of forming interlocus hybrids in AT lymphocytes. The exaggeration of hybrid gene formation in AT is not restricted to T cells. There is also an increase of Igκ-IgH hybrids (corresponding to t(2;14) translocations[150]) in the B-cell population of these patients.[50] This "exaggeration" in AT of V(D)J recombinase–mediated chromosomal aberration extends from hybrid gene formation to the formation of translocations and inversions frankly associated with abnormal proliferation and malignancy. Over time, patients with AT can develop a clonal proliferation within their T-cell population that is associated with the formation of an inversion or translocation of chromosome 14: inv(14)(q11.2q32.1) or t(14;14)(q11.2;q32.1). Much more rarely, this clonal proliferation is associated with a t(X;14) translocation. Carrying one or another of these aberrations, a particular T-cell clone can persist or proliferate in the peripheral blood of a patient with AT to the point where it constitutes essentially 100 per cent of the peripheral T-cell population.[151] At this point, the overall white blood cell count of the individual can still be within a normal range and there may be no evidence or stigmata of lymphoid malignancy. However, a percentage of such patients with these clonal proliferations will subsequently develop a T-cell malignancy in which the malignant cell contains the marker inv(14) or t(14;14). Cloning of the chromosomal breakpoints in these cells[152, 153] has revealed site-specific recombination between TCRα J segments and a region within chromosomal band 14q32.1 in which a growth-effecting gene is presumed to reside but in which no such gene has been found as yet. A cytogenetically identical aberration has been associated with the development of T-cell prolymphocytic leukemia, a relatively virulent malignancy that is seen most commonly in older males.[154] Cloning studies of these malignancies in patients without AT have revealed an identical V(D)J contributory mechanism, but still no target gene on 14q32.1.[155, 156]

Other Targets for the V(D)J Recombinase

The V(D)J recombinase is a powerful mechanism for rearranging DNA. In the presence of this enzyme complex, accessible signal sequences are targeted for structural reconfiguration. The usual targets are the immune receptor loci, but any accessible signal sequence is at risk for rearrangement. Thus, two loci, Sil and Scl, that either fortuitously or for reasons yet to be discovered carry within their loci appropriate signal recognition signals have been shown to be rearranged with each other by the V(D)J recombinase, although neither is an immune receptor locus.[49] The Sil locus encodes a product that bears a eukaryotic topoisomerase I active site.[157] Scl is a putative transcription factor that likely functions at a nodal point in hematopoietic differentiation.[158] The V(D)J recombinase–mediated interstitial deletion that unites these two loci is seen in the malignant cells of 20 to 30 per cent of all patients with T-cell-ALL.[159, 160]

Section Summary

In summary, the immune receptor loci are the most characteristic targets of the chromosomal aberrations associated with the development of lymphoid malignancies. In the usual case, a chromosomal aberration juxtaposes one or another growth-effecting gene with an immune receptor that is being highly expressed in the particular lymphocyte. The current view is that such juxtaposition places the control of the growth-effecting gene under those factors driving immune receptor expression. This situation leads to inappropriate, dysregulated, and often increased expression of the growth-effecting gene, which results in abnormal growth and contributes to malignant translocation. The entire process could be viewed as a random process. In that view, chromosomes would be presumed to be constantly breaking and rejoining, but only when the particular growth-effecting gene–immune receptor juxtaposition was achieved would that particular cell have a selective growth advantage and thus emerge from the general population of all cells undergoing chromosomal reconfigurations. This view is probably too simplistic and may be frankly incorrect. The cell-type specificity of particular chromosomal aberrations suggests that not all genes and not all parts of the genome are equally susceptible in a particular type of cell to participate in a chromosomal aberration and transforming event. Chromatin structure and DNA accessibility may have a strong influence on the predisposition to gene rearrangement. Furthermore, lymphocytes elaborate powerful systems for rearranging DNA, namely, the "switch" and V(D)J recombinase complexes. Those parts of the genome that are accessible and that contain recognition signals for these complexes are likely to be at much greater risk for rearrangement.

THE USE OF POLYMERASE CHAIN REACTION TO FOLLOW CHROMOSOMAL ABERRATIONS

Earlier in this chapter, we described the use of PCR analysis for immunoglobulin and TCR rearrangements to follow minimal residual disease in patients with leukemia or lymphoma. All of the steps described then could be applied in the analysis of chromosomal aberrations, but often they are not all necessary. Thus, the assay can sometimes be made simpler. Part of the reason for this is that there are a group of leukemia-associated chromosomal aberrations that are of leukemic type but *not* patient specific, so that a single set of primers can be applied to every patient whose cells carry the aberration and there is not always a need to develop a clonogenic probe unique for each patient. The very presence of an amplified product is indicative of the presence of chromosomal aberration. The primers must be oriented so that at the genomic DNA or cDNA level an amplified product of between 200 and 2000 bp will be generated. One primer comes from one side of the aberration and the other from the other side. By definition, normally the two primers are too far apart (or even on two different chromosomes), so that amplification of a DNA segment that lies between them is impossible. Only when the aberration has occurred is an amplified product generated. The premise for the use of this assay in minimal residual disease determination is that the juxtaposition of the two chromosomal regions that makes amplification possible *occurs only in the leukemic cells.* Although this appears to be generally true (and, indeed, is part of the basis for the study of cancer-associated chromosomal aberrations as a means of identifying genes that can contribute to malignant transformation), it may not be correct in every case. For example, it is now known that the t(14;18) translocation associated with adult follicular lymphoma can be identified in the reactive tonsils or lymph nodes of a significant number (20–40 per cent) of normal children.[161]

IMMUNE RECEPTOR GENE DELETIONS/ALTERATIONS AND DISEASE

Heavy Chain Diseases

This class of diseases is characterized by lymphoproliferation of varying degree and severity in which the proliferative clone produces an aberrant, usually truncated IgH chain *unlinked* to an immunoglobulin light chain. The truncated chain can be of any heavy chain subclass.[162] An analysis of a case of μ heavy chain disease revealed that a DNA insertion/deletion had removed a J_H splice donor site from the rearranged J segment, leading to splicing of the leader sequence to the constant segment.[163] It has been speculated that continued synthesis of immunoglobulin might be important for optimum viability of the cell but that absence of V segment peptides might allow the cell to escape idiotypic control.[164] It is also possible that this truncated IgH segment, lacking a V segment and therefore unresponsive to antigen, but theoretically capable of membrane emplacement, might provide an aberrant stimulus to proliferation of the lymphocyte on which it was anchored. It might be that an analogy

could be drawn between this effect and the presumed proliferative effect on fibroblasts of a truncated epidermal growth factor, erbB.[165] Cases of α heavy chain disease have been observed in which the cells bear surface α chain but do not secrete it.[166] Cases of α and γ heavy chain disease have been associated with deletions within the variable and part of the constant segments.[166–168]

Immunodeficiency

The bulk of immunodeficiency syndromes defined to date do not appear to have as their root cause deletion of the immune receptor loci. Although rare individuals have been identified who lacked immunoglobulin subclasses on the basis of deletions of a part of the IgH locus,[169] most such immunodeficiencies appear to have a regulatory rather than a structural basis.[170, 171] Studies of individuals heterozygous for alleles that carry IgH deletions have revealed that the level of immunoglobulin subclass production from the remaining genes was variable. One such study of individuals heterozygous for a large deletion stretching from ψγ-α2 revealed essentially normal IgG production but below-normal IgA2 levels. This finding was postulated to reflect a dosage and switching defect.[172]

SUMMARY

Genomic DNA is unstable and dynamic, not static and immutable. This ability of primary genetic material to undergo reconfiguration is one of the keys to the rapidity of evolutionary development. Structural realignments of DNA also provide the fundamental basis of our ability to mount an almost infinitely diverse immune response. The mechanism that causes "innocent" or malignant lymphocyte-specific chromosomal aberrations is often just a variation on the physiologic mechanism of V(D)J or "switch" recombination. The elucidation of this mechanism was one of the early successes of recombinant DNA research, but the fine mechanistic details of the recombination events are still at the stage of model and speculation. Understanding recombination at this refined level will not only give us crucial insight into the necessary and sufficient features for immune responsiveness but also will provide a conceptual basis for viewing all mutation and rearrangement of DNA and thus yield insight into development, cancer and carcinogenesis, and aging. In the meantime, techniques based on recognition of DNA alterations from germline status are expanding our knowledge and pinpointing steps of lymphocyte lineage differentiation. They are also providing a basis for the diagnosis, classification, staging, and tracking of a variety of hematological diseases.

REFERENCES

1. Vitetta, E. S., Fulton, R. J., May, R. D., Till, M., and Uhr, J. W.: Redesigning nature's poisons to create anti-tumor reagents. Science 238:1098, 1987.
2. Suresh, M. R., Cuello, A. C., and Milstein, C.: Advantages of bispecific hybridomas in one-step immunocytochemistry and immunoassays. Proc. Natl. Acad. Sci. USA 83:7989, 1986.
3. Tramontano, A., Janda, K. D., and Lerner, R. A.: Catalytic antibodies. Science 234;1566, 1986.
4. Pollack, S. J., Jacobs, J. W., and Schultz, P. G.: Selective chemical catalysis by an antibody. Science 234:1570, 1986.
5. Potter, M.: Immunoglobulin-producing tumors and myeloma proteins of mice. Physiol. Rev. 62:631, 1972.
6. Nathans, D., and Smith, H.: Restriction endonucleases in the analysis and restructuring of DNA molecules. Annu. Rev. Biochem. 46:273, 1975.
7. Landsteiner, K.: The Specificity of Serologic Reactions. Cambridge, Mass., Harvard University Press, 1945.
8. Dreyer, W. J., and Bennett, J. C.: The molecular basis of antibody formation. Proc. Natl. Acad. Sci. USA 54:864, 1965.
9. Kabat, E. A., Wu, T. T., Perry, H. M., Gottesman, K. S., and Foeller, C.: Sequences of Proteins of Immunological Interest. 5th ed. Washington, D.C., Department of Health and Human Services, U.S. Public Health Service, 1991.
10. Davies, D. R., and Metzgar, H.: Structural basis of antibody function. Annu. Rev. Immunol. 1:87, 1983.
11. Amit, A. G., Mariuzza, R. A., Phillips, S. E. V., and Poljak, R. J.: Three-dimensional structure of an antigen-antibody complex at 2.8Å resolution. Science 233:747, 1986.
12. Capra, J. D., and Edmundson, A. B.: The antibody combining site. Sci. Am. 236:50, 1977.
*13. Darnell, J., Lodish, H., and Baltimore, D.: Molecular Cell Biology. 2nd ed. Chapter 25, Immunity. New York, W. H. Freeman and Co., 1990.
14. Watson, J. D., Hopkins, N. H., Roberts, J. W., Steitz, J. A., Weiner, A. M.: Molecular Biology of the Gene. 4th ed. Chapter 23, The generation of immunological specificity. Menlo Park, Calif. The Benjamin-Cummings Publishing Co., 1987.
15. Lewin, B.: Genes IV. Chapter 36, Generation of immune diversity involves reorganization of the genome. Oxford, England, Oxford University Press, Cambridge, Mass., and Cell Press, 1990.
16. Max, E. E.: Immunoglobulins: Molecular genetics. In Paul, W. E.: Fundamental Immunology. 2nd ed. New York, Raven Press, 1989.
17. Malissen, M., McCoy, C., Blanc, D., Trucy, J., Devaux, C., Schmitt-Verhulst, A. M., Fitch, F., Hood, L., and Malissen, B.: Direct evidence for chromosomal inversion during T-cell receptor beta-gene rearrangements. Nature 319:28, 1986.
18. Okazaki, K., Davis, D. D., and Sakano, H. T.: Cell receptor beta gene sequences in the circular DNA of thymocyte nuclei: Direct evidence for intramolecular DNA deletion in V-D-J joining. Cell 49:477, 1987.
19. Kronenberg, M., Goverman, J., Haars, R., Malissen, M., Kraig, E., Phillips, L., Delovitch, T., Suciu-Foca, N., and Hood, L.: Rearrangement and transcription of the beta-chain genes of the T-cell antigen receptor in different types of murine lymphocytes. Nature 313:647, 1985.
20. Tycko, B., Palmer, J. D., and Sklar, J.: T-cell receptor gene transrearrangements: Chimeric γ-δ genes in normal lymphoid tissues. Science 245:1242, 1989.
21. Lipkowitz, S., Stern, M.-H., and Kirsch, I. R.: Hybrid T cell receptor genes formed by interlocus recombination in normal and ataxia-telangiectasia lymphocytes. J. Exp. Med. 172:409, 1990.
22. Lieber, M. R., Hesse, J., Mizuuchi, K., and Gellert, M.: Lymphoid V(D)J recombination: Nucleotide insertion at signal joints as well as coding joints. Proc. Natl. Acad. Sci. USA 85:8588, 1988.
23. Altenburger, W., Steinmetz, M., and Sachau, H. G.: Functional and nonfunctional joining in immunoglobulin light chain genes of a mouse myeloma. Nature 287:603, 1980.
24. Bernard, O., Gough, N. M., and Adams, J. M.: Plasmacytomas with more than one immunoglobulin kappa mRNA: Implications for allelic exclusion. Proc. Natl. Acad. Sci. USA 78:5812, 1981.
25. Lafaille, J. J., DeCloux A., Bonneville, M., Takagaki, Y., and Tonegawa, S.: Junctional sequences of T cell receptor γδ T cell lineages and for a novel intermediate of V-(D)-J joining. Cell 59:859, 1989.
26. Alt, F., and Baltimore, D.: Joining of immunoglobulin heavy chain gene segments: Implications from a chromosome with evidence of three D-J$_H$ fusions. Proc. Natl. Acad. Sci. USA 79:4118, 1982.
27. Blackwell, T. K., and Alt, F. W.: Molecular characterization of the lymphoid V(D)J recombination activity. J. Biol. Chem. 264:10327, 1989.
28. Landau, N. R., Schatz, D. G., Rosa, M., and Baltimore, D.: Increased frequency of N-region insertion in a murine pre-B-cell line infected with a terminal deoxynucleotidyl transferase retroviral expression vector. Mol. Cell. Biol. 7:3237, 1987.
28a. Gu, H., Foster, I., and Rajewsky, K.: Sequence homologies, N sequence insertion and JH gene utilization in VDJ joining: Implications for the joining mechanism and the ontogenetic timing of Ly1 B cell and B-CLL progenitor generation. EMBO J. 9:2133, 1990.
29. Levy, N. S., Malipero, U. V., Lebecque, S. G., and Gearhart, P. J.: Early onset of somatic mutation in immunoglobulin V$_H$ genes during the primary immune response. J. Exp. Med. 169:2007, 1989.
30. McKean, D., Huppi, K., Bell, M., Staudt, L., Gerhard, W., and Weigert, M.: Generation of antibody diversity in the immune response of BALB/c mice to influenza virus hemagglutinin. Proc. Natl. Acad. Sci. USA. 81:3180, 1984.
31. Lebecque, S. G., and Gearhart, P. J.: Boundaries of somatic mutation in rearranged immunoglobulin genes: 5' Boundary is near the promoter, and 3' boundary is ~1 kb from V(D)J gene. J. Exp. Med. 172:1717, 1990.
32. Schatz, D. G., Oettinger, M. A., and Baltimore, D.: The V(D)J recombination activating gene, RAG-1. Cell 59:1035, 1989.
33. Oettinger, M. A., Schatz, D. G., Gorka, C., and Baltimore, D.: RAG-1 and RAG-2, adjacent genes that synergistically activate V(D)J recombination. Science 248:1517, 1990.
34. Bosma, G. C., Custer, R. P., and Bosma, M. J.: A severe combined immunodeficiency mutation in the mouse. Nature 301:527, 1983.
35. Schuler, W., Weiler, I. J., Schuler, A., et al.: Rearrangement of antigen receptor genes is defective in mice with severe combined immune deficiency. Cell 46:963, 1986.
36. Lieber, M. R., Hesse, J. E., Lewis, S., Bosma, G. C., Rosenberg, N., Mizuuchi, K., Bosma, M. J., and Gellert, M.: The defect in murine severe combined immune deficiency: Joining of signal sequences but not coding segments in V(D)J recombination. Cell 55:7, 1988.
37. Malynn, B. A., Blackwell, T. K., Fulop, G. M., Rathbun, G. A., Furley, A. J., Ferrier, P., Heinke, L. B., Phillips, R. A., Yancopoulos, G. D., and Alt, F. W.: The scid defect affects the final step of the immunoglobulin VDJ recombinase mechanism. Cell 54:453, 1988.
38. Okazaki, K., Nishikawa, S., and Sakano, H.: Aberrant immunoglobulin gene rearrangement in scid mouse bone marrow cells. J. Immunol. 141:1348, 1988.

---

*In regard to references 13 to 16, an enormous amount of work and numerous investigators have contributed to our current understanding of the organization and structure of the immunoglobulin and T-cell antigen receptor loci. The data generated in this area have indeed now achieved a textbook acceptability. Among the many excellent textbook treatments of this material are these four references, which provided useful examples in the preparation of this chapter.

39. Giblett, E. R., Anderson, J. E., Cohen, I., Pollara, B., and Mewissen, J. H.: Adenosine-deaminase deficiency in two patients with severely impaired cellular immunity. Lancet 2:1067, 1972.

40. Giblett, E. R., Ammann, A. J., Wara, D. W., Sandman, R., and Diamond, L. K.: Nucleoside-phosphorylase deficiency in a child with severely defective T-cell immunity and normal B-cell immunity. Lancet 1:1010, 1974.

41. Rosen, F. S., Gitlin, D., and Janeway, C. A.: Alymphocytosis, agammaglobulinemia, homografts, and delayed hypersensitivity: Study of a case. Lancet 2:380, 1962.

42. Gelfand, E. W., and Dosch, H. M.: Diagnosis and classification of severe combined immunodeficiency disease. Birth Defects 19:65, 1983.

43. Chang, L. M. S., and Bollum, F. J.: Molecular biology of terminal transferase. Crit. Rev. Biochem. 21:27, 1986.

44. Matsunami, N., Hamaguchi, Y., Yamamoto, Y., Kuze, K., Kangawa, K., Matsuo, H., Kawaichi, M., and Honjo, T.: A protein binding to the Jκ recombination sequence of immunoglobulin genes contains a sequence related to the integrase motif. Nature 342:934, 1989.

45. Hesse, J. E., Lieber, M. R., Mizuuchi, K., and Gellert, M.: V(D)J recombination: A functional definition of the joining signals. Genes Dev. 3:1053, 1989.

46. Yancopoulos, G. D., and Alt, F. W.: Developmentally controlled and tissue specific expression of unrearranged V_H gene segments. Cell 40:271, 1985.

47. Blackwell, T. K., Moore, M. W., Yancopoulos, G. D., Suh, H., Lutzker, S., Selsing, E., and Alt, F. W.: Recombination between immunoglobulin variable region segments is enhanced by transcription. Nature 324:585, 1986.

48. Yancopoulos, G. D., Blackwell, T. K., Suh, H., Hood, L., and Alt, F.: Introduced T cell receptor variable region gene segments recombine in pre-B cells: Evidence that B and T cells use a common recombinase. Cell 44:251, 1986.

49. Aplan, P. D., Lombardi, D. P., Ginsberg, A. M., Cossman, J., Bertness, V. L., and Kirsch, I. R.: Disruption of the human SCL locus by "illegitimate" V(D)J recombinase activity. Science 250:1426, 1990.

50. Kirsch, I. R., Brown, J. A., Lawrence, J., Korsmeyer, S., and Morton, C. C.: Translocations that highlight chromosomal regions of differentiated activity. Cancer Genet. Cytogenet. 18:159, 1985.

51. Boehm, T., Mengle-Gaw, L., Kees, U. R., Spurr, N., Lavenir, I., Forster, A., and Rabbitts, T. H.: Alternating purine-pyrimidine tracts may promote chromosomal translocations seen in a variety of human lymphoid tumors. EMBO J. 8:2621, 1989.

52. Staudt, L. M., and Lenardo, M. J.: Immunoglobulin gene transcription. Annu. Rev. Immunol. 9:373, 1991.

53. Winoto, A., and Baltimore, D.: αβ Lineage-specific expression of the α T cell receptor gene by nearby silencers. Cell 59:649, 1989.

54. Li, Q., Zhou, B., Powers, P., Enver, T., and Stamatoyannopoulos, G.: β-Globin locus activation regions: Conservation of organization, structure, and function. Proc. Natl. Acad. Sci. USA 87:8207, 1990.

55. Schlissel, M. S., Corcoran, L. M., and Baltimore, D.: Virus-transformed pre-B cells show ordered activation but not inactivation of immunoglobulin gene rearrangement and transcription. J. Exp. Med. 173:711, 1991.

56. Blackwell, T. K., and Alt, F. W.: Mechanism and developmental program of immunoglobulin gene rearrangement in mammals. Annu. Rev. Genet. 23:605, 1989.

57. Gu, H., Kitamura, D., and Rajewsky, K.: B cell development regulated by gene rearrangement: Arrest of maturation by membrane-bound Dμ protein and selection of D_H element reading frames. Cell 65:47, 1991.

58. Raynal, M., Liu, Z., Hirano, T., Mayer, L., Kishimoto, T., and Chen-Kiang, S.: Interleukin 6 induces secretion of IgG1 by coordinated transcriptional activation and differential mRNA accumulation. Proc. Natl. Acad. Sci. 86:8024, 1989.

59. Dariavach, P., Williams, G. T., Campbell, K., Pettersson, S.,

and Neuberger, M. S.: The mouse IgH 3′-enhancer. Eur. J. Immunol. 21:1499, 1991.

60. Strominger, J. L.: Developmental biology of T cell receptors. Science 244:943, 1989.

61. Boehm, T., and Rabbitts, T. H.: The human T cell receptor genes are targets for chromosomal abnormalities in T cell tumors. FASEB J. 3:2344, 1989.

62. Hedrick, S. M.: T lymphocyte receptors. In Paul, W. E.: Fundamental Immunology. 2nd ed. New York, Raven Press, 1989.

63. Davis, M. M.: T cell receptor gene diversity and selection. Annu. Rev. Biochem. 59:475, 1990.

64. Ashwell, J. D., and Klausner, R. D.: Genetic and mutational analysis of the T-cell antigen receptor. Annu. Rev. Immunol. 8:139, 1990.

65. Strominger, J. L.: The γδ T cell receptor and class 1b MHC-related proteins: Enigmatic molecules of immune recognition. Cell 57:895, 1989.

66. Allison, J. P., and Havran, W. L.: The immunobiology of T cells with invariant γδ antigen receptors. Annu. Rev. Immunol. 9:679, 1991.

67. Chan, A., and Mak, T. W.: Genomic organization of the T cell receptor. Cancer Detect. Prev. 14:261, 1989.

68. Lai, E., Wilson, R. K., and Hood, L. E.: Physical maps of the mouse and human immunoglobulin-like loci. Adv. Immunol. 46:1, 1989.

69. Wells, F. B., Gahm, S., Hedrick, S. M., Bluestone, J. A., Dent, A., and Matis, L. A.: Requirement for positive selection of γδ receptor–bearing T cells. Science 253:903, 1991.

70. Dent, A. L., Matis, L. A., Hooshmand, F., Widacki, S. M., Bluestone, J. A., and Hedrick, S. M.: Self-reactive γδ T cells are eliminated in the thymus. Nature 343:714, 1990.

71. Bonneville, M., Ishida, I., Itohara, S., Verbeek, S., Berns, A., Kanagawa, O., Haas, W., and Tonegawa, S.: Self-tolerance to transgenic γδ T cells by intrathymic inactivation. Nature 344:163, 1990.

72. Fowlkes, B. J., and Pardoll, D. M.: Molecular and cellular events of T cell development. Adv. Immunol. 44:207, 1989.

73. Sprent, J.: T lymphocytes and the thymus. In Paul, W. E.: Fundamental Immunology. 2nd ed. New York, Raven Press, 1989.

74. Von Boehmer, H.: Developmental biology of T cells in T cell–receptor trangenic mice. Annu. Rev. Immunol. 8:531, 1990.

75. Ishida, I., Verbeek, S., Bonneville, M., Itohara, S., Berns, A., and Tonegawa, S.: T-cell receptor γδ and γ transgenic mice suggest a role of a γ gene silencer in the generation of αβ T cells. Proc. Natl. Acad. Sci. USA 87:3067, 1990.

76. Winoto, A., and Baltimore, D.: Separate lineages of T cells expressing the αβ and γδ receptors. Nature 338:430, 1989.

77. Takeshita, S., Toda, M., and Yamagishi, H.: Excision products of the T cell receptor gene support a progressive rearrangement model of the α/δ locus. EMBO J. 8:3261, 1989.

78. Turka, L. A., Schatz, D. G., Oettinger, M. A., Chun, J. J. M., Gorka, C., Lee, K., McCormack, W. T., and Thompson, C. B.: Thymocyte expression of RAG-1 and RAG-2: Termination by T cell receptor cross-linking. Science 253:778, 1991.

79. Hasemann, C. A., and Capra, J. D.: Immunoglobulins: Structure and function. In Paul, W. E.: Fundamental Immunology. 2nd ed. New York, Raven Press, 1989.

80. Honjo, T., Shimizu, A., and Yaoita, Y.: Constant-region genes of the immunoglobulin heavy chain and the molecular mechanism of class switching. In Honjo, T., Alt, F. W., Rabbitts, T. H. (eds): Immunoglobulin Genes. New York, Academic Press, 1989, p. 123.

81. Wall, R., and Kuehl, M.: Biosynthesis and regulation of immunoglobulins. Annu. Rev. Immunol. 1:393, 1983.

82. Rolink, A., and Melchers, F.: Molecular and cellular origins of B lymphocyte diversity. Cell 66:1081, 1991.

83. Rathbun, G., Berman, J., Yancopoulos, G., and Alt, F. W.: Organization and expression of the mammalian heavy-chain variable-region locus. In Honjo, T., Alt, F. W., and Rabbitts, T. H. (eds): Immunoglobulin Genes. New York, Academic Press, 1989, p. 63.

83a. Matsuda, F., Shin, E. K., Nagaoka, H., Matsumura, R., Haino, M., Fukita, Y., Taka-ishi, S., Imai, T., Riley, J. H., Anand, R., et al.: Structure and physical map of 64 variable segments in the 3' 0.8-megabase region of the human immunoglobulin heavy-chain locus. Nature Genetics 3:88, 1993.

84. Koshland, M. E.: The immunoglobulin helper: The J chain. *In* Honjo, T., Alt, F. W., and Rabbitts, T. H.: Immunoglobulin Genes. New York, Academic Press, 1989, p. 345.

85. Venkitaraman, A. R. J., Williams, G. T., Dariavach, P., and Neuberger, M. S.: The B-cell antigen receptor of the five immunoglobulin classes. Nature 352:777, 1991.

86. Graininger, W. B., Goldman, P. L., Morton, C. C., O'Brien, S. J., Korsmeyer, S. J.: The κ-deleting element: Germline and rearranged, duplicated and dispersed forms. J. Exp. Med. 167:488, 1988.

87. Bauer, S. R., Kudo, A., and Melchers, F.: Structure and pre-B lymphocyte restricted expression of the VpreB gene in humans and conservation of its structure in other mammalian species. EMBO J. 7:111, 1988.

88. Bauer, S. R., Huebner, K., Budarf, M., Finan, J., Erikson, J., Emanuel, B. S., Nowell, P. C., Croce, C. M., and Melchers, F.: The human Vpre-B gene is located on chromosome 22 near a cluster of Vλ₁ gene segments. Immunogenetics 28:328, 1988.

89. Chang, H., Dmitrovsky, E., Hieter, P. A., Mitchell, K., Leder, P., Turoczi, L., Kirsch, I. R., and Hollis, G. F.: Identification of three new Igλ–like genes in man. J. Exp. Med. 163:425, 1986.

90. Hollis, G. F., Evans, R. J., Stafford-Hollis, J. M., Korsmeyer, S. J., and McKearn, J. P.: Immunoglobulin λ light-chain–related genes 14.1 and 16.1 are expressed in pre-B cells and may encode the human immunoglobulin ω light-chain protein. Proc. Natl. Acad. Sci. USA 86:5552, 1989.

91. Toda, M., Hirama, T., Takashita, S., and Yamagishi, H.: Excision products of immunoglobulin gene rearrangements. Immunol. Lett. 21:311, 1989.

92. Ott, D. E., Alt, F. W., and Marcu, K. B.: Immunoglobulin heavy chain switch region recombination within a retroviral vector in murine pre-B cells. EMBO J. 6:577, 1987.

93. Reth, M., Gehrmann, P., Petrac, E., and Wiese, P.: A novel V_H to VDJ_H joining mechanism in heavy-chain–negative (null) pre-B cells results in heavy-chain production. Nature 322:840, 1986.

94. McCormack, W. T., Tjoelker, L. W., and Thompson, C. B.: Avian B-cell development: Generation of an immunoglobulin repertoire by gene conversion. Annu. Rev. Immunol. 9:219, 1991.

95. Cooper, M. D., and Burrows, P. D.: B-cell differentiation. *In* Honjo, T., Alt, F. W., and Rabbitts, T. H. (eds.): Immunoglobulin Genes. New York, Academic Press, 1989, p. 1.

96. Okun, F. M.: Regulation of human B-cell ontogeny. Blood 76:1908, 1990.

97. Storb, U., Engler, P., Hagman, J., Gollahon, K., Manz, J., Roth, P., Rudin, C., Doglio, L., Hackett, J., Haasch, D., Chaplin, D., Lo, D., and Brinster, R.: Control of expression of immunoglobulin genes. Prog. Immunol. 7:316, 1989.

98. Rose, S. M., Smith, G. P., and Kuehl, W. M.: Cloned MPC 11 myeloma cells express two kappa genes: A gene for a complete light chain and a gene for a constant region polypeptide. Cell 12:453, 1977.

99. Alt, F. W., Rosenberg, N., Lewis, S., Thomas, E., and Baltimore, D.: Organization and reorganization of immunoglobulin genes in A-MuLV–transformed cells: Rearrangement of heavy but not light chain genes. Cell 27:381, 1981.

100. Hendershot, L., Bole, D., Kohler, G., and Kearney, J. F.: Assembly and secretion of heavy chains that do not associate posttranslationally with immunoglobulin heavy chain–binding protein. J. Cell Biol. 104:761, 1987.

101. Pillai, S., and Baltimore, D.: Formation of disulphide-linked $\mu_2\omega_2$ tetramers in pre-B cells by the 18K ω-immunoglobulin light chain. Nature 329:172, 1987.

102. Karasuyama, H., Kudo, A., and Melchers, F.: The proteins encoded by the VpreB and λ5 pre-B cell–specific genes can associate with each other and with μ heavy chain. J. Exp. Med. 172:969, 1990.

103. Tsubata, T., and Reth, M.: The products of pre-B cell–specific genes (γ5 and VpreB) and the immunoglobulin μ chain form a complex that is transported onto the cell surface. J. Exp. Med. 172:973, 1990.

104. Cherayil, B. J., and Pillai, S.: The ω/λ5 surrogate immunoglobulin light chain is expressed on the surface of transitional B lymphocytes in murine bone marrow. J. Exp. Med. 173:111, 1991.

105. Nishimoto, N., Kubagawa, H., Ohno, T., Gartland, G. L., Stankovid, A. K., and Cooper, M. D.: Normal pre-B cells express a receptor complex of μ heavy chains and surrogate light-chain proteins. Proc. Natl. Acad. Sci. USA 88:6284, 1991.

106. Neuberger, M. S., Caskey, H. M., Pettersson, S., Williams, G. T., and Surani, M. A.: Isotype exclusion and transgene down-regulation in immunoglobulin-γ transgenic mice. Nature 338:350, 1989.

107. Guise, J. W., Galli, G., Nevins, J. R., and Tucker, P. W.: Developmental regulation of secreted and membrane forms of immunoglobulin μ chain. *In* Honjo, T., Alt, F. W., and Rabbitts, T. H. (eds.): Immunoglobulin Genes. New York, Academic Press, 1989, p. 275.

108. Gritzmacher, C. A.: Molecular aspects of heavy-chain class switching. Crit. Rev. Immunol. 9:173, 1989.

109. Esser, C., and Radbruch, A.: Immunoglobulin class switching: Molecular and cellular analysis. Annu. Rev. Immunol. 8:717, 1990.

109a. Ravetch, J. V., Kirsch, I. R., and Leder, P.: An evolutionary approach to the question of immunoglobulin heavy chain switching: Evidence from cloned human and mouse genes. Proc. Natl. Acad. Sci. USA 77:6734, 1980.

110. Hans-Martin, J., McDowell, M., Steinberg, C. M., and Wabl, M.: Looping out and deletion mechanism for the immunoglobulin heavy-chain class switch. Proc. Natl. Acad. Sci. USA 85:1581, 1988.

111. Matsuoka, M., Yoshida, K., Maeda, T., Usuda, S., and Sakano, H.: Switch circular DNA formed in cytokine-treated mouse splenocytes: Evidence for intramolecular DNA deletion in immunoglobulin class switching. Cell 62:135, 1990.

112. Durdick, J., Gerstein, R. M., Rath, S., Robbins, P. F., Nisonoff, and Selsing, E.: Isotype switching by a microinjected μ immunoglobulin heavy chain gene in transgenic mice. Proc. Natl. Acad. Sci. USA 86:2346, 1989.

113. Kuze, K., Shimizu, A., and Honjo, T.: Characterization of the enhancer region for germline transcription of the gamma 3 constant region gene of human immunoglobulin. Int. Immunol. 3:647, 1991.

114. Kocks, C., and Rajewsky, K.: Stable expression and somatic hypermutation of antibody V regions in B-cell developmental pathways. Annu. Rev. Immunol. 7:537, 1989.

115. MacLennan, I.: The centre of hypermutation. Nature 354:352, 1991.

116. Cleary, M. I., Warnke, R., and Sklar, J.: Monoclonality of lymphoproliferative lesions in cardiac transplant recipients. N. Engl. J. Med. 310:477, 1984.

117. Weiss, L. M., Wood, G. S., Nickoloff, B. J., and Sklar, J.: Gene rearrangement studies in lymphoproliferative disorders of skin. Adv. Dermatol. 3:141, 1988.

118. Weiss, L. M., Hu, E., Wood, G. S., Moulds, C., Cleary, M. L., Warnke, R., and Sklar, J.: Clonal rearrangements of the T cell receptor gene in mycosis fungoides and dermatopathic lymphadenopathy. N. Engl. J. Med. 313:539, 1985.

119. Korsmeyer, S. J., Hieter, P. A., Ravetch, J. V., Poplack, D. G., Waldmann, T. A., and Leder, P.: Developmental hierarchy of immunoglobulin gene rearrangements in human leukemic pre-B-cells. Proc. Natl. Acad. Sci. USA 78:7096, 1981.

120. Sklar, J., Cleary, M. L., Thielemans, K., Gralow, J., Warnke, R., and Levy, R.: Biclonal B-cell lymphoma. N. Engl. J. Med. 311:20, 1984.

121. Korsmeyer, S. J., Arnold, A., Bakhshi, A., Ravetch, J. V., Siebenlist, U., Hieter, P. A., Sharrow, S. O., LeBien, T. W., Kersey, J. H., Poplack, D. G., et al.: Immunoglobulin gene

rearrangement and cell surface antigen expression in acute lymphocytic leukemias of T cell and B cell precursor origins. J. Clin. Invest. 71:301, 1983.

122. Waldmann, T. A., Korsmeyer, S. J., Bakhshi, A., Arnold, A., and Kirsch, I. R.: Molecular genetic analyses of human lymphoid neoplasms: Immunoglobulin genes and c-myc oncogene. A combined clinical staff conference. Ann. Intern. Med. 102:497, 1985.

123. Felix, C. A., Poplack, D. G., Reaman, G. H., Steinberg, S. M., Cole, D. E., Taylor, B. J., Begley, C. G., and Kirsch, I. R.: Characterization of immunoglobulin and T-cell receptor gene patterns in B-cell precursor acute lymphoblastic leukemia of childhood. J. Clin. Oncol. 8:431, 1990.

124. Bertness, V., Kirsch, I., Hollis, G., Johnson, B., and Bunn, P. A.: T-cell receptor gene rearrangements as clinical markers of human T-cell lymphomas. N. Engl. J. Med. 313:534, 1985.

125. Flug, F., Pelicci, P. G., Bonetti, R., Knowles, D. M., and Dalla-Favera, R.: T-cell receptor gene rearrangements as markers of lineage and clonality in T-cell neoplasms. Proc. Natl. Acad. Sci. USA 82:3460, 1985.

126. Kitchingman, G. R., Rovigatti, U., Mauer, A. M., Melvin, S., Murphy, S. B., and Stass, S.: Rearrangement of immunoglobulin heavy chain genes in T cell acute lymphoblastic leukemia. Blood 65:725, 1985.

127. Pelicci, P.-G., Knowles, D. M., and Dalla-Favera, R.: Lymphoid tumors displaying rearrangements of both immunoglobulin and T cell receptor genes. J. Exp. Med. 162:1015, 1985.

128. Siegelman, M., Cleary, M. L., Warnke, R., and Sklar, J.: Frequent biclonality and immunoglobulin gene alterations among B cell lymphomas that show multiple histologic forms. J. Exp. Med. 161:850, 1985.

129. Erlich, H. A. (ed.): PCR Technology. New York, Stockton Press, 1989.

130. Sasavage, N.: Are clinical labs ready for PCR? J. NIH Res. 3:47, 1991.

131. Bourguin, A., Tung, R., Galili, N., and Sklar, J.: Rapid, nonradioactive detection of clonal T-cell receptor gene rearrangements in lymphoid neoplasms. Proc. Natl. Acad. Sci. USA 87:8536, 1990.

132. Myers, R. M., Maniatis, T., and Lerman, L. S.: Detection and localization of single base changes by denaturing gradient gel electrophoresis. Methods Enzymol. 155:501, 1986.

133. Yamada, M., Wasserman, R., Lange, B., Reichard, B., Womer, R., and Rovera, G.: Minimal residual disease in childhood B-lineage lymphoblastic leukemia. N. Engl. J. Med. 323:448, 1990.

134. Billadeau, D., Blackstadt, M., Griepp, P., Kyle, R. A., Oken, M. M., Kay, N., and Van Ness, B.: Analysis of B-lymphoid malignancies using allele-specific polymerase chain reaction: A technique for sequential quantitation of residual disease. Blood 78:3021, 1991.

135. Macintyre, E., D'Auriol, L., Duparc, N., Leverger, G., Galibert, F., and Sigaux, F.: Use of oligonucleotide probes directed against T cell antigen receptor gamma delta variable-(diversity)-joining junctional sequences as a general method for detecting minimal residual disease in acute lymphoblastic leukemias. J. Clin. Invest. 86:2125, 1990.

136. Yokota, S., Hansen-Hagge, T. E., Ludwig, W.-D., Reiter, A., Raghavachar, A., Kleihauer, E., and Bartram, C. R.: Use of polymerase chain reaction to monitor minimal residual disease in acute lymphoblastic leukemia patients. Blood 77:331, 1991.

137. Van Dongen, J. J. M., Breit, T. M., Adriaansen, H. J., Beishuizen, A., and Hooijkaas, H.: Detection of minimal residual disease in acute leukemia by immunological marker analysis and polymerase chain reaction. Leukemia 6(suppl):47, 1992.

138. Shen-Ong, G. L. C., Keath, E. J., Piccoli, S. P., and Cole, M. D.: Novel c-myc oncogene RNA from abortive immunoglobulin gene recombination in mouse plasmacytomas. Cell 31:443, 1982.

139. Dalla-Favera, R., Bregni, M., Erikson, J., Patterson, D., Gallo, R. C., and Croce, C. M.: Human c-myc oncogene is located on the region of chromosome 8 that is translocated in Burkitt lymphoma cells. Proc. Natl. Acad. Sci. USA 79:7824, 1982.

140. Taub, R., Kirsch, I., Morton, C., Lenoir, G., Swan, D., Tronick, S., Aaronson, S., and Leder, P.: Translocation of the c-myc gene into the immunoglobulin heavy chain locus in human Burkitt lymphoma and murine plasmacytoma cells. Proc. Natl. Acad. Sci. USA 79:7837, 1982.

141. Magrath, I.: The pathogenesis of Burkitt's lymphoma. Adv. Cancer Res. 55:133, 1990.

142. Ohno, H., Takimoto, G., and McKeithan, T. W.: The candidate proto-oncogene bcl-3 is related to genes implicated in cell lineage determination and cell cycle control. Cell 60:991, 1990.

143. Begley, C. G., Aplan, P. D., Davey, M. P., Nakahara, K., Tchorz, K., Kurtzberg, J., Hershfield, M. S., Haynes, B. F., Cohen, D. I., Waldmann, T. A., et al.: Chromosomal translocation in a human leukemic stem cell line disrupts the TCRD δ region and results in a previously unreported fusion transcript. Proc. Natl. Acad. Sci. USA 86:2031, 1989.

144. Boehm, T., Mengle-Gaw, L., Kees, U. R., Spurr, N., Lavenir, I., Forster, A., and Rabbitts, T. H.: Alternating purine-pyrimidine tracts may promote chromosomal translocations seen in a variety of human lymphoid tumors. EMBO J. 8:2621, 1989.

145. Smith, G. R.: Chi hotspots of generalized recombination. Cell 34:709, 1983.

146. Krowczynska, A. M., Rudders, R. A., and Krontiris, T. G.: The human minisatellite consensus at breakpoints of oncogene translocations. Nucleic Acids Res. 18:1121, 1989.

147. Aurias, A., Couturier, J., Dutrillaux, A.-M., Dutrillaux, B., Herpin, F., Lamoliatte, E., Lombard, M., Muleris, M., Paravatou, M., Prieur, M., et al.: Inversion 14(q12qter) or (q11.2q32.3): The most frequently acquired rearrangement in lymphocytes. Hum. Genet. 71:19, 1985.

148. Denny, C. T., Hollis, G. F., Hecht, F., Morgan, R., Link, M. P., Smith, S. D., and Kirsch, I. R.: Common mechanism of chromosomal inversion in B and T cell tumors: Relevance to lymphocyte development. Science 234:197, 1986.

149. Jäck, H.-M., Berg, J., and Wabl, M.: Translation affects immunoglobulin mRNA stability. Eur. J. Immunol. 19:843, 1989.

150. Sonnier, J. A., Buchanan, G. R., Howard-Peebles, P. N., Rutledge, J., and Smith, R. G.: Chromosomal translocation involving the immunoglobulin kappa-chain and heavy-chain loci in a child with chronic lymphocytic leukemia. N. Engl. J. Med. 309:590, 1983.

151. Aurias, A., Croquette, M. F., Nuyts, V. P., Griscelli, C., and Dutrillaux, B.: New data on clonal anomalies of chromosome 14 in ataxia-telangiectasia: tct(14;14) and inv(14). Hum. Genet. 72:22, 1986.

152. Davey, M. P., Bertness, V., Nakahara, K., Johnson, J. P., McBride, O. W., Waldmann, T. A., and Kirsch, I. R.: Juxtaposition of the T-cell receptor α-chain locus (14q11) and a region (14q32) of potential importance in leukemogenesis by a 14;14 translocation in a patient with T-cell chronic lymphocytic leukemia and ataxia-telangiectasia. Proc. Natl. Acad. Sci. USA 85:9287, 1988.

153. Russo, G. M., Isobe, M., Gatti, R., Finan, J., Batuman, O., Huebner, K., Nowell, P. C., and Croce, C. M.: Molecular analysis of a t(14;14) translocation in leukemic T-cells of an ataxia-telangiectasia patient. Proc. Natl. Acad. Sci. USA 86:602, 1989.

154. Brito-Babapulle, V., Pomfret, M., Matutes, E., and Catovsky, D.: Cytogenetic studies on prolymphocytic leukemia. II. T cell prolymphocytic leukemia. Blood 70:926, 1987.

155. Baer, R., Heppell, A., Taylor, A. M. R., Rabbitts, P. H., Boullier, B., and Rabbitts, T. H.: The breakpoint of an inversion chromosome 14 in a T cell leukemia: Sequence downstream of the immunoglobulin heavy chain locus implicated in tumorigenesis. Proc. Natl. Acad. Sci. USA 84:9069, 1987.

156. Bertness, V. L., Felix, C. A., McBride, O. W., Morgan, R., Smith, S. D., Sandberg, A. A., and Kirsch, I. R.: Characterization of the breakpoint of a t(14;14)(q11.22) from the

leukemic cells of a patient with T-cell acute lymphoblastic leukemia. Cancer Genet. Cytogenet. 44:47, 1990.

157. Aplan, P. D., Lombardi, D. P., and Kirsch, I. R.: Structural characterization of SIL, a gene frequently disrupted in T-cell acute lymphoblastic leukemia. Mol. Cell. Biol. 11:5462, 1991.

158. Aplan, P. D., Begley, C. G., Bertness, V., Nussmeier, M., Ezquerra, A., Coligan, J., and Kirsch, I. R.: The SCL gene is formed from a transcriptionally complex locus. Mol. Cell. Biol. 10:6426, 1990.

159. Brown, L., Cheng, J.-T., Chen, Q., Siciliano, M. J., Crist, W., Buchanan, G., and Baer, R.: Site-specific recombination of the *tal-1* gene is a common occurrence in human T cell leukemia. EMBO J. 9:3343, 1990.

160. Aplan, P. D., Lombardi, D. P., Reaman, G. H., Sather, H. N., Hammond, G. D., and Kirsch, I. R.: Involvement of the putative hematopoietic transcription factor SCL in T-cell acute lymphoblastic leukemia. Blood 79:1327, 1992.

161. Limpens, J., de Jong, D., van Krieken, J. H., Price, C. G., Young, B. D., van Ommen, G. J., and Kluin, P. M.: Bcl-2/J$_H$ rearrangments in benign lymphoid tissues with follicular hyperplasia. Oncogene 6:2271, 1991.

162. Seligmann, M., Mihaesco, E., Preud'homme, J.-L., Danao, F., and Brouet, J.-C.: Heavy chain disease: Current findings and concepts. Immunol. Rev. 48:145, 1979.

163. Bakhshi, A., Guglielmi, P., Siebenlist, U., Ravetch, J. V., Jensen, J. P., and Korsmeyer, S. J.: A DNA insertion/deletion necessitates an aberrant RNA splice accounting for a human μ heavy chain disease protein. Proc. Natl. Acad. Sci. USA 83:2689, 1986.

164. Cogné, M., Preud'homme, J.-L., and Guglielmi, P.: Immunoglobulin gene alterations in human heavy chain diseases. Res. Immunol. 140:487, 1989.

165. Downward, J., Yarden, Y., Mayes, E., Scrace, G., Totty, N., Stockwell, P., Ullrich, A., Schlessinger, J., and Waterfield, M. D.: Close similarity of epidermal growth factor receptor and v-*erb*-B oncogene protein sequences. Nature 307:521, 1984.

166. Brouet, J. C., Mason, D. Y., Danon, F., Preud'homme, J. L., Seligmann, M., Reyes, F., Navab, F., Galian, A., Rene, E., and Rambaud, J. C.: Alpha-chain disease: Evidence for a common clonal origin of intestinal immunoblastic lymphoma and plasmacytic proliferation. Lancet 1:861, 1977.

167. Alexander, A., Steinmetz, M., Barritault, D., Frangione, B., Franklin, E. C., Hood, L., and Buxbaum, J. N.: γ Heavy chain disease in man: cDNA sequence supports partial gene deletion model. Proc. Natl. Acad. Sci. USA 79:3260, 1982.

168. Guglielmi, P., Bakhshi, A., Miahesco, E., Broudet, J., Waldmann, T. A., and Korsmeyer, S. J.: DNA deletion in human gamma heavy chain disease. Clin. Res. 32:348A, 1984.

169. LeFranc, M. P., LeFranc, G., and Rabbitts, T. H.: Inherited deletion of immunoglobulin heavy chain constant region genes in normal human individuals. Nature 300:760, 1982.

170. Keyeux, G., LeFranc, M. P., Chevailler, A., and LeFranc, G.: Molecular analysis of the IgHA and MHC class III region genes in human IgA and C4 deficiencies. Exp. Clin. Immunogenet. 7:170, 1990.

171. Rosen, F. S.: Genetic deficiencies in specific immune responses. Semin. Hematol. 27:333, 1990.

172. Hendricks, R. W., vanTol, M. J., deLange, G. G., and Schuurman, R. K.: Inheritance of a large deletion within the human immunoglobulin heavy chain constant region gene complex and immunological implications. Scand. J. Immunol. 29:535, 1989.

173. Lieber, M. R.: Site-specific recombination in the immune system. FASEB J. 5:2934, 1991.

174. Felix, C. A., Reaman, G. H., Korsmeyer, S. J., Hollis, G. F., Dinndorf, P. A., Wright, J. J., and Kirsch, I. R.: Immunoglobulin and T-cell receptor gene configuration in acute lymphoblastic leukemia of infancy. Blood 70:536, 1987.

Lymphopoiesis

Barton F. Haynes and Stephen M. Denning

INTRODUCTION

The lymphoid lineage is one of the most extensively studied cell types in man and animals. Interest in lymphoid differentiation has been stimulated by the remarkable diversity generated by rearranging antigen receptor genes during lymphoid cell differentiation, by the accessibility of lymphoid cells for study, and by the critical roles that lymphoid cells play in the maintenance of health and in the pathogenesis of autoimmune and immunodeficiency diseases. In humans, the lymphoid system comprises *primary lymphoid organs,* which are the bone marrow and thymus, and *secondary lymphoid organs,* which are the spleen, lymph node, tonsil, Peyer's patches of the gut, and foci of lymphoid cells in the peribronchial areas of the lung. The types of lymphocytes that circulate in secondary lymphoid organs are thymus-derived (T) lymphocytes, bone marrow—derived (B) lymphocytes, and large granular lymphocytes (LGL), also termed natural killer (NK) cells.

The functions of primary lymphoid organs in man are to provide lymphoid precursors capable of developing into T, B, or NK lymphocytes; to provide the microenvironments that are capable of promoting lineage-specific differentiation of precursors into immunocompetent effector cells; and to appropriately regulate the availability and number of mature lymphocytes produced in bone marrow and thymus. Other functions of primary and secondary lymphoid organs are to serve as a unified system to collect diverse populations of antigen-specific lymphocytes throughout the body, to ensure contact of antigen-specific lymphocytes with invading foreign antigens, and to promote intercellular interactions of developing or mature lymphocytes.[1] Finally, both primary and secondary lymphoid organs limit the activation and development of autoreactive lymphocytes.

In this chapter, we describe how the normal human immune system develops during fetal ontogeny, characterize the primary and secondary lymphoid microenvironments, define the roles of immune system microenvironments in lymphoid cell differentiation, and review the molecular basis of lymphoid cell migration and recirculation in man.

OVERVIEW OF DEVELOPMENT OF THE HUMAN LYMPHOID SYSTEM

The establishment of the immune system during fetal development involves the organogenesis of the primary and secondary lymphoid organs and is followed by continuing differentiation of T, B, and NK lymphocytes postnatally from hematopoietic stem cells. Both processes involve a myriad of lymphocyte and microenvironment cell surface structures and have necessitated the development of a nomenclature of human cell surface lymphocyte differentiation antigens.

The Cluster of Differentiation (CD) Classification of Human Lymphocyte Differentiation Antigens

The development of monoclonal antibody technology led to the discovery, functional characterization, purification, and cloning of an extraordinary number of new leukocyte surface molecules. The First International Workshop on Leukocyte Differentiation Antigens was held in 1982 to establish a nomenclature for cell surface molecules of human white blood cells.[2] From this and subsequent workshops has come the CD classification of leukocyte antigens[3–5] (Table 12–1). Initially developed for human cell surface antigens, this system is now widely used for mouse, sheep, and other animal species. The data presented in Table 12–1 represent a tool, as well as establishing a context, to help sort through the extraordinarily complex series of events that transpire during normal human immune system development.

Lymphopoiesis in Human Fetal Development

Studies in animals and man have demonstrated that lymphocyte development in the mammalian embryo develops as a consequence of hematopoietic stem cell migration.[6–9] Immunohistological analyses of lymphoid populations in developing human fetal tissues, taken together with a large body of experimental work in birds and mice, have provided a composite view of the sequence of events that transpire during fetal lymphoid system development (reviewed in references 10 to 13) (Fig. 12–1).

HEMATOPOIETIC EVENTS IN FETAL YOLK SAC AND LIVER. Elegant studies in the mouse have demonstrated that hematopoietic stem cells (HSCs) and their progeny are derived from totipotent embryonic stem cells from the inner cell mass of the embryonic blastocyst.[6] In the human yolk sac, early hematopoiesis begins in blood islands at 2.5 to 3 weeks of gestational age and continues until 9 to 10 weeks.[9, 12] HSCs in the fetal yolk sac, chorion, and stalk migrate to the fetal liver at 5 weeks of gestation.[9, 12] Hematopoiesis occurs in the human fetal liver at 6 weeks.[9, 12] B-cell development first begins in man in the fetal liver, with cytoplasmic immunoglobulin M (cIgM) (μ) heavy chain expression present in B-cell progenitors (pre-B cells) at 7 weeks of gestation.[9, 14] Surface IgM (sIgM) and sIgG+ B cells are present in fetal liver soon after the appearance of pre-B cells (7 to 11 weeks), whereas fetal liver sIgD+ and sIgA+ B cells are present at 12 to 13 weeks.[14–19] Surface T-cell receptor (sTCR)+ T cells do not appear in the human fetal liver until 10.5 to 11 weeks.[20]

MIGRATION OF HEMATOPOIETIC STEM CELLS TO PRIMARY AND SECONDARY LYMPHOID ORGANS. From fetal liver, and perhaps from yolk sac, HSCs seed the human thymic rudiment (8 weeks), seed fetal bone marrow (8 to 10 weeks), and at 8 weeks migrate to the developing spleen[12] (Fig. 12–1). HSCs seed bone marrow and give rise to regenerating myeloid, erythroid, megakaryocytoid, B-cell, and NK lineages that function throughout life (reviewed in reference 21). HSC seeding of bone marrow also gives rise to a regenerating bone marrow HSC population capable of seeding the thymus after fetal liver hematopoietic function ceases in the third trimester.

By analogy with elegant studies of T-cell development in birds and mice, stem cell colonization of the human thymic rudiment is thought to take place in waves.[6–8] From studies in mice, it has been estimated that it takes approximately 3 weeks for stem cells to migrate through the thymus and emerge as mature T cells ready for exportation to peripheral lymphoid organs.[22] Much of the HSC traffic from fetal liver and bone marrow to thymus occurs in early life, with postthymic T cells that colonize secondary lymphoid organs retaining self-renewal capacities.[23, 24] In the thymus, HSCs differentiate into mature T cells that first colonize fetal lymph nodes, gut, and spleen at 12 weeks[12, 25] (Fig. 12–1).

In the spleen, HSCs from the fetal liver establish an initial wave of myeloid hematopoiesis at 8 weeks, as well as initiate B-cell development.[14] Pre-B and sIg+ B cells are present in the spleen by 12.5 weeks.[14] From 12 weeks on in gestation, sTCR+ T cells are present in the fetal spleen.[26]

At 14 to 15 weeks, thymus emigrants colonize developing tonsils and other peripheral lymphoid tissues.[12, 25] By 20 weeks, the immune system is sufficiently established in primary and secondary lymphoid organs that the fetus can mount B-cell antibody responses to congenital infections that occur in utero[27, 28] and T cells are capable of responding to foreign

TABLE 12–1.   CD CLASSIFICATION OF HUMAN LYMPHOCYTE SURFACE MOLECULES

CD	OTHER NAMES	MOLECULAR MASS (Daltons)	MOLECULAR STRUCTURE	TISSUE/LINEAGE	FUNCTION
CD1a	T6	49,000	Ig superfamily associated with β_2-microglobulin (β_2M)	Cortical thymocytes, Langerhans' cells, interdigitating cells	Antigen presentation to TCR$\gamma\delta$ cells
CD1b	—	45,000	Ig superfamily associated with β_2M	Same as CD1a	Same as CD1a
CD1c	—		Ig superfamily associated with β_2M	Cortical thymocyte, Langerhans' cells, subset of B cells	Same as CD1a
CD2	T11, LFA-3 receptor ϵ-rosette receptor	50,000	Ig superfamily	CD3$\gamma,\delta,\epsilon,\zeta,\eta$, T lymphocytes, cytoplasmic CD3ϵ, NK cells	Binds LFA-3 (CD58) on red blood cells (RBCs), monocytes, thymic epithelial cells; alternative pathway of T-cell activation
CD3	T3, CD3 complex, Leu4	CD3γ—26,000 CD3δ—20,000 CD3ϵ—20,000 CD3ζ—16,000 CD3η—28,000	CD3, γ,δ,ϵ Ig superfamily; CD3 η,ζ; homologous to each other and with FcRϵ ζ chain comprise λ family of signal transducers	T lymphocytes	T-cell–associated molecules; transduces signals from T-cell receptors
CD4	T4, Leu3a	59,000	Ig superfamily	T lymphocytes, monocytes, tissue macrophages, microglial cells, Epstein-Barr virus (EBV)–transformed B lymphocytes	Receptor for HIV env gp120; binds to HLA class II; associated with p56 *lck* tyrosine kinase
CD5	T1	67,000	Ig superfamily	T lymphocytes, B-lymphocyte subset	Co-mitogenic for T lymphocytes; ligand for CD72
CD6	T12	100,000	Scavenger receptor type I superfamily	Subset of T and B lymphocytes	?
CD7	3A1, Leu9	40,000	Ig superfamily	T lymphocytes, NK cells; on subsets of T, B, and myeloid precursors	Co-mitogenic for T lymphocytes; Ca^{2+}-inducible gene
CD8	T8, Leu2a	CD8α—38,000, CD8β—38,000	CD8 α, β, Ig superfamily	T-cell subset	Receptor for MHC class I; associated with p56 *lck* tyrosine kinase
CD9	p24	24,000		Pre-B cells, monocytes, platelets	Mediates platelet activation; ?receptor-associated ion channel
CD10	J5, common acute lymphoblastic leukemia antigen (CALLA), neutral endopeptide	100,000	Endopeptidase enzyme	B lymphoid progenitor cells	Peptide cleavage
CD11a	LFA-1α chain	180,000	Integrin	T, B, NK lymphocytes, monocytes	With β_2 integrin, ligand for ICAM-1 (CD54) and ICAM-2; mediates leukocyte adhesion and leukocyte-endothelial adherence
CD11b	MAC-1, MO-1α chain, CR3	165,000	Integrin	NK cells, polymorphonuclear neutrophils (PMNs), monocytes	With β_2 integrin, receptor for C3bi, fibrinogen, factor X
CD11c	gp150/95 α chain, CR4	150,000	Integrin	NK cells, PMNs, monocytes	With β_2 integrin, mediates cell binding to C3bi
CD15	Sialyl Lewis X (sLe^x)	Carbohydrate	Neu Acα 2–3 Gal β1–4 (Fucα1-3) GlcNac	Granulocytes; cryptic form of CD15 is on T cells (cutaneous lymphocyte antigen CLA)	Ligand for ELAM-1 on endothelial cells; CLA mediates T-cell homing to skin
CD16	Fc receptor (FcR) for IgG (low affinity) FcγIII	50,000–65,000	Ig superfamily, PI and TM forms	NK cells, PMNs, monocytes	FcR for IgG
CD18	LFA-1β chain	95,000	Integrin	T, B, NK lymphocytes, monocytes	Ligand for ICAM-1 (CD54) and ICAM-2; mediates leukocyte-endothelial interactions
CD19	B4	90,000	Ig superfamily	B lymphocytes	Regulates B-cell activation
CD20	B1, Bp35	35,000–37,000	—	B lymphocytes	Mediates B-cell activation
CD21	B2	140,000	Complement regulatory protein family	B lymphocytes	C3d/EBV receptor; complement receptor 2 (CR2)
CD22	Bgp135	135,000	Ig superfamily, homology with N-CAM, myelin-associated glycoprotein (MAG)	B lymphocytes	Co-mitogenic for B-cell activation; interacts with CD45RO on T cells and with CD75 on B cells
CD23	Low-affinity receptor for IgE FcϵRII	45,000–50,000	Homology with asialoglycoprotein receptor (lectin)	Activated B lymphocytes, thymic epithelial cells, macrophages, eosinophils, platelets	FcϵRII; soluble CD23 activates immature T cells
CD24	BA-1	38,000–41,000	PI-linked gp	B lymphocytes, PMNs	?Regulates calcium fluxes
CD25	TAC, IL-2 receptor α chain	55,000		Activated T and B lymphocytes, monocytes	Low-affinity receptor for IL-2

Table continued on following page

TABLE 12–1. CD CLASSIFICATION OF HUMAN LYMPHOCYTE SURFACE MOLECULES *Continued*

CD	OTHER NAMES	MOLECULAR MASS (Daltons)	MOLECULAR STRUCTURE	TISSUE/LINEAGE	FUNCTION
CD26	Dipeptidyl-peptidase IV, gp120	120,000	Dipeptidyl-peptidase IV enzyme	Activated T and B lymphocytes, monocytes	Serine exopeptidase; binds collagen
CD27	—	55,000	Homodimer	T lymphocytes	
CD28	Tp44	44,000	Ig superfamily	T lymphocytes and activated B cells	Co-mitogenic for T lymphocytes; regulates T-cell cytokine stability; ligand for B7 molecule
CD29	Integrin β1 chain; common β subset of VLA-1-6	130,000	Integrin	Panhematopoietic, many other cell types	Ligand for many extracellular matrix molecules
CD31	PECAM-1	130,000	Ig superfamily, homology with FcRγ	T, B, NK cells, platelets	Adhesion molecule
CD32	gp40 FCγRII	40,000	Ig superfamily, homology with FcRγ	B cells, macrophages, PMNs, eosinophils	FcR for IgG
CD34	MY10	105,000–120,000	Sialomucin with unique protein sequence	T lymphocyte, other hematopoietic precursors	?
CD35	CR1, C3b receptor	160,000–250,000	—	B cells, subset of NK cells, PMNs, monocytes, RBCs	Binds immune complexes
CD37	gp40–52	40,000–52,000	TAPA-1 family, three transmembrane domains	B cells, epithelial cells	? Receptor-associated ion channel
CD38	OKT10, T10	45,000	Single-chain glycoprotein	Activated lymphocytes, immature B cells	?
CD39	gp80	70,000–100,000	—	Activated B lymphocytes, T lymphocytes, and NK cells	Mediates homotypic adhesion of B cells
CD40	gp50	44,000–48,000	Homology with nerve growth factor receptor, fas (APO-1), and TNF receptor	B cells, follicular dendritic cells, macrophages	B-cell activation; homotypic adhesion
CD43	Leukosialin, sialophorin, leukocyte sialoglycoprotein	95,000	Cell surface sialomucin	T, B, and NK cells, monocytes	Involved in leukocyte activation; deficient in Wiskott-Aldrich syndrome; ligand for ICAM-1
CD44	Pgp-1, In(Lu)-related p80, Hermes, extracellular matrix receptor III	80,000–120,000	Cartilage link protein, core proteoglycan homology; multiple isoforms generated by alternative splicing	T, B, and NK cells, monocytes, RBCs	Transmembrane hyaluronate receptor; promotes leukocyte adhesion; co-mitogenic for T cells; mediates leukocyte-endothelial binding
CD45	Leukocyte common antigen, T200	CD45RO—180,000; CD45RA—220,000; CD45RB—220,000, 205,000, 190,000	Multiple isoforms generated by alternative splicing	Leukocytes	Cytoplasmic domain is a tyrosine phosphatase, regulates lymphocyte activation; CD45RO in T cells is a ligand for CD22 on B cells
CD49b	VLA-2α chain	170,000	Integrin	Activated T cells, platelets	With β_1 integrin, binds collagen
CD49d	VLA-4α chain	150,000	Integrin	T and B lymphocytes, monocytes	With β_1 integrin, is the receptor for endothelial VCAM-1; mediates leukocyte–endothelial cell binding in Peyer's patches
CD54	ICAM-1	40,000	Ig superfamily	Endothelial cells, activated lymphocytes	Ligand for LFA-1, rhinoviruses, *Plasmodium falciparum* malaria, CD43
CD56	N-CAM, NKH-1	140,000	Ig superfamily, homology with N-CAM	NK cells	Mediates NK cell homotypic adhesion
CD57	HNK1, Leu7	110,000	—	NK cells, subset of T cells	?
CD58	LFA-3	40,000–65,000	Ig superfamily	Widespread; activated lymphocytes	Ligand for CD2
CD69	Activation inducer molecule, EA-1, gp34/28	28,000, 34,000	Homodimer	Activated B, T, and NK cells, monocytes	Ligand binding to CD69 triggers cytolytic activity of NK and TCRγδ T cells
CD71	T9, transferrin receptor	95,000	Heterodimer	Activated T and B lymphocytes, monocytes, proliferating cells of many types	Binds transferrin
CD72	—	39,000, 43,000	Heterodimer	B cells	Ligand for CD5 molecule
CD73	Ecto-5′-nucleotidase	69,000	Nucleotidase enzyme	Subsets of B and T lymphocytes	Regulates uptake of nucleotides
CD74	MHC Class II invariant chain	41,35, 33,000	Homology with thyroglobulin	B cells, monocytes	Regulates intracellular transport of MHC Class II molecules and processing of antigen
CD75	α2–6 Sialyltransferase	53,000	Protein enzyme	B cells	Ligand for CD22; catalyzes transfer of sialic acids

Data from CD references cited throughout the chapter and from Knapp, W., et al.: Leucocyte Typing IV: White Cell Differentiation Antigens. Oxford, England, Oxford University Press, 1991.

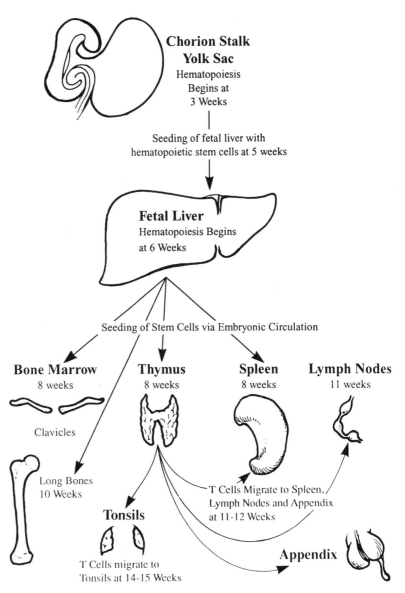

Chorion Stalk
Yolk Sac
Hematopoiesis
Begins at
3 Weeks

Seeding of fetal liver with
hematopoietic stem cells at 5 weeks

Fetal Liver
Hematopoiesis Begins
at 6 Weeks

FIGURE 12–1. Migration patterns of hematopoietic stem cells and mature lymphocytes during human fetal development.

Seeding of Stem Cells via Embryonic Circulation

Bone Marrow
8 weeks

Thymus
8 weeks

Spleen
8 weeks

Lymph Nodes
11 weeks

Clavicles

Long Bones
10 Weeks

T Cells Migrate to Spleen,
Lymph Nodes and Appendix
at 11-12 Weeks

Tonsils

Appendix

T Cells migrate to
Tonsils at 14-15 Weeks

antigens.[29] From the end of the fifth month of gestation to birth, the primary lymphoid organs, thymus and bone marrow, undergo rapid expansion in size and evolve functional maturity related to expansion of diversity in T- and B-cell antigen receptor repertoires. However, at birth, the immune system is not completely functional but continues to undergo maturation postnatally, driven by the contact of T and B lymphocytes with foreign antigens in peripheral lymphoid organs.[23, 24]

Lymphopoiesis in Human Postnatal Development

B lymphocytes are continually generated throughout postnatal life. In the mouse, approximately 50 million B cells are generated each day from B-lineage precursors in bone marrow. Of these, 2 to 3 million enter the peripheral pools of mature B cells (reviewed in reference 30). On the basis of the size of peripheral B-cell pools in mice (5×10^8 cells), approximately 1/200 of the peripheral B-cell pool is replaced each day.[30] From bone marrow, B cells or B-cell precursors continually circulate and home to secondary lymphoid tissue.[31] In contrast, the peripheral T-cell pool is established early in fetal and early postnatal life, with post-thymic T cells in secondary lymphoid organs having self-renewal capacities[23, 24] (Figs. 12–2 and 12–3). Although the thymus continues to be seeded and produce emigrants throughout life, the number of mature thymic emigrants is reduced in postnatal immune system development, and thymectomy of humans after birth does not result in demonstrable immunodeficiencies[32, 33] (Fig. 12–2).

Once the T-cell receptors (TCR) repertoire of the peripheral T-cell pool is established, the recirculating nature of T cells provides an efficient surveillance system for ensuring that T cells expressing appropriate TCR come in contact with antigen-presenting cells containing foreign antigens.

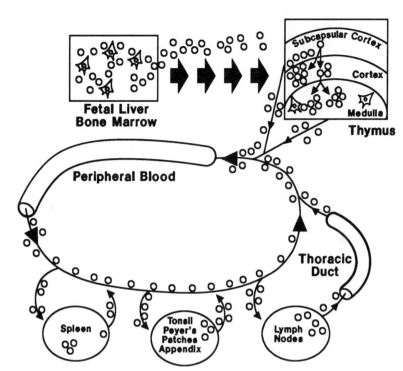

FIGURE 12–2. T-cell maturation during human fetal development.

DEVELOPMENT OF HEMATOPOIETIC STEM CELLS

Hematopoietic stem cells have two major characteristics: self-renewal capacity and the ability to differentiate into all hematopoietic cell types (reviewed in references 21 and 34) (Fig. 12–4). The search for HSCs began in 1961 with the identification of murine spleen colony-forming units (CFU-S) containing pre-dominantly myeloid and erythroid lineages.[35] Recent studies have demonstrated that CFU-S progenitors are heterogeneous and contain both myeloid progenitors and pluripotent HSCs (pre–CFU-S) with self-renewing potential (reviewed in references 21 and 34). By infecting bone marrow cells with retroviral vectors carrying selectable genes as markers, it has been demonstrated that a single HSC gives rise to both lymphoid and myeloerythroid cell lineages.[36, 37]

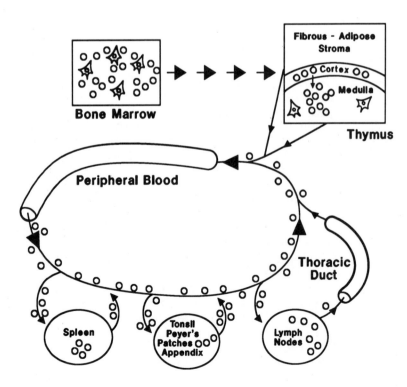

FIGURE 12–3. T-cell maturation during human adult life.

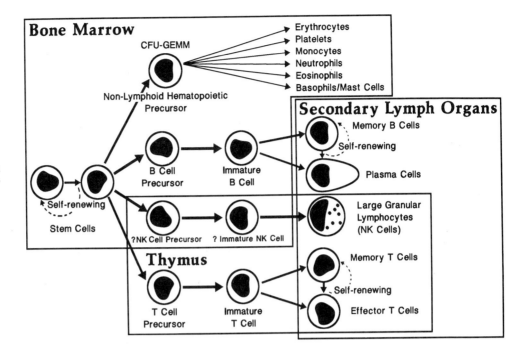

FIGURE 12–4. Lymphopoiesis in bone marrow, thymus, and secondary lymphoid organs.

Phenotypic and Functional Characterization of Hematopoietic Stem Cells in Mice

In general, HSC-enriched populations do not express most of the lineage-specific cell surface antigens of mature myeloid, T-cell, B-cell, and NK cell types. HSC-enriched populations of adult bone marrow and fetal liver have been purified using the criteria of low Thy-1 antigen expression (Thy-1lo+); the absence of myeloid, erythroid, T-cell (other than Thy-1), B-cell, and NK lineage markers (lin−); and high expression of stem cell antigen-1 (Sca-1)[21, 34, 38–45] (Table 12–2). This population of cells is enriched 2000-fold for the ability to reconstitute irradiated animals with all hematopoietic lineages.[21] By using the fluorescent vital dye rhodamine 123, which stains mitochondrial membranes in rapidly dividing cells, subsets of the Thy-1lo, lin−, Sca-1+ cells can be isolated that are rhodamine 123lo+ (~25 per cent of cells) or rhodamine 123hi+ (~50 per cent of cells).[46] Both rhodamine 123hi+ and lo+ cells contain multipotent cells capable of reconstituting the myeloerythroid and the T-cell lineages. However, the rhodamine 123lo+ subset of cells contains a 20-fold higher level of precursors for CFU-S and is more active in repopulating hematopoietic tissues of irradiated animals.[46] Recent studies have demonstrated the presence of CFU-S in a large number of bone marrow subsets other than Thy-1lo+, lin−, Sca1+ cells, whereas HSC with renewal and pluripotent capacities are present only in the Thy-1lo+, lin−, Sca-1+ bone marrow or fetal liver subset.[45]

Phenotypic and Functional Characterization of Hematopoietic Stem Cells in Humans

Progress in the identification of human pluripotent populations has come from advances in human bone marrow transplantation,[47–49] studies using primates as recipients of hematopoietic stem cell populations,[50] the identification of leukemias of multipotent progenitor cells,[51–54] and the development of the SCID/Hu mouse as an in vivo animal model of human HSC development[55, 56] (see Table 12–2).

SBA−, ER− bone marrow cells successfully reconstitute human patients with SCID, and this population of bone marrow is enriched for CD7+ and CD34+, lin− cells.[57] CD7 is a 40,000 dalton glycoprotein member of the immunoglobulin superfamily,[58–60] whereas CD34 is a 115,000 dalton sialoglycoprotein that bears extensive O-linked glycosylation characteristic of cell-associated mucins[61, 62] (see Table 12–1). Expression of

TABLE 12–2. PHENOTYPE OF CELL POPULATIONS THAT ARE ENRICHED IN HEMATOPOIETIC STEM CELLS

HEMATOPOIETIC PROGENITOR CELL TYPE	HUMAN	MOUSE
Multipotent stem cell	CD45+ (CD45RA+, CD45Ro−) CD34+ CD38− Thy-1lo+ CD17+/− Lin− P glycoprotein+ Rhodamine 123lo+ CD44+ c-kit+/− HLA-DR−	CD45+ Sca-1 (Ly6 A/E)+ Thy-1lo+ Lin− Rhodamine 123lo+ P glycoprotein+ CD44+ c-kit+ VLA-4+

+/− = Antigen present on a subset but not all cells; − = antigen not expressed; lo+ = dull expression as determined by flow cytometry analysis; + = antigen present; sCD3+ = surface CD3 expression; cCD3+ = cytoplasmic CD3 expression; Lin− = cells do not express antigens of mature myeloid, B, T, or NK cells.

CD34 is limited to a minor subset of bone marrow and fetal liver cells and to small vessel endothelium,[61, 62] whereas CD7 is expressed on early hematopoietic cells (including a subset of CD34+ bone marrow cells), as well as on immature and mature T and NK cells (reviewed in references 63 and 64). CD34+ bone marrow cells are devoid of lineage-specific antigens of mature myeloid, T, B, and NK cells, and both in vitro and in vivo studies in humans and primates have demonstrated that myeloerythroid progenitors are present in the CD34+ subset.[65–72] Using SCID mice engrafted with human hematopoietic microenvironments (SCID/Hu mice), Weissman, McCune, and colleagues showed that human CD34+, lin−, rhodamine 123lo+ bone marrow and fetal liver cells contain precursors of T, B, and myeloerythroid lineages and are capable of reconstituting these lineages for long periods[55, 56] (see Table 12–2). Others have suggested that the most primitive HSCs in man are human leukocyte antigen (HLA)–DR−,[68] CD38−,[73] CD45RA+,[74] and CD7−[56, 75–77] (see Table 12–2). Maturation to rapidly dividing or more differentiated stages of HSCs as they begin to enter various hematopoietic lineages (see Fig. 12–4) is associated with expression of HLA-DR[68]; lack of CD45RA expression and expression of a second isoform of CD45, CD45RO[74]; gradual expression of CD38[73]; CD7 expression on subsets of early T, B, and myeloid progenitor cells[13, 20, 63, 64, 78–81]; and a decrease in the levels of CD34.[73] Also associated with initial HSC differentiation is a high uptake of rhodamine 123 dye, resulting from a decrease in expression in HSCs of the multidrug efflux pump, P-glycoprotein.[82]

Although little is known about HSCs with regard to their role as receptors needed for adherence of HSCs to microenvironments, recent data suggest that both human and mouse HSCs express the transmembrane receptor for hyaluronic acid, CD44,[83–87] and fibronectin receptors.[88] Both CD44 and fibronectin receptors have been implicated in bone marrow progenitor interaction with stromal cells,[87–89] and it has been suggested that CD44 mediates migration of HSCs to the thymus.[85]

Recent studies in humans have demonstrated the presence of HSCs in cord peripheral blood, and cord blood mononuclear cells have been successfully used as a source for bone marrow transplants.[90–92]

Stem Cell Leukemias in Man

In 1984, Hershfield and colleagues described a patient with an acute lymphoblastic leukemia (ALL) syndrome and a malignant cell phenotype of CD7+, CD2+, CD3−, CD4−, CD8−, B lineage−, and myeloid lineage−.[51] Although containing TCR gene rearrangements, leukemic blasts had the remarkable capacity of differentiating in vitro into any of the T, B, or myeloerythroid lineages.[51] On the basis of the phenotype of CD7+, CD4−, CD8−, CD3− (triple negative, or TN), leukemic cells in the setting of ALL, multiple cases of CD7+, lin− ALL with multipotent

differentiating capacities in vitro and in vivo have been described (reviewed in reference 52). From this work on stem cell leukemias, and from studies of CD7 expression in fetal hematopoietic tissues, it was postulated that CD7 was expressed on T-cell precursors, and perhaps on earlier hematopoietic cell precursors (reviewed in references 63 and 64).

Cytokines That Regulate Embryonic Stem Cell Differentiation into Hematopoietic Stem Cells

Schmitt and associates have studied cytokine genes and receptors that are activated in embryonic stem cell cultures.[93] Steel factor (SLF), also known as stem cell factor (SCF), is deficient in the Steel (Sl/Sl^d) mouse with severe anemia and mast cell deficiency (reviewed in reference 21). Early in embryonic stem cell cultures, SCF is upregulated as HSCs differentiate from embryonic stem cells.[93] The receptor for SCF is the product of the c-kit proto-oncogene, a transmembrane tyrosine kinase that functions in cell signaling and is deficient in the W/W^v mouse (reviewed in reference 21). Hematopoietic defects present in the W/W^v mouse are similar to those in the Steel mouse. Like SCF, the product of c-kit is expressed on undifferentiated embryonic stem cells and HSCs throughout the in vitro culture of embryonic stem cells.[93] Over 8 days in culture, embryonic stem cells sequentially express messenger RNA (mRNA) for the erythropoietin receptor, erythropoietin, interleukin-4 (IL-4) receptor, macrophage colony-stimulating factor (M-CSF), IL-6, and IL-4. From day 8 until day 24, all of the above-mentioned cytokines continue to be expressed, and sequential expression of the IL-1 receptor, CD45 (transmembrane tyrosine phosphatase), granulocyte colony-stimulating factor (G-CSF) receptor, IL-1β, and G-CSF occurs. Thus, a complex series of cytokines and cytokine receptors are sequentially expressed during embryonic stem cell differentiation into HSCs, suggesting cytokine regulation of the process.[93]

Cytokine Regulation of Pluripotent Hematopoietic Stem Cell Proliferation and Differentiation

Once differentiated from embryonic stem cells, most HSCs enter a quiescent phase, with only a few HSCs at any one time escaping an active process of inhibition of cell growth (reviewed in reference 93). Two factors maintain HSC quiescence: stem cell inhibitor-1 (SCI-1) and transforming growth factor β (TGFβ)[94, 95] (Table 12–3). These two cytokines are thought to regulate the entry of the appropriate number of cells into the hematopoietic lineages to avoid excess cell growth.

Because Steel mice have normal numbers of HSCs in fetal liver and bone marrow, it has been suggested that c-kit receptor/SCF interactions are not essential for the initiation of hematopoiesis and the self-renewal of fetal HSCs.[96] What SCF does appear to do is to synergize with leukemia inhibitory factor (LIF), IL-3, IL-6, IL-11, G-CSF, and granulocyte-macrophage colony-stimulating factor (GM-CSF), for HSC survival and entry into the cell cycle.[96-101] Similarly, IL-4 has been shown to synergize with IL-11, and basic fibroblast growth factor β (FGFβ) synergizes with both IL-3 and GM-CSF, for HSC proliferation[69, 102, 103] (see Table 12–3).

LYMPHOPOIESIS IN BONE MARROW

B-Cell Development

B-lymphocyte development can be separated into two phases: antigen-independent and antigen-dependent B-cell development. Antigen-independent B-cell development occurs in primary lymphoid organs, including fetal liver and bone marrow, and includes all stages of B-cell maturation up to the sIg+ mature B cell.[104] Antigen-dependent B-cell maturation is driven by the interaction of antigen with B-cell sIg, leading to memory B-cell induction and plasma cell formation.[105, 106] The late antigen-dependent stages of B-cell maturation occur in secondary lymphoid organs, including lymph node, spleen, and Peyer's patches.[107] Antigen-independent B-cell development is discussed here, and antigen-dependent B-cell development is discussed below under Lymphopoiesis in Secondary Lymphoid Organs.

ANTIGEN-INDEPENDENT B-CELL DEVELOPMENT. A primary component of antigen-independent B-cell development involves the generation of immunoglobulin diversity and the expression of a unique immunoglobulin structure on the B-cell surface. During B-cell development, diversity of the antigen-binding variable region of the immunoglobulin is generated by an ordered set of immunoglobulin gene rearrangements. First, the process brings diversity (D) segments to joining (J) segments and then brings a variable (V) gene segment and constant (C) segments to yield a functional immunoglobulin heavy chain gene (V-D-J-C). During later stages, a functional κ or λ light chain gene is generated by rearrangement of a V segment to a J segment, ultimately yielding an intact immunoglobulin molecule comprising heavy and light chains.[104-106] (See Chapter 11.)

At each maturation step, immunoglobulin rearrangements may be productive or non-productive.[30] Since B cells lacking surface immunoglobulin are not present in peripheral lymphoid organs, cells lacking productively rearranged genes are eliminated within the bone marrow or fetal liver microenvironments.[30, 108] The mechanisms of stromal cell elimination of non-productively rearranged B cells are not well understood, but *apoptosis*, or the process of programmed cell death mediated by an endogeneous nuclease, has been implicated.[108, 109]

A series of stages of B-cell development have been defined based on immunoglobulin gene rearrangement patterns[108, 110] (Table 12–4). The *pro-B cell* is defined as the earliest committed B-cell progenitor with germline Ig genes.[108, 110] The first step of B-cell maturation involves rearrangement of immunoglobulin genes prior to expression of immunoglobulin heavy or light chains and is termed the *pre-pre-B cell.* IgM (μ) heavy chains are first produced in *pre-B cells* and are expressed only in the cytoplasm, since no light chains are produced at the pre-B stage.[30] Late in the pre-B stage, μ heavy chains in combination with a

TABLE 12–3. CYTOKINES THAT REGULATE MULTIPOTENT OR PLURIPOTENT HEMATOPOIETIC STEM CELL PROLIFERATION AND DIFFERENTIATION

CYTOKINE	OTHER NAMES/ABBREVIATION	EFFECT ON STEM CELLS
Interleukin-1α,β	IL-1αβ	Indirectly stimulates HSCs by inducing IL-6 production from bone marrow (BM) stromal cells
Interleukin-3	IL-3	Promotes survival of HSCs; synergizes with IL-11, LIF, and SCF for entry of HSCs into cell cycle; effect of IL-3 potentiated by fibrinogen
Interleukin-4	IL-4, B-cell differentiating factor (BCDF)	Synergizes with IL-11 for entry of HSCs into cell cycle
Interleukin-6	IL-6	Synergizes with IL-3 for HSC differentiation into myeloid lineages
Interleukin-11	IL-11	Synergizes with IL-3 and SCF for entry of HSCs into cell cycle
Stem cell factor	SCF, c-*kit* ligand, Steel factor (SLF), mast cell differentiating factor	Synergizes with IL-3, IL-6, IL-11, G-CSF, and GM-CSF for HSC proliferation
Basic fibroblast growth factor	βFGF	Synergizes with IL-3 and GM-CSF for HSC activation
Granulocyte colony-stimulating factor	G-CSF	Stimulates HSC entry into cell cycle
Granulocyte-monocyte/macrophage colony-stimulating factor	GM-CSF	Synergizes with SCF, IL-11, IL-3 for HSC activation
Leukemia inhibitory factor	LIF, HILDA, DIA	Inhibits proliferation of HSC
Macrophage inflammatory protein-1α	MIP1α, stem cell inhibitor 1 (SCI-1)	Inhibits proliferation of embryonic stem cells but synergizes with SCF entry of HSCs into cell cycle
Transforming growth factor β	TGFβ	Inhibits proliferation of HSCs

TABLE 12–4. DEVELOPMENTAL STAGES OF HUMAN B CELLS

Antigen-Indepenent

Pro-B cell	Immunoglobulin genes are germline; first descendent of pluripotent stem cell that is committed to B lineage
Pre-pre-B cell	Immunoglobulin genes are rearranged; no cytoplasmic μ heavy chains or surface IgM
Pre-B cell	Immunoglobulin genes are rearranged; cytoplasmic expression of μ heavy chains but no surface IgM
Immature B cell	Immunoglobulin genes are rearranged; both μ heavy chains and surface IgM are expressed; no surface IgD
Mature B cell	Immunoglobulin genes are rearranged; surface IgM and IgD are expressed
Virgin or naive B cell	sIg+ mature B cell prior to contact with antigen

Antigen-Dependent

Memory B cell	sIg+ mature B cell after antigen stimulation
Plasma cell	sIg−, immunoglobulin-secreting cell

pseudo (ψ) light chain (LC) complex are expressed on the surface.[111] κ and λ light chain expression occurs at the next stage of B-cell development, with *immature B cells* expressing μ heavy chains and surface IgM. Finally, with further B-cell maturation, *mature B cells* express both sIgM and sIgD.[110]

The process of early B-cell maturation initially gives rise to a repertoire normally skewed toward autoreactive antibody production.[111–115] Schroeder has reported that fetal liver B cells transcribe only a limited fraction of the total repertoire of heavy chain V genes and that two of the expressed genes correspond to genes encoding rheumatoid factor heavy chains.[112] Others have demonstrated that early human B cells express poly-

reactive IgM antibodies that can bind to a variety of different autoantigens[114, 115] and may play important roles in selection of the early B-cell repertoire.[111]

B-Cell Surface Antigens. The maturation of human B-cell precursors into mature B cells proceeds through a highly regulated process involving the coordinated acquisition and loss of B-lineage functional molecules (Fig. 12–5; Tables 12–1 and 12–5). More than 20 distinct differentiation antigens have been identified on B-lineage cells (Table 12–1).[110, 116, 117] Major functional categories of B-lineage surface molecules include membrane-associated enzymes, B-cell activation structures, and cell surface ligands that mediate intercellular interactions (see Table 12–5). Membrane-associated enzymes include CD10, a neutral endopeptidase that regulates receptor binding of cytokines[118]; CD45, a family of transmembrane protein tyrosine phosphatases[119]; and CD73, an ecto-5′-nucleotidase that regulates the uptake of purines by B cells.[120]

CD19, CD20, and CD21 antigens participate in the transduction of sIg-mediated activation signals in mature B cells.[116, 117] CD21 and CD19 are complement component receptors and signal-transducing subunits that form a complex on the B-cell surface.[110, 121, 122] The CD20 antigen regulates B-cell transmembrane calcium fluxes and serves as a substrate for protein kinase C, thus playing an essential regulating role in B-cell activation.[123]

Other molecules of particular importance to human B-cell development include CD22, B7, VLA-4, CD44, E-selectin (LAM-1), and CD11a/18 (see Tables 12–1 and 12–5). The CD22 antigen has homology to myelin-associated glycoprotein and mediates B-cell adhesion to T cells and monocytes via CD45RO.[124] The B7 antigen serves as a ligand for the CD28 T-cell

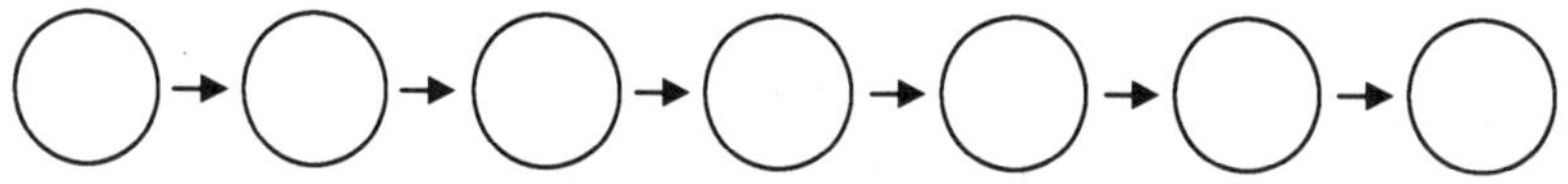

	Stem Cell	Pro-B	Pre-Pre-B	Pre-Pre-B	Pre-B	Immature B	Mature B
	CD34	CD34	CD34	CD34	-	-	-
		CD10	CD10	CD10	-	-	-
			CD19	CD19	CD19	CD19	CD19
			CD40	CD40	CD40	CD40	CD40
				CD73	CD73	CD73	CD73
				CD22	CD22	CD22	CD22
				CD24	CD24	CD24	CD24
				CD38	CD38	-	-
					CD21	CD21	CD21
							CD23
IL-7 Receptor	-	+	+	-	-	-	-
IL-3 Receptor	-	+	+	+	+	-	-
IL-4 Receptor	-	-	-	-	+	+	+
Immunoglobulin Gene Rearrangement	-	-	+	+	+	+	+
IgM Expression	-	-	-	-	cytoplasm	surface	surface
IgD Expression	-	-	-	-	-	-	surface

FIGURE 12–5. Antigen-independent human B-cell development.

TABLE 12–5. FUNCTIONALLY IMPORTANT CLASSES OF HUMAN B-CELL SURFACE MOLECULES

Membrane-Associated Enzymes	Ig Superfamily Activation Structures
CD10	CD19
CD45	CD20
CD73	CD21
Cell Surface Ligands	**Regulatory Proteins/Cytokine Receptors**
CD22	CD23
CD44	CD40
B7	
VLA-4 (CDw49)	
CD11a/CD18	
E-Selectin (LAM-1)	

antigen.[125, 126] Adhesion between B-cell B7 and T-cell CD28 molecules is thought to mediate T-cell regulation of antigen-specific B-cell activation, particularly in germinal centers.[110, 117] The VLA-4, CD44, E selectin, and CD11a/18 molecules mediate B-cell adhesion to bone marrow stromal cells and to components of the lymph node microenvironment.[30, 127]

Finally, CD23, the low-affinity Fc receptor for IgE (FCεRII), and CD40 have been postulated to be receptors for as yet undefined ligands.[117] CD40 has homology to nerve growth factor receptor[128, 129] and is coupled to at least two transmembrane signaling pathways: the adenylate cyclase–cyclic AMP (cAMP)–protein kinase A cascade and the phospholipase C–inositol triphosphate–protein kinase C cascade.[130] CD23 exists in both transmembrane and soluble forms.[131] sCD23+ stimulates the activation of T-cell precursors and may also play a role in B-cell–regulated proliferation of progenitor T cells in bone marrow.[132]

ONTOGENY OF HUMAN B CELLS. The most immature B-cell precursors (pro-B cells) express surface CD10 and CD34 and nuclear terminal deoxynucleotidyl transferase (TdT); lack B-lineage–specific antigens CD19 and CD22; and are cIg− and sIg− (see Fig. 12–5). At this stage, immunoglobulin genes are germline, and CD10 expression on CD34 + HSCs is thought to be an initial event in B-cell development.[110, 133] Recently, it has been suggested that CD10 is on a subset of bone marrow pre-T cells as well as pre-B cells.[134, 135] Thus, it is not clear at what stage non-reversible B-lineage commitment occurs.[110]

The next stage in B-cell development, the pre-pre-B cell, is marked by the acquisition of CD19 and CD22 B-cell antigens.[110, 134, 136] Immunoglobulin genes undergo rearrangement in pre-pre-B cells, but immunoglobulin heavy chain protein is not expressed. Late in the pre-pre-B-cell stage, CD38 and CD40 antigens are expressed.[110] The hallmark of the next maturation stage, the pre-B cell, is expression of cμ heavy chain.[14–16] In association with the appearance of cμ, CD73 and CD21 are expressed.[110, 134, 136] At the pre-B-cell stage, expression of CD34 and CD10 ceases and nuclear TdT is no longer present.[30, 110] Later in pre-B cells, a pseudo LC complex, ψLC, is produced

without light chain rearrangement, and a subset of pre-B cells express surface μ heavy chain–ψLC complexes.[30, 111, 137] The genes encoding the proteins of the ψLC complex are conserved in both mice and humans, and their restricted expression pattern in both species suggests a critical role in B-cell development.[30, 111] Burrows and Cooper have suggested that the μ heavy chain–ψLC complex may serve as an indicator of successful immunoglobulin heavy chain gene rearrangement and is involved in mechanisms that eliminate B cells with defective immunoglobulin gene rearrangements generated during B-cell development.[111]

Immature B cells have rearranged immunoglobulin light chain genes and express sIg.[110] As immature B cells develop into mature B cells, sIgD is expressed, as well as sIgM and CD23.[108, 110] At this point, B-lineage development in bone marrow is complete, and B cells exit into the peripheral circulation and migrate to secondary lymphoid organs[30, 104] (see Fig. 12–5).

BONE MARROW–STROMAL B-CELL PROGENITOR CELL INTERACTIONS. Elements of the bone marrow microenvironment, collectively known as bone marrow stroma, include reticular dendritic cells, endothelial cells, fibroblasts, macrophages, adipocytes, and extracellular matrix.[138] Long-term cultured B-lineage cells proliferating in the Whitlock-Witte mouse bone marrow culture system include B-lineage progenitor cells capable of reconstitution of B-lineage lymphopoiesis and restoration of humoral immunity in immunodeficient mice.[138–142] Studies of cell-cell interactions in Whitlock-Witte cultures have demonstrated that physical association with bone marrow stromal cells is required for the development of immature B cells from B-cell progenitor cells[143, 144] (Fig. 12–6).

Two adhesion-ligand pairs are important in progenitor B-cell interaction with stromal cells: CD44 (hyaluronate receptor–hyaluronate) and VLA-4 (CD49, integrin-fibronectin).[88, 145–147] Monoclonal antibodies to CD44 inhibit B-cell maturation in long-term Whitlock-Witte cultures,[88] and CD44 on B-cell progenitors mediates adhesion to stromal cells via stromal cell hyaluronate.[145] VLA-4 is also an important mediator of precursor cell–stromal cell contact necessary for normal hematopoiesis.[146, 147] Studies performed with human VLA-4 have described two potential ligands: fibronectin on stromal cells and macrophages and VCAM-1 on endothelial cells.[148–150] VLA-4 recognizes the connecting segment-1 (CS-1) domain of fibronectin,[151] and pre-B-cell lines and bone marrow B cells bind to fibronectin fragments.[152] Moreover, monoclonal antibodies to the fibronectin receptor inhibit the activation of pre-B cells by stromal cells.[153] VCAM-1 mediates adhesion of leukocytes to endothelium and bone marrow stromal cells[148, 150] and may be involved in B-cell migration from bone marrow, as well as homing of B cells to Peyer's patches.[154] Monoclonal antibodies produced against murine stromal cell lines that inhibit B-cell lymphopoiesis in long-term bone marrow cultures recognize a 107 kDa molecule that likely is the murine homologue of VCAM-1.[147]

CYTOKINES THAT REGULATE B-CELL DEVELOP-

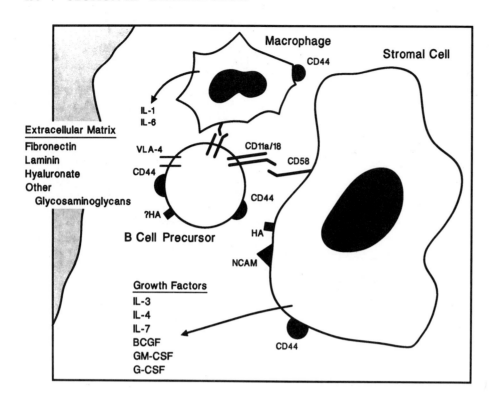

FIGURE 12–6. Bone marrow stromal–B-cell interactions.

MENT. Initial studies of cloned bone marrow stromal cell lines revealed the production of a variety of cytokines, including M-CSF, G-CSF, GM-CSF, IL-6, IL-7, and TGFβ[138–141] (see Fig. 12–6). Although multiple cytokines are thought to contribute to HSC differentiation or proliferation (see Table 12–3), few cytokines have been demonstrated to influence antigen-independent B-lineage lymphopoiesis. Stromal cell– and T cell–derived interleukin-7 (IL-7) drives the earliest stages of B-cell differentiation.[155–157] IL-7 receptors are expressed in pro-B and pre-pre-B-cell stages[110] and show a marked proliferative response to IL-7.[156] IL-7–mediated progenitor B-cell proliferation is associated with stimulation of phosphoinositol turnover and intracellular calcium mobilization.[158] Pre-pre-B cells in long-term stromal cell cultures supplemented with IL-7 predominantly have heavy chain DJ rearrangements with no productive VDJ rearrangements, and therefore do not produce μ heavy chains.[159–161] Removal of IL-7 or stromal cells from the proliferating pre-pre-B cell leads to induction of heavy chain V to DJ rearrangements, LC rearrangements, and the appearance of sIg+ B cells.

Low molecular weight B-cell growth factor (BCGF), purified from lectin-stimulated T lymphocytes, induces marked proliferation of leukemic as well as normal B-cell precursors.[162–164] BCGF binds to high-affinity receptors expressed on all B-cell precursors except pro-B cells.[110, 163] IL-3 receptors are present on pre-pre-B cells and pre-B cells.[110, 165] Recombinant IL-3 induces proliferation of both leukemic and normal pre-B cells in a dose-dependent fashion.[165] Although IL-4 receptors are present in multiple early stages of

B-cell maturation (see Fig. 12–5), IL-4 does not induce B-cell precursor proliferation.[166]

Large Granular Lymphocyte Development and Function

Large granular lymphocytes that mediate natural killer (NK) activity constitute 10 to 15 per cent of human peripheral blood lymphocytes.[167–169] The ability of NK cells to lyse target cells without prior sensitization and without restriction by major histocompatibility complex (MHC) antigens serves many purposes in vivo, including destruction of tumor cells, early resistance to viral infections, and regulation of hematopoiesis.[168, 169] Studies of immune function in lower animal species suggest that the development of cells mediating NK activity preceded the evolution of immune cells with immunological memory.[168]

SURFACE ANTIGENS OF NATURAL KILLER CELLS. Whereas NK cells are defined by their functional capability of non–MHC-restricted cytotoxicity, phenotypic definition of a discrete cell subset has proved difficult. Only 60 to 80 per cent of LGLs exhibit NK activity or characteristic NK cell surface antigens,[170] and some NK cells do not demonstrate LGL morphology.[171] The antigens used most extensively as NK cell markers are CD56 and CD16.[168] The CD56 antigen is expressed by essentially all human peripheral blood cells capable of non–MHC-restricted cytotoxicity[168, 171] and is identical to neural cell adhesion molecule (NCAM), which mediates homotypic adhesion between neural and muscle cells.[172] CD16, the low-affinity receptor for IgG, binds IgG in immune complexes.[173]

Approximately 10 per cent of normal peripheral blood NK cells are CD16−.[171]

Other cell surface antigens expressed on NK cells include CD57, a 110 kDa protein expressed on 50 to 60 per cent of peripheral blood NK cells.[174] CD7 and CD2 are present on 70 to 90 per cent of NK cells, whereas CD8 is expressed on 30 to 40 per cent of NK cells (reviewed in reference 168). Approximately 80 per cent of NK cells[168, 169] express CD11b (C3b receptor) and 30 to 60 per cent express CD11c.[168] Essentially all NK cells express the CD11a and CD18 chains of the lymphocyte function associated antigen–1 (LFA-1) complex, and 85 to 90 per cent of NK cells express the ligand for CD2, CD58 (LFA-3) (reviewed in reference 168).

ONTOGENY OF NATURAL KILLER CELLS. NK cell activity has been reported in human fetal liver cells at 8 to 11 weeks of gestation,[175] with CD57+ cells first seen in the fetal liver at 7 weeks[176] and NK activity first appearing in fetal peripheral blood at 27 to 28 weeks.[177]

Data in both humans and animals indicate that NK cells are derived from bone marrow precursors (reviewed in reference 169) (see Fig. 12–4). Bone marrow grafts can reconstitute NK cells in lethally irradiated mice.[178] After human bone marrow transplantation, NK cells are the first lymphocyte population to reconstitute the recipient and may represent more than 50 per cent of circulating lymphocytes at 30 to 50 days after transplantation.[179]

The relationship of NK cells to T and myeloid lineages remains unclear. Detailed characterization of leukocyte cell surface antigens has not allowed an unambiguous lineage designation because NK cells share surface antigens with T cells and myeloid cells (reviewed in references 166 to 168).

Studies of immunodeficient SCID mice lacking normal recombinase activity have revealed normal NK-cell activity.[180, 181] Mice homozygous for the beige mutation with defects in lysosomal membrane functions have markedly depressed NK cell activity.[182] Rare patients with complete absence of NK cells have been described; these patients lack both NK activity and CD56+, CD16+ lymphocytes but have normal T- and B-cell function.[183, 184] NK cell hyporesponsiveness is observed in patients with the Chédiak-Higashi syndrome, an autosomal recessive disease associated with fusion of cytoplasmic granules and defective degranulation of neutrophil lysosomes.[185, 186] In Chédiak-Higashi syndrome, humoral immunity and T-cell responses are normal.[185] Patients with various types of congenital B-cell deficiencies have normal NK cells and NK activity.[169, 187] Finally, patients with the DiGeorge syndrome and absence of T-cell function have normal NK cell activity.[168] Thus, studies of both human and murine immunodeficiency states indicate that NK cell development does not depend on the normal development of T- or B-cell lineages.[168, 169] Nor does T- and B-cell development depend on normal NK cell development.[168]

Although NK cells arise from a bone marrow precursor,[188, 189] it is not clear that NK cell differentiation occurs entirely in bone marrow. Most data, especially studies of SCID mice, suggest that thymic processing is not required (reviewed in reference 169). Normal thymus contains few NK cells, and fresh thymocytes express little cytotoxic activity.[190] However, studies of human thymocytes have demonstrated CD16+ NK cells arising during in vitro culture of either CD7+ TN (CD3−, CD4−, CD8−, or triple negative) thymocytes[191, 192] or CD7+, CD8+, CD4−, sCD3− thymocytes.[193] Studies in birds have demonstrated sTCR− NK cells within the thymus.[194] NK cells constitute approximately 30 per cent of thymic lymphocytes in SCID mice.[195] Together, these data suggest that NK cell development may also occur within the thymus as well as within bone marrow (see Fig. 12–4).

After being released from bone marrow, NK cells circulate in the peripheral blood or migrate to the spleen, with few NK cells in peripheral lymph nodes. The mechanisms regulating peripheral blood recirculation and splenic localization of NK cells are poorly understood but likely involve specific NK cell–endothelial cell interactions. The life span of mature NK cells is not well characterized but has been reported to range from a few days to several months.[168, 169] At least some mature peripheral blood NK cells retain proliferative capability.[195]

Recently, a series of elegant studies have suggested that NK cells can specifically recognize normal allogeneic cells in a clonal fashion.[196–200] Studies of multiple NK cell clones have defined a novel family of 58 kDa surface molecules that may serve as NK cell receptor molecules.[197] Four distinct NK cell subsets, each with a specific pattern of allogeneic reactivity, have been defined. Investigations of allogeneic target cells suggest that the genetic locus controlling NK alloantigen lysis is different from conventional MHC products, is inherited as an autosomal recessive trait, and has been mapped to chromosome 6 in the region of the MHC class I genes.[199–201]

LYMPHOPOIESIS IN THE THYMUS

Cloning of the genes for the T-cell receptor for antigen,[202, 203] determination of the structure of HLA molecules,[204] and discovery of the accessory molecules involved in the interaction of T cells with antigen-presenting cells and thymic epithelial cells (reviewed in references 64 and 205) have provided a basis for understanding the molecular and cellular events that occur during intrathymic T-cell maturation. Within the thymus, TCR gene rearrangements are initiated in intrathymic T-cell precursors that culminate in thymocyte surface expression of either TCRαβ or TCRγδ heterodimers. Cellular selection of TCR+ thymocytes occurs whereby thymocytes able to recognize antigen in the context of self-HLA antigens are retained (*positive selection*) and autoreactive thymocytes that have high-affinity TCR for self-antigens are eliminated *(negative selection)*.

Ontogeny of the Human Thymic Microenvironment

The thymic microenvironment develops early during human fetal gestation.[10, 11, 13, 206] At 4 weeks of gestation, the thymic rudiment is formed from ectoderm of the third pharyngeal cleft and endoderm of the third pharyngeal pouch[207, 208] (Fig. 12–7). A number of monoclonal antibodies that define components of the human thymic microenvironment have been generated.[13, 206, 209–211] Postnatal thymic epithelium (TE) consists of ectoderm-derived subcapsular cortical and medullary epithelium (TE4/p19/A2B5+) surrounding endoderm-derived TE3+ cortical epithelium[206, 210] (see Fig. 12–7). The subcapsular cortical (SCC) TE zone is phenotypically distinct in that SCC TE cells also express the human homologue of the rodent Thy-1 molecule.[212] Hassall's bodies are swirls of terminally differentiated medullary epithelial cells located in the thymic medulla that are first seen at 16 to 18 weeks of gestation.[13, 213] Hassall's bodies express keratins and epithelial cell surface markers that are also expressed in terminally differentiated stratum granuloma and stratum corneum of skin.[214, 215]

Macrophages are present in the fetal human thymus by at least 10 weeks of fetal gestation (reviewed in reference 13), and in rodents they have been postulated to mature simultaneously with T-cell precursors in the thymus in response to IL-3/GM-CSF production by developing thymocytes.[216] In the postnatal thymus, macrophages are located throughout the thymic cortex and medulla and frequently are clustered at the corticomedullary junction.[13] Langerhans' cells with phenotypic (CD1+, S100+) and morphological (intercellular Birbeck granules) similarities to Langerhans' cells in skin are present in the thymus at 9 to 10 weeks of gestation[217] and in postnatal thymus are scattered about the thymic medulla.[218]

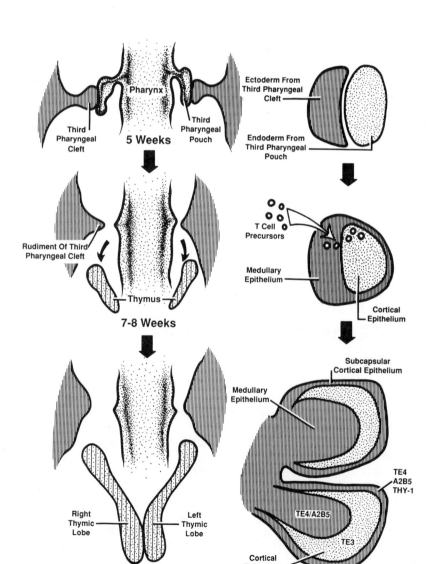

FIGURE 12–7. Development of the human thymic microenvironment during the first trimester of gestation. (From Haynes, B. F.: Human thymic epithelium and T cell development. Current issues and future development. Thymus 16:143, 1990; with permission.)

T-Cell Surface Molecules

CD45, CD34, and CD7 are expressed on multipotent progenitor populations and continue to be expressed in the earliest stages of the T lineage in fetal liver and bone marrow before the migration of T-cell precursors to the thymus[55, 56, 63, 64, 78, 218] (see Table 12–1). CD4 and CD8 molecules are adhesion molecules of the immunoglobulin gene superfamily that serve to stabilize TCR interactions with HLA molecules and antigen peptides on bone marrow–derived antigen-presenting cells or on TE cells.[205] CD4 and CD8 molecules also directly interact with HLA molecules, with CD4 binding to HLA class II molecules and CD8 binding to HLA class I molecules.[219, 220] Finally, CD4 and CD8 molecules are directly involved in the regulation of T-cell activation and are physically linked intracellularly to the *lck* protein tyrosine kinase.[221] The CD3 complex of signal-transducing molecules is composed of $\gamma,\delta,\epsilon,\zeta$, and η subunits (reviewed in reference 222) (Fig. 12–8). During intrathymic T-cell maturation, molecules of the CD3 complex become functionally and physically linked to either the $\alpha\beta$ or the $\gamma\delta$ TCR heterodimer (reviewed in references 222 and 223). (See Chapters 11 and 13.)

CD5 is an immunoglobulin superfamily member that is expressed on T-cell precursors and is maintained throughout ontogeny.[224] The function of CD5 on thymocytes is unknown; on peripheral T cells, CD5 serves as an adhesion molecule that mediates T-cell binding to B cells via B-cell CD72 molecules.[224] CD1 comprises three chains—CD1a, CD1b, and CD1c—that are associated with β_2-microglobulin on cortical thymocytes.[225] CD1 is also expressed on Langerhans' cells in the thymic medulla and has been proposed as an antigen-presenting molecule for TCR$\gamma\delta$ cells.[226] CD2 and CD11/18 (LFA-1) are cell surface adhesion molecules that stabilize TCR-HLA interactions and mediate TCR − immature thymocyte interactions with TE cells[205, 227–230] (see Fig. 12–8). The ligand on TE cells and monocytes for LFA-1 is CD54 (ICAM-1) and for CD2 is CD58 (LFA-3) (reviewed in references 64 and 205). CD28 is an immunoglobulin superfamily member and binds to the B7 molecule on B cells and fibroblasts.[231] Ligand binding to CD28 augments peripheral T-cell and thymocyte activation by prolongation of T-cell cytokine mRNA half-life.[231]

Identification of Extrathymic T-Cell Precursors

Pro-T cells (T-cell progenitors with germline TCR genes) are thought to be CD45 +, CD7 +, CD34 + and express low levels of human Thy-1 (Thy-1lo).[13, 20, 21, 52, 55, 56, 63, 64, 78, 218] CD7 is expressed on CD45 + hematopoietic cells in fetal thorax at 7 weeks of gestation prior to the time of colonization of the thymic epithelial rudiment with fetal HSC.[63, 64, 78, 218] From 7 to 10 weeks, the only fetal liver cells expressing antigens shared with the T-cell lineage are CD7 +, CD45 + cells that express cytoplasmic CD3ϵ (cCD3ϵ).[20, 78, 218] A sim-

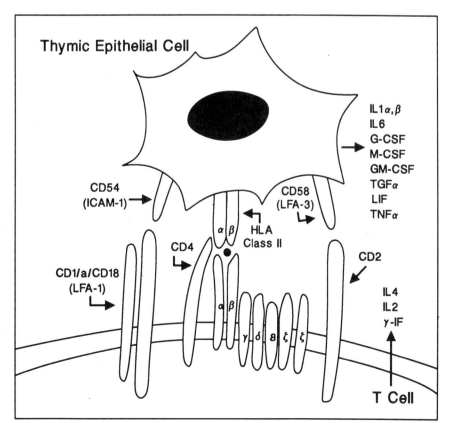

FIGURE 12–8. Molecules that mediate thymic epithelial–thymocyte interactions.

ilar population of CD7+ cells has been identified in bone marrow and postulated to be a pro-T cell prior to migration to the thymus.[232] Precursors of NK cells have been found in the thymus that are CD7+ and express cCD3ε but not cCD3δ,[191–193, 197] whereas cCD3δ expression is thought to be characteristic of commitment to the T-cell lineage.[233] Whether CD7+, CD45+, cCD3ε+ cells identified in 7 to 10 week fetal thorax are also CD3δ+ is not known. However, Hori and associates have cloned CD7+, cCD3ε+, cCD3δ+ cells from 17 week human fetal liver.[233]

The phenotype of human T-cell precursors from human bone marrow,[234, 235] peripheral blood,[236] and fetal liver[218] has been studied by determining the ability of putative T-cell progenitors to differentiate in vitro in the presence of T-cell–conditioned media and other cytokines. Surprisingly, a uniform observation has been that human bone marrow or fetal liver CD7+, CD34+/−, CD2−, sCD3−, CD4− or lo+, CD8− cells can mature into TCRαβ+ cells in vitro in the absence of the thymus.

A large body of work in both mouse and humans suggests that the precursors of T cells in fetal liver and bone marrow do not express molecules of mature T cells, such as surface CD3/TCR, CD4, and CD8, and can be identified by expression of CD34, CD7, cCD3ε, and CD44 (Table 12–6).

Migration of T-Cell Precursors to the Thymus

Although no information regarding patterns of human HSC traffic to the thymus is available, initial seeding of the avian and mouse thymus with fetal liver HSCs occurs in waves.[6–8] In birds, it has been shown that the thymus secretes a soluble form of β2-microglobulin, thymotaxin, that is secreted coincident with the observed waves of HSC migration to the thymic rudiment.[237] In mice, bone marrow cells destined to home to the thymus express certain isoforms of the CD44 molecule,[85] and CD44 antibodies inhibit the homing of bone marrow T-cell precursors to the

thymus.[85] Presumably, hyaluronic acid production by endothelial cells in thymic vessels plays an important role in the binding of bone marrow T-cell progenitors to murine thymic vessels.[85]

The issue of when and where T-cell precursors undergo lineage commitment to T cells remains unresolved.[11] Data in animals suggest the existence of a committed lymphoid stem cell capable of giving rise to T cells and B cells, but not giving rise to myeloerythroid lineages.[238] In humans, isolation and culture of the presumed earliest cell immigrants in the thymus (CD7+, CD34+/−, sCD3−, CD4lo+, CD8−, TN cells) yielded either mature T cells or mature myeloerythroid cells in vitro, suggesting that intrathymic CD7+, TN cells are not irreversibly committed to the T lineage.[239] An important recent study isolated CD7+ pro-T cells from human thymus and demonstrated the absence of an important early rearrangement event that is known to precede TCRα rearrangement and deletion of the TCRδ gene, the δRec-ψJα rearrangement.[240] (See Chapter 11.) In the presence of soluble CD23 and IL-1, CD7 pro-T cells underwent the δRec-ψJα rearrangement in vitro and matured to TCRαβ+ T cells.[240] De Villartay and colleagues proposed that soluble CD23 and IL-1 from activated T cells are the primary cytokine stimuli during the differentiation of intrathymic TE-cell precursors to the TCRαβ lineage.[240]

Maturation Pathways of Developing Thymocytes

T-CELL MATURATION DURING FETAL DEVELOPMENT. Table 12–7 summarizes the phenotypic changes that occur in the thymus during the earliest stages of human fetal T-cell development.[20, 26, 218, 241, 242] At 8 to 9.5 weeks, approximately 20 per cent of thymocytes are sCD3+, and 40 to 60 per cent express CD4 and CD8. At 9.5 weeks, more than 95 per cent of thymocytes are CD7+, CD2+, CD4+, CD8+, and cCD3+, whereas approximately 30 per cent of thymocytes expressed the CD1 inner cortical thymocyte antigen. At 10 to 11 weeks, about 30 per cent of fetal thymocytes are sCD3+. By 13 weeks, a definite thymic medulla has formed, and single positive (SP) CD4+ and SP CD8+ cells are present (see Table 12–7).

At the earliest stages studied for TCR expression in the human thymus, TCRδ is expressed at 9.5 weeks (11 per cent of thymocytes) and rapidly falls to fewer than 1 per cent of thymocytes at 15 weeks (see Table 12–7).[241] Although the predominant thymic TCRδ type from 15 weeks of gestation until birth is Vδ1+, the initial wave of TCRδ cells seen from 9.5 to 12.75 weeks is Vδ2+.[243, 244] The ratio of Vδ2/Vδ1 TCRδ cells in the thymus changes from approximately 100:1 at 9.5 weeks to approximately 25:75 at 15 weeks.[243] Parker and associates suggest that the wave of TCR Vδ2+ cells seen early in human fetal thymic development seeds the periphery and is the population of

TABLE 12–6. PHENOTYPE OF T PROGENITOR (PRO-T) CELLS

HUMAN	MOUSE
CD34+/−	CD4lo+
CD10+/−	CD5lo+
CD38+	sCD3γ,δ,ε−
CD7+	CD8−
CD5lo	Thy-1+
CD2+/−	CD44+
sCD3γ,δ,ε−	H2+
cCD3ε+/−	Ia−
?cCD3δ+	sTCR−
CD4lo+/−	HSAhi+
CD8−	Rhodamine 123hi+
CD44+	
?c-kit+/−	
sTCR−	

HSA = Heat-stable antigen.

TABLE 12–7. PHENOTYPE OF THYMOCYTES IN FETAL THYMUS TISSUES AS DETERMINED BY IMMUNOHISTOLOGICAL ANALYSIS OF TISSUE SECTIONS OR THYMOCYTES IN SUSPENSIONS

GESTATIONAL AGE (WK)	MARKER										
	CD45	CD7	CD2	CD4*	CD8	CD1	cCD3ε	sCD3ε†	TCRδ‡	TCRβ	TCRαβ
					(% of Cells Positive)						
7	0	0	0	0	0	0	0	NA	NA	NA	NA
9.5	>95	>95	>95	>95	>95	~30	>95	18	11	30	0
10	>95	>95	>95	>95	>95	~30	>95	34	4	45	25
12.75	>95	>95	>95	>95	>95	>50	>95	50	1	70	70
15	>95	>95	>95	>90	>90	>50	>95	50	≤1	90	80
1.0 postnatal	>95	>95	>95	>90	>90	>85	>95	90	≤1	>95	>95

*Lipofuscin-containing thymic macrophages also were CD4+.
†sCD3ε = Surface CD3ε expression; from references 20 and 26, determined by immunofluorescence assays on fetal thymocytes in suspension.
‡The initial wave of TCRγδ cells are Vδ2 cells. At 15 weeks, the predominant TCRγδ type in human thymus is Vδ1.
cCD3ε = Cytoplasmic CD3ε expression; NA = not applicable.
Other data summarized from references 217 and 240, determined by immunofluorescence assays on tissue sections.

TCRγδ cells that expands throughout postnatal life in response to antigen stimulation.[245]

Cytoplasmic TCRβ expression can be detected in approximately 30 per cent of thymocytes at 9.5 weeks, in 45 per cent at 10 weeks, and in 90 per cent at 15 weeks.[241] TCRαβ expresssion is not detected at 9.5 weeks and gradually rises to expression in more than 95 per cent of thymocytes postnatally.[241] Taken together, these data suggest that TCR gene rearrangement begins immediately after seeding of the thymus by HSCs, and establishment of the TCR repertoire in man begins at 8 to 10 weeks of gestational age.

Two genes that encode components of the V(D)J recombinase, RAG-1 and RAG-2, have been cloned.[246] Co-expression of RAG-1 and RAG-2 is both necessary and sufficient to induce V(D)J TCR recombination, and the postulate has been made that RAG-1 and RAG-2 control TCR recombination during T-cell ontogeny.[246] RAG-1 and RAG-2 genes are selectively expressed in the subcapsular cortex and inner cortex of mouse thymus, but not in the thymic medulla.[246]

George and Schroeder have presented recent evidence that TCRβ rearrangements begin as early as 8 weeks in the human thymus, with low levels of TdT detected at 8 weeks.[247] Early human fetal thymocytes expressed a limited set of TCR D-J transcripts and generated a TCRβ repertoire of limited diversity.[247] During fetal gestation, an increase occurred both in the percentage of DJ and VDJ TCR transcripts with N regions and in the average number of inserted nucleotides per transcript.[247]

T-CELL DEVELOPMENT IN THE POSTNATAL THYMUS. Figure 12–9 shows proposed maturation pathways of human T cells based on surface and cytoplasmic antigen expression of human thymocytes (reviewed in references 63, 64, 248, and 249). Evidence for the T-cell maturation events has been obtained from extrapolating from studies in animal models[250, 251]; from studies injecting T-cell precursor populations intrathymically in human thymus, in SCID/Hu mice,[55, 56] or in mouse thymic lobes in vitro[252]; and from studies of in vitro maturation properties of human thymocyte populations.[253–261]

Because cells within the CD7+, CD3−, CD4−, CD8−, or TN, subset of thymocytes can be infected with human immunodeficiency virus (HIV), it was found that most cells in this subset are CD4lo+.[260] In the mouse, Wu and associates have defined the earliest postnatal intrathymic pro-T cell as CD4lo+, CD8−, sCD3−, Sca−2+, rhodamine hi+ cells[238, 261] (see Table 12–6). In man, CD7+, CD34+/−, cCD3+ *pre-T cells* (T progenitors that have begun to rearrange TCR but without surface TCR expression) are the next identifiable T-cell precursors isolated from postnatal thymus.[255, 258, 259] In vitro, putative intrathymic pre-T cells give rise to TCRγδ, to NK cells, and to a small percentage of TCRαβ cells.[253–262]

In the thymus, pre-T cells undergo a series of differentiation events whereby CD4 and CD8 expression is upregulated. It has been suggested that in the mouse CD4− or lo+ pre-T cells express CD8 as an intermediate to becoming CD4+ and CD8+ inner cortical thymocytes.[263] In man, a CD4+, CD8α+, β− (expressing the CD8α chain but not expressing the CD8β chain) TCRαβ+ intermediate stage has been proposed,[264] although in vitro culture of this thymocyte subset has yielded primarily CD16+, TCR− cells with NK activity.[265] In summary, studies of both human and mouse TN populations of thymocytes have demonstrated that cells within these subsets give rise either in vivo and in vitro to both CD4+, CD8+ double positive (DP) and CD4+ or CD8+ SP thymocytes of both the TCRαβ and the TCRγδ lineages, as well as to CD16+ TCR− cells with NK activity.

The transient or sequential expression of a number of other thymocyte molecules listed in Table 12–1 and Figure 12–9 is important for understanding the functional capabilities of T cells acquired during intrathymic T-cell development. These molecules include CD1, CD11a/CD18 (LFA-1), CD28, CD29, CD44, CD58 (LFA-3), and isoforms of CD45 (see Fig. 12–9) (reviewed in reference 64). It is interesting that CD29, CD44, and CD58, as well as the CD45 180 kDa isoform (CD45RO), are all markers of memory T cells, with an increase in, or de novo expression of, these molecules occurring after antigen-induced activation of naive T cells in the periphery (see Fig. 12–9).

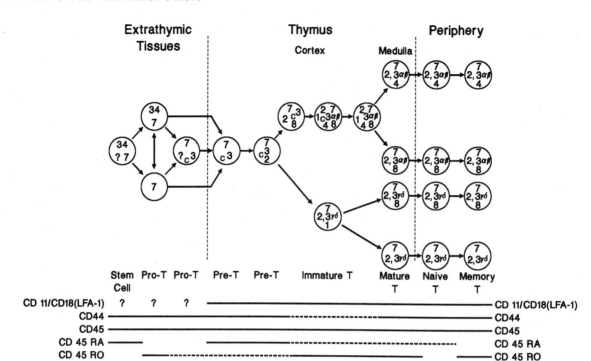

FIGURE 12–9. Human intrathymic T-cell maturation pathways. (Adapted from Haynes, B. F., Denning, S. M., Le, P. T., and Singer, K. H.: Human intrathymic T cell differentiation. Semin. Immunol. 2:67, 1990; with permission.)

Cytokines That Regulate Intrathymic T-Cell Development

A myriad of cytokines produced by thymocytes and non-lymphoid cells of the thymic microenvironment have been proposed to play important roles in coordinating the complex events that transpire during intrathymic T-cell maturation (Table 12–8) (reviewed in reference 64). An important concept is that adhesion molecules mediate TE-thymocyte interactions, both in the presence and in the absence of sTCR thymocyte expression, and adhesion molecule–mediated interactions of TE cells with thymocytes induce cytokine production by both TE cells and thymocytes[266] (see Fig. 12–8).

Human TE cells bind to all resting thymocyte subsets via CD2 on thymocytes and CD58 (LFA-3) molecules on TE cells.[227–230] Thymocyte binding to TE cells induces IL-1α and IL-1β production by TE cells[266] and, in the case of TN thymocytes, leads to TN thymocyte activation.[228] In vivo, TE cells express high levels of MHC class II and CD54 (ICAM-1) molecules.[207, 229] After in vitro culture of TE cells, expression of TE ICAM-1 and MHC class II molecules decreases but can be induced by the culture of TE cells in vitro with interferon-γ (IFN-γ).[267] ICAM-1 + TE cells bind LFA-1 + (CD11, CD18)–activated thymocytes.[229] These observations have led to the proposal that during the course of CD2/LFA-3–mediated TE-thymocyte interactions, thymocytes are stimulated by TE cytokines to produce IFN-γ, leading to local upregulation of TE-cell ICAM-1 and MHC class II antigen expression.[64, 208, 268]

Humoral factors produced by TE cells have long been postulated to play important roles in T-cell maturation. Originally thought to drive intrathymic maturation, the thymic hormones thymosin-α1, facteur thymique serique (FTS), and thymopoietin have been found to be most active on mature T cells (reviewed in reference 269).

Human TE cells are rich sources of myeloerythroid-stimulating activity and constitutively produce IL-1α, IL-1β, TGFα, G-CSF, M-CSF, GM-CSF, LIF, and IL-6 in vitro[270–272] (see Fig. 12–8). Cortical TE cells provide the activation signals that drive TN thymocyte proliferation, and TE-cell–mediated TN thymocyte activation depends on IL-1 and GM-CSF.[228] With the use of indirect immunofluorescent analysis of thymus sections, production of IL-1[270] and G-CSF (B.F. Haynes, unpublished data) has been confirmed in vivo.

Physical interactions of developing thymocytes with cortical TE cells, cortical macrophages, and medullary dendritic cells have been demonstrated. Specialized forms of subcapsular cortical (SCC) epithelial thymocyte complexes are called *thymic nurse cells*, with developing thymocytes contained within Thy-1 + SCC TE cells.[273]

In man, TE-TN thymocyte interactions upregulate TN thymocyte IL-2 receptor expression and upregulate the ability of TN thymocytes to respond to IL-2,

TABLE 12–8. ROLES OF CYTOKINES IN T-CELL PROLIFERATION AND DIFFERENTIATION*

CYTOKINE	SOURCE WITHIN THYMUS	FUNCTION
IL1α,β	Macrophages, TE cells, fibroblasts, endothelial cells, dendritic cells	Induces proliferation of thymocytes; induces production of other cytokines (i.e., IL-6, GM-CSF); with sCD23, induces TCR$\alpha\beta$ maturation in T-cell precursors
IL-2	Activated T cells	Induces proliferation of mature and immature thymocytes
IL-4	T cells	Induces proliferation of thymocytes; inhibits growth of TE cells
IL-5	Activated T cells	Induces cytotoxic T-cell differentiation
IL-6	Activated T cells, macrophages, fibroblasts, TE cells, endothelial cells	Synergizes with mitogen or IL-1 for T-cell/thymocyte proliferation
IL-7	Fibroblasts, BM stromal cell line	Co-mitogenic factor for thymocytes and T cells
IL-8	Monocytes/macrophages	Chemotactic for T cells
IL-9 (p40)	Helper T cell line (mouse)	Drives proliferation of helper T cells (mouse)
IL-10	Fetal and postnatal thymocytes, B cells (mouse)	Co-stimulant for immature and mature thymocyte proliferation and maturation (mouse)
Thymotaxin (β_2-microglobulin)	TE cells (rat)	Chemotactic for T-cell precursors (rat)
Soluble CD 23 (FcϵRII)	TE cells, B cells	With IL-1, induces TCR$\alpha\beta$ maturation in T-cell precursors
GM-CSF	Activated T cells, fibroblasts, endothelial cells, T cells	Promotes growth of early T-cell leukemias; promotes proliferation of immature thymocytes
G-CSF	TE cells, macrophages, fibroblasts	?Mitogenic for immature thymocytes
M-CSF	TE cells, monocytes, fibroblasts, endothelial cells	Supports differentiation of progenitors committed to the monocyte/macrophage lineages; ?mitogenic for immature thymocytes
LIF	TE cells, activated cells	?Prevents multilineage differentiation of intrathymic stem cells prior to signal to become T-cell precursors
IFN-γ	Activated T cells, thymocytes	Upregulates expression of TE, fibroblast, and macrophage CD54 (ICAM-1) and MHC class II; anti-proliferative effect on thymocytes via adenylate cyclase pathway
TNFα	Macrophages, activated T cells, thymocytes	IL-1–like effects
TGFα	Activated macrophages, TE cells	Regulates production of other cytokines (IL-1 and IL-6) by TE cells; drives TE-cell proliferation and/or differentiation via EGF receptor
TGFβ	?TE cells, T cells	Regulates expression of several oncogenes; suppresses lymphocyte responses to other cytokines; ?inhibits TE-cell proliferation
EGF	?Monocytes/macrophages, ?fibroblasts ?TE cells	Drives TE-cell proliferation

*Unless otherwise stated, effect reported or postulated (?) is in humans.
TE = Thymic epithelial; BM = bone marrow; IFN-γ = interferon-γ; TNFα = tumor necrosis factor α; EGF = epidermal growth factor.
Adapted from Haynes, B. F., Denning, S. M., Le, P. T., and Singer, K. H.: Human intrathymic T cell differentiation. Semin. Immunol. 2:67, 1990; with permission.

as well.[228] Another TE cytokine, G-CSF, has been shown in rodents to be required for the initiation of cell division in HSCs.[96–100] Thus, multiple cytokines produced within the thymus may have synergistic or competitive effects on intrathymic T-cell activation and differentiation. It seems likely that the ordered progression of T-cell receptor expression that occurs during fetal thymic development must involve the sequential induction of a series of cytokines within the thymic microenvironment that modulates T-cell recombinase activity.[64]

Functional Sequelae of Normal Thymic Development

In mice, the TCR$\gamma\delta$ cell lineage develops early in the thymus and seeds the skin and other peripheral epithelial microenvironments.[274] Subsets of murine epithelial-associated TCR$\gamma\delta$ and TCR$\alpha\beta$ cells can differentiate and select for functional cells in the absence of the thymus.[274–277] However, in humans a comparable epithelial distribution of TCR$\gamma\delta$ cells has not been observed.[278]

As immature cortical thymocytes begin to express sTCR, a remarkable selection process of thymocytes takes place. Autoreactive thymocytes are destroyed (negative selection), thymocytes with TCR capable of interacting with foreign antigens in the context of HLA self-antigens are activated and develop to maturity (positive selection), and thymocytes with TCR that are incapable of binding to self-MHC die of attrition (no selection) (reviewed in references 279 and 280). Mature thymocytes that survive the selection process either are CD4+, CD8− TCRαβ helper T, or HLA class II–restricted cytotoxic T lymphocyte (CTL), or are CD4−, CD8+ TCRαβ cells destined to become MHC class I–restricted CTL. (See Chapter 13.) Intrathymic TCRγδ cells also undergo positive selection.[281] For T cells to be HLA class I or class II restricted means that T cells recognize antigen peptide fragments as immunogenic only when they are presented in the notch of the HLA antigens expressed by the thymic microenvironment.[279–282] (See Chapters 11 and 13.) In the normal situation, the HLA antigens that present antigens capable of positively selecting developing T cells are autologous HLA antigens that are the same as those expressed on the T cells themselves. In HLA-mismatched bone marrow transplantation, it is possible for T cells to be restricted to recognize foreign antigen only when presented in the context of HLA antigens that are different from the HLA antigens of the T cells but are the HLA antigens of the host thymic microenvironment that selected the T cells during T-cell development after bone marrow transplantation.[47, 48]

It is thought that thymic selection processes occur sequentially.[283] The earliest immature thymocytes that have just begun to express low levels of sTCR (sTCRlo+) first undergo positive selection while still refractory to negative selection, and then later in T-cell development, autoreactive T cells are deleted via the negative selection process.[283]

ADHESION MOLECULES AND THYMIC MICROENVIRONMENT CELL TYPES THAT MEDIATE THYMOCYTE SELECTION. Positive selection is in large part mediated by cortical TE cells.[279, 283] Thus, for the positive selection of human CD8+ T cells, T-cell CD8 and TCR interact with self-HLA class I molecules on the surface of cortical TE cells and receive signals that lead to thymocyte survival. Similarly, the positive selection of CD4+ T cells involves TCR and CD4 binding to HLA class I molecules on the surface of cortical TE cells[279, 283] (Fig. 12–10). It is not known if CD4+ and

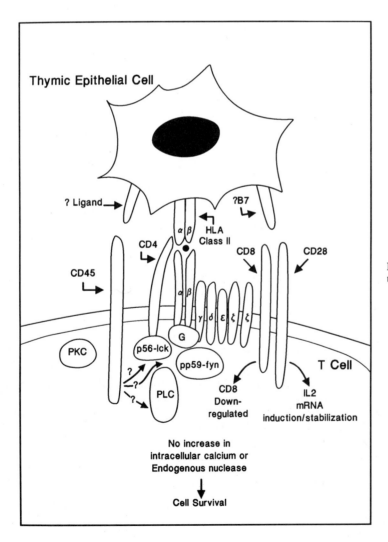

FIGURE 12–10. Factors involved in the positive selection of thymocytes.

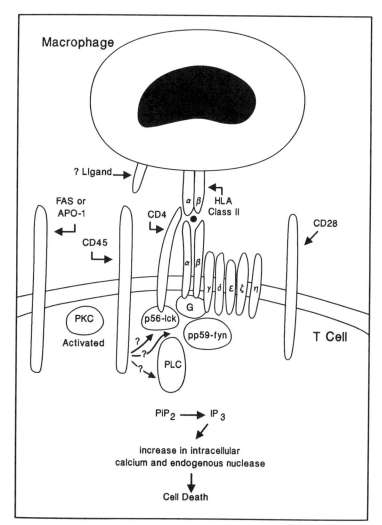

FIGURE 12–11. Factors involved in the negative selection of thymocytes.

CD8+ cell binding to TE cells is via TE-cell HLA molecules with the normal repertoire of self-peptides or, rather, if cortical TE cells present a unique repertoire of peptides.

Once through the positive selection process, the remaining thymocytes undergo changes that protect selected cells from spontaneous cell death. Surviving thymocytes are next subjected to negative selection, to remove those potentially pathological autoreactive T cells that recognize self-peptides in the context of self-HLA molecules or that recognize self-antigens with a high affinity.[279–283] Negative selection of thymocytes is mediated by bone marrow–derived thymic macrophages, dendritic cells, and perhaps B cells, probably located in the thymic cortex at the corticomedullary junction.[279, 283] Some investigators have suggested that medullary TE cells also participate in tolerance induction of medullary thymocytes.[284] In contrast to thymocyte binding to cortical TE cells (which results in a signal that promotes survival and prevents programmed thymocyte death), thymocyte binding to thymic macrophages during the process of negative selection leads to the induction of programmed thymocyte death (apoptosis) and prevention of thymocyte survival.[284] Again, CD4 interaction with macrophage class II and CD8 interaction with macrophage class I molecules are critical to the process of negative selection for the elimination of autoreactive CD4+ and CD8+ thymocytes[280–284, 285] (Fig. 12–11).

Other adhesion molecules that likely participate in the positive and negative selection processes are CD54 (ICAM-1) and CD58 (LFA-3) molecules on TE cells and their ligands on thymocytes, CD11a/CD18 (LFA-1) and CD2 (see Fig. 12–8).[64, 208]

MOLECULAR MECHANISMS OF SELECTION OF THYMOCYTES. Whereas cross-linking the CD3/TCR of peripheral T cells in vitro or in vivo leads to T-cell activation and clonal expansion, cross-linking immature human and mouse thymocytes with anti-CD3 or TCR monoclonal antibodies generates a signal that induces thymocyte apoptosis.[286–290] A key feature of the induction of thymocyte apoptosis is the generation of high levels of intracellular calcium, as calcium ionophores can also mediate thymocyte death.[286, 287]

Positive selection of thymocytes is thought to take place first in the thymus at a time when engagement of TCR by HLA molecules is not capable of leading to signals that mediate thymocyte death.[283] The precise mechanisms of protection of early immature TCR+ thymocytes from TCR engagement–mediated apoptosis are not known. Figure 12–10 outlines some of the factors thought to be important for mediation of the positive selection of CD4+ thymocytes (reviewed in reference 283).

Finkel and associates have proposed that TCR crosslinking does not generate a Ca^{2+} flux in positively selected thymocytes, whereas in non-selected immature thymocytes, a Ca^{2+} flux occurs and leads to endonuclease activation and thymocyte death.[283] In this model, DP thymocytes lack appropriate coupling of CD3 to TCRαβ molecules, leading to lack of inositol triphosphate generation that is necessary for the elevation of intracellular calcium.[283]

T cells with the CD3ζη heterodimer undergo TCR ligation–induced apoptosis, whereas T cells with the CD3ζζ homodimer do not undergo TCR-mediated apoptosis.[291] Thus, the form of CD3 components present in the TCR/CD3 complex may be a factor in the outcome of a TCR-mediated signal.

A critical discovery regarding mechanisms of lymphocyte triggering was the recognition that the cytoplasmic tail of CD45 isoforms is a tyrosine phosphatase capable of regulating T-cell signal transduction events.[292] The p56-*lck* tyrosine kinase associated with CD4 and CD8 has been shown to be a substrate for CD45 phosphatase activity,[293] and mechanisms have been proposed whereby CD45 could upregulate or downregulate T-cell triggering.[292–294] Gillitzer and Pilarski have suggested that thymocytes destined to die in the thymic cortex do not express the CD45RA isoform.[295]

Turka and associates have proposed that the interaction of CD28 with thymic microenvironment B7 during thymocyte selection is an important determinant of thymocyte survival.[231] In concert with CD3 or CD2 ligation of thymocytes, ligation of CD28 leads to thymocyte proliferation and inhibition of apoptosis.[231]

Positively selected thymocytes migrate to the thymic corticomedullary area to undergo the negative selection process. Recent data have suggested that the maturation of DP to CD4+ or CD8+ SP thymocytes is an event whereby positively selected thymocytes are instructed to shut off either CD4 or CD8 expression following TCR ligation.[296] Thus, if CD4/TCR was bound to class II on a TE cell, CD8 would be downregulated (see Fig. 12–10); if CD8/TCR was bound to class I on a TE cell, expression of CD4 would be inhibited.[296]

Figure 12–11 summarizes some of the factors postulated to be relevant for the induction of apoptosis in immature thymocytes during negative selection.[279, 280, 283–285] Unlike the immature thymocyte that undergoes positive selection, the pool of thymocytes able to undergo negative selection has undergone a maturation step whereby TCR ligation leads to inositol triphosphate generation and an increase in intracellular calcium.[283] The specific roles that *fyn* and *lck* tyrosine kinases play in regulating these events are not known, although data demonstrate that both are critical for T-cell activation via the TCR.[283, 297] (See Chapter 13.) Finkel and associates suggest that during negative

selection the CD3 complex is effectively "coupled" to the TCRαβ heterodimer, and in Figure 12–11, this is represented by the presence of a CD3ζη heterodimer.[283] Finally, two molecules have been reported to be expressed on cells suceptible to apoptosis, Fas and Apo-1[298, 299] (see Fig. 12–11). Whether there is selective expression of either of these molecules on thymocytes undergoing negative selection is not known. Another gene product, bcl-2, a cytoplasmic protein of mitochondria, has been reported to protect thymocytes and other cell types from apoptosis.[300, 301] In mouse thymus, bcl-2 is selectively expressed only in medullary thymocytes and may be involved in terminating the negative selection process.[300]

Thymocytes either are eliminated in the inner cortex by thymic macrophages or are eliminated in localized swirls of medullary TE cells, termed Hassall's bodies[1] (Fig. 12–12).

SUPERANTIGENS IN T-CELL DEVELOPMENT. Recently, a new class of molecules, termed superantigens, has been described; these molecules are capable of activating up to 20 per cent of the peripheral T-cell pool, whereas conventional antigens activate fewer than 1 in 10,000 T cells.[302–306] T-cell superantigens include staphylococcal enterotoxins, other bacterial products, and the murine minor lymphocyte stimulatory antigens (MLS-1a and MLS-2a) (reviewed in references 302 and 303).

Conventional antigens bind to HLA class II molecules in the groove of the αβ heterodimer and bind to T cells via CDR3 V regions of both TCRα and β chains.[307] In contrast, superantigens bind directly to TCRβ chains and HLA class II β chains at sites that differ from those associated with conventional antigen peptides.[304] In mice, the superantigens MLS-1a and MLS-1b are molecules that are capable of negatively selecting entire TCRβ familes during murine intrathymic T-cell maturation.[302, 303] Remarkably, these antigens have been found to be encoded by mouse mammary tumor viruses (MMTV) that have been integrated into the murine germline as DNA proviruses.[302, 303] Although viral superantigens have been shown to play a major role in shaping the Vβ TCR repertoire in mice, a role for endogenous superantigens in thymic selection has not, to date, been demonstrated in other animals or in man. However, superantigen stimulation of human peripheral T cells does occur and is the cause of the staphylococcal toxic shock syndrome.[305] Moreover, superantigen-driven autoimmune disease has been postulated to occur in rheumatoid arthritis.[308] Finally, HIV has been postulated to contain proteins that act as superantigens and stimulate peripheral deletion of Vβ TCR families in the acquired immunodeficiency syndrome (AIDS).[309]

KINETICS OF THYMOCYTE DEVELOPMENT. Although little is known of the kinetics of T-cell maturation in humans, the kinetics of thymocyte development have been elegantly studied in mice.[310–318] An extrapolated picture of the kinetics of human T-cell development can be drawn (Table 12–9). Approximately 100 HSCs seed the neonatal murine thymus daily.[312] The time

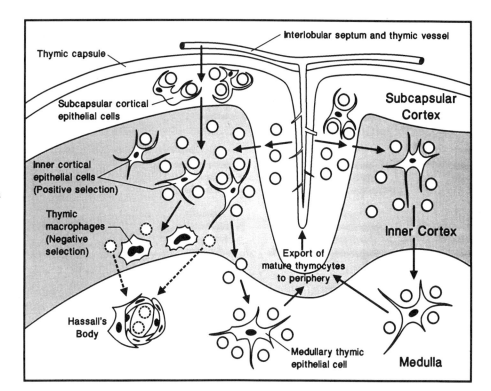

FIGURE 12–12. Intrathymic migration patterns of developing thymocytes.

taken by a HSC and its progeny to traverse the thymus is approximately 21 days.[312] During the first 8 days, 100 stem cells increase 500-fold to 50,000 TN thymocytes. By 2 weeks after seeding the thymus, HSCs have multiplied 100,000-fold to become 10 million DP cortical thymocytes. Over a 3 day period, the selection process occurs, whereby approximately one third of the total cortical thymocyte pool per day either is not selected or is actively eliminated during negative selection. Thus, during thymocyte selection, 97 per cent of all cortical thymocytes die, and the 3 per cent of surviving cells are SP for either CD4 or CD8.[312–318] Overall, 1 HSC gives rise to approximately 3000 mature medullary thymocytes.

EXPORT OF THYMOCYTES TO THE PERIPHERY. Once mature thymocytes reach the thymic medulla, they are exported to the periphery and home to various lymphoid organs, such as the spleen, lymph nodes, tonsils, Peyer's patches, appendix, and lungs.

The precise mechanisms and location of egress of mature thymocytes from the thymus are not known. Chaffin and Perlmutter constructed an *lck*-pertussin toxin (PT) transgenic mouse that selectively expressed PT in thymocytes.[319] Although CD3/TCR-mediated signaling in the T cells of PT transgenic mice was normal (suggesting that G proteins were not directly involved in TCR-mediated triggering), the export of medullary thymocytes to peripheral lymphoid organs was deficient in these animals in spite of the normal expression of Mel-14, and CD11a/CD18.[319] These data indicated that G protein–coupled signaling is required for a critical event controlling thymocyte emigration from the thymus.

LYMPHOPOIESIS IN SECONDARY LYMPHOID ORGANS

The Molecular Basis of Lymphocyte Homing

The control of lymphocyte trafficking between blood stream and lymphoid organs operates at the

TABLE 12–9. THYMOCYTE PROGENY FROM ONE DAY'S INPUT OF STEM CELLS

DAY	NUMBER AND TYPE OF CELL	PHENOTYPE OF ANALOGOUS HUMAN THYMOCYTE SUBSET*
1	100 stem cells	CD7+, CD8−, CD4−, CD3−, CD44+
8	50,000 pre-T cells (cortex)	CD7+, CD8−, CD4−, CD3−, CD44lo+
16	10,000,000 cortical thymocytes	CD7+, CD8+, CD4+, CD3+, TCR+, CD44lo+
17	6,700,000 cortical thymocytes	Same
18	3,300,000 cortical thymocytes	Same
19	300,000 medullary thymocytes	CD7+, CD4+, CD3+, TCR+, CD44+
		or
		CD7+, CD8+, CD3+, TCR+, CD44+

*Data are from studies in mice, whereas human thymocyte phenotypes are inferred from the pathway in Figure 12–9.

level of lymphocyte–endothelial cell interactions to control the specificity of lymphocyte subset entry into organs.[320-325] Adhesion molecules also regulate the retention and subsequent egress of lymphocytes within tissue sites of antigenic stimulation, delaying cell exit from tissue and preventing re-entry into the circulating lymphocyte pool. All types of lymphocyte migration begin with the attachment of lymphocytes to specialized regions of vessels, termed high endothelial venules (HEV).[320, 322, 324]

The first stage of leukocyte–endothelial cell interactions, *reversible adhesion,* occurs when leukocytes leave the central stream of flowing blood cells in a postcapillary venule and roll along the endothelial lining of the venules.[326] Leukocyte rolling is mediated by the L-selectin molecule (LECAM-1, LAM-1)[327, 328] (Table 12–10). L-selectin presents oligosaccharide ligands (sialylated derivatives of the Lewis X oligosaccharide) to endothelial cell E-selectin (ELAM-1) and P-selectin (GMP-140).[329] L-selectin is constitutively functional and is present at high levels on circulating resting leukocytes.[330, 331] Leukocyte rolling markedly slows transit time through venules, allowing time for leukocyte activation.[326, 328]

The second stage of leukocyte recognition, *leukocyte activation,* requires chemoattractant or endothelial cell–derived cytokine stimulation.[326] Factors thought to participate in leukocyte activation include members of the IL-8–intercrine family, platelet activation factor, leukotriene B_4, and C5a.[326, 332, 333] Following activation by chemoattractants, leukocytes shed L-selectin from the cell surface and upregulate CD11b/18 (Mac-1).[326, 334]

Whereas lymphocyte homing to peripheral lymph nodes involves the primary adhesion of L-selectin with carbohydrate of peripheral node HEV addressin,[326, 335] homing to intestinal Peyer's patches involves adhesion of L-selectin to the mucosal vascular addressin.[326] The α4 integrins (CD49d/CD29, VLA-4) also participate in lymphocyte binding to Peyer's patch HEVs and participate as well in the interaction of memory T cells with endothelial cells in multiple organs.[336-338]

A high-affinity CD11a/CD18 (LFA-1) form is induced on activated leukocytes[323] and promotes CD11a/CD18 interaction with CD54 (ICAM-1) on endothelial cells. Similarly, CD44 interacts with hyaluronate on cells of HEVs.[339] Whereas the selectins and their ligands are important in the initial stages of leukocyte–endothelial cell interactions, CD11a/CD18, CD54, CD44-hyaluronate interactions, and other integrin-ligand pairs are important in the later phases of leukocyte-HEV binding and in the promotion of leukocyte migration through endothelial cell layers into tissue perivascular areas (reviewed in references 326, 332, 337, and 340).

Post–Bone Marrow Antigen-Dependent B-Cell Maturation

After expression of sIgM and sIgD, B cells leave bone marrow and enter the peripheral circulation.

Naive sIg+ B lymphocytes recirculate among lymph nodes, gut-associated Peyer's patches, and splenic white pulp.[107, 320, 322] Both the size and the composition of the secondary B-cell compartment are tightly controlled[30, 341, 342]; antiproliferative cytokines such as LIF and TGFβ may play a role in this process.[94, 95]

B-cell follicles in peripheral lymphoid organs in which no antigen-driven processes are taking place are termed *primary follicles* and consist of a network of follicular dendritic cells in close apposition to recirculating sIgM+, sIgD+ small B cells.[107, 342] Primary follicles are present in lymph nodes early in human fetal development.[107, 342] *Secondary follicles* develop after birth and contain activated B cells triggered by foreign antigens.[107, 342, 343] Secondary follicles are characterized by the presence of discrete clusters of rapidly dividing B cells (germinal centers) formed in association with specific antigen deposits on follicular dendritic cells.[107, 342, 344] Secondary follicle formation and germinal center formation are antigen dependent and characteristically require T-cell help.[341, 342]

The initiation of a B-cell immune response in lymph nodes occurs outside the follicle in T-cell areas and involves interactions of naive B cells with helper T cells and interdigitating dendritic cells in the T-cell areas.[107, 345, 346] Upon binding of specific antigen to sIg, B-cell triggering occurs and surface expression of receptors for, and response to, IL-1, IL-2, IL-4, IL-5, and IL-6 occurs.[110]

Antigen-activated B cells give rise to antibody-forming plasma cells, memory B cells, or secondary follicle centroblasts.[107, 341, 342] A wave of B-cell activation and cell division occurring 1 to 2 days after antigen exposure is the earliest measurable response to antigen.[1, 30, 341] Antibody-secreting plasma cells producing IgM antibodies appear 3 to 4 days after antigen exposure. Plasma cells continue to express sIgM but no longer express sIgD or the major B-lineage antigens CD19, CD20, CD21, or CD22.[107]

B-cell blasts fill lymph node germinal centers 4 to 6 days after antigen exposure.[107, 342] At this stage, primary B-cell blasts migrate to one edge of the germinal center follicular network, termed the *dark zone* (Fig. 12–13). The blasts, now termed centroblasts, exhibit surface phenotypic changes, including the loss of immunoglobulin, E-selectin, and CD44, and cease expression of receptors for IL-1, IL-2, IL-3, IL-4, IL-5, and IL-6.[110] Centroblasts give rise to non-dividing centrocytes that express sIg. Centrocytes enter the dense follicular dendritic cell network of the follicle *(light zone)* of the germinal center.

Recruitment of naive B cells into T-cell–dependent antibody responses occurs only in the first few days after exposure to antigen[347]; sustained antibody responses are maintained by memory B-cell clones. Initial antibody produced in response to antigen is low-affinity IgM.[341, 342] During antibody maturation, a wave of somatic mutation events occurs within rearranged immunoglobulin genes.[104-106] Immunoglobulin V region–directed mutation is induced in cells that have already been stimulated by antigen and generates

TABLE 12-10. LEUKOCYTE–ENDOTHELIAL CELL ADHESION MOLECULES

LEUKOCYTE MOLECULE	DISTRIBUTION	LIGAND	FUNCTIONS
Selectin Family			
E-selectin (LECAM-1, LAM-1)	Leukocyte	Lymph node addressin	Regulates leukocyte binding to inflamed endothelium; lymph node homing receptor
P-selectin (GMP-140)	Endothelial cells, α granules of platelets	Sialylated derivatives of Lewis X oligosaccharides	Involved in initial leukocyte–endothelial cell interactions
L-selectin (ELAM-1)	Endothelial cells	Sialylated derivatives of Lewis X oligosaccharides	Involved in initial leukocyte–endothelial cell interactions
Integrin Family			
α1β1 (VLA-1, CD49a)	Activated T cells, monocytes, endothelial cells	Laminin, collagen	Activation-dependent adhesion receptor; marker for memory T cells
α2β1 (VLA-2, CD49b)	Leukocytes, endothelial cells widespread	Collagen	Activation-dependent adhesion receptor
α3β1 (VLA-3, CD49c)	Leukocytes, endothelial cells widespread	Fibronectin, collagen, laminin	Activation-dependent adhesion receptor
α4β1 (VLA-4, CD49d)	Leukocytes	VCAM-1, fibronectin fragment, vascular addressin	Involved in organ-specific homing; activation upregulates adhesion
α5β1 (VLA-5, CD49e)	Leukocytes, endothelial cells widespread	Fibronectin	Activation-dependent adhesion receptor; marker for memory T cells
α6β1 (VLA-6, CD49f)	Widespread	Laminin	Adhesion to endothelial cells
αLβ2 (LFA-1, CD11a)	Leukocytes	ICAM-1, ICAM-2	Activation-dependent adhesion receptor
αMβ2 (MAC-1, CD11a)	Myeloid, NK cells	ICAM-1, C3bi, factor X	Activation-dependent adhesion receptor; mediates adhesion of myeloid cells to endothelial cells
αXβ1 (p150, 95, CD11c)	Myeloid cells, subset of lymphocytes	?	Activation-dependent adhesion receptor; mediates binding of myeloid cells to ligands derived from complement cascade
Immunoglobulin Gene Superfamily			
CD2	T cells, NK cells	CD58 (LFA-3)	Activation-dependent adhesion receptor; can transmit proliferation signal
CD54 (ICAM-1)	Activated lymphocytes, thymic epithelium, cytokine (IL-1, TNFα, IFN-γ)–stimulated endothelial cells	LFA-1, rhinoviruses, *P. falciparum*	Upregulated expression on many tissues; mediates endothelial-leukocyte adherence
ICAM-2	Endothelial cells	LFA-1	Mediates leukocyte-endothelial adherence
ICAM-3	All resting leukocytes	LFA-1	Leukocyte-leukocyte interactions prior to leukocyte activation
CD58 (LFA-3)	Most tissue cell types	CD2	Upregulated expression in lymphoid tissues; involved in cytotoxic T lymphocytes (CTL): target cell interactions
VCAM-1 (InCAM-110)	TNFα-stimulated and IL-1–stimulated endothelial cells, follicular dendritic cells	VLA-4 (α4β1)	Mediates homing of VLA-4 + leukocytes to Peyer's patches; mediates binding of B cells to germinal centers
Cartilage Link Protein Family			
CD44 (Hermes, Pgp1, EcMRIII)	Leukocytes, widespread	Hyaluronate	Mediates leukocyte adhesion to endothelial cells, probably by activation-dependent adhesion

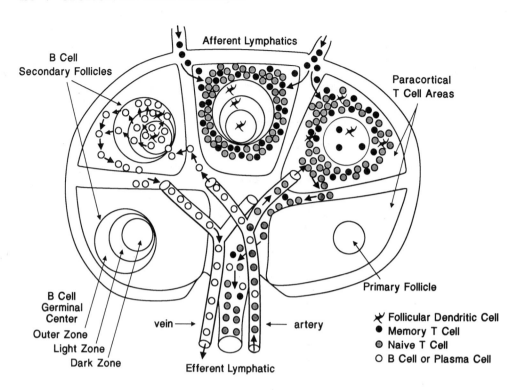

FIGURE 12–13. T- and B-cell migration routes in peripheral lymph nodes.

Labels on figure:

Afferent Lymphatics

B Cell Secondary Follicles

Paracortical T Cell Areas

B Cell Germinal Center
Outer Zone
Light Zone
Dark Zone

vein → ← artery

Efferent Lymphatic

Primary Follicle

⚕ Follicular Dendritic Cell
● Memory T Cell
◉ Naive T Cell
○ B Cell or Plasma Cell

further diversity of the B-cell repertoire.[105] Large numbers of B cells are produced by the mutation process during the centroblast stage, and germinal center B cells with low-affinity sIg are lost by apoptosis, whereas high-affinity sIg+ B cells survive. Thus, the high death rate of B cells in the light zone of the germinal center reflects a selection process of cells with high-affinity sIg for antigen.[107, 348]

B cells that are selected for a high affinity for antigen migrate outward in the germinal center light zone to an area termed the *apical light zone*. Here, B cells encounter CD23+ follicular dendritic cells. Antigen-selected B cells may receive paracrine signals delivered through CD23 and IL1.[107] Interaction of CD40 with its natural ligand may also promote B-cell survival at this stage.[107, 349] Cells stimulated through either the B-cell receptor complex, CD23 plus IL-1, or the CD40 antibody express the protein product of the bcl-2 gene that inhibits B-cell apoptosis and allows cell survival (reviewed in reference 30). Expression of the bcl-2 protein is also a marker for B cells that leave the germinal center.

The B-cell activation process results in two different B-cell types: memory B cells and plasmablasts. Memory B cells are non-dividing cells that re-enter the circulating lymphocyte pool and provide the ability for high-affinity secondary antigen responses.[107, 341, 350] Recent data have demonstrated the retention of antigen in follicular dendritic cells for up to 12 months and have shown that long-lived memory in both B and T cells depends on persistent antigen stimulation in lymph node and spleen.[351, 352] Plasmablasts produced from follicular B-cell blasts migrate to the bone marrow or the lamina propria of the gut, where they also give rise to plasma cells.[107] Plasma cells continue to produce antigen-specific antibody in the bone marrow or lamina propria for approximately 4 weeks. It has been postulated that B cells stimulated via CD23 in the light zone give rise to plasmablasts, whereas B cells stimulated via CD40 or other pathways develop into memory B cells.[353]

Post-thymic Antigen-Dependent T-Cell Maturation

Naive post-thymic T lymphocytes are CD45RA+, CD44lo+, CD58lo+ or −, CD2lo+, and CD11a/18lo+.[354–358] In contrast, following contact with antigen, memory T cells express high levels of a number of adhesion molecules and are CD45ROhi+, CD44hi+, CD58hi+, CD2hi+, and CD11a/CD18hi+ and have high expression of the fibronectin or laminin receptors, VLA4, VLA5, and VLA6.[354–358] In cord blood, all T cells initially are CD45RO− or lo+, and the percentage of CD45ROhi+ T cells increases with age.[245] Cross-linking many of the adhesion receptors on memory T cells is a potent co-mitogenic signal for CD3/TCR-mediated T-cell triggering and has been postulated to enhance T-cell activation when adhesion molecules are bound to their ligands, such as fibronectin, laminin, and hyaluronic acid, in vivo.[359–362]

Both in mice and in humans, maintenance of the peripheral lymphoid pool is not solely dependent on thymus exports but rather is dependent on antigen-driven expansion of peripheral T cells.[23, 24, 356] Studies in mice have clearly shown that post-thymic peripheral T cells have the capacity to repopulate the T-cell pool in irradiated and thymectomized animals (reviewed in reference 24).

Like negative selection in the thymus, clonal deletion of self-reactive T cells can occur in the periphery against self-antigens that are expressed only in peripheral lymphoid organs.[280] Non-reactivity to self-antigens can also be maintained by clonal anergy in the peripheral lymphoid organs, whereby contact with self-antigens induces downregulation of TCR expression and abrogates the response of T cells to antigen without killing the self-reactive T cell.[280]

Both T and B lymphocytes recirculate in the long-lived lymphocyte pool. Most of the lymphocytes in thoracic duct lymph are T cells.[356] It has been thought for years that after contact with antigen, memory T cells are generated and circulate for 4 to 6 months in the blood, lymph node, efferent lymph, thoracic duct route.[356, 357] Recent data are challenging this view and suggest that long-lived circulating T cells are CD45RA+ naive T cells that arrive in lymph nodes via adhesion to HEV, whereas CD45RO+ memory T cells recirculate through a blood, tissue, afferent lymphatic, lymph node route[340, 356, 357] (see Fig. 12–13). Once in the lymph node, only a minority of memory T cells leave the node by efferent lymph and enter the long-lived recirculating pool of lymphocytes.[340, 356] Data now support the idea that T-cell memory is maintained by repeated stimulation of T cells by retained antigen in antigen-presenting cells (reviewed in references 340, 356, and 357). Thus, many memory T cells likely die in secondary lymphoid organs rather than recirculate on a long-term basis.

DISEASES OF DISORDERED LYMPHOPOIESIS

General Overview

Overreactive immune responses to foreign or self-antigens manifest clinically as inflammatory, allergic, or autoimmune disease syndromes. Overproduction of immune cells is seen in leukemias and lymphomas, and underproduction or destruction of immune cells occurs in congenital and acquired immunodeficiency syndromes. Although it is beyond the scope of this chapter to review all of the clinical manifestations of disordered lymphopoiesis, immune dysfunction in AIDS will be discussed as an example of how the normal processes discussed above can go awry and lead to dysfunction of the lymphopoietic system.

Immune Dysfunction in the Acquired Immunodeficiency Syndrome

Human immunodeficiency virus infection in humans in most cases leads to progressive loss of the CD4+ T-cell pool, premature destruction of the thymus, and eventually death due to either overwhelming infections or malignancies (reviewed in reference 363). Loss of CD4+ T cells leads to defects in the generation of specific antibody responses to antigen, defects in antiviral cytolytic T-cell function, and loss of normal

immune surveillance mechanisms that control the expansion of malignant cells.[363] The cellular receptor for HIV is the CD4 molecule that is expressed on T cells, monocytes, and all varieties of tissue macrophages (glial cells, synovial lining cells, liver Kupffer's cells, skin Langerhans' cells, and lymph node antigen-presenting dendritic cells).[364, 365] Thus, not only are CD4+ T cells infected with HIV but all of the cell types in the body that express even low levels of CD4 can be infected with HIV as well. Table 12–11 shows the potential sites of damage to the immune system in HIV infection.

HIV DAMAGE TO BONE MARROW. Macrophages, monocytes, and megakaryocytes all express varying levels of CD4 and have been shown to be infectable with HIV.[364, 366] In some patients with HIV infection, bone marrow CD34+ cells have been isolated and shown to contain HIV.[367] It is not known if bone marrow stromal cells are infectable with HIV, but the generative bone marrow microenvironment does not function normally in HIV infection.[368]

THYMIC DAMAGE IN HIV INFECTION. The thymus in AIDS undergoes several pathological changes.[369] Thymic atrophy is common owing to an inordinate decrease in TE and thymocyte number.[369] Foci of necrotic TE cells are frequently present. In the early stages of HIV infection, B-cell follicles and germinal centers, multinucleated giant cells, and plasma cell infiltrates are common in the thymus.[369] Later in HIV infection, the thymus shows a dysplastic morphology with loss of cortex and medullary zones and a decrease in the number of Hassall's bodies as well as calcification of these bodies.[369] An anti–TE-cell antibody response in HIV has been implicated by the finding of antibody and complement on the remaining TE cells in the thymus.[370]

The implications of the thymic histopathology in AIDS are that normal T-cell maturation is disrupted and, similarly, that TE-cell maturation and function are also disrupted. The lack of thymocytes in the AIDS-affected thymus signifies that the normal seeding of the thymus by postnatal bone marrow HSCs has been interrupted, by HIV-induced dysfunction of

TABLE 12–11. POTENTIAL SITES OF DAMAGE TO IMMUNE CELLS IN AIDS

Bone Marrow
  Infection of T-cell precursors
  Infection of macrophage/monocytes/megakaryocytes
  ?Infection of BM stroma
Thymus
  Infection of T-cell precursors
  Infection of developing thymocytes
  Infection of macrophage/monocytes
  Infection of medullary dendritic cells
  Disruption of TE-thymocyte interactions, leading to disordered TE-cell cytokine secretion
Peripheral Pool of Hematopoietic Cells
  Infection of T cells
  Infection of macrophage/monocytes
  Infection of peripheral microenvironment dendritic cells

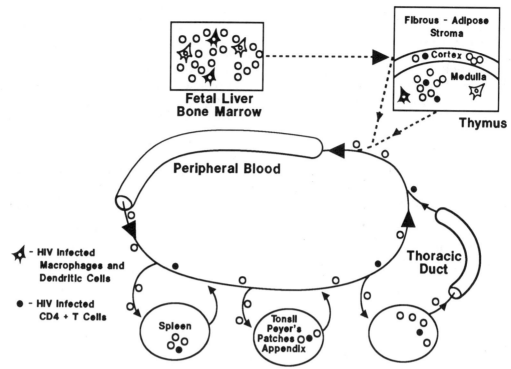

FIGURE 12–14. T-cell maturation in AIDS.

either the thymus or the bone marrow. Because normal thymocyte maturation is disrupted, normal migration of mature T cells from the thymus does not occur. Finally, disordered TE-cell function is implied by antibody-mediated TE-cell damage.[370]

In humans, intrathymic T-cell precursors express low levels of CD4 and are capable of being infected with HIV in vitro.[260] Certainly, the more mature developing thymocytes that are DP CD4+ and SP CD4+ cells are capable of being infected with HIV.[260] However, of perhaps equal importance is the fact that thymic macrophages and thymic dendritic cells are CD4+ and are also capable of supporting HIV infection. Thus, damage to the generative microenvironments of bone marrow and thymus may be a central feature of the inability of the T-cell arm of the immune system to regenerate in AIDS.

DAMAGE TO THE PERIPHERAL IMMUNE SYSTEM IN AIDS. Although a small number of peripheral T cells can be shown to be infected with HIV,[365] the level of infection does not explain the profound T-cell lymphopenia that occurs in the terminal stages of AIDS. It has recently been proposed that peripheral T cells from patients with AIDS are inordinately susceptible to undergoing apoptosis following T-cell activation.[371] Lymph node dendritic cells as well as lymph node T cells are infected with HIV in vivo, and given the importance of antigen-driven expansion of the peripheral T-cell pool for maintaining the level of T lymphocytes in the periphery postnatally, HIV-induced dysfunction and destruction of antigen-presenting cells in lymph node and in other peripheral immune microenvironments likely also contributes to progres-

sive CD4+ T-cell lymphopenia.[363] Figure 12–14 summarizes the state of the immune system during the later stages of active HIV infection in man.

CONCLUSIONS AND FUTURE DIRECTIONS

Understanding the molecular basis of the normal function of the immune system has provided remarkable insights into the pathophysiological abnormalities present in immune-mediated diseases and in immunodeficiency syndromes. In the not-so-distant future, immunologists will be identifying pathogenic clones of T and B cells that overreact to cause the various autoimmune diseases and inflammatory disease syndromes. Sequencing of immunoglobulin and T-cell receptors will provide the sequences needed for development of interventional immunotherapeutic strategies for autoimmune diseases targeted toward idiotypic determinants on T and B cells. Similarly, understanding the molecular basis of lymphocyte interactions, responses to cytokines, and lymphocyte homing has provided multiple new sites of therapeutic interventions for autoimmune and lymphoproliferative diseases. For autoimmune diseases, new therapies are being devised, using recombinant adhesion molecules to inhibit normal immune cell interactions and to inhibit the homing of inflammatory cells to the sites of organ-specific tissue damage. Recombinant hematopoietic cytokine therapy is already a clinically proven effective therapy for various deficiencies of myeloid cell lines and for boosting NK and T-cell responses to tumor antigens. For the immunodeficiency syndromes, the rapid progress made in identifying HSCs and the precursors of the T and B lineages has made immune reconstitution of multiple hematopoietic lineages a reality.

Thus, recent research advances have provided a remarkable view of how the human immune system develops and functions and has set the stage for extraordinary advances to be made in the treatment of diseases of disordered lymphopoiesis. Although much remains to be understood regarding the mechanisms of normal lymphopoiesis, a firm foundation has been laid to ensure rapid progress.

REFERENCES

1. Butcher, E. C., and Weissman, I. L.: Lymphoid tissues and organs. *In* Paul, W. (ed.): Fundamental Immunology. New York, Raven Press, 1989, pp. 117–137.
2. Bernard, A., Boumsell, L., Dausset, J., Milstein, C., and Schlossman, S.: Proceedings of the First International Workshop and Conference on Human Leukocyte Differentiation Antigens. Heidelberg, Germany, Springer-Verlag, 1984.
3. Reinherz, E., Haynes, B. F., Nadler, L., and Bernstein, L.: Proceedings of the Second International Workshop and Conference on Human Leukocyte Differentiation Antigens. Heidelberg, Germany, Springer-Verlag, 1986.
4. McMichael, A. J.: Leukocyte Typing III. Oxford, England, Oxford University Press, 1987.
5. Knapp, W., Dorken, B., Gilks, W. R., Rieber, E. P., Schmidt, R. E., Stein, H., and von dem Borne, A. E. G.: Leucocyte Typing IV: White Cell Differentiation Antigens. Oxford, England, Oxford University Press, 1991.
6. Moore, M. A., and Metcalf, D.: Ontogeny of the haemopoietic system: Yolk sac origin of *in vivo* and *in vitro* colony forming cells in the developing mouse embryo. Br. J. Haematol. 18:279, 1970.
7. Jotereau, F. V., and LeDouarin, N. M.: Demonstration of a cycle renewal of the lymphocyte precursor cells in the quail thymus during embryonic and perinatal life. J. Immunol. 129:1809, 1982.
8. Coltey, M., Bucy, R. P., Chen, C. H., Cihak, J., Losch, U., Char, D., LeDouarin, N. M., and Cooper, M. D.: Analysis of the first two waves of thymus homing stem cells and their T cell progeny in chick-quail chimeras. J. Exp. Med. 170:543, 1989.
9. Bloom, W., and Bartelmez, G. W.: Hematopoiesis in young human embryos. Am. J. Anat. 67:21, 1940.
10. Moore, M. A. S., and Owen, J. J. T.: Experimental studies on the development of the thymus. J. Exp. Med. 126:715, 1967.
11. Owen, J. J. T., and Jenkinson E. J.: Early events in T lymphocyte genesis in the fetal thymus. Am. J. Anat. 170:301, 1984.
12. Kelemen, E., Calvo, W., and Fliedner, T.: Atlas of Human Hemopoietic Development. Berlin, Springer-Verlag, 1979.
13. Lobach, D. F., and Haynes, B. F.: Ontogeny of the human thymus during fetal development. J. Clin. Immunol. 7:81, 1987.
14. Gathings, W. E., Lawton, A. R., and Cooper, M. D.: Immunofluorescent studies of the development of pre-B cells, B lymphocytes and immunoglobulin isotype diversity in humans. Eur. J. Immunol. 7:804, 1977.
15. Kamps, W. A., and Cooper, M. D.: Microenvironmental studies of pre-B and B cell development in human and mouse fetuses. J. Immunol. 129:526, 1982.
16. Kamps, W. A., and Cooper, M. D.: Development of lymphocyte subpopulations identified by monoclonal antibodies in human fetuses. J. Clin. Immunol. 4:36, 1984.
17. Rosenthal, P., Rimm, I. J., Umiel, T., Griffin, J. D., Osathanondh, R., Schlossman, S. F., and Nadler, L. M.: Ontogeny of human hematopoietic cells: Analysis utilizing monoclonal antibodies. J. Immunol. 31:232, 1983.

18. Uckun, F. M., Gajl-Peczalska, K., Myers, D. E., Jaszcz, W., Haissig, S., and Ledbetter, J. A.: Temporal association of CD40 antigen expression with discrete stages of human B-cell ontogeny and the efficacy of anti-CD40 immunotoxins against clonogenic B-lineage acute lymphoblastic leukemia as well as B-lineage non-Hodgkin's lymphoma cells. Blood 76:2449, 1990.
19. Dosch, H., Lam, P., Hui, M. F., and Hibi, T.: Concerted generation of Ig isotype diversity in human fetal bone marrow. J. Immunol. 143:2464, 1989.
20. Campana, D., Janossy, G., Coustan-Smith, E., Amlot, P. L., Tian, W., Ip, S., and Wong, L.: The expression of T cell receptor–associated proteins during T cell ontogeny in man. J. Immunol. 142:57, 1989.
21. Ikuta, K., Uchida, N., Friedman, J., and Weissman, I. L.: Lymphocyte development from stem cells. Annu. Rev. Immunol. 10:759, 1992.
22. Shortman, K., Egeston, M., Spangrude, G. J., and Scollay, R.: The generation and fate of thymocytes. Semin. Immunol. 2:3, 1990.
23. Stutman, O.: Postthymic T cell development. Immunol. Rev. 91:159, 1986.
24. Miller, R. A., and Stutman, O.: T cell repopulation from functionally restricted splenic progenitors: 10,000-fold expansion documented by using limiting dilution analyses. J. Immunol. 133:2925, 1984.
25. Horst, E., Meijer, C. J., Duijvestijn, A. M., Hartwig, N., Van der Harten, J. H., and Pals, S. T.: The ontogeny of human lymphocyte recirculation: High endothelial cell antigen (HECA-452) and CD44 homing receptor expression in the development of the immune system. Eur. J. Immunol. 20:1483, 1990.
26. Royo, C., Touraine, J. L., and DeBouteiller, O.: Ontogeny of T lymphocyte differentiation in the human fetus: Acquisition of phenotype and functions. Thymus 10:57, 1987.
27. Silverstein, A. M., and Lukes, R. J.: Fetal response to antigenic stimulus: Plasmacellular and lymphoid reactions in the human fetus to intrauterine infection. Lab. Invest. 11:918, 1962.
28. Hayward, A. R., and Ezer, G.: Development of lymphocyte populations in the human foetal thymus and spleen. Clin. Exp. Immunol 17:169, 1974.
29. Toivanen, P., Uksila, J., Leino, A., Lassila, O., Hirvonen, T., and Ruuskanen, O.: Development of mitogen responding T cells and natural killer cells in the human fetus. Immunol. Rev. 57:89, 1981.
30. Rolink, A., and Melchers, F.: Molecular and cellular origins of B lymphocyte diversity. Cell 66:1081, 1991.
31. Mackay, C. R., Kimpton, W. G., Brandon, M. R., and Cahill, R. N. P.: Lymphocyte subsets show marked differences in their distribution between blood and the afferent and efferent lymph of peripheral lymph nodes. J. Exp. Med. 167:1755, 1988.
32. Scollay, R. G., Butcher, E. C., and Weissman, I. L.: Thymus cell migration quantitative aspects of cellular traffic from the thymus to the periphery in mice. Eur. J. Immunol. 10:210, 1980.
33. Kendall, M. D.: Have we underestimated the importance of the thymus in man? Experientia 40:1181, 1984.
34. Spangrude, G. J., Smith, L., Uchida, N., Ikuta, K., Heimfeld, S., Friedman, J., and Weissman I. L.: Mouse hematopoietic stem cells. Blood 78:1395, 1991.
35. Till, J. E., and McCullooch, E. A.: A direct measurement of the radiation sensitivity of normal mouse bone marrow cells. Radiat. Res. 14:213, 1961.
36. Keller, G., Paige, C., Gilboa, E., and Wagner, E. F.: Expression of a foreign gene in myeloid and lymphoid cells derived from multipotent haematopoietic precursors. Nature 318:149, 1985.
37. Lemischka, I. R., Raulet, D. H., and Mulligan, R. C.: Developmental potential and dynamic behavior of hematopoietic stem cells. Cell 45:917, 1986.
38. Muller-Sieburg, C. E., Townsend, K., Weissman, I. L., and Rennick, D.: Proliferation and differentiation of highly

enriched mouse hematopoietic stem cells and progenitor cells in response to defined growth factors. Science 241:1825, 1988.

39. Spangrude, G. J., Heimfeld, S., and Weissman, I. L.: Purification and characterization of mouse hematopoietic stem cells. Science 241:58, 1988.

40. Heimfeld, S., Guidos, C. J., Holzmann, B., Siegelman, M. H., and Weissman I. L.: Development analysis of the mouse hematolymphoid system. Cold Spring Harb. Symp. Quant. Biol. 54:75, 1989.

41. Spangrude, G. J., Klein, J., Heimfeld, S., Aihara, Y., and Weissman, I. L.: Two monoclonal antibodies identify thymic-repopulating cells in mouse bone marrow. J. Immunol. 142:425, 1989.

42. Heimfeld, S., Hudak, S., Weissman, I. L., and Rennick, D.: The in vitro response of phenotypically defined mouse stem cells and myeloerythroid progenitors to single or multiple growth factors. Proc. Natl. Acad. Sci. USA 88:9902, 1991.

43. Smith, L. G., Weissman, I. L., and Heimfeld, S.: Clonal analysis of hematopoietic stem-cell differentiation *in vivo*. Proc. Natl. Acad. Sci. USA 88:2788, 1991.

44. Heimfeld, S., and Weissman, I. L.: Development of mouse hematopoietic lineages. Curr. Top. Dev. Biol. 25:155, 1991.

45. Uchida, N., and Weissman, I. L.: Searching for hematopoietic stem cells: Evidence that Thy-1.1lo Lin-Sca-1 + cells are the only stem cells in C57BL/Ka-Thy.1.1 bone marrow. J. Exp. Med. 175:175, 1992.

46. Spangrude, G. J., and Johnson, G. R.: Resting and activated subsets of mouse multipotent hematopoietic stem cells. Proc. Natl. Acad. Sci. USA 87:7433, 1990.

47. Schiff, S., and Buckley, R. H: Modified responses to recipient and donor B cells by genetically donor T cells from human haploidentical bone marrow chimeras. J. Immunol. 138:2088, 1987.

48. Roncarolo, M. G., Yssel, H., Touraine, J. L., et al.: Antigen recognition by MHC-incompatible cells of a human mismatched chimera. J. Exp. Med. 168:2139, 1988.

49. Berenson, R. J., Bensinger, W. I., Hill, R. S., Andrews, R. G., Garcia-Lopes, J., Kalamasz, D. F., Still, B. J., Spitzer, G., Buckner, C. D., Bernstein, I. D., and Thomas, E. D.: Engraftment after infusion of CD34+ marrow cells with breast cancer and neuroblastoma. Blood 77:1717, 1991.

50. Berenson, R. J., Andrews, R. G., Bensinger, W. I., Kalamasz, D., Knitter, G., Buckner, C. D., and Bernstein, I. D.: CD34+ marrow cells engraft lethally irradiated baboons. J. Clin. Invest. 81:951, 1988.

51. Hershfield, M. S., Kurtzberg, J., Harden, E., Moore, J. O., Whang-Peng, J., and Haynes, B. F.: Conversion of a stem cell leukemia from a T-lymphoid to a myeloid phenotype induced by the adenosine deaminase inhibitor 2'-deoxycoformycin. Proc. Natl. Acad. Sci. USA 81:253, 1984.

52. Kurtzberg, J., Waldmann, T. A., Davey, M. P., Bigner, S. H., Moore, J. O., Hershfield, M. S., and Haynes, B. F.: CD7+, CD4−, Cd8-acute leukemia: A syndrome of malignant pluripotent lymphohematopoietic cells. Blood 73:381, 1989.

53. Griesinger, F., Arthur, D. C., Brunning, R., Parkin, J. L., Ochoa, A. C., Miller, W. J., Wilkowski, C. W., Greenberg, J. M., Hurwitz, C., and Kersey, J. H.: Mature T-lineage leukemia with growth factor–induced multilineage differentiation. J. Exp. Med. 169:1101, 1989.

54. O'Connor, R., Cesano, A., Kreider, B. L., Lange, B., Clark, S. C., Nowell, P. C., Finan, J., Rovera, G., and Santoli, D.: Growth factor–dependent differentiation along the myeloid and lymphoid lineages in an immature acute T lymphocytic leukemia. J. Immunol. 145:3779, 1990.

55. Peault, B., Weissman, I. L., Baum, C., McCune, J. M., and Tsukamoto, A.: Lymphoid reconstitution of the human fetal thymus in SCID mice with CD34+ precursor cells. J. Exp. Med. 174:1283, 1991.

56. Baum, C. M., Weissman, I. L., Tsukamoto, A. S., Buckle, A., and Peault, B.: Isolation of a candidate human hematopoietic stem cell population. Proc. Natl. Acad. Sci. USA 89:2804, 1992.

57. Schiff, S. E., Kurtzberg, J., and Buckley, R. H.: Studies of

human bone marrow treated with soybean lectin and sheep erythrocytes: Stepwise analysis of cell morphology, phenotype and function. Clin. Exp. Immunol. 68:685, 1987.

58. Haynes, B. F., Eisenbarth, G. S., and Fauci, A. S.: Human lymphocyte antigens. Production of a monoclonal antibody which defines functional thymus derived lymphocyte subsets. Proc. Natl. Acad. Sci. USA 76:5829, 1979.

59. Aruffo, A., and Seed, B.: Molecular cloning of two CD7 (T cell leukemia antigen) cDNAs by a COS cell expression system. EMBO J. 6:3313, 1987.

60. Ware, R. E., Scearce, R. M., Dietz, M. A., Starmer, C. F., Palker, T. J., and Haynes, B. F.: Characterization of the surface topography and putative tertiary structure of the human CD7 molecule. J. Immunol. 143:3632, 1989.

61. Civin, C. I., Strauss, L. C., Brovall, C., Fackler, M. J., Schwartz, J. F., and Shaper, J. H.: Antigenic analysis of hematopoiesis: A hematopoietic progenitor cell surface antigen defined by a monoclonal antibody raised against KG-1a cells. J. Immunol. 133:157, 1984.

62. Simmons, D. L., Satterthwaite, A. B., Tenen, D. G., and Seed, B.: Molecular cloning of a cDNA encoding CD34, a sialomucin of human hematopoietic stem cells. J. Immunol. 148:267, 1992.

63. Haynes, B. F., Denning, S. M., Singer, K. H., and Kurtzberg, J.: Ontogeny of T cell precursors: A model for the initial stages of human T-cell development. Immunol. Today 10:87, 1989.

64. Haynes, B. F., Denning, S. M., Le, P. T., and Singer, K. H.: Human intrathymic T cell differentiation. Semin. Immunol. 2:67, 1990.

65. Brandt, J., Baird, N., Lu, L., Srour, E., and Hoffman, R.: Characterization of a human hematopoietic progenitor cell capable of forming blast cell containing colonies in vitro. J. Clin. Invest. 82:1017, 1988.

66. Andrews, R. G., Singer, J. W., and Bernstein, I. D.: Precursors of colony-forming cells in humans can be distinguished from colony-forming cells by expression of the CD33 and CD34 antigens and light scatter properties. J. Exp. Med. 169:1721, 1989.

67. Sutherland, H. J., Eaves, C. J., Eaves, A. C., Dragowska, W., and Lansdorp, P. M.: Characterization and partial purification of human marrow cells capable of initiating long-term hematopoiesis in vitro. Blood 74:1563, 1989.

68. Verfaillie, C., Blakolmer, K., and McGlave, P.: Purified primitive human hematopoietic progenitor cells with long-term in vitro repopulating capacity adhere selectively to irradiated bone marrow stroma. J. Exp. Med. 172:509, 1990.

69. Gabbianelli, M., Sargiacomo, M., Pelosi, E., Testa, U., Isacchi, G., and Peschle, C.: "Pure" human hematopoietic progenitors: Permissive action of basic fibroblast growth factor. Science 249:1561, 1990.

70. Andrews, R. G., Singer, J. W., and Bernstein, I. D.: Human hematopoietic precursors in long-term culture: Single CD34+ cells that lack detectable T cell, B cell, and myeloid cell antigens produce multiple colony-forming cells when cultured with marrow stromal cells. J. Exp. Med. 172:355, 1990.

71. Bernstein, I. D., Andrews, R. G., and Zsebo, K. M.: Recombinant human stem cell factor enhances the formation of colonies by CD34+ and CD34+lin- cells, and the generation of colony-forming cell progeny from CD34+lin- cells cultured with interleukin-3, granulocyte colony-stimulating factor, or granulocyte-macrophage colony-stimulating factor. Blood 77:2316, 1991.

72. Bernstein, I. D., Leary, A. G., Andrews, R. G., and Ogawa, M.: Blast colony-forming cells and precursors of colony-forming cells detectable in long-term marrow culture express the same phenotype (CD33− CD34+). Exp. Hematol. 19:680, 1991.

73. Terstappen, W. M. M., Huang, S., Safford, M., and Lansdorp, P. M. L.: Sequential generations of hematopoietic colonies derived from single nonlineage-committed CD34+CD38− progenitor cells. Blood 77:1, 1991.

74. Lansdorp, P. M., Sutherland, H. J., and Eaves, C. J.: Selective

expression of CD45 isoforms on functional subpopulations of CD34+ hemopoietic cells from human bone marrow. J. Exp. Med. 172:363, 1990.

75. Stong, R. C., Uckun, F., Youle, R. J., Kersey, J. H., and Vallera, D. A.: Use of multiple T cell–directed intact ricin immunotoxins for autologous bone marrow transplantation. Blood 66:627, 1985.

76. Herve, P., Cahn, J. Y., Flesch, M., Plouvier, E., Noir, R. A., Couteret, Y., Goldstein, C. G., Bernard, A., Lenys, R., Bresson, J. L., Leconte des Floris, R., and Peters, A.: Successful graft versus host disease prevention without graft failure in 32 HLA-identical allogeneic bone marrow transplantations with marrow depleted of T cells by monoclonal antibodies and complement. Blood 69:388, 1987.

77. Preijers, W. M. B., DeWitte, T., Wessels, J. M. C., DeGast, G. C., Van Leeuwen, E., Capel, P. J. A. and Haanen, C.: Autologous transplantation of bone marrow purged in vitro with anti-CD7−(WT1−) ricin A immunotoxin in T cell lymphoblastic leukemia and lymphoma. Blood 74:1152, 1989.

78. Lobach, D. F., Hensley, L. L., Ho, W., and Haynes, B. F.: Human T cell antigen expression during the early stages of fetal thymic maturation. J. Immunol. 135:1752, 1985.

79. Grumayer, E. V., Griesinger, F., Hummell, D. S., Brunning, R. D., and Kersey, J. H.: Identification of novel B-lineage cells in human fetal bone marrow that co-express CD7. Blood 77:64, 1991.

80. Seremetis, S. V., Pelicci, P., Tabilio, A., Ubriaco, A., Grignani, F., Cuttner, J., Winchester, R. J., Knowles, D. M., and Dalla-Favera, R.: High frequency of clonal immunoglobulin or T cell receptor gene rearrangements in acute myelogenous leukemia expressing terminal deoxyribonucleotidyltransferase. J. Exp. Med. 165:1703, 1987.

81. Jensen, A. W., Hokland, M., Jorgensen, H., Justesen, J., Ellegaard, J., and Hokland, P.: Solitary expression of CD7 among T-cell antigens in acute myeloid leukemia: Identification of a group of patients with similar T-cell receptor β and γ rearrangements and course of disease suggestive of poor prognosis. Blood 78:1292, 1991.

82. Chaudhary, P. M. R., and Roninson, I. B.: Expression and activity of P-glycoprotein, a multidrug efflux pump, in human hematopoietic stem cells. Cell 66:85, 1991.

83. Bauman, J. G. J., Wagemaker, G., and Visser, J. W. M.: A fractionation procedure of mouse bone marrow cells yielding exclusively pluripotent stem cells and committed progenitors. J. Cell. Physiol. 128:133, 1986.

84. Kelly, K., Shortman, K., and Scollay, R.: The surface phenotype of activated T lymphocytes. Immunol. Cell Biol. 66:297, 1988.

85. O'Neill, H. C.: Antibody which defines a subset of bone marrow cells that can migrate to thymus. Immunology 68:59, 1989.

86. Lewinsohn, D. M., Nagler, A., Ginzton, N., Greenberg, P., and Butcher, E. C.: Hematopoietic progenitor cell expression of the H-CAM (CD44) homing-associated adhesion molecule. Blood 75:589, 1990.

87. Spangrude, G. J., and Scollay, R.: A simplified method for enrichment of mouse hematopoietic stem cells. Exp. Hematol. 18:920, 1990.

88. Williams, D. A., Rios, M., Stephens, C., and Patel, V. P.: Fibronectin and VLA-4 in haematopoietic stem cell–microenvironment interactions. Nature 352:438, 1991.

89. Miyake, K., Medina, K. L., Hayashi, S., Ono, S., Hamaoka, T., and Kincade, P. W.: Monoclonal antibodies to Pgp-1/CD44 block lympho-hemopoiesis in long-term bone marrow cultures. J. Exp. Med. 171:477, 1990.

90. Gluckman, E., Broxmeyer, H. E., Auerbach, A. D., Friedman, H. S., Devergie, A., Esperou, H., Thierry, D., Socie, G., Lehn, P., Cooper, S., English, P., Kurtzberg, J., Bard, J., and Boyse, E. A.: Hematopoietic reconstitution in a patient with Fanconi's anemia by means of umbilical-cord blood from an HLA-identical sibling. N. Engl. J. Med. 321:1174, 1989.

91. Broxmeyer, H. E., Douglas, G. W., Hangoc, G., Cooper, S.,

Bard, J., English, D., Arny, M., Thomas, L., and Boyse, E. A.: Human umbilical cord blood as a potential source of transplantable hematopoietic stem/progenitor cells. Proc. Natl. Acad. Sci. USA 86:3828, 1989.

92. Broxmeyer, H. E., Hangoc, G., Cooper, S., Ribeiro, R. C., Graves, V., Yoder, M., Wagner, J., Vadhan-Raj, S., Benninger, L., Rubinstein, P., and Broun, E. R.: Growth characteristics and expansion of human umbilical cord blood and estimation of its potential for transplantation of adults. Proc. Natl. Acad. Sci. USA 89:4109, 1992.

93. Schmitt, R. M., Bruyns, E., and Snodgrass, H. R.: Hematopoietic development of embryonic stem cells in vitro: Cytokine and receptor gene expression. Genes Dev. 5:728, 1991.

94. Dexter, T. M., and White, H.: Growth without inflation. Nature 344:380, 1990.

95. Hatzfeld, J., Li, M., Brown, E. L., Sookdeo, H., Levesque, J. P., O'Toole, T., Gurney, C., Clark, S. C., and Hatzfeld, A.: Release of early human hematopoietic progenitors from quiescence by antisense transforming growth factor β1 or Rb oligonucleotides. J. Exp. Med. 174:925, 1991.

96. Ikuta, K., and Weissman, I. L.: Evidence that hematopoietic stem cells express c-kit, but do not depend on Steel factor for their generation. Proc. Natl. Acad. Sci. USA 89:1502, 1992.

97. Tsuji, K., Zsebo, K. M., and Ogawa, M.: Murine mast cell colony formation supported by IL3, IL4, and recombinant rat stem cell factor, ligand for c-kit. J. Cell. Physiol. 148:362, 1991.

98. Carow, C. E., Hangoc, G., Cooper, S. H., Williams, D. E., and Broxmeyer, H. E.: Mast cell growth factor (c-kit ligand) supports the growth of human multipotential progenitor cells with a high replating potential. Blood 78:2216, 1991.

99. Tsuji, K., Zsebo, K. M., and Ogawa, M.: Enhancement of murine blast cell colony formation in culture by recombinant rat stem cell factor, ligand for c-kit. Blood 78:1223, 1991.

100. Ogawa, M.: Humoral regulation of early hemopoiesis studied in culture. In Murphy, M. J. (ed.): Blood Cell Growth Factors: Their Present and Future Use in Hematology and Oncology. Proceedings of the Beijing Symposium. Dayton, Ohio, AlphaMed Press, 1991.

101. Leary, A. G., Zeng, H. Q., Clark, S. C., and Ogawa, M.: Growth factor requirements for survival in Go and entry into the cell cycle of primitive human hemopoietic progenitors. Proc. Natl. Acad. Sci. USA 89:4013, 1992.

102. Musashi, M., Clark, S. C., Sudo, T., Urdal, D. L., and Ogawa, M.: Synergistic interactions between interleukin-11 and interleukin-4 in support of proliferation of primitive hematopoietic progenitors of mice. Blood 78:1448, 1991.

103. Musashi, M., Yang, Y., Paul, S. R., Clark, S. C., Sudo, T., and Ogawa, M.: Direct and synergistic effects of interleukin 11 on murine hemopoiesis in culture. Proc. Natl. Acad. Sci. USA 88:765, 1991.

104. Alt, F. W., Blackwell, T. K., and Yancopoulos, G. D.: Development of the primary antibody repertoire. Science 238:1079, 1987.

105. Tonegawa, S.: Somatic generation of antibody diversity. Nature 302:575, 1983.

106. Rajewsky, K., Forster, I., and Cumano, A.: Evolutionary and somatic selection of the antibody repertoire in the mouse. Science 238:1088, 1987.

107. Liu, Y., Johnson, G. D., Gordon, J., and MacLennan, I. C. M.: Germinal centres in T cell dependent antibody responses. Immunol. Today 13:17, 1992.

108. Osmond, D. G.: B cell development in the bone marrow. Semin. Immunol. 2:173, 1990.

109. Gallagher, R. B., and Osmond, D. G.: To B, or not to B: That is the question. Immunol. Today 12:1, 1991.

110. Uckun, F. M.: Regulation of human B-cell ontogeny. Blood 76:1908, 1990.

111. Burrows, P. D., and Cooper, M. D.: Regulated expression of cell surface antigens during B cell development. Semin. Immunol. 2:189, 1990.

112. Schroeder, H. W., Hillson, J. L., and Perlmutter, R. M.: Early

restriction of the human antibody repertoire. Science 238:791, 1987.

113. Cuisiner, A., Guigou, V., Boubli, L., Fougereau, M., and Tonnelle, C.: Preferential expression of VH5 and VH6 immunoglobulin genes in early human B-cell ontogeny. Scand. J. Immunol. 30:493, 1989.

114. Lydyard, P. M., Quartey-Papafio, R., Broker, B., Mackenzie, L., Jouquan, J., Blaschek, M. A., Steele, J., Petrou, M., Collins, P., Isenberg, D., and Youinou, P. Y.: The antibody repertoire of early human B cells. Scand J. Immunol 31:33, 1990.

115. Lydyard, P. M., Quartey-Papafio, R. P., Broker, B. M., Mackenzie, L., Hay, F. C., Youinou, P. Y., Jefferis, Y., and Mageed, R. A.: The antibody repertoire of early human B cells. III. Expression of cross-reactive idiotopes characteristic of certain rheumatoid factors and identifying VkIII, VHI and VHIII gene family products. Scand. J. Immunol. 32:709, 1990.

116. Clark, E. A., and Ledbetter, J. A.: Structure, function, and genetics of human B cell associated surface molecules. Adv. Cancer Res. 52:81, 1989.

117. Clark, E. A., and Lane, P. J. L.: Regulation of human B-cell activation and adhesion. Annu. Rev. Immunol. 9:97, 1991.

118. Letarte, M., Vera, S., Tran, R., Addis, J. B., Onizuka, R. J., Quackenbush, E. J., Jongeneel, C. V., and McInnes, R. R.: Common acute lymphocytic leukemia antigen is identical to neutral endopeptidase. J. Exp. Med. 168:1247, 1988.

119. Clark, E. A., and Ledbetter, J. A.: Leukocyte cell surface enzymology: CD45 (LCA, T200) is a protein tyrosine phosphatase. Immunol. Today 10:225, 1989.

120. Knapp, W., Rieber, P., Dorken, B., Schmidt, R. E., Stein, H., and Borne, A. E. G.: Towards a better definition of human leucocyte surface molecules. Immunol. Today 10:253, 1989.

121. Pesando, J. M., Bouchard, L. S., and McMaster, B. E.: CD19 is functionally and physically associated with surface immunoglobulin. J. Exp. Med. 170:2159, 1989.

122. Cooper, N. R., Moore, M. D., and Newerow, G. R.: Immunobiology of CR2, the B lymphocyte receptor for Epstein-Barr virus and the C3d complement component. Annu. Rev. Immunol. 6:85, 1988.

123. Einfeld, D. A., Brown, J. P., and Valentine, M. A.: Molecular cloning of the human B cell CD20 receptor predicts a hydrophobic protein with multiple transmembrane domains. EMBO J. 7:711, 1988.

124. Stamenkovic, I., Sgroi, D., Aruffo, A., Sy, M. S., and Anderson, T.: The B lymphocyte adhesion molecule CD22 interacts with leukocyte common antigen CD45RO on T cells and α2-6 sialyltransferase, CD75, on B cells. Cell 66:1133, 1991.

125. Linsley, P. S., Clark, E. A., and Ledbetter, J. A.: T-cell antigen CD28 mediates adhesion with B cells by interacting with activation antigen B7/BB-1. Proc. Natl. Acad. Sci. USA 87:5031, 1990.

126. Freeman, G. J., Freedman, A. S., Segil, J. M., Lee, G., Whitman, J. F., and Nadler, L. M.: B7, a new member of the Ig superfamily with unique expression on activated and neoplastic B cells. J. Immunol. 143:2714, 1989.

127. Kansas, G. S., and Dailey, M. O.: Expression of adhesion structures during B cell development in man. J. Immunol. 142:3058, 1989.

128. Clark, E. A.: CD40: A cytokine receptor in search of a ligand. Tissue Antigens 35:33, 1990.

129. Paulie, S., Rosen, A., Ehlin-Hendriksson, B., Braesch-Andersen, S., Jakobson, E., Koho, H., and Perlmann, P.: The human B lymphocyte and carcinoma antigen, CDw40, is a phosphoprotein involved in growth signal transduction. J. Immunol. 142:590, 1989.

130. Uckun, F. M., Gajl-Peczalska, K. J., Waddick, K. G., Hupke, M., Hanson, M., Langlie, M. C., Myers, D., and Ledbetter, J. A.: Expression and function of CD40/BP50 human B-cell receptor. Blood, Vol. 282, Supplement 1 (abstract), 1989.

131. Delespesse, G., Suter, U., Mossalayi, D., Bettler, B., Sarfati, M., Hofstetter, H., Kilcherr, E., Debre, P., and Dalloul, A.: Expression, structure, and function of the CD23 antigen. Adv. Immunol. 49:149, 1991.

132. Mossalayi, M. D., Dalloul, A. H., Fourcade, C., Arock, M., and Debre, P.: Soluble CD23 is a potent cytokine for early human haematopoietic precursors. Bull. Inst. Pasteur 89:139, 1991.

133. LeBien, T. W., Wormann, B., Villablanca, J. G., Law, C., Steinberg, L. M., Shah, V. O., and Loken, M. R.: Multiparameter flow cytometric analysis of human fetal bone marrow B cells. Leukemia 4:354, 1990.

134. Loken, M. R., Shah, V. O., Dattilio, K. L., and Civin, C. I.: Flow cytometric analysis of human bone marrow. II. Normal B lymphocyte development. Blood 70:1316, 1987.

135. Hokland, P., Hokland, M., Daley, J., and Ritz, J.: Identification and cloning of a prethymic precursor T lymphocyte from a population of common acute lymphoblastic leukemia antigen (CALLA)–positive fetal bone marrow cells. J. Exp. Med. 165:1749, 1987.

136. LeBien, T. W., Elstrom, R. L., Moseley, M., Kersey, J. H., and Griesinger, F.: Analysis of immunoglobulin and T cell receptor gene rearrangements in human fetal bone marrow B lineage cells. Blood 76:1196, 1990.

137. Nishimoto, N., Kubagawa, H., Ohno, T., Gartland, G. L., Stankovic, A. K., and Cooper, M. D.: Normal pre-B cells express a receptor complex of μ heavy chains and surrogate light-chain proteins. Proc. Natl. Acad. Sci. USA 88:6284, 1991.

138. Dorshkind, K.: Regulation of hemopoiesis by bone marrow stromal cells and their products. Annu. Rev. Immunol. 8:111, 1990.

139. Whitlock, C. A., Robertson, D., and Witte, O. N.: Murine B cell lymphopoiesis in long term culture. J. Immunol. Methods 67:353, 1984.

140. Henderson, A. J., and Dorshkind, K.: In vitro models of B lymphocyte development. Semin. Immunol. 2:181, 1990.

141. Kincade, P. W., Lee, G., Pietrangeli, C. E., Hayashi, S., and Gimble, J. M.: Cells and molecules that regulate B lymphopoiesis in bone marrow. Annu. Rev. Immunol. 7:111, 1989.

142. Dorshkind, K.: In vitro differentiation of B lymphocytes from primitive hemopoietic precursors present in long-term bone marrow cultures. J. Immunol. 136:422, 1986.

143. Kierney, P. C., and Dorshkind, K.: B lymphocyte precursors and myeloid progenitors survive in diffusion chamber cultures but B cell differentiation requires close association with stromal cells. Blood 70:1418, 1987.

144. Witte, P. L., Robinson, M., Henley, A., Low, M. G., Stiers, D. L., Perkins, S., Fleischman, R. A., and Kincade, P. W.: Relationships between B-lineage lymphocytes and stromal cells in long-term bone marrow cultures. Eur. J. Immunol. 17:1473, 1987.

145. Miyake, K., Underhill, C. B., Lesley, J., and Kincade, P. W.: Hyaluronate can function as a cell adhesion molecule and CD44 participates in hyaluronate recognition. J. Exp. Med. 172:69, 1990.

146. Miyake, K., Weissman, I. L., Greenberger, J. S., and Kincade, P. W.: Evidence for a role of the integrin VLA-4 in lymphohemopoiesis. J. Exp. Med. 173:599, 1991.

147. Kina, T., Majumdar, A. S., Heimfeld, S., Kaneshima, H., Holzmann, B., Katsura, Y., and Weissman, I. L.: Identification of a 107kd glycoprotein that mediates adhesion between stromal cells and hematolymphoid cells. J. Exp. Med. 173:373, 1991.

148. Springer, T. A.: Adhesion receptors of the immune system. Nature 346:425, 1990.

149. Osborn, L., Hession, C., Tizard, R., Vassallo, C., Luhowskyj, S., Chi-Rosso, G., and Lobb, R.: Direct expression cloning of vascular cell adhesion molecule 1, a cytokine-induced endothelial protein that binds to lymphocytes. Cell 59:1203, 1989.

150. Elices, M. J., Osborn, L., Takada, Y., Crouse, C., Luhowskyj, S., Hemler, M. E., and Lobb, R.: VCAM-1 on activated endothelium interacts with the leukocyte integrin VLA-4 at a site distinct from the VLA-4/fibronectin binding site. Cell 60:577, 1990.

151. Wayner, E. A., Garcia-Pardo, A., Humphries, M. J., McDonald, J. A., and Carter, W. G.: Identification and characterization of the lymphocyte adhesion receptor for an alternative cell

attachment domain in plasma fibronectin. J. Cell Biol. 109:1321, 1989.

152. Bernardi, P., Patel, V. P., and Lodish, H. F.: Lymphoid precursor cells adhere to two different sites on fibronectin. J. Cell Biol. 105:489, 1987.

153. Lemoine, F. M., Dedhar, S., Lima, G. M., and Eaves, C. J.: Transformation-associated alterations in interactions between pre-B cells and fibronectin. Blood 76:2311, 1990.

154. Holzmann, B., McIntyre, B. W., and Weissman, I. L.: Identification of a murine Peyer's patch–specific lymphocyte homing receptor as an integrin molecule with an α chain homologous to human VLA-4α. Cell 56:37, 1989.

155. Gunji, Y., Sudo, T., Suda, J., Yamaguchi, Y., Nakauchi, H., Nishikawa, S., Yanai, N., Obinata, M., Yanagisawa, M., Miura, Y., and Suda, T.: Support of early B-cell differentiation in mouse fetal liver by stromal cells and interleukin-7. Blood 77:2612, 1991.

156. Saeland, S., Duvert, V., Pandrau, D., Caux, C., Durand, I., Wrighton, N., Wideman, J., Lee, F., and Banchereau, J.: Interleukin-7 induces the proliferation of normal human B cell precursors. Blood 78:2229, 1991.

157. McNiece, I. K., Langley, K. E., and Zsebo, K. M.: The role of recombinant stem cell factor in early B cell development: Synergistic interaction with IL7. J. Immunol. 146:3785, 1991.

158. Uckun, F. M., Dibirdik, I., Smith, R., Tuel-Ahlgren, L. T., Chandan-Langlie, M., Schieven, G. L., Waddick, K. G., Hanson, M., and Ledbetter, J. A.: Interleukin 7 receptor ligation stimulates tyrosine phosphorylation, inositol phospholipid turnover, and clonal proliferation of human B-cell precursors. Proc. Natl. Acad. Sci. USA 88:3589, 1991.

159. Hayashi, S., Kunisada, T., Ogawa, M., Sudo, T., Kodama, H., Suda, T., Nishikawa, S., and Nishikawa, S.: Stepwise progression of B lineage differentiation supported by interleukin 7 and other stromal cell molecules. J. Exp. Med. 171:1683, 1990.

160. Era, T., Ogawa, M., Nishikawa, S., Okamoto, M., Honjo, T., Akagi, K., Miyazaki, J., and Yamamura, K.: Differentiation of growth signal requirement of B lymphocyte precursor is directed by expression of immunoglobulin. EMBO J. 10:337, 1991.

161. Rolink, A., Kudo, A., Karasuyama, H., Kikuchi, Y., and Melchers, F.: Long-term proliferating early pre B cell lines and clones with the potential to develop to surface Ig-postive mitogen reactive B cells in vitro and in vivo. EMBO J. 10:327, 1991.

162. Uckun, F. M., and Ledbetter, J. A.: Immunobiologic differences between normal and leukemic human B-cell precursors. Proc. Natl. Acad. Sci. USA 85:8603, 1988.

163. Uckun, F. M., Fauci, A. S., Heerema, N. A., Song, C. W., Mehta, S. R., Gajl-Peczalska, K., Chandan, M., and Ambrus, J. L.: B-cell growth factor receptor expression and B-cell growth factor response of leukemic B cell precursors and B lineage lymphoid progenitor cells. Blood 870:1020, 1987.

164. Wormann, B., Mehta, S. R., Maizel, A. L., and LeBien, T. W.: Low molecular weight B cell growth factor induces proliferation of human B cell precursor acute lymphoblastic leukemias. Blood 70:132, 1987.

165. Wormann, B., Gesner, T. G., Mufson, R. A., and LeBien, T. W.: Proliferative effect of interleukin 3 on normal and leukemic human B cell precursors. Leukemia 3:399, 1989.

166. Law, C., Armitage, R. J., Vallablanca, J. G., and LeBien, T. W.: Expression of interleukin-4 receptors on early human B-lineage cells. Blood 78:703, 1991.

167. Ritz, J., Schmidt, R. E., Michon, J., Hercend, T., and Schlossman, S. F.: Characterization of functional surface structures on human natural killer cells. Adv. Immunol. 42:181, 1988.

168. Robertson, M. J., and Ritz, J.: Biology and clinical relevance of human natural killer cells. Blood 76:2421, 1990.

169. Trinchieri, G.: Biology of natural killer cells. Adv. Immunol. 47:187, 1989.

170. Timonen, T., Ortaldo, J. R., and Herberman, R. B.: Characteristics of human large granular lymphocytes and relationship to natural killer and K cells. J. Exp. Med. 153:569, 1981.

171. Lanier, L. L., Le, A. M., Civin, C. I., Loken, M. R., and Phillips, J. H.: The relationship of CD16 (LEU-11) and Leu-19 (NKH-1) antigen expression on human peripheral blood NK cells and cytotoxic T lymphocytes. J. Immunol. 136:4480, 1986.

172. Lanier, L. L., Testi, R., Bindl, J., and Phillips, J. H.: Identity of Leu-19 (CD56) leukocyte differentiation antigen and neural cell adhesion molecule. J. Exp. Med. 169:2233, 1989.

173. Perussia, B., Acuto, O., Terhorst, C., Faust, J., Lazarus, R., Fanning, V., and Trinchieri, G.: Human natural killer cells analyzed by B73.1, a monoclonal antibody blocking Fc receptor functions. J. Immunol. 130:2142, 1983.

174. Lanier, L. L., Le, A. M., Phillips, J. H., Warner, N. L., and Babcock, G. F.: Subpopulations of human natural killer cells defined by expression of the Leu7 (HNK-1) and Leu-11 (NK-15) antigens. J. Immunol. 131:1789, 1983.

175. Uksila, J., Lassila, O., Hirvonen, T., and Toivanen, P.: Natural killer cell activity of human fetal liver cells after allogeneic stimulation. Scand. J. Immunol. 22:433, 1985.

176. Phan, D. T., Mihalik, R., Benczur, M., Domotori, J., Kiss, C., Petranyi, G. G., and Hollan, S. R.: Expression of NK-cell associated antigen on human fetal liver cells. Thymus 11:253, 1988.

177. Ueno, Y., Miyawaki, T., Seki, H., Matsuda, A., Taga, K., Sato, H., and Taniguchi, N.: Differential effects of recombinant human interferon-γ and interleukin 2 on natural killer cell activity of peripheral blood in early human development. J. Immunol. 135:180, 1985.

178. Haller, O., Kiessling, R., Orn, A., and Wigzell, H.: Generation of natural killer cells: An autonomous function of the bone marrow. J. Exp. Med. 145:1411, 1977.

179. Ault, K. A., Antin, J. H., Ginsburg, D., Orkin, S. H., Rappeport, J. M., Keohan, M. L., Martin, P., and Smith, B. R.: Phenotype of recovering lymphoid cell populations after marrow transplantation. J. Exp. Med. 161:1483, 1985.

180. Dorshkind, K., Pollack, S. B., Bosma, M. J., and Phillips, R. A.: Natural killer (NK) cells are present in mice with severe combined immunodeficiency (SCID) 1. J. Immunol. 134:3798, 3801, 1985.

181. Hackett, J., Bosma, G. C., Bosma, M. J., Bennett, M., and Kumar, V.: Transplantable progenitors of natural killer cells are distinct from those of T and B lymphocytes. Proc. Natl. Acad. Sci. USA 83:3427, 1986.

182. Roder, J., and Duwe, A.: The beige mutation in the mouse selectively impairs natural killer cell function. Nature 278:451, 1979.

183. Fleisher, G., Starr, S., Koven, N., Kamiya, H., Douglas, S. D., and Henle, W.: A non–X linked syndrome with susceptibility to severe Epstein-Barr virus infections. J. Pediatr. 100:727, 1982.

184. Biron, C. A., Byron, K. S., and Sullivan, J. L.: Severe herpesvirus infections in an adolescent without natural killer cells. N. Engl. J. Med. 320:1731, 1989.

185. Roder, J., Haliotis, T., Klein, M., Korec, S., Jett, J. R., Ortaldo, J., Heberman, R. B., Katz, P., and Fauci, A. S.: A new immunodeficiency disorder in humans involving NK cells. Nature 284:553, 1980.

186. Abo, T., Roder, J. C., Abo, W., Cooper, M. D., and Balch, C. M.: Natural killer (HNK-1+) cells in Chédiak-Higashi patients are present in normal numbers but are abnormal in function and morphology. J. Clin. Invest. 70:193, 1982.

187. Lipinski, M., Virelizier, J., Tursz, T., and Griscelli, C.: Natural killer and killer cell activities in patients with primary immunodeficiencies or defects in immune interferon production. Eur. J. Immunol. 10:246, 1980.

188. van den Brink, M. R. M., Boggs, S. S., Herberman, R. B., and Hiserodt J. C.: The generation of natural killer (NK) cells from NK precursor cells in rat long-term bone marrow cultures. J. Exp. Med. 172:303, 1990.

189. van den Brink, M. R. M., Herberman, R. B., and Hiserodt, J. C.: Generation of natural killer cells from Thy 1.1+ bone marrow precursor cells in the rat. Blood 78:2392, 1991.

190. Michon, J. M., Caligiuri, M. A., Hazanow, S. M., Levine, H., Schlossman, S. F., and Ritz, J.: Induction of natural killer effectors from human thymus with recombinant IL2. J. Immunol. 140:3660, 1988.

191. Poggi, A., Biassoni, R., Pella, N., Paolieri, F., Bellomo, R., Bertolini, A., Moretta, L., and Mingari, M. C.: In vitro expansion of CD3/TCR− human thymocyte populations that selectively lack CD3g gene expression: A phenotypic and functional analysis. J. Exp. Med. 172:1409, 1990.

192. Denning, S. M., Jones, D. M., Ware, R. E., Weinhold, K. J., Brenner, M. B., and Haynes, B. F.: Analysis of clones derived from human CD7+CD4−CD8−CD3− thymocytes. Int. Immunol. 3:1015, 1991.

193. Denning, S. M., Jones, D. M., Ware, R. E., and Haynes, B. F.: Definition of new stages of human intrathymic T cell development by analysis of clonal progeny of CD3−, CD4−CD8− thymocytes. Clin. Res. 38:390, 1991.

194. Bucy, R. P., Chen, C. H., and Cooper, M. D.: Development of cytoplasmic CD3+/T cell receptor–negative cells in the peripheral lymphoid tissues of chickens. Eur. J. Immunol. 20:1345, 1990.

195. Garni-Wagner, B. A., Witte, P. L., Tutt, M. M., Kuziel, W. A., Tucker, P. W., Bennett, M., and Kumar, V.: Natural killer cells in the thymus: Studies in mice with severe combined immune deficiency. J. Immunol. 144:796, 1990.

196. Trinchieri, G., Matsumoto-Kobayashi, M., Clark, S. C., Seehra, J., London, L., and Perussia, B.: Response of resting human peripheral blood natural killer cells to interleukin 2. J. Exp. Med. 160:1147, 1984.

197. Moretta, A., Ciccone, E., Pantaleo, G., Tambussi, G., Bottino, C., Melioli, G., Mingari, C., and Moretta, L.: Surface molecules involved in the activation and regulation of T or natural killer lymphocytes in humans. Immunol. Rev. 111:145, 1989.

198. Moretta, A., Tambussi, G., Bottino, C., Tripodi, G., Merli, A., Ciccone, E., Pantaleo, G., and Moretta, L.: A novel surface antigen expressed by a subset of human CD3-CD16+ natural killer cells: Role in cell activation and regulation of cytolytic function. J. Exp. Med. 171:695, 1990.

199. Moretta, A., Bottino, C., Pende, D., Tripodi, G., Tambussi, G., Viale, O., Orengo, A., Barbaresi, M., Merli, A., Ciccone, E., and Moretta, L.: Identification of four subsets of human CD3−CD16+ natural killer (NK) cells by the expression of clonally distributed functional surface molecules: Correlation between subset assignment of NK clones and ability to mediate specific alloantigen recognition. J. Exp. Med. 172:1589, 1990.

200. Ciccone, E., Pende, D., Viale, O., Tambussi, G., Ferrini, S., Biassoni, R., Longo, A., Guardiola, J., Moretta, A., and Moretta, L.: Specific recognition of human CD3−CD16+ natural killer cells requires the expression of an autosomic recessive gene on target cells. J. Exp. Med. 172:47, 1990.

201. Ciccone, E., Moretta, A., and Moretta, L.: Specific functions of human NK cells. Immunol. Lett. 31:99, 1992.

202. Hedrick, S. M., Cohen, D. I., Nelson, E. A., and Davis, M. M.: Isolation of cDNA clones encoding T cell–specific membrane-associated proteins. Nature 308:149, 1984.

203. Yanagi, Y., Yoshikai, Y., and Leggett, K., Clark, S. P., Aleksander, I., and Mak, T. W.: A human T cell specific cDNA clone encodes a protein having extensive homology to immunoglobulin chains. Nature 308:145, 1984.

204. Bjorkman, P. J., Saper, M. A., Samraoui, B., Bennett, W. S., Strominger, J. L., and Wiley, D. C.: The foreign antigen binding site and T cell recognition regions of class I histocompatibility antigens. Nature 329:506, 1987.

205. Bierer, B. E., Sleckman, B. P., Ratnofsky, S. E., and Burakoff, S. J.: The biologic roles of CD2, CD4 and CD8 in T cell activation. Annu. Rev. Immunol. 7:579, 1989.

206. Haynes, B. F., Scearce, R. M., Lobach, D. F., and Hensley, L. L.: Phenotypic characterization and ontogeny of mesodermal-derived and endocrine epithelial components of the human thymic microenvironment. J. Exp. Med. 159:1149, 1984.

207. Weller, G. L.: Development of the thyroid, parathyroid and thymus gland in man. Contrib. Embryol. Carnegie Inst. 22:95, 1933.

208. Haynes, B. F.: Human thymic epithelium and T cell development. Current issues and future development. Thymus 16:143, 1990.

209. Haynes, B. F.: The human thymic microenvironment. Adv. Immunol. 36:87, 1984.

210. MacFarland, E. J., Scearce, R. M., and Haynes, B. F.: The human thymic microenvironment: Cortical thymic epithelium is an antigenically distinct region of the thymic microenvironment. J. Immunol. 133:1241, 1984.

211. Demaagd, R. A., MacKenzie, W. A., Schuurman, H.-J., Ritter, M. A., Price, K. M., Broekhuizen, R., and Kater, L.: The human thymus microenvironment: Heterogeneity detected by monoclonal anti-epithelial cell antibodies. Immunology 54:745, 1985.

212. Ritter, M. A., Sauvage, C. A., and Cotmore, C. R.: The human thymus microenvironment in vivo identification of thymic mouse cells and other antigenically distinct subpopulations of epithelial cells. Immunology 44:439, 1981.

213. Lobach, D. F., Scearce, R. M., and Haynes, B. F.: The human thymic microenvironment. Phenotypic characterization of Hassall's bodies with the use of monoclonal antibodies. J. Immunol. 134:250, 1985.

214. Lobach, D. F., Itoh, T., Singer, K. H., and Haynes, B. F.: The thymic microenvironment. Demonstration of thymic epithelial cell differentiation in vitro. Differentiation 34:50, 1987.

215. Laster, A. J., Itoh, T., Palker, T. J., and Haynes, B. F.: The human thymic microenvironment: Thymic epithelium contains specific keratins associated with early and late stages of epidermal keratinocyte maturation. Differentiation 31:67, 1986.

216. Papiernik, M., Lepault, F., and Pontoux, C.: Synergistic effect of colony-stimulating factors and IL2 on prothymocyte proliferation linked to the maturation of macrophage/dendritic cells within L3T4- Lyt2-, Ia-, Mac- cells. J. Immunol. 140:1431, 1988.

217. Krause, V. B., Harden, E. A., Wittles, B., Moore, J. O., and Haynes, B. F.: Demonstration of phenotypic abnormalities of thymic epithelium in thymoma including two cases with abundant Langerhans' cells. Am. J. Pathol. 132:552, 1988.

218. Haynes, B. F., Martin, M. E., Kay, H. H., and Kurtzberg, J.: Early events in human T cell ontogeny: Phenotypic characterization and immunohistologic localization of T cell precursors in early human fetal tissues. J. Exp. Med. 168:1061, 1988.

219. Doyle, C., and Strominger, J. L.: Introduction between CD4 and Class II MHC molecules mediates cell adhesion. Nature 330:256, 1987.

220. Norment, A. M., Salter, R. D., Parham, P., and Englehard, V. H.: Cell-cell adhesion mediated by CD8 and MHC class I molecules. Nature 336:79, 1988.

221. Turner, J. M., Brodsky, M. H., Irving, B. A., Levin, S. D., Perlmutter, R. M., and Littman, D. R.: Interaction of the unique N-terminal region of tyrosine kinase p56 lck with cytoplasmic domains of CD4 and CD8 is mediated by cysteine motifs. Cell 66:755, 1990.

222. Klausner, R. D., and Samelson, L. E.: T cell antigen receptor activation pathways: The tyrosine kinase connection. Cell 64:875, 1991.

223. Finkel, T. H., Cambier, J. C., Kubo, R. T., Born, W. K., Marrack, P., and Kappler J. W.: The thymus has two functionally distinct populations of immature αβ+ T cells: One population is deleted by ligation of αβ TCR. Cell 58:1047, 1989.

224. Kantor, A. B.: The development and repertoire of B-1 cells (CD5 B cells). Immunol. Today 12:389, 1991.

225. Amiot, H., Dastot, H., Fabbi, M., Degos, L., Bernard, A., and Boumsell, L.: Intermolecular complexes between three human CD1 molecules on normal thymus cells. Immunogenetics 27:187, 1988.

226. Poncelli, S., Brenner, M. B., Greenstein, J. L., Balk, S. P., Terhorst, C., Bleicher, P. A.: Recognition of differentiation

l antigens by human CD4−8− cytolytic T lymphocytes. Nature 341:447, 1989.

227. Denning, S. M., Dustin, M. L., Springer, T. A., Singer, K. H., and Haynes B. F.: Purified LFA-3 antigen activates human thymocytes via the CD2 pathway. J. Immunol. 141:2980, 1988.

228. Denning, S. M., Kurtzberg, J., Le, P. T., Tuck, D. T., Singer, K. H., and Haynes, B. F.: Human thymic epithelial cells directly induce activation of autologous immature thymocytes. Proc. Natl. Acad. Sci. USA 85:3125, 1988.

229. Singer, K. H., Denning, S. M., Whichard, L. P., and Haynes, B. F.: Thymocyte LFA-1 and thymic epithelial cell ICAM-1 molecules mediate binding of activated human thymocytes to thymic epithelial cells. J. Immunol. 143:3944, 1986.

230. Vollger, L. W., Tuck, D. T., Springer, T. A., Haynes, B. F., and Singer, K. H.: Thymocyte binding to human thymic epithelial cells is inhibited by monoclonal antibodies to CD2 and LFA3 antigens. J. Immunol. 138:358, 1987.

231. Turka, L. A., Linsley, P. S., Paine, R., Schieven, G. L., Thompson, C. B., and Ledbetter, J. A.: Signal transduction via CD4, CD8, and CD28 in mature and immature thymocytes. J. Immunol. 146:1428, 1991.

232. Van Dongen, J. J. M., Hooijkaas, H., Comans-Bitter, M., Hahlen, K., de Klein, A., van Zanen, G. E., van' T Veer, M. B., Abels, J. and Benner, R.: Human bone marrow cells positive for terminal deoxynucleotidyl transferase (TDT), HLA-DR, and A T cell marker may represent prothymocytes. J. Immunol. 135:3144, 1985.

233. Hori, T., Malefyt, R., Duncan, B. W., Harrison, M. R., Roncarolo, M. G., and Spits, H.: Cloning of a novel cell type from human fetal liver expressing cytoplasmic CD3 δ and ε but not membrane CD3. Int. Immunol. 3:353, 1991.

234. Bertho, J. M., Mossalayi, M. D., Dalloul, A. H., Mouterde, G., and Debre, P.: Isolation of an early T cell precursor (CFU-TL) from human bone marrow. Blood 75:1064, 1990.

235. Mossalayi, D., Dalloul, A. H., Bertho, J., Lecron, J., de Laforest, P. G., and Debre, P.: In vitro differentiation and proliferation of purified human thymic and bone marrow CD7+CD2− T cell precursors. Exp. Hematol. 18:326, 1990.

236. Preffer, F. I., Kim, C. W., Fischer, K. H., Sabga, E. M., Kradin, R. L., and Colvin, R. B.: Identification of pre-T cells in human peripheral blood: Extrathymic differentiation of CD7+CD3− cells into CD3+ γ/δ+ or α/β+ T cells. J. Exp. Med. 170:177, 1989.

237. Imof, B. A., Dengnier, M. A., Girault, J. M., Champion, S., Damaif, C., Itoh, T., and Thiery, J. P.: Thymotaxin: A thymic epithelial peptide chemotactic from T cell precursors. Proc. Natl. Acad. Sci. USA 85:7699, 1988.

238. Wu, L., Antica, M., Johnson, G. R., Scollay, R., and Shortman, K.: Development potential of the earliest precursor cells from the adult mouse thymus. J. Exp. Med. 174:1617, 1991.

239. Kurtzberg, J., Denning, S. M., Nycum, N. M., Singer, K. H., and Haynes, B. F.: Immature human thymocytes can be driven to differentiate into nonlymphoid lineages by cytokines from thymic epithelial cells. Proc. Natl. Acad. Sci. USA 86:7575, 1989.

240. De Villartay, J., Mossalayi, D. M., de Chasseval, R., Dolloul, A. H., and Debre, P.: Induction of the T cell receptor δ gene deletional rearrangement by soluble CD23 in human prothymocytes. Int. Immunol 3:1301, 1991.

241. Haynes, B. F., Singer, K. H., Denning, S. M., and Martin, M. E.: Analysis of expression of CD2, CD3, and T cell antigen receptor molecules during early human fetal thymic development. J. Immunol. 141:3776, 1988.

242. Asma, G. M., Van Den Bergh, L., and Vossen, J. M.: Use of monoclonal antibodies in a study of the development of T lymphocytes in the human fetus. Clin. Exp. Immunol. 53:429, 1983.

243. Haynes, B. F., and Brenner, M. B.: The first wave of TCRγδ cells in human fetal thymus are Vδ2+ (submitted for publication).

244. Krangel, M. S., Yssel, H., Brocklehurst, C., and Spits, H.: A distinct wave of human T cell receptor gd lymphocytes in the early fetal thymus: Evidence for controlled gene rearrangement and cytokine production. J. Exp. Med. 172:847, 1990.

245. Parker, C. M., Groh, V., Band, H., Porcelli, S. A., Mortia, C., Fabbi, M., Glass, D., Strominger, J. L., and Brenner, M. B.: Evidence for extrathymic changes in the T cell receptor gd repertoire. J. Exp. Med. 171:1597, 1990.

246. Turka, L. A., Schatz, D. G., Oettinger, M. A., Chun, J. J. M., Gorka, C., Lee, K., McCormack, W. T., and Thompson, C. B.: Thymocyte expression of RAG-1 and RAG-2: Termination by T cell receptor cross-linking. Science 253:778, 1991.

247. George, J. F., and Schroeder, H.: Developmental regulation of Dβ reading frame and functional diversity in T cell receptor−β transcripts from human thymus. J. Immunol. 148:1230, 1992.

248. Reinherz, E. L., Goldstein, G., Levey, R. H., and Schlossman, S. F.: Discrete stages of human intrathymic differentiation analysis of normal thymocytes and leukemic lymphoblasts of T lineage. Proc. Natl. Acad. Sci. USA 77:1588, 1980.

249. Terstappen, L. W. M., Huang, S., and Picker, L. J.: Flow cytometric assessment of human T-cell differentiation in thymus and bone marrow. Blood 79:1, 1992.

250. Fowlkes, B. J., and Pardoll, D. M.: Molecular and cellular events of T cell development. Adv. Immunol. 44:207, 1989.

251. Scollay, R., Smith, J., and Stauffer, V.: Dynamics of early T cells: Prothymocyte migration and proliferation in the adult mouse thymus. Immunol. Rev., 91:129, 1986.

252. Fisher, A. G., Larsson, L., Goff, L. K., Restall, D. E., Happerfield, L., and Merkenschlager, M.: Human thymocyte development in mouse organ cultures. Int. Immunol. 2:571, 1990.

253. Toribo, M. L., Martinez, A. C., Marcos, M. A. R., Marquez, C., Cabrero, E., and de la Hera, A.: A role for T3+, 4−6−8− transitional thymocytes in the differentiation of mature and functional T cells from human prothymocytes. Proc. Natl. Acad. Sci. USA 83:6985, 1986.

254. Furley, A. J., Mizutani, S., Weibaecher, K., Dhaliwai, H. S., Ford, A. M., Chan, L. C., Molgaard, H. V., Toyonaga, B., Mak, T., van den Elsen, P., Gold, D., Terhorst, C., and Greaves, M. F.: Developmentally regulated rearrangement and expression of genes encoding the T cell receptor−T3 complex. Cell 46:75, 1986.

255. de la Hera, A., Marston, W., Aranda, C., Toribio, M., and Martinez, A. C.: Thymic stroma is required for the development of human T cell lineages in vitro. Int. Immunol. 1:471, 1989.

256. Dalloul, A. H., Mossalayi, M. D., Dellagi, K., Bertho, J., and Debre, P.: Factor requirements for activation and proliferation steps of human CD2+, CD3−, CD4−CD8− early thymocytes. Eur. J. Immunol. 19:1985, 1989.

257. Mossalayi, M. D., Lecron, J., Dalloul, A. H., Sarfati, M., Bertho, J., Hofstetter, H., Delespesse, G., and Debre, P.: Soluble CD23 (FceRII) and interleukin 1 synergistically induce early human thymocyte maturation. J. Exp. Med. 171:959, 1990.

258. Groh, V., Fabbi, M., and Strominger, J. L.: Maturation or differentiation of human thymocyte precursors in vitro. Proc. Natl. Acad. Sci. USA 87:5973, 1990.

259. Denning, S. M., Kurtzberg, J., Leslie, D. S., and Haynes, B. F.: Human postnatal CD4−CD8−CD3− thymic T cell precursors differentiate in vitro into T cell receptor δ−bearing cells. J. Immunol. 142:2988, 1989.

260. Schnittman, S. M., Denning, S. M., Greenhouse, J. J., Justement, J. S., Baseler, M., Kurtzberg, J., Haynes, B. F., and Fauci, A. S.: Evidence for susceptibility of intrathymic T-cell precursors and their progeny carrying T-cell antigen receptor phenotypes TCRαβ+ and TCRγδ+ to human immunodeficiency virus infection: A mechanism for CD4+ (T4) lymphocyte depletion. Proc. Natl. Acad. Sci. USA 87:7727, 1990.

261. Wu, L., Scollay, R., Egerton, M., Pearse, M., Spangrude, G. J., and Shortman, K.: CD4 expressed on earliest T-lineage precursor cells in the adult murine thymus. Nature 349:71, 1991.

262. Hori, T., and Spits, H.: Clonal analysis of human CD4 − CD8 − CD3 − thymocytes highly purified from post-natal thymus. J. Immunol. 146:2116, 1991.

263. Guidos, G. J., Weissman, I. L., and Adkins, B.: Intrathymic maturation of murine T lymphocytes from CD8 + precursors. Proc. Natl. Acad. Sci. USA 86:7542, 1989.

264. Hori, T., Cupp, J., Wrighton, N., Lee, F., and Spits, H.: Identification of a novel human thymocyte subset with phenotype of CD3 − CD4 + CD8α + β-1. J. Immunol. 146:4078, 1991.

265. Denning, S. M., and Haynes, B. F.: Human CD4 − CD8 + CD3 − thymocytes give rise to NK cells in vitro (submitted for publication).

266. Le, P. T., Vollger, L. W., Haynes, B. F., and Singer, K. H.: Ligand binding to the LFA-3 cell adhesion molecule induced IL1 production by human thymic epithelium cells. J. Immunol. 144:4541, 1990.

267. Berrih, S., Arenzana-Seisoedos, F., Cohen, S., Devos, R., Charron, D., and Virelizier, J. L.: Interferon-γ modulates Class II antigen expression on cultured human thymic epithelial cells. J. Immunol. 135:1165, 1986.

268. Haynes, B.: Phenotypic characterization and ontogeny of the human thymic microenvironment. Clin. Res. 32:500, 1984.

269. Goldstein, A. L. (ed.): Thymic Hormones and Lymphokines. Basic Chemistry and Clinical Applications. New York, Plenum Press, 1984.

270. Le, P. T., Tuck, D. T., Dinarello, C. A., Haynes, B. F., and Singer, K. H.: Human thymic epithelial cells produce interleukin-1. J. Immunol. 138:2520, 1988.

271. Le, P. T., Lazorick, S., Whichard, L. P., Haynes, B. F., and Singer, K. H.: Regulation of cytokine production in the human thymus: Epidermal growth factor and transforming growth factor α regulate mRNA levels of thymic epithelial cells at a post-transcriptional level. J. Exp. Med. 174:1147, 1991.

272. Le, P. T., Lazorick, S., Whichard, L. P., Yang, Y. C., Clark, S. C., Haynes, B. F., and Singer, K. H.: Human thymic epithelial cells produce IL6 GM-CSF and leukemia inhibitory factor (LIF). J. Immunol. 145:3310, 1990.

273. Werkerle, H., Ketelsen, U., and Ernst, M.: Thymic nurse cells. Lymphoepithelial cell complexes in murine thymuses: Morphological and serological characterization. J. Exp. Med. 151:925, 1980.

274. Allison, J. P., and Raulet, D. H.: The immunobiology of γδ + T cells. Semin. Immunol. 2:59, 1990.

275. Lefrancois, L.: Extrathymic differentiation of intraepithelial lymphocytes: Generation of a separate and unequal T-cell repertoire? Immunol. Today 12:426, 1991.

276. Bandeira, A., Itohara, S., Bonneville, M., Burlen-Defranoux, O., Mota-Santos, T., Coutinho, A., and Tonegawa, S.: Extrathymic origin of intestinal intraepithelial lymphocytes bearing T-cell antigen receptor γδ. Proc. Natl. Acad. Sci. USA 88:43, 1991.

277. Lefrancois, L., LeCorre, R., Mayo, J., Bluestone, J. A., and Goodman, T.: Extrathymic selection of TCRγδ + T cells by class II major histocompatibility complex molecules. Cell 63:333, 1990.

278. Spits, H.: Human T cell receptor γδ + T cells. Semin. Immunol. 3:119, 1991.

279. Kisielow, P., and von Boehmer, H.: Negative and positive selection of immature thymocytes: Timing and the role of the ligand for αβ T cell receptor. Semin. Immunol. 2:35, 1990.

280. Marrack, P., and Kappler, J.: T cell tolerance. Semin. Immunol. 2:45, 1990.

281. Itohara, S., and Tonegawa, S.: Selection of γδ T cell with canonical T-cell antigen receptors in fetal thymus. Proc. Natl. Acad. Sci. USA 87:7935, 1990.

282. Nikolic-Zugic, J.: Phenotypic and functional stages in the intrathymic development of αβ T cells. Immunol. Today 12:65, 1991.

283. Finkel, T. H., Kubo, R. T., and Cambier, J. C.: T-cell development and transmembrane signaling: Changing biological responses through an unchanging receptor. Immunol. Today 12:79, 1991.

284. Boyd, R. L., and Hugo, P.: Towards an integrated view of thymopoiesis. Immunol. Today 12:71, 1991.

285. Rothenberg, E. V.: Death and transfiguration of cortical thymocytes: A reconsideration. Immunol. Today 11:116, 1990.

286. Smith, C. A., Williams, G. T., Kingston, R., Jenkinson, E. J., and Owen, J. J. T.: Antibodies of CD3/T-cell receptor complex induce death by apoptosis in immature T cells in thymic cultures. Nature 337:181, 1989.

287. McConkey, D. J., Hartzell, P., Amador-Perez, J. F., Orrenius, S., and Jondal, M.: Calcium-dependent killing of immature thymocytes by stimulation via the CD3/T cell receptor complex. J. Immunol. 143:1801, 1989.

288. Nieto, M. A., Gonzalez, A., Lopez-Rivas, A., Diaz-Espada, F., and Gambon, F.: IL2 protects against anti-CD3 induced cell death in human medullary thymocytes. J. Immunol. 145:1364, 1990.

289. Janssen, O., Wesselborg, S., Heckl-Ostreicher, B., Pechhold, K., Bender, A., Schondelmaier, S., Moldenhauer, G., and Kabelitz, D.: T cell receptor/CD3-signaling induces death by apoptosis in human T cell receptor γδ + T cells. J. Immunol. 146:35, 1991.

290. Riegel, J. S., Richie, E. R., and Allison, J. P.: Nuclear events after activation of CD4 + 8 + thymocytes. J. Immunol. 144:3611, 1990.

291. Mercep, M., Weissman, A. M., Frank, S. J., Klausner, R. D., and Ashwell, J. D.: Activation-driven programmed cell death and T cell receptor ζη expression. Science 246:1162, 1989.

292. Fischer, E. H., Chabonneau, H., and Tonks, N. K.: Protein tyrosine phosphatases: A diverse family of intracellular and transmembrane enzymes. Science 253:401, 1991.

293. Ostergaard, H. L., and Trowbridge, I. S.: Coclustering CD45 with CD4 or CD8 alters the phosphorylation and kinase activity of p56lck. J. Exp. Med. 172:347, 1990.

294. Iivanainen, A. V., Lindqvist, C., Mustelin, T., and Anderson, L. C.: Phosphotyrosine phosphatases are involved in reversion of T lymphoblastic proliferation. Eur. J. Immunol. 20:2509, 1990.

295. Gillitzer, R., and Pilarski, L. M.: In situ localization of CD45 isoforms in the human thymus indicates a medullary location for the thymic generative lineage. J. Immunol. 144:66, 1990.

296. Robey, E. A., Fowlkes, B. J., Gordon, J. W., Kioussi, D., von Boehmer, H., Ramsdell, F., and Axel, R.: Thymic selection in CD8 transgenic mice supports an instructive model for commitment to a CD4 or CD8 lineage. Cell 64:99, 1991.

297. Cooke, M. P., Abraham, K. M., Forbush, K. A., and Perlmutter, R. M.: Regulation of T cell receptor signaling by a src family protein-tyrosine kinase (p59fyn). Cell 65:281, 1991.

298. Itoh, N., Yonehara, S., Ishii, A., Yonehara, M., Mizushima, S., Sameshima, M., Hase, A., Seto, Y., and Nagata, S.: The polypeptide encoded by the cDNA for human cell surface antigen fas can mediate apoptosis. Cell 66:233, 1991.

299. Trauth, B. C., Klas, C., Peters, A. M. J., Matzku, S., Moller, P., Falk, W., Debatin, K., and Krammer, P. H.: Monoclonal antibody-mediated tumor regression by induction of apoptosis. Science 21:301, 1989.

300. Sentman, C. L., Shutter, J. R., Hockenbery, D., Kanagawa, O., and Korsmeyer, S. J.: bcl-2 inhibits multiple forms of apoptosis but not negative selection in thymocytes. Cell 67:879, 1991.

301. Strasser, A., Harris, A. W., and Cory, S.: bcl-2 transgene inhibits T cell death and perturbs thymic self-censorship. Cell 67:889, 1991.

302. Acha-Orbea, H., and Palmer, E.: Mls-a retrovirus exploits the immune system. Immunol. Today 12:356, 1991.

303. Janeway, C.: Mls: Makes a little sense. Nature 349:459, 1991.

304. Dellabona, P., Peccoud, J., Kappler, J., Marrack, P., Benoist, C., and Mathis, D.: Superantigens interact with MHC class II molecules outside of the antigen groove. Cell 62:1115, 1990.

305. Herman, A., Croteau, G., Sekaly, P., Kappler, J., and Marrack, P.: HLA-DR alleles differ in their ability to present staphylococcal enterotoxins to T cells. J. Exp. Med. 172:709, 1990.

306. Marrack, P., Kushnir, E., and Kappler, J.: A maternally inherited superantigen encoded by a mammary tumor virus. Nature 349:524, 1991.
307. Jorgensen, J. L., Esser, U., Fazekas de St. Groth, B., Reay, P. A., and Davis, M. M.: Mapping T-cell receptor–peptide contacts by variant peptide immunization of single-chain transgenics. Nature 355:224, 1992.
308. Paliard, X., West, S. G., Lafferty, J. A., Clements, J. R., Kappler, J. W., Marrack, P., and Kotzin, B. L.: Evidence for the effects of a superantigen in rheumatoid arthritis. Science 253:325, 1991.
309. Imberti, L., Sottini, A., Bettinardi, A., Puoti, M., and Primi, D.: Selective depletion in HIV infection of T cells that bear specific T cell receptor Vβ sequences. Science 254:860, 1991.
310. Jotereau, F., Heuze, F., Salomon-Vie, V., and Gascan, H.: Cell kinetics in the fetal mouse thymus: Precursor cell input, proliferation, and emigration. J. Immunol. 138:1026, 1987.
311. Sharp, A., Kukulansky, T., and Globerson, A.: In vitro analysis of age-related changes in the development potential of bone marrow thymocyte progenitors. Eur. J. Immunol. 20:2541, 1990.
312. Shortman, K., Egerton, M., Spangrude, G. J., and Scollay, R.: The generation and fate of thymocytes. Semin. Immunol. 2:3, 1990.
313. Egerton, M., Scollay, R., and Shortman, K.: Kinetics of mature T-cell development in the thymus. Proc. Natl. Acad. Sci. USA 87:2579, 1990.
314. Spangrude, G. J., and Scollay, R.: Differentiation of hematopoietic stem cells in irradiated mouse thymic lobes. J. Immunol. 145:3661, 1990.
315. Egerton, M., Shortman, K., and Scollay, R.: The kinetics of immature murine thymocyte development in vivo. Int. Immunol. 2:501, 1990.
316. Lepault, F., Coffman, R. L., and Weissman, I. L.: Characteristics of thymus-homing bone marrow cells. J. Immunol. 131:64, 1983.
317. Spangrude, G. J., and Scollay, R.: Differentiation of hematopoietic stem cells in irradiated mouse thymic lobes. J. Immunol. 145:3661, 1990.
318. Penit, C.: In vivo thymocyte maturation, BudR labeling of cycling thymocytes and phenotypic analysis of their progeny support the single lineage model. J. Immunol. 137:2115, 1986.
319. Chaffin, K. E., and Perlmutter, R. M.: A pertussis toxin–sensitive process controls thymocyte emigration. Eur. J. Immunol. 21:2565, 1991.
320. Butcher, E. C.: The regulation of lymphocyte traffic. Curr. Top. Microbiol. Immunol. 128:86, 1986.
321. Woodruff, J. J., and Clarke, L. M.: Specific cell-adhesion mechanisms determining migration pathways of recirculating lymphocytes. Annu. Rev. Immunol. 5:201, 1987.
322. Yenock, T. A., and Rosen, S. D.: Lymphocyte homing. Adv. Immunol. 44:313, 1989.
323. Dustin, M. L., and Springer, T. A.: Role of lymphocyte adhesion receptors in transient interactions and cell locomotion. Annu. Rev. Immunol. 9:27, 1991.
324. Duijvestiijn, A., and Hamann, A.: Mechanisms and regulation of lymphocyte migration. Immunol. Today 10:23, 1989.
325. Stoolman, L. M.: Adhesion molecules controlling lymphocyte migration. Cell 56:907, 1989.
326. Butcher, E. C.: Leukocyte–endothelial cell recognition: Three (or more) steps to specificity and diversity. Cell 67:1033, 1991.
327. Ley, K., Gaehtgens, P., Fennie, C., Singer, M. S., Lasky, L. A., and Rosen, S. D.: Lectin-like cell adhesion molecule 1 mediates leukocyte rolling in mesenteric venules in vivo. Blood 77:2553, 1991.
328. Lawrence, M. B., and Springer, T. A.: Leukocytes roll on a selectin at physiologic flow rates: Distinction from a prerequisite for adhesion through integrins. Cell 65:859, 1991.
329. Picker, L. J., Warnock, R. A., Burns, A. R., Doerschuk, C. M., and Butcher, B. C.: The neutrophil selectin LECAM-1 presents carbohydrate ligands to the vascular selectins ELAM-1 and GMP-140. Cell 66:921, 1991.
330. Tedder, T. F., Penta, A. C., Levine, H. B., and Freedman, A. S.: Expression of the human leukocyte adhesion molecule, LAM1: Identity with the TQ1 and Leu-8 differentiation antigens. J. Immunol. 144:532, 1990.
331. Kishimoto, T. K., Jutila, M. A., and Butcher, E. C.: Identification of a human peripheral lymph node homing receptor: A rapidly down-regulated adhesion molecule. Proc. Natl. Acad. Sci. USA 87:2244, 1990.
332. Pober, J. S., and Cotran, R. S.: The role of endothelial cells in inflammation. Transplantation 50:537, 1990.
333. Nathan, C., and Sporn, M.: Cytokines in context. J. Cell Biol. 113:981, 1991.
334. Kishimoto, T. K., Jutila, M. A., Berg, E. L., and Butcher, E. C.: Neutrophil Mac-1 and MEL-14 adhesion proteins inversely regulated by chemotactic factors. Science 245:1238, 1989.
335. Imai, K., Singer, M. S., Fennie, C., Lasky, L. A., and Rosen, S. D.: Identification of a carbohydrate-based endothelial ligand for a lymphocyte homing receptor. J. Cell Biol. 113:1213, 1991.
336. Hemler, M. E.: VLA proteins in the integrin family: Structures, functions, and their role on leukocytes. Annu. Rev. Immunol. 8:365, 1990.
337. Albelda, S. M., and Buck, C. A.: Integrins and other cell adhesion molecules. FASEB J. 4:2868, 1990.
338. Shimizu, Y., Newman, W., Gopal, T. V., Horgan, K. J., Graber, N., Beall, L. D., van Seventer, G. A., and Shaw, S.: Four molecular pathways of T cell adhesion to endothelial cells: Roles of LFA-1, VCAM-1, and ELAM-1 and changes in pathway hierarchy under different activation conditions. J. Cell Biol. 113:1203, 1991.
339. Aruffo, A., Stamenkovic, I., Melnick, M., Underhill, C. B., and Seed, B.: CD44 is the principal cell surface receptor for hyaluronate. Cell 61:1303, 1990.
340. Mackay, C. R.: T-cell memory: The connection between function, phenotype and migration pathways. Immunol. Today 12:189, 1991.
341. MacLennan, C. M., and Gray, D.: Antigen-driven selection of virgin and memory B cells. Immunol. Rev. 91:61, 1986.
342. MacLennan, C. M. I., Oldfield, S., Liu, Y., and Lane, P. J. L.: Regulation of B-cell populations. Curr. Top. Microbiol. Immunol. 159:37, 1990.
343. Timens, W., Boes, A., Rozeboom-Uiterwijk, T., and Poppema, S.: Immaturity of the human splenic marginal zone in infancy. J. Immunol. 143:3200, 1989.
344. Tew, J. G., Kosco, M. H., Burton, G. F., and Szakal, A. K.: Follicular dendritic cells as accessory cells. Immunol. Rev. 117:185, 1990.
345. Gray, D.: Recruitment of virgin B cells into an immune response is restricted to activation outside lymphoid follicles. Immunology 65:73, 1988.
346. Rooijen, N. V.: Antigen processing and presentation in vivo: The microenvironment as a crucial factor. Immunol. Today 11:436, 1990.
347. Gray, D., MacLennan, I. C. M., and Lane, J. L.: Virgin B cell recruitment and lifespan of memory clones during antibody responses to 2, 4-dinitrophenylhemocyanin. Eur. J. Immunol. 16:641, 1986.
348. Berek, C., Berger, A., and Apel, M.: Maturation of the immune response in germinal centers. Cell 67:1121, 1991.
349. Liu, Y., Joshua, D. E., Williams, G. T., Smith, C. A., Gordon, J., and MacLennan, I. C. M.: Mechanism of antigen-driven selection in germinal centres. Nature 342:929, 1989.
350. MacLennan, I. C. M., Liu, Y. J., Oldfield, S., Zhang, J., and Lane, P. J. L.: The evolution of B-cell clones. Curr. Top. Microbiol. Immunol. 159:37, 1990.
351. Gray, D., Kosco, M., and Stockinger, B.: Novel pathways of antigen presentation for the maintenance of memory. Int. Immunol. 3:141, 1990.
352. Gray, D., and Leanderson, T.: Expansion, selection and maintenance of memory of B-cell clones. Curr. Top. Microbiol. Immunol. 159:1, 1990.
353. Liu, Y., Cairns, J. A., Holder, M. J., Abbot, S. D., Jansen, K. U., Bonnefoy, J., Gordon, J., and MacLennan, C. M.: Re-

combinant 25-kDa CD23 and interleukin 1a promote the survival of germinal center B cells: Evidence for bifurcation in the development of centrocytes rescued from apoptosis. Eur. J. Immunol. 21:1107, 1991.

354. Budd, R. C., Cerottini, J., Horvath, C., Bron, C., Pedrazzini, T., Howe, R. C., and MacDonald, H. R.: Distinction of virgin and memory T lymphocytes. J. Immunol. 138:3120, 1987.

355. Sanders, M. E., Makgoba, M., Sharrow, S. O., Stephany, D., Springer, T. A., Young, H. A., and Shaw, S.: Human memory T lymphocytes express increased levels of three cell adhesion molecules (LFA-3, CD2, and LFA-1) and three other molecules (UCHL1, CDw29, and Pgp-1) and have enhanced IFN-γ production. J. Immunol. 140:1401, 1988.

356. Mackay, C. R., Marston, W. L., and Dudler, L.: Naive and memory T cells show distinct pathways of lymphocyte recirculation. J. Exp. Med. 171:801, 1990.

357. Mackay, C. R., Klimpton, W. G., Brandon, M. R., and Cahill, R. N. P.: Lymphocyte subsets show marked differences in their distribution between blood, and afferent and efferent lymph draining peripheral lymph nodes. J. Exp. Med. 167:1755, 1988.

358. Bradley, L. M., Atkins, G. G., and Swain, S. L.: Long-term CD4+ memory T cells from the spleen lack MEL-14, the lymph node homing receptor. J. Immunol. 148:324, 1992.

359. Van Seventer, G. A., Newman, W., Shimizu, Y., Nutman, T. B., Tanaka, Y., Horgan, K. J., Gopal, T. V., Ennis, E., O'Sullivan, D., Grey, H., and Shaw, S.: Analysis of T cell stimulation by superantigen plus major histocompatibility complex class II molecules or by CD3 monoclonal antibody: Constitution by purified adhesion ligands VCAM-1, ICAM-1 but not ELAM-1. J. Exp. Med. 174:901, 1991.

360. De Sousa M., Tilney N. L., and Kupiec-Weglinski, J. W.: Recognition of self within self: Specific lymphocyte positioning and the extracellular matrix. Immunol. Today 12:262, 1991.

361. Denning, S. M., Le, P. T., Singer, K. H., and Haynes, B. F.: Antibodies against the CD44 p80 lymphocyte homing receptor augment human peripheral blood T cell activation. J. Immunol. 144:7, 1990.

362. Haynes, B. F., Telen, M. J., Hale, L. P., and Denning, S. M.: CD44—a molecule involved in leukocyte adherence and T-cell activation. Immunol. Today 10:423, 1989.

363. Haynes, B. F.: Immune responses to HIV. In DeVita, V. T., Hellman, S., and Rosenberg, S. A. (eds.): AIDS: Etiology, Diagnosis, Treatment and Prevention. 3rd ed., Philadelphia, J. B. Lippincott, 1991.

364. Robey, E., and Axel, R.: CD4: Collaborator in immune recognition and HIV infection. Cell 60:697, 1990.

365. Schnittman, S. M., Lane, H. C., Greenhouse, J., Justement, J. S., Baseler, M., and Fauci, A. S.: Preferential infection of CD4+ memory T cells by human immunodeficiency virus type 1: Evidence for a role in the selective T-cell functional defects observed in infected individuals. Proc. Natl. Acad. Sci. USA 87:6058, 1990.

366. Basch, R. S., Kouri, Y. H., and Karpatkin, S.: Expression of CD4 by human megakaryocytes. Proc. Natl. Acad. Sci. USA 87:8085, 1990.

367. Stanley, S. K., Kessler, S. W., Justement, J. S., Schnittman, S. M., Greenhouse, J. J., Brown, C. C., Musongela, L., Musey, K., Kapita, B., and Fauci, A. S.: CD34+ bone marrow cells are infected with the human immunodeficiency virus in a subset of seropositive individuals. J. Immunol. 149:689, 1992.

368. Freedman, A. R., Gibson, F. M., Fleming, S. C., Spry, C. J., and Griffin, G. E.: Human immunodeficiency virus infection of eosinophils in human bone marrow cultures. J. Exp. Med. 174:1661, 1991.

369. Schuurman, H., Krone, W. J. A., Broekhuizen, R., van Baarlen, J., van Veen, P., Goldstein, A. L., Huber, J., and Goudsmit, J.: The thymus in acquired immune deficiency syndrome. Am. J. Pathol. 134:1329, 1989.

370. Savino, W., Dardenne, M., Marche, C., Trophilme, D., Dupuy, J., Pekovic, D., Lapointe, N., and Bach, J.: Thymic epithelium in AIDS: An immunohistologic study. Am. J. Pathol. 122:302, 1985.

371. Ameisen, J. C., and Capron, A.: Cell dysfunction and depletion in AIDS: The programmed cell death hypothesis. Immunol. Today 12:102, 1991.

ACKNOWLEDGMENTS: The authors acknowledge Diane Bennett and Kim R. McClammy for expert secretarial assistance.

Antigen Processing and T-Cell Effector Mechanisms

Roger M. Perlmutter

INTRODUCTION

White blood cells exist to provide broad protection from parasitism. The effector mechanisms that constitute host defense operate with considerable vigor. This fact requires that strategies must also exist to permit satisfactory discrimination of potential pathogens from normal host cells. Not surprisingly, the cellular and molecular processes that permit this exquisitely subtle identification of non-self structures are highly sophisticated.

The pathway underlying a typical immune response to a typical protein antigen can be schematized as follows (Fig. 13–1). The primary B-cell repertoire is sufficiently large ($>10^8$ different species at the minimum) to permit binding of most proteins with some measurable affinity. (See Chapter 11.) Foreign proteins, bound to the surface immunoglobulins of a B lymphocyte, or simply ingested by a macrophage, are then internalized and digested in an endosomal compartment, yielding peptide fragments, some of which can bind to class II antigen presentation molecules. Peptide/class II complexes appear on the B-cell or macrophage surface, permitting recognition by T-cell

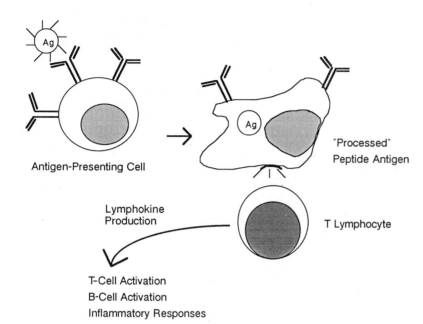

Antigen-Presenting Cell

"Processed" Peptide Antigen

Lymphokine Production

T Lymphocyte

T-Cell Activation
B-Cell Activation
Inflammatory Responses

FIGURE 13–1. A simplified schematic diagram of immune response physiology at the cellular level. Complex immunogens are processed by specialized antigen-presenting cells (a B lymphocyte in this case) to yield peptides that form stimulatory complexes with class I or class II antigen-presenting molecules that are recognized by T cells. Lymphokines produced by these cells regulate all other aspects of immune function.

antigen receptors. This recognition event in turn stimulates the elaboration of lymphokines, and T-cell replication. In this way, additional cells bearing receptors for the peptide/class II complex antigen are produced. B-cell replication and antibody production are also enhanced. Moreover, lymphokine expression by "helper" T lymphocytes encourages migration of additional inflammatory cells to the site of antigen contact. The process is maintained until all stimulatory antigen has been consumed and degraded.

Three simple lessons may be deduced from considering immune function in this schematic way. First, T lymphocytes regulate all immune responses. Antigen recognition by T cells permits elaboration of potent lymphokines that regulate the activity of phagocytic cells, B lymphocytes, and other T cells as well. Second, T lymphocytes recognize peptide antigens derived from the digestion of proteins within antigen-presenting cells. This means of recognition provides fundamental safeguards against the propagation of autoimmune responses and directly underlies self/non-self discrimination. Third, there exist both cellular (principally involving cytotoxic T cells and phagocytic cells) and humoral (principally involving antibodies and complement components) immune effector mechanisms, both types of which are required for satisfactory host defense against parasitism.

In the following discussion, the cellular effector mechanisms that mediate immune function are considered in detail, beginning with a description of the molecular features of antigen processing and presentation, proceeding to examine the biochemistry of lymphocyte activation, and finally evaluating the molecules elaborated by T cells that coordinate immune attack. Each of these areas has experienced dramatic advances in understanding during the past few years, resulting in a fairly comprehensive view of mammalian host defense mechanisms. Moreover, abnormalities in

the recognition and effector functions of T-cell immunity contribute to the pathogenesis of many inflammatory diseases.

ANTIGEN PROCESSING AND PRESENTATION

T Lymphocytes Recognize Peptides Associated with Major Histocompatibility Complex (MHC)–Encoded Proteins

Early studies of humoral immunity permitted identification of B lymphocytes as antibody-secreting cells that also bear cell surface antibody molecules.[1] In these cells, the recognition element (surface antibody) differs from the effector molecule simply by the presence of a membrane-spanning region at the carboxy-terminal end of two constituent polypeptides (the antibody heavy chains). Not surprisingly, binding of cognate antigen by B cells can be demonstrated directly.[2, 3]

This situation contrasts with that observed in the case of T lymphocytes. Such cells do not recognize polypeptide antigens in soluble form. Moreover, no binding of antigen to immune T cells can be demonstrated. Careful experiments conducted over a period of years revealed that T-cell recognition of protein antigens requires degradation of the antigen by a presenting cell, which then displays fragments of the protein in association with specialized dimeric glycoproteins, the class I and class II molecules. It is this complex of peptide fragment and cell surface presentation molecules that commands the attention of the T-cell antigen receptor, which must distinguish between self-polypeptides and foreign polypeptides that are presented simultaneously. The biochemical pathway that converts proteins to appropriate T-cell antigens is termed "antigen processing."

Differential Processing of Exogenous and Endogenous Antigens

Although pulsing of antigen-presenting cells with antigen is required to permit generation of a substrate capable of stimulating T cells, in some circumstances the antigenic molecule may be synthesized endogenously. This occurs, for example, in virally infected cells, where viral proteins synthesized on host ribosomes nevertheless yield antigenic determinants that can be recognized by T lymphocytes interacting with cell surface structures. Moreover, a variety of "self"-antigens are routinely presented to T cells and provide a mechanism for deleting or neutralizing clones of cells that might potentially mediate autoimmune responses.[4] Comprehensive studies over many years demonstrate that the distinction between exogenous antigens, acquired via phagocytosis, and endogenous antigens, which are synthesized directly by the presenting cell itself, is quite rigorous. They are processed in distinct compartments and are presented by different cell surface glycoproteins. Exogenous antigens appear on the cell surface in association with class II molecules, whereas endogenous antigens are presented in association with class I molecules. These two types of peptide-presenting proteins are structurally related and are encoded by linked genes.

Specialization of T Cells for Recognition of MHC Class I or Class II Structures

The restriction of antigen presentation to class I or class II pathways is mirrored by a similar specialization of T cells themselves. Although all T cells bear very similar antigen receptors on their surfaces, they differ with respect to the synthesis of two coreceptor structures. In healthy adults, about two thirds of peripheral T cells express the CD4 coreceptor molecule. These T cells are specialized to recognize exogenous antigens and to respond to antigen interaction by elaborating potent lymphokines. The remaining one third of circulating T cells instead express the CD8 coreceptor, and these cells usually recognize endogenous antigens. The response of CD8+ T cells to endogenous antigens presented in association with class I molecules also results in the production of lymphokines but in addi-

tion can stimulate the maturation of cytolytic pathways that permit the CD8-bearing cell to specifically lyse target cells bearing appropriate antigens.

In normal adult T cells, CD4 expression and CD8 expression are mutually exclusive, reflecting the subspecialization of T cells bearing these structures (Fig. 13–2). However, T cells of both types must be presented with a processed antigen. Many of the enzymes required for this processing to take place, as well as the class I and class II presentation molecules themselves, are encoded within a multigene complex, the human leukocyte antigen (HLA) region.

MOLECULAR BIOLOGY OF THE HUMAN LEUKOCYTE ANTIGEN COMPLEX

Classic experiments performed more than 50 years ago by Owen and by Medawar and colleagues defined a set of simple rules that govern the fate of tissue grafts exchanged between individuals.[5] A rapid, immune-mediated rejection is observed for virtually all such allografts (performed between members of the same species) unless identity exists in a genetic region that came to be called the *major histocompatibility complex.* Defined in all vertebrates, the MHC includes a set of codominantly inherited genes that function to permit appropriate antigen presentation to T lymphocytes. In man, the genes of the MHC were first identified using serological reagents that detect white blood cell antigens. Hence the MHC gene complex came to be known as the *human leukocyte antigen* or HLA locus.[6] During the past decade, energetic application of molecular genetic methods has resulted in the nearly complete dissection of genes that reside within the HLA complex and its mouse analogue, the H-2 complex. Included within the nearly 4 million base pairs (bp) that encompass the HLA complex are more than 76 genes, most of which exert direct effects on immune responsiveness.[7]

Class I Genes Encode Classical Transplantation Antigens

Traditionally, genes positioned within the HLA complex are divided into three classes. Class I genes

---

CD4+ T Cell

FIGURE 13–2. Subspecialization in the T-cell compartment. Mature T cells can be divided into two distinct populations, those that bear CD4 surface coreceptors and those that bear analogous CD8 polypeptides. The main functions of these two classes of cells are tabulated.

* Recognize peptide/class II complexes
* Produce IL-2, IL-3, IL-4, IL-5, IL-6, GM-CSF
* Regulate antibody production by B cells
* Regulate maturation of cytotoxic T cells

CD8+ T Cell

* Recognize peptide/class I complexes
* Produce interferon-gamma and IL-2
* Stimulate antigen presentation
* Activate inflammatory cells
* Directly mediate cytotoxicity

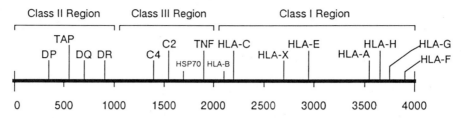

FIGURE 13–3. Genetic structure of the HLA locus. Some of the 76 known genes that reside within this genetic region that spans more than 4 million base pairs (bp) on chromosome 6 are indicated. The positions of these genes are indicated along a scale calibrated in kilobase pairs. The centromere is at the left. TNF = Tumor necrosis factor; HLA = human leukocyte antigen. (Data from Trowsdale, J., Ragoussis, J., and Campbell, R. D.: Map of the human MHC. Immunol. Today 12:443, 1991.)

are expressed in all nucleated cells and encode proteins that present peptide antigens to CD8-bearing T cells. The HLA-A, HLA-B, and HLA-C subregions include those genes that encode human class I molecules. The class II molecules are structurally related and are encoded within the HLA-D region. A third set of molecules, encoded within the class III region, includes the complement components C2, C4, and factor B. More recently, additional genes have been identified that encode components of the intracellular antigen-processing machinery. Figure 13–3 presents a diagram of the human HLA locus indicating the approximate positions of the various genetic elements and the subregions into which these are grouped. Cosmid-based chromosomal walking techniques have provided physical map information for much of the HLA complex.[8-11] Nevertheless, numerous regions remain only partially characterized. Hence the 76 genes already defined within the HLA locus together provide only a minimal estimate of the total number of functional elements. An up-to-date listing of the known HLA genes is presented in Table 13–1.

The class I molecules define targets for recognition by cytotoxic T lymphocytes (CTLs) and hence are

TABLE 13–1. HLA GENES

CLASS II REGION	CLASS III REGION	CLASS I REGION
KE3(D6S219)	G18(X6)(G6S214E)	1.7p
RING1(D6S111E)	G17(D6213E)	HLA-B
RING2(D6S112E)	G16(X5)(D6S212E)	HLA-C
KE4	G15(X4)(D6S211E)	HLA-X
KE5(D6S218)	G14(X3)(D6S210E)	HLA-E(6.2)
COL11A2	G13(X1,X2)D6S209E)	cda12(D6S203)(5.9p)
HLA-DPB2	G12(D6S208E)	HLA-A
HLA-DPA2	OSG(opposite strand gene/D6S103E)	HLA-H(H/AR/12.4)
HLA-DPB1	CYP21B(CYP21)	HLA-G(6.0)
HLA-DPA1	C4B	7.5p and 9p(X)
HLA-DNA(DZα/DOα)	CYP21A(CYP21P)	HLA-F(5.4)
Y5	C4A	
RING3(D6113E/Y4)	G11(D6S60E)	
RING6(DMA)	RD(D6S45)	
RING7(DMB)	Bf (factor B)(BF)	
RING12	C2	
RING4(D6S114E/Y3/PSF1)	G10(BAT9)(D6S59E)	
RING9(D6S215)	G9a(BAT8)	
RING10(Y2)(D6S216E)	G9(BAT7)(D6S58E)	
RING11(Y1/PSF2)(D6S217E)	G8(D6S57E)	
HLA-DOB	Hsp70-2(HSPA1L)	
HLA-DQB2	Hsp70-1(HSP70)(HSPA1)	
HLA-DQA2	Hsp70-HOM	
DQB3(DVβ/D6S205)	G7a(BAT6)(valyl-tRNA synthetase)(VARS2)	
HLA-DQB1	G7(D6S56E)	
HLA-DQA1	G6(D6S55E)	
HLA-DRB	BAT5(D6S82E)	
β1ψ-PSEUDOGENE(β-1 exon)	G5(BAT4)(D6S54E)	
HLA-DRA	G4(D6S53E)	
	G3(BAT3)(D6S52E)	
	G2(BAT2)(D6S51E)	
	G1(D6S50E)	
	B144(D6S49)	
	TNFA(tumor necrosis factor-α)	
	TNFB(lymphotoxin)	
	BAT1(D6S81E)	

often called classical transplantation antigens. Typical representatives of the extended family of immunoglobulin-like cell surface molecules, the class I proteins exist on the surfaces of all nucleated cells as noncovalently linked heterodimers of a 44 kDa heavy chain, the HLA-A, -B, or -C product, and a 12 kDa polypeptide, β_2-microglobulin, encoded separately on chromosome 15. Each class I heavy chain consists of three extracellular domains, $\alpha 1$, $\alpha 2$, and $\alpha 3$, fused to a membrane-spanning region and a short intracytoplasmic extension (Fig. 13–4). The $\alpha 1$ and $\alpha 2$ domains, each about 90 amino acids in length, fold to yield two parallel helical segments that form the boundaries of a groove that ordinarily accommodates peptide antigens.[12] The floor of the groove is formed by an eight-stranded antiparallel β-pleated sheet to which both the $\alpha 1$ and the $\alpha 2$ domains contribute. The $\alpha 3$ domain assumes a more conventional β-barrel structure, like that of other immunoglobulin superfamily members, and forms a stable interaction with β_2-microglobulin, itself similarly configured.[12] The $\alpha 3$ domain also includes a site that interacts with the CD8 coreceptor glycoprotein expressed on most T lymphocytes that recognize class I–presented antigens.[13] Figure 13–5 provides two views of the class I crystal structure first determined by Wiley and colleagues for an HLA-A molecule.[12] These investigators noted that positioned within the outward-facing groove was additional electron density, representing processed peptide antigens that copurify with class I proteins.[14] Indeed, persuasive evidence supports the view that stable assembly of class I proteins at physiological temperatures requires, in most cases, additional peptides that interact non-covalently and that result from intracellular proteolysis of autologous proteins.[15] It should be apparent from Figure 13–5 that variations in the structure of HLA class I proteins between individuals could potentially influence the efficiency with which certain peptides are bound. Such differences almost certainly account for some variations in immune responses to infections in the human population and also contribute to susceptibility to numerous autoimmune diseases (see below).

The HLA-A, -B, and -C proteins are all quite similar and are encoded by closely related genes (Fig. 13–6). In each case, the organization of exons parallels to a large extent the structure of the protein itself: Each exon defines a distinct protein domain. Control of HLA class I expression depends primarily on transcriptional regulatory mechanisms that direct the synthesis of HLA-A, -B, and -C transcripts simultaneously in virtually all cells.[16] Defects in this transcriptional regulation may in part explain certain cases of bare lymphocyte syndrome in which the class I gene products are absent.[17] Additional highly specialized class I genes have also been identified, such as the HLA-E, -F, and -G genes,[18] which encode structurally similar proteins that also associate with β_2-microglobulin. In the mouse, related atypical class I molecules encoded by the Tla gene have been shown to behave as specialized antigen presentation structures in gut epithelia, at least in some circumstances.[19] A similar role has been postulated for the human HLA-E, -F, and -G products. For example, HLA-G is expressed preferentially in human trophoblast cells[20] and may serve to provide a means of cell-cell recognition at this site.

Some atypical class I heavy chains are encoded outside the HLA locus. These polypeptides share overall organization with conventional HLA-A, -B, and -C molecules, and they associate with β_2-microglobulin to form typical class I proteins. Included in this group are the CD1 heavy chains, which may form recognition structures capable of presenting peptide antigens to γ/δ T cells, a rare T-cell subset.[21] In addition, an immunoglobulin F_c-binding transport protein, which assists in directing antibody secretion across epithelia, has recently been shown to consist of an atypical class I heavy chain interacting with β_2-microglobulin.[22]

Class II Genes Encode Regulators of Immune Responsiveness

Genetically determined differences in immune responsiveness between individuals of the same species frequently result from sequence variability in genes

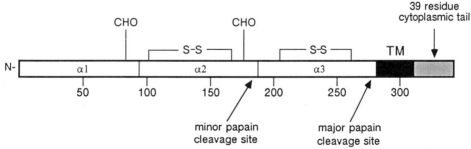

FIGURE 13–4. Structure of a class I molecule. Three extracellular domains are juxtaposed to a single transmembrane sequence and a short cytoplasmic tail. The presence of a dominant papain cleavage site near the outer membrane boundary has facilitated purification and crystallization of this molecule (see Fig. 13–5). The $\alpha 2$ and $\alpha 3$ domains contain typical immunoglobulin homology units (see reference 11), with centrally placed disulfide bonds. The positions of carbohydrate residues are indicated. Data used to generate this diagram were derived from the structure of a murine class I molecule (H-2K^b); the structures of all class I molecules are closely related (see reference 206 for details).

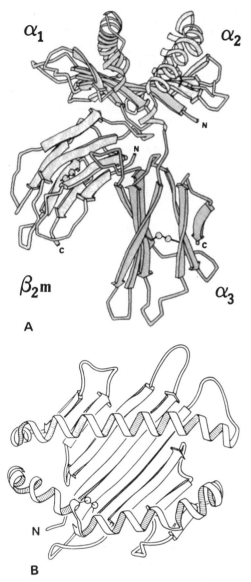

FIGURE 13–5. The three-dimensional structure of a class I molecule. Shown are ribbon diagrams illustrating the structure of HLA-A2. *Left panel,* Complete structure of the two-chain molecule seen from an axis perpendicular to the cell membrane. The free amino- and carboxy-termini of both the heavy chain and β₂-microglobulin are indicated. The β strands appear as thick arrows in the amino- to carboxy-terminal direction. Loops and helical regions are depicted as thin lines and ribbons, respectively. Disulfide bonds are indicated by small circles. The carboxy-terminus of the heavy chain has been truncated at a papain cleavage site (see Fig. 13–4) near the membrane. Processed peptides bind within the helical groove defined at the top of the figure. The CD8 molecule on T cells interacts with class I heavy chains via sequences on both faces of the β barrel of the α3 domain. *Right panel,* A second view of the HLA-A2 molecule locking down on the peptide-binding groove. This is the perspective that we imagine confronts a T-cell receptor molecule bent on antigen recognition. The T-cell receptor appears to make contacts with both the peptide and the class I molecule. (Redrawn by permission from Nature Vol. 329, pp. 506–512. Copyright © 1987, Macmillan Magazines Limited.)

encoding class II molecules.[23, 24] Early studies in inbred animals established that the immune response or IR loci mapped coordinately with class II specificities defined using lymphocyte proliferation assays.[24] In most cases, MHC-linked genetically determined nonresponsiveness displays recessive inheritance, although exceptions, apparent instances of MHC-encoded immunosuppression, have been widely (but not yet fruitfully) described.[25] Biochemical studies now provide a firm basis for understanding the immune response differences determined by class II genes. These elements encode cell surface proteins that present peptide antigens, derived via catabolism of ingested proteins, to CD4-bearing T lymphocytes.[26, 27] Hence allelic differences in class II gene structure almost certainly correspond directly to differences in the ability to present certain protein antigens properly.

Figure 13–7 provides a schematic representation of

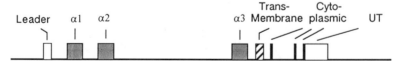

FIGURE 13–6. Organization of genes encoding class I molecules. The domain organization of these proteins is mirrored in the exon structures of the genes that encode them. Open boxes designate exons encoding the leader or the 3′ untranslated region. Three distinct exons (shown as filled areas) contribute to the synthesis of the 39 residue cytoplasmic domain. The sizes of the intervening sequences vary somewhat from element to element. (Data from Hood, L., Steinmetz, M., and Malissen, B.: Genes of the major histocompatibility complex of the mouse. Annu. Rev. Immunol. 1:529, 1988.)

FIGURE 13–7. Class I and class II MHC proteins share a common structure. The schematic organization of class I and class II proteins is compared, showing how β_2-microglobulin, interacting with the $\alpha3$ and $\alpha1$ domains of the class I heavy chain, could have come to take the place of the $\alpha2$ domain of the class II protein. (Adapted, with permission, from the Annual Reviews in Immunology, Vol. 8, pp. 23–63, © 1990 by Annual Reviews, Inc.)

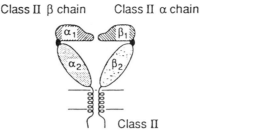
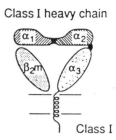

the structure of class II molecules. Each consists of two approximately 30 kDa glycoproteins, the α and β chains, which are both encoded within the HLA complex.[28] In man, at least seven functional α chain genes and a similar number of β chain genes have been directly identified by DNA sequencing. These are grouped by sequence relatedness and by physical organization into the HLA-DO, -DP, -DQ, and -DR families (Fig. 13–8). All class II molecules share the same general structure, reflecting their common antigen presentation function and a common evolutionary origin that they share with class I molecules.[29] At present, no class II structures have been visualized by physical methods; however, a detailed model based on the known structure of class I proteins has satisfactorily met some empirical challenges (Fig. 13–9).[30] The class II polypeptides consist of two extracellular "domains" linked to the cell surface by a transmembrane helix and a short cytoplasmic tail. Interaction between the $\alpha1$ and $\beta1$ domains is proposed to yield an antigen-binding cleft like that already visualized in class I molecules. The $\alpha2$ and $\beta2$ domains contain sequence motifs that probably direct them to fold as typical immunoglobulin homology units.[31] During intracellular assembly, class II molecules are associated with a non–MHC-encoded "invariant" chain (Ii or γ), which, as discussed below, is believed to assist in regulating intracellular transport of class II complexes.[32]

Regulation of Class II Gene Expression

The class II proteins are expressed on the surfaces of specialized antigen-presenting cells: B lymphocytes, macrophages, dendritic cells, thymic epithelia, and some other stromal cell types. Although the principal function of class II molecules manifestly is peptide presentation to T cells, considerable evidence supports the view that the cytoplasmic tails of class II proteins may provide signals to the antigen-presenting cell as well, perhaps signaling cognate recognition by an antigen-specific T cell.[33] The restricted expression of class II molecules by inflammatory cells provides a mechanism whereby immune function can be triggered most effectively at sites of parasite accumulation. In man, class II gene expression can also be induced in activated T lymphocytes.[34]

As in the case of class I genes, expression of the HLA class II genes is coordinately regulated. Transcriptional control regions for the class II genes have been defined in detail,[35] and nuclear factors that participate in regulating the expression of class II transcripts have been rigorously identified. Restriction of class II protein expression to specialized antigen-presenting cells appears to be important. For example, evidence exists to support the view that inappropriate class II expression in certain cell types stimulates a focused autoimmune response. Thus, for example, enhanced expression of class II molecules in the β cells of pancreatic islets may precipitate the development of diabetes in some cases.[36] Similarly, class II expression on thyroid follicular cells in autoimmune thyroiditis has been occasionally observed. However, these results may reflect the action of inflammatory cytokines that act to increase class II gene transcription in many cell types (see below).

Although controversy exists regarding the deleterious effects of inappropriate class II gene expression, the failure to transcribe class II genes produces unambiguous immune deficits. Since the class II genes are coordinately expressed, individuals lacking class II

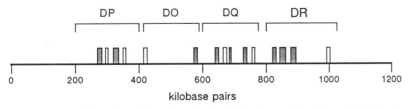

FIGURE 13–8. Structure of the class II region of the HLA locus. The four HLA-D subregions span approximately 1000 kb. Filled boxes denote Dβ genes, whereas the open boxes encode Dα genes. It is important to note that substantial polymorphism in HLA-D region organization exists in the human population. For example, although three DRβ genes are noted, the central gene is a pseudogene, and individuals with as few as one DRβ gene element (DR$\beta1$) or as many as four (with two central pseudogenes) have been identified. Additional class II genes have been tentatively positioned between DP and DO. (Redrawn from Trowsdale, J., Ragoussis, J., and Campbell, R. D.: Map of the human MHC. Immunol. Today 12:443, 1991; with permission.)

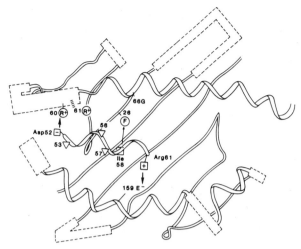

FIGURE 13–9. Hypothetical three-dimensional structure of a class II molecule. Shown is a model for the structure of a murine class II molecule (I-A^k) to which a peptide derived from hen egg lysozyme (residues 52 to 61), known to be presented by this class II protein, has been bound. The peptide is assumed to adopt a helical configuration. Within the peptide, boxes represent residues that by experimental criteria interact with the class II protein, and triangles represent those residues that interact with the T-cell receptor. Bold arrows indicate potential salt bridges. Although the structure has been modeled based on the known configuration of class I proteins and on the positioning of shared residues in these related proteins, significant differences must exist in the configurations of the peptide-binding clefts, since class I proteins bind short (8 or 9 residue) peptides, whereas class II molecules typically associate with much larger polypeptides (see text for details). (Adapted with permission from Nature Vol. 332, pp. 845–850. Copyright © 1988, Macmillan Magazines Limited.)

expression intact), reacquire expression of all class II proteins simultaneously after fusion with B cells from a normal individual.[37, 38] Such studies define four distinct complementation groups of genes regulating basal class II protein expression.[39]

In one special case, a transcription factor believed to be defective in at least some patients with bare lymphocyte syndrome was defined by molecular cloning.[40] However, the mechanisms responsible for most cases of defective class II protein synthesis remain undefined. As outlined in Chapter 12, failure to produce class II proteins results in the inability to support development of CD4-bearing T lymphocytes and hence a profound immunodeficiency.[41, 42]

Although class I protein expression can be adjusted to only a limited degree in most normal cells, class II expression is highly responsive to the presence of certain lymphokines, notably interferon-γ and interleukin-4 (IL-4).[43–45] In both of these cases, expression is regulated at the level of transcription initiation. Indeed, in most cell types, including several that do not ordinarily participate in antigen presentation, the addition of interferon-γ results in significant expression of class II molecules.[46] Since there is reason to believe that the proteolytic machinery responsible for antigen processing is widely distributed, the induction of class II transcription can suffice to promote effective antigen presentation by a variety of cells. An outline of the known transcriptional regulatory elements in typical class II genes is presented in Figure 13–10; one should note especially the presence of putative interferon-γ regulatory sequences.

ANTIGEN PROCESSING IN MOLECULAR DETAIL

Two fundamental types of antigens must gain access to antigen presentation molecules: products of intracellular synthesis and materials ingested through phagocytosis. Until very recently, the mechanisms that

protein were believed to have sustained mutations in a critical *trans*-acting factor that regulates all class II genes simultaneously. This hypothesis is borne out by somatic cell hybridization studies demonstrating that class II B cells from patients with bare lymphocyte syndrome, type II (the form in which class II gene expression is selectively abrogated, leaving class I gene

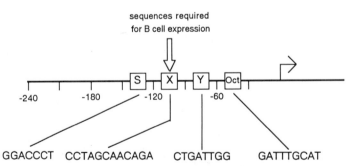

FIGURE 13–10. Sequences involved in regulating class II gene expression. The positions of regulatory elements within the DRα gene are indicated schematically, with the transcription start site (conventionally defined as +1) designated with an arrow at the right. Base pairs in the 5′ direction are indicated, preceded by a minus sign. A set of critical regulatory "boxes," representing the sequences noted at the bottom, determines class II gene expression and responsiveness to extracellular stimuli. In DRα, 5′ truncation to the X box depresses expression in B cells, but not in T cells or fibroblasts. Similarly, deletion of the X box markedly reduces B-cell expression.[207] The X box also appears to be involved in the response to interferon-γ[208] and is affected by the S and Y regions.[209] The DRα gene is unique in containing an "Oct" sequence, first defined in the immunoglobulin enhancer, that interacts with octamer-binding proteins, notably Oct-2, which is thought to be involved in B-cell expression.[210]

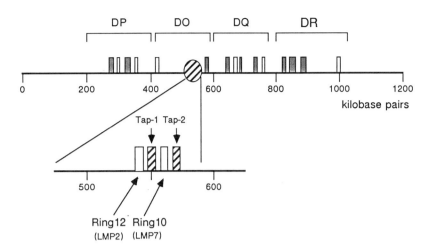

FIGURE 13–11. Components of a peptide-processing system are encoded within the HLA class II region. The position of two recently described members of the "ABC" family of transporter-encoding genes near the DOβ gene is shown. These two elements, now designated TAP-1 and TAP-2,[211] are almost certainly products of a gene duplication event that also included a component of the low molecular mass polypeptide (LMP) complex,[212, 213] such that two Tap transporter genes are interspersed with two LMP genes in a very short segment of germline DNA.

permit catabolism of protein antigens and those that direct interactions between peptides and MHC-encoded presentation molecules were enigmatic. Remarkably, it now appears that several crucial components of the antigen-processing apparatus are themselves encoded within the MHC (i.e., the HLA) complex.[47, 48] Moreover, refinements in microscale protein chemistry have led to the purification and characterization of processed peptides eluted from both class I and class II molecules.[49–51] With this information, it has become possible to distill a satisfactory working model of antigen-processing pathways.

Presentation of Endogenously Synthesized Proteins

Proteins encoded by most chromosomal genes, and those that are synthesized on cellular ribosomes using viral RNA templates, are presented in peptide form to CD8-bearing T lymphocytes by class I molecules. The basic steps in this process involve digestion by endogenous proteases, transport of peptides to an appropriate site for interaction with class I proteins, and movement of the class I/peptide complex to the cell surface. Since both the class I heavy chain and β₂-microglobulin are glycoproteins synthesized on membrane-bound polysomes, peptide binding to the nascent class I protein must occur either within the lumen of the endoplasmic reticulum or in the Golgi complex. However, since peptides derived from proteins synthesized on free polysomes are effectively presented by class I molecules, mechanisms must exist to transport peptides from the cytosol into the endoplasmic reticulum.[52] Indeed, elegant experiments by Bevan and colleagues demonstrated that soluble proteins, introduced into the cytoplasm of cells via hypotonic lysis of pinocytotic vesicles, can be cleaved to yield peptides that become associated with class I molecules. Hence the transport mechanism must act to "pump" peptides from the cytoplasm into secretory compartments, where assembly of class I molecules is achieved.[53]

At least some components of both the proteolytic apparatus and the peptide pump are encoded within the class II region of the HLA complex. Two components of a common multifunctional protease (the low molecular mass polypeptide or LMP complex, which represents a subset of the multifunctional protease structures known generally as proteasomes), expressed ubiquitously and highly conserved throughout eukaryotic evolution, are found here (LMP2 and LMP7; Fig. 13–11). Moreover, two genes (TAP-1 and TAP-2) that are closely related to the multidrug resistance gene (*mdr*) and therefore appear to act as peptide transporters also reside within the class II subregion.[47, 48] These putative transporters are members of a larger "ABC" family of ATP-binding transmembrane pumps. It is probable that the TAP-1 and TAP-2 proteins together form a heterodimeric transporter. Although definitive evidence linking proteasome-mediated proteolysis to antigen processing has not yet been adduced, there seems little doubt that at least some peptides are produced via this mechanism.[54]

Studies of mutant mouse and human cell lines that cannot present peptides in association with class I molecules strongly suggest that proper assembly of these structures requires association with peptides generated in situ.[15, 55] This finding is reflected in heightened thermal instability of the "empty" class I structures. Thus, intact class I molecules appear when such mutant cells are cultivated at low temperature, but they separate into constituent heavy and light chains when the temperature is raised to 37°C.[15, 56] The peptide-free class I structures can be stabilized by adding exogenous peptide. Proper folding of the class I molecule with peptides is probably facilitated by molecular chaperones. Indeed, two members of the heat shock protein (Hsp 70) family, believed to assist in this process, are encoded within the HLA complex.[10]

From a biochemical perspective, it is difficult to imagine that three major class I proteins, the HLA-A, -B, and -C molecules, can satisfactorily present the full range of viral peptides that might be necessary for immune defense. Similarly, it is difficult to imagine how satisfactory antigen presentation can be achieved when peptides derived via catabolism of host proteins

TABLE 13–2. CONSENSUS MOTIFS IN PEPTIDES ELUTED FROM MHC CLASS I MOLECULES*

SPECIES	CLASS I ALLELE	PEPTIDE SEQUENCE AT POSITION								
		1	**2**	**3**	**4**	**5**	**6**	**7**	**8**	**9**
Mouse	D^b	X	M L P V	I E Q V	K	**N** F	L	X	X	**M** I
Mouse	K^d	X	**Y**	N I L	P	M	K F	T N	X	**I** L
Mouse	K^b	X	X	Y	X	**F** Y	X	X	**L** M	
Human	HLA-A2	X	**L** M	X	E K	X	V	X	K	**V**
Human	HLA-B27	R K G	**R**	X	X	X	X	X	X	K R

*Shown are consensus sequences, in single-letter code, with "X" denoting any amino acid, of peptides eluted from immunoprecipitates containing the indicated class I molecule. In each case, multiple different peptides were purified by high-performance liquid chromatography, and alignment was achieved with reference to the few highly conserved residues. Assignments noted in boldface are those believed to be critical for binding to the indicated class I protein. Note that the class I protein encoded by the mouse K^b gene binds octamer sequences that differ dramatically from those nonamers found associated with the allelic K^d class I protein. See Falk et al.[59] and Jardetzky et al.[62] for additional information.

must certainly outnumber to a very large extent those encoded by intracellular parasites. Purification of the peptides associated with class I proteins from man and mouse provides some partial answers to these questions.[4, 49, 50] This strategy, first pursued by Rammensee and colleagues, has proved to be extraordinarily revealing. In general, papain-solubilized class I molecules are purified and the peptide components eluted using organic acid. These peptide products can be fractionated and characterized. Several general con-

clusions emerge from the studies. First, class I proteins bind peptides of quite specific length; only peptides composed of eight or nine amino acids are acceptable. X-ray crystallographic evidence supports the view that nonamer peptides bind to class I molecules in an expanded conformation in which both the amino- and the carboxyl-termini of the peptide fit within small pockets in the class I molecule–binding surface.[57, 58] Moreover, each class I molecule exhibits a distinct preference for peptides with certain primary structures.[59] This observation applies even to allelic class I proteins. Table 13–2 lists sets of peptides that have been found to be bound to representative class I molecules and distills a consensus sequence for binding based on these results. Simply by using the sequence rules inferred from such studies, it has been possible to correctly assign class I–presented peptides in whole-protein immunogens[60] and in proteins derived from parasites that reside intracellularly, such as *Listeria monocytogenes*.[61] Hence the weight of evidence supports the view that endogenously synthesized proteins are in part degraded by a proteasome-based proteolytic mechanism, yielding peptides that in aggregate can be transported to the lumen of the endoplasmic reticulum, and that simple affinity mechanisms select those peptides that bear appropriate residues and that fit within the class I peptide–binding groove. The entire process is illustrated schematically in Figure 13–12.

Can class I molecules bind sufficient peptides to permit recognition of the entire universe of potential pathogens? Determination of the permissible binding sequences for HLA-B27 (an allele of HLA-B) allows some inferences in this regard. Tabulating all of the identified amino acid residues at each of the eight variable sequence positions (position 2 is an invariant arginine) and assuming that all amino acid combinations are acceptable (an as yet untested assumption), we find that 13 million unique peptide sequences could

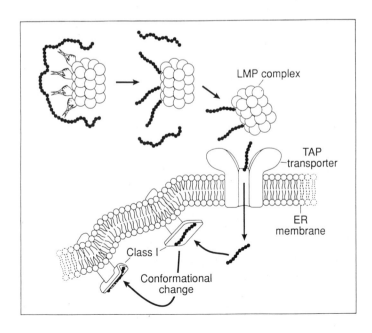

FIGURE 13–12. A model of class I antigen processing. Cytoplasmic proteins are degraded by the low molecular mass polypeptide (LMP) complex, which represents a subset of the cellular pool of proteasomes. Multiple peptides, believed confined primarily to 9 residue segments, can be generated from each polypeptide targeted for degradation. Peptides are delivered to the TAP transporter, probably composed of both TAP-1– and TAP-2–encoded proteins. Once within the lumen of the endoplasmic reticulum, peptides bind to class I molecules. Many believe that this binding precipitates a conformational change that permits transport to the cell surface. (Adapted from Monaco, J. J.: A molecular model of MHC class-I–restricted antigen processing. Immunol. Today 13:173, 1992; with permission.)

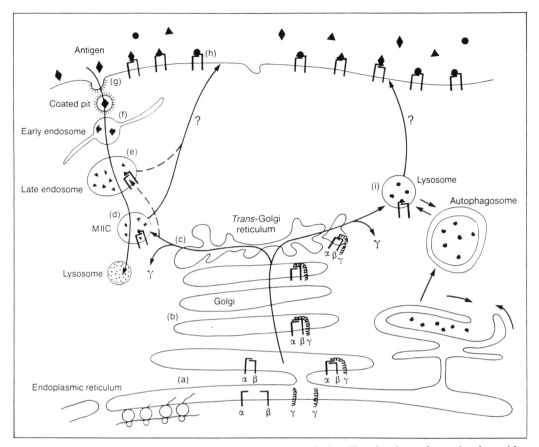

FIGURE 13–13. A schematic model of intracellular transport of class II molecules and associated peptides. Class II molecules are assembled from α and β chains, along with the invariant (or γ) chain, shown at step "a" in the endoplasmic reticulum. These are transported through the endoplasmic reticulum to the *trans*-Golgi as a complex. The γ chain assists in directing transport to the endocytic vesicle, where processed peptides arrive from coated pit–mediated internalization ("d" through "g" at the top of the figure). Cytosolic proteins can enter the class II pathway through autophagosomes. In either case, the resulting class II–peptide complex, lacking the γ chain that has been degraded, is transported to the surface by unknown mechanisms. (Adapted from Neefjes, J. J., and Ploegh, H. L.: Intracellular transport of MHC class II molecules. Immunol. Today 13:174, 1992.)

be accommodated. This should therefore provide an adequate mechanism for sampling, and presenting, the majority of significant protein antigens. Perhaps not surprisingly, most of those peptides that have been characterized in HLA-B27 eluates derive from very abundant cellular proteins, such as histones and ribosomal proteins.[62] Peptide abundance will in part determine the efficacy of expression; however, many studies suggest that there also exists a hierarchy for peptide binding. This observation has prompted a search for high-affinity binding peptides that could be used to block presentation of self-antigens, thereby interdicting immune activation in autoimmune diseases.[63, 64] Clearly, such "masking" peptides would have the potential to serve as broad-spectrum immunosuppressants.

Similar concepts apply in understanding the mechanisms responsible for presentation of peptide antigens in association with class II proteins. In this case, exogenous proteins are ingested and degraded within membrane-bound vesicles, either endosomes or lysosomes. During synthesis, class II polypeptides extrude within the lumen of the endoplasmic reticulum and become associated with the invariant chain. This 30 kDa protein, another immunoglobulin-like molecule, binds to class II proteins in the endoplasmic reticulum but becomes cleaved and dissociates when these molecules transit the Golgi apparatus.[65] It is believed that the invariant chain, the gene for which is coordinately regulated with class II genes,[66] prevents binding of peptides to class II molecules until Golgi-derived vesicles fuse with endosomes. This process is diagrammed in Figure 13–13. In addition, the invariant chain probably helps to sort newly synthesized class II polypeptides to the endocytic compartment.[32] Although the precise timing of the interaction of class II molecules with catabolyzed ingested protein is unknown, the association is favored at low pH, a condition like that which occurs in phagocytic vesicles.[67] The association between class II molecules and their cognate peptides is remarkably stable, even in vivo.[68] Hence one may think of the peptide as an integral component of the surface-expressed class II molecule. Mutant cell lines bearing intact class II genes that nevertheless fail to assemble class II/peptide complexes have been described, and again the defect in such cells maps within the class II subregion of the HLA locus.[69] The nature of the genetic defect in such cells has not yet been defined.

As in the case of class I proteins, peptides that normally associate with class II molecules can be eluted from immunopurified class II structures and characterized directly.[51, 70, 71] In this case, however, no simple consensus sequence can be derived by inspection of the amino acid sequences represented in the purified peptides (Table 13–3). Indeed, in contrast to the situation described for class I molecules, class II protein–associated peptides vary dramatically in length and amino acid content.[71] A more comprehensive tabulation of bound peptide sequences may provide the raw materials necessary to decode features of class II/peptide binding. In one interesting case, it has been possible to generate class II molecule–binding peptides that specifically block T-cell responses in an antigen-specific fashion.[72] These antigen antagonists might prove useful as pharmacological agents in that they offer the potential to block self-directed immune responses manifesting limited clonal heterogeneity.

ALLELIC VARIATION IN MAJOR HISTOCOMPATIBILITY COMPLEX GENES

One of the most striking features about both class I and class II genes is their extraordinary degree of sequence polymorphism. The unusually large number of MHC alleles, and the fact that no single allele predominates in most human populations, stimulated early interest in the MHC on the part of human geneticists. Assignment of this allelic variation to specific substitutions in gene sequences has provided a fairly comprehensive view of variability within the class I and class II genes.

In considering only the class I genes, it should first be noted that no special constraints dictate the precise number of such elements that exist in mammals. Thus, the rat MHC includes more than 60 classical and nonclassical class I genes, whereas the pig SLA locus includes perhaps as few as 6 such elements.[73, 74] Examination of the allelic differences among human HLA-A, -B, and -C genes, defined from complementary DNA (cDNA) cloning studies, shows that most variability is concentrated within the α1 and α2 domains that figure prominently in defining the peptide-binding site. Indeed, virtually all of the residues exhibiting high variability between alleles are believed to participate in peptide binding.[58, 74, 75] These are residues located within the groove-flanking α helices or the β-pleated sheet floor that display inwardly directed side chains (Fig. 13–14). Hence the polymorphism of the MHC genes almost certainly contributes directly to variations in the antigen presentation repertoire in man as previously suggested based on peptide elution analyses.[59] Recent studies indicate that this type of variation provides an important substrate for environmental selection. In particular, of the 50 known alleles at the HLA-B locus, the HLA-Bw53 allele is uniquely associated with a decreased risk of severe infection with *Plasmodium falciparum* malaria in West Africa.[76] Similarly, inheritance of a particular set of class II genes confers some protection from malarial disease. Both the HLA-Bw53 allele and the malaria-resistant class II haplotype are present at 10- to 15-fold increased frequency in West Africans compared with other ethnic groups, and the geographical distribution of these alleles follows that of the classically protective hemoglobin mutation Hb S.[76]

Polymorphisms in class I and class II sequences also contribute dramatically to susceptibilities to certain autoimmune diseases. Included among these are insulin-dependent diabetes mellitus, ankylosing spondylitis, and juvenile rheumatoid arthritis. As noted in Table 13–4, the proportion of affected individuals who inherit specific MHC alleles can be quite high. Although the mechanism responsible for disease susceptibility in these cases remains enigmatic, it is attractive to postulate that certain class I or class II binding specificities present a peptide that stimulates T cells capable of interacting with a self-antigen.[77] Analysis of the unique susceptibility to type I diabetes conferred by certain HLA-DR alleles has led to the hypothesis that the presence of a single amino acid within the β chain may confer a relatively resistant state.[78, 79]

Regardless of the precise mechanism involved, it is apparent that sequence variations in MHC genes can

TABLE 13–3. HETEROGENEOUS SEQUENCES ELUTED FROM THE MOUSE I-A^d CLASS II MOLECULE*

PEPTIDE	SEQUENCE	LENGTH	SOURCE
1	W A N L M E K I Q A S V A T N P I	17	APO-E
2	D A Y H S R A I Q V V R A R K Q	16	CYS-C
3	A S F E A Q G A L A N I A V D K A	17	I-E^d-α
4	E E Q T Q Q I R L Q A E I F Q A R	17	APO-E
5	K P V S Q M R M A T P L L M R P M	17	Ii
6	V P Q L N Q M V R T A A E V A G Q X	18	TF RCP

*Shown are sequences of six peptides eluted in good yield from a mouse class II molecule. Compared with class I–associated peptides (Table 13–2), these peptides vary in length from 16 to 18 residues and also vary dramatically in sequence. Perhaps not surprisingly, the most abundant peptides are derived from abundant cell surface molecules that have been either internalized after expression or processed coordinately with expression of the class II molecule. The sources, deduced by comparison with all known proteins, are as follows: APO-E, mouse apolipoprotein-E; CYS-C, rat cystatin-C; I-E^d-α, mouse class II protein; Ii, mouse class II invariant chain; TF RCP, rat transferrin receptor. Note that peptides derived from processing of a different class II protein (I-E^d) can associate with the I-A^d molecule. See Hunt et al.[215] for additional discussion.

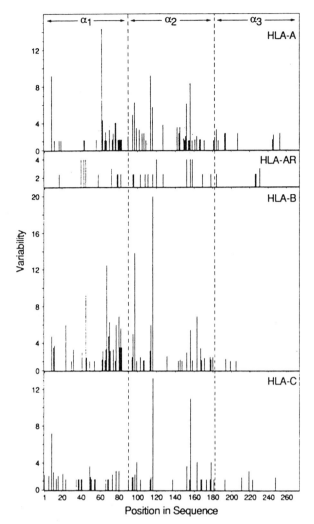

FIGURE 13–14. Polymorphisms are concentrated in the α1 and α2 domains of class I heavy chains. Deduced sequences of a series of 23 HLA-A, 6 HLA-AR, 30 HLA-B, and 11 HLA-C genes were aligned and variability was plotted in each case as the quotient of the number of amino acids found at the indicated sequence position divided by the frequency of the most common amino acid. Relative "hot spots," indicating sites that presumably define differences in the ability to present peptide antigens, are readily discernible. (Adapted, with permission, from the Annual Reviews in Immunology, Vol. 8, pp. 23–63, © 1990 by Annual Reviews, Inc.)

profoundly affect disease susceptibility. This observation in turn suggests that strong environmental selection, acting locally, is responsible for maintaining the high degree of polymorphism of MHC genes. But how does this sequence variation arise? Studies in mice suggest intriguing possibilities. Experimental selection of mutant mice that no longer accept skin grafts from isogenic donors, or that can no longer donate grafts capable of surviving without rejection, led to the isolation of a series of class I gene mutations generated via an unusual mechanism of intergenic gene conversion.[80] For example, the bm3, bm4, bm10, and bm11 mutations in the mouse H-2K class I gene almost certainly reflect a non-reciprocal genetic exchange process that substitutes short segments derived from different class I genes in place of the analogous seg-

ment in the H-2K gene.[81] Indeed, segmental intergenic gene conversion appears to predominate in generating sequence substitutions in the H-2K gene. Similar mechanisms may help to explain some examples of variation in the HLA-A, -B, and -C genes; however, the majority of observed variation in these elements occurs intragenically. Hence the HLA-A, -B, and -C loci retain their independent identities over evolutionary time. For example, some HLA-A alleles can be recognized within the background of variation observed in the chimpanzee,[74] an organism that shared a common ancestor with human beings at most 15 million years ago. These observations suggest two principal conclusions: first, that evolutionary selection, presumably reflecting susceptibility to childhood infectious diseases, acts on the accumulated allelic variation in the human population to maintain a high degree of polymorphism; and second, that from the perspective of the species, the presence of a large repertoire of MHC class I and class II specificities is highly desirable. Therefore, one consequence of the profound reduction in the numbers of certain mammalian species as a result of human interference will be the loss of a species-wide repertoire of potentially protective antigen presentation variants. All available evidence suggests that the cheetah, for example, no longer boasts any allelic variation in MHC class I or class II genes.[82] Intergenic gene conversion could provide a substrate for subsequent selection in this case.

An intriguing example of the rapidity with which

TABLE 13–4. A SAMPLING OF DISEASES FOR WHICH SUSCEPTIBILITY HAS BEEN LINKED TO CERTAIN HLA ALLELES*

DISEASE	SUSCEPTIBLE ALLELE	APPROXIMATE RELATIVE RISK
Ankylosing spondylitis	B27	210
Anterior uveitis	B27	8
Behçet's disease	B5	5
Celiac disease	DR3	12
Dermatitis herpetiformis	DR3	17
Goodpasture's syndrome	DR2	14
Hemochromatosis	A3	7
Narcolepsy	DR2	130
Psoriasis	B37	8
Reiter's syndrome	B27	37
Rheumatoid arthritis	DR4	5
Sjögren's syndrome	DW5	6

*Susceptibility to more than 500 different diseases has been noted to be associated with inheritance of certain HLA alleles or haplotypes. Some of the more significant examples are tabulated here. The mechanisms responsible for these disease associations almost certainly vary, but it is striking that many of those diseases for which the relative risk to individuals at least heterozygous for an HLA allele is very high are often believed to be autoimmune in nature. The most dramatic association remains one of the first to be discovered, that of HLA-B27 with susceptibility to ankylosing spondylitis. Different susceptibility patterns emerge in various racial backgrounds. In the case of narcolepsy, for example, susceptibility of individuals at least heterozygous for the HLA-DR2 allele is especially profound in Asians (relative risk >350). A comprehensive tabulation of these disease association data is presented in reference 216.

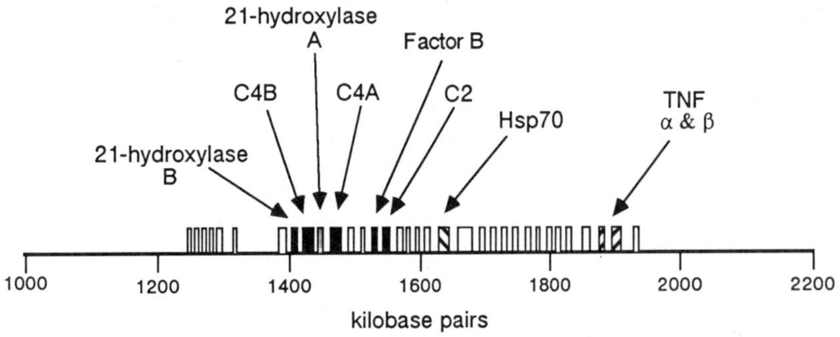

FIGURE 13–15. Gene organization in the HLA class III region. The positions of defined open reading frames (see Table 13–1) are indicated in a magnified view of Figure 13–3. Genes encoding components of the complement pathway (C4B, C4A, and factor B) are juxtaposed with those encoding enzymes of steroid biosynthesis (21-hydroxylase), elements that regulate protein folding (the heat shock protein Hsp 70), and potent cytokines (tumor necrosis factors [TNF]–α and –β). It is perhaps unsurprising that polymorphisms in genes that reside in this region may be in linkage disequilibrium with others that potently affect immune function. See text for details.

sequence heterogeneity can become fixed in the human class I genes has recently emerged through study of Native American populations. These peoples are believed to be descended from Asian immigrants who arrived relatively recently, certainly during the past 40,000 years. Remarkably, the HLA-B alleles of South American Indians are both novel and highly diverse, reflecting a pattern of interallelic segmental exchange that has occurred at very high frequency.[83–85] These data suggest that gene conversion contributes more to allelic variation in human class I sequences than does point mutation.

Polymorphism in Peptide Transporters

Although polymorphisms in the side-chain–binding pockets of class I molecules will alter the characteristics of peptide binding and hence promote allelic differences in the efficacy of presentation of some antigens, other genes undoubtedly influence this process. For example, there is reason to believe that the peptide transporters responsible for conveying products of proteolysis from the cytoplasm to the lumen of the endoplasmic reticulum may preferentially select certain peptide sequences. In one recent study, an allelic difference in a putative peptide transporter gene positioned within the class II locus of the rat (the mtp-2 gene, which is the TAP-2 gene in this species) proved responsible for variations in the representation of class I peptide complexes obtained when identical class I genes were present.[86] Similarly, variations in the efficacy of HLA-B27–restricted peptide presentation by different cell lines have been mapped to genes that reside in the human class II region, presumably either TAP-1 or TAP-2.[87] Some data support the view that polymorphisms in peptide transporters contribute to variations in susceptibility to autoimmune diseases, notably insulin-dependent diabetes mellitus.[88]

The Class III Region

The human MHC class III region comprises more than 1 million bp of DNA, within which at least 36 transcriptional units have been described.[7] Included among these are the genes encoding steroid 21-hy-droxylase (a P-450 enzyme[89]), Hsp70,[10] tumor necrosis factors (TNFs)–α and –β,[90] and the complement components C2, C4A, C4B, and factor B[91–93] (Fig. 13–15). The functions of the products of the remaining genes are at the moment unknown. Allelic variations in the structures of some class III genes have been defined, and there exists evidence suggesting that this genetic variation may influence susceptibility to some diseases. The C4A and C4B genes provide good examples. These two genes are 99 per cent similar, differing by only 14 nucleotides (nt), and encode classical pathway components involved in the formation of the C3 convertase.[94] Probably as a result of one amino acid difference, the C4A protein is most effective in interacting with antigen-antibody complexes, via the formation of an amide bond between C4A and free NH_2 groups on immune complex polypeptides, whereas the C4B protein forms ester bonds with carbohydrate moieties.[95] Approximately 35 per cent of individuals in most populations, irrespective of race, have at least one non-functional C4 allele. Persons inheriting MHC haplotypes that lack a full set of functional C4 genes are at considerably increased risk for a variety of autoimmune diseases. For example, the frequency of individuals with at least one C4A[null] allele is greatly increased in populations of those afflicted with systemic lupus erythematosus. Moreover, almost all patients with complete C4 deficiency manifest either systemic or discoid lupus erythematosus,[96] presumably resulting from a decreased ability to clear immune complexes. Deficiency of the C4A gene may occur in as much as 8 per cent of some populations and may be associated with a variety of immunodeficiency states. An intriguing recent report suggests that other genes within the class III complex may influence susceptibility to immunoglobulin A deficiency (the most common primary immunodeficiency disease) or common variable immunodeficiency.[97]

RECOGNITION OF ANTIGEN BY T LYMPHOCYTES

The response of T lymphocytes to appropriate antigen-presenting cells determines in a fundamental way all subsequent features of the immune response. T-cell–derived lymphokines regulate the influx of inflammatory cells, the maturation of antigen-specific B cells, and the recruitment of cytotoxic effector cells. The response of CD4-bearing helper T cells is therefore especially important, since these cells are the principal sources of lymphokines.

Mature peripheral T lymphocytes provide a highly mobile surveillance system, passing through the interstitial spaces of all organs and into secondary lymphoid sites. Throughout these migrations, T cells make frequent contacts with potential antigen-presenting cells. Adhesion molecules expressed on the T-cell surface provide a molecular basis for interactions between cells bearing class I and especially class II proteins and circulating T cells. Included among these cell surface proteins are specialized integrins, adhesion molecules of the immunoglobulin superfamily (e.g., N-CAM, L-CAM), and the lectin-like molecules called "selectins." Descriptions of these adhesion molecules are provided in Chapter 12. However, two key points regarding the interactions between T cells and antigen-presenting cells deserve special emphasis. First, variations in the expression of the adhesion structures can fundamentally alter the consequences of interaction between antigen-presenting cells and T lymphocytes. For example, loss of the β1 integrin LFA-1, a feature of patients with leukocyte adhesion deficiency, dramatically reduces T-cell responses.[98-101] Second, T-cell activation, usually stimulated by cross-linking of the T-cell antigen receptor, improves the avidity of the interaction between T cells and antigen-presenting cells. This phenomenon is again well illustrated in the case of LFA-1/ICAM-1 interactions, in which high-affinity binding results from productive stimulation of the T-cell antigen receptor.[102] Weak interactions between cell adhesion molecules on the T lymphocyte and its cognate presenting cell initially serve to juxtapose the antigen receptor with appropriate antigen presentation molecules. If the T-cell activation sequence is not initiated through this juxtaposition, deadhesion permits dissociation of the two cells. In contrast, if antigen receptor stimulation occurs, the avidity of the cell interaction rapidly increases through post-translational changes in the affinity of adhesion molecule pairs and through the synthesis of new adhesion molecules (e.g., the β4 integrin VLA-4). These mechanisms presumably act to ensure an adequate and prolonged T-cell response.[103, 104] Moreover, it has become apparent that simple cross-linking of the T-cell antigen receptor by cognate antigen is probably not sufficient, in most cases, to direct the full T-cell activation response. Improved adhesion resulting from T-cell receptor cross-linking probably serves to increase the likelihood that accessory stimuli, crucial for T-cell responses, are provided. Included among the latter are signals from the CD28 molecule[105] and perhaps from IL-1 receptors interacting with cell surface–bound IL-1.[106] However, the principal structure mediating T-cell activation is the T-cell antigen receptor itself.

ARCHITECTURE OF THE T-CELL RECEPTOR

As discussed in Chapter 11, the T-cell antigen receptor is a cell surface glycoprotein formed from two distinct polypeptide chains, usually termed α and β. A second isoform of T-cell receptor, composed of γ and δ chains, forms the antigen-binding structure on a small minority (usually fewer than 5 per cent) of circulating T lymphocytes.[107] The α and β chains (also γ and δ) are encoded by gene segments, positioned discontinuously in germline DNA, that become juxtaposed during intrathymic development. Combinatorial mechanisms permit the generation of an astonishingly large number ($>10^8$) of T-cell receptors from a relative small set of germline gene segments. The nature of these combinatorial strategies, coupled with a poorly defined feedback regulatory mechanism, ensures that each T lymphocyte expresses on its surface only a single type of receptor—the product of functional gene rearrangements driven to completion on only one allelic T-cell receptor gene copy.[108]

Each T-cell receptor polypeptide is a glycoprotein composed of two immunoglobulin-like extracellular domains linked to a transmembrane sequence that terminates in a quite short (about six amino acids) cytoplasmic tail. The T-cell receptor membrane-spanning domains are unusual in that they contain a single negatively charged residue positioned within an otherwise hydrophobic sequence. It is widely believed that this charge is masked through interaction with other cell surface proteins bearing positively charged transmembrane residues, and indeed the T-cell receptor heterodimer ordinarily associates with just such structures, the γ, δ, and ε chains of the CD3 complex.[109]

Structure of the CD3 Molecules and the Genes That Encode Them

The CD3γ, CD3δ, and CD3ε components were originally detected by using monoclonal antibodies that identified a surface structure capable of transmitting activation signals to naive T lymphocytes. Each is an immunoglobulin-like membrane-spanning single-chain glycoprotein with a basic residue positioned within the putative membrane-spanning helix. All three proteins are encoded by closely linked genes positioned on chromosome 11 (11q23) in man.[110] The CD3γ and δ genes reside within 2 kb of each other.[111] The human and mouse CD3 proteins are quite closely related and are expressed according to a similar developmental hierarchy. (See Chapter 12.) Compared with the T-cell receptor heterodimer, the CD3 chains boast comparatively long cytoplasmic extensions. Considerable evidence supports the view that these cytoplasmic domains constitute part of the signal transduction apparatus that links antigen recognition to the cell interior. Moreover, CD3 expression is absolutely required for appropriate assembly of the T-cell receptor protein complex.[112, 113] Immunoprecipitation of T-cell surface molecules with anti-CD3 reagents led to the discovery of a disulfide-linked homodimer, the ζ chain, which also forms part of the T-cell receptor complex.[114] Like the other CD3 components, the ζ homodimer must be present to permit efficient intracellular assembly of the T-cell receptor. Only 6 residues of the mature ζ polypeptide are displayed extracellularly, whereas the comparatively long (113 residue) cytoplasmic portion contributes to the machinery of T-cell receptor signal transduction.[115, 116] Figure 13–16 provides a schematic diagram of the structure of the T-cell receptor complex, indicating those molecules that interact directly at the cell surface and depicting several of the coreceptor and signal transduction components that contribute to T-cell signaling (see below). The enormous complexity of this cell surface receptor oligomer probably reflects a need to permit multiple different signal transduction responses to be activated selectively, depending on the nature of the stimulating cell. Recent evidence supports the view that a quite short sequence segment, minimally consisting of 18 amino acids, that exists in three copies in the ζ chain and in analogous forms in the CD3γ, δ, and ε chains, provides the link between the surface features of these signaling molecules and the signal transduction machinery at the cytoplasmic face of the cell membrane.[117–119] There is reason to believe that the related but distinct coupling motifs of these different CD3 polypeptides provide a means to deliver subtly different signals following antigen recognition.[117]

Binding of the T-Cell Receptor to Antigen Presentation Structures

The T-cell receptor heterodimer recognizes peptide antigens presented in the context of class I or class II HLA-encoded structures. With the use of highly purified class II molecules and a soluble form of the T-cell receptor (generated by producing a phosphatidylinositol-linked form of the α/β heterdimer and cleaving it from the surfaces of transfected cells, using phospholipases), it has been possible to study the characteristics of antigen recognition by T cells. These studies demonstrate that the T-cell receptor itself binds the class II/peptide complex and recognizes all three components (the peptide as well as both class II chains) together. Hence the specificity of antigen recognition is conferred by the T-cell receptor itself.[120] However, the binding affinity for this interaction is quite low, at least an order of magnitude below that which characterizes antigen/antibody binding.[121] Several features of this binding reaction merit attention. First, under normal circumstances, T cells are multivalent structures, and antigen receptor binding may well exhibit cooperative characteristics. Second, other accessory molecules help to stabilize the interaction between the T-cell receptor and its cognate antigen presentation structure. Included among these are the adhesion molecules; the accessory signaling molecules, as already mentioned; and the coreceptor structures

CD4 and CD8. These coreceptors play especially important roles in thymocyte development. (See Chapter 12.)

Coreceptor Structures Contributing to T-Cell Activation

Although the vast majority of thymocytes simultaneously express both CD4 and CD8 surface glycoproteins, mature T lymphocytes express these genes in a mutually exclusive fashion, reflecting two very distinct developmental programs. Thus, CD4+ cells recognize peptide antigens presented by class II proteins and, when activated, respond by elaborating lymphokines. In contrast, CD8+ cells recognize peptide antigens presented in association with class I antigen presentation molecules and respond to stimulation primarily by maturing into cytolytic effector cells (although some cytokines, particularly interferon-γ, are produced by these cells as well). The CD4 and CD8 coreceptor structures themselves are superficially similar products of unlinked genes that conform to the general outline of immunoglobulin superfamily members.[122] The CD4 protein is a monomer that recognizes monomorphic determinants present on all class II molecules.[123] It boasts a simple membrane-spanning domain and a short (28 residues) cytoplasmic tail. The CD8 structure is actually composed of two polypeptides, CD8α and CD8β, that are most often expressed as heterodimers but that can exist as homodimers as well.[124] Both forms of CD8 recognize determinants in the α3 domains of class I molecules.[13] Recent studies demonstrate that the CD8β chain contributes to the efficacy of T-cell signaling, since CD8α/β heterodimers serve as much more effective coreceptors than do α homodimers in a model system employing an antigen-specific T-cell hybridoma. The critical defining feature that determines CD8β chain activity appears to reside within the extracellular portion of the molecule.[125]

Despite the easily documented recognition of class I and class II proteins by CD8 and CD4, respectively, it is quite apparent that the structure of the T-cell receptor heterodimer by itself determines the recognition specificity of the T cell on which it is expressed. Experiments performed in hybridomas demonstrated persuasively that both nominal peptide antigen specificity and specificity for either class I or class II presentation molecules were discretely defined by the presence of the α and β T-cell receptor chains themselves.[120] Hence it was initially proposed that CD4 and CD8 might simply act to improve the affinity of interaction between T cells and antigen-presenting cells.[126] However, it soon became apparent that the CD4 molecule actually becomes incorporated into the antigen receptor complex during cognate recognition of appropriate ligands by T cells.[127] A similar situation applies in the case of CD8. Antibodies directed against these coreceptor structures usually block T-cell receptor–mediated activation. Nevertheless, it is apparent that the CD4 and CD8 coreceptors are not required

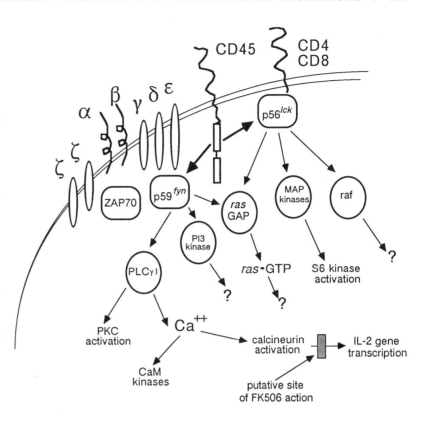

FIGURE 13–16. Structure of the T-cell receptor and of T-cell signaling pathways. The α/β heterodimer interacts with at least four other polypeptides to form the T-cell receptor/CD3 complex. At least three protein tyrosine kinases, ZAP-70, p59^{fyn}, and p56^{lck}, all of which could potentially be regulated by the CD45 phosphotyrosine phosphatase, couple to the receptor. In the case of p56^{lck}, this is probably achieved through its association with the CD4 and CD8 coreceptor molecules. Although the precise functions that are regulated by these protein tyrosine kinases have not been elucidated, the phosphatidylinositol–specific phospholipase PLCγ1 is an apparent target. The involvement of the P-I-3 kinase, the GTPase regulator of *ras*, *ras*-GAP, the mitogen-activated MAP kinases, and the *raf*-encoded serine/threonine kinase represents speculation based on results obtained in other signaling systems. These enzymes in turn regulate various aspects of intracellular metabolism. The central role of early increases in intracellular calcium is in part illustrated by the importance of the calcium-sensitive phosphatase calcineurin, which is a target for the inhibitory function of FK506 when bound to its cognate binding protein, FKBP.

for T-cell signaling, since there exist T lymphocytes, particularly those bearing γ/δ T-cell receptors, that do not express either coreceptor structure. Experiments performed using gene transfection methods to direct coreceptor expression in T-cell lines that are CD4$^-$8$^-$ indicate that given a T-cell receptor with complementary specificity, the presence of coreceptor structures dramatically improves the efficiency of T-cell activation in response to a minimal antigen dose.[128] Possible mechanisms for this effect are described below.

THE BIOCHEMISTRY OF T-CELL SIGNALING

Ligand occupancy of the T-cell antigen receptor leads to a series of readily measured biochemical changes that evolve over a period of hours and culminate in cell replication. Experiments performed using antibodies to the T-cell receptor complex as surrogate activators suggest that, as in the case of B-cell immunoglobulin, cross-linking of the receptor is absolutely required to permit a full activation response. Monovalent T-cell receptor ligands are ineffective.[129] Studies performed using purified MHC class I molecules embedded in artificial membranes support the view that as few as 50 to 300 class I protein molecules can efficiently trigger a T-cell–bearing receptor of the appropriate specificity.[130, 131] Similar estimates derive from analyses of antigen-presenting cells themselves.[132, 133] Although in most cases antigen-presenting cells will display more than 10,000 class I or class II molecules per cell, only a small fraction of these, perhaps fewer than 1 per cent, can be expected

to contain a given processed peptide. Thus, there is reason to believe that non-specific adhesive interactions linking stimulator/responder cell pairs are necessary to permit the juxtaposition of sufficient T-cell receptor structures with appropriate cognate antigen presentation molecules.

Within seconds following T-cell receptor stimulation, it is possible to observe the accumulation of protein substrates that have become phosphorylated on tyrosine.[134, 135] Although the complete range of phosphotyrosine-containing substrates is unknown, several potentially important signaling molecules have been identified among the newly appearing phosphoproteins (see Fig. 13–16). These include a phosphotidylinositol-specific phospholipase C[136, 137] and members of the *erk* family of mitogen-stimulated kinases.[138] In addition, the *ras*-GAP protein that regulates GTPase activity of *ras*-type small molecular weight GTP-binding proteins is believed to be affected.[139] These substrates resemble quite closely those that become phosphorylated after stimulation of growth factor receptor protein tyrosine kinases, suggesting a congruence between the signal transduction pathways employed by these very different types of receptor structure.

Within 30 seconds after cross-linking of T-cell antigen receptors, mobilization of intracellular calcium stores is observed. As a result, cytosolic free calcium levels rise from mean basal concentrations of 100 nM to values exceeding 500 nM.[140] It should be emphasized that calcium accumulation in individual cells followed serially through time exhibits regular oscillations in stimulated T cells. These oscillations probably reflect the behavior of T-cell–specific calcium

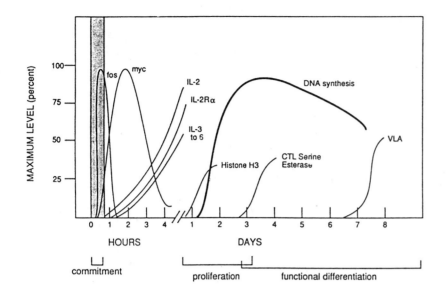

FIGURE 13–17. The biochemistry of T-cell activation. Shown is a sequence of biochemical changes induced in a hypothetical T cell after antigen activation. In most cells, the first hour of ligand occupancy of the receptor induces an irreversible commitment to the subsequent activation sequence. Effects are represented on an approximate time line, with the magnitude of the effect graded in per cent on the ordinate. (Adapted, with permission, from the Annual Reviews in Immunology, Vol. 8, pp. 421–452, © 1990 by Annual Reviews, Inc.)

channels.[141, 142] After the initial rise in intracellular free calcium concentrations, there follows a series of contingent regulatory events, including the accumulation of p21^{ras} in its GTP-bound form,[143] augmented transcription of the IL-2 receptor α chain gene,[144] augmented translation of ornithine decarboxylase transcripts,[145] and the synthesis of IL-2 itself.[146] DNA synthesis commences after about 24 hours, and replication occurs within 48 hours.[147]

Figure 13–17 outlines the biochemical events associated with T-cell receptor–stimulated T-cell activation, placing these along an arbitrary time line. In most cases, T-cell activation can be fully achieved via artificial treatment with a calcium ionophore and an activator of protein kinase C. This observation suggested a two-signal model of T-cell activation wherein T-cell receptor stimulation would stimulate membrane phospholipid breakdown, leading to production of inositol phosphate second messengers that could trigger the release of calcium from intracellular stores.[148] Simultaneously, activation of protein kinase C would strongly promote alterations in transcriptional regulatory molecules. More recent studies have focused on the protein tyrosine phosphorylation events that occur at the very beginning of the lymphocyte activation

sequence.[149] Indeed, it now appears that these changes in the activity of protein tyrosine kinases or phosphotyrosine phosphatases (or both) lie at the very heart of the lymphocyte response to antigen.

Protein Tyrosine Kinases Mediating Lymphocyte Activation

The enzymes responsible for phosphorylating inositol-specific phospholipase Cγ1 following T-cell stimulation are unknown. However, attention has increasingly focused on two members of the *src* family of non-receptor protein tyrosine kinases, p56^{lck} and p59^{fyn}, which physically associate with components of the T-cell receptor complex and appear to relay signals directly after antigen recognition.

The *lck* gene encodes a lymphocyte-specific membrane-associated protein tyrosine kinase that is expressed in T lymphocytes at all stages of development and at much lower levels in some B-lineage cells.[150] Natural killer (NK) cells also contain high levels of p56^{lck} protein.[151] Like other members of the *src* family, p56^{lck} is myristoylated at its amino-terminus and boasts three discrete sequence "domains" (Fig. 13–18): a

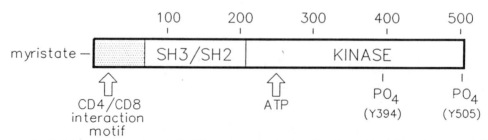

FIGURE 13–18. Schematic structure of the *lck*-encoded protein tyrosine kinase. The shaded amino-terminal region defines a "domain" that differs markedly among the otherwise closely related *src* family protein tyrosine kinases. The SH3 and SH2 motifs appear to be involved in binding substrates or regulatory molecules. The kinase domain contains sites involved in interacting with ATP, as well as two tyrosine phosphorylation sites. The carboxy-terminal of these (Tyr505) defines a potent regulatory element in that phosphorylation of this site dramatically reduces in vivo activity. See reference 152 for details.

carboxy-terminal kinase domain occupying more than half of the 509 residues; a central domain containing so-called "src homology" motifs (SH2 and SH3 regions); and a unique amino-terminal domain, spanning about 70 amino acids, which differs for each of the eight well-characterized src family kinases but is conserved between species when analogous kinase genes are examined.[152] This amino-terminal segment, in the case of p56^{lck}, directs the interaction of the kinase with the carboxy-terminal cytoplasmic tails of the CD4 and CD8 coreceptor molecules.[153] Immunoprecipitation of either CD4 or CD8 from lymphocyte membranes results in coprecipitation of p56^{lck} kinase activity.[154] Two pairs of cysteine residues surrounded by seemingly complementary basic (in CD4 and CD8) or acidic (in p56^{lck}) amino acids form the highly specific binding sites that link coreceptor and kinase together. Since the association can be disrupted by certain chelating agents (e.g., orthophenanthroline) and since elimination of any of the four cysteine residues also prevents association,[153] it is possible that the interaction between these two molecules requires tetravalent coordination of a metal ion, probably Zn^{2+}. Whatever the mechanism, antibody-mediated cross-linking of CD4 provokes readily observable increases in p56^{lck} kinase activity.[155] These observations suggest a straightforward model for T-cell activation wherein interaction of T-cell receptors with antigen-presenting molecules results in juxtaposition of the T-cell receptor complex with either CD4 or CD8 coreceptors, and hence the intracellular apposition of the T-cell receptor CD3 components with the p56^{lck} protein tyrosine kinase, now in an activated form (see Fig. 13–16).

Evidence supporting this model derives from two types of experiments. First, in a T-cell line that absolutely requires CD4 coreceptor expression to sustain a signaling response, mutations in this coreceptor that compromise the interaction with p56^{lck} also compromise antigen-induced activation.[128] Second, introduction of an artificially activated form of p56^{lck}, bearing a mutation in a regulatory phosphorylation site (Tyr505) positioned near the carboxy-terminus (see Fig. 13–18), into some T cell lines yields cells that respond more vigorously to antigenic challenge.[156] It is also intriguing that the lck gene is rearranged in at least two examples of human acute lymphocytic leukemia[157] and that overexpression of the lck gene in transgenic mice induces rapid lymphomagenesis.[158] Nevertheless, T lymphocytes lacking both CD4 and CD8 respond appropriately to antigen. Hence other signaling molecules must be capable of initiating the normal T-cell activation sequence. Since T-cell activation can be effectively blocked by protein tyrosine kinase inhibitors,[159] signaling that does not require coreceptor input probably proceeds via an alternative mechanism of p56^{lck} activation or via stimulation of another similar protein tyrosine kinase.

Involvement of p59^{fyn} in T-Cell Receptor Signaling

Among the candidate kinases that might couple T-cell receptor–derived signals to the cell interior, evidence supporting a role for p59^{fyn} is especially strong. The fyn gene is expressed at high levels in neuronal cells[160] and in T lymphocytes and directs the synthesis of slightly different proteins in these two cell types. This situation results from mutually exclusive alternative splicing of a single pair of fyn exons (exons 7A and 7B) to yield transcripts differing only in a central 150 nt sequence.[161] In human[162] and murine developing thymocytes, p59^{fyn} expression correlates with the acquisition of signal transduction capability by the T-cell antigen receptor.[163] Moreover, overexpression of p59^{fyn} in the thymocytes of transgenic mice yields cells that exhibit hyperstimulable phenotypes when exposed to T-cell receptor–specific triggering events.[163] The T-cell form of p59^{fyn} proved especially capable of mediating this effect when expressed in an insulin-reactive T-cell line.[164] These results provide evidence favoring a functional coupling of p59^{fyn} with the T-cell receptor complex. In fact, a small fraction of total cellular p59^{fyn} protein can be shown to associate with the T-cell antigen receptor complex itself.[165] Overexpression of a catalytically inactive form of p59^{fyn} blocks T-cell receptor–induced proliferation of mature thymocytes,[163] suggesting that p59^{fyn} activity is required for antigen-stimulated responses in these cells. This result has recently been confirmed in mice that lack a functional fyn gene, which were produced via gene targeting methods.[166] Therefore, both genetic evidence and biochemical evidence favor the view that p59^{fyn} is a critical regulator of T-cell receptor signaling.

Almost certainly, other protein tyrosine kinases participate in controlling T-cell receptor signaling. For example, shortly after T-cell stimulation, a novel kinase becomes associated with the CD3 ζ chain. This zeta-associated protein, ZAP-70, exhibits protein tyrosine kinase activity and probably forms part of a signal transduction complex that may include p56^{lck} and p59^{fyn} as well.[167] Other similarly sized T-cell protein tyrosine kinases have been identified by molecular cloning (e.g., syk).[168] Although the precise functions of these kinases remain to be determined, it is of interest that although thymocytes from mice bearing a homozygous mutation in the fyn gene fail to proliferate in response to T-cell receptor–derived signals, the mature T cells in these animals exhibit near-normal stimulatory characteristics.[166] Activation of these cells nevertheless proceeds via a protein tyrosine kinase–mediated pathway, perhaps involving ZAP-70, the syk-encoded protein, or other T-cell kinases.

Control of T-Cell Activation by Phosphotyrosine Phosphatases

One important feature of the protein tyrosine kinases in general is that they themselves often receive critical regulatory input from other protein tyrosine kinases. For example, the src-like protein tyrosine kinases all possess tyrosine residues near their carboxyl-termini that, when phosphorylated, act as negative regulators of kinase activity, perhaps by serving as pseudosubstrates (see Fig. 13–18). Phosphorylation

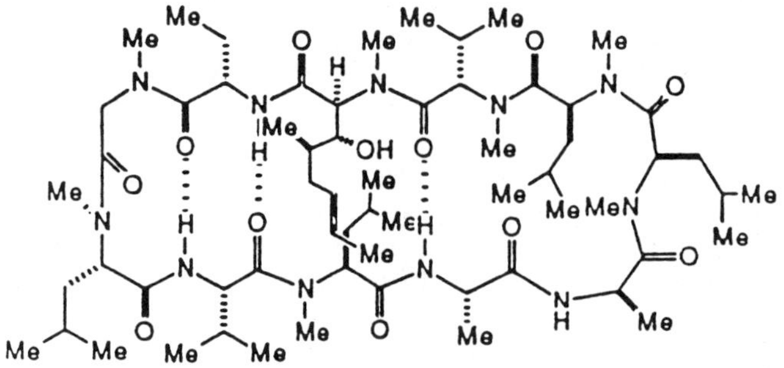

FIGURE 13–19. Structures of three potent immunosuppressants that bind *cis-trans* prolyl isomerases. (Adapted from Schreiber, S. L.: Chemistry and biology of the immunophilins and their immunosuppressive ligands. Science 251:283, 1991; with permission. Copyright 1991 by the American Association for the Advancement of Science.)

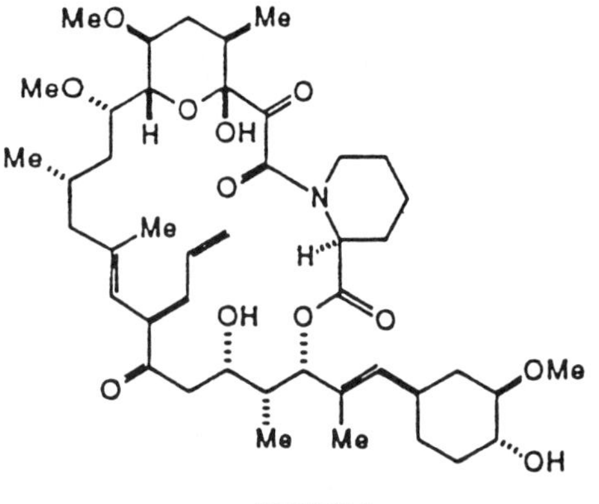

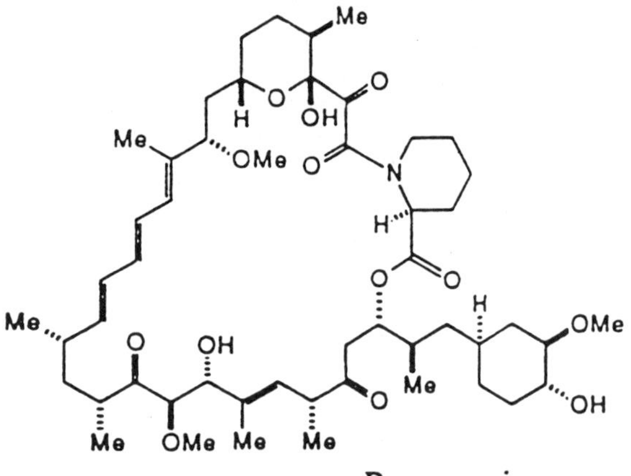

of this site is probably mediated by *c-src* kinase (CSK), a protein tyrosine kinase.[169] Hence protein phosphorylation is achieved in the context of a regulatory cascade. Not surprisingly, dephosphorylation plays a critical role in the control of kinase signaling pathways. The importance of phosphotyrosine phosphatases in T-cell signaling became apparent with the discovery that the so-called leukocyte common antigen CD45 contains two intracellular phosphotyrosine phosphatase domains.[170] The CD45 molecule is an extremely abundant protein on most leukocytes (>100,000 molecules per cell) and can be found in multiple different forms as a result of alternative splicing of exons that encode extracellular portions of the molecule.[171] Although some evidence favors the view that the CD22 molecule can serve as a ligand for at least one form of CD45 (CD45RO), definitive identification of ligands for other CD45 extracellular structures has not yet been achieved.[172] Remarkably, CD45 function is required for normal T-cell activation. Mutant T-cell lines lacking CD45 expression no longer sustain activation signals from the T-cell antigen receptor.[173, 174] Moreover, CD45 can be shown to act to dephosphorylate the carboxy-terminal phosphotyrosine (Tyr505) of p56[lck] in a relatively specific fashion.[175] That is, dephosphorylation of this carboxy-terminal site proceeds

more efficiently than does dephosphorylation of a second, internally positioned phosphotyrosine residue (Tyr394; see Fig. 13–18). These observations further refine models for the control of T-cell activation via T-cell receptor signaling. If, as has been proposed, antigen recognition induces coaggregation of T-cell receptors, coreceptor structures, and CD45, activation of the p56[lck] and p59[fyn] protein tyrosine kinases might result from dephosphorylation of their carboxy-termini. These in turn could phosphorylate, and presumably activate, phospholipases and other protein kinases that would provide the necessary signals to permit activation to proceed.

Insights into T-Cell Signaling Derived from the Study of Immunophilin Ligands

Additional features of the signal transduction pathways regulating T-cell activation have emerged through study of a set of clinically useful drugs that suppress allograft rejection. The first of these, cyclosporine, is a fungal product that binds an abundant intracellular protein called cyclophilin.[176] A structurally unrelated compound called FK506 (Fig. 13–19) exhibits a similar spectrum of activities but binds a quite different target, one or more of a group of FK506-binding proteins (FKBPs). Cyclosporine and FK506 act quite early in the T-cell activation process (within the first few hours) and block subsequent proliferation in large part by preventing transcription of lymphokine genes, particularly IL-2.[177] This effect seems to result from the failure to correctly assemble critical transcription factors required for IL-2 expression.[178]

Remarkably, both cyclophilin and the FKBPs behave as *cis-trans* prolyl isomerases.[176] That is, these relatively abundant proteins appear to participate in regulating protein folding in various cellular compartments. Cyclophilin and FK506 block the isomerase activities of their respective ligands, which naturally suggested that the isomerization process was in some fashion crucial to T-cell activation. Recent studies suggest, however, that drug/protein complexes form the active principles that abrogate signaling from the T-cell antigen receptor. For example, structural analogues of FK506 that retain the ability to inhibit prolyl isomerization by their respective ligands, but that no longer block T-cell activation, have been generated.[179] Moreover, the amount of drug required to inhibit T-cell function falls far below that which would be required to saturate even 50 per cent of the cellular binding sites for each.[176] These observations have prompted several groups to attempt to define additional signaling molecules that might interact with the complex of cyclosporine plus cyclophilin. One such protein is the calcium-sensitive phosphoserine-specific phosphatase calcineurin.[180] Although it remains to be seen whether alteration of calcineurin activity contributes to the pharmacological potency of cyclosporine, recent experiments demonstrate a calcineurin-induced activation of IL-2 gene transcription that is blocked by FK506 binding to FKBP in vitro.[181, 182]

One interesting feature of both cyclosporine and FK506 is that although they effectively block T-cell activation stimulated from the T-cell antigen receptor, signaling from some other cell surface structures (notably CD28; see below) remains intact. This observation emphasizes the underlying complexity of T-cell signaling pathways. Similarly, the macrolide rapamycin, which closely resembles FK506 in structure (see Fig. 13–19), fails to block T-cell receptor–mediated signaling but instead acts to prevent proliferation by interfering with lymphokine receptor–linked activation pathways. Clearly, the immunophilin ligands promise to provide remarkably specific tools with which to dissect the circuitry of lymphocyte signaling.

Alternative Outcomes of T-Cell Stimulation: Activation, Anergy, and Apoptosis

Not all interactions between T-cell receptor and cognate antigen-presenting molecules stimulate mitogenesis. Indeed, under some circumstances signaling from the T-cell antigen receptor not only fails to deliver an activation signal but also induces a state of relative refractoriness to subsequent antigenic challenge.[183] This phenomenon, termed clonal anergy, can be readily demonstrated in transgenic mouse models in which a self-reactive T-cell antigen receptor is deliberately expressed in all developing T lymphocytes.[184] Depending on the nature of the receptor genes used, two distinct outcomes have been observed. First, self-reactive thymocytes may be deleted during development through an active process known as apoptosis.[185, 186] Cells undergoing apoptosis activate a nuclear DNase that cleaves chromatin into nucleosome-sized fragments.[187] In some cases, however, thymocytes bearing a self-reactive receptor survive to populate secondary lymphoid organs, where they remain for the most part unresponsive to signals from their antigen receptors.[184] This phenomenon is felt to reflect a kind of fail-safe mechanism that ordinarily prevents T-cell activation in the absence of accessory signals normally provided by antigen-presenting cells.

In vitro systems that model the clonal anergy phenomenon suggest that a single signal derived from the T-cell antigen receptor in isolation probably produces a refractory state in most cases.[188] Appropriate second signals can be provided using fresh accessory cells and appear to result from cell-to-cell contact.[184] Although numerous candidates exist for relaying second signals, evidence supporting such a role for the CD28 molecule is especially strong. Expressed on virtually all T cells, CD28 interacts effectively with the B7/BB1 molecule on B lymphocytes.[190] Hence B cells, which are extremely efficient antigen-presenting cells, can supply a second signal through CD28 that will prevent anergy induction and permit proliferative responses.[105] Almost certainly, other molecules capable of delivering an accessory stimulus also exist.

In summary, T-cell interactions with antigen-presenting cells are initiated through relatively non-specific adhesion events that are stabilized as activation proceeds. The T-cell stimulation pathway requires recognition of cognate antigen by the T-cell antigen receptor, which results in the activation of intracellular protein tyrosine kinases and a series of subsequent biochemical events leading ultimately to lymphokine secretion and proliferation. Satisfactory propagation of a T-cell receptor–derived stimulus requires additional signals that ordinarily result from interactions between surface structures present on the antigen-presenting cell and the responding T lymphocyte. In the absence of such accessory signals, an anergic state may result. It is easy to predict that a more detailed understanding of these signaling processes should permit the therapeutic manipulation of immune responses to reduce the risk of allograft rejection or autoimmune disease activity.

T-CELL EFFECTOR MECHANISMS

Antigen recognition by mature CD4+ T cells results in the elaboration of lymphokines that regulate all other immune phenomena. For example, TNF and the related molecule lymphotoxin (LT) help to stimulate inflammatory cells and epithelial cells. Similarly, IL-4 and IL-2 both can act on B lymphocytes as well as on T cells themselves. Thus, products of activated CD4$^+$ T cells stimulate both specific and non-specific immunity. However, within the CD4$^+$ T-cell population there exist subsets of more specialized cells that differ with respect to cytokine repertoire. Initially defined in the mouse, it is now apparent that human T cells exhibit similar specialization. Among CD4$^+$ T cells, the Th1 cells secrete primarily IL-2 and IFN-γ, when activated, and subserve the function of stimulating cellular immune responses.[191] IFN-γ acts to stimulate macrophage phagocytic activity and to augment expression of both class I and class II molecules. In contrast, Th2 cells secrete primarily IL-4, IL-5, and IL-6 and are potent regulators of B-cell responses to antigen.[192] Variations in the representation of Th1 and Th2 subsets may be responsible for different manifestations of common infectious syndromes. For example, recent evidence indicates that lepromatous and tuberculoid responses to infection with *Mycobacterium leprae* result from a relative preponderance of Th2 and Th1 cells, respectively.[193]

Similar distinctions exist in the variable response to *Leishmania* infection in humans and mice.[194] Infection of most inbred mouse strains with *L. major* produces a cutaneous lesion that heals spontaneously, whereas progressive fatal infection is observed in a few strains. This difference in outcome appears to reflect the action of either Th1 or Th2 CD4$^+$ cells in strains that respectively recover or succumb to the infectious process.[195] Differential outcomes of infection with *Plasmodium* and with various helminths have also been reported to depend on the relative extent to which Th1 versus Th2 cells are activated.[196] The mechanisms responsible for the preponderance of one response compared with another are unknown; however, it is of interest that the cytokines released by each subset are mutually inhibitory for cytokine production in cells of the other subset.[196, 197] This observation may explain the phenomenon of conditioning of immune responses, whereby a previously established Th1 response, for example, renders subsequent Th2 responses less likely.

Effector Properties of CD8$^+$ Cells

Like CD4$^+$ T lymphocytes, mature CD8-bearing T cells exert part of their effector function through the release of cytokine molecules that activate other cell populations. Stimulated CD8$^+$ T cells in particular release IFN-γ, which both stimulates phagocytic cells and promotes the expansion of B cells secreting certain immunoglobulin (IgG) isotypes, and TNF. However, CD8$^+$ T lymphocytes also participate directly in the destruction of foreign targets through a contact-dependent, cell-mediated cytolysis mechanism. In general, cytolytic effector cells are CD8$^+$ T cells that specifically lyse membrane-enclosed targets following stimulation of their antigen receptors. The lytic proc-

ess has been resolved into three steps involving (1) Mg^{2+}-dependent binding; (2) delivery of a "lethal hit," a calcium- and temperature-dependent phenomenon; and (3) disintegration of the target. The precise molecular features of CTL-mediated cell lysis remain controversial; however, there exists a coherent model, supported by much experimental evidence, linking target cell destruction to the release of specific toxins from CTL granules via a calcium-requiring exocytotic process.[198]

The potential importance of granules in CD8$^+$ T cells first became apparent when ultrastructural studies revealed the presence of pore-like structures in CTL targets undergoing lysis. These pores resembled those produced by the membrane attack complex, the terminal components in the complement cascade.[199] Systematic evaluation of the contents of CTL granules provided a candidate molecule that may mediate pore formation. This protein, perforin, shares sequence similarity with complement components C6 to C9.[200, 201] Purified perforin is a 65 to 70 kDa protein that readily polymerizes to form polyperforin. Perforin will also directly lyse target cells when applied in solution, presumably by polymerizing to form pore structures.[202] In addition to perforin, the granules of CD8$^+$ CTLs, and of NK cells as well, contain both serine esterases and lysosomal enzymes believed to assist in disrupting the integrity of target cells. Table 13–5 provides an updated list of those enzymes known to reside in the granules of CTLs.

It should be mentioned that other mechanisms that permit activated CD8$^+$ T cells to destroy stimulating cells may exist. For example, DNA fragmentation, analogous to that seen in apoptotic cells, can occur in CTL targets during the prelytic period.[203] Moreover, in some cases CTL-mediated lysis can be demonstrated even in calcium-depleted media that do not permit granule release.[204, 205] Regardless of the precise mechanism, the end result of stimulation of CD8-bearing cytolytic effector cells is the rapid destruction of membrane-enclosed targets, a process that can occur re-

TABLE 13–5. COMPONENTS OF CYTOPLASMIC GRANULES IN CYTOTOXIC T LYMPHOCYTES

MOLECULE	FUNCTION
Perforin	Pore formation
Granzyme A	Trypsin-like protease
Granzyme B	Protease (cleaves after methionines)
Granzyme C	Protease
Granzyme D	Protease
Granzyme E	Protease
Granzyme F	Protease
Granzyme G	Protease
Chondroitin sulfate A	Carrier molecule?
Leukolexin	Lymphokine (resembles TNF)
Cathepsin D	Lysosomal enzyme
Arylsulfatase	Lysosomal enzyme
β-Glucuronidase	Lysosomal enzyme
β-Hexosaminidase	Lysosomal enzyme

Adapted, with permission, from the Annual Reviews in Immunology, Vol. 8, pp. 279–302, © 1990 by Annual Reviews, Inc.

peatedly without obvious damage to the CTL itself. Hence a complete description of the action of these CTLs must explain the surprising directionality of this lethal hit.

SUMMARY

Progressively more thorough application of micro-scale biochemical and molecular biological methods has resulted in the coalescence of findings into a fairly comprehensive view of immune function. Mechanisms that permit processing and presentation of foreign antigens, recognition by T lymphocytes, activation of these T cells, and the subsequent elaboration of potent effector molecules acting to stimulate, or in some cases to eliminate, target cells are now understood in considerable molecular detail. The impact of these discoveries is just being felt in a clinical setting. In particular, the biochemical basis of disease susceptibility, both for autoimmune processes and for decreased resistance to infectious agents, has become apparent in many cases. Successful defense against the universe of all potential pathogens requires a recognition mechanism capable of extraordinarily subtle discrimination, as well as effector mechanisms of substantial power. In the future, improved understanding of both of these processes will permit the design of novel therapeutic strategies. Competitive peptides capable of blocking specific antigen presentation have already emerged, and more powerful immune blockers based on this line of attack will almost certainly appear. Similarly, the immunophilin ligands, which capably interdict lymphocyte signaling pathways, will soon share clinical duties with potent inhibitors of phosphotyrosine metabolism, some of which target the protein tyrosine kinases of lymphoid cells with considerable specificity. An equally bright future can be predicted for agonists and antagonists of T-cell–derived cytokines. Indeed, modulation of the regulatory circuitry that dictates release of, and response to, these molecules holds special promise for immune intervention. Careful manipulation of these various strategies should permit substantial improvement in the prevention and treatment of autoimmune diseases without global compromise in immune responsiveness. Moreover, a detailed understanding of immune function should someday permit much more effective implementation of tissue transplantation. Finally, advances in understanding of immune recognition and effector mechanisms have already had a profound effect on the design of vaccines, which in many cases provide the most cost-effective means of protecting human health. The successful eradication of human immunodeficiency virus (HIV)–mediated diseases, and of the parasitic diseases of underdeveloped countries, will depend on progress in each of these areas of immune system physiology.

REFERENCES

1. Nossal, G. J. V., Szenberg, A., Ada, G. L., and Austin, C. M.: Single cell studies on 19S antibody production. J. Exp. Med. 119:485, 1964.
2. Naor, D., and Sulitzeanu, D.: Binding of radioiodinated bovine serum albumin to mouse spleen cells. Nature 214:687, 1967.
3. Davie, J. M., and Paul, W. E.: Receptors on immunocompetent cells. IV. Direct measurement of avidity of cell receptors and cooperative binding of multivalent ligands. J. Exp. Med. 135:643, 1972.
4. Udaka, K., Tsomides, T. J., and Eisen, H. N.: A naturally occurring peptide recognized by alloreactive CD8+ cytotoxic T lymphocytes in association with a class I MHC protein. Cell 69:989, 1992.
5. Medawar, P. B.: The behavior and fate of skin autografts and skin homografts in rabbits. J. Anat. 78:176, 1947.
6. Dausset, J.: Iso-Leuco-anticorps. Acta Haematol. 20:156, 1958.
7. Trowsdale, J., Ragoussis, J., and Campbell, R. D.: Map of the human MHC. Immunol. Today 12:443, 1991.
8. Auffray, C., and Strominger, J. L.: Molecular genetics of the human major histocompatibility complex. Adv. Hum. Genet. 15:197, 1986.
9. Spies, T., Blanck, G., Bresnahan, M., Sands, J., and Strominger, J. L.: A new cluster of genes within the human major histocompatibility complex. Science 243:214, 1989.
10. Spies, T., Bresnahan, M., and Strominger, J. L.: Human major histocompatibility complex contains a minimum of 19 genes between the complement cluster and HLA-B. Proc. Natl. Acad. Sci. USA 86:8955, 1989.
11. Carroll, M. C., Katzman, P., Alicot, E. M., Koller, B. H., Geraghty, D. E., Orr, H. T., Strominger, J. L., and Spies, T.: Linkage map of the human major histocompatibility complex including the tumor necrosis factor genes. Proc. Natl. Acad. Sci. USA 84:8535, 1987.
12. Bjorkman, P. J., Saper, M. A., Samraoui, B., Bennett, W. S., Strominger, J. L., and Wiley, D. C.: Structure of the human class I histocompatibility antigen, HLA-A2. Nature 329:506, 1987.
13. Salter, R. D., Benjamin, R. J., Wesley, P. K., Buxton, S. E., Garrett, T. P., Clayberger, C., Krensky, A. M., Norment, A. M., Littman, D. R., and Parham, P.: A binding site for the T-cell coreceptor CD8 on the alpha 3 domain of HLA-A2. Nature 345:41, 1990.
14. Bjorkman, P. J., Saper, M. A., Samraoui, B., Bennett, W. S., Strominger, J. L., and Wiley, D. C.: The foreign antigen binding site and T cell recognition regions of class I histocompatibility antigens. Nature 329:512, 1987.
15. Ljunggren, H. G., Stam, N. J., Ohlen, C., Neefjes, J. J., Hoglund, P., Heemels, M. T., Bastin, J., Schumacher, T. N., Townsend, A., Karre, K., et al.: Empty MHC class I molecules come out in the cold. Nature 346:476, 1990.
16. David-Watine, B., Israel, A., and Kourilsky, P.: The regulation and expression of MHC class I genes. Immunol. Today 11:286, 1990.
17. Touraine, J. L., Betuel, H., Sovillet, G., and Jeune, M.: Combined immunodeficiency disease associated with absence of cell surface HLA-A and -B antigens. J. Pediatr. 93:47, 1978.
18. Geraghty, D. E., Pei J., Lipsky, B., Hansen, J. A., Taillon-Miller, P., Broson, S. K., and Chaplin, D. D.: Cloning and physical mapping of the HLA class I region spanning the HLA-E to HLA-F interval by using artificial chromosomes. Proc. Natl. Acad. Sci. USA 89:2669, 1992.
19. Hershberg, R., Eghtesady, P., Sydora, B., Brorson, K., Cheroutre, H., Modlin, R., and Kronenberg, M.: Expression of the thymus leukemia antigen in mouse intestinal epithelium. Proc. Natl. Acad. Sci. USA 87:9727, 1990.
20. Calderon, J., Sheehan, K. C., Chance, C., Thomas, M. L., and Schreiber, R. D.: Purification and characterization of the human interferon-gamma receptor from placenta. Proc. Natl. Acad. Sci. USA 85:4837, 1988.
21. Porcelli, S., Brenner, M. B., Greenstein, J. L., Balk, S. P., Terhorst, C., and Bleicher, P. A.: Recognition of cluster of differentiation 1 antigens by human CD4−CD8− cytolytic T lymphocytes. Nature 341:447, 1989.
22. Simister, N. E., and Mostov, K. E.: An Fc receptor structurally related to MHC class I antigens. Nature 337:184, 1989.
23. Klein, J., Figueroa, F., and Nagy, Z. A.: Genetics of the major

histocompatibility complex: The final act. Annu. Rev. Immunol. 1:119, 1982.

24. McDevitt, H. O., Deak, B. D., Shreffler, D. C., Klein, J., Stimpfling, J. H., and Snell, G. D.: Genetic control of the immune response. Mapping of the *Ir*-1 locus. J. Exp. Med. 135:1259, 1972.

25. Watanabe, H., Matsushita, S., Kamikawaji, N., Hirayama, K., Okumura, M., and Sasazuki, T.: Immune suppression gene on HLA-Bw54-DR4-DRw53 haplotype controls nonresponsiveness in humans to hepatitis B surface antigen via CD8+ suppressor T cells. Hum. Immunol. 22:9, 1988.

26. Harding, C. V., Leyva Cobian, F., and Unanue, E. R.: Mechanisms of antigen processing. Immunol. Rev. 106:77, 1988.

27. Buus, S., Sette, A., and Grey, H. M.: The interaction between protein-derived immunogenic peptides and Ia. Immunol. Rev. 98:115, 1987.

28. Blanck, G., and Strominger, J. L.: Molecular organization of the DQ subregion (DO-DX-DV-DQ) of the human MHC and its evolutionary implications. J. Immunol. 141:1734, 1988.

29. Hood, L., Steinmetz, M., and Malissen, B.: Genes of the major histocompatibility complex of the mouse. Annu. Rev. Immunol. 1:529, 1983.

30. Brown, J. H., Jardetzky, T., Saper, M. A., Samraoui, B., Bjorkman, P. J., and Wiley, D. C.: A hypothetical model of the foreign antigen binding site of Class II histocompatibility molecules. Nature 332:845, 1988.

31. Williams, A. F., and Barclay, A. N.: The immunoglobulin superfamily—domains for cell surface recognition. Annu. Rev. Immunol. 6:381, 1988.

32. Lotteau, V., Teyton, L., Peleraux, A., Nilsson, T., Karlsson, L., Schmid, S. L., Quaranta, V., and Peterson, P. A.: Intracellular transport of class II MHC molecules directed by invariant chain. Nature 348:600, 1990.

33. Lane, P. J. L., McConnell, F. M., Schieven, G. L., Clark, E. A., and Ledbetter, J. A.: The role of class II molecules in human B cell activation. Association with phosphatidyl inositol turnover, protein tyrosine phosphorylation, and proliferation. J. Immunol. 144:3684, 1990.

34. Benoist, C., and Mathis, D.: Regulation of major histocompatibility complex genes: X,Y, and other letters of the alphabet. Annu. Rev. Immunol. 8:681, 1990.

35. Glimcher, L. H., and Kara, C. J.: Sequences and factors: A guide to MHC class-II transcription. Annu. Rev. Immunol. 10:13, 1992.

36. Bottazzo, G. F., Dean, B. M., McNally, J. M., MacKay, E. H., Swift, P. G. F., and Gamble, D. R.: In situ characterization of autoimmune phenomena and expression of HLA molecules in the pancreas in diabetic insulitis. N. Engl. J. Med. 313:353, 1985.

37. Hume, C. R., and Lee, J. S.: Congenital immunodeficiencies associated with absence of HLA class II antigens on lymphocytes result from distinct mutations in *trans*-acting factors. Hum. Immunol. 26:288, 1989.

38. Yang, Z., Accolla, R. S., Pious, D., Zegers, B. J. M., and Strominger, J. L.: Two distinct genetic loci regulating class II gene expression are defective in human mutant and patient cell lines. EMBO J. 7:1965, 1988.

39. Benichou, B., and Strominger, J. L.: Class II-antigen–negative patient and mutant B-cell lines represent at least three, and probably four, distinct genetic defects defined by complementation analysis. Proc. Natl. Acad. Sci. USA 88:4285, 1991.

40. Reith, W., Satola, S., Herrero Sanchez, C., Amaldi, I., Lisowska-Grospierre, B., Griscelli, C., Hadam, M. R., and Mach, B.: Congenital immunodeficiency with a regulatory defect in MHC class II gene expression lacks a specific HLA-DR promoter binding protein, RF-X. Cell 53:897, 1988.

41. Cosgrove, D., Gray, D., Dierich, A., Kaufman, J., Lemeur, M., Benoist, C., and Mathis, D.: Mice lacking MHC class II molecules. Cell 66:1051, 1991.

42. Grusby, M. J., Johnson, R. S., Papaioannou, V. E., and Glimcher, L. H.: Depletion of CD4+ T cells in major histocompatibility complex class II–deficient mice. Science 253:1417, 1991.

43. Blanar, M. A., Boettger, E. C., and Flavell, R. A.: Transcriptional activation of HLA-DRa by interferon-γ requires a *trans*-acting protein. Proc. Natl. Acad. Sci. USA 85:4672, 1988.

44. Amaldi, I., Reither, W., Berte, C., and Mach, B.: Induction of HLA class II genes by IFN-γ is transcriptional and requires a *trans*-acting protein. J. Immunol. 142:999, 1989.

45. Boothby, M., Gravallese, E., Liou, H.-C., and Glimcher, L. H.: A DNA binding protein regulated by IL-4 and by differentiation in B cells. Science 242:1559, 1988.

46. Rosa, F, M., and Fellous, M.: Regulation of HLA-DR gene by IFN-γ. J. Immunol. 140:1660, 1988.

47. Bahram, S., Arnold, D., Bresnahan, M., Strominger, J. L., and Spies, T.: Two putative subunits of a peptide pump encoded in the human major histocompatibility complex class II region. Proc. Natl. Acad. Sci. USA 88:10094, 1991.

48. Trowsdale, J., Hanson, I., Mockridge, I., Beck, S., Townsend, A., and Kelly, A.: Sequences encoded in the class II region of the MHC related to the "ABC" superfamily of transporters. Nature 348:741, 1990.

49. Rötzschke, O., Falk, K., Deres, K., Schild, H., Norda, M., Metzger, J., Jung, G., and Rammensee, H.-G.: Isolation and analysis of naturally processed viral peptides as recognized by cytotoxic T cells. Nature 348:252, 1990.

50. Falk, K., Rötzschke, O., and Rammensee, H.-G.: Cellular peptide composition governed by major histocompatibility complex class I molecules. Nature 348:248, 1990.

51. Rudensky, A. Y., Preston-Hurlburt, P., Murphy, D. B., and Janeway, C. A., Jr.: On the complexity of self. Nature 353:660, 1991.

52. Bevan, M. J.: Class discrimination in the world of immunology. Nature 325:192, 1987.

53. Moore, M. W., Carbone, F. R., and Bevan, M. J.: Introduction of soluble protein into the class I pathway of antigen processing and presentation. Cell 54:777, 1988.

54. Martinez, C. K., and Monaco, J. J.: Homology of proteasome subunits to a major histocompatibility complex–linked LMP gene. Nature 353:664, 1991.

55. Spies, T., Cerundolo, V., Colonna, M., Cresswell, P., Townsend, A., and DeMars, R.: Presentation of viral antigen by MHC class I molecules is dependent on a putative peptide transporter heterodimer. Nature 355:644, 1992.

56. Elliott, T., Cerundolo, V., Elvin, J., and Townsend, A.: Peptide-induced conformational change of the class I heavy chain. Nature 351:402, 1991.

57. Madden, D. R., Gorga, J. C., Strominger, J. L., and Wiley, D. C.: The structure of HLA-B27 reveals nonamer self-peptides bound in an extended conformation. Nature 353:321, 1991.

58. Garrett, T. P., Saper, M. A., Bjorkman, P. J., Strominger, J. L., and Wiley, D. C.: Specificity pockets for the side chains of peptide antigens in HLA-Aw68. Nature 342:692, 1989.

59. Falk, K., Rötzschke, O., Stevanovic, S., Jung, G., and Rammensee, H.-G.: Allele-specific motifs revealed by sequencing of self-peptides eluted from MHC molecules. Nature 351:290, 1991.

60. Rötzschke, O., Falk, K., Stevanovic, S., Jung, G., Walden, P., and Rammensee, H.-G.: Exact prediction of a natural T cell epitope. Eur. J. Immunol. 21:2891, 1991.

61. Pamer, E. G., Harty, J. T., and Bevan, M. J.: Precise prediction of a dominant class I MHC–restricted epitope of *Listeria monocytogenes*. Nature 353:852, 1991.

62. Jardetzky, T. S., Lane, W. S., Robinson, R. A., Madden, D. R., and Wiley, D. C.: Identification of self peptides bound to purified HLA-B27. Nature 353:326, 1991.

63. Smilek, D. E., Lock, C. B., and McDevitt, H. O.: Antigen recognition and peptide-mediated immunotherapy in autoimmune disease. Immunol. Rev. 118:37, 1990.

64. Sinha, A. A., Lopez, M. T., and McDevitt, H. O.: Autoimmune diseases: The failure of self tolerance. Science 248:1380, 1990.

65. Roche, P. A., and Cresswell, P.: Invariant chain association

with HLA-DR molecules inhibits immunogenic peptide binding. Nature 345:615, 1990.

66. Rahmsdorf, H. J., Harth, N., Eades, A.-M., Litfin, M., Steinmetz, M., Forni, L., and Herrlich, P.: Interferon-γ, mitomycin C, and cycloheximide as regulatory agents of MHC class II–associated invariant chain expression. J. Immunol. 136:2293, 1986.

67. Wettstein, D. A., Boniface, J. J., Reay, P. A., Schild, H., and Davis, M. M.: Expression of a class II major histocompatibility complex (MHC) heterodimer in a lipid-linked form with enhanced peptide/soluble MHC complex formation at low pH. J. Exp. Med. 174:219, 1991.

68. Lanzavecchia, A., Reid, P. A., and Watts, C.: Irreversible association of peptides with class II MHC molecules in living cells. Nature 357:249, 1992.

69. Mellins, E., Kempin, S., Smith, L., Monji, T., and Pious, D.: A gene required for class II–restricted antigen presentation maps to the major histocompatibility complex. J. Exp. Med. 174:1607, 1991.

70. Rudensky, A. Y., Preston-Hurlburt, P., Hong, S.-C., Barlow, A., and Janeway, C. A., Jr.: Sequence analysis of peptides bound to MHC class II molecules. Nature 353:622, 1991.

71. Sette, A., Buus, S., Colon, S., Miles, C., and Grey, H. M.: Structural analysis of peptides capable of binding to more than one Ia antigen. J. Immunol. 142:35, 1989.

72. DeMagistris, M. T., Alexander, J., Coggeshall, M., Altman, A., Gaeta, F. C. A., Grey, H. M., and Sette, A.: Antigen analog–major histocompatibility complexes act as antagonists of the T cell receptor. Cell 68:625, 1992.

73. Rogers, J. H.: Mouse histocompatibility-related genes are not conserved in other mammals. EMBO J. 4:749, 1985.

74. Lawlor, D. A., Zemmour, J., Ennis, P. D., and Parham, P.: Evolution of class-I MHC genes and proteins: From natural selection to thymic selection. Annu. Rev. Immunol. 8:23, 1990.

75. Bjorkman, P. J., Strominger, J. L., and Wiley, D. C.: Crystallization and X-ray diffraction studies on the histocompatibility antigens HLA-A2 and HLA-A28 from human cell membranes. J. Mol. Biol. 186:205, 1985.

76. Hill, A. V. S., Allsopp, C. E. M., Kwiatkowski, D., Anstey, N. M., Twumasi, P., Rowe, P. A., Bennett, S., Brewster, D., McMichael, A. J., and Greenwood, B. M.: Common West African HLA antigens are associated with protection from severe malaria. Nature 352:595, 1991.

77. Wraith, D. C., Smilek, D. E., Mitchell, D. J., Steinman, L., and McDevitt, H. O.: Antigen recognition in autoimmune encephalomyelitis and the potential for peptide-mediated immunotherapy. Cell 59:247, 1989.

78. Todd, J. A., Bell, J. I., and McDevitt, H. O.: HLA antigens and insulin-dependent diabetes. Nature 333:710, 1988.

79. Todd, J. A., Bell, J. I., and McDevitt, H. O.: HLA-DQ beta gene contributes to susceptibility and resistance to insulin-dependent diabetes mellitus. Nature 329:599, 1987.

80. Hemmi, S., Geliebter, J., Zeff, R. A., Melvold, R. W., and Nathenson, S. G.: Three spontaneous H-2Db mutants are generated by genetic micro-recombination (gene conversion) events. Impact on the H-2-restricted immune responsiveness. J. Exp. Med. 168:2319, 1988.

81. Geliebter, J., and Nathenson, S. G.: Microrecombinations generate sequence diversity in the murine major histocompatibility complex: Analysis of the Kbm3, Kbm4, Kbm10, and Kbm11 mutants. Mol. Cell. Biol. 8:4342, 1988.

82. O'Brien, S. J., Roelke, M. E., Marker, L., Newman, A., Winkler, C. A., Meltzer, D., Colly, L., Evermann, J. F., Bush, M., and Wildt, D. E.: Genetic basis for species vulnerability in the cheetah. Science 227:1428, 1985.

83. Watkins, D. I., McAdam, S. N., Liu, Z., Strang, C. R., Milford, E. L., Levine, C. G., Garber, T. L., Dogon, A. L., Lord, C. I., Ghim, S. H., Troup, G. M., Hughes, A. L., and Letvin, N. L.: New recombinant HLA-B alleles in a tribe of South American Amerindians indicate rapid evolution of MHC class I loci. Nature 357:329, 1992.

84. Belich, M. P., Madrigal, J. A., Hildebrand, W. H., Zemmour, J., Williams, R. C., Luz, R., Petzl-Erler, M. L., and Parham, P.: Unusual HLA-B alleles in two tribes of Brazilian Indians. Nature 357:326, 1992.

85. Howard, J.: Fast forward in the MHC. Nature 357:284, 1992.

86. Powis, S. J., Deverson, E. V., Coadwell, W. J., Ciruela, A., Huskisson, N. S., Smith, H., Butcher, G. W., and Howard, J. C.: Effect of polymorphism of an MHC-linked transporter on the peptides assembled in a class I molecule. Nature 357:211, 1992.

87. Pazmany, L., Rowland-Jones, S., Huet, S., Hill, A., Sutton, J., Murray, R., Brooks, J., and McMichael, A.: Genetic modulation of antigen presentation by HLA-B27 molecules. J. Exp. Med. 175:361, 1992.

88. Faustman, D., Li, X., Lin, H. Y., Fu, Y., Eisenbarth, G., Avruch, J., and Guo, J.: Linkage of faulty major histocompatibility complex class I to autoimmune diabetes. Science 254:1756, 1991.

89. White, P. C., Grossberger, D., Onufer, B. J., Chaplin, D. D., New, M. I., Dupont, B., and Strominger, J. L.: Two genes encoding steroid 21-hydroxylase are located near the genes encoding the fourth component of complement in man. Proc. Natl. Acad. Sci. USA 82:1089, 1985.

90. Spies, T., Morton, C. C., Nedospasov, S. A., Fiers, W., Pious, D., and Strominger, J. L.: Genes for the tumor necrosis factors alpha and beta are linked to the human major histocompatibility complex. Proc. Natl. Acad. Sci. USA 83:8699, 1986.

91. Carroll, M. C., Palsdottir, A., Belt, K. T., and Porter, R. R.: Deletion of complement C4 and steroid 21-hydroxylase genes in the HLA class III region. EMBO J. 4:2547, 1985.

92. Woods, D. E., Edge, M. D., and Colten, H. R.: Isolation of a complementary DNA clone for the human complement protein C2 and its use in the identification of a restriction fragment length polymorphism. J. Clin. Invest. 74:634, 1984.

93. Morley, B. J., and Campbell, R. D.: Internal homologies of the Ba fragment from human complement component factor B, a class III MHC antigen. EMBO J. 3:153, 1984.

94. Yu, C. Y., Belt, K. T., Giles, C. M., Campbell, R. D., and Porter, R. R.: Structural basis of the polymorphism of human complement components C4A and C4B: Gene size, reactivity and antigenicity. EMBO J. 35:2873, 1986.

95. Isenman, D. E., and Young, J. R.: The molecular basis for the difference in immune hemolysis activity of the Chido and Rodgers isotypes of human complement C4. J. Immunol. 132:3019, 1984.

96. Colten, H. R., and Rosen, F. S.: Complement deficiencies. Annu. Rev. Immunol. 10:809, 1992.

97. Volanakis, J. E., Zhu, Z.-B., Schaffer, F. M., Macon, K. J., Palermos, J., Barger, B. O., Go, R., Campbell, R. D., and Schroeder, H. W., Jr.: Major histocompatibility complex class III genes and susceptibility to immunoglobulin A deficiency and common variable immunodeficiency. J. Clin. Invest. 89:1914, 1992.

98. Hibbs, M. L., Wardlaw, A. J., Stacker, S. A., Anderson, D. C., Lee, A., Roberts, T. M., and Springer, T. A.: Transfection of cells from patients with leukocyte adhesion deficiency with an integrin beta subunit (CD18) restores lymphocyte function–associated antigen-1 expression and function. J. Clin. Invest. 85:674, 1990.

99. Kishimoto, T. K., Larson, R. S., Corbi, A. L., Dustin, M. L., Staunton, D. E., and Springer, T. A.: The leukocyte integrins. Adv. Immunol. 46:149, 1989.

100. Kishimoto, T. K., and Springer, T. A.: Human leukocyte adhesion deficiency: Molecular basis for a defective immune response to infections of the skin. Curr. Probl. Dermatol. 18:106, 1989.

101. Voss, L. M., Abraham, R. T., Rhodes, K. H., Schoon, R. A., and Leibson, P. J.: Defective T-lymphocyte signal transduction and function in leukocyte adhesion deficiency. J. Clin. Immunol. 11:175, 1991.

102. Dustin, M. L., and Springer, T. A.: T-cell receptor cross-linking transiently stimulates adhesiveness through LFA-1. Nature 341:619, 1989.

103. Hibbs, M. L., Xu, H., Stacker, S. A., and Springer, T. A.:

Regulation of adhesion of ICAM-1 by the cytoplasmic domain of LFA-1 integrin beta subunit. Science 251:1611, 1991.

104. Larson, R. S., and Springer, T. A.: Structure and function of leukocyte integrins. Immunol. Rev. 114:181, 1990.

105. Harding, F. A., McArthur, J. G., Gross, J. A., Raulet, D. H., and Allison, J. P.: CD28-mediated signalling co-stimulates murine T cells and prevents induction of anergy in T-cell clones. Nature 356:607, 1992.

106. Rogers, H. W., Sheehan, K. C., Brunt, L. M., Dower, S. K., Unanue, E. R., and Schreiber, R. D.: Interleukin 1 participates in the development of anti-Listeria responses in normal and SCID mice. Proc. Natl. Acad. Sci. USA 89:1011, 1992.

107. Groh, V., Porcelli, S., Fabbi, M., Lanier, L. L., Picker, L. J., Anderson, T., Warnke, R. A., Bhan, A. K., Strominger, J. L., and Brenner, M. B.: Human lymphocytes bearing T cell receptor gamma/delta are phenotypically diverse and evenly distributed throughout the lymphoid system. J. Exp. Med. 169:1277, 1989.

108. Kronenberg, M., Siu, G., and Hood, L. E.: The molecular genetics of the T-cell antigen receptor and T-cell antigen recognition. Annu. Rev. Immunol. 4:529, 1986.

109. Ashwell, J. D., and Klausner, R. D.: Genetic and mutational analysis of the T-cell antigen receptor. Annu. Rev. Immunol. 8:139, 1990.

110. Tunnacliffe, A., Buluwela, L., and Rabbitts, T. H.: Physical linkage of three CD3 genes on human chromosome 11. EMBO J. 6:2953, 1987.

111. Clevers, H. C., Dunlap, S., Wileman, T. E., and Terhorst, C.: Human CD3-e gene contains three miniexons and is transcribed from a non-TATA promoter. Proc. Natl. Acad. Sci. USA 85:8156, 1988.

112. Bonifacino, J. S., Chen, C., Lippincott-Schwartz, J., Ashwell, J. D., and Klausner, R. D.: Subunit interactions within the T cell antigen receptor: Clues from the study of partial complexes. Proc. Natl. Acad. Sci. USA 85:6929, 1988.

113. Berkhout, B., Alarcon, B., and Terhorst, C.: Transfection of genes encoding the T cell receptor–associated CD3 complex into COS cells results in assembly of the macromolecular structure. J. Biol. Chem. 263:8528, 1988.

114. Weissman, A. M., Baniyash, M., Hou, D., Samelson, L. E., Burgess, W. H., and Klausner, R. D.: Molecular cloning of the zeta chain of the T cell antigen receptor. Science 239:1018, 1988.

115. Frank, S. J., Niklinska, B. B., Orloff, D. G., Mercep, M., Ashwell, J. D., and Klausner, R. D.: Structural mutations of the T cell receptor a chain and its role in T cell activation. Science 249:174, 1990.

116. Irving, B. A., and Weiss, A.: The cytoplasmic domain of the T cell receptor a chain is sufficient to couple to receptor-associated signal transduction pathways. Cell 64:891, 1991.

117. Letourneur, F., and Klausner, R. D.: Activation of T cells by a tyrosine kinase activation domain in the cytoplasmic tail of CD3ε. Science 255:79, 1992.

118. Wegener, A.-M. K., Letourneur, F., Hoeveler, A., Brocker, T., Luton, F., and Malissen, B.: The T cell receptor/CD3 complex is composed of at least two autonomous transduction modules. Cell 68:83, 1992.

119. Romeo, C., and Seed, B.: Cellular immunity to HIV activated by CD4 fused to T cell or Fc receptor polypeptides. Cell 64:1037, 1991.

120. Kappler, J. W., Skidmore, B., White, J., and Marrack, P.: Antigen-inducible, H-2 restricted interleukin-2–producing T cell hybridomas. Lack of independent antigen and H-2 recognition. J. Exp. Med. 153:1198, 1981.

121. Matsui, K., Boniface, J. J., Reay, P. A., Schild, H., Fazekas de St Groth, B., and Davis, M. M.: Low affinity interaction of peptide-MHC complexes with T cell receptors. Science 254:1788, 1991.

122. Littman, D. R.: The structure of the CD4 and CD8 genes. Annu. Rev. Immunol. 5:561, 1987.

123. Doyle, C., and Strominger, J. L.: Interaction between CD4 and class II MHC molecules mediates cell adhesion. Nature 330:256, 1987.

124. Norment, A. M., and Littman, D. R.: A second subunit of CD8 is expressed in human T cells. EMBO J. 7:3433, 1988.

125. Wheeler, C. J., von Hoegen, P., and Parnes, J. R.: An immunological role for the CD8 β-chain. Nature 357:247, 1992.

126. Sleckman, B. P., Peterson, A., Jones, W. K., Foran, J. A., Greenstein, J. L., Seed, B., and Burakoff, S. J.: Expression and function of CD4 in a murine T-cell hybridoma. Nature 328:351, 1987.

127. Rojo, J. M., Saizawa, K., and Janeway, C. A., Jr.: Physical association of CD4 and the T cell receptor can be induced by anti-T cell receptor antibodies. Proc. Natl. Acad. Sci. USA 86:3311, 1989.

128. Glaichenhaus, N., Shastri, N., Littman, D. R., and Turner, J. M.: Requirement for association of p56lck with CD4 in antigen-specific signal transduction in T cells. Cell 64:511, 1991.

129. Janeway, C. A., Jr.: The T cell receptor as a multicomponent signalling machine: CD4/CD8 coreceptors and CD45 in T cell activation. Annu. Rev. Immunol. 10:645, 1992.

130. Brian, A. A., and McConnell, H. M.: Allogeneic stimulation of cytotoxic T cells by supported planar membranes. Proc. Natl. Acad. Sci. USA 81:6159, 1984.

131. Watts, T. H., and McConnell, H. M.: Biophysical aspects of antigen recognition by T cells. Annu. Rev. Immunol. 5:461, 1987.

132. Harding, C. V., and Unanue, E. R.: Quantitation of antigen-presenting cell MHC class II/peptide complexes necessary for T-cell stimulation. Nature 346:574, 1990.

133. Demotz, S., Grey, H. M., and Sette, A.: The minimal number of class II MHC–antigen complexes needed for T cell activation. Science 249:1028, 1990.

134. Samelson, L. E., Patel, M. D., Weissman, A. M., Harford, J. B., and Klausner, R. D.: Antigen activation of murine T cells induces tyrosine phosphorylation of a polypeptide associated with the T cell antigen receptor. Cell 46:1083, 1986.

135. June, C. H., Fletcher, M. C., Ledbetter, J. A., and Samelson, L. E.: Increases in tyrosine phosphorylation are detectable before phospholipase C activation after T cell receptor stimulation. J. Immunol. 144:1591, 1990.

136. Secrist, J. P., Karnitz, L., and Abraham, R. T.: T-cell antigen receptor ligation induces tyrosine phosphorylation of phospholipase C-g1. J. Biol. Chem. 266:12135, 1991.

137. Weiss, A., Koretzky, G., Schatzman, R. C., and Kadlecek, T.: Functional activation of the T-cell antigen receptor induces tyrosine phosphorylation of phospholipase C-gamma 1. Proc. Natl. Acad. Sci. USA 88:5484, 1991.

138. Ettehadieh, E., Sanghera, J. S., Pelech, S. L., Hess Bienz, D., Watts, J., Shastri, N., and Aebersold, R.: Tyrosyl phosphorylation and activation of MAP kinases by p56lck. Science 255:853, 1992.

139. Izquierdo, M., Downward, J., Graves, J. D., and Cantrell, D. A.: Role of protein kinase C in T-cell antigen receptor regulation of p21ras: Evidence that two p21ras regulatory pathways coexist in T cells. Mol. Cell. Biol. 12:3305, 1992.

140. Imboden, J., Weiss, A., and Stobo, J. D.: The antigen receptor on a human T cell line initiates activation by increasing cytoplasmic free calcium. J. Immunol. 134:663, 1985.

141. Lewis, R. S., and Cahalan, M. D.: Ion channels and signal transduction in lymphocytes. Annu. Rev. Physiol. 52:415, 1990.

142. Lewis, R. S., and Cahalan, M. D.: Mitogen-induced oscillations of cytosolic Ca^{++} and transmembrane Ca^{++} current in human leukemic cells. Cell. Reg. 1:99, 1989.

143. Downward, J., Graves, J. D., Warne, P. H., Rayter, S., and Cantrell, D. A.: Stimulation of p21ras upon T-cell activation. Nature 346:719, 1990.

144. Kronke, M., Leonard, W. J., Depper, J. M., and Green, W. C.: Sequential expression of genes involved in human T lymphocyte growth and differentiation. J. Exp. Med. 161:1593, 1985.

145. Abrahamsen, M. S., and Morris, D. R.: Cell type–specific mechanisms of regulating expression of the ornithine de-

carboxylase gene after growth stimulation. Mol. Cell. Biol. 10:5525, 1990.

146. Shaw, J. P., Utz, P., Durand, D. B., Toole, J. J., Emmel, E. A., and Crabtree, G. R.: Identification of a putative regulator of early T cell activation genes. Science 241:202, 1988.

147. Ullman, K. S., Northrop, J. P., Verweij, C. L., and Crabtree, G. R.: Transmission of signals from the T lymphocyte antigen receptor to the genes responsible for cell proliferation and immune function: The missing link. Annu. Rev. Immunol. 8:421, 1990.

148. Wiskocil, R., Weiss, A., Imboden, J., Kamin-Lewis, R., and Stobo, J.: Activation of a human T cell line: A two stimulus requirement in the pretranslational events involved in the coordinate expression of IL-2 and gamma interferon gene. J. Immunol. 134:1599, 1985.

149. Altman, A., Coggeshall, K. M., and Mustelin, T.: Molecular events mediating T cell activation. Adv. Immunol. 48:227, 1990.

150. Marth, J. D., Peet, R., Krebs, E. G., and Perlmutter, R. M.: A lymphocyte-specific protein-tyrosine kinase is rearranged and overexpressed in the murine T cell lymphoma LSTRA. Cell 43:393, 1985.

151. Biondi, A., Paganin, C., Rossi, V., Benvestito, S., Perlmutter, R. M., Mantovani, A., and Allavena, P.: Expression of lineage-restricted protein tyrosine kinase genes in human natural killer cells. Eur. J. Immunol. 21:843, 1991.

152. Perlmutter, R. M., Marth, J. D., Ziegler, S. F., Garvin, A. M., Pawar, S., Cooke, M. P., and Abraham, K. M.: Specialized protein tyrosine kinase proto-oncogenes in hematopoietic cells. Biochem. Biophys. Acta 948:245, 1988.

153. Turner, J. M., Brodsky, M. H., Irving, B. A., Levin, S. D., Perlmutter, R. M., and Littman, D. R.: Interaction of the unique N-terminal region of the tyrosine kinase p56^{lck} with the cytoplasmic domains of CD4 and CD8 is mediated by cysteine motifs. Cell 60:755, 1990.

154. Veillette, A., Bookman, M. A., Horak, E. M., and Bolen, J. B.: The CD4 and CD8 T cell surface antigens are associated with the internal membrane tyrosine protein kinase p56^{lck}. Cell 55:301, 1988.

155. Veillette, A., Bookman, M. A., Horak, E. M., Samelson, L. E., and Bolen, J. B.: Signal transduction through the CD4 receptor involves the activation of the internal membrane tyrosine-protein kinase p56^{lck}. Nature 338:257, 1989.

156. Abraham, N., Miceli, M. C., Parnes, J. R., and Veillette, A.: Enhancement of T cell responsiveness by the lymphocyte-specific tyrosine protein kinase p56^{lck}. Nature 350:62, 1991.

157. Tycko, B., Smith, S. D., and Sklar, J.: Chromosomal translocations joining LCK and TCRB loci in human T cell leukemia. J. Exp. Med. 174:867, 1991.

158. Abraham, K. M., Levin, S. D., Marth, J. D., Forbush, K. A., and Perlmutter, R. M.: Thymic tumorigenesis induced by overexpression of p56^{lck}. Proc. Natl. Acad. Sci. USA 88:3977, 1991.

159. Mustelin, T., Coggeshall, K. M., Isakov, N., and Alman, A.: T cell antigen receptor–mediated activation of phospholipase C requires tyrosine phosphorylation. Science 247:1584, 1990.

160. Ingraham, C. A., Cooke, M. P., Chuang, Y.-N., Perlmutter, R. M., and Maness, P. F.: Cell type and developmental regulation of the *fyn* proto-oncogene in neural retina. Oncogene 7:95, 1992.

161. Cooke, M. P., and Perlmutter, R. M.: Expression of a novel form of the *fyn* proto-oncogene in hematopoietic cells. New Biol. 1:66, 1989.

162. Sancho, J., Silverman, L. B., Castigli, E., Ahern, D., Laudano, A. P., Terhorst, C., Geha, R. S., and Chatila, T. A.: Developmental regulation of transmembrane signaling via the T cell antigen receptor/CD3 complex in human T lymphocytes. J. Immunol. 148:1315, 1992.

163. Cooke, M. P., Abraham, K. M., Forbush, K. A., and Perlmutter, R. M.: Regulation of T cell receptor signalling by a *src* family protein-tyrosine kinase (p59^{fyn}). Cell 65:281, 1991.

164. Davidson, D., Chow, L. M., Fournel, M., and Veillette, A.: Differential regulation of T cell antigen responsiveness by

isoforms of the src-related tyrosine protein kinase p59^{fyn}. J. Exp. Med. 175:1483, 1992.

165. Samelson, L. E., Phillips, A. F., Luong, E. T., and Klausner, R. D.: Association of the *fyn* protein tyrosine kinase with the T cell antigen receptor. Proc. Natl. Acad. Sci. USA 87:4358, 1990.

166. Appleby, M. W., Gross, J. A., Cooke, M. P., Levin, S. D., Qian, X., and Perlmutter, M. D.: Defective T cell receptor signaling in mice lacking the thymic isoform of p59^{fyn}. Cell 70:751, 1993.

167. Chan, A. C., Irving, B. A., Fraser, J. D., and Weiss, A.: The ζ chain is associated with a tyrosine kinase and upon T-cell antigen receptor stimulation associates with ZAP-70, a 70-kDa tyrosine phosphoprotein. Proc. Natl. Acad. Sci. USA 88:9160, 1991.

168. Taniguchi, T., Kobayashi, T., Kondo, J., Takahashi, K., Nakamura, H., Suzuki, J., Nagai, K., Yamada, T., Nakamura, S-I., and Yamamura, H.: Molecular cloning of a porcine gene *syk* that encodes a 72-kDa protein-tyrosine kinase showing high susceptibility to proteolysis. J. Biol. Chem. 266:15790, 1991.

169. Nada, S., Okada, M., MacAuley, A., Cooper, J., and Nakagawa, H.: Cloning of a complementary DNA for a protein-tyrosine kinase that specifically phosphorylates a negative regulatory site of p60^{c-src}. Nature 351:69, 1991.

170. Fischer, E. H., Charbonneau, H., and Tonks, N. K.: Protein tyrosine phosphatases: A diverse family of intracellular and transmembrane enzymes. Science 253:401, 1991.

171. Fernandez Luna, J. L., Matthews, R. J., Brownstein, B. H., Schreiber, R. D., and Thomas, M. L.: Characterization and expression of the human leukocyte–common antigen (CD45) gene contained in yeast artificial chromosomes. Genomics 10:756, 1991.

172. Stamenkovic, I., Sgroi, D., Aruffo, A., Sy, M. S., and Anderson, T.: The B lymphocyte adhesion molecule CD22 interacts with leukocyte common antigen CD45RO on T cells and α2–6 sialyltransferase, CD75, on B cells. Cell 66:1133, 1991.

173. Koretzky, G. A., Picus, J., Thomas, M. L., and Weiss, A.: Tyrosine phosphatase CD45 is essential for coupling T-cell antigen receptor to the phosphatidyl inositol pathway. Nature 346:66, 1990.

174. Weaver, C. T., Pingel, J. T., Nelson, J. O., and Thomas, M. L.: CD8 + T-cell clones deficient in the expression of the CD45 protein tyrosine phosphatase have impaired responses to T-cell receptor stimuli. Mol. Cell. Biol. 11:4415, 1991.

175. Mustelin, T., and Altman, A.: Dephosphorylation and activation of the T cell tyrosine kinase pp56^{lck} by the leukocyte common antigen (CD45). Oncogene 5:809, 1990.

176. Schreiber, S. L.: Chemistry and biology of the immunophilins and their immunosuppressive ligands. Science 251:283, 1991.

177. Tocci, M. J., Matkovich, D. A., Collier, K. A., Kwok, P., Dumont, F., Lin, S., Degudicibus, S., Siekierka, J. J., Chin, J., and Hutchinson, N. I.: The immunosuppressant FK506 selectively inhibits expression of early T cell activation genes. J. Immunol. 143:718, 1989.

178. Emmel, E. A., Verweij, C. L., Durand, D. B., Higgins, K. M., Lacy, E., and Crabtree, G. R.: Cyclosporin A specifically inhibits function of nuclear proteins involved in T cell activation. Science 246:1617, 1989.

179. Bierer, B. E., Somers, P. K., Wandless, T. J., Burakoff, S. J., and Schreiber, S. L.: Probing immunosuppressant action with a nonnatural immunophilin ligand. Science 250:556, 1990.

180. Liu, J., Farmer, J. D., Jr., Lane, W. S., Friedman, J., Weissman, I., and Schreiber, S. L.: Calcineurin is a common target of cyclophilin–cyclosporin A and FKBP-FK506 complexes. Cell 66:807, 1991.

181. O'Keefe, S. J., Tamura, J., Kincaid, R. L., Tocci, M. J., and O'Neill, E. A.: FK-506- and CsA-sensitive activation of the interleukin-2 promoter by calcineurin. Nature 357:692, 1992.

182. Clipstone, N. A., and Crabtree, G. R.: Identification of calci-

neurin as a key signalling enzyme in T-lymphocyte activation. Nature 357:695, 1992.

183. Schwartz, R. H.: A cell culture model for T lymphocyte clonal anergy. Science 248:1349, 1990.

184. Blackman, M. A., Gerhard-Burgert, H., Woodland, D. L., Palmer, E., Kappler, J. W., and Marrack, P.: A role for clonal inactivation in T cell tolerance to Mls-1a. Nature 345:540, 1990.

185. Von Boehmer, H., and Kisielow, P.: Self-nonself discrimination by T cells. Science 248:1369, 1990.

186. Blackman, M., Kappler, J., and Marrack, P.: The role of the T cell receptor in positive and negative selection of developing T cells. Science 248:1335, 1990.

187. Swat, W., Ignatowicz, L., von Boehmer, H., and Kisielow, P.: Clonal deletion of immature CD4$^+$8$^+$ thymocytes in suspension culture by extrathymic antigen-presenting cells. Nature 351:150, 1991.

188. Jenkins, M. K., and Schwartz, R. H.: Antigen presentation by chemically modified splenocytes induces antigen specific T cell unresponsiveness in vitro and in vivo. J. Exp. Med. 165:302, 1987.

189. Jenkins, M. K., Ashwell, J. D., and Schwartz, R. H.: Allogeneic non-T spleen cells restore the responsiveness of normal T cell clones stimulated with antigen and chemically modified antigen-presenting cells. J. Immunol. 140:3324, 1988.

190. Linsley, P. S., Clark, E. A., and Ledbetter, J. A.: T-cell antigen CD28 mediates adhesion with B cells by interacting with activation antigen B7/BB-1. Proc. Natl. Acad. Sci. USA 87:5031, 1990.

191. Swain, S. L., Bradley, L. M., Croft, M., Tonkonogy, S., Atkins, G., Weinberg, A. D., Duncan, D. D., Hedrick, S. M., Dutton, R. W., and Huston, G.: Helper T-cell subsets: Phenotype, function and the role of lymphokines in regulating their development. Immunol. Rev. 123:115, 1991.

192. Finkelman, F. D., Holmes, J., Katona, I. M., Urban, J. F., Jr., Beckmann, M. P., Park, L. S., Schooley, K. A., Coffman, R. L., Mosmann, T. R., and Paul, W. E.: Lymphokine control of in vivo immunoglobulin isotype selection. Annu. Rev. Immunol. 8:303, 1990.

193. Yamamura, M., Uyemura, K., Deans, R. J., Weinberg, K., Rea, T. H., Bloom, B. R., and Modlin, R. L.: Defining protective responses to pathogens: Cytokine profiles in leprosy lesions. Science 254:277, 1991.

194. Liew, F. Y.: Functional heterogeneity of CD4$^+$ T cells in leishmaniasis. Immunol. Today 10:40, 1989.

195. Heinzel, F. P., Sadick, M. D., Mutha, S. S., and Locksley, R. M.: Production of IFN-gamma, IL-2, IL-4 and IL-10 by CD4$^+$ lymphocytes in vivo during healing and progressive murine leishmaniasis. Proc. Natl. Acad. Sci. USA 88:7011, 1991.

196. Sher, A., and Coffman, R. L.: Regulation of immunity to parasites by T cells and T cell–derived cytokines. Annu. Rev. Immunol. 10:385, 1992.

197. Salgame, P., Abrams, J. S., Clayberger, C., Goldstein, H., Convit, J., Modlin, R. L., and Bloom, B. R.: Differing lymphokine profiles of functional subsets of human CD4 and CD8 T cell clones. Science 254:279, 1991.

198. Tschopp, J., and Nabholz, M.: Perforin-mediated target cell lysis by cytolytic T lymphocytes. Annu. Rev. Immunol. 8:279, 1990.

199. Podack, E. R., and Dennert, G.: Assembly of two types of tubules with putative cytolytic function by cloned natural killer cells. Nature 302:442, 1983.

200. Podack, E. R., Young, J. D.-E., and Cohn, Z. A.: Isolation and biochemical and functional characterization of perforin 1 from cytolytic T-cell granules. Proc. Natl. Acad. Sci. USA 82:8629, 1985.

201. Zalman, L. S., Martin, D. E., Jung, G., and Müller-Eberhard, H. J.: The cytolytic protein of human lymphocytes related to the ninth component (C9) of human complement: Isolation from anti-CD3–activated peripheral blood mononuclear cells. Proc. Natl. Acad. Sci. USA 84:2426, 1987.

202. Young, J. D.-E., Hengartner, H., Podack, E. R., and Cohn, Z. A.: Purification and characterization of a cytolytic pore-forming protein from granules of cloned lymphocytes with natural killer activity. Cell 44:849, 1986.

203. Duke, R. C., Persechini, P. M., Chang, S., Liu, C.-C., Cohen, J. J., and Young, J. D.-E.: Self recognition by T cells. I. Bystander killing of target cells bearing syngeneic MHC antigens. J. Exp. Med. 170:1451, 1987.

204. Ostergaard, H. L., Kane, K. P., Mescher, M. F., and Clark, W. R.: Cytotoxic T lymphocyte mediated lysis without release of serine esterase. Nature 330:71, 1987.

205. Trenn, G., Takayama, H., and Sitkovsky, M. V.: Exocytosis of cytolytic granules may not be required for target cell lysis by cytotoxic T-lymphocytes. Nature 330:72, 1987.

206. Coligan, J. E., Kindt, T. J., Uehara, H., Martinko, J., and Nathenson, S. G.: Primary structure of a murine transplantation antigen. Nature 291:35, 1981.

207. Sherman, P. A., Basta, P. V., and Ting, J. P.-Y.: Upstream DNA sequences required for tissue-specific expression of the HLA-DRa gene. Proc. Natl. Acad. Sci. USA 84:4254, 1987.

208. Tsang, S. Y., Nakanishi, M., and Peterlin, B. M.: B-cell–specific and interferon-gamma–inducible regulation of the HLA-DRa gene. Proc. Natl. Acad. Sci. USA 85:8598, 1988.

209. Tsang, S. Y., Nakanishi, M., and Peterlin, B. M.: Mutational analysis of the DRA promoter: cis-acting sequence and trans-acting factors. Mol. Cell. Biol. 10:711, 1990.

210. Sherman, P. A., Basta, P. V., Heguy, A., Wloch, M. K., Roeder, R. G., and Ting, J. P.-Y.: The octamer motif is a B-lymphocyte–specific regulatory element of the HLA-DRa gene promoter. Proc. Natl. Acad. Sci. USA 86:6739, 1989.

211. Monaco, J. J.: A molecular model of MHC class-I–restricted antigen processing. Immunol. Today 13:173, 1992.

212. Glynne, R., Powis, S. H., Beck, S., Kelly, A., Kerr, L.-A., and Trowsdale, J.: A proteasome-related gene between the two ABC transporter loci in the class II region of the human MHC. Nature 353:357, 1991.

213. Ortiz-Navarret, V., Seelig, A., Gernold, M., Frentzel, S., Kloetzel, P. M., and Hammerling, G. J.: Subunit of the "20S" proteasome (multicatalytic proteinase) encoded by the major histocompatibility complex. Nature 353:662, 1991.

214. Neefjes, J. J., and Ploegh, H. L.: Intracellular transport of MHC class II molecules. Immunol. Today 13:174, 1992.

215. Hunt, D. F., Michel, H., Dickinson, T. A., Shabanowitz, J., Cox, A. L., Sakaguchi, K., Appella, E., Grey, H. M., and Sette, A.: Peptides presented to the immune system by the murine class II major histocompatibility complex molecule 1-A^d. Science 256:1817, 1992.

216. Tiwari, J. L., and Terasaki, P. I.: HLA and Disease Associations. New York, Springer-Verlag, 1985, pp. 32–48.

ACKNOWLEDGMENTS: I thank Kathi Prewitt for help in preparing this manuscript, Dr. Stephen Jameson for advice, and the Howard Hughes Medical Institute for generous support.

SECTION IV

WHITE CELLS

Genetic Disorders of Phagocyte Function

John T. Curnutte, Stuart H. Orkin, and Mary C. Dinauer

INTRODUCTION

Phagocytes serve as major effector cells of the host defense against invading bacteria, fungi, and parasites. This subset of marrow-derived cells is equipped with specialized machinery enabling them to seek out, ingest, and kill microorganisms. The phagocyte system has two principal limbs: granulocytes (neutrophils, eosinophils, and basophils) and mononuclear phagocytes (monocytes and tissue macrophages). Granulocytes circulate in the blood stream until encountering specific chemotactic signals that promote adhesion to the vascular endothelium, diapedesis, and migration to sites of microbial invasion. In contrast, mononuclear phagocytes spend only a brief time in the intravascular compartment and function primarily as resident cells in certain tissues, such as lung, liver, spleen, and peritoneum. At those sites, they perform a surveillance role in antimicrobial protection and also interact closely with lymphocytes in the immune response. Both groups of phagocytes destroy appropriately opsonized targets by engulfing and sequestering them within intracellular vacuoles. Destruction of the target is mediated by the release of hydrolytic enzymes and bactericidal antibiotic proteins from storage granules and by the generation of highly reactive oxygen derivatives from the respiratory burst pathway.

Clinical disorders in which phagocyte dysfunction leads to a propensity for infection are relatively rare, which probably reflects a redundancy within the pathways that operate in each step of phagocyte antimicrobial activity. This chapter focuses on two inherited disorders that affect distinct aspects of phagocyte function. In leukocyte adhesion deficiency (LAD), phagocytes from affected individuals are deficient in cell surface proteins important for normal adhesion, chemotaxis, and phagocytosis. These functions are normal in chronic granulomatous disease (CGD), a disorder in which defects in the respiratory burst lead to impaired microbial killing. In each disorder, the investigation of the molecular basis of the clinical syndrome has made major contributions to our understanding of normal phagocyte function.

INFLAMMATION AND REPAIR

Inflammation is the reaction of vascularized living tissue to local injury, whether it be caused by microbial infection, trauma, burns, hypoxia, or a variety of immunological reactions. The acute phase of inflammation is fairly stereotypical regardless of the inciting agent, lasts for several hours to days, and is characterized by the accumulation of neutrophils and a proteinaceous exudate in the affected tissue. If the acute response is unsuccessful, chronic inflammation ensues, with the infiltration of mononuclear leukocytes and the proliferation of fibroblasts and small blood vessels. The process of repair is closely related to the inflammatory response and begins soon after the injurious agent has been neutralized. Phagocytes play critical roles in both acute inflammation and repair, as evidenced by the clinical manifestations of LAD and CGD. In both disorders, infections are poorly controlled and wounds are slow to heal.

The inflammatory response also has a darker side. In some circumstances, the vigor of the response and the potency of the microbicidal agents can cause severe damage to normal tissues.[1] Thus, the inflammatory and repair processes are subject to elaborate control mechanisms that serve to balance the beneficial and injurious consequences. On the one hand, they enable the host to recognize an almost limitless variety of pathogens and injuries and respond with remarkable quickness. On the other hand, these regulatory mechanisms serve to contain and limit the response, albeit imperfectly, so that damage to normal tissue is minimized. During the past decade, tremendous insights have been gained into the molecular basis of the inflammatory response, its regulation, and the inherited disorders in which it goes awry. This section focuses on the molecules and genes that mediate the phagocyte response during inflammation.

In addition to the need for precise regulation of the inflammatory response, one other logistical problem must be overcome by the host: The major effector cells, primarily phagocytes during the early stages of inflammation, are present largely in the circulation and not in the tissues where injury and infection frequently occur. Therefore, it is necessary that signals be sent promptly from these sites to attract neutrophils and to induce the extravasation of serum proteins critical for phagocyte function (opsonic antibodies and complement). As is discussed below, a diverse group of diffusible chemicals and proteins serve as mediators of inflammation. These include vasoactive amines, eicosanoids, plasma proteins, platelet-activating factor (PAF), cytokines, growth factors, and free radicals (nitric oxide [NO] and superoxide [O_2^-]). Except for the free radicals, each of these mediators has its own specialized receptor (or receptors) on one or more target cells.

For purposes of discussion, the acute inflammatory response can be subdivided into six phases as follows: (1) changes in vascular flow and permeability; (2) margination and adhesion of phagocytes; (3) transendothelial migration and chemotaxis; (4) recognition and ingestion of microbes and damaged cells; (5) degranulation; and (6) activation of microbicidal pathways in phagocytes. The first five steps are reviewed in this section, followed by a discussion of LAD and related disorders. In the second half of the chapter, the activation of microbicidal pathways in phagocytes is reviewed, and the major clinical disorder affecting this part of the inflammatory response, CGD, is discussed.

Changes in Vascular Flow and Permeability

Soon after a tissue is injured or invaded by pathogenic microorganisms, arterioles and microvascular beds in the vicinity vasodilate, increase the flow of blood, and cause the characteristic *rubor* and *calor* of inflammation. One of the key pathways leading to vasodilation is shown in Figure 14–1, a schematic diagram of the acute inflammatory response initiated by bacteria (in this case, a gram-negative organism). The host defense alarm system is tripped when bacteria activate sentinel tissue macrophages to release a wide variety of inflammatory mediators. Two of these, monocyte chemoattractant peptide–1 (MCP-1) and RANTES (*r*egulated upon *a*ctivation, *n*ormal *T* cell *e*xpressed and presumably *s*ecreted), cause basophils and tissue mast cells to release histamine, which in turn causes vasodilation in the microcirculation, mainly through H_1-type receptors.[2-4] In addition, PAF from activated macrophages and mast cells causes platelets to degranulate and release not only histamine but also another vasoactive amine capable of inducing vasodilation, serotonin.[5, 6] Prostaglandin E and prostacyclin generated by the cyclooxygenase pathway in activated macrophages (as well as by other cells) are also potent vasodilators and probably play a major role in vivo. Finally, nitric oxide released by endothelial and smooth muscle cells in large blood vessels may

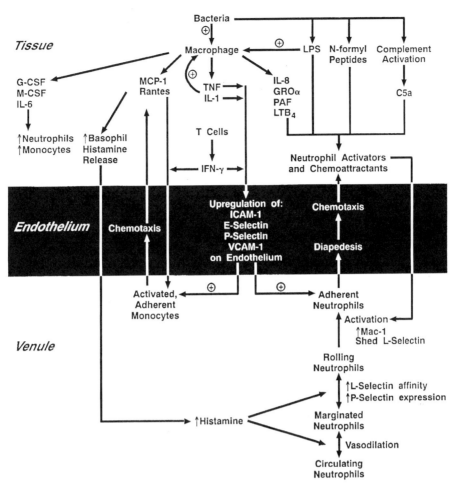

FIGURE 14–1. Initiation of the acute inflammatory response by bacteria. This scheme shows some of the major steps involved in recruiting neutrophils (and eventually monocytes) to sites of bacterial infection. The host defense alarm system is tripped when bacteria activate sentinel tissue macrophages to release (1) hematopoietic growth factors (e.g., G-CSF) that increase the production of neutrophils and monocytes in the bone marrow; (2) protein and lipid chemoattractants for neutrophils and monocytes (e.g., IL-8 and LTB$_4$); and (3) proinflammatory cytokines (TNF and IL-1) that serve to activate other immune cells and upregulate the expression of a series of endothelial adhesion molecules in nearby postcapillary venules. As a result of vasodilatation and other rheological changes in the blood (mediated in part by histamine release from basophils and mast cells), circulating neutrophils marginate in the venule and begin to roll along the endothelium in a process mediated by selectins. Neutrophils become firmly adherent to the cytokine-stimulated endothelium by means of the β_2 integrins, which increase their affinity for their counterreceptors upon activation of the neutrophils by agents that include macrophage-derived chemoattractants (e.g., IL-8, PAF), bacteria-derived N-formyl peptides, lipopolysaccharide (LPS), and complement fragment C5a. Once firmly bound to the endothelium, the neutrophils undergo diapedesis and directed migration (chemotaxis) along the chemotactic gradient emanating from the site of infection. A similar, but slower, process occurs with monocytes in response to cytokines derived from macrophages (MCP-1, RANTES) and T cells (INF-γ). C5a = Complement component 5 fragment a; G-CSF = granulocyte colony-stimulating factor; ICAM-1 = intercellular adhesion molecule–1; IFN-γ = interferon-gamma; IL-1 (−6, −8) = interleukin-1 (−6, −8); LTB$_4$ = leukotriene B$_4$; LPS = lipopolysaccharide; MCP-1 = monocyte chemoattractant peptide–1; M-CSF = macrophage colony-stimulating factor; PAF = platelet-activating factor; RANTES = regulated upon activation, normal T cell expressed and presumably secreted; TNF = tumor necrosis factor; VCAM-1 = vascular cell adhesion molecule–1. The "+" symbol indicates stimulation of a cell or enhancement of a function, and the "↑" denotes increased expression, affinity, release, or concentration as indicated.

mediate the lowering of arterial blood pressure seen clinically during gram-negative septicemia or following the administration of cytokines.[7–9]

The other early hallmark of the acute inflammatory response is an increase in the permeability of small arterioles, capillaries, and venules. As a result, plasma proteins and fluid leak into the surrounding tissues, forming the characteristic edema (*tumor*) of inflammation. As mentioned above, this process allows immunoglobulins and complement components necessary for opsonizing invading microbes to penetrate the tissues. A variety of inflammatory mediators play a key role in vivo in increasing vascular permeability. These include histamine, serotonin, PAF, and leukotrienes (LT) C_4, D_4, and E_4.[5, 10] The complement fragments C3a and C5a generated by complement activation at the site of inflammation further enhance vascular permeability by inducing mast cells to release additional histamine. Finally, bradykinin generated as a result of Hageman factor activation is capable of causing enhanced vascular permeability as well as pain (the *dolor* of inflammation).

Margination and Adhesion of Phagocytes

Under conditions of normal blood flow in the microvasculature, erythrocytes and leukocytes are confined to the center of the vessel where the flow is greatest. During acute inflammation, circulation slows in these vessels owing to both vasodilation and the increased viscosity of the blood brought about by the exudation of plasma proteins. As stasis develops, neutrophils begin to accumulate along the vessel wall where the flow rate is even lower. Under these conditions, neutrophils begin to interact loosely with the endothelium (particularly in the postcapillary venules) and roll along the vessel wall in the direction of blood flow. Rolling greatly diminishes the transit time of neutrophils through the venules and allows them to sample the local environment for activating or chemoattractant signals. In the absence of the appropriate inflammatory mediators, the rolling leukocytes eventually become detached from the endothelium and reenter the circulation. If the neutrophils do encounter activating signals, they become firmly adherent to the endothelium in ever increasing numbers. Eventually, the wall of the venule is lined with a single layer of phagocytes, a phenomenon known as pavementing.[11-15] This remarkable series of events was described in exquisite detail by Julius Cohnheim more than a century ago, a description based on his microscopic observations of how the microvasculature in the frog tongue and mesentery reacts to injury or treatment with a strong irritant such as croton oil (for a review, see reference 16). Cohnheim hypothesized that there was a molecular change in the vessel wall induced by the inflammatory stimulus that promoted the adherence of leukocytes. It took nearly a century to prove the Cohnheim hypothesis. We now know that at least three families of adhesion receptors mediate the interactions of leukocytes with the endothelium—the selectin, immunoglobulin-related, and integrin receptor families.

The properties of the selectin family of adhesion receptors are summarized in Table 14–1.[11, 17-36] The first selectin identified was a lymphocyte homing receptor that recognized a counterreceptor in the high endothelial venules of peripheral lymph nodes (for reviews, see references 18, 19, and 37). The observation that this binding was Ca^{2+} dependent and could be inhibited by polysaccharides rich in fucose sulfate suggested that the receptor on lymphocytes was a Ca^{2+}-dependent (C-type) lectin. A similar type of surface protein was identified in platelets and endothelial cells

exposed to histamine or thrombin. Yet another related molecule was identified in endothelial cells exposed to either lipopolysaccharide (LPS) or any one of several inflammatory cytokines (interferon-γ [IFN-γ], tumor necrosis factor [TNF], and interleukin-1 [IL-1]).[12, 15, 18, 19, 25] These three lectin-like adhesion molecules were originally referred to by a wide variety of names (see Table 14–1), but when it was discovered that they were closely related in both structure and function, a consensus nomenclature was adopted, and the term *selectin* was used to designate this family of adhesion receptors. As shown in Table 14–1, there are three known members of this family: L-selectin (the lymphocyte homing receptor that is also present in neutrophils), P-selectin (expressed in platelets and endothelium), and E-selectin (expressed on cytokine-activated endothelium). The finding that the genes encoding the three selectins have similar structures and are closely linked on the long arm of human chromosome 1 at position q21–24[24] suggests that they arose by gene duplication. Each of the three selectins is an integral membrane protein with a positively charged carbohydrate-binding domain situated near the extracellular N-terminus of the protein. The extracellular domain also contains a single epidermal growth factor–like module and two to nine short consensus repeats (~62 residues each) characteristic of complement-binding proteins followed by a transmembrane segment and a short cytoplasmic tail (see Table 14–1).[18, 25]

L-selectin is the only member of the selectin family known to be expressed on neutrophils and monocytes, where it is present constitutively. Its counterreceptor is present on endothelial cells and undergoes upregulation in response to inflammatory mediators such as IL-1, TNF, IFN-γ, and LPS, thus promoting the accumulation of phagocytes in areas of infection or injury (Figs. 14–1 and 14–2).[22, 23, 26] The identity of the L-selectin counterreceptor has not been established, although it likely contains sialic acid and either a fucose sulfate or a mannose phosphate moiety. The apparent requirement for sialic acid is consistent with the observation that the carbohydrate-binding domains of the selectins contain many positively charged amino acids. The affinity of L-selectin on lymphocytes and neutrophils for its counterreceptor appears to be enhanced by lineage-specific cell activators (e.g., granulocyte colony-stimulating factor [G-CSF] in neutrophils).[23] As discussed below, this provides yet another mechanism for targeting neutrophils to areas of inflammation. Soon after activation, leukocytes shed L-selectin by proteolytic cleavage of the molecule near the transmembrane domain.[23, 38] This process appears to be important in converting the neutrophil from a loosely adherent, rolling cell to one that is firmly bound to the endothelium. E-selectin is present on endothelial cells and undergoes de novo synthesis and increased surface expression within 1 to 8 hours after exposure to IL-1, TNF, IFN-γ, and LPS (see Figs. 14–1 and 14–2 and Table 14–1).[15, 18, 19, 39] E-selectin binds to a sialyl–Lewis X (SLe^x) carbohydrate ligand

TABLE 14–1.   PROPERTIES OF THE SELECTIN FAMILY OF ADHESION RECEPTORS

PROPERTY	L-SELECTIN	P-SELECTIN	E-SELECTIN
CD number	—	CD62	—
Synonyms	LAM-1 Leu 8 LECCAM-1 LECAM-1 MEL-14 TQ1 DREG.56 gp90^{mel} LHR	GMP-140 PADGEM	ELAM-1 LECAM-2
Molecular weight (kDa)	90	140	115
Chromosome	1q21–24	1q21–24	1q21–24
Complement-binding repeat domains	2	9	6
Cell distribution	Lymphocytes Neutrophils Monocytes	Platelets (α granules) Endothelium (Weibel-Palade bodies)	Endothelium
Upregulation of binding activity	↑ Affinity with cell stimulation (e.g., G-CSF) (minutes)	Translocates to membrane in response to thrombin, histamine, C5b-9 complex, and peroxides (minutes)	*De novo* synthesis in response to LPS, IFN-γ, TNF-α, IL-1β (hours)
Ligand/counterreceptor	Vascular addressins	Sialyl–Lewis X Lewis X (CD15) (weak) Sulfatides	Sialyl–Lewis X Sialyl–Lewis A (weak) Lewis X (CD15)
Cell distribution of ligand/counterreceptor	High endothelial venules in lymph nodes Endothelium	Neutrophils Monocytes Tumor cells	Neutrophils Monocytes Tumor cells
Function	Binding of neutrophils to endothelium Binding of lymphocytes to lymph nodes ("homing")	Binding of platelets to neutrophils	Binding of neutrophils to endothelium

G-CSF = Granulocyte colony-stimulating factor; LPS = lipopolysaccharide; IFN-γ = interferon-gamma; IL-1β = interleukin-1-beta; TNF-α = tumor necrosis factor–alpha.
Data from references 11 and 17 to 36.

(NeuAcα2 → 3Galβ1→4[Fucα1→3]GlcNAc→R) present in its counterreceptor on myeloid and tumor cells.[28–31, 33] Neutrophils are rich in glycoproteins and glycolipids containing SLe$^×$ and are therefore able to bind to inflamed endothelial cells expressing E-selectin.[25] Unlike the other two selectins, P-selectin is stored within intracellular organelles (the α granule in the platelet and the Weibel-Palade body in endothelial cells) and rapidly translocates to the cell surface as a result of the fusion of these organelles with the plasma membrane induced by histamine or thrombin (see Fig. 14–2).[8] P-selectin recognizes SLe$^×$ as well as Lewis X(Le$^×$; CD15) (Galβ1→4[Fucα1→3]GlcNac→R) carbohydrate domains on its counterreceptor present on myeloid cells (see Table 14–1).[21, 27, 32–36] Thus, all three selectins are involved in the enhanced adhesion of neutrophils and monocytes to endothelial cells (and platelets) during inflammation. Evidence now exists that both L-selectin and P-selectin mediate the early adherence of unstimulated neutrophils to endothelial cells in postcapillary venules, whereas E-selectin participates at a later stage after its upregulation by cytokines (see Figs. 14–1 and 14–2).[11, 12, 15, 40–42] As discussed below, a second form of LAD has recently been described in which neutrophils from two unrelated children exhibit a deficiency in the SLe$^×$ carbohydrate structure and are unable to adhere to E-selectin (and possibly other selectins) on activated endothelial cells.[43]

Selected members of the immunoglobulin gene superfamily of proteins constitute the second group of adhesion receptors that play a key role in the inflammatory response (Table 14–2).[13, 19, 20, 44] These adhesion molecules contain anywhere from two to six immunoglobulin domains and are present on endothelial cells, T cells, and a variety of other cell types. Intracellular adhesion molecule–1 (ICAM-1; CD54) and ICAM-2 are of particular importance in mediating the binding of neutrophils and other leukocytes to the endothelium, since they serve as counterreceptors for the leukocyte integrins (see Fig. 14–2 and discussion below). ICAM-2 is constitutively expressed on endothelial cells, whereas ICAM-1 is synthesized in increased amounts in response to inflammatory stimuli such as IL-1, TNF, IFN-γ, and LPS.[13, 19, 45–47] As is the case with E-selectin and the L-selectin counterreceptor, enhanced expression of ICAM-1 under these conditions allows phagocytes to be captured on the wall of

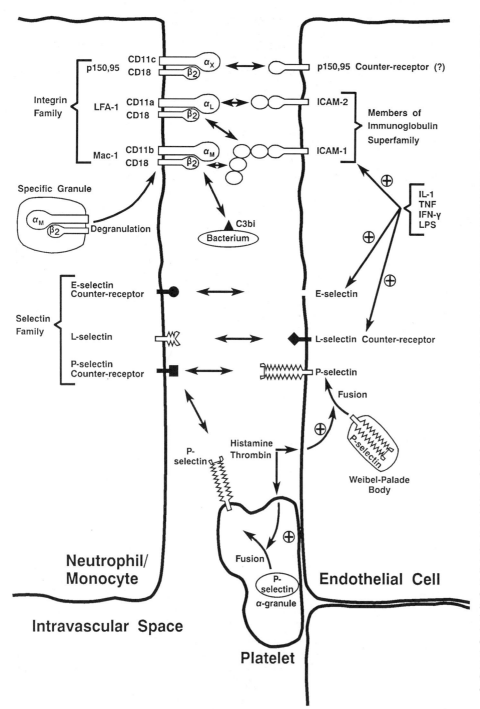

FIGURE 14–2. Integrins and selectins that mediate neutrophil or monocyte attachment to vascular endothelial cells. The leukocyte (β_2) integrins bind to their counterreceptors on endothelial cells that include ICAM-1 (CD54) and ICAM-2, both members of the immunoglobulin superfamily. ICAM-2 is constitutively expressed, whereas ICAM-1 is synthesized in increased amounts in response to inflammatory stimuli (IL-1, TNF, IFN-γ, LPS), a process that allows phagocytes to be attracted to areas of inflammation. The Mac-1 integrin also serves as the receptor for C3bi-opsonized microbes and can be expressed in high levels on the neutrophil surface through fusion of specific granules (which contain an intracellular pool of Mac-1) with the plasma membrane. Adherence to vascular endothelium, is also mediated by the three lectin-like proteins of the selectin family (L-selectin [LAM-1], E-selectin [ELAM-1], and P-selectin [GMP-140]). LAM-1 is the only selectin known to be expressed on neutrophils, where it is present constitutively but is rapidly shed upon cell stimulation. The LAM-1 counterreceptor is present on endothelial cells. The other two selectins are present on endothelial cells and undergo increased surface expression in response to inflammatory mediators (in the case of E-selectin) or to histamine and thrombin (in the case of P-selectin). P-selectin is also present in the α-granules of platelets and is expressed in increased amounts on the platelet surface following thrombin stimulation. ICAM-1 (or -2) = Intercellular cell adhesion molecule–1 (or –2); IL-1 =interleukin-1; TNF =tumor necrosis factor; IFN-γ = interferon gamma; LPS = lipopolysaccharide; ELAM-1 = endothelial leukocyte adhesion molecule–1; GMP-140 = granule membrane protein of 140 kDa (cluster designation, CD62); LAM-1 = lectin adhesion molecule–1. For reviews, see references 18 to 20, 44, and 49. (Adapted from Curnutte, J. T.: Disorders of granulocyte function and granulopoiesis. *In* Nathan, D. G., and Oski, F. A. [eds.]: Hematology of Infancy and Childhood. Philadelphia, W. B. Saunders Co., 1992, p. 908.)

the venule in areas of inflammation (see Fig. 14–1). Vascular cell adhesion molecule–1 (VCAM-1) is another member of the immunoglobulin superfamily that undergoes similar upregulation on endothelial cells (see Fig. 14–1). This adhesion molecule serves as a counterreceptor for a different integrin, VLA-4, that is expressed on lymphocytes and monocytes. Thus, VCAM-1 may play a role in promoting adherence of monocytes to the endothelium during inflammation.[13]

The third, and most diverse, group of adhesion receptors comprises the integrins (Table 14–3).[13, 14, 19, 20, 44, 48–50] Integrins are α/β heterodimers consisting of

an α chain (ranging in size between 120 and 180 kDa) non-covalently linked to a single β subunit (90 to 110 kDa). To date, a total of 22 distinct integrin subunits have been described—14 α chains and 8 β chains. Although this number of subunits could theoretically give rise to more than 100 different heterodimer combinations, it appears that many of the α subunits associate with only a single β subunit, since only about 20 different integrins have thus far been identified (see Table 14–3). Therefore, integrins are typically subcategorized according to their β subunit, as shown in Table 14–3. The majority of integrins are expressed

TABLE 14–2. SELECTED MEMBERS OF THE IMMUNOGLOBULIN (IG) SUPERFAMILY THAT FUNCTION AS ADHESION RECEPTORS

RECEPTOR	Ig DOMAINS	CELL DISTRIBUTION	UPREGULATION	COUNTER-RECEPTORS	FUNCTION
ICAM-1 (CD54)	5	Endothelium Many others	TNF-α, IL-1 IFN-γ, LPS	LFA-1, Mac-1 Rhinovirus	Leukocyte adhesion
ICAM-2	2	Endothelium	No	LFA-1	Leukocyte adhesion
VCAM-1	6	Endothelium	TNF-α, IL-1 LPS	VLA-4	Lymphocyte/monocyte adhesion
LFA-2 (CD2)	2	T cells	No	LFA-3 (CD58)	T-cell adhesion
LFA-3 (CD58)	2	Widespread	No	LFA-2 (CD2)	T-cell adhesion

ICAM = Intracellular adhesion molecule; IFN-γ = interferon-gamma; IL-1 = interleukin-1; LFA = lymphocyte function–related antigen; LPS = lipopolysaccharide; TNF-α = tumor necrosis factor–alpha; VCAM = vascular cell adhesion molecule.
Data from references 13, 19, 20, and 44.

on a wide variety of cells, and their most common function is to mediate attachment to extracellular matrices by serving as receptors for matrix proteins. For example, the $\alpha_5\beta_1$ integrin is a major fibronectin receptor, whereas $\alpha_v\beta_3$ and $\alpha_5\beta_5$ are key vitronectin receptors. Other integrins are involved in coagulation, such as $\alpha_{IIb}\beta_3$ (also known as glycoprotein IIb/IIIa) on platelets that bind fibrinogen, fibronectin, von Willebrand factor, and thrombospondin. Finally, several of the integrins play critical roles in cell-cell adhesion events, most notably the β_2 integrins that mediate the attachment of various leukocytes to endothelial cells. There are three β_2 integrins: $\alpha_L\beta_2$ (CD11a/CD18; lymphocyte function-related antigen–1 [LFA-1]), $\alpha_M\beta_2$ (CD11b/CD18; Mac-1), and $\alpha_x\beta_2$ (CD11c/CD18; p150,95) (see Table 14–3 and Fig. 14–2). As discussed below, LAD is caused by mutations in the β_2 subunit gene, with the result that the expression of all three

TABLE 14–3. THE INTEGRIN FAMILY OF ADHESION RECEPTORS

INTEGRIN SUBUNITS		OTHER DESIGNATIONS FOR THE INTEGRIN COMPLEX	LIGANDS AND COUNTERRECEPTORS	BINDING SITE*	CELL DISTRIBUTION OF INTEGRIN
β	α				
β_1 (CD29)	α_1 (CD49a)	VLA-1	Collagens, LN	—	Fibroblasts
	α_2 (CD49b)	VLA-2, gpIa/IIa	Collagens, LN	DGEA	
	α_3 (CD49c)	VLA-3	FN, LN, collagens	RGD(?)	
	α_4 (CD49d)	VLA-4	FN, VCAM-1	EILDV	
	α_5 (CD49e)	VLA-5, gpIc/IIa FN receptor	FN	RGD	Lymphocytes Platelets
	α_6 (CD49f)	VLA-6, gpIc/IIa	LN	—	Endothelium
	α_7	—	LN	—	Monocytes (VLA-4)
	α_8	—	?	—	
	α_v (CD51)	VN receptor–β_1	VN, FN(?)	RGD	
β_2 (CD18)	α_L (CD11a)	LFA-1	ICAM-1 (CD54) ICAM-2	—	B cells, T cells, monocytes, macrophages, granulocytes, NK cells
	α_M (CD11b)	Mac-1, Mo1, CR3	C3bi, ICAM-1 Factor X, FB	—	Monocytes, macrophages, granulocytes, NK cells
	α_X (CD11c)	p150,95 CR4	FB C3bi (?)	GPRP	Monocytes/macrophages, granulocytes, NK cells, some activated lymphocytes
β_3 (CD61)	α_{IIb} CD41b	gpIIb/IIIa CD41a	FB, FN, vWF VN, TSP	RGD	Platelets Endothelium
	α_v (CD51)	VN receptor–β_3	VN, FB, vWF TSP, FN, collagen	RGD	Endothelium
β_4	α_6 (CD49f)	—	LN(?)	—	Epithelial cells
β_5	α_v (CD51)	VN receptor–β_5	VN	RGD	Epithelial cells
β_6	α_v (CD51)	—	FN	RGD	—
β_7	α_4 (CD49d)	—	FN, VCAM-1	EILDV	Lymphocytes
β_8	α_v (CD51)	—	?	—	—

*Recognition sequences are given using single-letter amino acid code.
CR3 (and 4) = Complement receptor 3 (and 4); C3bi = complement fragment C3bi; FB = fibrinogen; FN = fibronectin; ICAM-1 (and -2) = intracellular adhesion molecule–1 (and -2); LFA-1 = lymphocyte function–related antigen–1; LN = laminin; NK = natural killer cells; TSP = thrombospondin; VCAM-1 = vascular cell adhesion molecule–1; VLA = very late activation antigen; VN = vitronectin; vWF = von Willebrand factor.
Data from references 13, 14, 19, 20, 44, and 48 to 50.

β_2 integrins on leukocytes is greatly diminished. Monocytes express one of the β_1 integrins, $\alpha_4\beta_1$ (CD49d/CD29; VLA-4), which may play a role in mediating adhesion of monocytes to endothelial cells that express its VCAM-1 counterreceptor (see Tables 14–2 and 14–3).

The properties of the leukocyte integrin subunits are summarized in Table 14–4.[13, 19, 20, 44, 51–60] The subunits are synthesized as precursor proteins (α', β') containing high-mannose N-linked oligosaccharides. The α' and β' subunits associate in the Golgi apparatus, where further processing to complex-type N-linked oligosaccharide occurs.[44] The mature heterodimer (α/β) is then transported to the cell surface or to intracellular granules. The α subunits are typical integral membrane glycoproteins with a leader sequence of 15 to 25 amino acids, an extracellular domain of approximately 1000 amino acids, a C-terminal single transmembrane domain of about 26 amino acids, and a short cytoplasmic tail with 19 to 53 residues (see Table 14–4). This structure is based on the amino acid sequences predicted from the cDNA clones for the three human α subunits.[54, 56, 57] Seven homologous tandem repeats (each about 60 amino acids) are present in the N-terminal half of the extracellular domain, three of which (between amino acids 412 and 616) contain divalent cation-binding motifs (DXXDXGXXD; D = aspartic acid, G = glycine, and X = any amino acid) that must be occupied by Ca^{2+} or Mg^{2+} for ligand binding to occur.[44, 48, 60] The transmembrane regions are highly conserved (88 per cent identity) among the leukocyte integrin α subunits, in contrast to the cytoplasmic domains, which have very different sequences. On the basis of studies with chimeric α subunits, it appears that different cytoplasmic domains trigger different functions[61] and that this is accomplished, at least in part, through interactions with the cytoskeleton.[48] The α subunit cytoplasmic domains also have different (and multiple) potential phosphorylation sites that may also be important in regulating function (see Table 14–4).[48, 60] The genes for α_L, α_M, and α_X are clustered on chromosome 16p11.1–p13,[55, 62] which, together with the striking similarities in amino acid sequences (36 to 61 per cent overall identity) and exon/intron boundaries, suggests that these subunits arose by gene duplication (see Table 14–4). The nucleotide sequence of the human CD18 cDNA has also been determined[51, 52] and has been used to construct a probable protein structure as shown in Figure 14–3. The N-terminal portion of CD18 is extracellular and consists of 678 amino acids (after cleavage of a 22 amino acid signal peptide) with six potential N-glycosylation sites as indicated by the triangles in Figure 14–3. Two highly conserved domains are also present: a stretch of 250 amino acids beginning at residue 111 (47 to 70 per cent homology with other β subunits) and a group of four cysteine-rich tandem repeats located between Cys 459 and Cys 615 that appear to confer a rigid structure on this extracellular portion of CD18. It is interesting that most of the mutations that have been identified in LAD occur in these two highly conserved regions, as discussed below. A single transmembrane domain of 23 residues is followed by a cytoplasmic tail consisting of 46 amino acids[49, 51, 63] that include a tyrosine and several serines and threonines that are phosphorylated upon β_2 integrin activation (see Table 14–4).[48, 60, 64, 65] The functional importance of CD18 phosphorylation, however, is not clear.[65] Like the α integrin subunits, the cytoplasmic domain of CD18 interacts with cytoskeletal proteins, such as talin, vinculin, and α-actinin.[48, 64, 66, 67]

The cellular distribution of the three β_2 integrins is shown in Table 14–3. They are expressed only on leukocytes, but to varying degrees on each cell type. For example, only LFA-1 ($\alpha_L\beta_2$) is expressed in large amounts on B cells and T cells, whereas granulocytes, monocytes, and macrophages express all three. The

TABLE 14–4. PROPERTIES OF THE LEUKOCYTE INTEGRIN SUBUNITS

INTEGRIN SUBUNIT	α_L	α_M	α_X	β_2
CD designation	CD11a	CD11b	CD11c	CD18
Amino acids	1063	1136	1114	747
Molecular weight (kDa)				
Precursor form	165	160	145	89
Mature form	180	170	150	95
Potential glycosylation sites (N-linked)	10	18	12	6
Amino acids in cytosolic domain (C-terminus)	53	19	29	46
Potential cytoplasmic phosphorylation sites	Serine Threonine	Serine	Serine Threonine	Tyrosine Serine Threonine
Homology	←————————— 37% —————————→			
	←——— 36% ———→	←——— 61% ———→		
mRNA	5.2 kb	4.8 kb	4.7 kb	3.0 kb
Chromosome	16p11.1–p13	16p11.1–p13	16p11.1–p13	21q22.3
Monoclonal antibodies that recognize subunit	Ts1/22 TS2/14	OKM-1 OKM-10 Mo1 Leu-15 904	S-HCL-3 Leu M5	IB4 TS1/18 60.3

Data from references 13, 19, 20, 44, and 51 to 60.

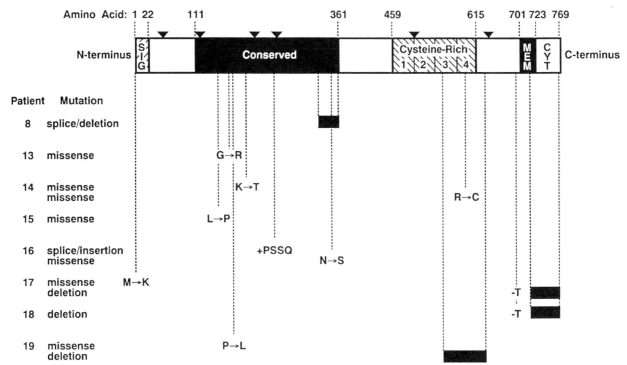

FIGURE 14–3. Schematic diagram of the structure of CD18 and location of mutations identified in patients with leukocyte adhesion deficiency (LAD). The N-terminus of the CD18 is extracellular and has a 22 residue signal peptide (SIG) followed by a 250 residue domain highly conserved among integrin β subunits (shaded region between Gln 111 and Asn 361). Four cysteine-rich repeats (1 to 4) reside between Cys 459 and Cys 615. A single transmembrane domain (MEM) of 23 residues begins at Ile 701, followed by a 46 residue cytoplasmic tail (CYT) at the C-terminus of CD18. Six potential *N*-glycosylation sites are shown by the solid triangles. Patient numbers are the same as used in Table 14–8, in which further details about each mutation are provided. Note the clustering of mutations in the conserved region and in the cysteine-rich domains. See Table 14–8 for references. (Data from Arnaout,[49] Kishimoto et al.,[51] and Nelson et al.[63])

ligands and counterreceptors for the β_2 integrins are indicated in Table 14–3 as well as in Figure 14–2. LFA-1 recognizes both ICAM-1 and ICAM-2 (members of the immunoglobulin superfamily; Table 14–2) and serves to facilitate binding of cytolytic T cells and NK cells to their targets. Recent studies suggest there may be a third counterreceptor for LFA-1, at least in a T-cell lymphoma cell line.[45] Mac-1 ($\alpha_M\beta_2$) is more restricted and recognizes ICAM-1 on endothelial cells (see Fig. 14–2). This interaction is of particular importance in the acute inflammatory response, since it is in large part responsible for the eventual anchoring of rolling neutrophils to the walls of venules near sites of inflammation. Since both Mac-1 and ICAM-1 are upregulated by inflammatory mediators, neutrophils are trapped only in those areas of the microvasculature where they are needed. As mentioned earlier, the surface expression of ICAM-1 on endothelial cells is low but substantially increases in the presence of TNF, IL-1, and IFN-γ (see Figs. 14–1 and 14–2).[46, 47] Mac-1, on the other hand, is upregulated differently. One mechanism involves the translocation of intracellular Mac-1 to the plasma membrane following exposure of neutrophils to any of a variety of activating agents that include *N*-formyl peptides, TNF, C5a, LTB$_4$, and even increases in ambient temperature.[13, 68–70] The intracellular site of Mac-1 is the specific granule, which readily

fuses with the plasma membrane upon stimulation.[71] Despite the fact that the increased surface expression of Mac-1 is temporally correlated with the enhanced adherence of neutrophils to endothelial cells, it now appears that a second mechanism may be much more important. Mac-1 is capable of undergoing reversible increases in its affinity for its ligands or counterreceptors following exposure to a number of neutrophil stimulants and inflammatory mediators.[69] LFA-1 in neutrophils undergoes a similar transient increase in binding affinity in response to phorbol esters. Activation of these two leukocyte integrins appears to be accompanied by conformational changes that can be detected as neo-epitopes recognized by specific monoclonal antibodies.[48, 72] One recent report describes a soluble 340 dalton lipid, termed integrin-modulating factor–1 (IMF-1), that can increase the binding affinity of Mac-1 and LFA-1.[73] IMF-1 is not present in unstimulated neutrophils but transiently increases in concentration following cell activation. Addition of IMF-1 to either intact cells or purified Mac-1 enhances the binding of the ligand 3Cbi.[73] Thus, IMF-1 appears to act as an energy-independent allosteric activator of Mac-1 that can function in either an autocrine or a paracrine fashion. In addition to its important role in localizing phagocytes to inflamed endothelium, Mac-1 serves as the major receptor for C3bi and is therefore often referred to as complement receptor 3 (CR3).[74] C3bi is deposited on microbes and other surfaces through the activation of either the classical or the alternative pathway of complement activation and functions as a critical opsonin for phagocytes. Relatively little is known about the ligands and function of the third leukocyte integrin, p150,95 ($\alpha_x\beta_2$). It is believed to play an important role in cell adherence in granulocytes, monocytes or macrophages, natural killer (NK) cells, and some activated lymphocytes. The integrin p150,95 has been reported to bind C3bi coupled to sepharose columns and, as a result, has been termed the complement receptor 4 (CR4).[44]

At least two important questions arise from the flood of new information regarding the structure, function, and regulation of the three classes of adhesion receptors involved in inflammation. First, how is specificity achieved in a system in which individual receptors often participate in multiple leukocyte-endothelial interactions? For example, both neutrophils and lymphocytes express L-selectin, yet only lymphocytes bind to the counterreceptor in the venules in the peripheral lymph nodes. Second, how are the multiple interactions coordinated—are they simply redundant mechanisms, or do they function during specific phases of the inflammatory response? There is growing evidence that leukocyte adhesion to endothelium at sites of inflammation is a multistep process that utilizes only certain adhesion receptors at each stage and relies on cell-specific activation steps to confer specificity.[11, 12, 14, 15, 40, 48, 64] The first step, mediated by L-selectin and P-selectin, appears to be the loose binding of neutrophils to the endothelium and their subsequent rolling along the venule wall.[11, 40–42] The neutrophil is poised to initiate binding, since both the P-selectin counterreceptor and L-selectin are constitutively expressed on its surface. The endothelium, on the other hand, must upregulate both of the corresponding complementary structures. As depicted in Figure 14–2, P-selectin is rapidly translocated to the endothelial surface upon exposure to histamine or thrombin,[18, 21, 75] whereas the L-selectin counterreceptor is expressed after exposure to inflammatory cytokines such as IL-1, TNF, IFN-γ.[22, 40, 41] As discussed above, the initial binding of neutrophils (but not lymphocytes) is further enhanced by the transient increase in the affinity of L-selectin for its ligand following exposure to a variety of activators such as G-CSF.[23] E-selectin also appears to be important in this process, although its upregulation on the endothelial surface takes longer, since it must be synthesized de novo[15, 39] (see Table 14–1). Thus, the role of the selectins is to "catch" marginated leukocytes with sufficient adhesive force to initiate a slow rolling process that can withstand the shear stress of the blood flow in the venule. The second major step in leukocyte–endothelial cell recognition involves the activation of leukocytes by cell-specific agonists generated as part of the inflammatory reaction. Once tethered to the endothelium via selectins, neutrophils and other leukocytes can sample the local environment for activation signals and chemoattractants that can

cause the rapid shedding of L-selectin[38, 40] and the concomitant activation of the β_2 integrins (see Fig. 14–1). As discussed in the next section, a wide variety of neutrophil-activating agents are generated during the acute inflammatory response. The third and final step in this process is the establishment of tight binding of the leukocytes to the endothelium, mediated by the interactions of activated Mac-1 and LFA-1 with ICAM-1. Consistent with this model is the finding that monoclonal antibodies to the integrin β_2 subunit have no effect on neutrophil rolling in inflamed venules but do cause the cells to return eventually to the circulation without ever undergoing stable attachment to the endothelium.[14] In contrast, antibodies to L-selectin greatly attenuate the rolling process.[40–42] Moreover, a monoclonal antibody to P-selectin has been found to block acute lung injury induced by cobra venom factor by inhibiting neutrophil adherence to pulmonary vascular endothelium.[76] Thus, there is an adhesive cascade leading to tight leukocyte binding to the endothelium via β_2 integrins only in the appropriate locations in the microvasculature and only after preliminary selectin-mediated adherence. Various adhesion receptors play specialized roles at different stages in this cascade. Specificity comes primarily from the activation-dependent steps that are triggered by cell-specific agonists. In LAD caused by mutations in the gene for the β_2 subunit, neutrophils roll normally along the endothelium; it is the subsequent firm attachment of phagocytes to the vessel wall that fails to occur. In the recently described second form of LAD, the earlier selectin-mediated steps in adhesion are abnormal owing to a defect in the synthesis of fucose-containing carbohydrates that affect the E-selectin and P-selectin counterreceptors.[43] In both diseases, neutrophils fail to emigrate to sites of inflammation.

Transendothelial Migration and Chemotaxis

Once firmly adherent, leukocytes move slightly along the wall of the venule and insert large pseudopods into the widened junctions between endothelial cells. The β_2 integrins are necessary for this process of transendothelial migration (diapedesis), as evidenced by the failure of LAD neutrophils to migrate across endothelial cell monolayers in response to chemotactic stimuli.[77] A similar defect in transendothelial migration is also seen when normal neutrophils are treated with certain monoclonal antibodies to the β_2 (CD18) subunit.[14, 78] The β_2 integrins (and ICAM-1) are necessary for transendothelial migration even when granulocytes adhere by an integrin-independent mechanism,[79] suggesting that they provide more than just a mechanism for phagocytes to stick to the endothelium.

The migration of leukocytes from the endothelium into the tissues is not a passive process; that is, the cells do not leak out of the inflamed vessel along with plasma proteins. Rather, the phagocytes respond to a complex set of chemotactic signals generated at the inflammatory focus and propel themselves in that direction. The orientation of chemotactic gradient is sensed by a series of chemotactic receptors that, once engaged, generate second messengers that regulate the contractile apparatus within the cell. The major neutrophil and monocyte chemoattractants in humans are summarized in Table 14–5.[2–6, 10, 12, 80–108] These agents are chemically diverse (lipids, complement fragments, peptides, and cytokines) and are generated by a wide variety of cells (or by the complement pathways) under the influence of bacterial products (N-formyl peptides, LPS) or certain inflammatory mediators (IL-1, TNF). Although functional redundancies in the system undoubtedly exist, the diversity of agents and cellular sources ensures that leukocytes will be attracted to sites of tissue injury or infection regardless of the initiating insult. Moreover, some of the chemotactic factors operate only on granulocytes, such as IL-8, whereas others are recognized only by monocytes, such as monocyte chemotactic protein–1 (MCP-1). This selectivity is responsible, in part, for the staggered appearance of neutrophils and monocytes at inflammatory sites. Generally speaking, neutrophils predominate during the first 6 to 24 hours and then are gradually replaced by monocytes (and eventually lymphocytes) within the next 24 hours. It is also important to note that the molecules in Table 14–5 serve not only as chemoattractants but also as activators of phagocytes. As discussed in the previous section, tight adherence of phagocytes to the endothelial surface requires that the β_2 integrins undergo conformational changes to increase their affinity for counterreceptors on the endothelium. The intracellular signals generated by the binding of these chemoattractants to their appropriate receptors trigger this change in the integrins and also cause the fusion of specific granules with the plasma membrane.[81, 82] This results in the transfer to the phagocyte surface of complement receptor type 1 (CR1) as well as the β_2 integrins Mac-1 and p150,95. Another consequence of the fusion of specific granules with the plasma membrane is the release of a variety of soluble proteins that include plasminogen activator, cobalamin-binding protein, lactoferrin, and metalloproteinases capable of degrading collagen (collagenase and gelatinase) that are used by the phagocyte to penetrate the endothelial basement membrane and extravascular connective tissue.[1] Finally, these chemoattractants cause a rapid, brief activation of the respiratory burst and the generation of low levels of (O_2^-), hydrogen peroxide (H_2O_2), and hypochlorous acid (HOCl). HOCl serves to activate collagenase and gelatinase, which are stored and released from the specific granules as zymogens, and to inactivate their antagonists, certain serine proteinase inhibitors (serpins) that include α_1-proteinase inhibitor $(\alpha_1 PI)$.[1, 109, 110] Other roles for respiratory burst products during this early stage of acute inflammation have not been established. It is important to note that this transient activation of the burst by chemoattractants does not preclude its subsequent reactivation by opsonized microbes.

The way in which phagocyte chemoattractants are

TABLE 14–5. NEUTROPHIL AND MONOCYTE CHEMOATTRACTANTS IN HUMANS

CHEMOATTRACTANT	SOURCE	UPREGULATORS	TARGET CELLS	RECEPTORS	REFERENCES
Lipids					
PAF	N, E, B, P, M Endothelium	Calcium ionophores	N, E	Cloned; 7-TMS	83–85, 87 5, 6, 88, 89
LTB$_4$	N, M	Microbial pathogens, N-formyl peptides	N, M, E	G protein coupled	88 10, 90
Intercrines (α subfamily)					
IL-8	M, endothelium, many other cells	LPS, IL-1, TNF, IL-3	N, B	Cloned; 7-TMS	81, 82, 91–93 3, 94, 95
GRO α, β, γ (MGSA)	M, endothelium, many other cells	IL-1, TNF	N	IL-8 receptor; 7-TMS	82, 95–97
NAP-2	P*	Platelet activators	N	IL-8 receptor; 7-TMS	82, 86, 95, 96, 98
Intercrines (β subfamily)					
MCP-1 (MCAF)	M, endothelium, many other cells	IL-1, TNF, LPS, PDGF	M	Not cloned	3, 4, 99–101
RANTES	M	IL-1, TNF, Anti-CD3	M	Not cloned	2, 102
Other					
N-formyl peptides	Bacteria Mitochondria	No	N, M	Cloned; 7-TMS	103–106
C5a	Complement activation	Complement activation	N	Cloned; 7-TMS	105, 107, 108

*Platelets, when activated, secrete platelet basic protein (PBP) and connective tissue–activating peptide–III (CTAP-III), which are cleaved to NAP-2 by cathepsin.

General references include 3, 12, and 80 to 82.

B = Basophil; E = eosinophil; F = fibroblast; IL-1 (-3, -8) = interleukin-1 (-3, -8); K = keratinocyte; LPS = lipopolysaccharide; LTB$_4$ = leukotriene B$_4$; M = monocyte; MCAF = monocyte chemotactic and activating factor; MCP-1 = monocyte chemoattractant protein–1; MGSA = melanoma growth-stimulating activity; N = neutrophil; NAP-2 = neutrophil-activating peptide–2; P = platelet; PAF = platelet-activating factor; PDGF = platelet-derived growth factor; RANTES = regulated upon activation, normal T cell expressed and presumably secreted; 7-TMS = family of G protein–coupled receptors with transmembrane segments; T = T lymphocyte; TNF = tumor necrosis factor.

generated during an acute gram-negative bacterial infection is depicted in Figure 14–1. Several important molecules are derived from the bacterium itself, including peptides that contain an *N*-formylmethionine residue, lipids (including arachidonate metabolites), and LPS. *N*-formylmethionyl proteins are also present in mitochondria, and their release from damaged tissue cells may play a role in the accumulation of phagocytes at sites of inflammation.[103] Bacteria also cause complement activation by either the classical or the alternative pathway, with the generation of C5a, an extremely potent chemotactic agent for neutrophils. The interaction of the invading bacteria with tissue macrophages results in the release of a host of inflammatory mediators, many of which serve as chemoattractants or phagocyte activators or both (see Fig. 14–1). TNF and IL-1 released by activated macrophages function in an autocrine fashion to enhance further the ability of the macrophage to generate these molecules. IL-1 also triggers temperature elevation and, along with TNF, causes the upregulation of adhesion receptors and their counterreceptors on nearby endothelial cells that recruit additional phagocytes from the blood. PAF is a phospholipid with an *O*-alkyl ether group at the *sn*-1 position, an acetate at the *sn*-2 position, and a phosphocholine moiety at the *sn*-3 position. It is generated by a variety of cells, including macrophages, upon activation.[5, 6, 83–85, 87–89] In addition to serving as a strong chemoattractant for neutrophils and eosinophils, PAF triggers platelet aggregation and granule release. Macrophage activation also results in the release of free arachidonic acid from its usual esterified position in membrane phospholipids so that it can be metabolized by both the cyclooxygenase and the lipoxygenase pathways. The former results in the synthesis of prostaglandins that serve as potent vasodilators (see above), and the latter generates leukotrienes that increase vascular permeability (leukotrienes C_4, D_4, E_4) or attract phagocytes (leukotriene B_4).[10, 88, 90] The remaining major chemoattractants are members of the intercrine subfamily of cytokines. These molecules have molecular masses in the 8 to 10 kDa range and share areas of homology in their amino acid sequences.[3] All of the intercrines have four cysteine residues, which form two disulfide bridges. In the α intercrine subfamily, the first two cysteines are separated by one amino acid (C–X–C), whereas in the β intercrines, the first two cysteines are adjacent to each other (C–C). The genes for the α intercrines are all located on chromosome 4q12–21, and those for the β subfamily are on chromosome 17q11–32.[3, 81] Not all members of the α intercrine subfamily are capable of activating neutrophils—for example, platelet basic protein (PBP), connective tissue–activating peptide–III (CTAP-III), and IFN-γ inducible protein (IP10). Only those members with a Glu-Leu-Arg (ELR) motif near the N-terminus—IL-8, GROα, GROβ, GROγ, and neutrophil-activating peptide-2 (NAP-2)—have neutrophil-activating properties. The ELR-containing α intercrines are also strongly chemotactic for neutrophils except for NAP-

2. IL-8 and the GRO cytokines are produced by monocytes, macrophages, and a wide variety of mesenchymal cells following exposure to inflammatory mediators such as IL-1 and TNF. NAP-2, which is not chemotactic but certainly a strong neutrophil activator, is generated in a different manner. Platelets, when activated, secrete PBP and CTAP-III, which are then cleaved to NAP-2 by cathepsin G from monocytes and neutrophils.[86]

Among the β intercrines, the two most important molecules involved in the recruitment of phagocytes are MCP-1 and RANTES.[2, 3, 99–102] Like IL-8, MCP-1 is produced by macrophages and a wide variety of other cells that have been exposed to inflammatory stimuli.[101] The production of RANTES is more restricted, with only macrophages reported to generate this cytokine. MCP-1 is highly selective for monocytes and induces chemotaxis and activation of the respiratory burst.[100] RANTES is chemotactic for both monocytes and memory T cells.[3, 102] Both MCP-1 and RANTES also interact with human basophils and cause the release of histamine.[2, 4] As discussed above, histamine release induced by this macrophage-derived cytokine plays an important role in the early stages of the acute inflammatory response (see Fig. 14–1).

The complementary DNAs (cDNAs) for the receptors for four of the chemoattractants listed in Table 14–5 have now been cloned and sequenced: PAF,[83–85, 87] IL-8,[91, 92, 94] *N*-formyl peptides,[104–106] and C5a.[107, 108] All of these receptors are structurally related to rhodopsin and are members of the seven-transmembrane segment (7-TMS) receptor family.[80] These receptors have seven hydrophobic α-helical segments that span the lipid bilayer and utilize intracellular guanine nucleotide-binding regulatory proteins (G proteins) to transduce signals. The chemotactic receptors, like many other members of the 7-TMS family, share the ability to be desensitized; that is, the receptor becomes refractory to further stimulation after an initial response, despite the continued presence of the stimulus.[95, 111, 112] Following exposure to agonists, these receptors are rapidly uncoupled from their G proteins and often sequestered from the cell surface.[80, 113] One of the consequences of desensitization is that it serves to limit the duration of the respiratory burst induced by phagocyte chemoattractants.

The signal transduction pathways linking neutrophil chemotactic receptors with the various functions they trigger have been partially characterized. Like other members of the 7-TMS receptor family, they are coupled to *Bordetella pertussis* toxin–sensitive heterotrimeric G protein consisting of α (39 to 52 kDa), β (35 to 36 kDa), and γ (7 to 10 kDa) subunits.[114–116] In the unstimulated neutrophil, the heterotrimeric G protein has GDP bound to the α subunit and is associated with the plasma membrane. Binding of the chemoattractant results in a conformational change in the receptor that promotes the exchange of GTP for GDP, which in turn leads to the dissociation of the α subunit from the β-γ complex. The β-γ subunits of the G protein then stimulate a phosphatidylinositol (PI)–specific phospholipase C (PLC) that catalyzes the hydrolysis of phosphatidylinositol 4,5-bisphosphate (PIP$_2$) to yield inositol 1, 4, 5-triphosphate (IP$_3$) and diacylglycerol (DAG) (Fig. 14–4).[117–122] As is the case in many cell types, calcium released from intracellular stores by IP$_3$[123] works in conjunction with DAG to activate the several isozymes of protein kinase C (PKC).[117, 124–126] As shown in Figure 14–4, DAG is also generated through the sequential action of phospholipase D (PLD) on phosphatidylcholine (PC) and phosphatidic acid (PA) phosphohydrolase on PA.[119, 121, 127–131] The mechanisms responsible for regulating PLD activity are not known, although recent evidence indicates that a PKC-dependent pathway may be involved.[119, 121, 127, 132, 133] Arachidonate can be generated by several pathways, including phospholipase A$_2$ (PLA$_2$)–catalyzed hydrolysis of PA, PC, PI, or DAG.[121, 134–136] Arachidonate serves as a precursor for a wide range of eicosanoids that include prostaglandins, thromboxanes, prostacyclin, leukotrienes, and lipoxins, as discussed above. Arachidonate may also function as a second messenger in its own right.[137]

The mechanisms by which these second messengers cause respiratory burst activation, granule fusion, and cell movement are only beginning to come to light. Arachidonic acid can activate the pivotal enzyme of the respiratory burst, NADPH oxidase, both in intact cells and in cell-free systems.[137, 138] It is not clear, however, whether sufficiently high concentrations of free arachidonate can be achieved in stimulated neutrophils to activate the oxidase. PA is also a potent activator of the oxidase and does so at concentrations that are reached in stimulated phagocytes.[139–141] Protein kinase C, or some other kinase activated by PKC, phosphorylates one of the NADPH oxidase subunits, p47-*phox*, an event correlated with the acquisition of catalytic activity.[142] The mechanisms regulating the fusion of lysosomal granules in the neutrophil with the plasma membrane are poorly understood. It is believed that increases in the intracellular concentration of free Ca^{2+} are necessary, but not sufficient, for degranulation to occur.[120, 143, 144] One recent study suggests that a fusogenic protein present in neutrophil cytosol, annexin I, modulates Ca^{2+}-dependent membrane fusion.[144] Calcium may also facilitate granule fusion by participating in the disassembly of actin filaments that would normally impede collision between granules in the plasma membrane.[145, 146] Finally, the motility of neutrophils is largely determined by the assembly and disassembly of cytoplasmic actin. The regulation of actin polymerization is exceedingly complex and involves the participation of more than a dozen actin-binding proteins. (See Chapter 15.) Second messengers thought to be important in actin polymerization include Ca^{2+}, PIP$_2$, and phosphatidylinositol phosphate (PIP).[145]

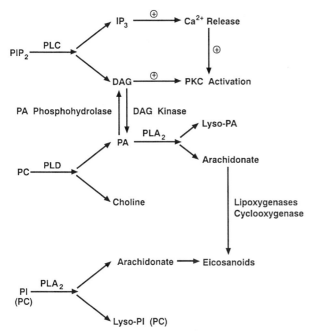

FIGURE 14–4. Signal transduction pathways in human neutrophils. A wide range of lipid second messengers are generated in neutrophils by phospholipases C (PLC), D (PLD), and A$_2$ (PLA$_2$) and by a series of kinases, phosphohydrolases, lipases, esterases, lipoxygenases, and cyclooxygenases. The binding of chemoattractant molecules to their receptors (e.g., IL-8 to its receptor) or counterreceptors/ligands to their corresponding adhesion receptors (e.g., C3bi to Mac-1) leads to the activation of one or more of the phospholipases shown. In the case of phospholipase C, activation is mediated by a heterotrimeric pertussis toxin–sensitive GTP-binding protein. Phospholipase C–catalyzed hydrolysis of phosphatidylinositol 4,5-bisphosphate (PIP$_2$) yields inositol 1,4,5-triphosphate (IP$_3$) and diacylglycerol (DAG). Calcium released by IP$_3$ works in conjunction with DAG to activate the several isozymes of protein kinase C (PKC), which in turn affect multiple cellular functions either directly or indirectly. The release of Ca^{2+} also plays a role in the regulation of the cytoskeleton (and hence, motility) as well as degranulation. DAG is also generated indirectly through the sequential action of PLD on phosphatidylcholine (PC) and of phosphatidic acid phosphohydrolase on phosphatidic acid (PA). There is growing evidence that PA itself may be an important lipid second messenger capable of activating critical functions such as the respiratory burst. Arachidonate can be generated by several pathways, including PLA$_2$-catalyzed hydrolysis of PA, PC, or phosphatidylinositol (PI). Arachidonate may function as a second messenger in its own right and serves as the precursor for a wide range of eicosanoids that include prostaglandins, thromboxanes, prostacyclin, leukotrienes, and lipoxins. The "+" symbol indicates stimulation of a function or enzyme activity.

Recognition and Ingestion

Unambiguous recognition of microbes, irreversibly damaged cells, and foreign particulate matter by phagocytes at sites of inflammation is a crucial step in the acute inflammatory response. Given the potency of their microbicidal and proteolytic systems, it is essential that phagocytes be discriminating in their selection of targets. Moreover, rapidly dividing microbes must be efficiently recognized and sequestered within phagocytes before they quantitatively overwhelm the recruited leukocytes and eventually the host. This logistical problem of having to mount a highly selective response to a diverse array of potential targets is accomplished through a series of receptors and humoral opsonins. Since the tissue macrophage is often the first cell to encounter potentially injurious agents, it must have receptors capable of recognizing a variety of ligands even in the absence of opsonins. These include the mannose receptor and the scavenger receptor.[147–150] The macrophage mannose receptor in the mouse, for example, recognizes *Pneumocystis carinii* and mediates its ingestion. The scavenger receptor has remarkably broad binding specificities and likely plays an important role in the clearance of diverse foreign materials.[150] Neutrophils and monocytes are not able to recognize most microorganisms, however, unless they are first coated with immunoglobulin (Ig) or complement or both—a process termed *opsonization*. The key humoral components of this system are IgM, IgG-1, IgG-3, and C3 complement fragments C3b and C3bi. Target cells are opsonized by the deposition of IgG onto the surfaces via the Fab portion of the antibody or by the accumulation of C3b and C3bi on their surfaces by means of the classical or alternative complement pathways.[74] IgM antibodies, although not opsonic by themselves, play an important role in recognition and ingestion by activating complement.

The opsonins are recognized by specific receptors on the membranes of phagocytic cells (Table 14–6). IgG molecules are bound by three distinct classes of Fc receptors (FcγR):FcγRI, FcγRII, and FcγRIII.[74, 151, 152]

The FcγR proteins are members of the immunoglobulin supergene family and have evolved from a common precursor through gene duplication and alternative splicing.[152] The functions of each of the three FcγR subtypes have not been clearly delineated, although it appears that they all can function as opsonic receptors (FcγRII and FcγRIII also interact with insoluble immune complexes).[153] Each is expressed at different levels, depending on the type of phagocytic cell. For example, FcγRI is not expressed on neutrophils unless they have been exposed to INF-γ or G-CSF.[152, 154] In contrast, only neutrophils appear to express FcγRIIIB, the only FcγR receptor that is anchored in the membrane by a glycosyl-phosphatidylinositol (GPI) moiety instead of a transmembrane domain. Neutrophils from patients with paroxysmal nocturnal hemoglobinuria (PNH), an acquired clonal stem cell disorder characterized by a defect in the biosynthesis of the GPI anchor, show a marked deficiency in FcγRIIIB.[151, 155] The signal transduction pathways triggered by the FcγRs have not been fully characterized, although it is known that their engagement results in a rise in the concentration of intracellular Ca^{2+}, suggesting the involvement of a PLC-mediated pathway, as in the case of the chemotactic receptors (see Fig. 14–4). The human phagocyte C3b receptor (CR1) is a high molecular weight, single-

TABLE 14–6. HUMAN PHAGOCYTE Fcγ AND COMPLEMENT RECEPTORS

	FcγRI	FcγRII	FcγRIII	CR1	CR3
CD designation	CD64	CD32	CD16	CD35	CD11b/CD18
Molecular weight (kDa)	72	40	50–80	160–250	CD11b:170 CD18:95
Genes	1	3 (A, B, C)	2 (A, B)	1	1/1
Chromosome	1q	1q23	1q23	1q32	16p11–13/21q22.3
Alleles	2	2 for FcγRIIA	2 for FcγRIIIB (NA-1, NA-2)	10	1/1
Cell distribution	Monocytes Macrophages IFN-γ–treated neutrophils	Monocytes Neutrophils Macrophages Eosinophils B lymphocytes Platelets	Neutrophils* Eosinophils Macrophages NK cells	Monocytes Macrophages Neutrophils Erythrocytes B lymphocytes	Monocytes Macrophages Monocytes
Inducers	IFN-γ G-CSF	—	—	—	—
Ligands	Monomeric IgG ($G_1 = G_3 > G_4 >> G_2$)	Complexed IgG ($G_1 = G_3 >> G_2, G_4$)	Complexed IgG ($G_1 = G_3 >> G_2, G_4$)	C3b C4b	C3bi ICAM-1 ICAM-2
Affinity	High	Low	Low	Moderate	Moderate
Function	ADCC	ADCC Trigger respiratory burst	Immune complex clearance Phagocytosis	Phagocytosis (opsonin receptor)	Phagocytosis (opsonin receptor) Cell adherence
Monoclonal antibodies	32.2, FR51 10.1, 44.1	IV.3 KU79 2E1 41H.16	3G8 4F7 Leu 11a, b B73.1	Anti-CR1	Leu 15 Mo1 OKM-1

*Only FcγRIIIB is found in neutrophils and is anchored to the outer leaflet of the plasma membrane by a glycosylphosphatidylinositol moiety. FcγRIIIB is not expressed in monocytes, macrophages, and NK cells. In these cells, FcγRIIIA is expressed and has a conventional transmembrane domain.

ADCC = Antibody-dependent cellular cytotoxicity; G-CSF = granulocyte colony-stimulating factor; IFN-γ = interferon-gamma; FcγR = Fc receptor for IgG; CR = complement receptor; ICAM = intracellular adhesion molecule.

Data from references 74, 151, 152, 156, and 157.

subunit glycoprotein that shows substantial heterogeneity in size owing to the presence in the human population of four distinct alleles that encode proteins of 160, 190, 220, and 250 kDa[74, 156, 157] (see Table 14–6). CR1 is responsible for the binding of C3b-opsonized particles and for initiating their ingestion. The other major opsonic receptor, CR3, recognizes particles opsonized by C3bi. This receptor is the same as the β_2 integrin Mac-1 (CD11/CD18) discussed in detail above. Binding of C3bi-opsonized particles to CR3 triggers both phagocytosis and the respiratory burst. Both of these processes are severely defective in patients with LAD caused by mutations in the β (CD18) subunit of Mac-1/CR3.

Engagement of any of the opsonic receptors initiates the phagocytosis of the opsonized particles. Pseudopods flow around the object to be engulfed, eventually resulting in the complete enclosure of the particle. The molecular details of how pseudopod formation is regulated and how the contractile proteins in the cytosol assemble and disassemble in an orderly fashion have not been fully elucidated. It seems likely that the same mechanisms that result in cell movement when chemotactic receptors are engaged are also involved in the ingestion of opsonized particles. (See Chapter 15.)

Degranulation

Neutrophils contain two broad classes of lysosomes—specific granules and azurophil granules. As discussed above, the specific granules deliberately secrete their contents into the extracellular medium when chemotactic agents such as C5a, PAF, and LTB_4 bind to their respective receptors.[120] The fusion of specific granules with the plasma membrane results not only in the release of the contents of the granules but also in the transfer of the proteins and lipids in the granule membrane to the plasma membrane. In this manner, the surface expression of the C5a receptor, Mac-1, p150,95, and cytochrome b_{558} (a redox component of NADPH oxidase discussed below), can be increased during chemotaxis.[68, 70, 71, 158–160] The release of lactoferrin and cobalamin-binding protein serves to bind ferric (Fe^{3+}) iron and a wide variety of corrinoids, respectively, whereas two metalloproteinases, collagenase and gelatinase, appear to facilitate the movement of neutrophils through the endothelial basement membrane and surrounding connective tissue.[1, 161] The contents of the azurophil granules are used almost exclusively for the disposal of ingested microorganisms and other cellular debris. Therefore, these granules generally do not undergo exocytosis but instead fuse with the phagocytic vacuoles containing the ingested microbes. The azurophil granules contain a variety of microbicidal agents that include defensins, bactericidal/permeability-increasing protein (BPI), lysozyme, and myeloperoxidase.[162–164] Azurophil granules also have a battery of hydrolytic enzymes that act on a wide variety of substrates, including proteins, nucleic acids, polysaccharides, and lipids. These enzymes include neutral proteases (elastase, cathepsin G, proteinase III) and acid hydrolases (cathepsin D, lysozyme, RNase). The importance of these lysosomal proteins in the microbicidal activities of phagocytes is discussed in greater detail below.

LEUKOCYTE ADHESION DEFICIENCY

Clinical Features

Leukocyte adhesion deficiency is a rare autosomal recessive disorder in which phagocyte adhesion, chemotaxis, and ingestion of C3bi-opsonized microbes are severely impaired. Approximately 60 patients with this disorder have been described in the literature to date.[49, 60, 165–170] The clinical hallmark of LAD is the occurrence of repeated, and sometimes widespread, bacterial and fungal infections without the production of pus despite a persistent granulocytosis that can increase to levels as high as 100,000 neutrophils per cubic millimeter during acute infections (Table 14–7).

TABLE 14–7. CLINICAL PRESENTATIONS OF LEUKOCYTE ADHESION DEFICIENCY*

CHRONIC CONDITIONS	ACUTE INFECTIONS	INFECTING ORGANISMS
Persistent granulocytosis (12,000–100,000/mm²)	Cutaneous abscesses and cellulitis (possibly invasive)	*Staphylococcus aureus*
Failure to form pus	Gingivitis and periodontitis	*Escherichia coli*
Delayed umbilical cord separation	Facial cellulitis and stomatitis	*Pseudomonas aeruginosa*
Patent urachus	Otitis media	*Pseudomonas* spp.
Impaired wound healing	Omphalitis	*Proteus*
Hepatosplenomegaly	Perirectal abscesses and cellulitis (possibly invasive)	*Klebsiella*
	Sepsis	*Candida albicans*
	Pneumonia/laryngotracheitis	*Aspergillus* spp.
	Peritonitis/necrotizing enterocolitis	Viruses (slightly increased risk)
	Bronchitis	
	Sinusitis	
	Esophagitis/erosive gastritis	
	Appendicitis	
	Aseptic meningitis	

*Each list is arranged in approximate order of frequency based on reviews summarizing various series of patients with leukocyte adhesion deficiency.[49, 60, 165, 167–170]

The disease is caused by mutations in the gene encoding the common β_2 subunit of the leukocyte integrins. Depending on the nature of the mutation, leukocytes express anywhere between 0 and 20 per cent of the normal levels of each of the three β_2 integrins. The clinical severity of LAD is largely determined by the level of integrin expression—those patients with expression of less than 2 per cent of normal are most severely affected. Since neutrophils and other phagocytes are unable to emigrate to the soft tissues, any area of the body exposed to pathogens from the outside world is susceptible to infection. LAD usually manifests shortly after birth with omphalitis and delayed separation of the umbilical cord. Cutaneous and perirectal infections are common and tend to form abscesses devoid of pus. These lesions heal poorly and sometimes evolve into chronic ulcerative lesions that can spread to deeper tissues and the blood stream. Necrotizing enterocolitis and peritonitis have also been observed in severe cases owing to the presence of gram-negative bacteria in the bowel. Ulcerative lesions of the tongue and pharynx are common, as is an unusually aggressive form of gingivitis and periodontitis. Laryngotracheitis, bronchitis, sinusitis, pneumonia, and otitis media are also encountered because of the poor acute inflammatory response to upper respiratory tract pathogens. The majority of infections are caused by *Staphylococcus aureus* and a host of gram-negative bacteria, including *Pseudomonas aeruginosa* (and related species), *Escherichia coli*, and *Proteus* species. Fungal pathogens are also encountered, particularly *Candida albicans* and *Aspergillus* species. It is interesting that viral infections are not generally problematical in LAD.

Molecular Basis of Leukocyte Adhesion Deficiency

The molecular basis of LAD was first suggested by Crowley and colleagues, who found that the particulate fraction of neutrophils from a patient with this clinical syndrome lacked a high molecular weight glycoprotein.[171] Since the patient's neutrophils neither adhered to plastic surfaces nor underwent an oxidative burst when exposed to serum-opsonized particles, it was hypothesized that the missing glycoprotein was responsible both for adhesion and for cell-particle interactions. A similar glycoprotein was subsequently found to be missing in several other patients[172, 173] and was eventually identified as the α subunit of Mac-1. During this same period, the structure and function of a variety of integrins were being characterized. The availability of monoclonal antibodies to α and β integrin subunits led to the finding that in LAD the levels of LFA-1 ($\alpha_L\beta_2$), Mac-1 ($\alpha_M\beta_2$), and p150,95 ($\alpha_X\beta_2$) were either undetectable or severely deficient.[44, 60, 165, 168, 169] Since all three of these integrins share a common β_2 chain, it was hypothesized that the molecular defect might involve this integrin subunit. In support of this hypothesis was the finding that in a mouse-human

LAD somatic cell hybrid, the mouse β_2 subunit (CD18) was able to associate with the human (LAD) CD11a and become expressed on the cell surface as a CD11a/CD18 complex.[58] In contrast, the human CD18 could not associate with the mouse CD11a. In other experiments, Springer and colleagues directly showed there were normal levels of the LFA-1 α_L subunit (CD11a) precursors in lymphoid cell lines from three patients with LAD.[58, 174] Finally, Epstein-Barr virus (EBV)–transformed cell lines from four LAD patients that had been transfected with a normal β_2 subunit cDNA were found to express the LFA-1 heterodimer on the cell surface.[175]

More than a dozen patients with LAD have now been characterized at the molecular genetic level. In each case, a mutation in the gene encoding the β_2 subunit has been identified. Thus far, α subunit mutations have not been reported to cause LAD. Table 14–8 summarizes published data on 19 cases of LAD.[51, 63, 167, 176–181] Patients 1 to 7 were among the first to be studied at the molecular level and were found to exhibit two CD18 mRNA phenotypes.[167, 176] Patients 1 to 3 had undetectable CD18 mRNA, whereas patients 4 to 7 had low levels. There was a correlation between the amount of mRNA and the levels of β precursor protein (β') and the mature α-β dimer. As discussed earlier, the β subunit is synthesized in a precursor form that associates with an α subunit precursor (α') to form an α'-β' complex. This precursor complex is then processed to a mature α-β form and transported to the specific granule and plasma membranes. In patients 4 to 7, small amounts of β' appeared to be incorporated into α-β dimers that were expressed at levels sufficient to confer a moderate clinical phenotype on this group of patients. In contrast, patients 1 to 3 failed to express any α-β dimer and had severe disease. In both sets of patients, the CD18 gene mutations leading to the abnormal mRNA levels have not been reported.

Patients 8 to 11 in Table 14–8 are related and have a splice mutation that leads to the moderate clinical phenotype.[167, 168, 176, 177] A third-position mutation in a 5' splice site (gtga → gtca) results in the abnormal splicing of two non-consecutive exons and the loss of a single 90 nucleotide (nt) exon. The level of CD18 mRNA in these patients was found to be normal, although 97 per cent of the message had the in-frame 90 nt deletion. The β' subunit translated from this defective message was abnormally small and apparently unable to associate normally with the α' subunit. Roughly 3 per cent of the CD18 mRNA, however, was found to be normally spliced and was probably responsible for the low level of α-β dimer expression in the patients' leukocytes and the moderate clinical phenotype. As shown in Figure 14–3, the splice mutation and the predicted 30 amino acid deletion are located in one of the most highly conserved regions of the β_2 protein.

Patient 12 is unique among the 19 summarized in Table 14–8 in that an abnormally large β precursor was identified in the patient's cells.[167, 176] The protein

TABLE 14–8. β_2 SUBUNIT (CD18) MUTATIONS IN LEUKOCYTE ADHESION DEFICIENCY

PATIENT	MUTATION TYPE*	mRNA LEVELS	PROTEIN EXPRESSION		CLINICAL SEVERITY	MUTATIONS IDENTIFIED*		REFERENCES
			β Precursor	α/β Dimer		Nucleotide†	Amino Acid Change‡	
1–3	NR	0	0	0	Severe	Not reported		167, 176
4–7	NR	Low	0–Trace	0–Low	Moderate	Not reported		167, 176
8–11	Splice/deletion (homozygous)	Normal	Abnormally small	Low	Moderate	g → c at position 3 of 5′ splice site of intron following exon containing nt 1066–1155, causing 90 nt deletion in 97% of mRNA	30 AA deletion (residues 332–361)	167, 176, 177
12	NR	Normal	Abnormally large	0	Severe	Not identified; appears to cause an extra N-glycosylation site		167, 176
13	1. Missense 2. NR	Normal	Normal	0	Severe	1. G-577 → A 2. Not identified (? homozygous)	1. Gly 169 → Arg 2. Not expressed	178
14	1. Missense 2. Missense	Normal	Normal	10–20%	Moderate	1. A-659 → C 2. C-1849 → T	1. Lys 196 → Thr 2. Arg 593 → Cys	179
15	1. Missense 2. NR	Normal	Normal	Low	Moderate	1. T-517 → C 2. Not identified (probably after nt 965)	1. Leu 149 → Pro 2. Not identified	178
16	1a. Splice/ insertion	Normal	Normal	10–20%	Moderate	1a. C → a in intron 6 forming aberrant splice site and insertion of 12 nt after nt 813	1a. In-frame insertion of PSSQ after Pro 247	63
	1b. Missense					1b. C-1828 → T (? polymorphism)	1b. Arg 586 → Trp	
	2. Missense					2. A-1124 → G	2. Asn 351 → Ser	
17	1. Missense	Low	Low	9%	Moderate	1. T-74 → A (initiation codon)	1. Delete Met-1; low-level initiation at codon 2 (Leu)	180
	2. Deletion					2. Deletion T-2142	2. Frameshift with premature stop codon predicting loss of last 56 AA	
18	1. Deletion	NR	NR	0	Severe	1. Deletion T-2142	1. Frameshift with premature stop codon predicting loss of last 56AA	180
	2. NR					2. Not identified	2. Not identified	
19	1. Missense 2. Deletion	Normal	NR	NR	NR	1. C-605 → T 2. Deletion nt 1729–1959	1. Pro 170 → Leu 2. Loss of 78AA (residues 553–630) and then frameshift	181

*The two alleles are indicated by numbers 1 and 2.
†Nucleotides are numbered according to Kishimoto and colleagues, beginning with the 5′ end of the β_2 subunits cDNA.[51]
‡Predicated from nucleotide change.
0 = Undetectable level; AA = amino acid; NR = not reported.

appeared to be excessively glycosylated, and a mutant extra N-glycosylation site was hypothesized. The abnormal β' subunit does not associate with the α' subunit, leading to an absence of β_2 integrins and a severe clinical phenotype.

Patient 13 represents an example of a CD18 missense mutation leading to severe disease.[178] An A → G substitution at nucleotide 577 predicts the incorporation of arginine instead of glycine at amino acid residue 169 (see Table 14–8). COS cells transfected with the mutant β cDNA were found to contain a β precursor of normal size and stability, suggesting that the absence of mature α-β dimers in the patient's leukocytes was due to a disruption of a β' site critical for association with the α' subunits. As shown in Figure 14–3, this missense mutation is present in one of the extracellular domains that is highly conserved among the integrin β subunits. In contrast to patient 13, patient 14 (a compound heterozygote) has at least one missense mutation that permits low-level expression of the β_2 integrin proteins (see Table 14–8).[178, 179] One of the mutations (Lys 196 → Thr) lies in the conserved region affected in the previously discussed patients, whereas the other (Arg 593 → Cys) is in the fourth cysteine-rich repeat, a domain that is also highly conserved among the integrin β subunits (see Fig. 14–3). Transfection experiments with COS cells indicated that the β precursors encoded by both mutant alleles were normal in amount and size. This finding suggests that the mutations affect regions in β' required for association with α′ subunits. At least one of the mutations, however, must not completely disrupt α′-β′ interactions, since the patient's neutrophils expressed 10 to 20 per cent of normal levels of β_2 integrins (see Table 14–8). Patients 15 and 16 are also compound heterozygotes with moderate clinical phenotypes who have missense and splice mutations affecting the highly conserved extracellular domain nearest the N-terminus of CD18 (see Table 14–8 and Fig. 14–3).[63, 178]

The only CD18 mutation that has thus far been seen in unrelated LAD patients is a deletion of T-2142 (see Table 14–8, patients 17 and 18). It results in a frameshift that predicts a premature stop codon and the formation of a truncated β_2 subunit lacking the last 56 amino acids that normally constitute the cytosolic domain of the protein (see Fig. 14–3). As might be expected, this mutation results in the severe clinical phenotype with undetectable levels of β_2 integrin.[180] In patient 17, the allele not containing the T-2142 deletion has an abnormality in the initiation codon (T-74 → A). It is of interest that this patient has a moderate clinical phenotype with the expression of approximately 9 per cent of normal levels of the α-β dimer. Since the T-2142 mutation results in failure to express β_2 integrins (based on patient 18 in Table 14–8), it appears that the moderate phenotype in patient 17 is due to low-level translation of the CD18 mRNA with initiation of protein synthesis at the second codon.[180]

Functional Consequences of Mutations in CD18

Phagocytes from patients with LAD synthesize normal leukocyte integrin α subunit precursor (α_L', α_M', and α_X'). In the absence of a normal β_2 subunit precursor (β_2'), the α′ chains do not associate into normal α′-β′ complexes and are not expressed on the cell surface. In some patients, the β_2 precursor protein is either undetectable (patients 1 to 3 in Table 14–8) or synthesized in a mutant form that is unable to associate with the three α subunits (patient 13). In both situations, β_2 integrin expression on leukocytes is undetectable, and the clinical symptoms are severe. In other cases, the β_2 precursor protein is made either in low levels (patients 8 to 11 and 17) or in a mutant form that can still undergo some association with the three α subunit precursors (patients 14, 15, and 16). If the level of surface expression of the β_2 integrins exceeds approximately 2.5 per cent of normal, then the patients exhibit a more moderate clinical picture.

The diminished or absent expression of all three β_2 integrins in LAD leukocytes results in a series of severe abnormalities in adhesion-dependent functions in vivo and in vitro (Table 14–9). One of the most striking abnormalities in LAD is the failure of phagocytes to emigrate from the blood stream to sites of inflammation in the tissue. The observation that allogeneic leukocytes transfused into patients with LAD accumulate at sites of infection indicates that the defect resides in the leukocyte.[173] The early stages of phagocyte binding to the endothelium, processes mediated by selectins and their counterreceptors, occur normally in LAD. It is the tight adherence of neutrophils and monocytes to cytokine-activated endothelium that is severely defective in LAD, since these interactions are mediated by the β_2 integrins. Transendothelial migration is also severely impaired in these patients, since it, too, depends on normal β_2 integrin expression.[14] These phenomena can be reproduced in vitro using endothelial cell monolayers (see Table 14–9). Prior to stimulation, LAD neutrophils adhere normally to the cultured endothelium. Following stimulation, however, the patient's cells fail to undergo the dramatic increase in tight adherence that is seen with normal neutrophils.[14] The persistent granulocytosis seen in LAD is likely due to this abnormality in integrin-mediated adherence to endothelial cells. It is interesting that patients with LAD have a normal "marginated" pool of granulocytes—that is, those cells that are not in the circulating pool but that are rapidly released during stress or following the administration of epinephrine. It appears that the marginated pool represents granulocytes transiently sequestered in pulmonary capillary beds and that this subset of neutrophils is normal in LAD.[182]

The other major functional defect in LAD is the failure of neutrophils and monocytes to interact normally with C3bi-opsonized particles. Mac-1 is the major receptor for C3bi (see Table 14–6). Microbes that are primarily opsonized with C3bi bind poorly to LAD neutrophils and monocytes, are not ingested, and fail to trigger degranulation and the respiratory burst (see Table 14–9).[60, 168, 169, 171, 183] LAD phagocytes, however, do not have an intrinsic defect in either of these critical cellular functions. Following exposure to other types of stimuli, such as phorbol myristate acetate, they degranulate normally and undergo a vigorous respiratory burst. Moreover, LAD phagocytes can recognize and ingest particles opsonized with IgG and C3b, since the receptors for these opsonins are expressed normally. This redundancy in the mechanisms used to recognize microbes probably lessens the clinical impact of not having a receptor for C3bi. This is evidenced in in vitro bacterial killing assays, in which LAD neutrophils have been found to kill serum-opsonized Staphylococcus aureus normally.[168, 173, 184] Nonetheless, microbes that are primarily recognized via C3bi in vivo would be expected to be problematical in LAD.

Neutrophil-mediated antibody-dependent cellular cytotoxicity (ADCC) is abnormal in LAD. For example, the number of herpes simplex virus–infected ^{51}Cr-labeled Chang liver target cells killed by neutrophils from patients with severe LAD was only 20 per cent of normal.[168] This defect in ADCC appears to be causally related to defective neutrophil–target cell binding that is normally mediated by the three β_2 integrins (see Table 14–9).

Defects in lymphocyte functions dependent on LFA-1 have been observed in many patients with LAD in vitro (see Table 14–9). Proliferative responses, T-

TABLE 14–9. LEUKOCYTE FUNCTION IN LEUKOCYTE ADHESION DEFICIENCY

FUNCTION	LEVEL OF FUNCTION	β_2 INTEGRIN RESPONSIBLE FOR FUNCTION
Neutrophils/Monocytes (in vitro)		
Adherence/spreading/chemotaxis		
Glass	↓	CD11a, b, c
Endothelium	↓	CD11b, CD11a
Endothelium (cytokine-activated)	↓	CD11a, b, c
Aggregation	↓	CD11a, b
Phagocytosis		
IgG-opsonized	N	(Fc receptors)
C3-opsonized	↓	CD11b
Degranulation		
Soluble stimuli (FMLP, PMA)	N	(FMLP receptor; PMA bypasses β_2 integrins)
C3-opsonized	↓	CD11b
Respiratory burst O_2^- production)		
Soluble stimuli (FMLP, PMA)	N	(FMLP receptor; PMA bypasses β_2 integrins)
C3-opsonized	↓	CD11b
Bacterial killing	N	(Fc receptors; CR1)
ADCC	↓	CD11a, b, c
Lymphocytes (in vitro)*		
Antigen/mitogen–induced proliferation	↓	CD11a
Cytotoxic T-cell function	↓	CD11a
NK function	↓	CD11a, b, c
ADCC	↓	CD11a
Adherence to cytokine-activated endothelium	N	(possibly β_1 integrin VLA-4)

*These in vitro defects are not generally manifested in vivo, as patients with LAD exhibit normal production of specific antibodies and undergo normal delayed cutaneous hypersensitivity reactions.
ADCC = Antibody-dependent cellular cytotoxicity; FMLP = N-formyl peptide; N = normal; ↓ = decreased function; PMA = phorbol myristate acetate.
Data from references 60, 165, 169, 171, 172, 183, 186, and 392.

lymphocyte–mediated killing, natural killing, and antibody-dependent killing by the patient's lymphocytes have all been found to be defective.[185–189] In one report, severe hypoplasia of lymphoid tissues was observed in two siblings with LAD, suggesting that lymphocyte homing to the thymus, lymph nodes, and spleen may be defective.[190] Despite these histological and functional abnormalities, most patients with LAD have relatively few problems with lymphocyte function in vivo. They exhibit normal delayed cutaneous hypersensitivity reactions and are not unusually susceptible to viral infections. It has been observed, however, that these patients do not respond well to repeated vaccinations with new antigens such as tetanus and poliovirus.[165, 168, 190]

Animal Models of Leukocyte Adhesion Deficiency

A syndrome resembling LAD has been identified in both dogs[191, 192] and Holstein cattle.[193–195] The canine form was first characterized in a female Irish setter that was born of a mother-son mating and suffered from recurrent bacterial infections, persistent granulocytosis, impaired formation of pus, and delayed wound healing.[192] Neutrophils from the affected dog were found to have undetectable levels of CD11b and CD18 and failed to adhere normally to glass and plastic surfaces. In young Holstein calves, the disorder presents as recurrent pneumonia, ulcerative stomatitis, periodontitis, delayed wound healing, and persistent granulocytosis.[193–195] It is interesting that all of the affected calves studied to date can be traced to a common sire and appear to have inherited the disorder in an autosomal recessive manner.[194] Their neutrophils have greatly diminished expression of the α and β subunits of the β_2 integrins (approximately 2 per cent of normal).

Diagnosis and Treatment

The diagnosis of LAD should be suspected in any infant or child who presents with unusually severe bacterial infections accompanied by a striking granulocytosis. Although this clinical picture may simply represent a leukemoid reaction in an otherwise immunologically normal infant, the diagnosis of LAD should nonetheless be considered, especially if there is a relative absence of neutrophils at the affected sites or if there has been delayed separation of the umbilical cord. The diagnosis of LAD can be made by demonstrating a severe deficiency of the β_2 subunit on neutrophils and other leukocytes. This is best accomplished by flow cytometry using commercially available monoclonal antibodies to CD18 (see Table 14–4). Alternatively, monoclonal antibodies to CD11a, CD11b, or CD11c can be used to demonstrate a deficiency in any one of the α subunits. In vitro assays of phagocyte function can be used to confirm the diagnosis of LAD. As discussed above, LAD neutrophils show striking defects in adherence; chemotaxis; ADCC; and C3bi-mediated ingestion, degranulation, and respiratory burst activation. Carriers of LAD can be identified by flow cytometry, since their leukocytes express β_2 integrins at levels that are approximately 50 per cent of normal.[168] Prenatal diagnosis of LAD can be made by one of two methods. In those families in which the mutations in the two CD18 alleles are known, chorionic villus or amniocyte DNA can be analyzed for the presence of the mutations. In the absence of knowing the family-specific mutations, fetal blood granulocytes can be assayed for the expression of β_2 integrins, using flow cytometry.[167, 196]

The treatment of LAD is largely dictated by the clinical severity of the disease. In one review of 46 patients with LAD, 22 exhibited an exceptionally severe phenotype characterized by aggressive bacterial infections and the high probability of death by the age of 2 years (6 of the 22 patients).[167] The remaining 24 patients had a more moderate phenotype in which bacterial infections were less frequent and usually less severe. Death during the first decade of life was uncommon in this latter group, although 75 per cent of the patients died between the ages of 12 and 32 years.[167] As discussed above, the level of expression of the β_2 integrins on neutrophils can be used to predict the clinical course. Patients with the severe phenotype have β_2 integrin levels less than 2 per cent of normal (often in the 0 to 0.3 per cent range), whereas those with the moderate form of LAD express β_2, α_M, and α_X at levels 2.5 to 10 per cent of normal.[60, 165, 167–169] Given the grim prognosis in severe LAD, bone marrow transplantation is recommended for these patients. In a series of six patients who received transplants in Paris, 2 of 3 human leukocyte antigen (HLA)–matched and 3 of 3 mismatched transplants were successful.[167, 189, 197] In the one unsuccessful transplantation, the patient died of chronic graft-versus-host disease following engraftment of the donor myeloid cells. A heavy conditioning regimen is apparently required in LAD to ablate hyperactive myeloid elements in the recipient bone marrow.[167, 198] In each of the three HLA–non-identical transplants, the donor marrow was depleted of T cells and the recipient was treated with a 60-day course of cyclosporin A.[197] It is interesting that all three of the patients who received mismatched transplants have done well with immunosuppressive therapy 19 to 57 months after transplantation, without evidence of graft rejection. It appears that patients severely deficient in LFA-1 readily accept HLA-mismatched bone marrow, possibly because the LFA-1–deficient lymphocytes are unable to bind and kill the HLA-incompatible cells. The management of severe LAD prior to bone marrow transplant (or in those patients who do not have a suitable donor) requires the aggressive, and often anticipatory, use of parenteral antibiotics. Granulocyte transfusions may also be helpful in some cases, although their long-term use is limited because of the development of alloantibodies. Prophylactic antibiotics, such as trimethoprim-sulfamethoxasole, may also be helpful in preventing infections or in slowing their progression. Particular attention must be paid to the severe gingival and periodontal disease observed in all patients with LAD, regardless of whether they have a severe or moderate phenotype.[165] In contrast to the situation in severe LAD, guidelines for bone marrow transplantation in moderately severe LAD have not been established, since conservative medical management results in substantially longer survival in this subset of patients with LAD.

Because LAD is caused by a defect in a unique gene, it is possible that the introduction of a normal CD18 gene into a patient's hematopoietic stem cells could correct the defect. Moreover, complete gene reconstitution may not be necessary to achieve substantial clinical benefits. As discussed above, patients who have residual β_2 integrin expression (5 to 10 per cent of normal) have a much milder clinical phenotype. Therefore, if transfected myeloid cells from patients with severe LAD could express even low levels of β_2 integrins, clinical improvement might be appreciable. Moreover, results of allogeneic bone marrow transplants indicate that partial engraftment (7 to 34 per cent of donor cells) is associated with dramatic clinical improvement. The technical feasibility of gene replacement therapy in LAD has now been demonstrated by several groups.[175, 199, 200] In these experiments, EBV-transformed B-lymphocyte cell lines from patients with LAD were transfected with normal CD18 cDNA, using retroviruses or an EBV-based vector. In two of the reports, normal quantities of CD11a (α_L) and CD18 were expressed on the cell surface of the lymphocytes, and LFA-1–dependent functions were fully reconstituted.[175, 200] One of the major obstacles standing between these exciting results and the eventual use of gene replacement therapy for LAD is the development of techniques for retrovirus-mediated gene transfer into human hematopoietic stem cells.

OTHER DISORDERS OF LEUKOCYTE ADHESION

Neutrophil Actin Dysfunction

In 1974, Boxer and colleagues described a clinically severe disorder in a male infant who suffered from recurrent vesicular skin lesions infected with *Staphylococcus aureus* and a cutaneous-cecal fistula complicated by *Streptococcus faecalis* sepsis.[201] The sites of infection were unusual in that they healed slowly and were devoid of neutrophils despite a marked granulocytosis. The patient's neutrophils showed markedly diminished chemotaxis in vitro and a decreased capacity to ingest serum-opsonized particles. The underlying defect appeared to involve neutrophil actin, as it was found to polymerize abnormally in the presence of 0.6 M potassium chloride. This finding suggested that the chemotactic defect was due to a qualitative abnormality in the actin or some actin-associated protein, a hypothesis supported by the finding that neutrophils from the patient's father, mother, and sister had actin that polymerized half as well as did that from controls.[202] The disorder was therefore termed *neutrophil actin dysfunction* (NAD). The clinical and laboratory similarities between the patient with NAD and those subsequently described with LAD raised the possibility that the two disorders might be related. Unfortunately, the NAD patient succumbed to infection shortly after a bone marrow transplant (the marrow from a histocompatible sibling did engraft[198]). Neutrophils from the surviving family members were analyzed for β_2 integrin expression and were found to have intermediate levels of Mac-1 (CD11b/CD18), suggesting that they were heterozygote carriers of LAD.[203] The relationship between NAD and LAD was complicated, however, by the finding that not all patients with LAD had an abnormality in actin polymerization. Neutrophils from seven LAD patients (two with severe disease and five with the moderate phenotype) were all found to have normal actin filament assembly.[171, 203] On the basis of the currently available evidence, it appears that NAD represents a special subset of LAD. As discussed above, there is good evidence that the cytoplasmic domains of the integrin α and β chains associate with cytoskeletal proteins such as talin, vinculin, and α-actinin.[48, 66, 67] In light of the heterogeneity of the mutations that have been identified in LAD (see Table 14–8 and Fig. 14–3), it is possible that only certain types of mutations lead to an associated defect in actin function, such as those that affect the cytoplasmic domain of CD18.

Leukocyte Adhesion Deficiency Due to a Deficiency in Sialyl–Lewis X (LADII)

A clinical syndrome closely related to LAD, but caused by a defect in selectin-mediated adhesion events, has recently been described in two unrelated boys of Moslem Arab origin and has been termed *LADII*.[43] The patients were offspring of consanguineous matings, suggesting that the defect was inherited in an autosomal recessive manner. As in LAD, the two children suffered from recurrent episodes of bacterial infections, periodontitis, otitis media, and cellulitis without infiltration of neutrophils despite blood granulocyte counts between 60,000 and 150,000/mm³. Unique clinical features included short stature, severe mental retardation, and the Bombay (hh) blood phenotype. Neutrophils from the patients exhibited markedly diminished chemotaxis in vitro (10 per cent of control) toward zymosan-activated serum and an *E. coli* bacterial filtrate. Unlike patients with LAD, however, their neutrophils had normal levels of CD18 and were able to phagocytize serum-opsonized particles.

The finding that the erythrocytes of the two unrelated patients not only exhibited the rare Bombay phenotype but also were secretor negative and Lewis antigen negative suggested that the synthesis of carbohydrate structures containing fucose was defective. The Bombay and non-secretor phenotypes are caused by the deficient formation of Fucα1 $\rightarrow$ 2 Gal linkages in the ABO blood group core antigens, whereas the absence of Lewis antigens is due to the failure to synthesize Fucα1 $\rightarrow$ 4 GlcNAc and Fucα1 $\rightarrow$ 3 GlcNAc carbohydrate structures. It was therefore hypothesized that the patients might not express Sialyl–Lewis X (which also contains fucose, as discussed above), the ligand recognized by E-selectin and P-selectin. As predicted, neutrophils from both boys were devoid of immunoreactive Sialyl–Lewis X structures and were unable to adhere to human umbilical cord endothelial cells activated with IL-1β to induce E-selectin expression. Thus, the failure of LADII neutrophils to migrate to sites of inflammation in vivo appears to be caused by a loss of selectin-mediated binding due to the absence of Sialyl–Lewis X structures on the neutrophil selectin counterreceptors. Since the patients exhibit deficiencies in multiple fucosylated carbohydrates that depend on distinct fucosyl transferase genes, it is likely that they suffer from some fundamental defect in fucose metabolism.

MICROBICIDAL PATHWAYS IN PHAGOCYTES

Once localized by the phagocyte, the microbial invader is destroyed by a combination of oxidative and non-oxidative mechanisms. The existence of multiple microbicidal pathways is not surprising, given the crucial importance of this aspect of host defense. The basic features of these pathways and associated genetic disorders are summarized in this section. The two following sections then focus in detail on the respiratory burst oxidase and inherited defects in CGD.

Oxygen-Dependent Mechanisms

The unstimulated neutrophil relies primarily on glycolysis for energy and hence consumes relatively little oxygen.[204] Within seconds after contacting appropriately opsonized microorganisms or certain soluble factors, oxygen consumption increases dramatically, often by more than 100-fold. This phenomenon, referred to as the "respiratory burst," represents the non-mitochondrial conversion of oxygen to the radical O_2^- by the transfer of a single electron from NADPH (Fig. 14–5, Reaction 1).[204, 205] This reaction and related pathways are summarized in Figure 14–5.

The production of O_2^- is mediated by a phagocyte-specific NADPH oxidase, also referred to as the respiratory burst oxidase, that is associated with the plasma membrane and phagocytic vacuoles.[206] As detailed in the following section, the active oxidase complex is formed by both cytosolic and membrane proteins and includes a flavoprotein and a *b*-type cytochrome serving as electron carriers.[205, 207, 208] Superoxide, although not an important microbicidal agent by itself, is the precursor to a family of potent oxidants.[204, 205] The O_2^- radical is first converted, either spontaneously or by means of superoxide dismutase, into H_2O_2 (Reaction 2 in Fig. 14–5). Myeloperoxidase (MPO), in the presence of halides, catalyzes the conversion of H_2O_2 to HOCl (Reaction 4 in Fig. 14–5).

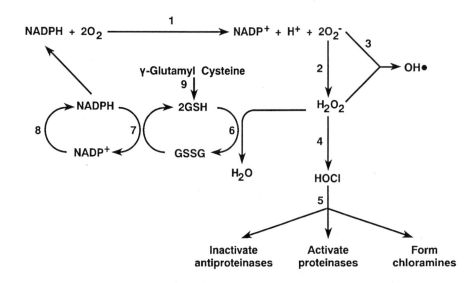

FIGURE 14–5. Reactions of the respiratory burst pathway. The enzymes responsible for Reactions 1 to 9 are as follows: (1) the respiratory burst oxidase (NADPH oxidase); (2) superoxide dismutase or spontaneous; (3) non-enzymatic, Fe^{2+}-catalyzed; (4) myeloperoxidase; (5) spontaneous; (6) glutathione peroxidase; (7) glutathione reductase; (8) glucose-6-phosphate dehydrogenase; (9) glutathione synthetase. (Adapted from Curnutte, J. T.: Disorders of phagocyte function. *In* Hoffman, R., Benz, E. J., Jr., Shattil, S. J., Furie, B., and Cohen, H. J. [eds.]: Hematology: Basic Principles and Practice. New York, Churchill Livingstone, 1991, pp. 571–589; with permission.)

Hydrogen peroxide may also be converted into the hydroxyl radical (OH•) in a non-enzymatic reaction with O_2^- catalyzed by either iron or copper ions (Reaction 3 in Fig. 14–5).[209] Hydrogen peroxide, HOCl, and OH• are all strong oxidants[210] that are important for effective microbial killing within the phagocytic vacuole. In addition, reactive oxidants modulate phagocyte proteolytic activity by activating latent phagocyte metalloproteinases (such as collagenase and gelatinase) and inactivating plasma antiproteinases.[1] Enhanced phagocyte proteolysis at localized sites may be important for facilitating cellular migration from the blood stream into tissues, removal of cellular debris, and destruction of microbes.

Other enzymatic pathways related to the production of oxidants include the detoxification of excess H_2O_2 by glutathione peroxidase and reductase (Reactions 6 and 7, Fig. 14–5).[204, 210] Glutathione is produced from γ-glutamyl cysteine by the enzyme glutathione synthetase (Reaction 9, Fig. 14–5). Other important antioxidant systems present in phagocytes and other tissues include catalase, which catalyzes the conversion of H_2O_2 into oxygen and water; ascorbic acid; and α-tocopherol (vitamin E).[210] The generation of NADPH is important in providing a source of reducing equivalents for the glutathione detoxification pathway as well as the respiratory burst oxidase itself. NADPH is replenished from $NADP^+$ by the action of leukocyte glucose-6-phosphate dehydrogenase (G6PD; Reaction 8, Fig. 14–5) in the hexose monophosphate shunt.

Oxygen-Independent Mechanisms

Oxidant-mediated destruction by phagocytes is supplemented by non-oxidative antimicrobial systems.[161, 162, 211] In addition to providing another avenue of attack, oxygen-independent mechanisms enable effective killing under the adverse conditions of hypoxia and acidosis often encountered locally at the site of infection. Neutrophils store an array of degradative enzymes and antimicrobial proteins within both the primary (azurophil) and the secondary (specific) granules.[161] The best characterized "antibiotic" proteins are listed in Table 14–10.[212] Lysozyme hydrolyzes the cell wall of saprophytic gram-positive organisms and may also assist in the non-lytic killing of other microbes. The iron-binding glycoprotein lactoferrin has bactericidal properties both related and unrelated to the chelation of iron compounds required for bacterial metabolism. In addition, lactoferrin may participate in the non-enzymatic formation of OH• radicals during the respiratory burst (Reaction 3, Fig. 14–5).[213] BPI, cathepsin G, and the defensins[162] are an important group of microbicidal polypeptides localized to azurophilic granules. These cationic, amphipathic proteins

TABLE 14–10. NEUTROPHIL GRANULE MICROBICIDES

NEUTROPHIL ANTIMICROBIAL GRANULE COMPONENTS	MOLECULAR WEIGHT (kDa)	LOCATION	CONCENTRATION IN NEUTROPHILS ($\mu g/10^6$ cells)
Lysozyme	14.4	Azurophil and specific granules	3
Lactoferrin	80	Specific granules	2–6
Bactericidal- and permeability-increasing factor	58	Azurophil granules	<1
Cathepsin G	25–29	Azurophil granules	1–2
Defensins	3.6–4.0	Azurophil granules	4–6

Reproduced, with permission, from Lehrer, R. I., Ganz, T., Selsted, M. E., Babior, B. M., and Curnutte, J. T.: Neutrophils and host defense. Ann. Intern. Med. 1988; 109:127–141.

kill susceptible bacteria, fungi, and viruses by damaging microbial cytoplasmic membranes.[211]

Regulation of Antimicrobial Activity

Although critical for effective killing of pathogens, the toxic antimicrobial molecules produced by phagocytic cells have the potential for causing damage to normal tissues.[214] The cellular release of microbicidal products is therefore coupled to specific receptor-mediated events and is largely confined to protected intracellular compartments.

The respiratory burst oxidase is quiescent in the resting phagocyte. Oxidase activation involves the translocation of a complex of cytosolic proteins to the plasma membrane, with the latter containing the redox carriers cytochrome b and flavin adenine dinucleotide (FAD)[207, 208] (see next section). The physical separation of various oxidase components in the resting cell may be an important "fail-safe" means of preventing inappropriate oxidase activity. As discussed above, oxidase assembly can be triggered by receptor-mediated binding of many soluble chemotactic agents, such as N-formylated peptides, IL-8, and C5 complement fragments.[111] Note that stimulation of the respiratory burst requires higher concentrations of these molecules compared with initiation of chemotaxis. The binding of opsonized microorganisms to phagocyte Fcγ[151] and C3bi[44, 169] receptors is another major physiological trigger of the respiratory burst that can be activated at localized sites of microbial contact.[215] As detailed in a previous section, receptor-mediated signal transduction in phagocytes is accomplished by a molecular cascade of second messengers, including inositol phosphates, PA, DAG, intracellular calcium, and activated protein kinases.[216] Many aspects of phagocyte function, such as cell movement and degranulation, are regulated by these pathways. The specific molecules that interface these common signals with activation of the respiratory burst oxidase have not been clearly defined.

Another means by which phagocyte antimicrobial products are restricted to sites of infection or inflammation depends on localization to specific cellular compartments. Degradative lysosomal enzymes and antibiotic peptides are sequestered within azurophil granules until phagocytosis triggers degranulation. The contents of the azurophil granules are incorporated into the phagocytic vacuole, with little actually released into the extracellular space.[161, 211] The activated oxidase, assembled in the plasma membrane, is also incorporated into phagolysosomes during ingestion. Since release of O_2^- occurs largely at the extracellular side of the membrane[205, 206] (but see also reference 217), oxidants are restricted to the extracellular space at sites of microbial contact or within the phagocytic vacuole. Indeed, the interaction of granule contents and respiratory burst products within the phagosome potentiates their microbicidal effects. For example, azurophil granules provide myeloperoxidase

for catalysis of HOCl production.[218] The degranulation and membrane fusion of specific granules, which contain the majority of cytochrome b in the neutrophil,[160] may contribute to a sustained respiratory burst.

Genetic Defects in Phagocyte Antimicrobial Pathways

Myeloperoxidase deficiency is the most common inherited disorder of phagocytes, with complete deficiency seen in approximately 1 in 4000 individuals and partial deficiency in approximately 1 in 2000 (reviewed in reference 218). The MPO gene is located on chromosome 17 at q22–23, and a variety of specific gene defects associated with MPO deficiency are now being identified.[219, 220] Despite the pivotal role of MPO in the production of HOCl, affected persons are notable for the lack of symptoms. In vitro neutrophil killing is slower than normal, but eventually complete.[218] A more active and sustained respiratory burst, coupled with the toxic effects of other oxidants and non-oxidative killing mechanisms, may account for the lack of clinical manifestations in the majority of cases of MPO deficiency. Disseminated fungal infections, however, have been described in patients who suffer from both MPO deficiency and diabetes mellitus.

Chronic granulomatous disease occurs at a frequency of approximately 1 in 500,000 to 1,000,000[204] and is characterized by the deficient production of O_2^-. This disorder results from inherited defects in any of four different genes that encode components of the respiratory burst oxidase[207, 208] and is discussed in detail in the following section. The very rare condition of severe X-linked G6PD deficiency, in which extremely low steady-state levels of NADPH are associated with hemolytic anemia even in the absence of redox stress, exhibits a similar clinical pattern because NADPH is the required substrate for the respiratory burst oxidase.[204] It is distinguished by the presence of very low levels of G6PD and congenital hemolytic anemia. A few cases of autosomal recessive inheritance of severe deficiencies in glutathione reductase or glutathione synthetase that can be associated with a CGD-like syndrome have been reported[221, 222] (see Fig. 14–5). The oxidase can be activated in the absence of glutathione but is soon damaged by oxidants, resulting in premature termination of the respiratory burst.[223]

Two inherited disorders of granule function that affect primarily non-oxidative killing have also been described. Chédiak-Higashi syndrome is an uncommon autosomal recessive disorder characterized by giant cytoplasmic granules in multiple tissues and cells throughout the body.[161, 224–227] The abnormal granules are associated with defects in phagocyte and platelet function, and partial oculocutaneous albinism results from uneven pigment distribution by giant melanosomes. The underlying etiology is unknown but may be related to abnormal granule morphogenesis. A variety of functional neutrophil defects have been noted in this disorder and contribute to an enhanced susceptibility to bacterial infections of the skin, mucous membranes, and respiratory tract. These include abnormal adherence and chemotaxis, delayed degranulation, and slow killing of ingested microorganisms. Specific granule deficiency is another exceedingly rare disorder affecting phagocyte granule function and has been described in only five patients.[161, 228] It is presumed to be autosomal recessive, and the underlying gene or genes involved are unknown. Affected patients have suffered from recurrent infections, primarily involving the skin and lungs. Normal-appearing specific granules are absent, and deficiencies in proteins of both azurophil (defensins) and specific granules (lactoferrin, cobalamin-binding protein, gelatinase) have been observed.[227, 229, 230] The underlying defect may be specific to the regulation of granule protein synthesis in the myeloid lineage, as lactoferrin was secreted normally in glandular epithelium in these patients.[230] Circulating neutrophils commonly have bilobed nuclei similar to those seen in the Pelger-Huët anomaly; how this relates to granule defects is unknown.

THE RESPIRATORY BURST OXIDASE

Overview

The "extra respiration of phagocytosis" was first observed in 1933,[231] but not until more than 20 years later was it appreciated that this process was insensitive to mitochondrial poisons and hence not directly related to increased energy demands.[232] Subsequent enzymological studies established that what is now referred to as the NADPH or respiratory burst oxidase is associated with the plasma and phagolysosomal membranes and catalyzes the transfer of an electron from NADPH to molecular oxygen, thereby forming O_2^-.[204, 233, 234] As described in the preceding section, O_2^- is the precursor to a family of toxic oxidants important for efficient microbial killing. The importance of this pathway to normal host defense was underscored by the discovery that phagocytes obtained from patients with "fatal granulomatosus of childhood" (CGD), first described in 1956,[235, 236] lack detectable respiratory burst oxidase activity.[237, 238] In the initial reports of CGD, affected patients were males who appeared to inherit the disorder in an X-linked recessive manner. Subsequently, females with an identical clinical syndrome and pedigree consistent with autosomal recessive inheritance were described.[204, 239] That at least three different gene products were required for intact oxidase function was elegantly demonstrated by the functional analysis of monocyte heterokaryons derived from different patients with CGD.[240, 241] This genetic heterogeneity hinted at the complexity of the active oxidase, which was originally viewed as a single "enzyme."

A series of rapid advances in the past several years has now led to a clearer picture of the respiratory burst oxidase as a complex of membrane-bound and soluble proteins. These resulted from a remarkable convergence of biochemical and molecular genetic approaches, both benefiting greatly from the analysis of patients with CGD. Four polypeptides that are essential for respiratory burst function have now been identified and their cDNAs cloned. Mutations in the corresponding genes are responsible for the four different genetic subgroups of CGD now recognized. The oxidase subunit proteins have been given the designation "phox" (abbreviated from phagocyte oxidase) and are referred to by the apparent molecular mass of the component (in kilodaltons) and a letter indicating whether it is a protein (p) or glycoprotein (gp). The properties of the four established oxidase components are summarized in Table 14–11 and reviewed in detail in the following portions of this section.[208] A phagocyte-specific b-type cytochrome heteromer, formed by the gp91-phox and p22-phox polypeptides,[242, 243] is located in the plasma and specific granule membranes and is the terminal electron carrier of the oxidase.[205, 206] Two other oxidase components, p47-phox and p67-phox,[244-246] are located in the cytosol of unstimulated cells but translocate to the membrane upon oxidase activation.[247, 248] A flavin-binding protein, believed to be the initial electron acceptor in the transport of electrons from NADPH to oxygen,[206, 249, 250] remains uncharacterized. Two recent reports suggest that the FAD redox center may actually be part of cytochrome b.[251, 252] The regulation of oxidase assembly by receptor-ligand–initiated intracellular second messengers is also poorly defined but may involve low molecular weight G proteins.[253-256]

Cytochrome b

An unusual low-potential b-type cytochrome was first described in horse neutrophils[205, 257] and subsequently identified in membranes of human neutrophils, monocytes, macrophages, and eosinophils.[258, 259] Because the wavelength of the α band of light absorption is at 558 nm, this cytochrome has often been referred to as cytochrome b_{558}. It has also been called cytochrome b_{-245}, in reference to its midpoint potential of −245 mV, which is the lowest reported for any mammalian cytochrome.[206, 260] Its redox properties suggested that this cytochrome might be the terminal electron carrier in respiratory burst oxidase, according to the following scheme[205]:

$$NADPH \rightarrow flavoprotein \rightarrow cytochrome\ b \rightarrow O_2 \rightarrow O_2^-$$
$$-330\ mV \quad -256\ mV \quad -245\ mV \quad -160\ mV$$

Further suspicion that cytochrome b might be a component of the respiratory burst oxidase resulted from the discovery that its characteristic heme spectrum was absent in neutrophils obtained from patients with X-linked CGD, whereas normal levels were detected in those with the autosomal recessive disease.[261] However, a few patients with X-linked CGD had detectable neutrophil cytochrome b,[204, 262] and certain autosomal recessive patients did not.[241, 263, 264] Furthermore, ad-

TABLE 14–11. PROPERTIES OF THE PHAGOCYTE RESPIRATORY BURST OXIDASE (phox) COMPONENTS

PROPERTY	gp91-phox	p22-phox	p47-phox	p67-phox
Synonyms	β chain Heavy chain	α chain Light chain	NCF-1 SOC II C4	NCF-2 SOC III C2
Amino acids	570	195	390	526

Molecular weight (kDa)
  Predicted
  As seen by PAGE
  Glycosylation
  Phosphorylation
	65.0
	91
	Yes (N-linked)
	No
		20.9
		22
		No
		No
			44.6
			47
			No
			Yes
				60.9
				67
				No
				No*

pI	9.7	10.0	9.5	5.8
mRNA	4.7 kb	0.8 kb	1.4 kb	2.4 kb
Gene locus	CYBB Xp21.1	CYBA 16q24	NCF1 7q11.23	NCF2 1q25
Exons/span	13/30 kb	6/8.5 kb	9/18 kb	16/37 kb
Cellular location in resting neutrophil	Specific granule membrane Plasma membrane	Specific granule membrane Plasma membrane	Cytosol Cytoskeleton	Cytosol Cytoskeleton
Level in neutrophil (pmol/10^6 cells)	3.3–5.3	3.3–5.3	3.3	1.2
Tissue specificity	Myeloid, B lymphocytes	mRNA in all cells tested; protein only in myeloid cells	Myeloid, B lymphocytes	Myeloid, B lymphocytes
Functional domains	Carboxy-terminus may bind cytosolic oxidase components; heme-binding domain and FAD-binding domains	Heme-binding domain	6–9 potential serine phosphorylation sites; cytoskeleton binding sites	Cytoskeleton binding sites
Homologies	Ferredoxin-NADP⁺ reductase (FNR)	Polypeptide I of cytochrome c oxidase (weak homology)	SH3 domain of src; p67-phox	SH3 domain of src; p47-phox

*There are tyrosine residues in p67-phox that could potentially be phosphorylated.

phox = phagocyte oxidase component; NCF = neutrophil cytosol factor; SOC = soluble oxidase component; C = component; PAGE = polyacrylamide gel electrophoresis; SH3 = src homology domain 3.

Reproduced from Curnutte, J. T.: Molecular basis of the autosomal recessive forms of chronic granulomatous disease. Immunodef. Rev. 3:149, 1992; with permission.

ditional biochemical abnormalities in X-linked CGD neutrophils had also been observed. For example, membrane flavoprotein concentrations were consistently about half those of normal neutrophils.[206, 249, 252] Indeed, whether the cytochrome actually was part of the respiratory burst complex at all was controversial.[204] Hence, it was uncertain whether the absence of the cytochrome b spectrum represented the primary genetic defect in X-linked CGD.

Two independent experimental approaches finally established that the product of the X-linked "CGD" gene was in fact a subunit of cytochrome b, and, as such, an essential component of the respiratory burst oxidase. One approach relied on a genetic strategy, whereby the gene mutated in X-linked CGD was identified and cloned on the basis of its chromosomal location at Xp21.1.[265, 266] Antibodies raised to the predicted polypeptide sequence reacted with the 91 kDa glycoprotein (gp91-phox) of cytochrome b,[267] which upon conventional purification appeared to be a complex of two tightly associated integral membrane polypeptides.[242, 243] This approach represented the first

example in which the protein defect responsible for a human disease was identified by "reverse genetics" (positional cloning), a strategy that has also been applied with notable success to an increasing number of inherited diseases, such as Duchenne muscular dystrophy,[268] neurofibromatosis,[269, 270] and cystic fibrosis.[271–273] The development of a purification scheme for the cytochrome led to the independent identification of its larger subunit as the product of the X-linked CGD locus. The N-terminal amino acid sequence of purified gp91-phox[274] corresponded to that predicted by the cDNA derived from the identified locus at Xp21.1.

The identification of cytochrome b as an oligomer composed of 91 kDa and 22 kDa subunits provided an explanation for the observation that neutrophil cytochrome b is also absent in some cases of autosomal recessive CGD. The hypothesis that mutations in the gene for p22-phox lead to this form of CGD proved correct based on DNA sequence analysis of affected patients.[275]

Expression of the gp91-phox gene is restricted almost exclusively to mature phagocytic cells of the myeloid lineage[266] (see Table 14–11). RNA transcripts for gp91-*phox* have also been seen in EBV-transformed B-lymphocyte cell lines in which at least a subpopulation appears to be capable of mounting a respiratory burst.[276, 277] Recently, gp91-*phox* (or a form thereof) was also detected in renal mesangial cells, in which low rates of O_2^- production have been detected.[278] In contrast to this relative tissue specificity, p22-*phox* mRNA is constitutively expressed in a wide variety of cell types.[279] However, it appears that coordinate synthesis of both subunits is required for normal intracellular stability of each polypeptide chain. Only trace amounts of the p22-*phox* subunit are detectable in nonphagocytic cells, which lack the gp91-*phox* transcript,[279] or in neutrophils obtained from patients with X-linked CGD who are genetically deficient in gp91-*phox*.[242, 243, 279, 280] Conversely, gp91-*phox* is absent in neutrophils from patients with autosomal recessive CGD who are genetically deficient in p22-*phox*.[275, 280] These observations are reminiscent of those made for the leukocyte adhesion β_2 integrins and other oligomeric membrane protein complexes, in which steady-state levels of each subunit are dependent on interchain association during biosynthesis.[51, 281]

In resting neutrophils, the majority (up to 80 per cent) of cytochrome *b* resides in specific granules, with the remainder in the plasma membrane.[160, 204] The specific granule pool may serve as a reservoir to maintain sustained respiratory burst activity. Cytochrome *b* is also incorporated into the phagosomal membrane during phagocytosis.[258, 282]

Little detailed information is available on the overall structure of cytochrome *b* and the relative function of the two subunits during the respiratory burst. The hydrodynamic mass of the cross-linked cytochrome is most consistent with a heterodimer.[283] The deduced primary amino acid sequences[266, 279] of both gp91-*phox* and p22-*phox* have no obvious homology to other polypeptides, including other cytochromes, with two exceptions (see Table 14–11). One region in p22-*phox* has some resemblance to heme-binding domains in other heme-bearing polypeptides,[279] whereas a small portion of gp91-*phox* is homologous to an FAD-binding motif seen in ferredoxin-NADP$^+$ reductase.[251, 252] The gp91-*phox* polypeptide contains 570 amino acids and includes a number of hydrophobic domains as well as five potential *N*-glycosylation sites.[284] The smaller p22-*phox* cytochrome subunit, composed of 195 residues, contains hydrophobic sequences concentrated in the N-terminal half and a proline-rich, basic C-terminus.[279]

Quantitative analysis of the heme content in purified preparations suggests a stoichiometry of two heme groups per cytochrome *b*.[279, 285] The actual location of the protoporphyrin IX ring[286] has been in doubt. Indirect evidence based on radiation-inactivation target analysis and sedimentation equilibrium studies suggests that p22-*phox* may contain a heme group.[287] Another group has purified a heme-bearing polypeptide from neutrophils that was thought to be p22-*phox*, yet its amino acid composition[288] did not resemble that

predicted from the cDNA sequence.[279] Detailed spectroscopy of partially purified cytochrome is suggestive of imidazole or imidazolate axial ligation,[286] which would require a pair of histidine residues. Since the p22-*phox* sequence contains only one invariant histidine (a second histidine predicted by the original cDNA clone[279] proved to be polymorphic with tyrosine[275]), the heme groups must interact with histidine residues in gp91-*phox*.

The topological organization of the cytochrome within the membrane has been explored with antibodies raised against the two subunits. The C-terminal portions of both gp91-*phox*[289, 290] and p22-*phox*[291] reside at the cytoplasmic face of the membrane, as shown using indirect immunofluorescence localization of antibody binding. This finding correlates with other evidence that links the carboxy-terminal domain of at least gp91-*phox* with functional interactions with other oxidase components (see below). A monoclonal antibody raised to the cytochrome binds to the external face of the plasma membrane[292]; however, the epitope to which this antibody is directed is uncertain. The gp91-*phox* subunit must have at least one external domain, as it is heavily glycosylated with the N-linked oligosaccharides.[243, 293] A tentative topological model that incorporates antibody localization data and predictions based on the amino acid sequence of each cytochrome subunit is shown in Figure 14–6.[294]

Cytosolic Components

The development of a cell-free assay of oxidase activity in the mid-1980s was a major breakthrough that led directly to the recognition that cytosol-derived proteins were absolutely required for catalytic activity of the membrane-associated, activated oxidase.[138, 295–297] In this assay, the addition of certain anionic amphiphiles (such as sodium dodecyl sulfate [SDS] or arachidonic acid) to mixtures of membrane and cytosol fractions isolated from resting neutrophils elicits oxidase activity at rates comparable to those observed in intact cells. The capacity to reconstitute the oxidase in this manner has proved to be a powerful tool for the analysis of specific oxidase components.

The identification of two cytosol-derived oxidase components was greatly facilitated by the discovery that neutrophil cytosol obtained from autosomal recessive CGD patients with normal cytochrome *b* levels could not reconstitute the oxidase in the presence of normal membranes.[298] Subsequent complementation studies using cytosols from different cytochrome-positive autosomal recessive patients indicated that there were at least two distinct cytosolic defects, each involving a different oxidase component.[245, 246] One proved to be a highly basic 47 kDa phosphoprotein (p47-*phox*)[244–246] that was already a suspected oxidase component because of the absence of its phosphorylation pattern in cytochrome-positive autosomal recessive CGD patients[206, 299] (see Table 14–11). The other complementing cytosolic oxidase component was iden-

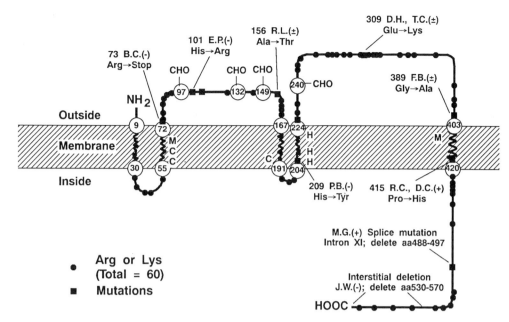

FIGURE 14–6. Proposed protein conformation of gp91-*phox*. Locations of deduced amino acid changes or deletions in patients with X-linked chronic granulomatous disease are shown. (+) denotes that the gp91-*phox* protein is still detectable by immunoblot, whereas (−) denotes its absence and (±) indicates that it is diminished in quantity. Numbers in circles indicate amino acid residue numbers. In the transmembrane domains, M = methionine, C = cysteine, and H = histidine. (Adapted from Hopkins, P. J., Bemiller, L. S., and Curnutte, J. T.: Chronic granulomatous disease: Diagnosis and classification at the molecular level. Clin. Lab. Med. 12:277, 1992; with permission.)

tified as a 67 kDa species (p67-*phox*) that is slightly acidic.[244–246] The corresponding cDNAs for both p47-*phox* and p67-*phox* were subsequently cloned, and the recombinant proteins were shown to restore oxidase activity to either p47-*phox*– or p67-*phox*–deficient cytosol, respectively.[300–302] The expression of p47-*phox* and p67-*phox* is restricted to mature myelomonocytic cells and B lymphocytes,[303] similar to what is observed for gp91-*phox*.

Little is known regarding the actual function of p47-*phox* and p67-*phox* in the respiratory burst oxidase. Although p47-*phox* and p67-*phox* are present in the cytosol of resting neutrophils, probably as a complex,[264, 304] both become associated with the membrane upon oxidase activation.[247, 248] In studies performed with CGD neutrophils deficient in either p47-*phox* or p67-*phox*, p47-*phox* appeared to be essential for the translocation process.[248] Thus, although p47-*phox* could associate with the membrane in the absence of p67-*phox*, p67-*phox* translocation failed to occur in p47-*phox*–deficient cells. Translocation also depends on the presence of cytochrome *b*, as it fails to occur in neutrophils obtained from cytochrome-negative CGD patients.[248, 305] There is indirect evidence that the cytosol factor membrane-binding site may involve the extreme C-terminus of the gp91-*phox* subunit of the cytochrome. A peptide derived from the sequence corresponding to this region blocks oxidase activation both in electrically permeabilized cells and in the cell-free system.[289, 290]

Oxidase activation is accompanied by the stepwise phosphorylation of multiple sites on p47-*phox*.[306–308] The initial modifications occur in the cytosol, but complete phosphorylation depends on membrane binding and requires cytochrome *b*. In studies performed on intact neutrophils activated by phorbol myristate acetate (a direct activator of protein kinase C), inhibition of p47-*phox* phosphorylation by staurosporine blocked p47-*phox* and p67-*phox* translocation

to neutrophil membranes. This finding suggests that phosphorylation by protein kinase C or another staurosporine-sensitive kinase may be an important regulatory signal for translocation and oxidase activation under these conditions.[309] However, p47-*phox* phosphorylation is not required for oxidase activity per se, as O_2^- production in the cell-free assay is independent of phosphorylation.[264, 310, 311]

Although analyses of the predicted amino acid sequences of p47-*phox* and p67-*phox* are generally unrevealing, both proteins contain a pair of sequences that have some homology to SH3 (src homology region 3) domains (Fig. 14–7),[300–302, 312] which have been implicated in protein association at the inner face of the plasma membrane. SH3 domains were first described in non-receptor tyrosine kinases and subsequently detected in a variety of other proteins, including non-erythroid α-spectrin, myosin IB, and guanosine triphosphatase–activating proteins (GAP), that constitute or can be associated with the cytoskeleton and membrane.[313] The SH3 domains noted in p47-*phox* and p67-*phox* may be important for membrane translocation during oxidase activation.

Other Oxidase Components

Flavoproteins

Many lines of evidence suggest that the oxidase contains a flavoprotein that functions as the initial electron acceptor from NADPH, using FAD as the cofactor.[205, 206] Although a confusing array of potential candidates have been proposed, a protein with the appropriate characteristics has not been identified with certainty. Reaction of neutrophil membranes with photoaffinity or reactive dialdehyde NADPH congeners labels a protein of approximately 66 kDa.[314–316] In other studies, a 45 kDa flavin-binding polypeptide

```
                *  *  *    *              *  * *      * *   * *  * * *       *       *              *    *    * *  * * * *

p47-phox   163  A I A D Y E K T S G S E - M A L S T G D - V V E K S E K S E S G W W F C Q M K - - A K R G W I P A S F L E

p47-phox   233  A I K A Y T A V E G D E - V S L L E G E - A V E V I H K L L D G W W V I R   K D D - V T G Y F P S M Y L Q

p67-phox   247  V L F G F V P E T K E E - L Q V M P G N - I V F V L K K G N D N W A T V M F N - - G Q K G L V P C N Y L E

p67-phox   464  A L F S Y E A T Q P E D - L E F Q E G D - I I L V L S K V N E E W L E G E C K - - G K V G I F P K V F V E

GAP        286  A I L P Y T K V P D T D E I S F L K G D - M F I V H N E L K D G W M W V T N L R T D E Q G L I V E D L V E

α spectrin 974  A L Y D Y Q E K S P R E - V T M K K G D - I L T L L N S T N K D W W K V E - V N D R Q - G F V P A A Y V K

ABP1       539  A E Y D Y D A A E D N E - L T F V E N D K I I - N I E F V D D D W W L G E L E K D G S K G L F P S N Y V S

myoIB      983  A L Y D F A A E N P D E - L T F N E G A - V V T V I N K S N P D W W E G E L - - N G Q R G V F P A S Y V E

myoI Dict. 1060 A L Y D Y D A S S T D E - L S F K E G D - I I F I V Q K D N G G W T Q G E L K - S G Q K G W A P T N Y L Q

c-src      88   A L Y D Y E S R T E T D - L S F K K G E - R L Q I V N N T E G D W W L A H S L T T G Q T G Y I P S N Y V A
```

FIGURE 14–7. *The SH3 domains of p47-phox and p67-phox aligned with those of other proteins.* GAP = GTPase activating protein; α-spectrin = human non-erythroid α-spectrin; ABP-1 = yeast actin-binding protein; myoIB = *Acanthamoeba* myosin IB; myoI Dict. = *Dictyostelium* myosin I; c-src = human src-like non-receptor tyrosine kinase. Letters in bold type (asterisked) represent residues where the level of homology (identical plus highly conserved amino acids) is 70 per cent or more within this group of 10 SH3 domains. Numbers refer to the first amino acid in each sequence. (From Heyworth, P. G., Peveri, P., and Curnutte, J. T.: Cytosolic components of NADPH oxidase: Identity-function and role in regulation of oxidase activity. *In* Cochrane, C. G., and Gimbrone, M. A., Jr. [eds.]: Biological Oxidants—Generation and Injurious Consequences. San Diego, Academic Press, 1992; with permission.)

was shown to bind diphenylene iodonium, a potent oxidase inhibitor.[317] This species is located both in cytosol and in membrane fractions, and antibodies raised against it partially inhibit oxidase activity in a cell-free assay.[317] Other workers have identified an approximately 32 kDa NADPH-binding protein in resting neutrophil cytosol that translocates to the membrane with oxidase activation and whose inactivation by NADPH dialdehyde inhibits oxidase activity.[318] Recent evidence suggests that the FAD redox center is bound to gp91-*phox*.[251, 252] Resolution of which, if any, of the above species correspond to the flavoprotein component of the oxidase will require demonstration of functional oxidase reconstitution, using well-characterized components.

Low Molecular Weight G Proteins

A substantial number of low molecular weight guanine nucleotide-binding proteins (LMWG) with homology to Ras have been identified in recent years.[319] All share common features of size (~21 to 26 kDa), slow spontaneous exchange of GDP and GTP, and intrinsic GTPase activity. Most LMWG also undergo a post-translational attachment of polyisoprenoid units at the carboxy-terminus that results in localization to the membrane. Like other guanine nucleotide-binding proteins, LMWG are thought to serve as molecular "switches" via changes in conformation as the protein cycles between inactive GDP- and active GTP-bound forms (Fig. 14–8).[312] The relative levels of the two forms may be modulated by other proteins that regulate guanine nucleotide exchange or GTP hydrolysis (GAP proteins).[312, 320] Although the specific functions of most LMWG are unknown, different subfamilies have been implicated in receptor-mediated signal transduction, cytoskeletal organization, intracellular vesicle transport, and secretion.[116, 319, 321–323] A number of recent studies have suggested that one or more LMWG also participate in regulation of respiratory burst oxidase activity.[253–256, 324–329] The involvement of low molecular weight G proteins in the regulation of oxidase activity provides an attractive explanation for the observation that the oxidase has an absolute requirement for GTP.[310, 311, 330]

Cytochrome *b* purified from solubilized neutrophil membranes by either conventional column chromatography or immunoaffinity matrices is associated with approximately equimolar amounts of a 22 kDa polypeptide known as Rap 1 (or Krev-1) that is about 55 per cent homologous to the Ras.[256] Rap 1 is a ubiquitously expressed protein with two closely related forms, Rap 1A and Rap 1B, which are 95 per cent identical at the amino acid level.[331, 332] Rap 1A appears to be the predominant form in neutrophils,[333] and its stoichiometric association with cytochrome *b* is inhibited by Rap 1A phosphorylation by cAMP-dependent protein kinase.[326] The latter observation is intriguing in light of the inhibition of neutrophil activation and O_2^- production by hormones that increase the intracellular concentration of cyclic adenosine monophosphate (cAMP).[334] However, the specific role played by Rap 1A in respiratory burst function remains to be clarified. It has been reported that immunodepletion of Rap 1 in the cell-free system abolishes oxidase activity, which is reversed by the addition of a truncated form of recombinant Rap 1A.[255] However, others have found that full-length recombinant Rap 1A does not stimulate oxidase activity under similar conditions (see reference 254).

Recent studies have also implicated one or more cytosol-derived LMWG in playing a role in oxidase activation. Attempts to isolate cytosolic proteins that stimulate the oxidase have consistently yielded a fraction distinct from those containing p47-*phox* and p67-*phox*, variously called neutrophil cytosolic factor (NCF)

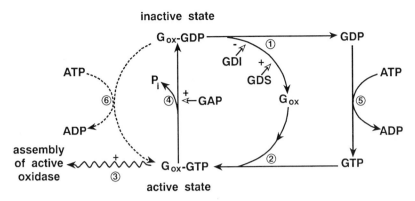

FIGURE 14–8. GDP and GTP cycling of an NADPH oxidase–related low molecular mass GTP-binding protein (G_{ox}). G_{ox} can represent Rac 1, Rac 2, Rac 1A, or an as yet unknown GTP-binding protein. In the GDP-bound form, G_{ox} is in its inactive state. The release of GDP (1) is modulated by GDP dissociation inhibitor (GDI) and GDP dissociation stimulator (GDS). Binding of GTP (2) converts the protein to the active state, in which it can activate the assembly and/or catalytic activity of NADPH oxidase (3). Hydrolysis of GTP to GDP (4) causes G_{ox} to revert to its inactive form. By analogy with other low molecular mass GTP-binding proteins, this step is likely to be regulated by a GTPase activating protein (GAP). Freed GDP can be phosphorylated by nucleoside diphosphate kinase (NDPK) to GTP (5). There is also recent evidence that GDP bound to GTP-binding proteins can be phosphorylated by NDPK (6), although in this scheme this step is entirely speculative. (From Heyworth, P. G., Peveri, P., and Curnutte, J. T.: Cytosolic components of NADPH oxidase: Identity, function and role in regulation of oxidase activity. *In* Cochrane, C. G., and Gimbrone, M. A., Jr. [eds.]: Biological Oxidants—Generation and Injurious Consequences. San Diego, Academic Press, 1992; with permission.)

3,[245] C3,[246] soluble oxidase component (SOC) 1,[335] or Sigma 1.[336] The combination of neutrophil membranes, NCF-3, and recombinant forms of p47-*phox* and p67-*phox* is necessary and sufficient for oxidase activity in the cell-free system.[337]

The active component of Sigma 1, as isolated from guinea pig macrophages, contains two proteins identified by microsequencing to be Rac 1, a 21 kDa polypeptide, and a 26 kDa GDP-dissociation inhibitor known as rhoGDI, a regulator of guanine nucleotide exchange in Rho, another LMWG.[253] Partially purified or recombinant Rac 1 enhances oxidase activity in the cell-free system.[253, 328] Another group has isolated Rac 2, a closely related species (92 per cent identical to Rac 1) from human neutrophil cytosol on the basis of its GTP-binding and oxidase-stimulatory activities.[254] Rac 2 is expressed almost exclusively in myeloid cells, whereas Rac 1 appears to have a ubiquitous distribution.[338] Rac proteins are closely related to Rho, a group of LMWG that have been implicated in controlling cytoskeletal organization.[319, 321, 322] It appears likely that the active component or components in SOC1, C3, and NCF-3 will also prove to include a Rac species. The pI of C3, for example, is nearly identical to that for Rac 2.[254]

Assembly of the Active Oxidase Complex

With the identification and characterization of many of the oxidase components accomplished, the next phase of oxidase research will move toward defining how these polypeptides function together in the regulated production of O_2^-. A provisional model of the respiratory burst oxidase is shown in Figure 14–9.

Membrane-associated components include the integral membrane protein complex of gp91-*phox* and p22-*phox*, which forms cytochrome *b*, and possibly an FAD-containing flavoprotein as electron carriers (see above and Fig. 14–8 legend). The cytochrome is at least physically associated with Rap 1A, a low molecular weight G protein. The cytosolic oxidase components exist as a preformed complex of approximately 260 kDa, which contains the p47-*phox* and p67-*phox* subunits, as well as possibly Rac 1/Rac 2.[264, 304] The translocation of the complex to the membrane is triggered in response to chemotactic factors or binding of opsonized microbes. The specific second messenger signals that interface receptor-mediated events at the cell surface with assembly of the catalytically active oxidase complex are not known with certainty but likely involve PA, DAG, arachidonic acid, and Ca^{2+} (see Fig. 14–4 and discussion above). The stepwise phosphorylation of p47-*phox* by protein kinase C or a related kinase may be a signal for translocation in the intact cell.[309, 339] Binding of cytosolic oxidase factors may involve direct binding to the carboxy-terminus of the gp91-*phox* subunit of cytochrome *b*.[289, 290] Changes in the association of cytochrome *b*, p47-*phox*, and p67-*phox* with the submembranous cytoskeleton have also been observed with oxidase assembly.[309, 340]

Kinetic analysis has suggested that cytosolic factors are incorporated as subunits into the oxidase complex.[341] Cytosolic factors may form part of the catalytically active portion of the complex and/or modify the membrane redox carriers so that electron flow can proceed efficiently. The observation that respiratory burst activation can result in low levels of intracellular oxidants in CGD patients deficient in p47-*phox* suggests that the latter may be the case.[217] The role of LMWG

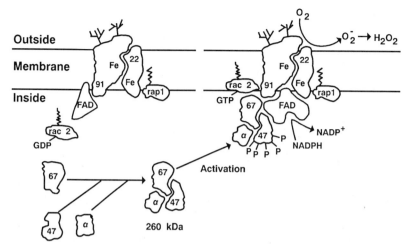

FIGURE 14–9. Hypothetical model of NADPH oxidase activation. Current knowledge of the oxidase suggests that in its dormant state (left side of figure) it is composed of both membrane-bound and cytosolic components. The former include the gp91-*phox* and p22-*phox* subunits of cytochrome b_{558} (and possibly Rap 1A). Recent evidence suggests that the flavin adenine dinucleotide (FAD) redox center is bound to gp91-*phox*,[251, 252] but since this has not been conclusively established, the FAD is shown bound to a distinct oxidase subunit in the membrane. The cytosolic components include p47-*phox* and p67-*phox*, which appear to exist in a preformed complex of 260 kDa.[264, 304] It is likely this complex contains at least one other additional component (as yet undetermined), labeled in this model as "α." The low molecular mass GTP-binding protein, Rac 2, is also present in the cytosol in its inactive state (with GDP bound), presumably complexed with a GDP dissociation inhibitor (GDI; not shown) that serves to keep Rac 2 in its inactive state. Upon stimulation, the p47-*phox*/p67-*phox* complex translocates to the membrane. This process may be under the control of the active (GTP-bound) form of Rac 2 and further regulated by phosphorylation of p47-*phox*. In its active state, the FAD redox center accepts electrons from NADPH and passes them on to molecular oxygen via the heme groups in cytochrome b_{558}. Two heme groups are believed to be present in each cytochrome b_{558} heterodimer.[279, 285, 286]

proteins in oxidase function is also likely to involve modulation of oxidase assembly or activity rather than a direct role in electron transport.

Many phagocytic antimicrobial functions can be potentiated or "primed" by prior exposure to various agents that include LPS, chemotactic peptides, and cytokines (e.g., granulocyte-macrophage colony-stimulating factor, IL-1, IFN-γ) (reviewed in reference 342). Priming of the respiratory burst is a complex phenomenon that is poorly understood. Depending on the agent and duration of exposure, effects on both the rapidity of oxidase activation and the rate of O_2^- production can be observed. The underlying molecular mechanisms may involve changes in the transcription of oxidase subunit mRNAs[342] as well as modifications in the pathways that regulate oxidase assembly.

CHRONIC GRANULOMATOUS DISEASE

Clinical Features

Chronic granulomatous disease is a rare, genetically heterogeneous disorder that occurs in approximately 1 in 500,000 to 1,000,000 individuals and is characterized by inherited defects in the phagocyte respiratory burst oxidase.[204] A respiratory burst of 1 to 10 per cent of normal is detectable in approximately 5 per cent of remaining patients, who are said to have "variant" CGD.[207, 208, 343, 344] In all cases of CGD studied

at the molecular level to date, genetic defects have been identified in one of the four oxidase components summarized in Table 14–11.

The CGD phenotype provides direct evidence for the in vivo importance of the phagocyte respiratory burst pathway. Affected patients develop severe, recurrent bacterial and fungal infections, often by organisms not ordinarily considered pathogens.[345, 346] The majority of patients with CGD manifest symptoms within the first year of life. Table 14–12 summarizes the types of infections and infecting organisms associated with CGD.[346, 347] The most common pathogens include *Staphylococcus aureus*, *Aspergillus* species, and a variety of gram-negative bacilli, including *Serratia marcescens*, *Pseudomonas cepacia*, and various *Salmonella* species. It has long been recognized that patients with CGD are particularly susceptible to organisms that contain catalase, which prevents the CGD phagocyte from scavenging microbial-generated H_2O_2 for phagosomal killing.[204]

Chronic conditions associated with CGD are responsible for many of the major complications of CGD and are also summarized in Table 14–12. These include the formation of granulomas, another hallmark of this disorder, which is believed to reflect a chronic inflammatory response to inadequate phagocytic killing or digestion. These lesions contain lymphocytes and pigmented, lipid-containing macrophages.[236, 348] Granuloma formation can lead to obstructive symptoms in

TABLE 14–12. CLINICAL PRESENTATION OF CHRONIC GRANULOMATOUS DISEASE

CHRONIC CONDITIONS*	INFECTIONS*	INFECTING ORGANISMS*
Lymphadenopathy	Pneumonia	*Staphylococcus aureus*
Hepatomegaly	Lymphadenitis	*Klebsiella* spp.
Splenomegaly	Cutaneous abscesses/impetigo	*Serratia marcescens*
Anemia of chronic disease	Perirectal abscesses	*Escherichia coli*
Dermatitis	Hepatic abscesses	*Aspergillus* spp.
Aphthous stomatitis	Osteomyelitis	*Pseudomonas cepacia*
Restrictive lung disease	Sepsis	*Candida albicans*
Gingivitis	Conjunctivitis	*Salmonella* spp.
Hydronephrosis	Sinusitis	Other enteric bacteria
Persistent diarrhea	Pyelonephritis (often due to	Rare, but important:
Gastric antral narrowing	obstruction)	*Nocardia* spp.
(infants and children)	Rare, but important:	Myobacteria
	Pericarditis	*Pneumocystis carinii*
	Brain abscesses	
	Meningitis	

*Each list is arranged in approximate order of frequency based on 35 patients followed at The Scripps Research Institute and on a review of the literature by Forrest and colleagues.

From Curnutte, J. T.: Disorders of phagocyte function. *In* Hoffman, R., Benz, E. J., Jr., Shattil, S. J., Furie, B., and Cohen, H. J. (eds.): Hematology: Basic Principles and Practice. New York, Churchill Livingstone, 1991, pp. 571–589; with permission.

the upper gastrointestinal tract and urinary tract, as well as to a chronic ileocolitis syndrome resembling Crohn's disease.[349, 350]

Molecular Basis of Chronic Granulomatous Disease

A modern classification of CGD groups the type of CGD according to the oxidase component that is affected (Table 14–13). Nomenclature has also been adopted for an abbreviated designation within each major group and includes the mode of inheritance, oxidase component by molecular weight, and level of *phox* protein expression. Overall, defects in the X-linked gene for the gp91-*phox* subunit of cytochrome *b* account for approximately 60 per cent of CGD, whereas autosomal recessive defects in the p22-*phox* cytochrome subunit are rare (5 per cent).[343, 351] Autosomal recessive deficiencies in the cytosolic factors p47-

phox and p67-*phox* represent approximately 30 per cent and 5 per cent of cases, respectively.[343, 351]

Mutations in Cytochrome b

The gp91-*phox* gene (termed CYBB) that encodes the large subunit of cytochrome *b* contains 13 exons and spans approximately 30 kilobases (kb) in the Xp21.1 region of the X chromosome.[265, 266, 352] Defects in the gene are heterogeneous, as listed in Table 14–14.[265, 266, 353–361] Relatively large deletions in Xp21.1 involving X-linked CGD and other adjacent loci have been described in a few rare patients (Cases 1 to 4, Table 14–14). These individuals have complex phenotypes that include CGD and McLeod's syndrome (a mild hemolytic anemia associated with depressed levels of Kell antigens due to defects in the red cell antigen K_x), with or without concomitant Duchenne muscular dystrophy and retinitis pigmentosa.[284] Partial gp91-*phox* gene deletions have been found in two other

TABLE 14–13. CLASSIFICATION OF CHRONIC GRANULOMATOUS DISEASE

COMPONENT AFFECTED	INHERITANCE	SUBTYPE*	CYTOCHROME *b* SPECTRUM	NBT SCORE (% POSITIVE)	FREQUENCY (% OF CASES)	IMMUNOBLOT LEVELS†				ACTIVITY IN CELL-FREE SYSTEM	
						gp91	p22	p47	p67	Membrane	Cytosol
gp91-*phox*	X	X91⁰	0	0	50	0	0–Trace	N	N	0	N
		X91⁻	Low	80–100 (weak)	3	Low	Low	N	N	Trace	N
		X91⁺	N	0	3	N	N	N	N	0	N
p22-*phox*	A	A22⁰	0	0	5	0	0	N	N	0	N
		A22⁺	N	0	1	N	N	N	N	0	N
p47-*phox*	A	A47⁰	N	0	33	N	N	0	N	N	0
p67-*phox*	A	A67⁰	N	0	5	N	N	N	0	N	0

*In this nomenclature, the first letter represents the mode of inheritance (X-linked [X] or autosomal recessive [A]), whereas the number indicates the *phox* component that is generally affected. The superscript symbols indicate whether the level of protein of the affected component is undetectable (⁰), diminished (⁻), or normal (⁺) as measured by immunoblot analysis.

†Defined by immunoblotting with component-specific antibodies.

X = X-linked inheritance; A = autosomal recessive inheritance; N = normal level of protein; 0 = undetectable level of protein activity.

From Curnutte, J. T.: Molecular basis of the autosomal recessive forms of chronic granulomatous disease. Immunodef. Rev. 3:149, 1992; with permission.

TABLE 14–14. SUMMARY OF gp91-*phox* MUTATIONS IDENTIFIED IN 21 CASES OF X91 CHRONIC GRANULOMATOUS DISEASE*

CASE/SEX	MUTATION TYPE	O_2^-	CYTOCHROME *b*			NUCLEOTIDE CHANGE	AMINO ACID CHANGE	CGD TYPE	REFERENCES
			Protein	*Spectrum*	*mRNA*				
1. M	Deletion	(0)	(0)	(0)	(0)	≈5000 kb deletion	N/A	X91⁰	353
2. M	Deletion	(0)	(0)	(0)	(0)	≈4000 kb deletion	N/A	X91⁰	265, 266, 354
3. M	Deletion	0	0	0	ND	≈800 kb deletion	N/A	X91⁰	355
4. M	Deletion	0	(0)	0	ND	ND	ND	X91⁰	356
5. M	Deletion	0	0	0	N	≈1 kb deletion from intron XII to 3′UT	C-terminal 41 amino acid deletion	X91⁰	266
6. M	Deletion	(0)	(0)	0	0	≈10 kb deletion	N/A	X91⁰	357
7. M	Splice/deletion	6%	N	N	N	Splice ag→gg at 3′ end of intron XI	Delete 10 AA amino acids in exon 12 (then in frame)	X91⁺	358
8. M	Splice/deletion	0	0	0	Slight ↓ in size	Splice gt→ga at start of intron VII	Deletion of exon 7, then frameshift	X91⁰	359
9. M	Splice/deletion	0	0	0	Slight ↓ in size	Splice gta→gtt at start of intron V	Deletion of exon 5, then stop	X91⁰	359
10. M	Splice/deletion	0	0	0	N	Splice gtaag→gtaaa at start of intron III	Deletion of exon 3	X91⁰	359
11. M	Splice/deletion	0	0	0	ND	Splice ag→gg at 3′ end of intron II	ND	X91⁰	Scripps
12. M	Splice/deletion	(0)	(0)	(0)′	ND	Splice gt→gc at 5′ end of intron V	ND	(X91⁰)	Scripps
13. 2M	Missense	0	N	N	N	C-1256→A	Pro 415→His	X91⁺	360
14. 2M	Missense	3%–9%	<10%	10%–15%	N	G-937→A	Glu 309→Lys	X91⁻	Scripps
15. M	Missense	±	0	±	N	G-1178→C	Gly 389→Ala	X91⁻	361
16. M	Missense	±	0†	±	N	G-743→C	Cys 244→Ser	X91⁻	361
17. M	Missense	±	0	±	N	G-478→A	Ala 156→Thr	X91⁻	361
18. M	Missense	0	0	0	N	C-637→T	His 209→Tyr	X91⁰	361
19. F	Missense	0	0	0	N	A-314→G	His 101→Arg	X91⁰	361
20. M	Nonsense	0	0	0	N	C-229→T	Arg 73→stop	X91⁰	361
21. M	Nonsense	0	0	0	ND	C-481→T	Arg 157→stop	X91⁰	Scripps
22. M	Nonsense	0	0	0	ND	C-880→T	Arg 290→stop	X91⁰	Scripps
23. M	Nonsense	0	0	0	ND	C-283→T	Arg 91→stop	X91⁰	Scripps
24. M	Nonsense	0	0	0	ND	C-880→T	Arg 290→stop	X91⁰	Scripps
25. M	Nonsense	0	0	0	ND	Insert G after G-207 in exon 3	Stop codon in exon 4	X91⁰	Scripps

*Values in parentheses are presumed from the nature of the mutation. Nucleotide residues are numbered according to the system of Orkin.[284] Case 13 represents two brothers, and Case 14 describes two boys who are first maternal cousins. Case 19 is a female with extreme lyonization (2 to 5 per cent NBT-positive cells).

†p22-*phox* appeared normal on immunoblot.

N = Normal in appearance; ± = diminished level (quantitative data not presented); N/A = not applicable; ND = not determined; Scripps = case analyzed at The Scripps Research Institute (Cases 11, 12, 14, 21 to 25) and at University of Massachusetts (Case 14) but not yet published.

patients (Cases 5 and 6, Table 14–14), including one that predicts the synthesis of a truncated protein (see Fig. 14–6, patient J.W.).[266] The gp91-*phox* gene, however, appears grossly normal by Southern blot analysis in the majority of patients with X-linked CGD. Many of these patients have absent or markedly deficient gp91-*phox* RNA transcripts,[284] presumably due to mutations that adversely affect RNA transcription, mRNA processing, and/or mRNA stability. The specific mutations in this group of patients are largely unknown. Most mutations so far characterized have been identified by DNA sequence analysis of gp91-*phox* coding sequences amplified by the polymerase chain reaction. As summarized in Table 14–14, these are all point mutations that affect mRNA splicing (Cases 7 to 12) or that alter coding sequence by introducing missense (Cases 13 to 19) or nonsense mutations (Cases 20 to 25). Some of these mutations are depicted in the gp91-*phox* model in Figure 14–6.

Of particular interest are mutations identified in the subgroup of "variant" patients with residual oxidase function associated with small amounts of cytochrome *b* (X91⁻ CGD). In one example, a missense mutation (Glu 309 → Lys) results in normal levels of gp91-*phox* mRNA and low, but detectable, levels of cytochrome *b* (X91⁻ CGD) and residual oxidase activity (Case 14, Table 14–14; also shown at amino acid residue 309 in Fig. 14–6). The two affected cousins have enjoyed a relatively mild clinical course. The Glu 309 → Lys mutation must reduce the stability of gp91-*phox* in some manner distinguishable from other missense mutations associated with X91⁰ CGD (Cases 18 and 19 in Table 14–14; also shown in Fig. 14–6 at amino acid residues 209 and 101). Three other examples of X91⁻ variant CGD with missense mutations (Cases 15 to 17) have also been reported (Fig. 14–6, mutations at residues 389 and 156).[344, 361] Another subset of patients with X91⁻ CGD have markedly reduced levels of neutrophil gp91-*phox* mRNA (e.g., the patient described by Ezekowitz and colleagues[362]) and must carry mutations that affect RNA transcription or stability, such as defects involving promoter sequences in the gp91-*phox* gene.

Two patients with X-linked CGD presented in Table 14–14 have normal levels of a dysfunctional cytochrome *b*, in contrast to the usual situation of markedly reduced or absent cytochrome. In one example, abnormal mRNA splicing due to an A → G mutation in an acceptor splice site leads to the in-frame deletion of 30 nt in exon 12 (Case 7, Table 14–14; patient M.G. in Fig. 14–6).[358] The splicing defect predicts the deletion of 10 amino acids in the middle of the large intracytoplasmic carboxy-terminal domain of gp91-*phox*.[289] Although the level and spectral characteristics of cytochrome *b* are unaffected, rates of O_2^- production are only 6 per cent of normal. This finding may reflect an impaired ability of gp91-*phox* to interact with cytosolic oxidase factors.[358] This patient had no history of significant infections until the age of 69; however, his grandson died at the age of 5 years of *Pseudomonas cepacia* sepsis. In a second case of X91⁺ CGD (Case 13, Table 14–14), a point mutation resulted in a Pro 415 → His substitution[360] predicted to be near the membrane-intracytoplasmic junction of the carboxy-terminus of gp91-*phox* (see amino acid residue 415 in Fig. 14–6). Affected patients have no residual oxidase activity and have exhibited a moderately severe clinical course. The mechanism by which this mutation disables oxidase function is unknown. The spectral and redox characteristics of the cytochrome are normal,[286] as is translocation of the cytosolic oxidase subunits p47-*phox* and p67-*phox*.[248]

Mutations in the gene for the p22-*phox* subunit of cytochrome *b* are an uncommon cause of CGD. The p22-*phox* gene (termed CYBA) resides at 16q24 and contains six exons that span 8.5 kb.[275] The genetic defects that have been identified are heterogeneous and range from a large interstitial gene deletion (Case 1, Table 14–15)[275, 363] to point mutations associated with missense, frameshift, or RNA splicing defects (Cases 2 to 7, Table 14–15).[275, 291, 307, 364, 365] Owing to consanguinity, all but one of the cases are homozygous for the specific mutation. A mutation associated with normal levels of cytochrome *b* and a dysfunctional oxidase (A22⁺ CGD, Case 7 in Table 14–15),[291] analogous to the cases of X91⁺ CGD described above, has been reported. The Pro 156 → His mutation occurs in the intracytoplasmic carboxy-terminus of p22-*phox*; the underlying basis for the profound effect on oxidase activity is unknown at this time.

Mutations in Cytosolic Factors

The gene for p47-*phox*, termed NCF1, resides on chromosome 7 at q11.23[366] and contains nine exons spanning 18 kb.[367] Mutations at this locus are associated with one third of all cases of CGD. In contrast to the variety of mutations seen in X91 and A22 CGD, only three different mutations have been identified thus far among nine unrelated patients with p47-*phox* defects.[367, 368] The most common mutant allele bears deletion of a GT dinucleotide at the beginning of exon 2 (Table 14–16), which results in a frameshift and premature translational termination after the synthesis of a 50 residue protein. This mutation was identified in all nine patients, and six are homozygous despite no history of consanguinity. The remaining three patients are compound heterozygotes, with the other defective allele carrying point mutations that predict a missense substitution in the coding sequence (Thr 53 → Ala in Case 7, Lys 135 → Glu in Cases 8 and 9). Levels of p47-*phox* mRNA are normal in all cases, but p47-*phox* (or a truncated derivative) is undetectable in neutrophil extracts. Hence, it appears that all three mutant alleles direct the synthesis of an unstable protein.

The gene for p67-*phox*, termed NCF2, is located on the long arm of chromosome 1 at position q25.[366] Its structure has been reported in abstract form to span 37 kb and contain 16 exons.[369] Mutations have not yet been described in association with the relatively uncommon A67⁰ form of CGD. Defects in other poly-

TABLE 14–15.   SUMMARY OF p22-*phox* MUTATIONS IN 7 PATIENTS WITH CHRONIC GRANULOMATOUS DISEASE

CASE/SEX	MUTATION TYPE	O_2^-	CYTOCHROME *b* Protein	Spectrum	mRNA	NUCLEOTIDE CHANGE	AMINO ACID CHANGE	CGD TYPE	REFERENCES
1. F	≥10 kb del. (homozygous)	0	0	0	0	N/A	N/A	A22⁰	275, 363
2. M	1. Deletion 2. Missense	0	0	0	N	C-272 del. G-297→A	Frameshift Arg 90→Gln	A22⁰	275, 307, 364
3. F	Missense (homozygous)	0	0	0	N	C-382→A	Ser 118→Arg	A22⁰	275
4. 2F, 1M	Missense (homozygous)	0	0	0	N	G-297→A	Arg 90→Gln	A22⁰	241, 365
5. M	Splice/deletion (homozygous)	0	0	0	N	Splice gtga→atga at start of intron 4	Deletion of exon 4	A22⁰	365
6. F	Missense (homozygous)	0	0	0	N	A-309→G	His 94→Arg	A22⁰	365
7. F	Missense (homozygous)	0	N	N	N	C-495→A	Pro 156→Gln	A22⁺	291

N = Normal in appearance; 0 = undetectable level; N/A = not applicable; del. = deletion. Patient 2 is the male sibling of a female patient with CGD who was previously reported and is now deceased.[364]

peptides recently implicated in oxidase function, such as Rac 1, Rac 2, and Rap 1A, have not been identified.

Molecular Basis of Clinical Heterogeneity

The classification of CGD according to specific gene defects provides an explanation for many of the previously confusing aspects of this disorder. Identification of specific mutations by DNA sequence analysis may also help to clarify the basis for some of the variability in clinical severity. Patients with "variant" X-linked CGD who have low but detectable respiratory burst activity usually, but not always, have a milder clinical course. Many of these patients have had mu-

tations associated with a residual level of cytochrome *b* (e.g., X91⁻, Cases 14 to 17, Table 14–14). Molecular analysis has not yet been reported on members of another rare subset of variant X-linked CGD who have undetectable levels of neutrophil cytochrome *b* yet some residual oxidase activity (reviewed in reference 204; see also references 370 to 373). The K_m of the oxidase complex for NADPH has been studied in broken cell preparations obtained from such patients and found to be 20 to 70 times higher than the normal level of 40 μM. Whether an alternative pathway is used for electron transport in the absence of cytochrome *b* or whether a tiny amount of cytochrome *b* is able to maintain some oxidase function is unknown.

TABLE 14–16.   SUMMARY OF p47-*phox* MUTATIONS IN 9 PATIENTS WITH A47 CGD

PATIENT/SEX	MUTATION TYPE	O_2^-	p47-*phox* Protein	mRNA	NUCLEOTIDE CHANGE	AMINO ACID CHANGE	CGD TYPE	REFERENCES
1–3/M	Deletion/ frameshift (homozygous)	NR	0	N	Deletion of G-95 and T-96 at beginning of exon 2	Frameshift with substitution of 25 incorrect amino acids (residues 26–50) before premature stop codon	A47⁰	368
4–6/2M,1F	Deletion/ frameshift (homozygous)	0	0	N	Same as Patients 1–3		A47⁰	367
7/F	1. Deletion/ frameshift 2. Missense	0–1%	0	N	1. Same as Patients 1–3 2. A-179→G	Thr 53→Ala	A47⁰	367
8,9/M	1. Deletion/ frameshift 2. Missense	0–1%	0	N	1. Same as Patients 1–3 2. A-425→G	Lys 135→Glu	A47⁰	367

Nucleotide residues are numbered per Casimir and colleagues, beginning with the 5′ end of the p47-*phox* cDNA.[368]
Abbreviations are as defined in tables 14–14 and 14–15. NR = Not reported.
From Curnutte, J. T.: Disorders of granulocyte function and granulopoiesis. *In* Nathan, D. G., and Oski, F. A. (eds.): Hematology of Infancy and Childhood. Philadelphia, W. B. Saunders Co., 1992, p. 928.

Patients with defects in cytosolic oxidase components have often been noted to exhibit milder disease compared with those with X-linked CGD.[346, 374–376] A recent report suggests this may be related to low levels of intracellular oxidant production in A47[0] (and in some A67[0]) neutrophils, as detected using a sensitive intracellular fluorescent probe in activated neutrophils.[217] In contrast, none of the patients studied with X91[0] CGD had measurable levels of neutrophil fluorescence in this assay.

It is likely that other factors affecting the clinical severity of CGD are related to the ability of auxiliary microbicidal systems to maintain an effective host defense. Indeed, the efficacy of INF-γ treatment in CGD appears to be mediated by these auxiliary pathways[375, 377] (see following section).

Diagnosis and Treatment

The diagnosis of CGD is suggested by the characteristic clinical features or by a family history of the disease. In light of the variable severity of symptoms among different patients, the diagnosis of CGD should still be considered in adolescents and adults who present with an unusual infection typical of CGD (see Table 14–12). The diagnostic feature of CGD is an absent or greatly diminished neutrophil respiratory burst. Numerous assays have been used to quantitate respiratory burst activity (reviewed in reference 378). The simplest, and most commonly used, is the nitroblue tetrazolium (NBT) test, in which the water-soluble, yellow tetrazolium dye is reduced to a blue, insoluble formazan pigment by O_2^- generated by the activated oxidase complex.[204, 207] A typical example is shown in Figure 14–10. Figure 14–10A shows the normal positive heavy staining of a group of seven peripheral blood neutrophils and one monocyte; the staining is absent in cells obtained from a patient with X91[0] CGD, as shown in Figure 14–10B. The NBT test is also helpful in diagnosing the female carrier state in X-linked CGD, in which cells will stain positive or negative, depending on random X-chromosome inactivation. This feature is demonstrated in an obligate carrier female in Figure 14–10C. Since X-linked CGD may arise by a de novo germline mutation in a parent, NBT-negative cells are not always seen in the mother of a child with X-linked CGD.[379] The NBT test is normal in carriers of autosomal recessive forms of CGD. Light staining with formazan deposits in an NBT test may suggest the presence of variant forms of CGD with low levels of respiratory burst function.

With the exception of classic X-linked disease in a male, identification of the specific oxidase protein component affected in an individual patient with CGD generally requires immunoblot analysis of neutrophil extracts, or, alternatively, spectral assay in the case of cytochrome b.[378] In a male with absent cytochrome b without clear evidence for a maternal carrier, it would be necessary to identify the mutation directly by DNA sequencing or other analysis of the gp91-phox and p22-

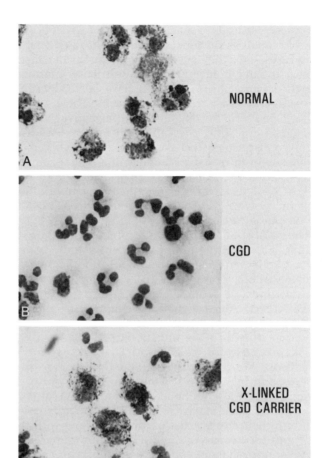

FIGURE 14–10. Nitroblue tetrazolium (NBT) slide test. Peripheral blood neutrophils and monocytes from a drop of fresh whole blood were made adherent to glass slides and stimulated with phorbol myristate acetate in the presence of NBT. *A*, Normal neutrophils and monocytes, all of which are NBT positive. *B*, Neutrophils and monocytes from a patient with X-linked CGD, which are all NBT negative. *C*, A mixture of NBT-positive and NBT-negative neutrophils from the X-linked carrier mother of the patient in *B*. (From Curnutte, J. T.: Disorders of phagocyte function. *In* Hoffman, R., Benz, E. J., Jr., Shattil, S. J., Furie, B., and Cohen, H. J. [eds.]: Hematology: Basic Principles and Practice. New York, Churchill Livingstone, 1991, pp. 571–589; with permission.)

phox genes. In the rare case in which all four known oxidase components were present at the protein level, functional analysis of membrane and cytosol fractions would be helpful[378] (e.g., the A22[+] and X91[+] forms of CGD in Table 14–13[291, 360]).

Until somatic genetic therapy becomes a realistic therapeutic option, classification of the specific CGD subgroup is useful primarily for purposes of genetic counseling and prenatal diagnosis. In utero fetal blood sampling and NBT slide test analysis of fetal blood neutrophils has been used for prenatal diagnosis (reviewed in reference 294). An alternative approach that may prove useful in cytochrome b–negative forms of CGD involves a monoclonal antibody for cytochrome b that gives positive immunocytochemical staining of normal chorionic villus macrophages (Hofbauer cells).[380] DNA analysis of amniotic fluid cells or chorionic villus biopsy provides another option for earlier and more accurate prenatal diagnosis of CGD. Southern blot analysis of gene structure will be normal in most cases, since the majority of CGD-associated alleles appear to have point mutations. Restriction fragment length polymorphisms (RFLPs) have been identified for gp91-*phox*[357, 381, 382] and p67-*phox*[383] (Table 14–17) and will be useful for diagnosis in informative families. The gene for gp91-*phox* also contains at least two highly polymorphic $(GT/AC)_n$ repeats, which can be diagnostic in informative families in a manner analogous to RFLPs.[384] Alleles differing in the number of $(GT/AC)_n$ repeats can be identified by amplification with the polymerase chain reaction, using very little DNA (nanograms).

The most specific approach to prenatal diagnosis is to first determine the family-specific mutation or mutations and then analyze fetal DNA for the specific mutation. Polymerase chain reaction amplification of individual exons from genomic DNA, followed by single-strand conformation polymorphism (SSCP) analysis on denaturing gels, is proving to be a rapid way of identifying point mutations.[294]

The prognosis for patients with CGD has continued to improve over the years since the disorder was first described in the 1950s, at which time the majority of patients died in childhood. With newer treatment strategies, a large majority of patients should survive well into their adult years, particularly those with the A47[0] and A67[0] forms of the disease. The key elements in current management of CGD include:(1) prevention and early treatment of infections; (2) aggressive use of parenteral antibiotics, augmented by surgical drainage or resection of recalcitrant infections; (3) use of prophylactic trimethoprim-sulfamethoxazole or dicloxacillin; and (4) the use of prophylactic recombinant human IFN-γ (rIFN-γ).[375] Use of cortisteroids should be avoided except in severe asthma or in the management of refractory granulomatous lesions in the gastrointestinal or urinary tract.[385]

Recombinant human IFN-γ has recently been shown to be an effective and well-tolerated treatment that reduces the incidence of serious infections in patients in all four genetic subgroups of CGD.[375] IFN-γ enhances many aspects of normal phagocyte function, including microbial killing and rates of H_2O_2 production.[386, 387] Augmentation of oxidant production appears, in part, to be related to increased levels of gp91-*phox* mRNA[362] and has prompted attempts to correct the functional deficiency in CGD phagocytes with rIFN-γ. Initial studies demonstrated that rIFN-γ led to some improvement in O_2^- production and bacterial killing by CGD neutrophils both in vitro and in vivo.[362, 388, 389] This effect was most dramatic in patients with variant X-linked CGD (X91⁻, Table 14–13). These encouraging results prompted a double-blind, placebo-controlled phase III trial to evaluate whether prophylactic rIFN-γ could reduce the incidence of serious infections in different genetic forms of CGD.[375] The key results of this study are summarized in Table 14–18. The group receiving rIFN-γ had significantly fewer patients who developed at least one serious infection (14 versus 30). The total number of serious infections (20 versus 56) and the total number of days in the hospital (497 versus 1493) were also markedly reduced in the rIFN-γ cohort. The beneficial effects were independent of age, mode of inheritance, and concomitant use of prophylactic antibiotics. Treatment (50 μg/m² three times a week, given subcutaneously) was well tolerated and easy to administer. Surprisingly, there was no difference in neutrophil O_2^- production and *Staphylococcus aureus* killing between the rIFN-γ and placebo groups.[375, 377] This finding suggests that the beneficial effect of rIFN-γ in most patients with CGD is achieved by enhancing non-oxidative microbicidal mechanisms or other aspects of phagocyte function. This observation raises the possibility of a more general role for rIFN-γ as an adjunct to conventional antimicrobial therapy in other clinical settings.

Since CGD results from genetic defects in specific phagocyte oxidase proteins whose cDNAs have been cloned, the disorder should, in principle, be correctable by gene transfer into bone marrow hematopoietic stem cells. However, experimental barriers to achieving long-term expression of exogenous genes in transduced marrow cells must be overcome for this approach to become a realistic clinical option. The first step toward reaching this goal has been the successful

TABLE 14–17.   RESTRICTION FRAGMENT LENGTH POLYMORPHISMS (RFLP) IN NADPH OXIDASE COMPONENT GENES

GENE	RESTRICTION ENZYME	ALLELE	BAND SIZE (kb)	FREQUENCY IN NORMAL POPULATIONS (%)
gp91-*phox*	*Nsi*I	A1	2.9	19
		A2	2.5	81
gp91-*phox*	*Nsi*I	B1	1.7	90
		B2	1.3	10
p67-*phox*	*Hind*III	C1	3.8	80
		C2	2.1	20

See text for details and references.
From Hopkins, P. J., Bemiller, L. S., and Curnutte, J. T.: Chronic granulomatous disease: Diagnosis and classification at the molecular level. Clin. Lab. Med. 12:277, 1992; with permission.

TABLE 14–18. SUMMARY OF THE PHASE III STUDY ESTABLISHING THE EFFICACY OF rIFN-γ FOR INFECTION PROPHYLAXIS IN CGD*

VARIABLE	TREATMENT GROUP		P VALUE
	Interferon	Placebo	
Number of patients	63	65	
X-linked	45	41	
Autosomal recessive	18	24	
Age ± SD (yr)	14.3 ± 10.1	15.0 ± 9.6	
Number of patients with at least one serious infection(%)	14 (22%)	30 (46%)	0.0006
Total number of serious infections	20	56	<0.0001
Total hospital days	497	1493	0.02
Average hospital stay (days)	32	48	

The table shows a summary of the final results of a phase III randomized, double-blind, placebo-controlled study in which 128 patients with chronic granulomatous disease received either rIFN-γ (50 μg/m²/dose) or placebo by subcutaneous injections three times per week for an average duration of 8.9 months.[375] The major endpoints of the study were the time to the first serious infection and the number of such infections. A serious infection was defined as an event requiring hospitalization and parenteral antibiotics.

retroviral expression of p47-*phox* in EBV-transformed B lymphocytes from patients with A47⁰ CGD.[390, 391]

REFERENCES

1. Weiss S. J.: Mechanisms of disease. Tissue destruction by neutrophils. N. Engl. J. Med. 320:365, 1989.
2. Kuna, P., Reddigari, S. R., Schall, T. J., Rucinski, D., Viksman, M. Y., and Kaplan, A. P.: RANTES, a monocyte and T lymphocyte chemotactic cytokine releases histamine from human basophils. J. Immunol. 149:636, 1992.
3. Oppenheim, J. J., Zachariae, C. O., Mukaida, N., and Matsushima, K.: Properties of the novel proinflammatory supergene "intercrine" cytokine family. Annu. Rev. Immunol. 9:617, 1991.
4. Alam, R., Lett-Brown, M. A., Forsythe, P. A., Anderson-Walters, D. J., Kenamore, C., Kormos, C., and Grant, J. A.: Monocyte chemotactic and activating factor is a potent histamine-releasing factor for basophils. J. Clin. Invest. 89:723, 1992.
5. Snyder, F.: Biochemistry of platelet-activating factor: A unique class of biologically active phospholipids. Proc. Soc. Exp. Biol. Med. 190:125, 1989.
6. Prescott, S. M., Zimmerman, G. A., and McIntyre, T. M.: Platelet-activating factor. J. Biol. Chem. 120:17381, 1992.
7. Nathan, C.: Nitric oxide as a secretory product of mammalian cells. FASEB J. 6:3051, 1992.
8. Lowenstein, C. J., and Snyder, S. H.: Nitric oxide, a novel biologic messenger. Cell 70:705, 1992.
9. Moncada, S.: Nitric oxide gas: Mediator, modulator, and pathophysiologic entity. J. Lab. Clin. Med. 120:187, 1992.
10. Lewis, R. A., Austen, K. F., and Soberman, R. J.: Leukotrienes and other products of the 5-lipoxygenase pathway. Biochemistry and relation to pathobiology in human diseases. N. Engl. J. Med. 323:645, 1990.
11. Lawrence, M. B., and Springer, T. A.: Leukocytes roll on a selectin at physiologic flow rates: Distinction from and prerequisite for adhesion through integrins. Cell 65:859, 1991.
12. Butcher, E. C.: Leukocyte–endothelial cell recognition: Three (or more) steps to specificity and diversity. Cell 67:1033, 1991.
13. Carlos, T. M., and Harlan, J. M.: Membrane proteins involved in phagocyte adherence to endothelium. Immunol. Rev. 114:5, 1990.
14. Schwartz, B. R., and Harlan, J. M.: Consequences of deficient granulocyte-endothelium interactions. *In* Gordon, J. L. (ed.): Vascular Endothelium: Interactions with Circulating Cells.

New York, Elsevier Science Publishers B. V., 1992, pp. 231–252.
15. Zimmerman, G. A., Prescott, S. M., and McIntyre, T. M.: Endothelial cell interactions with granulocytes: Tethering and signaling molecules. Immunol. Today 13:93, 1992.
16. Tauber, A. I., and Chernyak, L.: Metchnikoff's emerging concept of inflammation. *In* Metchnikoff and the Origins of Immunology. From Metaphor to Theory. New York, Oxford University Press, 1991, pp. 101–134.
17. Bevilacqua, M., Butcher, E., Furie, B., Gallatin, M., Gimbrone, M., Harlan, J., Kishimoto, K., Lasky, L., McEver, R., Paulson, J., Rosen, S., Seed, B., Siegelman, M., Springer, T., Stoolman, L., Tedder, T., Varki, A., Wagner, D., Weissman, I., and Zimmerman, G.: Selectins: A family of adhesion receptors. Cell 67:233, 1991.
18. McEver, R. P.: Selectins: Novel receptors that mediate leukocyte adhesion during inflammation. Thromb. Haemost. 65:223, 1991.
19. Springer, T. A.: Adhesion receptors of the immune system. Nature 346:425, 1990.
20. Albelda, S. M., and Buck, C. A.: Integrins and other cell adhesion molecules. FASEB J. 4:2868, 1990.
21. Larsen, E., Celi, A., Gilbert, G. E., Furie, B. C., Erban, J. K., Bonfanti, R., Wagner, D. D., and Furie, B.: PADGEM protein: A receptor that mediates the interaction of activated platelets with neutrophils and monocytes. Cell 59:305, 1989.
22. Spertini, O., Luscinskas, F. W., Kansas, G. S., Munro, J. M., Griffin, J. D., Gimbrone, M. A., Jr., and Tedder, T. F.: Leukocyte adhesion molecule–1 (LAM-1, L-selectin) interacts with an inducible endothelial cell ligand to support leukocyte adhesion. J. Immunol. 147:2565, 1991.
23. Spertini, O., Kansas, G. S., Munro, J. M., Griffin, J. D., and Tedder, T. F.: Regulation of leukocyte migration by activation of the leukocyte adhesion molecule–1 (LAM-1) selectin. Nature 349:691, 1991.
24. Watson, M. L., Kingsmore, S. F., Johnston, G. I., Siegelman, M. H., Le Beau, M. M., Lemons, R. S., Bora, N. S., Howard, T. A., Weissman, I. L., McEver, R. P., and Seldin, M. F.: Genomic organization of the selectin family of leukocyte adhesion molecules on human and mouse chromosome 1. J. Exp. Med. 172:263, 1990.
25. Springer, T. A., and Lasky, L. A.: Sticky sugars for selectins. Nature 349:196, 1991.
26. Jutila, M. A., Rott, L., Berg, E. L., and Butcher, E. C.: Function and regulation of the neutrophil MEL-14 antigen *in vivo*: Comparison with LFA-1 and MAC-1. J. Immunol. 143:3318, 1989.
27. Larsen, E., Palabrica, T., Sajer, S., Gilbert, G. E., Wagner, D. D., Furie, B. C., and Furie, B.: PADGEM-dependent adhe-

sion of platelets to monocytes and neutrophils is mediated by a lineage-specific carbohydrate, LNF III (CD15). Cell 63:467, 1990.

28. Phillips, J. L., Nudelman, E., Caeta, F. C. A., Perez, M., Singhal, A. K., Hakomori, S.-I., and Paulson, J. C.: ELAM-1 mediates cell adhesion by recognition of a carbohydrate ligand, Sialyl-Le^x. Science 250:1130, 1990.

29. Walz, G., Aruffo, A., Kolanus, W., Bevilacqua, M., and Seed, B.: Recognition by ELAM-1 of the Sialyl-Le^x determinant on myeloid and tumor cells. Science 250:1132, 1990.

30. Tyrrell, D., James, P., Rao, N., Foxall, C., Abbas, S., Dasgupta, F., Nashed, M., Hasegawa, A., Kiso, M., Asa, D., Kidd, J., and Brandley, B. K.: Structural requirements for the carbohydrate ligand of E-selectin. Proc. Natl. Acad. Sci. USA 88:10372, 1991.

31. Berg, E. L., Robinson, M. K., Mansson, O., Butcher, E. C., and Magnani, J. L.: A carbohydrate domain common to both sialyl Le^a and sialyl Le^x is recognized by the endothelial cell leukocyte adhesion molecule ELAM-1. J. Biol. Chem. 266:14869, 1991.

32. Handa, K., Nudelman, E. D., Stroud, M. R., Shiozawa, T., and Hakomori, S.: Selectin GMP-140 (CD62; PADGEM) binds to sialosyl-Le^a and sialosyl-Le^x, and sulfated glycans modulate this binding. Biochem. Biophys. Res. Commun. 181:1223, 1991.

33. Polley, M. J., Phillips, M. L., Wayner, E., Nudelman, E., Singhal, A. K., Hakomori, S.-I. and Paulson, J. C.: CD62 and endothelial cell–leukocyte adhesion molecule 1 (ELAM-1) recognize the same carbohydrate ligand, sialyl-Lewis X. Proc. Natl. Acad. Sci. USA 88:6224, 1991.

34. Aruffo, A., Kolanus, W., Walz, G., Fredman, P. and Seed, B.: CD62/P-selectin recognition of myeloid and tumor cell sulfatides. Cell 67:35, 1991.

35. Picker, L. J., Warnock, R. A., Burns, A. R., Doerschuk, C. M., Berg, E. L., and Butcher, E. C.: The neutrophil selectin LECAM-1 presents carbohydrate ligands to the vascular selectins ELAM-1 and GMP-140. Cell 66:921, 1991.

36. Zhou, Q., Moore, K. L., Smith, D. F., Varki, A., McEver, R. P., and Cummings, R. D.: The selectin GMP-140 binds to sialylated, fucosylated lactosaminoglycans on both myeloid and nonmyeloid cells. J. Cell Biol. 115:557, 1991.

37. Stoolman, L. M.: Adhesion molecules controlling lymphocyte migration. Cell 56:907, 1989.

38. Kishimoto, T. K., Jutila, M. A., Berg, E. L., and Butcher, E. C.: Neutrophil Mac-1 and MEL-14 adhesion proteins inversely regulated by chemotactic factors. Science 245:1238, 1989.

39. Bevilacqua, M. P., Stengelin, S., Gimbrone, M. A., Jr., and Seed, B.: Endothelial leukocyte adhesion molecule 1: An inducible receptor for neutrophils related to complement regulatory proteins and lectins. Science 243:1160, 1989.

40. Smith, C. W., Kishimoto, T. K., Abbass, O., Hughes, B., Rothlein, R., McIntire, L. V., Butcher, E., and Anderson, D. C.: Chemotactic factors regulate lectin adhesion molecule 1 (LECAM-1)–dependent neutrophil adhesion to cytokine-stimulated endothelial cells in vitro. J. Clin. Invest. 87:609, 1991.

41. Von Adrian, U. H., Chambers, J. D., McEvoy, L. M., Bargatze, R. F., Arfors, K.-E., and Butcher, E. C.: Two-step model of leukocyte–endothelial cell interaction in inflammation: Distinct roles for LECAM-1 and the leukocyte β_2 integrins in vivo. Proc. Natl. Acad. Sci. USA 88:7538, 1991.

42. Ley, K., Gaehtgens, P., Fennie, C., Singer, M. S., Lasky, L. A., and Rosen, S. D.: Lectin-like cell adhesion molecule 1 mediates leukocyte rolling in mesenteric venules in vivo. Blood 77:2553, 1991.

43. Etzioni, A., Frydman, M., Pollack, S., Avidor, I., Phillips, M. L., Paulson, J. C., and Gershoni-Baruch, R.: A syndrome of leukocyte adhesion deficiency (LAD II) due to deficiency of Sialyl-Lewis-X, a ligand for selectins. N. Engl. J. Med. 327:1789, 1992.

44. Larson, R. S., and Springer, T. A.: Structure and function of leukocyte integrins. Immunol. Rev. 114:181, 1990.

45. De Fougerolles, A. R., Stacker, S. A., Schwarting, R., and

Springer, T. A.: Characterization of ICAM-2 and evidence for a third counter-receptor for LFA-1. J. Exp. Med. 174:253, 1991.

46. Bevilacqua, M. P., Pober, J. S., Wheeler, M. E., Cotran, R. S., and Gimbrone, M. A., Jr.: Interleukin 1 acts on cultured human vascular endothelium to increase the adhesion of polymorphonuclear leukocytes, monocytes, and related leukocyte cell lines. J. Clin. Invest. 76:2003, 1985.

47. Pober, J. S., Gimbrone, M. A., Jr., Lapierre, L. A., Mendrick, D. L., Fiers, W., Rothlein, R., and Springer, T. A.: Overlapping patterns of activation of human endothelial cells by interleukin 1, tumor necrosis factor, and immune interferon. J. Immunol. 137:1893, 1986.

48. Hynes, R. O.: Integrins: Versatility, modulation, and signaling in cell adhesion. Cell 69:11, 1992.

49. Arnaout, M. A.: Structure and function of the leukocyte adhesion molecules CD11/CD18. Blood 75:1037, 1990.

50. Ruosahti, E.: Integrins. J. Clin. Invest. 87:1, 1991.

51. Kishimoto, T. K., O'Connor, K., Lee, A., Roberts, T. M., and Springer, T. A.: Cloning of the beta subunit of the leukocyte adhesion proteins: Homology to an extracellular matrix receptor defines a novel supergene family. Cell 48:681, 1987.

52. Law, S. K. A., Gagnon, J., Hildreth, J. E. F., Wells, C. E., Willis, A. C., and Wong, A. J.: The primary structure of the beta-subunit of the cell surface adhesion glycoproteins LFA-1, CR-3, and p150,95 and its relationship to the fibronectin receptor. EMBO J. 6:915, 1987.

53. Corbi, A. L., Garcia-Aguilar, J., and Springer, T. A.: Genomic structure of an integrin alpha subunit, the leukocyte p150,95 molecule (erratum JBC 265:12750, 1990). J. Biol. Chem. 265:2782, 1990.

54. Corbi, A. L., Kishimoto, T. K., Miller, L. J., and Springer, T. A.: The human leukocyte adhesion glycoprotein Mac-1 (Complement receptor type 3, CD11b) alpha subunit: Cloning, primary structure, and relation to the integrins, von Willebrand factor and factor B. J. Biol. Chem. 263:12403, 1988.

55. Corbi, A. L., Larson, R. S., Kishimoto, T. K., Springer, T. A., and Morton, C. C.: Chromosomal location of the genes encoding the leukocyte adhesion receptors LFA-1, Mac-1, and p150,95. Identification of a gene cluster involved in cell adhesion. J. Exp. Med. 167:1597, 1988.

56. Corbi, A. L., Miller, L. J., O'Connor, K., Larson, R. S., and Springer, T. A.: cDNA cloning and complete primary structure of the alpha subunit of a leukocyte adhesion glycoprotein, p150,95. EMBO J. 6:4023, 1987.

57. Larson, R. S., Corbi, A. L., Berman, L., and Springer, T. A.: Primary structure of the LFA-1 alpha subunit: An integrin with an embedded domain defining a protein superfamily. J. Cell Biol. 108:703, 1989.

58. Marlin, S. D., Morton, C. C., Anderson, D. C., and Springer, T. A.: LFA-1 immunodeficiency disease: Definition of the genetic defect and chromosomal mapping of alpha and beta subunits by complementation in hybrid cells. J. Exp. Med. 164:855, 1986.

59. Nathan, C., Srimal, S., Fraber, C., Sanchez, E., Kabbash, L., Asch, A., Gailit, J., and Wright, S. D.: Cytokine-induced respiratory burst of human neutrophils: Dependence on extracellular matrix proteins and CD11/CD18 integrins. J. Cell Biol. 109:1341, 1989.

60. Arnaout, M. A.: Leukocyte adhesion molecules deficiency: Its structural basis, pathophysiology and implications for modulating the inflammatory response. Immunol. Rev. 114: 145, 1990.

61. Chan, B. M. C., Kassner, P. D., Schiro, J. A., Byers, R., Kupper, T. S., and Hemler, M. E.: Distinct cellular functions mediated by different VLA integrin α subunit cytoplasmic domains. Cell 68:1051, 1992.

62. Arnaout, M. A., Remold-O'Donnell, E., Pierce, M. W., Harris, P., and Tenen, D. G.: Molecular cloning of the alpha subunit of human and guinea pig leukocyte adhesion glycoprotein Mo1: Chromosomal localization and homology to the alpha

subunits of integrins. Proc. Natl. Acad. Sci. USA 85:2776, 1988.

63. Nelson, C., Rabb, H., and Arnaout, M. A.: Genetic cause of leukocyte adhesion molecule deficiency. Abnormal splicing and a missense mutation in a conserved region of CD18 impair cell surface expression of β2 integrins. J. Biol. Chem. 267:3351, 1992.

64. Pardi, R., Inverardi, L., and Bender, J. R.: Regulatory mechanisms in leukocyte adhesion: Flexible receptors for sophisticated travelers. Immunol. Today 13:224, 1992.

65. Hibbs, M. L., Jakes, S., Stacker, S. A., Wallace, R. W., and Springer, T. A.: The cytoplasmic domain of the integrin lymphocyte function–associated antigen 1 β subunit: Sites required for binding to intercellular adhesion molecule 1 and the phorbol ester–stimulated phosphorylation site. J. Exp. Med. 174:1227, 1991.

66. Horwitz, A., Duggan, E., Buck, C., Beckerle, M. C., and Burridge, K.: Interaction of plasma membrane fibronectin receptor with talin—a transmembrane linkage. Nature 320:531, 1986.

67. Marcantonio, E. E., Guan, J. L., Trevithick, J. E., and Hynes, R. O.: Mapping of the functional determinants of the integrin β_1 cytoplasmic domain by site-directed mutagenesis. Cell Regul. 1:597, 1990.

68. Petrequin, P. R., Todd, R. F., III, Devall, L. J., Boxer, L. A., and Curnutte, J. T.: Association between gelatinase release and increased plasma membrane expression of the Mo1 glycoprotein. Blood 69:605, 1987.

69. Lo, S. K., Detmers, P. A., Levin, S. M., and Wright, S. D.: Transient adhesion of neutrophils to endothelium. J. Exp. Med. 169:1779, 1989.

70. Miller, L. J., Bainton, D. F., Borregaard, N., and Springer, T. A.: Stimulated mobilization of monocyte Mac-1 and p150,95 adhesion proteins from an intracellular vesicular compartment to the cell surface. J. Clin. Invest. 80:535, 1987.

71. Bainton, D. F., Miller, L. J., Kishimoto, T. K., and Springer, T. A.: Leukocyte adhesion receptors are stored in peroxidase-negative granules of human neutrophils. J. Exp. Med. 166:1641, 1987.

72. Altieri, D. C., and Edgington, T. S.: A monoclonal antibody reacting with distinct adhesion molecules defines a transition in the functional state of the receptor CD11b/CD18 (Mac-1). J. Immunol. 141:2656, 1988.

73. Hermanowski-Vosatka, A., Van Strijp, J. A. G., Swiggard, W. J., and Wright, S. D.: Integrin modulating factor–1: A lipid that alters the function of leukocyte integrins. Cell 68:341, 1992.

74. Unkeless, J. C., and Wright, S. D.: Phagocytic cells: Fc-gamma and complement receptors. In Gallin, J. I., Goldstein, I. M., and Snyderman, R. (eds.) Inflammation: Basic Principles and Clinical Correlates. New York, Raven Press, 1988, pp. 343–362.

75. Garcia, J. G. N.: Molecular mechanisms of thrombin-induced human and bovine endothelial cell activation. J. Lab. Clin. Med. 120:513, 1992.

76. Mulligan, M. S., Polley, M. J., Bayer, R. J., Nunn, M. F., Paulson, J. C., and Ward, P. A.: Neutrophil-dependent acute lung injury. Requirement for P-selectin (GMP-140). J. Clin. Invest. 90:1600, 1992.

77. Harlan, J. M.: Leukocyte-endothelial interactions. Blood 65:513, 1985.

78. Arfors, K. E., Lundberg, C., Lindborn, L., Lundberg, K., Beatty, P. G., and Harlan, J. M.: A monoclonal antibody to the membrane glycoprotein complex CD18 inhibits polymorphonuclear leukocyte accumulation and plasma leakage in vivo. Blood 69:338, 1987.

79. Smith, C. W., Rothlein, R., Hughes, B. J., Mariscalco, M. M., Rudloff, H. E., Schmalstieg, F. C., and Anderson, D. C.: Recognition of an endothelial determinant for CD18-dependent human neutrophil adherence and transendothelial migration. J. Clin. Invest. 82:1746, 1988.

80. Dohlman, H. G., Thorner, J., Caron, M. G., and Lefkowitz, R. J.: Model systems for the study of seven-transmembrane-segment receptors. Annu. Rev. Biochem. 60:653, 1991.

81. Baggiolini, M., Dewald, B., and Walz, A.: Interleukin-8 and related chemotactic cytokines. In Gallin, J. I., Goldstein, I. M., and Snyderman, R. (eds.) Inflammation: Basic Principles and Clinical Correlates. New York, Raven Press 1992, pp 247–263.

82. Baggiolini, M., and Clark-Lewis, I.: Interleukin-8, a chemotactic and inflammatory cytokine. FEBS Lett. 307:97, 1992.

83. Kunz, D., Gerard, N. P., and Gerard, C.: The human leukocyte platelet-activating factor receptor. cDNA cloning, cell surface expression, and construction of a novel epitope-bearing analog. J. Biol. Chem. 267:9101, 1992.

84. Nakamura, M., Honda, Z., Izumi, T., Sakanaka, C., Mutoh, H., Minami, M., Bito, H., Seyama, Y., Matsumoto, T., Noma, M., and Shimizu, T.: Molecular cloning and expression of platelet-activating factor receptor from human leukocytes. J. Biol. Chem. 266:20400, 1991.

85. Ye, R. D., Prossnitz, E. R., Zou, A., and Cochrane, C. G.: Characterization of a human cDNA that encodes a functional receptor for platelet activating factor. Biochem. Biophys. Res. Commun. 180:105, 1991.

86. Walz, A., and Baggiolini, M.: Generation of the neutrophil-activating peptide NAP-2 from platelet basic protein or connective tissue–activating peptide III through monocyte proteases. J. Exp. Med. 171:449, 1990.

87. Honda, Z., Nakamura, M., Miki, I., Minami, M., Watanabe, T., Seyama, Y., Okado, H., Toh, H., Ito, K., Miyamoto, T., and Shimizu, T.: Cloning by functional expression of platelet-activating factor receptor from guinea-pig lung. Nature 349:342, 1991.

88. Rola-Pleszczynski, M.: LTB_4 and PAF in the cytokine network. Adv. Exp. Med. Biol. 314:205, 1991.

89. Bussolino, F., Sironi, M., Bocchietto, E., and Mantovani, A.: Synthesis of platelet-activating factor by polymorphonuclear neutrophils stimulated with interleukin-8. J. Biol. Chem. 267:14598, 1992.

90. Ford-Hutchinson, A. W.: Leukotriene B_4 in inflammation. Crit. Rev. Immunol. 10:1, 1990.

91. Murphy, P. M., and Tiffany, H. L.: Cloning of complementary DNA encoding a functional human interleukin-8 receptor. Science 253:1280: 1991.

92. Holmes, W. E., Lee, J., Kuang, W.-J., Rice, G. C., and Wood, W. I.: Structure and functional expression of a human interleukin-8 receptor. Science 253:1278, 1991.

93. Peveri, P., Walz, A., Dewald, B., and Baggiolini, M.: A novel neutrophil-activating factor produced by human mononuclear phagocytes. J. Exp. Med. 167:1547, 1988.

94. Thomas, K. M., Taylor, L., and Navarro, J.: The interleukin-8 receptor is encoded by a neutrophil-specific cDNA clone, F3R. J. Biol. Chem. 266:14839, 1991.

95. Moser, B., Schumacher, C., von Tscharner, V., Clark-Lewis, I., and Baggiolini, M.: Neutrophil-activating peptide 2 and gro/melanoma growth-stimulatory activity interact with neutrophil-activating peptide 1/interleukin 8 receptors on human neutrophils. J. Biol. Chem. 266:10666, 1991.

96. Walz, A., Meloni, F., Clark-Lewis, I., von Tscharner, V., and Baggiolini, M.: [Ca2 +]i changes and respiratory burst in human neutrophils and monocytes induced by NAP-1/interleukin-8, NAP-2, and gro/MGSA. J. Leukoc. Biol. 50:279, 1991.

97. Haskill, S., Peace, A., Morris, J., Sporn, S. A. Anisowicz, A., Lee, S. W., Smith, T., Martin, G., Ralph, P., and Sager, R.: Identification of three related human GRO genes encoding cytokine functions. Proc. Natl. Acad. Sci. USA 87:7732, 1990.

98. Leonard, E. J., Yoshimura, T., Rot, A., Noer, K., Walz, A., Baggiolini, M., Walz, D. A., Goetzl, E. J., and Castor, C. W.: Chemotactic activity and receptor binding of neutrophil attractant/activation protein–1 (NAP-1) and structurally related host defense cytokines: Interaction of NAP-2 with NAP-1 receptor. J. Leukoc. Biol. 49:258, 1991.

99. Zachariae, C. O., Anderson, A. O., Thompson, H. L., Appella, E., Mantovani, A., Oppenheim, J. J., and Matsushima, K.: Properties of monocyte chemotactic and activating factor

(MCAF) purified from a human fibrosarcoma cell line. J. Exp. Med. 171:2177, 1990.

100. Rollins, B. J., Walz, A., and Baggiolini, M.: Recombinant human MCP-1/JE induces chemotaxis, calcium flux, and the respiratory burst in human monocytes. Blood 78:1112, 1991.

101. Baggiolini, M., and Dewald, B.: Cytokine regulation of mononuclear phagoctye activation. Curr. Opin. Hematol. p. 133, 1993.

102. Schall, T. J., Bacon, K., Toy, K. J., and Goeddel, D. V.: Selective attraction of monocytes and T lymphocytes of the memory phenotype by cytokine RANTES. Nature 347:669, 1990.

103. Carp, H.: Mitochondrial N-formylmethionyl proteins as chemoattractants for neutrophils. J. Exp. Med. 155:264, 1982.

104. Boulay, F., Tardif, M., Brouchon, L., and Vignais, P.: The human N-formyl peptide receptor. Characterization of two cDNA isolates and evidence for a new subfamily of G-protein—coupled receptors. Biochemistry 29:11123, 1990.

105. Bao, L., Gerard, N. P., Eddy, R. L., Jr., Shows, T. B., and Gerard, C.:Mapping of genes for the human C5a receptor (C5AR), human FMLP receptor (FPR), and two FMLP receptor homologue orphan receptors (FPRH1, FPRH2) to chromosome 19. Genomics 13:437, 1992.

106. Boulay, F., Tardif, M., Brouchon, L., and Vignais, P.: Synthesis and use of a novel N-formyl peptide derivative to isolate a human N-formyl peptide receptor cDNA. Biochem. Biophys. Res. Commun. 168:1103, 1990.

107. Boulay, F., Mery, L., Tardif, M., Brouchon, L., and Vignais, P.: Expression cloning of a receptor for C5a anaphylatoxin on differentiated HL-60 cells. Biochemistry 30:2993, 1991.

108. Gerard, N. P., and Gerard, C.: The chemotactic receptor for human C5a anaphylatoxin. Nature 349:614, 1991.

109. Desrochers, P. E., Mookhtiar, K., Van Wart, H. E., Hasty, K. A., and Weiss, S. J.: Proteolytic inactivation of α_1-proteinase inhibitor and α_1-antichymotrypsin by oxidatively activated human neutrophil metalloproteinases. J. Biol. Chem. 267:5005, 1992.

110. Desrochers, P. E., Jeffrey, J. J., and Weiss, S. J.: Interstitial collagenase (matrix metalloproteinase–1) expresses serpinase activity. J. Clin. Invest. 87:2258, 1991.

111. Allen, R. A., Traynor, A. E., Omann, G. M., and Jesaitis, A. J.: The chemotactic peptide receptor: A model for future understanding of chemotactic disorders. In Curnutte, J. T. (ed.): Hematology/Oncology Clinics of North America. Phagocytic Defects I, Vol. 2. Philadelphia, W. B. Saunders, Co., 1988, pp. 33–59.

112. Didsbury, J. R., Uhing, R. J., Tomhave, E., Gerard, C., Gerard, N., and Snyderman, R.: Receptor class desensitization of leukocyte chemoattractant receptors. Proc. Natl. Acad. Sci. USA 88:11564, 1991.

113. Jesaitis, A. J., Bokoch, G. M., Tolley, J. O., and Allen, R. A.: Lateral segregation of neutrophil chemotactic receptors into actin- and fodrin-rich plasma membrane microdomains depleted in guanyl nucleotide regulatory proteins. J. Cell Biol. 107:921, 1988.

114. Gilman, A. G.: G proteins: Transducers of receptor-generated signals. Annu. Rev. Biochem. 56:615, 1987.

115. Kaziro, Y., Itoh, H., Kozasa, T., Nakafuku, M., and Satoh, T.: Structure and function of signal-transducing GTP-binding proteins. Annu. Rev. Biochem. 60:349, 1991.

116. Bourne, H. R., Sanders, D. A., and McCormick, F.: The GTPase superfamily: Conserved structure and molecular mechanism. Nature 349:117, 1991.

117. Berridge, M. J., and Irvine, R. F.: Inositol phosphates and cell signalling. Nature 341:197, 1989.

118. Camps, M., Hou, C., Sidiropoulos, D., Stock, J. B., Jakobs, K. H., and Gierschik, P.: Stimulation of phospholipase C by guanine-nucleotide—binding protein β gamma subunits. Eur. J. Biochem. 206:821, 1992.

119. English, D.: Involvement of phosphatidic acid, phosphatidate phosphohydrolase, and inositol-specific phospholipase D in neutrophil stimulus-response pathways. J. Lab. Clin. Med. 120:520, 1992.

120. Smolen, J. E.: Neutrophil signal transduction: Calcium, kinases, and fusion. J. Lab. Clin. Med. 120:527, 1992.

121. Dennis, E. A., Rhee, S. G., Billah, M. M., and Hannun, Y. A.: Role of phospholipases in generating lipid second messengers in signal transduction. FASEB J. 5:2068, 1991.

122. Serhan, C. N., Broekman, M. J., Korchak, H. M., Marcus, A. J., and Weissmann, G.: Endogenous phospholipid metabolism in stimulated neutrophils: Differential activation by FMLP and PMA. Biochem. Biophys. Res. Commun. 107:951, 1982.

123. Bradford, P. G., Wang, X., Jin, Y., and Hui, P.: Transcriptional regulation and increased functional expression of the inositol trisphosphate receptor in retinoic acid–treated HL-60 cells. J. Biol. Chem. 267:20959, 1992.

124. Nishizuka, Y.: The molecular heterogeneity of protein kinase C and its implications for cellular regulation. Nature 334:661, 1988.

125. Majumdar, S., Rossi, M. W., Fujiki, T., Phillips, W. A., Disa, S., Queen, C. F., Johnston, R. B., Jr., Rosen, O. M., Corkey, B. E., and Korchak, H. M.: Protein kinase C isotypes and signaling in neutrophils: Differential substrate specificities of a translocatable, calcium- and phospholipid-dependent beta-protein kinase C and a novel calcium-independent, phospholipid-dependent protein kinase which is inhibited by long chain fatty acyl coenzyme A. J. Biol. Chem. 266:9285, 1991.

126. Kanoh, H., Yamada, K., and Sakane, F.: Diacylglycerol kinase: A key modulator of signal transduction? TIBS 15:47, 1990.

127. Perry, D. K., Hand, W. L., Edmondson, D. E., and Lambeth, J. D.: Role of phospholipase D–derived diradylglycerol in the activation of the human neutrophil respiratory burst oxidase. J. Immunol. 149:2479, 1992.

128. Agwu, D. E., McPhail, L. C., Chabot, M. C., Daniel, L. W., Wykle, R. L., and McCall, C. E.: Choline-linked phosphoglycerides. A source of phosphatidic acid and diglycerides in stimulated neutrophils. J. Biol. Chem. 264:1405, 1989.

129. Wang, P., Anthes, J. C., Siegel, M. I., Egan, R. W., and Billah, M. M.: Existence of cytosolic phospholipase D. Identification and comparison with membrane-bound enzyme. J. Biol. Chem. 266:14877, 1991.

130. Billah, M. M., Eckel, S., Mullmann, T. J., Egan, R. W., and Siegel, M. I.: Phosphatidylcholine hydrolysis by phospholipase D determines phosphatidate and diglyceride levels in chemotactic peptide-stimulated human neutrophils. Involvement of phosphatidate phosphohydrolase in signal transduction. J. Biol. Chem. 264:17069, 1989.

131. Truett, A. P., III, Bocckino, S. B., and Murray, J. J.: Regulation of phosphatidic acid phosphohydrolase activity during stimulation of human polymorphonuclear leukocytes. FASEB J. 6:2720, 1992.

132. Reinhold, S. L., Prescott, S. M., Zimmerman, G. A., and McIntyre, T. M.:Activation of human neutrophil phospholipase D by three separable mechanisms. FASEB J. 4:208, 1990.

133. Mullmann, T. J., Siegel, M. I., Egan, R. W., and Billah, M. M.: Phorbol-12-myristate-13-acetate activation of phospholipase D in human neutrophils leads to the production of phosphatides and diglycerides. Biochem. Biophys. Res. Commun. 1707:1197, 1990.

134. Balsinde, J., Diez, E., and Mollinedo, F.: Arachidonic acid release from diacylglycerol in human neutrophils. Translation of diacylglycerol-deacylating enzyme activities from an intracellular pool to plasma membrane upon cell activation. J. Biol. Chem. 266:15638, 1991.

135. Balsinde, J., Diez, E., Schuller, A., and Mollinedo, F.: Phospholipase A_2 activity in resting and activated human neutrophils. Substrate specificity, pH dependence, and subcellular localization. J. Biol. Chem. 263:1929, 1988.

136. Walsh, C. E., Dechatelet, L. R., Chilton, F. H., Wykle, R. L., and Waite, M.: Mechanisms of arachidonic acid release in human polymorphonuclear leukocytes. Biochim. Biophys. Acta 750:32, 1983.

137. Badwey, J. A., Curnutte, J. T., Robinson, J. M., Berde, C. B., Karnovsky, M. J., and Karnovsky, M. L.: Effects of free

fatty acids on release of superoxide and on change of shape by human neutrophils: Reversibility by albumin. J. Biol. Chem. 259:7870, 1984.

138. Curnutte, J. T.: Activation of human neutrophil nicotinamide adenine dinucleotide phosphate, reduced (triphosphopyridine nucleotide, reduced) oxidase by arachidonic acid in a cell-free system. J. Clin. Invest. 75:1740, 1985.

139. Agwu, D. E., McPhail, L. C., Sozzani, S., Bass, D. A., and McCall, C. E.: Phosphatidic acid as a second messenger in human polymorphonuclear leukocytes. Effects on activation of NADPH oxidase. J. Clin. Invest. 88:531, 1991.

140. Peveri, P., and Curnutte, J. T.: Phosphatidic acid may be a physiologic activator of human neutrophil NADPH oxidase (abstract). Blood 76:190a, 1990.

141. Agwu, D. E., McPhail, L. C., Wykle, R. L., and McCall, C. E.: Mass determination of receptor-mediated accumulation of phosphatidate and diglycerides in human neutrophils measured by coomassie blue staining and densitometry. Biochem. Biophys. Res. Commun. 159:79, 1989.

142. Heyworth, P. G., and Badwey, J. A.: Protein phosphorylation associated with the stimulation of neutrophils. Modulation of superoxide production by protein kinase C and calcium. J. Bioenerg. Biomembr. 22:1, 1990.

143. Jacking, M. E. E., Lew, P., Carpentier, J. L., Magnusson, K. E., Sjorgren, M., and Stendahl, O.: Cytosolic free calcium elevation mediates the phagosome-lysosome fusion during phagocytosis in human neutrophils. J. Cell Biol. 110:1555, 1990.

144. Francis, J. W., Balazovich, K. J., Smolen, J. E., Margolis, D. I., and Boxer, L. A.: Human neutrophil annexin I promotes granule aggregation and modulates Ca^{2+}-dependent membrane fusion. J. Clin. Invest. 90:537, 1992.

145. Stossel, T. P.: From signal to pseudopod: How cells control cytoplasmic actin assembly. J. Biol. Chem. 264:18261, 1989.

146. Howard, T. H., Chaponnier, C., Yin, H., and Stossel T. P.: Gelsolin-actin interaction and actin polymerization in human neutrophils. J. Cell Biol. 110: 1983, 1990.

147. Ezekowitz, R. A., Sastry, K., Bailly, P., and Warner, A.: Molecular characterization of the human macrophage mannose receptor: Demonstration of multiple carbohydrate recognition-like domain and phagocytosis of yeasts in Cos-1 cells. J. Exp. Med. 172:1785, 1990.

148. Sastry, K., Zahedi, K., Lelias, J. M., Whitehead, A. S., and Ezekowitz, R. A.: Molecular characterization of the mouse mannose-binding proteins. The mannose-binding protein A but not C is an acute phase reactant. J. Immunol. 147:692, 1991.

149. Ezekowitz, R. A., Williams, D. J., Koziel, H., Armstrong, M. Y., Warner, A., Richards, F. F., and Rose, R. M.: Uptake of *Pneumocystis carinii* is mediated by the macrophage mannose receptor. Nature 351:155, 1991.

150. Krieger, M.: Molecular flypaper and atherosclerosis: Structure of the macrophage scavenger receptor. TIBS 17:141, 1992.

151. Unkeless, J. C.: Function and heterogeneity of human Fc receptors for immunoglobulin G. J. Clin. Invest. 83:355, 1989.

152. Ravetch, J. V., and Kinet, J.-P.:Fc receptors. Annu. Rev. Immunol. 9:457, 1991.

153. Brunkhorst, B. A., Strohmeier, G., Lazzari, K., Weil, G., Melnick, D., Fleit, H. B., and Simons, E. R.: Differential roles of Fc-gamma-RII and Fc-gamma-RIII in immune complex stimulation of human neutrophils. J. Biol. Chem. 267:20659, 1992.

154. Repp, R., Valerius, Th., Sendler, A., Gramatzki, M., Iro, H., Kalden, J. R., and Platzer, E.: Neutrophils express the high affinity receptor for IgG (Fc-gamma-RI, CD64) after *in vivo* application of recombinant human granulocyte colony-stimulating factor. Blood 78:885, 1991.

155. Selvaraj, P., Rosse, W. F., Silber, R., and Springer, T. A.: The major Fc receptor in blood has a phosphatidylinositol anchor and is deficient in paroxysmal nocturnal haemoglobinuria. Nature 333:565, 1988.

156. Klickstein, L. B., Wong, W. W., Smith, J. A., Weis, J. H., Wilson, J. G., and Fearon, D. T.: Human C3b/C4b receptor

(CR1). Demonstration of long homologous repeating domains that are composed of the short consensus repeats characteristic of C3/C4 binding proteins. J. Exp. Med. 165:1095, 1987.

157. Wong, W. W., Kennedy, C. A., Bonaccio, E. T., Wilson, J. G., Klickstein, L. B., Weis, J. H., and Fearon, D. T.: Analysis of multiple restriction fragment length polymorphisms of the gene for the human complement receptor type I. Duplication of genomic sequences occurs in association with a high molecular mass receptor allotype. J. Exp. Med. 164:1531, 1986.

158. Berger, M., Birx, D. L., Wetzler, E. M., O'Shea, J. J., Brown, E. J., and Cross, A. S.: Calcium requirements for increased complement receptor expression during neutrophil activation. J. Immunol. 135:1342, 1985.

159. Todd, R. F., III, Arnaout, M. A., Rosin, R. E., Crowley, C. A., Peters, W. A., and Babior, B. M.: Subcellular localization of the large subunit of Mo1 (Mo1 alpha; formerly gp 110), a surface glycoprotein associated with neutrophil adhesion. J. Clin. Invest. 74:1280, 1984.

160. Borregaard, N., Heiple, J. M., Simons, E. R., and Clark, R. A.: Subcellular localization of the *b*-cytochrome component of the human neutrophil microbicidal oxidase: Translocation during activation. J. Cell Biol 97:52, 1983

161. Boxer, L. A., and Smolen, J. E.: Neutrophil granule constituents and their release in health and disease. *In* Curnutte, J. T. (ed.): Hematology/Oncology Clinics of North America. Phagocytic Defects I, Vol. 2. Philadelphia, W. B. Saunders Co., 1988, pp. 101–134.

162. Lehrer, R. I., and Ganz, T.: Antimicrobial polypeptides of human neutrophils. Blood 76:2169, 1990.

163. Lehrer, R. I., Ganz, T., and Selsted, M. E.:Defensins: Endogenous antibiotic peptides of animal cells. Cell 64:229, 1991.

164. Klebanoff, S. J.: Myeloperoxidase–halide–hydrogen peroxide antibacterial system. J. Bacteriol. 95:2131, 1968.

165. Anderson, D. C., Smith, C. W., and Springer, T. A.: Leukocyte adhesion deficiency and other disorders of leukocyte motility. *In* Scriver, C. R., Beaudet, A. L., Sly, W. S., and Valle, D. (eds.): The Metabolic Basis of Inherited Disease. New York, McGraw-Hill, 1989, pp. 2751–2777.

166. Anderson, D. C., and Springer, T. A.: Leukocyte adhesion deficiency: An inherited defect in the Mac-1, LFA-1 and p150,95 glycoproteins. Annu. Rev. Med. 38:175, 1987.

167. Fischer, A., Lisowska-Grospierre, B., Anderson, D. C., and Springer, T. A.: Leukocyte adhesion deficiency: Molecular basis and functional consequences. Immunodef. Rev. 1:39, 1988.

168. Anderson, D. C., Schmalstieg, F. C., Finegold, M. J., Hughes, B. J., Rothlein, R., Miller, L. J., Kohl, S., Tosi, M. F., Jacobs, R. L., Waldrop, T. C., Goldman, A. S., Shearer, W. T., and Springer, T. A.: The severe and moderate phenotypes of heritable Mac-1, LFA-1 deficiency: Their quantitative definition and relation to leukocyte dysfunction and clinical features. J. Infect. Dis. 152:668, 1985.

169. Todd, R. F., III, and Freyer, D. R.: The CD11/CD18 leukocyte glycoprotein deficiency. *In* Curnutte, J. T. (ed.): Hematology/Oncology Clinics of North America. Phagocytic Defects I, Vol. 2. Philadelphia, W. B. Saunders Co., 1988, pp. 13–31.

170. Schmalstieg, F. C.: Leukocyte adherence defect. Pediatr. Infect. Dis. J. 7:867, 1988.

171. Crowley, C. A., Curnutte, J. T., Rosin, R. E., Andre-Schwartz, J., Gallin, J. I., Klempner, M., Snyderman, R., Southwick, F. S., Stossel, T. P., and Babior, B. M.: An inherited abnormality of neutrophil adhesion: Its genetic transmission and its association with a missing protein. N. Engl. J. Med. 302: 1163, 1980.

172. Arnaout, M. A., Pitt, J., Cohen, H. J., Melamed, J., Rosen, F. S., and Colten, H. R.: Deficiency of a granulocyte-membrane glycoprotein (gp150) in a boy with recurrent bacterial infections. N. Engl. J. Med. 306:693, 1982.

173. Bowen, T. J., Ochs, H. D., Altman, L. C., Price, T. H., Van Epps, D. E., Brautigan, D. L., Rosin, R. E., Perkins, W. D., Babior, B. M., Klebanoff, S. J., and Wedgwood, R. J.: Severe

recurrent bacterial infections associated with defective adherence and chemotaxis in two patients with neutrophils deficient in a cell-associated glycoprotein. J. Pediatr. 101: 932, 1982.

174. Springer, T. A., Thompson, W. S., Miller, L. J., and Anderson, D. C.: Inherited deficiency of the Mac-1, LFA-1, p150,95 glycoprotein family and its molecular basis. J. Exp. Med. 160:1901, 1984.

175. Hibbs, M. L., Wardlaw, A. J., Stacker, S. A., Anderson, D. C., Lee, A., Roberts, T. M., and Springer, T. A.: Transfection of cells from patients with leukocyte adhesion deficiency with an integrin β subunit (CD18) restores lymphocyte function–associated antigen-1 expression and function. J. Clin. Invest. 85:674, 1990.

176. Kishimoto, T. K., Hollander, N., Roberts, T. M., Anderson, D. C., and Springer, T. A.: Heterogenous mutations of the beta subunit common to the LFA-1, Mac-1, and p150,95 glycoproteins cause leukocyte adhesion deficiency. Cell 50:193, 1987.

177. Kishimoto, T. K., O'Connor, K., and Springer, T. A.: Leukocyte adhesion deficiency: Aberrant splicing of a conserved integrin sequence causes a moderate deficiency phenotype. J. Biol. Chem. 264:3588, 1989.

178. Wardlaw, A. J., Hibbs, M. L., Stacker, S. A., and Springer, T. A.: Distinct mutations in two patients with leukocyte adhesion deficiency and their functional correlates. J. Exp. Med. 172:335, 1990.

179. Arnaout, M. A., Dana, N., Gupta, S. K., Tenen, D. G., and Fathallah, D. M.: Point mutations impairing cell surface expression of the common β subunit (CD18) in a patient with leukocyte adhesion molecule (Leu-CAM) deficiency. J. Clin. Invest. 85:977, 1990.

180. Sligh, J. E., Jr., Hurwitz, M. Y., Zhu, C., Anderson, D. C., and Beaudet, A. L.: An initiation codon mutation in CD18 in association with the moderate phenotype of leukocyte adhesion deficiency. J. Biol. Chem. 267:714, 1992.

181. Back, A. L., and Hickstein, D. D.: Two different CD18 mutations in a child with severe leukocyte adhesion deficiency (LAD) (abstract). Blood 76:176a, 1990.

182. Buchanan, M. R., Crowley, C. A., Rosin, R. E., Gimbrone, M. A., and Babior, B. M.: Studies on the interaction between GP-180 deficient neutrophils and vascular endothelium. Blood 60:160, 1982.

183. Beller, D. I., Springer, T. A., and Schreiber, R. D.: Anti-Mac-1 selectively inhibits the mouse and human type three complement receptor. J. Exp. Med. 156:1000, 1982.

184. Anderson, D. C., Schmalstieg, F. C., Kohl, S., Arnaout, M. A., Tosi, M. F., Dana N., Buffone, G. J., Hughes, B. J., Brinkley, B. R., Dickey, W. D., Abramson, J. S., Springer, T., Boxer, L. A., Hollers, J. M., and Smith, C. W.: Abnormalities of polymorphonuclear leukocyte function associated with a heritable deficiency of high molecular weight surface glycoproteins (GP138): Common relationship to diminished cell adherence. J. Clin. Invest. 74:563, 1984.

185. Kohl, S., Springer, T. A., Schmalstieg, F. C., Loo, L. S., and Anderson, D. C.: Defective natural killer cytotoxicity and polymorphonuclear leukocyte antibody-dependent cellular cytotoxicity in patients with LFA-1/OKM-1 deficiency. J. Immunol. 133:2972, 1984.

186. Kohl, S., Loo, L. S., Schmalstieg, F. C., and Anderson, D. C.: The genetic deficiency of leukocyte surface glycoprotein Mac-1, LFA-1, p150,95 in humans is associated with defective antibody-dependent cellular cytotoxicity in vitro and defective protection against herpes simplex virus infection in vivo. J. Immunol. 137:1688, 1986.

187. Krensky, A. M., Sanchez-Madrid, F., Robbins, E., Nagy, J. A., Springer, T. A., and Burakoff, S. J.: The functional significance, distribution, and structure of LFA-1, LFA-2, LFA-3: Cell surface antigens associated with CTL-target interactions. J. Immunol. 131:611, 1983.

188. Weisman, S. J., Berkow, R. L., Plautz, G., Torres, M., McGuire, W. A., Coates, T. D., Haak, R. A., Floyd, A., Jersild, R., and Baehner, R. L.: Glycoprotein-180 deficiency: Genetics and abnormal neutrophil activation. Blood 65:696, 1985.

189. Fischer, A., Descamps-Latscha, B., Gerota, I., Scheinmetzler, C., Virelizier, J. L., Trung, P. H., Lisowska-Grospierre, B., Perez, N., Durandy, A., and Griscelli, C.: Bone marrow transplantation for inborn error of phagocytic cells associated with defective adherence, chemotaxis and oxidative response during opsonized particle phagocytosis. Lancet 2:473, 1983.

190. Nunoi, H., Yanabe, Y., Higuchi, S., Tsuchiya, H., Yamamoto, J., Matsuda, I., Naito, M., Takahashi, K., Fujita, K., Uchida, M., Kobayashi, K., Jono, J., and Malech, H.: Severe hypoplasia of lymphoid tissues in Mo1 deficiency. Hum. Pathol. 19:753, 1988.

191. Renshaw, H. W., and Davis, W. C.: Canine granulocytopathy syndrome: An inherited disorder of leukocyte function. Am. J. Pathol. 95:731, 1979.

192. Giger, U., Boxer, L. A., Simpson, P. J., Lucchesi, B. R., and Todd, R. F., III: Deficiency of leukocyte surface glycoproteins Mo1, LFA-1, and Leu M5 in a dog with recurrent bacterial infections: An animal model. Blood 69:1622, 1987.

193. Hagemoser, W. A., Roth, J. A., Lofstedt, J., and Fagerland, J. A.: Granulocytopathy in a Holstein heifer. J. Am. Vet. Med. Assoc. 183:1093, 1983.

194. Kehrli, M. E., Schmalstieg, F. C., Anderson, D. C., Van Der Maaten, M. J., Hughes, B. J., Ackerman, M. R., Wilhelmsen, C. L., Brown, G. B., Stevens, M. G., and Whetstone, C. A.: Molecular definition of the bovine granulocytopathy syndrome: Identification of deficiency of the Mac-1 (CD11b/CD18) glycoprotein. Am. J. Vet. Res. 51:1826, 1990.

195. Kehrli, M. E., Ackermann, M. R., Shuster, D. E., Van Der Maaten, M. J., Schmalstieg, F. C., Anderson, D. C., and Hughes, B. J.: Animal model of human disease. Bovine leukocyte adhesion deficiency. β2 integrin deficiency in young Holstein cattle. Am. J. Pathol. 140:1489, 1992.

196. Weisman, S. J., Mahoney, M. J., Anderson, D. C., Krause, P. J., and Grannum, P. A.: Prenatal diagnosis for Mo1 (CDw18) deficiency (abstract). Clin. Res. 35:435a, 1987.

197. Le Deist, F., Blanche, S., Keable, H., Gaud, C., Pham, H., Descamp-Latscha, B., Wahn, V., Griscelli, C., and Fischer, A.: Successful HLA nonidentical bone marrow transplantation in three patients with the leukocyte adhesion deficiency. Blood 74:512, 1989.

198. Camitta, B. M., Quesenberry, P. J., Parkman, R., Boxer, L. A., Stossel, T. P., Cassady, J. R., Rappeport, J. M., and Nathan, D. G.: Bone marrow transplantation for an infant with neutrophil dysfunction. Exp. Hematol. 5:109, 1977.

199. Back, A. L., Kwok, W. W., Adam, M., Collins, S. J., and Hickstein, D. D.: Retroviral-mediated gene transfer of the leukocyte integrin CD18 subunit. Biochem. Biophys. Res. Commun. 171:787, 1990.

200. Wilson, J. M., Ping, A. J., Krauss, J. C., Mayo-Bond, L., Rogers, C. E., Anderson, D. C., and Todd, R. F., III: Correction of CD18-deficient lymphocytes by retrovirus-mediated gene transfer. Science 248:1413, 1990.

201. Boxer, L. A., Hedley-Whyte, E. T., and Stossel, T. P.: Neutrophil actin dysfunction and abnormal neutrophil behavior. N. Engl. J. Med. 291:1093, 1974.

202. Southwick, F. S., Dabiri, G. A., and Stossel, T. P.: Neutrophil actin dysfunction is a genetic disorder associated with partial impairment of neutrophil actin assembly in three family members. J. Clin. Invest. 82:1525, 1988.

203. Southwick, F. S., Howard, T. H., Holbrook, T., Anderson, D. C., Stossel, T. P., and Arnaout, M. A.: The relationship between CR3 deficiency and neutrophil actin assembly. Blood 73:1973, 1989.

204. Curnutte, J. T., and Babior, B. M.: Chronic granulomatous disease. In Harris, H., and Hirschhorn, K. (eds.): Advances in Human Genetics. New York, Plenum Publishing Corporation, 1987, pp. 229–297.

205. Cross, A. R., and Jones, O. T. G.: Enzymic mechanisms of superoxide production. Biochim. Biophys. Acta 1057:281, 1991.

206. Segal, A. W.: The electron transport chain of the microbicidal oxidase of phagocytic cells and its involvement in the molec-

ular pathology of chronic granulomatous disease. J. Clin. Invest. 83:1785, 1989.

207. Smith, R. M., and Curnutte, J. T.: Molecular basis of chronic granulomatous disease. Blood 77:673, 1991.

208. Curnutte, J. T.: Molecular basis of the autosomal recessive forms of chronic granulomatous disease. Immunodef. Rev. 3:149, 1992.

209. Halliwell, B.: Reactive oxygen species in living systems: Source, biochemistry, and role in human disease. Am. J. Med. 91 (Suppl 3) 14s, 1991.

210. Bast, A., Haenen, G. R. M. M., and Doelman, C. J. A.: Oxidants and antioxidants: State of the art. Am. J. Med. 91(Suppl 3): 2s, 1991.

211. Spitznagel, J. K.: Antibiotic proteins of human neutrophils. J. Clin. Invest. 86:1381, 1990.

212. Lehrer, R. I., Ganz, T., Selsted, M. E., Babior, B. M., and Curnutte, J. T.: Neutrophils and host defense. Ann. Intern. Med. 109:127, 1988.

213. Ambruso, D. R., and Johnston, R. B., Jr.: Lactoferrin enhances hydroxyl radical production by human neutrophils, neutrophil particulate fractions, and an enzymatic generating system. J. Clin. Invest. 67:352, 1981.

214. Cochrane, C. G.: Cellular injury by oxidants. Am. J. Med. 91(Suppl 3): 23s, 1991.

215. Ohno, Y. I., Hirai, K. I., Kanoh, T., Uchino, H., and Ogawa, K.: Subcellular localization of hydrogen peroxide production in human polymorphonuclear leukocytes stimulated with lectins, phorbol myristate acetate, and digitonin: An electron microscope study using $CeCl_3$. Blood 60:1195, 1982.

216. Sadler, K. L., and Badwey, J. A.: Second messengers involved in superoxide production by neutrophils: Function and metabolism. In Curnutte, J. T. (ed.): Hematology/Oncology Clinics of North America. Phagocytic Defects II, Vol. 2. Philadelphia, W. B. Saunders Co., 1988, pp. 185–200.

217. Bemiller, L. S., Rost, J. R., Ku-Balai, T. L., and Curnutte, J. T.: The production of intracellular oxidants by stimulated neutrophils correlates with the clinical severity of chronic granulomatous disease (CGD) (abstract). Blood 78:377a, 1991.

218. Nauseef, W. M.: Myeloperoxidase deficiency. In Curnutte, J. T. (ed.): Hematology/Oncology Clinics of North America. Phagocytic Defects I, Vol. 2. Philadelphia, W. B. Saunders Co., 1988, pp. 135–143.

219. Nauseef, W. M.: Aberrant restriction endonuclease digests of DNA from subjects with hereditary myeloperoxidase deficiency. Blood 73:290, 1989.

220. Tobler, A., Selsted, M. E., Miller, C. W., Johnson, K. R., Novotny, M. J., Rovera, G., and Koeffler, H. P.: Evidence for a pretranslational defect in hereditary and acquired myeloperoxidase deficiency. Blood 73:1980, 1989.

221. Roos, D., Weening, R. S., Voetman, A. A., van Schaik, M. L. J., Bot, A. A. M., Meerhof, L. J., and Loos, J. A.: Protection of phagocytic leukocytes by endogenous glutathione: Studies in a family with glutathione reductase deficiency. Blood 53:851, 1979.

222. Spielberg, S. P., Garrick, M. D., Corash, L. M., Butler, J. D., Tietze, F., Rogers, L., and Schulman, J. D.: Biochemical heterogeneity in glutathione synthetase deficiency. J. Clin. Invest. 61:1417, 1978.

223. Whitin, J. C., and Cohen, H. J.:Disorders of respiratory burst termination. In Curnutte, J. T. (ed.): Hematology/Oncology Clinics of North America. Phagocytic Defects II, Vol. 2. Philadelphia, W. B. Saunders Co., 1988, pp. 289–299.

224. Blume, R. S., and Wolff, S. M.: The Chédiak-Higashi syndrome: Studies in four patients and a review of the literature. Medicine (Baltimore) 51:247, 1972.

225. Wolff, S. M., Dale, D. C., Clark, R. A., Root, R. K., and Kimball, H. R.: The Chédiak-Higashi syndrome: Studies of host defenses. Ann. Intern. Med. 76:293, 1972.

226. Witkop, C. J., Jr., Quevedo, W. C., Jr., Fitzpatrick, T. B., and King, R. A.: Albinism. In Scriver, C. R., Beaudet, A. L., Sly, W. S., and Valle, D. (eds.): The Metabolic Basis of Inherited Disease. New York, McGraw-Hill, 1989, pp. 2905–2947.

227. Ganz, T., Metcalf, J. A., Gallin, J. I., Boxer, L. A., and Lehrer, R. I.: Microbicidal/cytotoxic proteins of neutrophils are deficient in two disorders: Chédiak-Higashi syndrome and "specific" granule deficiency. J. Clin. Invest. 82:552, 1988.

228. Gallin, J. I.: Neutrophil specific granule deficiency. Annu. Rev. Med. 36:263, 1985.

229. Boxer, L. A., Coates, T. D., Haak, R. A., Wolach, J. B., Hoffstein, S., and Baehner, R. L.: Lactoferrin deficiency associated with altered granulocyte function. N. Engl. J. Med. 307:404, 1982.

230. Lomax, K. J., Gallin, J. I., Rotrosen, D., Raphael, G. D., Kaliner, M. A., Benz, E. J., Jr., Boxer, L. A., and Malech, H. L.: Selective defect in myeloid cell lactoferrin gene expression in neutrophil specific granule deficiency. J. Clin. Invest. 83:514, 1989.

231. Baldridge, C. W., and Gerard, R. W.: The extra respiration of phagocytosis. Am. J. Physiol. 103:235, 1933.

232. Sbarra, A. J., and Karnovsky, M. L.: The biochemical basis of phagocytosis. I. Metabolic changes during the ingestion of particles by polymorphonuclear leukocytes. J. Biol. Chem. 234:1355, 1959.

233. Babior, B. M.: Oxygen-dependent microbial killing by phagocytes. N. Engl. J. Med. 298:659, 1978.

234. Babior, B. M., Kipnes, R. S., and Curnutte, J. T.: Biological defense mechanisms: The production by leukocytes of superoxide, a potential bactericidal agent. J. Clin. Invest. 52:741, 1973.

235. Berendes, H., Bridges, R. A., and Good, R. A.: Fatal granulomatosus of childhood: Clinical study of new syndrome. Minn. Med. 40:309, 1957.

236. Landing, B. H., and Shirkey, H. S.: Syndrome of recurrent infection and infiltration of viscera by pigmented lipid histiocytes. Pediatrics 20:431, 1957.

237. Quie, P. G., White, J. G., Holmes, B., and Good R. A.: In vitro bactericidal capacity of human polymorphonuclear leukocytes: Diminished activity in chronic granulomatous disease of childhood. J. Clin. Invest. 46:668, 1967.

238. Curnutte, J. T., Whitten, D. M., and Babior, B. M.: Defective superoxide production by granulocytes from patients with chronic granulomatous disease. N. Engl. J. Med. 290:593, 1974.

239. Azimi, P. H., Bodenbender, J. G., Hintz, R. L., and Kontras, S. B.: Chronic granulomatous disease in three female siblings. JAMA 206:2865, 1968.

240. Hamers, M. N., de Boer, M., Meerhof, L. J., Weening, R. S., and Roos, D.: Complementation in monocyte hybrids revealing genetic heterogeneity in chronic granulomatous disease. Nature 307:553, 1984.

241. Weening, R. S., Corbeel, L., de Boer, M., Lutter, R., van Zwieten, R., Hamers, M. N., and Roos, D.: Cytochrome b deficiency in an autosomal form of chronic granulomatous disease. A third form of chronic granulomatous disease recognized by monocyte hybridization. J. Clin. Invest. 75:915, 1985.

242. Segal, A. W.: Absence of both cytochrome b_{-245} subunits from neutrophils in X-linked chronic granulomatous disease. Nature 326:88, 1987.

243. Parkos, C. A., Allen, R. A., Cochrane, C. G., and Jesaitis, A. J.: Purified cytochrome b from human granulocyte plasma membrane is comprised of two polypeptides with relative molecular weights of 91,000 and 22,000. J. Clin. Invest. 80:732, 1987.

244. Volpp, B. D., Nauseef, W. M., and Clark, R. A.: Two cytosolic neutrophil oxidase components absent in autosomal chronic granulomatous disease. Science 242:1295, 1988.

245. Nunoi, H., Rotrosen, D., Gallin, J. I., and Malech, H. L.: Two forms of autosomal chronic granulomatous disease lack distinct neutrophil cytosol factors. Science 242:1298, 1988.

246. Curnutte, J. T., Scott, P. J., and Mayo, L. A.: Cytosolic components of the respiratory burst oxidase: Resolution of four components, two of which are missing in complementing types of chronic granulomatous disease. Proc. Natl. Acad. Sci. USA 86:825, 1989.

247. Clark, R. A., Volpp, B. D., Leidal, K. G., and Nauseef, W. M.: Two cytosolic components of the human neutrophil respiratory burst oxidase translocate to the plasma membrane during cell activation. J. Clin. Invest. 85:714, 1990.

248. Heyworth, P. G., Curnutte, J. T., Rosen, H., Nauseef, W. M., Volpp, B. D., Pearson, D. W., and Clark, R. A.: Neutrophil nicotinamide adenine dinucleotide phosphate oxidase assembly. Translocation of p47-*phox* and p67-*phox* requires interaction between p47-*phox* and cytochrome b_{558}. J. Clin. Invest. 87:352, 1991.

249. Cross, A. R., Jones, O. T. G., Garcia, R., and Segal, A. W.: The association of FAD with the cytochrome b_{-245} of human neutrophils. Biochem. J. 208:759, 1982.

250. Gabig, T. G.: The NADPH-dependent O_2-generating oxidase from human neutrophils. Identification of a flavoprotein component that is deficient in a patient with chronic granulomatous disease. J. Biol. Chem. 258:6352, 1983.

251. Rotrosen, D., Yeung, C. L., Leto, T. L., Malech, H. L., and Kwong, C. H.: Cytochrome b_{558}. The flavin-binding component of the phagocyte NADPH oxidase. Science 256:1459, 1992.

252. Segal, A. W., West, I., Wientjes, F., Nugent, J. H. A., Chavan, A. J., Haley, B., Garcia, R. D., Rosen, H., and Scrace, G.: Cytochrome b_{-245} is a flavocytochrome containing FAD and the NADPH-binding site of the microbicidal oxidase of phagocytes. Biochem. J. 284:781, 1992.

253. Abo, A., Pick, E., Hall, A., Totty, N., Teahan, C. G., and Segal, A. W.: Activation of the NADPH oxidase involves the small GTP-binding protein $p21^{rac1}$. Nature 353:668, 1991.

254. Knaus, U. G., Heyworth, P. G., Evans, T., Curnutte, J. T., and Bokoch, G. M.: Regulation of phagocyte oxygen radical production by the GTP-binding protein Rac 2. Science 254:1512, 1991.

255. Eklund, E. A., Marshall, M., Gibbs, J. B., Crean, C. D., and Gabig, T. G.: Resolution of a low molecular weight G protein in neutrophil cytosol required for NADPH oxidase activation and reconstitution by recombinant Krev-1 protein. J. Biol. Chem. 266:13964, 1991.

256. Quinn, M. T., Parkos, C. A., Walker, L., Orkin, S. H., Dinauer, M. C., and Jesaitis, A. J.: Association of a Ras-related protein with cytochrome b of human neutrophils. Nature 342:198, 1989.

257. Hattori, H.: Studies on the labile, stable NADI oxidase and peroxidase staining reactions in the isolated particles of horse granulocyte. Nagoya J. Med. Sci. 23:362, 1961.

258. Segal, A. W., and Jones, O. T.: Novel cytochrome b system in phagocytic vacuoles of human granulocytes. Nature 30:515, 1978.

259. Segal, A. W., Garcia, R., Goldstone, A. H., Cross, A. R., and Jones, O. T. G.: Cytochrome b_{-245} of neutrophils is also present in human monocytes, macrophages, and eosinophils. Biochem. J. 196:363, 1981.

260. Cross, A. R., Jones, O. T. G., Harper, A. M., and Segal, A. W.: Oxidation-reduction properties of the cytochrome b found in the plasma-membrane fraction of human neutrophils. Biochem. J. 194:599, 1981.

261. Segal, A. W., Cross, A. R., Garcia, R. C., Borregaard, N., Valerius, N., Soothill, J. F., and Jones, O. T. G.: Absence of cytochrome b_{-245} in chronic granulomatous disease: A multicenter European evaluation of its incidence and relevance. N. Engl. J. Med. 308:245, 1983.

262. Borregaard, N., Staehr-Johansen, K., Taudorff, E., and Wandall, J. H.: Cytochrome b is present in neutrophils from patients with chronic granulomatous disease. Lancet 1:949, 1979.

263. Ohno, Y., Buescher, E. S., Roberts, R., Metcalf, J. A., and Gallin, J. I.: Reevaluation of cytochrome b and flavin adenine dinucleotide in neutrophils from patients with chronic granulomatous disease and description of a family with probable autosomal recessive inheritance of cytochrome b deficiency. Blood 67:1132, 1986.

264. Curnutte, J. T., Kuver, R., and Scott, P. J.: Activation of neutrophil NADPH oxidase in a cell-free system. Partial purification of components and characterization of the activation process. J. Biol. Chem. 262:5563, 1987.

265. Baehner, R. L., Kunkel, L. M., Monaco, A. P., Haines, J. L., Conneally, P. M., Palmer, C., Heerema, N., and Orkin, S. H.: DNA linkage analysis of X chromosome–linked chronic granulomatous disease. Proc. Natl. Acad. Sci. USA 83:3398, 1986.

266. Royer-Pokora, B., Kunkel, L. M., Monaco, A. P., Goff, S. C., Newburger, P. E., Baehner, R. L., Cole, F. S., Curnutte, J. T., and Orkin, S. H.: Cloning the gene for an inherited human disorder—chronic granulomatous disease—on the basis of its chromosomal location. Nature 322:32, 1986.

267. Dinauer, M. C., Orkin, S. H., Brown, R., Jesaitis, A. J., and Parkos, C. A.: The glycoprotein encoded by the X-linked chronic granulomatous disease locus is a component of the neutrophil cytochrome b complex. Nature 327:717, 1987.

268. Darras, B. T.: Molecular genetics of Duchenne and Becker muscular dystrophy. J. Pediatr. 117:1: 1990.

269. Marchuk, D. A., Saulino, A. M., Tavakkol, R., Swaroop, M., Wallace, M. R., Andersen, L. B., Mitchell, A. L., Gutmann, D. H., Boguski, M., and Collins, F.S.: cDNA cloning of the type 1 neurofibromatosis gene: Complete sequence of the NF1 gene product. Genomics 11:931, 1991.

270. Gutmann, D. H., and Collins, F. S.: Recent progress toward understanding the molecular biology of von Recklinghausen neurofibromatosis. Ann. Neurol. 31:555, 1992.

271. Rommens, J. M., Iannuzzi, M. C., Kerem, B.-S., Drumm, M. L., Melmer, G., Dean, M., Rozmahel, R., Cole, J. L., Kennedy, D., Hidaka, N., Zsiga, M., Buchwald, M., Riordan, J. R., Tsui, L.-C., and Collins, F. S.: Identification of the cystic fibrosis gene: Chromosome walking and jumping. Science 245:1059, 1989.

272. Riordan, J. R., Rommens, J. M., Kerem, B.-S., Alon, N., Rozmahel, R., Grzelczak, Z., Zielensi, J., Lok, S., Plavsic, N., Chou J.-L., Drumm, M. L., Iannuzzi, M. C., Collins, F. S., and Tsui, L.-C.: Identification of the cystic fibrosis gene: Cloning and characterization of complementary DNA. Science 245: 1066, 1989.

273. Kerem, B.-S., Rommens, J. M., Buchanan, J. A., Markiewicz, D., Cox, R. K., Chakravarti, A., Buchwald, M., and Tsui, L.-C.: Identification of the cystic fibrosis gene: Genetic analysis. Science 245:1073, 1989.

274. Teahan, C., Rowe, P., Parker, P., Totty, N., and Segal, A. W.: The X-linked chronic granulomatous disease gene codes for the beta-chain of cytochrome b-245. Nature 327:720, 1987.

275. Dinauer, M. C., Pierce, E. A., Bruns, G. A. P., Curnutte, J. T., and Orkin, S. H.: Human neutrophil cytochrome b light chain (p22-*phox*): Gene structure, chromosomal location, and mutations in cytochrome-negative autosomal recessive chronic granulomatous disease. J. Clin. Invest. 86:1729, 1990.

276. Volkman, D. J., Buescher, E. S., Gallin, J. I., and Fauci, A. S.: B cell lines as models for inherited phagocytic diseases: Abnormal superoxide generation in chronic granulomatous disease and giant granules in Chédiak-Higashi syndrome. J. Immunol. 133:3006, 1984.

277. Maly, F. E., Cross, A. R., Jones, O. T. G., Wolf-Vorbeck, G., Walker, C., Dahinden, C. A., and DeWeck, A. L.: The superoxide generating system of B cell lines: Structural homology with the phagocytic oxidase and triggering via surface Ig. J. Immunol. 140:2334, 1988.

278. Radeke, H. H., Cross, A. R., Hancock, J. T., Jones, O. T. G., Nakamura, M., Kaever, V., and Resch, K.: Functional expression of NADPH oxidase components (alpha and beta subunits of cytochrome b_{558} and 45-kDa flavoprotein) by intrinsic human glomerular mesangial cells. J. Biol. Chem. 266: 21025, 1991.

279. Parkos, C. A., Dinauer, M. C., Walker, L. E., Allen, R. A., Jesaitis, A. J., and Orkin, S. H.: Primary structure and unique expression of the 22-kilodalton light chain of human neutrophil cytochrome b. Proc. Natl. Acad. Sci. USA 85:3319, 1988.

280. Parkos, C. A., Dinauer, M. C., Jesaitis, A. J., Orkin, S. H., and

Curnutte, J. T.: Absence of both the 91kD and 22kD subunits of human neutrophil cytochrome *b* in two genetic forms of chronic granulomatous disease. Blood 73:1416, 1989.

281. Minami, Y., Weissman, A. M., Samelson, L. E., and Klausner, R. D.: Building a multichain receptor: Synthesis, degradation, and assembly of the T-cell antigen receptor. Proc. Natl. Acad. Sci. USA 84:2688, 1987.

282. Jesaitis, A. J., Buescher, E. S., Harrison, D., Quinn, M. T., Parkos, C. A., Livesey, S., and Linner, J.: Ultrastructural localization of cytochrome *b* in the membranes of resting and phagocytosing human granulocytes. J. Clin. Invest 85:821, 1990.

283. Parkos, C. A., Allen, R. A., Cochrane, C. G., and Jesaitis, A. J.: The quaternary structure of the plasma membrane b-type cytochrome of human granulocytes. Biochim. Biophys. Acta 932:71, 1988.

284. Orkin, S. H.: Molecular genetics of chronic granulomatous disease. Annu. Rev. Immunol. 7:277, 1989.

285. Quinn, M. T., Mullen, J. L., and Jesaitis, A. J.: Human neutrophil cytochrome *b* contains multiple hemes. Evidence for heme associated with both subunits. J. Biol. Chem. 267:7303, 1992.

286. Hurst, J. K., Loehr, T. M., Curnutte, J. T., and Rosen, H.: Resonance Raman and electron paramagnetic resonance structural investigations of neutrophil cytochrome b_{558}. J. Biol. Chem. 266:1627, 1991.

287. Nugent, J. H. A., Gratzer, W., and Segal, W.: Identification of the haem-binding subunit of cytochrome b_{-245}. Biochem. J. 264:921, 1989.

288. Yamaguchi, T., Hayakawa, T., Kaneda, M., Kakinuma, K., and Yoshikawa, A.: Purification and some properties of the small subunit of cytochrome b_{558} from human neutrophils. J. Biol. Chem. 264:112, 1989.

289. Rotrosen, D., Kleinberg, M. E., Nunoi, H., Leto, T., Gallin, J. I., and Malech, H. L.: Evidence for a functional cytoplasmic domain of phagocyte oxidase cytochrome b_{558}. J. Biol. Chem. 265:8745, 1990.

290. Kleinberg, M. E., Mital, D., Rotrosen, D., and Malech, H. L.: Characterization of a phagocyte cytochrome b_{558} 91-kilodalton subunit functional domain: Identification of peptide sequence and amino acids essential for activity. Biochemistry 31:2686, 1992.

291. Dinauer, M. C., Pierce, E. A., Erickson, R. W., Muhlebach, T. J., Messner, H., Orkin, S. H., Seger, R. A., and Curnutte, J. T.: Point mutation in the cytoplasmic domain of the neutrophil p22-*phox* cytochrome *b* subunit is associated with a nonfunctional NADPH oxidase and chronic granulomatous disease. Proc. Natl Acad. Sci. USA 88:11231, 1991.

292. Nakamura, M., Sendo, S., van Zwieten, R., Koga, T., Roos, D., and Kanegasaki, S.: Immunocytochemical discovery of the 22- to 23-Kd subunit of cytochrome b_{558} at the surface of human peripheral phagocytes. Blood 72:1550, 1988.

293. Harper, A. M., Dunne, M. J., and Segal, A. W.: Purification of cytochrome b_{-245} from human neutrophils. Biochem. J. 219:519, 1984.

294. Hopkins, P. J., Bemiller, L. S., and Curnutte, J. T.: Chronic granulomatous disease: Diagnosis and classification at the molecular level. Clin. Lab. Med. 12:277, 1992.

295. Bromberg, Y., and Pick, E.: Unsaturated fatty acids stimulate NADPH-dependent superoxide production by cell-free system derived from macrophages. Cell. Immunol. 88:213, 1984.

296. Heyneman, R. A., and Vercauteren, R. E.: Activation of a NADPH oxidase from horse polymorphonuclear leukocytes in a cell-free system. J. Leukoc. Biol. 36:751, 1984.

297. McPhail, L. C., Shirley, P. S., Clayton, C. C., and Snyderman, R.: Activation of the respiratory burst enzyme from human neutrophils in a cell-free system. J. Clin. Invest. 75:1735, 1985.

298. Curnutte, J. T., Berkow, R. L., Roberts, R. L., Shurin, S. B., and Scott, P. J.: Chronic granulomatous disease due to a defect in the cytosolic factor required for nicotinamide adenine dinucleotide phosphate oxidase activation. J. Clin. Invest. 81:606, 1988.

299. Segal, A. W., Heyworth, P. G., Cockcroft, S., and Barrowman, M. M.: Stimulated neutrophils from patients with autosomal recessive chronic granulomatous disease fail to phosphorylate a Mr-44,000 protein. Nature 316:547, 1985.

300. Lomax, K. J., Leto, T. L., Nunoi, H., Gallin, J. I., and Malech, H. L.: Recombinant 47 kD cytosol factor restores NADPH oxidase in chronic granulomatous disease. Science 245:409, 1989.

301. Volpp, B. D., Nauseef, W. M., Donelson, J. E., Moser, D. R., and Clark, R. A.: Cloning of the cDNA and functional expression of the 47-kilodalton cytosolic component of the human neutrophil respiratory burst oxidase. Proc. Natl. Acad. Sci. USA 86:7195, 1989.

302. Leto, T. L., Lomax, K. J., Volpp, B. D., Nunoi, H., Sechler, J. M. G., Nauseef, W. M., Clark, R. A., Gallin, J. I., and Malech, H. L.: Cloning of a 67-kDa neutrophil oxidase factor with similarity to a non-catalytic region of p60$^{c\text{-}src}$. Science 248:727, 1990.

303. Rodaway, A. R., Teahan, C. G., Casimir, C. M., Segal, A. W., and Bentley, D. L.: Characterization of the 47-kilodalton autosomal chronic granulomatous disease protein: Tissue-specific expression and transcriptional control by retinoic acid. Mol. Cell. Biol. 10:5388, 1990.

304. Heyworth, P. G., Tolley, J. O., Smith, R. M., and Curnutte, J. T.: The cytosolic components of the NADPH oxidase system exist as two complexes in the unstimulated neutrophil (abstract). Blood 76:183a, 1990.

305. Heyworth, P. G., Shrimpton, C. F., and Segal, A. W.: Localization of the 47 kDa phosphoprotein involved in the respiratory-burst NADPH oxidase of phagocytic cells. Biochem. J. 260:243, 1989.

306. Okamura, N., Curnutte, J. T., Roberts, R. L., and Babior, B. M.: Relationship of protein phosphorylation to the activation of the respiratory burst in human neutrophils. Defects in the phosphorylation of a group of closely related 48K proteins in two forms of chronic granulomatous disease. J. Biol. Chem. 263:6777, 1988.

307. Okamura, N., Malawista, S. E., Roberts, R. L., Rosen, H., Ochs, H. D., Babior, B. M., and Curnutte, J. T.: Phosphorylation of the oxidase-related 48K phosphoprotein family in the unusual autosomal cytochrome-negative and X-linked cytochrome-positive types of chronic granulomatous disease. Blood 72:811, 1988.

308. Rotrosen, D., and Leto, T. L.: Phosphorylation of neutrophil 47-kDa cytosolic oxidase factor: Translocation to membrane is associated with distinct phosphorylation events. J. Biol. Chem. 265:19910, 1990.

309. Nauseef, W. M., Volpp, B. D., McCormick, S., Leidal, K. G., and Clark, R. A.: Assembly of the neutrophil respiratory burst oxidase: Protein kinase C promotes cytoskeletal and membrane association of cytosolic oxidase components. J. Biol. Chem. 266:5911, 1991.

310. Peveri, P., Heyworth, P. G., and Curnutte, J. T.: Absolute requirement for GTP in the activation of the human neutrophil NADPH oxidase in a cell-free system. Role of ATP in regenerating GTP. Proc. Natl. Acad. Sci. USA 89:2494, 1992.

311. Uhlinger, D. J., Burnham, D. N., and Lambeth, J. D.: Nucleoside triphosphate requirements for superoxide generation and phosphorylation in a cell-free system from human neutrophils. Sodium dodecyl sulfate and diacylglycerol activate independently of protein kinase C. J. Biol. Chem. 266:20990, 1991.

312. Heyworth, P. G., Peveri, P., and Curnutte, J. T.: Cytosolic components of NADPH oxidase: Identity, function and role in regulation of oxidase activity. *In* Cochrane, C. G., and Gimbrone, M. A., Jr. (eds.): Biological Oxidants—Generation and Injurious Consequences. San Diego, 1992, pp. 43–81.

313. Koch, C. A., Anderson, D., Moran, M. F., Ellis, C., and Pawson, T.: SH2 and SH3 domains: Elements that control interac-

tions of cytoplasmic signaling proteins. Science 252:668, 1991.

314. Doussiere, J., Laporte, F., and Vignais, P. V.: Photolabeling of an O_2^- generating protein in bovine polymorphonuclear neutrophils by an arylazido $NADP^+$ analog. Biochem. Biophys. Res. Commun. 139:85, 1986.

315. Takasugi, S. I., Ishida, K., Takeshige, K., and Minakami, S.: Effect of 2', 3'-dialdehyde NADPH on activation of superoxide-producing NADPH oxidase in a cell-free system of pig neutrophils. J. Biochem. 105:155, 1989.

316. Umei, T., Takeshige, K., and Minakami, S.: NADPH-binding component of the superoxide-generating oxidase in unstimulated neutrophils and the neutrophils from the patients with chronic granulomatous disease. Biochem. J. 243:467, 1987.

317. Yea, C. M., Cross, A. R., and Jones, O. T. G.: Purification and some properties of the 45 kDa diphenylene iodonium–binding flavoprotein of neutrophil NADPH oxidase. Biochem. J. 265:95, 1990.

318. Umei, T., Babior, B. M., Curnutte, J. T., and Smith, R. M.: Identification of the NADPH-binding subunit of the respiratory burst oxidase. J. Biol. Chem. 266:6019, 1991.

319. Hall, A.: The cellular functions of small GTP-binding proteins. Science 249:635, 1990.

320. Hall, A.: Signal transduction through small GTPases—a tale of two GAPs. Cell 69:389, 1992.

321. Ridley, A. J., and Hall, A.: The small GTP-binding protein rho regulates the assembly of focal adhesions and actin stress fibers in response to growth factors. Cell 70:389, 1992.

322. Ridley, A. J., Peterson, H. F., Johnston, C. L., Diekmann, D., and Hall, A.: The small GTP-binding protein rac regulates growth factor–induced membrane ruffling. Cell 70:401, 1992.

323. Haubruck, H., and McCormick, F.: Ras p21: Effects and regulation. Biochim. Biophys. Acta 1072:215, 1991.

324. Quinn, M. T., Mullen, M. L., Jesaitis, A. J., and Linner, J. G.: Subcellular distribution of the Rap1A protein in human neutrophils. Colocalization and cotranslocation with cytochrome b_{559}. Blood 79:1563, 1992.

325. Mizuno, T., Kaibuchi, K., Ando, S., Musha, T., Hiraoka, K., Takaishi, K., Asada, M., Nunoi, H., Matsuda, I., and Takai, Y.: Regulation of the superoxide-generating NADPH oxidase by a small GTP-binding protein and its stimulatory and inhibitory GDP/GTP exchange proteins. J. Biol. Chem. 267:10215, 1992.

326. Bokoch, G. M., Quilliam, L. A., Bohl, B. P., Jesaitis, A. J., and Quinn, M. T.: Inhibition of Rap1A binding to cytochrome b_{558} of NADPH oxidase by phosphorylation of Rap1A. Science 254:1794, 1991.

327. Bokoch, G. M., and Prossnitz, V.: Isoprenoid metabolism is required for stimulation of the respiratory burst oxidase of HL-60 cells. J. Clin. Invest. 89:402, 1992.

328. Abo, A., Boyhan, A., West, I., Thrasher, A. J., and Segal, A. W.: Reconstruction of neutrophil NADPH oxidase activity in the cell-free system by four components: p67-*phox*, p47-*phox*, p21*rac*1, and cytochrome b_{-245}. J. Biol. Chem. 267:16767, 1992.

329. Knaus, U. G., Heyworth, P. G., Kinsella, B. T., Curnutte, J. T., and Bokoch, G. M.: Purification and characterization of Rac 2: A cytosolic GTP-binding protein that regulates human neutrophil NADPH oxidase. J. Biol. Chem. 267:23575, 1992.

330. Gabig, T. G., English, D., Akard, L. P., and Schell, M. J.: Regulation of neutrophil NADPH oxidase activation in a cell-free system by guanine nucleotides and fluoride. J. Biol. Chem. 262:1685, 1987.

331. Pizon, V., Chardin, P., Lerosey, I., Olofsson, B., and Tavitian, A.: Human cDNAs rap1 and rap2 homologous to the Drosophila gene Dras3 encode proteins closely related to ras in the "effector" region. Oncogene 3:201, 1988.

332. Pizon, V., Lerosey, I., Chardin, P., and Tavitian, A.: Nucleotide sequence of a human cDNA encoding a ras-related protein (rap1B). Nucleic Acids Res. 16:7719, 1988.

333. Quilliam, L. A., Mueller, H., Bohl, B. P., Prossnitz, V., Sklar, L. A., Der, C. J., and Bokoch, G. M.: Rap1A is a substrate for cyclic AMP-dependent protein kinase in human neutrophils. J. Immunol. 147:1628, 1991.

334. Mueller, H., Motulsky, H. J., and Sklar, L. A.: The potency and kinetics of the beta-adrenergic receptors on human neutrophils. Mol. Pharmacol. 34:347, 1988.

335. Bolscher, B. G. J. M., Denis, S. W., Verhoeven, A. J., and Roos, D.: The activity of one soluble component of the cell-free NADPH: O_2 oxidoreductase of human neutrophils depends on guanosine 5'-O-(3-Thio) triphosphate. J. Biol. Chem. 265:15782, 1990.

336. Pick, E., Kroizman, T., and Abo, A.: Activation of the superoxide-forming NADPH oxidase of macrophages requires two cytosolic components—one of them is also present in certain nonphagocytic cells. J. Immunol. 143:4180, 1989.

337. Kwong, C. H., Malech, H. L., and Leto, T. L.: Three cytosolic proteins are necessary and sufficient for reconstituting NADPH oxidase in neutrophil membrane (abstract). Clin. Res. 39:273a, 1991.

338. Didsbury, J., Weber, R. F., Bokoch, G. M., Evans, T., and Snyderman, R.: *rac*, a novel *ras*-related family of proteins that are botulinum toxin substrates. J. Biol. Chem. 264:16378, 1989.

339. Ding, J., and Badwey, J. A.: Effects of antagonists of protein phosphatases on superoxide release by neutrophils. J. Biol. Chem. 267:6442, 1992.

340. Woodman, R. C., Ruedi, J. M., Jesaitis, A. J., Okamura, N., Quinn, M. T., Smith, R. M., Curnutte, J. T., and Babior, B. M.: The respiratory burst oxidase and 3 of 4 oxidase-related polypeptides are associated with the cytoskeleton of human neutrophils. J. Clin. Invest. 87:1345, 1991.

341. Babior, B. M., Kuver, R., and Curnutte, J. T.: Kinetics of activation of the respiratory burst oxidase in a fully soluble system from human neutrophils. J. Biol. Chem. 263:1713, 1988.

342. Newburger, P. E., Dai, Q., and Whitney, C.: *In vitro* regulation of human phagocyte cytochrome *b* heavy chain and light chain gene expression by bacterial lipopolysaccharide and recombinant human cytokines. J. Biol. Chem. 266:16171, 1991.

343. Casimir, C., Chetty, M., Bohler, M.-C., Garcia, R., Fischer, A., Griscelli, C., Johnson, B., and Segal, A. W.: Identification of the defective NADPH-oxidase component in chronic granulomatous disease: A study of 57 European families. Eur. J. Clin. Invest. 22:403, 1992.

344. Roos, D., de Boer, M., Borregaard, N., Bjerrum, O. W., Valerius, N. H., Seger, R. A., Muhlebach, T., Belohradsky, B. H., and Weening, R. S.: Chronic granulomatous disease with partial deficiency of cytochrome b_{558} and incomplete respiratory burst: Variants of the X-linked, cytochrome b_{558}-negative form of the disease. J. Leukoc. Biol. 51:164, 1992.

345. Tauber, A. I., Borregaard, N., Simons, E., and Wright, J.: Chronic granulomatous disease: A syndrome of phagocyte oxidase deficiencies. Medicine 62:286, 1983.

346. Forrest, C. B., Forehand, J. R., Axtell, R. A., Roberts, R. L., and Johnston, R. B., Jr.: Clinical features and current management of chronic granulomatous disease. *In* Curnutte, J. T. (ed.): Hematology/Oncology Clinics of North America. Phagocyte Defects II, Vol. 2. Philadelphia, W. B. Saunders Co., 1988, pp. 253–266.

347. Curnutte, J. T.: Disorders of phagocyte function. *In* Hoffman, R., Benz, E. J., Jr., Shattil, S. J., Furie, B., and Cohen, H. J. (eds.): Hematology: Basic Principles and Practice. New York, Churchill Livingstone, 1991, pp. 571–589.

348. Curnutte, J. T.: Disorders of granulocyte function and granulopoiesis. *In* Nathan, D. G., and Oski, F. A. (eds.): Hematology of Infancy and Childhood. Philadelphia, W. B. Saunders Co., 1992, pp. 904–977.

349. Mulholland, M. W., Delaney, J. P., and Simmons, R. L.: Gastrointestinal complications of chronic granulomatous disease: Surgical implications. Surgery 94:569, 1983.

350. Isaacs, D., Wright, V. M., Shaw, D. G., Raafat, F., and Walker-Smith, J. A.: Case report: Chronic granulomatous disease

mimicking Crohn's disease. J. Pediatr. Gastroenterol. Nutr. 4: 498, 1985.

351. Clark, R. A., Malech, H. L., Gallin, J. I., Nunoi, H., Volpp, B. D., Pearson, D. W., Nauseef, W. M., and Curnutte, J. T.: Genetic variants of chronic granulomatous disease: Prevalence of deficiencies of two cytosolic components of the NADPH oxidase system. N. Engl. J. Med. 321:647, 1989.

352. Skalnik, D. G., Strauss, E. C., and Orkin, S. H.: CCAAT displacement protein as a depressor of the myelomonocytic specific gp91-*phox* promoter. J. Biol. Chem. 266:16736, 1991.

353. Francke, U., Ochs, H. D., De Martinville, B., Giacalone, J., Lindgren, V., Disteche, C., Pagon, R. A., Hofker, M. H., van Ommen, G.-J. B., Pearson, P. L., and Wedgwood, R. J.: Minor Xp21 chromosome deletion in a male associated with expression of Duchenne muscular dystrophy, chronic granulomatous disease, retinitis pigmentosa, and McLeod syndrome. Am. J. Hum. Genet. 37:250, 1985.

354. Kousseff, B.: Linkage between chronic granulomatous disease and Duchenne's muscular dystrophy. Am. J. Dis. Child. 135:1149, 1981.

355. Frey, D., Machler, M., Seger, R., Schmid, W., and Orkin, S. H.: Gene deletion in a patient with chronic granulomatous disease and McLeod syndrome: Fine mapping of the Xk gene locus. Blood 71:252, 1988.

356. De Saint-Basile, G., Bohler, M. C., Fischer, A., Cartron, J., Dufier, J. L., Griscelli, C., and Orkin, S. H.: Xp21 DNA microdeletion in a patient with chronic granulomatous disease, retinitis pigmentosa, and McLeod phenotype. Hum. Genet. 80:85, 1988.

357. Pelham, A., O'Reilly, M.-A. J., Malcolm, S., Levinsky, R. J., and Kinnon C.: RFLP and deletion analysis for X-linked chronic granulomatous disease using the cDNA probe: Potential for improved prenatal diagnosis and carrier determination. Blood 76:820, 1990.

358. Schapiro, B. L., Newburger, P. E., Klempner, M. S., and Dinauer, M. C.: Chronic granulomatous disease presenting in a 69-year-old man. N. Engl. J. Med. 325:1786, 1991.

359. De Boer, M., Bolscher, B. G. J. M., Dinauer, M. C., Orkin, S. H., Smith, C. I. E., Ahlin, A., Weening, R. S., and Roos, D.: Splice site mutations are a common cause of X-linked chronic granulomatous disease. Blood 80:1553, 1992.

360. Dinauer, M. C., Curnutte, J. T., Rosen, H., and Orkin, S. H.: A missense mutation in the neutrophil cytochrome *b* heavy chain in cytochrome-positive X-linked chronic granulomatous disease. J. Clin. Invest. 84:2012, 1989.

361. Bolscher, B. G. J. M., de Boer, M., de Klein, A., Weening, R. S., and Roos, D.: Point mutations in the β-subunit of cytochrome b_{558} leading to X-linked chronic granulomatous disease. Blood 77:2482, 1991.

362. Ezekowitz, R. A. B., Orkin, S. H., and Newburger, P. E.: Recombinant interferon gamma augments phagocyte superoxide production and X-chronic granulomatous disease gene expression in X-linked variant chronic granulomatous disease. J. Clin. Invest. 80:1009, 1987.

363. Baehner, R. L., and Nathan, D. G.: Quantitative nitroblue tetrazolium test in chronic granulomatous disease. N. Engl. J. Med. 278:971, 1968.

364. Quie, P. G., Kaplan, E. L., Page, A. R., Gruskay, F. L., and Malawista, S. E.: Defective polymorphonuclear-leukocyte function and chronic granulomatous disease in two female children. N. Engl. J. Med. 278:976, 1968.

365. De Boer, M., de Klein, A., Hossle J.-P., Seger, R., Corbeel, L., Weening, R. S., and Roos, D.: Cytochrome b_{558}-negative, autosomal recessive chronic granulomatous disease: Two new mutations in the cytochrome b_{558} light chain of the NADPH oxidase (p22-*phox*). Am. J. Hum. Genet. 41:1127, 1992.

366. Francke, U., Hsieh, C.-L., Foellmer, B. E., Lomax, K. J., Malech, H. L., and Leto, T. L.: Genes for two autosomal recessive forms of chronic granulomatous disease assigned to 1q25 (NCF2) and 7q11.23 (NCF1). Am. J. Hum. Genet. 47:483, 1990.

367. Chanock, S. J., Barrett, D. M., Curnutte, J. T., and Orkin, S. H.: Gene structure of the cytosolic component, *phox*-47 and mutations in autosomal recessive chronic granulomatous disease (abstract). Blood 78:165a, 1991.

368. Casimir, C. M., Bu-Ghanim, H. N., Rodaway, A. R. F., Bentley, D. L., Rowe, P., and Segal, A. W.: Autosomal recessive chronic granulomatous disease caused by deletion at a dinucleotide repeat. Proc. Natl. Acad. Sci. USA 88:2753, 1991.

369. Kenney, R. T., Malech, H. L., and Leto, T. L.: Structural characterization of the p67-*phox* gene (abstract). Clin. Res. 40:261a, 1992.

370. Lew, D. P., Southwick, F. S., Stossel, T. P., Whitin, J. C., Simons, E., and Cohen, H. J.: A variant of chronic granulomatous disease: Deficient oxidative metabolism due to a low affinity NADPH-oxidase. N. Engl. J. Med. 305:1329, 1981.

371. Seger, R. A., Tiefenauer, L., Matsunaga, T., Wildfeuer, A., and Newburger, P. E.: Chronic granulomatous disease due to granulocytes with abnormal NADPH oxidase activity and deficient cytochrome-*b*. Blood 61:423, 1983.

372. Styrt, B., and Klempner, M. S.: Late-presenting variant of chronic granulomatous disease. Pediatr. Infect. Dis. J. 3:556, 1984.

373. Newburger, P. E., Luscinskas, F. W., Ryan, T., Beard, C. J., Wright, J., Platt, O. S., Simons, E. R., and Tauber, A. I.: Variant chronic granulomatous disease: Modulation of the neutrophil by severe infection. Blood 68:914, 1986.

374. Weening, R. S., Adriaansz, L. H., Weemaes, C. M. R., Lutter, R., and Roos, D.: Clinical differences in chronic granulomatous disease in patients with cytochrome *b*–negative or cytochrome *b*–positive neutrophils. J. Pediatr. 107:102, 1985.

375. Gallin, J. I., Malech, H. L., Weening, R. S., Curnutte, J. T., Quie, P. G., Ezekowitz, R. A. B., et al.: A controlled trial of interferon gamma to prevent infection in chronic granulomatous disease. N. Engl. J. Med. 324:509, 1991.

376. Margolis, D. M., Melnick, D. A., Alling, D. W., and Gallin, J. I.: Trimethoprim-sulfamethoxazole prophylaxis in the management of chronic granulomatous disease. J. Infect. Dis. 162:723, 1990.

377. Woodman, R. C., Erickson, R. W., Rae, J., Jaffe, H. S., and Curnutte, J. T.: Prolonged recombinant interferon-gamma therapy in chronic granulomatous disease: Evidence against enhanced neutrophil oxidase activity. Blood 79:1558, 1992.

378. Curnutte, J. T.: Classification of chronic granulomatous disease. Hematol. Oncol. Clin. North Am. 20:241, 1988.

379. Curnutte, J. T., Hopkins, P. J., Kuhl, W., and Beutler, E.: Studying X inactivation. Lancet 339:749, 1992.

380. Nakamura, M., Imajoh-Ohmi, S., Kanegasaki, S., Kurozumi, H., Sato, K., Kato, S., and Miyazaki, Y.: Prenatal diagnosis of cytochrome-deficient chronic granulomatous disease (letter to the editor). Lancet 336:118, 1990.

381. Battat, L., and Francke, U.: Nsi I RFLP at the X-linked chronic granulomatous disease locus (CYBB). Nucleic Acids Res. 17:3619, 1989.

382. Muhlebach, T. J., Robinson, W., Seger, R. A., and Machler, M.: A second NsiI RFLP at the CYBB locus. Nucleic Acids Res. 18:4966, 1990.

383. Kenney, R. T., and Leto, T. L.: A *Hind*III polymorphism in the human NCF2 gene. Nucleic Acids Res. 18:7193, 1990.

384. Gorlin, J.: Identification of (CA/GT)$_n$ polymorphisms within the X-linked chronic granulomatous disease (X-CGD) gene: Utility for prenatal diagnosis (abstract). Blood 78:433a, 1991.

385. Quie, P. G., and Belani, K. K.: Corticosteroids for chronic granulomatous disease. J. Pediatr. 111:393, 1987.

386. Nathan, C. F., Murray, H. W., Wiebe, M. E., and Rubin, B. Y.: Identification of interferon gamma as the lymphokine that activates human macrophage oxidative metabolism and antimicrobial activity. J. Exp. Med. 158:670, 1983.

387. Murray, H. W.: Interferon-gamma, the activated macrophage, and host defense against microbial challenge. Ann. Intern. Med. 108:595, 1988.

388. Ezekowitz, R. A. B., Dinauer, M. C., Jaffe, H. S., Orkin, S. H., and Newburger, P. E.: Partial correction of the phagocyte defect in patients with X-linked chronic granulomatous disease by subcutaneous interferon gamma. N. Engl. J. Med. 319:146, 1988.

389. Sechler, J. M. G., Malech, H. L., White, C. J., and Gallin, J. I.: Recombinant human interferon gamma reconstitutes defective phagocyte function in patients with chronic granulomatous disease of childhood. Proc. Natl. Acad. Sci. USA 85:4874, 1988.

390. Cobbs, C. S., Malech, H. L., Leto, T. L., Freeman, S. M., Blaese, R. M., Gallin, J. I., and Lomax, K. J.: Retroviral expression of recombinant p47^{phox} protein by Epstein-Barr virus–transformed B lymphocytes from a patient with autosomal chronic granulomatous disease. Blood 79:1829, 1992.

391. Thrasher, A., Chetty, M., Casimir, C., and Segal, A. W.: Restoration of superoxide generation to a chronic granulomatous disease–derived B-cell line by retrovirus mediated gene transfer. Blood 80:1125, 1992.

15

The Molecular Basis of White Blood Cell Motility

Thomas P. Stossel

INTRODUCTION

Chapter 14 described the general features of white blood cell functions. Many of these functions, such as locomotion, phagocytosis, and secretion by exocytosis, involve active cell motility. This chapter reviews the subject of white blood cell motility from the standpoint of molecules within the cell that underlie these motile functions and how this information is beginning to be used to address diseases involving white blood cells.

The elements of white blood cell motility include motility-inducing *agonists* such as chemoattractants, opsonins, and secretagogues; externally disposed plasma membrane *receptors* for these agonists; *second messengers (signals)* modulated by channels; pumps and metabolic pathways generated by agonist-receptor engagement; *adhesin receptors;* and the proteins composing the *cytoskeleton* that are responsible for the mechanical forces driving these movements.

EXTRACELLULAR FACTORS THAT INDUCE WHITE BLOOD CELL MOTILITY (Table 15–1)

In keeping with the importance of leukocyte motility to the survival of the host, many agents have the capacity to stimulate this activity. These include the chemoattractants that derive from the systems that come into action during infection, inflammation, and specific immunological reactions. Products of the complement and coagulation systems, products of membrane lipid (eicosanoid) metabolism, and a growing list of cytokines elaborated by a variety of cells induce white blood cell motility. In some cases the effects are

Supported by United States Public Health Service Grants HL19429 and HL07680 and by the Edwin S. Webster Foundation.

541

TABLE 15–1. MOLECULES THAT ATTRACT LEUKOCYTES (CHEMOATTRACTANTS)

SOURCE	MOLECULES
Complement system (Plasma and Mononuclear phagocytes [MNP])	C5a, C5a-des-arg + Vitamin D–binding protein
Membrane phospholipids	Leukotriene B_4 (LTB_4), lipoxin A, B, acetylglycerophosphatidylcholine, (platelet-activating factor [PAF]), diacylglycerol, lysophosphatidylcholine
Coagulation system (plasma and platelets)	Thrombin,* fibrinopeptides A, Bb 1–42, platelet factor 4, platelet-derived growth factor (PDGF), urokinase, heparin cofactor II reaction products, interleukin-8 (IL-8)–like peptide derived from platelet factor 4 by monocyte proteinases
Mononuclear phagocytes Tumor cells Endothelial cells Lymphocytes Epithelial cells	IL-8 (monocyte-derived chemotactic factor, [MDFC]), ? tumor necrosis factor (TNF), ? colony-stimulating factor–1 (CSF-1) (colony-stimulating factor–macrophages [CSF-M]), oxidized low-density lipoprotein (LDL), macrophage inflammatory proteins 1 and 2 (MIP-1, MIP-2), KC/gro-related protein, neutrophil attractant protein–1†
Neutrophils	Defensins*
Altered proteins	Maleyl albumin, casein, collagen fragments, elastase-α-1-proteinase inhibitor complex
Bacteria, mitochondria	N-formyl oligopeptides
Metabolites, alkaloids	Adenosine, nicotine

*Reportedly chemotactic only for monocytes.
†Only for neutrophils.

general for many leukocyte types, and in others they are relatively specific. These agents can either increase the speed of random locomotion (chemokinetic factors) or focus the direction of movement (chemotactic factors). Related to chemoattractants are the opsonins, factors that when bound to particulate objects elicit localized movements within the membrane of leukocytes that result in ingestion (phagocytosis) of these objects. These agonists work by effects of specific membrane receptors. Other agents, however, such as diacylglycerol analogues (e.g., tumor-promoting phorbol esters), become incorporated into the plasma membrane bilayer.

THE MOTILE CORTEX OF THE WHITE BLOOD CELL AND LEUKOCYTE MOTILITY

The anatomical focus of white blood cell motility is the plasma membrane and the cytoplasm immediately beneath it, designated the cell cortex. The primacy of this region of the cell has long been appreciated by microscopists observing white blood cell motility who documented the invariable *polarity* of leukocytes during locomotion.[1] The morphological basis of this polarity is the extension of the cell cortex into one or more pleats (called pseudopodia, lamellae, or lamellipodia) in the direction of locomotion or around par-

ticles undergoing phagocytosis. Similar pleats (called ruffles) appear on the dorsal surface of white blood cells, especially on cells undergoing mitogenic stimulation, such as lymphocytes exposed to activating agonists. The sufficiency of the cell cortex in these functions is exemplified by experiments in which peripheral cellular fragments, separated from the nucleus and most internal organelles of the cell, exhibit chemotaxis and rudimentary phagocytosis,[2, 3] indicating that the cell periphery contains the sensory and motor structures for the execution of at least temporary cell motility. Even these cellular amputees, however, exhibit polarity when they move, in that the front edge is wider than the back.

Striking and consistent changes visible to the observer with the light microscope occur in the cortex during locomotion of leukocytes (Fig. 15–1A). In the absence of chemoattractants or other agonists, the cells remain relatively round. Following the addition of a chemoattractant, leukocytes begin to spread on the underlying substrate, and they extend ruffles from the dorsal surface. This initial response has been termed "cringing." Subsequently, within minutes, the general spreading is replaced by the polarized extension of cortical substance mentioned above, and locomotion begins.

When the cell moves in a particular direction, the

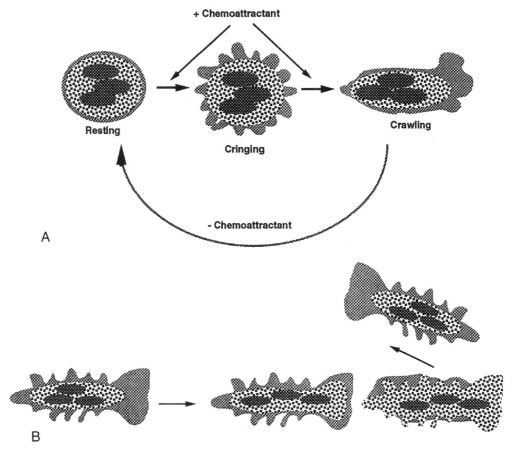

FIGURE 15–1. *A*, Changes in the leukocyte surface in response to chemoattractants. *B*, Changes in the leukocyte surface during random locomotion: As the leukocyte moving from left to right slows, granules move to the previous leading front, the original leading lamella dissolves, and a new one appears in the new direction of movement.

leading edge of the lamella generates many ruffles. Some of these fall forward and lie parallel to the substrate; others rise and move, like waves, at about 0.1 to 1.0 μm per second backward across the lamella toward the cell body and then disappear. Agents that cross-link surface receptors at the leading edge move backward at the same rate and collect in a protuberance at the rear of the cell (the uropod or tail), a phenomenon known as *capping*.

Observations with interference reflection microscopy have suggested that the region at the interface between the cell body and the lamella is where the cell is most tightly adherent to the substrate during locomotion.[4] Hence the front of the lamella may be more important for exploration and establishment of directionality rather than for providing frictional force for translocational movement. As the cell moves forward, the cell body tends to acquire indentations, especially at the junction of the cell body and the lamellae and at the rear of the cell, that give the appearance of originating from localized contraction of the cell surface. Internal organelles flow through these narrowings as if compressed by such contraction,[5] and it has been proposed that these "contraction waves" participate in the creation of cell polarity during locomotion.[6]

The leading lamella, like the cortex in general, tends

to exclude organelles visible in the light microscope, such as the nucleus and large secretory granules. In addition, mechanical measurements on the processes extended from activated leukocytes have indicated that these structures have elastic properties characteristic of solids. From these observations, it has long been inferred that the extended cortex is in a "gelled" state, relative to the rest of the cell.[7] This conclusion cannot be strictly true, since the cortex is obviously dynamic, and explaining how this structure can have both liquid and solid properties has been a major challenge.

Leukocytes move with their characteristic polarity toward the source of a gradient of chemoattractants. If the observer removes chemoattractant from such cells, the extended lamellae rapidly dissolve. The first events are cessation of forward movement and dissipation of the anterior organelle exclusion, and granules move to the former leading edge, which then retracts toward the cell body (Fig. 15–1*B*). If the experimenter reverses the gradient, the cells prefer to make a U turn by extending the pre-existing lamellae at angles to the side of the original direction, rather than rounding up and starting new lamellae. This tendency of the cell to retain its original polarity, even in the absence of the agonist gradient that initiated the polarity is termed *persistence*. If chemoattractant molecules are present but in the absence of a defined gradient, leukocytes meander randomly about, exhibiting both forms of behavior—making U turns or extending new lamellae in new directions as they retract old ones—but again they clearly demonstrate persistence.[6, 8, 9]

DIVERSE RECEPTORS MEDIATE LEUKOCYTE MOTILITY

One of the puzzles of leukocyte motility is the fact that the characteristic surface changes described above arise from perturbation of structurally diverse receptors that appear to generate different intracellular signal cascades (Fig. 15–2). One class of chemoattractants exemplified by *C5a, N-formyl-methionyl-leucyl phenylalanine, platelet-activating factor,* and *interleukin-8* bind to receptors with structures predicted to span the membrane bilayer seven times.[10–15] These receptors require pertussis toxin–sensitive *heterotrimeric GTP-binding proteins* to mediate their effects, which are often associated with waves of increased intracellular free calcium and with polyphosphoinositide turnover. The changes in calcium and in lipid turnover are mediated in part by the activation of phospholipase C. This activation follows binding to the enzyme of the GTP-complexed α subunit of the heterotrimeric G protein and leads to hydrolysis of phosphatidylinositol 4,5-bisphosphate, which generates inositol 3-phosphate and diacylglycerol. Inositol 3-phosphate releases calcium from intracellular stores, and diacylglycerol activates *protein kinase C.*[16]

By contrast, *platelet-derived growth factor (PDGF)* and *tumor growth factor β (TGFβ)* are chemoattractants in addition to being mitogens for proliferation-competent cells,[17] and their receptors are single-spanning polypeptides with tyrosine kinase activity. Engagement of these receptors by ligands causes autophosphorylation of tyrosine residues in the cytoplasmic tails of the receptors, and the phosphorylated residues are parts of binding sites for the g isoform of phospholipase C and for phosphatidylinositol 3-kinase.[18] Chemotaxis mediated by these receptors is not pertussis toxin sensitive and not clearly associated with changes in intracellular calcium levels. On the other hand, GTP-binding proteins related to the oncogene *ras* (e.g., *rho* and *rac*), GTP hydrolysis-activating factors acting on these proteins (e.g., GTPase-activating protein [GAP]), and GDP-GTP exchange factors required to complete the cycle of activity of these so-called small G proteins are implicated in signaling through this class of receptors.[19]

Receptors mediating phagocytosis, such as the re-

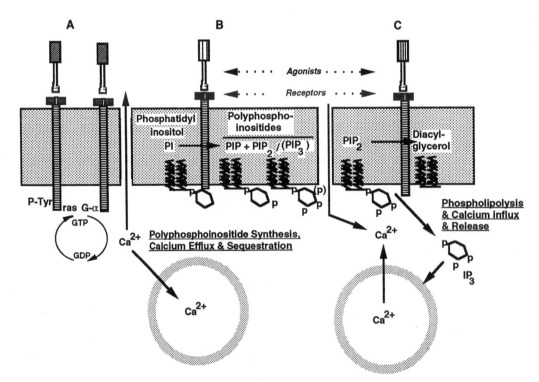

FIGURE 15–2. Signal transduction pathways potentially important for leukocyte motility. *A,* Some ligated receptors initiate phosphorylation cascades beginning with phosphorylation of the cytoplasmic tail of the receptor, which leads to downstream effects involving small G proteins; others interact with heterotrimeric G proteins. *B,* Ligated receptors bind enzymes (phospholipid kinases) that catalyze the phosphorylation of phosphatidylinositol to generate polyphosphoinositides. Under these circumstances, calcium is extruded from the cytoplasm. *C,* Ligated receptors bind phospholipase C, which hydrolyzes phosphatidylinositol 4,5-bisphosphate (PIP$_2$) to diacylglycerol and inositol 3-phosphate. These events are associated with cytosolic accumulation of calcium. The timing and placement of ligand binding, association of the receptor with cofactors such as G proteins, and unknown factors determine whether the receptor mediates events associated with *B* or *C.*

ceptors for the Fc domain of immunoglobulin G (IgG), the receptor for C3b, or the integrin receptors of leukocytes, have very different amino acid sequences in their cytoplasmic domains, and the signals by which they mediate their effects are not as well characterized as for the receptors discussed above. Calcium transients and changes in phosphoinositide turnover are frequently associated with their engagement by relevant agonists,[20–26] as is phosphorylation of tyrosine residues,[20, 27, 28] and studies with chimeric Fc receptors have identified specific cytoplasmic amino acid sequences required for ligand-induced capping or for endocytosis.[29, 30]

THE "CYTOSKELETON"

Definition

"Cytoskeleton" is a poorly descriptive term encompassing three protein polymer systems: *actin* and *tubulin*, which are highly conserved phylogenetically, and the tissue-specific *intermediate filament proteins*, named *desmin* in muscle cells, *keratin* in epithelial cells, *glial fibrillary acidic protein* in neuronal cells, and *vimentin* in mesenchymal cells, including leukocytes. An additional actin-related cytoskeletal element is a system of proteins related to *spectrin* (sometimes called *fodrin*), best characterized in erythrocytes (see Chapter 7), which laminate the inner surface of the plasma membrane.

General Features of the "Cytoskeleton" and the Particular Importance of Actin in White Blood Cell Cortical Structure and Function

Aside from relative abundance and the attribute of self-association, the polymerizing cytoskeletal molecules share relatively few similarities. Actin and tubulin have in common that they bind and hydrolyze nucleotides—adenine nucleotides in the case of actin and guanine nucleotides in the case of tubulin—and that they interact in their polymerized states with so-called motor proteins—actin with two types of *myosins* and tubulin with *dynein, dynamin,* and *kinesin.* These motor proteins can move themselves along the polymers in one direction or alternatively move the polymers in opposite directions.

The three cytoskeletal polymers differ, however, in their mechanical, pharmacological, and distributive properties. The intermediate filaments are very flexible yet highly resistant to rupture by deformation; actin filaments, on the other hand, are extremely stiff and break when bent beyond a critical point. Tubulin polymers (microtubules) have mechanical properties intermediate between those of the other two polymer types.[31]

The cytoskeletal systems also vary in the domains where they principally reside in the cell. Actin tends to have a peripheral location, microtubules radiate from the centriole near the nucleus of interphase cells

and form the mitotic spindle, and intermediate filaments usually have a perinuclear disposition, although they also participate in specialized junctional structures in epithelial cells. Thus, actin is the principal component in the principal site of motility, the cell cortex, where it exists in close to millimolar concentrations. Associated with actin are numerous actin-binding proteins, including many that bind both actin and components of the plasma membrane.

The cytoskeletal systems also have different susceptibilities to toxins and drugs. Fungal (the cytochalasins and chaetoglobosins), plant (the phallotoxins), bacterial (*Clostridium botulinum* C or iota toxins), and marine (latrunculins) toxins modify the function of actin yet have no effects on the other cytoskeletal proteins. Conversely, colchicine, nocodazole, vinca alkaloids, and griseofulvin inhibit tubulin assembly without affecting actin, and no known toxins interact with intermediate filaments. Consistent with the primacy of actin in white blood cell motility, toxins affecting actin drastically affect white blood cell motile functions,[32] whereas, in comparison, tubulin-active drugs have relatively subtle effects or none at all.[33, 34]

In summary, anatomical and pharmacological evidence implicates actin and actin-related proteins as the principal cytoskeletal molecules involved in leukocyte motility. Microtubules assemble and disassemble in leukocytes[35] and become tyrosinolated following stimulation of leukocytes by agonists,[36] and the long-term stability of leukocytes, membrane trafficking, and the efficient delivery of granules from the centriolar region to the periphery probably involve tubulin and tubulin-binding proteins.[34, 37–39] Microtubule-associated proteins may also play a role in the "priming" phenomenon of leukocytes, in which cytokines increase the rate of onset of effector responses such as superoxide release.[40] The role of intermediate filaments in leukocyte motility is unknown, although phosphorylation of vimentin by a cyclic GMP (cGMP)–dependent protein kinase following chemoattractant stimulation of neutrophils has been observed.[41, 42]

"CYTOSKELETAL" ACTIN IN RESTING AND ACTIVATED WHITE BLOOD CELLS

One frequently applied operational definition of the cytoskeleton is the material that resists extraction with non-ionic detergents. This conceptual view of the cytoskeleton is incomplete, however, because only the intermediate filaments are completely detergent insoluble, as are cellular components with no obvious relationship to the cytoskeletal polymer systems. Approximately one third to one half of the actin in unstimulated white blood cells is "cytoskeletal" according to this definition.

Actin filament cross-linking proteins are responsible for the stabilization of actin filaments in different configurations, and many of these proteins also link actin filaments to membranes. These actin filament–binding proteins are responsible for the incredible diversity of shapes that the linear actin polymer can confer on cells, depending on the circumstances.

Such polymeric actin, stabilized by actin cross-linking proteins, therefore constitutes a true cytoskeleton that invests the cortex of the resting leukocyte, although little is known about its organization. The actin skeleton of the resting cell presumably maintains the round shape of leukocytes circulating in the blood and may also arrange the display of selectins and other receptors that mediate the rolling of cells that represents the first response to inflammatory changes on the postcapillary venule endothelium.[43]

Agonists that activate blood cells cause remodeling of the actin organization in the resting cell into a new cytoskeletal structure, and this transformation causes the surface changes characteristic of the motile cell. The veils, pleats, and pseudopodia extended by activated white blood cells contain a delicate orthogonal actin network (Fig. 15–3), and filopodia that reside on the dorsal surface of macrophages and some lymphoid cells contain one or more long actin filaments. These actin-rich (cytoskeletal) structures account for the organelle exclusion and rigidity (gel-like state) of cortical processes. Agonists such as chemoattractants added to leukocytes can induce a net increase in this cytoskeletal actin, and the temporal change in total cytoskeletal actin corresponds to the cringing response. When the cells acquire polarity and begin to undergo locomotion after exposure to chemoattractants, their total cytoskeletal actin level may fall to the basal value.

DYNAMIC ACTIN IN WHITE BLOOD CELLS

The detergent-soluble actin in white blood cells is involved in cytoskeletal actin remodeling. It consists

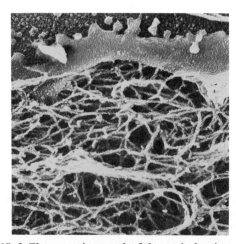

FIGURE 15–3. Electron micrograph of the cortical actin network of a leukocyte. The cell was adherent to a surface when a polylysine-coated coverslip was placed on top of it and removed, thereby ripping off parts of the dorsal membrane. Soluble contents floated out, and myosin subfragment 1 was perfused in. The myosin bound the cytoskeletal actin filaments, decorating them with arrowheads. The specimen was then fixed, rapidly frozen, etched, rotary shadowed with platinum-tungsten, and photographed (120,000× magnification) in the electron microscope. (Micrograph prepared by Dr. John H. Hartwig.)

of short filaments as well as monomers[44–46] and can, under appropriate conditions, be made to assemble into polymer gels in the extracts.[47, 48]

The remodeling of cortical actin that controls leukocyte motility depends on the fact that actin cycles between soluble (sol) and insoluble (gel) states, and the rate at which actin cycles between states is as important as or more important than any change in the net balance between soluble and cytoskeletal actin. Induction of phagocytosis in macrophages—for example, induction of capping of cross-linked cell surface receptors in lymphocytes or of exocytosis of granules in basophils—leads to extensive rearrangements in the morphology of cortical actin filaments, and the cytochalasins, which block actin assembly, inhibit phagocytosis and capping and enhance exocytosis. Nevertheless, these events occur without detectable changes in the absolute quantity of polymerized cellular actin.[49, 50] The remodeling of the actin architecture of these structures by this cycle, which accounts for leukocyte movements, is the secret to the mystery of cortical dynamics—the simultaneous solidity and liquidity of the peripheral cytoplasm.

These actin dynamics are responses to instructions initiated by agonists acting on cell membrane receptors, and the way that these signals control a cycle of linear actin assembly and disassembly and the reversible aggregation of the assembled actin filaments into three-dimensional "cytoskeletal" networks with regulated linkages to cell membranes (Fig. 15–4) is beginning to become clear at the molecular level.

THE ACTIN CYCLE

Fundamentals of Actin Assembly and Disassembly

LINEAR ASSEMBLY AND DISASSEMBLY OF ACTIN. Actin filaments (F-actin) disassemble by loss of monomers (G-actin) from their ends or by fragmentation (see Fig. 15–4); the annealing of fragments or the addition of monomers to the ends causes assembly. Monomers may also aggregate de novo, thereby starting new filaments, but this spontaneous *nucleation* reaction is very inefficient. F-actin has a polarity conventionally defined by the terms "barbed" and "pointed," because actin filaments saturated with proteolytic actin-binding fragments of myosin appear in the electron microscope as if adorned with a series of arrowheads. F-actin in the presence of myosin and ATP moves from the barbed to the pointed direction as defined by the arrowheads. The exchange of monomers with the barbed end is rapid (essentially diffusion limited) but an order of magnitude slower at the pointed end. One consequence of this polarity of actin assembly is, therefore, that *barbed actin filament ends can act as the nuclei for new actin assembly in cells and that in large part the temporal and spatial control of actin assembly can derive from the cell's use of proteins that block monomer exchange with this end in a regulated way.* Actin toxins such as the

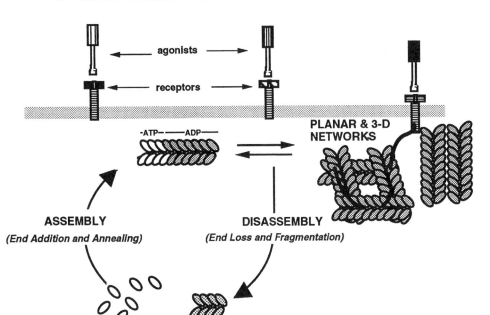

FIGURE 15–4. The actin cycle. The open actin monomers contain ATP, and the shaded monomers contain ADP. See text and Figure 15–5.

cytochalasins work principally by blocking addition of monomers to the barbed filament end.

ATP HYDROLYSIS AND EXCHANGE: ACTIN AS A TIME CLOCK. Adenine nucleotide binding to actin and hydrolysis by actin are important for actin assembly[51, 52] (Fig. 15–5). In the millimolar ATP concentrations usually existing in cells, each actin monomer binds one ATP molecule complexed to Mg^{2+}, and in this condition the actin monomers bind avidly ($K_d = 0.1\ \mu M$) to the barbed ends of actin filaments (step 1). Once incorporated within a filament, the actins slowly hydrolyze the ATP to ADP and orthophosphate (Pi) (step 2). The Pi leaches slowly off the filament (step 3), and this dissociation is inhibited by high Pi concentrations. When actin monomers containing ADP dissociate from the ends of filaments (step 4) (usually the barbed ends because of the faster exchange rate at those ends), these ADP monomers are about eightfold less efficient than ATP monomers in adding back onto the barbed ends of F-actin. Because actin monomers bind ATP with higher affinity than ADP, ADP monomers acquire ATP by exchange of their ADP for ATP in the medium (step 5). This exchange is relatively slow, however, so that ADP monomers accumulate under conditions of rapid actin depolymerization.

ATP-actin monomers therefore favor polymerization, and hydrolysis converts the ATP monomers in the filament to ADP protomers, which, when dissociated from the filaments, promote depolymerization. Accordingly, like GTP-binding proteins (G proteins) involved in signal transduction, actin can act as a time-delay switch. A newly assembled filament containing ATP monomers may also be functionally different from an old filament containing mostly ADP monomers, as amplified below.

Scheme for the Control of the Actin Cycle in White Blood Cells

Signals generated when agonists perturb leukocyte membranes run the actin cycle through the intermediary of actin-binding proteins (Fig. 15–6). The proteins of relevance for the actin cycle are molecules that interact with actin monomers and with actin filaments in a coordinated manner to promote the assembly or disassembly of actin by the mechanisms summarized above. These molecules in turn respond to signals elicited by agonist-receptor interaction. A noteworthy feature of the control of the actin cycle is that many of the proteins described below that are responsible for its regulation are multifunctional, promoting either actin assembly or disassembly, depending on the regulatory signals affecting them at particular times and places within the cell.

A scheme for regulation of the actin cycle that accommodates most available facts is possible, because identified signal mechanisms control the activities of these actin-binding proteins in vitro, and studies with intact cells by and large are consistent with this scheme,

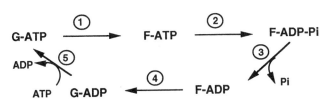

FIGURE 15–5. The actin cycle and adenine nucleotide exchange and hydrolysis.

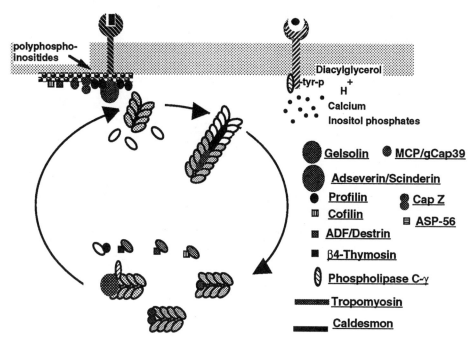

FIGURE 15–6. Regulation of actin assembly and disassembly in the actin cycle by second messengers and actin-modulating proteins. Open monomers indicate ATP-actin, and shaded monomers, ADP-actin. Gelsolin, MCP/gCap39, and Cap Z disassemble actin filaments by severing and/or barbed end capping when activated by calcium or hydrolysis of membrane polyphosphoinositides. Profilin, cofilin, ADF/destrin, and β_4 thymosin promote actin depolymerization by monomer sequestration. Gelsolin, MCP/gCap39, and Cap Z promote actin assembly following interaction with membrane polyphosphoinositides, which uncaps actin filament barbed ends. Profilin, cofilin, and actin-depolymerizing factor (ADF)/destrin desequester actin monomers following interaction with membrane phospholipids; in addition, profilin charges actin monomers by catalyzing ADP-ATP exchange. Tropomyosin and caldesmon bind elongating filaments and stabilize them. Gelsolin-actin complexes also bind phospholipase C-γ and carry it to its membrane substrates. Tyrosine phosphorylation of receptors may facilitate subsequent hydrolysis of phospholipids by this enzyme.

although gaps and inconsistencies invite considerable additional research. The following sections summarize the available evidence.

ACTIN-BINDING PROTEINS AND SIGNALS MEDIATING DISASSEMBLY OF ACTIN IN WHITE BLOOD CELLS. Removal of chemoattractant stimulation from locomoting leukocytes causes actin in the lamellipodia of the moving cell to disaggregate rapidly, at a rate approximating depolymerization of linear filaments by 10 μm per second.[53] The most efficient mechanism for such rapid cytoskeletal actin disassembly is the *fragmentation of actin filaments*. A fragmenting event shortens actin filament much more than loss of a monomer from the end, and it is a powerful mechanism for dissolving a network—a gel to sol transformation (see Fig. 15–6). Accordingly, a specific agent responsible in blood cells (and others) for this activity is the protein *gelsolin*, named for its ability to cause a gel to sol transformation of actin by rapidly severing the non-covalent bonds between actin monomers in a filament.[54, 55] *Calcium,* an important signal ion that accumulates in cytosol to average concentrations approaching 1 μM in response to membrane receptor perturbation, activates gelsolin for this actin-fragmenting function. Protons also activate gelsolin independently of calcium.[55a] Gelsolin binds ADP- but not ATP-actin,[55b] and this discrimination, as explained below, is important for the smooth control of the actin cycle in the cell.

After severing an actin filament, gelsolin remains firmly affixed to the barbed end of the shortened filaments, where it prevents either exchange of monomers with the barbed filament end or the annealing of filament fragments.[54, 55] Another protein, named *macrophage capping protein (MCP), MHb-1, or gelsolin-related capping protein 39 (gCap39)*, is abundant in myeloid cells.[56–58] It is structurally related to gelsolin, and like gelsolin, it binds tightly to (caps) filament barbed ends when activated by calcium, but it has no filament-severing activity.[59] This protein has also been shown to localize within the nucleus as well as the cytoplasm.[60, 60a] *Cap Z* is a heterodimeric protein isolated from muscle cells that has constitutive actin filament barbed end capping activity and, if present in blood cells, may also have a role in blockading their actin filament barbed ends.[61]

Several proteins in blood cells can bind actin monomers with affinities in the millimolar range and impair their ability to add onto filaments, particularly onto their pointed ends; the presence of these so-called monomer-sequestering proteins, named *profilin, cofilin, destrin,* and β_4 *thymosin*, helps to keep cellular actin depolymerized.[62–66] In contrast to gelsolin and MCP, calcium does not directly activate these proteins for binding to actin. Cofilin's actin-binding activity, however, is affected by pH; cofilin binds monomeric actin only at pH values above 7.5. Cytoplasmic alkalinization occurs transiently during certain cell activations, so that this pH control may be physiologically important. Cofilin and destrin (also called actin-depolymerizing factor [ADF]) have some actin filament–binding activity and weak severing activity.

FACTORS REGULATING ASSEMBLY OF ACTIN IN WHITE BLOOD CELLS. Following addition of chemoattractants to neutrophils, actin assembles in lamellipodia at a rate of approximately 10 μm per second.[67, 68] The poor spontaneous nucleation of actin monomers, especially ADP monomers, affords the cell a strategy for controlling the place and time of such rapid filament growth by inducing nucleation. The actin filament–binding proteins, gelsolin, MCP, and Cap Z, have varying degrees of actin filament–nucleating activity, detectable as a shortening of the lag time that reflects the inefficient spontaneous nucleation of purified actin. Because of the orientation of these proteins to the barbed ends of the actin filaments, the filaments grow in the pointed direction. Not only is pointed end growth slow, but also, as indicated below, cellular actin assembly is predominantly in the barbed direction. A key ingredient, therefore, in the scheme for regulation of actin assembly (see Fig. 15–6) is *the uncapping of actin oligomers with their barbed ends blocked, and the apparent nucleation activity of actin filament end–blocking proteins, according to this scheme, is to create actin oligomers for subsequent unblocking.*[69] This maneuver allows the oligomers to anneal or exposes sites that are efficient nuclei for monomer addition. Also inferred in this assembly mechanism is *a simultaneous lowering of the affinity of actin monomer–binding proteins for actin (desequestration),* which provides monomers competent to add onto the unblocked barbed filament ends.

An additional important factor in promoting the ability of monomers to polymerize is the *charging* of G-actin, catalysis of the exchange of ADP- for ATP-binding actin monomers (step 5 in Fig. 15–4), by profilin.[70, 70a] Not only do ATP-actin monomers add more efficiently onto the barbed ends of actin filaments than do ADP monomers, but also once attached they remain with greater stability than ADP filaments.[51] Moreover, the delay in hydrolysis of ATP by monomers within a filament creates a domain in the filament that is more resistant to the action of actin filament–severing proteins.

A central factor in this regulation of assembly is the accumulating evidence that membrane *polyphosphoinositides,* a class of lipids that turn over during cellular signal transduction, bind to actin filament–capping proteins and actin monomer–binding proteins, lower their affinities for actin, and free filament barbed ends and monomers for assembly.[71–79] The polyphosphoinositides shown to have these effects are principally phosphatidylinositol 4-phosphate (PIP) and phosphatidylinositol 4,5-bisphosphate (PIP_2); other members of this lipid class have not been available in sufficient quantities to test, but many other phospholipids and polyphosphate compounds are inactive. PIP and PIP_2 molecules must aggregate appropriately to interact with the actin-binding proteins, and the chemical environment strongly affects this aggregation state.[73] *Just as a diffusible messenger (e.g., calcium, pH) makes sense for rapid regional disassembly of a cortical actin network, a signal localized in the plane of the plasma (or other) membranes is reasonable for targeting precisely where actin filament growth is to occur.*

A recently proposed variation on the theme of membrane lipid control of actin assembly is based on the observed stimulation of actin monomer nucleation in *Dictyostelium discoideum* amoeba membranes stripped of proteins and exposed to diacylglycerol or diacylglycerol analogues.[80] Although diacylglycerols are activators of protein kinase C activity, protein kinase C was not included in the experimental system, and inhibitors of the enzyme did not block the nucleation effect. Therefore, diacylglycerol must act on a yet undefined component in the amoeba cell membrane. This nucleating activity has not been described in white blood cells, although diacylglycerol analogues induce slow and sustained shape changes, primarily extreme flattening without defined polarity, in leukocytes.[81, 82] These alterations correlate with increased net cytoskeletal actin in differentiated leukocytes,[83–85] although diacylglycerol analogue results in decreased cytoskeletal actin in undifferentiated white blood cells.[86] As observed for diacylglycerol actions on *Dictyostelium* membranes, the effects of diacylglycerol analogues on leukocyte actin assembly may not be mediated by protein kinase C activation.[87, 88]

NETWORK FORMATION OF ACTIN FILAMENTS IN WHITE BLOOD CELLS. A number of proteins in leukocytes promote actin bundle formation in vitro. These proteins are α-actinin, L-plastin, and *fimbrin.* In contrast, *actin-binding protein (ABP),* also called *filamin,* promotes high-angle branching of actin filaments characteristic of the leading edge of locomoting white blood cells[89] and in phagocytic cups surrounding particles being ingested.[90, 91] Bundles and gels form spontaneously when actin elongates in the presence of appropriate actin filament cross-linking proteins, but regulation of cross-linking by other factors is also possible. Calcium, for example, inhibits bundling of actin filaments by α-actinin.

PROTEINS MEDIATING MEMBRANE BINDING OF ACTIN FILAMENTS IN WHITE BLOOD CELLS. At a minimum, a physical contact between an underlying dynamic actin cytoskeleton can serve to stabilize the otherwise weak lipid bilayer of the plasma membrane. Under some circumstances, it is advantageous, in addition, for the leukocyte to have firm connections between the underlying actin cytoskeleton and the plasma membrane, as when, for example, the cell retracts extended processes. A large and growing number of such contacts have been identified. The extensive planar spectrin-based lamina of erythrocytes (see Chapter 17) and platelets[92] has not been observed in leukocytes, although these cells contain spectrin and spectrin-binding proteins, which in turn bind certain membrane adhesion receptors.[93–98] Another high-affinity actin-membrane connection in leukocytes is mediated by ABP, the actin cross-linking protein described above, which also binds FcgR1 (CD64), the high-affinity immunoglobulin receptor of leukocytes.[99]

As described in Chapter 14, β$_2$ integrins are important adhesion molecules of leukocytes. Studies with cultured cells have identified complex connections between the invariant β chain of these integrins and actin-associated proteins in structures known as adhesion plaques. In these membrane-spanning spot welds between the actin skeleton and the extracellular matrix, the integrin subunits bind actin through the intermediary of α-actinin or indirectly through a series of proteins—*talin, vinculin,* and α-actinin and *radixin*—in tandem.[100–102] Other proteins found in these adhesion complexes include *tensin*, a phosphoprotein with an SH-2 domain,[103] pp60[src],[104] and a pp60[src] substrate named pp120 or pp125[FAK].[28] Leukocytes do not tend to make structures with the high density of adhesion plaques, but the adhesion plaque–associated proteins are detectable in leukocytes in discrete dot-like structures representing cell-substrate interactions. These adhesion structures, sometimes called podosomes, are also characteristic of transformed fibroblasts in tissue culture.[105, 106] *Myristoylated arginine-rich protein C kinase substrate (MARCKS)* is also localized in podosomes and mediates a direct membrane-actin connection.[107, 108] LSP-1, a lymphocyte-specific membrane protein, has recently been shown to find F-actin as well.[109]

REGULATION OF ACTIN FILAMENT–MEMBRANE ASSOCIATIONS. When leukocyte membranes undergo protrusive activity, it may be advantageous to destabilize connections between the bilayer and the underlying actin system. Severing of actin filaments by proteins such as gelsolin, cofilin, or destrin is one mechanism for this dissociation. It is also possible that regulation of the membrane connections themselves could lead to loss of associations between them and actin. Ligation of FcgR1 by IgG dissociates ABP from this receptor in myeloid cells.[99] Phosphorylation on serines in the middle of the MARCKS polypeptide by protein kinase C or binding of calcium-calmodulin to a stretch near the phosphorylation sites dissociates MARCKS from plasma membranes, suggesting that transmembrane signaling controls the association between MARCKS, actin, and the membrane.[107, 108]

MYOSIN-BASED MOVEMENT OF ACTIN IN WHITE BLOOD CELLS. Assembled actin filaments and actin filament networks are also potentially subject to movement induced by the mechanochemical protein *myosin*. Different myosin isoforms are now recognized, of which there are two general classes, designated *myosin I* and *myosin II*. In recent years, there has been little study of leukocyte myosins, so that the following summary primarily represents inferences from research on blood platelets or other myosins.

Myosin II is the sarcomeric myosin, a hexameric protein comprising two heavy and four light subunits. The large subunits have globular head domains that interact with actin filaments and helical tails that aggregate to form characteristic bipolar filaments. The interaction of the myosin II heads with actin is regulated by the state of phosphorylation of a subset of the light chains, which in turn is controlled by a specific *myosin light chain kinase (MLCK)*. MLCK is activated by the calcium-binding protein *calmodulin* when bound to calcium. Myosin light chain dephosphorylation is mediated by a *type 1 protein phosphatase* or occurs when *protein kinase C* phosphorylates serine residues adjacent to the MLCK sites. Phosphorylation of these residues counteracts the activating effect of MLCK-induced phosphorylation.[110, 111] Phosphorylation of the myosin light chains, and possibly the heavy chains, may also regulate the aggregation of the myosin tails into bipolar filaments,[112] although evidence of such control has not been researched in the case of leukocyte myosins.

Two actin filament–binding proteins, *tropomyosin* and *caldesmon*, also modulate the interaction between phosphorylated myosin and actin. This interaction is usually measured by myosin's ATPase activity in the presence of actin, which transduces force in the form of the sliding of myosin heads along an actin filament. Caldesmon inhibits this activity, and calcium-calmodulin overcomes this inhibition; tropomyosin enhances the interaction.[113–115]

Myosin I represents a class of trimeric or hexameric myosins of lower molecular weight than myosin II, many of which do not form bipolar filaments. Myosin I binds phosphatidylserine in membrane vesicles and is therefore proposed to be another actin-membrane linkage protein. Originally discovered in amoebas in which there are multiple myosin I isoforms, this myosin class has been identified in mammalian epithelial cells, but not yet in white blood cells.[116, 117]

Cellular, Biochemical, and Histochemical Evidence for the Regulation Scheme of the Actin Cycle in Leukocytes

The scheme for regulation of remodeling of the leukocyte actin cytoskeleton is not a simple reversible assembly process but rather a cycle driven at different points by different signals, although some of the control proteins act at various points within the cycle. The cycle permits remodeling to be controlled in both space and time, thereby accounting for the fluidity characteristic of the cortical response to agonists approaching it at different parts of the cell surface as a function of time.

The proposal for regulation of actin monomer– and actin filament–binding proteins by messengers, however, originated from studies of these proteins with actin in vitro. The effects, for example, of calcium and of polyphosphoinositides on the activities of the actin regulatory proteins in vitro have been reproducible in many laboratories, and the chemical basis of the way in which these messengers affect the target proteins is becoming increasingly clear. Such information, nevertheless, indicates only that regulation of actin assembly *could* occur this way in the cell, not that it *does*. Evidence in support of this formulation at the cellular level, however, comes from correlative studies relating changes in signals to the state of actin assembly and from observations of cells expressing different concentrations of the regulatory proteins as a result of changes in endogenous expression or of genetic transfection.

CORRELATIONS BETWEEN SIGNALING EVENTS AND NET ACTIN ASSEMBLY IN STIMULATED CELLS. A role for calcium in leukocyte motility is suggested by the fact that many motility-inducing agonists raise the levels of free cytosolic calcium by opening transmembrane channels and by releasing calcium from intracellular stores. The intracellular calcium concentration of electrically permeabilized neutrophils can be adjusted to a particular level by the calcium content in the suspending medium. The cytoskeletal actin level of the electrically permeabilized cells varies inversely with the calcium concentration, being low at high calcium levels and high at low calcium levels. At the low (~ nanomolar) but not the high (~ millimolar) range of calcium values, addition of a chemotactic peptide increases the cytoskeletal actin content.[118] These results are consistent with calcium promoting actin disassembly through its effects on gelsolin and on MCP and with some other mechanism not directly related to calcium-inducing actin assembly. That this other mechanism is the accumulation of polyphosphoinositides is indicated by the finding that activation of neutrophils by chemoattractants increases, in isolated plasma membranes, the specific activity of enzymes that catalyze the phosphorylation of polyphosphoinositide precursors to the relevant polyphosphoinositides.[119–121]

Correlations between levels of signals such as calcium and actin assembly, however, are not always straightforward or consistent with the proposed scheme. Diacylglycerol analogues induce modest and sustained increments of actin assembly in leukocytes, and $TGF\beta_1$ elicits large increases without measurable changes in cytosolic calcium.[122] Neutrophils loaded with intracellular calcium chelators fail to have the customary rise in $Ca^{2+}i$ induced by agonists. Nevertheless, the agonists still cause increases in net actin assembly and protrusive activity, and the cells undergo locomotion on some surfaces.[123–125] In the chelated state, however, they cannot detach from integrin receptor ligands,[126] and their exocytic response is inhibited.[127] Human neutrophils and murine macrophages have been shown to demonstrate normal phagocytosis of yeast particles, oil droplets, or IgG-coated erythrocytes associated with localized actin assembly within pseudopodia surrounding the red cells undergoing ingestion under conditions in which cytosolic calcium was kept at nanomolar levels by intracellular chelators[128–130]; another study, however, has ascribed some of these results to methodological problems and reported an absolute correlation between intracellular calcium transients and phagocytosis.[131]

Worth considering is that the reduction and clamping of the average cytosolic calcium concentration by chelators does not represent a critical test of the role of calcium, because calcium-binding proteins could theoretically abstract calcium from vesicular pools, especially if it is bound to polyphosphoinositides in vesicular membranes. Gelsolin molecules have, in fact, been localized to vesicular structures inside cells.[132] Transfer of calcium from a vesicle to a binding protein could take place without affecting the average calcium content of the cell reported by chelating indicator compounds.

Increases in bulk cellular PIP or PIP_2 levels also do not correlate precisely with induced net actin assembly in agonist-treated cells.[133] Changes in a quantitatively minor polyphosphoinositide, *phosphatidylinositol 3,4,5-triphosphate (PIP₃)*, correlate better temporally with transient cytoskeletal actin accumulation in stimulated leukocytes,[134–136] but PIP_3 has not been available in sufficient quantities to determine if it interacts with actin regulatory proteins in vitro. As mentioned above, the aggregation state of the polyphosphoinositides is important in their interaction with the actin regulatory proteins, so that changes in the membrane environment where agonists interact with receptors may be more important than bulk concentrations of particular lipid species for the expression of their effects. Morphological studies, described below, are consistent with this idea.

EVIDENCE FOR CAPPED ACTIN OLIGOMERS IN LEUKOCYTES AS SUBSTRATES FOR ACTIN ASSEMBLY. If linear actin assembly results primarily from uncapping of filament barbed ends, such capped ends must be available in the resting cell, even in the absence of a calcium transient. Gelsolin is an example of an actin regulatory protein that is almost completely detergent extractable. A significant proportion of the gelsolin in extracts of resting neutrophils and macrophages is complexed to actin filaments in the extracts, indicative of a source of capped barbed filament ends available in the cell to nucleate actin assembly during stimulation.[137, 138] The proportion of gelsolin complexed to actin falls following stimulation with chemoattractants, indicating uncapping of some of the actin oligomers.[133, 137, 139] Short actin filaments with their barbed ends at the cytoplasmic face of adherent macrophage membranes are detectable, and gelsolin caps the barbed ends, as documented by gold bead conjugated antibodies.[132]

Conversely, actin filament nucleation activity, detectable as acceleration of the slow, spontaneous assembly of purified actin, exists in extracts of resting neutrophils, and this nucleation activity is in the barbed direction. This barbed end nucleation activity in extracts of both resting and stimulated cells decays rapidly as the extracts are left standing, and the actin filament–stabilizing alkaloid, phalloidin, inhibits this decay, pointing to short filaments with free barbed ends as the cause of the nucleating activity in the neutrophil extracts. The number of these filaments increases markedly in extracts of chemoattractant-stimulated cells, which is what would be predicted if gelsolin- or MCP-capped oligomers uncapped and elongated on stimulation.[45, 46] Finally, growth of actin filaments is demonstrable at the leading edge of permeabilized cells, and this growth is inhibitable by the addition of cytochalasins or actin filament barbed end capping proteins, indicating that uncapped barbed filament ends exist as potential nuclei for growth of actin filaments at the protrusive region of the cell.[140]

The uncapping mechanism requires that actin monomers be available for addition onto the uncapped filament ends. Profilin molecules in clusters on the cytoplasmic face of macrophage membranes have been documented by immunohistochemistry, a finding consistent with the involvement of profilin in desequestering actin and charging it by exchanging ATP for ADP at particular sites on the plasma membrane.[141, 142]

CHANGES IN CELL BEHAVIOR AS A RESULT OF ALTERATIONS IN THE EXPRESSION OF ACTIN-REGULATING PROTEINS. Compelling evidence for the proposed actin cycle and its control has come from recent studies involving genetic regulation of levels of gelsolin and ABP in cells. Increasing the levels of gelsolin in murine fibroblasts by genetic transfection of human gelsolin complementary DNA (cDNA) had no effect on gross cellular morphology or actin organization but enhanced chemotactic responsiveness of the cells in proportion to gelsolin concentrations expressed.[143] This result is expected if a regulatory component of the cycle is rate limiting and capable, as gelsolin is predicted to be, of controlling either disassembly or assembly in response to different signals.

Tumor cell lines from three unrelated patients with malignant melanoma were found to lack ABP, and cells from these lines, in contrast to four others that expressed ABP, were very deficient in translational locomotion and chemotaxis. Whereas ABP-containing cells responded to serum containing growth and chemotactic factors by assuming an asymmetrical shape and by extending veils and pleats, the ABP-negative cells remained polygonal and displayed striking circumferential blebbing. Transfection of ABP cDNA into one of the ABP-deficient cell lines yielded seven sublines expressing ABP levels below, above, and in the range detectable in wild-type ABP-expressing cells. All but the lines with the lowest ABP contents were asymmetrical in shape and did not have the sustained peripheral blebbing and ABP expression up to the wild-type level correlated with marked improvements in chemotactic responsiveness.[144]

The findings with the melanoma cells are explicable in terms of the actin cycle. ABP expression per se does not directly influence the linear assembly of actin that takes place under control of the actin filament and monomer-binding proteins involved in the scheme for linear assembly. Without the efficient gelation activity of ABP, however, the assembly phase of the scheme is abortive. Not only is the membrane unstable, as evidenced by the blebbing, but also filament mass is not localized efficiently by cross-linking or binding to membranes, and the dissipation of actin mass is responsible for the lack of polarity in the ABP-deficient cells.

COORDINATION OF SIGNALS IN THE CONTROL SCHEME FOR THE ACTIN CYCLE OF LEUKOCYTES. The control of the actin cycle at various points with different regulatory mechanisms allows actin assembly and disassembly to occur at different times and places, depending on need. A simple antagonism, however, between, for example, calcium and membrane polyphosphoinositides would probably be too crude for the smooth control of cell surface motility required for events such as chemotaxis and phagocytosis and would not account for the persistence phenomenon associated with leukocyte locomotion. A more complex coordination is required, particularly because it is unlikely that a cell undergoing multiple stimulatory events could precisely regulate its intracellular calcium in both space and time.

As mentioned above, gelsolin may sever domains of actin filaments containing ADP but not ATP. Since ATP hydrolysis lags behind actin polymerization, the growing region of a filament would be resistant to the action of gelsolin, even if the calcium level rose locally. In addition, gelsolin's initial binding to actin filaments is relatively slow.[145] Another stabilizing factor during the assembly of leukocyte actin may be actin cross-linking, which increases the resistance of actin filaments to depolymerization.[46, 144]

An additional way in which stability may be conferred is if the receptor-initiated transducing factors leading to actin assembly, such as enzymes that synthesize polyphosphoinositides, are activated by protein complexes involving GTP-binding proteins,[32, 146–150] GDP-GTP exchange-enhancing proteins, membrane-binding proteins requiring acylation,[151] and others. Once assembled, these complexes may require time to dissociate and therefore continue to induce polymerization even for a time after an agonist has been removed. Related to the foregoing control mechanism is if actin regulatory proteins also are involved in the regulation of membrane signal generation. Consistent with this hypothesis are the observations that profilin inhibits phospholipase C-γ activity by binding to the lipid substrate and that phospholipase C-γ associated with an activated, tyrosine autophosphorylated growth factor receptor overcomes the inhibition.[152] Phospholipase C-γ also binds actin-gelsolin complexes, suggesting that gelsolin-capped actin oligomers might carry the enzyme to the membrane where signal generation takes place.[153]

Another mechanism for localizing the site of actin assembly is if the assembled actin network concentrates membrane in the region of filament growth. Since the distribution of agonist receptors is constant per unit of membrane area,[154] localizing membrane by creating pleats and infoldings at one pole of the cell thereby raises the number of agonist receptors available in that domain for engagement by agonists. Transient fluctuations, therefore, in chemotactic gradients would not impede directed motility toward the gradient source. Control of receptor function and distribution may also reside in the transient binding of the receptors to stable (cytoskeletal) actin filaments in the cell periphery; such binding for formyl peptide receptors has in general been associated with receptors that bind ligands with slow off-rates and that do not stimulate locomotion as well as unbound receptors with fast off-rates for peptide ligands.[155] The biochemical basis of this chemotactic receptor-actin connection is unknown. Receptor recycling, with insertion at the front and capping and endocytosis at the rear of the cell, is another way to maintain persistence in the face of unstable gradients of activators.

MECHANISMS OF SPECIFIC LEUKOCYTE MOVEMENTS

Locomotion

Considerable evidence implicates actin assembly originating at the plasma membrane at the leading edge of the lamella in the extension of processes by activated leukocytes. First, inhibition of cellular energy metabolism depletes peripheral actin polymers, and following restoration of this metabolism, new filaments appear from the membrane inward.[156] Second, inhibition of actin filament assembly by cytochalasins also depletes peripheral filamentous actin, and, again, new filaments fill in from the plasma membrane.[157] Third, addition of monomeric actin to permeabilized spreading cells results in the formation of new actin filaments at the leading edge, consistent with a concentration of actin filament nuclei at that location.[140] Fourth, labeled actin monomers microinjected into cells accumulate initially at the leading edge of a moving cell and then move backward toward the cell body at the same rate as ruffles.[158, 159]

Although these studies were not all performed with leukocytes, the similarities in behavior among different cell types suggest that the mechanisms are grossly conserved and that actin nucleates and elongates at the advancing plasma membrane where agonists may induce polyphosphoinositide synthesis that promotes monomer desequestration and filament uncapping, leading to actin assembly. Disassembly occurs primarily at the rear of the lamella, where calcium levels may be sufficiently high to activate gelsolin and polyphosphoinositides unavailable to promote assembly. The actin cycle, therefore, drives locomotion by building the actin network at the leading edge of the lamella and dissipating it at the rear of the lamella. The propensity of moving cells to retain a distinct polarity even as they turn may be a result of the various stabilizing factors mentioned above that keep actin assembly localized to where it initiates.

Actin assembly, however, need not be limited to the leading edge, inasmuch as microinjected actin containing a photoactivatable label can assemble and disassemble all over the leading lamella,[160] although it can be biased toward the leading edge.[140] This finding is consistent with the lamella as a system of short actin filaments branched by ABP that turn over with great rapidity linked in parallel with a system of relatively stable actin filaments that migrate from the leading front of the cell toward the cell body. The stable component of the actin network may represent the cytoskeletal actin detectable in resting cells. This actin may interact with the plasma membrane through one or more of the membrane attachment proteins described above. This stable actin, which is prominent around the perimeter of the cell body, may also be contracted by myosin II molecules or filaments, accounting for the focal narrowings occasionally observed on moving cells.

Several theories have been advanced to account for how signal- and actin-modulating protein-mediated actin assembly at the leading edge of an advancing cell results in membrane protrusion. In one, thermal fluctuations of the membrane allow monomers to add onto filaments at the membrane-filament interface, permitting the membrane to ratchet forward.[161] In another, localized disruption of the submembrane actin network leads to swelling, which drives the membrane outward; reconstitution of the network by polymerization and cross-linking then consolidates the forward advance.[162] In a third, membrane-associated myosin I molecules move centrifugally on submembrane actin filaments, causing the leading edge to move forward.[163] It is not possible at present to decide between these alternatives, all of which may operate under particular circumstances.

One can also now only speculate about how the cell glides forward. One possible mechanism is a process coupled to an actin assembly-disassembly cycle whereby adhesion molecules, primarily integrins, bind to the substrate and serve as pinions around which actin-based assemblies, including the many adhesion plaque proteins, cluster. As the lamellar network moves forward in response to the assembly cycle, the actin surrounding the pinion turns over, and finally, as the cell body approaches the pinion, the actin coating dissipates; this step could be a signal to trigger internalization of the receptor, thereby releasing the adhesion. The finding that calcium depletion inhibits de-adhesion by neutrophils is consistent with a role for calcium-activated gelsolin-mediated actin severing in the clearing of actin from the internal part of adhesion sites.[126]

A second possibility is that myosins have a role in gliding movements. The finding that *Dictyostelium discoideum* amoebas genetically deprived of myosin II molecules were able to exhibit locomotion[164, 165] has focused the speculation on myosin I in this role, although a similar experiment has not been done with white blood cells. A role for myosin II in leukocyte motility is implied by its presence in lamellae extended by the cells,[166, 167] and by experiments in which both overphosphorylation and underphosphorylation of the 20 kDa myosin light chain were effected, respectively, by microinjection of anti-MLCK antibodies and unregulated, constitutively active MLCK fragments into macrophages. In both cases, macrophage motility was inhibited, implying an optimal range requirement of myosin light chain phosphorylation for movement.[168]

It is possible theoretically that membrane-associated

myosin I molecules attach to transmembrane proteins adherent to the substrate and motor the lamellar actin network forward; similar myosin molecules at the top of the lamella motor cross-linked membrane proteins toward the cell body. This mechanism demands correctly polarized actin filament tracks, and although long actin filaments with the proper polarity have been observed in cultured fibroblasts and murine macrophages,[169, 170] they have not been found in neutrophils. A small number of stable filaments, however—perhaps the cytoskeletal filaments of the resting cell—might be sufficient for facilitating myosin-mediated motility and might be hard to visualize. The fact that tropomyosin and caldesmon stabilize actin filaments against fragmentation by gelsolin in addition to regulating actin interactions with myosin[171, 172] supports the idea that a stable population of actin filaments is the scaffolding for gliding movement in white blood cells, while the actin cycle controls the guidance for this movement.

Phagocytosis

In many ways, phagocytosis by white blood cells morphologically appears to be a special form of locomotion in which the cell simply crawls around a micrometer-sized or larger object. As described in Chapter 14, phagocytosis by white cells depends on the expression of certain receptors for opsonins deposited on target objects, specifically the β_2 integrin CD11b/CD18, which recognizes C3bi; the type 1 complement receptor CR1 (CD35), which binds C3b; and receptors for the Fc domain of IgG, FcgRI (CD64), FcgRIIA and B (CD32), and FcgRIII (CD16). Ingestion of unopsonized microorganisms is mediated by β_1 integrins, by a β-glucan receptor,[173] or by mannose receptors.[174]

Consistent with the similarity between locomotion and phagocytosis, actin-rich lamellae extend from the cell and progress around the surface of particles. In addition, many of the same membrane-derived signals, such as those of calcium and diacylglycerols, appear in response to phagocytic stimuli of white blood cells. Cytochalasins inhibit phagocytosis as they inhibit locomotion.[175, 176] In addition, the actin-associated proteins—myosin, ABP, gelsolin, and talin—are identifiable in the phagocytic lamellae.[166, 167, 177] Presumably, the mechanism by which the lamellae advance over a field of ligands is similar to the protrusion of lamellae in the direction of locomotion. During ingestion of *Yersinia enterocolitica*, cells display prominent blebbing at the region where internalization occurs,[177] suggesting that the osmotic swelling mechanism of protrusion may be operational during this process.

When lamellae investing phagocytic particles come together, they fuse to form a phagocytic vesicle (phagosome), which buds off the plasma membrane. The mechanism of this fusion is unknown. The interaction of many actin-modulating proteins with plasma membrane lipids raises the possibility that modification of these lipids so as to disorder membrane structure

might play a role in the mixing of lipids that must underlie the fusion mechanism. One set of proteins implicated in this fusion mechanism comprises the *annexins*, a family of calcium- and actin-binding phosphoproteins, some of which have been shown to induce fusion of membranes in vitro.[178–180]

Phagocytosis is a specialized form of receptor-mediated endocytosis. The latter encompasses the uptake of fluid and surface-bound ligands by a process that does not involve the cytoskeleton as defined here but rather occurs by invagination of small vesicles through the action of protein assemblies, predominantly clathrin around coated pits that mediate interiorization of substances such as lipoproteins and transferrin or caveolin that mediate the uptake of folate conjugates.

Secretion

The actin cortex of the leukocyte plays a permissive role in the control of the exocytosis of large granules that accompanies phagocytosis (degranulation) and the agonist-induced secretion of similar granules by basophils, mast cells, and other leukocytes that leads to immediate hypersensitivity responses and other inflammatory reactions. During phagocytosis, the characteristic organelle exclusion of the cortex attenuates at the base of the forming phagosome, and granules fuse with the vacuole membrane, leading to the creation of a phagolysosome. The finding that preventing a rise in cytosolic calcium levels during phagocytosis inhibits degranulation[127, 181] suggests that gelsolin might play a role in severing actin filaments at the base of the vacuole to explain the movement of granules toward the phagosomal membrane at that location. Secretion by exocytosis of small vesicles is not affected by the cortical actin gel, because the secretory organelles are small enough to diffuse through its interstices. The fusion of these vesicles with the plasmalemma, like receptor-mediated endocytosis, appears to work by a different mechanism than does exocytosis of large granules[182] unrelated to the cytoskeleton as defined here. Microtubule integrity, however, may be required for proper trafficking of these vesicles to the cell surface.[39]

MOTILITY-RELATED WHITE BLOOD CELL DISORDERS

Chapter 14 described the molecular and clinical features of diseases caused by genetic deficiency of leukocyte adhesion molecules. In addition to these well-characterized genetic conditions caused by impaired leukocyte motility, the molecules of the cortical cytoplasm may also contribute to cellular alterations resulting in disease states.

Neutrophil Actin Dysfunction

In 1974, Boxer and colleagues reported the case of an infant with chronic peripheral blood neutrophilic leukocytosis who presented with recurrent severe pyogenic infections since birth and whose neutrophils were markedly deficient in locomotion and phagocytosis. Actin in extracts of the patient's neutrophils failed to polymerize under conditions that polymerized actin in control neutrophil extracts.[183] The neutrophil defects were corrected by allogeneic bone marrow transplantation, although the patient died of complications of the procedure. Subsequently, the patient's family was investigated, and it was found that a fraction of actin in extracts of parental neutrophils was deficient in polymerization. Actin purified from parental neutrophils polymerized normally, however, and treatment of neutrophils with the elastase inhibitor di-isopropylfluorophosphate prior to extraction corrected the abnormal behavior of actin in neutrophil extracts, suggesting that an actin-modulating factor was responsible.[184] The picture was complicated by the finding that paternal neutrophils expressed low levels of the β_2-integrin CD11b/CD18 (see Chapter 14), although further work established that abnormal actin assembly is not frequently associated with CD11b/CD18 deficiency.[185] With the exception of this family, and another subsequently encountered,[186] no defects of the actin system have been associated with congenital leukocyte disorders, although diminished actin polymerization in response to chemoattractants has been associated with defective locomotion of neonatal and of chronic myelogenous leukemic neutrophils.[187, 188]

Listeriosis

Many infectious diseases associated with intracellular parasitism begin by phagocytic penetration of cells by microorganisms, and this entry involves the molecules of the cellular cortex involved in phagocytosis in general.[177] Recently, it has been recognized that the actin system participates in a unique and striking way in the pathogenesis of intracellular parasitism involving leukocytes. The gram-positive bacterial microorganism *Listeria monocytogenes* enters macrophages (and other cells) by phagocytosis and then escapes the phagocytic vacuole by elaboration of a phospholipase and proceeds to move around the cytoplasm to the periphery, where it enters extended surface projections of the phagocyte and uses them to spread to adjacent cells. The movements of the microbe in the cytoplasm are rapid, on the order of 0.1 μm per second, and are mediated by its ability to take over the host cell's actin-based motile machinery.

A cloud of actin filaments begins to appear at one pole of the bacterium, and as the microorganism proceeds to move, these filaments trail behind the advancing microbe in a configuration that has been likened to a comet's tail; the filaments immediately adjacent to the bacterial surface orient their barbed ends toward it,[189] and actin assembly takes place at the point where the actin tail originates at the bacterial surface.[190] This fact and the finding that cytochalasins

or microinjection of actin monomer–sequestering proteins into the host cell stops assembly and bacterial movement[191] indicate that actin assembly initiated at the bacterial membrane drives the movement of the bacterium through the cytoplasm. The most likely mechanism for actin assembly and movement is that actin monomer desequestration and charging and filament uncapping occur at the bacterial membrane; filaments are generated, separated from the bacterium, and cross-linked in its immediate vicinity,[192] and it is the accumulation of a column of cross-linked actin behind the bacterium that drives its forward motion. Involvement of profilin and gelsolin in this process is suggested by the concentration of profilin at the bacterial-actin interface and by the observation that the rate of bacterial motion is proportional to the gelsolin content of cells. A *Listeria* protein with sequence motifs resembling the actin-binding protein vinculin is required for the bacterial induction of host cell actin assembly.[193]

Leukocyte Proliferation, Differentiation, and Neoplasia

In contrast to leukocyte motility, in which its role is relatively minor, the tubulin system is extremely important in leukocyte proliferation. In particular, tubulin is the principal constituent of the mitotic spindle on which chromosomes separate during cell division. Microtubules and microtubule-associated proteins also are implicated in signal transduction that occurs as cells respond to mitogens. Growth factors activate a cascade of protein serine/threonine kinases, including one that phosphorylates microtubule-associated proteins *(MAP-kinase)*,[194] and microtubule length and number increase following mitogenic stimulation.[195]

Anomalies of the actin system have been associated with neoplasia in general and with hematological malignancies in particular. One observation is that the hyporesponsiveness of chronic lymphatic leukemia B cells to mitogenic stimulation can be enhanced by cytochalasins,[196, 197] although the basis of these findings remains unknown and puzzling in light of cytochalasin's inhibition of some normal responses of lymphoid cells (see below).

It is almost certain that the invasiveness of neoplastic cells resides in part in their ability to disaggregate and to undergo active locomotion, both processes being dependent on the actin system. A consistent finding with regard to cells in culture has been the tendency of transformed cells not to lay down actin filaments on their ventral surfaces in bundles, sometimes called stress fibers, in contrast to their untransformed counterparts, implying differences in the organization of actin—hence in the action of actin-associated proteins—between transformed and untransformed cells. One explanation offered for these morphological distinctions has been the reduced expression in transformed cells of the actin filament stabilizing protein tropomyosin or the expression of tropomyosin variants with lowered affinity for binding to actin.[198, 199] Another interesting observation is the finding that the chronic myelogenous leukemia–associated oncogene, a fusion of chromosome 22–derived *bcr* with chromosome 9–derived *abl* genes, encodes *bcr/abl* fusion proteins, which, in addition to having tyrosine kinase activity, associate with actin filaments in transformed cells.[200]

Cells capable of mitosis, including myeloid progenitors exposed to proliferation-inducing cytokines such as colony-stimulating factor–1 (CSF-1) or platelet-derived growth factor, exhibit ruffling at the cell surface and rearrangements of cortical actin as well.[201–204] The small G protein c-*rac* has been implicated in the regulation of these cell surface changes.[150] Stimulation of human B lymphocytes with mitogens causes actin assembly through a mechanism involving a pertussis toxin–sensitive G protein, and inhibition of this assembly by cytochalasins, pertussis toxin, or botulinum C_2 toxin also prevents cellular proliferation.[205, 206] Another mitogen, phorbol myristate acetate, induces actin assembly in T lymphocytes.[85]

Actin content changes little during differentiation of myeloid cell lines HL-60 and U937,[207, 208] and profilin content changes hardly at all,[209] but there is significant upregulation of β_4 thymosin,[210, 211] of myosin heavy chain,[212] and of ABP, as well as very markedly increased expression of gelsolin, although the extent of elevation depends on the differentiating agent.[209] The appearance of these regulatory proteins may explain changes in the ability of developing myeloid cells to respond to agonists by polymerizing cellular actin,[207, 213–215] since this responsiveness correlates poorly with agonist receptor expression during myeloid maturation.[86, 216]

The increase in gelsolin expression as a function of myeloid differentiation[209] is interesting in light of other observations that the expression levels of this protein fall in neoplastic cells. For example, gelsolin is the major downregulated protein in simian virus 40 (SV40)–transformed cell lines.[217] Conversely, a mutant gelsolin is the major upregulated polypeptide in NIH 3T3 fibroblasts transformed with H-*ras* but that have undergone mutagen-induced reversion to a non-neoplastic phenotype.[218, 219] Invasive breast carcinoma cells in histological sections of human mammary cancer have barely detectable gelsolin by immunohistochemical reactivity, in contrast to brightly staining duct epithelium from which the cancers arose.[220] It is interesting that the murine variant of the gelsolin-related actin filament capping protein gCap 39/MCP/MHb-1 has also been shown to have sequences predicted to interact with the c-*myc* oncoprotein and was localized to the nucleus of fibroblasts by immunofluorescence microscopy.[60]

These preliminary results require follow-up research, but it is possible to speculate on what they might mean. Recent information has implicated polyphosphoinositides as signals involved in driving the phenotype of malignant transformation. In particular, kinases producing PI_3-P and $PI_{3,4}$-P_2 have been asso-

ciated with transforming oncogenes of SV40 middle T and with the *src* family of non-receptor tyrosine kinases.[221] It is possible that gelsolin and related proteins, being polyphosphoinositide-binding proteins, have the capacity to bind to these relatively minor phospholipid species in a way that inhibits their oncogenic expression, such that the cell that is to gain a selective advantage must first downregulate the interfering proteins. Exploration of this possibility may yield new insights into the physiology of malignant transformation and possible therapeutic strategies.

REFERENCES

1. Schultze, M.: Ein Heizbarer objekttisch und seine Verwendung bei Untersuchung des Blutes. Arch Mikrosk Anat. 1:1, 1965.
2. Keller, H., and Bessis, M.: Migration and chemotaxis of anucleate cytoplasmic fragments. Nature 258:723, 1975.
3. Malawista, S., and Boisfleury Chevance, A.: The cytokineplast: Purified, stable, and functional motile machinery from human blood polymorphonuclear leukocytes: Possible formative role of heat-induced centrosomal dysfunction. J. Cell Biol. 95:960, 1982.
4. Rinnerthaler, G., Geiger, B., and Small, J.: Contact formation during fibroblast locomotion: Involvement of membrane ruffles and microtubules. J. Cell Biol. 106:747, 1988.
5. DeBruyn, P.: The amoeboid movement of the mammalian leukocyte in tissue culture. Anat. Rec. 95:177, 1946.
6. Shields, J., and Haston, W.: Behaviour of neutrophil leucocytes in uniform concentrations of chemotactic factors: Contraction waves, cell polarity and persistence. J. Cell Sci. 74:75, 1985.
7. Evans, E., and Dembo, M.: Physical model for phagocyte motility: Local growth of a contractile network from a passive body. *In* Akkas, N. (ed.): Biomechanics of Active Movement and Deformation. Berlin/Heidelberg, Springer Verlag, 1990.
8. Gerisch, G., and Keller, H.: Chemotactic orientation of granulocytes stimulated with micropipettes containing fMet-Leu-Phe. J. Cell Sci. 52:1, 1981.
9. Keller, H., Zimmerman, A., and Cottier, H.: Crawling-like movements, adhesion to solid substrata and chemokinesis of neutrophil granulocytes. J. Cell Sci. 64:89, 1983.
10. Thomas, K., Pyun, H., and Navarro, J.: Molecular cloning of the f-met-leu-phe receptor from neutrophils. J. Biol. Chem. 265:20061, 1990.
11. Nakamura, M., Honda, Z.-I., Izumi, T., Sakanaka, C., Mutoh, H., Minami, M., Blto, H., Seyama, Y., Matsumoto, T., Noma, M., and Shimuzu, T.: Molecular cloning and expression of platelet-activating factor receptor from human leukocytes. J. Biol. Chem. 266:20400, 1991.
12. Murphy, P., and Tiffany, H.: Cloning of complementary DNA encoding a functional human interleukin-8 receptor. Science 253:1280, 1991.
13. Gerard, N., and Gerard, C.: The chemotactic receptor for human C5a anaphylatoxin. Nature 349:614, 1991.
14. Brandes, M., Mai, U., Ohura, K., and Wahl, S.: Type 1 transforming growth factor-β receptors on neutrophils mediate chemotaxis to transforming growth factor-β. J. Immunol. 147:1600, 1991.
15. Boulay, F., Mery, L., Tardif, M., Brouchon, L., and Vignais, P.: Expression cloning of a receptor for C5a anaphylatoxin on differentiated HL-60 cells. Biochemistry 30:2993, 1991.
16. Sha'afi, R., and Molski, T.: Activation of the neutrophil. Progr Allergy 42:1, 1988.
17. Holmes, W., Lee, J., Kuang, W.-J., Rice, G., and Wood, W.: Structure and functional expression of a human interleukin-8 receptor. Science 253:1278, 1991.
18. Ullrich, A., and Schlesinger, J.: Signal transduction by receptors with tyrosine kinase activity. Cell 61:203, 1990.

19. Hall, A.: The cellular function of small GTP-binding proteins. Science 249:635, 1990.

20. Bonnerot, C., Amigorena, S., Choquet, D., Pavlovich, R., Choukroun, V., and Fridman, W.: Role of associated γ-chain in tyrosine kinase activation via murine FcγRIII. EMBO J. 11:2747, 1992.

21. Huang, M.-M., Indik, Z., Brass, L., Hoxie, J., Schreiber, A., and Brugge, J.: Activation of FcγRII induces tyrosine phosphorylation of multiple proteins including FcγRII. J. Biol. Chem. 267:5467, 1992.

22. Koolwijk, P., Van de Winkel, J., Pfefferkorn, L., Jacobs, C., Otten, I., Spierenburg, G., and Bast, B.: Induction of intracellular Ca²⁺ mobilization and cytotoxity by hybrid mouse monoclonal antibodies. FcγRII regulation of FcγRI-triggered functions or signalling? J. Immunol. 147:595, 1991.

23. Liao, F., Shin, H., and Rhee, S.: Tyrosine phosphorylation of phospholipase C-γ1 induced by cross-linking of the high affinity or low affinity Fc receptor for IgG in U937 cells. Proc. Natl. Acad. Sci. USA 89:3659, 1992.

24. Rosales, C., and Brown, E.: Signal transduction by neutrophil immunoglobulin G Fc receptors. Dissociation of intracytoplasmic calcium concentration rise from inositol 4,5-trisphosphate. J. Biol. Chem. 267:5265, 1992.

25. Wirthmueller, U., Kurosaki, T., Murakami, M., and Ravetch, J.: Signal transduction by FcγRIII (CD16) is mediated through the γ chain. J. Exp. Med. 175:1381, 1992.

26. Hynes, R.: Integrins: Versatility, modulation, and signaling in cell adhesion. Cell 69:11, 1992.

27. Scholl, P., Ahern, D., and Geha, R.: Protein tyrosine phosphorylation induced via the IgG receptors FcγRI and FcγRII in the human monocytic cell lines THP-1. J. Immunol. 149:1751, 1992.

28. Guan, J.-L., and Shalloway, D.: Regulation of focal adhesion-associated protein tyrosine kinase by both cellular adhesion and oncogenic transformation. Nature 358:690, 1992.

29. Odin, J., Edberg, J., Painter, C., Kimberly, R., and Unkeless, J.: Regulation of phagocytosis and [Ca²⁺]ᵢ flux by distinct regions of an Fc receptor. Science 254:1785, 1991.

30. Amigorena, S., Bonnerot, C., Drake, J., Choquet, D., Hunziker, W., Guillet, J.-G., Webster, P., Sautes, C., Mellman, I., and Fridman, W.: Cytoplasmic domain heterogeneity and functions of IgG Fc receptors in B lymphocytes. Science 256:1808, 1992.

31. Janmey, P.: Mechanical properties of cytoskeletal polymers. Curr. Opin. Cell. Biol. 3:4, 1991.

32. Grimminger, F., Sibelius, U., Aktories, K., Just, I., and Seeger, W.: Suppression of cytoskeletal rearrangement in activated human neutrophils by Botulinum C2 toxin. Impact on cellular signal transduction. J. Biol. Chem. 266:19276, 1991.

33. Keller, H., Naef, A., and Cottier, H.: Effects of colchicine, vinblastine and nocodazole on polarity, motility, chemotaxis and cAMP levels of human polymorphonuclear leukocytes. Exp. Cell. Res. 153:173, 1984.

34. Bornens, M., Paintrand, M., and Celati, C.: The cortical microfilament system of lymphoblasts displays periodic oscillatory activity in the absence of microtubules: Implications for cell polarity. J. Cell Biol. 109:1071, 1989.

35. Cassimeris, L., Wadsworth, P., and Salmond, E.: Dynamics of microtubule depolymerization in monocytes. J. Cell Biol. 102:2023, 1986.

36. Nath, J., Powledge, A., and Wright, D.: Studies of signal transduction in the respiratory burst–associated stimulation of fMet-Leu-Phe–induced tubulin tyrosinolation and phorbol-12-myristate 13-acetate–induced posttranslational incorporation of tyrosine into multiple proteins in activated neutrophils and HL-60 cells. J. Biol. Chem. 264:848, 1989.

37. Singer, S., and Kupfer, A.: The directed migration of eukaryotic cells. Annu. Rev. Cell. Biol. 2:337, 1986.

38. Swanson, J., Bushnell, A., and Silverstein, S.: Tubular lysosome morphology and distribution within macrophages depend on the integrity of cytoplasmic microtubules. Proc. Natl. Acad. Sci. USA 84:1921, 1987.

39. Hollenbeck, P., and Swanson, J.: Radial extension of macro-

40. Gomez-Cambronero, J., Huang, C.-K., Gomez-Cambronero, T., Waterman, W., Becker, E., and Sha'afi, R.: Granulocyte-macrophage colony-stimulating factor–induced protein tyrosine phosphorylation of microtubule-associated protein kinase in human neutrophils. Proc. Natl. Acad. Sci. USA 89:7551, 1992.

41. Huang, C.-K., Hill, J., Jr., Bormann, B., Mackin, W., and Becker, E.: Chemotactic factors induced vimentin phosphorylation in rabbit peritoneal neutrophils. J. Biol. Chem. 259:1386, 1984.

42. Wyatt, T., Lincoln, T., and Pryzwansky, K.: Vimentin is transiently colocalized with and phosphorylated by cyclic GMP-dependent protein kinase in formyl-peptide–stimulated neutrophils. J. Biol. Chem. 266:21274, 1991.

43. Lawrence, M., and Springer, T.: Leukocytes roll on a selectin at physiologic flow rates: Distinction from and prerequisite for adhesion through integrins. Cell 65:859, 1991.

44. Amato, P., Unanue, E., and Taylor, D.: Distribution of actin in spreading macrophages: A comparative study on living and fixed cells. J. Cell Biol. 96:750, 1983.

45. Cano, M., Lauffenburger, D., and Zigmond, S.: Kinetic analysis of F-actin depolymerization in polymorphonuclear leukocyte lysates indicates that chemoattractant stimulation increases actin filament number without altering the filament length distribution. J. Cell Biol. 115:677, 1991.

46. Cano, M., Cassimeris, L., Fechheimer, M., and Zigmond, S.: Mechanisms responsible for F-actin stabilization after lysis of polymorphonuclear leukocytes. J. Cell Biol. 116:1123, 1992.

47. Stossel, T., and Hartwig, J.: Interactions of actin, myosin and an actin-binding protein of rabbit pulmonary macrophages. II. Role in cytoplasmic movement and phagocytosis. J. Cell Biol. 68:602, 1976.

48. Boxer, L., and Stossel, T.: Isolation and properties of actin, myosin and a new actin-binding protein of chronic myelogenous leukemia leukocytes. J. Clin. Invest. 57:5696, 1976.

49. Apgar, J.: Regulation of the antigen-induced F-actin response in rat basophilic leukemia cells by protein kinase C. J. Cell Biol. 112:1157, 1991.

50. Jackman, W., and Burridge, K.: Polymerization of additional actin is not required for capping of surface antigens in B-lymphocytes. Cell Motility Cytoskeleton 12:23, 1989.

51. Carlier, M.-F.: Actin: Protein structure and filament dynamics. J. Biol. Chem. 266:1, 1991.

52. Estes, J., Selden, L., Kinosian, H., and Gershman, L.: Tightly-bound divalent cation of actin. J. Muscle Res. Cell Motil. 13:272, 1992.

53. Cassimeris, L., McNeill, H., and Zigmond, S.: Chemoattractant-stimulated polymorphonuclear leukocytes contain two populations of actin filaments that differ in their spatial distributions and relative stabilities. J. Cell Biol. 110:1067, 1990.

54. Yin, H. L., and Stossel, T. P.: Control of cytoplasmic actin gel-sol transformation by gelsolin, a calcium-dependent regulatory protein. Nature 281:583, 1979.

55. Yin, H. L.: Gelsolin. A calcium- and polyphosphoinositide-regulated actin-modulating protein. BioEssays 7:176, 1987.

55a. Lamb, J., Allen, P., Tuan, B., and Janmey, P.: Modulation of gelsolin function: Activation at low pH overrides Ca²⁺ requirement. J. Biol. Chem. 268:8999, 1993.

55b. Laham, L., Lamb, J., Allen, P., and Janmey, P.: Selective binding of gelsolin to actin monomers containing ADP. J. Biol. Chem. 268:14202, 1993.

56. Southwick, F. S., and DiNubile, M. J.: Rabbit alveolar macrophages contain a Ca²⁺-sensitive, 41,000-dalton protein which reversibly blocks the "barbed" ends of actin filaments but does not sever them. J. Biol. Chem. 261:14191, 1986.

57. Young, C., Southwick, F., and Weber, A.: Kinetics of the interaction of a 41-kDa macrophage capping protein with actin: Promotion of nucleation during prolongation of the lag period. Biochemistry 29:2232, 1990.

58. Dabiri, G., Young, C., Rosenbloom, J., and Southwick, F.:

Molecular cloning of human macrophage capping protein cDNA. A unique member of the gelsolin/villin family expressed primarily in macrophages. J. Biol. Chem. 267:16545, 1992.

59. Yu, F., Johnston, P. A., Suedhof, T. C., and Yin, H. L.: gCap39, a calcium ion– and polyphosphoinositide–regulated actin capping protein. Science 250:1413, 1990.

60. Prendergast, G., and Ziff, E.: Mbh1: A novel gelsolin/severin-related protein which binds actin *in vitro* and exhibits nuclear localization *in vivo*. EMBO J. 10:757, 1991.

60a. Onoda, K., and Yin, H.: gCap39 is phosphorylated. Stimulation by okadaic acid and preferential association with nuclei. J. Biol. Chem. 268:4106, 1993.

61. Heiss, S., and Cooper, J.: Regulation of CapZ, an actin capping protein of chicken muscle, by anionic phospholipids. Biochemistry 30:8753, 1991.

62. Carlsson, L., Nystrom, L. E., Sundkvist, I., Markey, F., and Lindberg, U.: Actin polymerizability is influenced by profilin, a low molecular weight protein in non-muscle cells. J. Mol. Biol. 115:465, 1977.

63. Safer, D., Elzinga, M., and Nachmias, V.: Thymosin β4 and Fx, an actin-sequestering peptide, are indistinguishable. J. Biol. Chem. 266:4029, 1991.

63a. Cassimeris, L., Safer, D., Nachmias, V., and Zigmond, S.: Thymosin β$_4$ sequesters the majority of G-actin in resting human polymorphonuclear leukocytes. J. Cell. Biol. 119:1261, 1992.

63b. Yu, F.-X., Lin, S.-C., Morrison-Bogorad, M., Atkinson, M., and Yin, H.: Thymosin β10 and thymosin β4 are both actin monomer–sequestering proteins. J. Biol. Chem. 268:502, 1993.

64. Adams, M. E., Minamide, L. S., Duester, G., and Bamburg, J. R.: Nucleotide sequence and expression of a cDNA encoding chick brain actin depolymerizing factor. Biochemistry 29:7414, 1990.

65. Moriyama, K., Nishida, E., Yonezawa, N., Sakai, H., Matsumoto, S., Iida, K., and Yahara, I.: Destrin, a mammalian actin-depolymerizing protein, is closely related to cofilin. Cloning and expression of porcine brain destrin cDNA. J. Biol. Chem. 265:5768, 1990.

66. Yonezawa, N., Nishida, E., and Sakai, H.: pH control of actin polymerization by cofilin. J. Biol. Chem. 260:14410, 1985.

67. Wallace, P., Wersto, R., Packman, C., and Lichtman, M.: Chemotactic peptide-induced changes in neutrophil actin conformation. J. Cell. Biol. 99:1060, 1984.

68. White, J., Naccache, P., and Sha'afi, R.: Stimulation by chemotactic factor of actin association with the cytoskeleton in rabbit neutrophils. Effects of calcium and cytochalasin B. J. Cell. Biol. 258:14041, 1983.

69. Stossel, T.: From signal to pseudopod. How cells control cytoplasmic actin assembly. J. Biol. Chem. 264:18261, 1989.

70. Goldschmidt-Clermont, P., Machesky, L., Doberstein, S., and Pollard, T.: Mechanism of interaction of human platelet profilin with actin. J. Cell. Biol. 113:1081, 1991.

70a. Goldschmidt-Clermont, P., Furman, M., Wachstock, D., Safer, D., Nachmias, V., and Pollard, T.: The control of actin nucleotide exchange by thymosin β4 and profilin. A potential regulatory mechanism for actin polymerization in cells. Mol. Biol. Cell. 3:1015, 1992.

71. Janmey, P. A., Iida, K., Yin, H. L., Stossel, T. P.: Polyphosphoinositide micelles and polyphosphoinositide-containing vesicles dissociate endogenous gelsolin-actin complexes and promote actin assembly from the fast-growing end of actin filaments blocked by gelsolin. J. Biol. Chem. 262:12228, 1987.

72. Janmey, P. A., and Stossel, T. P.: Modulation of gelsolin function by phosphatidylinositol-4,5-bisphosphate. Nature 325:362, 1987.

73. Janmey, P. A., and Stossel, T. P.: Gelsolin-polyphosphoinositide interaction. Full expression of gelsolin-inhibiting function by polyphosphoinositides in vesicular form and inactivation by dilution, aggregation, or masking of the inositol head group. J. Biol. Chem. 264:4825, 1989.

74. Lassing, I., and Lindberg, U.: Specific interaction between

75. Lassing, I., and Lindberg, U.: Specificity of the interaction between phosphatidylinositol 4,5-bisphosphate and the profilin:actin complex. J. Cell. Biochem. 37:255, 1988.

76. Yonezawa, N., Nishida, E., Iida, K., Yahara, I., and Sakai, H.: Inhibition of the interactions of cofilin, destrin, and deoxyribonuclease I with actin by phosphoinositides. J. Biol. Chem. 265:8382, 1990.

77. Janmey, P., Lamb, J., Allen, P., and Matsudaira, P.: Phosphoinositide-binding peptides derived from the sequences of gelsolin and villin. J. Biol. Chem. 267:11818, 1992.

78. Yu, F.-X., Sun, H.-Q., Janmey, P., and Yin, P.: Identification of a polyphosphoinositide-binding sequence in an actin monomer-binding domain of gelsolin. J. Biol. Chem. 267:14616, 1992.

79. Machesky, L. M., Goldschmidt-Clermont, P. J., and Pollard, T. D.: The affinities of human platelet and Acanthamoeba profilin isoforms for polyphosphoinositides account for their relative abilities to inhibit phospholipase C. Cell Regul. 1:937, 1990.

80. Shariff, A., and Luna, E.: Diacylglycerol-stimulated formation of actin nucleation sites at plasma membranes. Science 256:245, 1992.

81. Roos, F., Zimmerman, A., and Keller, H.: Effect of phorbol myristate acetate and the chemotactic peptide fNLPNTL on shape and movement of human neutrophils. J. Cell Sci. 88:399, 1987.

82. Phaire-Washington, L., Silverstein, S., and Wang, E.: Phorbol myristate acetate stimulates microtubule and 10-nm filament extension and lysosome redistribution in mouse macrophages. J. Cell Biol. 86:641, 1980.

83. Sheterline, P., Rickard, J., Boothroyd, B., and Richards, R.: Phorbol ester induces rapid actin assembly in neutrophil leucocytes independently of changes in $[Ca^{2+}]_i$ and pH_i. J. Muscle Res. Cell Motil. 7:405, 1986.

84. Howard, T., and Wang, D.: Calcium ionophore, phorbol ester, and chemotactic peptide-induced cytoskeleton reorganization in human neutrophils. J. Clin. Invest. 79:1359, 1987.

85. Phatak, P., Packman, C., and Lichtman, M.: Protein kinase C modulates actin conformation in human T lymphocytes. J. Immunol. 141:2929, 1988.

86. Sham, R., Packman, C., Abboud, C., and Lichtman, M.: Signal transduction and the regulation of actin conformation during myeloid maturation: Studies in HL60 cells. Blood 77:363, 1991.

87. Niggli, V., and Keller, H.: On the role of protein kinases in regulating neutrophil actin association with the cytoskeleton. J. Biol. Chem. 266:7927, 1991.

88. Downey, G., Chan, C., Lea, P., Takai, A., and Grinstein, S.: Phorbol ester–induced actin assembly in neutrophils: Role of protein kinase C. J. Cell Biol. 116:695, 1992.

89. Hartwig, J. H., and Shevlin, P.: The architecture of actin filaments and the ultrastructural location of actin-binding protein in the periphery of lung macrophages. J. Cell Biol. 103:1007, 1986.

90. Hartwig, J., and Kwiatkowski, D.: Actin-binding proteins. Curr. Opin. Cell Biol. 3:87, 1991.

91. Matsudaira, P.: Modular organization of actin crosslinking proteins. Trends Biochem. Sci. 16:87, 1991.

92. Hartwig, J., and DeSisto, M.: The cytoskeleton of the resting human blood platelet: Structure of the membrane skeleton and its attachment to actin filaments. J. Cell Biol. 112:407, 1991.

93. Stevenson, K. B., Clark, R. A., and Nauseef, W. M.: Fodrin and band 4.1 in a plasma membrane–associated fraction of human neutrophils. Blood 74:2136, 1989.

94. Bourguignon, L., Kalomiris, E., and Lokeshwar, V.: Acylation of the lymphoma transmembrane glycoprotein, GP85, may be required for GP85-ankyrin interaction. J. Biol. Chem. 266:11761, 1991.

95. Lokeshwar, V., and Bourguignon, L.: Post-translational modification and expression of ankyrin-binding site(s) in GP85 (Pgp-1/CD44) and its biosynthetic precursors during T-

lymphoma membrane biosynthesis. J. Biol. Chem. 266: 17983, 1991.

96. Gregorio, C., Kubo, R., Bankert, R., and Repasky, E.: Translocation of spectrin and protein kinase C to a cytoplasmic aggregate upon lymphocyte activation. Proc. Natl. Acad. Sci. USA 89:4947, 1992.

97. Black, J., Koury, S., Bankert, R., and Repasky, E.: Heterogeneity in lymphocyte spectrin distribution: Ultrastructural identification of a new spectrin-rich cytoplasmic structure. J. Cell Biol. 106:97, 1988.

98. Pauly, J. L., Bankert, R. B., and Repasky, E. A.: Immunofluorescent patterns of spectrin in lymphocyte cell lines. J. Immunol. 136:246, 1986.

99. Ohta, Y., Stossel, T., and Hartwig, J.: Ligand-sensitive binding of actin-binding protein (ABP) to immunoglobulin G Fc receptor I(FcγRI, CD64). Cell 67:275, 1991.

100. Otey, C., Pavalko, F., and Burridge, K.: An interaction between a-actinin and the β1 integrin subunit in vitro. J. Cell Biol. 111:721, 1990.

101. Greenberg, S., Burridge, K., and Silverstein, S. C.: Colocalization of F-actin and talin during Fc receptor–mediated phagocytosis in mouse macrophages. J. Exp. Med. 172:1853, 1990.

102. Sato, N., Yonemura, S., Obinata, T., Tsukita, S., and Tsukita, S.: Radixin, a barbed end-capping actin-modulating protein, is concentrated at the cleavage furrow during cytokinesis. J. Cell Biol. 113:321, 1991.

103. Davis, S., Lu, M., Lo, S., Lin, S., Butler, J., Druker, B., Roberts, T., An, Q., and Chen, L.: Presence of an SH2 domain in the actin-binding protein tensin. Science 252:712, 1991.

104. Sobue, K.: Involvement of the membrane cytoskeletal proteins and the src gene product in growth cone adhesion and movement. Neurosc. Res. Suppl. 13:S80, 1990.

105. Marchisio, P., Cirillo, D., Teti, A., Zambonin-Zallone, A., and Tarone, G.: Rous sarcoma virus–transformed fibroblasts and cells of monocytic origin display a peculiar dot-like organization of cytoskeletal proteins involved in microfilament-membrane interactions. Exp. Cell Res. 169:202, 1987.

106. Allavena, P., Paganin, C., Martin-Padura, I., Peri, G., Gaboli, M., Dejana, E., Marchisio, P., Mantovani, A.: Molecules and structures involved in the adhesion of natural killer cells to vascular endothelium. J. Exp. Med. 173:439, 1991.

107. Hartwig, J., Thelen, M., Rosen, A., Janmey, P., Nairn, A., and Aderem, A.: MARCKS is an actin filament crosslinking protein regulated by protein kinase C and calcium-calmodulin. Nature 356:618, 1992.

108. Thelen, M., Rosen, A., Nairn, A., and Aderem, A.: Regulation by phosphorylation of reversible association of a myristoylated protein kinase C substrate with the plasma membrane. Nature 351:320, 1991.

109. Jongstra-Bilen, J., Janmey, P., Hartwig, J., Galea, S., and Jongstra, J.: The lymphocyte-specific protein LSP-1 binds to F-actin and to the cytoskeleton through its COOH-terminal basic domain. J. Cell Biol. 118:1443, 1993.

110. Fernandez, A., Brautigan, D., Mumby, M., and Lamb, N.: Protein phosphatase type-1, not type-2a, modulates actin microfilament integrity and myosin light chain phosphorylation in living nonmuscle cells. J. Cell Biol. 111:103, 1990.

111. Ikebe, M., and Reardon, S.: Phosphorylation of bovine platelet myosin by protein kinase C. Biochemistry 29:2713, 1990.

112. Tan, J., Ravid, S., and Spudich, J.: Control of nonmuscle myosins by phosphorylation. Annu. Rev. Biochem. 61:721, 1992.

113. Hayashi, K., Fujio, Y., Kato, I., and Sobue, K.: Structural and functional relationships between h- and l-caldesmons. J. Biol. Chem. 266:355, 1991.

114. Sellers, J. R.: Regulation of cytoplasmic and smooth muscle myosin. Curr. Opin. Cell Biol. 3:98, 1991.

115. Sobue, K., and Sellers, J.: Caldesmon, a novel regulatory protein in smooth muscle and nonmuscle actomyosin systems. J. Biol. Chem. 266:12115, 1991.

116. Korn, E., and Hammer, J. I.: Myosin I. Curr. Opin. Cell Biol. 2:57, 1990.

117. Pollard, T., Doberstein, S., and Zot, H.: Myosin-I. Annu. Rev. Physiol. 53:653, 1991.

118. Downey, G., Chan, C., Trudel, S., and Grinstein, S.: Actin assembly in electropermeabilized neutrophils: Role of intracellular calcium. J. Cell Biol. 110:1975, 1990.

119. Pike, M., Bruck, M., Arndt, C., and Lee, C.-S.: Chemoattractants stimulate phosphatidylinositol-4-phosphate kinase in human polymorphonuclear leukocytes. J. Biol. Chem. 265:1866, 1990.

120. Pike, M., Costello, K., and Southwick, F.: Stimulation of human polymorphonuclear leukocyte phosphatidylinositol-4 kinase by concanavalin A and formyl-methionyl-leucyl-phenylalanine is calcium independent. Correlation with maintenance of actin assembly. J. Immunol. 147:2270, 1991.

121. Pike, M., Costello, K., and Lamb, K.: IL-8 stimulates phosphatidylinositol-4-phosphate kinase in human polymorphonuclear leukocytes. J. Immunol. 148:3158, 1992.

122. Reibman, J., Meixler, S., Lee, T., Gold, L., Cronstein, B., Haines, K., Kolasinski, S., and Weissmann, G.: Transforming growth factor β1, a potent chemoattractant for human neutrophils, bypasses classic signal-transduction pathways. Proc. Natl. Acad. Sci. USA 88:6805, 1991.

123. Bengtsson, T., Stendahl, O., and Andersson, T.: The role of the cytosolic free Ca^{2+} transient for fMet-Leu-Phe induced actin polymerization in human neutrophils. Eur. J. Cell Biol. 42:338, 1986.

124. Sha'afi, R. I., and Molski, T. F. P.: Signalling for increased cytoskeletal actin in neutrophils. Biochem. Biophys. Res. Commun. 145:934, 1987.

125. Marks, P., and Maxfield, F.: Transient increases in cytosolic free calcium appear to be required for the migration of adherent human neutrophils. J. Cell Biol. 110:43, 1990.

126. Marks, P., Hendley, B., and Maxfield, F.: Attachment to fibronectin or vitronectin makes human neutrophil migration sensitive to alterations in cytosolic free calcium concentration. J. Cell Biol. 112:149, 1991.

127. Jaconi, M., Lew, D., Carpentier, J.-L., and Magnusson, K.: Cytosolic free calcium elevation mediates phagosome-lysosome fusion during phagocytosis in human neutrophils. J. Cell Biol. 110:1555, 1990.

128. Lew, P. D., Andersson, T., Hed, J., Di Virgilio, F. D., Pozzan, T., and Stendahl, O.: Ca^{2+}-dependent and Ca^{2+}-independent phagocytosis in human neutrophils. Nature 315:509, 1985.

129. Di Virgilio, F., Meyer, B. C., Greenberg, S., and Silverstein, S. C.: Fc receptor–mediated phagocytosis occurs in macrophages at exceedingly low cytosolic Ca^{2+} levels. J. Cell Biol. 106:657, 1988.

130. Greenberg, S., El Khoury, J., Di Virgilio, F., Kaplan, E., and Silverstein, S.: Ca^{2+}-independent F-actin assembly and disassembly during Fc receptor–mediated phagocytosis in mouse macrophages. J. Cell Biol. 113:757, 1991.

131. Hishikawa, T., Cheung, J., Yelamarty, R., and Knutson, D.: Calcium transients during Fc receptor–mediated and nonspecific phagocytosis by murine peritoneal macrophages. J. Cell Biol. 115:59, 1991.

132. Hartwig, J. H., Chambers, K. A., and Stossel, T. P.: Association of gelsolin with actin filaments and cell membranes of macrophages and platelets. J. Cell Biol. 108:467, 1989.

133. Dadabay, C., Patton, E., Cooper, J., and Pike, L.: Lack of correlation between changes in polyphosphoinositide levels and actin/gelsolin complexes in A431 cells treated with epidermal growth factor. J. Cell Biol. 112:1151, 1991.

134. Eberle, M., Traynor-Kaplan, A., Sklar, L., and Norgauer, J.: Is there a relationship between phosphatidylinositol trisphosphate and F-actin polymerization in human neutrophils? J. Biol. Chem. 265:16725, 1990.

135. Stephens, L., Hughes, K., and Irvine, R.: Pathway of phosphatidylinositol(3,4,5)-trisphosphate synthesis in activated neutrophils. Nature 351:33, 1991.

136. Dobos, G., Norgauer, J., Eberle, M., Schollmeyer, P., and Traynor-Kaplan, A.: C5a reduces formyl peptide–induced actin polymerization and phosphatidylinositol(3,4,5)trisphosphate formation, but not phosphatidylinositol(4,5)bis-

phosphate hydrolysis and superoxide production, in human neutrophils. J. Immunol. 149:609, 1992.

137. Howard, T., Chaponnier, C., Yin, H., and Stossel, T.: Gelsolin-actin interaction and actin polymerization in human neutrophils. J. Cell Biol. 110:1983, 1990.

138. Watts, R., and Howard, T.: Evidence for a gelsolin-rich, labile F-actin pool in human polymorphonuclear leukocytes. Cell Motil. Cytoskeleton 21:25, 1992.

139. Chaponnier, C., Yin, H. L., and Stossel, T. P.: Reversibility of gelsolin/actin interaction in macrophages. J. Exp. Med. 165:97, 1987.

140. Symons, M., and Mitchison, T.: Control of actin polymerization in live and permeabilized fibroblasts. J. Cell Biol. 114:503, 1991.

141. Hartwig, J. H., Chambers, K. A., Hopcia, K. L., and Kwiatkowski, D. J.: Association of profilin with filament-free regions of human leukocyte and platelet membranes and reversible membrane binding during platelet activation. J. Cell Biol. 109:1571, 1989.

142. Buss, F., Temm-Grove, C., Henning, S., and Jockusch, B.: Distribution of profilin in fibroblasts correlates with the presence of highly dynamic actin filaments. Cell Motil. Cytoskeleton 22:51, 1992.

143. Cunningham, G., Stossel, T., and Kwiatkowski, D.: Enhanced motility in NIH 3T3 fibroblasts that overexpress gelsolin. Science 251:1233, 1991.

144. Cunningham, C., Gorlin, J., Kwiatkowski, D., Hartwig, J., Janmey, P., Byers, H., and Stossel, T.: Actin-binding protein requirement for cortical stability and efficient locomotion. Science 255:325, 1992.

145. Schoepper, B., and Wegner, A.: Gelsolin binds to polymeric actin at a low rate. J. Biol. Chem. 267:13924, 1992.

146. Särndahl, E., Lindroth, M., Bengtsson, T., Fällman, M., Gustavsson, J., Stendahl, O., and Andersson, T.: Association of ligand-receptor complexes with actin filaments in human neutrophils: A possible regulatory role for a G-protein. J. Cell Biol. 109:2791, 1989.

147. Bengtsson, T., Särndahl, E., Stendahl, O., and Andersson, T.: Involvement of GTP-binding proteins in actin polymerization in human neutrophils. Proc. Natl. Acad. Sci. USA 87:2921, 1990.

148. Therrien, S., and Naccache, P.: Guanine nucleotide-induced polymerization of actin in electropermeabilized neutrophils. J. Cell Biol. 109:1125, 1989.

149. Ridley, A., and Hall, A.: The small GTP-binding protein rho regulates the assembly of focal adhesions and actin stress fibers in response to growth factors. Cell 70:389, 1992.

150. Ridley, A., Paterson, H., Johnston, C., Diekmann, D., and Hall, A.: The small GTP-binding protein rac regulates growth factor–induced membrane ruffling. Cell 70:401, 1992.

151. Fenton, R., Kung, H.-F., Longo, D., and Smith, M.: Regulation of intracellular actin polymerization by prenylated cellular proteins. J. Cell Biol. 117:347, 1992.

152. Goldschmidt-Clermont, P., Kim, J., Machesky, L., Rhee, S., and Pollard, T.: Regulation of phospholipase C-γ by profilin and tyrosine phosphorylation. Science 251:1231, 1991.

153. Banno, Y., Nakashima, T., Kumada, T., Ebisawa, K., Nonomura, Y., and Nozawa, Y.: Effects of gelsolin on human platelet cytosolic phosphoinositide–phospholipase C isozymes. J. Biol. Chem. 267:6488, 1992.

154. Pytowski, B., Maxfield, F., and Michl, J.: Fc and C3bi receptors and the differentiation antigen BH2-Ag are randomly distributed in the plasma membrane of locomoting neutrophils. J. Cell Biol. 110:661, 1990.

155. Jesaitis, A., Naemura, J., Sklar, L., Cochrane, C., and Painter, R.: Rapid modulation of N-formyl chemotactic peptide receptors on the surface of human granulocytes: Formation of high-affinity ligand-receptor complexes in transient association with the cytoskeleton. J. Cell Biol. 98:1378, 1984.

156. Svitkina, T., Neyfakh, A., Jr., and Bershadsky, A.: Actin cytoskeleton of spread fibroblasts appears to assemble at the cell edges. J. Cell Sci. 82:235, 1986.

157. Forscher, P., and Smith, S.: Actions of cytochalasins on the organization of actin filaments and microtubules in a neuronal growth cone. J. Cell Biol. 107:1505, 1988.

158. Okabe, S., and Hirokawa, N.: Incorporation and turnover of biotin-labeled actin microinjected into fibroblastic cells: An immunoelectron microscopic study. J. Cell Biol. 109:1581, 1989.

159. Sanders, M., and Wang, Y.-L.: Assembly of actin-containing cortex occurs at distal regions of growing neurites in PC12 cells. J. Cell Sci. 100:771, 1991.

160. Theriot, J., and Mitchison, T.: Actin microfilament dynamics in locomoting cells. Nature 352:126, 1991.

161. Córdova, N., Ermentrout, B., and Oster, G.: Dynamics of single-motor molecules: The thermal ratchet model. Proc. Natl. Acad. Sci. USA 89:339, 1992.

162. Oster, G.: Biophysics of the leading lamella. Cell Motil. Cytoskeleton 10:164, 1988.

163. Sheetz, M., Wayne, D., and Pearlman, A.: Extension of filopodia by motor-dependent actin assembly. Cell Motil. Cytoskeleton 22:160, 1992.

164. DeLozanne, A., and Spudich, J.: Disruption of the Dictyostelium myosin heavy chain gene by homologous recombination. Science 236:1086, 1987.

165. Knecht, D., and Loomis, W.: Antisense RNA inactivation of myosin heavy chain gene expression in *Dictyostelium discoideum*. Science 236:1081, 1987.

166. Valerius, N., Stendahl, O., Hartwig, J., and Stossel, T.: Distribution of actin-binding protein and myosin in polymorphonuclear leukocytes during locomotion and phagocytosis. Cell 24:195, 1981.

167. Stendahl, O. I., Hartwig, J. H., Brotschi, E. A., and Stossel, T. P.: Distribution of actin-binding protein and myosin in macrophages during spreading and phagocytosis. J. Cell Biol. 84:215, 1980.

168. Wilson, A., Gorgas, G., Claypool, W., and de Lanerolle, P.: An increase or a decrease in myosin II phosphorylation inhibits macrophage motility. J. Cell Biol. 114:277, 1991.

169. Karlsson, R., Lassing, I., Hoglund, A.-S., and Lindberg, U.: The organization of microfilaments in spreading platelets: A comparison with fibroblasts and glial cells. J. Cell. Physiol. 121:96, 1984.

170. Rinnerthaler, G., Herzog, M., Klappacher, M., Kunka, H., and Small, J.: Leading edge movement and ultrastructure in mouse macrophages. J. Struct. Biol. 106:1, 1991.

171. Fattoum, A., Hartwig, J. H., and Stossel, T. P.: Isolation and some structural and functional properties of macrophage tropomyosin. Biochemistry 22:1187, 1983.

172. Ishikawa, R., Yamashiro, S., and Matsumura, F.: Differential modulation of actin-severing activity of gelsolin by multiple isoforms of cultured rat cell tropomyosin. Potentiation of protective ability of tropomyosins by 83-kDa nonmuscle caldesmon. J. Biol. Chem. 264:7490, 1989.

173. Czop, J., and Kay, J.: Isolation and characterization of β-glucan receptors on human mononuclear phagocytes. J. Exp. Med. 173:1511, 1991.

174. Ezekowitz, R., Williams, D., Koziel, H., Armstrong, M., Warner, A., Richards, F., and Rose, R.: Uptake of *Pneumocystis carinii* mediated by macrophage mannose receptor. Nature 351:155, 1991.

175. Allison, A., Davies, P., and DePetris, S.: Subplasmalemmal microfilaments in macrophage movement and endocytosis. Nature 232:153, 1971.

176. Axline, S., and Reaven, E.: Inhibition of phagocytosis and plasma membrane mobility of cultivated macrophage by cytochalasin B. Role of subplasmalemmal microfilaments. J. Cell Biol. 62:647, 1974.

177. Young, V., Falkow, S., and Schoolnik, G.: The invasin protein of *Yersinia enterocolitica*: Internalization of invasin-bearing bacteria by eukaryotic cells is associated with reorganization of the cytoskeleton. J. Cell Biol. 116:197, 1992.

178. Blackwood, R., and Ernst, J.: Characterization of Ca^{2+}-dependent phospholipid binding, vesicle aggregation and membrane fusion by annexins. Biochem. J. 266:195, 1990.

179. Francis, J., Balazovich, K., Smolen, J., Margolis, D., and Boxer, L.: Human neutrophil annexin I promotes granule aggre-

gation and modulates Ca^{2+}-dependent membrane fusion. J. Clin. Invest. 90:537, 1992.

180. Jones, P., Moore, G., and Waisman, D.: A nonapeptide to the putative F-actin binding site of annexin-II tetramer inhibits its calcium-dependent activation of actin filament bundling. J. Biol. Chem. 267:13993, 1992.

181. Jacking, M., Lew, D., Carpentier, J., Magnussion, K., Sjogren, M., and Stendahl, O.: Cytosolic free calcium elevation mediates the phagosome-lysosome fusion during phagocytosis in human neutrophils. J. Cell Biol. 110:1555, 1990.

182. Diaz, R., Mayorga, L. S., Weidman, P. J., Rothman, J. E., and Stahl, P. D.: Vesicle fusion following receptor-mediated endocytosis requires a protein active in Golgi transport. Nature 339:398, 1989.

183. Boxer, L., Hedley-Whyte, E., and Stossel, T.: Neutrophil actin dysfunction and abnormal neutrophil behavior. N. Engl. J. Med. 291:1093, 1974.

184. Southwick, F., Dabiri, N., and Stossel, T.: Neutrophil actin dysfunction is a genetic disorder associated with partial impairment of neutrophil actin assembly in three family members. J. Clin. Invest. 82:1525, 1988.

185. Southwick, F., Howard, T., Holbrook, T., Anderson, D., Arnaout, M., and Stossel, T.: The relationship between CR3 deficiency and neutrophil actin dysfunction. Blood 73:1973, 1989.

186. Coates, T., Torkildson, J., Torres, M., Ja, C., and Howard, T.: An inherited defect of neutrophil motility and microfilamentous cytoskeleton associated with abnormalities in 47-Kd and 89-Kd proteins. Blood 78:1338, 1991.

187. Hilmo, A., and Howard, T.: F-actin content of neonatal and adult neutrophils. Blood 69:945, 1987.

188. Naik, N., Bhisey, A., and Advani, S.: Flow cytometric studies on actin polymerization in PMN cells from chronic myeloid leukemia (CML) patients. Leuk. Res. 14:921, 1990.

189. Tilney, L., and Portnoy, D.: Actin filaments and the growth, movement, and spread of the intracellular bacterial parasite, *Listeria monocytogenes*. J. Cell Biol. 109:1597, 1989.

190. Theriot, J., Mitchison, T., Tilney, L., and Portnoy, D.: The rate of actin-based motility of intracellular *Listeria monocytogenes* equals the rate of actin polymerization. Nature 357:257, 1992.

191. Dabiri, G., Sanger, J., Portnoy, D., and Southwick, F.: *Listeria monocytogenes* moves rapidly through the host cell cytoplasm by inducing directional actin assembly. Proc. Natl. Acad. Sci. USA 87:6068, 1990.

192. Tilney, L., DeRosier, D., and Tilney, M.: How *Listeria* exploits host cell actin to form its own cytoskeleton. I. Formation of a tail and how that tail might be involved in movement. J. Cell Biol. 118:71, 1992.

193. Domann, E., Wehland, J., Rohde, M., Pistor, S., Hartl, M., Goebel, W., Leimeister-Wächter, M., Wuenscher, M., and Chakrabarty, T.: A novel bacterial virulence gene in *Listeria monocytogenes* required for host cell microfilament interaction with homology to the proline-rich region of vinculin. EMBO J. 11:1981, 1992.

194. Robbins, D., Cheng, M., Zhen, E., Vanderbilt, C., Feig, L., and Cobb, M.: Evidence for a Ras-dependent extracellular signal-regulated protein kinase (ERK) cascade. Proc. Natl. Acad. Sci. USA 89:6924, 1992.

195. Anand, B., and Chou, I.-N.: Microtubules and microtubule-associated proteins in resting and mitogenically activated normal human peripheral blood T cells. J. Biol. Chem. 267:10716, 1992.

196. Rothstein, T.: Antiimmunoglobulin in combination with cytochalasin stimulates proliferation of murine B lymphocytes. J. Immunol. 135:106, 1985.

197. Van Haelst, C., and Rothstein, T.: Cytochalasin stimulates phosphoinositide metabolism in murine B lymphocytes. J. Immunol. 140:1256, 1988.

198. Reinach, F. C., and MacLeod, A. R.: Tissue-specific expression of the human tropomyosin gene involved in the generation of the trk oncogene. Nature 322:648, 1986.

199. Takenaga, K., Nakamura, Y., and Sakiyama, S.: Differential expression of a tropomyosin isoform in low- and high-metastatic Lewis lung carcinoma cells. Mol. Cell. Biol. 8:3934, 1988.

200. McWhirter, J., and Wang, J.: Activation of tyrosine kinase and microfilament-binding functions of c-abl by bcr sequences in bcr/abl fusion proteins. Mol. Cell. Biol. 11:1553, 1991.

201. Tushinski, R., Oliver, I., Guilbert, L., Tynan, P., Warner, J., and Stanley, E.: Survival of mononuclear phagocytes depends on a lineage-specific growth factor that the differentiated cells selectively destroy. Cell 28:71, 1982.

202. Mellstrom, K., Hoglund, A.-S., Nister, M., Heldin, K.-E., Westermark, B., and Lindberg, U.: The effect of platelet-derived growth factor on morphology and motility of human glial cells. J. Muscle Res. Cell Motil. 4:589, 1983.

203. Nister, M., Hammacher, A., Mellstrom, K., Siegbahn, A., Ronnstrand, L., Westermark, B., and Heldin, C.-H.: A glioma-derived PDGF A chain homodimer has different functional activities from a PDGF AB heterodimer purified from human platelets. Cell 52:791, 1989.

204. Boocock, C., Jones, J., Stanley, E., and Pollard, J.: Colony stimulating factor-1 induces rapid behavioral responses in the mouse macrophage cell line BAC1.2F5. J. Cell Sci. 93:447, 1989.

205. Matsuyama, T., Yamada, A., Deusch, K., Sleasman, J., Daley, J., Torimoto, Y., and Abe, T.: Cytochalasins enhance the proliferation of CD4 cells through the CD3-Ti antigen receptor complex or the CD2 molecule through an effect on early events of activation. J. Immunol. 146:3736, 1991.

206. Melamed, I., Downey, G., Aktories, K., and Roifman, C.: Microfilament assembly is required for antigen-receptor–mediated activation of human B lymphocytes. J. Immunol. 147:1139, 1991.

207. Nagata, K., Sagara, J., and Ichikawa, Y.: Changes in contractile proteins during differentiation of myeloid leukemia cells. I. Polymerization of actin. J. Cell Biol. 85:273, 1980.

208. Hoffman-Liebermann, B., and Sachs, L.: Regulation of actin and other proteins in the differentiation of myeloid leukemic cells. Cell 14:825, 1978.

209. Kwiatkowski, D. J.: Predominant induction of gelsolin and actin-binding protein during myeloid differentiation. J. Biol. Chem. 263:13857, 1988.

210. Shimamura, R., Kudo, J., Kondo, H., Dohmen, K., Gondo, H., Okamura, S., Ishibashi, H., and Niho, Y.: Expression of the thymosin β4 gene during differentiation of hematopoietic cells. Blood 76:977, 1990.

211. Gondo, H., Kudo, J., White, J., Barr, C., Selvanayagam, P., and Saunders, G.: Differential expression of the human thymosin-β4 gene in lymphocytes, macrophages and granulocytes. J. Immunol. 139:3840, 1987.

212. Toothaker, L., Gonzalez, D., Tung, N., Lemons, R., Le Beau, M., Arnaout, M., Clayton, L., and Tenen, D.: Cellular myosin heavy chain in human leukocytes: Isolation of 5′ cDNA clones, characterization of the protein, chromosomal localization, and upregulation during myeloid differentiation. Blood 78:1826, 1991.

213. Meyer, W., and Howard, T.: Changes in actin content during induced myeloid maturation of human promyelocytes. Blood 62:308, 1983.

214. Meyer, W., and Howard, T.: Actin polymerization and its relationship to locomotion and chemokinetic response in maturing human promyelocytic leukemia cells. Blood 70:363, 1987.

215. Nagata, K., Sagara, J., and Ichikawa, Y.: Changes in contractile proteins during differentiation of myeloid leukemia cells. II. Purification and characterization of actin. J. Cell Biol. 93:470, 1982.

216. Rao, K., Currie, M., Ruff, J., and Cohen, H.: Lack of correlation between induction of chemotactic peptide receptors and stimulus-induced actin polymerization in HL-60 cells treated with dibutyryl cyclic adenosine monophosphate or retinoic acid. Cancer Res. 48:6721, 1988.

217. Vanderkerckhove, J., Bauw, G., Vancompernolle, K., Honore, B., and Celis, J.: Comparative two-dimensional gel analysis and microsequencing identifies gelsolin as one of the most

prominent downregulated markers of transformed human fibroblast and epithelial cells. J. Cell Biol. 111:95, 1990.

218. Fujita, H., Suzuki, H., Kuzumaki, N., Müllauer, L., Ogiso, Y., Oda, Y., Ebisawa, K., Sakurai, T., Nonomura, Y., and Kijimoto-Ochiai, S.: Specific protein, p92, detected in flat revertants derived from NIH/3T3 transformed by human activated c-Ha-ras oncogene. Exp. Cell Res. 186:115, 1990.

219. Müllauer, L., Fujita, H., Suzuki, H., Katabami, M., Hitomi, Y., Ogiso, Y., and Kuzumaki, N.: Elevated gelsolin and α-actin expression in a flat revertant R1 of Ha-ras oncogene–transformed NIH/3T3 cells. Biochem. Biophys. Res. Commun. 171:852, 1990.

220. Chaponnier, C., and Gabbiani, G.: Gelsolin modulation in epithelial and stromal cells of mammary carcinoma. Am. J. Pathol. 134:597, 1989.

221. Cantley, L., Auger, K., Carpenter, C., Duckworth, B., Graziani, A., Kapeller, R., and Soltoff, S.: Oncogenes and signal transduction. Cell 64:281, 1991.

SECTION V

HEMOSTASIS

Vitamin K–Dependent Proteins

Johan Stenflo and Björn Dahlbäck

INTRODUCTION

Prothrombin activation is the final step in a series of zymogen activations resulting in precisely regulated generation of thrombin at the site of injury.[1-6] This sequence of reactions can proceed by either the *intrinsic* or the *extrinsic* pathway. In the intrinsic pathway, factor XI is activated by thrombin or by contact phase factors (factor XII, prekallikrein, and high molecular weight kininogen). Active factor XI (factor XIa) then activates factor IX by limited proteolysis, and factor IXa activates factor X (Fig. 16–1). Although the contact phase factors initiate coagulation in vitro, when blood is exposed to negatively charged surfaces, they appear to be of little or no significance for the initiation of blood coagulation in vivo. However, the intrinsic pathway is important to maintain fibrin formation once the coagulation cascade is activated. Initiation of blood coagulation results from activation of the extrinsic pathway, also referred to as the *tissue factor* (TF) pathway, a set of reactions triggered by the interaction of factor VII/VIIa with TF.[5, 6] This insight, largely gained during the past decade, is founded on an abundance of biochemical and clinical evidence. Factor VII bound to TF is activated either by trace amounts of factors VIIa, IXa, or Xa or thrombin or by some enzyme released from damaged cells. It has also been suggested that the binding of factor VII to TF induces a conformational alteration in factor VII, endowing it with proteolytic activity, although this is debated.[5, 6]

Intrinsic Pathway   **Extrinsic Pathway**

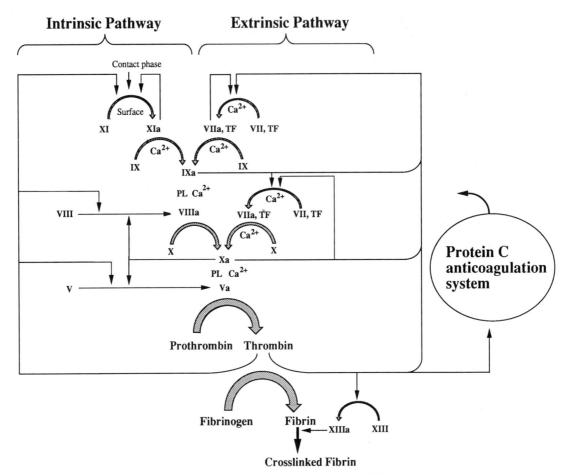

FIGURE 16–1. Schematic diagram of the *intrinsic* and *extrinsic* pathways of blood coagulation. The coagulation cascade is initiated via the extrinsic pathway as a result of tissue damage and the exposure of blood to tissue factor (TF). The two pathways converge when factor X is activated. The active forms of the serine proteases and of the two cofactors V and VIII are indicated by lowercase a; for example, X denotes the zymogen factor X, and Xa the active enzyme factor Xa. The activation of factors V and VIII by thrombin and by factor Xa is denoted, as well as the initiation of the *intrinsic* pathway by thrombin-mediated activation of factor XI. Thrombin also activates factor XIII and protein C of the protein C anticoagulant system. PL = Phospholipid.

The physiological substrates of factor VIIa are factors IX and X. The intrinsic and extrinsic pathways converge when factor X is activated by either factor VIIa or factor IXa. In the following step, factor Xa activates prothrombin to thrombin.

Among the proteins involved in blood coagulation, factors VII, IX, and X, prothrombin, and protein C are zymogens of serine proteases, which require vitamin K for normal biosynthesis.[2, 6–8] Protein S is a vitamin K–dependent cofactor of activated protein C.[7] Some properties of these proteins, collectively referred to as the vitamin K–dependent coagulation factors, are shown in Table 16–1.

A characteristic property of the vitamin K–dependent serine proteases is the very low activity against the physiological substrates in the absence of their respective cofactor.[1–3] The cofactors of factors IXa and Xa are factors VIIIa and Va, respectively. The two

TABLE 16–1.   VITAMIN K–DEPENDENT PLASMA PROTEINS

PROTEIN	PLASMA CONCENTRATION (mg/l)	MOLECULAR WEIGHT	AMINO ACIDS	SIZE OF GENE	EXONS	REFERENCE
Prothrombin (factor II)	100	72,000	579	21 kb	14	30, 305
Factor VII	0.5	48,000	406	13 kb	8	31, 306, 307
Factor IX	4	57,000	415	38 kb	8	32, 281, 305
Factor X	8	59,000	448	22 kb	8	33, 305
Protein C	4	56,000	417	11 kb	9	34, 35, 232
Protein S	20	75,000	635	>80 kb	15	49, 36
Protein Z	2	62,000	360	?	?	45, 46

homologous cofactors are high molecular weight proteins present as inactive precursors in plasma. They are activated by trace amounts of thrombin or factor Xa. Activation results in the assembly of biologically active macromolecular complexes, the factor Xase complex, and the prothrombinase complex. The factor Xase complex consists of factors IXa and VIIIa, negatively charged phospholipid, and calcium ions; the prothrombinase complex consists of factors Xa and Va, negatively charged phospholipid, and calcium ions. Factor Xa is 10^5- to 10^6-fold more active when it is part of the prothrombinase complex than in the absence of phospholipid and factor Va. Factors VIIIa and Va are substrates of activated protein C and are biologically inactive after cleavage.[2, 7] Protein C is activated by thrombin in complex with the endothelial cell cofactor thrombomodulin (TM). This set of reactions is a regulatory, anticoagulant counterpart to the blood coagulation cascade, known as the protein C anticoagulant pathway.

It is noteworthy that the cofactors of factor VIIa and thrombin are integral membrane proteins.[5–8] Neither of them requires proteolytic activation to be biologically active. However, whereas TM is expressed on the surface of endothelial cells, TF is normally inaccessible to blood, as it is located on fibroblasts in the adventitia of blood vessels and exposed to blood only as a result of tissue damage.[5, 8]

Findings in recent studies of the assembly of the enzymatically active macromolecular complexes that constitute the blood coagulation cascade,[1–6, 8] and the protein C anticoagulant system,[2, 7, 9] dovetail with those of structural studies of isolated modules of vitamin K–dependent proteins.[10–21] (Note: Rather than domain, the term *module*, suggested by Patthy[11] and by Baron and colleagues,[12] is used throughout this chapter.) The three-dimensional structures of prothrombin fragment 1, consisting of a γ-carboxyglutamic acid (Gla)–containing module and a kringle module,[13, 19, 20] and of thrombin[21] have been determined with X-ray diffraction methods. Modules homologous to the epidermal growth factor (EGF) have been identified in all but one of the vitamin K–dependent clotting factors.[10–12, 22–25] The structure of the NH2-terminal EGF module in factor X has been determined by two-dimensional nuclear magnetic resonance (NMR) spectroscopy,[14–16] as has the corresponding module of factor IX.[17, 18] Both EGF modules and kringle modules have been found in many non–vitamin K–dependent proteins with diverse functions.[11, 22–25]

A rational approach to the diagnosis and treatment of hemorrhagic and thrombotic diseases presupposes an understanding in molecular detail of the biochemical properties and metabolism not only of the traditional blood clotting factors but also of several cell surface receptors and complex polysaccharides. Elucidating structure-function relationships of proteins involved in blood clotting thus poses a formidable but worthwhile challenge. In this chapter we describe the structure of the vitamin K–dependent proteins involved in these reactions, with emphasis on the mod-

ular design of the proteins and on structure-function relationships. Mutations are discussed only when they shed light on structure-function relationships. For a comprehensive discussion of factor IX and protein C, the reader is referred to Chapters 19 and 17, respectively.

MODULAR ORGANIZATION OF VITAMIN K–DEPENDENT PLASMA PROTEINS

Seven plasma proteins require vitamin K for normal biosynthesis.[26–29] They contain 406 to 635 amino acids, and the size of their genes ranges from 11 kilobases (kb) to more than 80 kb (see Table 16–1).[30–38] Accordingly, the exons are short, as in most other extracellular proteins, and are separated by introns of variable length.[39–42] On the basis of their modular structure, three types of vitamin K–dependent coagulation factors can be discerned (Fig. 16–2). Factors VII, IX, and X and protein C form one group, whereas prothrombin and protein S have a unique modular structure.[22] The NH2-terminal module in all of these proteins contains 9 to 12 Gla residues, formed by vitamin K–dependent carboxylation of Glu residues.[26–29] A characteristic feature of the first group is that the Gla module is followed by two modules that are homologous to the EGF precursor, whereas the serine protease part is COOH-terminal. Protein Z, a vitamin K–dependent plasma protein of unknown function, should also belong to this group, as it is similar in structure to factors VII, IX, and X and protein C.[43–46] However, it has no amidolytic activity, as two of the residues in the catalytic triad have been mutated. In prothrombin there is a tetradecapeptide with a disulfide loop COOH-terminal of the Gla module. It is encoded by a separate exon.[30, 42] This region is followed by the two kringle modules, and the COOH-terminal half of the protein is occupied by the serine protease module. In protein S, the Gla module is followed by the thrombin-sensitive region, a short peptide stretch with an internal disulfide bond and two arginyl bonds, which are susceptible to cleavage by thrombin, and by four EGF-like modules.[47–50] The COOH-terminal part of protein S is not homologous to the serine proteases, but to the sex hormone–binding globulin (SHBG) of human plasma and to the androgen-binding protein in rat testis.[51, 52]

The family of vitamin K–dependent plasma proteins is representative of the view that complex genes in eukaryotes have been assembled via intron-mediated recombinations of exons.[11, 39–41] The exons encode intact functional units, modules, or smaller structural elements. A module in the protein may thus be coded for by one or more exons, such as the kringle modules in prothrombin.[30, 42] According to this view, the exons are remnants of primordial genes that in the course of evolution have been shuffled between genes and duplicated, giving rise to proteins of complex modular design.[11, 39–41] In this scenario, the coagulation proteins are derived from simple primordial serine proteases

Factor X

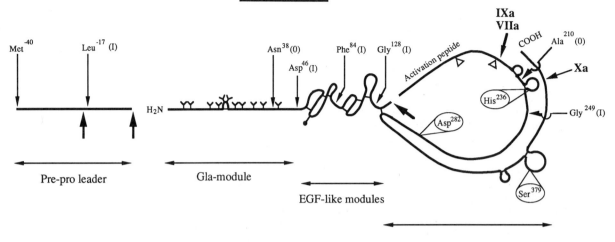

Prothrombin

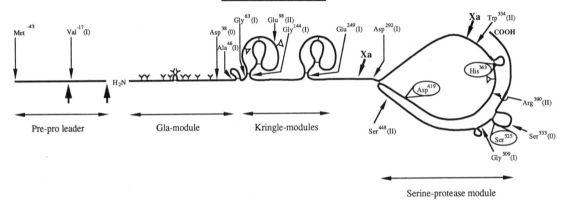

Protein S

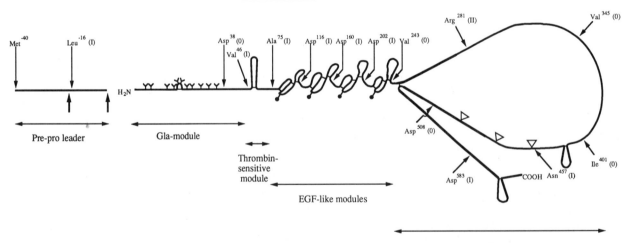

FIGURE 16–2. Modular structure of the vitamin K–dependent plasma proteins. The structure of factor X also represents the closely related factors VII and IX, protein C, and protein Z. The pre-pro leader sequences are shown to the left. Open triangles denote carbohydrate side chains. Cleavages in factor X and prothrombin that are mediated by factor VIIa or IXa and by factor Xa, respectively, are denoted by arrows. The remaining thick arrows denote, from left to right, cleavages that release the pre or signal sequence; the pro sequence; and, in factor X, the four residues that connect the light and heavy chains in the factor X precursor. Thin arrows denote the location of introns and the corresponding amino acid. The type of splice junction is given in parentheses. The residues in the active site of factor X and prothrombin are shown within ovals. The symbol **Y** denotes γ-carboxyglutamic acid, whereas a "lollipop" symbol on an EGF-like module denotes a β-hydroxyaspartic acid or β-hydroxyasparagine residue. EGF = Epidermal growth factor; SHBG = sex hormone–binding globulin.

that contained a signal peptide required for secretion and a COOH-terminal serine protease module.[11, 40] Exons were recruited to the genes encoding these simple proteins and inserted into the intron separating the exon that encoded the signal peptide from the exon that encoded the serine protease module. In some instances, the exons were then duplicated. The recruitment of exons and the exon duplications led to an increase in size of the NH_2-terminal, non-catalytic regions that account for approximately half of each of the vitamin K–dependent serine protease zymogens. These non-catalytic modules have important functions relating to protein secretion, postribosomal modification, cofactor interaction, and regulation of the coagulation response at the site of injury.

A characteristic feature of the non-catalytic modules of these proteins is that the exons encoding separate modules are symmetrical in the sense that they have introns of the same phase class on either side.[40] The exons that have been shuffled in the vitamin K–dependent proteins, as well as in related proteins, are surrounded by introns of phase class 1 (i.e., the intron is between the first and second nucleotide of a codon).[40, 42] Phase class 2 introns are located between the second and third nucleotides of the codon, and phase class 0 introns are found between codons. Symmetry of the exons with respect to phase class is thought to be a prerequisite for exon shuffling, since otherwise, insertion or duplication of an exon (e.g., with phase 1 in the 5′ end and phase 2 in the 3′ end) would lead to a disruption of the reading frame. It has been suggested that the preference for phase 1 introns between modules, in the proteins of the blood coagulation, fibrinolysis, and complement systems, has an origin in a separation of the exon encoding the signal peptide and the exon encoding the serine protease module in an ancestral protease by a phase 1 intron that has since served as the recipient for exons with class 1 splice junctions on either side.[11, 39–42]

In the precursors of the vitamin K–dependent proteins, the propeptide and the Gla module constitute a functional unit that is encoded by two exons.[30–37] The intron separates the exon encoding the propeptide and the non-helical NH_2-terminal part of the Gla module from the exon encoding the COOH-terminal α-helical part of the Gla module (see Fig. 16–2). The exon encoding the α-helical region has a type 0 phase splice junction in its 5′ end and a type 1 splice junction in its 3′ end. Thus, the two exons encoding the Gla module appear to have been recruited en bloc to the gene of an ancestral protease prior to the divergence of the vitamin K–dependent blood coagulation zymogens. The exon on the 5′ end of the propeptide encodes the signal peptide, and the exon on the 3′ end encodes a small disulfide loop peptide in prothrombin; EGF modules in factors VII, IX, and X and protein C[30–35, 42]; and the thrombin-sensitive region in protein S.[36–38] The propeptide region is recognized by the vitamin K–dependent carboxylase and is removed by proteolytic cleavage *after* carboxylation of appropriate Glu residues but *prior to* or concomitant with

secretion (see below). The first kringle module in prothrombin is encoded by two exons, and the second by one exon.[30, 42] Again, the phase of the splice junctions suggests that the two exons encoding the first kringle module have been recruited en bloc and that an intron was subsequently lost. However, it is also possible that introns have been inserted into the exons encoding the Gla and kringle modules after they were recruited to an ancestor of the vitamin K–dependent proteins. It is assumed that two kringle modules were recruited from a plasminogen ancestor to prothrombin in separate events rather than one kringle that was subsequently duplicated.[11, 42]

It is noteworthy that the locations of introns are conserved in vitamin K–dependent proteins of comparable modular structure. For instance, the three first introns in factors VII, IX, and X and prothrombin are located at precisely the same positions, whereas in protein C the first intron is moved 6 base pairs (bp) upstream, probably as a result of an intron sliding mechanism.[30–35] Each of the EGF-like modules is encoded by a single exon. The first exon of the serine protease part of each of these proteins has a type 1 splice junction in its 5′ end, allowing recombination by exon shuffling. In prothrombin, the serine protease part is encoded by six exons, with the residues of the catalytic triad, His 363, Asp 419, and Ser 525 (numbering as in reference 30), on different exons as in most other serine proteases. The positioning of the introns in the prothrombin gene is unique and has no counterpart in any of the other serine proteases. In the serine protease parts of factors VII, IX, and X and protein C,[31–35] the positions of the two introns are conserved. The large exon that encodes the COOH-terminal part contains both the active site Asp and Ser residues. The intron-exon organization of factors VII, IX, and X and protein C is compatible with an evolutionary process whereby the archetype of these proteins, formed by exon shuffling, later developed by gene duplication and point mutations.

Gla-CONTAINING MODULES

Structure of Gla-Containing Modules

The Gla modules are homologous and contain approximately 47 amino acids (Fig. 16–3). In this region, all 9 to 12 Glu residues are carboxylated to Gla in vitamin K–dependent reactions.[26–29, 53–58] The 10 COOH-terminal residues of each Gla module form an α-helical portion (residues 35 to 45 in prothrombin) that is encoded by a separate exon.[22, 30–37, 42] There is one Gla residue in this region in factors IX and X and protein Z, but not in factor VII, prothrombin, protein C, or protein S.[20] The remaining 9 to 11 Gla residues are located between residues 6 and 39. Three pairs of Gla residues are conserved in all proteins, as are the Gla residues in positions corresponding to 14, 16, and 29 in prothrombin. The Gla residues occur singly and in pairs, with either charged or hydrophobic residues

```
                        10                20                30         O        40        I
             ┌──────────────────────────────────────────────────────┐↓                  ↓
Prothrombin  A N T - F L Y Y V R K G N L Y R Y C V Y Y T C S Y Y Y A F Y A L Y S - S T A T D V F W A K Y T
Factor VII   A N A - F L Y Y C K R P G S L Y R Y C K Y Q C S F Y Y A R Y I F K D - A Y R T K L F W I S Y S
Factor IX    Y N S G K L Y Y F V Q G N L Y R Y C M Y Y K C S F Y Y A R Y V F Y N - T Y R T T Y F W K Q Y V
Factor X     A N S - F L Y Y M K K G H L Y R Y C M Y Y T C S Y Y Y A R Y V F Y D - S D K T N Y F W N K Y K
Protein C    A N S - F L Y Y L R H S S L Y R Y C I Y Y I C D F Y Y A K Y I F Q N - V D D T L A F W S K H V
Protein S    A N S - L L Y Y T K Q G N L Y R Y C I Y Y L C N K Y Y A R Y V F Y N D P Y - T D Y F Y P K Y L
Protein Z    A G S Y L L Y Y L F Y G N L Y K Y C Y Y Y I C V Y Y Y A R Y V F Y N - Y V V T D Y F W R R Y K
```

FIGURE 16–3. Amino acid sequences in the Gla modules of the human vitamin K–dependent plasma proteins. The numbering is that of human prothrombin. O denotes the position (and type of splice junction) of the intron that separates the two exons that encode the Gla module. The aromatic cluster is formed by Phe,[40] Trp,[41] and Tyr.[44] Residues are shaded when at least four of seven are identical. Point mutations leading to the synthesis of proteins with, in most cases, low biological activity are boxed (see the text). The sequences are prothrombin,[30] factor VII,[31] factor IX,[32] factor X,[33] protein C,[34] protein S,[36] and protein Z.[45]

adjacent, which raises questions about the substrate recognition mechanism for carboxylation.

The role of Gla in Ca^{2+} binding became evident when it was demonstrated that normal prothrombin contains Gla and binds Ca^{2+}, whereas abnormal prothrombin, synthesized under the influence of such vitamin K–antagonistic drugs as warfarin, contains Glu in the corresponding positions, does not bind Ca^{2+}, has no phospholipid affinity, and lacks biological activity.[26, 59–65] In factor Xa–mediated prothrombin activation, the addition of negatively charged phospholipid in the presence of Ca^{2+} results in a reduction of the K_m for prothrombin by more than two orders of magnitude.[2, 3] This effect is not obtained with uncarboxylated prothrombin. Warfarin administration also leads to the synthesis of forms of prothrombin with intermediate degrees of carboxylation.[66] In these partially carboxylated forms of prothrombin, the degree of carboxylation appears to be more severely reduced at the COOH-terminal end of the Gla module than at the NH$_2$-terminal end.[67] A marked reduction in phospholipid binding and activation is observed already with the loss of 3 or 4 of the 10 Gla residues in prothrombin.[66] Similar results have been obtained with prothrombin from patients with hereditary vitamin K–dependent carboxylation abnormalities.[68]

The recent determination of the three-dimensional structure of bovine prothrombin fragment 1 by X-ray crystallography[13, 19, 20, 69] represents an important step toward an understanding of the function of the Gla module in Ca^{2+} binding and provides a structural basis for future studies aimed at elucidation of the interactions of vitamin K–dependent plasma proteins with biological membranes and protein cofactors.

Fragment 1, formed during limited proteolysis of bovine or human prothrombin by thrombin, consists of the NH$_2$-terminal 156 or 155 amino acids, respectively. It contains the Gla module, the tetradecapeptide disulfide loop, and the NH$_2$-terminal kringle module.[13, 20, 70–72] Residue numbers in the following refer to human fragment 1.[30] The α-helical part of the Gla module, residues 35 to 45, forms three turns of α helix, such that the side chains of Phe 40, Trp 41, and Tyr 44 form an aromatic cluster that is adjacent to the disulfide bond connecting Cys 17 and Cys 22. In crystals of fragment 1 obtained in the absence of Ca^{2+}, the part of the Gla module NH$_2$-terminal to the α-helical segment appears to be random except for the structure imposed by the single disulfide bond. If crystallization is carried out in the presence of Ca^{2+}, the structure of the NH$_2$-terminal part of the Gla module is organized and has been solved at 2.25 Å resolution (Fig. 16–4).[13, 69] The gross structure of the module is discoid. Calcium ions interact with the carboxylate groups of Gla residues and seem to cross-link parts of the module that are fairly remote in the linear sequence.[13, 69] The carboxylate groups of Gla residues 16, 25, 26, and 29 form a negatively charged surface within the module apposing another negatively charged surface formed by the carboxylate groups of Gla residues 6 and 7. Four or five calcium ions are interposed between the two negatively charged surfaces. Each ion interacts with at least two carboxylate groups. Gla residues 14, 19, and 20 form a negatively charged cluster adjacent to the tetradecapeptide disulfide loop peptide. Two calcium ions have been identified in this region. Of the seven identified calcium ions, three seem to be inaccessible to solvent.

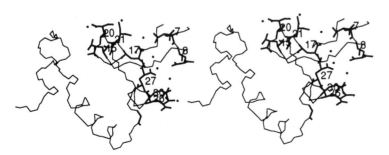

FIGURE 16–4. Stereoview of the structure of the Gla module in bovine prothrombin fragment 1. The polypeptide backbone is shown, as well as the side chains of the Gla residues. The solid circles denote calcium ions. Bovine prothrombin has a Gly residue in position 4 that has no counterpart in human prothrombin. Gla 7 and 8 in the figure thus correspond to Gla 6 and 7 in human prothrombin in Figure 16–3 and so forth. (From Tulinsky, A.: The structures of domains of blood proteins. Thromb. Haemost. 66: 16, 1991; with permission.)

The detailed coordination of the calcium ions is now under investigation.[69] Only six carboxylate oxygen atoms appear to be accessible for phospholipid binding mediated by bridging Ca^{2+} ions. The NH_2-terminal residues in the Gla module are folded in an Ω-like fashion, such that the amino group of Ala 1 is buried and makes ion pair interactions with Gla residues. It is also noteworthy that the Gla residue in position 14 forms an ion pair with Arg 54 in the tetradecapeptide disulfide loop.

Owing to the pronounced sequence similarity, it is assumed that the Gla modules in the other vitamin K–dependent plasma proteins are folded in a manner similar to that of the Gla module in fragment 1. There is also direct experimental evidence to support this hypothesis. For instance, the amino group of the NH_2-terminal Ala residue in the Gla module of prothrombin can be modified by reductive methylation in the absence of calcium ions.[73] The membrane binding of the modified protein is greatly impaired. If the chemical modification is carried out in the presence of Ca^{2+}, the Ala residue is not modified and the membrane binding of the modified prothrombin is normal. A similar observation was made when the amino-terminal residues of factors IX and X were modified.[74] It thus seems safe to infer that the NH_2-terminus of each of these proteins forms an ion pair with a conserved Gla residue, as in prothrombin.[13, 69] Similarity of structure in the Gla modules of several vitamin K–dependent clotting factors has also been inferred from studies with a monoclonal antibody that binds to a common epitope in all these proteins in a metal ion– and conformation–dependent manner.[75] Finally, the calcium ion–induced spectroscopic perturbations observed in Gla module–containing proteins and in fragments of these proteins are quite similar, attesting to the structural similarity of the Gla modules.[76–84]

Calcium- and Phospholipid-Binding Properties of Gla-Containing Modules

The conversion of 9 to 12 Glu residues to Gla in each of the vitamin K–dependent plasma proteins endows them with Ca^{2+}-binding properties at physiologic Ca^{2+} concentrations (1 to 2 mM). A monocarboxylic acid such as acetic acid binds Ca^{2+} with $K_d \approx 300$ mM, whereas malonic acid (a dicarboxylic acid similar to Gla) binds Ca^{2+} with higher affinity, $K_d \approx 30$ mM, but still far above the concentration of Ca^{2+} in plasma.[76] Binding of Ca^{2+} to prothrombin and prothrombin fragment 1, as well as to the other vitamin K–dependent plasma proteins, is characterized by a pronounced positive cooperativity in the binding of the first two or three Ca^{2+}, giving rise to characteristic bell-shaped binding curves in Scatchard plots (Fig. 16–5).[65, 76, 85, 86] The cooperative Ca^{2+} binding is consistent with the complex structure of the Gla module and the role of Ca^{2+} in its folding to a native conformation. Although metal ion–binding studies provided clear evidence of Ca^{2+}-induced conformational changes,

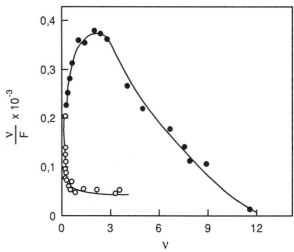

FIGURE 16–5. Binding of Ca^{2+} to normal (*solid circles*) and uncarboxylated (*open circles*) prothrombin. The data have been plotted according to Scatchard, and v is (mol Ca^{2+}/mol prothrombin) and F is the molar concentration of free Ca^{2+}. The upward convexity denotes a positive cooperativity in the binding of Ca^{2+} (Modified from Stenflo, J., and Ganrot, P.: Binding of Ca^{2+} to normal and dicumarol-induced prothrombin. Biochem. Biophys. Res. Commun. 50: 98, 1974; with permission.)

interpretation of the binding data has been confounded by the metal ion–induced dimerization, for instance, of prothrombin fragment 1.[76] The Ca^{2+}-binding properties of these proteins are interesting in the light of the three-dimensional structure of prothrombin fragment 1, in which Ca^{2+} serves to cross-link Gla residues that are remote in the linear sequence, thus illustrating the role of the metal ion in the folding of Gla modules to their native conformation. This situation is clearly quite different from Ca^{2+} binding to many intracellular proteins, such as calmodulin, in which the metal ion binds to a preformed pocket to trigger a biological response.[87] The vitamin K–dependent plasma proteins also bind other divalent cations, such as Mg^{2+}, Mn^{2+}, and Sr^{2+}, that do not, however, substitute for Ca^{2+} in blood coagulation and at best induce conformations similar to those induced by Ca^{2+}.[76, 86, 88, 89]

In addition to the recently determined three-dimensional structure of fragment 1, several lines of evidence indicate that Ca^{2+} induces folding of the Gla module not only in prothrombin fragment 1 but also in proteolytic fragments from factors IX and X and protein C that consist of the Gla module and one or two EGF modules.[74, 76, 77, 82–86] This process, which can be followed by measuring the metal ion–induced fluorescence emission quenching, has been studied in detail, particularly in prothrombin and in prothrombin fragment 1.[76, 78, 90] A proteolytic fragment from factor X, consisting of the Gla module and the first EGF module, has only one Trp residue (position 41).[84, 91] The fluorescence emission quenching that occurs on Ca^{2+} binding to this fragment can thus be linked to the conserved Trp residue in the aromatic cluster adjacent to the disulfide bond linking Cys 17 and Cys 22 (inferred from the X-ray structure of fragment 1).[13, 69] In pro-thrombin fragment 1, where the Gla module is linked to the disulfide-bonded hexadecapeptide and the krin-gle module, and in the fragments of factors IX and X and protein C, where the Gla modules are linked to one or two EGF modules, the fluorescence quenching occurs in the same range of Ca^{2+} concentrations as in the intact proteins.[82-86] This finding suggests that cal-cium ions induce similar conformational changes in the various fragments and that they contain sufficient structural information for normal folding of the Gla modules. Gla modules, cleaved in the aromatic cluster of the α-helical connecting peptide but otherwise in-tact, can be isolated after limited chymotryptic diges-tion of factors IX and X and protein C.[80, 83, 84, 91-94] The isolated cleaved Gla modules from factor X (res-idues 1 to 44), factor IX (residues 1 to 43), and prothrombin (residues 1 to 45) bind Ca^{2+} with lower affinity than does the Gla module in the intact pro-tein.[74, 83, 84, 95] Other properties of the isolated Gla modules, such as the comparatively low solubility in the presence of Ca^{2+}, also indicate that they do not have a native conformation.[74, 95] Nevertheless, they bind to negatively charged phospholipid vesicles, albeit at higher Ca^{2+} concentrations than those required to mediate the binding, for instance, of prothrombin fragment 1.[74] It thus appears as if the α-helical con-necting peptide is a nucleation site for the folding of the Gla module in the presence of Ca^{2+}. It is also possible that the tetradecapeptide disulfide loop (resi-dues 47 to 60) in prothrombin fragment 1 and the EGF modules in factors IX and X and protein C function as scaffolds for the normal folding of the Gla modules. This interpretation derives support from the fact that direct contact exists between the Gla module and neighboring modules; that is, Gla in position 14 of fragment 1 forms an ion pair with Arg 54.[13, 69]

The folded Gla module also protects susceptible peptide bonds in the α-helical aromatic cluster region in factors IX and X from proteolysis, suggesting a similar folding.[83, 84, 93] In the presence of Ca^{2+}, there is virtually no proteolytic cleavage in this region in a factor IX fragment consisting of the Gla module and the two EGF modules, whereas in the absence of Ca^{2+}, there is a rapid cleavage COOH-terminal of Lys 43.[83] Interaction between the Gla module and the adjacent modules was also inferred from studies of the Ca^{2+}-binding properties of protein S in which the thrombin-sensitive bond had been cleaved. In cleaved protein S, the Gla module is linked to the remainder of the molecule by a disulfide bond. The Gla module in the cleaved protein appears to have lower Ca^{2+} affinity than that in intact protein S, and the cleaved molecule has no biological activity.[7, 9, 49, 50]

Although other models have been proposed, the interaction of vitamin K–dependent proteins with neg-atively charged phospholipid membranes has gener-ally been assumed to be mediated by calcium ions bridging between Gla residues in the proteins and negatively charged groups on the phospholipid sur-face.[96] Recent findings demonstrating that high cal-cium ion concentrations tend to dissociate the proteins from the membrane surfaces have supported the no-tion that the interaction is purely ionic in nature and have been taken to be tentative support for a calcium ion bridging model.[74] However, the three-dimensional structure of fragment 1 suggests the possibility that very high calcium ion concentrations separate the two negatively charged surfaces within the Gla module, between which calcium ions are sandwiched, leading to incorrect folding of the Gla module, presumably destroying a phospholipid binding site.[74] Recently pub-lished evidence suggests that the Gla module of factor VII/VIIa is indispensable for a normal interaction with phospholipid-bound TF.[97] The function of Ca^{2+} in the interactions between Gla modules and negatively charged biological membranes, on the one hand, and protein cofactors, on the other, will have to be re-evaluated in the light of the now available three-dimensional structure of prothrombin fragment 1.

Mutations in Gla Modules

Several mutations that give rise to hemophilia B have been identified in the Gla module of factor IX.[98] Only a few are point mutations that result in the synthesis of an abnormal protein with low biological activity (see Chapter 19). So far none of these abnor-mal factor IX species has been isolated and character-ized. However, some properties of the factor IX mu-tant Oxford b1 (Cys 23 → Tyr; see Fig. 16–3) have been studied; it appears in plasma at 19 per cent of the normal concentration, whereas its biological activ-ity is below 1 per cent.[99] Defective adsorption of the mutant factor IX to alumina and its weak interaction with a monoclonal antibody that recognizes a Ca^{2+}-dependent epitope suggest that Ca^{2+} binding to the mutant molecule is impaired. Factor IX Zutphen (Cys 18 → Arg) has a normal plasma concentration, but its biological activity is below 1 per cent.[98, 100, 101] It does not bind Ca^{2+} normally. Moreover, Cys 18 (which is linked by a disulfide bond to Cys 23 in normal factor IX) appears to be linked to another polypeptide by a disulfide bridge. In contrast, the mutant designated Oxford b2 (Gla 7 → Ala) seems to be fully active, as there is a parallel reduction in plasma concentration and biological activity.[99] There are two point mutations of Gla 27 in factor IX. Factor IX Seattle 3 is Gla 27 → Lys, and factor IX Chongqing is Gla 27 → Val.[102, 103] Both mutations lead to severe hemophilia. Finally, the two mutations Arg 29 → Gin and Gla 33 → Asp are associated with hemophilia of mild and moderate severity, respectively.[104] Results of site-directed muta-genesis studies in factor IX have suggested that the various Gla residues are not functionally equivalent. Substitution of Gla 15 or Gla 20 by Asp resulted in only a slight reduction of the clotting activity, whereas the mutant with Asp instead of Gla in position 7 was reported to be almost completely inactive.[105]

In factor X Voralberg, Gla 14 is mutated to Lys.[106] The rate of activation of mutant factor X was only 15 per cent of that of normal factor X on activation by factor VIIa/TF, but 75 per cent of normal on activation with factor IXa/factor VIIIa. On activation with the factor X activator from Russell's viper venom, it was fully active. The reason for the different activation rates is unknown. Factor Xa Voralberg activated prothrombin at a normal rate, although a higher than normal concentration of Ca^{2+} was required. Site-specific mutagenesis has been used to alter the Gla residues in recombinant protein C. A mutant in which both Gla 6 and Gla 7 were replaced with Asp possessed less than 5 per cent of the activity of wild-type recombinant activated protein C toward its substrate, factor VIIIa.[107] Two other recombinant protein C species have been characterized: one in which Gla 19 and Gla 20 were mutated to Asp and one in which Cys 22 was mutated to Ser.[108] Both activated protein C species displayed less than 1 per cent of the activity of recombinant wild-type activated protein C in the activated partial thromboplastin assay and in the inactivation of purified factor VIIIa.

The functional defects of proteins with point mutations in the Gla modules (naturally occurring or recombinant mutant proteins) clearly establish that the Gla residues are not functionally equivalent. Studies of the mutant proteins (factor IX Oxford b1, factor IX Zutphen, and the recombinant protein C mutant Cys 22 → Ser) demonstrated that the structural integrity of the hexapeptide disulfide loop in the Gla module is necessary for normal biological activity and Ca^{2+} binding.[98, 99, 100, 107, 108] This finding is consistent with the observation that reduction and alkylation of the Cys residues in this disulfide loop result in a reduced Ca^{2+} affinity.[85]

Function of Gla in the Secretion of Vitamin K–Dependent Proteins

The post-translational carboxylation of Glu to Gla is required not only for normal Ca^{2+} binding and membrane interaction of the proteins but also for normal transport of the vitamin K–dependent proteins from the rough endoplasmic reticulum of the hepatocytes to the blood plasma.[26, 27] Treatment of patients with vitamin K–antagonistic coumarin anticoagulants such as warfarin results in an approximately 50 per cent reduction of the plasma prothrombin concentration.[59, 60] The abnormal prothrombin in plasma, either uncarboxylated or undercarboxylated, manifests defective Ca^{2+} binding and membrane interaction.[26, 27, 61–66] The coupling of carboxylation to secretion is particularly striking in the rat, in which uncarboxylated vitamin K–dependent proteins accumulate in the rough endoplasmic reticulum of the liver in vitamin K deficiency, with a concomitant reduction of the plasma concentration to very low values.[109–112] The same effect is observed with such vitamin K–antagonistic drugs as warfarin. This finding suggests a microsomal transport protein capable of distinguishing between carboxylated and uncarboxylated proteins, a protein that may well be the carboxylase itself.

Warfarin treatment of rats leads to the accumulation of several isoelectric forms of the prothrombin precursor in the endoplasmic reticulum of the liver. The precursors are rich in mannose and are susceptible to cleavage by endoglycosidase H.[113, 114] However, glycosylation does not appear to be coupled to carboxylation, as tunicamycin, which inhibits core glycosylation, does not affect the degree of carboxylation. Recently, it was suggested that there are different binding proteins for prothrombin and factor X in the microsomal membrane.[115]

Propeptides

In the Gla module, 9 to 12 Glu residues are carboxylated to Gla (see Fig. 16–3). It is noteworthy that there are no obvious sequences in the Gla modules that can constitute carboxylase recognition sites. There are three Gla-Gla sequences as well as Gla residues that occur singly, sometimes with adjacent hydrophobic residues and sometimes with a neighboring Arg residue. This finding suggests a substrate recognition mechanism of the vitamin K–dependent carboxylase that is fundamentally different from those of other enzymes that carry out postribosomal modifications, such as prolyl-4-hydroxylase, which recognizes proline in the sequence Gly-Xxx-Pro,[116] and N-glycosylating enzymes that recognize Asn in the sequence Asn-Xxx-Ser/Thr.[117] An intricate substrate recognition mechanism was also inferred from early experiments, which demonstrated that uncarboxylated prothrombin is a poor substrate for the carboxylase, whether it has been synthesized in vivo under the influence of such vitamin K–antagonistic drugs as warfarin or formed by heat decarboxylation of normal plasma prothrombin.[118] The synthetic peptide Phe-Leu-Glu-Glu-Leu and similar synthetic peptides have been used as substrates in many studies of the carboxylase.[27] However, these peptides are poor substrates, with K_m values in the millimolar range, that is, far higher than can be obtained with the uncarboxylated forms of prothrombin and related proteins that are substrates in vivo. In contrast to the synthetic peptides and the uncarboxylated prothrombin, the prothrombin precursor purified from rat liver is an excellent substrate for the carboxylase and has a K_m value in the micromolar range.[27, 29]

The determination of the complementary DNA (cDNA) sequences of vitamin K–dependent plasma proteins and the use of synthetic peptides as substrate for the carboxylase have provided insight into the mechanism by which the enzyme recognizes its substrates.[27–29, 119–122] Like other secreted proteins, the vitamin K–dependent plasma proteins have an NH_2-terminal hydrophobic extension, a signal peptide, that is removed by a signal peptidase.[123] The signal peptides have no structural features to set them apart from similar peptides in other secreted proteins. Each vitamin K–dependent protein contains a propeptide that is an immediate NH_2-terminal extension of the Gla module in the precursor.[27-29] In the propeptides, several residues are conserved between the vitamin K–dependent proteins, whereas others have been changed by conservative mutations (Fig. 16–6). Two Gla-containing proteins from mineralized tissues are particularly interesting in this respect: osteocalcin, or bone Gla protein that contains three Gla residues, and matrix Gla protein that contains five Gla residues.[124-126] There is no apparent sequence similarity between the mature Gla-containing proteins from mineralized tissue and the vitamin K–dependent plasma proteins. However, osteocalcin contains an NH_2-terminal propeptide with a sequence that is clearly related to corresponding regions of the vitamin K–dependent plasma proteins (see Fig. 16–6).[124, 125] Moreover, in the matrix Gla–containing protein, the sequence segment containing residues 15 to 30 appears to be homologous to the propeptides of the vitamin K–dependent plasma proteins.[126] It is noteworthy that this sequence in the matrix Gla protein is not removed by proteolytic cleavage prior to secretion. In addition, there is one Gla residue NH_2-terminal to this propeptide-related peptide segment in the matrix Gla protein. These results have established that not only the Gla residues but also the propeptides are common structural denominators of vitamin K–dependent proteins, whether in blood plasma or in bone.

Recently, the function of the propeptides as structural elements recognized by the vitamin K–dependent carboxylase has been amply documented by the expression of recombinant vitamin K–dependent proteins.[127-130] The proteins are secreted by eukaryotic cells and are carboxylated if the messenger RNA (mRNA) encodes the propeptide region and vitamin K is present, whereas no carboxylation occurs in the absence of the propeptide. Moreover, synthetic peptides that contain the propeptide region and the NH_2-terminal amino acids of the mature protein (residues -18 to $+10$) are excellent substrates for the carboxylase in in vitro carboxylation assays, with K_m values between 1 and 10 μM, whereas the corresponding peptides lacking the propeptide region are poor substrates, with K_m values three orders of magnitude higher.[27, 121] It is also noteworthy that the isolated propeptide stimulates carboxylation of small peptides containing glutamic acid, such as Phe-Leu-Glu-Glu-Leu.[119] The mechanism is unknown. It has been suggested that amino acids in the Gla region of the mature protein (Glu-Xxx-Xxx-Xxx-Glu-Xxx-Cys, residues 16 to 22 of human prothrombin) constitute a second site recognized by the carboxylase, although findings in other studies provide no support for this theory.[28, 126] Although the propeptide is the structure recognized by the vitamin K–dependent carboxylase, it remains an enigma how the carboxylase, while binding to the propeptide region, moves along the peptide chain and modifies consecutive Glu residues, in the matrix Gla protein apparently on either side of the propeptide region.

Comparison of sequences of propeptides of vitamin K–dependent proteins shows certain residues to be conserved.[28] The Phe residue in position -16 is present in all propeptides; Ala in position -10 is found in the plasma proteins, whereas bone Gla protein has Gly in this position. The hydrophobic amino acids in positions -6, -7, and -17 are conserved in most cases or replaced by other hydrophobic amino acids. Site-directed mutagenesis of factor IX and prothrombin, as well as studies using synthetic peptides as substrates for the carboxylase in vitro, indicate that residues -10, -15, -16, -17, and -18 are crucial for substrate recognition by the carboxylase.[28, 121, 128] In contrast, mutation of the residues in positions -14, -8, and -1 in factor IX does not affect the degree of carboxylation. Site-directed mutagenesis studies suggest that some differences exist between the vitamin K–dependent proteins. In factor IX, mutation of Ala at -10 completely abolished γ-carboxylation, whereas in protein C deletion of residues -1 to -12 had relatively little effect on the γ-carboxylation.[128-130] It has been proposed that the propeptide region in the coagulation factors forms an α helix in solution, with the residues that appear to be crucial for recognition by the carboxylase on one side of the helix.[131]

		-25					-20					-15					-10					-5					-1
Prothrombin	L	C	S	L	V	H	S	Q	H	V	F	L	A	P	Q	Q	A	R	S	L	L	Q	R	V	R	R	-
FVII	M	P	W	K	P	G	P	H	R	V	F	V	T	Q	E	E	A	H	G	V	L	H	R	R	R	R	-
FIX	G	Y	L	L	S	A	E	C	T	V	F	L	D	H	E	N	A	N	K	I	L	N	R	P	K	R	-
FX	A	G	L	L	L	L	G	E	S	L	F	I	R	R	E	Q	A	N	N	I	L	A	R	V	T	R	-
Protein C	S	G	T	P	A	P	L	D	S·V		F	S	S	S	E	R	A	H	Q	V	L	R	I	R	K	R	-
Protein S	L	L	V	L	P	V	S	E	A	N	F	L	S	K	Q	Q	A	S	Q	V	L	V	R	K	R	R	-
Bone Gla protein	K	P	S	G	A	E	S	S	K	A	F	V	S	K	Q	E	G	S	E	V	V	K	R	P	R	R	-
Matrix Gla protein	E	S	M	E	S	Y	E	L	N	P	F	I	N	R	R	N	A	N	T	F	I	S	P	Q	Q	R	-

FIGURE 16–6. **Sequence similarity in the propeptide regions of the vitamin K–dependent plasma proteins and the two vitamin K–dependent bone proteins osteocalcin and matrix Gla protein.** Residues are shaded when at least six of the eight residues are identical. In factor IX, the signal peptidase cleavage site (*arrowhead*) is between residues -19 and -18; in factor X, it is between residues -18 and -17; and in protein C, it is between residues -25 and -24. The residues mutated in factor IX Oxford and San Dimas (Arg $-4 \rightarrow$ Gln),[132, 133] factor IX Cambridge (Arg $-1 \rightarrow$ Ser),[134] and factor X Santo Domingo (Gly $-20 \rightarrow$ Arg)[135] are boxed, as well as the Arg $-1 \rightarrow$ His mutation in protein C.[135a] The sequences are from prothrombin,[30] factor VII,[31] factor IX,[32] factor X,[33] protein C,[34] protein S,[36] and bone Gla protein and matrix Gla protein.[124]

The signal peptidase cleavage site has been localized in factors IX and X and protein C.[129, 132–135] In factor IX, cleavage is between residues −19 and −18[132, 133]; in protein C, between residues −25 and −24[129]; and in factor X, between residues −18 and −17.[135] The four residues in the propeptide that immediately precede the mature protein (residues −1 to −4) constitute the recognition site for the propeptide-processing enzyme (Fig. 16–6). In all vitamin K–dependent plasma proteins, at least two of the four residues are Arg, and in factor VII all four are Arg. Position −1 is always an Arg residue. Similar sequences are present in the propeptides of many other secreted proteins, such as serum albumin.[136]

Recently, proteolytic enzymes that cleave at sites comprising pairs of basic amino acids have been identified. Such dibasic sites occur in numerous extracellular proteins in addition to the vitamin K–dependent proteins.[137] These proteolytic enzymes, which belong to the subtilisin family, may be responsible for the removal of propeptides from the vitamin K–dependent proteins. However, so far no enzyme has been stringently connected with the proteolytic removal of the propeptides in the vitamin K–dependent proteins.

Mutations in Propeptides

Several mutations have been identified in the propeptide region.[98] In factor IX Oxford[132] and in factor IX San Dimas, [133]Arg −4 is mutated to Gln; and in factor IX Cambridge, Arg −1 is mutated to Ser[134]. In either case, the propeptide is not cleaved, and accordingly the mature proteins are secreted with an 18 residue long NH₂-terminal extension. Both mutant forms of factor IX appear to be partially carboxylated and have low biological activity. Synthetic peptides with these point mutations are equally good substrates for the carboxylase as a peptide with the wild-type sequence, indicating that the basic residue region is not involved in the substrate recognition of the carboxylase.[120] The reason for the low biological activity of these mutant factor IX molecules is unresolved so far. However, presumably the propeptide prevents the residue that is NH₂-terminal in the mature protein from making an ion pair interaction with a Gla residue as it does in prothrombin fragment 1 (see Fig. 16–4).

Recently, a factor X mutation called factor X Santo Domingo (Gly −20 → Arg) was described. When the mutant factor X was expressed, no protein was produced despite normal mRNA levels in the cells. Since signal peptidase cleaves between residues −18 and −17 in factor X, it was suggested that the mutation prevented this cleavage, leading to a defective secretion of the mutant protein.[135]

Vitamin K–Dependent Carboxylase

Vitamin K–dependent carboxylase activity was first identified in rat liver microsomes.[26, 27, 138, 139] The enzyme has now been found in many tissues.[26, 124, 140] Most of the early studies of the carboxylase were performed on crude fractions obtained from either rat or bovine liver.[26, 27, 138, 139] Rat liver was particularly useful, as the uncarboxylated vitamin K–dependent proteins accumulate in the rough endoplasmic reticulum, forming a pool of endogenous substrate.[109] The vitamin K–dependent carboxylase is an integral microsomal membrane protein that catalyzes the incorporation of CO_2 from HCO_3- into glutamate residues (Fig. 16–7).[26–29] When exogenous substrates such as synthetic peptides are used,[27, 139] rather than the endogenous precursors of the vitamin K–dependent proteins, the endoplasmic reticulum has to be solubilized with detergents. For reasons that have already been discussed, the peptides, such as the commonly used pentapeptide Phe-Leu-Glu-Glu-Leu, are characterized by high K_m values.[27] By measuring the incorporation of $^{14}CO_2$ from $H^{14}CO_3$ into glutamate residues in the endogenous microsomal precursor, or into the appropriate synthetic peptide, enzyme activity is readily measured.[138, 141] The product of the reaction, γ-carboxyglutamic acid, has been chemically characterized in detail.[26, 27, 138] A characteristic feature of Gla is that, like malonic acid, it is decarboxylated when heated under acidic conditions, forming glutamic acid.[53] Standard conditions of acid hydrolysis of Gla-containing proteins thus result in the conversion of Gla to Glu. Gla is stable in alkali, however, and is determined after base hydrolysis of the proteins.[53]

The vitamin K–dependent carboxylase requires molecular oxygen[142] and uses CO_2 rather than HCO_3- in the carboxylation reaction.[143] ATP is not involved in the reaction, nor is biotin.[26] The biologically active form of vitamin K in the carboxylation is the reduced, hydroquinone form, which is oxidized to 2,3-epoxide in the reaction (see Fig. 16–7).[144–146] In crude microsomal preparations, the hydroquinone form of the vitamin is regenerated by microsomal reductases if they are supplied with NAD(P)H or dithiols. Alternatively, the chemically reduced, hydroquinone form of the vitamin can be used.[27] The enzymatic epoxide reduction occurs in two steps. First, the vitamin K epoxide is reduced to the corresponding quinone, and in a second step the quinone is reduced to the biologically active hydroquinone form of vitamin K. Both reductase activities are strongly inhibited by 4-hydroxy-coumarin derivatives, such as the widely used anticoagulant warfarin.[27] It is not yet known if the two reductions are carried out by one or two reductases. The anticoagulant drugs thus inhibit the recycling of the vitamin in the liver rather than the carboxylase itself.

The reaction mechanism for the vitamin K–dependent carboxylase has not yet been completely elucidated, primarily because the enzyme has been difficult to purify to homogeneity. Present knowledge is based on studies using crude microsomal preparations or partially purified preparations in which the active carboxylase is still a very minor part of the total protein. The vitamin K–dependent step in the carbox-

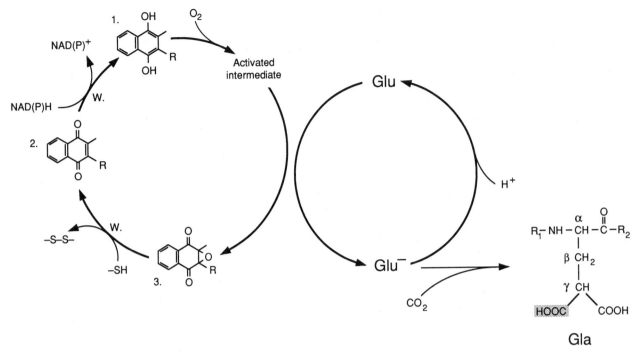

FIGURE 16–7. Gla formation and the vitamin K cycle. The vitamin K–dependent cleavage of a γ CH bond in peptide-bound glutamate and the addition of a carboxyl group at the γ position are shown to the right in the figure. In the absence of CO_2, Glu is regenerated. To the left, vitamin K (2) is reduced by a quinone reductase to vitamin KH_2 (1), the active form of the vitamin. Vitamin KH_2 and O_2 form an activated intermediate, the nature of which is uncertain, that abstracts a proton from the γ carbon atom of Glu. Carboxylation is coupled to the formation of the 2,3-epoxide of vitamin K. Vitamin K is then regenerated in a reaction catalyzed by a vitamin K epoxide reductase. W = The two reactions that are inhibited by warfarin and related anticoagulants.

ylation reaction is the removal of a hydrogen atom from the γ carbon of glutamic acid.[147] This step was deduced from experiments in which the peptide Phe-Leu-Glu-Glu-Leu with ^{3}H in the γ carbon of each glutamic acid residue was used as a substrate for the enzyme. In the absence of CO_2, the enzyme catalyzed an O_2- and vitamin K hydroquinone–dependent abstraction of [3]H. If the carboxylation reaction cannot proceed—for instance, when the bicarbonate concentration is severely depleted—the activated glutamic acid residue will again be protonated in the γ position, rather than forming adducts with other components in the reaction mixture. Accordingly, in the presence of the hydroquinone form of vitamin K, the carboxylase catalyzed an O_2-dependent exchange of ^{3}H from [3]H_2O into the γ position of glutamic acid in a peptide substrate.[148, 149] The vitamin K epoxide formation is coupled to the carboxylation.[148] Under reaction conditions in which the glutamyl substrate concentration is high, the ratio of vitamin K epoxide to Gla formed approaches unity. However, at low peptide concentrations, the vitamin is epoxidated and recycled to the hydroquinone form far more rapidly than the carboxylation event occurs. The currently favored hypothesis regarding the mode of action of vitamin K assumes that an oxygenated intermediate of vitamin K, such as a 2- or 3-hydroperoxide, provides the energy for the cleavage of the bond between the γ carbon and the

hydrogen atom and that this intermediate is on the pathway of epoxide formation (see Fig. 16–7).[27]

The vitamin K–dependent carboxylase was recently purified to apparent homogeneity by affinity chromatography.[150] The immobilized affinity ligand was a 59 residue peptide corresponding to residues −18 to 41 of human factor IX, with two mutations, Arg-4 → Gln and Arg-1 → Ser, to inhibit any proteolytic processing of the immobilized peptide. The recombinant peptide had been produced in *Escherichia coli* and thus had Glu in positions where plasma factor IX has Gla. The overall recovery of carboxylase activity was 34 per cent and the purification 7000-fold. The purified carboxylase consists of a single polypeptide chain with a molecular weight of approximately 94,000. The carboxylase has now been cloned and the cDNA sequence determined.[151] The carboxylase has 758 amino acids but has no amino-terminal signal peptide. In the NH_2-terminal part of the molecule, there are three hydrophobic putative transmembrane structural motifs. Comparison of the carboxylase sequence with that of soybean lipoxygenase revealed a 19 per cent identity. The enzymatic properties of the purified carboxylase have not yet been reported.

EPIDERMAL GROWTH FACTOR–LIKE MODULES

Epidermal growth factor is a small protein (53 amino acids) with six Cys residues linked by disulfide bonds in a characteristic pattern, 1—3, 2—4 and 5—6.[10, 12, 24, 152–156] EGF and the structurally related growth factor, transforming growth factor–α (TGF-α), are released from membrane-bound precursor molecules by limited proteolysis.[157] The EGF receptor is a transmembrane protein to which EGF and TGF-α bind with similar affinity. The ligands endow the receptor with protein tyrosine kinase activity. Activation of the receptor elicits a host of proliferative and developmental responses.

Modules homologous to EGF have been found in many extracellular proteins and membrane proteins.[10–12, 22–25] These proteins include the vitamin K–dependent plasma proteins, which all, except prothrombin, contain EGF-like modules. There are two EGF modules in factors VII, IX, and X, protein C, and protein Z, whereas protein S contains four. Each of the EGF modules is encoded by a separate exon. One of the modules in protein S manifests pronounced sequence similarity to one of the modules of the EGF precursor.[47, 48]

Structure of Epidermal Growth Factor–like Modules in Vitamin K–Dependent Proteins

In EGF-like modules from non–vitamin K–dependent proteins, the pairing of disulfide bonds has generally been inferred from the sequence similarity. However, in factor X the disulfide bond pairing has been demonstrated experimentally to be identical to that of EGF.[158] The EGF-like modules in the vitamin K–dependent proteins contain four types of postribosomal amino acid modifications. Postribosomal hydroxylation of Asp or Asn residues to *erythro*-β-hydroxyaspartic acid and *erythro*-β-hydroxyasparagine, respectively, was identified in protein C, factor X, and protein S (see below).[159–161] In the COOH-terminal EGF module of protein C, there is a carbohydrate chain linked by an *N*-glycosidic bond.[162] Recently, disaccharide and trisaccharide units linked by *O*-glycosidic bonds were identified in human and bovine factors VII and IX and protein Z.[163, 164] The disaccharide units were found in the human proteins and the trisaccharide units in the bovine proteins. The structure of the trisaccharide unit in bovine factor IX is D-Xyl*p*α 1-3-D-Xyl*p*α 1-3-D-Glc β1-*O*-Ser-53.[164] The disaccharide units in the human proteins lack the terminal Xyl residue.[163] The Ser residue to which the carbohydrate side chain is attached is located between the first and second Cys where the consensus sequence Cys-Xxx-Ser-Xxx-Pro-Cys (corresponding to residues 51 to 56 in bovine factor IX; see Fig. 16–11) has been identified. Factor X and protein C do not have the corresponding Ser residue and lack the carbohydrate chain. The consensus sequence has also been found in EGF modules of many non–vitamin K–dependent plasma proteins. In this context, it is noteworthy that the disaccharide chain has been isolated from human urine in amounts that are larger than can be accounted for by the vitamin K–dependent plasma proteins,

suggesting that at least some of these proteins have the carbohydrate side chain.[165] The glycosylating enzyme (or enzymes) has not yet been identified, and the function of the carbohydrate moiety is unknown.

The NH₂-terminal EGF-like modules of factors IX and X have been chemically synthesized and expressed in yeast and shown to fold spontaneously to their respective native conformation.[166, 167] Intact EGF-like modules have been isolated in a preparative scale from proteolytic digests of factors IX and X, protein C, and, in smaller amounts, protein S.[82–84, 91, 168] The structure of the NH₂-terminal EGF module from factor X (corresponding to residues 45 to 86 in bovine factor X) has been determined by two-dimensional NMR spectroscopy.[14–16] As it was isolated from an enzymatic digest of intact factor X, Asp 63 was hydroxylated to β-hydroxyaspartic acid. The overall structure was found to be similar to those of human and murine EGF,[152–156] which is noteworthy, as only 11 residues (including 6 Cys residues) of 42 are identical between factor X and EGF. The structure is dominated by β sheets (Fig. 16–8). The largest one is antiparallel and encompasses residues 59 to 64 and 67 to 72, which are linked by a β turn, residues 64 to 67. In murine and human EGF, the amino acids NH₂-terminal to the first Cys residue form a triple-stranded β sheet with the major antiparallel β sheet at least part of the time. In the factor X module, this part of the molecule appears to be freely mobile in the absence of Ca^{2+}. There is no evidence of triple-stranded sheet formation, perhaps because of electrostatic repulsion caused by the two Asp residues (positions 46 and 48 in factor X) that are conserved in factors VII, IX, and X and in protein C.[14, 15] The pleated sheet structures and β turns in the COOH-terminal part of the molecule occur in the same positions in human and in murine EGF. The NH₂-terminal EGF module from factor X and factor IX and at least two of the EGF modules in protein S bind Ca^{2+}.[16, 91, 166–168] Recently, a preliminary structure for the NH₂-terminal EGF module of human factor IX was reported.[17, 18] It was found to be more closely related to that of the NH₂-terminal EGF module of bovine factor X than to human EGF, as is consistent with the sequence similarity (above 60 per cent) between the two clotting factor modules.

β-Hydroxyaspartic Acid and β-Hydroxyasparagine

Erythro-β-hydroxyaspartic acid (Hya) was first described as a constituent of the NH₂-terminal EGF module of human and bovine vitamin K–dependent coagulation factors.[159–161, 169, 170] In human factor IX, the hydroxylation is partial (about 30 per cent), whereas bovine factor IX is fully hydroxylated in this position.[170] Human factor VII has no Hya.[171] *Erythro*-β-hydroxyasparagine (Hyn) was identified in the second, third, and fourth EGF modules of protein S.[161] Free Hya and Hyn, also in the *erythro* form, have been isolated from urine in amounts larger than can

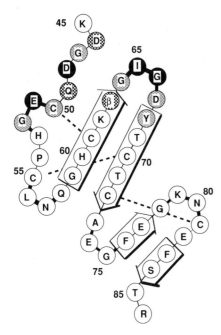

FIGURE 16–8. Secondary structure of the NH₂-terminal EGF module from bovine factor X (residues 45 to 86). *Top*, Schematic diagram of the secondary structure of the EGF-like module. The ^{1}H nuclear magnetic resonance (NMR) shift changes between the Ca^{2+} and apo forms of the fragment are indicated for each residue. Residues with $\Delta\delta$ more than 0.30 ppm are black (large difference between Ca^{2+} and apoform), those with $\Delta\delta$ 0.30 to 0.20 are checkered (intermediate difference between Ca^{2+} and apoform), and those with $\Delta\delta$ 0.20 to 0.10 are indicated by wavy lines (small difference between Ca^{2+} and apoform). The remaining residues are not influenced by Ca^{2+}. Disulfide bonds are displayed as broken lines. *Bottom*, Stick representation in stereo of the Ca^{2+}-loaded (*A*) and apo (*B*) forms of the EGF module as determined by two-dimensional NMR and simulated folding. The NH₂-terminal residue is at the top. (Modified from Selander, M., Ullner, M., Persson, E., Teleman, O., Stenflo, J., and Drakenberg, T.: Structure of the Ca^{2+} binding site in the β-hydroxyaspartic acid–containing EGF module of coagulation factor X (J. Biol. Chem. 267:19642, 1992; with permission.)

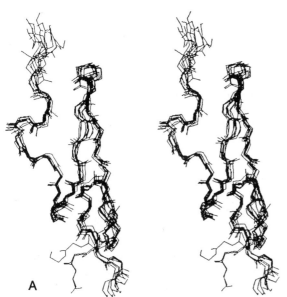

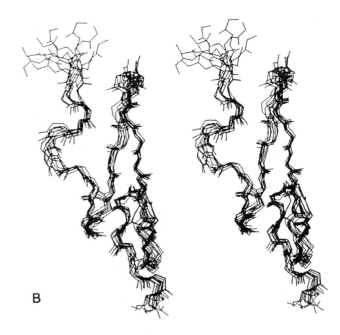

be accounted for by the turnover of vitamin K–dependent coagulation factors,[172] which may be explained by the fact that both postribosomal modifications are present in many non–vitamin K–dependent proteins, such as Hyn in the complement proteins C1r and C1s.[173] The two amino acids have been found only in EGF modules. They are positioned between the third and fourth Cys residues in the module (corresponding to residues 62 to 69 in bovine factor X; (Fig. 16–9) where the consensus sequence Cys-Xxx-Asp*/Asn*-Xxx-Xxx-Xxx-Xxx-Tyr/Phe-Xxx-Cys has been identified (the hydroxylated residues are denoted with an asterisk).[161, 174] This part constitutes the major antiparallel β sheet in the EGF module, the size of which appears to be crucial for recognition by the hydroxylase, as there are always eight residues between the

two Cys residues. The hydroxylated Asp/Asn residue is in juxtaposition to the Tyr/Phe residue. The lack of Hya in human factor VII that has the consensus sequence and the partial hydroxylation of human factor IX indicate that the β sheet structure and the consensus sequence do not constitute a sufficient structural requirement for the hydroxylase.

Many EGF module–containing extracellular proteins and membrane proteins contain the consensus sequence required by the hydroxylase; among these proteins are the complement proteins C1r and C1s already mentioned,[173] as well as the TGF-β–binding protein,[175] the EGF precursor,[176] fibrillin,[177, 178] and products of homeotic genes in *Drosophila melanogaster* and *Caenorhabditis elegans* that control the developmental fate of cells.[25] Among the *Drosophila melanogaster*

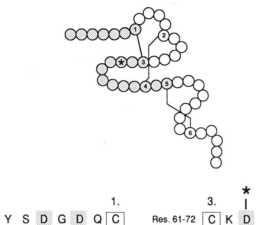

Factor	VII	Res. 44-50	Y	S	D	G	D	Q	C
Factor	IX	45-51	Y	V	D	G	D	Q	C
Factor	X	44-50	Y	K	D	G	D	Q	C
Protein	C	44-50	H	V	D	G	D	Q	C
Protein S	1.	74-80	N	A	I	P	D	Q	C
	2.	114-120	E	F	D	I	N	E	C
	3.	158-164	C	K	D	V	D	E	C
	4.	200-206	C	E	D	I	D	E	C
Protein	Z	45-51	Y	K	G	G	S	P	C

			3.						*			4.	5.	
Res. 61-72	C	K	D	Q	L	Q	S	Y	I	C	F	C
62-73	C	K	D	D	I	N	S	Y	E	C	W	C
61-72	C	K	D	G	L	E	E	Y	T	C	T	C
69-80	C	I	D	G	I	G	S	F	S	C	D	C
93-104	C	K	D	G	K	A	S	F	T	C	T	C
134-145	C	D	N	T	P	G	S	Y	H	C	S	C
176-187	C	K	N	I	L	G	D	F	E	C	E	C
215-228	C	V	N	Y	P	G	G	H	T	C	Y	C
62-73	C	Q	D	S	I	W	G	Y	T	C	T	C

FIGURE 16–9. Alignment of the amino acid sequences of the NH$_2$-terminal EGF module from factors VII, IX, and X, protein C and protein Z, and the four EGF modules of protein S. The sequences amino-terminal to the first Cys residue are shown to the left, and the sequences between the third, fourth, and fifth Cys residues are shown to the right. Asp/Hya/Glu residues are shaded. The hydroxylated Asp/Asn residues are denoted by * (the residue in factor VII is not hydroxylated).[171] The sequences are from the references given in the legend to Figure 16–3.

proteins are those encoded by the Notch,[179] Delta,[180] Crumbs,[181] and Slit[182] loci, which are integral membrane proteins that contain multiple EGF modules arranged in tandem. The Notch protein contains 36 EGF modules in tandem, 22 of which have the consensus sequence required by the Asp/Asn-β-hydroxylase. In fibrillin, a component of elastin-associated microfibrils, all 34 EGF modules have the hydroxylase consensus sequence.[177, 178] Although most of these gene products have been characterized only at the cDNA level, the TGF-β–binding protein has been purified and shown to contain Hya/Hyn.[175] A human homologue of the protein encoded by the *Drosophila* Notch locus was recently identified.[183] The locus was termed TAN-1, an acronym for translocation-associated Notch homologue. In three cases of human T lymphoblastic leukemia, translocations have been identified in which the breakpoints occurred in the TAN-1 locus. Many of the EGF modules in the protein encoded by the TAN-1 locus have the consensus sequence required by the aspartyl-β-hydroxylase.

Asp/Asn-β-Hydroxylase

Asp/Asn-β-hydroxylase is a 2-oxoglutarate–dependent dioxygenase.[184–186] It thus belongs to the same group of enzymes as prolyl-4-hydroxylase, prolyl-3-hydroxylase, lysyl hydroxylase, and γ-butyrobetaine hydroxylase.[116, 187] The NH$_2$-terminal EGF-like module in factors IX and X, protein C, and protein Z is substrate for the enzyme.[185, 186] In the reaction, one hydroxyl group is attached to the β carbon atom of Asp, forming Hya. The oxygen atom in the hydroxyl group derives from O$_2$. The other oxygen atom of O$_2$ emerges in succinate, which is formed from the cosubstrate 2-oxoglutarate—hence the term dioxygenase (Fig. 16–10). In addition to succinate, CO$_2$ is formed from the 2-oxoglutarate. Structural analysis of a hydroxylated EGF module has established that the Hya residue is localized to the position predicted by the consensus sequence (see Fig. 16–9).[159, 186] The three-dimensional structure of the EGF module appears to be crucial for substrate recognition by the enzyme, as linear peptides with the appropriate sequence do not stimulate 2-oxoglutarate decarboxylation.[185] The metal ion requirement of both prolyl-4-hydroxylase and Asp/Asn-β-hydroxylase is satisfied by Fe^{2+}.[116, 187, 188]

Of the 2-oxoglutarate–dependent dioxygenases, prolyl-4-hydroxylase has been studied in the greatest detail.[116] Analogues of 2-oxoglutarate, such as 2,4-dicarboxypyridine, which inhibit prolyl-4-hydroxylase, also inhibit Asp-β-hydroxylase. This compound (2,4-dicarboxypyridine) also inhibits hydroxylation of the appropriate Asp residue in recombinant factor IX expressed in mammalian tissue culture.[184] Unlike pro-

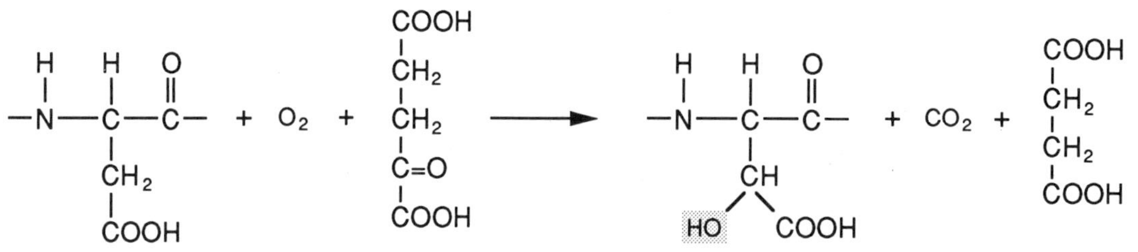

FIGURE 16–10. Hydroxylation of an aspartyl residue by Asp/Asn-β-hydroxylase to form *erythro*-β-hydroxy-aspartic acid. The enzyme is a dioxygenase that requires molecular oxygen and a cosubstrate, 2-oxoglutarate (α-ketoglutarate). The cosubstrate is decarboxylated to succinate.

lyl-4-hydroxylase, the Asp/Asn-β-hydroxylase does not require ascorbate or other reducing agents in vitro. It has also been demonstrated that the Hya content of the vitamin K–dependent proteins purified from severely scorbutic guinea pigs is normal.[189] Asp/Asn hydroxylation does not require vitamin K.[189a]

Asp/Asn-β-hydroxylase has been purified to homogeneity from bovine liver microsomes.[188, 190] The predominant form of the enzyme is a monomer with an apparent molecular weight of 52,000. It appears to hydroxylate both Asp- and Asn-containing substrates.[188]

Calcium Binding to Epidermal Growth Factor–like Modules

Attempts to elucidate structure-function relationships in the EGF modules of vitamin K–dependent serine proteins, including studies of the Ca^{2+}-binding properties, have exploited the modular organization of the non-catalytic parts of the proteins in four ways. First, modules have been isolated from limited proteolytic digests of the proteins. This approach was introduced when the Gla module in factor X was removed after careful chymotryptic cleavage of the intact protein.[92, 93] The products of the reaction were the Gla module cleaved in the aromatic cluster (COOH-terminal of Tyr 44) and the intact COOH-terminal remainder of the protein, known as Gla-domainless factor X. After activation, the latter had full amidolytic activity against low molecular weight substrates. The Gla module can now easily be removed from factors VII, IX, and X, protein C, and protein Z.[80, 94, 97, 191] Subsequently, methods were developed to isolate one or two intact EGF modules with or without the Gla module attached.[82–84, 91] This approach has the advantage that the modules presumably are native and contain postribosomal modifications. In the second approach, individual recombinant modules have been expressed in yeast[167, 192] or chemically synthesized.[166] In either case, the Hya residue has been replaced with an Asp residue. In the third approach, EGF modules have been exchanged between recombinant proteins.[193–196] For instance, recombinant factor IX, with

the NH₂-terminal EGF modules exchanged for the corresponding module in factor X, has been expressed in mammalian tissue culture. Finally, recombinant factor IX and protein C with point mutations have been expressed in mammalian tissue culture, purified to homogeneity and used to study the role of individual amino acids in, for instance, Ca^{2+} binding.[197, 198] Analysis of factor IX from hemophilia B patients with point mutations in the EGF modules has served the same purpose (see below).

The Gla-domainless forms of factors VII, IX, and X and protein C have one or two metal ion–binding sites that bind Ca^{2+} with apparent dissociation constants from 40 to 200 μM.[79, 80, 94, 199, 200] Ca^{2+} binding to these sites seems to induce global conformational changes in the proteins.[80, 94] The functional significance of Gla-independent Ca^{2+} binding became evident when it was demonstrated that Gla-domainless protein C was much more rapidly activated by thrombin-thrombomodulin in the presence of Ca^{2+} than in its absence.[79, 94] Gla-domainless protein Z does not bind Ca^{2+}.[191]

One of the Gla-independent Ca^{2+} sites has been located in the NH₂-terminal EGF module in factors IX and X and in protein C.[16, 91, 167, 192, 198] The dissociation constant for Ca^{2+} binding to this site varies from 200 μM to 2 mM, depending on which module is studied, the pH, and the ionic strength. There is no Ca^{2+} binding to the COOH-terminal EGF-like module in factors VII, IX, and X and in protein C. In factor X, Ca^{2+} binding has been studied using ¹H NMR spectroscopy.[16, 91] It is noteworthy that metal ion binding induced a chemical shift of aromatic protons in Tyr 68—that is, the residue that is located opposite to Hya in the major pleated sheet—suggesting a nearby location of the metal ion–binding site (see Fig. 16–8). The K_d for Ca^{2+} binding to this site was found to be 0.8 mM at pH 7.5, in the absence of NaCl, and 2 mM in the presence of 0.15 M NaCl. In the intact protein, K_d for Ca^{2+} binding to this site was approximately 0.1 mM.[84] The metal ion affinity of the site was pH dependent, which was attributed to two nearby His residues. The Ca^{2+}-binding site of an EGF module of factor IX, expressed in yeast, had a K_d of 200 to 300 μM.[167] This module has also been chemically synthesized and found to bind Ca^{2+}.[166] As it has Asp instead of Hya corresponding to position 64 in the intact protein, the hydroxyl group of Hya does not seem to be crucial to Ca^{2+} binding. However, no detailed comparison of the Ca^{2+}-binding properties of an EGF module with those of Hya has been made with a module that has Asp in this position but is otherwise identical. It is thus possible that the hydroxyl group alters the affinity of the metal ion–binding site for Ca^{2+} or that it affects the Ca^{2+}-Mg^{2+} ion selectivity of the metal ion–binding site.

Epidermal growth factor–like modules that bind Ca^{2+} have two conserved Asp residues, corresponding to positions 46 and 48 in factor X, that are located opposite to the conserved Hya/Asp residue in the major pleated sheet.[14–16, 91] It has been suggested that these three negatively charged residues are ligands for the Ca^{2+} ion.[153] This proposal has obtained support from the observation that the Gla-domainless form of protein Z that has Gly and Ser instead of the two conserved Asp residues does not have a Gla-independent Ca^{2+}-binding site.[191] Recent studies, using site-directed mutagenesis to change the residues in the NH_2-terminal EGF module of factor IX, have shed some light on the nature of the Ca^{2+}-binding site. The mutant factor IX species (Asp 47 → Lys or Gly; Asp 49 → Glu; and Asp/Hya 64 → Lys, Val, or Gly) were secreted by the eukaryotic cell line and shown to have biological activities of 1 to 8 per cent in factor IX clotting assays (Fig. 16–11).[197] Although the amounts of protein produced did not allow direct Ca^{2+} binding measurements, the results are compatible with the proposed location of the Ca^{2+}-binding site. In subsequent experiments, recombinant EGF modules from factor IX with point mutations in positions 47, 50, and 64 were shown to have severely reduced Ca^{2+} affinities. It was also found that mutation of the Gln residue in position 50 to Glu resulted in an increased affinity for Ca^{2+}.[192] In protein C, the Asp residue that becomes hydroxylated has been mutated to Glu, which led to a reduction of the biological activity to 10 per cent of normal.[198] Moreover, the mutant protein was not recognized by a monoclonal antibody that recognizes a Ca^{2+}-dependent epitope in the NH_2-terminal EGF module, suggesting an involvement of the Hya residue in Ca^{2+} binding. However, in evaluating these studies, it should be borne in mind that the mutations may have had inadvertent consequences.

Recently, two-dimensional NMR studies of the Ca^{2+}-saturated form of the NH_2-terminal EGF module of factor X have demonstrated that the chemical shifts corresponding to residues in the major β sheet and the residues NH_2-terminal to the first Cys (residues 45 to 49) are influenced by the metal ion (see Fig. 16–8).[16, 91] The backbone carbonyls of Gly 47 and Gly 64 are well-defined ligands to the Ca^{2+}, as well as the side-chain carbonyl of Gln 49 and one of the carboxyl oxygens of Hya 63.[16] In contrast, the residues in the COOH-terminal part of the module appear not to be involved in the metal ion binding.

In protein S, the NH_2-terminal EGF module has one Hya residue, whereas the three following modules have partially hydroxylated Asn residues. Acid hydrolysates of human protein S contain an average of

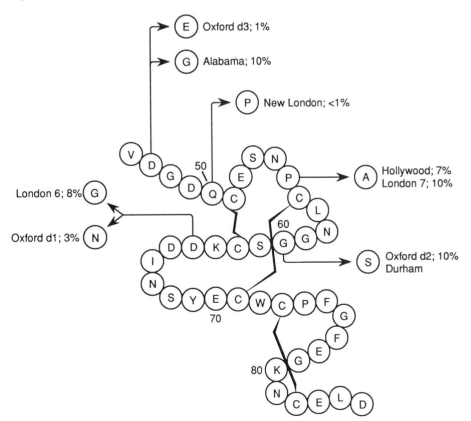

FIGURE 16–11. Mutations causing hemophilia B in the amino-terminal EGF module of factor IX. The mutations and the clotting activity of the mutant factor IX molecules are denoted. For details see the text.

2.2 mol of Hya per mole of protein.[48] Protein S has four sites with very high Ca^{2+} affinity, the values determined being $K_{d1} < 1 \times 10^{-8}$ M, $K_{d2} = 3 \times 10^{-8}$ M, $K_{d3} = 2.5 \times 10^{-7}$ M, and $K_{d4} = 1 \times 10^{-6}$ M.[168] These sites appear to be located in the EGF-like modules. From proteolytic digests, a fragment containing the two COOH-terminal EGF modules was isolated and found to retain very high affinity Ca^{2+}-binding sites. It is noteworthy that the Ca^{2+} affinities of the sites in protein S are two to four orders of magnitude greater than those of corresponding sites in factors IX and X and in protein C.[91, 168, 200, 201] Two of the protein S modules have the sequence Asp-Val/Ile-Asp-Glu-Cys, corresponding to residues 46 to 50 in factor X. Although the structural basis for the high Ca^{2+} affinity of the EGF modules in protein S has not yet been elucidated, it has been hypothesized that it is caused by the additional negative charge NH_2-terminal to the first Cys residue in modules 3 and 4 (Glu 163 and 205; see Fig. 16–9).[168] Moreover, the hydrophobic side chain of the Val/Ile residue in these modules probably increases the Ca^{2+} affinity by lowering the dielectric constant.[16] The Asp-Val/Ile-Asp-Glu-Cys sequence has recently been identified in EGF-like modules that have the consensus sequence for hydroxylation seen in many non–vitamin K–dependent proteins. Among these proteins are the gene products of the Notch[179] and Crumbs[181] loci in *Drosophila melanogaster,* the TGF-β–binding protein[175] and fibrillin[177, 178] (the protein implicated in the Marfan syndrome), and the protein coded by the TAN-1 locus.[183] Although many of the non–vitamin K–dependent proteins that have EGF modules containing the consensus sequence recognized by the Asp/Asn hydroxylase have been characterized only at the cDNA level, it seems safe to infer that many of them have Ca^{2+}-binding sites with very high affinity.

Mutations in Epidermal Growth Factor–like Modules

Mutations in the EGF modules have been found in factor IX in several patients with hemophilia B and in one patient with protein C deficiency (His 66 → Asn).[98, 202] A comprehensive review of factor IX mutations is given in Chapter 19. In this chapter, only point mutations that result in the secretion of a functionally defective molecule are considered. All but one of these mutations are in the NH_2-terminal EGF module. Positions of mutations and biological activities of the mutant factor IX are shown in Figure 16–11. Mutations involving amino acids that have been implicated in Ca^{2+} binding are factor IX Alabama (Asp 47 → Gly),[203, 204] factor IX Oxford d3 (Asp 47 → Glu),[99] factor IX Oxford d1 (Asp/Hya 64 → Asn),[99] and factor IX London 6 (Asp/Hya 64 → Gly).[205] The biological activity of the defective factor IX molecules varies between less than 1 per cent and 10 per cent. Of the mutant factor IX molecules, factor IX Alabama has been studied in most detail. Metal ion–binding studies

with factor IX Alabama have been interpreted to suggest that Asp 47 in normal factor IX coordinates with the bound Ca^{2+} ion, inducing a conformational change in the molecule. Factor IX New London (Gln 50 → Pro) causes severe hemophilia B.[206] Its Ca^{2+}-binding properties have not been studied. In general, the results of these studies corroborate those obtained by means of site-directed mutagenesis. Recently, the amino acids in factor X that correspond to Asp 47, Gln 50, and Asp/Hya 64 in factor IX were shown to be Ca^{2+} ligands.[16] The Pro 55 → Ala and Gly 60 → Ser mutations presumably cause a reduction in the biological activity of factor IX by affecting the tertiary structure of the EGF-like module.

Factor IX Fukuoka (Asn 92 → His) is a mutation in the second EGF module.[207] The factor IX antigen concentration is 64 per cent, and the coagulant activity is 3 per cent of normal. Although factor IX Fukuoka has normal amidolytic activity against low molecular weight substrates, V_{max} for the activation of factor X is 10-fold lower than normal. It was suggested that this is due to defective interaction of the second EGF module with factor VIIIa or factor X or both.

Function of Epidermal Growth Factor–like Modules

The EGF modules of the vitamin K–dependent proteins do not have the residues required for binding of EGF and TGF-α to the EGF receptor.[25, 152] It has also been experimentally demonstrated that the NH_2-terminal EGF module in human factor IX does not bind to the EGF receptor and has no growth factor activity.[166] In urokinase, the single EGF module mediates binding of urokinase to a cell surface receptor, and in thrombomodulin it has been demonstrated that the EGF modules bind thrombin.[7, 208–212] The affinities of these interactions are similar to that of EGF for its receptor ($K_d = 10^{-9}$ to 10^{-10} M).

Except for Ca^{2+} binding, information pertaining to the function of these modules is sparse. However, the NH_2-terminal EGF module would appear to affect the conformation and Ca^{2+}-binding properties of the Gla module. Accordingly, the Gla modules of factors IX and X do not have normal Ca^{2+}-binding properties, unless they are linked to the NH_2-terminal EGF module. This finding may be due to the proteolytic cleavage in the COOH-terminal aromatic cluster region of the Gla module, but it is also possible that the NH_2-terminal EGF module, together with this region, functions as a scaffold for the folding of the Gla module.[83, 84]

One function of the EGF modules in the vitamin K–dependent proteins is as a spacer between the Gla modules and the serine protease parts. This theory is illustrated by the recently estimated distance of 69 Å from the active site of factor Xa to the phospholipid surface, thought to be in direct contact with the Gla module.[213] The EGF modules in protein S may have a similar spacer function, a hypothesis that gains support from the observation that EGF module–containing proteins often are elongated molecules, such as fibrillin.[214]

Hybrids between factor IX and factor X have been expressed in mammalian tissue culture to gain insight into the function of these modules.[193, 194, 196] In factor IX, either the NH$_2$-terminal EGF module was exchanged for the corresponding module in factor X or both EGF modules were exchanged for the corresponding factor X modules. Factor IXa with only the NH$_2$-terminal EGF module from factor X had near-normal biological activity in clotting assays. However, a hybrid in which both EGF modules in factor IX had been exchanged for the modules in factor X had only 4 per cent of the normal clotting activity. Several interpretations are possible; for example, the EGF modules may interact directly with the cofactor, factor VIIIa, or the substrate factor X. It is also possible that the COOH-terminal EGF module is required for normal folding of the serine protease part. Recently, chimeric proteins composed of modules from factors VII and IX have been prepared and tested for their ability to bind to human TF.[195] The results indicate that the high-affinity interaction is between the EGF-like module(s) in factor VII(a) and TF, whereas the Gla module and the serine protease part appear not to participate. These conclusions have been corroborated by experiments in which a monoclonal antibody that interacted with the first EGF-like module in factor VII was found to inhibit the interaction between TF and factor VIIa.[214a]

Recombinant factor IXa's in which the amino acids implicated in Ca^{2+} binding in the NH$_2$-terminal EGF module have been mutated have low biological activity, possibly because of defective enzyme-cofactor or enzyme-substrate interaction. These mutant factor IX molecules, as well as the naturally occurring mutant factor IX Alabama, were activated at normal rates by factor XIa in the presence of Ca^{2+}. There was a small difference between mutant and normal factor IXa in the ability to activate factor X in the presence of phospholipid. In the presence of factor VIIIa *and* phospholipid, normal factor IXa activated factor X much more rapidly than did any of the mutant factor IXa molecules.[197] Although these effects may be due to a defective Ca^{2+} binding, affecting the interaction between the EGF module and either the cofactor or the substrate, an induced conformational change in a distant part of the molecule is also possible. A direct interaction between the EGF modules of factor IXa and the substrate factor X was proposed by the finding that a fragment containing the two EGF modules from factor IX inhibits the factor IXa–mediated activation of factor X in the absence of both phospholipid and factor VIIIa as well as in their presence.[215] The interaction between the EGF module and the substrate or cofactor, albeit weak, may be significant on the phospholipid surface.

KRINGLE MODULES

The determination of the amino acid sequence of prothrombin and the pairing of its cysteine residues, reported in 1974, established the presence of two regions within the molecule that display a high degree of sequence similarity and identical disulfide bond pairing (see Fig. 16–2).[58] Each region encompasses 80 to 85 amino acids and has 6 Cys residues that are paired 1—6, 2—4, and 3—5. The sequence identity between the two is approximately 35 per cent. The structure is reminiscent of a Danish pastry, called *kringle*—hence its name.[58] The identification of the two kringle modules in prothrombin demonstrated that the immunoglobulins were not unique in being composed of structural motifs judged to be homologous owing to pronounced sequence similarity. Moreover, from the structure of prothrombin, it was evident that a protein could be composed of modules of different type; that is, prothrombin contains, in addition to the two kringle modules, an NH$_2$-terminal Gla module and a COOH-terminal serine protease module. The NH$_2$-terminal kringle of prothrombin is encoded by two exons, and the COOH-terminal one by a single exon.[30, 42] The splice junctions at the intron/exon boundaries on either side of the two kringles are of phase 1, whereas the single intron within the NH$_2$-terminal kringle is of phase 2, suggesting assembly of the gene by duplication and exon shuffling.

Prothrombin is the only vitamin K–dependent protein that contains kringle modules.[11, 22] However, kringles have been found in several other plasma proteins. Plasminogen contains five kringles, urokinase and factor XII contain one each, tissue-type plasminogen activator contains two, and the hepatocyte growth factor contains four.[11, 216, 217] Apolipoprotein-A is remarkable in that it contains 38 kringles in tandem.[218] Like the first kringle in prothrombin, the kringles in urokinase, tissue-type plasminogen activator, and factor XII all contain an internal intron localized at a conserved position, attesting to their phylogenetic relationship.[11, 22, 30, 40, 42]

The structure of isolated kringle modules from plasminogen has been determined by X-ray crystallography and NMR spectroscopy, and the structure of prothrombin fragment 1, which contains one kringle, has been ascertained by X-ray crystallography.[13, 69, 219-221] The backbone of the kringles studied so far is folded in much the same way, despite considerable differences in amino acid sequence.[13] The overall shape of a kringle is discoid, with the approximate dimensions of 15 × 30 × 30 Å. It contains three disulfide bonds, the first of which links Cys 1 and Cys 6, keeping the NH$_2$- and COOH-termini in close proximity, whereas the disulfide bonds that link Cys 2 and 4 and 3 and 5 are buried in the interior of the kringle, apparently inaccessible to solvent. The peptide segments linked by the disulfide bonds protrude from the center as antiparallel β strands connected by β turns (for details of the structure, the reader is referred to references 13 and 219 to 221).

Kringles 1 and 4 in plasminogen and kringle 2 in tissue-type plasminogen activator have physiologically important fibrin-binding sites that also bind lysine, ε-aminocaproic acid, and similar ω-carboxylic acids.[13, 219, 221] The kringles in prothrombin do not bind ε-aminocaproic acid with measurable affinity.[13] Kringle 2 (fragment 2) from bovine prothrombin is thought to interact with factor Va, although no quantitative data have been reported for the interaction.[222] It also interacts with α thrombin with a K_d of 7.7×10^{-10} M and with prethrombin 2 with a $K_d = 1.3 \times 10^{-10}$ M, suggesting that fragment 2 is associated with α thrombin in vivo.[223] Fragment 2 has been reported to bind four calcium ions with comparatively low affinity.[224] The fragment has no effect on the clotting activity of α thrombin. Nothing is known about the function of the first kringle in prothrombin.

A MODULE IN PROTEIN S WITH THROMBIN-SENSITIVE BONDS

Protein S contains a unique module with two thrombin-sensitive bonds located between the Gla module and the four EGF modules (see Fig. 16–2). It is 29 amino acids long (Val 46 to Asn 74) and is encoded by a separate exon. There is no apparent sequence similarity with the peptide in prothrombin (residues 47 to 63) that links the Gla module and the NH_2-terminal kringle module. Thrombin cleaves the bovine protein S module at Arg 70.[50] A second cleavage at Arg 52 results in the release of a peptide 18 amino acids long. The thrombin cleavage sites are conserved in human protein S.[48] The module contains two Cys residues (positions 47 and 72) linked by a disulfide bond. The Gla module thus remains attached to the remainder of the molecule after cleavage. The peptide bond at Arg 70 is much more accessible to thrombin cleavage in the absence of Ca^{2+} than in the presence of the metal ion.[49] In experiments with monoclonal antibodies, Ca^{2+}-dependent epitopes have been identified in this region of the molecule.[225]

Compared with intact protein S, the Gla module in the thrombin-cleaved molecule appears to have a lower affinity for Ca^{2+}.[49] Moreover, its affinity for negatively charged phospholipid vesicles is low at 1 to 2 mM Ca^{2+}, suggesting that the Gla module in the cleaved molecule cannot attain the native conformation.[74] However, at higher Ca^{2+} concentrations (10 mM), the phospholipid interaction of cleaved protein S appears to be normal. Thrombin-cleaved protein S does not function as a cofactor to activated protein C.[226, 227] It is thus apparent that Ca^{2+} has a profound effect upon the structure of this part of the protein S molecule and that thrombin cleavage at Arg 70 results in structural alterations in the protein S molecule that preclude normal Ca^{2+} binding and cofactor activity. Whether thrombin cleavage of protein S is a regulatory step of physiological significance remains to be elucidated.

SERINE PROTEASE MODULES

The vitamin K–dependent serine proteases and the proteases of the fibrinolytic and complement systems are similar in that each has a large NH_2-terminal non-catalytic assemblage with modular organization.[11] The non-catalytic modules are regulatory elements; they bind Ca^{2+} and interact with phospholipid and with their respective cofactors, receptors, and substrates. At the molecular level, regulation of the coagulation system stems from the finely tuned assembly and subsequent inactivation of enzymatically active macromolecular complexes, such as the factor Xase and prothrombinase complexes, the factor VIIa–tissue factor complex, and the thrombin-thrombomodulin complex.[1–7] The substrate specificities of the active enzymes, which are much narrower than those of the archetype serine proteases chymotrypsin and trypsin, also contribute to the precise regulation of each step in the coagulation cascade. The coagulation enzymes are specific for Arg in the P1 position (nomenclature of Schechter and Berger[228]) of the substrate. Among the many arginyl bonds, only one or two are cleaved during zymogen activation. In comparison, trypsin cleaves most peptide bonds with Arg or Lys in the P1 position (except Arg/Lys-Pro) and would cleave several arginyl and lysyl bonds in the serine protease zymogens. The substrates of factor VIIa are factors VII, IX, and X; the substrates of factor IXa are factors VII and X; the substrates of factor Xa are factor VII, prothrombin, and factors V and VIII, whereas the substrates of activated protein C are factors Va and VIIIa. Although the specificities of the enzymes overlap to some extent, no other substrates of physiological significance have been found for these enzymes. In addition to initiating the fibrinogen to fibrin conversion, thrombin cleaves certain peptide bonds in other substrates (see Fig. 12–1).[4] The discrete cleavages in factors XI, V, and VIII are important to initiate and maintain the coagulation cascade,[4, 229, 230, 230a] whereas activation of factor XIII is a prerequisite for the covalent cross-linking of fibrin.[4, 231] Thrombin also downregulates the coagulation cascade by activating protein C.[7, 232] Finally, thrombin is a potent cellular stimulator and elicits secretion and arachidonic acid metabolism in platelets and endothelial cells.[233] The recently elucidated thrombin-mediated cleavage of the platelet thrombin receptor has revealed an interesting novel mechanism of receptor/substrate activation of potential future therapeutic significance.[234–237] Most mammalian cell types (except erythrocytes) respond to thrombin. The structural basis of the narrow substrate specificity of thrombin and of the active forms of the other coagulation enzymes is now beginning to be unraveled. Determination of the three-dimensional structure of thrombin by X-ray crystallography represents a crucial step in this direction.[21, 237a]

All the vitamin K–dependent serine proteases are synthesized as single-chain molecules, but the plasma forms of factor X and protein C have been processed to two chain forms prior to secretion (although approximately 15 percent of single-chain protein C remains in plasma).[232] On activation by limited proteolysis, full amidolytic and clotting activity is obtained after cleavage of one or two polypeptide bonds in prothrombin and factors VII, IX, and X and protein C. Although the serine proteases are homologous, profound structural differences exist between factors VIIa, IXa, and Xa and activated protein C on the one hand and thrombin on the other. In the former enzymes, the non-catalytic NH_2-terminal parts remain bound to the active serine protease modules by a disulfide bond, which ensures that factors VIIa, IXa, and Xa and activated protein C all retain their phospholipid affinity. On activation of prothrombin, however, the non-catalytic NH_2-terminal modules are released as activation peptides or remain non-covalently associated with thrombin.[1–3, 223] The 36 residue thrombin A chain is linked to the serine protease B chain by a disulfide bond.[30, 58] During prothrombin activation, intermediates possessing an active site are formed. Thrombin lacks affinity for the phospholipid and factors Va and VIIIa and leaves the prothrombinase complex by diffusion. This is reflected by the fact that thrombin, in addition to the cleavage of four peptide bonds in the soluble fibrinogen molecule, has several other seemingly diverse effects that are central to hemostasis.[233–235]

The Serine Protease Modules of Factors IXa and Xa Interact with Factors VIIIa and Va

The factor Xase and prothrombinase complexes are the result of binary protein-protein, protein-Ca^{2+}, and protein-phospholipid interactions. Factors V and VIII, the inactive precursors of factors Va and VIIIa, can be regarded as circulating precursors that upon activation by limited proteolysis are inserted into anionic phospholipid, thus forming complex receptors for factors Xa and IXa, respectively.[2, 3, 230] Since the K_d for the binding of factor Xa to factor Va is approximately 1×10^{-6} M (the stoichiometry is 1:1), the interaction between the two proteins is too weak to promote complex formation in solution at physiological concentrations.[238] However, factor Va interacts with phospholipid having a K_d of approximately 3×10^{-9} M,[239] and factor Xa interacts with phospholipid having a K_d of approximately 2×10^{-6} M.[2, 3] In the presence of Ca^{2+}, the interaction of factor IXa with factor VIIIa–phospholipid is characterized by a K_d of approximately 0.5×10^{-9} M[240, 241] and the interaction of factor Xa with factor Va–phospholipid by a K_d of approximately 0.7×10^{-9} M.[2, 3, 242] It is noteworthy that the affinity of factor Va for phospholipid is not influenced by factor Xa.[239] Although the role of the phospholipid surface in the assembly of the prothrombinase and factor Xase complexes is multifaceted, one of the effects is that the concentrations of the reactants adjacent to or on the surface are high enough to promote complex formation between enzyme and cofactor.[1–3]

The Gla modules of factors IXa and Xa bind Ca^{2+} and interact with phospholipid but do not interact with their cofactors, factors VIIIa and Va, with high affinity. Whether the EGF modules contribute to the interactions between enzymes and cofactors is still controversial. However, several lines of evidence suggest that most of the binding energy is accounted for by interactions between the serine protease parts of factors IXa and Xa and their respective cofactor.[2, 3] This theory has been inferred, for instance, from the fact that factor Xa interacts with a platelet receptor (factor Va) with high affinity, whereas the affinity between the zymogen and the receptor is not measurable and accordingly several orders of magnitude lower.[243–245] The specificity is explained by the major conformational change in the serine protease parts that results from the activation of factors IX and X.[246, 247] In comparison, the conformational changes in the Gla and EGF modules of factor X that accompany activation appear negligible. Furthermore, a monoclonal antibody with the epitope in the serine protease part of factor IXa inhibits the interaction between enzyme and cofactor.[248] Similarly, several peptides corresponding to the serine protease part of factor Xa inhibit the interaction between factor Xa and factor Va.[249]

Intermediates in the Activation of Prothrombin to Thrombin

In the activation of prothrombin to thrombin by factor Xa, two peptide bonds are cleaved, Arg 271—Thr 272 and Arg 320—Ile 321 (in bovine prothrombin the cleaved bonds are Arg 274—Thr 275 and Arg 323—Ile 324).[1, 2, 250, 251] If the Arg 320—Ile 321 bond is cleaved first, meizothrombin is formed (Fig. 16–12). In a subsequent step, meizothrombin is cleaved at the bond between Arg 271—Thr 272, leading to the formation of α thrombin and fragment 1–2. If the initial factor Xa–mediated cleavage is between Arg 271—Thr 272, fragment 1–2 and prethrombin 2 are intermediates. Subsequent cleavage of prethrombin 2 by factor Xa generates α thrombin. Activation can proceed by either pathway, depending on the reaction conditions. The pathway with meizothrombin as an intermediate is favored when the reaction is catalyzed by the intact prothrombinase complex.[250–253] In the absence of factor Va, activation proceeds via both pathways.[254] Cleavage of the Arg 320—Ile 321 bond appears to facilitate subsequent cleavage of the Arg 271—Thr 272 bond. In addition to the Arg 271—Thr 272 bond, the nearby Arg 284—Thr 285 bond in human prothrombin is susceptible to cleavage by thrombin or factor Xa or both.[252, 253] In plasma, the factor Xa–mediated cleavage appears to occur predominantly at Arg 284 rather than Arg 271.[252] The Arg 155—Ser 156 bond in fragment 1–2 can be cleaved by meizothrombin or thrombin. Cleavage of meizothrombin at Arg 155 yields meizothrombin(des fragment 1) and fragment 1; cleavage of fragment 1–2 yields fragment 1 and fragment 2; cleavage of prothrombin yields prethrombin 1 and fragment 1. The high-affinity interaction of bovine fragment 2 with thrombin ($K_d = 7.7 \times 10^{-10}$ M) suggests that the product of either activation pathway to a large extent

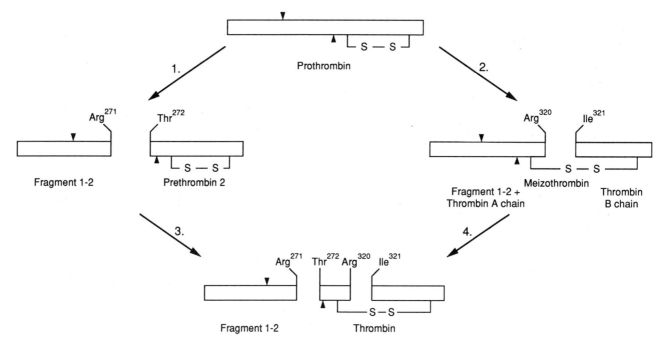

FIGURE 16–12. Schematic diagram showing the pathways for human prothrombin activation. Factor Xa catalyzes two peptide bond cleavages in prothrombin: between Arg 271 and Thr 272 and between Arg 320 and Ile 321. Pathway 1 yields fragment 1–2 and prethrombin 2, whereas pathway 2 yields meizothrombin. Prethrombin 2 can be cleaved to give thrombin (3), and meizothrombin is cleaved to give fragment 1–2 and thrombin (4). The thrombin-mediated cleavage that can separate fragment 1 from fragment 2 (between residues Arg 155 and Ser 156) is denoted by an arrowhead pointing downward. When prothrombin is cleaved, the products are fragment 1 and prethrombin 1; when fragment 1–2 is cleaved, the products are fragment 1 and fragment 2. The thrombin/factor Xa–mediated cleavage between Arg 284 and Thr 285 is denoted by an arrowhead pointing upward. The amino acids are numbered as in reference 30.

is a non-covalent complex of α thrombin and fragment 1–2.[223] The complex probably remains reversibly associated with the phospholipid surface. Subsequent cleavage at Arg 155—Ser 156 would release fragment 2 in complex with α thrombin from the membrane surface. In studies of the activation of prethrombin 1 by factor Xa alone, both the prethrombin 2–fragment 2 and the meizothrombin(des fragment 1) pathways were observed.[254] The relative importance of the two pathways of prothrombin activation under physiological conditions has not yet been resolved.

The amidolytic activities of meizothrombin and meizothrombin(des fragment 1) against chromogenic substrates are identical to that of α thrombin, whereas their proteolytic activities against fibrinogen, factor V, and the platelet thrombin receptor are only about 1 per cent and 10 per cent, respectively, of that of α thrombin.[255] The parallel decrease in the procoagulant activity of each intermediate suggests that the binding sites for fibrinogen, factor V, and the platelet receptor are related.

The rates of protein C activation by meizothrombin and thrombin have been reported to be identical in the presence of thrombomodulin and phospholipid (75 per cent phosphatidylcholine and 25 per cent phosphatidylserine).[255] Recently, however, meizothrombin was prepared from recombinant prothrombin in which the active site Ser residue (Ser 205, thrombin B chain numbering) had been mutated to

Ala to preclude autocatalytic activation of the meizothrombin to thrombin.[256] The recombinant meizothrombin did not bind to thrombomodulin, whereas recombinant thrombin with Ala in position 205 bound with the same affinity as did wild-type thrombin. The function of meizothrombin and its role in the microcirculation thus remain to be established.

Prothrombin can be activated not only by factor Xa but also by a bacterial protein, *staphylocoagulase*.[257, 258] Staphylocoagulase forms a complex with prothrombin and induces a conformational change in prothrombin, exposing its active site, which thus expresses amidolytic and clotting activity without prior cleavage of any peptide bond. The complex is therefore an "active zymogen." The Gla module is not involved in complex formation between staphylocoagulase and prothrombin. Prothrombin is also activated by enzymes from the venoms of the snakes *Echis carinatus*[259] and *Oxyuranus scutellatus*,[260] whereas factors IX and X and protein C are activated by the venom from *Vipera russelli*.[2, 261] The venom from *Oxyuranus scutellatus* also activates human factor VII.[262]

Structure of Thrombin

Human α thrombin is a glycoprotein that consists of two disulfide-linked polypeptide chains, an A chain of 36 amino acids (49 amino acids if there has been

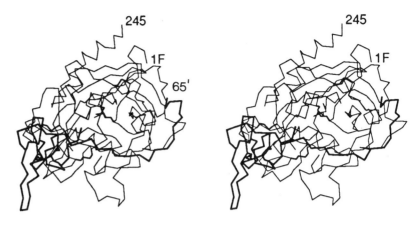

FIGURE 16–13. Stereoview of the polypeptide backbone of the complex between hirudin and thrombin. Hirudin is shown in bold. (From Tulinsky, A.: The structures of domains of blood proteins. Thromb. Haemost. 66: 16, 1991; with permission.)

no autocatalytic cleavage at Arg 284; see Fig. 16–12) and a B chain of 259 residues.[21, 30, 233, 237a] The thrombin molecule has an isoelectric point of approximately 7.4 and thus has no net charge at physiological pH. It is sparingly soluble and readily adheres to negatively charged and apolar surfaces.[263] The B chain of thrombin is closely related to chymotrypsin, the archetype serine protease, with a sequence identity of approximately 65 per cent.[21, 264, 265] A remarkable feature is that although thrombin has no net charge at physiological pH, it has an unusually large number of charged residues (twice as many as trypsin and chymotrypsin), many of which are located on the surface of the molecule.[21, 265]

The structure of active site–inhibited human α thrombin has been determined by X-ray crystallography to a resolution of 1.9 Å[21] and that of the hirudin-thrombin complex to 2.3 Å.[266–268] Knowledge of the detailed atomic structure of thrombin provides a wealth of important information. The thrombin molecule is almost spherical, with the dimensions 45 × 45 × 50 Å. The polypeptide backbone of the B chain is folded in the manner characteristic of trypsin, chymotrypsin, and other serine proteases. The A chain, a disulfide-bonded activation peptide with unknown function, is linked to the B chain on the side of the molecule opposite the active site. The major difference between the α thrombin B chain and chymotrypsin is the insertion of several loops in thrombin that change the surface topography of the molecule. The most conspicuous loops are nine residues, Tyr 47 to Thr 55 (numbering for thrombin B chain),[30] and five residues between Glu 146 and Val 152 that protrude around the active site.

The active site residues of the so-called charge-relay system are arranged as in trypsin and chymotrypsin.[21] However, this region, together with the substrate-binding region, has a most conspicuous elongated and kinked canyon-like cleft, which accommodates residues both NH₂- and COOH-terminal to the substrate's cleavage site. In trypsin and chymotrypsin, the active site cleft is less well demarcated and appears to be more easily accessible. The sides of the cleft in thrombin are lined primarily with hydrophobic residues, whereas its bottom contains several charged residues. The nine residue loop formed by residues Tyr 47 to

Thr 55, together with Trp 148, restricts accessibility to the active site cleft. In the Aα chain of fibrinogen, a hydrophobic motif, Phe 8, Leu 9, Val 15, preceding the scissile peptide bond (Arg 16—Gly 17) probably interacts with this hydrophobic region in thrombin. This theory would also explain why it is favorable to have a tosyl group NH₂-terminal to Gly in the P3 position in substrates such as Tos-Gly-Pro-Arg-pNA. The active site groove in thrombin extends far beyond the active site adjoining P' subsites. It is coated with positively charged amino acids, including Lys 21 Lys 52, Arg 62, Arg 70, and Arg 73, and is commonly referred to as the anion-binding exosite (see reference 21 and Fig. 16–4). This region appears to provide remarkable specificity for fibrinogen as well as some other thrombin substrates. Thrombomodulin and the leech anticoagulant hirudin compete with fibrinogen and factor V for binding to the exosite,[13, 265–269] whereas heparin seems to interact with a different site.[270] Therefore, either the thrombomodulin-binding site overlaps to some extent with the anion-binding exosite, or its binding to thrombin interferes sterically with the interaction between thrombin and fibrinogen. This competition is noteworthy in view of the modulation of thrombin from a procoagulant to an anticoagulant enzyme upon binding to thrombomodulin.

Hirudin consists of 65 amino acids and has three disulfide bonds. Its solution structure has been determined with two-dimensional NMR techniques, which also revealed that the 18 COOH-terminal residues have no defined structure.[271, 272] In the complex between thrombin and hirudin, the NH₂-terminal disulfide bridge–containing part of hirudin interacts with the catalytic site region of thrombin, whereas the COOH-terminal 18 residue tail adopts an extended conformation, which wraps around the thrombin molecule within the anion-binding exosite (Fig. 16–13).[266, 267] This tail region makes more electrostatic and hydrophobic interactions with the thrombin molecule than occur in other protease-inhibitor complexes. In the complex between trypsin and bovine pancreatic trypsin inhibitor, the area of contact has been estimated to be 475 Å²², whereas in the complex between thrombin and hirudin, the contact area is approximately 1400 Å².[267] The large contact area presumably contributes to the extraordinarily high affinity of hirudin for thrombin ($K_d \approx 10^{-14}$ M). In this context, it is noteworthy that the platelet receptor for thrombin contains a structural motif that resembles the COOH-terminal tail of hirudin and is thought to interact with the anion-binding exosite on thrombin.[234, 235]

Cleavage at the exposed Arg 73 in thrombin leads to the formation of β thrombin with greatly reduced clotting activity. It is assumed that this cleavage makes the fibrinogen-binding exosite more flexible and non-functioning, accounting for the loss of clotting activity.[20, 273] The surface loop formed by residues Ala 150 to Lys 154 in thrombin corresponds to the "autolysis loop" of α chymotrypsin and harbors residues susceptible to proteolytic cleavage. Cleavage of β thrombin by trypsin at the lysyl residue in position 154 yields γ thrombin with clotting activity less than 0.1 per cent of that for thrombin.[21, 273] Although both β thrombin and γ thrombin have lost clotting activity, they have full amidolytic activity.[265, 269] Pancreatic elastase and elastase from neutrophil granulocytes both cleave thrombin at a single site. Hydrolysis by elastase following Ala 150 yields ε thrombin,[265, 269, 273] and cathepsin G cleavage at the adjacent Trp 148 gives ζ thrombin.[274] There is only a partial loss of fibrinogen clotting activity in both ε thrombin and ζ thrombin, with retention of amidolytic activity. During blood coagulation, α thrombin is incorporated into the clot owing to its fibrin(ogen) affinity, which is mediated by the anionic exosite, whereas γ thrombin, lacking the exosite, is not, nor is the α thrombin–hirudin complex.[265] It is conceivable that α thrombin in the clot is degraded by granulocyte elastase and that the elastase-degraded forms, with low clotting activity, retain other activities and may provide a potent stimulus for fibrinolysis by releasing tissue-type plasminogen activator from the endothelial cells.

A Calcium-Binding Site in the Serine Protease Module of Coagulation Enzymes

Trypsin and trypsinogen bind a single Ca^{2+} ($K_d \approx$ 400 μM).[275] In addition, trypsinogen binds a Ca^{2+} with low affinity in the activation peptide region. The determination of the trypsin structure with X-ray crystallography allowed identification of the ligands to the metal ion.[275, 276] The side chains of Glu 52 and Glu 62 are ligands, whereas the side chain of Glu 59 seems to interact with the Ca^{2+} by means of an H_2O molecule that is sandwiched between the side-chain carboxylate group and the metal ion (Fig. 16–14; amino acids are numbered beginning with the residue that is NH_2-terminal in the serine protease module after activation). The backbone carbonyls of Asn 54 and Val 57 are also ligands to the Ca^{2+}. This Ca^{2+}, which is 21 Å from the active site Ser residue, stabilizes the trypsin molecule and inhibits its degradation by autodigestion.

Recently, binding of a monoclonal antibody directed against the serine protease part of factor IX was found to be Ca^{2+} dependent.[277, 278] By comparison with the Ca^{2+}-binding site in trypsin, it was inferred that the binding site is located at residues 54 to 66. A peptide corresponding to residues 51 to 85 was synthesized and found to bind Ca^{2+} with moderate affinity ($K_d \approx$ 500 μM). Figure 16–14 illustrates that the residues contributing side-chain ligands to the Ca^{2+} in trypsin are conserved. Whether the serine protease modules of factors VII and X and protein C bind Ca^{2+} with an affinity that is physiologically significant is not yet known. However, thrombin that does not bind Ca^{2+} has Lys and Ile corresponding to the two Glu residues that are ligands in trypsin and do not bind Ca^{2+}.

Mutations in Serine Protease Modules

Genetic defects that affect the serine protease regions range from complete gene deletions to point mutations that lead to the secretion of mutant proteins having low specific activity.[98] Most of these mutations have been identified in factor IX and cause hemophilia B (see Chapter 19). A few point mutations that shed light on the function of these proteins are discussed here.

One group of mutations involve the activation cleav-

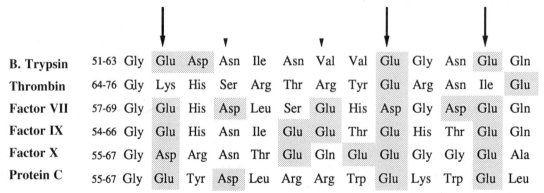

		Gly	Glu	Asp	Asn	Ile	Asn	Val	Val	Glu	Gly	Asn	Glu	Gln
B. Trypsin	51-63	Gly	Glu	Asp	Asn	Ile	Asn	Val	Val	Glu	Gly	Asn	Glu	Gln
Thrombin	64-76	Gly	Lys	His	Ser	Arg	Thr	Arg	Tyr	Glu	Arg	Asn	Ile	Glu
Factor VII	57-69	Gly	Glu	His	Asp	Leu	Ser	Glu	His	Asp	Gly	Asp	Glu	Gln
Factor IX	54-66	Gly	Glu	His	Asn	Ile	Glu	Glu	Thr	Glu	His	Thr	Glu	Gln
Factor X	55-67	Gly	Asp	Arg	Asn	Thr	Glu	Gln	Glu	Glu	Gly	Gly	Glu	Ala
Protein C	55-67	Gly	Glu	Tyr	Asp	Leu	Arg	Arg	Trp	Glu	Lys	Trp	Glu	Leu

FIGURE 16–14. Amino acid sequence in the Ca^{2+}-binding region of bovine trypsin and sequences in the corresponding regions of vitamin K–dependent serine proteases. Glu and Asp residues are shaded. Residues with backbone carbonyl oxygens that are ligands in trypsin are denoted with arrowheads, and residues with side-chain carboxyl groups that are ligands are denoted with arrows.[275, 276] Among the vitamin K–dependent plasma proteins, a calcium ion–binding site in this region has so far been identified only in factor IX. Amino acids are numbered beginning with the residue that is NH_2-terminal in the serine protease module *after* activation.

age sites. In prothrombin Barcelona/Madrid (Arg 271 → Cys; numbering begins with the first residue in the intact protein),[30] the factor Xa–mediated cleavage of meizothrombin to fragment 1–2 and thrombin is prevented (see Fig. 16–12).[279, 280] Subsequent factor Xa–thrombin–mediated cleavage at Arg 284 may yield thrombin, explaining the modest bleeding tendency associated with the defect. Single-chain factor IX is activated in two steps by factor XIa–Ca^{2+}–or factor VIIa–tissue factor–Ca^{2+}–mediated cleavage of the Arg 145—Ala 146 bond, followed by cleavage of the Arg 180—Val 181 bond.[32, 281] (See Chapter 19.) Amidolytic and clotting activity is obtained when the Arg 180—Val 181 bond is cleaved. If only the Arg 145—Ala 146 bond is cleaved, factor IXα is obtained, which has no amidolytic activity. Subsequent cleavage of the Arg 180—Val 181 bond yields biologically active factor IXαβ. The factor X activator from Russell's viper venom cleaves only the Arg 180—Val 181 bond, yielding factor IXαα. The specific activity of factor IXαα is only slightly lower than that of factor IXαβ in coagulation assays.[281] Two mutations of Arg 145 have been described; in factor IX Chapel Hill, the Arg residue is replaced by His (mild hemophilia B),[282] and in factor IX Cardiff, it is replaced by Cys (moderate hemophilia B).[283] Since the Arg 145—Ala 146 cleavage normally occurs before the Arg 180—Val 181 cleavage, the low specific activity of the two mutant factor IX species may be due to slow cleavage of the Arg 180-Val 181 bond in the single-chain factor IX mutants. There are also two mutations of Arg 180, both causing severe hemophilia B. Factor IX B$_M$ Nagoya is an Arg 180 → Trp mutation, and factor IX Hilo is an Arg 180 → Gln mutation.[284, 285] Neither mutant factor IX is activated by factor XIa–Ca^{2+}, but factor IX B$_M$ Nagoya can be activated by chymotrypsin. In the factor IX mutant labeled Kashihara, there is a Val 182 → Phe mutation (position 2 in the active enzyme).[32, 286] The mutant factor IX is not activated by factor XIa–Ca^{2+} or the factor X activator from Russell's viper venom. Mutations around position 180 are usually associated with a normal plasma concentration of factor IX with low biological activity.

Factor IX B$_M$ Lake Elsinore is Ala 210 → Val (numbering begins with the first residue in the heavy chain of the active enzyme), that is, immediately COOH-terminal of the last Cys residue in factor IX.[287] Factor IX Vancouver, identified in several patients with hemophilia B, is an Ile 217 → Thr mutation.[288–290] In both these types of mutations, the amidolytic activity of the mutant factor IXa is normal, whereas factor X activation is slow, suggesting that the mutations disrupt secondary binding sites for the substrate, factor X. Another mutation in this region, Gly 216 → Arg (factor IX Angers), gives rise to severe hemophilia B.[291] This mutation, as well as the other mutations in this region, is associated with an approximately normal concentration of a dysfunctioning protein. In factor X Friuli, a Pro 149 → Ser mutation in the serine protease module, the mutant protein has low activity against both low molecular weight substrates and its physiological substrate prothrombin.[292]

Recent studies employing site-directed mutagenesis of residues in the anion-binding exosite in thrombin have demonstrated that it is possible, at least to some extent, to dissociate the fibrinogen-clotting and thrombomodulin-binding activities of thrombin.[293] An alternative approach to alter the specificity of thrombin was based on the observation that thrombin (and protein C) has Glu in position 202, whereas most serine proteases have Gln or Met.[294] Mutation of Glu 202 → Gin allows thrombin to better accommodate the P3 Asp residue of protein C in the absence of thrombomodulin than occurs in the wild-type thrombin. k$_{cat}$ for protein C activation (in the absence of thrombomodulin) was 22-fold higher for the mutant than for native thrombin.

Three amino acid substitutions have been identified in congenitally mutant thrombins: thrombin Quick I, thrombin Quick II, and thrombin Tokushima. Thrombin Quick I, Arg 62 → Cys, has very low fibrinogen-clotting activity but an almost normal activity against low molecular weight substrates.[295] The k$_{cat}$/K$_m$ for release of fibrinopeptide A by thrombin Quick I is 100-fold lower than that for thrombin. In this context, it is noteworthy that Arg 62 is one of the positively charged residues in the anion-binding exosite that is thought to interact with fibrinogen. Thrombin Quick I also has a markedly reduced affinity for thrombomodulin, which presumably also interacts with the anion-binding exosite.[296] Thrombin Quick II results from a Gly 238 → Val mutation. Gly 238 is a conserved residue within the primary substrate-binding pocket. This mutant lacks catalytic activity toward thrombin substrates but binds diisopropyl fluorophosphate (DFP) stoichiometrically.[297] Thrombin Tokushima is an Arg 98 → Trp mutation.[298] This residue is adjacent to the Asp of the catalytic triad, and its mutation results in reduced activity against both low molecular weight substrates and the physiological substrate fibrinogen.

A MODULE IN PROTEIN S RESEMBLING SEX HORMONE–BINDING GLOBULIN

The COOH-terminal half of protein S (residues 245 to 635) is homologous to SHBG[51] and to rat androgen-binding protein (see Fig. 16–2).[51, 299] SHBG consists of two identical non-covalently linked subunits and binds a single steroid hormone molecule.[300, 301] SHBG with bound hormone interacts with a cell surface receptor.[302] Intron/exon boundaries in protein S and SHBG are in homologous positions.[303] The Cys residues in the SHBG-like part of protein S are paired as in SHBG, that is, Cys 247 to Cys 527, Cys 408 to Cys 434, and Cys 598 to Cys 625.[47, 48] It is noteworthy, however, that the part of SHBG that has been implicated in steroid hormone binding, a hydrophobic region with alternating leucine residues, is not found in protein S.[47, 48, 304] There is no evidence of dimer formation in protein S. The SHBG-like module of protein S has been implicated in the binding of protein S to C4b-binding protein (see Chapter 19).

REFERENCES

1. Jackson, C. M., and Nemerson, Y.: Blood coagulation. Annu. Rev. Biochem. 49:765, 1980.
2. Mann, K. G., Jenny, R. J., and Krishnaswamy, S.: Cofactor proteins in the assembly and expression of blood clotting enzyme complexes. Annu. Rev. Biochem. 57:915, 1988.
3. Mann, K. G., Nesheim, M. E., Church, W. R., Haley, P., and Krishnaswamy, S.: Surface-dependent reactions of the vitamin K–dependent enzyme complexes. Blood 76:1, 1990.
4. Davie, E. W., Fujikawa, K., and Kisiel, W.: The coagulation cascade: Initiation, maintenance, and regulation. Biochemistry 30:10363, 1991.
5. Nemerson, Y.: Tissue factor and hemostasis. Blood 71:1, 1988.
6. Rapaport, S. I.: The extrinsic pathway inhibitor: A regulator of tissue factor–dependent blood coagulation. Thromb. Haemost. 66:6, 1991.
7. Esmon, C. T.: The roles of protein C and thrombomodulin in the regulation of blood coagulation. J. Biol. Chem. 264:4743, 1989.
8. Edgington, T. S., Mackman, N., Brand, K., and Ruf, W.: The structural biology of expression and function of tissue factor. Thromb. Haemost. 66:67, 1991.
9. Dahlbäck B.: Protein S and C4b-binding protein: Components involved in the regulation of the protein C anticoagulant system. Thromb. Haemost. 66:49, 1991.
10. Stenflo J.: Structure-function relationships of epidermal growth factor modules in vitamin K–dependent clotting factors. Blood 78:1637, 1991.
11. Patthy, L.: Evolution of the proteases of blood coagulation and fibrinolysis by assembly from modules. Cell 41:657, 1985.
12. Baron, M., Norman, D. G., and Campbell, I. D.: Protein modules. Trends Biochem. Sci. 16:13, 1991.
13. Tulinsky, A.: The structures of domains of blood proteins. Thromb. Haemost. 66:16, 1991.
14. Selander, M., Persson, E., Stenflo, J., and Drakenberg, T.: ^{1}H NMR assignment and secondary structure of the Ca^{2+}-free form of the amino-terminal epidermal growth factor like domain in coagulation factor X. Biochemistry 29:8111, 1990.
15. Ullner, M., Selander, M., Persson, E., Stenflo, J., Drakenberg, T., and Teleman, O.: Three-dimensional structure of the NH_2-terminal EGF-homologous module of blood coagulation factor X as determined by NMR spectroscopy and simulated folding. Biochemistry 31:5974, 1992.
16. Selander-Sunnerhagen, M., Ullner, M., Persson, E., Teleman, O., Stenflo, J., and Drakenberg, T.: Structure of the Ca^{2+} binding site in the β-hydroxyaspartic acid–containing EGF module of coagulation factor X. J. Biol. Chem. 267:19642, 1992.
17. Huang, L. H., Cheng, H., Pardi, A., Tam, J., and Sweeny, W. V.: Sequence-specific ^{1}H NMR assignments, secondary structure, and location of the calcium binding site in the first epidermal growth factor like domain of blood coagulation factor IX. Biochemistry 30:7402, 1991.
18. Baron, M., Norman, D. G., Harvey, T. S., Handford, P. A., Mayhew, M., Tse, A. G. D., Brownlee, G. G., and Campbell, I. D.: The three-dimensional structure of the first EGF-like module of human factor IX: Comparison with EGF and TGF-α. Protein Sci. 1:81, 1992.
19. Tulinsky, A., Park, C. H., and Skrzypczak-Jankun, E.: Structure of prothrombin fragment 1 refined at 2.8 Å resolution. J. Mol. Biol. 202:885, 1988.
20. Soriano-Garcia, M., Park, C. H., Tulinsky, A., Ravichandran, K. G., and Skrzypczak-Jankun, E.: Structure of Ca^{2+} prothrombin fragment 1 including the conformation of the Gla domain. Biochemistry 28:6605, 1989.
21. Bode, W., Mayr, I., Baumann, U., Huber, R., Stone, S. R.,

and Hofsteenge, J.: The refined 1.9 Å crystal structure of human α-thrombin: Interaction with D-Phe-Pro-Arg chloromethylketone and significance of the Tyr-Pro-Pro-Trp insertion segment. EMBO J. 8:3467, 1989.
22. Furie, B., and Furie, B. C.: The molecular basis of blood coagulation. Cell 53:505, 1988.
23. Appella, E., Weber, I. T., and Blasi, F.: Structure and function of epidermal growth factor–like regions in proteins. FEBS Lett. 231:1, 1988.
24. Engel, J.: EGF-like domains in extracellular matrix proteins: Localized signals for growth and differentiation. FEBS Lett. 251:1, 1989.
25. Carpenter, G., and Wahl, M. I.: The epidermal growth factor family. In Sporn, M. B., and Roberts, A. B. (eds.): Handbook of Experimental Pharmacology. Vol. 95. New York, Springer-Verlag, 1990, pp. 69–171.
26. Stenflo, J., and Suttie, J. W.: Vitamin K–dependent formation of γ-carboxyglutamic acid. Annu. Rev. Biochem. 46:157, 1977.
27. Suttie, J. W.: Vitamin K–dependent carboxylase. Annu. Rev. Biochem. 54:459, 1985.
28. Furie, B., and Furie, B. C.: Molecular basis of vitamin K–dependent γ-carboxylation. Blood 75:1753, 1990.
29. Vermeer, C.: γ-Carboxyglutamate-containing proteins and the vitamin K–dependent carboxylase. Biochem. J. 266:625, 1990.
30. Friezner Degen, S. J., and Davie, E. W.: Nucleotide sequence of the gene for human prothrombin. Biochemistry 26:6165, 1987.
31. O'Hara, P. J., Grant, F. J., Haldeman, B. A., Gray, C. L., Insley, M. Y., Hagen, F. S., and Murray, M. J.: Nucleotide sequence of the gene coding for human factor VII, a vitamin K–dependent protein participating in blood coagulation. Proc. Natl. Acad. Sci. USA 84:5158, 1987.
32. Yoshitake, S., Schach, B. G., Foster, D. C., Davie, E. W., and Kurachi, K.: Nucleotide sequence of the gene for human factor IX. Biochemistry 24:3736, 1985.
33. Leytus, S. P., Foster, D. C., Kurachi, K., and Davie, E. W.: Gene for human factor X: A blood coagulation factor whose gene organization is essentially identical with that of factor IX and protein C. Biochemistry 25:5098, 1986.
34. Foster, D. J., Yoshitake, S., and Davie, E. W.: The nucleotide sequence of the gene for human protein C. Proc. Natl. Acad. Sci. USA 82:4673, 1985.
35. Plutzky, J., Hoskins, J. A., Long, G. L., and Crabtree, G. R.: Evolution and organization of the human protein C gene. Proc. Natl. Acad. Sci. USA 83:546, 1986.
36. Schmidel, D. K., Tatro, A. V., Phelps, L. G., Tomczak, J. A., and Long, G. L.: Organization of the human protein S gene. Biochemistry 29:7845, 1990.
37. Ploos van Amstel, H. K., Reitsma, P. H., van der Logt, P. E., and Bertina, R. M.: Intro-exon organization of the active human protein S gene PSα and its pseudogene PSβ: Duplication and silencing during primate evolution. Biochemistry 29:7853, 1990.
38. Edenbrandt, C.-M., Lundwall, Å., Wydro, R., and Stenflo, J.: Molecular analysis of the gene for vitamin K–dependent protein S and its pseudogene. Cloning and partial gene organization. Biochemistry 29:7861, 1990.
39. Gilbert, W.: Why genes in pieces? Nature 271:501, 1978.
40. Patthy, L.: Intron-dependent evolution: Preferred types of exons and introns. FEBS Lett. 214:1, 1987.
41. Traut, T. W.: Do exons code for structural or functional units in proteins? Proc. Natl. Acad. Sci. USA 85:2944, 1988.
42. Irwin, D. M., Robertson, K. A., and MacGillivray, R. T. A.: Structure and evolution of the bovine prothrombin gene. J. Mol. Biol. 200:31, 1988.
43. Prowse, C. W., and Esnouf, M. P.: The isolation of a new warfarin-sensitive protein from bovine plasma. Biochem. Soc. Trans. 5:255, 1977.
44. Höjrup, P., Jensen, M. S., and Petersen, T. E.: Amino acid sequence of bovine protein Z: A vitamin K–dependent serine protease homolog. FEBS Lett. 184:333, 1985.
45. Sejima, H., Hayashi, T., Deyashiki, Y., Nishioka, J., and

Suzuki, K.: Primary structure of vitamin K–dependent human protein Z. Biochem. Biophys. Res. Commun. 171:661, 1990.

46. Ichinose, A., Takeya, H., Espling, E., Iwanaga, S., Kisiel, W., and Davie, E. W.: Amino acid sequence of human protein Z, a vitamin K–dependent plasma glycoprotein. Biochem. Biophys. Res. Commun. 172:1139, 1990.

47. Dahlbäck, B., Lundwall, Å., and Stenflo, J.: Primary structure of bovine vitamin K–dependent protein S. Proc. Natl. Acad. Sci. USA 83:4199, 1986.

48. Lundwall, Å., Dackowski, W., Cohen, E., Shaffer, M., Mahr, A., Dahlbäck, B., Stenflo, J., and Wydro, R.: Isolation and sequence of the cDNA for human protein S, a regulator of blood coagulation. Proc. Natl. Acad. Sci. USA 83:6716, 1986.

49. Dahlbäck, B.: Purification of human vitamin K–dependent protein S and its limited proteolysis by thrombin. Biochem. J. 209:837, 1983.

50. Dahlbäck, B., Lundwall, Å., and Stenflo, J.: Localization of thrombin cleavage sites in the amino-terminal region of bovine protein S. J. Biol. Chem. 261:5111, 1986.

51. Gershagen, S., Fernlund, P., Lundwall, Å.: A cDNA coding for human sex hormone binding globulin. Homology to vitamin K–dependent protein S. FEBS Lett. 220:129, 1987.

52. Baker, M. E., French, F. S., and Joseph, D. R.: Vitamin K–dependent protein S is similar to androgen-binding protein. Biochem. J. 243:293, 1987.

53. Stenflo, J., Fernlund, P., Egan, W., and Roepstorff, P.: Vitamin K dependent modifications of glutamic acid residues in prothrombin. Proc. Natl. Acad. Sci. USA 71:2730, 1974.

54. Nelsestuen, G. L., Zytkovicz, T. H., and Howard, J. B.: The mode of action of vitamin K. Identification of γ-carboxyglutamic acid as a component of prothrombin. J. Biol. Chem. 249:6347, 1974.

55. Magnusson, S., Sottrup-Jensen, L., Petersen, T. E., Morris, H. R., and Dell, A.: Primary structure of the vitamin K–dependent part of prothrombin. FEBS Lett. 44:189, 1974.

56. Fernlund, P., Stenflo, J., Roepstorff, P., and Thomsen, J.: Vitamin K and the biosynthesis of prothrombin. 5. γ-Carboxyglutamic acids, the vitamin K–dependent structures in prothrombin. J. Biol. Chem. 250:6125, 1975.

57. Stenflo, J., Fernlund, P., and Roepstorff, P.: Structure of a vitamin K–dependent portion of prothrombin. In Reich, E., Rifkin, D. B., and Shaw, E. (eds.): Proteases and Biological Control. Cold Spring Harbor, N.Y., Cold Spring Harbor Laboratory, 1975, pp. 111–122.

58. Magnusson, S., Petersen, T. E., Sottrup-Jensen, L., and Claeys, H.: Complete primary structure of prothrombin: Structure and reactivity of ten carboxylated glutamic acid residues and regulation of prothrombin activation by thrombin. In Reich, E., Rifkin, D. B., and Shaw, E. (eds.): Proteases and Biological Control. Cold Spring Harbor, N. Y., Cold Spring Harbor Laboratory, 1975, pp. 123–149.

59. Ganrot, P.-O., and Niléhn, J.-E.: Plasma prothrombin during treatment with dicumarol. 2. Demonstration of an abnormal prothrombin fraction. Scand. J. Clin. Lab. Invest. 22:23, 1968.

60. Reekers, P. P., Lindhout, M. J., Kop-Klaassen, B. H. M., and Hemker, H. C.: Demonstration of three anomalous plasma proteins induced by a vitamin K–antagonist. Biochim. Biophys. Acta 317:559, 1973.

61. Stenflo, J.: Dicumarol-induced prothrombin in bovine plasma. Acta Chem. Scand. 24:3762, 1970.

62. Stenflo, J., and Ganrot, P.: Vitamin K and the biosynthesis of prothrombin. 1. Identification and purification of a dicumarol-induced abnormal prothrombin from bovine plasma. J. Biol. Chem. 247:8160, 1972.

63. Nelsestuen, G. L., and Suttie, J. W.: The purification and properties of an abnormal prothrombin protein produced by dicumarol-treated cows. Comparison to normal prothrombin. J. Biol. Chem. 247:8176, 1972.

64. Nelsestuen, G. L., and Suttie, J. W.: Mode of action of vitamin K. Calcium binding properties of bovine prothrombin. Biochemistry 11:961, 1972.

65. Stenflo, J., and Ganrot, P.: Binding of Ca^{2+} to normal and dicumarol-induced prothrombin. Biochem. Biophys. Res. Commun. 50:98, 1974.

66. Malhotra, O. P., Nesheim, M. E., and Mann, K. G.: The kinetics of activation of normal and γ-carboxyglutamic acid–deficient prothrombins. J. Biol. Chem. 260:279, 1985.

67. Liska, D. A., and Suttie, J. W.: Location of γ-carboxyglutamyl residues in partially carboxylated prothrombin preparations. Biochemistry 27:8636, 1988.

68. Borowski, B., Furie, B. C., Goldsmith, G. H., and Furie, B.: Metal and phospholipid binding properties of partially carboxylated human prothrombin variants. J. Biol. Chem. 260:9258, 1985.

69. Soriano-Garcia, M., Padmanabhn, K., deVos, A. M., and Tulinsky, A.: The Ca^{2+} ion and membrane binding structure of the Gla-domain of Ca^{2+}-prothrombin fragment 1. Biochemistry 31:2554, 1992.

70. Gitel, S. N., Owen, W. G., Esmon, C. T., and Jackson, C. M.: A polypeptide region of bovine prothrombin specific for binding to phospholipids. Proc. Natl. Acad. Sci. USA 70:1344, 1973.

71. Stenflo, J.: Vitamin K and the biosynthesis of prothrombin. 3. Structural comparison of an NH_2-terminal fragment from normal and from dicumarol-induced prothrombin. J. Biol. Chem. 248:6325, 1973.

72. Morita, T., Iwanaga, S., Suzuki, T., and Fujikawa, K.: Characterization of amino-terminal fragment liberated from bovine prothrombin by activated factor X. FEBS Lett. 36:313, 1973.

73. Welsh, D. J., Pletcher, C. H., and Nelsestuen, G. L.: Chemical modification of prothrombin fragment 1: Documentation of sequential, two-stage loss of protein function. Biochemistry 27:4933, 1988.

74. Schwalbe, R. A., Ryan, J., Stern, D. M., Kisiel, W., Dahlbäck, B., and Nelsestuen, G. L.: Protein structural requirements and properties of membrane binding by γ-carboxyglutamic acid–containing plasma proteins and peptides. J. Biol. Chem. 264:20288, 1989.

75. Church, W. R., Boulanger, L. L., Meissier, T. L., and Mann, K. G.: Evidence for a common metal ion–dependent transition in the 4-carboxyglutamic acid domains of several vitamin K–dependent proteins. J. Biol. Chem. 264:17882, 1989.

76. Jackson, C. M.: Calcium ion binding to γ-carboxyglutamic acid–containing proteins from the blood clotting system: What we still don't understand. In Suttie, J. W. (ed.): Current Advances in Vitamin K Research. New York, Elsevier, 1988, pp. 305–324.

77. Nelsestuen, G. L.: Role of γ-carboxyglutamic acid. An unusual protein transition required for the calcium-dependent binding of prothrombin to phospholipid. J. Biol. Chem. 251:5648, 1976.

78. Bloom, J. W., and Mann, K. G.: Metal ion induced conformational transitions of prothrombin and prothrombin fragment 1. Biochemistry 17:4430, 1978.

79. Johnson, A. E., Esmon, N. L., Laue, T. M., and Esmon, C. T.: Structural changes required for activation of protein C are induced by Ca^{2+} binding to a high affinity site that does not contain γ-carboxyglutamic acid. J. Biol. Chem. 258:5554, 1983.

80. Morita, T., Isaacs, B. S., Esmon, C. T., and Johnson, A. E.: Derivative of blood coagulation factor IX containing a high affinity Ca^{2+}-binding site that lacks γ-carboxyglutamic acid. J. Biol. Chem. 259:5698, 1984.

81. Skogen, W. F., Bushong, D. S., Johnson, A. E., and Cox, A. C.: The role of the Gla domain in the activation of bovine coagulation factor X by the snake venom protein XCP. Biochem. Biophys. Res. Commun. 111:14, 1983.

82. Öhlin, A.-K., Björk, I., and Stenflo, J.: Proteolytic formation and properties of a fragment of protein C containing the γ-carboxyglutamic acid rich region and the EGF-like region. Biochemistry 29:644, 1990.

83. Astermark, J., Björk, I., Öhlin, A.-K., and Stenflo, J.: Structural requirements for Ca^{2+} binding to the γ-carboxyglutamic acid and epidermal growth factor–like regions of

factor IX. Studies using intact domains isolated from controlled proteolytic digests of bovine factor X. J. Biol. Chem. 266:2430, 1991.

84. Persson, E., Björk, I., and Stenflo, J.: Protein structural requirements for Ca^{2+} binding to the light chain of factor X. Studies using isolated intact fragments containing the γ-carboxyglutamic acid region and/or the epidermal growth factor–like domains. J. Biol. Chem. 266:2444, 1991.

85. Henriksen, R. A., and Jackson, C. M.: Cooperative calcium binding by the phospholipid binding region of bovine prothrombin: A requirement for intact disulfide bridges. Arch. Biochem. Biophys. 170:149, 1975.

86. Prendergast, F. G., and Mann, K. G.: Differentiation of metal ion–induced transitions of prothrombin fragment 1. J. Biol. Chem. 252:840, 1977.

87. Kretsinger, R. H.: Calcium coordination and the calmodulin fold: Divergent versus convergent evolution. Cold Spring Harb. Symp. Quant. Biol. 52:499, 1987.

88. Deerfield, D. W., Olson, D. L., Berkowitz, P., Byrd, P. A., Koehler, K. A., Pedersen, L. G., and Hiskey, R. G.: Mg(II) binding by bovine prothrombin fragment 1 via equilibrium dialysis and the relative roles of Mg (II) and (CaII) in blood coagulation. J. Biol. Chem. 262:4017, 1987.

89. Borowski, M., Furie, B. C., Bauminger, S., and Furie, B.: Prothrombin requires two sequential metal-dependent conformational transitions to bind phospholipid. Conformation-specific antibodies directed against the phospholipid-binding site on prothrombin. J. Biol. Chem. 261:14969, 1986.

90. Marsh, H. C., Scott, M. E., Hiskey, R. G., and Koehler, K. A.: The nature of the slow metal ion–dependent conformational transition in bovine prothrombin. Biochem. J. 183:513, 1979.

91. Persson, E., Selander, M., Drakenberg, T., Öhlin, A.-K., and Stenflo, J.: Calcium binding to the isolated β-hydroxyaspartic acid–containing epidermal growth factor containing domain of bovine factor X. J. Biol. Chem. 264:16897, 1989.

92. Morita, T., and Jackson, C. M.: Structural and functional characteristics of a proteolytically modified "Gla domainless" bovine factor X and X$_a$ (des light chain residues 1–144). In Suttie, J. W. (ed.): Vitamin K Metabolism and Vitamin K–Dependent Proteins. Baltimore, Md., University Park Press, 1980, pp. 124–128.

93. Morita, T., and Jackson, C. M.: Preparation and properties of derivatives of bovine factor X and factor Xa from which the γ-carboxyglutamic acid containing domain has been removed. J. Biol. Chem. 261:4015, 1986.

94. Esmon, N. L., DeBault, L. E., and Esmon, C. Y.: Proteolytic formation and properties of γ-carboxyglutamic acid domainless protein C. J. Biol. Chem. 258:5548, 1983.

95. Pollock, J. S., Shephard, A. J., Weber, D. J., Olson, D. L., Klapper, D. G., Pedersen, L. G., and Hiskey, R. G.: Phospholipid binding properties of bovine prothrombin peptide residues 1–45. J. Biol. Chem. 263:14216, 1988.

96. Nelsestuen, G. L.: Basis for prothrombin-membrane binding. In Suttie, J. W. (ed.): Current Advances in Vitamin K Research. New York, Elsevier, 1988, pp. 335–339.

97. Sakai, T., Lund-Hansen, T., Thim, L., and Kisiel, W.: The γ-carboxyglutamic acid domain of human factor VIIa is essential for its interaction with cell surface tissue factor. J. Biol. Chem. 265:1890, 1990.

98. Gianelli, F., Green, P. M., High, K. A., Sommer, S., Lillicrap, D. P., Ludwig, M., Olek, K., Reitsma, P. H., Gossens, M., Yoshioka, A., and Brownlee, G. G.: Haemophilia B: Database of point mutations and short additions and deletions. Second edition. Nucleic Acids Res. 19:2193, 1991.

99. Winship, P. R., and Dragon, A. C.: Identification of haemophilia B patients with mutations in the two calcium binding domains of factor IX: Importance of a β-OH Asp 64 Asn change. Br. J. Haematol. 77:102, 1991.

100. Bertina, R. M., and Van Der Linden, I. K.: Factor IX Zutphen. A genetic variant of blood coagulation factor IX with an abnormally high molecular weight. J. Lab. Clin. Med. 100:695, 1982.

101. Bertina, R. M., and Veltkamp, J. J.: A genetic variant of factor IX with decreased capacity for Ca^{2+} binding. Br. J. Haematol. 42:623, 1979.

102. Chen, S.-H., Thompson, A. R., Zhang, M., and Scott, R. C.: Three point mutations in the factor IX genes of five hemophilia B patients. Identification strategy using localization by altered epitopes and their hemophilic proteins. J. Clin. Invest. 84:113, 1989.

103. Wang, N. S., Zhang, M., Thompson, A. R., and Chen, S.-H.: Factor IX Chongqing: a new mutation in the calcium-binding domain of factor IX resulting in severe hemophilia B. Thromb. Haemost. 63:24, 1990.

104. Koeberl, D. D., Bottema, C. D. K., Buerstedde, J.-M., and Sommer S. S.: Functionally important regions of the factor IX gene have a low rate of polymorphism and a high rate in the dinucleotide CpG. Am. J. Hum. Genet. 45:448, 1989.

105. Berkner, K. L., Walker, K., King, J., and Kumar, A. A.: Individual residues within the Gla domain of factor IX have different effects upon coagulant activity and upon overall Gamma-carboxylation. Thromb. Haemost. 62:1074, 1989.

106. Watzke, H. H., Lechner, K., Roberts, H. R., Reddy, S. V., Welch, D. J., Friedman, P., Mahr, G., Jagadeeswaran, P., Monroe, D. M., and High, K. A.: Molecular defect (Gla^{+14} Lys) and its functional consequences in a hereditary factor X deficiency (Factor X "Voralberg"). J. Biol. Chem. 265:11982, 1990.

107. Zhang, L., and Castellino, F. J.: A γ-carboxyglutamic acid (γ) variant (γ^{6}D, γ^{7}D) of human activated protein C displays greatly reduced activity as an anticoagulant. Biochemistry 29:19828, 1990.

108. Zhang, L., and Castellino, F. J.: Role of the hexapeptide disulfide loop present in the γ-carboxyglutamic acid domain of human protein C in its activation properties and in the in vitro anticoagulant activity of activated protein C. Biochemistry 30:6696, 1991.

109. Suttie, J. W.: Mechanism of action of vitamin K: Demonstration of a liver precursor of prothrombin. Science 179:192, 1973.

110. Corrigan, J. J., Jr., and Earnest, D. L.: Factor II antigen in liver disease and warfarin-induced vitamin K-deficiency: Correlation with coagulant activity using echis venom. Am. J. Hematol. 8:249, 1980.

111. Owens, M. R., Miller, L. L., and Cimino, C. D.: Synthesis of factor II antigen by isolated perfused rat livers. Biochem. Biophys. Acta 676:365, 1981.

112. Shah, D. V., Swanson, J. C., and Suttie J. W.: Abnormal prothrombin in the vitamin K–deficient rat. Thromb. Res. 35:451, 1984.

113. Swanson, J. C.: Prothrombin biosynthesis: Characterization of processing events in rat liver microsomes. Biochemistry 24:3890, 1985.

114. Graves, C. B., Grabau, G. G., Olson, R. E., and Munns, T. W.: Immunochemical isolation and electrophoretic characterization of precursor prothrombins in H-35 rat hepatoma cells. Biochemistry 19:266, 1980.

115. Wallin, R., and Martin, L. F.: Early processing of prothrombin and factor X by the vitamin K–dependent carboxylase. J. Biol. Chem. 263:9994, 1988.

116. Kivirikko, K. I., and Myllylä, R.: Recent developments in posttranslational modification: Intracellular processing. Methods Enzymol. 144:96, 1987.

117. Kornfeld, R., and Kornfeld, S.: Assembly of asparagine-linked oligosaccharides. Annu. Rev. Biochem. 54:631, 1985.

118. Shah, D. V., Swanson, J. C., and Suttie, J. W.: Vitamin K–dependent carboxylase: Effect of detergent concentrations, vitamin K status, and added protein precursor on activity. Arch. Biochem. Biophys. 222:216, 1983.

119. Knobloch, J. E., and Suttie, J. W.: Vitamin K-dependent carboxylase: Control of enzyme activity by the propeptide region of factor X. J. Biol. Chem. 262:15334, 1987.

120. Ulrich, M. M. M., Furie, B., Vermeer, C., and Furie, B. B.: Vitamin K–dependent carboxylation: A synthetic peptide based upon the γ-carboxylation recognition site sequence of the prothrombin propeptide is an active substrate for the carboxylase in vitro. J. Biol. Chem. 263:9697, 1988.

121. Jørgensen, M. J., Cantor, A. B., Furie, B. C., Brown, C. L., Shoemaker, C. B., and Furie, B.: Recognition site directing vitamin K–dependent γ-carboxylation resides on the propeptide of factor IX. Cell 48:185, 1987.

122. Hubbard, B. R., Jacobs, M., Ulrich, M. M. W., Furie, B., and Furie, B. C.: Vitamin K–dependent carboxylation: In vitro modification of synthetic peptides containing the γ-carboxylation recognition site. J. Biol. Chem. 264:14145, 1989.

123. Walter, P., and Lingappa, V. R.: Mechanism of protein translocation across the endoplasmic reticulum membrane. Annu. Rev. Cell Biol. 2:499, 1986.

124. Hauschka, P. A., Lian, J. B., Cole, D. E. C., and Gendberg, C. M.: Osteocalcin and matrix Gla protein: Vitamin K–dependent proteins in bone. Physiol. Rev. 69:990, 1989.

125. Pan, L. C., and Price, P. A.: The propeptide of rat bone γ-carboxyglutamic acid proteins shares homology with other vitamin K–dependent protein precursors. Proc. Natl. Acad. Sci. USA 82:6109, 1985.

126. Price, P. A., Fraser, J. D., and Metz-Virca, G.: Molecular cloning of matrix Gla protein: Implications for substrate recognition by the vitamin K–dependent γ-carboxylase. Proc. Natl. Acad. Sci. USA 84:8335, 1987.

127. Suttie, J. W., Hoskins, J. A., Engelke, J., Hopfgartner, A., Ehrlich, H., Bang, N. U., Belagaje, R. M., Schoner, B., and Long, G. L.: Vitamin K–dependent carboxylase: Possible role of the substrate "propeptide" as an intracellular recognition site. Proc. Natl. Acad. Sci. USA 84:634, 1987.

128. Rabiet, M.-J., Jorgensen, M. J., Furie, B., and Furie, B. C.: Effect of propeptide mutations on posttranslational processing of factor IX: Evidence that β-hydroxylation and γ-carboxylation are independent events. J. Biol. Chem. 262:14895, 1987.

129. Foster, D. C., Rudinski, M. S., Schach, B. G., Berkner, K. L., Kumar, A. A., Hagen, F. S., Sprecher, C. A., Insley, M. Y., and Davie, E. W.: Propeptide of human protein C is necessary for γ-carboxylation. Biochemistry 26:7003, 1987.

130. Wu, S.-M., Soute, B. A. M., Vermeer, C., and Stafford, D. W.: In vitro-carboxylation of a 59-residue recombinant peptide including the propeptide and the γ-carboxyglutamic acid domain of coagulation factor IX. Effect of mutation near the propeptide cleavage site. J. Biol. Chem. 265:13124, 1990.

131. Sanford, D. G., Kanagy, C., Sudmeier, J. L., Furie, B. C., Furie, B., and Bachovchin, W. W.: Structure of the propeptide of prothrombin containing the γ-carboxylation recognition site determined by two-dimensional NMR spectroscopy. Biochemistry 30:9835, 1991.

132. Bentley, A. K., Rees, D. J. G., Rizza, C., and Brownlee, G. G.: Defective propeptide processing of blood clotting factor IX caused by mutation of arginine to glutamine in position −4. Cell 45:343, 1986.

133. Ware, J., Diuguid, D. L., Liebman, H. L., Rabiet, M.-J., Kasper, C. K., Furie, B. C., Furie, B., and Stafford, D. W.: Factor IX San Dimas: Substitution of glutamine for arginine −4 in the propeptide leads to incomplete γ-carboxylation and altered phospholipid binding properties. J. Biol. Chem. 264:1401, 1989.

134. Diuguid, D. L., Rabiet, M. J., Furie, B. C., Liebman, H. A., and Furie, B.: Molecular basis of hemophilia B: A defective enzyme due to an unprocessed propeptide is caused by a point mutation in the factor IX precursor. Proc. Natl. Acad. Sci. USA 83:5803, 1986.

135. Watzke, H. H., Wallmark, A., Hamaguchi, N., Giardina, P., Stafford, D. W., and High, K. A.: Factor X Santo Domingo. Evidence that the severe clinical phenotype arises from a mutation blocking secretion. J. Clin. Invest. 88:1685, 1991.

135a. Gandrill, S., Alhene-Gelas, M., Goossens, M., and Aiach, M.: An abnormal protein C due to mutation at the cleavage site of the propeptide. Thromb. Haemost. 65:1196a, 1991.

136. Judah, J. D., Gamble, M., and Steadman, J. H.: Biosynthesis of serum albumin in rat liver. Evidence for the existence of "proalbumin." Biochem. J. 134:1083, 1973.

137. Barr, P. J.: Mammalian subtilisins: The long-sought dibasic processing endoproteases. Cell 66:1, 1991.

138. Esmon, C. T., Sadowski, J. A., and Suttie, J. W.: A new carboxylation reaction. The vitamin K–dependent incorporation of $H^{14}CO_3$ into prothrombin. J. Biol. Chem. 250:4744, 1975.

139. Sadowski, J. A., Esmon, C. T., and Suttie, J. W.: Vitamin K–dependent carboxylase. Requirements of the rat liver microsomal enzyme system. J. Biol. Chem. 251:2770, 1976.

140. Olivera, B. M., Rivier, J., Clark, C., Ramillo, C. A., Corpuz, G. P., Abogadie, F. C., Mena, E. E., Woodward, S. R., Hillyard, D. R., and Cruz, L. J.: Diversity of Conus neuropeptides. Science 249:257, 1990.

141. Suttie, J. W., Hageman, J. M., Lehrman, S. R., and Rich, D. H.: Vitamin K–dependent carboxylase. Development of a peptide substrate. J. Biol. Chem. 251:5827, 1976.

142. Suttie, J. W., Preusch, P. C., and McTigue, J. J.: Vitamin K–dependent carboxylase: Recent studies of the rat liver enzyme system. In Johnson, B. C.(ed.): Posttranslational Covalent Modification of Proteins. New York, Academic Press, 1983, pp. 253–279.

143. Jones, J. P., Gardner, E. J., Cooper, T. G., and Olson, R. E.: Vitamin K–dependent carboxylation of peptide-bound glutamate: The active species of CO_2 utilized by the membrane-bound preprothrombin carboxylase. J. Biol. Chem. 252:7738, 1977.

144. Bell, R. G.: Metabolism of vitamin K and prothrombin synthesis: Anticoagulants and the vitamin K–epoxide cycle. Fed. Proc. 37:599, 1978.

145. Suttie, J. W., Larson, A. E., Canfield, L. M., and Carlisle, T. L.: Relationship between vitamin K–dependent carboxylation and vitamin K epoxidation. Fed. Proc. 37:2605, 1978.

146. Larsson, A. E., Friedman, P. A., and Suttie, J. W.: Vitamin K–dependent carboxylase: Stoichiometry of carboxylation and vitamin K 2,3-epoxide formation. J. Biol. Chem. 256:11032, 1981.

147. Friedman, P. A., Shia, M. A., Gallop, P. M., and Griep, A. E.: Vitamin K–dependent γ-carbon-hydrogen bond cleavage and nonmandatory concurrent carboxylation of peptide-bound glutamic acid residues. Proc. Natl. Acad. Sci. USA 76:3126, 1979.

148. McTigue, J. J., and Suttie, J. W.: Vitamin K–dependent carboxylase: Demonstration of a vitamin K and O_2-dependent exchange of ^3H from ^3H_2O in glutamic acid residues. J. Biol. Chem. 258:12129, 1983.

149. Anton, D. L., and Friedman, P. A.: Fate of the activated γ-carbon-hydrogen bond in the uncoupled vitamin K–dependent γ-glutamyl carboxylation reaction. J. Biol. Chem. 258:14084, 1983.

150. Wu, S.-M., Morris, D. P., and Stafford, D. W.: Identification and purification to near homogeneity of the vitamin K–dependent carboxylase. Proc. Natl. Acad. Sci. USA 88:2236, 1991.

151. Wu, S.-M., Cheung, W.-F., Frazier, D., and Stafford, D. W.: Cloning and expression of the cDNA for human γ-glutamyl carboxylase. Science 254:1634, 1991.

152. Carpenter, G., and Cohen, S.: Epidermal growth factor. J. Biol. Chem. 265:7709, 1990.

153. Cooke, R. M., Wilkinson, A. J., Baron, M., Pastore, A., Tappin, M. J., Campbell, I. D., Gregory, H., and Sheard, B.: The solution structure of human epidermal growth factor. Nature 327:339, 1987.

154. Campbell, I. D., Cooke, R. M., Baron, M., Harvey, T. S., and Tappin, M. J.: The solution structure of epidermal growth factor and transforming growth factor alpha. Prog. Growth Factor Res. 1:13, 1989.

155. Montelione, G. T., Wüterich, K., Nice, E. C., Burgess, A. W., and Scheraga, H. A.: Solution structure of murine epidermal growth factor: Determination of the polypeptide backbone chain-fold by nuclear magnetic resonance and distance geometry. Proc. Natl. Acad. Sci. USA 84:5226, 1987.

156. Kline, T. P., Brown, F. K., Brown, S. C., Jeffs, P. W., Kopple, K. D., and Mueller, L.: Solution structure of human transforming growth factor α derived from ^1H NMR data. Biochemistry 29:7805, 1990.

157. Massagué, J.: Transforming growth factor–α. A model for

membrane-anchored growth factors. J. Biol. Chem. 265:21393, 1990.

158. Höjrup, P., and Magnusson, S.: Disulphide bridges of bovine factor X. Biochem. J. 245:887, 1987.

159. Drakenberg, T. P., Fernlund, P., Roepstorff, P., and Stenflo, J.: β-Hydroxyaspartic acid in vitamin K–dependent protein C. Proc. Natl. Acad. Sci. USA 80:1802, 1983.

160. McMullen, B. A., Fujikawa, K., Kisiel, W., Sasagawa, T., Howald, W. N., Kwa, E. Y., and Weinstein, B.: Complete amino acid sequence of the light chain of human blood coagulation factor X: Evidence for identification of residue 63 as β-hydroxyaspartic acid. Biochemistry 22:2875, 1983.

161. Stenflo, J., Lundwall, Å., and Dahlbäck, B.: β-Hydroxyasparagine in domains homologous to the epidermal growth factor precursor in vitamin K–dependent protein S. Proc. Natl. Acad Sci. USA 84:368, 1987.

162. Hase, S., Kawabata, S.-I., Nishimura, H., Takeya, H., Sueyoshi, T., Miyata, T., Iwanaga, S., Takao, T., Shimonishi, Y., and Ikenaka, T.: A new trisaccharide sugar chain linked to a serine residue in bovine coagulation factors VII and IX. J. Biochem. 104:867, 1988.

163. Nishimura, H., Kawabata, S.-I., Kisiel, W., Hase, S., Ikenaka, T., Takao, T., Shimonishi, Y., and Iwanaga, S.: Identification of a disaccharide (Xyl-Glc) and a trisaccharide (Xyl₂-Glc) O-glycosidically linked to a serine residue in the first epidermal growth factor–like domain of human factors VII and IX and protein Z and bovine protein Z. J. Biol. Chem. 264:20320, 1989.

164. Hase, S., Nishimura, H., Kawabata, S.-I., Iwanaga, S., and Ikenaka, T.: The structure of (xylose)₂ glucose-O-serine 53 found in the first epidermal growth factor–like domain of bovine blood clotting factor IX. J. Biol. Chem. 265:1858, 1990.

165. Lundblad, A., and Svensson, S.: Isolation and characterization of 3-O-α-D-Xylopranosyl-D-Glucose and 2-O-α-L-Fucopyranosyl-D-Glucose from normal human urine. Biochemistry 12:306, 1973.

166. Huang, L. H., Ke, X.-H., Sweeny, W., and Tam, J. P.: Calcium binding and putative activity of the epidermal growth factor domain of blood coagulation factor IX. Biochem. Biophys. Res. Commun. 160:133, 1989.

167. Handford, P. A., Baron, M., Mayhew, M., Wills, A., Beesley, T., Brownlee, G. G., and Campbell, I. D.: The first EGF-like domain from human factor IX contains a high-affinity calcium binding site. EMBO J. 9:475, 1990.

168. Dahlbäck, B., Hildebrand, B., and Linse, S.: Novel type of very high affinity calcium binding sites in β-hydroxyasparagine-containing epidermal growth factor–like domains in vitamin K–dependent protein S. J. Biol. Chem. 265:18481, 1990.

169. McMullen, B. A., Fujikawa, K., and Kisiel, W.: The occurrence of β-hydroxyaspartic acid in the vitamin K–dependent blood coagulation zymogens. Biochem. Biophys. Res. Commun. 115:8, 1983.

170. Fernlund, P., and Stenflo, J.: β-Hydroxyaspartic acid in vitamin K–dependent proteins. J. Biol. Chem. 258:12509, 1983.

171. Thim, L., Bjoern, S., Christensen, M., Nicolaisen, E. M., Lund-Hansen, T., Pedersen, H., and Hedner, U.: Amino acid sequence and posttranslational modifications of human factor VIIₐ from plasma and transfected baby hamster kidney cells. Biochemistry 27:7785, 1988.

172. Ikegami, T.: Studies on the metabolism of β-hydroxyaspartic acid. Acta Med. Okayama 29:241, 1975.

173. Przysiecki, C. T., Staggers, J. E., Rajmit, H. G., Musson, D. G., Stern, A. M., Bennet, C. D., and Friedman, P. A.: Occurrence of β-hydroxylated asparagine residues in non–vitamin K–dependent proteins containing epidermal growth factor–like domains. Proc. Natl. Acad. Sci. USA 84:7856, 1987.

174. Stenflo, J., Öhlin, A.-K., Owen, W. G., and Schneider, W. J.: β-Hydroxyaspartic acid or β-hydroxyasparagine in bovine low density lipoprotein receptor and in bovine thrombomodulin. J. Biol. Chem. 263:21, 1988.

175. Kanazaki, T., Olofsson, A., Morén, A., Wernstedt, C., Hellman, U., Miyazono, K., Claesson-Welsh, L., and Heldin, C.-H.: TGF-β1 binding protein: A component of the large latent complex of TGF-β1 with multiple repeat sequences. Cell 61:1051, 1990.

176. Gray, A., Dull, T. J., and Ullrich, A.: Nucleotide sequence of epidermal growth factor cDNA predicts a 128,000-molecular weight protein precursor. Nature 303:722, 1983.

177. Lee, B., Godfrey, M., Vitale, E., Hori, H., Mattei, M.-G., Sarfarazi, M., Tsipouras, P., Ramirez, F., and Hollister, D. W.: Linkage of Marfan syndrome and a phenotypically related disorder to two different fibrillin genes. Nature 352:330, 1991.

178. Maslen, C. L., Corson, G. M., Maddox, B. K., Glanville, R. W., and Sakai, L. Y.: Partial sequence of a candidate gene for the Marfan syndrome. Nature 352:334, 1991.

179. Wharton, K. A., Johansen, K. M., Xu, T., and Artavanis-Tsakonas, S.: Nucleotide sequence for the neurogenic locus notch implies a gene product that shares homology with proteins containing EGF-like repeats. Cell 43:567, 1985.

180. Vässin, H., Bremer, K. A., Knust, E., and Campus-Ortega, J. A.: The neurogenic gene delta of *Drosophila melanogaster* is expressed in neurogenic territories and encodes a putative transmembrane protein with EGF-like repeats. EMBO J. 6:3431, 1987.

181. Tepass, U., Theres, C., and Knust, E.: *Crumbs* encodes an EGF-like protein expressed on apical membranes of Drosophila epithelial cells and required for organization of epithelia. Cell 61:787, 1990.

182. Knust, E., Dietrich, U., Tepass, U., Bremer, K. A., Weigel, D., Vässin, H., and Campus-Ortega, J. A.: EGF homologous sequence encoded in the genome of *Drosophila melanogaster* and their relation to neurogenic genes. EMBO J. 6:761, 1987.

183. Ellisen, L. W., Bird, J., West, D. C., Soreng, A. L., Reynolds, T. C., Smith, S. D., and Sklar, J.: TAN-1, the human homolog of the Drosophila *Notch* gene, is broken by chromosomal translocations in T lymphoblastic neoplasms. Cell 66:649, 1991.

184. Derian, C. K., VanDusen, W., Przysieck, C. T., Walsh, P. N., Berkner, K. L., Kaufman, R. J., and Friedman, P. A.: Inhibitors of 2-ketoglutarate-dependent dioxygenases block aspartyl β-hydroxylation of recombinant human factor IX in several mammalian expression systems. J. Biol. Chem. 264:6615, 1989.

185. Stenflo, J., Holme, E., Lindstedt, S., Chandramouli, N., Tsai Huang, L. H., Tam, J., and Merrifield, R. B.: Hydroxylation of aspartic acid in domains homologous to the epidermal growth factor precursor is catalyzed by a 2-oxoglutarate-dependent dioxygenase. Proc. Natl. Acad. Sci. USA 86:444, 1989.

186. Gronke, R. S., VanDusen, W. J., Garsky, V. M., Jacobs, J. W., Saranda, M. K., Stern, A. M., and Friedman, P. A.: Aspartyl β-hydroxylase: *In vitro* hydroxylation of a synthetic peptide based on the structure of the first growth factor–like domain of human factor IX. Proc. Natl. Acad. Sci. USA 86:3609, 1989.

187. Hayaishi, O., Nozaki, M., and Abbott, M. T.: Oxygenases: dioxygenases. The Enzymes 12:119, 1975.

188. Wang, Q., VanDusen, W. J., Petroski, C. J., Garsky, V. M., Stern, A. M., and Friedman, P. A.: Bovine liver aspartyl β-hydroxylase. Purification and characterization. J. Biol. Chem. 266:14004, 1991.

189. Stenflo, J., and Fernlund, P.: β-Hydroxyaspartic acid in vitamin K–dependent plasma proteins from scorbutic and warfarin-treated guinea pigs. FEBS Lett. 168:287, 1984.

189a. Sugo, T., Persson, U., and Stenflo, J.: Protein C in bovine plasma after warfarin treatment. Purification, partial characterization, and β-hydroxyaspartic acid content. J. Biol. Chem. 260:10453, 1985.

190. Gronke, R. S., Welsh, D. J., VanDusen, W. J., Garsky, V. M., Sardana, M., Stern, A. M., and Friedman, P. A.: Partial purification and characterization of bovine liver aspartyl β-hydroxylase. J. Biol. Chem. 265:8558, 1990.

191. Morita, T., Kaetsu, H., Mizuguchi, J., Kawabata, S.-I., and

Iwanaga, S.: A characteristic property of vitamin K–dependent plasma protein Z. J. Biochem. 104:368, 1988.

192. Handford, P. A., Mayhew, M., Baron, M., Winship, P. R., Campbell, I. D., and Brownlee, G. G.: Key residues involved in calcium-binding motifs in EGF-like domains. Nature 351:184, 1991.

193. Lin, S.-W., Smith, K. J., Welsch, D., and Stafford, D. W.: Expression and characterization of human factor IX and factor IX-factor X chimeras in mouse C127 Cells. J. Biol. Chem. 265:144, 1990.

194. Cheung, W.-F., Straight, D. L., Smith, K. J., Lin, S.-W., Roberts, H., and Stafford, D. W.: The role of the epidermal growth factor-1 and hydrophobic stack domains of human factor IX in binding to endothelial cells. J. Biol. Chem. 266:8797, 1991.

195. Toomey, J. R., Smith, K. J., and Stafford, D. W.: Localization of the human tissue factor recognition determinant of human factor VIIa. J. Biol. Chem. 266:19198, 1991.

196. Herzberg, M. S., Ben-Tal, O., Furie, B., and Furie, B. C.: Construction, expression, and characterization of a chimera of factor IX and factor X. The role of the second epidermal growth factor domain and serine protease domain in factor Va binding. J. Biol. Chem. 267:14759, 1992.

197. Rees, D. J. G., Jones, I. M., Handford, P. A., Walter, S. J., Esnouf, M. P., Smith, K. J., and Brownlee, G. G.: The role of β-hydroxyaspartate and adjacent carboxylate residues in the first EGF domain of human factor IX. EMBO J. 7:2053, 1988.

198. Öhlin, A.-K., Landes, G., Bourdon, P., Oppenheimer, C., Wydro, R., and Stenflo, J.: β-Hydroxyaspartic acid in the first epidermal growth factor–like domain of protein C. Its role in Ca²⁺ binding and biological activity. J. Biol. Chem. 263:19240, 1988.

199. Sugo, T., Björk, I., Holmgren, A., and Stenflo, J.: Calcium-binding properties of bovine factor X lacking the γ-carboxyglutamic acid–containing region. J. Biol. Chem. 259:5705, 1984.

200. Morita, T., and Kisiel, W.: Calcium binding to a human factor IXₐ derivative lacking γ-carboxyglutamic acid: Evidence for two high-affinity sites that do not involve β-hydroxyaspartic acid. Biochem. Biophys. Res. Commun. 130:841, 1985.

201. Öhlin, A.-K., Linse, S., and Stenflo, J.: Calcium binding to the epidermal growth factor homology region of bovine protein C. J. Biol. Chem. 263:7411, 1988.

202. Tsay, W., Greengard, J. S., Montgomery, R., and Griffin, J. H.: Five previously undescribed mutations in protein C (PC) that identify elements critical for gene and protein activity. Blood (Suppl.) 78:184a, 1991.

203. Davis, L. M., McGraw, R. A., Ware, J. L., Roberts, H., and Stafford, D. W.: Factor IX Alabama: A point mutation in a clotting protein results in hemophilia B. Blood 69:140, 1987.

204. McCord, D. M., Monroe, D. M., Smith, K. J., and Roberts, H. R.: Characterization of the functional defect in factor IX Alabama. Evidence for a conformational change due to high affinity calcium binding in the first epidermal growth factor domain. J. Biol. Chem. 265:10250, 1990.

205. Green, P. M., Montandon, A. J., Ljung, R., Bentley, D. R., Nilsson, I.-M., Kling, S., and Giannelli, F.: Haemophilia B mutations in a complete Swedish population sample: A test of new strategy for the genetic counselling of diseases with high mutational heterogeneity. Br. J. Haematol. 78:390, 1991.

206. Lozier, J. N., Monroe, D. M., and Stanfield-Oakley, S. A.: Factor IX New London: Substitution of proline for glutamine at position 50 causes severe hemophilia B. Blood 75:1097, 1990.

207. Miyata, T., Nishimura, H., Suehiro, K., Takeya, H., Okamura, T., Murakawa, M., Niho, Y., and Iwanaga, S.: The 2nd EGF-like domain in factor IX is required for interaction with factor VIII. Thromb. Haemost. 65:471, 1991.

208. Blasi, F., Vassalli, J. D., and Dano, K.: Urokinase-type plasminogen activator: Proenzyme, receptor, and inhibitors. J. Cell. Biol. 104:801, 1987.

209. Roldan, A. L., Cubellis, M. V., Masucci, M. T., Behrendt, N., Lund, L. R., Danö, K., Appella, E., and Blasi, F.: Cloning and expression of the receptor for human urokinase plasminogen activator, a central molecule in cell surface, plasmin dependent proteolysis. EMBO J. 9:467, 1990.

210. Kurosawa, S., Stearns, D. J., Jackson, K. W., and Esmon, C. T.: A 10-kDa cyanogen bromide fragment from the epidermal growth factor homology domain of rabbit thrombomodulin contains the primary thrombin binding site. J. Biol. Chem. 263:5993, 1988.

211. Zushi, M., Gomi, K., Yamamoto, S., Maruyama, I., Hayashi, T., and Suzuki, K.: The last three consecutive epidermal growth factor–like structures of human thrombomodulin comprise the minimum functional domain for protein C–activating cofactor activity and anticoagulant activity. J. Biol. Chem. 264:10351, 1989.

212. Stearns, D. J., Kurosawa, S., and Esmon, C. T.: Microthrombomodulin. Residues 310–486 from the epidermal growth factor precursor homology domain of thrombomodulin will accelerate protein C activation. J. Biol. Chem. 264:3352, 1989.

213. Husten, E. J., Esmon, C. T., and Johnson, A. E.: The active site of blood coagulation factor Xa. Its distance from the phospholipid surface and its conformational sensitivity to components of the prothrombinase complex. J. Biol. Chem. 262:12953, 1987.

214. Sakai, L. Y., Keene, D. R., Glanville, R. W., and Bächinger, H. P.: Purification and partial characterization of fibrillin, a cysteine-rich structural component of connective tissue microfibrils. J. Biol. Chem. 266:14763, 1991.

214a. Clarke, B. J., Ofosu, F. A., Sridhara, S., Bona, R. D., Rickles, F. R., and Blajchman, M. A.: The first epidermal growth factor domain of human coagulation factor VII is essential for binding with tissue factor. FEBS Lett. 298:206, 1992.

215. Astermark, J., Björk, I., Hogg, P. J., and Stenflo, J.: Effects of γ-carboxyglutamic acid and epidermal growth factor–like modules of factor IX on factor X activation. Studies using proteolytic fragments of bovine factor IX. J. Biol. Chem. 267:3249, 1992.

216. Gardell, S. J., Duong, L. T., Diehl, R. E., York, J. D., Hare, T. R., Register, B. R., Jacobs, J. W., Dixon, R. A. F., and Friedman, P. A.: Isolation, characterization and cDNA cloning of vampire bat salivary plasminogen activator. J. Biol. Chem. 264:17947, 1989.

217. Nakamura, T., Nishizawa, T., Hagiya, M., Seki, T., Shimonishi, M., Sugimura, A., Tashiro, K., and Shimizu, S.: Molecular cloning and expression of human hepatocyte growth factor. Nature 342:440, 1989.

218. McLean, J. M., Tomlinson, J. E., Kuang, W.-J., Eaton, D. L., Chen, E. Y., Fless, G. M., Scanu, A. M., and Lawn, R. M.: cDNA sequence of human apolipoprotein(a) is homologous to plasminogen. Nature 300:132, 1987.

219. Mulichak, A. M., and Tulinsky, A.: Structure of the lysine-fibrin binding subsite of human plasminogen kringle 4. Blood Coag. Fibrinol. 1:673, 1990.

220. Williams, R. J. P.: NMR studies of mobility within protein structure. Eur. J. Biochem. 183:479, 1989.

221. Seshadri, T. P., Tulinsky, A., Skrzypczak-Jankun, E., and Park, C. H.: Structure of bovine prothrombin fragment 1 refined at 2.25 Å resolution. J. Mol. Biol. 220:481, 1991.

222. Esmon, C. T., and Jackson, C. M.: The conversion of prothrombin to thrombin. IV. The function of the fragment 2 region during activation in the presence of factor V. J. Biol. Chem. 249:7791, 1974.

223. Myrmel, K. H., Lundblad, R. L., and Mann, K. G.: Characteristics of the association between prothrombin fragment 2 and α-thrombin. Biochemistry 15:1767, 1976.

224. Bajaj, S. P., Butkowski, R. L., and Mann, K. G.: Prothrombin fragments. Ca²⁺ binding and activation kinetics. J. Biol. Chem. 250:2150, 1975.

225. Dahlbäck, B., Hildebrand, B., and Malm, J.: Characterization of functionally important domains in human vitamin K–dependent protein S using monoclonal antibodies. J. Biol. Chem. 265:8127, 1990.

226. Suzuki, K., Nishioka, J., and Hashimoto, S.: Regulation of

activated protein C by thrombin-modified protein S. J. Biochem. 94:699, 1983.

227. Walker, F. J.: Regulation of vitamin K–dependent protein S. Inactivation with thrombin. J. Biol. Chem. 259:10335, 1984.

228. Schechter, I., and Berger, A.: On the size of the active size of papain. Biochem. Biophys. Res. Commun. 2:157, 1967.

229. Naito, K., and Fujikawa, K.: Activation of human blood coagulation factor XI independent of factor XII. Factor XI is activated by thrombin and factor XIa in the presence of negatively charged surfaces. J. Biol. Chem. 266:7353, 1991.

230. Kane, W. H., and Davie, E. W.: Blood coagulation factors V and VIII: Structural and functional similarities and their relationship to hemorrhagic and thrombotic disorders. Blood 71:539, 1988.

230a. Gailani, D., and Broze, G. J.: Factor XI activation in a revised model of blood coagulation. Science 253:909, 1991.

231. Lorand, L.: Activation of blood coagulation factor XIII. Ann. N. Y. Acad. Sci. 485:144, 1986.

232. Stenflo, J.: The biochemistry of protein C. *In* Bertina, R. M. (ed.): Protein C and Related Proteins. Biochemical and Clinical Aspects. London, Churchill Livingstone, 1988, pp. 21–54.

233. Walz, D. A., Fenton, J. W., II, and Shuman, M. A. (eds.): Bioregulatory functions of thrombin. Ann. N. Y. Acad. Sci. Vol. 485, 1986.

234. Vu, T.-K. H., Hung, D. T., Wheaton, V. I., and Coughlin, S. R.: Molecular cloning of a functional thrombin receptor reveals a novel proteolytic mechanism of receptor activation. Cell 64:1057, 1991.

235. Vu, T.-K. H., Wheaton, V. I., Hung, D. T., Charo, I., and Coughlin, S. R.: Domains specifying thrombin-receptor interaction. Nature 353:674, 1991.

236. Hung, D. T., Vu, T.-K. H., Nelken, N. A., and Coughlin, S. R.: Thrombin-induced events in non–platelet cells are mediated by the unique proteolytic mechanism established for the cloned platelet thrombin receptor. J. Cell Biol. 116:827, 1992.

237. Coughlin, S. R., Vu, T.-K. H., Hung, D. T., and Wheaton, V. I.: Characterization of a functional thrombin receptor. Issues and opportunities. J. Clin. Invest. 89:351, 1992.

237a. Bode, W., Turk, D., and Karshikov, A.: The refined 1.9-Å X-ray structure of D-Phe-Pro-Arg chloromethylketone-inhibited human α-thrombin: Structure analysis, overall structure, electrostatic properties, detailed active-site geometry, and structure-function relationships. Protein Science 1:426, 1992.

238. Pryzdial, E. L. G., and Mann, K. G.: The association of coagulation factor Xa and factor Va. J. Biol. Chem. 266:8969, 1991.

239. Krishnaswamy, S., and Mann, K. G.: The binding of factor Va to phospholipid vesicles. J. Biol. Chem. 263:5714, 1988.

240. Van Dieijen, G., Tans, G., Rosing, J., and Hemker, H. C.: The role of phospholipid and factor VIIIa in the activation of bovine factor X. J. Biol. Chem. 256:3433, 1981.

241. Ahmed, S. S., Rawala-Sheikh, R., and Walsh, P. N.: Comparative interactions of factor IX and factor IXa with human platelets. J. Biol. Chem. 264:3244, 1989.

242. Krishnaswamy S.: Prothrombin complex assembly. Contributions of protein-protein and protein-membrane interactions toward complex formation. J. Biol. Chem. 265:3708, 1990.

243. Miletich, J. P., Jackson, C. M., and Majerus, P. W.: Interaction of coagulation factor Xa with human platelets. Proc. Natl. Acad. Sci. USA 74:4033, 1977.

244. Miletich, J. P., Jackson, C. M., and Majerus, P. W.: Properties of the factor Xa binding site on human platelets. J. Biol. Chem. 253:6908, 1978.

245. Dahlbäck, B., and Stenflo, J.: Binding of bovine coagulation factor Xa to platelets. Biochemistry 17:4938, 1978.

246. Keyt, B., Furie, B. C., and Furie, B.: Structural transitions in bovine factor X associated with metal binding and zymogen activation. Studies using conformation-specific antibodies. J. Biol. Chem. 257:8687, 1982.

247. Persson, E., Valcarce, C., and Stenflo, J.: The γ-carboxyglutamic acid and epidermal growth factor–like domains of

Factor X. Effects of isolated domains on prothrombin activation and endothelial cell binding of factor X. J. Biol. Chem. 266:2453, 1991.

248. Bajaj, S. P., Rapaport, S. I., and Maki, S. L.: A monoclonal antibody to factor IX that inhibits the factor VIII:Ca potentiation of factor X activation. J. Biol. Chem. 260:11574, 1985.

249. Chattopadhya, A., and Fair, D. S.: A limited number of regions on factor Xa are involved in prothrombin activation. Blood 74:1102, 1989.

250. Rosing, J., Zwaal, R. F. A., and Tans, G.: Formation of meizothrombin as intermediate in factor Xa–catalyzed prothrombin activation. J. Biol. Chem. 261:4224, 1986.

251. Krishnaswamy, S., Mann, K. G., and Nesheim, M. E.: The prothrombinase-catalyzed activation of prothrombin proceeds through the intermediate meizothrombin in an ordered, sequential reaction. J. Biol. Chem. 261:8997, 1986.

252. Rabiet, M. J., Blashill, A., Furie, B., and Furie, B. C.: Prothrombin fragment 1.2.3, a major product of prothrombin activation in human plasma. J. Biol. Chem. 261:13210, 1986.

253. Krishnaswamy, S., Church, W. R., Nesheim, M. E., and Mann, K. G.: Activation of human prothrombin by human prothrombinase. Influence of factor Va on the reaction mechanism. J. Biol. Chem. 262:3291, 1987.

254. Carlisle, T. L., Bock, P. E., and Jackson, C. M.: Kinetic intermediates in prothrombin activation. Bovine prethrombin 1 conversion to thrombin by factor X. J. Biol. Chem. 265:22044, 1990.

255. Doyle, M. F., and Mann, K. G.: Multiple active forms of thrombin. IV. Relative activities of meizothrombins. J. Biol. Chem. 265:10693, 1990.

256. Wu, Q., Tsiang, M., Lentz, S. R., and Sadler, J. E.: Ligand specificity of human thrombomodulin. Equilibrium binding of human thrombin, meizothrombin, and factor Xa to recombinant thrombomodulin. J. Biol. Chem. 265:7983, 1992.

257. Kawabata, S. I., Morita, T., Iwanaga, S., and Igarashi, H.: Staphylocoagulase-binding region in human prothrombin. J. Biochem. 97:325, 1985.

258. Kawabata, S. I., Morita, T., Iwanaga, S., and Igarashi, H.: Difference in enzymatic properties between α-thrombin–staphylocoagulase complex and free α-thrombin. J. Biochem. 97:1073, 1985.

259. Morita, T., and Iwanaga, S.: Prothrombin activator from *Echis carinatus* venom. Methods Enzymol. 80:303, 1981.

260. Spijer, H., Govers-Riemslag, J. W. P., Zwaal, R. F. A., and Rosing, J.: Prothrombin activation by an activator from the venom of *Oxyuranus scutellatus* (Taipan snake). J. Biol. Chem. 261:13258, 1986.

261. Kisiel, W., Hermodson, M. A., and Davie, E. W.: Factor X activating enzyme from Russell's viper venom: Isolation and characterization. Biochemistry 15:4901, 1976.

262. Nakagaki, T., Lin, P., and Kisiel, W.: Activation of human factor VII by the prothrombin activator from the venom of *Oxyuranus scutellatus* (Taipan snake). Thromb. Res. 65:105, 1992.

263. Fenton, J. W., II, Fasco, M. J., Stackrow, A. B., Aronson, D. L., Young, A. M., and Finlayson, J. S.: Human thrombins. Production, evaluation, and properties of α-thrombin. J. Biol. Chem. 252:3587, 1977.

264. Stenflo, J., and Fernlund, P.: Amino acid sequence of the heavy chain of bovine protein C. J. Biol. Chem. 257:12180, 1982.

265. Fenton, J. W., II: Thrombin. Ann. N. Y. Acad. Sci. USA 485:5, 1986.

266. Rydel, T. J., Ravichandran, K. G., Tulinsky, A., Bode, W., Huber, R., Roitsch, C., and Fenton, J. W., II: The structure of a complex of recombinant hirudin and human α-thrombin. Science 249:277, 1990.

267. Grütter, M. G., Priestle, J. P., Rahuel, J., Grossenbacher, H., Bode, W., Hofstenge, J., and Stone, R. S.: Crystal structure of the thrombin-hirudin complex: A novel mode of serine protease inhibition. EMBO J. 9:2361, 1990.

268. Skrzypczak-Jankun, E., Carperos, V. E., Ravichandran, K. G.,

and Tulinsky, A.: Structure of the hirugen and hirulog 1 complexes of α-thrombin. J. Mol. Biol. 221:1379, 1991.

269. Hofstenge, J., Braun, P. J., and Stone, S. R.: Enzymatic properties of proteolytic derivatives of human α-thrombin. Biochemistry 27:2144, 1988.

270. Church, F. C., Pratt, C. W., Noyes, C. M., Kalayanmit, T., Sherrill, G. B., Tobin, R. B., and Meade, J. B.: Structural and functional properties of human α-thrombin, phospho-pyridoxylated α-thrombin, and γ_T-thrombin. Identification of lysyl residues in α-thrombin that are critical for heparin and fibrin(ogen) interactions. J. Biol. Chem. 264:18419, 1989.

271. Folkers, P. J. M., Clore, G. M., Driscol, D. C., Dodt, J., Kohler, S., and Gronenborn, A. M.: Solution structure of recombinant hirudin and the Lys 47-Glu mutant: a nuclear magnetic resonance and hybrid geometry–dynamical stimulated annealing study. Biochemistry 28:2601, 1989.

272. Haruyama, H., and Wüterich, K.: Conformation of recombinant desulfatohirudin in aqueous solution determined by nuclear-magnetic resonance. Biochemistry 28:4301, 1989.

273. Fenton, J. W., II, and Bing, D. H.: Thrombin active-site regions. Semin. Thromb. Hemost. 12:200, 1986.

274. Brezniak, D. V., Brown, M. S., Witting, J. I., Walz, D. A., and Fenton, J. W., II: Human α- to ξ-thrombin cleavage occurs with neutrophil cathepsin g or chymotrypsin while fibrinogen clotting activity is retained. Biochemistry 29:3536, 1990.

275. Bode, W., and Schwager, P.: The single calcium-binding site of crystalline bovine β-trypsin. FEBS Lett. 56:139, 1975.

276. Bode, W., and Schwager, P.: The refined crystal structure of bovine β-trypsin at 1.8 Å resolution. II. Crystallographic refinement, calcium binding site, benzamidine binding site and active site at pH 7.0. J. Mol. Biol. 98:693, 1975.

277. Bajaj, S. P., Sabharwal, A. K., Gorka, J., and Birktoft, J. J.: Use of antibodies and factor IX variants in probing conformational transitions in the protease domain of factor IX. Thromb. Haemost. 65:293, 1991.

278. Bajaj, S. P., Sabharwal, A. K., Gorka, J., and Birktoft, J. J.: Antibody-probed conformational transitions in the protease domain of human factor IX upon calcium binding and zymogen activation: Putative high-affinity Ca²⁺-binding site in the protease domain. Proc. Natl. Acad. Sci. USA 89:152, 1992.

279. Rabiet, M.-J., Furie, B. C., and Furie, B.: Molecular defect of prothrombin Barcelona. Substitution of cysteine for arginine at residue 273. J. Biol. Chem. 261:15045, 1986.

280. Diuguid, D. L., Rabiet, M.-J., Furie, B. C., and Furie, B.: Molecular defects of factor IX Chicago-2 (Arg 145 → His) and prothrombin Madrid (Arg 271 → Cys): Arginine mutations that preclude zymogen activation. Blood 74:193, 1989.

281. Bertina, R. M., and Veltkamp, J. J.: Physiology and biochemistry of factor IX. In Bloom, A. L., and Thomas, D. P. (eds): Haemostasis and Thrombosis. London, Churchill Livingstone 1987, pp. 116–130.

282. Noyes, C. M., Griffith, M. J., Roberts, H. R., and Lundblad, R. L.: Identification of the molecular defect in factor IX Chapel Hill: Substitution of histidine for arginine at position 145. Proc. Natl. Acad. Sci. USA 80:4200, 1983.

283. Liddell, M. B., Peake, I. R., Taylor, S. A. M., Lillicrap, D. P., Giddings, J. C., and Bloom, A. L.: Factor IX Cardiff: A variant factor IX protein that shows abnormal activation is caused by an arginine to cysteine substitution at position 145. Br. J. Haematol. 72:556, 1989.

284. Suehiro, K., Kawabata, S.-I., Miyata, T., Takeya, H., Takamutsu, J., Ogata, K., Kamiya, T., Saito, H., Niho, Y., and Iwanaga, S.: Blood clotting factor IX B_M Nagoya. Substitution of arginine 180 by tryptophan and its activation by α-chymotrypsin and rat mast cell chymase. J. Biol. Chem. 264:21257, 1989.

285. Huang, M.-N., Kasper, C. K., Roberts, H. R., Stafford, D. W., and High, K. A.: Molecular defect in factor IX Hilo, a hemophilia B_m variant: Arg → Gln at the carboxyterminal cleavage site of the activation peptide. Blood 73:718, 1989.

286. Sakai, T., Yoshioka, A., Yamamoto, K., Niinomi, K., Fujimura, Y., Fukui, H., Miyata, T., and Iwanaga, S.: Blood clotting factor IX Kashihara: Amino acid substitution of valine-182 by phenylalanine. J. Biochem. 105:756, 1989.

287. Spitzer, S. G., Pendurti, U. R., Kasper, C. K., and Bajaj, S. P.: Molecular defect in factor IX_Bm Lake Elsinore. Substitution of Ala 390 by Val in the catalytic domain. J. Biol. Chem. 263:10545, 1988.

288. Ware, J., Davis, L., Frazier, D., Bajaj, P. S., and Stafford, D. W.: Genetic defect responsible for the dysfunctional protein: Factor IX Long Beach. Blood 72:820, 1988.

289. Geddes, V. A., Le Bonniec, B. F., Louie, G. V., Brayer, G. D., Thompson, A. R., and MacGillivray, R. T. A.: A moderate form of hemophilia B is caused by a novel mutation in the protease domain of factor IX Vancouver. J. Biol. Chem. 264:4689, 1989.

290. Spitzer, S. G., Warnewr-Cramer, B. J., Kasper, C. K., and Bajaj, S. P.: Replacement of isoleucine-397 by threonine in the clotting proteinase factor IXa (Los Angeles and Long Beach variants) affects macromolecular catalysis but not L-tosylarginine methyl ester hydrolysis. Biochem. J. 265:219, 1990.

291. Attree, O., Vidaud, D., Vidaud, M., Amselm, S., Lavergne, J.-M., and Goossens, M.: Mutations in the catalytic domain of human coagulation factor IX: Rapid characterization by direct genomic sequencing of DNA fragments displaying an altered melting behavior. Genomics 4:266, 1989.

292. James, H. L., Girolami, A., and Fair, D. S.: Molecular defect in coagulation factor X Friuli results from a substitution of serine for proline at position 343. Blood 77:317, 1991.

293. Wu, Q., Sheehan, J. P., Tsiang, M., Lentz, S. R., Birktoft, J. J., and Sadler, J. E.: Single amino acid substitutions dissociate fibrinogen-clotting and thrombomodulin-binding activities of human thrombin. Proc. Natl. Acad. Sci. USA 88:6775, 1991.

294. Le Bonniec, B. F., and Esmon, C. T.: Glu-192 → Gln substitution in thrombin mimics the catalytic switch induced by thrombomodulin. Proc. Natl. Acad. Sci. USA 88:7371, 1991.

295. Henriksen, R. A., and Mann, K. G.: Identification of the primary structure defect in the dysthrombin thrombin quick I: Substitution of cysteine for arginine-392. Biochemistry 27:9160, 1988.

296. Jakubowski, H. H., and Owen, W. G.: Macromolecular specificity determinants on thrombin for fibrinogen and thrombomodulin. J. Biol. Chem. 264:11119, 1989.

297. Henriksen, R. A., and Mann, K. G.: Substitution of valine for glycine in the congenital dysthrombin thrombin quick II alters primary substrate specificity. Biochemistry 20:2078, 1989.

298. Miyata, T., Morita, T., Inomoto, T., Kawauchi, S., Shirakami, A., and Iwanaga, S.: Prothrombin Tokushima, a replacement of arginine-418 by tryptophan that impairs the fibrinogen clotting activity of derived thrombin Tokushima. Biochemistry 26:1117, 1987.

299. Joseph, D. R., Hall, S. H., and French, F. S.: Rat androgen-binding protein: Evidence for identical subunits and amino acid sequence homology with human sex hormone–binding globulin. Proc. Natl. Acad. Sci. USA 84:339, 1987.

300. Petra, P. H., Kumar, S., Hayes, R., Ericsson, L. H., and Titani, K.: Molecular organization of the sex steroid–binding protein (SBP) of human plasma. J. Steroid Biochem. 24:45, 1986.

301. Hammond, G. L., Robinson, P. A., Sugino, H., Ward, D. N., and Finne, J.: Physicochemical characteristics of human sex hormone binding globulin: Evidence for two identical subunits. J. Steroid Biochem. 24:815, 1986.

302. Hryb, D. J., Kahn, M. S., Romas, N. A., and Rosner, W.: The control of the interaction of sex hormone–binding globulin with its receptor by steroid hormones. J. Biol. Chem. 265:6048, 1990.

303. Gershagen, S., Fernlund, P., and Edenbrandt, C.-M.: The genes for SHBG/ABP and the SHBG-like region of vitamin K–dependent protein S have evolved from a common ancestral gene. J. Steroid Biochem. Molec. Biol. 40:763, 1991.

304. Petra, P. H., Que, B. G., Namkung, P. C., Ross, J. B. A.,

Charbonneau, H., Walsh, K. A., Griffin, P. R., Shabanowitz, J., and Hunt, D. F.: Affinity labelling, molecular cloning, and comparative amino acid sequence analyses of sex steroid–binding protein of plasma. Ann. N. Y. Acad. Sci. 538:10, 1988.

305. Miletich, J. P., Broze, G. J., and Majerus, P. W.: Purification of human coagulation factors II, IX, and X using sulfated dextran beads. Methods Enzymol. 80:221, 1981.

306. Bajaj, S. P., Rapaport, S. I., and Brown, S. F.: Isolation and characterization of human factor VII. Activation of factor VII by factor Xa. J. Biol. Chem. 256:253, 1981.

307. Hagen, F. S., Gray, C. L., O'Hara, P., Grant, F. J., Saari, G. C., Woodbury, R. G., Hart, C. E., Insley, M., Kisiel, W., Kurachi, K., and Davie, E. W.: Characterization of a cDNA coding for human factor VII. Proc. Natl. Acad. Sci. USA 83:2412, 1986.

The Protein C Anticoagulant System

Björn Dahlbäck and Johan Stenflo

INTRODUCTION

Blood coagulation is rapidly activated in response to vascular injury. A cascade of zymogen activations leads to the formation of thrombin, a multifunctional serine protease that activates platelets and converts soluble fibrinogen to a fibrin network.[1, 2] Thrombin also stimulates the coagulation cascade by feedback activation of the two regulatory proteins, factors V and VIII (Fig. 17–1). The multiple zymogen activations of the coagulation cascade provide the potential for explosive amplification, resulting in local generation of high thrombin concentrations and coagulation in response to a triggering event. In vivo, the coagulation system is carefully regulated to ensure precise delivery of thrombin at the site of the lesion, without clot propagation leading to occlusion of the circulatory system. Under normal conditions, the balance between procoagulant and anticoagulant activities is shifted in favor of anticoagulation. The endothelial cells are crucial for the inhibition of clot formation, that is,

they synthesize and secrete prostacyclin, several potent vessel wall–relaxing factors, and tissue-type plasminogen activator.[3] Two other anticoagulant mechanisms involve close interactions between plasma proteins and the endothelial cell surface. One depends on the presence of heparin-like molecules on the endothelial cell surface, which accelerate antithrombin III (AT III)–dependent inactivation of coagulation proteases.[4] The second involves the endothelial cell membrane protein thrombomodulin (TM), which binds thrombin with high affinity and changes its substrate specificity. When thrombin binds to TM, its procoagulant properties are lost, and it is converted into a potent activator of protein C, which is the key component in a physiologically important anticoagulant system, commonly referred to as the protein C anticoagulant system.[5–13]

PROTEIN C

Protein C was purified from bovine plasma in 1976 and described as a previously unknown vitamin K–

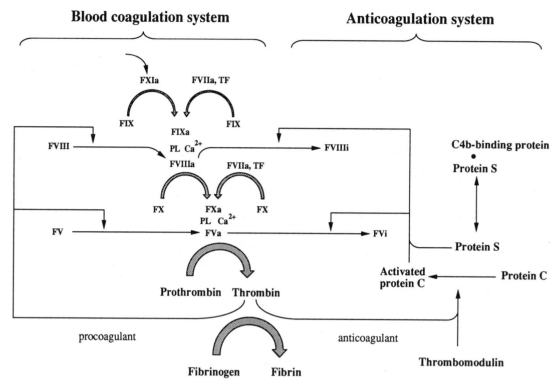

Blood coagulation system

Anticoagulation system

FIGURE 17–1. **A simplified scheme showing most of the reactions of blood coagulation and those of the protein C anticoagulant system.** The reactions leading to the formation of factor XIa have not been included in the coagulation cascade (see reference 1 and Chapter 16), nor are the feedback activations of factors V, VII, and VIII by factor Xa shown. The scheme emphasizes the balance between the procoagulant and anticoagulant mechanisms of thrombin and the specificity of activated protein C (APC). APC degrades factors Va and VIIIa when they are bound to phospholipid (PL). The binding of protein S to C4b-binding protein results in inhibition of its anticoagulant properties. TF denotes tissue factor, which triggers the reactions involving factor VII.

dependent protein.[7] It was soon found to be a zymogen of a serine protease with anticoagulant properties.[8] A few years later, protein C was also isolated from human plasma.[9] The rapid elucidation of the functions of activated protein C (APC) was facilitated by the discovery that it was identical to autoprothrombin II-A, a strong anticoagulant described already in 1960.[11] Autoprothrombin II-A activity was formed upon incubation of "prothrombin complex" with thrombin and was originally believed to be derived from the prothrombin molecule. In the early 1970s, it was shown that the precursor protein of autoprothrombin II-A was distinct from prothrombin.[12] Protein C is activated on the surface of endothelial cells by thrombin bound to TM. Together with its cofactor, vitamin K–dependent protein S, APC catalyzes the proteolytic degradation of the membrane-bound thrombin-activated forms of coagulation factors V and VIII (Va and VIIIa) (see Fig. 17–1). This mechanism is of crucial importance for the regulation of blood coagulation in vivo.[5–13] The cofactor, protein S, is unrelated to the serine protease family. In human plasma, approximately 40 per cent of protein S is free, the remaining 60 per cent circulating bound to C4b-binding protein (C4BP), an inhibitor of the classical complement pathway.[14, 15] Only free protein S has APC cofactor activity. APC is slowly neutralized in vivo by

at least three protease inhibitors, the protein C inhibitor (PCI), α_1-antitrypsin, and α_2-macroglobulin.[16–21] The physiological importance of the protein C anticoagulant system is most clearly demonstrated by the massive thrombotic complications occurring in infants with homozygous protein C or S deficiency.[22]

Factors Va and VIIIa, Substrates for Activated Protein C

The two substrates for APC, factors Va and VIIIa, are homologous high molecular weight plasma glycoproteins.[13, 23] The inactive procofactors factors V and VIII are converted to factors Va and VIIIa through limited proteolysis by thrombin or factor Xa (Fig. 17–2). Factor VIII is described in detail in Chapter 19. Factor V is a single-chain high molecular weight glycoprotein (Mr = 330,000) occurring in human plasma at a concentration of approximately 7 mg/l. In addition, platelets contain approximately 30 per cent of the factor V in human blood. After its activation by thrombin or factor Xa, factor Va, together with negatively charged phospholipid and Ca^{2+}, functions as a high-affinity receptor for factor Xa (K_d, approximately 1×10^{-10} M).[13, 23, 24] This membrane-bound macromolecular complex, the so-called prothrombinase com-

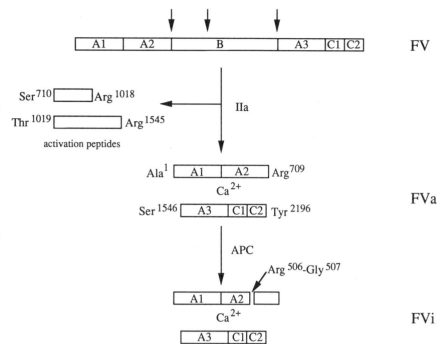

FIGURE 17–2. Schematic model of factor V. Factor V is composed of three A modules, one B module, and two C modules. Thrombin cleaves three peptide bonds, as indicated by the arrows. The heavy (residues 1–709) and light (residues 1546–2196) chains form a calcium-dependent complex, constituting factor Va. APC inactivates factor Va by cleavage of the heavy chain (Arg 506—Gly 507). Several other peptide bonds in the heavy chain are also cleaved by APC, but they have not been identified and are not indicated in the figure. A single peptide bond in the light chain of factor Va is cleaved by APC, but it is not associated with the loss of factor Va activity.

plex, can be assembled on the surface of activated platelets, platelet microparticles, macrophages, and endothelial cells. The intact prothrombinase complex activates prothrombin 10^5- to 10^6-fold more rapidly than does factor Xa alone. The rate enhancement has two causes: 1, a lowering of the K_m for prothrombin mediated by phospholipid; and 2, an increase in the V_{max} for prothrombin activation mediated by factor Va.[13, 24] The latter effect accounts for an approximately 10^3-fold increase in the rate of prothrombin activation. The potent anticoagulant activity of APC is in part mediated by the degradation of factor Va, resulting in inhibition of the prothrombinase activity. Factor VIIIa has a function analogous to that of factor Va in the factor Xase complex (factor VIIIa, phospholipid, Ca^{2+}, and factor IXa), and its activity is regulated in a similar fashion by APC.[1, 2, 13, 23, 24]

Factor V (comprising 2196 amino acid residues) and factor VIII appear to have evolved from a common ancestral protein.[13, 23] Both contain two types of internal repeats, three A modules and two C modules (see Fig. 17–2). A modules also appear in ceruloplasmin, a copper-binding protein in plasma. The amino acid sequences of the A modules in factor V, factor VIII, and ceruloplasmin are approximately 30 per cent identical. Factor V contains one copper ion, the function of which is unknown. Whether factor VIII also contains copper has yet to be elucidated. In factor V, two A modules occupy the amino-terminal region (residues 1 to 709), whereas the third A module and the two C modules constitute the carboxy-terminal part of the molecule (residues 1546 to 2196). The amino acid sequences of the two C modules in each of factors V and VIII are 35 to 50 per cent identical. These modules share approximately 20 per cent amino acid sequence identity with the first 150 amino acids

of discoidin I, a tetrameric galactose-binding lectin, essential for cell adhesion in the slime mold (*Dictyostelium discoidium*).[13, 23] Factor V is very rich in carbohydrate and contains both *N*- and *O*-linked sugars. The central portion of factor V, the B module, contains most of the 37 potential *N*-linked carbohydrate attachment sites in factor V and has been found to be highly glycosylated. The B module of factor VIII is also rich in carbohydrate but manifests no significant amino acid sequence similarity to the B module of factor V.[13, 23]

During thrombin activation of factor V, three peptide bonds are cleaved, Arg 709—Ser 710, Arg 1018—Thr 1019, and Arg 1545—Ser 1546, yielding four major fragments.[13, 23] The heavy chain (residues 1 to 709) forms a calcium-dependent, non-covalent complex with the light chain (residues 1546 to 2196), and together they constitute factor Va. The two fragments that are derived from the B module are activation peptides of unknown function. The light chain of factor Va contains the phospholipid-binding site. It has been localized to amino acid residues 1667 to 1765 in the middle of the A3 module.[25] Both chains support the interaction with factor Xa, whereas only the heavy chain appears to interact with prothrombin.[13, 24, 26]

APC is specific in that it efficiently degrades factors Va and VIIIa but cleaves intact factors V and VIII very slowly.[5–10, 23, 27] In vivo, the high specificity of APC is illustrated by the fact that the plasma concentrations of factors V and VIII are unaffected by APC infusion.[28–30] APC cleaves three peptide bonds in the heavy chain of factor VIIIa: Arg 336—Met 337, Arg 562—Gly 563, and Arg 740—Ser 741.[27] The cleavage between Arg 562 and Gly 563 appears to correlate best with the loss of factor VIIIa activity. Several peptide bonds in the heavy chain of factor Va are cleaved by APC, but so far only one of them has been identified (Arg 506—Gly 507).[13, 23] This cleavage correlates with the loss of factor Va activity, and the cleaved heavy chain does not interact with prothrombin and factor Xa.[13, 23, 24, 26] The light chain is also cleaved by APC, but this does not affect factor Va activity.[10, 23] Factor Xa and APC compete for binding sites on the light chain of factor Va. Accordingly, the binding of factor Xa to factor Va is associated with protection of factor Va from degradation by APC.[5–10, 13, 23, 24] The protective effect of factor Xa is abrogated by protein S, which may be one of the mechanisms by which this anticoagulant protein functions.[31] The binding of APC to negatively charged phospholipid is characterized by a K_d of approximately 7×10^{-8} M.[32, 33] The presence of protein S on the surface enhances the affinity of the APC binding approximately 10-fold.[32] In a system with purified components, factor Va has a similar effect and increases the affinity of APC for the membrane approximately 10-fold.[33] Intact factor V gives a fivefold increase in the affinity of APC for the membrane, suggesting that APC may interact with both factor Va and factor V. Even though APC seems to interact with factor V, it is much more efficient in cleaving factor Va than factor V.[5–10, 13, 23, 24] The structural basis for the specificity of this reaction is unknown. Nor is it known whether the positive effects of protein S and factor Va on APC binding to phospholipid are additive.

Activated Protein C and Fibrinolysis

It has been reported that APC possesses profibrinolytic activity.[34–41] When infused into dogs, APC was found to enhance clot lysis and increase the level of circulating plasminogen activator.[35, 36] It was concluded that the accelerating effect of APC on fibrinolysis was mediated by a second messenger and that both cells and plasma were required for the generation of this messenger. A profibrinolytic effect of APC has also been found in cats.[38] In contrast, neither APC infusion nor activation of endogenous protein C in squirrel monkeys increased the fibrinolytic activity.[40] Moreover, an essentially normal fibrinolytic system in homozygous protein C–deficient patients argues against an important function of protein C in the fibrinolytic system.[42] In vitro, profibrinolytic effects of APC can be demonstrated using blood clot lysis, plasma lysis, or euglobulin clot lysis.[37, 39–41] In vitro, the profibrinolytic effects of APC are due at least in part to complex formation between APC and the endothelial cell–related plasminogen activator inhibitor (PAI-1).[41] Although findings in several studies suggest a profibrinolytic effect of APC, the results are conflicting and difficult to evaluate, and the in vivo function of protein C in fibrinolysis in humans remains to be established.

Inhibition of Activated Protein C

Activated protein C is slowly neutralized in plasma, and its half-life in the circulation is 15 to 20 minutes.[28,]

[30, 43, 44] Both in vivo and in vitro, APC is inhibited by two serpins, PCI and α_1-antitrypsin.[16–19] Recently, α_2-macroglobulin has also been found to inhibit APC.[20, 21] The APC-PCI interaction is stimulated by heparin, whereas the inhibition of APC by α_1-antitrypsin is heparin independent. α_1-Antitrypsin and α_2-macroglobulin are major protease inhibitors in blood, circulating at concentrations of approximately 1.4 g/l (25 μM) and 2 g/l (2.5 μM), respectively. The plasma concentration of PCI, a single-chain glycoprotein with a molecular weight of 57,000, is much lower, 5 mg/l (90 nM).[16] Recently, it was found that the concentration of PCI is approximately 40-fold higher in seminal plasma, where it is an important inhibitor of serine proteases from the prostatic gland.[45, 46] Complementary DNA (cDNA) cloning showed that the mature PCI molecule contains 387 amino acid residues.[16] The sequence identities with both α_1-antitrypsin and α_1-antichymotrypsin are approximately 42 per cent. The reactive site for APC is Arg 354—Ser 355. In the absence of heparin, PCI is a slow inhibitor of APC. Once complexes are formed between APC and PCI, they are rapidly cleared from the circulation. The complexes between APC and α_1-antitrypsin have a much longer in vivo half-life than do the APC-PCI complexes.[43, 47] The long half-life of APC and its specificity for the activated forms of factors V and VIII are prerequisites for the proper function of APC as a circulating anticoagulant in vivo.

Structure-Function Relationships

Protein C is a zymogen of a serine protease with a plasma concentration of 3 to 5 μg/ml.[5–10] It is synthesized in the liver as a 461 amino acid single-chain precursor that contains a signal peptide and a propeptide.[48–50] Prior to secretion, the 42 amino acid preproleader sequence is removed by two proteolytic cleavages, first by a signal peptidase at Gly −25 and then by the propeptide-processing enzyme at Arg −1.[51] The propeptide in protein C is similar to propeptides in the other vitamin K–dependent proteins and is recognized by the vitamin K–dependent carboxylase. (See Chapter 16.) Single-chain protein C is cleaved between Arg 157 and Thr 158 by an enzyme with trypsin-like specificity, in the Golgi apparatus. In a subsequent step, presumably in plasma, Arg 157 and Lys 156 (numbering from the NH_2-terminus of the mature single-chain protein) are removed by an as yet unidentified enzyme with carboxypeptidase B–like specificity.[52] Similar removal of basic residues by a carboxypeptidase B–like enzyme occurs in several other plasma proteins, such as in factor X, and in the complement proteins C3 and C4.[53–56] In human plasma, approximately 85 per cent of protein C consists of two polypeptide chains linked by a single disulfide bridge, whereas the remaining 15 per cent is single-chain protein C.[57] Single- and two-chain protein C both appear to have equal biological activities after activation. The light and heavy chains of protein C in plasma contain 155 and 262 amino acids, respectively, and the apparent molecular weight of the mature protein is approximately 62,000. The molecular weight calculated from the amino acid sequence of the apoprotein is 47,456. The carbohydrate content is approximately 23 per cent divided among four N-linked carbohydrate side chains, one in the light chain and three in the heavy chain. The amino acid sequence identity between human and bovine protein C is 74 per cent, and the identity between the two species at the nucleotide level is 82 per cent.[10, 48–50, 58]

The mature protein C molecule contains a Gla module, two epidermal growth factor (EGF)–like modules and a serine protease module (Fig. 17–3). The Gla module in human protein C contains 9 Gla residues and that of bovine protein C 11.[48–50, 58] Although its three-dimensional structure has not been determined, the pronounced sequence similarity to the Gla module in prothrombin suggests that both its three-dimensional structure and its Ca^{2+}-binding properties are similar to those of prothrombin fragment 1.[59] In its calcium-saturated conformation, the Gla module interacts with negatively charged phospholipid, but during activation of protein C, the Gla module appears to interact directly with TM.[5, 60, 61] In vitro mutagenesis studies have shown that Gla residues at positions 6, 7, 19, and 20 are important for the anticoagulant properties of APC. Replacement of the Gla residues with Asp yielded molecules with low anticoagulant activity.[62, 63] The integrity of the hexapeptide disulfide loop present in the Gla module was also found to be crucial for the anticoagulant function of APC. The first EGF-like module in protein C is unique in that it contains two cysteine residues (at positions 59 and 64), which have no counterpart in other EGF-like modules. These cysteines presumably form a disulfide loop. The Asp residue in position 71 of protein C—that is, in the first EGF-like module—is hydroxylated to erythro-β-hydroxyaspartic acid (Hya).[64] The Hya residue has been implicated in the Ca^{2+} binding of the NH$_2$-terminal EGF module. Mutation of the Hya residue to Glu results in a functionally defective molecule with low calcium affinity and low biological activity.[65] In the second EGF-like module, there is an N-linked carbohydrate side chain at Asn 97 immediately NH$_2$-terminal of the first cysteine residue. In vitro mutation of this residue to Gln has shown the glycosylation at Asn 97 to be critical for efficient secretion of protein C and to affect the degree of glycosylation at Asn 329.[66] On the basis of indirect evidence, it has been suggested that the first EGF-like module in protein C interacts with the thrombin-sensitive region and the first EGF module in protein S.[65, 67] During protein C activation by the thrombin-TM complex, the Gla module and the two EGF-like modules account for most of the binding energy of protein C for the thrombin-TM complex.[68] In a recent report, it was demonstrated that in experiments using analytical ultracentrifugation the Gla module of protein C binds directly to TM and to the thrombin-TM complex.[69]

Thrombin activates human protein C by cleavage of the peptide bond between Arg 169 and Leu 170.[10] The 12 amino acid residue long activation peptide (residues 158 to 169 of the intact molecule) is rapidly eliminated from the circulation.[70] Recently, a mutant recombinant protein C was expressed, in which the activation peptide was replaced by an octapeptide derived from the insulin receptor precursor protein: Pro-Arg-Pro-Ser-Arg-Lys-Arg-Arg.[71] This peptide is cleaved COOH-terminal of the four basic residues when the insulin receptor precursor is converted to the two-chain form. The expected processing on the COOH-terminal end of the four basic residues also occurred in protein C, resulting in the secretion of active enzyme.

The heavy chain of protein C contains seven cysteine residues. Cys 277 forms a disulfide bridge with Cys 141 of the light chain.[10] There are intrachain disulfide bridges between Cys 196 and Cys 212, Cys 331 and Cys 345, and Cys 356 and Cys 384, positions conserved among the serine proteases. The heavy chain of human protein C contains three N-linked carbohydrate side chains at positions Asn 248, Asn 313, and Asn 329.[49, 50] The glycosylation site on Asn 329 is unusual

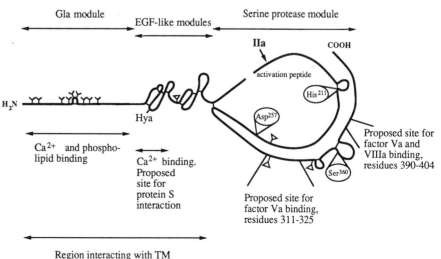

FIGURE 17–3. Human protein C. Schematic model demonstrating the modular composition of protein C. The arrow indicates the thrombin (IIa) cleavage site, leading to activation of protein C. The amino acid residues in the catalytic triad are enclosed in the ovals. Human protein C contains nine Gla residues (Y) and four potential sites for N-linked glycosylation (Y).

in that it appears in the sequence Asn-X-Cys rather than the commonly encountered Asn-X-Ser/Thr.[72] A similar glycosylation pattern has been found in von Willebrand factor.[73] Approximately 30 per cent of protein C in human plasma is not glycosylated at Asn 329.[74] This so-called β form of protein C has lower molecular weight than does fully glycosylated protein C, but the biological activities of the two forms are similar. It has been suggested that the degree of glycosylation of Asn 329 is partly determined by the rate of disulfide bond formation during protein folding.[74]

The catalytic triad in human protein C comprises His 211, Asp 257, and Ser 360.[10, 49, 50] The heavy chain of protein C is homologous to the other serine proteinases, with sequence identities ranging from 60 to 70 per cent vis-à-vis chymotrypsin, trypsin, and factors IX and X.[72] After activation, Leu 170 occupies the NH_2-terminus of the heavy chain, and it probably forms an ion pair with Asp 359. In this respect, protein C is unusual, as all other serine proteases have Val or Ile in the N-terminal position of the activated enzyme. By analogy with other serine proteases,[75] Asp 354 probably is located in the S1 site (nomenclature as in reference 76). APC cleaves substrates with Arg in the P1 position. The natural substrates, factors Va and VIIIa, have Arg, Glu, Leu, or Pro in the P2 position, whereas the P3 position is Gln, Asp, or Glu.[13, 23, 27] Factor Va and VIIIa are the only known physiologically important substrates for APC. It is not known which structural features give APC this narrow specificity, but it probably involves an interaction between the substrate and a secondary binding site on APC located outside the catalytic center, as in factor IX and thrombin. Recently, a synthetic peptide corresponding to residues 311 to 325 of protein C was demonstrated to inhibit APC-mediated degradation of factor Va, suggesting that this region in APC provides the binding site for factor Va.[77] In another report, the same authors have identified a sequence of human APC (residues 390 to 404) that is essential for its anticoagulant activity.[78] Monovalent cations stimulate the amidolytic activity of APC. Cs^+ is a more effective stimulator than Li^+ or Na^+, suggesting that the stimulatory effect increases with increasing ionic radius.[10, 79, 80] In addition, Ca^{2+} has a moderate stimulatory effect on the amidolytic activity of protein C.[79]

Gene Structure

Protein C synthesis appears to be confined to the liver.[10, 48–50, 81] The messenger RNA (mRNA) for human protein C is 1800 to 1850 nucleotides (nt) long, with a minor species (<10 per cent) that is approximately 200 nt shorter.[49] The protein C mRNA contains a short 5' untranslated region of 75 nt. The 461 amino acid precursor protein is encoded by 1383 nt, and the 3' non-coding region contains 296 nt. The polyadenylation signal AATAAA is 19 nt upstream of the polyadenylation segment. An alternative polyadenylation recognition sequence (ATTAAA) is located 229 nt upstream of this region. The smaller mRNA species may result from utilization of the latter polyadenylation signal.[49, 81]

The protein C gene is located on chromosome 2, position q14–q21, and is approximately 11 kilobases (kb) long.[82–87] The transcription start site has been identified 10,772 nt upstream of the polyadenylation site.[86] The gene is composed of 9 exons and 8 introns.[86] All the intron/exon boundaries follow the GT/AG rule. In protein C, as in factors VII, IX, and X, the modules in the non-catalytic part of the protein are encoded by separate exons. (See Chapter 16.) Exon 1 encodes the 5' untranslated segment and exon 2 the signal peptide (Met −42 to Gly −25) and six amino acids of the propeptide. Exon 3 encodes the rest of the propeptide and the Gla module (Asp −19 to Thr 37). The connecting segment between the Gla module and the EGF module is encoded by exon 4, and the two EGF modules are encoded by exons 5 and 6. The serine protease part is encoded by three exons corresponding to those observed in factors VII, IX, and X. The splice-junction types are also conserved between the four genes. Exon 7 encodes the C-terminal part of the light chain, the activation peptide, and the first 27 amino acids of the heavy chain. Exon 8 encodes Val 185 to Leu 223 in the heavy chain, and exon 9 the COOH-terminal part of the heavy chain. Sequence similarities between protein C and factors VII, IX, and X (35 to 40 per cent), as well as the conservation of intron locations and splice-junction types, attest to the common evolutionary origin of these proteins. However, there are no similarities in sequence or size between the introns of the four genes.[86, 87]

THROMBOMODULIN

Thrombin is in itself a poor activator of protein C, and it was not until the discovery of TM that its physiological role as the activator of protein C was fully appreciated and the concept of a protein C anticoagulant system emerged.[5–10] In the experiments that led to the discovery of TM, the coronary circulation in a so-called Langendorff heart preparation (an isolated rabbit heart) was simultaneously perfused with thrombin and protein C.[88] During its passage through the capillary system, protein C was rapidly activated by thrombin reversibly bound to a high-affinity receptor on the endothelium. This receptor was named thrombomodulin, since binding of thrombin to TM is associated with a dramatic change in the specificity of thrombin. Bound thrombin is a potent activator of protein C but has lost its procoagulant properties, including the ability to coagulate fibrinogen and to activate platelets and factors V, VIII, and XIII.[5–10, 89–93] Soon after the initial description, TM was solubilized with detergents and isolated from rabbit lung endothelium using thrombin-affinity chromatography.[94] It was later purified from human placenta and from bovine, mouse, and rat lung.[93, 95–97] The structures of bovine, human, and mouse TM, known from cDNA cloning, are highly conserved; the amino acid sequence of mouse TM is, for instance, 68 per cent identical to its human counterpart.[98–103]

Structure-Function Relationships

Thrombomodulin is a multimodular membrane-spanning protein, with an extracellular amino-terminus (Fig. 17–4). After proteolytic removal of a signal peptide 18 amino acid residues long, the mature single-chain human glycoprotein contains 557 amino acid residues.[99–101] The molecular weight of the apoprotein is 60,300. From its NH_2-terminus, TM contains a lectin-like module (residues 1 to 154), a hydrophobic region (residues 155 to 222), six EGF-like modules (residues 223 to 462), a Ser/Thr-rich region (residues

463 to 497), a transmembrane module 23 amino acid residues long (residues 498 to 521), and a cytoplasmic tail 35 amino acid residues long (residues 522 to 557). Human TM contains five potential sites for N-linked carbohydrate side-chain attachment and seven potential O-glycosylation sites (Ser/Thr-X-X-Pro sequence).[99] Three of the potential O-glycosylation sites are in the Ser/Thr-rich region, two in the hydrophobic region (residues 155 to 222), and two in the EGF modules. The Ser/Thr-rich region, in addition, has a consensus sequence for the attachment of a sulfated glycosaminoglycan (Ser-Gly-X-Gly; Ser 472—Gly 475).[104, 105]

The amino-terminal 154 residues of TM are homologous to the lectin modules in the hepatic asialoglycoprotein receptor, the IgE receptor, and members of the selectin family, including ELAM-1 (endothelial leukocyte adhesion molecule–1), LAM-1 (leukocyte adhesion molecule–1), and GMP-140 (granule membrane protein of 140 kDa).[106–108] It is not known whether TM has any lectin-like properties. The lectin module of TM contains eight cysteines, and the pairing of three disulfide bridges is suggested from the lectin homology: Cys 12—Cys 17, Cys 34—Cys 149, and Cys 119—Cys 140.[107] Cys 78 is probably linked to Cys 115, as most other lectins lack cysteines in corresponding positions, but it cannot be excluded that these cysteines form disulfide bridges with Cys 157 and Cys 206. We find it more likely, however, that the two cysteines that are located in the 68 residue long hydrophobic region form a disulfide bridge.

The six tandem EGF modules contain sites for thrombin binding and protein C interaction. The function of the EGF-like modules in TM was suggested when an elastase fragment, consisting of the six EGF-like modules, was found to catalyze thrombin activation of protein C.[61] A 10 kDa cyanogen bromide fragment (designated CB3), composed of the fifth and sixth EGF-like modules (residues 389 to 468), was later found to bind thrombin with high affinity but had no cofactor activity.[109] It functioned as an inhibitor in protein C activation by the thrombin-TM complex by competing with TM for binding to thrombin. The CB3 fragment also lowered the rate of thrombin-catalyzed fibrinopeptide release from fibrinogen, indicating that the fifth and sixth EGF modules contain enough structural information to alter the substrate specificity of thrombin. Thrombin binding to TM is inhibited by two linear peptides derived from the sequence of the latter half of the fifth EGF-like module, suggesting that the thrombin-binding site is located on this module.[110, 111] In human, mouse, and bovine TM, the fifth EGF-like module contains an N-linked carbohydrate side chain. It does not influence thrombin binding, and its function is unknown. A fragment (CB23), containing the third to the sixth EGF modules (residues 292 to 468), binds thrombin and in addition accelerates protein C activation.[112] The third or fourth EGF-like module thus seems to interact with protein C. Experiments using recombinant TM have corroborated that thrombin binds to the fifth EGF module and that the site for protein C interaction

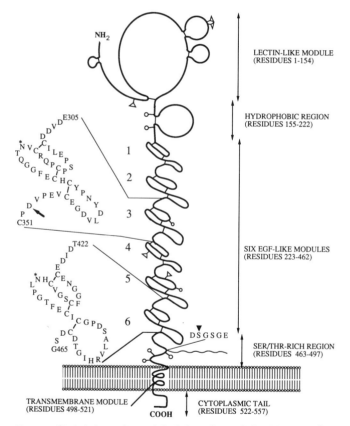

FIGURE 17–4. Schematic model of thrombomodulin (TM). TM is a single-chain membrane protein composed of different modules, as indicated in the figure. The organization of the disulfide bonds is tentative and based on homology with other proteins, in which disulfide bond locations have been experimentally determined (see the text). The amino acid sequences of the third and sixth EGF-like modules are shown, as their sequences suggest that they contain very high-affinity calcium-binding sites. The asterisks denote the positions of potential β-hydroxylated asparagines. The arrow indicates Asp 349, which has been implicated in the interaction of TM with the Gla module of protein C. The wavy line in the Ser/Thr-rich region symbolizes the glycosaminoglycan, and the probable site for its attachment is shown. Ser 472 is indicated by the arrowhead. The positions of the potential O- (♀) and N-linked (Y) carbohydrate side chains are indicated.

is on the fourth EGF module.[110, 113, 114] Deletion mutants of TM containing EGF modules 4 to 6 express full cofactor activity in thrombin-catalyzed protein C activation.[110] When TM fragments or recombinant deletion mutants of TM were used as cofactors to thrombin, intact protein C was found to be activated more rapidly than protein C lacking the Gla module.[61, 110, 113–115] This finding suggests that the Gla module of protein C is involved in the calcium-dependent interaction between protein C and EGF-like modules in TM. In vitro mutagenesis experiments recently demonstrated that Asp 349—that is, the beginning of the fourth EGF-like module of TM—is crucial for this calcium-dependent interaction.[116]

The third and sixth EGF modules of TM contain the consensus sequence for post-translational modification of asparagine to β-hydroxyasparagine (Hyn).[117] There is also a partial hydroxylation of the appropriate Asn residue (or residues).[118] Recently, the side-chain carboxyl group of the β-hydroxylated aspartic acid residue in the NH$_2$-terminal EGF module of factor X was found to be a Ca^{2+} ligand.[119] In intact factor X, this site binds Ca^{2+} with a K$_d$ of approximately 50 μM. The Hyn-containing EGF modules in protein S bind calcium with much higher affinity (K$_d$ in the nanomolar range).[120] The amino acids implicated in the high-affinity Ca^{2+} binding in protein S are conserved in the third and sixth EGF modules of TM (see Fig. 16–4).[99–101] It is therefore likely that these EGF modules in TM contain very high-affinity calcium-binding sites. In protein S, high-affinity calcium-binding sites must be saturated to ensure a native conformation and stability of the EGF modules.[120] The putative calcium-binding sites in TM presumably fulfill similar functions. A recently described monoclonal antibody, which reacted with a Ca^{2+}-dependent epitope in TM, lends support to the hypothesis that Ca^{2+} is required for TM to attain a native conformation.[121] The interactions between calcium and TM and their functional significance have, however, not been studied in detail.

The 34 amino acid residue long Ser/Thr-rich segment, located between the EGF modules and the membrane-spanning region, contains three to four potential sites for O-linked carbohydrate side chains.[99–101] A sulfated glycosaminoglycan, important for the expression of full anticoagulant activity, is located in this region.[122–127] The site for attachment is presumably Ser 472, as the Ser-Gly-Ser-Gly sequence (positions 472 to 475) is consistent with the consensus sequence for glycosaminoglycan attachment (Ser-Gly-X-Gly).[104, 105] The glycosaminoglycan has been isolated from rabbit TM and chemically characterized as a chondroitin sulfate.[128, 129] The importance of the sulfated glycosaminoglycan for TM to express full anticoagulant activity was first demonstrated in rabbit TM and more recently in recombinant human TM.[115, 122, 125–129] When the chondroitin sulfate side chain is released from TM, as, for instance, by chondroitin ABC-lyase digestion, the molecular weight of TM decreases by about 10,000, and its affinity for thrombin is reduced by a factor of 2 to 3.[115, 122, 130, 131] The glycosaminoglycan

moiety thus contributes, albeit little, to the binding of thrombin to TM. It has indirect anticoagulant effects as it stimulates the inhibition of thrombin by AT III. The chondroitin sulfate chain also appears to be important for the direct (AT III–independent) anticoagulant activity of TM, as recombinant soluble TM lacking the glycosaminoglycan moiety has relatively small inhibitory effect on thrombin-induced platelet activation and fibrinogen clotting.[115, 130, 131] The glycosaminoglycan is not directly involved in protein C activation but affects the calcium dependence of the reaction (see below). The chondroitin sulfate moiety is important for TM to express full anticoagulant activity on the cell surface. Thus, endothelial cells treated with β-D-xyloside (inhibits glycosaminoglycan attachment) manifest a thrombin-TM interaction with threefold to fivefold lower affinity than that found on untreated cells, paralleled by a reduction in the rate of protein C activation on the cell surface.[132]

The transmembrane part of TM is the region where sequence conservation between species is most pronounced.[98–103] Whether this feature reflects a signaling function is unknown. The cytoplasmic tail is short and has potential phosphorylation sites. Mouse TM is phosphorylated in hemangioma cells after treatment with phorbol myristate acetate (PMA) or dimethyl sulfoxide.[102] The phosphorylation event is associated with increased endocytosis and degradation of TM.

Location of Thrombomodulin

Thrombomodulin is present on the vascular surface of endothelial cells of arteries, veins, capillaries, and lymphatic vessels.[133, 134] In humans, it is present in all blood vessels, with the notable exception of vessels in the central nervous system, where it has been difficult to identify.[135] However, recently, regional distribution of TM in human brain was reported.[136] Hepatic sinusoids and postcapillary venules of lymph nodes do not appear to contain TM.[133] TM is present at low levels in platelets, approximately 60 molecules per platelet.[137] It has been found on squamous epithelium of the epidermis, on a variety of cultured cells, and on endothelial cell neoplasms.[138, 139] A soluble form, presumably a proteolytic product, has been identified in human plasma at approximately 20 ng/ml and in urine.[140] The physiological function of soluble TM is not known.

Function of the Thrombin-Thrombomodulin Complex

Protein C is rapidly activated on the endothelial cell surface by the thrombin-TM complex and possibly also by factor Xa, although the functional significance of the latter reaction remains to be elucidated.[5–10, 88, 94, 141–143] In addition, it has been reported that human factor Va, and its isolated light chain, can function as cofactors in thrombin-mediated activation of protein

C.[144] The activity of the factor Va light chain as thrombin cofactor was approximately 1/20 that of TM, and the in vivo functional significance of this activity is unknown.[145] Thrombin binds TM with high affinity ($K_d = 0.2 - 0.5 \times 10^{-9}$ M) in the formation of a 1:1 complex (Fig. 17–5).[88, 141] It has been demonstrated that bovine meizothrombin (a prothrombin activation intermediate) binds TM with the same affinity as thrombin and that protein C is efficiently activated by the meizothrombin-TM complex.[146] In a more recent study, a human prothrombin mutant, S205A, in which the active-site serine was replaced with alanine, was used to generate stable but catalytically inactive human thrombin and meizothrombin. Meizothrombin S205A did not demonstrate any affinity for TM, whereas thrombin S205A was found to bind to recombinant human TM with the same affinity as normal thrombin.[147] These results suggest that human meizothrombin is unlikely to be an important TM-dependent protein C activator. The active site of the thrombin molecule is approximately 65 Å away from the membrane surface when it is bound to TM, as estimated with a fluorescence energy transfer technique.[148] Activation of protein C by thrombin alone is very slow, but the formation of the thrombin-TM complex results in a more than 20,000-fold increase in the activation rate.[5, 6, 88, 141] The K_m for protein C in this system is approximately 0.5 μM. On binding to TM, thrombin is converted from a procoagulant to an anticoagulant enzyme. It loses its ability to clot fibrinogen and to activate factors V, VIII, and XIII and platelets.[5, 6, 89–93] These effects have been demonstrated with rabbit

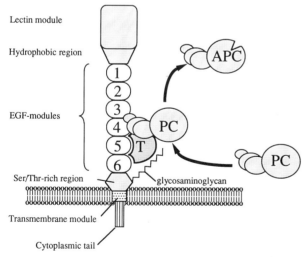

FIGURE 17–5. Modular organization of TM and schematic representation of the molecular interactions occurring during protein C activation. The single high-affinity thrombin (T)-binding site in TM is located in the fifth EGF-like module. The glycosaminoglycan side chain of TM appears to interact with the bound thrombin. It is important for expression of full anticoagulant activity of TM and is also required for stimulation of antithrombin III (AT III)–dependent inhibition of bound thrombin. Most experimental results suggest that protein C (PC) interacts with the fourth EGF-like module of TM. The light chain of protein C, containing the Gla module and the two EGF-like modules, accounts for most of the binding energy of protein C for TM.

Labels on figure: Lectin module; Hydrophobic region; EGF-modules; Ser/Thr-rich region; Transmembrane module; Cytoplasmic tail; glycosaminoglycan; APC; PC; T; 1 2 3 4 5 6

and bovine TM but have not been found with human TM purified from placenta.[149, 150] However, recent results suggest that purified human TM often is contaminated with the multifunctional plasma protein vitronectin, which may bind to the glycosaminoglycan and affect the anticoagulant activity of TM.[122] Consistent with this interpretation, a soluble recombinant form of human TM that contained the glycosaminoglycan side chain but no contaminating vitronectin was found to inhibit the procoagulant and platelet-activating activities of thrombin.[115, 130, 131] Thrombin bound to rabbit TM can be inactivated by AT III, a reaction catalyzed by the glycosaminoglycan present on TM. This effect, which has not been demonstrated with TM isolated from bovine[93, 96] and human[95, 149–151] sources, is, however, expressed by recombinant human TM.[130, 131] Modulation of the activity of thrombin by TM is crucial for proper function of the protein C anticoagulant system and for the regulation of blood coagulation in vivo.[5, 6, 152, 153]

There are 0.3 to 1.0 × 10[5] TM molecules per endothelial cell.[154] Within the circulation, the endothelial cell surface area per unit of blood volume increases dramatically as the blood passes from the larger vessels to the capillaries.[155] Assuming the number of TM molecules per endothelial cell to be independent of vessel diameter, the concentration of solid-phase TM in the microcirculation is more than 1000-fold higher than in the major vessels, ensuring that thrombin will be bound to endothelial TM, even at thrombin concentrations that are nonthrombogenic. In larger vessels, thrombin will be free, but as soon as the blood enters the microcirculation, it will encounter TM, and protein C will be activated. In this context, it should be noted that the half-life of APC in vivo is approximately 20 minutes because of the slow rate of inhibition by protease inhibitors.[5, 6, 28, 29, 43] Owing to the accumulation of thrombin in the microvasculature, the TM-mediated modulation of thrombin from a procoagulant to an anticoagulant enzyme is crucially important. In vivo, thrombin bound to TM will be either inhibited by AT III or removed by endocytosis of the thrombin-TM complex, and the half-life of the thrombin-TM compex on the cell membrane is less than 15 seconds.[5] The balance between the procoagulant and anticoagulant effects of thrombin in vivo is delicate, as illustrated by the dramatic thrombotic disorder accompanying homozygous protein C deficiency.[22]

The role of Ca^{2+} in the activation of protein C by thrombin is complex. On the one hand, it inhibits activation by thrombin alone, and on the other, it is required for activation of protein C by the thrombin-TM complex.[88, 94, 141, 156] Although protein C activation by the thrombin-TM complex is Ca^{2+} dependent, recent experiments demonstrate that binding of thrombin or protein C to TM does not require calcium.[69, 94] Both TM and protein C contain different types of Ca^{2+}-binding sites, which are important for protein C activation. Binding of Ca^{2+} to an intact Gla module of protein C is required for optimal activation of protein C, not only by the phospholipid-bound thrombin-TM complex but also by thrombin bound either to soluble TM fragments or to recombinant deletion mutants of TM containing the fourth to sixth EGF-like modules.[61, 113–115, 157–159] The requirement of the Gla module of protein C for rapid activation by thrombin bound to the soluble TM derivatives indicates that the Gla module of protein C interacts directly with the EGF-like modules of TM.[113, 114] A direct interaction between the Gla module of protein C and the elastase fragment of TM was recently demonstrated in experiments using ultracentrifugation.[69]

Further support for the hypothesis that the Gla module interacts with TM rather than with the phospholipid membrane derives from findings in phospholipid reconstitution experiments. Incorporation of rabbit TM into neutral phosphatidylcholine phospholipid vesicles reduced the K_m for protein C from 7.6 μM to 0.7 μM, but membrane incorporation had no effect on activation of protein C lacking the Gla module.[159] The K_m for protein C on phosphatidylcholine vesicles was similar to that observed on endothelial cells, suggesting that the Gla module does not interact with the negatively charged phospholipid but with TM. It was proposed that the incorporation of TM into neutral phospholipid results in the exposure of a binding site for the Gla module of protein C on the TM molecule, a binding site that is also exposed on soluble TM fragments.[110, 112–114, 116, 159] The observation that the activation of protein C does not require the exposure of negatively charged phospholipid may be physiologically important, as TM is present on the vessel wall surface of intact endothelial cells, where negatively charged phospholipid is not normally exposed. However, it should be borne in mind that rabbit and human TM may be different in the requirement for acidic phospholipid, because in phospholipid reconstitution experiments using human TM, protein C was found to be more rapidly activated on acidic phospholipid vesicles than on neutral vesicles.[160]

Activation of protein C on intact endothelium, or on phospholipid vesicles with reconstituted TM, is optimal at 2 mM of calcium. When either soluble TM fragments or recombinant deletion mutants of TM (containing the fourth to sixth EGF-like modules) were used as cofactors and the rate of protein C activation was plotted as a function of the Ca^{2+} concentration, a bell-shaped curve with a maximum at 0.3 mM of Ca^{2+} was obtained.[5, 6, 156, 159, 160] This type of curve was seen only when intact protein C and TM lacking the glycosaminoglycan were used, suggesting that the glycosaminoglycan somehow affects the site on TM that interacts with the protein C Gla module.[61, 113–115] Asp 349 is part of this site, as site-directed mutagenesis to Ala resulted in loss of the typical bell-shaped Ca^{2+} titration curve, which was replaced by a curve with a hyperbolic shape.[116]

Saturation of Gla-independent Ca^{2+}-binding sites in protein C is also important for rapid protein C activation, as reflected in the calcium requirement by the thrombin-TM complex for activation of protein C lacking the Gla module.[157, 158] The location of this calcium-binding site has not been unraveled. The NH_2-terminal EGF-like module of protein C binds Ca^{2+}, but whether this is relevant to the activation process is unknown.[157, 161] Protein C may also contain another Ca^{2+}-binding site of unknown physiological importance in its heavy chain. (See Chapter 16.) Moreover, Ca^{2+} binding to protein C affects the conformation of the activation peptide close to the thrombin cleavage site either directly or indirectly. In vitro mutagenesis of Asp 167 in protein C (P3 position in the thrombin cleavage site) to either Gly or Phe alters the calcium response of the mutant protein C.[162] In the presence of calcium, the activation rates of these mutants by thrombin alone were fivefold to eightfold higher than that of wild-type protein C. Mutant protein C was also more rapidly activated by the thrombin-TM complex. Asp 167 in the activation peptide is thus important for the calcium-induced inhibition of protein C activation by thrombin. The importance of calcium for protein-protein interactions involving the activation peptide has been illustrated by results obtained with a monoclonal antibody (HPC4), which reacts with an epitope spanning residues Glu 163 to Lys 174. The interaction between this epitope and the antibody is calcium dependent, even though neither the antibody nor the peptide alone binds calcium. Thus, both protein C and the antibody appear to contribute ligands to the calcium ion.[163]

Thrombomodulin Modulates the Substrate Specificity of Thrombin

Binding of TM to a site on the thrombin molecule that is distinct from its catalytic center modulates the substrate specificity of thrombin in an anticoagulant direction.[10, 101, 11, 165–171] This is due both to steric hindrance restricting the accessibility of the active site of thrombin and to allosteric conformational changes in the active site of thrombin. The steric barrier caused by TM binding to thrombin is evident from experiments showing direct competition between TM, fibrinogen, hirudin, and factor V for binding to thrombin.[111] The TM-binding site on thrombin seems to overlap, at least in part, with the so-called anion-binding exosite, which also interacts with fibrinogen, hirudin, factors, V, VIII, and XIII, and the recently characterized platelet receptor for thrombin.[164] By using spin-labeled active site inhibitors to thrombin, it was demonstrated that TM binding induces allosteric conformation changes in the active site of thrombin.[165, 166] Similar changes are induced by acidic synthetic peptides corresponding to segments of several nonhomologous thrombin inhibitors.[167]

The binding site for TM on thrombin appears to be discontinuous, involving at least two different regions. A monoclonal antibody against an epitope located between Thr 147 and Asp 175 (the number indicates position in the linear amino acid sequence of the B chain) of thrombin was found to block the thrombin-TM interaction, and a synthetic peptide corresponding to Thr 147 to Ser 158 inhibited the binding of thrombin to TM.[168] The peptide also inhibited the procoagulant activity of thrombin, suggesting that it contained a fibrinogen-binding site.[169] Other investigators have suggested that the region comprising residues Arg 62 to Arg 73 of the B chain of thrombin, which is in the so-called anion-binding exosite, interacts not only with fibrinogen and hirudin but also with TM.[170, 171] The three-dimensional structure of thrombin is similar to that of other trypsin-like proteases, but with loops protruding around the active site, narrowing the substrate-binding cleft.[172–174]

Recent site-directed mutagenesis studies have revealed that mutation of either Arg 68 or Arg 70 in thrombin to Glu compromises TM binding and reduces the rate of protein C activation.[175] Both these residues contribute to the positive charge of the anion-binding exosite of thrombin.[172–174] It is interesting that the Arg 68 to Glu mutation lost the ability to clot fibrinogen and activate platelets, whereas the Arg 70 mutant was normal in both respects. The results suggest that the TM- and fibrinogen-binding sites on thrombin overlap but are not identical.[175] Protein C has Asp residues in both positions 167 and 172, which correspond to the P3 and P'3 positions in relation to the thrombin cleavage site. Unlike trypsin, thrombin is a poor enzyme for cleavage of peptides with acidic residues in these positions. This was recently demonstrated to be at least partly due to Glu 202 (Glu 192 according to the chymotrypsinogen numbering[172]) in thrombin, which is located three residues from the active site Ser 205. Most trypsin-like proteases have Gln in this position, and site-directed mutagenesis of Glu202 to Gln yielded a thrombin that was more efficient in activating protein C.[176] The increased efficiency was more pronounced in the absence of TM (22-fold) than in its presence (2-fold). The thrombin-catalyzed release of fibrinopeptide A was not influenced. It was concluded that Glu 202 in thrombin is important in restricting the substrate specificity of thrombin and that TM binding to thrombin alters the enzyme-substrate interaction near this residue.[176] The Asp residues in the P3 position and in the P'3 position appear to contribute to slow activation of protein C by thrombin in the absence of TM, as the rate of thrombin cleavage of a peptide that corresponded to P7 to P'5 in protein C (residues 163 to 174) was 30 times lower than the cleavage rate of a similar peptide, but with Gly residues replacing the Asp residues at the P3 and P'3 positions.[176, 177]

Gene Structure and Regulation of Expression

A single TM gene in the human genome is located on chromosome 20, position p12-cen.[100, 101, 178, 179] The TM gene is unusual in that it contains no introns. Northern blotting of human endothelial and placental RNA revealed a single mRNA species 3.7 kb long.[100] Human full-length cDNA clones contain an approximately 150 nt long 5' untranslated segment, a coding region of 1725 bp, and a 1779 bp long 3' untranslated segment.[91, 100] The 3' untranslated region is highly conserved between mouse, human, and bovine TM.[98–103] All three species contain the sequence TTATTTAT, which has been suggested to be associated with short mRNA half-lives.[180] However, since the half-life of TM mRNA in the mouse is about 9 hours, the sequence does not appear to have this effect in the TM mRNA.

Thrombomodulin is one of several important anticoagulant activities expressed on the surface of endothelial cells, and the level of TM expression is regulated by a variety of mechanisms. It has been proposed that the TM level on endothelium is regulated by internalization and degradation and that internalization is induced by the binding of thrombin.[154] The thrombin in the complex is believed to be transported to the lysosomes, where it is released and degraded, whereas TM is recirculated to the cell surface. This endocytosis has been found to be inhibited by protein C.[181] A similar recycling of TM has been found on A549 lung cancer cells, whereas no internalization and recycling of TM was found when endothelial cells from human saphenous veins or an endothelial cell line, EA.hy 926, were studied.[182] Inflammatory mediators such as endotoxin, interleukin 1 (IL-1), and tumor necrosis factor (TNF) decrease the surface expression of TM.[183–188] A decrease in the surface concentration of TM has also been observed after exposure of cultured endothelial cells to hypoxia and in association with a viral infection (herpes simplex) of endothelial cell cultures.[189, 190] In parallel to the decreasing TM expression, inflammatory mediators, hypoxia, and herpes simplex infections increased the surface activity of tissue factor (TF). In an in vivo situation, such a shift in the balance between procoagulant and anticoagulant mechanisms favors coagulation and might contribute to the pathogenesis of disseminated intravascular coagulation in gram-negative septicemia. Recently, interleukin-4, a product of activated T cells that exerts anti-inflammatory effects on endothelial cells, was shown to neutralize the downregulation of TM by IL-1, TNF, and endotoxin.[191]

Tumor necrosis factor inhibits transcription of the TM gene in endothelial cells, resulting in decreased mRNA levels and TM synthesis.[188, 191–193] Whether TM internalization and degradation increases after TNF stimulation is controversial. PMA is a potent activator of protein kinase C. In hemangioma cells, it was found to induce endocytosis and degradation after short-term incubation (<6 hours).[102] Under these conditions, TM was not phosphorylated. In vivo, mouse TM was found to be phosphorylated on serine residues, though this is believed not to be due to protein kinase C activity but rather to the action of another phosphorylating enzyme, possibly protein kinase A. Longer incubations with PMA (>6 hr) reversed the down regulation effect by increasing mRNA levels for TM and enhancing surface expression.[194]

Thrombomodulin expression in human umbilical vein endothelial cells, in a human megakaryoblastic leukemia cell line, and in mouse hemangioma cells was found to be upregulated by different agents that increase the intracellular cyclic AMP (cAMP) levels.[194–196] Such agents include dibutyryl cAMP, pentoxifylline, forskolin, and isobutylmethylxanthine. Increased mRNA levels accompanied the increased surface expression, suggesting that cAMP regulates TM gene transcription. Agents that upregulated TM transcription counteracted the effects of IL-1 and TNF. Mouse TM was recently reported to be identical to fetomodulin, a glycoprotein that has been postulated to be involved in developmental organogenesis via quantitative modulation mediated by alterations in intracellular cAMP levels.[197] A recent report demonstrated upregulation of TM expression by activation of histamine H_1 receptors in human umbilical vein endothelial cells in vitro. This effect was not mediated by increased cAMP.[198]

Transcription of the TM gene was increased after treatment of mouse hemangioma cells with cycloheximide and thrombin.[199] Cycloheximide, an inhibitor of protein synthesis, enhanced the TM transcription approximately fourfold. Between a twofold and sevenfold increase in transcription was induced by thrombin, but the effects of thrombin and cycloheximide were not additive. Treatment of the cells with thrombin increased the mRNA levels by approximately 50 per cent, accompanied by a concomitant 50 per cent increase in TM synthesis. The increased transcription in response to cycloheximide has been interpreted as an indication of the existence of a labile protein repressor of TM transcription. The stimulatory effect of thrombin may be mediated by such a repressor. In contrast to the results obtained with hemangioma cells, there was no effect of thrombin on TM expression when human saphenous vein endothelial cells were studied.[185]

Thrombomodulin in Clinical Medicine

Deficiency of TM or functionally defective TM has not yet been found, probably owing to the obvious difficulties in measuring the activity of TM, as it is a membrane protein. A C/T dimorphism in the TM gene predicting an Ala 455 to Val replacement (in the sixth EGF module) was recently described.[200] The allelic frequencies were found to be 82 per cent (Ala) and 18 per cent (Val) in a normal population. In a group of persons with unexplained thrombophilia, the allelic frequencies were found to be the same as in the normal population, indicating that with respect to thrombophilia, the dimorphism is neutral. Lupus anticoagulants—which are antibodies against phospholipid that may be present in the plasma of patients with SLE, for example—have occasionally been found to inhibit TM function in vitro.[201–205] Lupus anticoagulants are more often associated with thrombosis than with bleeding, and inhibition of protein C activation may contribute to the thrombotic tendency in these patients. Lupus anticoagulants can also inhibit other

reactions in the protein C anticoagulant system, and it has been reported that they may inhibit the function of APC or protein S or both.[206] Methods for measuring soluble TM in blood and in the urine have recently been devised.[138, 140, 152, 207] Although the plasma concentration of soluble TM increases when endothelium is injured, the clinical usefulness of TM measurements has not yet been established. Recombinant soluble TM or TM derivatives may become useful therapeutic anticoagulant agents; for example, TM has been used successfully to inhibit thrombin-induced thromboembolism in mice and rats.[97, 208, 209]

PROTEIN S

A Cofactor to Activated Protein C

The concentration of protein S in plasma is 20 to 25 mg/l (0.26 to 0.30 μM).[14, 210] It functions as a cofactor to APC in the degradation of factors Va and VIIIa, although its mechanism of action is unknown.[5, 6, 23, 211–219] However, several mechanisms have been proposed. Protein S has the highest affinity for negatively charged phospholipids among the vitamin K–dependent proteins, and it has been shown to increase the affinity of APC for negatively charged phospholipid.[213, 214, 220] The K_d for APC binding to the phospholipid was estimated to be 1.5×10^{-7} M in the absence of protein S and 1.4×10^{-8} M in its presence.[213] Although it has not been possible to demonstrate an interaction between protein S and APC in fluid phase, they appear to form a complex with 1:1 stoichiometry on the lipid surface.[213, 214] The binding sites on the two proteins may be expressed only after binding to the phospholipid. Factor Xa and APC compete for the same binding site on factor Va, and this is believed to be the mechanism for the factor Xa–mediated protection of factor Va from degradation.[5–10] Protein S has been reported to abrogate the protective effect of factor Xa.[31] Protein S and APC interact on the surface of platelets, on platelet microparticles, and on endothelial cells.[215–217, 221] Protein S binds to cultured bovine endothelial cells ($K_d \approx 10^{-8}$ M), and the presence of APC increases its binding affinity more than 10-fold ($K_d \approx 2 \times 10^{-10}$ M).[217]

Protein S may be involved in the regulation of the classical pathway of the complement system, as approximately 60 per cent of the protein in human plasma occurs in a high molecular weight, non-covalent complex with C4b-binding protein (C4BP) (see below).[14] Only the free form of protein S functions as an APC cofactor.[222–224] The functional significance of this is illustrated by the relationship found between the inherited deficiency of free protein S and the occurrence of thrombosis.[5, 6, 14, 223, 225] Bovine plasma differs from its human counterpart in that it does not contain the complex between protein S and C4BP.[222] It has been reported that bovine plasma contains a protein S–binding protein, distinct from C4BP, which

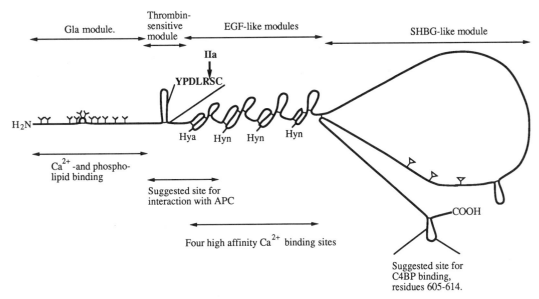

FIGURE 17–6. Schematic representation of human protein S. Human protein S is a single-chain molecule, 635 amino acids long, composed of different modules. The thrombin (IIa) cleavage site, which is conserved in human and bovine protein S, is detailed. The positions of the Hya and the three Hyn residues are shown. Human protein S contains 11 Gla residues (**Y**) and three potential *N*-linked glycosylation sites (**γ**).

functions by increasing the anticoagulant activity of protein S.[226] It is unknown whether there is a human counterpart to this protein.

The Protein S Molecule

Protein S is synthesized in the liver, by endothelial cells, and by testicular Leydig cells.[227–230] It is present at low concentrations in platelets, and it is synthesized by megakaryocytic cell lines.[231, 232] The primary structures of human and bovine protein S have been determined by protein sequencing and cDNA cloning.[233–236] Bovine liver contains one mRNA species of approximately 2.4 kb, whereas its human counterpart is 3.5 kb.[233, 234] The difference between human and bovine mRNA resides in the 3′ untranslated region, which is 826 bp longer in human mRNA. Human protein S is synthesized as a precursor protein with 676 amino acids, of which 41 form a leader sequence that is cleaved off before secretion.[233–236] Mature human protein S is a single-chain glycoprotein (7 to 8 per cent carbohydrate) with 635 amino acids, the bovine counterpart being 1 amino acid shorter.[233–236] The molecular weight of human protein S, calculated from the amino acid composition, is 70,690. Three types of modified amino acids are found in protein S as well as *N*-linked carbohydrate side chains.[117, 237–239] The nucleic acid sequence identity between human and bovine protein S is 87.5 per cent, and the amino acid sequence identity is 81.6 per cent. The function of protein S is species specific; that is, human protein S does not work as a cofactor of bovine APC.[212, 222]

The human genome contains two protein S genes (PSα and PSβ).[240–242] The chimpanzee and gorilla also have two protein S genes, whereas the orangutan,

rhesus monkey, and African green monkey have one.[241] It has been concluded that the gene duplication event occurred after the branching of the orangutan from the African apes. The PSα gene is expressed, whereas the PSβ gene is a pseudogene. Both protein S genes are located on chromosome 3 close to the centromere (band q11.2).[243–245] The sequence identity between the exons of the two genes is 96.5 per cent. The PSα gene is more than 80 kb long and contains 15 exons and 14 introns.

Mature protein S is a mosaic protein composed of multiple modules (Fig. 17–6).[233–236] Starting from the NH₂-terminus, it contains a Gla module, a thrombin-sensitive region, four EGF-like modules, and a carboxy-terminal region that is unrelated to the serine proteases but homologous to sex hormone–binding globulin (SHBG) and to rat androgen-binding protein (ABP).[246, 247] The modular structure of protein S correlates with the intron/exon organization of the gene and suggests that it has evolved through a combination of exon shuffling and gene duplication events.[240–242] The regions in protein S that are encoded by exons I to VIII (except the exon encoding the thrombin-sensitive module) are homologous to the other vitamin K–dependent coagulation proteins. Residues −41 to −18 constitute the hydrophobic signal peptide responsible for transport across the endoplasmic reticulum. The signal peptide cleavage site between Ala −18 and Asn −17 is tentative. The −17 amino acid long propeptide (residues Asn −17 to Arg −1) contains the recognition site for the vitamin K–dependent carboxylase and is homologous to corresponding structures in the other vitamin K–dependent proteins. Both the signal peptide and the propeptide are removed by proteolytic cleavage before secretion of protein S from the cell. The 5′ untranslated region and the signal peptide are encoded by the first exon.[240–242] The second exon encodes the propeptide and the Gla module. Residues Ala 1 to Thr 37 constitute the Gla module, which contains 11 Gla residues. It binds multiple Ca^{2+} ions, and the Ca^{2+}-stabilized structure has a high affinity for negatively charged phospholipid membranes.[210, 220, 237, 239] The Gla module is followed by a short connecting hydrophobic segment (residues 38 to 46), encoded by a separate exon.[240–242] The thrombin-sensitive region (exon IV; residues 46 to 75) contains two cysteines, forming a disulfide bridge. Two peptide bonds in this region are sensitive to proteolysis by thrombin: Arg 52—Ala 53 and Arg 70—Ser 71 in bovine protein S.[248] Human protein S has similar thrombin sensitivity and Arg 70 is conserved, whereas the human equivalent to the Arg 52—Ala 53 cleavage site is presumably Arg 49—Ser 50. After cleavage by thrombin, the Gla module remains attached to the rest of protein S via the disulfide bond (Cys 47—Cys 72), but in thrombin-cleaved protein S, the Gla module cannot undergo the calcium-mediated conformational change required for biological activity at physiologic Ca^{2+} concentration, suggesting that the thrombin-sensitive region is intimately involved in the folding of the Gla module.[210, 248] At this Ca^{2+} concentration (around 2 mM), thrombin-cleaved protein S does not bind negatively charged phospholipid membranes, whereas at a fivefold higher Ca^{2+} concentration, protein S binds to the phospholipid with the same affinity as uncleaved protein S.[249] The APC cofactor function of protein S is lost in the thrombin-cleaved form.[250, 251] This observation suggests that the thrombin-sensitive region interacts with APC on the phospholid surface, an interpretation deriving support from findings in experiments using monoclonal antibodies.[252]

Protein S is unique among the vitamin K–dependent proteins in containing four EGF-like modules (positions 76 to 242), each encoded by a separate exon (exons V to VIII).[240–242] The phase of the splice junctions (predominantly phase I) in this part of the protein S gene supports the idea of the gene's being formed by exon shuffling, with the notable exception of the exon encoding the fourth EGF-like module, which does not have the same splice-junction type in the 3' end as the others. The first EGF-like module contains a Hya, and the three following contain Hyn.[117] The Hyn-containing EGF-like modules of protein S contain very high-affinity Ca^{2+}-binding sites (K_d down to the nanomolar level).[120] The Ca^{2+} binding is important for protein S to attain protease resistance and a native conformation. It also appears to be important for the protein S–C4BP interaction, as the affinity of the interaction increases 100-fold in the presence of micromolar concentrations of calcium.[253, 254] Recently, it was reported that recombinant human protein S synthesized under conditions that inhibited the hydroxylation (the protein contains Asp and Asn instead of Hya and Hyn) still expressed full cofactor function and C4b-binding.[255] EGF-like modules with a consensus sequence for Hya/Hyn in other proteins, such as low density lipoprotein (LDL) receptor and TM, are involved in biologically important protein-protein in-

teractions. (See Chapter 16.)[109–114, 256] Whether very high-affinity calcium-binding sites and Hyn are important for their functions remains to be elucidated.

Exons IX to XV encode the carboxy-terminal half of protein S (amino acids 243 to 635), which is homologous to SHBG and ABP.[240–242, 246, 247] The intron/exon organization of this region of protein S is very similar to that of SHBG, including the positions of the introns and their splice-junction phases.[240–242, 257] The occurrence of all three intron phases in this part of the protein S gene suggests that it is not the result of exon shuffling and that the SHBG-like region as a whole may be considered a separate module. This module contains two small disulfide loops formed by internal disulfide bridges (Cys 408 to Cys 434 and Cys 597 to Cys 625),[233–236] each of which is encoded by a separate exon.[240–242] In human protein S, there are three potential N-linked glycosylation sites in the SHBG-like module, at Asn 458, at Asn 468, and at Asn 489, but it is not known whether all are occupied by carbohydrate side chains. Although the SHBG-like module is homologous to the steroid hormone–binding proteins, it does not appear to bind steroids.[230]

Interaction with C4b-Binding Protein

Protein S and C4BP form a 1:1 noncovalent complex, in which protein S has no anticoagulant cofactor function.[14, 15, 222, 223, 224, 258–260] The K_d is approximately 10^{-7} M in the absence of calcium and approximately 5×10^{-10} M in its presence.[253, 254, 259, 260] Calcium mainly enhances the rate of association, whereas the rate of dissociation is low, both in the presence and in the absence of calcium. The stimulating effect of calcium suggests that the EGF-like modules of protein S may be involved in the interaction. Despite the potentiating effect of calcium on the affinity between protein S and C4BP, the ratio of free to bound protein S is similar in plasma and in serum, indicating that other factors are involved in the regulation of the protein S–C4BP interaction in vivo.[253] This idea gains support from studies of a type of hereditary protein S deficiency that is characterized by normal total protein S concentrations and subnormal levels of free protein S.[223, 225, 261, 262, 312]

On the basis of results in experiments using synthetic peptides, it has been suggested that residues 605 to 614 within the loop between Cys 597 and Cys 625 contain the binding site for C4BP.[263] A mutant in which the entire Cys 597 to Cys 625 region was deleted still bound C4BP, albeit with lower affinity than did native protein S.[264] This finding is consistent with the location of a C4BP-binding site within the Cys 597 to Cys 625 region but indicates that binding may be complex and involve more than one site on the protein S molecule. It has also been suggested that the C4BP-binding site is located close to the middle of the SHBG-like module (the exact position is not given in the reference).[265]

C4b-BINDING PROTEIN

Structure-Function Relationships

C4b-binding protein is a regulator of the classical complement pathway.[266–271] It binds the activated complement protein C4b and is a cofactor to the serine protease factor I in C4b degradation. Moreover, it accelerates the natural decay of C2a from the C4bC2a complex (the classical pathway C3 convertase). C4BP is an acute phase protein, and in certain inflammatory disorders its concentration may increase to 400 per cent of normal.[272, 273] It is composed of seven identical 70 kDa α chains and a single 45 kDa β chain.[14, 266, 274, 275] Protein S interacts with the β chain, whereas each of the α chains contains a C4b-binding site. The binding sites for protein S and C4b on the C4BP molecule are thus distinct, and the protein S binding does not affect the function of C4BP as a regulator of the classical C3 convertase.[276] The C4BP molecule is spider or octopus shaped, as revealed by high-resolution electron microscopy (Fig. 17–7).[277, 278] Each α chain forms a thin (30 Å), extended (300 Å) tentacle that radiates from a central body. The β chain is considerably shorter than the α chains. The α and β chains contain 549 and 235 amino acids, respectively.[275, 279] Both chains are composed of internally homologous repeats, known as short consensus repeats (SCRs), complement control repeats (CCRs), or Suchi modules.[266, 280–283] In this discussion, they are referred to as SCRs. Each α chain contains eight SCRs, and the β chain three.[275, 279] The carboxy-terminal regions of the α and β chains contain two cysteines that are involved in interchain disulfide bridging and the formation of the central C4BP body. The sequence identity between the three β chain SCRs ranges from 26 to 34 per cent, and the identities with the α chain SCRs range from 17 to 35 per cent. The β chain has presumably evolved from the α chain during evolution through gene duplication. The β chain sequence contains five potential N-linked glycosylation sites, and most or all of them contain complex carbohydrate side chains.[275]

An SCR is approximately 60 amino acid residues long and contains a framework of conserved amino acid residues, including four cysteines, two prolines, one tryptophan, and several other partially conserved glycines and hydrophobic residues. A large number of complement regulatory proteins contain one or more SCRs.[266, 280–283] These proteins include factor H, the complement receptors 1 (CR1) and 2 (CR2), membrane cofactor protein (MCP), and decay-accelerating factor (DAF). Other complement proteins with SCRs are C1r, C1s, C2, factor B, C6, and C7. Each SCR constitutes a distinct protein module; the cysteines form two disulfide bridges linked 1–3 and 2–4, and with few exceptions, each SCR is encoded by a separate exon. The three-dimensional structure of an individual SCR from factor H has been resolved with two-dimensional nuclear magnetic resonance (NMR).[283, 284, 285] The SCR is a rather compact structure based on a β sandwich arrangement: one face made up of three β strands and the other face formed from two separate β strands.[285] The genes for MCP, CR1, CR2, DAF,

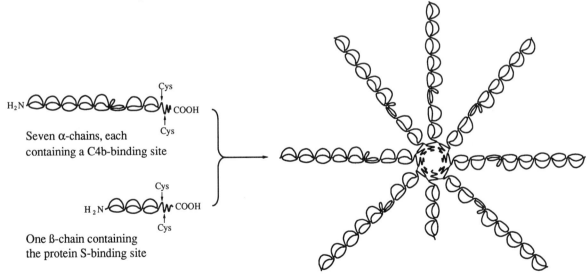

FIGURE 17–7. Subunit composition and assembly of C4b-binding protein (C4BP). Electron microscopy of C4BP reveals an octopus-like structure with multiple long tentacles. The distance from the center of the molecule to the peripheral end of an extended tentacle is 330 Å, and the diameter of a tentacle is 30 Å. C4BP contains two types of subunits, seven α chains and one β chain. Each of the α chains contains a C4b-binding site, whereas the protein S–binding site is located in the β chain. The subunits are linked by disulfide bridges, involving cysteine residues located in the COOH-terminal ends of both α and β chains. The major form of C4BP contains seven α chains and one β chain. (Modified from Hillarp, A., and Dahlbäck, B.: Cloning of cDNA coding for the β chain of human complement component of C4b-binding protein: Sequence homology with the α chain. Proc. Natl. Acad. Sci. USA 87:1183–1187, 1989; with permission.)

C4BP (α and β chains), and factor H are closely linked in a cluster of genes known as the regulator of complement activation (RCA) gene cluster, which is located on the long arm of chromosome 1, band q32.[286, 287] The α and β chain genes of C4BP are very close, only approximately 4 kb apart, in a head-to-tail orientation.[288, 289] SCRs are found not only in complement proteins but also in the B subunit of coagulation factor XIII, β2-glycoprotein 1, haptoglobin, and three cell adhesion molecules belonging to the selectin family (ELAM-1, MEL-14, and GMP-140).[108, 283] The function of the SCRs in these proteins has not been determined.

The β chain is required for protein S binding, but not for the polymerization of the C4BP chains during the assembly of the molecule. This is demonstrated by the observation that C4BP in blood is heterogeneous in subunit composition and protein S binding. Between 10 and 15 per cent of the C4BP molecules in plasma do not bind protein S and lack the β chain.[290] C4BP is unique in the group of SCR-containing proteins in being composed of two distinct SCR-containing subunits with different binding specificities, and the protein S binding to the β chain of C4BP is the only example of the binding of a vitamin K–dependent protein to an SCR-containing protein. The binding of protein S to C4BP suggests a link between the coagulation and complement systems.[14] C4BP regulates the expression of protein S anticoagulant activity, as binding of C4BP to protein S results in a loss of protein S cofactor activity. Protein S may affect the function of C4BP as a regulator of the classical complement pathway, as the C4BP–protein S complex binds to negatively charged phospholipid membranes through the protein S moiety.[254]

Interaction with Serum Amyloid P Component

The high-affinity binding of the serum amyloid P (SAP) component to C4BP is an interaction of unknown biological significance.[14, 291] SAP, which is homologous to the acute phase protein CRP, is a normal constituent in plasma and extravascular tissues and is also present in amyloid deposits.[292] It is a so-called pentraxin, composed of five identical subunits (molecular weight of 25,000) linked by non-covalent bonds. The biological function of SAP is not known. The stoichiometry of the SAP-C4BP interaction is 1:1, and it is optimal at 0.4 mM of calcium.[291] The self-association of SAP and its interactions with phospholipid or C4BP are mutually exclusive, its binding to C4BP being favored over self-association or its binding to phospholipid membranes. The binding sites for protein S and SAP on C4BP are independent. The macromolecular complex of C4BP, SAP, protein S, and C4b can bind to phospholipid membranes in the presence of calcium. The vitamin K–dependent part of protein S is required for membrane interaction of the complex.[291] It is possible that protein S localizes C4BP to anionic phospholipid surfaces, where blood

coagulation is activated, and that this provides local regulation of the complement system. Other SCR-containing proteins are known to regulate the complement system on cell membranes; that is, DAF is covalently linked to a glycolipid, whereas CR1, CR2, and MCP are integral membrane proteins with phospholipid-spanning regions.[266] Activation of complement results in a local inflammatory reaction, partly because of the release of anaphylatoxins and the attraction of leukocytes.[266] Inhibition of the complement system where blood coagulation occurs may be beneficial, as an inflammatory reaction at the same site may result in impaired regulation of coagulation (e.g., that due to the release of leukocyte proteases).

THE PROTEIN C ANTICOAGULANT SYSTEM, AN IMPORTANT REGULATOR OF BLOOD COAGULATION IN VIVO

The importance of the protein C anticoagulant system in vivo is most clearly illustrated by the severe thromboembolic disease that affects individuals with homozygous deficiency of either protein C or protein S.[22] The high incidence of thrombosis in people with heterozygous deficiency of either protein supports the idea that this anticoagulant system is important for the regulation of blood coagulation in vivo.[293–296] Under normal conditions, protein C appears to be slowly activated, as the protein C activation peptide can be detected in blood, albeit at very low concentration.[70] Activation of protein C is the result of a low-grade activation of coagulation with a constant slow generation of thrombin. Dramatically elevated levels of protein C activation peptides were found in patients with disseminated intravascular coagulation, deep vein thrombosis, and pulmonary embolism.[297] In addition to these clinical findings, studies in experimental animals have illustrated the functional role of the protein C anticoagulant system in vivo and have suggested that the protein C system may be involved in the host defense reactions occurring during such intravascular inflammatory challenges as sepsis.[298]

In vivo experiments using rabbits, dogs, or monkeys have shown protein C to be activated in response to the infusion of thrombin or a mixture of factor Xa and acidic phospholipid vesicles.[28, 30, 44, 299, 300] In a coronary artery occlusion model, using porcine hearts, ischemic insult induced rapid protein C activation in the coronary microcirculation, and recovery was impaired when protein C activation was blocked.[301] In humans, it has been shown that protein C is activated in response to thromboembolic events and during intravascular coagulation and that complexes between APC and either PCI or α1-antitrypsin inhibitor circulate during these conditions.[302–306]

Infusion of APC in experimental animals prolongs the activated partial thromboplastin time.[29, 40] However, the bleeding time is unaffected, and the plasma levels of factors V and VIII remain normal during and after the infusion.[28, 30] This is due to the high specificity of APC; that is, it degrades the phospholipid-bound forms of factors Va and VIIIa but does not cleave the circulating procofactors.[5–10, 23, 27] When administered in a baboon arterial thrombosis model, APC was found to inhibit platelet-dependent thrombus formation.[29] Other components of the protein C system are also powerful anticoagulants; for example, purified natural or recombinant TM has antithrombotic effects on thrombin-induced thromboembolism in vivo.[97, 208] This is mainly due to stimulation of protein C activation, but direct anticoagulant functions of TM may also be involved. It is possible that APC or TM or both will find therapeutic use in the future.

In addition to its important anticoagulant functions, the protein C system appears to play a major protective part in limiting tissue damage due to gram-negative septicemia.[298] In a baboon model, APC infusions prevented the coagulopathy and the *Escherichia coli*–induced shock that was fatal in untreated animals.[307] Active site–inhibited factor Xa (DEGR-Xa) blocked the disseminated intravascular coagulation initiated by *E. coli* but, in contrast to APC, did not prevent shock and organ damage.[308] This finding suggested that APC, in addition to blocking the formation of thrombin, has other protective, as yet unidentified functions. This hypothesis is consistent with other in vivo experiments in which inhibition of the intravascular coagulation response observed after *E. coli* infusion was obtained with heparin or with antibodies to tissue factor. These components, however, failed to protect the animals from the shock.[298]

Activation of protein C is critical in host defense from infection by *E. coli*, as borne out by the observation that inhibition of protein C activation by a monoclonal antibody exacerbated the shock response after the infusion of sublethal doses of *E. coli*. The APC cofactor function of protein S is also crucial for the APC-mediated protection. Thus, when the baboons were first given a monoclonal antibody against protein S, a lethal response was obtained after an otherwise sublethal dose of *E. coli*.[298] Monoclonal antibodies against protein S that blocked the APC cofactor activity produced the lethal response, whereas non-inhibitory antibodies did not. The functional importance of the free form of protein S was obvious, since infusion of C4BP prior to administration of the sublethal *E. coli* dose exacerbated the inflammatory response and made the outcome fatal. This did not happen when C4BP was given together with a slight excess of protein S.[309] These in vivo experiments clearly demonstrate that the protein C anticoagulant system plays an important protective part in host defense inflammatory reactions induced by septicemia, although the basic biochemical mechanisms remain unclear.

DEFICIENCY OF PROTEIN C

The frequency of heterozygous protein C deficiency in patients with thromboembolic disease is between 2 and 5 per cent.[310–312] In younger patients (<40 years) with recurrent thrombotic disease, the frequency may be as high as 10 to 15 per cent.[313, 314] Studies of Dutch and French families with protein C deficiency and thrombosis suggest that protein C deficiency is inherited as an autosomal dominant trait. Among affected family members, 50 per cent were found to have had thrombosis before the age of 30 years and 80 per cent before the age of 40 years.[295] In a large family in New England, approximately 50 per cent of the patients had their first thrombotic episode before the age of 50 years.[315] The strong correlation between protein C deficiency and thrombosis in these families suggests a causal relationship. The frequency of this type of protein C deficiency, the so-called clinically dominant form, has been estimated to be 1 in 16,000 in the western part of the Netherlands.[295] It was therefore surprising when heterozygous protein C deficiency was found to be rather common in the population as a whole. In one study, approximately 1 in 250 to 300 blood donors was found to have heterozygous protein C deficiency, but there was no family history of an increased incidence of thrombosis.[316] Apparently, protein C deficiency in a family without thrombophilia is not in itself a significant risk factor for thromboembolic disease. This type of protein C deficiency is designated clinically recessive, and only the homozygous form is associated with thromboembolic disease.[295] The difference between the dominant and the recessive forms of protein C deficiency is still enigmatic. It was recently reported that mutation of the codon for Arg 306 to a stop codon was present *both* in a family with clinically recessive and in a family with the clinically dominant form of protein C deficiency.[317] A possible explanation of this apparent paradox is that the clinically dominant form of protein C deficiency is associated with a defect in a gene that is closely linked to the protein C gene, suggesting that important regulatory factors remain to be discovered. Homozygous, or double heterozygous, protein C deficiency is a rare condition that is inherited as an autosomal recessive trait.[22, 318, 319] It leads to severe and fatal thrombosis in the neonatal period. The clinical picture is that of purpura fulminans, and the symptoms include necrotic skin lesions due to microvascular thrombosis. Other major symptoms are thrombosis in the brain and disseminated intravascular coagulation. Several cases have been successfully treated with fresh frozen plasma or with protein C concentrates.[22, 318, 320] When family members of individuals with homozygous protein C deficiency have been examined, the incidence of thrombosis has been found to be quite low (approximately 5 per cent), demonstrating that they have the clinically recessive type of protein C deficiency and that only the double heterozygotes (or true homozygotes) develop thrombotic disease.[22, 318, 319]

Two types of autosomal dominant protein C deficiency have been described.[295] In type I, there is a parallel reduction in protein C antigen and functional activity; that is, the protein C concentration is reduced in both immunological and functional assays. Type II protein C deficiency is characterized by a functional defect in the protein, and the plasma concentration of the protein may be normal. The majority of reported cases of autosomal dominant protein C deficiency belong to type I. The so-called clinically dominant form of protein C deficiency is mainly associated with deep venous thrombosis in the lower extremities. Superficial thrombophlebitis and pulmonary embolism are also common clinical manifestations. There are no indications that protein C deficiency constitutes a risk factor for the early development of arterial thrombosis.

Rarely, skin necrosis develops after initiation of anticoagulant therapy with such vitamin K antagonists as warfarin, and this condition has been found to be associated with protein C deficiency.[5–10, 22, 295, 321] Four of 118 Dutch and French patients with protein C deficiency developed skin necrosis during anticoagulant therapy.[295] It is believed that skin necrosis may develop as a result of transient severe protein C deficiency caused by a short biological half-life of the protein.[295, 322–324] During the induction phase of anticoagulant therapy, functional protein C levels decline more rapidly ($t\frac{1}{2} \approx 8$ hours) than do those of factors IX and X and prothrombin ($t\frac{1}{2} > 40$ hours). As a consequence, functional protein C levels can be very low during the first days of anticoagulant therapy, particularly in protein C–deficient patients, which increases the risk of microvascular thrombosis and skin necrosis. The occurrence of skin necrosis is not restricted to patients with protein C deficiency.[321, 325]

Few polymorphic sites that can be used for genetic linkage analysis have been identified in the protein C gene.[326] One Msp I polymorphism is reported to be located approximately 7 kb upstream of the protein C gene and to have allelic frequencies of 69 per cent and 31 per cent.[327] A second Msp I polymorphism is present in intron 8 of the protein C gene, and the allelic frequencies in the general population are 99 per cent and 1 per cent, making it less useful for linkage analysis.[328] However, it was observed that the rare allele of this restriction fragment length polymorphism (RFLP) was more frequent (7 per cent) in a panel of 22 Dutch families with protein C deficiency, and it coincided with a point mutation in the protein C gene, resulting in a stop codon at Arg 306.[329] A third neutral polymorphic site has been found in exon 6, at position Ser 99, which demonstrates a T/G variation in the third nucleotide of the codon for Ser. The allelic frequencies were found to be 82 per cent for T and 18 per cent for G in a Japanese population, and the corresponding values among Caucasians were 75 per cent and 25 per cent.[330] Recently, three other polymorphic sites that appear useful for segregation studies in protein C deficiency were reported. They were located at positions corresponding to Arg 87 (CGC/CGT, allelic frequencies of 87.5/12.5 per cent), Lys 156 (AAA/AAG, allelic frequencies of 64.3/35.7 per cent), and Asp 214 (GAT/GAC, allelic frequencies of 64/36 per cent).[331, 332]

There are many reports of protein C deficiency in patients, although the genetic defects have been characterized in only a few of them. The defects include both nonsense and mis-sense mutations. The majority of point mutations affect CpG dinucleotides, which is consistent with methylation-mediated deamination of 5-methylcytosine.[326] Thirty-two different mutations in the protein C gene have so far been reported in patients with clinically dominant heterozygous protein C deficiency of type I (Table 17–1). The majority of the mutations are located within the region coding for the mature protein and are point mutations causing a single amino acid substitution. These mutations probably result in unstable proteins that may not even be secreted. Two point mutations have also been found in the promotor region of the gene, one located at position −1533, in the predicted TATA box, and the other at position −1511, just upstream of the transcription initiation site.[333] The gene defects have been characterized in 11 cases of type II deficiency (see Table 17–1). The mutation changing Arg −1 to His is presumably associated with a defective cleavage of the propeptide, by analogy with similar mutations in factor IX.[334] Four type II deficiencies have mutations in the Gla module, and one is located in the EGF-like modules. This changes His 66, which is located in the first EGF-like module, to an Asn, which will be a potential carbohydrate attachment site. Whether this Asn actually contains a carbohydrate side chain remains to be elucidated. A C to T mutation changes Arg 169 to Trp, which destroys the activation cleavage site, yielding a molecule that cannot be activated. This molecular defect has been found in at least two independent families, in protein C Tochigi and in Protein C London 1.[335, 336] Four point mutations have been found in the serine protease module in association with type II deficiency. One of them, an Asp 359 to Asn mutation, occurs in an amino acid that is located next to the active site Ser 360.[333] Asp 359 has been predicted to form an ion pair with Leu 170 after activation, and the mutation leading to an Asn probably affects this interaction. The gene defects have been characterized in four cases of clinically recessive protein C deficiency. It it not apparent why these mutations are not associated with thromboembolic disease. In particular, it is noteworthy that the C to T mutation at nucleotide 8631 (Arg 306 to stop) is found in families with both recessive and dominant protein C deficiency.[317]

DEFICIENCY OF PROTEIN S

The frequency of hereditary protein S deficiency in a population of patients with thromboembolic disease was found to be similar to that of protein C deficiency.[310–312] The frequency of heterozygous protein S deficiency in the general population is not known. There are three recognizable types of inherited protein S deficiency.[296] As there is no consensus regarding the nomenclature of protein S deficiencies, the one used here (proposed by Dr. R.M. Bertina at the Inter-

TABLE 17–1. MUTATIONS IN THE PROTEIN C GENE

PATIENT	NUCLEOTIDE*	AMINO ACID*	CHANGE	REFERENCES
Type I Protein C Deficiency (Clinically Dominant Form)				
1	−1533, A–G	In TATA box		333
2	−1511, C–T	Just before transcription initiation		333
3	1380, △7	△Arg −3, Lys −2	Frameshift	337
4	1432, C–T	Arg 15	Trp	338
5	1433, G–A	Arg 15	Gln	338
6	3169, T–C	Phe 76	Leu	317
7	3217, G–T	Glu 92	Stop	339
8	3222, G–A	Donor splice site		317
9	3222, G–T	Donor splice site		317
10	3222, G–C	Donor splice site		317
11	3359, G–A	Cys 105	Tyr	317
12	3360, C–A	Cys 105	Stop	317
13	3402, C–G	Ser 119	Arg	317
14	3439, C–T	Gln 132	Stop	317
15	6134, T–C	Cys 141	Arg	317
16	6152, C–T	Arg 147	Trp	333
17	6153, △1	Arg 147	Frameshift	340, 341
18	6167, C–T	Arg 152	Cys	338
19	6182, C–T	Arg 157	Stop	338
20	6216, C–T	Pro 168	Leu	338
21	6245, C–T	Arg 178	Trp	317, 337, 340
22	6246, G–A	Arg 178	Gln	337–340
23	7253, C–T	Leu 223	Phe	317
24	8403, C–T	Arg 230	Cys	317, 339
25	8455, C–T	Pro 247	Leu	340
26	8491, C–T	Ala 259	Val	340
27	8589, G–A	Gly 292	Ser	317
28	8631, C–T	Arg 306	Stop	317, 340, 342
29	8678, △3	Ile 321, Lys 322	Met	337
30	8857, △1	Gly 381	Frameshift	343
31	8921, G–C	Trp 402	Cys	342
32	8924, C–G	Ile 403	Met	317
Type II Protein C Deficiency (Clinically Dominant Form)				
1	1388, G–A	Arg 1	His	344
2	1414, C–T	Arg 9	Cys	337
3	1432, C–G	Arg 15	Gly	345
4	1448, A–C	Glu 20	Ala	346
5	1489, G–A	Val 34	Met	346
6	3139, C–A	His 66	Asn	333
7	6218, C–T	Arg 169	Trp	335, 336, 338, 340
8	8400, C–T	Arg 229	Trp	337
9	8401, G–A	Arg 229	Gln	337
10	8470, G–A	Ser 252	Asn	337
11	8790, G–A	Asp 359	Asn	333
Clinically Recessive Protein C Deficiency				
1	3171, △18	△Ser 77–Ser 82		347
2	3174, △18	△Cys 78–Gly 83		347
3	6274, C–T	Intron G	Splice/junction	347
4	8403, C–T	Arg 230	Cys	317

*Nucleotide and amino acid numbering is as in Foster et al.[87]
The symbol △ denotes deletion.

national Society of Thrombosis and Haemostasis [ISTH] subcommittee meeting in 1991) is tentative. Type I is characterized by a reduction in the levels of both total and free protein S.[296, 348–352] Type II is due to a functionally defective molecule. The antigen levels of total and free protein S are normal in these patients, but the ratio between functional activity and the concentration of free protein S is below the normal range.[353] This condition appears to be very rare, which may be due to the difficulties in measuring protein S function. More common is type III, which is charac-

terized by an abnormal distribution of protein S between the free and C4BP complexed forms.[223, 225, 261, 262, 312] The concentration of free protein S is quite low in these cases, whereas the concentration of total protein S is normal. Typically, these patients have a normal C4BP concentration. The pathophysiological mechanisms responsible for the disequilibrium are not known, and it has not been determined whether such deficiencies are due to mutations in the protein S gene or in the C4BP gene or whether type III protein S deficiency is due to a defect in another gene. It should be borne in mind that in the original reports on protein S deficiency, this latter type was classified as type I, whereas the cases in which both total and free protein S was decreased were designated type II.[224, 225] The nomenclature we have used is more consistent with that used for deficiencies of other proteins in which type I deficiency usually means low protein concentrations and type II a functionally defective molecule.

Acquired protein S deficiency is associated with oral anticoagulation, nephrotic syndrome, disseminated intravascular coagulation, and pregnancy.[354–357] In nephrotic syndrome, the concentration of C4BP is high, since its molecular weight does not allow glomerular filtration. Accordingly, the concentration of the complexed form of protein S is increased.[355] Free protein S is lost to the urine, resulting in a decrease in the level of functionally active protein S. During normal pregnancy, the concentrations of both total and free protein S in plasma drop and reach levels found in heterozygous protein S–deficient patients.[356, 357] In particular, the levels of free protein S decrease. Whether this contributes to the thrombotic tendency during pregnancy is unknown.

The clinical manifestations of hereditary protein S deficiency are similar to those of dominant protein C deficiency.[296, 358] Hereditary protein S deficiency may also predispose to arterial thrombotic disease.[359] A few cases of warfarin-induced skin necrosis associated with protein S deficiency have been described.[22, 360–362] Purpura fulminans in the neonatal period has occurred in conjunction with homozygous protein S deficiency. The clinical manifestations are similar to those observed in homozygous protein C deficiency.[22, 363]

There are few reports on the genetic defects in protein S deficiency. Even though the protein S gene is large (80 kb), only one polymorphic site has been found.[364] This is a CCA/CCG (frequency of 52 per cent/48 per cent) neutral dimorphism in the codon for Pro 626. Four variant protein S alleles have been characterized. Protein S Heerlen is a variant that is caused by a Ser 460 to Pro substitution in the consensus sequence for *N*-linked glycosylation.[365] The variant molecule has a lower molecular weight, but full biological activity. It is not associated with thrombotic disease. A second type of protein S deficiency is linked to a mutation in the protein S β gene (the pseudogene), resulting in the disappearance of an Msp I restriction site.[366] The mutation is not the cause of the disease but is a linked genetic marker in this family. Two gene deletions have been found in type I protein S deficiency, one a 5.3 kb deletion including exon XIII of the protein S α gene, the other one a gene deletion of unknown size in the middle portion of the protein S coding sequence.[367, 368]

UPDATE

Table 17–1 reports protein C mutations that were known at the time this chapter was written. A compre-hensive database of protein C gene mutations has since been published.[369]

Another potentially important paper was recently published; this paper describes a previously unrecognized mechanism for familial thromboembolic disease characterized by poor anticoagulant response to APC.[370] The APC resistance was found to be inherited and could not be explained by the currently accepted scheme of the protein C anticoagulant system. The condition appeared to be best explained by a hypothesized inherited deficiency of a previously unrecognized cofactor to APC. More recent data obtained in the laboratory of one of the authors (BD) indicate this to be a frequent cause of familial thrombophilia.

REFERENCES

1. Davie, E. W., Fujikawa, K., and Kisiel, W.: The coagulation cascade: Initiation, maintenance and regulation. Biochemistry 30:10363, 1991.
2. Furie, B., and Furie, B. C.: The molecular basis of blood coagulation. Cell 33:505, 1988.
3. Gimbrone, M. A., Jr.: Vascular endothelium: Nature's blood container. *In* Gimbrone, M. A., Jr. (ed.): Vascular endothelium in hemostasis and thrombosis. Contemp. Issues Haemost. Thromb. 2:1, 1986.
4. Bauer, K. A., and Rosenberg, R. D.: Role of antithrombin III as a regulator of in vivo coagulation. Semin. Hematol. 28:10, 1991.
5. Esmon, C. T.: The roles of protein C and thrombomodulin in the regulation of blood coagulation. J. Biol. Chem. 264:4743, 1989.
6. Esmon, C. T.: The regulation of natural anticoagulant pathways. Science 235:1348, 1987.
7. Stenflo, J.: A new vitamin K–dependent protein. Purification from bovine plasma and preliminary characterization. J. Biol. Chem. 251:355, 1976.
8. Kisiel, W., Canfield, W. M., Ericsson, L. H., and Davie, E.: Anticoagulant properties of bovine plasma protein C following activation by thrombin. Biochemistry 16:5824, 1977.
9. Kisiel, W.: Human plasma protein C. Isolation, characterization, and mechanism of activation by α-thrombin. J. Clin. Invest. 64:761, 1979.
10. Stenflo, J.: The biochemistry of protein C. *In* Bertina, R. M. (ed.): Protein C and Related Proteins. London, Churchill Livingstone, Longman Group UK, 1988, pp. 21–54.
11. Seegers, W. H., Novoa, E., Henry, R. L., and Hassouna, H. I.: Relationship of "new" vitamin K–dependent protein C and "old" autoprothrombin II-A. Thromb. Res. 8:543, 1976.
12. Marcianik, E.: Inhibitor of human blood coagulation elicited by thrombin. J. Lab. Clin. Med. 79:921, 1972.
13. Mann, K. G., Jenny, R. J., and Krishnaswamy, S.: Cofactor proteins in the assembly and expression of blood clotting enzyme complexes. Annu. Rev. Biochem. 57:915, 1988.
14. Dahlbäck, B.: Protein S and C4b-binding protein: Components involved in the regulation of the protein C anticoagulant system. Thromb. Haemost. 66:49, 1991.
15. Hessing, M.: The interaction between complement component C4b-binding protein and the vitamin K–dependent protein S forms a link between blood coagulation and the complement system. Biochem. J. 277:581, 1991.
16. Suzuki, K., Deyashiki, Y., Nishioka, J., and Toma, K.: Protein C inhibitor: Structure and function. Thromb. Haemost. 61:337, 1989.
17. Van der Meer, F. J., van Tilburg, N., van Wijngaarden, A., van der Linden, I. K., Briet, E., and Bertina, R. M.: A second plasma inhibitor of activated protein C: α1-antitrypsin. Thromb. Haemost. 62:756, 1989.
18. Heeb, M. J., and Griffin, J. H.: Physiologic inhibition of human

activated protein C by alpha-1-antitrypsin. J. Biol. Chem. 263:11613, 1988.

19. Heeb, M. J., Espana, F., and Griffin, J. H.: Inhibition and complexation of activated protein C by two major inhibitors in plasma. Blood 73:446, 1989.

20. Hoogendoorn, H., Toh, C. H., Nesheim, M. E., and Giles, A. R.: α_2-macroglobulin binds and inhibits activated protein C. Blood 78:2283, 1991.

21. Heeb, M. J., Gruber, A., and Griffin, J. H.: Identification of different metal ion–dependent inhibition of activated protein C by alpha 2-macroglobulin and alpha 2-antiplasmin in blood and comparisons to inhibition of factor Xa, thrombin, and plasmin. J. Biol. Chem. 266:17606, 1991.

22. Marlar, R. A., and Neumann, A.: Neonatal purpura fulminans due to homozygous protein C or protein S deficiency. Semin. Thromb. Hemost. 16:299, 1990.

23. Kane, W. H., and Davie, E. W.: Blood coagulation factors V and VIII: Structural and functional similarities and their relationship to hemorrhagic and thrombotic disorders. Blood 71:539, 1988.

24. Mann, K. G., Nesheim, M. E., Church, W. R., Haley, P., and Krishnaswamy, S.: Surface-dependent reactions of the vitamin K–dependent enzyme complexes. Blood 76:1, 1990.

25. Kalifatis, M., Jenny, R. J., and Mann, K. G.: Identification and characterization of a phospholipid-binding site of bovine factor Va. J. Biol. Chem. 265:21580, 1990.

26. Guinto, E. R., and Esmon, C. T.: Loss of prothrombin and factor Xa–factor Va interactions upon inactivation of factor Va by activated protein C. J. Biol. Chem. 259:13986, 1984.

27. Fay, P. J., Smudzin, T. M., and Walker, F. J.: Activated protein C–catalyzed inactivation of factor VIII and VIIIa. J. Biol. Chem. 260:20139, 1991.

28. Comp, P. C., Jacobs, R. M., Ferrell, G. L., and Esmon, C. T.: Activation of protein C in vivo. J. Clin. Invest. 70:127, 1982.

29. Gruber, A., Hanson, S. R., Kelly, A. B., Yan, B. S., Bang, N. U., Griffin, J. H., and Harker, L. A.: Inhibition of thrombus formation by activated recombinant protein C in a primate model of arterial thrombosis. Circulation 82:578, 1990.

30. Comp, P. C.: Animal studies of protein C physiology. Semin. Thromb. Hemost. 10:149, 1984.

31. Solymoss, S., Tucker, M. M., and Tracy, P. B.: Kinetics of inactivation of membrane-bound factor V by activated protein C. J. Biol. Chem. 263:14884, 1988.

32. Walker, F. J.: Interactions of protein S with membranes. Semin. Thromb. Hemost. 14:216, 1988.

33. Krishnaswamy, S., Williams, E. B., and Mann, K. G.: The binding of activated protein C to factors V and Va. J. Biol. Chem. 261:9684, 1986.

34. De Fouw, N. J., Bertina, R. M., and Haverkate, F.: Activated protein C and fibrinolysis. In Bertina, R. M. (ed.): Protein C and related proteins. London, Churchill Livingstone, Longman Group UK, 1988, pp. 71–90.

35. Zolton, R. P., and Seegers, W. H.: Autoprothrombin II-A: Thrombin removal and mechanism of induction of fibrinolysis. Thromb. Res. 3:23, 1973.

36. Comp, P. C., and Esmon, C. T.: Generation of fibrinolytic activity by infusion of activated protein C in dogs. J. Clin. Invest. 68:1221, 1981.

37. Taylor, F. B., and Lockhart, M. S.: Whole blood clot lysis: In vivo modulation by activated protein C. Thromb. Res. 37:639, 1985.

38. Burdick, M. D., and Schaub, R. G.: Human protein C produces anticoagulation and increased fibrinolytic activity in the cat. Thromb. Res. 45:413, 1987.

39. Bajzar, L., Fredenburgh, J. C., and Nesheim, M. E.: The activated protein C–mediated enhancement of tissue-type plasminogen activator–induced fibrinolysis in a cell-free system. J. Biol. Chem. 265:16948, 1990.

40. Colucci, M., Stassen, J. M., and Collen, D.: Influence of protein C activation on blood coagulation and fibrinolysis in squirrel monkeys. J. Clin. Invest. 74:200, 1984.

41. Sakata, Y., Loskutoff, D. J., Gladson, C. L., Hekman, C. M., and Griffin, J. H.: Mechanism of protein C–dependent clot lysis: Role of plasminogen activator inhibitor. Blood 68:1218, 1986.

42. Aznar, J., Dasi, A., Espana, F., and Estellés, A.: Fibrinolytic study in a homozygous protein C dependent patient. Thromb. Res. 42:313, 1986.

43. Espana, F., Gruber, A., Heeb, M. J., Hanson, S. R., Harker, L. A., and Griffin, J. H.: In vivo and in vitro complexes of activated protein C with two inhibitors in baboons. Blood 77:1754, 1991.

44. Hoogendoorn, H., Nesheim, M. E., and Giles, A. R.: A qualitative and quantitative analysis of the activation and inactivation of protein C in vivo in a primate model. Blood 75:2164, 1990.

45. Laurell, M., Christensson, A., Abrahamsson, P.-A., Stenflo, J., and Lilja, H.: Protein C inhibitor in human body fluids; seminal plasma is rich in inhibitor antigen deriving from cells throughout the male reproductive system. J. Clin. Invest. 89:1094, 1992.

46. Espana, F., Gilabert, J., Estellés, A., Romeu, A., Aznar, J., and Cabo, A.: Functionally active protein C inhibitor/plasminogen activator inhibitor-3 (PCI/PAI-3) is secreted in seminal vesicles, occurs at high concentrations in human seminal plasma and complexes with prostate-specific antigen. Thromb. Res. 64:309, 1991.

47. Laurell, M., Stenflo, J., and Carlson, T. H.: Turnover of *I-protein C inhibitor and *I-alpha-1-antitrypsin and their complexes with activated protein C. Blood 76:2290, 1990.

48. Long, G. L., Belagaje, R. M., and MacGillivray, R. T. A.: Cloning and sequencing of liver cDNA coding for bovine protein C. Proc. Natl. Acad. Sci. USA 81:5653, 1984.

49. Beckman, R. J., Schmidt, R. J., Santerre, R. F., Plutzky, J., Crabtree, G. R., and Long, G. L.: The structure and evolution of a 461 amino acid human protein C precursor and its messenger RNA, based upon the DNA sequence of cloned human liver cDNA's. Nucleic Acids Res. 13:5233, 1985.

50. Foster, D. C., Yoshitake, S., and Davie, E. W.: Characterization of cDNA coding for human protein C. Proc. Natl. Acad. Sci. USA 81:4766, 1984.

51. Foster, D. C., Rudinski, M. S., Schack, B. G., Berkner, K. L., Kumar, A. A., Hagen, F. S., Sprecher, C. A., Insley, M. Y., and Davie, E. W.: Propeptide of human protein C is necessary for γ-carboxylation. Biochemistry 26:7003, 1987.

52. Foster, D. C., Holly, R. O., Sprecher, C. A., Walker, K. M., and Kumar, A. A.: Endoproteolytic processing of the human protein C precursor by the yeast kex 2 endopeptidase coexpressed in mammalian cells. Biochemistry 30:367, 1991.

53. Leytus, S. P., Foster, D. C., Kurachi, K., and Davie, E. W.: Gene for human factor X. A blood coagulation factor whose gene organization is essentially identical with that of factor IX and protein C. Biochemistry 25:5098, 1986.

54. Fung, M. R., Hay, C. W., and MacGillivray, R. T. A.: Characterization of an almost full-length cDNA coding for human blood coagulation factor X. Proc. Natl. Acad. Sci. USA 82:3591, 1985.

55. De Binijor, M. H. L., and Fey, G. H.: Human complement component C3: cDNA coding sequence and derived primary structure. Proc. Natl. Acad. Sci. USA 82:708, 1985.

56. Belt, K. T., Carroll, M. C., and Porter, R. R.: The structural basis of the multiple forms of human complement component C4. Cell 36:907, 1984.

57. Miletich, J. P., Leykam, J. F., and Broze, G. J., Jr.: Detection of single chain protein C in plasma. Blood (Suppl. I) 62:306a, 1983.

58. Fernlund, P., and Stenflo, J.: Amino acid sequence of the light chain of bovine protein C. J. Biol. Chem. 257:12170, 1982.

59. Tulinsky, A.: The structures of domains of blood proteins. Thromb. Haemost. 66:16, 1991.

60. Stenflo, J., and Suttie, J. W.: Vitamin K–dependent formation of γ-carboxyglutamic acid. Annu. Rev. Biochem. 46:157, 1977.

61. Kurosawa, S., Galvin, J. B., Esmon, N. L., and Esmon, C. T.: Proteolytic formation and properties of functional domains of thrombomodulin. J. Biol. Chem. 262:2206, 1987.

62. Zhang, L., and Castellino, F. J.: A γ-carboxyglutamic acid (γ)

variant (γ^6D, γ^7D) of human activated protein C displays greatly reduced activity as an anticoagulant. Biochemistry 29:10828, 1990.

63. Zhang, L., and Castellino, F. J.: Role of the hexapeptide disulfide loop present in the γ-carboxyglutamic acid domain of human protein C in its activation properties and in the in vitro anticoagulant activity of activated protein C. Biochemistry 30:6696, 1991.

64. Drakenberg, T. P., Fernlund, P., Roepstorff, P., and Stenflo, J.: β-Hydroaspartic acid in vitamin K–dependent protein C. Proc. Natl. Acad. Sci. USA 80:1802, 1983.

65. Öhlin, A.-K., Laudes, G., Bourdon, P., Oppenheimer, C., Wydro, R., and Stenflo, J.: β-Hydroxyaspartic acid in the first epidermal growth factor–like domain of protein C. J. Biol. Chem. 263:19240, 1988.

66. Grinnell, B. W., Walls, J. D., and Gerlitz, B.: Glycosylation of human protein C affects its secretion, processing, functional activities and activation by thrombin. J. Biol. Chem. 266:9778, 1991.

67. Öhlin, A.-K., Björk, I., and Stenflo, J.: Proteolytic formation and properties of a fragment of protein C containing the γ-carboxyglutamic acid rich domain of the EGF-like region. Biochemistry 29:644, 1990.

68. Hogg, P. J., Öhlin, A.-K., and Stenflo, J.: Identification of structural domains in protein C involved in its interaction with thrombin-thrombomodulin on the surface of endothelial cells. J. Biol. Chem. 267:703, 1992.

69. Olsen, P. H., Esmon, N. L., Esmon, C. T., and Laue, T. M.: Ca^{2+} dependence of the interactions between protein C, thrombin and the elastase fragment of thrombomodulin. Analysis by ultracentrifugation. Biochemistry 31:746, 1992.

70. Bauer, K. A., Kass, B. L., Beeler, D. L., and Rosenberg, R. D.: The detection of protein C activation in humans. J. Clin. Invest. 74:2033, 1984.

71. Ehrlich, H. J., Jashunas, S. R., Grinnell, B. W., Yan, S. B., and Bang, N. U.: Direct expression of recombinant activated human protein C, a serine protease. J. Biol. Chem. 264:14298, 1989.

72. Stenflo, J., and Fernlund, P.: Amino acid sequence of the heavy chain of bovine protein C. J. Biol. Chem. 257:12180, 1982.

73. Titani, K., Kumar, S., Takio, K., Ericsson, L. E., Wade, R. D., Ashida, K., Walsch, K. A., Chopek, M. W., Sadler, J. E., and Fujikawa, K.: Amino acid sequence of human von Willebrand factor. Biochemistry 25:3171, 1986.

74. Miletich, J. P., and Broze, G. J., Jr.: β-Protein C is not glycosylated at asparagine 329. J. Biol. Chem. 265:11397, 1990.

75. Bode, W., and Schwager, P.: The refined crystal structure of bovine β-trypsin at 1.8 Å resolution. II. Crystallografic refinement, calcium binding site, benzamidine binding site and active site at pH 7.0. J. Mol. Biol. 98:693, 1975.

76. Schechter, I., and Berger, A.: On the size of the active site in proteases. I. Papain. Biochem. Biophys. Res. Commun. 27:157, 1967.

77. Mesters, R. M., and Griffin, J. H.: Identification of a sequence in activated protein C (APC) essential for APC interaction with factor Va. Blood 78:277a, 1991.

78. Mesters, R. M., Houghten, R. A., and Griffin, J. H.: Identification of a sequence of human activated protein C (residues 390–404) essential for its anticoagulant activity. J. Biol. Chem. 266:24514, 1991.

79. Steiner, S. A., Amphlett, G. W., and Castellino, F. J.: Stimulation of the amidase and esterase activity of activated bovine plasma protein C by monovalent cations. Biochem. Biophys. Res. Commun. 94:340, 1980.

80. Hill, K. A. W., and Castellino, F. J.: The effect of monovalent cations on the pre-steady state reaction kinetics of bovine activated plasma protein C and des 1-41-light chain activated plasma protein C. J. Biol. Chem. 262:140, 1987.

81. Long, G. L.: The human protein C gene. In Bertina, R. M. (ed.): Protein C and Related Proteins. London, Churchill Livingstone, Longman Group UK, 1988, pp. 117–129.

82. Rocchi, M., Roncuzzi, L., Santamaria, R., Archidracono, N., Dente, L., and Romeo, G.: Mapping through somatic cell hybrids and cDNA probes of protein C to chromosome 2, factor X to chromosome 13 and α1-acid glycoprotein to chromosome 9. Hum. Genet. 74:30, 1986.

83. Long, G. L., Marshall, A., Gardner, J. C., and Naylor, S. L.: Genes for human vitamin K–dependent plasma proteins C and S are located on chromosome 2 and 3, respectively. Somat. Cell Mol. Genet. 14:93, 1988.

84. Kato, A., Miura, O., Sumi, Y., and Aoki, N.: Assignment of the human protein C gene (PROC) to chromosome region 2q14–q21 by in situ hybridization. Cytogenet. Cell Genet. 47:46, 1988.

85. Patracchini, P., Aiello, V., Palazzi, P., Calzolari, E., and Bernardi, F.: Sublocalization of the human protein C gene on chromosome 2 q 13–14. Hum. Genet. 81:191, 1989.

86. Plutsky, J., Hoskins, J. A., Long, G. L., and Crabtree, G. R.: Evolution and organization of the human protein C gene. Proc. Natl. Acad. Sci. USA 83:546, 1986.

87. Foster, D. C., Yoshitake, S., and Davie, E. W.: The nucleotide sequence of the gene for human protein C. Proc. Natl. Acad. Sci. USA 82:4673, 1985.

88. Esmon, C. T., and Owen, W. G.: Identification of an endothelial cell cofactor for thrombin catalyzed activation of protein C. Proc. Natl. Acad. Sci. USA 78:2249, 1981.

89. Esmon, C. T., Esmon, N. L., and Harris, K. W.: Complex formation between thrombin and thrombomodulin inhibits both thrombin catalyzed fibrin formation and factor V activation. J. Biol. Chem. 257:7944, 1982.

90. Esmon, N. L., Carroll, R. C., and Esmon, C. T.: Thrombomodulin blocks the ability of thrombin to activate platelets. J. Biol. Chem. 258:12238, 1983.

91. Hofsteenge, J., and Stone, S.: The effect of thrombomodulin on the cleavage of fibrinogen and fibrinogen fragments by thrombin. Eur. J. Biochem. 168:49, 1987.

92. Polgár, J., Léránt, I., Muszbek, L., and Machovich, R.: Thrombomodulin inhibits the activation of factor XIII by thrombin. Thromb. Haemost. 58:506a, 1987.

93. Jakubowski, H. V., Kline, M. D., and Owen, W. G.: The effect of bovine thrombomodulin on the specificity of bovine thrombin. J. Biol. Chem. 261:3876, 1986.

94. Esmon, N. L., Owen, W. G., and Esmon, C. T.: Isolation of a membrane-bound cofactor for thrombin-catalyzed activation of protein C. J. Biol. Chem. 257:859, 1982.

95. Salem, H. H., Maruyama, I., Ishii, H., and Majerus, P. W.: Isolation and characterization of thrombomodulin from human placenta. J. Biol. Chem. 259:12246, 1984.

96. Suzuki, K., Kusumoto, H., and Hashimoto, S.: Isolation and characterization of thrombomodulin from bovine lung. Biochem. Biophys. Acta 882:343, 1986.

97. Kumada, T., Dittman, W. A., and Majerus, P. W.: A role for thrombomodulin in the pathogenesis of thrombin-induced thromboembolism in mice. Blood 71:728, 1987.

98. Jackman, R. W., Beeler, D. L., vanDeWater, L., and Rosenberg, R. D.: Characterization of a thrombomodulin cDNA reveals structural similarity to the low density lipoprotein receptor. Proc. Natl. Acad. Sci. USA 83:8834, 1986.

99. Suzuki, K., Kusumoto, H., Deyashiki, Y., Nishioka, J., Maruyama, I., Zushi, M., Kawahara, S., Honda, G., Yamamoto, S., and Horiguchi, S.: Structure and expression of human thrombomodulin, a thrombin receptor on endothelium acting as a cofactor for protein C activation. EMBO J. 6:1891, 1987.

100. Wen, D., Dittman, W. A., Ye, R. D., Deaven, L. L., Majerus, P. W., and Sadler, J. E.: Human thrombomodulin: Complete cDNA sequence and chromosome localization of the gene. Biochemistry 26:4350, 1987.

101. Jackman, R. W., Beeler, D. L., Fritze, L., Soff, G., and Rosenberg, R. D.: Human thrombomodulin gene is intron depleted: Nucleic acid sequence of the cDNA and gene predict protein structure and suggest sites of regulatory control. Proc. Natl. Acad. Sci. USA 84:6425, 1987.

102. Dittman, W. A., Kumada, T., Sadler, J. E., and Majerus, P. W.: The structure and function of mouse thrombomodulin. J. Biol. Chem. 263:15815, 1988.

103. Dittman, W. A., and Majerus, P. W.: Sequence of a cDNA for mouse thrombomodulin and comparison of the predicted mouse and human amino acid sequences. Nucleic Acids Res. 17:802, 1988.

104. Zimmermann, D. R., and Ruoslahti, E.: Multiple domains of the large fibroblast proteoglycan versican. EMBO J. 8:2975, 1990.

105. Mann, D. M., Yamaguchi, Y., Bourdon, M. A., and Ruoslahti, E.: Analysis of glycosaminoglycan substitution in decorin by site-directed mutagenesis. J. Biol. Chem. 265:5317, 1990.

106. Petersen, T. E.: The amino-terminal domain of thrombomodulin and pancreatic stone protein homologous with lectins. FEBS Lett. 231:51, 1988.

107. Patthy, L.: Detecting distant homologies of mosaic proteins. Analysis of the sequences of thrombomodulin, thrombospondin complement components C9, C8 alpha and beta, vitronectin and plasma cell membrane glycoprotein PC-1. J. Mol. Biol. 202:689, 1988.

108. McEver, R. P.: Leukocyte interactions mediated by selectins. Thromb. Haemost. 66:80, 1991.

109. Kurosawa, S., Stearns, D. J., Jackson, K. W., and Esmon, C. T.: A 10-kDa cyanogen bromide fragment from the epidermal growth factor homology domain of rabbit thrombomodulin contains the primary thrombin binding site. J. Biol. Chem. 263:5993, 1988.

110. Hayashi, T., Zushi, M., Yamamoto, S., and Suzuki, K.: Further localization of binding sites for thrombin and protein C in human thrombomodulin. J. Biol. Chem. 265:20156, 1990.

111. Tsiang, M., Lentz, S. R., Dittman, W. A., Wen, D., Scarpati, E. M., and Sadler, J. E.: Equilibrium binding of thrombin to recombinant human thrombomodulin: Effect of hirudin, fibrinogen, factor Va and peptide analogues. Biochemistry 29:10602, 1990.

112. Stearns, D. J., Kurosawa, S., and Esmon, C. T.: Microthrombomodulin. J. Biol. Chem. 264:3352, 1989.

113. Suzuki, K., Hayashi, T., Nishioka, J., Kosaka, Y., Zushi, W., Honda, G., and Yamamoto, S.: A domain composed of epidermal growth factor–like structures of human thrombomodulin is essential for thrombin binding and for protein C activation. J. Biol. Chem. 264:4872, 1989.

114. Zushi, M., Gomi, K., Yamamoto, S., Maruyama, I., Hayashi, T., and Suzuki, K.: The last three consecutive epidermal growth factor–like structures of human thrombomodulin comprise the minimum functional domain for protein C–activating cofactor activity and anticoagulant activity. J. Biol. Chem. 264:10351, 1989.

115. Parkinson, J. F., Grinell, B. W., Moore, R. E., Hoskins, J., Vlakos, C. J., and Bang, N. U.: Stable expression of a secretable deletion mutant of recombinant human thrombomodulin in mammalian cells. J. Biol. Chem. 265:12602, 1990.

116. Zushi, M., Gomi, K., Honda, G., Kondo, S., Yamamoto, S., Hayashi, T., and Suzuki, K.: Aspartic acid 349 in the fourth epidermal growth factor–like structure of human thrombomodulin plays a role in its Ca^{2+}-mediated binding to protein C. J. Biol. Chem. 266:19886, 1991.

117. Stenflo, J., Lundwall, Å, and Dahlbäck, B.: β-Hydroxyasparagine in domains homologous to the epidermal growth factor precursor in vitamin K–dependent protein S. Proc. Natl. Acad. Sci. USA 84:368, 1987.

118. Stenflo, J., Öhlin, A.-K., Owen, W. G., and Schneider, W. J.: β-Hydroxyaspartic acid or β-hydroxyasparagine in bovine low density lipoprotein receptor and in bovine thrombomodulin. J. Biol. Chem. 263:21, 1988.

119. Selander-Sunnerhagen, M., Ullner, M., Persson, E., Teleman, O., Stenflo, J., and Drakenberg, T.: How an epidermal growth factor (EGF)–like domain binds calcium: High resolution NMR structure of the calcium form of the NH_2-terminal EGF–like domain in coagulation factor X. J. Biol. Chem. 267:19642, 1992.

120. Dahlbäck, B., Hildebrand, B., and Linse, S.: Novel type of very high affinity calcium-binding sites in β-hydroxyasparagine–containing epidermal growth factor–like domains in vitamin K–dependent protein S. J. Biol. Chem. 265:18481, 1990.

121. Kimura, S., Nagoya, S., and Aoki, N.: Monoclonal antibodies to human thrombomodulin whose binding is calcium dependent. J. Biochem. 105:478, 1989.

122. Preissner, K. T., Koyama, T., Müller, D., Tschopp, J., and Müller-Berghaus, G.: Domain structure of the endothelial cell receptor thrombomodulin as deduced from modulation of its anticoagulant functions. J. Biol. Chem. 265:4915, 1990.

123. Bourin, M.-C., Boffa, M.-C., Björk, I., and Lindahl, U.: Functional domains of rabbit thrombomodulin. Proc. Natl. Acad. Sci. USA 83:5924, 1986.

124. Hofsteenge, J., Taguchi, H., and Stone, S. R.: Effect of thrombomodulin on the kinetics of the interaction of thrombin with substrates and inhibitors. Biochem. J. 237:243, 1986.

125. Preissner, K. T., Delvos, U., and Müller-Berghaus, G.: Binding of thrombin to thrombomodulin accelerates inhibition of the enzyme by antithrombin III. Evidence for a heparin-independent mechanism. Biochemistry 26:2521, 1987.

126. Bourin, M.-C., Öhlin, A.-K., Lane, D. A., Stenflo, J., and Lindahl, U.: Relationship between anticoagulant activities and polyanionic properties of rabbit thrombomodulin. J. Biol. Chem. 263:8044, 1988.

127. Bourin, M.-C.: Effect of rabbit thrombomodulin on thrombin inhibition by antithrombin in the presence of heparin. Thromb. Res. 54:27, 1989.

128. Bourin, M.-C., Lundgren-Åkerlund, E., and Lindahl, U.: Isolation and characterization of the glycosaminoglycan component of rabbit thrombomodulin proteoglycan. J. Biol. Chem. 265:15424, 1990.

129. Nawa, K., Sakano, K., Fujiwara, H., Sato, Y., Sugiyama, N., Ternuchi, T., Iwamoto, M., and Murimoto, Y.: Presence and function of chondroitin-4-sulfate on recombinant human soluble thrombomodulin. Biochem. Biophys. Res. Commun. 171:729, 1990.

130. Koyma, T., Parkinson, J. F., Sie, P., Bang, N. U., Müller-Berghaus, G., and Preissner, K. T.: Different glycoforms of human thrombomodulin. Eur. J. Biochem. 198:563, 1991.

131. Koyma, T., Parkinson, J. F., Aoki, N., Bang, N. U., Müller-Berghaus, G., and Preissner, K. T.: Relationship between post-translational glycosylation and anticoagulant function of secretable recombinant mutants of human thrombomodulin. Br. J. Haematol. 78:515, 1991.

132. Parkinson, J. F., Garcia, J., and Bang, N. U.: Decreased thrombin affinity of cell-surface thrombomodulin following treatment of cultured endothelial cells with β-D-xyloside. Biochem. Biophys. Res. Commun. 169:177, 1990.

133. Maruyama, I., Bell, C. E., and Majerus, P. W.: Thrombomodulin is found on endothelium of arteries, veins, capillaries, and lymphatics, and on syncytiotrophoblast of human placenta. J. Cell Biol. 101:363, 1985.

134. DeBault, L. E., Esmon, N. L., Olson, J. R., and Esmon, C. T.: Distribution of the thrombomodulin antigen in the rabbit vasculature. Lab. Invest. 54:172, 1986.

135. Ishii, H., Salem, H. H., Bell, C. E., Laposata, E. A., and Majerus, P. W.: Thrombomodulin, an endothelial anticoagulant protein, is absent from the human brain. Blood 67:362, 1986.

136. Wong, V. L. Y., Hofman, F. M., Ishii, H., and Fisher, M.: Regional distribution of thrombomodulin in human brain. Brain Res. 556:1, 1991.

137. Suzuki, K., Nishioka, J., Hayashi, T., and Kosaka, Y.: Functionally active thrombomodulin is present in human platelets. J. Biochem. 104:628, 1988.

138. Yoshida, M., Kozaki, M., Ioya, N., Kaji, N., Tamaki, T., Hiraishi, S., Ishii, H., Kazama, M., Fukutomi, K., and Nagasawa, T.: Plasma thrombomodulin levels as an indicator of vascular injury caused by cyclosporine nephrotoxicity. Transplantation 50:1066, 1990.

139. Yonezawa, S., Maruyama, I., Sakae, K., Igata, A., Majerus, P. W., and Sato, E.: Thrombomodulin as a marker for vascular tumors: Comparative study with factor VIII and Ulex europaes 1 lectin. Am. J. Clin. Pathol. 88:405, 1987.

140. Ishii, H., and Majerus, P. W.: Thrombomodulin is present in human plasma and urine. J. Clin. Invest. 76:2178, 1985.

141. Owen, W. G., and Esmon, C. T.: Functional properties of an endothelial cell cofactor for thrombin-catalyzed activation of protein C. J. Biol. Chem. 256:5532, 1981.

142. Haley, P. E., Doyle, M. F., and Mann, K. G.: The activation of bovine protein C by factor Xa. J. Biol. Chem. 264:16303, 1989.

143. Freyssinet, J. M., Wiesel, M. L., Grunebaum, L., Pereillo, J. M., Gauchy, J., Schuhler, S., Freund, G., and Cazenave, J. P.: Activation of human protein C by blood coagulation factor Xa in the presence of anionic phospholipids. Enhancement by sulphated polysaccharides. Biochem. J. 261:341, 1989.

144. Salem, H. H., Broze, G. J., Miletich, J. P., and Majerus, P. W.: The light chain of factor Va contains the activity of factor Va that accelerates protein C activation by thrombin. J. Biol. Chem. 258:8531, 1983.

145. Salem, H. H., Esmon, N. L., Esmon, C. T., and Majerus, P. W.: Effects of thrombomodulin and coagulation factor Va-light chain on protein C activation in vitro. J. Clin. Invest. 73:968, 1984.

146. Doyle, M. F., and Mann, K. G.: Multiple active forms of thrombin. IV. Relative activities of meizothrombins. J. Biol. Chem. 265:10693, 1990.

147. Wu, Q., Tsiang, M., Lentz, S. R., and Sadler, J. E.: Ligand specificity of human thrombomodulin. Equilibrium binding of human thrombin, meizothrombin, and factor Xa to recombinant thrombomodulin. J. Biol. Chem. 267:7083, 1992.

148. Lu, R., Esmon, N. L., Esmon, C. T., and Johnson, A. E.: The active site of the thrombin-thrombomodulin complex. J. Biol. Chem. 264:12956, 1989.

149. Maruyama, I., Salem, H. H., Ishii, H., and Majerus, P. W.: Human thrombomodulin is not an efficient inhibitor of the procoagulant activity of thrombin. J. Clin. Invest. 75:987, 1985.

150. Kurosawa, S., and Aoki, N.: Preparation of thrombomodulin from human placenta. Thromb. Res. 37:353, 1985.

151. Hirahara, K., Koyama, M., Matsuishi, T., and Kurata, M.: The effect of human thrombomodulin on the inactivation of thrombin by human antithrombin III. Thromb. Res. 57:117, 1990.

152. Dittman, W. A., and Majerus, P. W.: Structure and function of thrombomodulin: A natural anticoagulant. Blood 75:329, 1990.

153. Freyssinet, J.-M., and Cazenave, J.-P.: Thrombomodulin. In Bertina, R. M. (ed.): Protein C and Related Proteins. London, Churchill Livingstone, Longman Group UK, 1988, pp. 91–105.

154. Maruyama, I., and Majerus, P. W.: The turnover of thrombin-thrombomodulin complex in cultured human umbilical vein endothelial cells and A549 lung cancer cells. J. Biol. Chem. 260:15432, 1985.

155. Busch, C., Cancilla, P., Debault, L. E., Goldsmith, J. C., and Owen, W. G.: Use of endothelium cultured on microcarriers as a model for the microcirculation. Lab. Invest. 47:498, 1982.

156. Esmon, C. T., and Esmon, N.: Protein C activation. Semin. Thromb. Hemost. 10:122, 1984.

157. Johnson, A. E., Esmon, N. L., Laue, T. M., and Esmon, C. T.: Structural changes required for activation of protein C are induced by Ca^{2+} binding to a high affinity site that does not contain γ-carboxyglutamic acid. J. Biol. Chem. 258:5554, 1983.

158. Esmon, N. L., DeBault, L. E., and Esmon, C. T.: Proteolytic formation and properties of γ-carboxyglutamic acid–domainless protein C. J. Biol. Chem. 258:5548, 1983.

159. Galvin, J. B., Kurosawa, S., Moore, K., Esmon, C. T., and Esmon, N. L.: Reconstitution of rabbit thrombomodulin into phospholipid vesicles. J. Biol. Chem. 262:2199, 1987.

160. Freyssinet, J. M., Gauchy, J., and Cazenave, J. P.: The effect of phospholipids on the activation of protein C by the human thrombin-thrombomodulin complex. Biochem. J. 238:151, 1986.

161. Öhlin, A.-K., Linse, S., and Stenflo, J.: Calcium binding to the epidermal growth factor homology region of bovine protein C. J. Biol. Chem. 263:7411, 1988.

162. Ehrlich, H. J., Grinnell, B. W., Jaskunas, S. R., Esmon, C. T., Yan, S. B., and Bang, N. U.: Recombinant human protein C derivatives: Altered response to calcium resulting in enhanced activation by thrombin. EMBO J. 9:2367, 1990.

163. Stearns, D. J., Kurosawa, S., Sims, P. J., Esmon, N. L., and Esmon, C. T.: The interaction of a Ca^{2+} dependent monoclonal antibody with the protein C activation peptide region. Evidence for obligatory Ca^{2+} binding to both antigen and antibody. J. Biol. Chem. 263:826, 1988.

164. Vu, T.-K. H., Wheaton, V. I., Hung, D. T., Charo, I., and Coughlin, S. R.: Domains specifying thrombin-receptor interaction. Nature 353:675, 1991.

165. Musci, G., Berliner, L. J., and Esmon, C. T.: Evidence for multiple conformational changes in the active center of thrombin induced by complex formation with thrombomodulin: An analysis employing nitroxide spin-labels. Biochemistry 27:769, 1988.

166. Ye, J., Esmon, N. L., Esmon, C. T., and Johnson, A. E.: The active site of thrombin is altered upon binding to thrombomodulin. Two distinct structural changes detected by fluorescence, but only one correlates with protein C activation. J. Biol. Chem. 266:23016, 1991.

167. Holtin, G. L., and Trimpe, B. L.: Allosteric changes in thrombin's activity produced by peptides corresponding to segments of natural inhibitors and substrates. J. Biol. Chem. 266:6866, 1991.

168. Suzuki, K., Nishioka, J., and Hayashi, T.: Localization of thrombomodulin-binding site within human thrombin. J. Biol. Chem. 265:13263, 1990.

169. Suzuki, K., and Nishioka, J.: A thrombin-based peptide corresponding to the sequence of the thrombomodulin-binding site blocks the procoagulant activities of thrombin. J. Biol. Chem. 266:18498, 1991.

170. Noé, G., Hofsteenge, J., Rovelli, G., and Stone, S. R.: The use of sequence-specific antibodies to identify a secondary binding site in thrombin. J. Biol. Chem. 263:11729, 1988.

171. Hofsteenge, J., Braun, P. J., and Stone, S. R.: Enzymatic properties of proteolytic derivatives of human α-thrombin. Biochemistry 27:2144, 1988.

172. Bode, W., Mayr, I., Bauman, Y., Huber, R., Stone, S. R., and Hofsteenge, J.: The refined 1.9 Å crystal structure of human α-thrombin: Interaction with D-Phe-Pro-Arg chloromethylketone and significance of the Tyr-Pro-Pro-Trp insertion segment. EMBO J. 88:3467, 1989.

173. Grütter, M. G., Priestle, J. P., Rahuel, J., Grossenbacher, H., Bode, W., Hofsteenge, J., and Stone, S. R.: Crystal structure of the thrombin-hirudin complex: A novel mode of serine protease inhibition. EMBO J. 9:2361, 1990.

174. Rydel, T. J., Ravichandran, K. G., Tulinsky, A., Bode, W., Huber, R., Roitsch, C., Fenton, J. W., II: The structure of a complex of recombinant hirudin and human α-thrombin. Science 249:277, 1990.

175. Wu, Q., Sheehan, J. P., Tsiang, M., Lentz, S. R., Birktoft, J. J., and Sadler, J. E.: Single amino acid substitutions dissociate fibrinogen-clotting and thrombomodulin-binding activities of human thrombin. Proc. Natl. Acad. Sci. USA 88:6775, 1991.

176. Le Bonniec, B. F., and Esmon, C. T.: Glu-192–Gln substitution in thrombin mimics the catalytic switch induced by thrombomodulin. Proc. Natl. Acad. Sci. USA 88:7371, 1991.

177. Le Bonniec, B. F., MacGillivray, R. T. A., and Esmon, C. T.: Thrombin Glu-39 restricts the P'3 specificity to nonacidic residues. J. Biol. Chem. 266:13796, 1991.

178. Shirai, T., Shiojiri, S., Ito, E., Yamamoto, S., Kusomoto, H., Deyashiki, Y., Maruyama, I., and Suzuki, K.: Gene structure of human thrombomodulin, a cofactor for thrombin-catalyzed activation of protein C. J. Biochem. 103:281, 1988.

179. Espinosa, R., III, Sadler, J. E., and LeBeau, M. M.: Regional localization of the human thrombomodulin gene to 20p12-cen. Genomics 5:649, 1989.

180. Shaw, G., and Kamen, R.: A conserved Au sequence from the

3′ untranslated region of GM-CSF mRNA mediates selective mRNA degradation. Cell 46:659, 1986.

181. Maruyama, I., and Majerus, P. W.: Protein C inhibits endocytosis of thrombin-thrombomodulin complexes in A549 lung cancer cells and human umbilical vein endothelial cells. Blood 69:1481, 1987.

182. Beretz, A., Freyssinet, J.-M., Gauchy, J., Schmitt, D. A., Klein-Soyer, C., Edgell, C.-J. S., and Cazenave, J.-P.: Stability of the thrombin-thrombomodulin complex on the surface of endothelial cells from human sapahenous vein and from the cell line EA.hy 926. Biochem. J. 259:35, 1989.

183. Moore, K. L., Andreoli, S. P., Esmon, N. L., Esmon, C. T., and Bang, N. U.: Endotoxin enhances tissue factor and suppresses thrombomodulin expression of human vascular endothelium in vitro. J. Clin. Invest. 79:124, 1987.

184. Nawroth, P. P., Handley, D. A., Esmon, C. T., and Stern, D. M.: Interleukin 1 induces endothelial cell procoagulant while suppressing cell-surface anticoagulant activity. Proc. Natl. Acad. Sci. USA 83:3460, 1986.

185. Archipoff, G., Beretz, A., Freyssinet, J.-M., Klein-Soyer, C., Brisson, C., and Cazenave, J.-P.: Heterogeneous regulation of constitutive thrombomodulin or inducible tissue-factor activities on the surface of human saphenous-vein endothelial cells in culture following stimulation by interleukin-1, tumor necrosis factor, thrombin or phorbol ester. Biochem. J. 272:679, 1991.

186. Nawroth, P. P., and Stern, D. M.: Modulation of endothelial cell hemostatic properties by tumor necrosis factor. J. Exp. Med. 163:740, 1986.

187. Moore, K. L., Esmon, C. T., and Esmon, N. L.: Tumor necrosis factor leads to the internalization and degradation of thrombomodulin from the surface of bovine aortic endothelial cells in culture. Blood 73:159, 1989.

188. Conway, E. M., and Rosenberg, R. D.: Tumor necrosis factor suppresses transcription of the thrombomodulin gene in endothelial cells. Mol. Cell. Biol. 8:5588, 1988.

189. Ogawa, S., Gerlach, H., Esposito, C., Pasagiau-Macaulay, A., Brett, J., and Stern, D.: Hypoxia modulates the barrier and coagulant function of cultured bovine endothelium. J. Clin. Invest. 85:1090, 1990.

190. Key, N. S., Vercellotti, G. M., Winkelmann, J. C., Moldo, C. F., Goodman, J. L., Esmon, N. L., Esmon, C. T., and Jacob, H. S.: Infection of vascular endothelial cells with herpes simplex virus enhances tissue factor activity and reduces thrombomodulin expression. Proc. Natl. Acad. Sci. USA 87:7095, 1990.

191. Kapotis, S., Besemer, J., Bevec, D., Valent, P., Bettelheim, P., Lechner, K., and Speiser, W.: Interleukin-4 counteracts pyrogen-induced downregulation of thrombomodulin in cultured human vascular endothelial cells. Blood 78:410, 1991.

192. Scarpati, E. M., and Sadler, J. E.: Regulation of endothelial cell coagulant properties: Modulation of tissue factor, plasminogen activator inhibitors and thrombomodulin by phorbol 12-myristate 13-acetate and tumor necrosis factor. J. Biol. Chem. 264:20705, 1989.

193. Lentz, S. R., Tsiang, M., and Sadler, J. E.: Regulation of thrombomodulin by tumor necrosis factor-α: Comparison of transcriptional and posttranscriptional mechanisms. Blood 77:542, 1991.

194. Hirokawa, K., and Aoki, N.: Up-regulation of thrombomodulin in human umbilical vein endothelial cells in vitro. J. Biochem. 108:839, 1990.

195. Ohdama, S., Tahano, S., Ohashi, K., Miyake, S., and Aoki, N.: Pentoxifylline prevents tumor necrosis factor induced suppression of endothelial cell surface thrombomodulin. Thromb. Res. 62:745, 1991.

196. Maruyama, I., Soejima, Y., Osame, M., Ito, T., Ogawa, K., Yamamoto, S., Dittman, W. A., and Saito, H.: Increased expression of thrombomodulin on the cultured human umbilical vein endothelial cells and mouse hemangioma cells by cyclic AMP. Thromb. Res. 61:301, 1991.

197. Imada, S., Yamaguchi, H., Nagumo, M., Katayanagi, S., Iwasaki, H., and Imada, M.: Identification of fetomodulin, a surface marker protein of fetal development, as thrombomodulin by gene cloning and functional assays. Dev. Biol. 140:113, 1990.

198. Hirokawa, K., and Aoki, N.: Up-regulation of thrombomodulin by activation of histamin H₁-receptors in human umbical-vein endothelial cells in vitro. Biochem. J. 276:739, 1991.

199. Dittman, W. A., Kumada, T., and Majerus, P. W.: Transcription of thrombomodulin mRNA in mouse hemangioma cells is increased by cycloheximide and thrombin. Proc. Natl. Acad. Sci. USA 86:7179, 1989.

200. Van der Welden, P. A., Krommenhoek-Van Es, T., Allaart, C. F., Bertina, R. M., and Reitsma, P. H.: A frequent thrombomodulin amino acid dimorphism is not associated with thrombophilia. Thromb. Haemost. 65:511, 1991.

201. Comp, P. C., DeBault, L. E., Esmon, N. L., and Esmon, C. T.: Human thrombomodulin is inhibited by IgG from two patients with nonspecific anticoagulants. Blood 62:299a, 1983.

202. Freyssinet, J. M., and Cazenave, J. P.: Lupus like anticoagulants, modulation of the protein C pathway and thrombosis. Thromb. Haemost. 58:679, 1987.

203. Cariou, R., Tobelem, G., Bellucci, S., Soria, J., Soria, C., Maclouf, J., and Caen, J.: Effect of lupus anticoagulant on antithrombogenic properties of endothelial cells—inhibition of thrombomodulin-dependent protein C activation. Thromb. Haemost. 60:54, 1988.

204. Ruiz-Arguelles, G. J., Ruiz-Arguelles, A., Deleze, M., and Alarcon-Segovia, D.: Acquired protein C deficiency in a patient with primary antiphospholipid syndrome. Relationship to reactivity of anticardiolipin antibody with thrombomodulin. J. Rheumatol. 16:381, 1989.

205. Tsakiris, D. A., Pettas, L., Makris, F. E., and Marbet, G. A.: Lupus anticoagulant-antiphospholipid antibodies and thrombophilia. Relation to protein C–protein S–thrombomodulin. J. Rheumatol. 17:785, 1990.

206. Malia, R. G., Kitchen, S., Greaves, M., and Preston, F. E.: Inhibition of activated protein C and its cofactor protein S by antiphospholipid antibodies. Br. J. Haematol. 76:101, 1990.

207. Takano, S., Kimura, S., Ohdama, S., and Aoki, N.: Plasma thrombomodulin in health and diseases. Blood 76:2024, 1990.

208. Gomi, K., Zushi, M., Honda, G., Kawakako, S., Matsuki, O., Kanabayashi, T., Yamamoto, S., Maruyama, I., and Suzuki, K.: Antithrombotic effect of recombinant human thrombomodulin on thrombin-induced thromboembolism in mice. Blood 75:1396, 1990.

209. Solis, M. M., Cook, C., Cook, J., Glaser, C., Light, D., Morser, J., Yu, S., Fink, L., and Eidt, J. F.: Intravenous recombinant soluble human thrombomodulin prevents venous thrombosis in a rat model. J. Vasc. Surg. 14:599, 1991.

210. Dahlbäck, B.: Purification of human vitamin K–dependent protein S and its limited proteolysis by thrombin. Biochem. J. 209:837, 1983.

211. Walker, F. J.: Regulation of activated protein C by a new protein. J. Biol. Chem. 255:5521, 1980.

212. Walker, F. J.: Regulation of bovine activated protein C by protein S. Thromb. Res. 22:321, 1981.

213. Walker, F. J.: Regulation of activated protein C by protein S. The role of phospholipid in factor Va inactivation. J. Biol. Chem. 256:11128, 1981.

214. Walker, F. J.: Interactions of protein S with membranes. Semin. Thromb. Hemost. 14:216, 1988.

215. Suzuki, K., Nishioka, J., Matsuda, J., Murayama, M., and Hashimoto, S.: Protein S is essential for the activated protein C–catalyzed inactivation of platelet-associated factor Va. J. Biochem. 96:455, 1984.

216. Harris, K. W., and Esmon, C. T.: Protein S is required for bovine platelets to support activated protein C binding and activity. J. Biol. Chem. 260:2007, 1985.

217. Stern, D. M., Nawroth, P. P., Harris, K., and Esmon, C. T.: Cultured bovine aortic endothelial cells promote activated protein C–protein S–mediated inactivation of factor Va. J. Biol. Chem. 261:713, 1986.

218. Koedam, J. A., Meijers, J. C. M., Sixma, J. J., and Bouma, B. N.: Inactivation of human factor VIII by activated protein C. J. Clin. Invest. 82:1236, 1988.

219. Walker, F. J., Chavin, S. I., and Fay, P. I.: Inactivation of factor VIII by activated protein C and protein S. Arch. Biochem. Biophys. 252:322, 1987.

220. Nelsestuen, G. L., Kisiel, W., and DiScipio, R. G.: Interaction of vitamin K dependent proteins with membranes. Biochemistry 17:2134, 1978.

221. Dahlbäck, B., Wiedmer, T., and Sims, P. J.: Binding of anticoagulant vitamin K–dependent protein S to platelet-derived microparticles. Biochemistry 31:12769, 1992.

222. Dahlbäck, B.: Inhibition of protein Ca cofactor function of human and bovine protein S by C4b-binding protein. J. Biol. Chem. 261:12022, 1986.

223. Comp, P. C., Nixon, R. R., Cooper, M. R., and Esmon, C. T.: Familial protein S deficiency is associated with recurrent thrombosis. J. Clin. Invest. 74:2082, 1984.

224. Bertina, R. M., van Wijngaarden, A., Reinalda-Poot, J., Poort, S. R., and Bom, V. J. J.: Determination of plasma protein S—the protein cofactor of activated protein C. Thromb. Haemost. 53:268, 1985.

225. Comp, P. C., Doray, D., Patton, D., and Esmon, C. T.: An abnormal distribution of protein S occurs in functional protein S deficiency. Blood 67:504, 1986.

226. Walker, F. J.: Identification of a new protein involved in the regulation of the anticoagulant activity of activated protein C. Protein S binding protein. J. Biol. Chem. 261:10941, 1986.

227. Fair, D. S., and Marlar, R. A.: Biosynthesis and secretion of factor VII, protein C, protein S, and the protein C inhibitor from a human hepatoma cell line. Blood 67:64, 1986.

228. Fair, D. S., Marlar, R. A., and Levin, E. G.: Human endothelial cells synthesize protein S. Blood 67:1168, 1986.

229. Stern, D., Brett, J., Harris, K., and Nawroth, P.: Participation of endothelial cells in the protein C–protein S anticoagulant pathway: The synthesis and release of protein S. J. Cell. Biol. 102:1971, 1986.

230. Malm, J., Abrahamsson, P.-A., and Dahlbäck, B.: Synthesis of vitamin K–dependent anticoagulant protein S by Leydig cells of human testis (in preparation).

231. Schwarz, H. P., Heeb, M. J., Wencel-Drake, J. D., and Griffin, J. H.: Identification and quantitation of protein S in human platelets. Blood 66:1452, 1985.

232. Ogura, M., Tanabe, N., Nishioka, J., Suzuki, K., and Saito, H.: Biosynthesis and secretion of functional protein S by a human megakaryoblastic cell line (MEG-01). Blood 70:301, 1987.

233. Dahlbäck, B., Lundwall, Å, and Stenflo, J.: Primary structure of bovine vitamin K–dependent protein S. Proc. Natl. Acad. Sci. USA 83:4199, 1986.

234. Lundwall, Å., Dackowski, W., Cohen, E., Shaffer, M., Mahr, A., Dahlbäck, B., Stenflo, J., and Wydro, R.: Isolation and sequence of the cDNA for human protein S, a regulator of blood coagulation. Proc. Natl. Acad. Sci. USA 83:6717, 1986.

235. Hoskins, J., Norman, D. K., Beckmann, R. J., and Long, G. L.: Cloning and characterization of human liver cDNA encoding a protein S precursor. Proc. Natl. Acad. Sci. USA 84:349, 1987.

236. Ploos van Amstel, H. K., van der Zanden, A. L., Reitsma, P. H., and Bertina, R. M.: Human protein S cDNA encodes Phe 16 and Tyr 222 in the consensus sequences for the post-translational processing. FEBS Lett. 22:186, 1987.

237. DiScipio, R. G., Hermodson, M. A., Yates, S. G., and Davie, E. W.: A comparison of human prothrombin, factor IX (Christmas factor), factor X (Stuart factor), and protein S. Biochemistry 16:698, 1977.

238. DiScipio, R. G., and Davie, E. W.: Characterization of protein S, a γ-carboxy-glutamic acid containing protein from bovine and human plasma. Biochemistry 18:899, 1979.

239. Stenflo, J., and Jönsson, M.: Protein S, a new vitamin K–dependent protein from bovine plasma. FEBS Lett. 101:377, 1979.

240. Edenbrandt, C.-M., Lundwall, Å., Wydro, R., and Stenflo, J.:

241. Ploos van Amstel, H. K., Reitsma, P. H., van der Logt, P. E., and Bertina, R. M.: Intron-exon organization of the active human protein S gene PSα and its pseudogene PSβ; duplication and silencing during primate evolution. Biochemistry 29:7853, 1990.

242. Schmidel, D. K., Tatro, A. V., Phelps, L. G., Tomczak, J. A., and Long, G. L.: Organization of the protein S genes. Biochemistry 29:7845, 1990.

243. Ploos van Amstel, H. K., van der Zanden, A. L., Bakker, E., Reitsma, P. H., and Bertina, R. M.: Two genes homologous with human protein S cDNA are located on chromosome 3. Thromb. Haemost. 58:982, 1987.

244. Watkins, P. C., Eddy, R., Fukushima, Y., Byers, M. G., Cohen, E. H., Dackowski, W. R., Wydro, R. M., and Shows, T. B.: The gene for protein S maps near the centromere of human chromosome 3. Blood 71:238, 1988.

245. Long, G. L., Marshall, A., Gardner, J. C., and Naylor, S. L.: Genes for human vitamin K–dependent plasma proteins C and S are located on chromosome 2 and 3, respectively. Somat. Cell Mol. Genet. 14:93, 1988.

246. Gershagen, S., Fernlund, P., and Lundwall, Å.: A cDNA coding for human sex hormone binding globulin. Homology to vitamin K–dependent protein S. FEBS Lett. 220:129, 1987.

247. Baker, M. E., French, F. S., and Joseph, D. R.: Vitamin K–dependent protein S is similar to rat androgen-binding protein. Biochem. J. 243:293, 1987.

248. Dahlbäck, B., Lundwall, Å., and Stenflo, J.: Localization of thrombin cleavage sites in the aminoterminal region of bovine protein S. J. Biol. Chem. 261:5111, 1986.

249. Schwalbe, R. A., Ryan, J., Stern, D. M., Kisiel, W., Dahlbäck, B., and Nelsestuen, G. L.: Protein structural requirements and properties of membrane binding by γ-carboxyglutamic acid–containing plasma proteins and peptides. J. Biol. Chem. 264:20288, 1989.

250. Suzuki, K., Nishioka, J., and Hashimoto, S.: Regulation of activated protein C by thrombin-modified protein S. J. Biochem. 94:699, 1983.

251. Walker, F. J.: Regulation of vitamin K–dependent protein S. Inactivation with thrombin. J. Biol. Chem. 259:10335, 1984.

252. Dahlbäck, B., Hildebrand, B., and Malm, J.: Characterization of functionally important domains in vitamin K–dependent protein S using monoclonal antibodies. J. Biol. Chem. 265:8127, 1990.

253. Dahlbäck, B., Frohm, B., and Nelsestuen, G.: High affinity interaction between C4b-binding protein and vitamin K–dependent protein S in the presence of calcium. Suggestion of third component in blood regulating the interaction. J. Biol. Chem. 265:16082, 1990.

254. Schwalbe, R., Dahlbäck, B., Hillarp, A., and Nelsestuen, G.: Assembly of protein S and C4b-binding protein on membranes. J. Biol. Chem. 265:16074, 1990.

255. Nelson, R. M., van Dusen, W. J., Friedman, P. A., and Long, G. L.: β-Hydroxyaspartic acid and β-hydroxyasparagine residues in recombinant human protein S are not required for anticoagulation cofactor activity or for binding to C4b-binding protein. J. Biol. Chem. 266:20586, 1991.

256. Davis, C. G., Goldstein, J. L., Südhof, T. C., Anderson, R. G. W., Russel, D. W., and Brown, M. S.: Acid-dependent ligand dissociation and recycling of LDL receptor mediated by growth factor homology region. Nature 326:760, 1987.

257. Gershagen, S., Lundvall, P., and Fernlund, P.: Characterization of the human sex hormone binding globulin (SHBG) gene and demonstration of two transcripts in both liver and testis. Nucleic Acids Res. 17:9245, 1989.

258. Dahlbäck, B., and Stenflo, J.: High molecular weight complex in human plasma between vitamin K–dependent protein S and complement component C4b-binding protein. Proc. Natl. Acad. Sci. USA 78:2512, 1981.

259. Dahlbäck, B.: Purification of human C4b-binding protein and

Molecular analysis of the gene for vitamin K–dependent protein S and its pseudogene. Cloning and partial characterization. Biochemistry 29:7861, 1990.

formation of its complex with vitamin K–dependent protein S. Biochem. J. 209:847, 1983.

260. Nelson, R. M., and Long, G. L.: Solution-phase equilibrium binding interaction of human protein S with C4b-binding protein. Biochemistry 30:2384, 1991.

261. Iijima, K., Inone, N., Nakamura, K., Fukuda, C., Ohgi, S., Okada, M., Mori, T., Nishioka, J., Hayashi, T., and Suzuki, K.: Inherited deficiency of functional and free form protein S. Acta Haematol. Jpn. 52:126, 1989.

262. Lauer, C. G., Reid, T. J. III, Wideman, C. S., Evatt, B. L., and Alving, B. M.: Free protein S deficiency in a family with venous thrombosis. J. Vasc. Surg. 12:541, 1990.

263. Walker, F. J.: Characterization of a synthetic peptide that inhibits the interaction between protein S and C4b-binding protein. J. Biol. Chem. 264:17645, 1989.

264. Chang, G. T. G., Maas, B. H. A., Ploos van Amstel, H. K., Reitsma, P. R., Bertina, R. M., and Bouma, B. N.: The carboxy terminal loop of human protein S is involved in the interaction with human C4b-binding protein. Blood (Suppl.)78:277a, 1991.

265. Fernández, J. A., and Griffin, J. H.: Identification of regions of protein S essential for binding to C4b-binding protein. Thromb. Haemost. 65:711a, 1991.

266. Law, S. K. A., and Reid, K. B. M.: Activation and control of the complement. In Male, D. (ed.): Complement. Oxford, United Kingdom, IRL Press, 1988, pp. 9–27.

267. Scharfstein, J., Ferreira, A., Gigli, I., and Nussenzweig, V.: Human C4b-binding protein. I. Isolation and characterization. J. Exp. Med. 148:207, 1978.

268. Fujita, T., Gigli, I., and Nussenzweig, V.: Human C4-binding protein. II. Role in proteolysis of C4b by C3b-inactivator. J. Exp. Med. 148:1044, 1978.

269. Fujita, T., and Nussenzweig, V.: The role of C4-binding protein and β1H in proteolysis of C4b and C3b. J. Exp. Med. 150:267, 1979.

270. Gigli, I., Fujita, T., and Nussenzweig, V.: Modulation of the classical pathway C3 convertase by plasma proteins C4 binding protein and C3b inactivator. Proc. Natl. Acad. Sci. USA 76:6596, 1979.

271. Nagasawa, S., Ichihara, C., and Stroud, R.: Cleavage of C4b by C3b inactivator: Production of a nicked form of C4b, C4b′, as an intermediate cleavage product of C4b by C3b inactivator. J. Immunol. 125:578, 1980.

272. Saeki, T., Hirose, S., Nakutsukam, M., Kusunoki, Y., and Nagasawa, S.: Evidence that C4b-binding protein is an acute phase protein. Biochem. Biophys. Res. Commun. 164:1446, 1989.

273. Barnum, S. R., and Dahlbäck, B.: C4b-binding protein, a regulatory component of the classical pathway of complement, is an acute phase protein and is elevated in systemic lupus erythematosus. Complement Inflamm. 7:711, 1990.

274. Hillarp, A., and Dahlbäck, B.: Novel subunit in C4b-binding protein required for protein S binding. J. Biol. Chem. 263:12759, 1988.

275. Hillarp, A., and Dahlbäck, B.: Cloning of cDNA coding for the β chain of human complement component of C4b-binding protein: Sequence homology with the α chain. Proc. Natl. Acad. Sci. USA 87:1183, 1989.

276. Dahlbäck, B., and Hildebrand, B.: Degradation of human complement component C4b in the presence of the C4b-binding protein–protein S complex. Biochem. J. 209:857, 1983.

277. Dahlbäck, B., Smith, C. A., and Müller-Eberhard, H. J.: Visualization of human C4b-binding protein and its complexes with vitamin K–dependent protein S and complement protein C4b. Proc. Natl. Acad. Sci. USA 80:3461, 1983.

278. Dahlbäck, B., and Müller-Eberhard, H. J.: Ultrastructure of C4b-binding protein fragments formed by limited proteolysis using chymotrypsin. J. Biol. Chem. 259:11631, 1984.

279. Chung, L. P., Bentley, D. R., and Reid, K. B. M.: Molecular cloning and characterization of the cDNA coding for C4b-binding protein, a regulatory protein of the classical pathway of the human complement system. Biochem. J. 230:133, 1985.

280. Reid, K. B. M., Bentley, D. R., Campbell, R. D., Chung, L. P., Sim, R. B., Kristensen, T., and Tack, B. F.: Complement system proteins which interact with C3b or C4b. A superfamily of structurally related proteins. Immunol. Today 7:230, 1986.

281. Kristensen, T., D'Eustachio, P., Ogata, R. T., Chung, L. P., Reid, K. B. M., and Tack, B. F.: The superfamily of C3b/C4b-binding proteins. Fed. Proc. 46:2463, 1987.

282. Reid, K. B. M., and Day, A. J.: Structure-function relationships of the complement components. Immunol. Today 10:177, 1989.

283. Baron, M., Norman, D. G., and Campbell, I. D.: Protein modules. TIBS 16:13, 1991.

284. Barlow, P. N., Baron, M., Norman, D. G., Day, A. J., Willis, A. C., Sim, R. B., and Campbell, I. D.: Secondary structure of a complement control protein module by two-dimensional ^{1}H NMR. Biochemistry 30:997, 1991.

285. Norman, D. G., Barlow, P. N., Baron, M., Day, A. J., Sim, R. B., and Campbell, I. D.: Three-dimensional structure of a complement control protein module in solution. J. Mol. Biol. 219:717, 1991.

286. Rey-Campos, J., Rubinstein, P., and Rodriguez de Cordoba, S.: A physical map of the human regulator of complement activation gene cluster linking the complement genes CR 1, CR 2, DAF and C4BP. J. Exp. Med. 167:664, 1988.

287. Carroll, M. C., Alicot, E. M., Katzman, P. J., Klickstein, L. B., Smith, J. A., and Fearon, D. T.: Organization of the genes encoding complement receptors type 1 and 2, decay-accelerating factor, and C4b-binding protein in the RCA locus on human chromosome 1. J. Exp. Med. 167:1271, 1988.

288. Andersson, A., Dahlbäck, B., Hanson, C., Hillarp, A., Levan, G., Szpirer, J., and Szpirer, C.: Genes for C4b-binding protein α- and β-chains (C4BPA and C4BPB) are located on chromosome 1, band 1q32, in humans and on chromosome 13 in rats. Somat. Cell Mol. Genet. 16:493, 1990.

289. Padro-Manuel, F., Rey-Campos, J., Hillarp, A., Dahlbäck, B., and Rodriguez de Cordoba, S.: Human genes for the α and β chains of complement C4b-binding protein are closely linked in a head-to-tail arrangement. Proc. Natl. Acad. Sci. USA 87:4529, 1990.

290. Hillarp, A., Hessing, M., and Dahlbäck, B.: Protein S binding in relation to the subunit composition of human C4b-binding protein. FEBS Lett. 259:53, 1989.

291. Schwalbe, R. A., Dahlbäck, B., and Nelsestuen, G. L.: Independent association of serum amyloid P component, protein S, and complement C4b with complement C4b-binding protein and subsequent association of the complex with membranes. J. Biol. Chem. 265:21749, 1990.

292. Skinner, M., and Cohen, A. S.: Amyloid P component. Methods Enzymol. 163:523, 1988.

293. Clouse, L. H., and Comp, P. C.: The regulation of hemostasis: The protein C system. N. Engl. J. Med. 20:1298, 1986.

294. Bertina, R. M.: Molecular basis of thrombosis. In Bertina, R. M. (ed.): Protein C and Related Proteins. London, Churchill Livingstone, Longman Group UK, 1988, pp. 1–20.

295. Broekmans, A. W., and Conard, J.: Hereditary protein C deficiency. In Bertina, R. M. (ed.): Protein C and Related Proteins. London, Churchill Livingstone, Longman Group UK, 1988, pp. 160–181.

296. Briët, E., Broekmans, A. W., and Engesser, L.: Hereditary protein S deficiency. In Bertina, R. M. (ed.): Protein C and Related Proteins. London, Churchill Livingstone, Longman Group UK, 1988, pp. 203–212.

297. Rosenberg, R. D.: Regulation of the hemostatic mechanism. In Stamatoyannopoulos, G., Nienhuis, A. W., Leder, P., and Majerus, P. W. (eds.): The Molecular Basis of Blood Disease. Philadelphia, W. B. Saunders, 1986, pp. 534–574.

298. Esmon, C. T., Taylor, F. B., and Snow, T. R.: Inflammation and coagulation: Linked processes potentially regulated through a common pathway mediated by protein C. Thromb. Haemost. 66:160, 1991.

299. Hyde, E., Wetmore, R., and Gurewich, V.: Isolation and characterization of an in vivo thrombin-induced anticoagulant activity. Scand. J. Haematol. 13:121, 1974.

300. Taylor, F. B., Jr., Chang, A., Hinshaw, L. B., Esmon, C. T., Archer, L. T., and Beller, B. K.: A model for thrombin protection against endotoxin. Thromb. Res. 36:177, 1984.

301. Snow, T. R., Deal, M. T., Dikey, D. T., and Esmon, C. T.: Protein C activation following coronary artery occlusion in the in situ porcine heart. Circulation 84:293, 1991.

302. Marlar, R. A., Endres-Brooks, J., and Miller, C.: Serial studies of protein C and its plasma inhibitor in patients with disseminated intravascular coagulation. Blood 66:59, 1985.

303. Espana, F., and Griffin, J. H.: Determination of functional and antigenic protein C inhibitor and its complexes with activated protein C in plasmas by ELISA's. Thromb. Res. 55:671, 1989.

304. Espana, F., Vicente, V., Scharrer, I., Tabernero, D., and Griffin, J. H.: Determination of plasma protein C inhibitor and of two activated protein C inhibitor complexes in normals and in patients with intravascular coagulation and thrombotic disease. Thromb. Res. 59:593, 1990.

305. Tabernero, D., Espana, F., Vicente, V., Estellés, A., Gilbert, J., and Aznar, J.: Protein C inhibitor and other components of the protein C pathway in patients with acute deep vein thrombosis during heparin treatment. Thromb. Haemost. 63:380, 1990.

306. Vicente, V., Espana, F., Tabernero, D., Estellés, A., Aznar, J., Hendl, S., and Griffin, J.: Evidence of activation of the protein C pathway during acute vascular damage induced by Mediterranean spotted fever. Blood 78:416, 1991.

307. Taylor, F. B., Jr., Chang, A., Esmon, C. T., D'Angelo, A., Vigano-D'Angelo, S., and Blick, K. E.: Protein C prevents the coagulopathic and lethal effects of Escherichia coli infusion in the baboon. J. Clin. Invest. 79:918, 1987.

308. Taylor, F. B., Jr., Chang, A. C. K., Peer, G. T., Mather, P. T., Blick, K., Catlett, R., Lockhart, M. S., and Esmon, C. T.: DEGR–factor Xa blocks disseminated intravascular coagulation initiated by Escherichia coli without preventing shock or organ damage. Blood 78:364, 1991.

309. Taylor, F. B., Jr., Chang, A., Ferrell, G., Mather, T., Catlett, R., Blick, K., and Esmon, C. T.: C4b-binding protein exacerbates the host response to Escherichia coli. Blood 78:357, 1991.

310. Tabernero, D., Tomas, J. F., Alberca, I., Orfao, A., Borrasca, A. L., and Vicente, V.: Incidence and clinical characteristics of hereditary disorders associated with venous thrombosis. Am. J. Hematol. 36:249, 1991.

311. Heijboer, H., Brandjes, D. P., Buller, H. R., Sturk, A., and ten Cate, J. W.: Deficiencies of coagulation-inhibiting and fibrinolytic proteins in outpatients with deep-vein thrombosis. N. Engl. J. Med. 323:1512, 1990.

312. Malm, J., Laurell, M., Nilsson, I. M., and Dahlbäck, B.: Thromboembolic disease—critical evaluation of laboratory investigation. Thromb. Haemost. 68:7, 1992.

313. Gladson, C. L., Scharrer, I., Hach, V., Beck, K. H., and Griffin, J. H.: The frequency of type I heterozygous protein S and protein C deficiency in 141 unrelated young patients with venous thrombosis. Thromb. Haemost. 59:18, 1988.

314. Broekmans, A. W., van der Linden, I. K., Jansen-Koeter, Y., and Bertina, R. M.: Prevalence of protein C (PC) and protein S (PS) deficiency in patients with thromboembolic disease. Thromb. Res. (Suppl.)6:135a, 1986.

315. Bovill, E. G., Bauer, K. A., Dickermann, J. D., Callas, P., and West, B.: The clinical spectrum of heterozygous protein C deficiency in a large New England kindred. Blood 73:712, 1989.

316. Miletich, J., Sherman, L., and Broze, G., Jr.: Absence of thrombosis in subjects with heterozygous protein C deficiency. N. Engl. J. Med. 317:991, 1987.

317. Reitsma, P. H., Poort, S. R., Allaart, C. F., Briët, E., and Bertina, R. M.: The spectrum of genetic defects in a panel of 40 Dutch families with symptomatic protein C deficiency type I: Heterogeneity and founder effects. Blood 78:890, 1991.

318. Marlar, R. A., Montgomery, R., and Broekmans, A.: Diagnosis and treatment of homozygous protein C–children. J. Pediatr. 114:528, 1989.

319. Seligsohn, U., Berger, A., Abend, A., Rubin, L., Attias, D., Zivelin, A., and Rapaport, S. I.: Homozygous protein C deficiency manifested by massive thrombosis in the newborn. N. Engl. J. Med. 310:559, 1984.

320. Dreyfus, M., Magny, J. F., Bridey, F., Schwarz, H. P., Planché, C., Dehan, M., and Tchernia, G.: Treatment of homozygous protein C deficiency and neonatal purpura fulminans with a purified protein C concentrate. N. Engl. J. Med. 325:1565, 1991.

321. Rose, V. L., Kwaan, H. C., Williamson, K., Hoppensteadt, D., Walenga, J., and Fareed, J.: Protein C antigen deficiency and warfarin necrosis. Am. J. Clin. Pathol. 86:653, 1986.

322. Vigano, S., Mannucci, P. M., Solinas, S., Bottasso, B., and Mariani, G.: Decrease in protein C antigen and formation of an abnormal protein soon after starting oral anticoagulant therapy. Br. J. Haematol. 57:213, 1984.

323. Epstein, D. J., Bergum, P. W., Bajaj, P., and Rapaport, S. I.: Radioimmunoassays for protein C and factor X. Plasma antigen levels in abnormal hemostatic states. Am. J. Clin. Pathol. 82:573, 1984.

324. Weiss, P., Soff, G. A., Halkin, H., and Seligsohn, U.: Decline of proteins C and S and factors II, VII, IX and X during the initiation of warfarin therapy. Thromb. Res. 45:783, 1987.

325. Rowbotham, B., Clouston, W., Kime, N., Rowell, J., and Exner, T.: Coumarin skin necrosis without protein C deficiency. Aust. N. Z. J. Med. 16:513, 1986.

326. Cooper, D. N.: The molecular genetics of familial venous thrombosis. Blood Rev. 5:55, 1991.

327. Te Lintel-Hekkert, W., Bertina, R. M., and Reitsma, P. H.: Two RFLPs 7 kb 5' of the human protein C gene. Nucleic Acids Res. 16:11849, 1988.

328. Koenhen, E., Bertina, R. M., and Reitsma, P. H.: MspI RFLP in intron 8 of the human protein C gene. Nucleic Acids Res. 17:8401, 1989.

329. Reitsma, P. H., te Linkel Hekkert, W., Koenhen, E., van der Velden, P. A., Allaart, C. F., Deutz-Terlouw, P. P., Poort, S. R., and Bertina, R. M.: Application of two neural Mspl DNA polymorphisms in the analysis of hereditary protein C deficiency. Thromb. Haemost. 64:239, 1990.

330. Yamamoto, K., Tanimoto, M., Matsushita, T., Kagami, K., Suguira, I., Hamaguchi, M., Takamatsu, J., and Saito, H.: Genotype establishments for protein C deficiency by use of a DNA polymorphism in the gene. Blood 77:2633, 1991.

331. Yamamoto, K., Takamatsu, J., and Saito, H.: Two novel sequence polymorphisms of the human protein C gene. Nucleic Acids Res. 19:6973, 1991.

332. Gandrille, S., and Alach, M.: Polymorphism in the protein C gene detected by denaturing gradient gel electrophoresis. Nucleic Acids Res. 19:6982, 1991.

333. Tsay, W., Greengard, J. S., Montgomery, R., and Griffin, J. H.: Five previously undescribed mutations in protein C (PC) that identify elements critical for gene and protein activity. Blood (Suppl.) 78:184a, 1991.

334. Diuguid, D. L., Rabiet, M. J., Furie, B. C., Liebman, H. A., and Furie, B.: Molecular basis of hemophilia B: A defective enzyme due to an unprocessed propeptide is caused by a point mutation in the factor IX precursor. Proc. Natl. Acad. Sci. USA 83:5803, 1986.

335. Matsuda, M., Sugo, T., Sakata, Y., Murayama, H., Mimuro, J., Tanabe, S., and Yoshitake, S.: A thrombogenic state due to an abnormal protein C. N. Engl. J. Med. 319:1265, 1988.

336. Grundy, C., Chitolie, A., Talbot, S., Bevan, D., Kakkar, V., and Cooper, D. N.: Protein C London 1: Recurrent mutation at Arg 169 (CGG-TGG) in the protein C gene causing thrombosis. Nucleic Acids Res. 17:10513, 1989.

337. Sala, N., Poort, S. R., Bertina, R. M., Soria, J. M., Fontcuberta, J., and Reitsma, P. H.: Identification of two deletions and four point mutations in the protein C gene of 6 unrelated Spanish patients with hereditary protein C deficiency. Blood (Suppl.) 78:184a, 1991.

338. Gandrille, S., Vidaud, M., Aiach, M., Alhene-Geias, M., Fischer, A. M., Gouault-Heilman, M., Toulon, P., and Goossens, M.: Six previously undescribed mutations in 9 families

with protein C quantitative deficiency. Thromb. Haemost. 65:646a, 1991.

339. Reitsma, P. H., Poort, S. R., and Bertina, R. M.: Genetic abnormalities in the protein C genes of homozygous and compound heterozygotes for protein C deficiency. Thromb. Haemost. 65:808a, 1991.

340. Grundy, C. B., Melissari, E., Kakkar, V. V., and Cooper, D. N.: A molecular genetic study of protein C deficiency. Thromb. Haemost. 65:646a, 1991.

341. Grundy, C., Plendl, H., Grote, W., Zoll, B., Kakkar, V. V., and Cooper, D. N.: A single base-pair deletion in the protein C gene causing recurrent thromboembolism. Thromb. Res. 61:335, 1991.

342. Romeo, G., Hassan, H. J., Staempfli, S., Roncuzzi, L., Cianetti, L., Leonardi, A., Vicente, V., Mannucci, P. M., Bertina, R. M., Peschle, C., and Cortese, R.: Hereditary thrombophilia: Identification of nonsense and missense mutations in the protein C gene. Proc. Natl. Acad. Sci. USA 84:2829, 1987.

343. Yamamoto, K., Tanimoto, M., Matsushita, T., Sugiura, I., Takamatsu, J., and Saito, H.: Hereditary protein C deficiency due to a frameshift mutation in exon IX of the protein C gene. Thromb. Haemost. 65:646a, 1991.

344. Gandrille, S., Alhene-Gelas, M., Goossens, M., and Aiach, M.: PC Malakoff: An abnormal protein C due to mutation at the cleavage site of the propeptide. Thromb. Haemost. 65:1196a, 1991.

345. Nakamura, K.: A new hereditary abnormal protein C (protein C Yonago) with a dysfunctional Gla-domain. Thromb. Haemost. 65:1197a, 1991.

346. Bovill, E. G., Tomczak, J., Grant, B., Pilimet, E., Rainville, I., and Long, G. L.: Association of two novel mutations in the Gla-domain (Glu_{20} to ALA and VAL_{34} to MET) with symptomatic type II protein C deficiency. Thromb. Haemost. 65:647a, 1991.

347. Tsuda, S., Reitsma, P., and Miletich, J.: Molecular defects causing heterozygous protein C deficiency in three asymptomatic kindreds. Thromb. Haemost. 65:647a, 1991.

348. Schwartz, H. P., Fischer, M., Hopmeier, P., Batard, M. A., and Griffin, J. H.: Plasma protein S deficiency in familial thrombotic disease. Blood 64:1297, 1984.

349. Comp, P. C., and Esmon, C. T.: Recurrent thromboembolism in patients with a partial deficiency of protein S. N. Engl. J. Med. 311:1525, 1984.

350. Kamiya, T., Sugihara, T., Ogata, K., Saito, H., Suzuki, K., Nishioka, J., Hashimoto, S., and Yamagata, K.: Inherited deficiency of protein S in a Japanese family with recurrent venous thrombosis: A study of three generations. Blood 67:406, 1986.

351. Broekmans, A. W., Bertina, R. M., Reinalda-Poot, J., Engesser, L., Muller, H. P., Leeuw, J. A., Michiels, J. J., Brommer, E. J. P., and Briët, E.: Hereditary protein S deficiency and venous thrombo-embolism. A study in three Dutch families. Thromb. Haemost. 53:273, 1985.

352. Bertina, R. M.: Hereditary protein S deficiency. Haemostasis 15:241, 1985.

353. Mannucci, P. M., Valsecchi, C., Krachmalnicoff, A., Faioni, E. M., and Tripodi, A.: Familial dysfunction of protein S. Thromb. Haemost. 62:763, 1989.

354. D'Angelo, A., Vigano-D'Angelo, S., Esmon, C. T., and Comp, P. C.: Acquired deficiencies of protein S. Protein S activity during oral anticoagulation, in liver disease, and in disseminated intravascular coagulation. J. Clin. Invest. 81:1445, 1988.

355. Vigano-D'Angelo, S., D'Angelo, A., Kaufman, M., Jr., Sholer, C., Esmon, C. T., and Comp, P. C.: Protein S deficiency occurs in the nephrotic syndrome. Ann. Intern. Med. 107:42, 1987.

356. Comp, P. C., Thurnau, G. R., Welsh, J., and Esmon, C. T.: Functional and immunological protein S levels are decreased during pregnancy. Blood 68:881, 1986.

357. Malm, J., Laurell, M., and Dahlbäck, B.: Changes in the plasma levels of vitamin K–dependent protein C and S and of C4b-binding protein during pregnancy and oral contraception. Br. J. Haematol. 68:437, 1988.

358. Engesser, L., Broekmans, A. W., Briët, E., Brommer, E. J. P., and Bertina, R. M.: Hereditary protein S deficiency: Clinical manifestations. Ann. Intern. Med. 106:677, 1987.

359. Allaart, C. F., Aronson, D. O., Ruys, T., Rosendaal, F. R., van Bockel, J. H., Bertina, R. M., and Briët, E.: Hereditary protein S deficiency in young adults with arterial occlusive disease. Thromb. Haemost. 22:206, 1990.

360. Craig, A., Taberner, D. A., Fisher, A. H., Foster, D. N., and Mitra, J.: Type I protein S deficiency and skin necrosis. Postgrad. Med. J. 66:389, 1990.

361. Grimaudo, V., Gueissaz, F., Hauert, J., Sarraj, A., Kruithof, E. K. O., and Bachmann, F.: Necrosis of skin induced by coumarin in a patient deficient in protein S. Br. Med. J. 298:233, 1989.

362. Goldberg, S. L., Orthner, C. L., Yalisove, B. L., Elgart, M. L., and Kessler, C. M.: Skin necrosis following prolonged administration of coumarin in a patient with inherited protein S deficiency. Am. J. Hematol. 38:64, 1991.

363. Mahasandana, C., Suvatte, V., Chuansumit, A., Marlar, R. A., Manco-Johnson, M. J., Jacobson, L. J., and Hathaway, W. E.: Homozygous protein S deficiency in an infant with purpura fulminans. J. Paediatr. 117:750, 1990.

364. Diepstraten, C. M., Ploos van Amstel, J. K., Reitsma, P. H., and Bertina, R. M.: aCCA/CCG neutral dimorphism in the codon for Pro 626 of the human protein S gene PSAplhpa (PROS1). Nucleic Acids Res. 19:5091, 1991.

365. Bertina, R. M., Ploos van Amstel, H. K., van Wijngaarden, A., Coenen, J., Leemhuis, M. P., Deutz-Terlow, P. P., van der Linden, I. K., and Reitsma, P. H.: Heerlen polymorphism of protein S, an immunologic polymorphism due to dimorphism of residue 460. Blood 76:538, 1990.

366. Ploos van Amstel, H. K., Reitsma, P. H., Hamulyak, K., de Die-Smulders, C. E., Mannucci, P. M., and Bertina, R. M.: A mutation in the protein S pseudogene is linked to protein S deficiency in a thrombophilic family. Thromb. Haemost. 62:897, 1989.

367. Schmidel, D. K., Nelson, R. M., Broxson, E. H., Jr., Comp, P. C., Marlar, R. A., and Long, G. L.: A 5.3-kb deletion including exon XIII of the protein S α gene occurs in two protein S–deficient families. Blood 77:551, 1991.

368. Ploos van Amstel, H. K., Huisman, M. V., Reitsma, P. H., ten Cate, J. W., and Bertina, R. M.: Partial protein S gene deletion in a family with hereditary thrombophilia. Blood 73:479, 1989.

369. Reitsma, P. H., Poort, S. R., Bernardi, F., Gandrille, S., Long, G. L., Sala, N., and Cooper, D. N.: Protein C deficiency: A database of mutations. Thromb. Haemost. 69:77, 1993.

370. Dahlbäck, B., Carlsson, M., and Svensson, P. J.: Familial thrombophilia due to a previously unrecognized mechanism characterized by poor anticoagulant response to activated protein C: Prediction of a cofactor to activated protein C. Proc. Natl. Acad. Sci. USA 90:1004, 1993.

Regulation of Blood Coagulation by Protease Inhibitors

George J. Broze, Jr., and Douglas M. Tollefsen

INTRODUCTION

Blood coagulation is part of the hemostatic response to injury and serves to maintain the integrity of the vascular system. Coagulation involves a complex series of interactions between protease zymogens, enzymes, and cofactors that leads to the generation of thrombin and a fibrin clot. (See Chapter 16.) This process is regulated to limit the extent of coagulation to the site of injury and to allow the eventual dissolution of fibrin concomitant with the healing process. The endogenous mechanisms for the regulation of coagulation include the inhibition of coagulation enzymes, the inactivation of coagulation cofactors (the protein C, protein S, thrombomodulin pathway; see Chapter 17), and fibrinolysis (see Chapter 21). Abnormalities in any of these control mechanisms may be associated with bleeding or thrombosis. This chapter describes the control of the initiation of coagulation by tissue factor pathway inhibitor (TFPI) and the regulation of thrombin by antithrombin and heparin cofactor II.

Owing to the influence of Schmidt[1] and Morawitz,[2] in the first half of this century it was widely accepted that the initiating event in blood coagulation was the exposure of plasma to damaged tissues. The substance in tissues responsible for this induction of coagulation was initially called tissue thromboplastin and later tissue factor (factor III).[3] Early studies suggesting the existence of an alternative pathway of coagulation that does not require tissue factor were initially rationalized to conform to the prevalent theory of Schmidt and Morawitz.[4–7] Mounting evidence, however—in particular, the observation that blood from hemophiliacs apparently clotted normally after the addition of tissue factor—eventually forced a reassessment of the coagulation mechanism.

In 1964, the cascade[8] and waterfall[9] hypotheses proposed an "intrinsic" pathway of coagulation (Fig. 18–1). In these theories, the exposure of the "contact" factors (factor XII, high molecular weight kininogen, and prekallikrein) in plasma to a surface leads to the activation of factor XI, which in turn activates factor IX. Factor IXa, in the presence of factor VIII, activates factor X; factor Xa, in the presence of factor V, then activates prothrombin (factor II) to thrombin, which subsequently cleaves fibrinogen (factor I) to fibrin. Mentioned only in passing was the "extrinsic" coagulation pathway, in which factor VIIa with tissue factor directly activated factor X. It was considered of little importance to hemostasis, since factors VIII and IX, whose deficiencies caused severe bleeding, lay in the "intrinsic" pathway.

The segregation of the known coagulation factors into the "intrinsic" and "extrinsic" pathways and the availability of assays to test each pathway (partial thromboplastin time and prothrombin time, respectively) proved invaluable in the diagnosis of hemorrhagic diseases. It became apparent, however, that the cascade/waterfall hypotheses fail to reflect hemostasis accurately. Individuals deficient in one of the "contact" factors required for the initiation of "intrinsic" coagulation are asymptomatic,[10–12] whereas individuals deficient in factor VII bleed abnormally.[13, 14] These clinical data and the laboratory observation of Osterud and Rapaport[15] that factor VIIa with tissue factor can activate factor IX of the "intrinsic" pathway as well as factor X produced a resurgence of interest in "extrinsic" coagulation and a renewed appreciation of the pivotal role of tissue factor in the initiation of coagulation.

If tissue factor provides the trigger for coagulation in vivo, and since the factor VIIa–tissue factor complex is a potent activator of factor X, why, then, do hemophiliacs bleed? Clues to the resolution of this dilemma were provided by early investigators who showed that when plasma is induced to clot by the addition of small amounts of tissue factor, the presence of factor VIII and factor IX is required for optimal coagulation.[16, 17] This result contrasts with that of the standard prothrombin time assay, in which relatively large quantities of tissue factor are used to initiate coagulation, and in which hemophiliac plasma, deficient in factor VIII or factor IX, is indistinguishable from normal plasma. The recently rediscovered and characterized inhibitor of tissue factor–induced coagulation, termed tissue factor pathway inhibitor, accounts for these in vitro observations and appears to explain the paradox of the severe hemorrhage that occurs in hemophiliacs in the face of an intact "extrinsic" pathway of coagulation.

INITIATION OF COAGULATION BY FACTOR VIIa–TISSUE FACTOR

Tissue Factor

Human tissue factor is a 45,000 molecular weight, integral membrane protein that acts as a cofactor to enhance the proteolytic activity of activated factor VII (factor VIIa) toward its substrates, factor IX and factor X.[18, 19] Tissue factor is a member of the cytokine/interferon receptor superfamily, and its extracellular domain is predicted to consist of two barrel-like structures that form a V-shaped, ligand-binding trough (Fig. 18–2).[20, 21] In contrast to the cytokine/interferon receptors, however, there is no evidence that tissue factor is involved in transmembrane signaling.

Immunohistochemical studies of normal human tissues have demonstrated that the cellular expression of tissue factor is selective and that cells normally in contact with plasma, the blood cells and the endothelium of blood vessels, are devoid of tissue factor.[22–24] Brain, lung, and placenta stain strongly for tissue factor, as do peripheral nerves, autonomic ganglia, the epithelium of the skin and mucosa, and the vascular adventitia. Similar studies in tissues affected by a range of pathological conditions have not been reported, but it has been shown that cells and extracellular material within atherosclerotic plaques contain tissue factor.[22, 25]

Two cells of particular interest are the monocyte

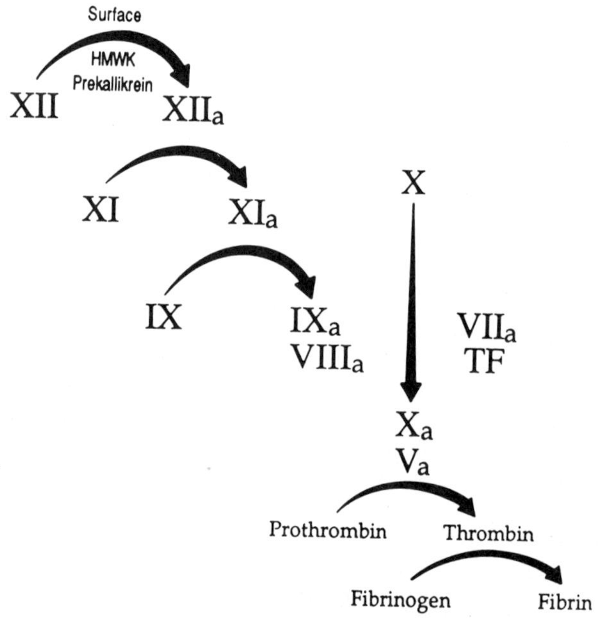

FIGURE 18–1. The cascade/waterfall hypothesis of blood coagulation. The intrinsic pathway of coagulation is initiated by exposure of the contact factors (factor XII, prekallikrein, and high molecular weight kininogen [HMWK]) to an appropriate surface with subsequent activation of factor XI by factor XIIa. The extrinsic pathway of coagulation is initiated by exposure of factor VIIa to tissue factor. The cofactors, factor V and factor VIII, are depicted in their activated forms, and the requirement for phospholipids and calcium ions for certain of the reactions is not included.

FIGURE 18–2. The factor VIIa–tissue factor catalytic complex. On the basis of sequence homology with other members of the cytokine/interferon receptor family of proteins, the extracellular region of tissue factor is depicted as two domains that form a V-shaped, ligand-binding trough. The transmembrane domain of tissue factor traverses the plasma membrane of a cell and is followed by a short cytoplasmic tail. Factor VIIa is shown bound to tissue factor, and factor X is shown in the process of being activated by the factor VIIa–tissue factor complex. The γ-carboxyglutamic acid (GLA), epidermal growth factor (EGF), and catalytic (CAT) domains of factor VIIa and factor X are depicted as globular structures, as is the activation peptide of factor X (AP). Calcium ion binding by the Gla domain in factor VIIa is required for factor VIIa binding to tissue factor, and the EGF domain in factor VIIa plays an important role in its interaction with tissue factor. Calcium ion binding by the Gla domain in factor X is required for its association with the phospholipid surface.

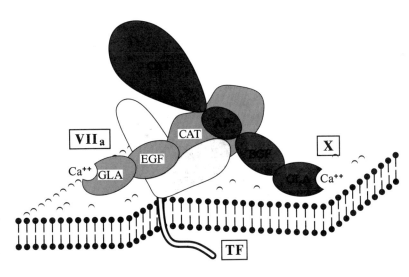

and the endothelial cell, which lack tissue factor activity when they are quiescent but express tissue factor in response to agents that may be physiologically relevant, including endotoxin,[26, 27] interleukin-1,[28] tumor necrosis factor,[29, 30] thrombin,[31, 32] activated complement factors,[33, 34] and immune complexes.[35, 36] In the case of monocyte activation, the response to certain stimuli requires or is enhanced by the presence of T lymphocytes.[37–43] The elaboration of many of these stimulatory agents has been demonstrated in a variety of clinical diseases, particularly those associated with inflammation. Thus, the local induction of coagulation at sites of inflammation and the systemic thrombotic propensity that accompanies these diseases may be due to aberrant production of tissue factor by these cells, which are normally not thrombogenic. Indirect evidence supports such a role for monocyte-generated tissue factor. Increased levels of tissue factor have been detected ex vivo in peripheral blood monocytes and tissue macrophages from animals and humans with a number of pathological states.

The phospholipid milieu surrounding the tissue factor apoprotein within the plasma membrane of a cell is critical for its function,[18, 44] and studies using purified phospholipids show that the functional activity of tissue factor is several-fold greater when it is inserted into micelles containing a combination of neutral and acidic phospholipids (e.g., 70 per cent phosphatidylcholine and 30 per cent phosphatidylserine) rather than neutral phospholipids alone.[45–47] The enhancement in cell surface tissue factor activity that accompanies the sublethal perturbation or disruption of many cells appears to reflect the redistribution of acidic phospholipids from the inner to the outer leaflet of their plasma membrane.[23, 48–52]

Factor VII

Human factor VII is a single-chain glycoprotein of about 50,000 molecular weight that is present in plasma at trace concentrations (10 nM, 500 ng/ml).[53–55] It is synthesized predominantly by the liver, although stimulated monocytes or macrophages may provide an important source of factor VII at local sites.[56–59] Factor VII is proteolytically activated in vitro by thrombin[60] and factor XIIa[61, 62] and by factor Xa and factor IXa in the presence of calcium ions and procoagulant phospholipids.[53, 60, 63, 64] Autoactivation of factor VII by factor VIIa has also been described.[65–67] Whether zymogen factor VII possesses a low level of intrinsic catalytic activity, albeit less than 1 per cent that of factor VIIa, is controversial[68]; recent studies suggest that it is inactive.[69–71]

Vitamin K is required for the post-translational γ carboxylation of a number of glutamic acid residues near the amino-termini of factor VII and the substrates for factor VIIa–tissue factor, factor IX, and factor X. (See Chapter 16.) Calcium ion binding mediated by these γ-carboxyglutamic acid (Gla) residues induces a conformational change in the proteins that leads to the expression of membrane- and cofactor-binding properties that are essential for their functional activity.[72–76] Thus, the binding of factor VIIa to the tissue factor on the surface of cells requires calcium ions and the presence of its Gla domain.[77, 78] Similarly, the Gla domains of factor IX and factor X are needed for the optimal interaction between these substrates and the catalytic factor VIIa–tissue factor complex.

Following the Gla domain, factor VII, factor IX, and factor X have a so-called epidermal growth factor (EGF) domain, which contains two modules that are homologous in structure to the EGF precursor. This domain appears to play an important role in mediating protein-protein interactions, and the EGF domain in factor VII, along with the peptide linking it to the Gla domain, appears to be critical for the binding of factor VII to tissue factor.[79, 80]

The catalytic domains of these coagulation factors are similar in structure to the prototype serine proteases trypsin and chymotrypsin. The proteolytic activation of the zymogen forms of these factors induces a conformational change in the molecules that converts them from inactive precursors to active enzymes. In the case of factor IX and factor X, a portion of the protein termed the activation peptide is proteolytically removed during the activation process. Factor VII is activated by proteolytic cleavage at a single site with the production of a two-chain, disulfide-bonded molecule.

Zymogen factor VII and factor VIIa bind to tissue factor with equal affinities, and this tissue factor binding dramatically affects their coagulant activities (see Fig. 18–2).[77, 81] First, zymogen factor VII bound to tissue factor, as opposed to that in solution, is rapidly and preferentially cleaved to factor VIIa by trace concentrations of factor Xa.[82, 83] Second, the enzymatic activity of factor VIIa is enhanced 5000-fold when it is bound to tissue factor.[84, 85] The substrates, factor IX and factor X, compete for the enzymatic factor VIIa–tissue factor complex.[86] Most,[86–90] but not all,[85] investigators have found factor X to be the preferred substrate for factor VIIa–tissue factor in vitro.

When compared with other activated coagulation factors, factor VIIa is remarkably stable in plasma, remaining in the circulation nearly as long as zymogen factor VII.[91] A potent inhibitor of factor VIIa has not been described, and antithrombin, even in the presence of heparin, inhibits factor VIIa slowly.[53, 92] Thus, physiologic regulation of tissue factor–initiated coagulation does not appear to be mediated at the level of the enzyme factor VIIa. Instead, TFPI, an inhibitor that targets the catalytic factor VIIa–tissue factor complex, appears to provide the endogenous means for regulating this pathway.

TISSUE FACTOR PATHWAY INHIBITOR

History

In 1947, Thomas[93] and Schneider[94] independently showed that the preincubation of crude tissue thromboplastin with serum prevented the lethal disseminated intravascular coagulation that occurs following thromboplastin infusion in animals. Thomas also noted that this inhibitory effect of serum required the presence of calcium ions, that the inhibitor appeared to bind to the thromboplastin, and that the inhibition could be reversed by calcium ion chelators. Later, Hjort[95] showed that the serum inhibitor recognized the factor VIIa–Ca^{2+}–tissue factor complex, which he called "convertin," rather than factor VIIa or tissue factor alone. About the same time, Biggs and her colleagues[16, 17] reported that coagulation was delayed and incomplete following the addition of low concentrations of tissue factor to hemophiliac plasma, but with the advent of the cascade[8] and waterfall[9] theories of coagulation, the possible connection between this observation and the previously described thromboplastin inhibitor was not explored further.

More than 20 years later, Marlar and colleagues[96] showed that when coagulation was induced by small amounts of tissue factor, much less factor X was activated in hemophiliac plasma, lacking either factor VIII or factor IX, than in normal plasma. Subsequently, Morrison and Jesty[97] noted that the activation of factor IX (and factor X) in plasma was also incomplete following the addition of tissue factor and that this apparent inhibition of factor VIIa–tissue factor enzymatic activity was directly related to the presence of factor X or to brief pretreatment of the plasma with factor Xa. In 1985, Sanders and associates[98] demonstrated that the presence of not only factor X but also an inhibitor present in the total lipoprotein fraction of plasma following density centrifugation was required for this apparent inhibition of tissue factor–directed coagulation. Additional studies from several groups confirmed these results and went on to show that the inhibition was reversed by chelation of calcium ions with ethylenediaminetetra-acetic acid (EDTA), with release of functionally active factor VIIa and tissue factor.[99–101] Thus, the rediscovered inhibitor appears to be identical to the "anticonvertin" studied by Hjort in 1957.[95] Previously referred to as lipoprotein-associated coagulation inhibitor (LACI) and extrinsic pathway inhibitor (EPI), in 1991 the inhibitor was renamed tissue factor pathway inhibitor by a subcommittee of the Scientific and Standardization Committee of the International Society of Thrombosis and Haemostasis.

Biochemistry and Molecular Biology of Tissue Factor Pathway Inhibitor

The primary structure of TFPI, based on complementary DNA (cDNA) sequencing,[102] is shown in Figure 18–3. After the proteolytic removal of a 24 or 28 amino acid leader sequence by the signal peptidase, the mature protein contains an acidic amino-terminal domain followed by three tandem Kunitz-type protease inhibitory modules and a basic carboxy-terminal domain. Ser 2 is partially phosphorylated, possibly through the action of casein kinase II, in the TFPI expressed by cells in tissue culture,[103] and one or more of the three potential sites for N-linked glycosylation (Asn 117, Asn 167, and Asn 228) are utilized.[104] The N-linked oligosaccharides in TFPI produced by endothelial and kidney cells in vitro are sulfated.[105, 106, 106a] What effect these post-translational modifications have on TFPI function or physiology is not known.

The TFPI gene contains nine exons and resides on the long arm of chromosome 2 (q31–q32.1).[107, 108, 108a] Exons 1 and 2 encode a 5′ untranslated sequence in the TFPI messenger RNA (mRNA), and exon 3 encodes the signal peptide and amino-terminus of the mature TFPI molecule. The three Kunitz-type domains are encoded by exons 4, 6, and 8, and the polypeptide sequences linking the Kunitz domains are encoded by exons 5 and 7. The carboxy-terminus of TFPI and a long 3′ untranslated region are encoded by exon 9. All the splice junctions between exons are of the same type (type 1), suggesting that the TFPI

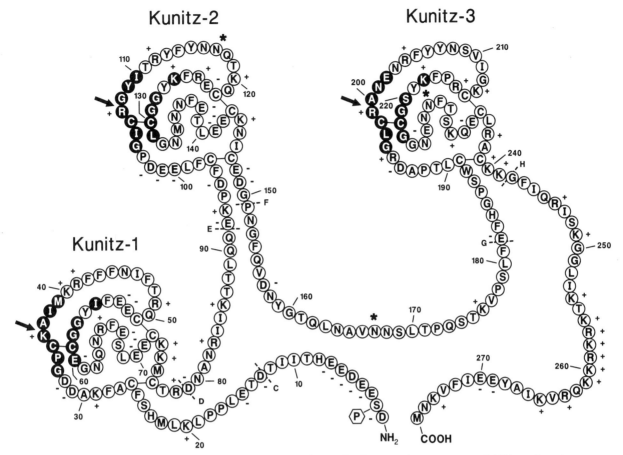

FIGURE 18–3. Structure of tissue factor pathway inhibitor. The three Kunitz-type protease inhibitory domains are labeled, and arrows indicate the location of their respective active site inhibitory clefts (P1–P1′). On the basis of the structure of the aprotinin-trypsin complex, residues within each Kunitz-type domain that would be in close contact with the catalytic domain of a target protease are shown as solid circles. Charged residues are indicated by plus (+) and minus (−) signs. Asterisks denote the potential sites for N-linked glycosylation; phosphorylation at Ser 2 is also shown. The sites of introns in the TFPI gene are labeled with capital letters.

gene was assembled during evolution through a process of gene duplication and exon shuffling.[109]

One NF-1[110] and two imperfect AP-1[111] sequences have been identified in the putative promoter region of the TFPI gene. In several other genes,[112, 113] AP-1–binding sites have been shown to act as protein kinase C–responsive elements, and the induction of TFPI expression in cultured monocytic cells (U937) following the administration of phorbol myristate acetate has been reported.[114] The 5′ DNA of the TFPI gene, however, does not contain a TATA box or CCAAT sequence, which may account for the apparent use of multiple, alternative transcriptional start sites.[107, 108] Alternative splicing of exon 2 in the untranslated region of the TFPI message occurs, and TFPI mRNAs of 1.4 and 4.0 kb arise through the use of alternative polyadenylation signals.[115] Preliminary evidence suggests that both the 1.4 and the 4.0 kb TFPI messages are relatively stable despite the presence in the 4.0 kb message of many AUUU and two UAAUUUAU sequences that have been associated with mRNA instability.[116, 117]

Kunitz-type Inhibitors

Whereas most inhibitors of the coagulation proteases are members of the serpin family, TFPI belongs to the Kunitz family of serine protease inhibitors. Other members of the Kunitz family of inhibitors that might be involved in hemostasis are certain forms of β amyloid precursor protein that inhibit factor XIa[118] and inter-α-trypsin inhibitor,[119] which contains two Kunitz-type domains. The most extensively characterized Kunitz-type inhibitor is bovine basic pancreatic trypsin inhibitor, or aprotinin (Trasylol).[120] The linear amino acid sequences of Kunitz-type inhibitory domains contain six specifically spaced cysteine residues, and the intramolecular disulfide bridges are presumably responsible for the observed functional stability of Kunitz-type inhibitors, despite treatment with a variety of physical and chemical denaturants, including sodium dodecyl sulfate.[120, 121] These inhibitors appear to act by the standard mechanism,[122] in which the inhibitor feigns to be a good substrate, but after the enzyme binds, subsequent cleavage at the active site cleft (P1–P1′) of the inhibitor occurs only very slowly or not at all. The P1 residue is an important determinant of inhibitory specificity, and alterations of the residue in the P1 position can profoundly alter the activity of Kunitz-type inhibitors. On the basis of the known structure of the prototype Kunitz inhibitor, aprotinin, and its interaction with trypsin, the disulfide bonds, the active site cleft, and the residues predicted to be in close contact with the catalytic domain in a target enzyme are depicted in Figure 18–3 for each of the three Kunitz domains of the TFPI molecule.

In kinetic terms, Kunitz-type inhibitors typically produce slow, tight-binding, competitive, and reversible inhibition of the following form:

$$E + I \underset{k_2}{\overset{k_1}{\rightleftharpoons}} EI \underset{k_4}{\overset{k_3}{\rightleftharpoons}} EI^*$$

where E = enzyme, I = inhibitor, EI is the initial collision complex with a $K_i(initial) = k_2/k_1$, and EI^* is the final complex that develops slowly from EI and is of higher affinity.[123, 124] The $K_i(final)$ of the final EI^* complex equals $K_i(initial)[k_4/(k_3 + k_4)]$. "Slow" implies that the final degree of inhibition does not occur immediately, and "tight-binding" refers to the fact that these inhibitors produce significant inhibition at concentrations near that of the enzyme being inhibited.

Inhibition of Factor Xa by Tissue Factor Pathway Inhibitor

Tissue factor pathway inhibitor inhibits factor Xa by binding at or near the active site of the enzyme.[125] This interaction has 1:1 stoichiometry, does not require calcium ions, and is reversed by treatment with sodium dodecyl sulfate or high concentrations of benzamidine, a competitive serine protease inhibitor. TFPI is also a potent inhibitor of trypsin, but this property is unlikely to be physiologically significant.[126]

The second Kunitz domain in TFPI is responsible for the inhibition of factor Xa,[127] but other regions of the TFPI molecule also participate in the formation of the factor Xa–TFPI complex. The very basic carboxy-terminal region of TFPI (residues 253 to 276) is required for a high-affinity interaction between factor Xa and TFPI in the initial encounter complex (EI) and overall optimal factor Xa inhibition.[128] Furthermore, a form of the TFPI molecule that lacks the amino-terminus and first Kunitz domain (residues 1 to 87) is a much less potent inhibitor of factor Xa than is full-length TFPI.[129]

Two forms of TFPI are isolated from the conditioned media of cultured cells. One is full-length TFPI, and the other is proteolytically truncated at its carboxy-terminus and lacks the highly basic domain that is required for high-affinity binding to factor Xa.[128, 130] The enzyme (or enzymes) in the conditioned media that is responsible for this carboxy-terminal truncation has not been identified, and it is not known whether similar proteolysis serves to modulate TFPI activity in vivo. Full-length TFPI binds to heparin-agarose with greater affinity than does carboxy-truncated TFPI. The addition of exogenous TFPI to plasma in vitro prolongs coagulation induced by tissue factor (prothrombin time). This effect, however, is predominantly due to the inhibition of factor Xa, rather than factor VIIa–tissue factor, by TFPI.[128]

Inhibition of the Factor VIIa–Tissue Factor Complex by Tissue Factor Pathway Inhibitor

Factor Xa–dependent inhibition of factor VIIa–tissue factor by TFPI involves the formation of a putative quaternary factor Xa–TFPI–factor VIIa–tissue factor complex.[125] This quaternary inhibitory complex could result from the binding of TFPI to a preformed factor Xa–factor VIIa–tissue factor complex, or, alternatively, TFPI could first bind factor Xa, with subsequent binding of the factor Xa–TFPI complex to factor VIIa–tissue factor. In the final quaternary complex, the second Kunitz domain of TFPI is responsible for binding factor Xa, and the first Kunitz domain of TFPI presumably binds factor VIIa[127] (Fig. 18–4). The functional role of the third Kunitz domain in TFPI is not known.

This proposed mechanism[125] explains the need for the persistent presence of factor Xa for effective factor VIIa–tissue factor inhibition[101] and also explains the requirement for catalytically active factor Xa,[100] since active site–inactivated factor Xa does not bind to TFPI.[125] Also consistent with the quaternary complex hypothesis is the fact that factor Xa lacking its amino-terminal Gla domain (GD-Xa) binds to and is inhibited by TFPI but that the subsequent GD-Xa–TFPI complex fails to inhibit factor VIIa–tissue factor.[125, 131] A chimeric molecule containing only the amino-terminal portion of factor Xa and the first Kunitz domain of TFPI inhibits the factor VIIa–tissue factor complex directly, suggesting that the binding of factor Xa to TFPI serves to juxtapose these domains on separate molecules, thereby producing a complex that binds to factor VIIa–tissue factor with high affinity.[132]

The requirement for factor Xa for the inhibition of factor VIIa–tissue factor by TFPI is not absolute,[133] and TFPI will inhibit the cleavage of factor IX by factor VIIa–tissue factor in the absence of factor Xa,[134] although 100-fold greater concentrations of TFPI are required to produce an effect equivalent to that when factor Xa is present.[135] This factor Xa–independent inhibition of factor VIIa–tissue factor by TFPI is of uncertain physiological relevance but could be important when TFPI is used as a therapeutic agent and plasma levels of TFPI reach 10- to 50-fold that of normal plasma.[136, 137]

Physiology of Tissue Factor Pathway Inhibitor

Greater than 90 per cent of the TFPI in plasma is bound to the lipoproteins: low density lipoproteins

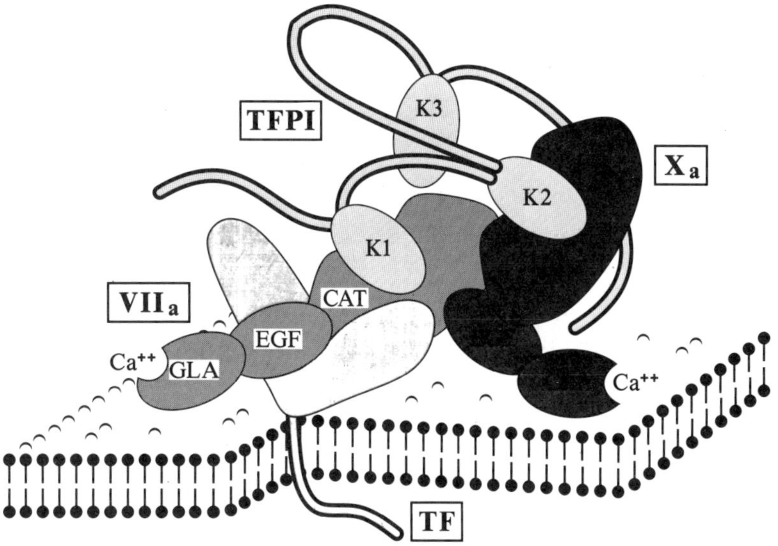

FIGURE 18–4. Model of the factor Xa–TFPI–factor VIIa–tissue factor quaternary inhibitory complex. As in Figure 18–2, factor VIIa is shown bound to tissue factor at the surface of a cell. Factor Xa is illustrated on the right. The Kunitz-1 domain of TFPI is bound at the catalytic site of factor VIIa, and the Kunitz-2 domain of TFPI is bound at the catalytic site of factor Xa. The γ-carboxyglutamic acid (GLA), epidermal growth factor (EGF), and catalytic (CAT) domains of factor VIIa and factor Xa, as well as the Kunitz domains (K1, K2, K3) of TFPI, are depicted as globular structures.

(LDL) > high density lipoproteins (HDL) >> very low density lipoproteins (VLDL).[104, 138] The predominant forms of TFPI in plasma have molecular weights of 34,000 and 40,000, although less abundant forms of higher molecular weight are also present. This size heterogeneity is due to the formation of mixed disulfide complexes between TFPI and apolipoprotein (apo) A-II.[104, 139] The major form of TFPI in LDL is 34,000 molecular weight, that in HDL is 40,000 molecular weight (TFPI + apo A-II), and VLDL contains both 34,000 and 40,000 molecular weight forms. The reason for the disparity in size between the TFPI in plasma and recombinant TFPI expressed by tissue culture cells (molecular weight of 42,000) may in part reflect differences in glycosylation.[104] The mechanism by which TFPI associates with lipoproteins is not known.

Platelets carry about 10 per cent of the total TFPI in blood and release this TFPI following stimulation by thrombin.[140] Platelet TFPI appears to represent an endogenous product of megakaryocytes, since TFPI mRNA has been detected in platelets and a megakaryocyte cell line.[140, 141] The contribution of platelet TFPI to the total TFPI concentration at the site of a wound, where platelets aggregate, could be substantial. Indeed, the TFPI concentration in plasma escaping from a superficial laceration (template bleeding time) reaches levels several-fold that of venous plasma obtained simultaneously by venipuncture.[140] This increase is presumably related to the release of platelet TFPI, although the contribution of other cells, including perhaps endothelial cells, cannot be excluded.

Plasma levels of TFPI increase following the infusion of heparin.[142, 143] As the ex vivo addition of heparin to blood or plasma does not change the TFPI level, the in vivo effect of heparin appears to be due to the release of TFPI from readily available intracellular or extracellular stores. The source of this additional TFPI is thought to be the endothelium, where TFPI may be bound to heparan sulfate or other

gylcosaminoglycans at the endothelial cell surface. The TFPI released by heparin in vivo is 42,000 molecular weight, binds tightly to heparin-agarose, and associates with plasma lipoproteins in vitro.[144]

The TFPI is synthesized by cultured cells derived from a variety of tissues, including liver,[145, 146] endothelium,[147] the monocytic cell line U937,[114] and lung, bladder, and kidney (D. Crecelius and G. J. Broze, unpublished data). It is not clear, however, that the production of TFPI by these cells in tissue culture accurately reflects the sites of endogenous TFPI expression. For example, primary cultures of hepatocytes do not produce TFPI,[141] and recent immunohistochemical studies have identified TFPI in the endothelium of capillaries, venules, and lymphatic channels but not in the endothelium of large vessels or in hepatocytes.[148]

A wide range of plasma TFPI concentrations exists in normal individuals, with a mean of approximately 2.5 nM (100 ng/ml).[142, 143, 149] Modest alterations in the plasma level of TFPI have been described in certain clinical conditions, but the physiological relevance of these differences between the plasma TFPI concentration in health and disease is uncertain.[143, 149–157] The several-fold increase in plasma TFPI following heparin treatment suggests that TFPI in plasma represents only a fraction of total TFPI that can be mobilized and raises the possibility that other physiological or pathological mechanisms may similarly affect the concentration of TFPI in plasma or at local sites. Furthermore, the TFPI presumably bound at the surface of the endothelium and in contact with plasma is likely a major contributor to overall TFPI action in vivo but is not reflected by the plasma TFPI concentration. The fact that individuals with abetalipoproteinemia have very low plasma TFPI levels (<20 per cent of normal) that increase to levels similar to those in normal individuals following heparin infusion,[143] and do not have an increased risk of thrombosis, suggests that plasma is not the most important reservoir of TFPI.

Although low levels of plasma TFPI are occasionally seen in septicemia and disseminated intravascular coagulation, more often the TFPI concentrations are normal.[134, 143, 147, 150, 156, 158] The progression of disseminated intravascular coagulation, in the face of a normal plasma level of TFPI, is consistent with the fact that TFPI, at physiologic concentrations, inhibits factor VIIa–tissue factor effectively only after factor Xa has been generated. Thus, TFPI dampens, but does not prevent, the coagulation process when generation of tissue factor is continued. Animal studies have shown that the depletion of endogenous TFPI sensitizes rabbits to the disseminated intravascular coagulation induced by tissue factor or endotoxin[159, 160] and that the infusion of high, therapeutic concentrations of TFPI lessens the intravascular coagulation induced by tissue factor.[136]

THE REVISED HYPOTHESIS OF BLOOD COAGULATION

The revised formulation of blood coagulation shown in Figure 18–5 takes into account the novel feedback inhibition of factor VIIa–tissue factor produced by TFPI. In this hypothesis, coagulation is initiated when damage to blood vessels at the site of a wound allows the exposure of blood to the tissue factor produced constitutively by cells beneath the endothelium. The factor VII or factor VIIa present in plasma then binds to this tissue factor, and the factor VIIa–tissue factor complex activates limited quantities of factor X and

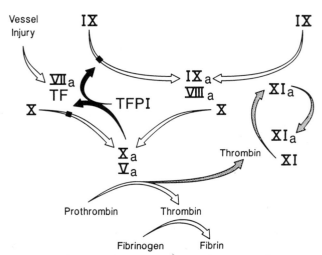

FIGURE 18–5. The revised hypothesis of blood coagulation. Hemostasis is initiated when factor VII or factor VIIa in plasma gains access to tissue factor at the site of blood vessel injury. Limited quantities of factor IXa and factor Xa are generated before there is feedback inhibition of the factor VIIa–tissue factor complex mediated by TFPI in concert with factor Xa. The generation of factor Xa is then amplified through the action of factor VIIIa and factor IXa, the latter produced initially by factor VIIa–tissue factor and supplemented by factor XIa. Factor XI activation may be produced by thrombin and autoactivation by factor XIa. The requirement for calcium ions and a phospholipid surface for certain of the reactions is not included in the figure.

factor IX. With the generation of factor Xa, however, the inhibitory effect of TFPI becomes manifest and prevents further production of factor Xa and factor IXa by factor VIIa—tissue factor. Additional factor Xa can then be produced only through the alternative pathway involving factor IXa and factor VIIIa.

The fact that individuals with factor XI deficiency have a variable but usually mild bleeding diathesis implies that under certain conditions the initial quantity of factor IXa produced by factor VIIa–tissue factor is insufficient and additional factor IXa generated by factor XIa is needed for normal hemostasis. The mechanism for the activation of factor XI is unclear; however, the model predicts that factor XI activation occurs "late" in the coagulation process, after the initial generation of factor Xa and thrombin through the action of factor VIIa–tissue factor. Recently, it has been shown that thrombin is capable of activating factor XI and that, in the presence of a polyanion (e.g., dextran sulfate, heparin, or sulfatides), this process is amplified through the autoactivation of additional factor XI by factor XIa.[161, 162] This pathway for factor XI activation is included in Figure 18–5, but it has not yet been demonstrated to occur in vivo, and its potential role in hemostasis remains controversial.[162a, 162b]

The revised hypothesis of blood coagulation differs from the cascade[8] and waterfall[9] theories in two major respects (see Fig. 18–1). First, it integrates all of the factors known to be involved in coagulation into a single pathway that is initiated by factor VIIa–tissue factor and in which the "contact" factors (factor XII, prekallikrein, and high molecular weight kininogen) are not required. Second, in contrast to the cascade and waterfall hypotheses, an integral tenet of the revised model is that the hemostatic process does not end with the initial generation of factor Xa and thrombin. Instead, the initial hemostatic response must be "consolidated" by the progressive local generation of factor Xa and thrombin. This phenomenon has been demonstrated in vivo[163] and presumably reflects the influence of inhibitors of the coagulation proteases (see below) and the competing process of fibrinolysis. (See Chapter 21.)

Thus, hemophiliacs bleed because the initial factor Xa generated through the action of factor VIIa–tissue factor, and dampened by TFPI, is insufficient to sustain hemostasis and must be amplified through the action of factor IXa and factor VIIIa.[125, 164] Similarly, factor XIa is required to supplement the factor IXa formed by factor VIIa–tissue factor, which is limited owing to the presence of TFPI. As a corollary to this hypothesis, it has been suggested that effective inhibition of TFPI could provide a novel means of alleviating the hemorrhagic manifestations in hemophiliacs.[125]

Tissue factor pathway inhibitor–induced feedback inhibition of factor VIIa–tissue factor can explain the clinical need for both the "extrinsic" and "intrinsic" (factors VIII, IX, and XI) coagulation pathways (see Fig. 18–1) and is consistent with in vitro results showing deficient factor Xa production in hemophiliac plasma induced to clot by small quantities of tissue factor.[96] In addition, present data are consistent with the idea that, in normal hemostasis at least, factor VIIa–tissue factor is responsible for the initial factor Xa generation. That ultimate and persistent hemostasis requires the continued production of factor Xa through the action of factor IXa and factor VIIIa is consistent with the bleeding, frequently delayed in onset, seen in hemophiliacs.

FUNCTIONS OF THROMBIN IN HEMOSTASIS

Factor Xa converts prothrombin to thrombin, a 36,000 molecular weight serine protease that plays a central role in hemostasis. Thrombin's substrates include the following: (1) the platelet thrombin receptor, which is cleaved to release a tethered peptide ligand that stimulates platelet aggregation and secretion[165]; (2) factors V and VIII, which are activated to factors Va and VIIIa and serve as non-enzymatic cofactors for factors Xa and IXa, respectively; (3) factor XI, which is converted to factor XIa[161, 162]; (4) fibrinogen, which is cleaved near the amino-terminal ends of the Aα and Bβ chains to produce fibrin monomers that polymerize to form the clot; and (5) factor XIII, a transglutaminase that cross-links polymerized fibrin to stabilize the clot. The first three reactions provide positive feedback loops that are presumed to accelerate thrombin generation at the site of a wound. Thrombin also has mitogenic[166–168] and chemotactic[169] activities that may be important in wound healing. If normal vascular endothelial cells are present, thrombin binds to the integral membrane protein thrombomodulin and activates protein C, which produces an anticoagulant effect by proteolytically inactivating factors Va and VIIIa.

Thrombin is inhibited by antithrombin and heparin cofactor II, plasma proteins that are homologous to α_1-antitrypsin and other serpins.[170] Both antithrombin and heparin cofactor II require the presence of a glycosaminoglycan such as heparin for maximal activity. In 1923, Howell used the term "heparin" to describe an aqueous extract of canine liver that inhibited coagulation of blood in vitro.[171] Similar extracts were shown later to consist of mixtures of sulfated polysaccharides containing uronic acid and glucosamine.[172] In 1939, Brinkhous and colleagues[173] discovered that the anticoagulant effect of heparin is mediated by an endogenous plasma component termed "heparin cofactor," and investigators in Canada and Sweden reported the use of heparin as a treatment for thrombosis and pulmonary embolism.[172, 174] Antithrombin was first purified from plasma by Abildgaard in 1968 and was shown to have heparin cofactor activity, that is, the ability to inhibit thrombin rapidly in the presence of heparin.[175] A separate thrombin inhibitor with heparin cofactor activity was observed in 1974[176]; this protein, termed heparin cofactor II, was later purified,

and its activity was shown to be stimulated by dermatan sulfate as well as by heparin.[177, 178]

The association between antithrombin deficiency and recurrent venous thromboembolism,[179, 180] first reported by Egeberg in 1965,[181] established the idea that antithrombin plays a critical role in regulating hemostasis. More recently, Rosenberg has suggested that heparan sulfate synthesized by vascular endothelial cells constitutively activates antithrombin to prevent thrombosis from occurring within normal blood vessels.[182]

ANTITHROMBIN

Biochemistry and Molecular Biology of Antithrombin

Antithrombin is a 58,000 molecular weight glycoprotein that consists of a single polypeptide chain (Fig. 18–6). The amino acid sequence of antithrombin, determined directly[183] and by cDNA sequencing,[184–186] is about 30 per cent identical to other serpins.[170] Antithrombin contains three disulfide bonds, one of which (Cys 8 to Cys 128) is required for heparin cofactor activity.[187] In addition, it contains three or four biantennary N-linked oligosaccharides.[188] No other post-translational modifications have been reported.

Two forms of antithrombin that differ in their carbohydrate content have been isolated from normal human plasma by heparin-agarose affinity chromatography.[189] The major form (α antithrombin), comprising approximately 90 per cent of the total antithrombin, is eluted from the affinity matrix with 1 M NaCl and appears to be fully glycosylated. The minor form (β antithrombin), which is eluted at a higher salt concentration, lacks the oligosaccharide unit linked to Asn 135 near the proposed heparin-binding site.[190] Both α antithrombin and β antithrombin inhibit thrombin rapidly in the presence of heparin. However, β antithrombin requires a lower concentration of heparin for full activity, consistent with its higher heparin affinity.

The antithrombin gene on human chromosome 1 (q23–25)[191, 192] contains seven exons distributed over approximately 19 kb of DNA.[193, 194] The 5' flanking sequence of the antithrombin gene lacks a TATA-like sequence at the expected location 25 to 30 bases upstream from the transcription initiation site.[195] In addition, a DNA length polymorphism of unknown significance has been identified, resulting from insertion of either 32 or 108 bp of DNA at the position 345 bases upstream from the translation initiation codon.[196] The 5' flanking region of the antithrombin gene also contains short sequences that are similar to an enhancer element found in the immunoglobulin Jκ-Cκ gene.[197] When the antithrombin enhancer element was ligated to the chloramphenicol acetyltransferase gene and transfected into cells, expression of chloramphenicol acetyltransferase activity was in-

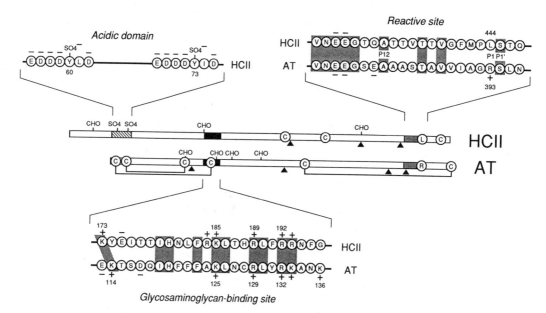

FIGURE 18–6. Structural features of antithrombin and heparin cofactor II. The heparin cofactor II (HCII) and antithrombin (AT) polypeptides are aligned according to amino acid sequence homology in the center of the figure. The positions of cysteine residues (C), P1 leucine (L) and arginine (R) residues, *N*-linked glycosylation sites (CHO), and sulfate groups (SO4) are indicated. The triangles show the positions of introns in the coding sequence of each gene. The amino-terminal acidic domain of heparin cofactor II (*cross-hatched box*) and the glycosaminoglycan-binding sites (*solid boxes*) and reactive sites (*stippled boxes*) of both proteins are enlarged to show details of the amino acid sequences. The numbers indicate the positions of residues in the polypeptide chains.

creased preferentially in Alexander hepatoma (liver) and Cos-1 (kidney) cells. Thus, the enhancer may be involved in tissue-specific expression of the antithrombin gene.

The mRNA for antithrombin is approximately 1500 nt in length. It codes for a signal peptide of 32 residues followed by the mature protein of 432 residues.[184–186] Antithrombin mRNA is present in the liver, and synthesis of antithrombin has been demonstrated in cultured human hepatoma cells.[198] Alternative splicing of the antithrombin mRNA has been demonstrated in the liver.[195] The alternative splicing event introduces a 42 base segment between codons −19 and −18 of the signal peptide. This segment of mRNA contains an in-frame termination codon such that the predicted protein product encoded by the alternatively spliced mRNA would be only 19 amino acids long. Although the alternatively spliced mRNA accounts for 20 to 40 per cent of the antithrombin mRNA in human liver, it is not known whether translation occurs. In the adult rat, antithrombin mRNA was detected in the kidney at a level about 20 per cent of that found in the liver.[199]

Little is known about the regulation of antithrombin biosynthesis. Biosynthesis of antithrombin by isolated rat hepatocytes is unaffected by the presence of protease-antithrombin complexes or by the supernatant medium of macrophages incubated with these complexes.[200] However, antithrombin biosynthesis is stimulated by the supernatant medium of macrophages incubated with endotoxin or fibrinogen fragment D. Under these conditions, fibrinogen and α_1-antitrypsin biosynthesis are stimulated concurrently.

Protease Inhibition by Antithrombin

Antithrombin inhibits the coagulation proteases thrombin, factor Xa, factor IXa, factor XIa, factor XIIa, and kallikrein.[201] It also inhibits the fibrinolytic protease plasmin.[202] Antithrombin has very little activity toward factor VIIa[53] or activated protein C.[203] In vitro experiments suggest that antithrombin is the major inhibitor of factors IXa and Xa and thrombin in plasma.[204–206] By contrast, factor XIa is inhibited primarily by α_1-antitrypsin,[207] factor XIIa by C1 inhibitor,[208] and plasmin by α_2-antiplasmin.[209] (See Chapter 21.)

Antithrombin forms an essentially irreversible, equimolar complex with each of its target proteases.[210] The serine residue at the active site of the protease is required for complex formation but thereafter becomes inaccessible to substrates. Furthermore, a small peptide is cleaved from the carboxy-terminus of antithrombin during complex formation.[211] Thrombin, factor Xa, and factor IXa cleave the same peptide bond in antithrombin (Arg 393 to Ser 394), which is termed the reactive site (see Fig. 18–6).[212] The antithrombin-protease complex resists dissociation in denaturing agents, suggesting that a covalent bond is formed between the two proteins. The complex can be dissociated by treatment with nucleophiles, which release the protease along with the cleaved form of antithrombin from the complex.[211, 213] These properties are consistent with the presence of an ester linkage between the active center serine hydroxyl group of thrombin and the α carbonyl group of Arg 393 in the reactive site of antithrombin (Fig. 18–7).

Antithrombin and other serpins undergo a striking conformational change after proteolytic cleavage at the reactive site. X-ray crystallography of intact ovalbumin suggests that the P1 to P12 residues amino-terminal to the cleavage site form an exposed loop on the surface of the molecule (Fig. 18–8).[214] This structure is consistent with the finding that the region immediately upstream from the reactive site in many serpins is susceptible to proteolytic cleavage by enzymes other than the target protease, resulting in loss of the serpin's inhibitory activity.[215] In α1-antitrypsin cleaved at P1–P1′, movement of the exposed loop about a "hinge" located near P12 allows residues P1 to P12 to become the fourth strand of a six-membered β sheet, separating the P1 and P1′ amino acids by 69 Å (see Fig. 18–8).[216] This conformational change results in greater thermal stability of the cleaved ("relaxed") form in comparison to the intact ("stressed") form of the serpin. Mutations of the "hinge" region (e.g., antithrombin Cambridge, P10 Ala → Pro) that may interfere with intercalation of the exposed reactive site loop into the β sheet prevent the "stressed" to "relaxed" conformational change and abolish the protease inhibitor activity of the serpin.[217]

Stimulation of Antithrombin by Heparin

The concentration of antithrombin in plasma (~ 2.6 μM, 150 μg/ml) greatly exceeds that of any of the target proteases generated during coagulation. Under these conditions, protease inhibition follows pseudo

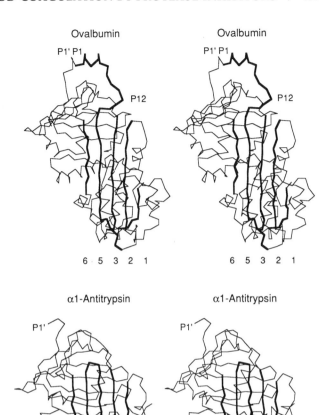

FIGURE 18–8. Structures of uncleaved and cleaved serpins. The structures of uncleaved ovalbumin[214] and cleaved α1-antitrypsin[358] were determined by X-ray crystallography. The α carbon tracing of the polypeptide backbone is shown for each protein. The P1 to P12 residues of ovalbumin form an exposed loop on the surface of the protein, which is susceptible to proteolytic attack. After cleavage, the P1 and P1′ amino acid residues of α1-antitrypsin are separated by 69 Å, and residues P1 to P12 are incorporated into a β sheet structure (thick lines; strands numbered according to α1-antitrypsin).

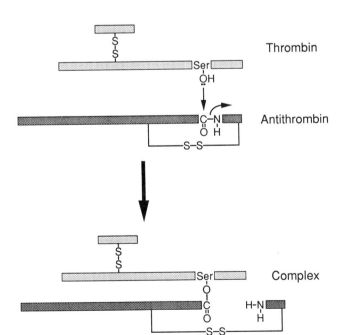

FIGURE 18–7. Model for protease-antithrombin complex formation. The active center serine hydroxyl group of the protease attacks the reactive site peptide bond in antithrombin, becoming trapped in an acyl ester linkage.

first-order kinetics. In the absence of heparin, thrombin and factor Xa are inhibited by antithrombin in plasma with t½ values of 0.5 to 1.5 minutes, whereas factor IXa is inhibited about 10 times more slowly.[218] Addition of heparin to plasma increases the rate of inhibition of thrombin, factor Xa, and factor IXa by antithrombin at least 1000-fold. As a result, inhibition of these proteases becomes essentially instantaneous (t½ = 10 to 60 msec).[218] Heparin also stimulates inhibition of XIa, XIIa, kallikrein, and plasmin, but the magnitude of the effect is much less.[201] Acceleration of antithrombin-protease reactions accounts for most of the anticoagulant effect produced by an intravenous infusion of heparin.

Heparin can be fractionated according to its ability to bind to antithrombin. Thus, approximately 30 per cent of heparin extracted from porcine intestinal mucosa binds to antithrombin with high affinity.[219–221] The high-affinity molecules account for virtually all the anticoagulant activity of the starting material, whereas the low-affinity molecules are inactive. Antithrombin binds to heparin with a dissociation constant of approximately 2×10^{-8} M.[222, 223] The binding is disrupted at high ionic strength, which implies that electrostatic interactions occur between basic amino acid residues on antithrombin and sulfate groups on the heparin molecule. The following observations point to regions of antithrombin that may be involved in heparin binding:

1. Chemical modification of several lysine residues in antithrombin, including Lys 107, Lys 114, Lys 125, and Lys 136, blocks heparin binding and heparin cofactor activity without affecting the thrombin inhibitory activity in the absence of heparin.[224, 225] As already mentioned, the presence of an oligosaccharide linked to Asn 135 decreases the affinity of α antithrombin for heparin relative to that of β antithrombin.[190]

2. Chemical modification of a single tryptophan residue, identified as Trp 49, blocks heparin binding to antithrombin.[226] Furthermore, structural analyses of inherited antithrombin variants that react normally with thrombin but lack the ability to bind heparin have revealed mutations of Arg 47 and Pro 41.[227–229] These studies suggest that Pro 41, Arg 47, and Trp 49 lie within or near the heparin-binding site of antithrombin. When the sequence of antithrombin is superimposed on the tertiary structure of the proteolytically cleaved form of α1-antitrypsin, it appears that Arg 47 and a cluster of basic amino acid residues surrounding Lys 125 occur in close proximity in the protein (Fig. 18–9).[170] If so, these residues could participate simultaneously in heparin binding.

3. An alternative model for the heparin-binding site is based on the denaturation of an α-helical domain in antithrombin by exposure to guanidine-HCl.[230] This treatment is accompanied by loss of heparin-binding activity, whereas the ability of antithrombin to react with thrombin is retained. The unstable α-helical domain of antithrombin has been tentatively identified as the segment containing Lys 290, Lys 294, and Lys 297 based on secondary structure modeling.

Heparin is found in the secretory granules of mast cells. It is synthesized from UDP-sugar precursors as a polymer of alternating D-glucuronic acid (linked β1 → 4) and N-acetyl-D-glucosamine (linked α1 → 4)[231] (Fig. 18–10). The glycosaminoglycan chains are built on a core structure consisting of one xylose and two galactose residues covalently attached to serine in a polypeptide backbone. About 10 to 15 glycosaminoglycan chains, each containing 200 to 300 monosaccharide units, are attached to a single core protein to yield a proteoglycan with a molecular weight of 750,000 to 1,000,000. As the glycosaminoglycan chains are being synthesized, they rapidly undergo a series of modification reactions that include the following[231]: (1) N-deacetylation of glucosamine residues, followed by sulfation of virtually all the free amino groups to yield N-sulfo-D-glucosamine; (2) epimerization at the C5 position of D-glucuronic acid to yield L-iduronic acid; (3) O-sulfation of iduronic acid residues at the C2 position; and (4) O-sulfation of glucosamine residues at the C6 position. In addition, several minor but important reactions occur, including O-sulfation of glucuronic acid at C2 and C3 and of glucosamine at C3. The reactions that modify the glycosaminoglycan chain appear to be catalyzed by membrane-bound enzymes in the endoplasmic reticulum or Golgi apparatus of the mast cell and are completed within minutes of synthesis of the core protein. Many of these reactions are regulated by modifications that have occurred on neighboring sugar residues. Furthermore, all the reactions, with the exception of N-sulfation, are incomplete, yielding heterogeneous oligosaccharide structures within the glycosaminoglycan chain. After the heparin proteoglycan has been transported to the mast cell secretory granules, an endo-β-D-glucuronidase catalyzes partial degradation of the glycosaminoglycan chains to fragments of 5,000 to 10,000 molecular weight over a period of hours.

Two other glycosaminoglycans, heparan sulfate and dermatan sulfate, possess anticoagulant activity in vitro.[232] Heparan sulfate is closely related to heparin and is found on the surface of most eukaryotic cells and in the extracellular matrix. Heparan sulfate proteoglycans vary considerably in structure. In general, they are smaller than the heparin proteoglycan, containing fewer glycosaminoglycan chains linked to a larger and more complex core protein. In some cases, the core protein has a hydrophobic domain that anchors the proteoglycan to the cell membrane. Heparan sulfate is synthesized from the same repeating disaccharide precursor (D-glucuronic acid linked to N-acetyl-D-glucosamine) as heparin.[233] However, heparan sulfate undergoes less polymer modification than does heparin and, therefore, contains higher proportions

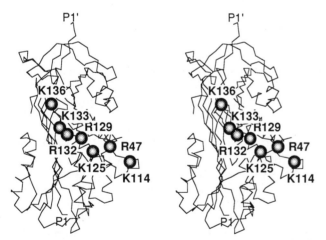

FIGURE 18–9. Structure of the proposed heparin-binding site of antithrombin. The polypeptide backbone shown in the diagram is that of α1-antitrypsin. The positions of residues in antithrombin thought to be involved in heparin binding are superimposed on this backbone. In comparison to Figure 18–8, the projection is rotated approximately 90° about the vertical axis.

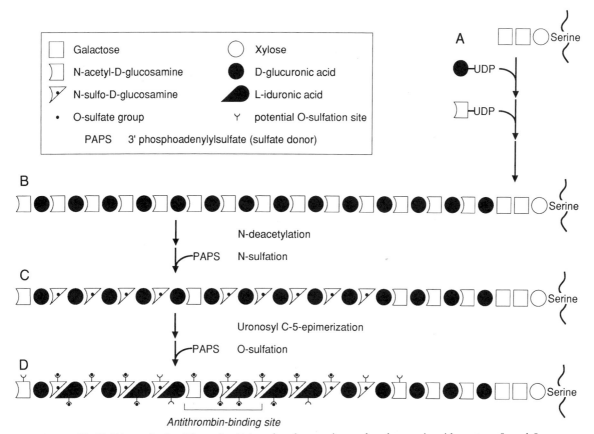

FIGURE 18–10. Biosynthesis of heparin. *N*-Acetyl-D-glucosamine and D-glucuronic acid are transferred from UDP-sugar precursors to a trisaccharide structure linked to a serine residue in the core protein (*A*), forming the unmodified glycosaminoglycan chain (*B*). *N*-Deacetylation of some of the *N*-acetyl-D-glucosamine residues then occurs, followed by *N*-sulfation of the free amino groups (*C*). Epimerization of D-glucuronic acid to L-iduronic acid and *O*-sulfation occur to a limited extent to yield the final product (*D*), which is then transported to the mast cell secretory granule. The structure of the antithrombin-binding site is shown in Figure 18–11. (Modified from Lindahl, U., Kusche, M., Lidholt, K., and Oscarsson, L.-G.: Biosynthesis of heparin and heparan sulfate. Ann. N. Y. Acad. Sci. 556:36, 1989; with permission.)

of glucuronic acid and *N*-acetylglucosamine and fewer sulfate groups. Dermatan sulfate is a repeating polymer of L-iduronic acid and *N*-acetyl-D-galactosamine (instead of glucosamine).[233] *O*-Sulfation of iduronic acid residues at the C2 position and of galactosamine residues at the C4 and C6 positions occurs to a variable extent. Like heparan sulfate, dermatan sulfate is a

component of proteoglycans on the cell surface and in the extracellular matrix.

The smallest fragment of heparin that binds to antithrombin with high affinity is the pentasaccharide shown in Figure 18–11.[234–236] This structure contains a 3-*O*-sulfate group that appears to be unique to the high-affinity binding site. Several of the sulfate groups

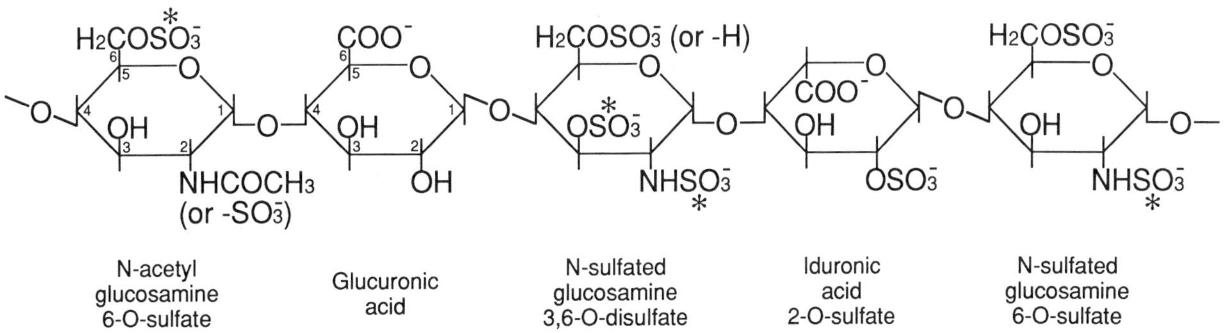

FIGURE 18–11. Structure of the antithrombin-binding pentasaccharide of heparin. Sulfate groups marked with asterisks are essential for high-affinity binding to antithrombin. The first residue may be either *N*-sulfated or *N*-acetylated, and the C6 position of the third residue may or may not be sulfated.

within the pentasaccharide are essential for binding to antithrombin, whereas others do not appear to be required. In commercial heparin preparations, approximately 30 per cent of the molecules contain this structure and bind to antithrombin with high affinity. An identical structure is thought to arise during the biosynthesis of heparan sulfate chains, although at a much lower frequency. Heparan sulfate chains that contain this structure bind to antithrombin and stimulate protease inhibition. Other glycosaminoglycans that lack the specific pentasaccharide structure (e.g., dermatan sulfate, chondroitin 4-sulfate, or chondroitin 6-sulfate) do not interact with antithrombin.[178]

Rapid kinetic analyses indicate that heparin binding induces a conformational change in antithrombin that locks the heparin molecule into place on the surface of the inhibitor.[223] The heparin-antithrombin complex then reacts with a target protease. Binding of a protease to antithrombin reduces the affinity of antithrombin for heparin, allowing the antithrombin-protease complex to dissociate from the heparin molecule.[237] Thus, heparin is able to function in a catalytic manner in the reaction.

Two models have been proposed to explain the mechanism by which heparin catalyzes the inhibition of proteases:

1. In the first model, heparin binding induces a conformational change that affects the reactive site of antithrombin, allowing target proteases to interact more rapidly with this site. This model is supported by the fact that conformational changes in antithrombin can be detected spectroscopically as a consequence of heparin binding.[238–241] Furthermore, the initial rate of protease inhibition increases in proportion to the amount of heparin-antithrombin complex formed at low heparin concentrations ($<1 \times 10^{-7}$ M).[218]

2. In the second model, heparin functions as a template to which both antithrombin and the target protease bind. Catalysis thus occurs mainly by an approximation effect. This model is supported by the fact that heparin molecules containing 18 or more sugar residues are required to catalyze the reaction of antithrombin with thrombin, even though smaller molecules bind with high affinity and induce a conformational change.[235, 242] Formation of ternary complexes that contain antithrombin, heparin, and thrombin is supported also by physical evidence.[243, 244] Kinetic analyses demonstrate that the rate of thrombin inhibition saturates at high protease concentrations; this finding has been interpreted to indicate that formation of a ternary complex is an obligate intermediate in the catalytic reaction.[245–247]

The relative importance of conformational and template phenomena in the inhibition of thrombin by antithrombin remains controversial.[182, 248] Nevertheless, the synthetic pentasaccharide that contains only the antithrombin-binding site of heparin catalyzes inhibition of factor Xa.[234] Since an oligosaccharide of this size is unlikely to function as a template, induction of a conformational change in the reactive site of antithrombin may be sufficient to catalyze factor Xa inhibition.

Several proteins competitively inhibit antithrombin binding to heparin. They include histidine-rich glycoprotein[249] and vitronectin (complement S protein),[250] both of which are present in plasma at micromolar concentrations. Whether these proteins regulate hemostasis remains to be determined. Platelet factor 4 is released from the α granules during platelet aggregation and binds tightly to heparin.[249] It is likely to promote local clot formation at the site of hemostasis by blocking the binding of antithrombin to heparan sulfate.

Activity of Antithrombin In Vivo

When radiolabeled thrombin is injected intravenously into an experimental animal, it appears rapidly in the circulation as a complex with antithrombin.[251] Similarly, formation of factor IXa–antithrombin complexes occurs rapidly in vivo.[205] Although thrombomodulin has been shown to serve as a receptor for internalization of thrombin by endothelial cells in vitro,[252] the importance of this pathway in the clearance of thrombin in vivo remains to be clarified. In contrast to thrombin and factor IXa, factor Xa has been reported to form complexes primarily with α_2-macroglobulin after intravenous injection.[253] Factor Xa is protected from inhibition by antithrombin in vitro when the protease is bound to platelets[254] or to the prothrombinase complex, which contains factor Va, prothrombin, and phospholipids.[255] It is not known whether these mechanisms also protect factor Xa from inhibition by antithrombin in vivo.

In experimental animals, antithrombin-protease complexes are removed from the circulation by hepatocytes with a t½ of 2 to 3 minutes.[205, 256] The hepatocyte uptake mechanism is saturable in vivo and recognizes the antithrombin-protease complex but not the free inhibitor. Complexes of proteases with α_1-antitrypsin competitively inhibit uptake of the antithrombin-protease complex and, therefore, are thought to be taken up by the same hepatocyte mechanism.[257]

Uptake of antithrombin-protease complexes and degradation to low molecular weight peptides by rat hepatocytes have been demonstrated in vitro.[258] Uptake by the hepatocyte receptor in vitro is saturable and is competitively inhibited by antithrombin-protease and α_1-antitrypsin–protease complexes, but not by free antithrombin, α_2-macroglobulin–methylamine, asialo-orosomucoid, fucosyl–bovine serum albumin, N-acetylglucosaminyl–bovine serum albumin, or mannosyl–bovine serum albumin. An abundant receptor (4.5×10^5 receptors per cell) with high affinity ($K_d = 4.0 \times 10^{-8}$ M) for serpin-enzyme complexes has been identified on human HepG2 cells and monocytes.[259] The receptor has been shown to mediate internalization and degradation of the complexes.[260] Binding of serpin-enzyme complexes to the receptor is blocked by a synthetic peptide (Phe-Val-Phe-Leu-Met) that corresponds to a highly conserved sequence found in the carboxy-terminal portion of serpins[261]; this sequence may represent a receptor-binding site that becomes exposed on the surface of the serpin after complex formation with a protease.

The distribution of ^{131}I-labeled antithrombin in vivo has been investigated in humans.[262] The data are compatible with a three-compartment model in which approximately 40 per cent of the antithrombin is distributed in the plasma, approximately 10 per cent in a non-circulating vascular pool, and approximately 50 per cent in an extravascular compartment. The fractional catabolic rates of the total intravascular pool and the extravascular pool are about 0.5 per day and about 0.2 per day, respectively. Thus, free antithrombin is cleared from the circulation much more slowly than its complexes with proteases.

Activation of Antithrombin by Endogenous Heparin-like Molecules

Under normal circumstances, heparin is not released from mast cells into the circulation and cannot be detected in plasma. However, a small amount of heparin may appear in the circulation of patients with systemic mastocytosis and may produce mild prolongation of the activated partial thromboplastin time.[263] Circulating heparan sulfate, apparently released from damaged tissues, has been reported to cause marked prolongation of the activated partial thromboplastin time and bleeding in a few severely ill patients with hematological malignancies.[264–266]

Glycosaminoglycans extracted from cloned endothelial cells possess anticoagulant activity.[267] Treatment of the extracts with heparinase abolishes the activity, indicating that the active moiety is heparin-like. De novo biosynthesis of heparan sulfate proteoglycans has been demonstrated by culturing endothelial cells in the presence of [^{35}S]sulfate.[268] Approximately 1 to 10 per cent of the labeled heparan sulfate from endothelial cells binds to immobilized antithrombin with high affinity, and this fraction possesses essentially all the anticoagulant activity of the cell extract. Structural analysis of the high-affinity heparan sulfate has revealed the presence of the 3-O-sulfated glucosamine residue that is characteristic of the antithrombin-binding structure of heparin.[268]

Direct binding of antithrombin to endothelial cells cloned from bovine aorta has been demonstrated. The inhibitor binds to approximately 60,000 sites per cell, with a dissociation constant of 12 nM.[268] Binding is diminished by pretreatment of the cells with heparinase. Similar results have been obtained with intact segments of bovine aorta.[269] However, the binding of antithrombin to intact rabbit aortic endothelium is weak, whereas antithrombin appears to bind more avidly to heparinase-sensitive components beneath the endothelial cell layer.[270] Electron microscopic autoradiography of ^{125}I-labeled antithrombin bound to en-

dothelial cells in culture or after perfusion of segments of rat aorta ex vivo indicates that more than 90 per cent of the antithrombin is associated with the extracellular matrix located in the subendothelium.[271] Binding to the subendothelial matrix is greatly increased after crush injury of the aorta, which removes most of the endothelial cells. Since the intact endothelium may be permeable to proteins, the interaction of coagulation proteases with antithrombin bound to subendothelial heparan sulfate proteoglycans may inhibit thrombosis.[271]

Evidence for the stimulation of antithrombin by vascular heparan sulfate in vivo has been more difficult to obtain. Marcum and associates[272] perfused a rodent hind limb preparation with thrombin until a constant concentration of the protease was present in the venous effluent. Then antithrombin was perfused through the preparation, and the amount of thrombin-antithrombin complex that formed was determined in comparison to the amount that formed during a similar period in vitro. A 15- to 19-fold increase in the rate of complex formation appeared to occur within the microvasculature, compared with in vitro incubations in the absence of heparin. The rate enhancement was diminished by prior perfusion of the hind limb preparation with heparinase or when Trp 49–modified antithrombin was used, suggesting that interaction of antithrombin with microvascular heparan sulfate was responsible for the effect.

A different process may occur when only a trace amount of thrombin is injected into the circulation. Under these circumstances, thrombin may become bound initially to thrombomodulin on the endothelial cell surface.[251] A modest (~ threefold) increase in the rate of thrombin inhibition by circulating antithrombin may then occur because of the altered substrate specificity of thrombin when it is bound to thrombomodulin.[273] In comparison to free thrombin, thrombin bound to thrombomodulin in vitro reacts less rapidly with fibrinogen, more rapidly with protein C, and at about the same rate with antithrombin. The net effect of these changes in substrate specificity is postulated to be a small increase in the rate of the thrombin-antithrombin reaction because of diminished competition from other substrates. According to this hypothesis, only when thrombomodulin becomes saturated with thrombin will the excess thrombin interact with antithrombin in a heparan sulfate–catalyzed reaction.

Antithrombin Deficiency

Antithrombin deficiency was the first inherited abnormality to be associated with a thrombotic tendency.[181] The diagnosis is usually made in patients who experience the onset of recurrent thromboembolic disease at an early age or in whom a positive family history of thromboembolic disease is obtained. The concentration of antithrombin in adult plasma is approximately 150 μg/ml (2.6 μM).[274] The range of concentrations is narrow in normal individuals, who

TABLE 18–1. ANTITHROMBIN MUTATIONS*

PATIENT	ANTIGEN (%)	ACTIVITY (%)	MUTATION	AMINO ACID CHANGE	COMMENTS	REFERENCES
Type Ia (Classical): Reduced Levels of Normal Antithrombin						
1 family	53	47	−T, codon 81	Frameshift	Met 89→stop	281
1 family	60	63	−T, codon 119	Frameshift	Stop codon 126	282
2 families	<60	<60	CGA→TGA	Arg 129→stop		283
1 family	<60	<60	+A, codon 228	Frameshift	Glu 232→stop	283a
1 family	<60	<60	2 bp del, codon 290–1	Frameshift	Asp 309→stop	283a
1 family	<60	<60	4 bp del, codon 308–9	Frameshift	Glu 313→stop	283a
1 family	<60	<60	+A, codon 408	Frameshift	Stop codon 432	283
Type Ib: Reduced Levels of Normal Antithrombin and the Presence of a Low Level of Variant						
Unnamed	<60	<60	G to A, intron 4	Frameshift	13 nt 5′ to exon V → new 3′ splice site, stop codon 285	284
Rosny	70	52	TTC→TGC	Phe 402→Cys		285
Torino	69	46	TTC→TCC	Phe 402→Ser		285
Oslo	40	58	GCC→ACC	Ala 404→Thr		286
Unnamed	70		AAC→AAG	Asn 405→Lys	Also Val (−3)→Glu	Unpublished
Kyoto (?)			AGG→ATG	Arg 406→Met		287
Utah	50	50	CCT→CTT	Pro 407→Leu		288
Budapest 5	100	70	CCT→ACT	Pro 407→Thr	Also protein C deficiency	Unpublished
Unnamed	75	52	+G, codon 423–4	Frameshift	Stop codon 432	281
Unnamed			9 bp del, codon 427–9	Frameshift	Stop codon 430; also Arg 47→His	289
Types IIa and IIb: Defects in the Reactive Site or Both the Reactive Site and the Heparin-Binding Site						
Glasgow III	121		AAC→AAA	Asn 187→Lys		Unpublished
Unnamed	98	55	AAC→GAC	Asn 187→Asp		Unpublished
Hamilton	100	50	GCA→ACA	Ala 382→Thr	Transformed into substrate	290, 291
Charleville	100	60	GCA→CCA	Ala 384→Pro	Transformed into substrate	292, 293
Cambridge II	103	75	GCA→TCA	Ala 384→Ser		293a
Stockholm			GGC→GAC	Gly 392→Asp		294
Northwick Park	162	65	CGT→TGT	Arg 393→Cys	Complex with albumin	295, 296
Glasgow	87	43	CGT→CAT	Arg 393→His	Increased heparin affinity	296
Pescara	100	62	CGT→CCT	Arg 393→Pro	Increased heparin affinity	297, 298
Denver	92	54	TCG→TTG	Ser 394→Leu	Increased clearance?	299
Budapest	75	20	CCT→CTT	Pro 429→Leu	Homozygous	299a
Type IIc: Defects Limited to the Heparin-Binding Site						
Rouen III			ATC→AAC	Ile 7→Asn	Additional carbohydrate	300
Whitechapel	92		ATG→ACG & TAT→TGT	Met 20→Thr & Trp 166→Cys	Double mutation	Unpublished
Rouen IV	105	56	CGC→TGC	Arg 24→Cys		301
Basel	104	60	CCG→CTG	Pro 41→Leu		229
Toyama	100	26	CGT→TGT	Arg 47→Cys	Homozygous	227
Rouen I	111	55	CGT→CAT	Arg 47→His		228
Rouen II	102	64	CGT→AGT	Arg 47→Ser		302
Geneva	100	50	CGA→CAA	Arg 129→Gln		303
Truro			GAA→AAA	Glu 237→Lys		Unpublished

*Only variants in which the mutation has been identified are listed. Data from Lane, D. A., Ireland, H., Olds, R. J., Thein, S. L., Perry, D. J., and Aiach, M.: Antithrombin III: A database of mutations. Thromb. Haemost. 66:657, 1991.

have heparin cofactor activities of 84 to 166 per cent (mean ± 2 SD) and antithrombin antigen concentrations of 72 to 128 per cent (mean ± 2 SD).[179] Healthy, full-term newborn infants have antithrombin antigen concentrations of 39 to 87 per cent of adult values.[275] The level gradually increases to the normal adult range by 3 months of age.

Classical (type Ia) antithrombin deficiency is inherited as an autosomal dominant trait. Affected heterozygotes have 25 to 60 per cent of the normal plasma levels of both antithrombin activity and antigen.[179] Total absence of antithrombin has not been reported and may be lethal in utero. Oral anticoagulant therapy may increase the antithrombin level in some deficient patients, making the diagnosis more difficult.[276] Clas-

sical antithrombin deficiency has been reported to result from deletion of one of the two antithrombin genes,[277] from a dysfunctional gene,[277, 278] or from mutations in the coding sequence that cause a frameshift or a premature stop codon (Table 18–1). The catabolic rate of infused radiolabeled antithrombin is normal in patients with inherited antithrombin deficiency, implying that the decreased plasma concentration is not caused by accelerated clearance of normal antithrombin.[279, 280] A patient whose plasma contains approximately 50 per cent of normal antithrombin activity and antigen, but in which a small amount of an abnormal antithrombin is also detectable, is classified as having type Ib deficiency. The mutations found in these patients (see Table 18–1) apparently cause decreased synthesis or accelerated clearance of the abnormal antithrombin.

Patients who have low antithrombin activity but normal antithrombin antigen have type II deficiencies. Variants of this type have provided important insights into the mechanism of action of antithrombin and can be grouped into several categories (see Table 18–1): type IIa, mutations that affect both the reactive site and the heparin-binding site; type IIb, mutations that are limited to the reactive site; and type IIc, mutations that are limited to the heparin-binding site. Type II variants appear to be synthesized at a normal rate and have a normal half-life in the circulation. Therefore, in most instances the plasma of an affected heterozygote has approximately equimolar amounts of normal and variant antithrombin. In contrast to type I antithrombin deficiency, homozygous patients with type II deficiency have been reported.[227, 305, 306] One report includes a child born to consanguineous parents, both of whom had antithrombin deficiency (antithrombin Fontainebleau).[306] The child was apparently homozygous, having undetectable heparin cofactor activity, and died at 3 years of age of massive intracardiac thrombosis while receiving oral anticoagulant therapy.

The prevalence of inherited antithrombin deficiency in the general population has been estimated to range from 1 per 2000 to 1 per 5000.[307, 308] However, in a recent study of 4189 healthy blood donors in Scotland, the prevalence was about 1 per 250, with most affected individuals having asymptomatic type IIc deficiency.[309] In a series of 752 patients with thromboembolic disease, inherited antithrombin deficiency was established in 13 (1.7 per cent) by family studies.[310] An additional 14 patients had "probable" inherited antithrombin deficiency. Thus, it appears that antithrombin deficiency is more common in patients with thromboembolic symptoms than in asymptomatic individuals, although this point has not been established rigorously.

Thromboembolic disease has been reported to occur equally in males and females with antithrombin deficiency and usually manifests as deep vein thrombosis of the lower extremities or as pulmonary embolism.[179, 180] Less frequently, thrombosis of the cerebral, renal, hepatic, or mesenteric veins occurs.[311, 312] These complications may be life threatening. Arterial thrombosis is rarely observed in patients with antithrombin deficiency. Thrombosis may occur spontaneously or after some predisposing condition such as trauma, surgery, or pregnancy.

The incidence of thromboembolism in patients with antithrombin deficiency has been estimated from retrospective reviews of published case reports.[179, 180] By 50 years of age, about 85 per cent of heterozygous individuals will have had at least one thromboembolic episode.[179] Typically, affected individuals present with thromboembolic disease after the age of 15. The median age of onset of symptoms is approximately 24 years. A history of recurrent thrombosis occurs in about 60 per cent of patients and is the factor that usually prompts a search for antithrombin deficiency. There may be great variability in the severity of

complications that arise in individuals within a single family. Therefore, it is presumed that antithrombin deficiency is but one of several factors that predispose to thrombosis in these patients. Patients with variant forms of antithrombin (type II) are difficult to distinguish clinically from those with classical antithrombin deficiency (type I). Nevertheless, it appears that heterozygous patients with variant antithrombin molecules have fewer thromboembolic complications.[305, 309, 313, 314]

Acquired antithrombin deficiency can occur in liver disease,[315] in the nephrotic syndrome,[316] and during disseminated intravascular coagulation.[317] Whether antithrombin deficiency contributes to the thrombotic complications reported in these conditions is unclear. Antithrombin is mildly decreased in patients taking estrogens.[318] A more profound decrease in antithrombin occurs in patients receiving L-asparaginase.[319] Despite the acquired antithrombin deficiency, a hypercoagulable state may not occur in these patients because the levels of procoagulant factors such as prothrombin are decreased concomitantly by L-asparaginase.[320]

HEPARIN COFACTOR II

Structure and Protease Specificity of Heparin Cofactor II

Heparin cofactor II is a glycoprotein that consists of a single polypeptide chain with a molecular weight of 66,000 (see Fig. 18–6).[177] The gene for heparin cofactor II on human chromosome 22 (q11) contains five exons distributed over approximately 16 kb of DNA.[321, 322] The positions of the introns are similar to those of the α_1-antitrypsin and angiotensinogen genes but differ from those of the antithrombin, plasminogen activator inhibitor-1, plasminogen activator inhibitor-2, and ovalbumin genes. No TATA or CAAT sequences (or a variety of other proposed regulatory elements) have been identified at the 5′ end of the gene, and transcription may initiate at several positions.[321] A 2200 base mRNA for heparin cofactor II was isolated from human liver,[323] and biosynthesis was demonstrated in cultured human hepatoma cells (HepG2).[324, 325] The amino acid sequence of heparin cofactor II has been determined by cDNA cloning.[323, 326] The protein contains 480 amino acid residues preceded by a signal peptide 19 residues in length, three potential N-linked glycosylation sites, and two tyrosine residues near the amino-terminus that become O-sulfated during biosynthesis (see Fig. 18–6).[325] Three cysteine residues are present that apparently do not form disulfide bonds.[327] Heparin cofactor II is about 30 per cent identical in sequence to other members of the serpin family, with the greatest similarity occurring in the carboxy-terminal two thirds of the protein. Heparin cofactor II contains an amino-terminal extension of about 80 amino acid residues that shares no homology with other serpins.

The reactive site of heparin cofactor II contains the peptide bond Leu 444 to Ser 445.[328] In part because of the leucine residue in the P1 position, heparin cofactor II differs from antithrombin with respect to its protease specificity. In the absence of a glycosaminoglycan, heparin cofactor II inhibits chymotrypsin more rapidly than it inhibits thrombin.[329] Furthermore, heparin cofactor II does not inhibit other proteases involved in coagulation or fibrinolysis that preferentially cleave substrates following basic amino acid residues.[330] Cleavage of the Leu 444 to Ser 445 bond occurs during inhibition of both thrombin and chymotrypsin.[329] Mutation of Leu 444 to arginine increases the basal rate of inhibition of thrombin in the absence of glycosaminoglycan approximately 100-fold and decreases the ability of heparin cofactor II to inhibit chymotrypsin.[331] These results emphasize the importance of the P1 residue in determining the rate of protease inhibition and suggest that heparin cofactor II has evolved to be essentially inactive toward thrombin in the absence of a glycosaminoglycan.

Stimulation of Heparin Cofactor II by Glycosaminoglycans

Approximately 10-fold higher concentrations of heparin and heparan sulfate are required to accelerate thrombin inhibition by heparin cofactor II in comparison to antithrombin.[178] The affinity of heparin cofactor II for heparin is lower than that of antithrombin, and heparin cofactor II does not require the specific pentasaccharide structure shown in Figure 18–11 for stimulation by heparin.[332, 333] However, the activity of heparin cofactor II is stimulated approximately 1000-fold by dermatan sulfate, which has no effect on the activity of antithrombin.[178] The high-affinity binding site for heparin cofactor II in dermatan sulfate is a tandem repeat of three iduronic acid-2-sulfate → N-acetylgalactosamine-4-sulfate disaccharide subunits, which appear to be clustered within the polymer.[334] Addition of dermatan sulfate to plasma in vitro causes prolongation of the thrombin time and the activated partial thromboplastin time,[232] and intravenous infusion of dermatan sulfate into experimental animals produces an antithrombotic effect.[335] Both of these effects appear to be mediated by heparin cofactor II.[178, 336]

The glycosaminoglycan-binding site of heparin cofactor II was identified, in part, by analysis of the mutation in heparin cofactor II Oslo (Arg 189 → His).[337] This mutation causes a marked decrease (~60-fold) in the affinity of heparin cofactor II for dermatan sulfate but does not affect the affinity of the inhibitor for heparin. The four basic amino acid residues between positions 185 and 193 of heparin cofactor II align perfectly with basic residues in antithrombin (see Fig. 18–6) but are poorly conserved in other serpins. Site-directed mutagenesis of basic amino acid residues in the vicinity of Arg 189 demonstrated that the binding sites for dermatan sulfate and heparin overlap

but are not identical; thus, mutations of Lys 173, Arg 184, and Arg 185 affect heparin binding, whereas mutations of Arg 184, Arg 185, Arg 189, Arg 192, and Arg 193 affect dermatan sulfate binding.[338–341] Arg 103, which may correspond to Arg 47 in antithrombin, does not appear to be involved in binding to either glycosaminoglycan.

The stimulatory effect of heparin and dermatan sulfate on thrombin inhibition depends on the presence of an acidic polypeptide domain near the amino-terminus of heparin cofactor II.[342] The acidic domain contains a tandem repeat of two nearly identical sequences (see Fig. 18–6), each of which is similar to the carboxy-terminal sequence of hirudin, a potent thrombin inhibitor in the saliva of the medicinal leech. The carboxy-terminal portion of hirudin binds with high affinity to anion-binding exosite I of thrombin, whereas the amino-terminal domain of hirudin occupies the catalytic site.[343, 344] A synthetic peptide corresponding to the acidic domain of heparin cofactor II competes with hirudin for binding to thrombin but does not affect the ability of thrombin to hydrolyze a tripeptide p-nitroanilide substrate.[345] Thus, binding of thrombin to the acidic domain of heparin cofactor II could facilitate covalent complex formation by bringing the active site of thrombin into approximation with the reactive site of heparin cofactor II.

Experiments with recombinant heparin cofactor II have established the importance of the amino-terminal acidic domain.[340–342] For example, deletion of the first acidic repeat (residues 1 to 67) or both acidic repeats (residues 1 to 74) does not affect the rate of inhibition of thrombin or chymotrypsin in the absence of a glycosaminoglycan. Deletion of the first acidic repeat, however, greatly diminishes the ability of dermatan sulfate or heparin to stimulate the inhibition of thrombin.[342] The deletion mutants also bind heparin more tightly, suggesting that the acidic domain occupies the glycosaminoglycan-binding site in native heparin cofactor II. These findings are consistent with the model for inhibition of thrombin by heparin cofactor II shown in Figure 18–12. In this model, a glycosaminoglycan displaces the amino-terminal acidic domain of heparin cofactor II from the glycosaminoglycan-binding site, enabling the acidic domain to interact with thrombin. Dermatan sulfate or heparin chains of sufficient length to bind thrombin and heparin cofactor II simultaneously may accelerate the inhibitory reaction further by a template mechanism.

Physiology of Heparin Cofactor II

The concentration of heparin cofactor II in normal human plasma is 1.2 ± 0.4 μM (mean ± 2 SD).[346] Several individuals with inherited partial deficiency of heparin cofactor II (~50 per cent of normal) were reported to have histories of thrombotic disease.[347, 348] In one series, however, 4 of 379 apparently healthy individuals had heparin cofactor II levels less than 60 per cent.[349] Thus, it is premature to conclude that

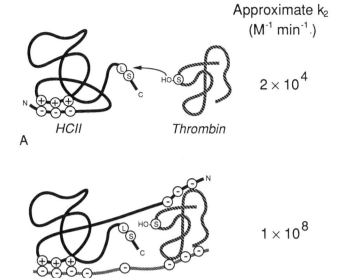

Approximate k_2
(M^{-1} min^{-1}.)

2×10^4

1×10^8

FIGURE 18–12. Model for inhibition of thrombin by heparin cofactor II. *A,* The active site serine (S) hydroxyl group of thrombin attacks the reactive site leucyl-serine (LS) peptide bond of heparin cofactor II to form a covalent complex. In the absence of a glycosaminoglycan, the amino-terminal acidic domain of heparin cofactor II (−) forms ionic bonds with the glycosaminoglycan-binding site (+) and is unable to interact with thrombin. *B,* A glycosaminoglycan chain displaces the amino-terminal acidic domain of heparin cofactor II from the glycosaminoglycan-binding site. The acidic domain then interacts with the anion-binding exosite I of thrombin. Binding of thrombin both to the amino-terminal acidic domain of heparin cofactor II and to the glycosaminoglycan template greatly increases the rate of covalent complex formation. Approximate second-order rate constants (k_2) for the thrombin-heparin cofactor II reaction are indicated. (From Van Deerlin, V. M. D., and Tollefsen, D. M.: The N-terminal acidic domain of heparin cofactor II mediates the inhibition of α-thrombin in the presence of glycosaminoglycans. J. Biol. Chem. 266:20223, 1991; with permission of the American Society for Biochemistry and Molecular Biology.)

heparin cofactor II deficiency is a risk factor for thrombosis. The concentration of heparin cofactor II is markedly decreased in some patients with liver disease, disseminated intravascular coagulation, and obstetric complications.[346, 350–352] In these situations, the heparin cofactor II and antithrombin levels are usually decreased to a similar degree. A moderately elevated concentration of heparin cofactor II is present in women who are pregnant or who use oral contraceptives.[353] Normal levels are present in patients taking oral anticoagulants, in the vast majority of patients with venous thromboembolic disease,[351, 352] and in symptomatic patients with inherited antithrombin deficiency.[350, 351, 354]

Cultured fibroblasts and vascular smooth muscle cells accelerate the inhibition of thrombin by heparin cofactor II.[355] In the case of fibroblasts, a dermatan sulfate proteoglycan was demonstrated to be responsible for this effect. These results suggest that heparin cofactor II could inhibit thrombin in the connective tissues rather than within the blood vessels. A derma-

tan sulfate proteoglycan appears during pregnancy in both the maternal and the fetal circulations, and it stimulates inhibition of thrombin by plasma heparin cofactor II approximately twofold.[356] The placenta is rich in dermatan sulfate[357] and may be the source of this proteoglycan. Thus, heparin cofactor II could be activated locally to inhibit coagulation within the placenta.

REFERENCES

1. Schmidt, A.: Zur Blutlehre. Vogel, Leipzig, 1892.
2. Morawitz, P.: Die Chemie der Blutzgerinnung. Ergeo. Physiol. 4:307, 1905.
3. Wright, I. S.: The nomenclature of blood clotting factors. Thromb. Diath. Haemorrh. 7:381, 1962.
4. Lister, J.: On the coagulation of the blood. Proc. R. Soc. Lond. 12:580, 1863.
5. Freund, E.: Ein Beitrag zur Kenntniss der Blutgerinnung. Medizinische Jahrbuch Wein 1:46, 1886.
6. Bordet, J., and Gengou, O.: Recherches sur la coagulation du sang et les serum anticoagulants. Ann. Inst. Pasteur 15:129, 1901.
7. Conley, C. L., Hartmann, R. C., and Morse, W. I., II: The clotting behavior of human "platelet free" plasma: Evidence for the existence of a "plasma thromboplastin." J. Clin. Invest. 28:340, 1949.
8. MacFarlane, R. G.: An enzyme cascade in the blood clotting mechanism, and its function as a biochemical amplifier. Nature 202:498, 1964.
9. Davie, E. W., and Ratnoff, O. D.: Waterfall sequence for intrinsic blood clotting. Science 145:1310, 1964.
10. Hathaway, W., Bilhasen, L., and Hathaway, H.: Evidence for a new plasma thromboplastin factor I: Case report, coagulation studies and physiological properties. Blood 26:521, 1965.
11. Nemerson, Y., and Furie, B.: Zymogens and cofactors of blood coagulation. CRC Crit. Rev. Biochem. 9:45, 1980.
12. Kaplan, A. P., and Silverberg, M.: The coagulation-kinin pathway of human plasma. Blood 70:1, 1987.
13. Ragni, M. V., Lewis, J. H., Spero, J. A., and Hasiba, U.: Factor VII deficiency. Am. J. Hematol. 10:79, 1981.
14. Triplett, D. A., Brandt, J. T., Batard, M. A. M., Dixon, J. L. S., and Fair, D. S.: Hereditary factor VII deficiency: Heterogeneity defined by combined functional and immunochemical analysis. Blood 66:1284, 1985.
15. Osterud, B., and Rapaport, S.: Activation of factor IX by the reaction product of tissue factor and factor VII. Additional pathway for initiating blood coagulation. Proc. Natl. Acad. Sci. USA 74:5260, 1977.
16. Biggs, R., and MacFarlane, R. G.: The reaction of hemophiliac plasma to thromboplastin. J. Clin. Invest. 4:445, 1951.
17. Biggs, R., and Nossel, H. L.: Tissue extract and the contact reaction in blood coagulation. Thromb. Diath. Haemorrh. 6:1, 1961.
18. Broze, G. J., Jr., Leykam, J. E., Schwartz, B. D., and Miletich, J. P.: Purification of human brain tissue factor. J. Biol. Chem. 260:10917, 1985.
19. Guha, A., Bach, R., Konigsberg, W., and Nemerson, Y.: Affinity purification of human tissue factor: Interaction of factor VII and tissue factor in detergent micelles. Proc. Natl. Acad. Sci. USA 83:299, 1986.
20. Bazan, J. F.: Structural design and molecular evolution of a cytokine receptor superfamily. Proc. Natl. Acad. Sci. USA 87:6934, 1990.
21. Bazan, J. F.: Haemopoietic receptors and helical cytokines. Immunol. Today 11:350, 1990.
22. Wilcox, J. N., Smith, K. M., Schwartz, S. M., and Gordon, D.: Localization of tissue factor in the normal vessel wall and in the atherosclerotic plaque. Proc. Natl. Acad. Sci. USA 86:2839, 1989.

23. Drake, T. A., Morrissey, J. H., and Edgington, T. S.: Selective cellular expression of tissue factor in human tissues: Implications for disorders of hemostasis and thrombosis. Am. J. Pathol. 134:1087, 1989.

24. Fleck, R. A., Rao, L. V. M., Rapaport, S. I., and Varki, N.: Localization of human tissue factor antigen by immunostaining with monospecific, polyclonal anti-human tissue factor antibody. Thromb. Res. 59:421, 1990.

25. Tipping, P. G., Malliaros, J., and Holdsworth, S. R.: Procoagulant activity expression by macrophages from atheromatous vascular plaques. Atherosclerosis 79:237, 1989.

26. Lerner, R. G., Goldstein, R. G., and Cummings, G.: Stimulation of leukocyte thromboplastic activity by endotoxin. Proc. Soc. Exp. Biol. Med. 138:145, 1971.

27. Stern, D., Nawroth, P., Handley, D., and Kisiel, W.: An endothelial cell–dependent pathway of coagulation. Proc. Natl. Acad. Sci. USA 82:2523, 1985.

28. Bevilacqua, M. P., Pober, J. S., Majeau, G. R., Cotran, R. S., and Gimbrone, M. A., Jr.: Interleukin-1 (IL-1) induces biosynthesis and cell surface expression of procoagulant activity in human vascular endothelial cells. J. Exp. Med. 160:618, 1984.

29. Bevilacqua, M. P., Pober, J. S., Majeau, G. R., Fiers, W., Cotran, R. S., and Gimbrone, M. A., Jr.: Recombinant tumor necrosis factor induces procoagulant activity in cultured human vascular endothelium: Characterization and comparison with the actions of interleukin 1. Proc. Natl. Acad. Sci. USA 83:4533, 1986.

30. Nawroth, P. P., and Stern, D. M.: Modulation of endothelial cell hemostatic properties by tumor necrosis factor. J. Exp. Med. 163:740, 1986.

31. Brox, J. H., Osterud, B., Bjorklid, E., and Fenton, J. W.: Production and availability of thromboplastin in endothelial cells: The effects of thrombin, endotoxin and platelets. Br. J. Haematol. 57:239, 1984.

32. Galdal, K. S., Lyberg, T., Evensen, S. A., Nilsen, E., and Prydz, H.: Thrombin induces thromboplastin synthesis in cultured vascular endothelial cells. Thromb. Haemost. 54:373, 1985.

33. Prydz, H., Allison, A. C., and Schorlemmer, H. U.: Further link between complement activation and blood coagulation. Nature 270:173, 1977.

34. Muhlfelder, T. W., Niemetz, J., Kreutzer, D., Beebe, D., Ward, P., and Rosenfeld, S. I.: C5 chemotactic fragment induces leukocyte production of tissue factor activity. J. Clin. Invest. 63:147, 1979.

35. Rothberger, H., Zimmerman, T. S., Spiegelberg, H. L., and Vaughan, J. H.: Leukocyte procoagulant activity. Enhancement of production in vitro by IgG and antigen-antibody complexes. J. Clin. Invest. 59:549, 1977.

36. Schwartz, B. S., and Edgington, T. S.: Immune complex–induced human monocyte procoagulant activity. I. Rapid undirectional lymphocyte-instructed pathway. J. Exp. Med. 154:892, 1981.

37. Edwards, R. L., Rickles, F. R., and Bobrove, A. M.: Mononuclear cell tissue factor: Cell of origin and requirements for activation. Blood 54:359, 1979.

38. Edwards, R. L., and Rickles, F. R.: The role of human T-cells (and T-cell products) for monocyte tissue factor generation. J. Immunol. 125:606, 1980.

39. Levy, G. A., Schwartz, B. S., and Edgington, T. S.: The kinetics and metabolic requirements for direct lymphocyte induction of human procoagulant monokines by bacterial lipopolysaccharide. J. Immunol. 127:357, 1981.

40. Gregory, S. A., and Edgington, T. S.: Tissue factor induction in human monocytes: Two distinct mechanisms displayed by different alloantigen-responsive T-cell clones. J. Clin. Invest. 76:2440, 1985.

41. Nakamura, S., Gotoh S., Takenaka, O., and Takahashi, K.: Monocyte thromboplastin (tissue factor): Complementary effect of lymphocytes upon its generation by endotoxin-stimulated monkey (Macaca fuscata) cells. J. Biochem. 97:1603, 1985.

42. Ryan, J., and Geczy, C. L.: Characterization and purification of mouse macrophage procoagulant inducing factor. J. Immunol. 137:2864, 1986.

43. Gregory, S. A., Kornbluth, R. S., Helin, H., Remold, H. G., and Edgington, T. S.: Monocyte procoagulant inducing factor: A lymphokine involved in the T-cell–instructed monocyte procoagulant response to antigen. J. Immunol. 137:3231, 1986.

44. Bach, R., Nemerson, Y., and Konigsberg, W.: Purification and characterization of bovine tissue factor. J. Biol. Chem. 256:8324, 1981.

45. Nemerson, Y.: The phospholipid requirement of tissue factor in blood coagulation. J. Clin. Invest. 47:72, 1968.

46. Pitlick, F. A., and Nemerson, Y.: Binding of the protein component of tissue factor to phospholipids. Biochemistry 9:5105, 1970.

47. Bjorklid, E., Storm, E., Osterud, B., and Prydz, H.: The interaction of the protein and phospholipid components of tissue thromboplastin (factor III) with the factors VII and X. Scand. J. Haematol. 14:65, 1975.

48. Bach, R., and Rifkin, D. B.: Expression of tissue factor procoagulant activity: Regulation by cytosolic calcium. Proc. Natl. Acad. Sci. USA 87:6995, 1990.

49. Maynard, J. R., Dryer, B. E., Stemerman, M. B., and Pitlick, F. A.: Tissue factor coagulant activity of cultured human endothelial and smooth muscle cells and fibroblasts. Blood 50:387, 1977.

50. Schorer, A. E., Kaplan, M. E., Rao, G. H. R., and Modlow, C. F.: Interleukin 1 stimulates endothelial cell tissue factor production and expression by a prostaglandin-independent mechanism. Thromb. Haemost. 56:256, 1986.

51. Carson, S. D., and Johnson, D. R.: Consecutive enzyme cascades: Complement activation at the cell surface triggers increased tissue factor activity. Blood 76:361, 1990.

52. Zwaal, R. F. A., Comfurius, P., and van Deenen, L. L. M.: Membrane asymmetry and blood coagulation. Nature 268:358, 1977.

53. Broze, G. J., Jr., and Majerus, P. W.: Purification and characterization of human coagulation factor VII. J. Biol. Chem. 150:1242, 1980.

54. Bajaj, S. P., Rapaport, S. I., and Brown, S. F.: Isolation and characterization of human factor VII. Activation of factor VII by factor Xa. J. Biol. Chem. 256:253, 1981.

55. Fair, D. S.: Quantitation of factor VII in the plasma of normal and warfarin-treated individuals by radioimmunoassay. Blood 62:784, 1983.

56. Tsao, B. P., Fair, D. S., Curtiss, L. K., and Edgington, T. S.: Monocytes can be induced by LPS triggered T-lymphocytes to express functional factor VII/VIIa protease activity. J. Exp. Med. 159:1042, 1984.

57. Chapman, H. A., Allen, C. L., and Stone, O. L.: Human alveolar macrophages synthesize factor VII in vitro: Possible role in interstitial lung disease. J. Clin. Invest. 75:2030, 1985.

58. Godfrey, H. P., Angadi, C. V., Haak-Frendscho, M., and Kaplan, A. P.: Concurrent production of macrophage agglutination factor and factor VII by antigen-stimulated human peripheral blood mononuclear cells. Immunology 57:77, 1986.

59. McGee, M. P., Devlin, R., Saluta, G., and Koren, H.: Tissue factor and factor VII messenger RNAs in human alveolar macrophages: Effects of breathing ozone. Blood 75:122, 1990.

60. Radcliffe, R., and Nemerson, Y.: Activation and control of factor VII by activated factor X and thrombin. J. Biol. Chem. 250:388, 1975.

61. Radcliffe, R., Bagdasarian, A., Colman, R., and Nemerson, Y.: Activation of bovine factor VII by Hageman factor fragments. Blood 50:611, 1977.

62. Kisiel, W., Fujikawa, K., and Davie, E. W.: Activation of bovine factor VII (proconvertin) by factor XIIa (activated Hageman factor). Biochemistry 16:4189, 1977.

63. Masys, D. R., Bajaj, P. S., and Rapaport, S. I.: Activation of human factor VII by activated factors IX and X. Blood 60:1143, 1982.

64. Wildgoose, P., and Kisiel, W.: Activation of human factor VII by factors IXa and Xa on human bladder carcinoma cells. Blood 73:1888, 1989.

65. Nakagaki, T., Foster, D. C., Berkner, K. L., and Kisiel, W.: Initiation of the extrinsic pathway of blood coagulation: Evidence for the tissue factor–dependent autoactivation of human coagulation factor VII. Biochemistry 30:10819, 1991.

66. Sakai, T., Lund-Hansen, T., Paborsky, L., Pedersen, A. H., and Kisiel, W.: Binding of human factors VII and VIIa to a human bladder carcinoma cell line (J82). J. Biol. Chem. 264:9980, 1989.

67. Pedersen, A., Lund-Hansen, T., Bisgaard-Frantzen, H., Olsen, F., and Petersen, L. C.: Autoactivation of human recombinant coagulation factor VII. Biochemistry 28:9331, 1989.

68. Zur, M., Radcliffe, R. D., Oberdick, J., and Nemerson, Y.: The dual role of factor VII in blood coagulation. Initiation and inhibition of a proteolytic system by a zymogen. J. Biol. Chem. 257:5623, 1982.

69. Rao, L. V. M., Rapaport, S. I., and Bajaj, S. P.: Activation of human factor VII in the initiation of tissue factor–dependent coagulation. Blood 68:685, 1986.

70. Williams, E. B., Krishnaswamy, S., and Mann, K. G.: Zymogen/enzyme discrimination using peptide chloromethyl ketones. J. Biol. Chem. 264:7536, 1989.

71. Wildgoose, P., Berkner, K. L., and Kisiel, W.: Synthesis, purification and characterization of an Arg 152–Glu site-directed mutant of recombinant human blood clotting factor VII. Biochemistry 29:3413, 1990.

72. Nelsestuen, G. L.: Role of γ-carboxyglutamic acid. An unusual transition required for calcium-dependent binding of pro-thrombin to phospholipid. J. Biol. Chem. 251:5648, 1976.

73. Prendergast, F. G., and Mann, K. G.: Differentiation of metal ion–induced transitions of prothrombin fragment 1. J. Biol. Chem. 252:840, 1977.

74. Borowski, M., Furie, B. C., Bauminger, S., and Furie, B.: Prothrombin requires two sequential metal-dependent conformational transitions to bind phospholipid. J. Biol. Chem. 261:14969, 1986.

75. Church, W. R., Messier, T., Howard, P. R., Amiral, J., Meyer, D., and Mann, K. G.: A conserved epitope on several human vitamin K–dependent proteins. Location of the antigenic site and influence of metal ions on antibody binding. J. Biol. Chem. 263:6259, 1988.

76. Church, W. R., Boulanger, L. L., Messier, T. L., and Mann, K. G.: Evidence for a common metal ion–dependent transition in the 4-carboxyglutamic acid domains of several vitamin K–dependent proteins. J. Biol. Chem. 264:17882, 1989.

77. Broze, G. J., Jr.: Binding of human factor VII and VIIa to monocytes. J. Clin. Invest. 70:526, 1982.

78. Sakai, T., Lund-Hansen, T., Thim, L., and Kisiel, W.: The γ-carboxyglutamic acid domain of human factor VIIa is essential for its interaction with cell surface tissue factor. J. Biol. Chem. 265:1890, 1990.

79. Kumar, A., Blumenthal, D. K., and Fair, D. S.: Identification of molecular sites on factor VII which mediate its assembly and function in the extrinsic pathway activation complex. J. Biol. Chem. 266:915, 1991.

80. Toomey, J. R., Smith, K. J., and Stafford, D. W.: Localization of the human tissue factor recognition determinant of human factor VIIa. J. Biol. Chem. 266:19198, 1991.

81. Bach, R., Gentry, R., and Nemerson, Y.: Factor VII binding to tissue factor in reconstituted phospholipid vesicles: Induction of cooperativity by phosphatidylserine. Biochemistry 25:4007, 1986.

82. Nemerson, Y., and Repke, D.: Tissue factor accelerates the activation of coagulation factor VII: The role of a bifunctional coagulation cofactor. Thromb. Res. 40:351, 1985.

83. Rao, L. V. M., and Rapaport, S. I.: Activation of factor VII bound to tissue factor: A key early step in the tissue factor pathway of blood coagulation. Proc. Natl. Acad. Sci. USA 85:6687, 1988.

84. Bom, J. J., and Bertina, R. M.: The contributions of Ca^{2+}, phospholipids and tissue-factor apoprotein to the activation of human blood-coagulation factor X by activated factor VII. Biochem. J. 265:327, 1990.

85. Komiyama, Y., Pedersen, A., and Kisiel, W.: Proteolytic activation of human factors IX and X by recombinant human factor VIIa: Effects of calcium, phospholipids, and tissue factor. Biochemistry 29:9418, 1990.

86. Jesty, J., and Silverberg, S. A.: Kinetics of the tissue factor–dependent activation of coagulation factors IX and X in a bovine plasma system. J. Biol. Chem. 254:12337, 1979.

87. Repke, D. I., MacLean, D., and Nemerson, Y.: Heparin affects the substrate specificity of the tissue factor pathway of coagulation (abstract). Fed. Proc. 40:274, 1981.

88. Zur, M., and Nemerson, Y.: Kinetics of factor IX activation via the extrinsic pathway. Dependence of Km on tissue factor. J. Biol. Chem. 255:5703, 1980.

89. Warn-Cramer, B. J., and Bajaj, S. P.: Intrinsic versus extrinsic coagulation. Kinetic considerations. Biochem. J. 239:757, 1986.

90. Almus, F. E., Rao, L. V. M., and Rapaport, S. I.: Functional properties of factor VIIa/tissue factor formed with purified tissue factor and with tissue factor expressed on cultured endothelial cells. Thromb. Haemost. 62:1067, 1989.

91. Seligsohn, U., Kasper, C. K., Osterud, B., and Rapaport, S. I.: Activated factor VII: Presence in factor IX concentrates and persistence in the circulation after infusion. Blood 53:828, 1979.

92. Kondo, S., and Kisiel, W.: Regulation of factor VIIa activity in plasma: Evidence that antithrombin III is the sole plasma protease inhibitor of human factor VIIa. Thromb. Res. 46:325, 1987.

93. Thomas, L.: Studies on the intravascular thromboplastin effect of tissue suspensions in mice: II. A factor in normal rabbit serum which inhibits the thromboplastin effect of the sedimentable tissue component. Bull. Johns Hopkins Hosp. 81:26, 1947.

94. Schneider, C. L.: The active principle of placental toxin: thromboplastin; its inactivator in blood: antithromboplastin. Am. J. Physiol. 149:123, 1947.

95. Hjort, P. F.: Intermediate reactions in the coagulation of blood with tissue thromboplastin. Scand. J. Clin. Lab. Invest. 9(Suppl. 27):1, 1957.

96. Marlar, R. A., Kleiss, A. J., and Griffin, J. H.: An alternative extrinsic pathway of human blood coagulation. Blood 60:1353, 1982.

97. Morrison, S. A., and Jesty, J.: Tissue factor–dependent activation of tritium-labeled factor IX and factor X in human plasma. Blood 63:1338, 1984.

98. Sanders, N. L., Bajaj, S. P., Zivelin, A., and Rapaport, S. I.: Inhibition of tissue factor/factor VIIa activity in plasma requires factor X and an additional plasma component. Blood 66:204, 1985.

99. Hubbard, A. R., and Jennings, C. A.: Inhibition of tissue thromboplastin-mediated blood coagulation. Thromb. Res. 42:489, 1986.

100. Broze, G. J., Jr., and Miletich, J. P.: Characterization of the inhibition of tissue factor in serum. Blood 69:150, 1987.

101. Rao, L. V. M., and Rapaport, S. I.: Studies of a mechanism inhibiting the initiation of the extrinsic pathway of coagulation. Blood 69:645, 1987.

102. Wun, T.-C., Kretzmer, K. K., Girard, T. J., Miletich, J. P., and Broze, G. J., Jr.: Cloning and characterization of a cDNA coding for the lipoprotein-associated coagulation inhibitor shows that it consists of three tandem Kunitz-type inhibitory domains. J. Biol. Chem. 263:6001, 1988.

103. Girard, T. J., McCourt, D., Novotny, W. F., MacPhail, L. A., Likert, K. M., and Broze, G. J., Jr.: Endogenous phosphorylation of the lipoprotein-associated coagulation inhibitor at serine-2. Biochem. J. 270:621, 1990.

104. Novotny, W. F., Girard, T. J., Miletich, J. P., and Broze, G. J., Jr.: Purification and characterization of the lipoprotein-associated coagulation inhibitor from human plasma. J. Biol. Chem. 264:18832, 1989.

105. Colburn, P., and Buonassisi, V.: Identification of an endothe-

lial cell product as an inhibitor of tissue factor activity. In Vitro Cell. Dev. Biol. 24:1133, 1988.

106. Warn-Cramer, B. J., Maki, S. L., and Rapaport, S. I.: A sulfated rabbit endothelial cell glycoprotein that inhibits factor VIIa/tissue factor is functionally and immunologically identical to rabbit extrinsic pathway inhibitor. Thromb. Res. 61:515, 1991.

106a. Smith, P. L., Skelton, T. P., Fiete, D., Dharmesh, S. M., Beranek, M. C., MacPhail, L., Broze, G. J., Jr., and Baenziger, J. U.: The asparagine-linked oligosaccharides on tissue factor pathway inhibitor terminate with SO_4–4GalNAcβ1, 4GlcNAcβ1, 2Manα. J. Biol Chem. 267:19140, 1992.

107. Van der Logt, C. P. E., Reitsma, P. H., and Bertina, R. M.: Intron-exon organization of the human gene coding for the lipoprotein-associated coagulation inhibitor: The factor Xa dependent inhibitor of the extrinsic pathway of coagulation. Biochemistry 30:1571, 1991.

108. Girard, T. J., Eddy, R., Wesselschmidt, R. L., MacPhail, L. A., Likert, K. M., Byers, M. G., Shows, T. B., and Broze, G. J., Jr.: Structure of the human lipoprotein-associated coagulation inhibitor gene: Intron/exon gene organization and localization of the gene to chromosome 2. J. Biol. Chem. 266:5036, 1991.

108a. Van der Logt, C. P., Kluck, P. M., Wiegant, J., Landegent, J. E., and Reitsma, P. H.: Refined regional assignment of the human tissue factor pathway inhibitor (TFPI) gene to chromosome band 2q32 by nonisotopic in situ hybridization. Hum. Genet. 89:577, 1992.

109. Patthy, L.: Intron-dependent evolution: Preferred types of exons and introns. FEBS Lett. 214:1, 1987.

110. Gronostajski, R. M.: Site-specific DNA binding of nuclear factor I: Effect of the spacer region. Nucleic Acids Res. 14:9117, 1987.

111. Lee, W., Haslinger, A., Karin, M., and Tjian, R.: Activation of transcription by two factors that bind promoter and enhancer sequences of the human metallothionein genes and SV40. Nature 325:368, 1987.

112. Lee, W., Mitchell, P., and Tjian, R.: Purified transcription factor AP-1 interacts with TPA inducible enhancer elements. Cell 49:741, 1987.

113. Angel, P., Baumann, I., Stein, B., Deliuw, H., Rahmsdorf, H. J., and Herrlick, P.: 12-O-tetradecanoyl-phorbol-13 acetate induction of the human collagenase gene is mediated by an inducible enhancer element located in the 5′ flanking region. Mol. Cell. Biol. 7:2256, 1987.

114. Rana, S. V., Reimers, H. J., Pathikonda, M. S., and Bajaj, S. P.: Expression of tissue factor and factor VIIa/TF inhibitory activity in endotoxin or phorbol ester stimulated U937 monocyte-like cells. Blood 71:259, 1988.

115. Girard, T. J., Warren, L. A., Novotny, W. F., Miletich, J. P., and Broze, G. J., Jr.: Identification of the 1.4 and 4.0 kb messages for the lipoprotein-associated coagulation inhibitor and expression of the encoded protein. Thromb. Res. 55:37, 1989.

116. Shaw, G., and Kamen, R.: A conserved AU sequence from the 3′ untranslated region of GM-CSF mRNA mediates selective mRNA degradation. Cell 46:659, 1986.

117. Caput, D., Beutler, B., Hartog, K., Thayer, R., Brown-Skinner, S., and Cerami, A.: Identification of a common nucleotide sequence in the 3′ untranslated region of mRNA molecules specifying inflammatory mediators. Proc. Natl. Acad. Sci. USA 83:1670, 1986.

118. Smith, R. P., Higuchi, D. A., and Broze, G. J., Jr.: Platelet coagulation factor XIa inhibitor, a form of Alzheimer amyloid precursor protein. Science 248:1421, 1990.

119. Pratt, C. W., Roche, P. A., and Pizzo, S. V.: The role of inter-alpha-trypsin inhibitor and other proteinase inhibitors in the plasma clearance of neutrophil elastase and plasmin. Arch. Biochem. Biophys. 258:591, 1987.

120. Gebhard, W., Tschesche, H., and Fritz, H.: Biochemistry of aprotinin and aprotinin-like inhibitors. In Barrett, A. J., and Salveson, G. (eds.): Proteinase Inhibitors. Amsterdam, Elsevier Science Publishers B. V., 1986, pp. 375–388.

121. Broze, G. J., Jr., and Miletich, J. P.: Isolation of the tissue factor inhibitor produced by HepG2 hepatoma cells. Proc. Natl. Acad. Sci. USA 84:1886, 1987.

122. Laskowski, M., Jr., and Kato, I.: Protein inhibitors of proteinases. Annu. Rev. Biochem. 49:593, 1980.

123. Morrison, J. F.: The slow-binding and slow, tight-binding inhibition of enzyme-catalyzed reactions. Trends Biochem. Sci. 7:102, 1982.

124. Antonini, E., Ascenzi, P., Menegatti, E., and Guarneri, M.: Multiple intermediates in the reaction of bovine β-trypsin with bovine pancreatic trypsin inhibitor (Kunitz). Biopolymers 22:363, 1983.

125. Broze, G. J., Jr., Warren, L. A., Novotny, W. F., Higuchi, D. A., Girard, J. J., and Miletich, J. P.: The lipoprotein-associated coagulation inhibitor that inhibits the factor VII–tissue factor complex also inhibits factor Xa: Insight into its possible mechanism of action. Blood 71:335, 1988.

126. Broze, G. J., Jr., Girard, T. J., and Novotny, W. F.: Regulation of coagulation by a multivalent Kunitz-type inhibitor. Biochemistry 29:7539, 1990.

127. Girard, T. J., Warren, L. A., Novotny, W. F., Likert, K. M., Brown, S. G., Miletich, J. P., and Broze, G. J., Jr.: Functional significance of the Kunitz-type inhibitory domains of lipoprotein-associated coagulation inhibitor. Nature 338:518, 1989.

128. Wesselschmidt, R. L., Girard, T. J., Likert, K. M., Wun, T.-C., and Broze, G. J., Jr.: Tissue factor pathway inhibitor: The carboxy-terminus is required for optimal inhibition of factor Xa. Blood 79:2004, 1992.

129. Higuchi, D., Wun, T.-C., Likert, K. M., and Broze, G. J., Jr.: The effect of leukocyte elastase on tissue factor pathway inhibitor. Blood 79:1712, 1992.

130. Nordfang, O., Bjorn, S. E., Valentin, S., Nielsen, L. S., Wildgoose, P., Beck, T. C., and Hedner, U.: The C-terminus of tissue factor pathway inhibitor is essential to its anticoagulant activity. Biochemistry 30:10371, 1991.

131. Warn-Cramer, B. J., Rao, L. V. M., Maki, S. L., and Rapaport, S. I.: Modifications of extrinsic pathway inhibitor (EPI) and factor Xa that affect the ability to interact and to inhibit factor VIIa/tissue factor: Evidence for a two-step model of inhibition. Thromb. Haemost. 60:453, 1988.

132. Girard, T. J., MacPhail, L. A., Likert, K. M., Novotny, W. F., Miletich, J. P., and Broze, G. J., Jr.: Inhibition of factor VIIa–tissue factor coagulation activity by a hybrid protein. Science 248:1421, 1990.

133. Pedersen, A. H., Nordfang, O., Norris, F., Wiberg, F. C., Christensen, P. M., Moeller, K. B., Meidahl-Pedersen, J., Beck, T. C., Norris, K., Hedner, U., and Kisiel, W.: Recombinant human extrinsic pathway inhibitor. Production, isolation, and characterization of its inhibitory activity on tissue factor–initiated coagulation reactions. J. Biol. Chem. 265:16786, 1990.

134. Rapaport, S. I.: The extrinsic pathway inhibitor: A regulator of tissue factor–dependent blood coagulation. Thromb. Haemost. 66:6, 1991.

135. Callander, N. S., Rao, L. V. M., Nordfang, O., Sandset, P. M., Warn-Cramer, B., and Rapaport, S. I.: Mechanisms of binding of recombinant extrinsic pathway inhibitor (rEPI) to cultured cell surfaces. J. Biol. Chem. 267:876, 1992.

136. Day, K. C., Hoffman, L. C., Palmier, M. O., Kretzmer, K. K., Huang, M. D., Pyla, E. Y., Spokas, E., Broze, G. J., Jr., Warren, T. G., and Wun, T.-C.: Recombinant lipoprotein-associated coagulation inhibitor inhibits tissue thromboplastin-induced intravascular coagulation in the rabbit. Blood 76:1538, 1990.

137. Haskel, E. J., Torr, S. R., Day, K. C., Palmier, M. O., Wun, T.-C., Sobel, B. E., and Abendschein, D. R.: Prevention of arterial reocclusion after thrombolysis with recombinant lipoprotein-associated coagulation inhibitor. Circulation 84:821, 1991.

138. Hubbard, A. R., and Jennings, C. A.: Inhibition of the tissue factor–factor VII complex: Involvement of factor Xa and lipoproteins. Thromb. Res. 46:527, 1987.

139. Warn-Cramer, B. J., Maki, S. L., Zivelin, A., and Rapaport, S. I.: Partial purification and characterization of extrinsic path-

way inhibitor (the factor Xa–dependent plasma inhibitor of factor VIIa/tissue factor). Thromb. Res. 48:11, 1987.

140. Novotny, W. F., Girard, T. J., Miletich, J. P., and Broze, G. J., Jr.: Platelets secrete a coagulation inhibitor functionally and antigenically similar to the lipoprotein-associated coagulation inhibitor. Blood 72:2020, 1988.

141. Bajaj, M. S., Kuppuswamy, M. N., Saito, H., Spitzer, S. G., and Bajaj, S. P.: Cultured normal human hepatocytes do not synthesize lipoprotein-associated coagulation inhibitor: Evidence that endothelium is the principal site of its synthesis. Proc. Natl. Acad. Sci. USA 87:8869, 1990.

142. Sandset, P. M., Abildgaard, U., and Larsen, M. L.: Heparin induces release of extrinsic coagulation pathway inhibitor (EPI). Thromb. Res. 50:803, 1988.

143. Novotny, W. F., Brown, S. G., Miletich, J. P., Rader, D. J., and Broze, G. J., Jr.: Plasma antigen levels of the lipoprotein-associated coagulation inhibitor in patient samples. Blood 78:387, 1991.

144. Novotny, W. F., Palmier, M., Wun, T.-C., Broze, G. J., Jr., and Miletich, J. P.: Purification and properties of heparin-releasable lipoprotein-associated coagulation inhibitor. Blood 78:394, 1991.

145. Broze, G. J., Jr., Warren, L. A., Girard, T. J., and Miletich, J. P.: Isolation of the lipoprotein-associated coagulation inhibitor produced by HepG2 (human hepatoma) cells using bovine factor Xa affinity chromatography. Thromb. Res. 48:253, 1987.

146. Wun, T.-C., Huang, M. D., Kretzmer, K. K., Palmier, M. O., Day, K. C., Bulock, J. W., Fok, K. F., and Broze, G. J., Jr.: Immunoaffinity purification and characterization of lipoprotein-associated coagulation inhibitors from HepG2 hepatoma, Chang liver, and SK hepatoma cells. A comparative study. J. Biol. Chem. 265:16096, 1990.

147. Bajaj, M. S., Rana, S. V., Wysolmerski, R. B., and Bajaj, S. P.: Inhibitor of the factor VIIa–tissue factor complex is reduced in patients with disseminated intravascular coagulation but not in patients with severe hepatocellular disease. J. Clin. Invest. 79:1874, 1987.

148. Werling, R. W., Zacharski, L. R., Kisiel, W., Bajaj, S. P., Memoli, V. A., and Rousseau, S. M.: Distribution of tissue factor pathway inhibitor in normal and pathologic human tissue (abstract). Blood 78(Suppl. 1):72, 1991.

149. Warr, T. A., Warn-Cramer, B. J., Rao, L. V. M., and Rapaport, S. I.: Human plasma extrinsic pathway inhibitor activity. I. Standardization of assay and evaluation of physiologic variables. Blood 74:201, 1989.

150. Abildgaard, U., Sandset, P. M., Andersson, T. R., Oldegaard, O. R., and Rosio, S.: The inhibitor of TF/VIIa in plasma measured with a sensitive chromogenic substrate assay: Comparison with antithrombin, protein C and heparin cofactor II in a clinical material. Folia Haematol. 115:274, 1988.

151. Sandset, P. M., and Andersson, T. R.: Coagulation inhibitor levels in pneumonia and stroke: Changes due to consumption and acute phase reaction. J. Intern. Med. 225:311, 1989.

152. Sandset, P. M., Sirnes, P. A., and Abildgaard, U.: Factor VII and extrinsic pathway inhibitor in acute coronary disease. Br. J. Haematol. 72:391, 1989.

153. Sandset, P. M., Rosio, O., Aasen, A. O., and Abildgaard, U.: Extrinsic pathway inhibitor in postoperative/post-traumatic septicemia: Increased levels in fatal cases. Haemostasis 19:189, 1989.

154. Sandset, P. M., Hogevold, H. E., Lyberg, T., Andersson, T. R., and Abildgaard, U.: Extrinsic pathway inhibitor in elective surgery: A comparison with other coagulation inhibitors. Thromb. Haemost. 62:856, 1989.

155. Sandset, P. M., Hellgren, U., Uvebrandt, M., and Bergstrom, H.: Extrinsic pathway inhibitor and heparin cofactor II during normal and hypertension pregnancy. Thromb. Res. 55:6645, 1989.

156. Warr, T. A., Rao, L. V. M., and Rapaport, S. I.: Human plasma extrinsic pathway inhibitor activity. II. Plasma levels

157. Lindahl, A. K., Sandset, P. M., Abildgaard, U., Andersson, T. R., and Harbitz, T. B.: High plasma levels of extrinsic pathway inhibitor and low levels of other coagulation inhibitors in advanced cancer. Acta Chir. Scand. 155:389, 1989.

158. Brandtzaeg, P., Sandset, P. M., Joo, G. B., Questebo, R., Abildgaard, U., and Kierfulf, P.: The quantitative association of plasma endotoxin, antithrombin, protein C, extrinsic pathway inhibitor and fibrinopeptide A in systemic meningococcal disease. Thromb. Res. 55:459, 1989.

159. Sandset, P. M., Warn-Cramer, B. J., Maki, S. L., and Rapaport, S. I.: Immunodepletion of extrinsic pathway inhibitor sensitizes rabbits to endotoxin-induced intravascular coagulation and the generalized Shwartzman reaction. Blood 78:1496, 1991.

160. Sandset, P. M., Warn-Cramer, B. J., Rao, L. V. M., Maki, S. L., and Rapaport, S. I.: Depletion of extrinsic pathway inhibitor (EPI) sensitizes rabbits to disseminated intravascular coagulation induced with tissue factor: Evidence supporting a physiologic role for EPI as a natural anticoagulant. Proc. Natl. Acad. Sci. USA 88:708, 1991.

161. Naito, K., and Fujikawa, K.: Activation of human blood coagulation factor XI independent of factor XII. Factor XI is activated by thrombin and factor XIa in the presence of negatively charged surfaces. J. Biol. Chem. 266:7353, 1991.

162. Gailani, D., and Broze, G. J., Jr.: Factor XI activation in a revised model of blood coagulation. Science 253:909, 1991.

162a. Scott, C. F., and Colman, R. W.: Fibrinogen blocks the autoactivation and thrombin-mediated activation of factor XI on dextran sulfate. Proc. Natl. Acad. Sci. USA 89:11189, 1992.

162b. Brunnee, T., La Porta, C., Reddigari, S. R., Salerno, V. M., Kaplan, A. P., and Silverberg, M.: Activation of factor XI in plasma is dependent on factor XII. Blood 81:580, 1993.

163. Vander Velden, P., and Giles, A. R.: A detailed morphological evaluation of the evolution of the haemostatic plug in normal, factor VII, and factor VIII deficient dogs. Br. J. Haematol. 70:345, 1988.

164. Repke, D., Gemmell, C. H., Guha, A., Turitto, V. T., Broze, G. J., Jr., and Nemerson, Y.: Hemophilia as a defect of the tissue factor pathway of blood coagulation: Effect of factors VIII and IX on factor X activation in a continuous-flow reactor. Proc. Natl. Acad. Sci. USA 87:7623, 1990.

165. Vu, T. K., Hung, D. T., Wheaton, V. I., and Coughlin, S. R.: Molecular cloning of a functional thrombin receptor reveals a novel proteolytic mechanism of receptor activation. Cell 64:1057, 1991.

166. Chen, L. B., and Buchanan, J. M.: Mitogenic activity of blood components. I. Thrombin and prothrombin. Proc. Natl. Acad. Sci. USA 72:131, 1975.

167. Glenn, K. C., Carney, D. H., Fenton, J. W., II, and Cunningham, D. D.: Thrombin active site regions required for fibroblast receptor binding and initiation of cell division. J. Biol. Chem. 255:6609, 1980.

168. Bar-Shavit, R., Kahn, A. J., Mann, K. G., and Wilner, G. D.: Identification of a thrombin sequence with growth factor activity on macrophages. Proc. Natl. Acad. Sci. USA 83:976, 1986.

169. Bar-Shavit, R., Kahn, A., Wilner, G. D., and Fenton, J. W., II: Monocyte chemotaxis: Stimulation by specific exosite region in thrombin. Science 220:728, 1983.

170. Carrell, R. W., and Boswell, D. R.: Serpins: The superfamily of plasma serine proteinase inhibitors. In Barrett, A. J., and Salveson, G. (eds.): Proteinase Inhibitors. Amsterdam, Elsevier Science Publishers B. V., 1986, pp. 403–420.

171. Howell, W. H.: Heparin, an anticoagulant. Am. J. Physiol. 63:434, 1923.

172. Jorpes, E.: Heparin: Its Chemistry, Physiology, and Application in Medicine. London, Oxford University Press, 1939.

173. Brinkhous, K. M., Smith, H. P., Warner, E. D., and Seegers, W. H.: The inhibition of blood clotting: An unidentified substance which acts in conjunction with heparin to prevent

the conversion of prothrombin into thrombin. Am. J. Physiol. 125:683, 1939.

174. Murray, G. D. W.: Heparin in thrombosis and embolism. Br. J. Surg. 27:567, 1939.

175. Abildgaard, U.: Highly purified antithrombin III with heparin cofactor activity prepared by disc electrophoresis. Scand. J. Clin. Lab. Invest. 21:89, 1968.

176. Briginshaw, G. F., and Shanberge, J. N.: Identification of two distinct heparin cofactors in human plasma. Separation and partial purification. Arch. Biochem. Biophys. 161:683, 1974.

177. Tollefsen, D. M., Majerus, D. W., and Blank, M. K.: Heparin cofactor II. Purification and properties of a heparin-dependent inhibitor of thrombin in human plasma. J. Biol. Chem. 257:2162, 1982.

178. Tollefsen, D. M., Pestka, C. A., and Monafo, W. J.: Activation of heparin cofactor II by dermatan sulfate. J. Biol. Chem. 258:6713, 1983.

179. Thaler, E., and Lechner, K.: Antithrombin III deficiency and thromboembolism. Clin. Haematol. 10:369, 1981.

180. Cosgriff, T. M., Bishop, D. T., Hershgold, E. J., Skolnick, M. H., Martin, B. A., Baty, B. J., and Carlson, K. S.: Familial antithrombin III deficiency: Its natural history, genetics, diagnosis and treatment. Medicine (Baltimore) 62:209, 1983.

181. Egeberg, O.: Inherited antithrombin deficiency causing thrombophilia. Thromb. Diath. Haemorrh. 13:516, 1965.

182. Rosenberg, R. D.: Regulation of the hemostatic mechanism. In Stamatoyannopoulos, G., Nienhuis, A. W., Leder, P., and Majerus, P. W. (eds.): The Molecular Basis of Blood Diseases. Philadelphia, W. B. Saunders Company, 1987, pp. 534–574.

183. Petersen, T. E., Dudek-Wojciechowska, G., Sottrup-Jensen, L., and Magnusson, S.: Primary structure of antithrombin-III (heparin cofactor). Partial homology between α1-antitrypsin and antithrombin-III. In Collen, D., Wiman, B., and Verstraete, M. (eds.): The Physiological Inhibitors of Coagulation and Fibrinolysis. Amsterdam, Elsevier/North Holland, 1979, pp. 43–54.

184. Bock, S. C., Wion, K. L., Vehar, G. A., and Lawn, R. M.: Cloning and expression of the cDNA for human antithrombin III. Nucleic Acids Res. 10:8113, 1982.

185. Prochownik, E. V., Markham, A. F., and Orkin, S. H.: Isolation of a cDNA clone for human antithrombin III. J. Biol. Chem. 258:8389, 1983.

186. Stackhouse, R., Chandra, T., Robson, K. J., and Woo, S. L.: Purification of antithrombin III mRNA and cloning of its cDNA. J. Biol. Chem. 258:703, 1983.

187. Sun, X. J., and Chang, J. Y.: Heparin binding domain of human antithrombin III inferred from the sequential reduction of its three disulfide linkages. An efficient method for structural analysis of partially reduced proteins. J. Biol. Chem. 264:11288, 1989.

188. Franzén, L.-E., Svensson, S., and Larm, O.: Structural studies on the carbohydrate portion of human antithrombin III. J. Biol. Chem. 255:5090, 1980.

189. Peterson, C. B., and Blackburn, M. N.: Isolation and characterization of an antithrombin III variant with reduced carbohydrate content and enhanced heparin binding. J. Biol. Chem. 260:610, 1985.

190. Brennan, S. O., George, P. M., and Jordan, R. E.: Physiological variant of antithrombin-III lacks carbohydrate sidechain at Asn 135. FEBS Lett. 219:431, 1987.

191. Kao, F. T., Morse, H. G., Law, M. L., Lidsky, A., Chandra, T., and Woo, S. L.: Genetic mapping of the structural gene for antithrombin III to human chromosome 1. Hum. Genet. 67:34, 1984.

192. Bock, S. C., Harris, J. F., Balazs, I., and Trent, J. M.: Assignment of the human antithrombin III structural gene to chromosome 1q23–25. Cytogenet. Cell Genet. 39:67, 1985.

193. Prochownik, E. V., Bock, S. C., and Orkin, S. H.: Intron structure of the human antithrombin III gene differs from that of other members of the serine protease inhibitor superfamily. J. Biol. Chem. 260:9608, 1985.

194. Jagd, S., Vibe-Pedersen, K., and Magnusson, S.: Location of two of the introns in the antithrombin-III gene. FEBS Lett. 193:213, 1985.

195. Prochownik, E. V., and Orkin, S. H.: In vivo transcription of a human antithrombin III "minigene." J. Biol. Chem. 259:15386, 1984.

196. Bock, S. C., and Levitan, D. J.: Characterization of an unusual DNA length polymorphism 5′ to the human antithrombin III gene. Nucleic Acids Res. 11:8569, 1983.

197. Prochownik, E. V.: Relationship between an enhancer element in the human antithrombin III gene and an immunoglobulin light-chain gene enhancer. Nature 316:845, 1985.

198. Fair, D. S., and Bahnak, B. R.: Human hepatoma cells secrete single chain factor X, prothrombin, and antithrombin III. Blood 64:194, 1984.

199. D'Souza, S. E., and Mercer, J. F.: Antithrombin III mRNA in adult rat liver and kidney and in rat liver during development. Biochem. Biophys. Res. Commun. 142:417, 1987.

200. Hoffman, M., Fuchs, H. E., and Pizzo, S. V.: The macrophage-mediated regulation of hepatocyte synthesis of antithrombin III and alpha 1-proteinase inhibitor. Thromb. Res. 41:707, 1986.

201. Rosenberg, R. D.: Biologic actions of heparin. Semin. Hematol. 14:427, 1977.

202. Highsmith, R. F., and Rosenberg, R. D.: The inhibition of human plasmin by human antithrombin-heparin cofactor. J. Biol. Chem. 249:4335, 1974.

203. Suzuki, K., Nishioka, J., and Hashimoto, S.: Protein C inhibitor: Purification from human plasma and characterization. J. Biol. Chem. 258:163, 1983.

204. Downing, M. R., Bloom, J. W., and Mann, K. G.: Comparison of the inhibition of thrombin by three plasma protease inhibitors. Biochemistry 17:2649, 1978.

205. Fuchs, H. E., Trapp, H. G., Griffith, M. J., Roberts, H. R., and Pizzo, S. V.: Regulation of factor IXa in vitro in human and mouse plasma and in vivo in the mouse. Role of the endothelium and the plasma proteinase inhibitors. J. Clin. Invest. 73:1696, 1984.

206. Gitel, S. N., Medina, V. M., and Wessler, S.: Inhibition of human activated Factor X by antithrombin III and alpha 1-proteinase inhibitor in human plasma. J. Biol. Chem. 259:6890, 1984.

207. Scott, C. F., Schapira, M., James, H. L., Cohen, A. B., and Colman, R. W.: Inactivation of factor XIa by plasma protease inhibitors: Predominant role of alpha 1-protease inhibitor and protective effect of high molecular weight kininogen. J. Clin. Invest. 69:844, 1982.

208. De Agostini, A., Lijnen, H. R., Pixley, R. A., Colman, R. W., and Schapira, M.: Inactivation of factor XII active fragment in normal plasma. Predominant role of C1-inhibitor. J. Clin. Invest. 73:1542, 1984.

209. Wiman, B., and Collen, D.: On the kinetics of the reaction between antiplasmin and plasmin. Eur. J. Biochem. 84:573, 1978.

210. Rosenberg, R. D., and Damus, P. S.: The purification and mechanism of action of human antithrombin-heparin cofactor. J. Biol. Chem. 248:6490, 1973.

211. Fish, W. W., and Björk, I.: Release of a two-chain form of antithrombin from the antithrombin-thrombin complex. Eur. J. Biochem. 101:31, 1979.

212. Björk, I., Jackson, C. M., Jörnvall, H., Lavine, K. K., Nordling, K., and Salsgiver, W. J.: The active site of antithrombin. Release of the same proteolytically cleaved form of the inhibitor from complexes with factor IXa, factor Xa, and thrombin. J. Biol. Chem. 257:2406, 1982.

213. Owen, W. G.: Evidence for the formation of an ester between thrombin and heparin cofactor. Biochim. Biophys. Acta 405:380, 1975.

214. Stein, P. E., Leslie, A. G. W., Finch, J. T., Turnell, W. G., McLaughlin, P. J., and Carrell, R. W.: Crystal structure of ovalbumin as a model for the reactive centre of serpins. Nature 347:99, 1990.

215. Carrell, R. W., and Owen, M. C.: Plakalbumin, α1-antitrypsin, antithrombin and the mechanism of inflammatory thrombosis. Nature 317:730, 1985.

216. Huber, R., and Carrell, R. W.: Implications of the three-dimensional structure of α1-antitrypsin for structure and function of serpins. Biochemistry 28:8951, 1989.

217. Perry, P. J., Harper, P. L., Fairham, S., Daly, M., and Carrell, R. W.: Antithrombin Cambridge, 384 Ala to Pro: A new variant identified using the polymerase chain reaction. FEBS Lett. 254:174, 1989.

218. Jordan, R. E., Oosta, G. M., Gardner, W. T., and Rosenberg, R. D.: The kinetics of hemostatic enzyme-antithrombin interactions in the presence of low molecular weight heparin. J. Biol. Chem. 255:10081, 1980.

219. Höök, M., Björk, I., Hopwood, J., and Lindahl, U.: Anticoagulant activity of heparin: Separation of high-activity and low-activity species by affinity chromatography on immobilized antithrombin. FEBS Lett. 66:90, 1976.

220. Andersson, L.-O., Barrowcliffe, T. W., Holmer, E., Johnson, E. A., and Sims, G. E. C.: Anticoagulant properties of heparin fractionated by affinity chromatography on matrix-bound antithrombin III and by gel filtration. Thromb. Res. 9:575, 1976.

221. Lam, L. H., Silbert, J. E., and Rosenberg, R. D.: The separation of active and inactive forms of heparin. Biochem. Biophys. Res. Commun. 69:570, 1976.

222. Jordan, R., Beeler, D., and Rosenberg, R.: Fractionation of low molecular weight heparin species and their interaction with antithrombin. J. Biol. Chem. 254:2902, 1979.

223. Olson, S. T., Srinivasan, K. R., Björk, I., and Shore, J. D.: Binding of high affinity heparin to antithrombin III. Stopped flow kinetic studies of the binding interaction. J. Biol. Chem. 256:11073, 1981.

224. Pecon, J. M., and Blackburn, M. N.: Pyridoxylation of essential lysines in the heparin-binding site of antithrombin III. J. Biol. Chem. 259:935, 1984.

225. Peterson, C. B., Noyes, C. M., Pecon, J. M., Church, F. C., and Blackburn, M. N.: Identification of a lysyl residue in antithrombin which is essential for heparin binding. J. Biol. Chem. 262:8061, 1987.

226. Blackburn, M. N., Smith, R. L., Carson, J., and Sibley, C. C.: The heparin-binding site of antithrombin III. Identification of a critical tryptophan in the amino acid sequence. J. Biol. Chem. 259:939, 1984.

227. Koide, T., Odani, S., Takahashi, K., Ono, T., and Sakuragawa, N.: Antithrombin III Toyama: Replacement of arginine-47 by cysteine in hereditary abnormal antithrombin III that lacks heparin-binding ability. Proc. Natl. Acad. Sci. USA 81:289, 1984.

228. Owen, M. C., Borg, J. Y., Soria, C., Soria, J., Caen, J., and Carrell, R. W.: Heparin binding defect in a new antithrombin III variant: Rouen, 47 Arg to His. Blood 69:1275, 1987.

229. Chang, J. Y., and Tran, T. H.: Antithrombin III Basel. Identification of a Pro-Leu substitution in a hereditary abnormal antithrombin with impaired heparin cofactor activity. J. Biol. Chem. 261:1174, 1986.

230. Villanueva, G. B.: Predictions of the secondary structure of antithrombin III and the location of the heparin-binding site. J. Biol. Chem. 259:2531, 1984.

231. Lindahl, U., Kusche, M., Lidholt, K., and Oscarsson, L.-G.: Biosynthesis of heparin and heparan sulfate. Ann. N. Y. Acad. Sci. 556:36, 1989.

232. Teien, A. N., Abildgaard, U., and Höök, M.: The anticoagulant effect of heparan sulfate and dermatan sulfate. Thromb. Res. 8:859, 1976.

233. Conrad, H. E.: Structure of heparan sulfate and dermatan sulfate. Ann. N. Y. Acad. Sci. 556:18, 1989.

234. Choay, J., Petitou, M., Lormeau, J. C., Sinay, P., Casu, B., and Gatti, G.: Structure-activity relationship in heparin: A synthetic pentasaccharide with high affinity for antithrombin III and eliciting high anti-factor Xa activity. Biochem. Biophys. Res. Commun. 116:492, 1983.

235. Lindahl, U., Thunberg, L., Bäckström, G., Riesenfeld, J., Nordling, K., and Björk, I.: Extension and structural variability of the antithrombin-binding sequence in heparin. J. Biol. Chem. 259:12368, 1984.

236. Atha, D. H., Lormeau, J. C., Petitou, M., Rosenberg, R. D., and Choay, J.: Contribution of monosaccharide residues in heparin binding to antithrombin III. Biochemistry 24:6723, 1985.

237. Olson, S. T., and Shore, J. D.: Transient kinetics of heparin-catalyzed protease inactivation by antithrombin III. The reaction step limiting heparin turnover in thrombin neutralization. J. Biol. Chem. 261:13151, 1986.

238. Einarsson, R., and Andersson, L.-O.: Binding of heparin to human antithrombin III as studied by measurements of tryptophan fluorescence. Biochim. Biophys. Acta 490:104, 1977.

239. Nordenman, B., and Björk, I.: Binding of low-affinity and high-affinity heparin to antithrombin. Ultraviolet difference spectroscopy and circular dichroism studies. Biochemistry 17:3339, 1978.

240. Olson, S. T., and Shore, J. D.: Binding of high affinity heparin to antithrombin III. Characterization of the protein fluorescence enhancement. J. Biol. Chem. 256:11065, 1981.

241. Stone, A. L., Beeler, D., Oosta, G., and Rosenberg, R. D.: Circular dichroism spectroscopy of heparin-antithrombin interactions. Proc. Natl. Acad. Sci. USA 79:7190, 1982.

242. Oosta, G. M., Gardner, W. T., Beeler, D. L., and Rosenberg, R. D.: Multiple functional domains of the heparin molecule. Proc. Natl. Acad. Sci. USA 78:829, 1981.

243. Pomerantz, M. W., and Owen, W. G.: A catalytic role for heparin. Evidence for a ternary complex of heparin cofactor, thrombin and heparin. Biochim. Biophys. Acta 535:66, 1978.

244. Danielsson, Å., Raub, E., Lindahl, U., and Björk, I.: Role of ternary complexes, in which heparin binds both antithrombin and proteinase, in the acceleration of the reactions between antithrombin and thrombin or factor Xa. J. Biol. Chem. 261:15467, 1986.

245. Griffith, M. J.: The heparin-enhanced antithrombin III/thrombin reaction is saturable with respect to both thrombin and antithrombin III. J. Biol. Chem. 257:13899, 1982.

246. Pletcher, C. H., and Nelsestuen, G. L.: Two-substrate reaction model for the heparin-catalyzed bovine antithrombin/protease reaction. J. Biol. Chem. 258:1086, 1983.

247. Nesheim, M. E.: A simple rate law that describes the kinetics of the heparin-catalyzed reaction between antithrombin III and thrombin. J. Biol. Chem. 258:14708, 1983.

248. Björk, I., and Danielsson, Å.: Antithrombin and related inhibitors of coagulation proteinases. In Barrett, A. J., and Salveson, G. (eds.): Proteinase Inhibitors. Amsterdam, Elsevier Science Publishers B. V., 1986, pp. 489–513.

249. Lane, D. A., Pejler, G., Flynn, A. M., Thompson, E. A., and Lindahl, U.: Neutralization of heparin-related saccharides by histidine-rich glycoprotein and platelet factor 4. J. Biol. Chem. 261:3980, 1986.

250. Preissner, K. T., and Muller-Berghaus, G.: S protein modulates the heparin-catalyzed inhibition of thrombin by antithrombin III. Evidence for a direct interaction of S protein with heparin. Eur. J. Biochem. 156:645, 1986.

251. Lollar, P., and Owen, W. G.: Clearance of thrombin from the circulation in rabbits by high-affinity binding sites on the endothelium. Possible role in the inactivation of thrombin by antithrombin III. J. Clin. Invest. 66:1222, 1980.

252. Maruyama, I., and Majerus, P. W.: The turnover of thrombin-thrombomodulin complex in cultured human umbilical vein endothelial cells and A549 lung cancer cells. Endocytosis and degradation of thrombin. J. Biol. Chem. 260:15432, 1985.

253. Fuchs, H. E., and Pizzo, S. V.: Regulation of factor Xa in vitro in human and mouse plasma and in vivo in mouse. Role of the endothelium and plasma proteinase inhibitors. J. Clin. Invest. 72:2041, 1983.

254. Miletich, J. P., Jackson, C. M., and Majerus, P. W.: Properties of the factor Xa binding site on human platelets. J. Biol. Chem. 253:6908, 1978.

255. Lindhout, T., Baruch, D., Schoen, P., Franssen, J., and Hemker, H. C.: Thrombin generation and inactivation in the presence of antithrombin III and heparin. Biochemistry 25:5962, 1986.

256. Shifman, M. A., and Pizzo, S. V.: The in vivo metabolism of antithrombin III and antithrombin III complexes. J. Biol. Chem. 257:3243, 1982.

257. Fuchs, H. E., Michalopoulos, G. K., and Pizzo, S. V.: Hepatocyte uptake of alpha 1-proteinase inhibitor–trypsin complexes in vitro: Evidence for a shared uptake mechanism for proteinase complexes of alpha 1-proteinase inhibitor and antithrombin III. J. Cell. Biochem. 25:231, 1984.

258. Fuchs, H. E., Shifman, M. A., Michalopoulos, G., and Pizzo, S. V.: Hepatocyte receptors for antithrombin III–proteinase complexes. J. Cell. Biochem. 24:197, 1984.

259. Perlmutter, D. H., Glover, G. I., Rivetna, M., Schasteen, C. S., and Fallon, R. J.: Identification of a serpin-enzyme complex receptor on human hepatoma cells and human monocytes. Proc. Natl. Acad. Sci. USA 87:3753, 1990.

260. Perlmutter, D. H., Joslin, G., Nelson, P., Schasteen, C., Adams, S. P., and Fallon, R. J.: Endocytosis and degradation of alpha 1-antitrypsin-protease complexes is mediated by the serpin-enzyme complex (SEC) receptor. J. Biol. Chem. 265:16713, 1990.

261. Joslin, G., Fallon, R. J., Bullock, J., Adams, S. P., and Perlmutter, D. H.: The SEC receptor recognizes a pentapeptide neodomain of alpha 1-antitrypsin–protease complexes. J. Biol. Chem. 266:11282, 1991.

262. Carlson, T. H., Simon, T. L., and Atencio, A. C.: In vivo behavior of human radioiodinated antithrombin III: Distribution among three physiologic pools. Blood 66:13, 1985.

263. Nenci, G. G., Berrettini, M., Parise, P., and Agnelli, G.: Persistent spontaneous heparinaemia in systemic mastocytosis. Folia Haematol. (Leipz.) 109:453, 1982.

264. Khoory, M. S., Nesheim, M. E., Bowie, E. J. W., and Mann, K. G.: Circulating heparan sulfate proteoglycan anticoagulant from a patient with a plasma cell disorder. J. Clin. Invest. 65:666, 1980.

265. Bussel, J. B., Steinherz, P. G., Miller, D. R., and Hilgartner, M. W.: A heparin-like anticoagulant in an 8-month-old boy with acute monoblastic leukemia. Am. J. Hematol. 16:83, 1984.

266. Palmer, R. N., Rick, M. E., Rick, P. D., Zeller, J. A., and Gralnick, H. R.: Circulating heparan sulfate anticoagulant in a patient with a fatal bleeding disorder. N. Engl. J. Med. 310:1696, 1984.

267. Marcum, J. A., and Rosenberg, R. D.: Heparin-like molecules with anticoagulant activity are synthesized by cultured endothelial cells. Biochem. Biophys. Res. Commun. 126:365, 1985.

268. Marcum, J. A., Atha, D. H., Fritze, L. M., Nawroth, P., Stern, D., and Rosenberg, R. D.: Cloned bovine aortic endothelial cells synthesize anticoagulantly active heparan sulfate proteoglycan. J. Biol. Chem. 261:7507, 1986.

269. Stern, D., Nawroth, P., Marcum, J., Handley, D., Kisiel, W., Rosenberg, R., and Stern, K.: Interaction of antithrombin III with bovine aortic segments. Role of heparin in binding and enhanced anticoagulant activity. J. Clin. Invest. 75:272, 1985.

270. Hatton, M. W., Moar, S. L., and Richardson, M.: On the interaction of rabbit antithrombin III with the luminal surface of the normal and deendothelialized rabbit thoracic aorta in vitro. Blood 67:878, 1986.

271. De Agostini, A. I., Watkins, S. C., Slayter, H. S., Youssoufian, H., and Rosenberg, R. D.: Localization of anticoagulantly active heparan sulfate proteoglycans in vascular endothelium: Antithrombin binding on cultured endothelial cells and perfused rat aorta. J. Cell Biol. 111:1293, 1990.

272. Marcum, J. A., McKenney, J. B., and Rosenberg, R. D.: Acceleration of thrombin-antithrombin complex formation in rat hindquarters via heparinlike molecules bound to the endothelium. J. Clin. Invest. 74:341, 1984.

273. Jakubowski, H. V., Kline, M. D., and Owen, W. G.: The effect of bovine thrombomodulin on the specificity of bovine thrombin. J. Biol. Chem. 261:3876, 1986.

274. Conard, J., Brosstad, F., Lie-Larsen, M., Samama, M., and Abildgaard, U.: Molar antithrombin concentration in normal human plasma. Haemostasis 13:363, 1983.

275. Andrew, M., Paes, B., Milner, R., Johnston, M., Mitchell, L., Tollefsen, D. M., and Powers, P.: Development of the human coagulation system in the full-term infant. Blood 70:165, 1987.

276. Marciniak, K., Farley, C. H., and DeSimone, P. A.: Familial thrombosis due to antithrombin III deficiency. Blood 43:219, 1974.

277. Prochownik, E. V., Antonarakis, S., Bauer, K. A., Rosenberg, R. D., Fearon, E. R., and Orkin, S. H.: Molecular heterogeneity of inherited antithrombin III deficiency. N. Engl. J. Med. 308:1549, 1983.

278. Bock, S. C., Harris, J. F., Schwartz, C. E., Ward, J. H., Hershgold, E. J., and Skolnick, M. H.: Hereditary thrombosis in a Utah kindred is caused by a dysfunctional antithrombin III gene. Am. J. Hum. Genet. 37:32, 1985.

279. Ambruso, D. R., Leonard, B. D., Bies, R. D., Jacobson, L., Hathaway, W. E., and Reeve, E. B.: Antithrombin III deficiency: Decreased synthesis of a biochemically normal molecule. Blood 60:78, 1982.

280. Knot, E. A., de Jong, E., ten Cate, J. W., Iburg, A. H., Henny, C. P., Bruin, T., and Stibbe, J.: Purified radiolabeled antithrombin III metabolism in three families with hereditary AT III deficiency: Application of a three-compartment model. Blood 67:93, 1986.

281. Olds, R. J., Lane, D. A., Ireland, H., Leone, G., De Stefano, V., Cazenave, J. P., Wiesel, M. L., and Thein, S. L.: Novel point mutations leading to type Ia antithrombin deficiency and thrombosis. Br. J. Haematol. 78:408, 1991.

282. Olds, R. J., Lane, D. A., Finazzi, G., Barbui, T., and Thein, S. L.: A frameshift mutation leading to type 1 antithrombin deficiency and thrombosis. Blood 76:2182, 1990.

283. Gandrille, S., Vidaud, D., Emmerich, J., Clauser, E., Sié, P., Fiessinger, J. N., Alhenc-Gelas, M., Priollet, P., and Aiach, M.: Molecular basis for hereditary antithrombin III quantitative deficiencies: A stop codon in exon IIIa and a frameshift in exon VI. Br. J. Haematol. 78:414, 1991.

283a. Vidaud, D., Emmerich, J., Sirieix, M. E., Sié, P., Alhenc-Gelas, M., and Aiach, M.: Molecular basis for antithrombin III type I deficiency: Three novel mutations located in exon IV. Blood 78:2305, 1991.

284. Vidaud, D., Gandrille, S., Emmerich, J., Sirieix, M. E., Alhenc-Gelas, M., Fiessinger, J. N., Sié, P., Gouault-Heilman, M., and Aiach, M.: Identifications of 6 novel mutations responsible for type I AT III deficiencies (abstract). Thromb. Haemost. 65:991, 1991.

285. Olds, R. J., Thein, S. L., Ireland, H., Lane, D. A., Boisclair, M., Conard, J., and Horellou, M. H.: Identification of 402 phenylalanine as a functionally important residue in antithrombin (abstract). Thromb. Haemost. 65:670, 1991.

286. Bock, S. C., Silberman, J. A., Wikoff, W., Abildgaard, U., and Hultin, M. B.: Identification of a threonine for alanine substitution at residue 404 of antithrombin III Oslo suggests integrity of the 404–407 region is important for maintaining normal inhibitor levels (abstract). Thromb. Haemost. 62:494, 1989.

287. Nakagawa, M., Tanaka, S., Tsuji, H., Takada, O., Uno, M., Hashimoto-Gotoh, T., and Wagatsuma, M.: Congenital antithrombin III deficiency (At-III Kyoto): Identification of a point mutation altering arginine-406 to methionine behind the reactive site. Thromb. Res. 64:101, 1989.

288. Bock, S. C., Marrinan, J. A., and Radziejewska, E.: Antithrombin III Utah: Proline 407 to leucine mutation in a highly conserved region near the inhibitor reactive site. Biochemistry 27:6171, 1988.

289. Vidaud, D., Sirieix, M. E., Alhenc-Gelas, M., Chadeuf, G., Aillaud, M. F., Juhan-Vague, I., and Aiach, M.: A double heterozygosity in 2 brothers with antithrombin (ATIII) deficiency due to the association of an Arg 47 to His mutation with a 9 base pair (bp) deletion in exon VI (abstract). Thromb. Haemost. 65:838, 1991.

290. Devraj-Kizuk, R., Chui, D. H. K., Prochownik, E. V., Carter, C. J., Ofosu, F. A., and Blajchman, M. A.: Antithrombin III Hamilton: A gene with a point mutation (guanine to aden-

ine) in codon 382 causing impaired serine protease reactivity. Blood 72:1518, 1988.

291. Ireland, H., Lane, D. A., Thompson, E., Walker, I. D., Blench, I., Morris, H. R., Freyssinet, J. M., Grunebaum, L., Olds, R., and Thein, S. L.: Antithrombin Glasgow II: Alanine 382 to threonine mutation in the serpin P12 position, resulting in a substrate reaction with thrombin. Br. J. Haematol. 79:70, 1991.

292. Mohlo-Sabatier, P., Aiach, M., Gaillard, I., Fiessinger, J. N., Fischer, A. M., Chadeuf, G., and Clauser, E.: Molecular characterization of antithrombin III (ATIII) variants using polymerase chain reaction. Identification of the ATIII Charleville as an Ala384 Pro mutation. J. Clin. Invest. 84:1236, 1989.

293. Caso, R., Lane, D. A., Thompson, E. A., Olds, R. J., Thein, S. L., Panico, M., Blench, I., Morris, H., Freyssinet, J. M., Aiach, M., Rodeghiero, F., and Finazzi, G.: Antithrombin Vicenza, Ala 384 to Pro (GCA to CCA) mutation transforming the inhibitor into a substrate. Br. J. Haematol. 77:87, 1990.

293a. Perry, D. J., Daly, M., Harper, P. L., Tait, R. C., Price, J., Walker, I. D., and Carrell, R. W.: Antithrombin Cambridge II, 384 Ala to Ser. Further evidence of the role of the reactive centre loop in the inhibitory function of the serpins. FEBS Lett. 285:248, 1991.

294. Blajchman, M. A., Fernandez-Rachubinski, F., Sheffield, W. P., Austin, R. C., and Schulman, S.: Antithrombin-III-Stockholm: A codon 392 (Gly → Asp) mutation with normal heparin binding and impaired serine protease reactivity. Blood 79:1428, 1992.

295. Erdjument, H., Lane, D. A., Ireland, H., Panico, M., DiMarzo, V., Blench, I., and Morris, H. R.: Formation of a covalent disulfide-linked antithrombin complex by an antithrombin variant, antithrombin Northwick Park. J. Biol. Chem. 262:13381, 1987.

296. Erdjument, H., Lane, D. A., Panico, M., DiMarzo, V., and Morris, H. R.: Single amino acid substitutions in the reactive site of antithrombin leading to thrombosis. Congenital substitution of arginine 393 to cysteine in antithrombin Northwick Park and to histidine in antithrombin Glasgow. J. Biol. Chem. 263:5589, 1988.

297. Lane, D. A., Erdjument, H., Thompson, E., Panico, M., DiMarzo, V., Morris, H. R., Leone, G., De Stefano, V., and Thein, S. L.: A novel amino acid substitution in the reactive site of a congenital variant antithrombin: Antithrombin Pescara, Arg 393 to Pro, caused by CGT to CCT mutation. J. Biol. Chem. 264:10200, 1989.

298. Owen, M. C., George, P. M., Lane, D. A., and Boswell, D. R.: P1 variant antithrombins Glasgow (393 Arg to His) and Pescara (393 Arg to Pro) have increased heparin affinity and are resistant to catalytic cleavage by elastase. Implications for the heparin activation mechanism. FEBS Lett. 280:216, 1991.

299. Stephens, A. W., Thalley, B. S., and Hirs, C. H. W.: Antithrombin-III Denver, a reactive site variant. J. Biol. Chem. 262:1044, 1987.

299a. Olds, R. J., Lane, D. A., Caso, R., Panico, M., Morris, H. R., Sas, G., Dawes, J., and Thein, S. L.: Antithrombin III Budapest: A single amino acid substitution (429 Pro to Leu) in a region highly conserved in the serpin family. Blood 79:1206, 1992.

300. Brennan, S. O., Borg, J. Y., George, P. M., Soria, C., Soria, J., Caen, J., and Carrell, R. W.: New carbohydrate site in mutant antithrombin (7 Ile–Asn) with decreased heparin affinity. FEBS Lett. 237:118, 1988.

301. Borg, J. Y., Brennan, S. O., Carrell, R. W., George, P., Perry, D. J., and Shaw, J.: Antithrombin Rouen IV 24 Arg to Cys. The amino terminal contribution to heparin binding. FEBS Lett. 266:163, 1990.

302. Borg, J. Y., Owen, M. C., Soria, C., Soria, J., Caen, J., and Carrell, R. W.: Arginine 47 is a prime heparin binding site in antithrombin. A new variant Rouen II, 47 Arg to Ser. J. Clin. Invest. 81:1292, 1988.

303. Gandrille, S., Aiach, M., Lane, D. A., Vidaud, D., Mohlo-

Sabatier, P., Caso, R., de Moerloose, P., Fiessinger, J. N., and Clauser, E.: Important role of Arg 129 in heparin binding site of antithrombin III: Identification of novel mutation Arg 129 to Gln. J. Biol. Chem. 265:18997, 1990.

304. Lane, D. A., Ireland, H., Olds, R. J., Thein, S. L., Perry, D. J., and Aiach, M.: Antithrombin III: A database of mutations. Thromb. Haemost. 66:657, 1991.

305. Fischer, A. M., Cornu, P., Sternberg, C., Meriane, F., Dautzenberg, M. D., Chafa, O., Beguin, S., and Desnos, M.: Antithrombin III Alger: A new homozygous AT III variant. Thromb. Haemost. 55:218, 1986.

306. Boyer, C., Wolf, M., Vedrenne, J., Meyer, D., and Larrieu, M. J.: Homozygous variant of antithrombin III: AT III Fontainebleau. Thromb. Haemost. 56:18, 1986.

307. Ødegård, O. R., and Abildgaard, U.: Antithrombin III: Critical review of assay methods. Significance of variations in health and disease. Haemostasis 7:127, 1978.

308. Rosenberg, R. D.: Actions and interactions of antithrombin and heparin. N. Engl. J. Med. 292:146, 1975.

309. Tait, R. C., Walker, I. D., Perry, D. J., Carrell, R. W., Islam, S. I. A., McCall, F., Mitchell, R., and Davidson, J. F.: Prevalence of antithrombin III deficiency subtypes in 4000 healthy blood donors (abstract). Thromb. Haemost. 65:839, 1991.

310. Vikydal, R., Korninger, C., Kyrle, P. A., Niessner, H., Pabinger, I., Thaler, E., and Lechner, K.: The prevalence of hereditary antithrombin-III deficiency in patients with a history of venous thromboembolism. Thromb. Haemost. 54:744, 1985.

311. Gruenberg, J. C., Smallridge, R. C., and Rosenberg, R. D.: Inherited antithrombin III deficiency causing mesenteric venous infarcton: A new clinical entity. Ann. Surg. 181:791, 1975.

312. Das, M., and Carroll, S. F.: Antithrombin III deficiency: An etiology of Budd-Chiari syndrome. Surgery 97:242, 1985.

313. Girolami, A., Fabris, F., Cappellato, G., Sainati, L., and Boeri, G.: Antithrombin III (AT III) Padua 2: A "new" congenital abnormality with defective heparin co-factor activities but no thrombotic disease. Blut 47:93, 1983.

314. Chasse, J. F., Esnard, F., Guitton, J. D., Mouray, H., Perigois, F., Fauconneau, G., and Gauthier, F.: An abnormal plasma antithrombin with no apparent affinity for heparin. Thromb. Res. 34:297, 1984.

315. Knot, E., ten Cate, J. W., Drijfhout, H. R., Kahle, L. H., and Tytgat, G. N.: Antithrombin III metabolism in patients with liver disease. J. Clin. Pathol. 37:523, 1984.

316. Kauffmann, R. H., Veltkamp, J. J., van Tilburg, N. H., and van Es, L. A.: Acquired antithrombin III deficiency and thrombosis in the nephrotic syndrome. Am. J. Med. 65:607, 1978.

317. Spero, J. A., Lewis, J. H., and Hasiba, U.: Disseminated intravascular coagulation. Findings in 346 patients. Thromb. Haemost. 43:28, 1980.

318. Fagerhol, M. K., Abildgaard, U., Bergsjø, P., and Jacobsen, J. H.: Oral contraceptives and low antithrombin III concentration. Lancet 1:1175, 1970.

319. Conard, J., Cazenave, B., Maury, J., Horellou, M. H., and Samama, M.: L-Asparaginase, antithrombin III, and thrombosis. Lancet 1:1091, 1980.

320. Bauer, K. A., Teitel, J. M., and Rosenberg, R. D.: L-Asparaginase induced antithrombin III deficiency: Evidence against the production of a hypercoagulable state. Thromb. Res. 29:437, 1983.

321. Ragg, H., and Preibisch, G.: Structure and expression of the gene coding for the human serpin hLS2. J. Biol. Chem. 263:12129, 1988.

322. Herzog, R., Lutz, S., Blin, N., Marasa, J. C., Blinder, M. A., and Tollefsen, D. M.: Complete nucleotide sequence of the gene for human heparin cofactor II and mapping to chromosomal band 22q11. Biochemistry 30:1350, 1991.

323. Ragg, H.: A new member of the plasma protease inhibitor gene family. Nucleic Acids Res. 14:1073, 1986.

324. Jaffe, E. A., Armellino, D., and Tollefsen, D. M.: Biosynthesis of functionally active heparin cofactor II by a human hep-

atoma-derived cell line. Biochem. Biophys. Res. Commun. 132:368, 1985.

325. Hortin, G., Tollefsen, D. M., and Strauss, A. W.: Identification of two sites of sulfation of human heparin cofactor II. J. Biol. Chem. 261:15827, 1986.

326. Blinder, M. A., Marasa, J. C., Reynolds, C. H., Deaven, L. L., and Tollefsen, D. M.: Heparin cofactor II: cDNA sequence, chromosome localization, restriction fragment length polymorphism, and expression in *Escherichia coli*. Biochemistry 27:752, 1988.

327. Church, F. C., Meade, J. B., and Pratt, C. W.: Structure-function relationships in heparin cofactor II: Spectral analysis of aromatic residues and absence of a role for sulfhydryl groups in thrombin inhibition. Arch. Biochem. Biophys. 259:331, 1987.

328. Griffith, M. J., Noyes, C. M., Tyndall, J. A., and Church, F. C.: Structural evidence for leucine at the reactive site of heparin cofactor II. Biochemistry 24:6777, 1985.

329. Church, F. C., Noyes, C. M., and Griffith, M. J.: Inhibition of chymotrypsin by heparin cofactor II. Proc. Natl. Acad. Sci. USA 82:6431, 1985.

330. Parker, K. A., and Tollefsen, D. M.: The protease specificity of heparin cofactor II. Inhibition of thrombin generated during coagulation. J. Biol. Chem. 260:3501, 1985.

331. Derechin, V. M., Blinder, M. A., and Tollefsen, D. M.: Substitution of arginine for Leu 444 in the reactive site of heparin cofactor II enhances the rate of thrombin inhibition. J. Biol. Chem. 265:5623, 1990.

332. Hurst, R. E., Poon, M.-C., and Griffith, M. J.: Structure-activity relationships of heparin. Independence of heparin charge density and antithrombin-binding domains in thrombin inhibition by antithrombin and heparin cofactor II. J. Clin. Invest. 72:1042, 1983.

333. Maimone, M. M., and Tollefsen, D. M.: Activation of heparin cofactor II by heparin oligosaccharides. Biochem. Biophys. Res. Commun. 152:1056, 1988.

334. Maimone, M. M., and Tollefsen, D. M.: Structure of a dermatan sulfate hexasaccharide that binds to heparin cofactor II with high affinity. J. Biol. Chem. 265:18263, 1990.

335. Fernandez, F., van Ryn, J., Ofosu, F. A., Hirsh, J., and Buchanan, M. R.: The haemorrhagic and antithrombotic effects of dermatan sulfate. Br. J. Haematol. 64:309, 1986.

336. Ofosu, F. A., Modi, G. J., Smith, L. M., Cerskus, A. L., Hirsh, J., and Blajchman, M. A.: Heparan sulfate and dermatan sulfate inhibit the generation of thrombin activity in plasma by complementary pathways. Blood 64:742, 1984.

337. Blinder, M. A., Andersson, T. R., Abildgaard, U., and Tollefsen, D. M.: Heparin cofactor II Oslo. Mutation of Arg-189 to His decreases the affinity for dermatan sulfate. J. Biol. Chem. 264:5128, 1989.

338. Blinder, M. A., and Tollefsen, D. M.: Site-directed mutagenesis of arginine 103 and lysine 185 in the proposed glycosaminoglycan-binding site of heparin cofactor II. J. Biol. Chem. 265:286, 1990.

339. Whinna, H. C., Blinder, M. A., Szewczyk, M., Tollefsen, D. M., and Church, F. C.: Role of lysine 173 in heparin binding to heparin cofactor II. J. Biol. Chem. 266:8129, 1991.

340. Ragg, H., Ulshöfer, T., and Gerewitz, J.: On the activation of human leuserpin-2, a thrombin inhibitor, by glycosaminoglycans. J. Biol. Chem. 265:5211, 1990.

341. Ragg, H., Ulshöfer, T., and Gerewitz, J.: Glycosaminoglycan-mediated leuserpin-2/thrombin interaction. Structure-function relationships. J. Biol. Chem. 265:22386, 1990.

342. Van Deerlin, V. M. D., and Tollefsen, D. M.: The N-terminal acidic domain of heparin cofactor II mediates the inhibition of α-thrombin in the presence of glycosaminoglycans. J. Biol. Chem. 266:20223, 1991.

343. Grutter, M. G., Priestle, J. P., Rahuel, J., Grossenbacher, H., Bode, W., Hofsteenge, J., and Stone, S. R.: Crystal structure of the thrombin-hirudin complex: A novel mode of serine protease inhibition. EMBO J. 9:2361, 1990.

344. Rydel, T. J., Ravichandran, K. G., Tulinsky, A., Bode, W., Huber, R., Roitsch, C., and Fenton, J. W. II: The structure of a complex of recombinant hirudin and human α-thrombin. Science 249:277, 1990.

345. Hortin, G. L., Tollefsen, D. M., and Benutto, B. M.: Antithrombin activity of a peptide corresponding to residues 54–75 of heparin cofactor II. J. Biol. Chem. 264:13979, 1989.

346. Tollefsen, D. M., and Pestka, C. A.: Heparin cofactor II activity in patients with disseminated intravascular coagulation and hepatic failure. Blood 66:769, 1985.

347. Sié, P., Dupouy, D., Pichon, J., and Boneu, B.: Constitutional heparin co-factor II deficiency associated with recurrent thrombosis. Lancet 2:414, 1985.

348. Tran, T. H., Marbet, G. A., and Duckert, F.: Association of hereditary heparin co-factor II deficiency with thrombosis. Lancet 2:413, 1985.

349. Andersson, T. R., Larsen, M. L., Handeland, G. F., and Abildgaard, U.: Heparin cofactor II activity in plasma: Application of an automated assay method to the study of a normal adult population. Scand. J. Haematol. 36:96, 1986.

350. Tran, T. H., and Duckert, F.: Heparin cofactor II determination—levels in normals and patients with hereditary antithrombin III deficiency and disseminated intravascular coagulation. Thromb. Haemost. 52:112, 1984.

351. Abildgaard, U., and Larsen, M. L.: Assay of dermatan sulfate cofactor (heparin cofactor II) activity in human plasma. Thromb. Res. 35:257, 1984.

352. Ezenagu, L. C., and Brandt, J. T.: Laboratory determination of heparin cofactor II. Arch. Pathol. Lab. Med. 110:1149, 1986.

353. Massouh, M., Jatoi, A., Gordon, E. M., and Ratnoff, O. D.: Heparin cofactor II activity in plasma during pregnancy and oral contraceptive use. J. Lab. Clin. Med. 114:697, 1989.

354. Griffith, M. J., Carraway, T., White, G. C., and Dombrose, F. A.: Heparin cofactor activities in a family with hereditary antithrombin III deficiency: Evidence for a second heparin cofactor in human plasma. Blood 61:111, 1983.

355. McGuire, E. A., and Tollefsen, D. M.: Activation of heparin cofactor II by fibroblasts and vascular smooth muscle cells. J. Biol. Chem. 262:169, 1987.

356. Andrew, M., Mitchell, L., Berry, L., Paes, B., Delorme, M., Ofosu, F., Burrows, R., and Khambalia, B.: An anticoagulant dermatan sulfate proteoglycan circulates in the pregnant woman and her fetus. J. Clin. Invest. 89:321, 1992.

357. Brennan, M. J., Oldberg, A., Pierschbacher, M. D., and Ruoslahti, E.: Chondroitin/dermatan sulfate proteoglycan in human fetal membranes: Demonstration of an antigenically similar proteoglycan in fibroblasts. J. Biol. Chem. 259:13742, 1984.

358. Loebermann, H., Tokuoka, R., Deisenhofer, J., and Huber, R.: Human α1-proteinase inhibitor. Crystal structure analysis of two crystal modifications, molecular model and preliminary analysis of the implications for function. J. Mol. Biol. 177:531, 1984.

Hemophilia A, Hemophilia B, and von Willebrand Disease

J. Evan Sadler and Earl W. Davie

INTRODUCTION

Most of our knowledge of the mechanism of hereditary bleeding disorders has been acquired only recently. What we know as hemophilia A apparently was recognized more than 1700 years ago, as documented in the Talmud,[1] and the genetics of the disease was described in detail by 1800.[2] However, the first correct description of the role of antihemophilic factor (factor VIII) in hemostasis was not published until 1937,[3] and the resolution of hemophilia into two distinct disorders, hemophilia A (factor VIII deficiency) and hemophilia B (factor IX deficiency), did not occur until 1952.[4, 5] The relationship between hereditary factor VIII deficiency and von Willebrand disease once was controversial because a deficiency of von Willebrand factor, which is autosomally inherited, is usually associated with some degree of factor VIII deficiency. Furthermore, factor VIII and von Willebrand factor tend to copurify. Classic hemophilia A, however, is an X chromosome–linked disease. Consequently, for almost three decades the term "factor VIII" (with varying suffixes) has been used to designate the protein that is defective in both hemophilia A and von Willebrand disease, depending on the context.

In this chapter, *factor VIII* refers to the protein, specified by an X chromosome–linked gene, that is defective in hemophilia A and accelerates the activation of factor X by factor IXa in the presence of calcium ions and phospholipid. Similarly, *von Willebrand factor* (vWF) refers to the protein, specified by an autosomal gene, that is defective in von Willebrand disease (vWD) and participates in normal platelet function as measured by the bleeding time. The complex of these proteins that occurs in vivo is referred to as the *factor VIII/vWF complex.*

FACTOR VIII AND HEMOPHILIA A

Purification and Structural Characterization of Factor VIII

Assays for Factor VIII

Antihemophilic factor (factor VIII) was first assayed as an activity that corrects the clotting defect in hemophilic plasma.[3] Assays based on this principle are still widely used. Factor VIII has no intrinsic enzyme activity but acts as a cofactor in a multicomponent reaction; furthermore, thrombin converts the cofactor to a much more active form that subsequently decays into an inactive form. The complex kinetics of activation and inactivation can make the measurement of factor VIII cofactor activity dependent on specific assay conditions. *One unit* of factor VIII is that amount of activity in 1 ml of pooled normal plasma, measured as shortening of the clotting time of hemophilia A plasma.[6]

When greater precision is necessary, a method based on the specific cofactor activity of factor VIII in a purified system can be employed: Factor VIII is activated by thrombin, and its cofactor activity for the activation of factor X is measured in the presence of factor IXa, phospholipid, and calcium ions. The resultant factor Xa activity in such assays can be determined by a plasma clotting assay,[7] by measuring the cleavage of a chromogenic peptide substrate for factor Xa (S-2222),[8] or by direct measurement of the factor IXa–mediated release of radiolabeled activation peptide from factor X.[9] The characteristics of these reactions are discussed in detail under Biological Function of Factor VIII (page 660).

Factor VIII protein can be measured by immunological methods. By several related assay methods, as little as 1 per cent of normal factor VIII antigen levels can be detected.[10–12]

Purification of Factor VIII

In blood, factor VIII is bound non-covalently to vWF. The plasma concentration of factor VIII is 100 to 200 ng/ml, or ~0.7 nM, assuming an average M_r of 280,000. This corresponds to ~2 per cent of the mass of circulating vWF. The vWF moiety of the factor VIII/vWF complex has many unusual physical properties, including large size and a tendency to polymerize, and in plasma it has molecular weights ranging from 500,000 to more than 10,000,000. By exploiting these peculiarities of vWF, human factor VIII can be extensively purified 7,000- to 10,000-fold as part of the factor VIII/vWF complex.[13, 14]

Further purification of factor VIII has been achieved after dissociation of the factor VIII/vWF complex in solutions of high ionic strength, such as ~1 M NaCl[15] or ~0.25 to 0.5 M CaCl$_2$.[16] Once dissociated, factor VIII can be resolved from vWF by a variety of chromatographic methods. The highest specific activities obtained for purified factor VIII are in the range of 2300 to 6000 U/mg for the human,[17, 18] bovine,[19] and porcine proteins.[20, 21] These values, however, may not correspond precisely to the specific activity of intact factor VIII, because factor VIII preparations often are a mixture of inactive precursor and activated and inactivated proteins.

Structure of Factor VIII

Factor VIII is derived from a primary translation product of 2351 amino acids.[22–25] After removal of a signal peptide of 19 amino acids, single-chain factor VIII consists of 2332 amino acids and has an M_r of 264,763. The protein also contains a total of 25 potential asparagine-linked carbohydrate-binding sites (Fig. 19–1). If all these Asn residues were glycosylated, the M_r for the glycoprotein would be ~330,000 (±20,000).

Factor VIII contains two types of repeated homologous domains (see Fig. 19–1). One (A domain) occurs twice in the amino-terminal region of the molecule (residues 1 to 329 and 380 to 711) and once in the carboxyl-terminal region of the molecule (residues 1649 to 2019). The second and third A domains are separated by a large 980 amino acid connecting peptide (B domain). The other repeated domain (C domain) occurs in tandem repeats of ~150 amino acids in the carboxyl-terminal region of the molecule. The A domains are ~30 per cent identical in amino acid sequence, whereas the C domains are ~40 per cent identical.[22, 23]

The A domains of factor VIII are also ~30 per cent identical to each of three similar domains of ceruloplasmin, a copper-binding protein in plasma.[26] The C domains of factor VIII are ~20 per cent identical to the first 150 amino acids of discoidin I, a galactose-

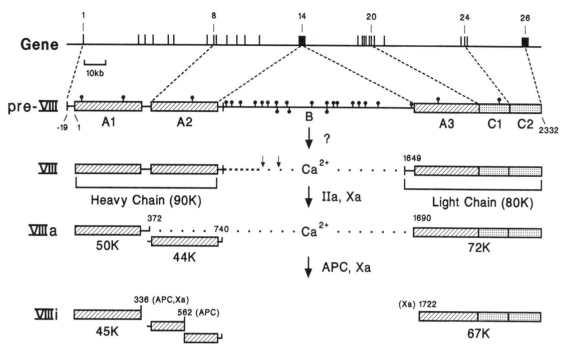

FIGURE 19–1. Structure of human factor VIII gene and protein. *Gene:* The region of the X chromosome containing the factor VIII gene is represented. Selected exons are numbered, and the scale in kilobases of DNA is shown. The relationship between segments of the gene and repeated domains of the protein is indicated by the dashed lines connecting the gene to pre-VIII. *Pre-VIII:* The primary translation product consists of a signal peptide (amino acid residues − 19 to 1) and single-chain precursor (amino acid residues 1 to 2332). Sites of *N*-linked glycosylation are indicated by ●, and structural domains of the protein are labeled. *VIII:* Factor VIII in plasma consists of one heavy chain and one light chain, stabilized by calcium ions. Unknown proteases (?) are responsible for generating the amino-terminus of the light chain and the carboxyl-terminal heterogeneity of the heavy chain. *VIIIa:* Thrombin (IIa) or factor Xa (Xa) can activate factor VIII by cleaving at the indicated amino acid residues. *VIIIi:* Activated protein C (APC) or factor Xa (Xa) can cleave and inactivate factor VIIIa at the sites indicated.

binding and phospholipid-binding protein of slime mold.[27] The C domains of factor VIII are also ~54 per cent identical in sequence to an ~300 amino acid segment of a mouse mammary epithelial surface protein that contains two tandemly repeated C-like domains.[28] Whether the C domains of factor VIII are responsible for binding to phospholipid or cell surfaces is not known.

Factor VIII is also homologous to factor V.[29–31] Both proteins share a similar organization into domains (A1-A2-B-A3-C1-C2), and corresponding A and C domains of factor VIII and factor V are ~40 per cent identical in amino acid sequence. In contrast, the connecting regions (B domains) show no significant sequence similarity. The evolutionary and structural similarities of factor V and factor VIII are reflected in their biological functions, which involve similar mechanisms as cofactors.

Although factor VIII is synthesized as a single polypeptide chain, almost all of the factor VIII in plasma is a heterodimer. During biosynthesis or in the circulation, factor VIII is cleaved after Arg 1648 to generate the amino-terminus of the M_r ~80,000 *light chain*. Additional cleavages within the connecting peptide region generate several species of *heavy chain* with an M_r of 90,000 to 210,000.[17, 18, 22, 23, 32, 33] The proteases

responsible for these reactions have not been identified, although thrombin can cleave after Arg 740 to give the smallest heavy chain fragment with an M_r of 90,000.[22] The subunits of factor VIII are not joined by disulfide bonds. Similar patterns have been described for bovine[19] and porcine[20, 21] factor VIII.

Both the heavy and light chains of human factor VIII contain *N*-linked[18, 19, 34] and *O*-linked[35] carbohydrate chains. The *N*-linked oligosaccharides on the heavy chain appear to be mainly of the hybrid or complex type, whereas some oligosaccharides on the light chain are of the high-mannose type.[35] Like two-chain factor Va,[36] the polypeptides of factor VIII are dissociated by high concentrations of ethylenediaminetetra-acetic acid (EDTA), with loss of procoagulant activity,[21] suggesting that metal ions are required for structural integrity.

Human factor VIII contains at least seven tyrosines associated with short acidic sequences that meet criteria for potential sites of tyrosine sulfation. The presence of tyrosine sulfate has been confirmed at Tyr 346[37]; at one or more of Tyr 718, Tyr 719, and Tyr 723[37, 38]; and at both Tyr 1664 and Tyr 1680.[37–39]

The structure and topography of factor VIII have been studied by ultracentrifugation, fluorescence energy transfer, and electron microscopy. Factor VIII is a very asymmetrical particle with M_r of 250,000 or 285,000.[40, 41] The A2 domain of the heavy chain and the A3 domain of the light chain are closely approximated[42] and form a compact globular core of 10 to 14 nm in diameter. The connecting region, or B domain, appears to form an elongated 5- to 14-nm extension from the core. This appendage is lost upon activation of factor VIII by thrombin.[43]

Association of Factor VIII with von Willebrand Factor

Factor VIII circulates in the blood as a non-covalent complex with vWF. The interaction is disrupted by high ionic strength[15, 16] or by phospholipids,[44, 45] suggesting that it involves both electrostatic and hydrophobic components. The binding site on factor VIII requires an acidic 41 amino acid segment at the amino-terminus of the light chain, particularly amino acid residues between Val 1670 and Glu 1684,[46, 47] and optimal binding requires sulfation of Tyr 1680.[37, 39]

Biosynthesis and Metabolism of Factor VIII

The liver is the major site of factor VIII synthesis, and liver transplantation corrects factor VIII deficiency due to hemophilia A.[48, 49] Factor VIII mRNA also has been detected in human liver, spleen, lymph node, pancreas, muscle, fetal heart, placenta, and kidney.[22, 50, 51] The physiological significance of these potential minor extrahepatic sites of factor VIII synthesis is not known.

Within the liver, which cell types synthesize factor VIII continues to be controversial. Human factor VIII appears to be synthesized in hepatocytes.[51–54] However, other studies report the detection of human factor VIII anigens in liver sinusoidal endothelial cells but not in hepatocytes.[55–57] Whether localization in human sinusoidal endothelium reflects uptake or synthesis is not known.

The synthesis of recombinant factor VIII in transfected cell lines appears to be fairly conventional. The factor VIII primary translation product is translocated into the endoplasmic reticulum, where N-linked glycosylation and disulfide bond formation are initiated. A substantial fraction of the molecules form a complex with immunoglobulin heavy chain–binding protein (BiP/GRP78) and are retained at least transiently in the endoplasmic reticulum. Some of this retained material appears to be degraded. The remainder is transported to the Golgi apparatus, where glycosylation is completed and selected tyrosine residues are sulfated. In the Golgi or a later compartment, the single-chain factor VIII precursor is cleaved after Arg 1648 to generate the amino-terminus of the light chain. Inclusion of vWF in the extracellular medium promotes the secretion of the factor VIII light chain and its metal ion–dependent association with the heavy chain. In the absence of vWF, the secreted free light and heavy chains do not form a stable complex and

are degraded. Thus, extracellular vWF may be required for optimal assembly of the factor VIII heavy and light chains into a stable complex.[58]

The normal metabolism of factor VIII depends on complex formation with vWF, which not only may promote the assembly of the factor VIII heavy and light chains but also stabilizes factor VIII in the circulation. Injected factor VIII/vWF complex is cleared from circulation with a half-disappearance time of about 12 hours.[59–61] The kinetics are actually biphasic and are identical to the clearance of the coadministered vWF.[61] In contrast, if factor VIII (containing only traces of vWF) is administered to patients with severe vWF deficiency, the factor VIII is rapidly eliminated, with a half-time of ~2.4 hours,[60] confirming the role of vWF in stabilizing factor VIII. Factor VIII and factor VIII/vWF complex show similar clearance patterns in patients with hemophilia A, demonstrating that exogenous factor VIII can associate with and be stabilized by endogenous vWF.[60]

Biological Function of Factor VIII

The role of factor VIII in blood coagulation has been defined over several decades of study.[31, 62, 63] Factor VIII is a component of the intrinsic pathway of blood coagulation, so called because all of the components required for blood clotting by this pathway are found in blood plasma; that is, they are "intrinsic" to the blood. Factor VIII does not have any known catalytic activity but participates as a cofactor in the proteolysis of factor X by factor IXa (Fig. 19–2). The reaction requires calcium ions and phospholipids (PL). The PL requirement is presumably met in vivo by platelet membranes or other cellular membranes. For in vitro clotting of plasma, PL vesicles suffice, and most of our knowledge of factor VIII biochemistry is derived from studies of clotting in solution containing PL.

Regulation of Factor VIIIa Activity

An enormous number of molecular reactions may directly or indirectly affect the procoagulant function of factor VIII. Factor VIII requires activation to participate optimally in the activation of factor X, and this is accomplished by limited proteolysis. Once gen-

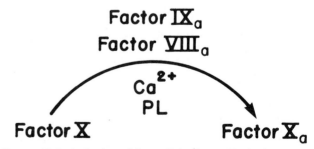

FIGURE 19–2. Activation of factor X by factor IXa in the presence of factor VIIIa, calcium ions, and phospholipid (PL).

erated, activated factor VIII (factor VIIIa) is inactivated by proteolytic and non-proteolytic mechanisms that may be influenced by many positive and negative effectors.

Proteolytic Activation of Factor VIII. Among the proteases known to activate factor VIII, thrombin has been the most thoroughly studied. Human factor VIII can be activated up to approximately 40-fold by digestion with thrombin.[9, 33, 64, 65] Upon thrombin activation, factor VIII dissociates from vWF.[66]

Two-chain factor VIII is rapidly cleaved by thrombin after Arg 740 to liberate carbohydrate-rich connecting peptide fragments of variable size (see Fig. 19–1). The product is a heterodimer consisting of fragments of M_r 90,000 (heavy chain) and ~80,000 (light chain), and it probably corresponds to the smallest form of unactivated factor VIII found in plasma. The connecting region or B domain may, therefore, be unnecessary for factor VIII function. In fact, deletion of the B domain is compatible with the biosynthesis of factor VIII species possessing apparently normal binding to vWF and procoagulant activity, at least in vitro.[67–69]

Upon further digestion, thrombin cleaves after Arg 372 of the 90,000 dalton heavy chain, between the A1 and A2 domains, to generate 50,000 dalton and 43,000 dalton fragments.[33] Thrombin also cleaves after Arg 1689, just before the A3 domain in the 80,000 dalton light chain, to give a 73,000 dalton fragment and an amino-terminal light chain fragment that probably dissociates from the complex.[33] This cleavage destroys or releases the binding site for vWF.[70] The final product, factor VIIIa, is a heterotrimer that consists of a 50,000 dalton A1 chain, a 43,000 dalton A2 chain, and a 73,000 dalton A3-C1-C2 chain[71–73] (see Fig. 19–1). Similar changes in structure accompany the activation of the homologous factor V by thrombin, except that factor V lacks a cleavage site between domains A1 and A2, so that factor Va is a heterodimer.[31]

The role of specific cleavages in the activation of factor VIII has been determined by using site-directed mutagenesis to make individual cleavage sites resistant to thrombin. Substitution of Arg 740 and Arg 1648 by isoleucine prevents cleavage at these sites by thrombin but does not prevent activation. Thus, proteolytic excision of the B domain apparently is unnecessary for activation of factor VIII. In contrast, mutation of either Arg 372 or Arg 1689 yields molecules with very low intrinsic factor VIIIa activity that are, however, resistant to activation by thrombin.[74]

Thrombin cleaves several bonds in factor VIII to generate factor VIIIa, and this product is not stable. Therefore, the kinetics of factor VIII activation by thrombin are complex. As the factor VIII concentration is increased, the rate of activation by low concentrations of thrombin shows saturation, with a half-maximal rate at approximately 0.086 U factor VIII/ml (~60 pM).[75] Because this value is ~10-fold lower than the average plasma concentration of factor VIII (1 U/ml, ~0.7 nM), under most conditions that initiate clotting in vivo, the concentration of factor VIII is never limiting. Thrombin generated in the course of clotting by either the intrinsic or the extrinsic pathway can, in principle, exert a positive feedback influence by activating additional factor VIII.

Factor Xa also activates factor VIII (see Fig. 19–1).[19, 64] Factor Xa acts at all of the sites that are cleaved by thrombin. Factor Xa probably also cleaves at the same site as activated protein C (APC), as well as at another site in the factor VIII light chain, after Arg 1719, that is not cleaved by either thrombin or APC.[33] The binding of factor VIII to vWF appears to inhibit activation of factor VIII by factor Xa but to have no effect on activation by thrombin.[76]

To summarize, either thrombin or factor Xa can activate factor VIII, and both proteases may play a critical role in the feedback amplification of clotting. In addition, factor IXa has been shown to activate factor VIII in vitro. However, very high concentrations of factor IXa are required, and the physiological significance of this activation mechanism is not known.[77]

Proteolytic and Non-proteolytic Inactivation of Factor VIIIa. Under most conditions, thrombin-activated factor VIIIa is intrinsically unstable, and factor VIIIa activity decays in what appears to be a first-order process without further proteolytic cleavage.[9, 40, 64, 78] This loss of activity apparently is accompanied by spontaneous dissociation of the 43 kDa A2 domain heavy chain fragment from the factor VIIIa A1/A2/A3-C1-C2 heterotrimer,[73] and active factor VIIIa can be reconstituted from purified inactive A1/A3-C1-C2 heterodimer and A2 domains. Dissociation of the A2 chain in inhibited at high concentrations of factor VIIIa, low ionic strength, and low pH.[72, 79] Under approximately physiological conditions, however, human factor VIIIa activity decays with a half-life of several minutes. Factor VIIIa is markedly stabilized by association with factor IXa and phospholipid.[80] The importance in vivo of the non-proteolytic loss of factor VIIIa activity, relative to proteolytic destruction, remains unknown.

Factor VIIIa is also degraded and inactivated by activated protein C (APC), as discussed in Chapter 16. Protein C is activated by thrombin,[81] in a reaction that is markedly accelerated by the endothelial cell surface cofactor thrombomodulin.[82, 83] Protein C deficiency is associated with severe thrombotic disease,[84] suggesting that this feedback mechanism for the inactivation of factor VIIIa and factor Va is physiologically important. This anticoagulant mechanism is discussed in Chapter 17.

APC can degrade factors V and VIII, as well as their activated forms, in a reaction that is stimulated about 50-fold by phospholipid and calcium.[19, 85, 86] However, thrombin-activated factors Va and VIIIa are much better substrates for APC than are the native factors.[81, 85, 87] APC cleaves either the heavy chain of factor VIII or the heavy chain–derived fragments of factor VIIIa, after Arg 336 at the carboxyl-end of domain A1 and Arg 562 within domain A2 (see Fig.

19–1).[87] Factor Xa also can cleave factor VIII after Arg 336, and this concordance may explain the ability of factor Xa to inactivate factor VIIIa.[33] APC also appears to cleave the heavy chain of factor VIII after Arg 740, which is the junction of domains A2 and B.[87] APC does not cleave the light chain of factor VIII or factor VIIIa.[33, 87]

Efficient cleavage of factor VIII or VIIIa by APC requires binding to a light chain site,[88] possibly to a segment including amino acids 2009 to 2018 within domain A3.[89] Association of the heavy chain with the light chain is necessary for recognition and cleavage of the heavy chain; free heavy chain is not a substrate for APC.[88]

The sensitivity to proteolysis of factor VIII and factor VIIIa may be regulated to some extent by interactions with other components of the factor X–activating complex and by other proteases that occur in the blood. For example, vWF inhibits the cleavage of factor VIII by APC,[90] and factor IXa protects factor VIII or VIIIa from degradation by APC.[91, 92] Granulocyte proteases destroy factor VIII or factor VIIIa in a reaction that is inhibited by the presence of factor IXa.[93] Plasmin destroys factor VIII,[94, 95] provided that the inhibition of α_2-antiplasmin is overcome, as may occur systemically in disseminated intravascular coagulation or locally in the clot environment. However, such an interaction between plasmin and factor VIII has not been demonstrated to affect clotting in vivo.

Coagulation on Artificial Surfaces

INTERACTIONS WITHIN THE INTRINSIC FACTOR X–ACTIVATING COMPLEX. The four known parts of the optimal factor Xa–generating complex are calcium ions, a phospholipid surface, factor IXa, and factor VIIIa. The role of each of these components can be illustrated by reconstructing the complete system in stages.

During clotting via the intrinsic pathway in vitro, factor IXa activates factor X by cleavage of a single specific peptide bond. The mechanism of factor IXa action is discussed under Biological Function of Factor IX (page 671). Factor VIIIa, phospholipid, and calcium ions act as cofactors that accelerate the rate of factor X cleavage. In the absence of cofactors, bovine factor IXa has a low but measurable activity toward factor X (Table 19–1). The addition of phospholipid alone has no effect on this reaction, and the addition of calcium ions alone results in a modest eightfold increase in the catalytic efficiency. If *both* calcium ions and phospholipid are added together, the K_m decreases dramatically by 3000- to 5000-fold into the range of plasma factor X concentrations (~0.2 μM), but the maximum rate of reaction increases only an additional twofold. However, if factor VIIIa is then added, the K_m for factor X stays roughly constant, whereas the catalytic rate (V_{max}) of the reaction increases more than 20,000-fold.[96] Qualitatively similar results have been reported for the human system.[97, 98] Presumably, the stoichiometric interaction between

TABLE 19–1. ACTIVATION OF BOVINE FACTOR X BY BOVINE FACTOR IXa

COMPOSITION OF REACTION	$K_m$app (μM)	V_{max} (mol Xa/mol IXa·min)	CATALYTIC EFFICIENCY (RELATIVE)
IXa	299	0.0022	[1]
IXa, Ca²⁺	181	0.0105	8
IXa, Ca²⁺, PL	0.058	0.0247	58,000
IXa, Ca²⁺, PL, VIIIa	0.063	500	1×10^9

Where indicated, reactions contained Ca^{2+}, ~10 mM; phospholipid (PL), 10 μM; factor VIIIa, 11 U/ml. Relative catalytic efficiency is V_{max}/K_m, normalized to the value for factor IXa above.

Adapted from Van Dieijen, G., et al.: The role of phospholipid and factor VIIIa in the activation of bovine factor X. J. Biol. Chem. 256:3433, 1981; with permission of the American Society for Biochemistry and Molecular Biology.

factors VIIIa and IXa[99] enhances the V_{max} of factor IXa, whereas the calcium-dependent binding of factors IXa and X to the phospholipid surface lowers the apparent K_m for factor X in the complete reaction system by increasing the local concentration of reactants.

PHOSPHOLIPID REQUIREMENT. Factor VIII and factor VIIIa bind tightly to phospholipid vesicles[44, 45]; the K_d for factor VIII binding to phosphatidylcholine (PC)/phosphatidylserine (PS) vesicles is ~2 nM.[100] This interaction is mediated by the factor VIII light chain[101] and appears to require a segment of domain C2.[102] Vesicles composed of pure PC, PS, or phosphatidylethanolamine (PE) usually have no procoagulant activity, nor do mixtures of PC and PE. In contrast, mixtures of PS/PC or PS/PE have significant procoagulant activity.[103, 104]

Coagulation on Biological Surfaces

During clotting in vivo, reactions that are moderately well understood in reconstituted solutions occur in the presence of cellular components that may profoundly alter them. In particular, platelets are normally quite inert until activated by thrombin. After thrombin activation, platelets demonstrate considerable procoagulant activity, perhaps serving the role in vivo that phospholipid vesicles fill for in vitro assays. In addition, the endothelial cell lining of the vascular system expresses both thrombogenic and anticoagulant properties that can be modulated by the adjacent plasma.

HEMOSTATIC REACTIONS AT THE PLATELET SURFACE. Platelets not only provide procoagulant phospholipid on demand but also have specific receptors for some clotting factors and secrete additional factors during the platelet release reaction. Hemostatic interactions of platelets are also discussed in Chapter 22.

The distribution of phospholipid types across the platelet plasma membrane is asymmetrical, with essentially all of the negatively charged PS confined to the cytoplasmic leaflet.[105] In the resting platelet, the phospholipid exposed to the blood is devoid of procoagulant activity, whereas that exposed to the cytoplasm is extremely active.[105, 106] Activation of platelets is claimed to result in redistribution of coagulantly active PS to the outer leaflet, although this mechanism has not been shown definitively to be physiologically significant.[106]

Binding of factor VIII to platelets is stimulated ~20-fold upon thrombin activation, and there are ~450 sites per platelet with a K_d of ~3 nM.[107] This binding affinity is similar to that of factor VIII binding to phospholipids, and phospholipids compete for binding of factor VIII to platelet-derived microparticles.[108] Factor V and factor VIII appear to bind with comparable affinity to different sites on activated platelets or platelet microparticles,[107, 108] although very high concentrations of factor Va can inhibit factor VIII binding.[108] vWF inhibits the binding of factor VIII to activated platelets, with an apparent dissociation constant of 0.44 nM for the factor VIII–vWF interaction.[109]

HEMOSTATIC REACTIONS AT THE ENDOTHELIAL CELL SURFACE. Endothelial cells can affect blood clotting on their surface through many mechanisms. They contain proteoglycans that accelerate the inactivation of thrombin by antithrombin III.[110, 111] Endothelial cells secrete prostacyclin, a potent inhibitor of platelet aggregation,[112] and tissue plasminogen activator, an initiator of fibrinolysis.[113] They also express thrombomodulin, a plasma membrane protein that binds thrombin, promoting the activation of protein C and inhibiting the procoagulant activities of thrombin. The protein C anticoagulant system is discussed in Chapter 17. Thus, the non-thrombogenic properties of endothelium are maintained by several independent pathways.

Several mechanisms by which endothelial cells might *enhance* rather than inhibit thrombosis have been described. Intact resting endothelium usually appears to lack tissue factor activity.[114] However, human umbilical vein endothelial cells can express tissue factor in response to stimulation with thrombin,[115] phorbol esters, phytohemagglutinin, or endotoxin[116] and therefore could mediate the activation of factor X by the extrinsic pathway under some conditions. In addition, several components of the intrinsic factor X–activating complex can bind to endothelial cells, which contain specific high-affinity surface receptors for factor IX/IXa and factor X.[117–119] As a consequence, most of the factor X–activating complex could be preassembled on the cell surface. If these clot-promoting activities of endothelium prove to occur in vivo, it will be interesting to learn how the opposing anticoagulant and thrombotic functions of the endothelium are regulated.

Molecular Biology of Factor VIII

The factor VIII gene is located near the tip of the long arm of the X chromosome at Xq28, just distal to the fragile site at Xq27.3,[120] and spans about 186 kb of DNA.[22, 24] Accordingly, it constitutes about 0.1 per cent of the X chromosome. The gene contains 25 introns, including one of 32.4 kb and three of about 22 kb in size, and 26 exons (see Fig. 19–1). The factor VIII gene is closely linked to the loci for deutan color blindness and glucose-6-phosphate dehydrogenase (G6PD) but is not closely linked to the nearby factor IX gene.[121, 122]

The factor VIII gene has an additional unusual structural feature. The largest intron, intron 22, contains another transcribed gene of unknown function. Two homologues of this "gene within a gene" are present within 1.1 megabase of the factor VIII gene. At least two of these genes are transcribed, and a homologous transcribed sequence is present in the mouse.[123]

Factor VIII Deficiency (Hemophilia A)

Clinical Features of Hemophilia A

So-called classical hemophilia, or hemophilia A, is an X-linked inherited disease characterized by deficient factor VIII activity. The prevalence of hemophilia A is approximately 100 per million males.[124] The residual factor VIII activity found in hemophilic plasma is variable. For clinical purposes, the factor VIII deficiency is classified as severe (<1 per cent), moderate (1 to 5 per cent), and mild (5 to 30 per cent) according to the percentage of factor VIII activity assayed relative to normal plasma.

Manifestations of hemophilia A include spontaneous bleeding into joints, muscles, and brain; delayed but prolonged bleeding from minor cuts; and severe bleeding from lacerations. Spontaneous bleeding is generally limited to patients with less than 5 per cent of normal factor VIII activity. Symptoms begin soon after birth and are lifelong but can be ameliorated by aggressive treatment of spontaneous or traumatic bleeding with various forms of factor VIII. The continuing evolution of home therapy for hemophilia has markedly decreased the dependence of hemophiliacs on hospital facilities.[124–126] Most patients with hemophilia can now lead relatively normal lives, handling routine bleeding by self-administration of factor VIII preparations. Before effective factor VIII concentrates were widely used, patients with frequent hemarthroses developed crippling joint deformities by their second decade. Although skeletal problems have been largely eliminated in patients participating in modern home-care programs, spontaneous intracranial bleeding and other internal bleeding still cause mortality.

Classification and Molecular Defects in Hemophilia A

Patients with hemophilia A have different degrees of factor VIII deficiency, but the severity of the deficiency varies little among those affected in any given hemophilia pedigree.[127] The qualitative heterogeneity of hemophilia was first directly demonstrated by the discovery of two classes of patients with severe factor VIII deficiency. About three fourths have no detectable factor VIII by both activity and antigen assays and are termed cross-reacting material negative (CRM−). The remainder have decreased or absent factor VIII activity with detectable factor VIII antigen. Patients with equal decrements of factor VIII antigen and activity are sometimes classified as CRM reduced (CRMred). Patients with disproportionately decreased factor VIII activity compared with antigen, consistent with the production of an immunologically recognizable but dysfunctional protein, are classified as CRM+.[10–12, 128–130]

The molecular basis for hemophilia A has been elucidated at the level of gene structure in many cases. These mutations are catalogued in a data base that is updated annually.[131] An astonishing number of patients, at least 2000, have been studied since 1984. The distinct mutations characterized include more than 60 large deletions, 7 small deletions, 6 insertions, 2 internal gene segment duplications, two splice-site mutations, 14 nonsense point mutations, and 66 missense mutations. Except for the missense mutations, most of these lesions appear to prevent the synthesis of detectable factor VIII antigen and cause severe CRM− hemophilia A. A detailed examination of all factor VIII exons in a small number of patients with hemophilia A suggests that approximately half of the causative mutations may lie outside factor VIII exons and splice junctions.[132] No potential mutations that reduce gene transcription have yet been found in the 5′ flanking region of the factor VIII gene.

Two families with hemophilia A were described in which the factor VIII gene was mutated by the insertion of a long interspersed element (LINE-1).[133] Approximately 50,000 to 100,000 of these repeats are distributed throughout the genome, and they apparently move to new sites by a process similar to the retrotransposition of retroviruses.[134] In both families, the LINE-1 insertions occurred de novo in the affected males, suggesting that they were derived from an actively transposing LINE-1 element. The probable functional progenitor LINE-1 element was subsequently identified on chromosome 22, cloned, and shown to encode a functional reverse transcriptase. Such functional LINE-1 elements were proposed to provide the reverse transcriptase necessary for the dispersal of various interspersed sequences with properties that suggest derivation from reverse transcripts, including LINE elements, *Alu* repeats, and processed pseudogenes.[135, 136]

Missense mutations are often compatible with the synthesis of significant, possibly normal, quantities of factor VIII proteins with variable functional defects. The resultant CRM+ hemophilia phenotype can sometimes be understood in terms of the known structure-function relationships of normal factor VIII. For example, mutations have been identified that substitute either His or Cys for Arg 372[137, 138] or Arg 1689[139, 140] and so prevent proteolytic activation by thrombin; these mutations cause mild to severe

CRM+ hemophilia A. As discussed under Association of Factor VIII with von Willebrand Factor, studies of recombinant mutant factor VIII, with the substitution Tyr 1680 → Phe, suggest that sulfation of Tyr 1680 is required for optimal binding to vWF.[37, 39] The identical mutation was found in a patient with mild hemophilia A.[141] The low factor VIII levels in this patient may be due partly to reduced binding to vWF, causing reduced stability of the mutant factor VIII in the circulation.

The distribution of observed mutations suggests some conclusions regarding the mechanism by which they occur. Deletions account for 2.5 to 10 per cent of mutations causing hemophilia A, depending on the sensitivity of the method employed to detect deletions. The remaining mutations are almost exclusively single nucleotide substitutions. No identical gene deletions have been found in unrelated patients, and no segment of the factor VIII gene appears to be strikingly susceptible to deletion or insertion events. In contrast, all but one of the known factor VIII nonsense mutations are C → T transitions occurring in CG dinucleotides, and identical mutations in some sites have occurred independently in many patients. Similarly, about two thirds of the known missense mutations in hemophilia A and all but one of the independently recurring mutations are due to CG → TG transitions. The cytidine residues in CG dinucleotides are frequently methylated in human genomic DNA,[142] and the resultant 5′-methylcytidine may undergo spontaneous deamination to yield thymidine.[143] This mechanism appears to explain why CG dinucleotides are hotspots for mutation in many genes, including the factor VIII gene. There are 69 CG dinucleotides in the coding region of the factor VIII cDNA sequence, and to date at least 60 apparently independent C → T transitions have been reported in 16 of them. In the factor VIII gene, the likelihood of mutation at CG dinucleotides is estimated to be increased 10- to 20-fold relative to other dinucleotides.[144]

Prenatal Diagnosis and Carrier Detection in Hemophilia A

At present, the best methods for the genetic analysis of hemophilia A are based on the detection of DNA sequence variations within or near the factor VIII gene. These typically employ DNA probes to identify the causative mutation itself, DNA sequence polymorphisms within the factor VIII gene, or restriction fragment length polymorphisms (RFLPs) at loci closely linked to the factor VIII gene. Completely informative DNA markers cannot be identified for all families, and a combination of DNA-based methods and assays of plasma factor VIII is often required for optimal carrier detection and prenatal diagnosis. Fetal samples for DNA extraction can be obtained by chorionic villus sampling at 8 to 11 weeks' gestation[145] or by amniocentesis in mid-trimester.[146] Factor VIII does not cross the placenta, and fetal blood suitable for factor VIII levels can be obtained by fetoscopy after 18 weeks' gestation.[147-150]

In the most favorable cases, the mutation in the factor VIII gene can be identified directly. Identification of the genetic lesion itself makes both carrier detection and prenatal diagnosis unambiguous. If the causative mutation is unknown, intragenic DNA sequence polymorphisms are the best alternative markers for genetic studies. At least nine polymorphisms have been reported within non-coding regions of the factor VIII gene.[151, 152] An additional nine sequence polymorphisms have been reported within factor VIII exons, among which four change the encoded amino acid sequence and the remainder are silent.[131] For these markers to be useful, a given pedigree must contain at least one affected male with a heterozygous mother. The likelihood of demonstrating heterozygosity increases with the number of available polymorphic markers. Most of the known factor VIII polymorphisms are in extreme linkage disequilibrium, however, and the use of several intragenic marker systems is often no more informative than one alone. There is some variation among races in the allelic frequencies of RFLPs, so no single combination of markers is necessarily optimal for all families. Nevertheless, analysis with the available intragenic polymorphisms has provided useful diagnostic information in approximately two thirds of women tested. This fraction may be increased substantially through use of the highly informative (CA)n marker in intron 13, for which the observed heterozygosity is 91 per cent.[151, 153]

If intragenic DNA markers are not informative, extragenic RFLPs can be used. Several highly polymorphic, extragenic RFLP marker systems are closely linked to the factor VIII locus, among which two or three have been used extensively for genetic analysis of hemophilia A.[151] For example, ~95 per cent of women are heterozygous at the St14(DXS52) locus, and this marker system is informative in almost all pedigrees. The utility of extragenic markers is limited by a significant probability (~5 per cent) of recombination between the polymorphic locus and the mutation in the factor VIII gene. To maximize the likelihood of identifying rare individuals in whom such recombination has occurred, diagnoses based upon extragenic RFLPs should be checked by assays of plasma factor VIII.

For families with a single sporadic case of hemophilia A, the use of linked DNA polymorphic markers has a fundamental limitation that can prevent the accurate tracking of mutant factor VIII alleles. Approximately one sixth of patients with hemophilia A are found in families with no known prior history of the disease.[154] This finding is consistent with the calculation of Haldane that about one third of cases of X-linked recessive disorders are due to spontaneous mutations, provided that the population is at equilibrium and affected persons have low fertility.[155] Sometimes the lack of family history must reflect inadequate historical information. Detailed genetic analysis suggests, however, that approximately one half of such cases are due to a spontaneous germline mutation in the mother or a grandparent of the affected child.[156] Such potential germline mosaicism destroys the correlation between inheritance of any factor VIII DNA marker pattern and inheritance of the hemophilia A allele. In the first subsequent generation, DNA marker studies can exclude carrier status or hemophilia A but generally cannot prove that a female is a carrier or that a male fetus will have hemophilia.

Because of this uncertainty, genetic counseling for these families may necessarily depend on the analysis of plasma factor VIII levels. Heterozygous carriers of hemophilia A often have plasma factor VIII levels intermediate between those of hemophiliacs and unaffected persons in their family, but several factors conspire to make factor VIII levels alone an unreliable index for distinguishing carriers from normal females. Factor VIII levels in carrier women may vary widely owing to differences in selective X-chromosome inactivation (lyonization) during development. A number of physiological mechanisms may cause transient or sustained elevations of factor VIII, and assays of factor VIII activity are also subject to significant uncertainty, complicating the interpretation of factor VIII levels for the purpose of genotype assignment. Even in normal males the level of factor VIII varies widely, and genetic analysis of this variation suggests that there are several normal alleles at the factor VIII locus, or linked to it, that cause inheritable differences in normal factor VIII activity.[122, 123] Non-linked modifiers of factor VIII activity also exist, such as ABO blood type.[157, 158] Consequently, even with the best available methods to measure and to analyze plasma factor VIII levels, between 6 and 20 per cent of women still are misclassified either as normal or as carriers.[158, 159]

The residual uncertainties in genetic analysis using RFLPs and factor VIII assays could be overcome, in principle, if the identification of hemophilia A mutations were feasible for all families. Potentially suitable methods have been described and tested on a few patients. These are based on polymerase chain reaction (PCR) amplification and analysis of factor VIII cDNA sequences, starting with the extremely low level of factor VIII mRNA that is present in peripheral blood cells. Once characterized, mutations can be detected in all potential carriers, and in male fetuses, by PCR assays.[160] If this experimental approach proves to be sufficiently rapid, reliable, and economical for routine clinical use, it should supplant less direct methods that make use of linked DNA markers and factor VIII assays.

Differential Diagnosis of Inherited Factor VIII Deficiency

SEVERE VON WILLEBRAND DISEASE. Patients with von Willebrand disease (vWD) type I ordinarily have a decrease in factor VIII levels that parallels their modest deficiency of vWF. Patients who have severe vWD type III occasionally have levels of factor VIII low enough to be classified as severe deficiency (<1 per cent). In contrast to hemophilia A, however, patients with severe vWD have extremely low levels of vWF antigen and ristocetin cofactor activity and markedly prolonged skin bleeding times. Severe vWD can also be distinguished from hemophilia A by its autosomal recessive mode of inheritance, but this is not possible in many families.

VON WILLEBRAND DISEASE NORMANDY. A recessive but autosomally inherited mimic of hemophilia A would occur if the factor VIII–binding site on vWF were altered without affecting other vWF functions. Recently, several unrelated patients with such defects were identified, and the condition was tentatively named vWD Normandy. This disorder is discussed in more detail on page 684.

COMBINED FACTOR V AND FACTOR VIII DEFICIENCY. Factor V and factor VIII deficiency may occur in the same individual through chance inheritance of both parahemophilia and hemophilia A.[161, 162] However, in most cases combined factor V and factor VIII deficiency apparently is due to a homozygous or compound heterozygous abnormality at a single autosomal locus.

Thirty-one apparently unrelated families with this combined deficiency have been described.[163–166] About half appear to have originated around the Mediterranean basin, and most of these are non-Ashkenazi Jews.[167] This is the fourth autosomal recessive bleeding disorder known to be relatively frequent in Jewish communities. The other diseases include factor XI deficiency in Ashkenazi Jews (frequency, 1 in 190), Glanzmann's thrombasthenia in Iraqi Jews (frequency, 1 in 6400), and factor VII deficiency with the Dubin-Johnson syndrome in Iranian, Moroccan, and Iraqi Jews.[163]

Heterozygous carriers of factor V/factor VIII deficiency are at worst mildly afflicted with bleeding tendencies and are generally indistinguishable from normal individuals by assays of factor V and factor VIII activity. Affected homozygotes usually have factor VIII activity less than 25 per cent of normal, with roughly equal deficiency of factor V activity.[163] Also, they have similar deficiencies of factor V and factor VIII antigens but normal levels of vWF.[165–171] The factor V and factor VIII molecules appear to be qualitatively normal, as judged by thrombin activation.[168]

The mechanism of combined factor V and factor VIII deficiency is unknown. Deficiency of a specific protein C inhibitor might cause such a disease because excessive activity of APC could degrade both factors simultaneously.[172] Most patients, however, have normal levels of protein C inhibitor.[164–166, 169, 171] Thus, there is no evidence that deficiency of protein C inhibitor is a major cause.

Treatment of Hemophilia A

Treatment of bleeding with factor VIII preparations carries many well-recognized risks. The major ones are the transmission of infectious agents and the development of alloantibody inhibitors of factor VIII activity. The risk of iatrogenic infection has been reduced markedly through improved methods to inactivate viruses in plasma-derived blood products and through the production of recombinant human factor VIII. New strategies also show considerable promise for the effective treatment of bleeding episodes in patients with factor VIII inhibitors.

VIRAL INFECTIONS IN HEMOPHILIA A. Before the application of viral inactivation methods to factor concentrates in 1985, nearly all transfused hemophiliacs had abnormal liver function tests or serological evidence of viral hepatitis,[173] and a substantial fraction had cirrhosis or chronic active hepatitis.[174] Most of this transfusion-associated liver disease appeared to be due to hepatitis C (non-A, non-B hepatitis).[175] Infection with the delta agent (a defective virus that can replicate only in the presence of hepatitis B virus) has been implicated as another cause of hepatitis in hemophiliacs.[176] Infection with human immunodeficiency virus (HIV) is also a transfusion-associated risk. In one study of 908 U.S. patients with hemophilia A who were transfused between 1978 and 1985, almost two thirds had serological evidence of HIV infection.[177]

Several methods have been used to inactivate hepatitis viruses and HIV in blood products. These include various forms of heating and treatment with detergents or organic solvents. In the United States, all plasma clotting factor preparations that are derived from large numbers of donors have been subjected to one or more such virucidal procedures. This includes factor VIII concentrates, highly purified factor VIII, prothrombin complex concentrates, and activated prothrombin complex concentrates, all of which may be manufactured from the pooled plasma of 10,000 or more donors. In contrast, virtually none of the products derived from single donors or from relatively small numbers of donors, such as cryoprecipitate, are so treated.

Current methods for heat treatment of factor VIII concentrates apparently prevent transmission of HIV viruses.[178, 179] Some virucidal methods also appear to prevent transmission of hepatitis B and C, although these viruses seem to be more resistant than HIV to inactivation.[180, 181] More clinical experience is required to determine whether the available plasma-derived products carry any residual risk of transmitting hepatitis.

FACTOR VIII PREPARATIONS FOR TREATMENT OF HEMOPHILIA A. Low-purity factor VIII concentrates may occasionally have other side effects, including skin test anergy[182] and decreased CD4 lymphocyte levels,[183] which have been attributed to the large variety and amount of contaminating proteins in such concentrates. Rarely, factor VIII concentrates have also been associated with allergic reactions or the development of pulmonary hypertension.[184]

Factor VIII preparations that are essentially free of extraneous proteins are now available. The plasma-derived products are prepared by immunoaffinity chromatography, using monoclonal antibodies to either factor VIII or vWF. The resultant "monoclonal-purified" factor VIII has a specific activity of more than ~2000 units/mg, exclusive of added albumin. Recombinant human factor VIII or similar purity has been evaluated in small clinical trials[185, 186] and soon may be available for general use.

ALTERNATIVES TO BLOOD PRODUCT THERAPY. Factor VIII levels in normal individuals and those with mild to moderate hemophilia A are elevated by a variety of stimuli, including estrogens, catecholamines, neurological stress, chronic inflammation, liver disease, and hyperthyroidism (reviewed by Bloom[187]). Consequently, pharmacological agents that mimic these effects have been sought. The most useful adjunct to factor replacement at present is 1-deamino-(8-D-arginine)-vasopressin (DDAVP), a synthetic analogue of antidiuretic hormone that lacks vasoconstrictor activity. DDAVP stimulates the release of pre-formed factor VIII and vWF from storage sites into the circulation, elevating plasma levels threefold to sixfold.[188] There are also transient increases in tissue plasminogen activator activity.[189] The reservoir of vWF is most likely endothelial cells located throughout the vasculature, but the source of factor VIII is unknown. The elevations in both factors are maximal at 30 to 90 minutes and decrease with variable rates over several hours to several days. Usually, but not uniformly, repeated administration of DDAVP elicits diminishing responses, which seem likely to reflect progressive depletion of stored factors rather than the desensitization of receptors.[190–192] In patients with severe vWD who have undetectable plasma vWF antigen, DDAVP does not cause an increase in factor VIII levels. Therefore, the factor VIII response obtained in patients with mild deficiency of either factor VIII or vWF probably is secondary to the induction of vWF release.[193] In suitable patients with either hemophilia A or vWD, DDAVP given intravenously, subcutaneously, or intranasally has been used successfully to treat hemarthroses and other spontaneous bleeding, as coverage for minor surgical procedures without the use of factor VIII concentrates.[194]

ANTIBODY INHIBITORS OF FACTOR VIII. In ~15 per cent of patients with hemophilia A, therapy is associated with the development of alloantibodies that inhibit factor VIII activity.[195, 196] Rarely, autoantibodies to factor VIII may occur in a non-hemophilic person, causing acquired factor VIII deficiency.

Alloantibody inhibitors of factor VIII occur mostly among patients with severe CRM− hemophilia A who have deletions or nonsense mutations in the factor VIII gene.[131] Although inhibitors do occur in patients with CRMred or CRM+ hemophilia A, in such patients they are more often transient or of low titer. The development of inhibitors clearly depends on more than the nature of the factor VIII mutation alone. The extent and location of a factor VIII gene deletion do not correlate with the occurrence of factor VIII inhibitors; patients with and without inhibitors have been found to have similar deletions. Similarly, patients with and without inhibitors have been found with identical nonsense mutations.

In patients who develop inhibitors, the nature of the antibody response appears to be at least partly under genetic control.[196–198] Patients fall into two major groups. Inhibitors developing in adults after life-long exposure to factor VIII are most often of low titer (<6 Bethesda U/ml), and marked increases in the inhibitor titer generally do not occur following treatment with factor VIII; these patients are classified as "low responders." More commonly, inhibitors develop after relatively brief exposure to factor VIII (<75 "exposure days") and occasionally after a single treatment with factor VIII. Most such inhibitors develop before the age of 30, with the greatest risk before the age of 5, are of high titer, and show dramatic increases in titer following additional treatment with factor VIII; such patients are classified as "high responders." Several studies have suggested an association between histocompatibility antigen patterns and the development of inhibitors[199, 200] (reviewed by Kasper[195]). In the United States, inhibitors are more common in black than in white patients with hemophilia A.[196] This could result from racial differences in factor VIII amino acid sequence polymorphisms, because plasma-derived factor VIII concentrates are prepared mainly from white donors. Alternatively, the increased prevalence of inhibitors among black patients could reflect inherited differences in immunological response.

Alloantibody inhibitors are most often of restricted polyclonal origin and are usually immunoglobulin G (IgG). The majority of inhibitors consist predominantly of subclass IgG4 antibodies and usually have at least one component of another IgG subclass.[201] Despite the large size of the factor VIII polypeptide, which offers many potential epitopes for the induction of antibody responses, a small subset of epitopes appear to be recognized by most of the clinically significant inhibitors. One major epitope is between amino acids 379 and 538 within domain A2 of the heavy chain, and another is between amino acids 2178 and 2332 within domain C2 of the light chain.[202]

There are no fully satisfactory methods to eliminate factor VIII antibodies (reviewed in Kasper[195]). Inhibitors have been suppressed in some patients by treatment with various combinations of corticosteroids, immunosuppressive drugs, and intravenous gamma globulin. Prolonged therapy with factor VIII, with or without accompanying immunosuppressive therapy, has been shown to induce immune tolerance to factor VIII in some patients. Extracorporeal absorption of inhibitor antibodies on protein A–agarose has been helpful in a few reported cases. The limited number of immunodominant factor VIII epitopes suggests a potential therapeutic use of recombinant factor VIII fragments either for the neutralization of inhibitor antibodies or for the induction of immune tolerance.

CIRCUMVENTION OF FACTOR VIII INHIBITORS. Very low titer inhibitors can be overcome by increased doses of factor VIII. If the antibodies are of sufficiently high titer, effective treatment of bleeding episodes with factor VIII concentrates becomes impossible.

Current methods for circumventing inhibitors fall into two categories: administration of animal factor VIII that does not react with human inhibitors, and "bypassing" inhibitors by generating fibrin through pathways that are independent of factor VIII.

Porcine Factor VIII. Alloantibody inhibitors of human factor VIII often are less potent inhibitors of heterologous factor VIII, and bovine or porcine preparations have been used sporadically for more than 35 years in the treatment of hemophilia A to circumvent these inhibitors.[203] Heterologous blood products have the additional potential advantage that they are not known to transmit viral diseases to humans. However, the vWF in most bovine or porcine factor VIII preparations aggregates human platelets in vivo, sometimes causing severe thrombocytopenia[203] or allergic reactions.[204]

These problems are reduced by the use of a highly purified concentrate of porcine factor VIII that is relatively free of vWF.[205, 206] Allergic reactions occur in up to half of treated patients. A transient decrease in platelet count occurs in some patients, occasionally with a nadir below 100,000/μl; this appears to be due to residual contamination with porcine vWF. Porcine factor VIII sometimes provokes the development of significant anti-porcine inhibitors.

Prothrombin Complex Concentrates. Examination of the intrinsic and extrinsic clotting cascades suggests that factor VIII deficiency might be bypassed by delivering either factor VIIa to activate factor X by the extrinsic mechanism or factor Xa itself or thrombin. So-called prothrombin-complex concentrates (PCCs) contain all of these components, as well as many unactivated zymogens (prothrombin, factors VII, IX, and X, and protein C) and variable amounts of factor VIII.[207, 208] These concentrates have been used for decades as a source of factor IX for the treatment of hemophilia B, and by the late 1960s they had been used sporadically to treat bleeding in patients with hemophilia A and factor VIII inhibitors. "Activated" prothrombin-complex concentrates (APCCs) that contain relatively more of the activated factors and less of their zymogens were prepared specifically for the treatment of patients with factor VIII inhibitors; APCCs also were reported to be effective.[209]

By 1981 the efficacy of both PCCs[210] and APCCs[211, 212] was demonstrated in blinded clinical trials. Since then, these agents have been widely used. Immediate complications are uncommon but have included thromboembolism[213] and disseminated intravascular coagulation.[214] Anamnestic rises of the factor VIII inhibitor titer occur in many patients.[215, 216]

Factor VIIa. Factor VIIa is one candidate for the effective component in PCCs. A large fraction of the factor VII in PCCs has been proteolytically activated, and this fraction is even higher in APCCs.[217] The procoagulant activity of factor VIIa depends on tissue factor, and factor VIIa does not combine with antithrombin III in the absence of heparin.[218] Therefore, injected factor VIIa might be able to reach a site of injury in an active form and combine there with liberated tissue factor. This could lead to the local activation of factor X by the extrinsic pathway, without causing significant systemic effects, and potentially could bypass the normal hemostatic requirement for factor VIII activity.

Limited clinical experience suggests that factor VIIa may be effective for the treatment of bleeding in patients with hemophilia A and high-titer factor VIII inhibitors. Purified plasma-derived human factor VIIa was shown to arrest bleeding in several such patients with muscle hematomas, oral bleeding, or hemarthroses.[219, 220] There were no immediate side effects and no evidence of systemic activation of the blood coagulation system. In additional patients, recombinant factor VIIa was similarly effective for the treatment of intracranial hemorrhage[221] and other spontaneous soft tissue bleeding[222, 223] and to control bleeding during a synovectomy.[224] It was not effective in one patient for the treatment of bleeding after a hernioplasty.[225] Several instances of mild bleeding at other sites were noted during therapy with recombinant factor VIIa.[221, 223]

FACTOR IX AND HEMOPHILIA B

Like factor VIII, factor IX participates in the middle phase of the intrinsic pathway of blood coagulation (see Fig. 19–2). It circulates in plasma as an inactive zymogen that is activated through proteolytic cleavage by factor XIa or by a complex of factor VIIa and tissue factor. Activated factor IXa then forms a complex with factor VIIIa, a phospholipid surface, and calcium to activate factor X. The clinical similarity of severe hemophilia A (factor VIII deficiency) and hemophilia B (factor IX deficiency) can therefore be rationalized as the result of deficient function of the intrinsic factor X–activating complex, arising by mutations affecting independent components of that complex.

Purification and Structural Characterization of Factor IX

Assays for Factor IX

Factor IX was first assayed as a component, present in both normal plasma and in plasma from patients with hemophilia A, that corrected the clotting in vitro of plasma from patients with hemophilia B.[4, 5] Unlike factor VIII, factor IX activity is not destroyed during clotting, and normal serum also corrects hemophilia B plasma. Synthetic peptide substrates with adequate specificity for factor IXa are not widely available. Consequently, assays for factor IX still generally involve a determination of the time required for a clot to form in factor IX–deficient plasma. This assay is relatively insensitive and not totally specific for factor

IX. One unit of factor IX activity is defined as the amount found in 1 ml of pooled normal plasma.[6]

Factor IXa can be assayed by modification of the factor VIII assays employing purified components, determining the factor IXa–mediated generation of factor Xa that is dependent on calcium, phospholipid, and factor VIII, as described in Assays for Factor VIII (page 658).

Heterologous polyclonal and monoclonal antibodies as well as alloantibodies to human factor IX have been reported. With the use of such reagents, assays of factor IX antigen by Laurell rocket, radiometric, and enzyme-linked immunoabsorbent methods have been described.[226]

Purification of Factor IX

Factor IX is difficult to purify for several reasons. The concentration of factor IX in plasma is low: ~2 to 3 μg/ml, or ~40 to 60 nM. The zymogen form of factor IX is susceptible to cleavage by several blood proteases that may be activated during the collection of blood or during purification procedures. In addition, factor IX belongs to a large family of proteins related to trypsin, many of which occur in blood plasma and tend to copurify. Among these, seven are known that have not only homologous protease-like domains, but also another homologous amino-terminal domain that contains 10 to 20 γ-carboxyglutamic acid (Gla) residues. These are discussed in Chapter 16 and include prothrombin, factor VII, factor X, protein C, protein S, and protein Z.

Purification of bovine[227] and human[228] factor IX to homogeneity with efficient resolution from factor VII, factor X, and prothrombin was first achieved by salt gradient elution from heparin-agarose, for which factor IX has the highest affinity. Pure factor IX has a specific activity of approximately 325 to 500 U/mg.[229]

Structure and Physical Properties of Factor IX

Human factor IX is composed of a single polypeptide chain of 415 amino acid residues and has a molecular weight of ~55,000, of which ~20 per cent is carbohydrate. There are only two potential N-glycosylation sites at asparagine residues 157 and 167, within the activation peptide.[230, 231] Oligosaccharides elsewhere in the protein are probably linked to Ser or Thr residues. One of these oligosaccharides has the unusual structure, (xylosyl)$_2$-glucose, attached to Ser 53 in the first epidermal growth factor (EGF)–like domain of the factor IX light chain.[232] Other sites of glycosylation and carbohydrate structures of human factor IX have not been determined.

Comparison of the factor IX amino acid sequence with other vitamin K–dependent clotting factors and with more distantly related serine proteases reveals striking similarities of sequence that reflect the evolution of this protein family from a common ancestor (see Chapter 16). On the basis of these homologies, factor IX can be considered to have four distinct domains. Starting at the amino-terminal tyrosine, these include (1) the Gla domain, (2) the growth factor domain, (3) the activation peptide domain, and (4) the catalytic domain (Fig. 19–3). In addition, the factor IX precursor contains a signal peptide (prepeptide) as well as a short propeptide that is required for efficient post-translational carboxylation of glutamic acid residues.

The Gla domain corresponds to amino acid residues 1 through 40. In this region, all 12 of the glutamic acid residues are carboxylated to yield Gla.[233] These residues are important for the calcium-binding function of normal factor IX.[234] The homologous Gla domains of other vitamin K–dependent proteins show considerable sequence conservation, which is consistent with the conserved calcium-binding function of this region in all of these proteins (Fig. 19–3). However, at least one high-affinity calcium-binding site in factor IX is outside the Gla domain[234] but instead is within the first EGF-like domain.[235]

The growth factor domain of factor IX corresponds approximately to residues 48 through 127 (Fig. 19–3). This section consists of two tandemly arranged segments that are homologous to EGF. Among serine proteases, similar EGF-like domains are found in factor X, tissue plasminogen activator, urokinase, protein C, and factor XII.[236, 237] However, prothrombin, which does have a homologous Gla domain and catalytic domain, has an unrelated domain in the position corresponding to the growth factor domain of factor IX. This segment of prothrombin is instead homologous to the "kringles" of plasminogen.[238, 239] Interestingly, factor XII,[237] tissue plasminogen activator,[240] and urokinase[241, 242] have *both* kringle *and* EGF-like domains. In addition, EGF-like domains are found in several other proteins that have no known role in hemostasis (reviewed in Massagué[243]). The corresponding gene segments appear to have been shuffled and rearranged in several ways to yield the domain patterns observed in these diverse proteins. The mechanisms underlying this evolutionary process as well as the function of most of these EGF-like domains remain unknown.

In addition to Gla, factor IX contains another unusual residue, β-hydroxyaspartic acid (Hya), present at position 64 in the first EGF-like domain.[244] This amino acid is produced by the post-translational hydroxylation of aspartic acid (Asp). About 25 per cent of human factor IX contains Hya at this position, and the remainder contains Asp. In bovine factor IX, however, there is one equivalent of Hya in the first growth factor domain. Hya or the similarly modified β-hydroxyasparagine (Hyn) has been found at the same location within the first EGF-like domains of many vitamin K–dependent proteins, and also in EGF-like domains of many otherwise unrelated proteins, as discussed in Chapter 16. The function of Hya and Hyn in these proteins is not known. In the case of factor IX, the first EGF-like domain binds calcium ions, and the presence of Asp 64 is necessary for high-

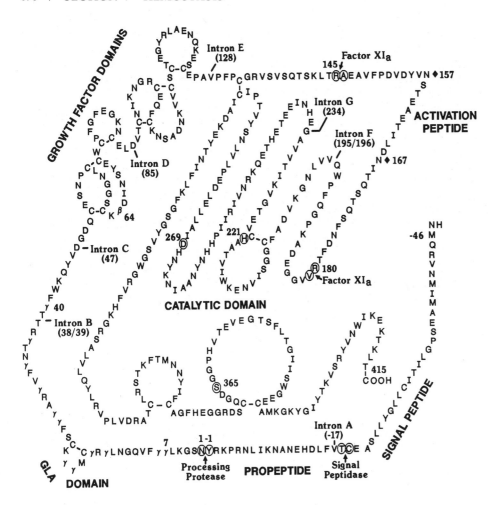

FIGURE 19–3. Structure of human profactor IX showing the location of the seven introns (A to G) of the factor IX gene. The factor IX precursor contains a 46 amino acid signal peptide and an 18 amino acid propeptide. The sites of cleavage by signal peptidase and a processing protease are indicated. The formation of factor IXa is due to the removal of an activation peptide following cleavage by factor XIa after Arg 145 and Arg 180. The amino acid residues of the catalytic triad, His 221, Asp 269, and Ser 365, are circled. The single-letter code for amino acids is used, plus γ for γ-carboxyglutamic acid and β for β-hydroxyaspartic acid. (Modified with permission from Yoshitake, S., et al.: Nucleotide sequence of the gene for human factor IX [antihemophilic factor B]. Biochemistry 24:3736, 1985. Copyright 1985, American Chemical Society.)

affinity binding; however, modification of Asp 64 to Hya is not required.[235, 245]

The activation peptide domain of factor IX contains 35 residues and is the least conserved domain among serine proteases. Variations in this region presumably allow the selective activation of these enzymes by proteases that recognize a specific amino acid sequence. Factor XIa cleaves factor IX at two sites in this region, after Arg 145 and Arg 180 (Fig. 19–3). Only the cleavage at the second site, however, results in expression of factor IXa catalytic activity. The sequence surrounding this arginine residue is the only highly conserved sequence in this domain among serine protease zymogens.

The catalytic domain of factor IX is a typical serine protease, and, like trypsin, the active site of factor IXa contains a catalytic triad composed of His 221, Asp 269, and Ser 365 (Fig. 19–3). The amino acid sequence surrounding these active site residues is highly conserved among this family of enzymes. As in trypsin, an acidic residue, Asp 359, is located in the bottom of the substrate-binding pocket and results in specificity for cleavage at basic amino acid residues. Many of the serine protease zymogens share a common mechanism of proteolytic activation. Cleavage of the Arg—Val bond after Arg 180 in the activation peptide of factor IX allows the new amino-terminal Val residue to

interact with Asp 364, which is adjacent to the active site Ser. This interaction causes a conformational change in the protein, increasing its catalytic activity.[246] Within the serine protease family, the similarities in protein structure and function are mirrored by features of gene organization, as discussed in Molecular Biology of Factor IX (page 672).

Biosynthesis and Metabolism of Factor IX

Factor IX is synthesized primarily in the liver.[230] In common with other secreted proteins, the initial factor IX translation product contains an amino-terminal extension that is present as a preproleader sequence containing 46 (or 41 or 39) amino acids. The prepeptide or signal peptide is cleaved during translation between amino acid residues −18 and −19 by a specific signal peptidase in the rough endoplasmic reticulum. Further proteolytic processing to remove the 18-amino acid propeptide generates the mature polypeptide found in plasma with amino-terminal tyrosine.

The factor IX propeptide functions as a recognition element for the vitamin K–dependent carboxylase, which catalyzes the conversion of glutamic acid residues to Gla. Certain features of the factor IX propeptide sequence are highly conserved among the vitamin K–dependent clotting factors and appear to be required for efficient carboxylation. These include amino acid residues Val −16, Ala −10, and (less dramatically) Leu −6.[247, 248] Additional conserved residues are required for efficient cleavage of the propeptide, and these include Arg −1,[249] Arg −4,[250] and also Leu −6.[248] The propeptide, therefore, may contain two independent, although possibly overlapping, recognition motifs: a region near the amino-terminus for the carboxylase and a region near the carboxyl-terminus for the propeptide processing protease.

The post-translational synthesis of β-hydroxyaspartic acid is independent of γ-carboxylation, because neither deletion of the factor IX propeptide nor inhibition of carboxylation by warfarin can prevent the hydroxylation of Asp 64 in the first growth factor domain.[251] On the basis of the alignment of EGF-like repeats that contain hydroxylated aspartic acid or asparagine residues, a consensus sequence has been proposed for the recognition of potential substrates by the hydroxylating machinery.[252] The hydroxylation reaction appears to be catalyzed by a 2-ketoglutarate–dependent dioxygenase.[253] Factor IX synthesized in the presence of suitable dioxygenase inhibitors does not contain β-hydroxyaspartic acid but nevertheless appears to have normal Gla content, blood-clotting activity, and cell-binding activity.[254] The function of Hya 64 remains, therefore, unknown.

Infusion of ^{125}I-labeled factor IX into patients with hemophilia B[255] shows a rapid initial clearance of factor IX with a t½ of approximately 50 minutes, consistent with distribution of the infused protein into a space approximately three times larger than the plasma volume. The rapid clearance phase is followed by slower disappearance, with a t½ of 24 to 30 hours for factor IX activity as seen in nonhemophilic patients who receive large doses of warfarin.[255] Unlabeled factor IX clearance in patients with hemophilia B shows a similar pattern.[256] Thus, these values may reflect the normal metabolism of factor IX, suggesting a daily turnover of 120 to 180 μg factor IX/kg body weight.

Biological Function of Factor IX

The interactions of factor IX in the intrinsic factor X–activating complex, in solution, and on cell surfaces are discussed in the preceding corresponding section for factor VIII.

The Role of Factor IXa in the Intrinsic Factor X–Activating Complex

Activated factor IXa specifically cleaves the heavy chain of factor X, generating factor Xa (see Fig. 19–2). The same site is cleaved during activation of factor X by the factor VIIa–tissue factor complex or by a Russell's viper venom protease, RVV-X. Factor Xa appears to be able to autocatalytically cleave this site as well, although this reaction is extremely slow and probably insignificant in vivo. However, in the absence of the cofactors, factor VIII, and tissue factor, the rate of autoactivation of factor X may be comparable to that of cleavage by factor IXa or factor VIIa.[257]

The K_m of factor IXa for its substrate, factor X, is lowered more than 5000-fold in the presence of both calcium ions and a suitable phospholipid surface (see Table 19–1). The addition of factor VIIIa causes little change in the K_m of the reaction but accelerates the (V_{max}) by a factor of more than 20,000. Thus, the complete factor X–activating complex, composed of factor IXa, factor VIIIa, phospholipid, and calcium, can activate factor X at a rate more than 10^9 times that of factor IXa alone, as shown with bovine reagents.[96] Under most conditions, the activation of factor X by this mechanism appears to be absolutely dependent on both factor VIIIa and factor IXa. Thus, it is not surprising that hemophilia A and hemophilia B are clinically indistinguishable.[257]

Proteolytic Activation of Factor IX

During activation of factor IX by limited proteolysis, two peptide bonds are cleaved, as shown in Figure 19–4. There are two possible routes to the final factor IXa product, but only one path appears to have a significant rate. When factor IX is activated by factor XIa or factor VIIa–tissue factor, the Arg 145—Ala bond is cleaved rapidly, generating a two-chain form of factor IX that is catalytically inactive and called factor IXα. The rate-limiting step in factor IX activation by either protease is the conversion of factor IXα to factor IXaβ by cleavage after Arg 180 in the activation peptide.[258, 259] The RVV-X protease from Russell's viper venom produces factor IXaα by cleaving only the Arg 180—Val bond. Activation of factor IX by either factor XIa or RVV-X requires the presence of divalent cations, such as calcium, which apparently interact in a complex manner with several metal-binding sites on factor IX.[260] High concentrations of factor Xa can apparently cleave factor IX at both sites, although so slowly that feedback activation of factor IX by factor Xa is not likely to be important in vivo.[261]

The two activated enzymes, factor IXaα and factor IXaβ, do not have equivalent coagulant properties. Although both have similar activity toward small synthetic substrates,[262] factor IXaα seems to interact with phospholipid less effectively than factor IXaβ. As a result, factor IXaα is far less active than factor IXaβ for the activation of factor X in a reaction containing factor VIIIa, calcium ions, and phospholipid.[257]

Whether factor VIIa or factor XIa is the most important activator of factor IX in vivo remains unknown. The kinetics of human factor IX activation by factor XIa and factor VIIa–tissue factor have been studied extensively in vitro,[259, 262–266] but detailed comparisons among studies are difficult because of methodological differences, and the results do not clearly show that activation by either mechanism is preferred. The plasma concentration of the substrate, factor IX, is well below the K_m for activation by either factor XIa

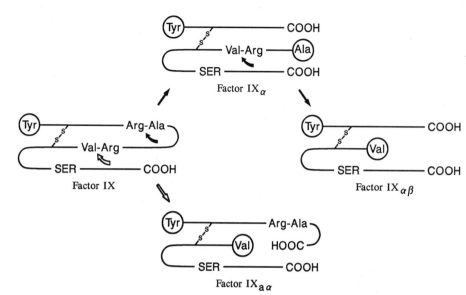

FIGURE 19–4. Proteolytic activation of factor IX. Amino-terminal residues of the heavy and light chains are shown in circles, and the active site serine residue is shown in large caps. The two polypeptide chains of factor IXa, factor IXaα and factor IXaβ, are joined by at least one disulfide bond. The reactions of the upper pathway are catalyzed either by factor XIa or by the factor VIIa–tissue factor complex in the presence of calcium ions. The reaction of the lower pathway is catalyzed by the RVV-X protease of Russell's viper venom, which cleaves the peptide bond indicated by the open curved arrow. (Adapted from Lindquist, P.A., et al.: Activation of bovine factor IX [Christmas factor] by factor XIa [activated plasma thromboplastin antecedent] and a protease from Russell's viper venom. J. Biol. Chem. 253:1902, 1978; with permission.)

(0.5 to 2 μM) or factor VIIa (0.25 to 0.54 μM), as determined in vitro. The concentration of circulating factor IX activation peptide in vivo is markedly reduced in congenital factor VII deficiency, but not in factor XI deficiency, suggesting that activation by factor VIIa–tissue factor is physiologically important.[267]

Inactivation of Factor IXa

The rate of clearance of factor IXa in humans has not been determined with precision. In mice, human factor IXa disappears from the circulation in a biphasic manner. Initially, there is rapid clearance of about 60 per cent of the injected dose in less than 5 minutes, perhaps reflecting rapid binding of factor IXa to endothelial cell receptors. The remaining factor IXa is cleared with a t½ similar to that of factor IX, which is about 24 hours in humans. However, within 2 minutes after injection, more than half of the circulating factor IXa is complexed to antithrombin III. These data indicate that the half-life of free, enzymatically active factor IXa is extremely short. Antithrombin III–factor IXa complexes are cleared primarily by the liver, through a receptor that apparently also binds to α1-antitrypsin–protease complexes.[268] In human plasma in vitro, factor IXa is rapidly inactivated by antithrombin III, and this reaction is markedly accelerated by heparin.[269] Among other plasma protease inhibitors, α1-antitrypsin and α2-macroglobulin do not react with factor IXa.[268] Binding of factor IXa to activated platelets appears to protect against inactivation by antithrombin III–heparin, whereas binding to phospholipid vesicles does not.[270]

Molecular Biology of Factor IX

The factor IX gene is located at the terminus of the long arm of the human X chromosome, closely linked to the q27.3 locus for the fragile-X mental retardation syndrome.[271, 272] In fact, the factor IX and factor VIII genes flank the fragile-X locus, with factor IX the more proximal of these loci.[120]

The factor IX gene (Fig. 19–5) is about 33.5 kb in length and consists of eight exons (I to VIII) separated by seven introns (A to G). The presumed promoter region does not have a classic TATA sequence in the usual position relative to the transcription initiation site, and the functional sequences in this region are not entirely clear.[273–275] The exons range in length from a very short 25 nucleotide (nt) (exon III) to a long 1935 nt (exon VIII). The introns range from 188 nt (intron B) to 9473 nt (intron F). The gene contains four *Alu* sequences, including one in intron A and three in intron F. A fifth *Alu* sequence is found immediately flanking the 3′ end of the gene. The positions of all seven introns within the coding sequence of the factor IX gene are similar to the seven introns of the genes for human protein C,[276] factor VII,[277] factor X,[278] and the first three introns of prothrombin.[231]

The introns divide the factor IX gene into regions that roughly correspond to structural or functional

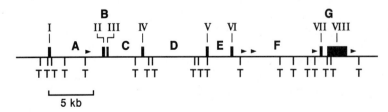

FIGURE 19–5. Map of the human factor IX gene. The region of the X chromosome containing the gene is represented. The scale is in kilobases of DNA. Exons are numbered (I to VIII), and introns are designated by letter (A to G). The location and orientation of *Alu* repeats are shown by arrowheads (▶). The location of restriction sites cleaved by *Taq*I are shown by T.

domains of the protein. Most of the hydrophobic signal sequence of factor IX is encoded by the first exon (see Fig. 19–3). However, cleavage sites for proteolytic processing are encoded by the second exon, which also encodes 11 of the 12 Glu residues that become carboxylated to Gla in the mature factor IX molecule. The twelfth Gla residue occurs in the 8 amino acid segment encoded by exon III.

The two growth factor domains of factor IX (and factor VII, factor X, and protein C) are each encoded by a single exon, which is compatible with the evolution of this region by tandem duplication of an ancestral gene segment that is in turn related to the gene for EGF. In fact, each homologous growth factor–like repeat of tissue plasminogen activator,[279] urokinase,[280] factor XII,[281] the EGF precursor, and the LDL receptor is also encoded by a single exon.[282]

The activation peptide domain, encompassing both factor XIa cleavage sites, is encoded by a single exon (exon VI), and the protease domain is encoded by two exons (VII and VIII). Exon VII contains the active site His 221, and exon VIII contains the remaining active site residues, Asp 269 and Ser 365. In contrast, many related serine protease genes possess a separate exon for each active site residue, including the genes for prothrombin,[231, 283] tissue plasminogen activator,[279] and trypsinogen,[284] among others. Furthermore, the positions of the other introns in the protease domain of the factor IX gene are frequently displaced relative to the corresponding introns in other genes within this family. Thus, introns appear to have been moved around and occasionally added to (or removed from) the factor IX gene during the evolution of the serine proteases.

Hemophilia B (Factor IX Deficiency)

Clinical Features of Hemophilia B

The X-linked inheritance of factor IX deficiency, or hemophilia B, is 10 to 20 per cent as common as hemophilia A, with a prevalence of 15 to 20 per million persons.[124] As in hemophilia A, the residual activity of factor IX in hemophilia B varies among affected kindreds, and the disease is classified as severe (<1 per cent), moderate (1 to 5 per cent), or mild (6 to 30 per cent), based on the per cent of normal factor IX activity assayed in the patient's plasma. About 80 per cent of affected kindreds have severe, 5 per cent have moderate, and 15 per cent have mild disease. As previously mentioned, the symptoms and clinical course of hemophilia B and hemophilia A are indistinguishable.

Replacement therapy for hemophilia B is similar in principle to that for hemophilia A. Antibodies to factor IX develop in less than 1 per cent of all treated patients with hemophilia B, or 2.5 per cent of those with severe disease.[285] For unknown reasons, the incidence of such inhibitors is much lower in hemophilia B than in hemophilia A.

Classification and Molecular Defects in Hemophilia B

As in hemophilia A, patients with hemophilia B can be divided into several immunologically defined groups. More than 50 per cent have no detectable factor IX antigen and are termed cross-reacting material negative (CRM− or hemophilia B−). The remaining patients possess some protein that can be recognized by one or more antibodies to normal factor IX and are therefore CRM+ or hemophilia B+. Both CRM+ and CRM− groups can be further subdivided, indicating that a wide variety of genetic lesions can produce factor IX deficiency. More than 230 different mutations causing hemophilia B have been characterized at the level of DNA sequence, and these provide insight into the mechanisms underlying spontaneous mutation, as well as the pathophysiology of hemophilia B. These mutations have been collected in a data base that is continuously updated.[286] Mutations have been identified in every class of gene structural element except for the poly(A) addition site. The known distinct factor IX mutations now outnumber those for either the thalassemias or the hemoglobinopathies.

Mutations causing severe CRM− hemophilia B tend to be caused by large gene deletions, frameshift mutations, splice site mutations, and nonsense mutations (causing premature termination of translation). The inability to synthesize part or all of the factor IX polypeptide appears to be associated with an increased risk for the development of factor IX inhibitors, probably because the appropriate epitopes are not expressed to establish tolerance. At least 29 patients with large partial or total gene deletions have been reported, among whom 15 have developed inhibitors.[287] Among patients with characterized frameshift, splice site, and nonsense mutations, inhibitors have been identified relatively frequently.[286] Among nearly 300 patients with known missense mutations, only 2 patients were found to have inhibitors[287, 288]; only 1 of these was CRM+.[288]

Among patients with CRM+ hemophilia B, a small minority (~5 per cent) shows an equal decrement of factor IX activity and antigen, and these variants are sometimes referred to as CRMred. This phenotype may be due to mutations that decrease the synthesis of an otherwise normal factor IX[289]; decreased factor IX secretion or increased catabolism are alternative mechanisms. Hemophilia B Leyden is an unusual CRMred variant in which the plasma level of factor IX is not stable. Affected males begin life with undetectable factor IX activity and antigen, and they suffer from typical spontaneous bleeding. Around the onset of puberty, factor IX levels begin to rise at 4 to 5 per cent per year, with subsequent cessation of bleeding. By adulthood, the factor IX level may be 20 to 60 per cent of normal, and the protein appears to be normal.[290] The mutations associated with the hemophilia B Leyden phenotype cluster within nucleotides −20 to +13, around a major transcription initiation site.[286] These mutations appear to cause abnormal developmental regulation of factor IX expression, although the mechanism of this effect is not known. Some of these mutations disrupt a functional binding site for CCAAT/enhancer-binding protein (C/EBP), between nucleotides +1 and +18.[291]

Most CRM+ patients have excess factor IX antigen, indicating that they produce a functionally defective factor IX. The characterization of these mutations has provided substantial information regarding the structure-function relationships of factor IX.

Propeptide cleavage is prevented by mutations at Arg −4 or Arg −1. These mutations result in moderate to severe hemophilia B, with mildly decreased to normal factor IX antigen levels. The presence of the uncleaved propeptide appears to interfere with the γ-carboxylation[249, 292] or function[250] of the adjacent Gla domain.

Several mutations within the Gla domain that interfere with calcium binding or function of this domain have been described.[286] Factor IX Zutphen contains an interesting mutation in this region, Cys 18 → Arg, that prevents the formation of the normal disulfide bond between Cys 18 and Cys 23.[286] The mutant protein circulates in the blood at normal antigen levels, with an uncharacterized peptide disulfide bonded probably to Cys 23.[293]

Mutations within the growth factor domains of factor IX often cause hemophilia B+ of varying severity; a few such mutations appear to cause equal decreases in factor IX antigen and activity (CRMred). In general, the mechanism by which mutations in these domains cause hemophilia B is not known, although several mutations in domain EGF-1 are suggested to alter either the binding of calcium ions or an important calcium-dependent protein conformation. Mutagenesis studies demonstrate that conserved residues Asp 47, Asp 49, Gln 50, Asp 64, and Tyr 69 contribute to high-affinity calcium ion binding by domain EGF-1[245]; except for Asp 49, substitutions have been identified at each of these residues in patients with hemophilia B.[286] The effect of mutations on calcium ion binding is not always predictable, however. The mutation Asp 47 → Glu causes severe hemophilia B[294] and moderately reduces the affinity of domain EGF-1 for calcium ions.[245] In contrast, the mutation Asp 47 → Gly causes mild hemophilia B but does not alter the affinity of calcium ion binding, and it is proposed to affect indirectly the interaction of factor IXa with factor VIIIa or factor X.[295]

Mutations within the activation peptide region confirm the importance for factor IX function of proteolytic cleavage after both Arg 145 and Arg 180. The substitution Arg 145 → His, first described in factor IX Chapel Hill,[296, 297] yields a protein that is activated slowly by factor XIa to a species resembling factor IXaα. Factor IX Chapel Hill has ~8 per cent of normal coagulant activity, and after activation to factor IXaα it has 20 to 33 per cent specific clotting activity compared with normal factor IXaβ.

Several mutations have been described that inhibit or prevent cleavage of the Arg 180–Val bond. These include Arg 180 → Gln, Arg 180 → Trp, Val 181 → Phe, Val 182 → Phe, and Val 182 → Leu.[286] Patients with these mutations have a surprising laboratory phenotype, referred to as hemophilia B$_M$. This variant was reported in 1967 by Hougie and Twomey,[298] who described two brothers with hemophilia B who had normal prothrombin times using human (or rabbit) brain thromboplastin as the source of tissue factor, but markedly prolonged prothrombin times using ox brain thromboplastin. Normal factor IX at similar concentrations does not prolong the ox brain prothrombin time. The variant was called hemophilia B$_M$, after the family name of the index cases—Murphy. This case provided the first evidence for heterogeneity in hemophilia B+, and ~10 per cent of hemophilia B+ can be classified as hemophilia B$_M$.[289, 299]

Several mutations in the catalytic domain of factor IX that destroy catalytic activity also prolong the ox brain prothrombin time and cause hemophilia B$_M$, indicating that this phenotype is genotypically rather heterogeneous. A common mechanism may explain the similar effects of these disparate mutations: The catalytically inactive abnormal factor appears to inhibit competitively the activation of factor X by the (human) factor VIIa–(ox brain) tissue factor complex.[300, 301]

Prenatal Diagnosis and Carrier Detection in Hemophilia B

The detection of female carriers of hemophilia B has many problems in common with the detection of carriers of hemophilia A, previously discussed. On the basis of assays of plasma factor IX alone, even the best statistical methods misclassify a fraction of prospective mothers.[158, 159] Prenatal diagnosis by fetoscopy has been successful but is complicated by the relatively low levels of factor IX even in normal fetal blood.[302]

Reliable genotype assignment for potential carriers and for prenatal diagnosis generally is accomplished by methods based upon detection of DNA sequence variations. The available marker systems include both intragenic and linked extragenic DNA sequence polymorphisms.[151] Strong linkage disequilibrium limits the utility of some of these polymorphisms. Certain polymorphisms show striking variations in frequency among ethnic groups, and the optimal choices among marker systems must take this into account. For an increasing number of patients, however, the precise molecular defect is known and can be detected directly; this permits unambiguous prenatal diagnosis and identification of carriers, without the need to identify informative matings in the pedigree. Methods employing the PCR permit rapid prenatal diagnosis of hemophilia B by amniocentesis[146] or biopsy of chorionic villi,[145] with less risk than is associated with fetoscopy.

Treatment of Hemophilia B

PCCs are widely used for the treatment of bleeding in hemophilia B. As discussed under Treatment of

Hemophilia A (page 666), these preparations contain a mixture of partially purified vitamin K–dependent blood clotting factors. PCCs are prepared with one or more virucidal treatments and do not appear to transmit HIV; the risk of transmission of viral hepatitis B and C also appears to be markedly reduced.[303–305] Treatment of hemophilia with PCCs has been associated with thrombotic complications, however, including myocardial infarction,[306] venous thrombosis,[213] and disseminated intravascular coagulation.[307] The pathophysiology of these complications is not known with certainty but may depend on the presence of large amounts of activated clotting factors or phospholipids. Highly purified factor IX concentrates containing very low concentrations of contaminating clotting factors recently have become available. Preliminary clinical studies suggest that these preparations have markedly decreased thrombogenicity compared with PCCs.[308, 309]

As for hemophilia A, recombinant DNA technology could provide a product for the treatment of hemophilia B that is free of the potential risks associated with human plasma derivatives. Active recombinant factor IX has been expressed in mammalian cell culture systems[310–312] and in transgenic animals.[313, 314] Factor IX activity depends on the carboxylation of glutamic acid to give 12 Gla residues in the amino-terminal Gla domain (see Fig. 19–3), but recombinant factor IX expressed in cultured mammalian cells often is incompletely carboxylated. Thus, an efficient factor IX expression system that correctly and quantitatively performs this modification is necessary before recombinant factor IX can become a practical therapeutic product.

The development of a factor IX inhibitor is rare in hemophilia B but can be an extremely serious problem. As discussed under Treatment of Hemophilia A, factor VIIa is effective for the treatment of bleeding in patients with factor VIII inhibitors. Recent experience in hemophilia B suggests that factor VIIa may be useful to circumvent factor IX inhibitors as well.[315]

Definitive correction of hemophilia B could be achieved, in principle, by the introduction of an active normal factor IX gene into some tissue of the patient. Hemophilia B is an attractive model disease for the development of such somatic cell gene therapy, because relatively modest levels of factor IX expression would significantly ameliorate bleeding symptoms, and organ-specific targeting of gene expression may not be required. Preliminary steps toward this goal have been achieved, including the expression of human factor IX by retroviral transduction of hepatocytes,[316] skin fibroblasts,[317, 318] and capillary endothelial cells.[319] Transient production of detectable human factor IX in blood plasma has been achieved by transplantation of transduced cells into mice and rats.[317, 318]

VON WILLEBRAND FACTOR AND VON WILLEBRAND DISEASE

In 1926, Eric von Willebrand described a bleeding disorder that differed from hemophilia by having an autosomal dominant mode of inheritance, a prolonged skin bleeding time, a normal platelet count, and severe mucocutaneous bleeding rather than spontaneous deep tissue bleeding.[320, 321] Von Willebrand and subsequent workers considered this to be a platelet or vessel wall disorder until 1953, when patients with von Willebrand disease were discovered to have reduced factor VIII activity, suggesting a plasma abnormality.[322–324] Subsequent transfusion studies confirmed that a factor in either normal or hemophilic plasma could correct the bleeding time in vWD.[325, 326] Thus, as in the hemophilias, vWF was first recognized through its absence in an inherited bleeding disease.

Purification and Structural Characterization of von Willebrand Factor

Assays for von Willebrand Factor

The first in vitro assay for vWF activity, described in 1963,[327, 328] was based on the retention of platelets by glass beads. In blood of normal individuals, most of the platelets adhere to glass, whereas in blood of patients with vWD only a small fraction adhere. This defect can be corrected by the addition of normal plasma. The glass bead retention assay is technically cumbersome, extremely sensitive to variations in technique, and not specific for vWF. Nevertheless, it was useful in the diagnosis of vWD and was the basis for the first documented purification of vWF in 1972.[329]

A more practical assay was developed in 1971, when Howard and Firkin discovered that the antibiotic ristocetin caused platelet aggregation in normal platelet-rich plasma but not in that from patients with vWD.[330] Normal vWF is now routinely assayed by measuring the ristocetin-induced aggregation of platelets. Ristocetin cofactor activity (vWF:RiCoF) is assayed by mixing a suitably diluted plasma sample, washed platelets (usually formalin-fixed), and a standard concentration of ristocetin. Platelet agglutination is followed by measuring the increase in light transmission through the platelet suspension as a function of time, and the slopes obtained are compared with those for dilutions of a reference plasma standard. One *unit* of ristocetin cofactor activity is the amount in 1 ml of normal plasma, and the sensitivity of this assay is approximately 0.03 U/ml.[331] In a variation of this principle, the ristocetin-induced platelet aggregation (RIPA) assay employs patient platelet-rich plasma; the rate and extent of platelet aggregation are determined at different concentrations of added ristocetin and compared with values obtained with normal platelet-rich plasma.

A component with similar platelet-aggregating activity has been identified in the venom of snakes belonging to the *Bothrops* genus, particularly *B. jararaca*.[332] This factor, termed *botrocetin*, acts by a different mechanism than ristocetin but can be used in similar assays of botrocetin cofactor activity (vWF:BoCoF).[333] In certain variants of vWD, either RIPA, vWF:RiCoF, or vWF:BoCoF may be paradoxically increased (see von Willebrand Disease, page 681).

Several immunoassay methods are commonly employed to quantitate vWF antigen (vWF:Ag). The Laurell rocket method can detect 0.01 to 0.03 U/ml of vWF, and a modification with ^{125}I-labeled antibody is 100-fold more sensitive.[334] Immunoassays using radiometric[335, 336] or enzymatic detection have been described with sensitivities of 0.002 to ~0.0002 U/ml.

For the assessment of the multimeric composition of vWF, two electrophoretic methods are commonly used. Crossed immunoelectrophoresis provides a qualitative assay of multimer distribution. A sample of plasma is electrophoresed through a strip of agarose to separate the multimers by size. The vWF is then detected by electrophoresis in a direction perpendicular to the first dimension, driving the proteins into a second agarose gel that contains anti-vWF antibody. The precipitin arc that forms is then a record of the separation achieved during electrophoresis in the first dimension. In most variants of vWD type II, the larger multimers that migrate more slowly are absent and the precipitin arc is displaced toward the anode.[337]

Precise information about multimer distribution in either plasma or platelets can be obtained by electrophoresis through agarose or agarose/acrylamide copolymer gels in the presence of the detergent sodium dodecyl sulfate (SDS). The separated vWF multimers are visualized by reaction with either ^{125}I-labeled antibody to vWF followed by autoradiography,[338–340] or by immunoenzymatic methods. The patterns observed for normal plasma and for several variants of vWD are shown in Figure 19–6.

Assays of vWF binding to collagen and to heparin have been described but are not widely used in clinical laboratories. Assays of factor VIII–vWF binding have identified several patients with defects in this interaction. Such patients can have symptomatic factor VIII deficiency, as discussed under von Willebrand Disease Normandy (page 684).

Purification of von Willebrand Factor

Factor VIII and vWF copurify through many different manipulations. Consequently, purification methods for these two proteins are quite similar. In most procedures, factor VIII and vWF are concentrated by cryoprecipitation and are copurified further by gel filtration chromatography on a 2 to 6 per cent agarose matrix. Both proteins co-elute in the void volume. If desired, factor VIII can be removed by rechromatography in 0.5 M $CaCl_2$.[341] Additional chromatography steps are required to remove contaminating fibrinogen and fibronectin. In this fashion, vWF can be purified from plasma about 10,000-fold to near homogeneity, in 50 per cent yield, with a specific activity of 150 to 200 vWF:Ag U/mg and ~110 vWF:RiCoF U/mg.[341]

Structure of von Willebrand Factor

Von Willebrand factor consists predominantly of a single type of subunit with an M_r of about 250,000.

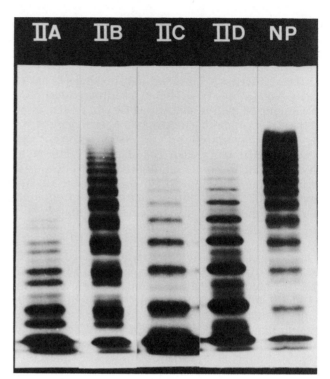

FIGURE 19–6. Sodium dodecyl sulfate (SDS)–agarose gel electrophoresis of human von Willebrand factor (vWF). Normal plasma (NP) and plasma from patients with von Willebrand disease (vWD) types IIA, IIB, IIC, and IID were electrophoresed in agarose gels. The vWF multimers were labeled by incubating the gel with ^{125}I–anti-vWF and visualized by autoradiography. The repeating triplet structure of normal vWF multimers is clearly visible. In type I disease, the pattern is normal, but the quantity of vWF is reduced. Type II variants typically lack large multimers and are distinguished by characteristic abnormal patterns. (Courtesy of Z.M. Ruggeri, from Holmberg, L., and Nilsson, I. M.: Von Willebrand disease. Clin. Haematol. 14:461, 1985; with permission.)

Minor components with lower molecular weight (mainly M_r 189,000, 176,000, 140,000, and 120,000) are present that are proteolytic fragments of the M_r 250,000 subunit.[341, 342]

Multimers of vWF differ in size by a constant number of subunits. This basic repeating unit is a dimer of M_r 250,000 subunits.[342–344] High-resolution electrophoresis methods show that each multimer of plasma vWF consists of a major band associated with several discrete but faint "satellite" bands; this heterogeneity appears to be due mostly to proteolytic degradation during circulation of vWF in the blood.[341, 342]

The vWF primary translation product is a precursor protein of 2813 amino acid residues (M_r ~360,000) that consists of a 22 amino acid signal peptide, a 741 amino acid (M_r ~95,000) propeptide, and the 2050 amino acid (M_r ~250,000) mature subunit (reviewed in Sadler[345]). The propeptide is also known as von Willebrand antigen II,[346] and it circulates in blood independently of vWF, possibly as a noncovalently associated homodimer.[347, 348] The amino acid residues of the prepropeptide region and the mature subunit are often numbered separately. The vWF precursor contains four types of repeated domain (A to D) that together account for more than 90 per cent of the sequence (Fig. 19–7).[345]

The amino acid composition of vWF is remarkable for the high percentage of half-cystine residues.[14, 349] These are clustered predominantly in two regions near the amino-terminus and carboxy-terminus of the subunit. The pairing of 52 half-cystine residues has been reported.[350] Dimers of vWF subunits contain interchain disulfide bonds between some of the 16 cysteine residues in the carboxyl-terminal 150 amino acid residues. Multimers are formed by interchain disulfide bonds involving some of the 3 cysteines between amino acids 459 and 464.

Von Willebrand factor contains ~15 to 19 per cent carbohydrate distributed among both Asn-linked and Thr/Ser-linked oligosaccharides.[351] At least five Asn-linked structures are present. One, constituting 60 per cent of the total N-linked carbohydrate, has been fully characterized. It is a typical biantennary structure similar to those found in other plasma glycoproteins.[352] Ten Thr/Ser- and 12 Asn-glycosylation sites have been identified in the mature vWF subunit[349] (see Fig. 19–7). Additional N-linked oligosaccharides may be attached to the four potential glycosylation sites in the propeptide.

Sulfate is a constituent of some vWF N-linked oligosaccharides, possibly restricted to those at Asn 384 and Asn 468 of the mature subunit. Additional sulfate is found on N-linked oligosaccharides of the propeptide.[353]

Von Willebrand factor in solution is extremely asymmetrical.[41] Electron micrographs show that vWF consists of long, flexible filaments containing small, regularly spaced nodules. The filaments range in length from 50 to 1150 nm, with a mean diameter of 2.5 nm[354] (Fig. 19–8).

Biosynthesis and Metabolism of von Willebrand Factor

Von Willebrand factor is synthesized by endothelial cells[355, 356] and also by megakaryocytes.[357] By immunochemical staining it is localized to endothelial cells, subendothelial connective tissue,[358, 359] syncytiotrophoblast of placenta,[360] and platelet α granules.[361] In severe vWD, both platelet and endothelial cell vWF is absent.[362–364] Transfusion studies in severe vWD suggest that there is no significant movement of plasma vWF into the subendothelium of intact blood vessels or into platelets.[193, 362] Thus, the observed tissue localization probably reflects local synthesis rather than absorption from plasma. Histochemical methods for the localization of vWF have been useful in the identification of endothelial cells and platelet precursors in normal and malignant tissues.

The biosynthesis of vWF is a complex process. In the endoplasmic reticulum, the signal peptide is cleaved from the primary translation product, N-linked glycosylation is initiated, and monomeric pro-vWF species rapidly form disulfide-bonded dimers. These pro-vWF dimers have free sulfhydryl groups

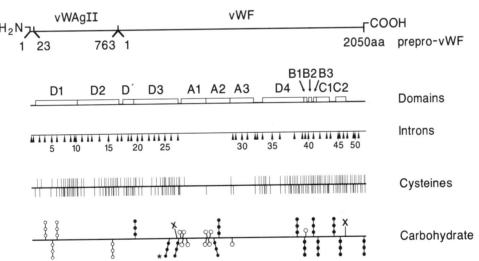

FIGURE 19–7. Structure of the human vWF precursor. *Prepro-vWF:* The signal peptide (SP) or prepeptide, the von Willebrand antigen II propeptide (vWAgII), and the mature subunit (vWF) are indicated. Amino acid residues in the prepropeptide are numbered consecutively 1 to 763; residues 1 to 22 are the signal peptide, and residues 23 to 763 are the propeptide. Amino acid residues (aa) in the mature subunit are separately numbered 1 to 2050. *Domains:* The repeated domains are labeled *D1, D2, D', D3, A1, A2, A3, D4, B1, B2, B3, C1,* and *C2. Introns:* The locations in the amino acid sequence of the 51 vWF introns are indicated by arrowheads. Every fifth intron is numbered. *Cysteines:* In regions of especially high cysteine content, one mark may represent more than 1 cysteine residue. Carbohydrate: Potential sites of N-glycosylation are indicated by open circles (ooo). N-glycosylation sites shown to be utilized are indicated by filled circles (●●●), and two potential sites that are not utilized are indicated by x. One site of N-glycosylation labeled with an asterisk (*) occurs in the sequence Asn-Ser-Cys. Sites of O-glycosylation are indicated by single open circles (o). (From Sadler, J. E.: Von Willebrand factor. J. Biol. Chem. 266:22777, 1991; with permission of the American Society for Biochemistry and Molecular Biology.)

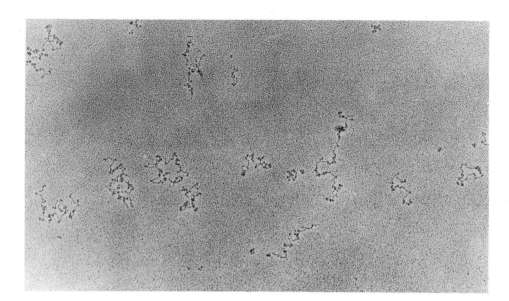

FIGURE 19–8. Rotary-shadowed electron micrograph of human vWF. The magnification is ×110,000. (From Ohmori, K., et al.: Electron microscopy of human factor VIII/ von Willebrand glycoprotein: Effect of reducing reagents on structure and function. Reproduced from the *Journal of Cell Biology*, 1982, Vol. 95, p. 632, by copyright permission of the Rockefeller University Press.)

that form disulfide bonds between dimers after transit to the Golgi apparatus.[365] vWF is the only protein known to form interchain disulfide bonds in such a "late" compartment, outside of the endoplasmic reticulum (reviewed in Wagner[366]).

Assembly into multimers coincides approximately with cleavage of the propeptide.[344, 365] This cleavage appears to be performed by a specific enzyme that cleaves after paired basic amino acid residues and is homologous to the family of subtilisin-like serine proteases.[367, 368] All vWF species except the intracellular dimer and monomer consist primarily of M_r ~250,000 subunits with only a few per cent of pro-vWF polypeptides. The final processing of complex-type *N*-linked oligosaccharides (including sulfation of some structures) and additional Ser/Thr-linked glycosylation also occur in the Golgi apparatus.[366]

Mature intracellular vWF is stored in subcellular organelles that are unique to endothelium, Weibel-Palade bodies (Fig. 19–9). These are elongated 0.1 × 2 to 3 μm vesicles with longitudinal striations that appear to be closely packed multimers of vWF. These organelles appear to be derived from the Golgi apparatus. Whether they participate actively in the assembly of vWF or are simply for storage is unknown.[369, 370] The propeptide may be required for targeting of vWF to the Weibel-Palade body[371]; the cleaved propeptide is packaged in this organelle together with vWF multimers, with a stoichiometry of one propeptide per mature subunit.[348]

Two pathways have been identified for vWF release from cultured endothelial cells. For convenience, these can be called the "constitutive" and the "regulated" pathways.[366] Constitutive secretion requires continuing protein synthesis and is not dependent on extracellular calcium ions or intracellular cyclic AMP levels.[372] In cultured endothelial cells, the majority of vWF is secreted constitutively and consists mainly of dimers and small multimers.[373]

Regulated secretion of vWF is stimulated by treatment of endothelial cells with either thrombin,[374] histamine,[375] fibrin,[376] complement proteins C5b-9,[377] the calcium ionophore A23187, or the tumor promoter phorbol myristate acetate (PMA).[372] vWF secreted by the regulated pathway consists of very large multimers and is associated with depletion of the Wiebel-Palade bodies.[373] In contrast to constitutive secretion, regulated secretion of vWF does not require protein synthesis and does depend on extracellular calcium influx.[372, 373]

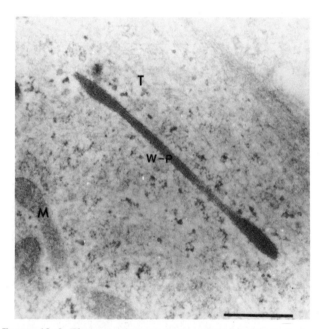

FIGURE 19–9. Electron micrograph of a Weibel-Palade body in a cultured human endothelial cell. The Weibel-Palade body (W-P) is 2 μm in length and shows typical longitudinal striations that readily distinguish it from mitochondria (M). The 25 nm microtubule (T) provides a convenient size comparison. The bar is 0.5 μm in length. (From Wagner, D.D., et al.: Immunolocalization of von Willebrand protein in Weibel-Palade bodies of human endothelial cells. Reproduced from the *Journal of Cell Biology*, 1982, Vol. 95, p. 355, by copyright permission of the Rockefeller University Press.)

Estrogen is reported to stimulate vWF synthesis, perhaps by affecting the constitutive mechanism. Some increase was detected at concentrations that occur during the normal menstrual cycle, pregnancy, and the administration of oral estrogens to postmenopausal women.[378] Consequently, this in vitro response may underlie the observed increase in vWF that occurs in pregnancy. A beneficial increase in vWF has been reported in some women with vWD following treatment with estrogens.[379, 380]

The plasma level of vWF antigen is about 10 μg/ml, but in normal individuals this level may range from 40 to 240 per cent of the mean.[381] Approximately 15 per cent of the total circulating protein is within platelets.[360] Plasma levels of vWF are significantly lower in persons of blood type O compared with all other ABO blood types, and this variation should be considered in the establishment and interpretation of normal ranges for the diagnosis of vWD. Additional smaller increases are correlated with age,[381] and variations may be associated with Lewis blood type (secretor status).[382]

A variety of physiological stresses are associated with transient changes in vWF and factor VIII levels. Most of these, such as exercise, trauma, or surgery, probably result from adrenergic stimulation. The vasopressin analogue, DDAVP, or growth hormone also causes an acute increase in plasma vWF, and the endogenous hormones may exert a similar influence in some diseases of the nervous system. Propranolol blocks the response to epinephrine but not to DDAVP, indicating that the DDAVP effect is not mediated by a β-adrenergic mechanism.[383] Sustained elevation of vWF or factor VIII has been noted in several chronic conditions, including pregnancy, oral estrogen therapy, hyperthyroidism, inflammatory states, renal disease, diabetes, cancer, liver disease, and atherosclerosis (reviewed by Bloom[187]).

The mechanism of vWF elevation is obscure in these conditions. The effect of epinephrine, which seems to be mediated by β₁ adrenoreceptors, is probably indirect, because cultured endothelium does not secrete vWF in response to epinephrine.[384] Similarly, DDAVP, 5-hydroxytryptamine, 2,3-DPG, cyclic AMP, thyroxine, corticosteroids, and growth hormone have no direct effect on the release of vWF from cultured endothelial cells.[384, 385]

Von Willebrand factor is removed from the circulation in a biphasic fashion. An initial rapid disappearance phase with an apparent half-time of ~4.5 hours is followed by slower clearance with a half-time of ~20 hours. These kinetics are observed in normal individuals as well as in patients with hemophilia A. In the latter group, the clearance of ¹²⁵I-labeled vWF parallels the clearance of factor VIII given as cryoprecipitate.[61] This is consistent with the observation that in vivo, vWF binds to factor VIII and protects it from catabolism.[60] The clearance of vWF depends to some extent on its multimeric state. Larger multimers (found in cryoprecipitate) disappear faster than do the dimer and small multimers (found in cryosuperna-

Biological Function of von Willebrand Factor

Von Willebrand factor has two well-characterized functions. It is a carrier in plasma for factor VIII, and it promotes platelet adhesion to damaged blood vessels.

Platelet adhesion can be observed and quantitated in vitro by perfusing a platelet suspension over a segment of blood vessel from which the endothelium has been removed.[386, 387] In this model system, platelet adhesion depends upon vWF in the perfusate. This is demonstrated most easily at high wall shear rates. At the lower shear rates characteristic of large veins and arteries, platelet adhesion is less dependent on vWF.[386–388] vWF already present in the subendothelium and that circulating in the perfusate both seem to be required for optimal platelet adhesion.[389, 390]

Von Willebrand factor acts as a bridge to connect two surfaces that otherwise may not interact—the platelet membrane and subendothelial connective tissue. Thus, the process of platelet adhesion to the blood vessel wall can be analyzed as two distinct binding interactions that imply separate protein functional domains and corresponding "receptors." The interactions of vWF with platelet membrane proteins are relatively well understood and are described in Chapter 22.

Interaction of von Willebrand Factor with the Vessel Wall

The primary physiological target for vWF in the subendothelium has not been identified with certainty. Indeed, there may be more than one. vWF, fibronectin, and collagen types III, IV, and V all seem to colocalize in the extracellular matrix.[391, 392] vWF binds to polymers of various purified collagens of types I, II, III, IV, V, and VI but not to denatured collagen (gelatin) or to elastin.[393–396] However, vWF appears to bind normally to extracellular matrix that is made deficient in fibrillar collagens either by digestion with collagenase or by treatment of cells with α, α'-dipyridyl, a collagen synthesis inhibitor.[391, 392] In addition, monoclonal antibodies to vWF have been identified that inhibit binding to collagen types I and III but not to subendothelial matrix. Conversely, monoclonal antibodies to vWF have been identified that inhibit binding to subendothelial matrix but not to fibrillar collagens.[397] Thus, some type of subendothelial collagen may be a receptor in vivo, but it may not be a fibrillar collagen. Collagen type VI is a logical candidate, because it contains large non-collagenous domains and is relatively resistant both to collagenase[398] and to α,α'-dipyridyl.[399]

Structure-Function Relationships of von Willebrand Factor

Von Willebrand factor has a number of binding functions and at least two types of intersubunit disulfide bonds. Furthermore, the degree of polymerization may influence the effectiveness of vWF both in vivo and in certain in vitro assays.

THE INFLUENCE OF MULTIMER SIZE ON VON WILLEBRAND FACTOR FUNCTION. Among the species present in plasma or concentrates, the vWF multimers that are the most active in ristocetin-induced platelet aggregation[400] and are preferentially adsorbed onto collagen[401] are composed of more than four or five dimers.[341] Furthermore, adhesion of platelets to subendothelium in perfusion chambers is promoted by the larger multimers in cryoprecipitate but not by the small multimers in commercial factor VIII concentrates.[402] Thus, for naturally occurring multimers, larger size correlates with higher binding activity, perhaps because of increased valency or steric constraints. However, the smaller multimers contain a higher proportion of proteolytic fragments of subunits than do larger multimers,[341] and this damage rather than small size per se may contribute to their decreased function. In this regard, it is interesting that small multimers can be derived from large multimers by partial reduction. These artificial small multimers appear to lose most of their ristocetin cofactor activity, but those with a minimal size of 2,000,000 daltons are reported to promote platelet adhesion to arterial subendothelium approximately as well as native vWF.[402] Thus, the relationship between the multimeric state, ristocetin cofactor activity, and function of vWF in hemostasis remains incompletely understood.

FUNCTIONAL DOMAINS OF THE VON WILLEBRAND FACTOR SUBUNIT. Binding sites on vWF for several macromolecules have been localized to discrete segments of the mature subunit polypeptide. In many cases, these binding sites appear to correlate with specific repeated domains (Fig. 19–10). The site that interacts with platelet GPIb is located between amino acid residues 449 and 728. A homodimeric tryptic fragment containing this sequence binds to platelet GPIb,[403, 404] and short segments within this fragment are proposed to mediate ristocetin-induced binding to platelet GPIb.[405] A smaller monomeric fragment that corresponds approximately to domain A1 (amino acid residues 480/481 to 718) binds to platelet GPIb in the presence of botrocetin and also binds directly to botrocetin.[406] Discrete sequences within the disulfide loop

defined by Cys 509 and Cys 695 are proposed to interact with botrocetin.[407] This same region contains binding sites for fibrillar collagens,[408] heparin,[404] and sulfatides.[409] Although both heparin and sulfatides contain sulfated carbohydrate moieties, they do not appear to bind competitively to the same site within domain A1.[409] The functional relationships between these clustered binding sites are not understood in detail.

A second collagen-binding site appears to be located in domain A3, between amino acid residues 944 and 998.[410] The vWF propeptide also has collagen-binding activity,[411] and one binding site appears to include propeptide amino acid residues 570 to 682 within domain D2.[412]

The vWF binding site for the GPIIb-IIIa complex of activated platelets is located near the carboxyl end of domain C1 and includes the tetrapeptide sequence Arg-Gly-Asp 1746.[413] Arg-Gly-Asp sequences also occur in fibronectin, fibrinogen, and vitronectin, and these proteins compete with vWF for binding to GPIIb-IIIa. Several integrin receptors besides GPIIb-IIIa also recognize ligands that contain Arg-Gly-Asp sequences but often exhibit striking specificity that depends on other structural features of the ligand. Arg-Gly-Asp–dependent interactions are required for the cell attachment activity of many integrins.[414]

The factor VIII–binding site is located within the amino-terminal 272 amino acids of the vWF subunit,[415] which includes domain D′ and part of domain D3. The epitope of a monoclonal antibody that inhibits factor VIII binding is localized between Thr 78 and Thr 98, suggesting that sequences within this segment interact directly with factor VIII.[416] The amino-terminal 272 amino acids of vWF also contain a heparin-binding site,[417] but this site may not be accessible in the intact protein.

THE FUNCTION OF CARBOHYDRATE PROSTHETIC GROUPS IN VON WILLEBRAND FACTOR. Some patients with vWD are reported to produce a vWF that is deficient in carbohydrate content, suggesting that the carbohydrate moieties might participate in the normal function of the protein.[418] Most of the N-linked and O-linked oligosaccharides of vWF terminate in sialic acid, with galactose as the penultimate residue. The highly charged sialic acid residues probably prevent

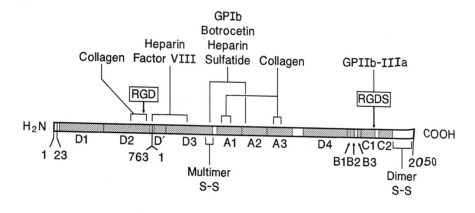

FIGURE 19–10. Structure-function relationships of vWF. Binding sites are indicated for collagen, heparin, factor VIII, platelet GPIb, botrocetin, sulfatide, and platelet GPIIb–IIIa. The locations of intersubunit disulfide bonds are shown. (From Sadler, J.E.: Von Willebrand factor. J. Biol. Chem. 266:22777, 1991; with permission of the American Society for Biochemistry and Molecular Biology.)

spontaneous platelet aggregation, because asialo-vWF aggregates platelets in the absence of ristocetin.[419] However, most of the *N*-linked oligosaccharides can be removed with no substantial effect on ristocetin cofactor activity[420] or vWF-dependent platelet adhesion.[421] Deglycosylated vWF shows increased susceptibility to proteases; therefore, one physiological role for the oligosaccharide moieties is to protect the native protein from proteolytic degradation.[420] Like other glycoproteins having terminal galactose residues, asialo-vWF is rapidly removed from circulation by a specific galactose-binding protein in the liver.[422]

Pathophysiology of von Willebrand Factor

ATHEROSCLEROSIS. Pigs with severe homozygous vWD show some resistance to diet-induced atherosclerosis of the abdominal aorta, whereas heterozygous pigs appear to be normally susceptible.[423, 424] In contrast, both normal and von Willebrand pigs develop similar coronary artery lesions in response to increased dietary cholesterol or catheter-induced injury.[424, 425] Despite having similar atherosclerotic lesions, however, von Willebrand pigs appear to be markedly less susceptible to occlusive thrombosis in a Goldblatt clamp model.[426] Thus, vWF may participate in the development of diet-induced atherosclerosis and thrombosis in pigs. Whether it does so in humans is unknown.

HEMOLYTIC UREMIC SYNDROME AND THROMBOTIC THROMBOCYTOPENIC PURPURA. Thrombotic thrombocytopenic purpura (TTP) is a disease of unknown cause characterized by microangiopathic hemolytic anemia, thrombocytopenia, and widespread small vessel thrombosis with ischemia. The hemolytic uremic syndrome (HUS) resembles TTP, but it tends to affect children rather than adults, and the vascular lesions tend to be limited to the kidneys, causing renal failure. Complex abnormalities of vWF multimer structure have been reported in TTP[427, 428] and HUS.[429] These observations have suggested the hypothesis that vWF may participate in the pathogenesis of these disorders. Alternatively, the abnormal vWF multimers may simply reflect endothelial cell injury, so that vWF may not play a causative role.

Molecular Biology of von Willebrand Factor

The gene for vWF is located near the tip of the short arm of chromosome 12 (12p12 → ter).[430] For most genes, the frequency of meiotic recombination is higher in females than in males, but the vWF gene lies within a short chromosomal interval for which recombination is higher in males.[431]

The vWF gene is ~180 kb in length and consists of 52 exons separated by 51 introns (see Fig. 19–7).[432] The gene contains at least 18 *Alu* repeats and one LINE-1 repeat. The 5′ flanking region contains an AT-rich sequence resembling a TATA element. Functional elements of the putative promoter have not been defined in detail. The exons range in length from 40 nt (exon 50) to 1379 nt (exon 28), and the introns range in length from 97 nt (intron 29) to ~19.9 kb (intron 6). Except for the A domains, segments of the vWF gene that encode homologous repeated domains tend to have similar intron-exon organization, and this is consistent with the evolution of this gene by repeated gene segment duplications.

Homologues of the vWF A domains have been found in at least 14 active genes belonging to six gene or protein superfamilies (reviewed in Colombatti and Bonaldo[433]). These are (1) the complement serine protease zymogens, factor B and complement component C2; (2) cartilage matrix protein; (3) collagens, including all three chains ($\alpha1$, $\alpha2$, $\alpha3$) of heterotrimeric collagen type VI, and the $\alpha1$ chains of homotrimeric collagen type XII[434]; (4) undulin, a collagen-binding constituent of connective tissue[435]; (5) a subset of integrin α subunits, including the α subunits of the leukocyte adhesion receptors Mac-1, p150,95, LFA-1, and the α subunits of the platelet collagen receptor $\alpha_2\beta_1$ (also known as GPIa-IIa), and another integrin collagen receptor $\alpha_1\beta_1$; and (6) vWF itself. Because the A domains in vWF perform several binding functions, it is tempting to speculate that A domains in other proteins could perform similar functions. In particular, the collagen-binding activity of undulin, integrin collagen receptors, cartilage matrix protein, and other collagens might be explained by the presence of homologous collagen-binding A domains. The presence of vWF A domains in so many otherwise unrelated proteins suggests that exon shuffling has contributed to the evolution of the corresponding protein superfamilies.

A partial unprocessed vWF pseudogene is located on chromosome 22q11-q13.[436] The pseudogene is 21 to 29 kb in length and corresponds to 12 exons (exons 23 to 34) and associated introns of the gene. The presence of splice site and nonsense mutations indicates that the vWF pseudogene cannot give rise to a functional transcript. The pseudogene has diverged from the gene ~3.1 per cent in nucleotide sequence, suggesting a recent evolutionary origin near the time of divergence of humans and apes from monkeys.

Von Willebrand Disease

Clinical Features of von Willebrand Disease

Von Willebrand disease appears to be the most common inherited bleeding disorder, although its prevalence is not known precisely. Inherited abnormalities of vWF can be detected by laboratory testing in approximately 8000 per million population, most of whom are asymptomatic.[437] Clinically significant vWD appears to affect approximately 125 persons per million population.[438] The recognition that vWD is relatively common has followed the discovery of many mildly affected persons, and the true prevalence is probably still higher because such cases may escape diagnosis.

The typical bleeding episodes in vWD are consistent with platelet dysfunction. The most common symptoms are bruising, epistaxis, metromenorrhagia, oral bleeding, and severe bleeding after trauma or surgery. Gastrointestinal bleeding is less common but may be recurrent and intractable. Unlike hemophilia A, deep tissue bleeding and hemarthrosis are uncommon.

Classification and Molecular Defects in von Willebrand Disease

A classification scheme that is widely employed today divides vWD according to whether the residual vWF is qualitatively normal (type I) or abnormal (type II); if the protein is essentially undetectable, the disease is classified as type III. In most cases, this classification correlates with the multimer pattern obtained upon SDS gel electrophoresis or counterimmunoelectrophoresis (Fig. 19–6 and Table 19–2). Each of these categories is heterogeneous, however, and this classification provides an imperfect guide to the identification of clinically significant patient subgroups. An excellent, comprehensive collection of almost all reported variants of vWD can be found in an article by Ruggeri.[439]

Many distinct mutations causing vWD have been characterized at the level of DNA sequence, and these have been collected in a data base that will be updated periodically.[440] Eventually, such knowledge may permit a comprehensive and systematic classification of vWD.

Amino acid sequence polymorphisms are quite common within vWF, and many occur close to mutations that cause vWD.[441] The high prevalence of polymorphisms must be considered when sequence changes identified in patients are proposed to be mutations that cause vWD.

VON WILLEBRAND DISEASE TYPE I. In vWD type I, all sizes of multimer are present, the vWF antigen is decreased (usually 5 to 30 per cent), and it appears to be structurally and functionally normal. This is the most common form of vWD, accounting for approximately three fourths of cases, and it is inherited as an autosomal dominant disorder. Most patients with vWD type I have mild or moderate bleeding symptoms.

Several subtypes of vWD type I that clearly are associated with abnormalities of protein structure or function have been proposed, thus blurring the correlation between a (superficially) normal multimer pattern and simple quantitative vWF deficiency. For example, in the subtype referred to as vWD type I Vicenza, the plasma multimer pattern contains larger than normal (supranormal) multimers.[442] Some subtypes show discrepancies between the plasma and platelet vWF antigen concentrations.[443, 444] Others exhibit discrepancies between plasma vWF antigen and ristocetin cofactor activity, associated with a full range of plasma vWF multimers that may show subtle structural abnormalities.[445, 446] In some patients with proposed variants of vWD type I, ristocetin-induced platelet aggregation is increased, and therapy with DDAVP causes thrombocytopenia.[447, 448] When the molecular defects are determined in such "type I" variants, some of them will require reclassification as "type II" (qualitative) disorders.

Although the recessive inheritance of severe vWD type III is logical, the basis for dominant inheritance of vWD type I remains obscure. Because a mildly reduced vWF level is adequate for normal hemostasis, heterozygous carriers of a gene that produces *no* vWF protein should be unaffected, whereas homozygosity for such a gene should cause severe deficiency and symptoms. However, to account for the more common dominant inheritance, a product of the abnormal gene might interfere with the biosynthesis, metabolism, or function of the normal factor.

Candidate mutations have been described in two

TABLE 19–2. A CLASSIFICATION OF SELECTED TYPES OF VON WILLEBRAND DISEASE

VON WILLEBRAND DISEASE	GENETICS	FACTOR VIII	vWF ANTIGEN	RISTOCETIN COFACTOR ACTIVITY	RIPA*	MULTIMER STRUCTURE
Type I	Dominant	Decreased	Decreased	Decreased	Decreased	Normal in plasma and platelets
Type IIA	Dominant	Decreased or normal	Decreased or normal	Markedly decreased	Markedly decreased	Large and intermediate multimers absent from plasma; variable in platelets
Type IIB	Dominant	Decreased or normal	Decreased or normal	Decreased or normal	Increased	Large multimers absent from plasma; normal in platelets
Normandy	Recessive	Moderately decreased	Normal	Normal	Normal	Normal in plasma and platelets
Type III	Recessive	Moderately to markedly decreased	Absent or trace	Absent	Absent	None or trace in plasma or platelets

*RIPA = Ristocetin-induced platelet aggregation in platelet-rich plasma.

families with apparent vWD type I. Affected members of one family were shown to have a 33 nt deletion in exon 28, resulting in a deletion of 11 amino acids.[449] Affected members of a second family were shown to have a potential missense mutation in exon 28, resulting in the substitution Phe 606 → Ile.[450] A causal relationship between this substitution and the disease phenotype was not conclusively demonstrated. If these findings are representative, however, a fraction of vWD type I may be caused by qualitative rather than quantitative abnormalities of vWF.

VON WILLEBRAND DISEASE TYPE II. Most qualitative abnormalities of vWF are associated with multimer patterns that are deficient in the large and intermediate multimers; some significant exceptions are discussed separately. Levels of vWF antigen may be decreased or normal. vWD type II is further divided into subtypes on the basis of specific laboratory tests. The most common subtypes, type IIA and type IIB, are distinguished mainly on the basis of RIPA. vWD type IIA is characterized by absent or markedly decreased RIPA, whereas vWD type IIB is characterized by a paradoxical gain of function with increased RIPA.[451]

Von Willebrand Disease Type IIA. vWD type IIA accounts for approximately three fourths of all vWD type II and is inherited as a dominant disorder. The multimer pattern in plasma is deficient in large mul-

timers, suggesting a polymerization defect.[338] The satellite band pattern of the remaining multimers is like that of normal plasma vWF, except that the fastest migrating satellite is relatively increased. The plasma vWF in these patients contains increased quantities of proteolytically degraded subunits.[452] For some patients with vWD type IIA, the protease-sensitive bond is between Tyr 842 and Met 843 in domain A2 of the vWF subunit.[453]

Heterogeneity of vWD type IIA was demonstrated by comparison of plasma and platelet multimers. In some patients the plasma and platelet multimers show a similar type II pattern, whereas in others the platelet multimer pattern is essentially normal.[443] The plasma multimer defect in the latter subgroup can be at least partially corrected by collection of plasma with appropriate protease inhibitors.[454, 455] Thus, at least two distinct mechanisms may contribute to the pathogenesis of vWD type IIA: defective biosynthesis of multimers and enhanced sensitivity of multimers to proteolysis.

The characterization of mutations indicates that each of these mechanisms can cause vWD type IIA. Nine missense mutations have been identified, and eight of them cluster within domain A2; the remaining mutation is in domain A1 (Fig. 19–11). Recombinant vWF biosynthesis in transfected COS cells was studied for five of these mutations, and they fell into two

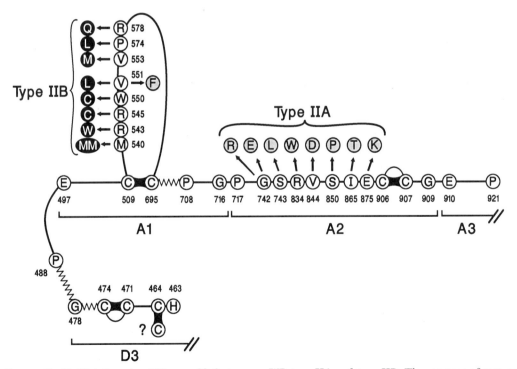

FIGURE 19–11. Mutations in vWF exon 28 that cause vWD type IIA and type IIB. The segment of mature vWF shown is encoded by exon 28 and includes amino acid residues 463 to 921. The positions of repeated domains D3, A1, A2, and A3 are indicated. The zigzag segments from Cys 474 to Pro 488 and Cys 695 to Pro 708 indicate regions proposed to interact directly with platelet GPIb.[405] Mutations reported to cause vWD type IIA (*shaded circles*) and type IIB (*black circles*) are indicated by brackets; one proposed type IIA mutation, Val 551 → Phe, occurs in the region of the type IIB mutations. (Adapted from Sadler, J. E.: Von Willebrand factor. J. Biol. Chem. 266:22777, 1991; with permission of the American Society for Biochemistry and Molecular Biology.)

groups. Group 1, which included the substitutions Val 844 → Asp, Ser 743 → Leu, and Gly 742 → Arg, was characterized by impaired biosynthesis with inefficient secretion of small multimers. Patients with these mutations had decreased large multimers in their platelet vWF. Group 2, which included the substitutions Arg 834 → Trp and Gly 742 → Glu, was characterized by efficient secretion of a full range of multimers. Patients with these mutations had normal platelet multimer patterns.[456]

At present, there is no explanation for the association of specific mutations with each group. Group 1 mutations result from either acidic, basic, or neutral substitutions over a segment of more than 100 amino acids in the vWF subunit. Group 2 mutations are also scattered over a large segment of the subunit, and one group 2 mutation, Gly 742 → Glu, occurs in the same codon as a group 1 mutation, Gly 742 → Arg.

Von Willebrand Disease Type IIB. Von Willebrand disease type IIB is relatively uncommon, accounting for less than ~20 per cent of vWD type II, or less than 5 per cent of all vWD. Like type IIA, vWD type IIB is a dominant disorder. Plasma vWF is deficient in large multimers, but the platelet multimer pattern is normal.[338] An important clinical feature of this variant is thrombocytopenia, which occasionally may be chronic[457] and often is exacerbated by the stress of pregnancy or surgery. The deficiency of large plasma multimers and the thrombocytopenia appear to be secondary effects of a gain-of-function mutation. The large plasma vWF multimers bind spontaneously to platelets[451] and are cleared[458]; the residual small multimers are not hemostatically effective. The administration of DDAVP causes the secretion of a full range of multimers that can be detected transiently in plasma.[458, 459] DDAVP can also induce transient severe thrombocytopenia.[192, 460]

Eight different candidate mutations have been identified in patients with vWD type IIB.[440] All of them cluster within a single disulfide loop of domain A1 (Fig. 19–11), within sequences that are proposed to interact with botrocetin.[407] Such mutations may induce a conformational change in vWF similar to the effect of botrocetin binding and thereby promote association with platelet GPIb. Five of these mutations are C → T transitions within CG dinucleotides, and four of them account for more than 90 per cent of the patients studied so far. Several of these mutations were expressed in recombinant vWF, and each caused increased binding to platelet GPIb. The restricted location and number of mutations suggest that direct detection of DNA sequence changes may be feasible for the rapid diagnosis of vWD type IIB.

Von Willebrand Disease Normandy. Factor VIII–vWF binding is required for normal factor VIII survival in the circulation, and a decrease in affinity between factor VIII and vWF would result in accelerated clearance of factor VIII. As discussed under Classification and Molecular Defects in Hemophilia A (page 663), the Tyr 1680 → Phe mutation, within the vWF binding site of the factor VIII light chain, appears to cause X chromosome–linked recessive mild hemophilia A by this mechanism.

A variant of vWD recently was identified that causes autosomal recessive factor VIII deficiency through a complementary mechanism, by inactivating the factor VIII binding site of vWF.[461, 462] The typical laboratory findings included normal values for vWF ristocetin cofactor activity, collagen-binding activity, antigen concentration, and multimer pattern. However, the binding of factor VIII to plasma vWF was markedly decreased or absent. Infusion of highly purified factor VIII was associated with low recovery and rapid clearance, whereas infusion of vWF almost devoid of factor VIII was associated with a delayed and sustained rise in factor VIII to normal levels. This disorder was tentatively named vWD Normandy, after the birthplace of one proband.[462]

At least nine unrelated patients with this phenotype have now been reported from the United States, France, the Netherlands, and Spain. Among these patients, three different missense mutations have been identified within the factor VIII–binding domain of vWF: Thr 28 → Met, Arg 53 → Trp, and Arg 91 → Gln. All of these are due to C → T transitions within CG dinucleotides. Recombinant vWF containing each of these mutations exhibits markedly decreased or absent factor VIII binding.[440]

Patients with vWD Normandy have been misdiagnosed with mild hemophilia A or as hemophilia A carriers with extreme lyonization. Correct diagnosis led to important changes in genetic counseling and therapy. The prevalence of vWD Normandy is not known, and it may be quite rare; nevertheless, this diagnosis should be considered in any patient with congenital factor VIII deficiency in whom the condition is not obviously X chromosome–linked.[463] Some patients have exhibited defective factor VIII binding combined with symptomatic decreases in other vWF functions. This intermediate phenotype may be due to co-inheritance of vWD type I and vWD Normandy defects, emphasizing the importance of compound heterozygosity in determining the clinical presentation of vWD variants.

Other von Willebrand Disease Type II Variants. There are many additional vWD type II variants, designated types IIC through IIH, most of which have been described in single case reports (reviewed by Ruggeri[439]). Phenotypically, these variants usually resemble vWD type IIA, with significantly decreased ristocetin cofactor activity and a deficiency of large multimers. They are distinguished by characteristic abnormalities of multimer structure, with either the loss of certain satellite bands or the presence of additional bands compared with normal plasma vWF. The recognition of these subtypes requires specialized high-resolution gel electrophoresis methods, and the prevalence of these variants may be underestimated.

Types IIC[464] and IIH[465] appear to be recessive disorders, and patients are presumably homozygous or compound heterozygous. A unique dominant variant that resembles vWD type IIC has been described;

in this variant, the characteristic type IIC multimer pattern is associated with extremely high levels of vWF antigen.[466] Types IID[467] and IIE[453] are autosomal dominant disorders. The mode of transmission of types IIF[468] and IIG[469] is unknown.

A variant called vWD type B,[470] represented by a single patient with a severe bleeding diathesis, shows an interesting dissociation between the ristocetin cofactor activity (absent) and the botrocetin cofactor activity (normal), with a normal level of plasma vWF antigen and factor VIII. The multimer pattern contains a full range of multimers. A missense mutation, Gly 561 → Ser, was identified in domain A1 of the vWF subunit, within the same disulfide loop that is affected by mutations in vWD type IIB. The corresponding mutant recombinant vWF reproduced the discrepancy between ristocetin and botrocetin cofactor activity.[440] Thus, these mediators appear to promote vWF binding to platelets by distinct mechanisms that can be dissociated by a point mutation.

VON WILLEBRAND DISEASE TYPE III. Von Willebrand disease type III is an autosomal recessive disorder with a very low prevalence of 0.5 to 3 per million; the rate is higher in Scandinavian countries and lower in western Europe.[471] The prevalence in the United States and in Israel may be intermediate, approximately 1.4 to 1.6 per million.[471, 472] Most patients presumably are compound heterozygous for mutant vWF alleles that cannot express significant quantities of the protein; homozygosity has been demonstrated in a few consanguineous families. Bleeding symptoms generally are severe and lifelong. Plasma vWF antigen usually is undetectable but may be present at low concentrations (1 to 5 per cent of normal). Sensitive electrophoretic assays have shown that some patients with vWD type III produce small amounts of qualitatively abnormal vWF.[473] The factor VIII level usually is less than 10 per cent and may be less than 1 per cent of normal, which is low enough to be associated with hemarthrosis and spontaneous soft tissue bleeding. The heterozygous parents of patients with vWD type III may have normal or mildly reduced levels of vWF, but usually they are asymptomatic.

Mutations have been characterized in a small number of patients with vWD type III.[440] These include three ostensibly unrelated patients with total gene deletions[474, 475] and one patient with a homozygous partial deletion spanning exon 42.[476] One patient was reported to have a deletion affecting one allele, with a normal restriction endonuclease pattern for the remaining allele by Southern blotting.[475] Nonsense mutations were reported in two alleles associated with vWD type III. One affected the codon for Arg 365 in the propeptide,[477] and the other affected the codon for Arg 1772.[478] Both of these changes represent C → T transitions within CG dinucleotides. Defects in vWF mRNA expression were found in some cases, but the structural basis for these effects is not known.[478, 479]

Prenatal Diagnosis and Genetic Counseling in von Willebrand Disease

Genetic counseling for vWD depends upon the accurate identification of mutant vWF alleles. Because of variable penetrance or expressivity, this can be difficult if based solely on assays of blood for vWF-dependent activities or protein antigens, particularly for families affected with mild vWD type I. Serial studies in the dominant forms of vWD frequently demonstrate one or more normal values among the bleeding time, factor VIII, vWF antigen, and ristocetin cofactor levels.[480]

If the causative mutation is not known, intragenic DNA sequence polymorphisms can be used to follow the inheritance of mutant vWF alleles. A large number of useful marker systems have been identified throughout the vWF gene,[441] and these have been used for linkage analysis and prenatal diagnosis. The most useful marker known is a highly polymorphic tetranucleotide repeat within intron 40. At least 98 alleles were identified, and the heterozygosity was calculated to be ~98 per cent in a European population.[481]

Differential Diagnosis of von Willebrand Disease

Inheritable symptomatic abnormalities of the structure, function, or concentration of vWF are grouped together as vWD. This diagnosis applies to patients with bleeding tendencies that range from trivial to life threatening, whose symptoms may be characteristic of platelet dysfunction or of hemophilia. Consequently, many conditions of quite different pathogenesis may resemble some form of vWD. These include a variety of congenital and acquired platelet disorders that may manifest with similar patterns of bleeding.

HEMOPHILIA A. Appropriate laboratory testing and family studies usually can exclude hemophilia A. However, mild hemophilia associated with aspirin ingestion may be easily confused with vWD. The similarities between hemophilia A and vWD Normandy have been discussed (pages 665 and 684).

ACQUIRED VON WILLEBRAND SYNDROME. More than 40 cases have been reported of spontaneous bleeding associated with decreased vWF occurring in adults without a prior personal or family history of abnormal bleeding.[482, 483] Most cases have occurred in the setting of a recognized autoimmune, lymphoproliferative, or myeloproliferative disease, suggesting an immunological basis for the syndrome. However, some patients do not have an underlying disease that is known to be associated with immune dysfunction, and antibodies to von Willebrand factor have been demonstrated in fewer than half.[482] The multimer pattern in plasma may be normal or may show absence of large multimers.[483] Aside from the patient's history, there may be no way to distinguish this syndrome from congenital vWD by assays of plasma factor VIII or vWF antigen or activity. However platelet-associated vWF is characteristically normal in quantity, ristocetin cofactor activity, and multimer distribution. Furthermore, both the endogenous vWF released by infusion of DDAVP and the exogenous vWF administered in cryoprecipitate have a shortened half-life in the acquired von Willebrand syndrome. The mechanisms of enhanced clearance are unknown, but the syndrome may disappear if the underlying illness is controlled.[483]

PLATELET-TYPE OR PSEUDO–VON WILLEBRAND DISEASE. Platelet-type or pseudo-vWD is nearly an exact mimic of vWD type IIB, but the defect is in the platelet rather than in the vWF.[484–486] It is autosomally inherited, and heterozygotes are clinically affected. The bleeding time is prolonged, and platelet adhesion to damaged endothelium is reduced. The vWF multimer pattern shows a decrease in large multimers, and ristocetin-induced platelet aggregation (RIPA) is increased in the patient's platelet-rich plasma. In addition, the platelet-associated vWF appears to be normal in quantity and multimer distribution. DDAVP induces an increase in large plasma multimers, but they are cleared rapidly, and thrombocytopenia may occur transiently.[487] However, the patient's plasma does not show disproportionately high ristocetin cofactor activity with normal platelets, whereas the patient's platelets spontaneously aggregate when added to normal or hemophilic plasma, and they adsorb normal vWF in the absence of ristocetin.[485, 486, 488] Mutations causing platelet-type or pseudo-vWD have been identified within the vWF-binding domain of platelet GPIbα.[440, 489]

OTHER DISORDERS. Patients with vWD type IIB may have chronic or intermittent thrombocytopenia associated with large platelets and decreased platelet survival with increased clearance by the spleen. This has led to the erroneous diagnosis of chronic autoimmune thrombocytopenia; two such patients were reported who were treated inappropriately with splenectomy.[457, 490] Thrombocytopenia associated with pregancy has been reported in at least eight patients with vWD type IIB; in four this was misdiagnosed as autoimmune thrombocytopenia and treated with corticosteroids[491, 492] or intravenous gamma globulin.[493, 494] vWD type IIB also is associated with postoperative thrombocytopenia[495] and has presented as thrombocytopenia in infancy.[496]

Treatment of von Willebrand Disease

The therapeutic response of bleeding in severe vWD emphasizes the different roles of factor VIII and vWF in hemostasis. Hemarthroses, soft tissue hemorrhage, and postoperative bleeding respond to elevations of factor VIII, whereas mucocutaneous bleeding responds to increases in vWF. Factor VIII levels usually are easy to support, because infusion of vWF generally results in a sustained rise of factor VIII. Correction of the platelet adhesion defect, as reflected in the bleeding time, is more difficult. Cryoprecipitate reliably stops bleeding in vWF but carries the risk of transmitting viral illnesses. Some virucidally treated intermediate-purity and high-purity factor VIII concentrates may be ineffective, probably because the vWF they contain has been denatured or degraded during preparation. However, certain specific commercial concentrates do retain larger multimers of vWF and are effective treatment for bleeding in

vWD.[497, 498] A very high purity, solvent/detergent–treated vWF concentrate, containing little factor VIII, was shown to be effective in small numbers of patients with vWD types I, IIA, IIB, and III.[499–501] This preparation is not yet widely available.

ANTIBODY INHIBITORS OF VON WILLEBRAND FACTOR. Among patients with vWD, antibodies to vWF develop very rarely. All of the reported examples have occurred in patients with severe von Willebrand disease type III. In this subgroup, the prevalence of alloantibodies is about 7.5 per cent,[482] which is similar to the prevalence of alloantibodies in hemophilia A. In contrast to hemophilia A and B, the inhibitors that develop in vWD tend to be polyclonal precipitating antibodies. The affected patients often suffer severe side effects from replacement therapy such as back pain, abdominal pain, and hypotension, consistent with acute serum sickness.[482]

Mucosal bleeding in such patients is often very difficult to control because infused vWF is rapidly neutralized.[482, 502] Elevation of factor VIII levels is easier to achieve, so that soft tissue and joint hemorrhages usually respond to therapy. A sustained elevation of factor VIII is not obtained, however, unless plasma vWF levels can be increased despite the presence of antibody.[503]

Deletions within the vWF gene appear to predispose patients to the development of alloantibody inhibitors. Deletions were reported in four patients with inhibitors[440, 474–476]; however, no deletions have been characterized among at least 100 patients with vWD type III who do not have inhibitors.

DDAVP. The use of DDAVP was discussed under Treatment of Hemophilia A (page 667), and the clinical experience in vWD was reviewed recently.[194, 504] In general, a favorable response to DDAVP appears to correlate with the presence in platelets of vWF with normal multimer distribution and normal function. This agent is usually effective in vWD type I but not in severe vWD type III. The therapeutic efficacy in vWD type II variants is variable, but patients who respond consistently can be identified by test infusions of DDAVP.[505] Some patients with type IIA disease respond, whereas others do not[188, 190, 192, 506]; this variation may correlate with specific mutations. As expected, administration of DDAVP to patients with vWD Normandy increases the level of vWF but does not significantly change the factor VIII level.[507]

In vWD type IIB, DDAVP causes transient thrombocytopenia that may be severe, with the appearance of circulating platelet aggregates,[460] and the bleeding time usually is not shortened.[458–460] These findings suggest that DDAVP might increase the risk of thrombosis and have led to the recommendation that DDAVP should not be used in vWD type IIB.[192, 460] Although thrombosis has occurred in a few patients with atherosclerosis who were treated with DDAVP, no such episodes have been reported in vWD type IIB, and the relative risk of thrombosis is not known. In a subset of type IIB patients, DDAVP is reported to be efficacious without causing clinically significant decrements in platelet count.[508, 509] Thus, the use of DDAVP may be appropriate in carefully selected patients with this variant.

REFERENCES

1. Rosner, F.: Hemophilia in the Talmud and Rabbinic writings. Ann. Intern. Med. 70:833, 1969.
2. Otto, J. E.: An account of an hemorrhagic disposition existing in certain families. Med. Repository 6:1, 1803.
3. Patek, A. J., Jr., and Taylor, F. H. L.: Hemophilia. II. Some properties of a substance obtained from normal human plasma effective in accelerating the coagulation of hemophilic blood. J. Clin. Invest. 16:113, 1937.
4. Aggeler, P. M., White, S. G., Glendenning, M. B., Page, E. W., Leake, T. B., and Bates, G.: Plasma thromboplastin component (PTC) deficiency: A new disease resembling hemophilia. Proc. Soc. Exp. Biol. Med. 79:692, 1952.
5. Biggs, R., Douglas, A. S., Macfarlane, R. G., Dacie, J. V., Pitney, W. R., Merskey, C., and O'Brien, J. R.: Christmas disease. Br. Med. J. 2:1378, 1952.
6. Rizza, C. R., and Rhymes, I. L.: Coagulation assay of VIIIC and IXC. In Bloom, A. L. (ed.): The Hemophilias. New York, Churchill Livingstone, 1982.
7. Barrowcliffe, T. W.: Methodology of the two-stage assay of factor VIII (VIII:C). Scand. J. Haematol. 33 (Suppl. 41):25, 1984.
8. Suomela, H., Blömback, M., and Blömback, B.: The activation of factor X evaluated by using synthetic substrates. Thromb. Res. 10:267, 1977.
9. Hultin, M. B., and Nemerson, Y.: Activation of factor X by factors IXa and VIII: A specific assay for factor IXa in the presence of thrombin-activated factor VIII. Blood 52:928, 1978.
10. Lazarchick, J., and Hoyer, L. W.: Immunoradiometric measurement of the factor VIII procoagulant antigen J. Clin. Invest. 62:1048, 1978.
11. Peake, I. R., Bloom, A. L., Giddings, J. C., and Ludlam, C. A.: An immunoradiometric assay for procoagulant factor VIII antigen: Results in haemophilia, von Willebrand's disease and fetal plasma and serum. Br. J. Haematol. 42:269, 1979.
12. Holmberg, L., Borge, L., Ljung, R., and Nilsson, I. M.: Measurement of antihaemophilic factor A antigen (VIII:CAg) with a solid phase immunoradiometric method based on homologous non-haemophilic antibodies. Scand. J. Haematol. 23:17, 1979.
13. Hershgold, E. J., Davison, A. M., and Janzen, M. E.: Isolation and some chemical properties of human factor VIII (antihemophilic factor). J. Lab. Clin. Med. 77:185, 1971.
14. Legaz, M. E., Schmer, G., Counts, R. B., and Davie, E. W.: Isolation and characterization of human factor VIII (antihemophilic factor). J. Biol. Chem. 248:3946, 1973.
15. Weiss, H. J., and Hoyer, L. W.: Von Willebrand factor: Dissociation from antihemophilic factor procoagulant activity. Science 182:1149, 1973.
16. Griggs, T. R., Cooper, H. A., Webster, W. P., Wagner, R. H., and Brinkhous, K. M.: Plasma aggregating factor (bovine) for human platelets: A marker for study of antihemophilic and von Willebrand factors. Proc. Natl. Acad. Sci. USA 70:2814, 1973.
17. Fulcher, C. A., and Zimmerman, T. S.: Characterization of the human factor VIII procoagulant protein with a heterologous precipitating antibody. Proc. Natl. Acad. Sci. USA 79:1648, 1982.
18. Fulcher, C. A., Roberts, J. R., and Zimmerman, T. S.: Thrombin proteolysis of purified factor VIII procoagulant protein: Correlation of activation with generation of a specific polypeptide. Blood 61:807, 1983.
19. Vehar, G. A., and Davie, E. W.: Preparation and properties of bovine factor VIII (antihemophilic factor). Biochemistry 19:401, 1980.
20. Fass, D. N., Knutson, G. J., and Katzmann, J. A.: Monoclonal antibodies to porcine factor VIII procoagulant and their use in the isolation of active coagulant protein. Blood 59:594, 1982.
21. Knutson, G. J., and Fass, D. N.: Porcine factor VIII:C prepared by affinity interaction with von Willebrand factor and heterologous antibodies: Sodium dodecyl sulfate polyacrylamide gel analysis. Blood 59:615, 1982.
22. Toole, J. J., Knopf, J. L., Wozney, J. M., Sultzman, L. A., Buecker, J. L., Pittman, D. D., Kaufman, R. J., Brown, E., Shoemaker, C., Orr, E. C., Amphlett, G. W., Foster, W. B., Coe, M. L., Knutson, G. J., Fass, D. N., and Hewick, R. M.: Molecular cloning of a cDNA encoding human antihaemophilic factor. Nature 312:342, 1984.
23. Vehar, G. A., Keyt, B., Eaton, D., Rodriquez, H., O'Brien, D. P., Rotblat, F., Oppermann, H., Keck, R., Wood, W. I., Harkins, R. N., Tuddenham, E. G. D., Lawn, R. M., and Capon, D. J.: Structure of human factor VIII. Nature 312:337, 1984.
24. Gitschier, J., Wood, W. I., Goralka, T. M., Wion, K. L., Chen, E. Y., Eaton, D. H., Vehar, G. A., Capon, D. G., and Lawn, R. M.: Characterization of the human factor VIII gene. Nature 312:326, 1984.
25. Wood, W. I., Capon, D. J., Simonsen, C. C., Eaton, D. L., Gitschier, J., Keyt, B., Seeburg, P. H., Smith, D. H., Hollingshead, P., Wion, K. L., Delwart, E., Tuddenham, E. G. D., Vehar, G. A., and Lawn, R. M.: Expression of active human factor VIII from recombinant DNA clones. Nature 312:330, 1984.
26. Takahashi, N., Ortel, T. L., and Putnam, F. W.: Single-chain structure of human ceruloplasmin: The complete amino acid sequence of the whole molecule. Proc. Natl. Acad. Sci. USA 81:390, 1984.
27. Poole, S., Firtel, R. A., Lamar, E., and Rowekamp, W.: Sequence and expression of the Discoidin I gene family in Dictyostelium discoideum. J. Mol. Biol. 153:273, 1981.
28. Stubbs, J. D., Lekutis, C., Singer, K. L., Bui, A., Yuzuki, D., Srinivasan, U., and Parry, G.: cDNA cloning of a mouse mammary epithelial cell surface protein reveals the existence of epidermal growth factor–like domains linked to factor VIII-like sequences. Proc. Natl. Acad. Sci. USA 87:8417, 1990.
29. Church W. R., Jernigan, R. L., Toole, J., Hewick, R. M., Knopf, J., Knutson, G. J., Nesheim, M. E., Mann, K. G., and Fass, D. N.: Coagulation factors V and VIII and ceruloplasmin constitute a family of structurally related proteins. Proc. Natl. Acad. Sci. USA 81:6934, 1984.
30. Fass, D. N., Hewick, R. M., Knutson, G. J., Nesheim, M. E., and Mann, K. G.: Internal duplication and sequence homology in factors V and VIII. Proc. Natl. Acad. Sci. USA 82:1688, 1985.
31. Kane, W. H., and Davie, E. W.: Blood coagulation factors V and VIII: Structural and functional similarities and their relationship to hemorrhagic and thrombotic disorders. Blood 71:539, 1988.
32. Fulcher, C. A., Roberts, J. R., Holland, L. Z., and Zimmerman, T. S.: Human factor VIII procoagulant protein. Monoclonal antibodies define precursor-product relationships and functional epitopes. J. Clin. Invest. 76:117, 1985.
33. Eaton, D., Rodriguez, H., and Vehar, G. A.: Proteolytic processing of human factor VIII. Correlation of specific cleavages by thrombin, factor Xa and activated protein C with activation and inactivation of factor VIII coagulant activity. Biochemistry 25:505, 1986.
34. Tuddenham, E. G. D., Trabold, N. C., Collins, J. A., and Hoyer, L. W.: The properties of factor VIII coagulant activity prepared by immunoadsorbent chromatography. J. Lab. Clin. Med. 94:40, 1979.
35. Kaufman, R. J., Wasley, L. C., and Dorner, A. J.: Synthesis, processing, and secretion of recombinant human factor VIII expressed in mammalian cells. J. Biol. Chem. 263:6352, 1988.
36. Esmon, C. T.: The subunit structure of thrombin-activated factor V. Isolation of activated factor V, separation of

subunits, and reconstitution of biological activity. J. Biol. Chem. 254:964, 1979.

37. Pittman, D. D., Wang, J. H., Michnick, D. A., Fass, D. N., and Kaufman, R. J.: Identification and functional importance of tyrosine-sulfate residues within human recombinant factor VIII. Blood 76 (Suppl. 1):433a, 1990.

38. Mikkelsen, J., Thomsen, J., and Ezban, M.: Heterogeneity in the tyrosine sulfation of Chinese hamster ovary cell produced recombinant FVIII. Biochemistry 30:1533, 1991.

39. Leyte, A., van Schijndel, H. B., Niehrs, C., Huttner, W. B., Verbeet, M. Ph., Mertens, K., and van Mourik, J. A.: Sulfation of Tyr1680 of human blood coagulation factor VIII is essential for the interaction of factor VIII with von Willebrand factor. J. Biol. Chem. 266:740, 1991.

40. Hoyer, L. W., and Trabold, N. C.: The effect of thrombin on human factor VIII. J. Lab. Clin. Med. 97:50, 1981.

41. Barlow, G. H., Martin, S. E., and Marder, V. J.: Sedimentation analysis of von Willebrand and factor VIIIC protein using partition cells in the analytical ultracentrifuge. Blood 63:940, 1984.

42. Fay, P. J., and Smudzin, T. M.: Intersubunit fluorescence energy transfer in human factor VIII. J. Biol. Chem. 264:14005, 1989.

43. Mossesson, M. W., Fass, D. N., Lollar, P., DiOrio, J. P., Parker, C. G., Knutson, G. J., Hainfeld, J. F., and Wall, J. S.: Structural model of porcine factor VIII and factor VIIIa molecules based on scanning transmission electron microscope (STEM) images and STEM mass analysis. J. Clin. Invest. 85:1983, 1990.

44. Andersson, L.-O., and Brown, J. E.: Interaction of factor VIII–von Willebrand factor with phospholipid vesicles. Biochem. J. 200:161, 1981.

45. Lajmanovich, A., Hudry-Clergeon, G., Freyssinet, J.-M., and Marguerie, G.: Human factor VIII procoagulant activity and phospholipid interaction. Biochim. Biophys. Acta 678:132, 1981.

46. Lollar, P., Hill-Eubanks, D. C., and Parker, C. G.: Association of the factor VIII light chain with von Willebrand factor. J. Biol. Chem. 263:10451, 1988.

47. Foster, P. A., Fulcher, C. A., Houghten, R. A., and Zimmerman, T. S.: An immunogenic region within residues Val1670-Glu1684 of the factor VIII light chain induces antibodies which inhibit binding of factor VIII to von Willebrand factor. J. Biol. Chem. 263:5230, 1988.

48. Marchioro, T. L., Hougie, C., Ragde, H., Epstein, R. B., and Thomas, E. D.: Hemophilia: Role of organ homografts. Science 163:188, 1969.

49. Lewis, J. H., Bontempo, F. A., Spero, J. A., Gorenc, T. J., Ragni, M. V., and Starzl, T. E.: Liver transplantation in a hemophilic. N. Engl. J. Med. 312:1189, 1981.

50. Rall, L. B., Bell, G. I., Caput, D., Truett, M. A., Masiarz, F. R., Najarian, R. C., Valenzuela, P., Anderson, H. D., Din, N., and Hansen, B.: Factor VIII:C synthesis in the kidney. Lancet 1:44, 1985.

51. Wion, K. L., Kelly, D., Summerfield, J. A., Tuddenham, E. G. D., and Lawn, R. M.: Distribution of factor VIII mRNA and antigen in human liver and other tissues. Nature 317:726, 1985.

52. Kelly, D. A., Summerfield, J. A., and Tuddenham, E. G. D.: Localization of factor VIIIC:antigen in guinea-pig tissues and isolated liver cell fractions. Br. J. Haematol. 56:535, 1984.

53. Zelechowska, M. G., van Mourick, J. A., and Brodniewicz-Proba, T.: Ultrastructural localization of factor VIII procoagulant antigen in human liver hepatocytes. Nature 317:729, 1985.

54. Ingerslev, J., Christiansen, B. S., Heickendorff, L., and Petersen, C. M.: Synthesis of factor VIII in human hepatocytes in culture. Thromb. Haemost. 60:387, 1988.

55. Stel, H. V., van der Kwast, Th. H., and Veerman, E. C. I.: Detection of factor VIII/coagulant antigen in human liver tissue. Nature 303:530, 1983.

56. Kadhom, N., Wolfrom, C., Gautier, M., Allain, J. P., and Frommel, D.: Factor VIII procoagulant antigen in human tissues. Thromb. Haemost. 59:289, 1988.

57. Shima, M., Yoshioka, A., Nakai, H., Tanaka, I., Fujikawa, T., Terada, S., Imai, S., and Fukui, H.: Factor VIII polypeptide specificity of monoclonal anti-factor VIII antibodies. Br. J. Haematol. 70:63, 1988.

58. Kaufman, R. J., Wasley, L. C., and Dorner, A. J.: Synthesis, processing, and secretion of recombinant human factor VII expressed in mammalian cells. J. Biol. Chem. 263:6352, 1988.

59. Douglas, A. S.: Antihemophilic globulin assay following plasma infusions in hemophilia. J. Lab. Clin. Med. 51:850, 1958.

60. Tuddenham, E. G. D., Lane, R. S., Rotblat, F., Johnson, A. J., Snape, T. J., Middleton, S., and Kernoff, P. B. A.: Response to infusions of polyelectrolyte fractionated human factor VIII concentrate in human haemophilia A and von Willebrand's disease. Br. J. Haematol. 52:259, 1982.

61. Over, J., Sixma, J. J., Doucet-de-Bruine, M. H. M., Trieschnigg, A. M. C., Vlooswijk, R. A. A., Beeser-Visser, N. H., and Bouma, B. N.: Survival of ^{125}iodine-labeled factor VIII in normals and patients with classic hemophilia. J. Clin. Invest. 62:223, 1978.

62. Vehar, G. A., and Eaton, D. L.: Factor VIII structure and function. In Zimmerman, T. S., and Ruggeri, Z. M. (eds.): Coagulation and Bleeding Disorders. The Role of Factor VIII and von Willebrand Factor. Hematology. Vol. 9. New York, Marcel Dekker, 1989.

63. Fass, D. N.: Factor VIII structure and function. Ann. N.Y. Acad. Sci. 614:76, 1991.

64. Rapaport, S. I., Schiffman, S., Patch, M. J., and Ames, S. B.: The importance of activation of antihemophilic globulin and proaccelerin by traces of thrombin in the generation of intrinsic prothrombinase activity. Blood 21:221, 1963.

65. Hultin, M. B., and Jesty, J.: The activation and inactivation of human factor VIII by thrombin: Effect of inhibitors of thrombin. Blood 57:476, 1981.

66. Cooper, H. A., Reisner, F. F., Hall, M., and Wagner, R. H.: Effects of thrombin treatment of preparations of factor VIII and Ca^{2+}-dissociated small active fragment. J. Clin. Invest. 56:751, 1975.

67. Burke, R. L., Pachl, C., Quiroga, M., Rosenberg, S., Haigwood, N., Nordfang, O., and Ezban, M.: The functional domains of coagulation factor VIII:C. J. Biol. Chem. 261:12574, 1986.

68. Toole, J. J., Pitman, D. D., Orr, E. C., Murtha, P., Wasley, L. C., and Kaufman, R. J.: A large region (~95 kDa) of human factor VIII is dispensible for in vitro procoagulant activity. Proc. Natl. Acad. Sci. USA 83:5939, 1986.

69. Eaton, D. L., Wood, W. I., Eaton, D., Hass, P. E., Hollingshead, P., Wion, K., Mather, J., Lawn, R. M., Vehar, G. A., and Gorman, C.: Construction and characterization of an active factor VIII variant lacking the central one-third of the molecule. Biochemistry 25:8343, 1986.

70. Bihoreau, N., Sauger, A., Yon, J. M., and Van de Pol, H.: Isolation and characterization of different activated forms of factor VIII, the human antihemophilic A factor. Eur. J. Biochem. 185:111, 1989.

71. Lollar, P., and Parker, C. G.: Subunit structure of thrombin-activated porcine factor VIII. Biochemistry 28:666, 1989.

72. Fay, P. J., Haidaris, P. J., and Smudzin, T. M.: Human factor VIIIa subunit structure. Reconstitution of factor VIIIa from the isolated A1/A3-C1-C2 dimer and A2 subunit. J. Biol. Chem. 266:8957, 1991.

73. Lollar, P., and Parker, E. T.: Structural basis for the decreased procoagulant activity of human factor VIII compared to the porcine homolog. J. Biol. Chem. 266:12481, 1991.

74. Pittman, D. D., and Kaufman, R. J.: Proteolytic requirements for thrombin activation of anti-hemophilic factor (factor VIII). Proc. Natl. Acad. Sci. USA 85:2429, 1988.

75. Broden, K., Andersson, L.-O., and Sandberg, H.: Kinetics of activation of human factor VIII by thrombin. Thromb. Res. 19:299, 1980.

76. Koedam, J. A., Hamer, R. J., Beeser-Visser, N. H., Bouma, B. N., and Sixma, J. J.: The effect of von Willebrand factor on

activation of factor VIII by factor Xa. Eur. J. Biochem. 189:229, 1990.

77. Rick, M. E.: Activation of factor VIII by factor IXa. Blood 60:744, 1982.

78. Switzer, M. E. P., and McKee, P. A.: Reactions of thrombin with human factor VIII/von Willebrand factor protein. J. Biol. Chem. 255:10606, 1980.

79. Lollar, P., and Parker, C. G.: pH-dependent denaturation of thrombin-activated porcine factor VIII. J. Biol. Chem. 265:1688, 1990.

80. Lollar, P., Knutson, G. J., and Fass, D. N.: Stabilization of thrombin-activated porcine factor VIII:C by factor IXa and phospholipid. Blood 63:1303, 1984.

81. Kisiel, W.: Human plasma protein C. Isolation, characterization, and mechanism of activation by α-thrombin. J. Clin. Invest. 64:761, 1979.

82. Esmon, C. T., and Owen, W. G.: Identification of an endothelial cell cofactor of thrombin-catalyzed activation of protein C. Proc. Natl. Acad. Sci. USA 78:2249, 1981.

83. Esmon, N. L., Owen, W. G., and Esmon, C. T.: Isolation of a membrane-bound cofactor for thrombin-catalyzed activation of protein C. J. Biol. Chem. 257:859, 1982.

84. Griffin, J. H., Evatt, B., Zimmerman, T. S., Kleiss, A. J., and Wideman, C.: Deficiency of protein C in congenital thrombotic disease. J. Clin. Invest. 68:1370, 1981.

85. Marlar, R. A., Kleiss, A. J., and Griffin, J. H.: Mechanism of action of human activated protein C, a thrombin-dependent anticoagulant enzyme. Blood 59:1067, 1982.

86. Kisiel, W., Canfield, W., Ericsson, L, and Davie, E.: Anticoagulant properties of bovine plasma protein C following activation by thrombin. Biochemistry 16:5824, 1977.

87. Fay, P. J., Smudzin, T. M., and Walker, F. J.: Activated protein C-catalyzed inactivation of human factor VIII and factor VIIIa. Identification of cleavage sites and correlation of proteolysis with cofactor activity. J. Biol. Chem. 266:20139, 1991.

88. Fay, P. J., and Walker, F. J.: Inactivation of human factor VIII by activated protein C: Evidence that the factor VIII light chain contains the activated protein C binding site. Biochim. Biophys. Acta 994:142, 1989.

89. Walker, F. J., Scandella, D., and Fay, P. J.: Identification of the binding site for activated protein C on the light chain of factors V and VIII. J. Biol. Chem. 265:1484, 1990.

90. Koedam, J. A., Meijers, J. C. M., Sixma, J. J., and Bouma, B. N.: Inactivation of human factor VIII by activated protein C. Cofactor activity of protein S and protective effect of von Willebrand factor. J. Clin. Invest. 82:1236, 1988.

91. Bertina, R. M., Cupers, R., and van Wijngaarden, A.: Factor IXa protects activated factor VIII against inactivation by activated protein C. Biochem. Biophys. Res. Commun. 125:177, 1984.

92. Walker, F. J., Chavin, S. I., and Fay, P. J.: Inactivation of factor VIII by activated protein C and protein S. Arch. Biochem. Biophys. 252:322, 1987.

93. Varadi, K., and Elodi, S.: Increased resistance of factor IXa–factor VIII complex against inactivation by granulocyte proteases. Thromb. Res. 19:571, 1980.

94. Donaldson, V. H.: Effect of plasmin in vitro on clotting factors in plasma. J. Lab. Clin. Med. 56:644, 1960.

95. Holmberg, L., Ljung, R., and Nilsson, I. M.: The effects of plasmin and protein C_a on factor VIII:C and VIII:CAg. Thromb. Res. 31:41, 1983.

96. Van Dieijen, G., Tans, G., Rosing, J., and Hemker, H. C.: The role of phospholipid and factor VIIIa in the activation of bovine factor X. J. Biol. Chem. 256:3433, 1981.

97. Griffith, M. J., Reisner, H. M., Lundblad, R. L., and Roberts, H. R.: Measurement of human factor IXa activity in an isolated factor X activation system. Thromb. Res. 27:289, 1982.

98. Hultin, M. B.: Role of human factor VIII in factor X activation. J. Clin. Invest. 69:950, 1982.

99. Van Dieijen, G., van Rijn, J. L. M. L., Govers-Riemslag, J. W. P., Hemker, H. C., and Rosing, J.: Assembly of the intrinsic factor X activating complex—Interactions between factor IXa, factor VIIIa and phospholipid. Thromb. Haemost. 53:396, 1985.

100. Gilbert, G. E., Furie, B. C., and Furie, B.: Binding of human factor VIII to phospholipid vesicles. J. Biol. Chem. 265:815, 1990.

101. Bloom, J. W.: The interaction of rDNA factor VIII, factor VIIIdes-797-1562, and factor VIIIdes-797-1562-derived peptides with phospholipid. Thromb. Res. 48:439, 1987.

102. Foster, P. A., Fulcher, C. A., Houghten, R. A., and Zimmerman, T. S.: Synthetic factor VIII peptides with amino acid sequences contained within the C2 domain of factor VIII inhibit factor VIII binding to phospholipids. Blood 75:1999, 1990.

103. Lundblad, R. L., and Davie, E. W.: The activation of antihemophilic factor (factor VIII) by activated Christmas factor (activated factor IX). Biochemistry 3:1720, 1964.

104. Broden, K., Brown, J. E., Carton, C., and Andersson, L.-O.: Effect of phospholipid on factor VIII coagulant activity and coagulant antigen. Thromb. Res. 30:651, 1983.

105. Zwaal, R. F. A.: Membrane and lipid involvement in blood coagulation. Biochim. Biophys. Acta 515:163, 1978.

106. Bevers, E. M., Comfurius, P., Van Rijn, J. L. M. L., Hemker, H. C., and Zwaal, R. F. A.: Generation of prothrombin-converting activity and the exposure of phosphatidylserine at the outer surface of platelets. Eur. J. Biochem. 122:429, 1982.

107. Nesheim, M. E., Pittman, D. D., Wang, J. H., Slonosky, D., Giles, A. R., and Kaufman, R. J.: The binding of ^{35}S-labeled recombinant factor VIII to activated and unactivated human platelets. J. Biol. Chem. 263:16467, 1988.

108. Gilbert, G. E., Sims, P. J., Wiedmer, T., Furie, B., Furie, B. C., and Shattil, S. J.: Platelet-derived microparticles express high affinity receptors for factor VIII. J. Biol. Chem. 266:17261, 1991.

109. Nesheim, M., Pittman, D. D., Giles, A. R., Fass, D. N., Wang, J. H., Slonosky, D., and Kaufman, R. J.: The effect of plasma von Willebrand factor on the binding of human factor VIII to thrombin-activated human platelets. J. Biol. Chem. 266:17815, 1991.

110. Teien, A. N., Abilgaard, U., and Hook, M.: The anticoagulant effect of heparan sulfate and dermatan sulfate. Thromb. Res. 8:859, 1976.

111. Hatton, M. W. C., Berry, L. R., and Regoeczi, E.: Inhibition of thrombin by antithrombin III in the presence of certain glycosaminoglycans found in the mammalian aorta. Thromb. Res. 13:655, 1978.

112. Weksler, B. B., Ley, C. W., and Jaffe, E. A.: Stimulation of endothelial cell prostacyclin production by thrombin, trypsin, and the ionophore A23187. J. Clin. Invest. 62:923, 1978.

113. Loskutoff, D. J., and Edgington, T. S.: Synthesis of a fibrinolytic activator and inhibitor by endothelial cells. Proc. Natl. Acad. Sci. USA 74:3903, 1977.

114. Rogers, G. M., Greenberg, C. S., and Shuman, M. A.: Characterization of the effects of cultured vascular cells on the activation of blood coagulation. Blood 61:1155, 1983.

115. Brox, J. H., Osterud, B., Bjorklid, E., and Fenton, J. W., II: Production and availability of thromboplastin in endothelial cells: The effects of thrombin, endotoxin and platelets. Br. J. Haematol. 57:239, 1984.

116. Lyberg, T., Galdal, K. S., Evensen, S. A., and Prydz, H.: Cellular cooperation in endothelial cell thromboplastin synthesis. Br. J. Haematol. 53:85, 1983.

117. Stern, D. M., Drillings, M., Kisiel, W., Nawroth, P., Nossel, H. L., and LaGamma, K. S.: Activation of factor IX bound to cultured bovine aortic endothelial cells. Proc. Natl. Acad. Sci. USA 81:913, 1984.

118. Stern, D. M., Drillings, M., Nossel, H. L., Hurlet-Jensen, A., LaGamma, K. S., and Owen, J.: Binding of factors IX and IX$_a$ to cultured vascular endothelial cells. Proc. Natl. Acad. Sci. USA 80:4119, 1983.

119. Heimark, R. L., and Schwartz, S. M.: Binding of coagulation factors IX and X to the endothelial cell surface. Biochem. Biophys. Res. Commun. 111:723, 1983.

120. Purrello, M., Alhadeff, B., Esposito, D., Szabo, P., Rocchi, M., Truett, M., Masiarz, F., and Siniscalco, M.: The human genes for hemophilia B flank the X chromosome fragile site of Xq27.3. EMBO J. 4:725, 1985.

121. Whittaker, D. L., Copeland, D. L., and Graham, J. B.: Linkage of color blindness to hemophilias A and B. Am. J. Hum. Genet. 14:149, 1962.

122. Filippi, G., Mannucci, P. M., Coppola, R., Farris, A., Rinaldi, A., and Siniscalco, M.: Studies on hemophilia A in Sardinia bearing on the problem of multiple allelism, carrier detection, and differential mutation rate in the two sexes. Am. J. Hum. Genet. 36:44, 1984.

123. Levinson, B., Kenwrick, S., Lakich, D., Hammonds, G., Jr., and Gitschier, J.: A transcribed gene in an intron of the human factor VIII gene. Genomics 7:1, 1990.

124. Kasper, C. K., and Dietrich, S. L.: Comprehensive management of hemophilia. Clin. Haematol. 14:489, 1985.

125. Smith, P. S., Keyes, N. C., and Forman, E. N.: Socioeconomic evaluation of a state-funded comprehensive hemophilia-care program. N. Engl. J. Med. 306:575, 1982.

126. Jones, P. K., and Ratnoff, O. D.: The changing prognosis of classic hemophilia (factor VIII "deficiency"). Ann. Intern. Med. 114:641, 1991.

127. Graham, J. B., McLendon, W. W., and Brinkhous, K. M.: Mild hemophilia: An allelic form of the disease. Am. J. Med. 225:46, 1953.

128. Reisner, H. M., Price, W. A., Blatt, P. M., Barrow, E. S., and Graham, J. B.: Factor VIII coagulant antigen in hemophilic plasma: A comparison of five alloantibodies. Blood 56:615, 1980.

129. Hoyer, L. W., and Breckenridge, R. T.: Immunologic studies of antihemophilic factor (AHF, factor VIII): Cross-reacting material in a genetic variant of hemophilia A. Blood 32:962, 1968.

130. Denson, K. W. E., Biggs, R., Haddon, M. E., Borrett, R., and Cobb, K.: Two types of haemophilia (A+ and A−): A study of 48 cases. Br. J. Haematol. 17:163, 1969.

131. Tuddenham, E. G. D., Cooper, D. N., Gitschier, J., Higuchi, M., Hoyer, L. W., Yoshioka, A., Peake, I. R., Schwaab, R., Olek, K., Kazazian, H. H., Lavergne, J.-M., Giannelli, F., and Antonarakis, S. E.: Haemophilia A: Database of nucleotide substitutions, deletions, insertions, and rearrangements of the factor VIII gene. Nucleic Acids Res. 19:4821, 1991.

132. Higuchi, M., Kazazian, H. H., Jr., Kasch, L, Warren, T. C., McGinnis, M. J., Phillips, J. A., III, Kasper, C., Janco, R., and Antonarakis, S. E.: Molecular characterization of severe hemophilia A suggests that about half the mutations are not within the coding regions and splice junctions of the factor VIII gene. Proc. Natl. Acad. Sci. USA 88:7405, 1991.

133. Kazazian, H. H., Jr., Wong, C., Youssoufian, H., Scott, A. F., Phillips, D. G., and Antonarakis, S. E.: Haemophilia A resulting from de novo insertion of L1 sequences represents a novel mechanism for mutation in man. Nature 332:164, 1988.

134. Fanning, T. G., and Singer, M. F.: LINE-1: A mammalian transposable element. Biochim. Biophys. Acta 910:203, 1987.

135. Dombroski, B. A., Mathias, S. L., Nanthakumar, E., Scott, A. F., and Kazazian, H. H., Jr.: Isolation of an active human transposable element. Science 254:1805, 1991.

136. Mathias, S. L., Scott, A. F., Kazazian, H. H., Jr., Boeke, J. D., and Gabriel, A.: Reverse transcriptase encoded by a human transposable element. Science 254:1808, 1991.

137. Arai, M., Inaba, H., Higuchi, M., Antonarakis, S. E., Kazazian, H. H., Jr., Fujimaki, M., and Hoyer, L. W.: Direct characterization of factor VIII in plasma: Detection of a mutation altering a thrombin cleavage site (arginine-372 → histidine). Proc. Natl. Acad. Sci. USA 86:4277, 1989.

138. Shima, M., Ware, J., Yoshioka, A., Fukui, H., and Fulcher, C. A.: An arginine to cysteine amino acid substitution at a critical thrombin cleavage site in a dysfunctional factor VIII molecule. Blood 74:1612, 1989.

139. Gitschier, J., Kogan, S., Levinson, B., and Tuddenham, E. G.

D.: Mutations of factor VIII cleavage sites in hemophilia A. Blood 72:1022, 1988.

140. Schwaab, R., Ludwig, M., Kochhan, L., Oldenburg, J., McVey, J. H., Egli, H., Brackmann, H. H., and Olek, K.: Detection and characterization of two missense mutations at a cleavage site in the factor VIII light chain. Thromb. Res. 71:225, 1991.

141. Higuchi, M., Wong, C., Kochhan, L., Olek, K., Aronis, S., Kasper, C. K., Kazazian, H. H., Jr., and Antonarakis, S. E.: Characterization of mutations in the factor VIII gene by direct sequencing of amplified genomic DNA. Genomics 6:65, 1990.

142. Bird, A. P.: DNA methylation and the frequency of CpG in animal DNA. Nucleic Acids Res. 8:1499, 1980.

143. Coulondre, C., Miler, J. H., Farabaugh, P. J., and Gilbert, W.: Molecular basis of base substitution hotspots in Escherichia coli. Nature 274:775, 1978.

144. Youssoufian, H., Antonarakis, S. E., Bell, W., Griffin, A. M., and Kazazian, H. H., Jr.: Nonsense and missense mutations in hemophilia A: Estimate of the relative mutation rate at CG dinucleotides. Am. J. Hum. Genet. 42:718, 1988.

145. Ward, H.: Review of the development and current status of techniques for monitoring embryonic and fetal development in the first trimester of pregnancy. Am. J. Med. Genet. 35:157, 1990.

146. Boehm, C. D., Stylianos, M. S., Antonarakis, E., Phillips, J. A., III, Stetten, G., and Kazazian, H. H., Jr.: Prenatal diagnosis using DNA polymorphisms. Report on 95 pregnancies at risk for sickle-cell disease or β-thalassemia. N. Engl. J. Med. 308:1054, 1983.

147. Cade, J. F., Hirsh, J., and Martin, M.: Placental barrier to coagulation factors: Its relevance to the coagulation defect at birth and to haemorrhage in the newborn. Br. Med. J. 2:281, 1969.

148. Firshein, S. I., Hoyer, L. W., Lazarchick, J., Forget, B. G., Hobbins, J. C., Clyne, L. P., Pitlick, F. A., Muir, W. A., Merkatz, I. R., and Mahoney, M. J.: Prenatal diagnosis of classic hemophilia. N. Engl. J. Med. 300:937, 1979.

149. Alter, B. P.: Advances in the prenatal diagnosis of hematologic diseases. Blood 64:329, 1984.

150. Hoyer, L. W., Carta, C. A., Golbus, M. S., Hobbins, J. C., and Mahoney, M. J.: Prenatal diagnosis of classic hemophilia (hemophilia A) by immunoradiometric assays. Blood 65:1312, 1985.

151. Peake, I.: Registry of DNA polymorphisms within or close to the human factor VIII and factor IX genes. Thromb. Haemost. 67:277, 1992.

152. Kogan, S., and Gitschier, J.: Mutations and a polymorphism in the factor VIII gene discovered by denaturing gradient gel electrophoresis. Proc. Natl. Acad. Sci. USA 87:2092, 1990.

153. Lalloz, M. R., McVey, J. H., Pattinson, J. K., and Tuddenham, E. G. D.: Haemophilia A diagnosis by analysis of a hypervariable dinucleotide repeat within the factor VIII gene. Lancet 338:207, 1991.

154. Barria, I., Cann, H. M., Cavalli-Sforza, L. L., Barbujani, G., and De Nicola, P.: Segregation analysis of hemophilia A and B. Am. J. Hum. Genet. 37:680, 1985.

155. Haldane, J. B. S.: The rate of spontaneous mutation of a human gene. J. Genet. 31:317, 1935.

156. Bernardi, F., Marchetti, G., Bertagnolo, V., Faggioli, L., Volinia, S., Patracchini, P., Bartolai, S., Vannini, F., Felloni, L., Rossi, L., Panicucci, F., and Conconi, F.: RFLP analysis in families with sporadic hemophilia A. Estimate of the mutation ratio in male and female gametes. Hum. Genet. 76:253, 1987.

157. Kerr, C. B., Preston, A. E., Barr, A., and Biggs, R.: Further studies on the inheritance of factor VIII. Br. J. Haematol. 12:212, 1966.

158. Graham, J. B., Rizza, C. R., Chediak, J., Mannucci, P. M., Briët, E., Llung, R., Kasper, C. K., Essien, E. M., and Green, P. P.: Carrier detection in hemophilia A: A cooperative international study. I. The carrier phenotype. Blood 67:1554, 1986.

159. Green, P. P., Mannucci, P. M., Briët, E., Llung, R., Kasper, C. K., Essien, E. M., Chediak, J., Rizza, C. R., and Graham, J. B.: Carrier detection in hemophilia A: A cooperative international study. II. The efficacy of a universal discriminant. Blood 67:1560, 1986.

160. Naylor, J. A., Green, P. M., Montandon, A. J., Rizza, C. R., and Giannelli, F.: Detection of three novel mutations in two haemophilia A patients by rapid screening of whole essential region of factor VIII gene. Lancet 337:635, 1991.

161. Sweeney, J., and Wenz, B.: Combined factor V and factor VIII deficiency. N. Engl. J. Med. 308:656, 1983.

162. Seligsohn, U.: Combined factor V and factor VIII deficiency. N. Engl. J. Med. 308:656, 1983.

163. Seligsohn, U., Zivelin, A., and Swang, E.: Combined factor V and factor VIII deficiency among non-Ashkenazi Jews. N. Engl. J. Med. 307:1191, 1982.

164. Suzuki, K., Nishioka, J., Hashimoto, S., Kamiya, T., and Saito, H.: Normal titer of functional and immunoreactive protein-C inhibitor in plasma of patients with congenital combined deficiency of Factor V and Factor VIII. Blood 62:1266, 1983.

165. Rahim Adam, K. A., El Seed, F. A. R., Karrar, Z. A., and Gader, A. M. A.: Combined factor V and factor VIII deficiency with normal protein C and protein C inhibitor. A family study. Scand. J. Haematol. 34:401, 1985.

166. Brown, J. M., Selik, N. R., Voelpel, M. J., and Mammen, E. F.: Combined factor V/VIII deficiency: A case report including levels of factor V and factor VIII coagulant antigen as well as protein C inhibitor. Am. J. Hematol. 20:401, 1985.

167. Seligsohn, U., Zivelin, A., and Zwang, E.: Decreased factor VIII clotting antigen levels in the combined factor V and VIII deficiency. Thromb. Res. 33:95, 1983.

168. Hultin, M. B., and Eyster, M. E.: Combined factor V-VIII deficiency: A case report with studies of factor V and VIII activation by thrombin. Blood 58:983, 1981.

169. Canfield, W. M., and Kisiel, W.: Evidence of normal functional levels of activated protein C inhibitor in combined factor V/VIII deficiency disease. J. Clin. Invest. 70:1260, 1982.

170. Tracy, P. B., Eide, L. L., Bowie, E. J. W., and Mann, K. G.: Radioimmunoassay of factor V in human plasma and platelets. Blood 60:59, 1982.

171. Giddings, J. C., Sugrue, A., and Bloom, A. L.: Quantitation of coagulant antigens and inhibition of activated protein C in combined factor V/VIII deficiency. Br. J. Haematol. 52:495, 1982.

172. Marlar, R. A., and Griffin, J. H.: Deficiency of protein C inhibitor in combined Factor V/VIII deficiency disease. J. Clin. Invest. 66:1186, 1980.

173. Schulman, S., and Wiechel, B.: Hepatitis, epidemiology and liver function in hemophiliacs in Sweden. Acta Med. Scand. 215:249, 1984.

174. Aledort, L. M., Levine, P. H., Hilgartner, M., Blatt, P., Spero, J. A., Goldberg, J. D., Bianchi, L., Desmet, V., Scheuer, P., Popper, H., and Berk, P. D.: A study of liver biopsies and liver disease among hemophiliacs. Blood 66:367, 1985.

175. Makris, M., Preston, F. E., Triger, D. R., Underwood, J. C. E., Choo, Q. L., Kuo, G., and Houghton, M.: Hepatitis C antibody and chronic liver disease in haemophilia. Lancet 335:1117, 1990.

176. Rizzetto, M., Morelio, C., Mannucci, P. M., Gocke, D. J., Spero, J. A., Lewis, J. H., van Thiel, D. H., Scaroni, C., and Peyretti, F.: Delta infection and liver disease in hemophilic carriers of hepatitis B surface antigen. J. Infect. Dis. 145:18, 1982.

177. Goedert, J. J., Kessler, C. M., Aledort, L. M., Biggar, R. J., Andes, W. A., White, G. C., II, Drummond, J. E., Vaidya, K., Mann, D. L., Eyster, M. E., Ragni, M. V., Lederman, M. M., Cohen, A. R., Bray, G. L., Rosenberg, P. S., Friedman, R. M., Hilgartner, M. W., Blattner, W. A., Kroner, B., and Gail, M. H.: A prospective study of human immunodeficiency virus type 1 infection and the development of AIDS in subjects with hemophilia. N. Engl. J. Med. 321:1141, 1989.

178. Schimpf, K., Brackmann, H. H., Kreuz, W., Kraus, B., Haschke, F., Schramm, W., Moesseler, J., Auerswald, G., Sutor, A. H., Koehler, K., Hellstern, P., Muntean, W., and Scharrer, I.: Absence of anti-human immunodeficiency virus type 1 and 2 seroconversion after the treatment of hemophilia A or von Willebrand's disease with pasteurized factor VIII concentrate. N. Engl. J. Med. 321:1148, 1989.

179. Brettler, D. B., and Levine, P. H.: Factor concentrates for treatment of hemophilia: Which one to choose? Blood 73:2067, 1989.

180. Mannucci, P. M., Zanetti, A. R., Colombo, M., Chistolini, A., De Biasi, R., Musso, R., and Tamponi, G., for the Study Group of the Fondazione dell'Emofilia: Antibody to hepatitis C virus after a vapour-treated factor VIII concentrate. Thromb. Haemost. 64:232, 1990.

181. Mannucci, P. M., Schimpf, K., Brettler, D. B., Ciavarella, N., Colombo, M., Haschke, F., Lechner, K., Lusher, J., Weissbach, G., and the International Study Group: Low risk for hepatitis C in hemophiliacs given a high-purity, pasteurized factor VIII concentrate. Ann. Intern. Med. 113:27, 1990.

182. Brettler, D. B., Forsberg, A. D., Sullivan, J. L., and Levine, P. H.: Delayed hypersensitivity in a group of hemophiliacs. Am. J. Med. 81:607, 1986.

183. Carr, R., Edmund, E., Precott, R. J., Veitch, S. E., Peutherer, J. F., Steel, C. M., and Ludlam, C. A.: Abnormalities of circulating lymphocyte subsets in haemophiliacs in an AIDS-free population. Lancet 1:1431, 1984.

184. Goldsmith, G. H., Bailey, R. G., Brettler, D. B., Davidson, W. R., Ballard, J. O., Driscol, T. E., Greenberg, J. M., Kasper, C. K., Levine, P. H., and Ratnoff, O. D.: Primary pulmonary hypertension in patients with classic hemophilia. Ann. Intern. Med. 108:797, 1988.

185. White, G. C., II, McMillan, C. W., Kingdon, H. S., and Shoemaker, C. B.: Use of recombinant antihemophilic factor in the treatment of two patients with classic hemophilia. N. Engl. J. Med. 320:166, 1989.

186. Schwartz, R. S., Abildgaard, C. F., Aledort, L. M., Arkin, S., Bloom, A. L., Brackmann, H. H., Brettler, D. B., Fukui, H., Hilgartner, M. W., Inwood, M. J., Kasper, C. K., Kernoff, P. B. A., Levine, P. H., Lusher, J. M., Mannucci, P. M., Scharrer, I., MacKenzie, M. A., Pancham, N., Kuo, H. S., Allred, R. U., and the Recombinant Factor VIII Study Group: Human recombinant DNA-derived antihemophilic factor (factor VIII) in the treatment of hemophilia A. N. Engl. J. Med. 323:1800, 1990.

187. Bloom, A. L.: The biosynthesis of factor VIII. Clin. Haematol. 8:53, 1979.

188. Mannucci, P. M., Ruggeri, Z. M., Pareti, F. I., and Capitanio, A.: 1-Deamino-8-D-arginine vasopressin: A new pharmacological approach to the management of haemophilia and von Willebrand's disease. Lancet 1:869, 1977.

189. Mannucci, P. M., Aberg, M., Nilsson, I. M., and Robertston, B.: Mechanism of plasminogen activator and factor VIII increase after vasoactive drugs. Br. J. Haematol. 30:81, 1975.

190. Theiss, W., and Schmidt, G.: DDAVP in von Willebrand's disease: Repeated administration and the behaviour of the bleeding time. Thromb. Res. 13:1119, 1978.

191. Mannucci, P. M., Canciani, M. T., Rota, L., and Donovan, B. S.: Response of factor VIII/von Willebrand factor to DDAVP in healthy subjects and patients with haemophilia A and von Willebrand's disease. Br. J. Haematol. 47:283, 1981.

192. De la Fuente, B., Kasper, C. K., Rickles, F. R., and Hoyer, L. W.: Response of patients with mild and moderate hemophilia A and von Willebrand's disease to treatment with desmopressin. Ann. Intern. Med. 103:6, 1985.

193. Mannucci, P. M., Pareti, F. I., Holmberg, L., Nilsson, I. M., and Ruggeri, Z. M.: Studies on the prolonged bleeding time in von Willebrand's disease. J. Lab. Clin. Med. 88:662, 1976.

194. Mannucci, P. M.: Desmopressin: A nontransfusional form of treatment for congenital and acquired bleeding disorders. Blood 72:1449, 1988.

195. Kasper, C. K.: The therapy of factor VIII inhibitors. In Zimmerman, T. S., and Ruggeri, Z. M. (eds.): Coagulation and Bleeding Disorders. The Role of Factor VIII and von Willebrand Factor. Hematology, Vol. 9. New York, Marcel Dekker, 1989.

196. Gill, F. M.: The natural history of factor VIII inhibitors in patients with hemophilia A. Prog. Clin. Biol. Res. 150:19, 1984.

197. Allain, J. P., and Frommel, D.: Antibodies to factor VIII. V. Patterns of immune response to factor VIII in hemophilia A. Blood 47:973, 1976.

198. McMillan, C. W., Shapiro, S. S., Whitehurst, D., Hoyer, L. W., Rao, A. V., Lazerson, J., and the Hemophilia Study Group: The natural history of factor VIII:C inhibitors in patients with hemophilia A: A national cooperative study. II. Observations on the initial development of factor VIII:C inhibitors. Blood 71:344, 1988.

199. Lippert, L. E., Fisher, L. Mc. A., and Schook, L. B.: Relationship of major histocompatibility complex class II genes to inhibitor antibody formation in hemophilia A. Thromb. Haemost. 64:564, 1990.

200. Aly, A. M., Aledort, L. M., Lee, T. D., and Hoyer, L. W.: Histocompatibility antigen patterns in haemophilic patients with factor VIII antibodies. Br. J. Haematol. 76:238, 1990.

201. Fulcher, C. A., Mahoney, S. deG., and Zimmerman, T. S.: FVIII inhibitor IgG subclass and FVIII polypeptide specificity determined by immunoblotting. Blood 69:1475, 1980.

202. Scandella, D., Mahoney, S. deG., Mattingly, M., Roeder, D., Timmons, L., and Fulcher, C. A.: Epitope mapping of human factor VIII inhibitor antibodies by deletion analysis of factor VIII fragments expressed in *Escherichia coli*. Proc. Natl. Acad. Sci. USA 85:6152, 1988.

203. Macfarlane, R. G., Mallam, P. C., Witts, L. J., Bidwell, E., Biggs, R., Fraenkel, G. J., Honey, G. E., and Taylor, K. B.: Surgery in haemophilia. The use of animal antihaemophilic globulin and human plasma in thirteen cases. Lancet 2:251, 1957.

204. Erskine, J. G., and Davidson, J. F.: Anaphylactic reaction to low-molecular-weight porcine factor VIII concentrates. Br. Med. J. 282:2011, 1981.

205. Brettler, D. B., Forsberg, A. D., Levine, P. H., Aledort, L. M., Hilgartner, M. W., Kasper, C. K., Lusher, J. M., McMillan, C., Roberts, H., and Cooperating Investigators: The use of porcine factor VIII concentrate (Hyate:C) in the treatment of patients with inhibitor antibodies to factor VIII. A multicenter US experience. Arch. Intern. Med. 149:1381, 1989.

206. Gringeri, A., Santagostino, E., Tradati, F., Giangrande, P. L. F., and Mannucci, P. M.: Adverse effects of treatment with porcine factor VIII. Thromb. Haemost. 65:245, 1991.

207. Mannucci, P. M., and Vigano, S.: Protein C concentrates for therapeutic use. Lancet 1:875, 1983.

208. Hultin, M. B.: Studies of factor IX concentrate therapy in hemophilia. Blood 62:677, 1983.

209. Kurczynski, E. M., and Penner, J. A.: Activated prothrombin concentrate for patients with factor VIII inhibitors. N. Engl. J. Med. 291:164, 1974.

210. Lusher, J. M., Shapiro, S. S., Palascak, J. E., Rao, A. V., Levine, P. H., Blatt, P. M., and the Hemophilia Study Group: Efficacy of prothrombin-complex concentrates in hemophiliacs with antibodies to factor VIII. A multicenter therapeutic trial. N. Engl. J. Med. 303:421, 1980.

211. Sjamsoedin, L. J. M., Heijnin, L., Mauser-Bucschoten, E. P., van Geijlswijk, J. L., van Houwelingen, H., van Asten, P., and Sixma, J. J.: The effect of activated prothrombin-complex concentrate (FEIBA) on joint and muscle bleeding in patients with hemophilia A and antibodies to factor VIII. A double-blind clinical trial. N. Engl. J. Med. 305:717, 1981.

212. Lusher, J. M., Blatt, P. M., Penner, J. A., Aledort, L. M., Levine, P. H., White, G. C., Warrier, A. I., and Whitehurst, D. A.: Autoplex versus Proplex: A controlled, double-blind study of effectiveness in acute hemarthroses in hemophiliacs with inhibitors to factor VIII. Blood 62:1135, 1983.

213. Abildgaard, C. F.: Hazards of prothrombin-complex concentrates in treatment of hemophilia. N. Engl. J. Med. 304:67, 1981.

214. Fukui, H., Fujimura, Y., Takahashi, Y., Mikami, S., and Yoshioka, A.: Laboratory evidence of DIC under FEIBA treatment of a hemophilic patient with intracranial bleeding and high titre factor VIII inhibitor. Thromb. Res. 22:177, 1981.

215. Hilgartner, M. W., Knatterud, G. L., and the FEIBA Study Group: The use of factor VIII inhibitor by-passing activity (FEIBA Immuno) product for treatment of bleeding episodes in hemophiliacs with inhibitors. Blood 61:36, 1983.

216. Kasper, C. K., and the Hemophilia Study Group: Effect of prothrombin complex concentrates on factor VIII inhibitor levels. Blood 54:1358, 1979.

217. Seligsohn, U., Kasper, C. K., Osterud, B., and Rapaport, S. I.: Activated factor VII: Presence in factor IX concentrates and persistence in the circulation after infusion. Blood 53:828, 1979.

218. Broze, G., and Majerus, P. W.: Human factor VII. Methods Enzymol. 80:228, 1981.

219. Hedner, U., and Kisiel, W.: Use of human factor VIIa in the treatment of two hemophilia A patients with high-titer inhibitors. J. Clin. Invest. 71:1836, 1983.

220. Hedner, U., Bjoern, S., Bernvil, S. S., Tengborn, L., and Stigendahl, L.: Clinical experience with human plasma-derived factor VIIa in patients with hemophilia A and high titer inhibitors. Hemostasis 19:335, 1989.

221. Schmidt, M. L., Gamerman, S., Smith, H. E., Scott, J. P., and DiMichele, D.: Recombinant activated factor VII (rVIIa) therapy for intracranial hemorrhage (ICH) in hemophilia A patients with inhibitors. Blood 78 (Suppl 1):62a, 1991.

222. Macik, B. G., Hohneker, J., Roberts, H. R., and Griffin, A. M.: Use of recombinant activated factor VII for treatment of a retropharyngeal hemorrhage in a hemophilic patient with a high titer inhibitor. Am. J. Hematol. 32:232, 1989.

223. Schmidt, M. L., Gamerman, S., Smith, H. E., Scott, J. P., and DiMichele, D.: Recombinant activated factor VII (rVIIa) therapy for muscle and soft tissue hemorrhage in factor VIII and IX-deficient patients with inhibitors. Blood 78 (Suppl 1):61a, 1991.

224. Hedner, U., Glazer, S., Pingel, K., Alberts, D. A., Blomback, M., Schulman, S., and Johnsson, H.: Successful use of recombinant factor VIIa in patient with severe haemophilia A during synovectomy. Lancet 2:1193, 1988.

225. Gringeri, A., Santagostino, E., and Mannucci, P. M.: Failure of recombinant activated factor VII during surgery in a hemophiliac with high-titer factor VIII antibody. Haemostasis 21:1, 1991.

226. Thompson, A. R.: Radioimmunoassay of factor IX. *In* Bloom, A. L. (ed.): The Hemophilias. New York, Churchill Livingstone, 1982.

227. Fujikawa, K., Thompson, A. R., Legaz, M. E., Meyer, R. G., and Davie, E. W.: Isolation and characterization of bovine factor IX (Christmas factor). Biochemistry 12:4938, 1973.

228. Andersson, L.-O., Borg, H., and Miller-Andersson, M.: Purification and characterization of human factor IX. Thromb. Res. 7:451, 1975.

229. DiScipio, R. G., Hermodson, M. A., Yates, S. G., and Davie, E. W.: A comparison of human prothrombin factor IX (Christmas factor), factor X (Stuart factor), and protein S. Biochemistry 16:698, 1977.

230. Kurachi, K., and Davie, E. W.: Isolation and characterization of a cDNA coding for human factor IX. Proc. Natl. Acad. Sci. USA 79:6461, 1982.

231. Davie, E. W., Degen, S. J. F., Yoshitake, S., and Kurachi, K.: Cloning of vitamin K–dependent clotting factors. *In* de Bernard, B., Scottocasa, G. L., Sandri, G., Carafoli, E., Taylor, A. N., Vanaman, T. C., and Williams, R. J. P. (eds.): Calcium-Binding Proteins. Amsterdam, Elsevier, 1983.

232. Nishimura, H., Kawabata, S., Kisiel, W., Hase, S., Ikenaka, T., Takao, T., Shimonishi, Y., and Iwanaga, S.: Identification of a disaccharide (Xyl-Glc) and a trisaccharide (Xyl_2-Glc) O-glycosidically linked to a serine residue in the first epidermal growth factor–like domain of human factors VII and IX and protein Z and bovine protein Z. J. Biol. Chem. 264:20320, 1989.

233. DiScipio, R. G., and Davie, E. W.: Characterization of protein S, a γ-carboxyglutamic acid containing protein from bovine and human plasma. Biochemistry 18:899, 1979.

234. Morita, T., Isaacs, B. S., Esmon, C. T., and Johnson, A. E.: Derivatives of blood coagulation factor IX contain a high affinity Ca²⁺-binding site that lacks γ-carboxyglutamic acid. J. Biol. Chem. 259:5698, 1984.

235. Handford, P. A., Baron, M., Mayhew, M., Willis, A., Beesley, T., Brownlee, G. G., and Campbell, I. D.: The first EGF-like domain from human factor IX contains a high-affinity calcium binding site. EMBO J. 9:475, 1990.

236. Banyai, L., Veradi, A., and Patthy, L.: Common evolutionary origin of the fibrin-binding structures of fibronectin and tissue-type plasminogen activator. FEBS Lett. 163:37, 1983.

237. McMullen, B. A., and Fujikawa, K.: Amino acid sequence of the heavy chain of human α-factor XIIa (activated Hageman factor). J. Biol. Chem. 260:5328, 1985.

238. Magnusson, S., Sottrup-Jensen, L., Petersen, T. E., Dudek-Wojciechoska, G., and Claeys, H.: Homologous "kringle" structures common to plasminogen and prothrombin. Substrate specificity of enzymes activating prothrombin and plasminogen. In Ribbons, D. W., and Brew, K. (eds.): Proteolysis and Physiological Regulation. New York, Academic Press, 1976.

239. Sottrup-Jensen, L., Claeys, J., Zajdel, M., Petersen, T. E., and Magnusson, S.: The primary structure of human plasminogen: Isolation of two lysine-binding fragments and one "Mini-" plasminogen (MW, 38,000) by elastase-catalyzed-specific limited proteolysis. In Davidson, J. F., Rowan, R. M., Samama, M. M., and Desnoyers, P. C. (eds.): Progress in Chemical Fibrinolysis and Thrombolysis. New York, Raven Press, 1978.

240. Pennica, D., Holmes, W. E., Kohr, W. J., Harkins, R. N., Vehar, G. A., Ward, C. A., Bennett, W. F., Yelverton, E., Seeburg, P. H., Heyneker, H. L., Goeddel, D. V., and Collen, D.: Cloning and expression of human tissue-type plasminogen activator cDNA in E. coli. Nature 301:214, 1983.

241. Gunzler, W. A., Steffens, G. J., Otting, F., Kim, S.-M.A., Frankus, E., and Flohe, L.: The primary structure of high molecular mass urokinase from human urine. The complete amino acid sequence of the A chain. Hoppe-Seylers Z. Physiol. Chem. 363:1155, 1982.

242. Steffens, G. J., Gunzler, W. A., Otting, F., Frankus, E., and Flohe, L.: The complete amino acid sequence of low molecular mass urokinase from human urine. Hoppe-Seylers Z. Physiol. Chem. 363:1043, 1982.

243. Massagué, J.: Transforming growth factor-α. A model for membrane-anchored growth factors. J. Biol. Chem. 265:21393, 1990.

244. McMullen, B. A., Fujikawa, K., and Kisiel, W.: The occurrence of β-hydroxyaspartic acid in the vitamin K-dependent blood coagulation zymogens. Biochem. Biophys. Res. Commun. 115:8, 1983.

245. Handford, P. A., Mayhew, M., Baron, M., Winship, P. R., Campbell, I. D., and Brownlee, G. G.: Key residues involved in calcium-binding motifs in EGF-like domains. Nature 351:164, 1991.

246. Sigler, P. B., Blow, D. M., Matthews, B. W., and Henderson, R.: Structure of crystalline α-chymotrypsin. II. A preliminary report including a hypothesis for the activation mechanism. J. Mol. Biol. 35:143, 1968.

247. Jorgensen, M. J., Cantor, A. B., Furie, B. C., Brown, C. L., Shoemaker, C. B., and Furie, B.: Recognition site directing vitamin K-dependent γ-carboxylation residues on the propeptide of factor IX. Cell 48:185, 1987.

248. Handford, P. A., Winship, P. R., and Brownlee, G. G.: Protein engineering of the propeptide of human factor IX. Protein Engineering 4:319, 1991.

249. Diuguid, D. L., Rabiet, M.-J., Furie, B. C., Liebman, H. A., and Furie, B.: Molecular basis of hemophilia B: A defective enzyme due to an unprocessed propeptide is caused by a point mutation in the factor IX precursor. Proc. Natl. Acad. Sci. USA 83:5803, 1986.

250. Bentley, A. K., Rees, D. J. G., Rizza, C., and Brownlee, G. G.: Defective propeptide processing of blood clotting factor IX caused by mutation of arginine to glutamine at position −4. Cell 45:343, 1986.

251. Rabiet, M.-J., Jorgensen, M. J., Furie, B., and Furie, B. C.: Effect of propeptide mutations on post-translational processing of factor IX. Evidence that β-hydroxylation and γ-carboxylation are independent events. J. Biol. Chem. 262:14895, 1987.

252. Stenflo, J., Lundvall, Å., and Dahlbäck, B.: β-Hydroxyasparagine in domains homologous to the epidermal growth factor precursor in vitamin K-dependent protein S. Proc. Natl. Acad. Sci. USA 84:368, 1987.

253. Gronke, R. S., VanDusen, W. J., Garsky, V. M., Jacobs, J. W., Sardana, M. K., Stern, A. M., and Friedman, P. A.: Aspartyl β-hydroxylase: In vitro hydroxylation of a synthetic peptide based on the structure of the first growth factor–like domain of human factor IX. Proc. Natl. Acad. Sci. USA 86:3609, 1989.

254. Derian, C. K., VanDusen, W., Przysiecki, C. T., Walsh, P. N., Berkner, K. L., Kaufman, R. J., and Friedman, P. A.: Inhibitors of 2-ketoglutarate-dependent dioxygenases block aspartyl β-hydroxylation of recombinant human factor IX in several mammalian expression systems. J. Biol. Chem. 264:6615, 1989.

255. Thompson, A. R.: Factor IX kinetics. In Seligsohn, U., Rimon, A., and Horoszowski, H. (eds.): Haemophilia. Kent, U.K., Castle House Publications, 1981.

256. Zauber, N. P., and Levin, J.: Factor IX levels in patients with hemophilia B (Christmas disease) following transfusion with concentrates of factor IX or fresh frozen plasma (FFP). Medicine 56:213, 1977.

257. Link, R. P., and Castellino, F. J.: Kinetic comparison of bovine blood coagulation factors IXaα and IXaβ toward bovine factor X. Biochemistry 22:4033, 1983.

258. Lindquist, P. A., Fujikawa, K., and Davie, E. W.: Activation of bovine factor IX (Christmas factor) by factor XIₐ (activated plasma thromboplastin antecedent) and a protease from Russell's viper venom. J. Biol. Chem. 253:1902, 1978.

259. Bajaj, S. P., Rapaport, S. I., and Russell, W. A.: Redetermination of the rate-limiting step in the activation of factor IX by factor XIa and by factor VIIa/tissue factor. Explanation for different electrophoretic radioactivity profiles obtained on activation of ³H- and ¹²⁵I-labeled factor IX. Biochemistry 22:4047, 1983.

260. Byrne, R., Amphlett, G. W., and Castellino, F. J.: Metal ion specificity of the conversion of bovine factors IX, IXα, and IXaα to bovine factor IXaβ. J. Biol. Chem. 255:1430, 1980.

261. Kalousek, F., Konigsberg, W., and Nemerson, Y.: Activation of factor IX by activated factor X: A link between the extrinsic and intrinsic coagulation systems. FEBS Lett. 50:382, 1975.

262. Link, R. P., and Castellino, F. J.: Kinetic properties of bovine blood coagulation factors IXaα and IXaβ toward synthetic substrates. Biochemistry 22:999, 1983.

263. Walsh, P. N., Bradford, H., Sinha, D., Piperno, J. R., and Tuszynski, G. P.: Kinetics of the factor XIa catalyzed activation of human blood coagulation factor IX. J. Clin. Invest. 73:1392, 1984.

264. Jesty, J., and Morrison, S. A.: The activation of factor IX by tissue factor-factor VII in a bovine plasma system lacking factor X. Thromb. Res. 32:171, 1983.

265. Bajaj, S. P.: Cooperative Ca²⁺ binding to human factor IX. Effects of Ca²⁺ on the kinetic parameters of the activation of factor IX by factor XIa. J. Biol. Chem. 257:4127, 1982.

266. Lawson, J. H., and Mann, K. G.: Cooperative activation of human factor IX by the human extrinsic pathway of blood coagulation. J. Biol. Chem. 266:11317, 1991.

267. Bauer, K. A., Kass, B. L., ten Cate, H., Hawiger, J. J., and Rosenberg, R. D.: Factor IX is activated in vivo by the tissue factor mechanism. Blood 78:731, 1990.

268. Fuchs, H. E., Trapp, H. G., Griffith, M. J., Roberts, H. R., and Pizzo, S. V: Regulation of factor IXa in vitro in human and mouse plasma and in vivo in the mouse. J. Clin. Invest. 73:1696, 1984.

269. Rosenberg, J. S., McKenna, P. W., and Rosenberg, R. D.: Inhibition of human factor IXa by human antithrombin. J. Biol. Chem. 250:8883, 1975.

270. Varadi, K., and Elodi, S.: Protection of platelet surface bound factors IXa and VIII against specific inhibitors. Thromb. Haemost. 47:32, 1982.

271. Chance, P. F., Dyer, K. A., Kurachi, K., Yoshitake, S., Ropers, H.-H., Wieacker, P., and Gartler, S. M.: Regional localization of the human factor IX gene by molecular hybridization. Hum. Genet. 65:207, 1983.

272. Camerino, G., Mattei, M. G., Mattei, J. F., Jaye, M., and Mandel, J. L.: Close linkage of fragile X–mental retardation syndrome to haemophilia B and transmission through a normal male. Nature 306:701, 1983.

273. Choo, K. H., Gould, K. G., Rees, D. J. G., and Brownlee, G. G.: Molecular cloning of the gene for human anti-haemophilic factor IX. Nature 299:178, 1982.

274. Anson, D. S., Choo, K. H., Rees, D. J. G., Giannelli, F., Gould, K., Huddleston, J. A., and Brownlee, G. G.: The gene structure of human anti-haemophilic factor IX. EMBO J. 3:1053, 1984.

275. Yoshitake, S., Schach, B. G., Foster, D. C., Davie, E. W., and Kurachi, K.: Nucleotide sequence of the gene for human factor IX (antihemophilic factor B). Biochemistry 24:3736, 1985.

276. Foster, D. C., Yoshitake, S., and Davie, E. W.: The nucleotide sequence of the gene for human protein C. Proc. Natl. Acad. Sci. USA 82:4673, 1985.

277. O'Hara, P. J., Grant, F. J., Haldeman, B. A., Gray, C. L., Insley, M. Y., Hagen, F. S., and Murray, M. J.: Nucleotide sequence of the gene coding for human factor VII, a vitamin K-dependent protein participating in blood coagulation. Proc. Natl. Acad. Sci. USA 84:5158, 1987.

278. Leytus, S. P., Foster, D. C., Kurachi, K., and Davie, E. W.: Gene for human factor X: A blood coagulation factor whose gene organization is essentially identical with that of factor IX and protein C. Biochemistry 25:5098, 1986.

279. Ny, T., Elgh, F., and Lund, B.: The structure of the human tissue-type plasminogen activator gene: Correlation of intron and exon structures to functional and structural domains. Proc. Natl. Acad. Sci. USA 81:5355, 1984.

280. Nagamine, Y., Pearson, D., Altus, M. S., and Reich, E.: cDNA and gene nucleotide sequence of porcine plasminogen activator. Nucleic Acids Res. 12:9525, 1984.

281. Cool, D. E., and MacGillivray, R. T. A.: Characterization of the human blood coagulation factor XII gene. Intron/exon gene organization and analysis of the 5'-flanking region. J. Biol. Chem. 262:13662, 1987.

282. Sudhof, T. C., Russell, D. W., Goldstein, J. L., Brown, M. S., Sanchez-Pescador, R., and Bell, G. I.: Cassette of eight exons shared by genes for LDL receptor and EGF precursor. Science 228:893, 1985.

283. Degen, S. J. F., and Davie, E. W.: Nucleotide sequence of the gene for human prothrombin. Biochemistry 26:6165, 1987.

284. Craik, C. S., Choo, Q.-L., Swift, G. H., Quinto, C., MacDonald, R. J., and Rutter, W. J.: Structure of two related rat pancreatic trypsin genes. J. Biol. Chem. 259:14255, 1984.

285. Rizza, C. R., and Spooner, R. J. D.: Treatment of haemophilia and related disorders in Britain and Northern Ireland during 1976-80: Report on behalf of the directors of haemophilia centres in the the United Kingdom. Br. Med. J. 286:929, 1983.

286. Giannelli, F., Green, P. M., High, K. A., Sommer, S., Lillicrap, D. P., Ludwig, M., Olek, K., Reitsma, P. H., Goossens, M., Yoshioka, A., and Brownlee, G. G.: Haemophilia B: Database of point mutations and short additions and deletions—second edition. Nucleic Acids Res. 19 (Suppl.):2193, 1991.

287. Thompson, A. R.: Molecular biology of the hemophilias. Prog. Hemost. Thromb. 10:175, 1991.

288. Ludwig, M., Sabharwal, A. K., Brackmann, H. H., Olek, K., Smith, K. J., Birktoft, J. J., and Bajaj, S. P.: Hemophilia B caused by five different nondeletion mutations in the protease domain of factor IX. Blood 79:1225, 1992.

289. Parekh, V. R., Mannucci, P. M., and Ruggeri, Z. M.: Immunological heterogeneity of haemophilia B: A multicentre study of 98 kindreds. Br. J. Haematol. 40:643, 1978.

290. Briet, E., Bertina, R. M., van Tilburg, N. H., and Veltkamp, J. J.: Hemophilia B Leyden. N. Engl. J. Med. 306:788, 1982.

291. Crossley, M., and Brownlee, G. G.: Disruption of a C/EBP binding site in the factor IX promoter is associated with haemophlia B. Nature 345:444, 1990.

292. Ware, J., Diuguid, D. L., Liebman, H. A., Rabiet, M.-J., Kasper, C. K., Furie, B. C., Furie, B., and Stafford, D. W.: Factor IX San Dimas. Substitution of glutamine for Arg-4 in the propeptide leads to incomplete γ-carboxylation and altered phospholipid binding properties. J. Biol. Chem. 264:11401, 1989.

293. Bertina, R. M., and van der Linden, I. K.: Factor IX Zutphen. A genetic variant of blood coagulation factor IX with an abnormally high molecular weight. J. Lab. Clin. Med. 100:695, 1982.

294. Bottema, C. D. K., Ketterling, R. P., Yoon, H.-S., and Sommer, S. S.: The pattern of factor IX germ-line mutation in Asians is similar to that of Caucasians. Am. J. Hum. Genet. 47:835, 1990.

295. McCord, D. M., Monroe, D. M., Smith, K. J., and Roberts, H. R.: Characterization of the functional defect in factor IX Alabama. Evidence for a conformational change due to high affinity calcium binding in the first epidermal growth factor domain. J. Biol. Chem. 265:10250, 1990.

296. Braunstein, K. M., Noyes, C. M., Griffith, M. J., Lundblad, R. L., and Roberts, H. R.: Characterization of the defect in activation of factor IX (Chapel Hill) by human factor XIa. J. Clin. Invest. 68:1420, 1981.

297. Noyes, C. M., Griffith, M. J., Roberts, H. R., and Lundblad, R. L.: Identification of the molecular defect in factor IX Chapel Hill: Substitution of histidine for arginine at position 145. Proc. Natl. Acad. Sci. USA 80:4200, 1983.

298. Hougie, C., and Twomey, J. J.: Haemophilia B$_M$: A new type of factor IX deficiency. Lancet 1:698, 1967.

299. Girolami, A., Dal Bo Zanon, R., Saltarin, P., Quaino, V., Altinier, G., Ripa, T., Marchetti, A., and Stocco, D.: Incidence, significance, and sugtypes of hemophilia B$_M$ in a large population of hemophilia B patients. Blut 44:41, 1982.

300. Osterud, B., Kasper, C. K., Lavine, K. K., Prodanos, C., and Rapaport, S. I.: Purification and properties of an abnormal blood coagulation factor IX (factor IX$_{Bm}$) kinetics of its inhibition of factor X activation by factor VII and bovine tissue factor. Thromb. Haemost. 45:55, 1981.

301. Bertina, R. M., van der Linden, I. K., Mannucci, P. M., Reinalda-Poot, H. H., Cupers, R., Poort, S. R., and Reitsma, P. H.: Mutations in hemophilia B$_m$ occur at the Arg^{180}-Val activation site or in the catalytic domain of factor IX. J. Biol. Chem. 265:10876, 1990.

302. Terwiel, J. Ph., Veltkamp, J. J., Bertina, R. M., and Muller, H. P.: Coagulation factors in the human fetus of about 20 weeks of gestational age. Br. J. Haematol. 45:641, 1980.

303. McDougal, J. S., Martin, L. S., Cort, S. P., Mozen, M., Heldebrant, C. M., and Evatt, B. L.: Thermal inactivation of the acquired immunodeficiency syndrome virus, T lymphotropic virus-III/lymphadenopathy–associated virus, with special reference to antihemophilic factor. J. Clin. Invest. 76:875, 1985.

304. Study group of the UK haemophilia centre directors on surveillance of virus transmission by concentrates: Effect of dry-heating of coagulation factor concentrates at 80°C for 72 hours on transmission of non-A, non-B hepatitis. Lancet 2:814, 1988.

305. Kreuz, W., Auerswald, G., Brückmann, C., Linde, R., Sutor, A. H., Schramm, W., Funk, M., Augerger, K., Zieger, B., Kröniger, A., Roggendorf, M., Schwarz, T., Doerr, H. W., and Kornhuber, B.: Virus safety of pasteurized clotting factor concentrates—an eleven year follow up. Thromb. Haemost. 65:824, 1991.

306. Agrawal, B. L., Zelkowitz, L., and Hleto, P.: Acute myocardial infarction in a young hemophiliac patient during therapy with factor IX concentrate and epsilon aminocaproic acid. J. Pediatr. 98:931, 1981.

307. Conlan, M. B., and Hoots, W. K.: Disseminated intravascular

coagulation and hemorrhage in hemophilia B following elective surgery. Am. J. Hematol. 35:203, 1990.

308. Mannucci, P. M., Bauer, K. A., Gringeri, A., Barzegar, S., Bottasso, B., Simoni, L., and Rosenberg, R. D.: Thrombin generation is not increased in the blood of hemophilia B patients after the infusion of a purified factor IX concentrate. Blood 76:2540, 1990.

309. Kim, H. C., McMillan, C. W., White, G. C., Bergman, G. E., Horton, M. W., and Saidi, P.: Purified factor IX using monoclonal immunoaffinity technique: Clinical trials in hemophilia B and comparison to prothrombin complex concentrates. Blood 79:568, 1992.

310. Anson, D. S., Austin, D. E. G., and Brownlee, G. G.: Expression of active human clotting factor IX from recombinant DNA clones in mammalian cells. Nature 315:683, 1985.

311. De la Salle, H., Altenburger, W., Elkaim, R., Dott, K., Dieterle, A., Drillien, R., Cazenave, J.-P., Tolstoshev, P., and Lecocq, J.-P.: Active γ-carboxylated human factor IX expressed using recombinant DNA techniques. Nature 316:268, 1985.

312. Busby, S., Kumar, A., Joseph, M., Halfpap, L., Insley, M., Berkner, K., Kurachi, K., and Woodbury, R.: Expression of active human factor IX in transfected cells. Nature 316:271, 1985.

313. Choo, K. H., Raphael, K., McAdam, W., and Peterson, M. G.: Expression of active human blood clotting factor IX in transgenic mice: Use of a cDNA with complete mRNA sequence. Nucleic Acids Res. 15:871, 1987.

314. Jallat, S., Perraud, F., Dalemans, W., Balland, A., Dieterle, A., Faure, T., Meulien, P., and Pavirani, A.: Characterization of recombinant human factor IX expressed in transgenic mice and in derived trans-immortalized hepatic cell lines. EMBO J. 9:3295, 1990.

315. Schmidt, M. L., Smith, H. E., Gamerman, S., DiMichele, D., Glazer, S., and Scott, J. P.: Prolonged recombinant activated factor VII (rFVIIa) treatment for severe bleeding in a factor-IX–deficient patient with an inhibitor. Br. J. Haematol. 78:460, 1991.

316. Armentano, D., Thompson, A. R., Darlington, G., and Woo, S. L. C.: Expression of human factor IX in rabbit hepatocytes by retrovirus-mediated gene transfer: Potential for gene therapy of hemophilia B. Proc. Natl. Acad. Sci. USA 87:6141, 1990.

317. St. Louis, D., and Verma, I. M.: An alternative approach to somatic cell gene therapy. Proc. Natl. Acad. Sci. USA 85:3150, 1988.

318. Palmer, T. D., Thompson, A. R., and Miller, A. D.: Production of human factor IX in animals by genetically modified skin fibroblasts: Potential therapy for hemophilia B. Blood 73:438, 1989.

319. Yao, S.-N., Wilson, J. M., Nabel, E. G., Kurachi, S., Hachiya, H. L., and Kurachi, K.: Expression of human factor IX in rat capillary endothelial cells: Toward somatic gene therapy for hemophilia B. Proc. Natl. Acad. Sci. USA 88:8101, 1991.

320. Von Willebrand, E. A.: Hereditär pseudohemofili. Finska Lakarsallskapets Handlingar 68:87, 1926.

321. Von Willebrand, E. A.: Über hereditäre pseudohämophilie. Acta Med. Scand. 76:521, 1931.

322. Alexander, B., and Goldstein, B.: Dual hemostatic defect in pseudohemophilia. J. Clin. Invest. 32:551, 1953.

323. Larrieu, M. J., and Soulier, J. P.: Deficit en facteur antihemophilique A chez une fille associée à un trouble saignement. Rev. Hematol. 8:61, 1953.

324. Quick, A. J., and Hussey, V. V.: Hemophilic condition in the female. J. Lab. Clin. Med. 42:929, 1953.

325. Nilsson, I. M., Blömback, M., and Von Francken, I.: On an inherited autosomal hemorrhagic diathesis with antihemophilic globulin (AHG) deficiency and prolonged bleeding time. Acta Med. Scand. 159:35, 1957.

326. Cornu, P., Larrieu, M. J., Caen, J., and Bernard, J.: Transfusion studies in von Willebrand's disease: Effect on bleeding time and factor VIII. Br. J. Haematol. 9:189, 1963.

327. Zucker, M. N.: In vitro abnormality of the blood in von Willebrand's disease correctable by normal plasma. Nature 197:601, 1963.

328. Salzman, E. W.: Measurement of platelet adhesiveness: A simple in vitro technique demonstrating an abnormality in von Willebrand's disease. J. Lab. Clin. Med. 62:724, 1963.

329. Bouma, B. N., Wiegerinch, Y., Sixma, J. J., van Mourik, J. A., and Mochtar, J. A.: Immunological characterization of purified antihaemophilic factor A (factor VIII) which corrects abnormal platelet retention in von Willebrand's disease. Nature (New Biol.) 236:104, 1972.

330. Howard, M. A., and Firkin, B. G.: Ristocetin: A new tool in the investigation of platelet aggregation. Thromb. Diath. Haemorrh. 26:362, 1971.

331. Macfarlane, D. E., and Zucker, M. B.: A method for assaying von Willebrand factor (ristocetin cofactor). Thromb. Diath. Haemorrh. 34:306, 1975.

332. Read, M. S., Shermer, R. W., and Brinkhous, K. M.: Venom coagglutinin: An activator of platelet aggregation dependent on von Willebrand factor. Proc. Natl. Acad. Sci. USA 75:4514, 1978.

333. Brinkhous, K. M., and Read, M. S.: Use of venom coagglutinin and lyophilized platelets in testing for platelet-aggregating von Willebrand factor. Blood 55:517, 1980.

334. Koutts, J., Walsh, P. N., Plow, E. F., Fenton, J. W., II, Bouma, B. N., and Zimmerman, T. S.: Active release of human platelet factor VIII–related antigen by adenosine diphosphate, collagen, and thrombin. J. Clin. Invest. 62:1255, 1978.

335. Hoyer, L. W.: Immunologic studies of antihemophilic factor (AHF, factor VIII). IV. Radioimmunoassay of AHF antigen. J. Lab. Clin. Med. 80:822, 1972.

336. Ruggeri, Z. M., Mannucci, P. M., Jeffcoate, S. L., and Ingram, G. I. C.: Immunoradiometric assay of factor VIII related antigen, with observations in 32 patients with von Willebrand's disease. Br. J. Haematol. 33:221, 1976.

337. Zimmerman, T. S., Roberts, J. R., and Ruggeri, Z. M.: Factor VIII–related antigen: Characterization by electrophoretic techniques. In Bloom, A. L. (ed.): The Hemophilias. Edinburgh, Churchill Livingstone, 1982.

338. Ruggeri, Z. M., and Zimmerman, T. S.: Variant von Willebrand's disease. Characterization of two subtypes by analysis of multimeric composition of factor VIII/von Willebrand factor in plasma and platelets. J. Clin. Invest. 65:1318, 1980.

339. Ruggeri, Z. M., and Zimmerman, T. S.: The complex multimeric composition of factor VIII/von Willebrand factor. Blood 57:1140, 1981.

340. Hoyer, L. W., and Chainoff, J. R.: Factor VIII–related protein circulates in normal human plasma as high molecular weight multimers. Blood 55:1056, 1980.

341. Chopek, M. W., Girma, J.-P., Fujikawa, K., Davie, E. W., and Titani, K.: Human von Willebrand factor: A multivalent protein composed of identical subunits. Biochemistry 25:3146, 1986.

342. Dent, J. A., Galbusera, M., and Ruggeri, Z. M.: Heterogeneity of plasma von Willebrand factor multimers resulting from proteolysis of the constituent subunit. J. Clin. Invest. 88:774, 1991.

343. Counts, R. B., Paskell, S. L., and Elgee, S. K.: Disulfide bonds and the quaternary structure of factor VIII/von Willebrand factor. J. Clin. Invest. 62:702, 1978.

344. Lynch, D. C., Zimmerman, T. S., Kirby, E. P., and Livingston, D. M.: Subunit composition of oligomeric human von Willebrand factor. J. Biol. Chem. 258:12757, 1983.

345. Sadler, J. E.: von Willebrand factor. J. Biol. Chem. 266:22777, 1991.

346. Fay, P. J., Kawai, Y., Wagner, D. D., Ginsburg, D., Bonthron, D., Ohlsson-Wilhelm, B. M., Chavin, S. I., Abraham, G. N., Handin, R. I., Orkin, S. H., Montgomery, R. R., and Marder, V. J.: Propolypeptide of von Willebrand factor circulates in blood and is identical to von Willebrand antigen II. Science 232:995, 1986.

347. Montgomery, R. R., and Zimmerman, T. S.: von Willebrand's disease antigen II: A new plasma and platelet antigen deficient in severe von Willebrand's disease. J. Clin. Invest. 62:1498, 1978.

348. Wagner, D. D., Fay, P. J., Sporn, L. A., Sinha, S., Lawrence,

S. O., and Marder, V. J.: Divergent fates of von Willebrand factor and its propolypeptide (von Willebrand antigen II) after secretion from endothelial cells. Proc. Natl. Acad. Sci. USA 84:1955, 1987.

349. Titani, K., Kumar, S., Takio, K., Ericsson, L. H., Wade, R. D., Ashida, K., Walsh, K. A., Chopek, M. W., Sadler, J. E., and Fujikawa, K.: Amino acid sequence of human von Willebrand factor. Biochemistry 25:3171, 1986.

350. Marti, T., Rösselet, S. J., Titani, K., and Walsh, K. A.: Identification of disulfide-bridged substructures within human von Willebrand factor. Biochemistry 26:8099, 1987.

351. Samor, B., Mazurier, C., Goudemand, M., Debeire, P., Fournet, B., and Montreuil, J.: Preliminary results on the carbohydrate moiety of factor VIII/von Willebrand factor (FVIII/vWF). Thromb. Res. 25:81, 1982.

352. Debeire, P., Montreuil, J., Samor, B., Mazurier, C., Goudemand, M., Van Halbeek, H., and Vliegenthart, J. F. G.: Structure determination of the major asparagine-linked sugar chain of human factor VIII–von Willebrand factor. FEBS Lett. 151:22, 1983.

353. Carew, J. A., Browning, P. J., and Lynch, D. C.: Sulfation of von Willebrand factor. Blood 76:2530, 1990.

354. Ohmori, K., Fretto, L. J., Harrison, R. L., Switzer, M. E. P., Erickson, H. P., and McKee, P. A.: Electron microscopy of human factor VIII/von Willebrand glycoprotein: Effect of reducing reagents on structure and function. J. Cell Biol. 95:632, 1982.

355. Jaffe, E. A., Hoyer, L. W., and Nachman, R. L.: Synthesis of antihemophilic factor antigen by cultured human endothelial cells. J. Clin. Invest. 52:2757, 1973.

356. Jaffe, E. A., Hoyer, L. W., and Nachman, R. L.: Synthesis of von Willebrand factor by cultured human endothelial cells. Proc. Natl. Acad. Sci. USA 71:1906, 1974.

357. Nachman, R., Levine, R., and Jaffe, E. A.: Synthesis of factor VIII antigen by cultured guinea pig megakaryocytes. J. Clin. Invest. 60:914, 1977.

358. Bloom, A. L., Giddings, J. C., and Wilks, C. J.: Factor VIII on the vascular intima: Possible importance in haemostasis and thrombosis. Nature (New Biol.) 241:217, 1973.

359. Hoyer, L. W., De Los Santos, R. P., and Hoyer, J. R.: Antihemophilic factor antigen. Localization in endothelial cells by immunofluorescent microscopy. J. Clin. Invest. 52:2737, 1973.

360. Maruyama, I., Bell, C. E., and Majerus, P. W.: Thrombomodulin is found on endothelium of arteries, veins, capillaries, and lymphatics, and on syncytiotrophoblast of human placenta. J. Cell Biol. 101:363, 1985.

361. Cramer, E. M., Meyer, D., le Menn, R., and Berton-Gorius, J.: Eccentric localization of von Willebrand factor in an internal structure of platelet α-granule resembling that of Weibel-Palade bodies. Blood 66:710, 1985.

362. Howard, M. A., Montgomery, D. C., and Hardisty, R. M.: Factor VIII–related antigen in platelets. Thromb. Res. 4:617, 1974.

363. Holmberg, L., Mannucci, P. M., Turesson, I., Ruggeri, Z. M., and Nilsson, I. M.: Factor VIII antigen in the vessel wall in von Willebrand's disease and haemophilia A. Scand. J. Haematol. 13:33, 1974.

364. Potter, E. V., Chediak, J., and Green, D.: Absence of ristocetin aggregation factor from the skin of a patient with von Willebrand's disease. Lancet 1:514, 1976.

365. Wagner, D. D., and Marder, V. J.: Biosynthesis of von Willebrand protein by human endothelial cells: Processing steps and their intracellular localization. J. Cell Biol. 99:2123, 1984.

366. Wagner, D. D.: Cell biology of von Willebrand factor. Annu. Rev. Cell. Biol. 6:217, 1990.

367. Wise, R. J., Barr, P. J., Wong, P. A., Kiefer, M. C., Brake, A. J., and Kaufman, R. J.: Expression of a human proprotein processing enzyme: Correct cleavage of the von Willebrand factor precursor at a paired basic amino acid site. Proc. Natl. Acad. Sci. USA 87:9378, 1990.

368. Van de Ven, W. J. M., Voorberg, J., Fonjijn, R., Pannekoek, H., van den Ouweland, A. M. W., van Duijnhoven, H. L.

P., Roebroek, A. J. M., and Siezen, R. J.: Furin is a subtilisin-like proprotein processing enzyme in higher eukaryotes. Mol. Biol. Rep. 14:265, 1990.

369. Wagner, D. D., Olmsted, J. B., and Marder, V. J.: Immunolocalization of von Willebrand protein in Weibel-Palade bodies of human endothelial cells. J. Cell Biol. 95:355, 1982.

370. Weibel, E. R., and Palade, G. E.: New cytoplasmic components in arterial endothelia. J. Cell Biol. 23:101, 1964.

371. Wagner, D. D., Saffaripour, S., Bonfanti, R., Sadler, J. E., Cramer, E. M., Chapman, B., and Mayadas, T. N.: Induction of specific storage organelles by von Willebrand factor propolypeptide. Cell 64:403, 1991.

372. Loesberg, C., Gonsalves, M. D., Zandbergen, J., Willems, C., Van Aken, W. G., Stel, H. V., Van Mourick, J. A., and De Groot, P. G.: The effect of calcium on the secretion of factor VIII–related antigen by cultured human endothelial cells. Biochim. Biophys. Acta 763:160, 1983.

373. Sporn, L. A., Marder, V. J., and Wagner, D. D.: Inducible secretion of large, biologically potent von Willebrand factor multimers. Cell 46:185, 1986.

374. Levine, J. D., Harlan, J. M., Harker, L. A., Joseph, M. L., and Counts, R. B.: Thrombin-mediated release of factor VIII antigen from human umbilical vein endothelial cells in culture. Blood 60:431, 1982.

375. Hamilton, K. K., and Sims, P. J.: Changes in cytosolic Ca^{2+} associated with von Willebrand factor release in human endothelial cells exposed to histamines. Study of microcarrier cell monolayers using the fluorescent probe indo-1. J. Clin. Invest. 79:600, 1987.

376. Ribes, J. A., Ni, F., Wagner, D. D., and Francis, C. W.: Mediation of fibrin-induced release of von Willebrand factor from cultured endothelial cells by the fibrin β-chain. J. Clin. Invest. 84:435, 1989.

377. Hattori, R., Hamilton, K. K., McEver, R. P., and Sims, P. J.: Complement proteins C5b-9 induce secretion of high molecular weight multimers of endothelial von Willebrand factor and translocation of granule membrane protein GMP-140 to the cell surface. J. Biol. Chem. 264:9053, 1989.

378. Harrison, R. L., and McKee, P. A.: Estrogen stimulates von Willebrand factor production by cultured endothelial cells. Blood 63:657, 1984.

379. Glueck, H. I., and Flessa, H. C.: Control of hemorrhage in von Willebrand's disease and a hemophiliac carrier with norethynodrelmestranol. Thromb. Res. 1:253, 1972.

380. Alperin, J. B.: Estrogens and surgery in women with von Willebrand's disease. Am. J. Med. 73:367, 1982.

381. Gill, J. C., Endres-Brooks, J., Bauer, P. J., Marks, W. J., Jr., and Montgomery, R. R.: The effect of ABO blood group on the diagnosis of von Willebrand disease. Blood 69:1691, 1987.

382. Ørstavik, K. H., Kornstad, L., Reisner, H., and Berg, K.: Possible effect of secretor locus on plasma concentration of factor VIII and von Willebrand factor. Blood 73:990, 1989.

383. Brommer, E. J. P., Derkx, F. H. M., Barrett-Bergshoeff, M. M., and Schalekamp, M. A. D. H.: The inability of propranolol and aspirin to inhibit the response of fibrinolytic activity and factor VIII-antigen to infusion of DDAVP. Thromb. Haemost. 51:42, 1984.

384. Tuddenham, E. G. D., Lazarchick, J., and Hoyer, L. W.: Synthesis and release of factor VIII by cultured human endothelial cells. Br. J. Haematol. 47:617, 1981.

385. Shearn, S. A. M., Peake, I. R., Giddings, J. C., Humphreys, J., and Bloom, A. L.: The characterization and synthesis of antigens related to factor VIII in vascular endothelium. Thromb. Res. 11:43, 1977.

386. Weiss, H. J., Turitto, V. T., and Baumgartner, H. R.: Effect of shear rate on platelet interaction with subendothelium in citrated and native blood. I. Shear rate-dependent decrease of adhesion in von Willebrand's disease and the Bernard-Soulier syndrome. J. Lab. Clin. Med. 92:750, 1978.

387. Sakariassen, K. S., Bolhuis, P. A., and Sixma, J. J.: Human blood platelet adhesion to artery subendothelium is mediated by factor VIII–von Willebrand factor bound to the subendothelium. Nature 279:636, 1979.

388. Badimon, L., Badimon, J. J., Turitto, V. T., and Fuster, V.: Role of von Willebrand factor in mediating platelet–vessel wall interaction at low shear rate; the importance of perfusion conditions. Blood 73:961, 1989.

389. Stel, H. V., Sakariassen, K. S., de Groot, P. G., van Mourik, J. A., and Sixma, J. J.: Von Willebrand factor in the vessel wall mediates platelet adherence. Blood 65:85, 1985.

390. Turitto, V. T., Weiss, H. J., Zimmerman, T. S., and Sussman, I. I.: Factor VIII/von Willebrand factor in subendothelium mediates platelet adhesion. Blood 65:823, 1985.

391. Hormia, M., Lehto, V.-P., and Virtanen, I.: Factor VIII–related antigen. A pericellular matrix component of cultured human endothelial cells. Exp. Cell. Res. 149:483, 1983.

392. Wagner, D. D., Urban-Pickering, M., and Marder, V. J.: von Willebrand protein binds to extracellular matrices independently of collagen. Proc. Natl. Acad. Sci. USA 81:471, 1984.

393. Santoro, S. A.: Adsorption of Willebrand factor/factor VIII by the genetically distinct interstitial collagens. Thromb. Res. 21:689, 1981.

394. Santoro, S. A., and Cowan, J. F.: Adsorption of von Willebrand factor by fibrillar collagen-implications concerning the adhesion of platelets to collagen. Coll. Relat. Res. 2:31, 1982.

395. Morton, L. F., Griffin, B., Pepper, D. S., and Barnes, M. J.: The interaction between collagens and factor VIII/von Willebrand factor: Investigation of the structural requirements for interaction. Thromb. Res. 32:545, 1983.

396. Rand, J. H., Patel, N. D., Schwartz, E., Zhou, S.-L., and Potter, B. J.: 150-kD von Willebrand factor binding protein extracted from human vascular subendothelium is type VI collagen. J. Clin. Invest. 88:253, 1991.

397. De Groot, P. G., Ottenhof-Rovers, M., van Mourik, J. A., and Sixma, J. J.: Evidence that the primary binding site of von Willebrand factor that mediates platelet adhesion on subendothelium is not collagen. J. Clin. Invest. 82:65, 1988.

398. Von der Mark, H., Sumailley, M., Wick, G., Fleischmajer, R., and Timpl, R.: Immunochemistry, genuine size and tissue localization of collagen VI. Eur. J. Biochem. 142:493, 1984.

399. Colombatti, A., and Bonaldo, P.: Biosynthesis of chick type VI collagen. II. Processing and secretion in fibroblasts and smooth muscle cells. J. Biol. Chem. 262:14461, 1987.

400. Martin, S. E., Marder, V. J., Francis, C. W., and Barlow, G. H.: Structural studies on the functional heterogeneity of von Willebrand protein polymers. Blood 57:313, 1981.

401. Aihara, M., Kimura, A., Chiba, Y., and Yoshida, Y: Plasma collagen cofactor correlates with von Willebrand factor antigen and ristocetin cofactor but not with bleeding time. Thromb. Haemost. 59:485, 1988.

402. Sixma, J. J., Sakariassen, K. S., Beeser-Visser, N. H., Ottenhof-Rovers, M., and Bolhuis, P. A.: Adhesion of platelets to human artery subendothelium: Effect of factor VIII–von Willebrand factor of various multimeric composition. Blood 63:128, 1984.

403. Martin, S. E., Marder, V. J., Francis, C. W., Loftus, L. S., and Barlow, G. H.: Enzymatic degradation of the factor VIII–von Willebrand protein: A unique tryptic fragment with ristocetin cofactor activity. Blood 55:848, 1980.

404. Mohri, H., Yoshioka, A., Zimmerman, T. S., and Ruggeri, Z. M.: Isolation of the von Willebrand factor domain interacting with platelet glycoprotein Ib, heparin, and collagen and characterization of its three distinct functional sites. J. Biol. Chem. 264:17361, 1989.

405. Mohri, H., Fujimura, Y., Shima, M., Yoshioka, A., Houghten, R. A., Ruggeri, Z. M., and Zimmerman, T. S.: Structure of the von Willebrand factor domain interacting with glycoprotein Ib. J. Biol. Chem. 263:17901, 1988.

406. Andrews, R. K., Gorman, J. J., Booth, W. J., Corino, G. L., Castaldi, P. A., and Berndt, M. C.: Cross-linking of a monomeric 39/34-kDa dispase fragment of von Willebrand factor (Leu-480/Val-481—Gly-718) to the N-terminal region of the α-chain of membrane glycoprotein Ib on intact platelets with bis(sulfosuccinimidyl) suberate. Biochemistry 28:8326, 1989.

407. Sugimoto, M., Mohri, H., McClintock, R. A., and Ruggeri, Z. M.: Identification of discontinuous von Willebrand factor

sequences involved in complex formation with botrocetin. A model for the regulation of von Willebrand factor binding to platelet glycoprotein Ib. J. Biol. Chem. 266:18172, 1991.

408. Pareti, F. I., Fujimura, Y., Dent, J. A., Holland, L. Z., Zimmerman, T. S., and Ruggeri, Z. M.: Isolation and characterization of a collagen binding domain in human von Willebrand factor. J. Biol. Chem. 261:15310, 1986.

409. Christophe, O., Obert, B., Meyer, D., and Girma, J.-P.: The binding domain of von Willebrand factor to sulfatides is distinct from those interacting with glycoprotein Ib, heparin, and collagen and resides between amino acid residues Leu 512 and Lys 673. Blood 78:2310, 1991.

410. Roth, G. J., Titani, K., Hoyer, L. W., and Hickey, M. J.: Localization of binding sites within human von Willebrand factor for monomeric type III collagen. Biochemistry 25:8357, 1986.

411. Takagi, J., Sekiya, F., Kasahara, K., Inada, Y., and Saito, Y.: Inhibition of platelet-collagen interaction by propolypeptide of von Willebrand factor. J. Biol. Chem. 264:6017, 1989.

412. Takagi, J., Fujisawa, T., Sekiya, F., and Saito, Y.: Collagen-binding domain within bovine propolypeptide of von Willebrand factor. J. Biol. Chem. 266:5575, 1991.

413. Berliner, S., Niiya, K., Roberts, J. R., Houghten, R. A., and Ruggeri, Z. M.: Generation and characterization of peptide-specific antibodies that inhibit von Willebrand factor binding to glycoprotein IIb-IIIa without interaction with other adhesive molecules. Selectivity is conferred by Pro1743 and other amino acid residues adjacent to the sequence Arg1744-Gly1745-Asp1746. J. Biol. Chem. 263:7500, 1988.

414. Rouslahti, E., and Pierschbacher, M. D.: New perspectives in cell adhesion: RGD and integrins. Science 238:491, 1987.

415. Foster, P. A., Fulcher, C. A., Marti, T., Titani, K., and Zimmerman, T. S.: A major factor VIII binding domain resides within the amino-terminal 272 amino acid residues of von Willebrand factor. J. Biol. Chem. 262:8443, 1987.

416. Bahou, W. F., Ginsburg, D., Sikkink, R., Litwiller, R., and Fass, D. N.: A monoclonal antibody to von Willebrand factor (vWF) inhibits factor VIII binding. Localization of its antigenic determinant to a nonadecapeptide at the amino terminus of the mature vWF polypeptide. J. Clin. Invest. 84:56, 1989.

417. Fretto, L. J., Fowler, W. E., McCaslin, D. R., Erickson, H. P., and McKee, P. A.: Substructure of human von Willebrand factor. Proteolysis by V8 and characterization of two functional domains. J. Biol. Chem. 261:15679, 1986.

418. Gralnick, H. R., Coller, B. S., and Sultan, Y.: Carbohydrate deficiency of the factor VIII/von Willebrand factor protein in von Willebrand's disease variants. Science 192:56, 1976.

419. De Marco, L., and Shapiro, S. S.: Properties of human asialo-factor VIII. A ristocetin-independent platelet-aggregating agent. J. Clin. Invest. 68:321, 1981.

420. Federici, A. B., Elder, J. H., DeMarco, L., Ruggeri, Z. M., and Zimmerman, T. S.: Carbohydrate moiety of von Willebrand factor is not necessary for maintaining multimeric structure and ristocetin cofactor activity but protects from proteolytic degradation. J. Clin. Invest. 74:2049, 1984.

421. Federici, A. B., De Romeuf, C., De Groot, P. G., Samor, B., Lombardi, R., D'Alessio, P., Mazurier, C., Mannucci, P. M., and Sixma, J. J.: Adhesive properties of the carbohydrate-modified von Willebrand factor (CHO-vWF). Blood 71:947, 1988.

422. Sodetz, J. M., Pizzo, S. V., and McKee, P. A.: Relationship of sialic acid to function and in vivo survival of human factor VIII/von Willebrand factor protein. J. Biol. Chem. 252:5538, 1977.

423. Fuster, V., Bowie, E. J. W., Lewis, J. C., Fass, D. N., Owen, C. A., Jr., and Brown, A. L.: Resistance to arteriosclerosis in pigs with von Willebrand's disease. Spontaneous and high cholesterol diet induced arteriosclerosis. J. Clin. Invest. 61:722, 1978.

424. Griggs, T. R., Reddick, R. L., Sultzer, D., and Brinkhous, K. M.: Susceptibility to atherosclerosis in aortas and coronary arteries of swine with von Willebrand's disease. Am. J. Pathol. 102:137, 1981.

425. Lamb, M. A., Manning, J. E., Reddick, R. L., and Griggs, T. R.: Smooth muscle cell proliferation in response to endothelial injury in coronary arteries of normal and von Willebrand's disease swine. Arteriosclerosis 4:84, 1984.

426. Nichols, T. C., Bellinger, D. A., Tate, D. A., Reddick, R. L., Read, M. S., Koch, G. G., Brinkhous, K. M., and Griggs, T. R.: von Willebrand factor and occlusive arterial thrombosis. A study in normal and von Willebrand's disease pigs with diet-induced hypercholesteremia and atherosclerosis. Arteriosclerosis 10:449, 1990.

427. Moake, J. L., Rudy, C. K., Troll, J. H., Weinstein, M. J., Colannino, N. M., Azocar, J., Seder, H. R., Hong, S. L., and Deykin, D.: Unusually large plasma factor VIII: von Willebrand factor multimers in chronic relapsing thrombotic thrombocytopenic purpura. N. Engl. J. Med. 307:1432, 1982.

428. Kelton, J. G., Moore, J., Santos, A., and Sheridan, D.: Detection of a platelet-agglutinating factor in thrombotic thrombocytopenic purpura. Ann. Intern. Med. 101:589, 1984.

429. Moake, J. L., Byrnes, J. J., Troll, J. H., Rudy, C. K., Weinstein, M. J., Colannino, N. M., and Hong, S. L.: Abnormal VIII:von Willebrand factor patterns in the plasma of patients with the hemolytic-uremic syndrome. Blood 64:592, 1984.

430. Ginsburg, D., Handin, R. I., Bonthron, D. T., Donlon, T. A., Bruns, G. A. P., Latt, S. A., and Orkin, S. H.: Human von Willebrand factor (vWF): Isolation of complementary DNA (cDNA) clones and chromosomal localization. Science 228:1401, 1985.

431. O'Connell, P., Lathrop, G. M., Law, M., Leppert, M., Nakamura, Y., Hoff, M., Kumlin, E., Thomas, W., Elsner, T., Ballard, L., Goodman, P., Azen, E., Sadler, J. E., Cai, G. Y., Lalouel, J.-M., and White, R.: A primary genetic linkage map for human chromosome 12. Genomics 1:93, 1987.

432. Mancuso, D. J., Tuley, E. A., Westfield, L. A., Worrall, N. K., Shelton-Inloes, B. B., Sorace, J. M., Alevy, Y. G., and Sadler, J. E.: Structure of the gene for human von Willebrand factor. J. Biol. Chem. 264:19514, 1989.

433. Colombatti, A., and Bonaldo, P.: The superfamily of proteins with von Willebrand factor type A-like domains: One theme common to components of extracellular matrix, hemostasis, cellular adhesion, and defense mechanisms. Blood 77:2305, 1991.

434. Yamagata, M., Yamada, K. M., Yamada, S. S., Shinomura, T., Tanaka, H., Nishida, Y., Obara, M., and Kimata, K.: The complete primary structure of type XII collagen shows a chimeric molecule with reiterated fibronectin type III motifs, von Willebrand factor A motifs, a domain homologous to a noncollagenous region of type IX collagen, and short collagenous domains with an Arg-Gly-Asp site. J. Cell Biol. 115:209, 1991.

435. Just, M., Herbst, H., Hummel, M., Dürkop, H., Tripier, D., Stein, H., and Schuppan, D.: Undulin is a novel member of the fibronectin-tenascin family of extracellular matrix glycoproteins. J. Biol. Chem. 266:17326, 1991.

436. Mancuso, D. J., Tuley, E. A., Westfield, L. A., Lester-Mancuso, T. L., Le Beau, M. M., Sorace, J. M., and Sadler, J. E.: Human von Willebrand factor gene and pseudogene: Structural analysis and differentiation by polymerase chain reaction. Biochemistry 30:253, 1991.

437. Rodeghiero, F., Castaman, G., and Dini, E.: Epidemiological investigation of the prevalence of von Willebrand's disease. Blood 69:454, 1987.

438. Holmberg, L., and Nilsson, I. M.: Von Willebrand disease. Clin. Haematol. 14:461, 1985.

439. Ruggeri, Z. M.: Structure and function of von Willebrand factor: Relationship to von Willebrand's disease. Mayo Clin. Proc. 66:847, 1991.

440. Ginsburg, D., and Sadler, J. E.: von Willebrand disease: A database of point mutations, insertions, and deletions. Thromb. Haemost. 69:177, 1993.

441. Sadler, J. E., and Ginsburg, D.: A database of polymorphisms in the von Willebrand factor gene and pseudogene. Thromb. Haemost. 69:185, 1993.

442. Mannucci, P. M., Lombardi, R., Castaman, G., Dent, J. A., Lattuada, A., Rodeghiero, F., and Zimmerman, T. S.: von Willebrand disease "Vicenza" with larger-than-normal (supranormal) von Willebrand factor multimers. Blood 71:65, 1988.

443. Weiss, H. J., Pietu, G., Rabinowitz, R., Girma, J.-P., Rogers, J., and Meyer, D.: Heterogeneous abnormalities in the multimeric structure, antigenic properties, and plasma-platelet content of factor VIII/von Willebrand factor in subtypes of classic (type I) and variant (type IIA) von Willebrand's disease. J. Lab. Clin. Med. 101:411, 1983.

444. Mannucci, P. M., Lombardi, R., Bader, R., Vianello, L., Federici, A. B., Solinas, S., Mazzucconi, M. G., and Mariani, G.: Heterogeneity of type I von Willebrand disease: Evidence for a subgroup with an abnormal von Willebrand factor. Blood 66:796, 1985.

445. Hoyer, L. W., Rizza, C. R., Tuddenham, E. G. D., Carta, C. A., Armitage, H., and Rotblat, F.: von Willebrand factor multimer patterns in von Willebrand's disease. Br. J. Haematol. 55:493, 1983.

446. Ciavarella, G., Ciavarella, N., Antonecchi, S., DeMattia, D., Ranieri, P., Dent, J., Zimmerman, T. S., and Ruggeri, Z. M.: High-resolution analysis of von Willebrand factor multimeric composition defines a new variant of type I von Willebrand disease with aberrant structure but presence of all size multimers (type IC). Blood 66:1423, 1985.

447. Holmberg, L., Berntorp, E., Donnér, M., and Nilsson, I. M.: von Willebrand's disease characterized by increased ristocetin sensitivity and the presence of all von Willebrand factor multimers in plasma. Blood 68:668, 1986.

448. Weiss, H. J., and Sussman, I. I.: A new von Willebrand variant (type I, New York): Increased ristocetin-induced platelet aggregation and plasma von Willebrand factor containing the full range of multimers. Blood 68:149, 1986.

449. Mancuso, D. J., Adam, P. A., Kroner, P. A., and Montgomery, R. R.: The molecular basis of a type I von Willebrand disease variant. Circulation 84:II-418, 1991.

450. Mancuso, D. J., Montgomery, R. R., and Adam, P.: The identification of a candidate mutation in the von Willebrand factor gene of patients with a variant form of type I von Willebrand disease. Blood 78(Suppl. 1):67a, 1991.

451. Ruggeri, Z. M., Pareti, F. I., Mannucci, P. M., Ciavarella, N., and Zimmerman, T. S.: Heightened interaction between platelets and factor VIII/von Willebrand factor in a new subtype of von Willebrand's disease. N. Engl. J. Med. 302:1047, 1980.

452. Zimmerman, T. S., Dent, J. A., Ruggeri, Z. M., and Nannini, L. H.: Subunit composition of plasma von Willebrand factor. Cleavage is present in normal individuals, increased in IIA and IIB von Willebrand disease, but minimal in variants with aberrant structure of individual oligomers (types IIC, IID, and IIE). J. Clin. Invest. 77:947, 1986.

453. Dent, J. A., Berkowitz, S. D., Ware, J., Kasper, C. K., and Ruggeri, Z. M.: Identification of a cleavage site directing the immunochemical detection of molecular abnormalities in type IIA von Willebrand factor. Proc. Natl. Acad. Sci. USA 87:6306, 1990.

454. Gralnick, H. R., Williams, S. B., McKeown, L. P., Maisonneuve, P., Jenneau, C., Sultan, Y., and Rick, M. E.: In vitro correction of the abnormal multimeric structure of von Willebrand factor in type IIA von Willebrand disease. Proc. Natl. Acad. Sci. USA 82:5968, 1985.

455. Batlle, J., Lopez Fernandez, M. F., Campos, M., Justica, B., Berges, C., Navarro, J. L., Diaz Cremades, J. M., Kasper, C. K., Dent, J. A., Rugger, Z. M., and Zimmerman, T. S.: The heterogeneity of type IIA von Willebrand's disease: Studies with protease inhibitors. Blood 68:1207, 1986.

456. Lyons, S. E., Bruck, M. E., Bowie, E. J. W., and Ginsburg, D.: Impaired intracellular transport produced by a subset of type IIA von Willebrand disease mutations. J. Biol. Chem. 267:4424, 1992.

457. Saba, H. I., Saba, S. R., Dent, J., Ruggeri, Z. M., and Zimmerman, T. S.: Type IIB Tampa: A variant of von Willebrand disease with chronic thrombocytopenia, circulating platelet

aggregates, and spontaneous platelet aggregation. Blood 66:282, 1985.

458. Ruggeri, Z. M., Lombardi, R., Gatti, L., Bader, R., Valsecchi, C., and Zimmerman, T. S.: Type IIB von Willebrand's disease: Differential clearance of endogenous versus transfused large multimer von Willebrand factor. Blood 60:1453, 1982.

459. Ruggeri, Z. M., Mannucci, P. M., Lombardi, R., Federici, A., and Zimmerman, T. S.: Multimeric composition of factor VIII/von Willebrand factor following administration of DDAVP: Implications for pathophysiology and therapy of von Willebrand's disease subtypes. Blood 59:1272, 1982.

460. Holmberg, L., Nilsson, I. M., Borge, L., Gunnarsson, M., and Sjorin, E.: Platelet aggregation induced by 1-desamino-8-D-arginine vasopressin (DDAVP) in type IIB von Willebrand's disease. N. Engl. J. Med. 309:816, 1983.

461. Nishino, M., Girma, J.-P., Rothschild, C., Fressinaud, E., and Meyer, D.: New variant of von Willebrand disease with defective binding to factor VIII. Blood 74:1591, 1989.

462. Mazurier, C., Dieval, J., Jorieux, S., Delobel, J., and Goudemand, M.: A new von Willebrand factor (vWF) defect in a patient with factor VIII (FVIII) deficiency but with normal levels and multimeric patterns of both plasma and platelet vWF. Characterization of abnormal vWF/FVIII interaction. Blood 75:20, 1990.

463. Mazurier, C., Gaucher, C., Jorieux, S., Parquet-Gernez, A., and Goudemand, M.: Evidence for a von Willebrand factor defect in factor VIII binding in three members of a family previously misdiagnosed mild haemophilia A and haemophilia A carriers: Consequences for therapy and genetic counselling. Br. J. Haematol. 76:372, 1990.

464. Ruggeri, Z. M., Nilsson, I. M., Lombardi, R., Holmberg, L., and Zimmerman, T. S.: Aberrant multimeric structure of von Willebrand factor in a new variant of von Willebrand's disease (Type IIC). J. Clin. Invest. 70:1124, 1982.

465. Federici, A. B., Mannucci, P. M., Lombardi, R., Lattuada, A., Colibretti, M. L., Dent, J. A., and Zimmerman, T. S.: Type IIH von Willebrand disease: New structural abnormality of plasma and platelet von Willebrand factor in a patient with prolonged bleeding time and borderline levels of ristocetin cofactor activity. Am. J. Hematol. 32:287, 1989.

466. Ledford, M. R., Rabinowitz, I., Sadler, J. E., Kent, J. W., and Civantos, F.: Genetic studies in a new variant of von Willebrand disease (vWD): Dominant vWD type IIC. Blood 78 (Suppl. 1):68a, 1991.

467. Kinoshita, S., Harrison, J., Lazerson, J., and Abilgaard, C. F.: A new variant of dominant type II von Willebrand's disease with aberrant multimeric pattern of factor VIII–related antigen (type IID). Blood 63:1369, 1984.

468. Mannucci, P. M., Lombardi, R., Federici, A. B., Dent, J. A., Zimmerman, T. S., and Ruggeri, Z. M.: A new variant of type II von Willebrand disease with aberrant multimeric structure of plasma but not platelet von Willebrand factor (type IIF). Blood 68:269, 1986.

469. Gralnick, H. R., Williams, S. B., McKeown, L. P., Maisonneuve, P., Jenneau, C., and Sultan, Y.: A variant of type II von Willebrand disease with an abnormal triplet structure and discordant effects of protease inhibitors on plasma and platelet von Willebrand factor structure. Am. J. Hematol. 24:259, 1987.

470. Howard, M. A., Salem, H. H., Thomas, K. B., Hau, L., Perkin, J., Coghlan, M., and Firkin, B. G.: Variant von Willebrand's disease type B-revisited. Blood 60:1420, 1982.

471. Mannucci, P. M., Bloom, A. L., Larrieu, M. J., Nilsson, I. M., and West, R. R.: Atherosclerosis and von Willebrand factor. I. Prevalence of severe von Willebrand's disease in Western Europe and Israel. Br. J. Haematol. 57:163, 1984.

472. Weiss, H. J., Ball, A. P., and Mannucci, P. M.: Incidence of severe von Willebrand's disease. N. Engl. J. Med. 307:127, 1982.

473. Zimmerman, T. S., Abildgaard, C. F., and Meyer, D.: The factor VIII abnormality in severe von Willebrand's disease. N. Engl. J. Med. 301:1307, 1979.

474. Shelton-Inloes, B. B., Chehab, F. F., Mannucci, P. M., Federici,

A. B., and Sadler, J. E.: Gene deletions correlate with the development of alloantibodies in von Willebrand disease. J. Clin. Invest. 79:1459, 1987.

475. Ngo, K. Y., Glotz, V. T., Koziol, J. A., Lynch, D. C., Gitschier, J., Ranieri, P., Ciavarella, N., Ruggeri, Z. M., and Zimmerman, T. S.: Homozygous and heterozygous deletions of the von Willebrand factor gene in patients and carriers of severe von Willebrand disease. Proc. Natl. Acad. Sci. USA 85:2753, 1988.

476. Peake, I. R., Liddell, M. B., Moodie, P., Standen, G., Mancuso, D. J., Tuley, E. A., Westfield, L. A., Sorace, J. M., Sadler, J. E., Verweij, C. L., and Bloom, A. L.: Severe type III von Willebrand's disease caused by deletion of exon 42 of the von Willebrand factor gene: Family studies that identify carriers of the condition and a compound heterozygous individual. Blood 75:654, 1990.

477. Bahnak, B. B., Lavergne, J.-M., Rothschild, C., and Meyer, D.: A stop codon in a patient with severe type III von Willebrand disease. Blood 78:1148, 1991.

478. Eikenboom, J. C. J., Briët, E., Reitsma, P. H., and Ploos van Amstel, H. K.: Severe type III von Willebrand's disease in the Dutch population is often associated with the absence of von Willebrand factor messenger RNA. Thromb. Haemost. 65:1127, 1991.

479. Nichols, W. C., Lyons, S. E., Harrison, J. H., Cody, R. L., and Ginsburg, D.: Severe von Willebrand disease due to a defect at the level of von Willebrand factor mRNA expression: Detection by exonic PCR-restriction fragment length polymorphism analysis. Proc. Natl. Acad. Sci. USA 88:3857, 1991.

480. Abildgaard, C. F., Suzuki, Z., Harrison, J., Jefcoat, K., and Zimmerman, T. S.: Serial studies in von Willebrand's disease. Variability versus "variants." Blood 56:712, 1980.

481. Mercier, B., Gaucher, C., and Mazurier, C.: Characterization of 98 alleles in 105 unrelated individuals in the F8VWF gene. Nucleic Acids Res. 19:4800, 1991.

482. Mannucci, P. M., and Mari, D.: Antibodies to factor VIII–von Willebrand factor in congenital and acquired von Willebrand's disease. In Hoyer, L. W. (ed.): Factor VIII Inhibitors. New York, Alan R. Liss, 1984.

483. Mannucci, P. M., Lombardi, R., Bader, R., Horellou, M. H., Finazzi, G., Besana, C., Conard, J., and Samama, M.: Studies of the pathophysiology of acquired von Willebrand's disease in seven patients with lymphoproliferative disorders or benign monoclonal gammopathies. Blood 64:614, 1984.

484. Takahashi, H.: Studies on the pathophysiology and treatment of von Willebrand's disease. IV. Mechanism of increased ristocetin-induced platelet aggregation in von Willebrand's disease. Thromb. Res. 19:857, 1980.

485. Miller, J. L., and Castella, A.: Platelet-type von Willebrand's disease: Characterization of a new bleeding disorder. Blood 60:790, 1982.

486. Weiss, H. J., Meyer, D., Rabinowitz, R., Pietu, G., Girma, J. P., Vicic, W. J., and Rogers, J.: Pseudo-von Willebrand's disease. An intrinsic platelet defect with aggregation by unmodified human factor VIII/von Willebrand factor and enhanced adsorption of its high-molecular-weight multimers. N. Engl. J. Med. 306:326, 1982.

487. Takahashi, H., Nagayama, R., Hattori, A., and Shibata, A.: Platelet aggregation induced by DDAVP in platelet-type von Willebrand's disease. N. Engl. J. Med. 310:722, 1984.

488. Miller, J. L., Boselli, B. D., and Kupinski, J. M.: In vivo interaction of von Willebrand factor with platelets following cryoprecipitate transfusion in platelet-type von Willebrand's disease. Blood 63:226, 1984.

489. Miller, J. L., Cunningham, D., Lyle, V. A., and Finch, C. N.: Mutation in the gene encoding the α chain of platelet glycoprotein Ib in platelet-type von Willebrand disease. Proc. Natl. Acad. Sci. USA 88:4761, 1991.

490. Sakariassen, K. S., Nieuwenhuis, H. K., and Sixma, J. J.: Differentiation of patients with subtype IIb–like von Willebrand's disease by means of perfusion experiments with reconstituted blood. Br. J. Haematol. 59:459, 1985.

491. Rick, M. E., Williams, S. B., Sacher, R. A., and McKeown, L.

P.: Thrombocytopenia associated with pregnancy in a patient with type IIB von Willebrand's disease. Blood 69:786, 1987.

492. Giles, A. R., Hoogendoorn, H., and Benford, K.: Type IIB von Willebrand's disease presenting as thrombocytopenia during pregnancy. Br. J. Haematol. 67:349, 1987.

493. Valster, F. A. A., Feijen, H. L. M., and Hutten, J. W. M.: Severe thrombocytopenia in a pregnant patient with platelet-associated IgM, and known von Willebrand's disease; a case report. Eur. J. Obstet. Gynecol. Reprod. Biol. 36:197, 1990.

494. Ieko, M., Sakurama, S., Sagawa, A., Yoshikawa, M., Satoh, M., Yasukouchi, T., and Nakagawa, S.: Effect of a factor VIII concentrate on type IIB von Willebrand's disease–associated thrombocytopenia presenting during pregnancy in identical twin mothers. Am. J. Hematol. 35:26, 1990.

495. Hultin, M. B., and Sussman, I. I.: Postoperative thrombocytopenia in type IIB von Willebrand disease. Am. J. Hematol. 33:64, 1990.

496. Donnér, M., Holmberg, L., and Nilsson, I. M.: Type IIB von Willebrand's disease with probable autosomal recessive inheritance and presenting as thrombocytopenia in infancy. Br. J. Haematol. 66:349, 1987.

497. Berntorp, E., and Nilsson, I. M.: Use of a high-purity factor VIII concentrate (Hemate P) in von Willebrand's disease. Vox Sang. 56:212, 1989.

498. Cumming, A. M., Fildes, S., Cumming, I. R., Wensley, R. T., Redding, O. M., and Burn, A. M.: Clinical and laboratory evaluation of National Health Service factor VIII concentrate (8Y) for the treatment of von Willebrand's disease. Br. J. Haematol. 75:234, 1990.

499. Mazurier, C., Jorieux, S., de Romeuf, C., Samor, B., and Goudemand, M.: In vitro evaluation of a very-high purity, solvent/detergent–treated, von Willebrand factor concentrate. Vox Sang. 61:1, 1991.

500. Lawrie, A. S., Goubran, H. A., Harrison, P., Holland, L. J., Weston-Smith, S. G., and Savidge, G. F.: Comparison of factor VIII concentrates and vWF:THP for the treatment of von Willebrand's disease. Thromb. Haemost. 65:1128, 1991.

501. Rothschild, C., Fressinaud, E., Wolf, M., Dreyfus, M., Laurian, Y., Peynaud-Debayle, E., Gazengel, C., Meyer, D., and Larrieu, M. J.: Unexpected results following treatment of patients with von Willebrand disease with a new highly purified von Willebrand factor concentrate. Thromb. Haemost. 65:1126, 1991.

502. Mannucci, P. M., Ruggeri, Z. M., Ciavarella, N., Kazatchine, M. D., and Mowbray, J. F.: Precipitating antibodies to factor VIII–von Willebrand factor in von Willebrand's disease: Effects on replacement therapy. Blood 57:25, 1981.

503. Bloom, A. L., Peake, I. R., Furlong, R. A., and Davies, B. L.: High potency factor VIII concentrate: More effective cryoprecipitate in a patient with von Willebrand's disease and inhibitor. Thromb. Res. 16:847, 1979.

504. Rodeghiero, F., Castaman, G., and Mannucci, P. M.: Clinical indications for desmopressin (DDAVP) in congenital and acquired von Willebrand disease. Blood Rev. 5:155, 1991.

505. Rodeghiero, F., Castaman, G., Di Bona, E., and Ruggeri, M.: Consistency of responses to repeated DDAVP infusions in patients with von Willebrand's disease and hemophilia A. Blood 74:1997, 1989.

506. Gralnick, H. R., Williams, S. B., McKeown, L. P., Rick, M. E., Maisonneuve, P., Jenneau, C., and Sultan, Y.: DDAVP in type IIa von Willebrand's disease. Blood 67:465, 1986.

507. López-Fernandez, M. F., Blanco-López, M. J., Castineira, M. P., and Batlle, J.: Further evidence for recessive inheritance of von Willebrand disease with abnormal binding of von Willebrand factor to factor VIII. Am. J. Hematol. 40:20, 1992.

508. Kyrle, P. A., Niessner, H., Dent, J., Panzer, S., Brenner, B., Zimmerman, T. S., and Lechner, K.: IIB von Willebrand's disease: Pathogenetic and therapeutic studies. Br. J. Haematol. 69:55, 1988.

509. Fowler, W. E., Berkowitz, L. R., and Roberts, H. R.: DDAVP for type IIB von Willebrand disease. Blood 74:1859, 1989.

20

The Molecular Biology of Fibrin

Russell F. Doolittle

INTRODUCTION

Fibrin is the primary material of blood clots. Its deposition is essential for preserving the integrity of the hemovascular system, but its inopportune occurrence can lead to stoppages that cause heart attacks, strokes, and other circulatory malfunctions. Clearly, its formation and destruction are matters of life and death. Its molecular countenance includes the soluble precursor called fibrinogen, the insoluble polymer itself, and the debris resulting from lysis referred to as "fibrin split products." These different states can be viewed in terms of a naturally regulated life cycle: the biosynthesis of the precursor, a dormant period before activation by thrombin, conversion to an insoluble polymer, dissolution of the polymeric fibrin gel by plasmin during the fibrinolytic stage, and the stim- ulation of biosynthesis by the resulting breakdown products.

In theory, we could begin our discussion at any stage of this cycle and continue around, but it seems logical to start with a consideration of the structure of the fibrinogen molecule. This provides a molecular frame of reference for all subsequent interactions. From there we can move forward to the details of fibrin formation, then to fibrinolysis, and finally return to biosynthesis and regulation. Throughout, we must remain aware of how these central components inter- act with the many other participants in the clotting process. Fibrinogen binds many coagulation proteins in advance of any need for clotting, for example. Fibrin, on the other hand, exhibits different binding sites that attract other interactants, and fibrin degra- dation products uniquely recognize receptors that are

701

TABLE 20–1. SOME PROPERTIES OF HUMAN FIBRINOGEN

Molecular mass	340,000
Per cent α helix	33
Molecular dimensions (approx.)	60×450 Å
Diffusion constant ($D_{20,w}$)	2.09×10^{-7} cm²/sec
Frictional coefficient (f/f_o)	2.34
Sedimentation coefficient ($S_{20,w}$)	7.9
Extinction coefficient	15.1
Partial specific volume	0.715
Isoelectric point	5.5
Calculated net charge at pH 7.3	-20
Per cent carbohydrate	3
Subunit formula	$\alpha_2 \, \beta_2 \, \gamma_2$

Adapted from Doolittle, R. F.: Structural aspects of the fibrinogen-fibrin conversion. Adv. Protein Chem. 27:1, 1973; with permission.

apparently ignored by fibrinogen and fibrin. Not every aspect of these many interactions is understood at present; our knowledge is still incomplete. Nonetheless, a quite reasonable scenario of events can be drawn. The reader must constantly keep in mind the overall aspect, even amid the morass of atomic detail.

The chapter also includes a brief review of variant human fibrinogens and a consideration of how these defective molecules help to elucidate many of the structure-function relationships discussed in the other sections. Some comments are also offered on recent successes in the expression of fibrinogen in recombinant systems and the potential for site-directed mutagenesis as a tool for addressing the same questions.

FIBRINOGEN: THE PRECURSOR OF FIBRIN

Fibrinogen is a large, complex glycoprotein that occurs in blood plasma at levels of 3 to 4 mg/ml (10^{-5} M). The molecular mass of the molecule found in humans is 340,000 daltons.* As we shall see, clotting depends on individual fibrinogen molecules colliding effectively after activation by thrombin. The data in Table 20–1 can be used to estimate that a volume increment of plasma measuring 100 nm on a side (one trillionth of a cubic millimeter) contains, on the average, eight or nine fibrinogen molecules. The nearest neighboring fibrinogens are only 50 to 100 nm apart, or as little as one or two molecular lengths. If no other macromolecules were in the way, each fibrinogen molecule would bump into another approximately every 5 msec. The volume increment described, however, contains about 500 albumin molecules and about 100 molecules of assorted other proteins, including—again on the average—one each of prothrombin and plasminogen (Table 20–2). The timely activation of these latter dictates the events of interest.

Size and Shape of Fibrinogen

The unraveling of the structure of fibrinogen over the course of the last half-century is a fascinating story, the early phases of which have been recounted elsewhere.[1-3] Here we offer only a brief outline of how a working model of fibrinogen was developed.

One of the earliest insights into the structure was accomplished by X-ray fiber diffraction. Concentrated solutions of fibrinogen are viscous enough that they can be drawn out to form fibers, and it was of interest

*It must be understood that fibrinogen and fibrin, like all proteins, differ to a degree from organism to organism. The focus in this chapter is on the proteins found in humans. It should be kept in mind, however, that much can be learned from comparisons with the equivalent proteins from other species. As a general rule, features found universally are likely to be more important than idiosyncratic differences. Accordingly, occasional comparisons are made to emphasize certain key structure-function relationships.

TABLE 20–2. RELATIVE CONCENTRATIONS OF SOME PROTEINS IN BLOOD PLASMA*

PROTEIN	MOLECULAR WEIGHT	µg/ml	MOLARITY	PER 1000 φ†
Albumin	70,000	40,000	6×10^{-4}	60,000
α_1-Antitrypsin	54,000	2900	5×10^{-5}	5000
Fibrinogen	340,000	3500	1×10^{-5}	1000
Antithrombin III	65,000	250	4×10^{-6}	400
α_2-Macroglobulin	730,000	2600	4×10^{-6}	350
Plasminogen	90,000	150	1.7×10^{-6}	170
Prothrombin	72,000	100	1.4×10^{-6}	140
α_2-Antiplasmin	70,000	70	1×10^{-6}	100
Fibronectin	440,000	350	8×10^{-7}	80
Factor X	56,000	10	2×10^{-7}	20
Factor XIII‡	320,000	30	1×10^{-7}	10
Factor IX	56,000	5	9×10^{-8}	10
Factor V‡	330,000	10	3×10^{-8}	3
Thrombospondin‡	450,000	8	2×10^{-8}	2
Factor VII	50,000	0.5	1×10^{-8}	1
Factor VIII	330,000	0.1	3×10^{-10}	(0.03)

*Taken from data presented in references 245 and 246.
†Molecules per 1000 molecules of fibrinogen.
‡Found in much higher concentrations in platelets.

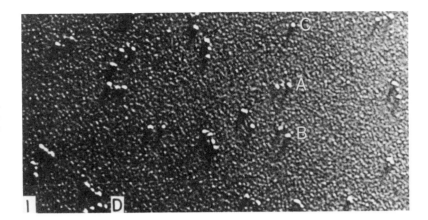

FIGURE 20–1. Metal-shadowed fibrinogen molecules. (From Hall, C. E., and Slayter, H. S.: The fibrinogen molecule: Its size, shape and mode of polymerization. J. Biophys. Biochem. Cytol. 5:11, 1959; with permission.)

to compare their diffraction patterns with those of fibrin. Indeed, the diffraction patterns of fibrinogen and fibrin were indistinguishable, suggesting that fibrin was nothing more than polymerized fibrinogen units.[4] Most surprising, however, the patterns were also the same as those observed for fibrous proteins like keratin and myosin. These diffraction patterns were subsequently found to be characteristic of α helices wound into "coiled coils."[5] When hydrodynamic studies were performed on fibrinogen, however, its character was found to be more globular than fibrous. When these data were taken together with some early electron microscope studies,[6] it was suggested that the data best fit a molecule with an extended nodular structure.[7]

The electron micrographs published by Hall and Slayter[8] in 1959 provided the first true representation of fibrinogen (Fig. 20–1). Those shadow-cast specimens revealed an extended triglobular structure about 475 ± 25 Å in length, the central globule of which was slightly smaller than the terminal ones. The regions connecting the globules could not be resolved, but it was conjectured that they might consist of the coiled α helices detected by the fiber diffraction study mentioned above.[9]

An important development in discovering the structure of fibrinogen was the purification of a set of stable core fragments generated by the action of plasmin.[10] When preparations of fibrinogen digested with plasmin were applied directly to a DEAE (diethylaminoethyl) cellulose column, a series of peaks emerged that were labeled A to E. Of these, D and E were found to account for the bulk of the mass; the mass ratio of D to E was approximately three to one. It was subsequently shown that short-term digestions with plasmin yielded transient intermediates, the principal ones of which were denoted X and Y.[11] This latter study led to the proposal that the stable core fragment E must correspond to the central module observed in the electron microscope and that the fragments D were the terminal ones (Fig. 20–2). Thus, fragment X is a degradation product in which two fragments D remain connected to an E, whereas fragment Y represents a further digested product in which a single fragment D is connected to the fragment E.[12] In retrospect, the

minor peaks A to C from the DEAE chromatography represented a variety of peptides chipped away from the native molecule. As much as two thirds of each α chain is lost during the conversion to fragment X,[13] an observation that gave rise to the notion of a pair of extended and easily removed polar protuberances.[2]

Subunit Arrangement

Each fibrinogen molecule is composed of three pairs of non-identical but homologous polypeptide chains,

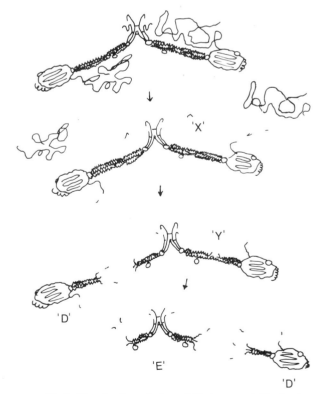

FIGURE 20–2. Plasmin degradation of fibrinogen yields the intermediate fragments denoted "X" and "Y" and the terminal fragments "D" and "E." Actually, numerous species of each occur, depending on the exact conditions of the digestion.

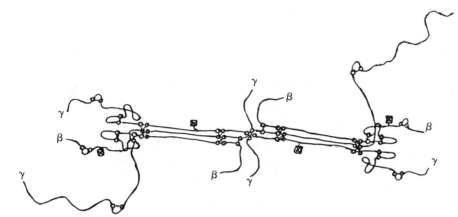

FIGURE 20–3. Arrangement of 29 disulfide bonds in human fibrinogen. (Modified with permission from Hoeprich, P. D., and Doolittle, R. F.: Dimeric half-molecules of human fibrinogen are joined through disulfide bonds in an antiparallel orientation. Biochemistry 22:2049, 1983. Copyright 1983, American Chemical Society.)

$\alpha_2\beta_2\gamma_2$,* the molecular masses of which are 67,000, 55,000, and 48,000 daltons, respectively.[14] The six chains are arranged in a manner such that all six amino-termini are gathered in the central part of the molecule (Fig. 20–3). All together, there are 29 disulfide bonds,[15] which fall into three classes: three connecting the two dimeric halves of the protein, two sets of seven *inter*chain bonds, and two other sets of six *intra*chain bonds. As yet, a crystal structure is not available for any fibrinogen, even though promising experiments have been in progress for a very long time.[16, 17] In the interim, models of fibrinogen have been fashioned on the basis of electron microscopy, physical chemistry, and a host of indirect biochemical studies.[18] As noted above, the protein has several well-defined regions† that can be visualized in the electron microscope (Fig. 20–4) and isolated by treating the native protein with appropriate proteases.

Amino Acid Sequence Studies

The proposal that fragments D and E correspond to the major globules of a trimodular molecule was completely borne out by biochemical and amino acid sequence studies. In particular, a fragment was obtained from fibrinogen treated with cyanogen bromide (which cleaves exclusively at methionine residues) that contained all six amino-terminals[19] and cross-reacted immunologically with fragment E.[20, 21] Subsequent amino acid sequence studies on the individual polypeptide chains revealed that each chain contains a

skein of amino acids with a rhythmic polarity characteristic of α helices, in each case bounded by braces of cysteines. It was proposed that these stretches, which amounted to about 110 amino acids in each chain, were the "coiled-coil" connectors.[22] Because an α helix translates 1.5 Å per residue, the lengths of the proposed connectors would be about 150 Å, in good agreement with the estimates made from electron microscopy. Models were built that showed how the three chains in each half of the molecule could be mutually bound by the disulfides at each end of the "coiled coils."[23]

The sequence of human fibrinogen was completed in 1979,[24–27] and the information was illuminating well

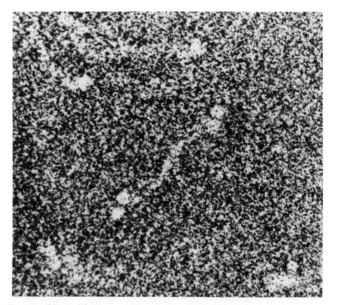

FIGURE 20–4. Electron micrograph of negative-stained fibrinogen molecule. Note the presence of two distinct domains in the terminal globule region. (From Williams, R. C.: Band patterns seen by electron microscopy in ordered arrays of bovine and human fibrinogen and fibrin after negative staining. Proc. Natl. Acad. Sci. USA 80:1570, 1983; with permission.)

---

*The combinations A α and B β are used by some to describe fibrinogen α and β chains with their fibrinopeptides still attached.

†Sometimes these fragments are referred to as "domains." Formally, a domain is defined as that part of a protein that can fold independently of neighboring sequences. In this chapter we will be less exacting and use the term casually for any definable region. We will also invoke the term *macrodomain* for large regions that are doubtless composed of more than one classic domain and *subdomain* for smaller regions associated with particular functions.

beyond the delineation of the regions corresponding to the "coiled coils" and the general boundaries of the major fragments. Most interesting was that it confirmed that the three non-identical chains were descended from a common ancestor (Fig. 20–5). In this regard, although the homology of the β and γ chains persists through their entire lengths (Fig. 20–6), the α chains are radically different in their carboxy-terminal two thirds (Fig. 20–7). Evidently some kind of crossing-over event or "exon shuffle" has occurred during the evolution of the α chain since the original gene duplications.

Carbohydrate Moieties

Most mammalian fibrinogens contain about 3 per cent carbohydrate. In the case of human fibrinogen, two asparagine-linked carbohydrate clusters occur in each half-molecule, one on the β chain at residue Asn 364, and another on the γ chain at residue Asn 52. In both instances the carbohydrate is a biantennary-type cluster composed of N-acetyl glucosamines, mannoses, galactoses, and terminal sialic acids.[28] The α chain actually contains a consensus sequence characteristic of carbohydrate attachment (Asn-Val-Ser at residues 400 to 402), but there is no evidence for its ever being substituted. Fibrinogens from other species have carbohydrate in various positions, however, including a cluster on the α chain of chicken fibrinogen[29] and clusters elsewhere on the β and γ chains of lamprey fibrinogen,[30, 31] and even its fibrinopeptide B.[32]

Calcium Binding

Fibrinogen has been found to have three "high-affinity" binding sites for calcium.[33, 34] High affinity for an extracellular protein means dissociation constants (K_d) of the order of 10^{-5} M. The extracellular concentration of calcium ions in vertebrate animals is of the order of 2.5×10^{-3} M, about one third of which is bound to assorted proteins at "low-affinity" sites that are only fractionally occupied. Under these conditions, the high-affinity sites ought to be fully occupied. Fibrinogen doubtless has low-affinity sites also, but we will not comment on them further.

Two of the (high-affinity) binding sites are situated on the two γ chains somewhere in the region encompassed by residues 300 to 350. The third site has not been determined with any certainty, but some circumstantial evidence suggests that it may involve the carboxy-terminal regions of α chains.[35] The basis for this conjecture is that fragment X apparently has only two high-affinity binding sites, although there is some dispute about this observation.[36] In contrast, the evidence linking calcium binding to large molecular weight fragment D takes several lines. First, when fibrinogen is digested by plasmin in the absence of calcium ions, the γ chain is degraded to a significantly greater extent than when calcium is present.[37] The portion removed in its absence amounts to the carboxy-terminal 109 residues. In addition, calcium ions tend to protect the intrachain disulfide involving γ chain residues 326 and 329 from reduction.[38] Finally, it has been reported that the cyanogen bromide fragment spanning residues 311 to 336 can bind terbium.[39]

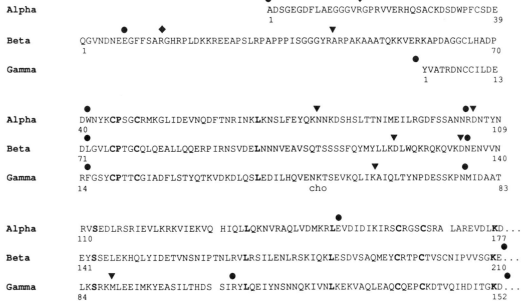

FIGURE 20–5. Alignment of amino-terminal portions of α, β and γ chains of human fibrinogen. Residues common to all three chains are emboldened. Intron positions, which further emphasize the common ancestry of the three chains, are indicated by solid circles. Solid diamonds mark thrombin cleavage points, and triangles indicate primary plasmin attack points. cho = carbohydrate cluster.

```
              (●)                                                    ●
Beta      ..CEEIIRKGGETSEMYLIQPDSSVKPYRVYCDMNTENGGWTVIQNRQDGSVDFGRKWDPYKQGFGNVATNT
          211
              (●)                                          ●
Gamma     ..CQDIANKGAKQSGLYFIKPLKANQQFLVYCEIDGSGNGWTVFQKRLDGSVDFKKNWIQYKEGFGHLSPTG
          153                                              200


                     ●
Beta      DGKNYCGLPGEYWLGNDKISQLTRMG  PTELLIEMEDWKGDKVKAHYGGFTVQNEANKYQISVNKYRGT
                            300
                                                 ●
Gamma        TTEFWLGNEKIHLISTQSAIPYALRVELEDWNGRTSTADYAMFKVGPEADKYRLTYAYFAGG



                            cho              ●
Beta      AGNALMDG ASQLMGENRTMTIHNGMFFSTYDRDNDGWLTSDPRKQCSKEDGGGWWYNRCHAANPNGRY
                                                          400
Gamma     DAGDA FDGFDFGDDPSDKFFTSHNGMQFSTWDNDNDKF    EGNCAEQDGSGWWMNKCHAGHLNGVY
                                 300



Beta      YWGGQYTWDMAKHGTDDGVVWMNWKGSWYSMRKMSMKIRPFFPQQ
                                                   461
                ●
Gamma     YQGGTYSKASTPNGYDNGIIWATWKTRWYSMKKTTMKIIPFNRLTIGEGQQHHLGGAKQAGDV    ●
                                                    400        411
```

FIGURE 20–6. **Alignment of carboxy-terminal regions of β and γ chains of human fibrinogen.** The sequences are approximately 50 per cent identical in this region, which constitutes the bulk of the terminal globule. Intron positions denoted with solid circles; cho = carbohydrate cluster.

```
                          ▼                  ▼
...YEDQQKQLEQVIAKDLLPSRDRQHLPLIKMKPVPDLVPGNFKSQLQKVPP
   178
   ▼       ▼         ▼
   EWKALTDMPQMRMELERPGGNEITRGGSTSYGTGSE..
   228

      ..TESPRNPSSAGSWNSGSSGPGSTGNRNPGSSGTGGTATW

      KPGSSGPGSTGSWNSGSSGTGSTGNQNPGSPRPGSTGTW

      NPGSSERGSAGHWTSESSVSGSTGQWHSESGSFRPDSPG

      SGNARPNNPD WGTFEEVSGNVSPGTRREYHTEKLVTS..
                                          ▼
                              ..KGDKELRTGK
                                418

   EKVTSGSTTTTRRSCSKTVTKTVIGPDGHKEVTKEVVTSEDGSDCPEAMD
   428

   LGTLSGIGTLDGFRHRHPDEAAFFDTASTGKTFPGFFSPMLGEFVSETES
   478

   RGSESGIFTNTKESSSHHPGIAEFPSRGKSSSYSKQFTSSTSYNRGDSTF
   528
   ▼
   ESKSYKMADEAGSEADHEGTHSTKRGHAKSRPV
   578                    610
```

FIGURE 20–7. **Amino acid sequence of carboxy-terminal two thirds of α chain from human fibrinogen, including region of 13-residue repeats (shown as four 39-residue segments).** There are no introns in this region of the gene. Plasmin attack points are denoted by solid triangles; the intrachain disulfide loop involves the emboldened cysteines (C).

Terbium (element number 65) is thought to bind to calcium-binding sites and has the advantage that under appropriate conditions it is fluorescent and easily detected. It is surprising, nonetheless, that a complex site involving multiple coordinate ligands can exist in the unfolded state usually found in small cyanogen bromide fragments, and these results should be regarded as tentative until other supporting data are forthcoming.

DNA Sequence Studies

The advent of recombinant DNA technology in the late 1970s set the stage for a surge of data that both confirmed the protein sequence determined for human fibrinogen, with some minor corrections,[40–43] and provided sequences for fibrinogens from a number of other species, including rat,[44] bovine,[45] chicken,[46, 47] frog,[48] and lamprey.[30, 31, 49] Moreover, the recombinant studies on human fibrinogen provided an explanation for a minor form of the γ chain and also uncovered a wholly unexpected α chain extension, two topics we will take up in our discussion of fibrinogen biosynthesis.

The comparative data have been very useful in assessing those features of fibrinogen most critical to its function. For example, in all cases save one, the bond cleaved by thrombin during the release of fibrinopeptides is an arginyl-glycine linkage. The exception is found in the case of the cleavage of fibrinopeptide B from chicken fibrinogen, in which case the bond is arginyl-alanine.[46] More important, the site exposed by the release of the fibrinopeptide A is universally Gly-Pro-Arg. Accordingly, one can expect that the complementary site for polymerization must also be highly conserved; possible regions in the terminal domains have been suggested on this basis.[31]

A Working Model of Fibrinogen

For the most part, the structures observed by electron microscopists are in accord with the results of peptide chemistry studies. One unresolved issue has to do with the precise localization of the carboxy-terminal regions of the α chains. The triglobular structure observed in electron micrographs corresponds well to what might be expected from a fragment X molecule, but where would the exposed carboxy-terminal regions of the α chains be? Initially, it was suggested that these regions, which account for a quarter of the mass of the native protein, were "free-swimming appendages," and in schematic depictions they are often drawn as randomly dispersed out and away from the terminal globules.[2, 18, 50] In support of this depiction, it can be noted that these regions are readily cleaved from fibrinogen by a variety of proteases,[13] they have little or no defined secondary structure,[51] and they vary greatly from species to species, both in sequence and in overall length.[2, 49] Also, at least one published electron micrograph shows chains extending from the terminal globules,[52] and in another immunostaining was used to show the α chain middle region lying out and away from the main body of the molecule.[53] Nevertheless, some investigators believe that these regions fold back on the triglobular molecule and either contribute to the central globule[54, 55] or form a fourth, less readily resolved module.[56] Also, an immunochemical study reports that these regions are at least partially shielded in the native molecule, new epitopes being revealed upon fibrinolysis.[57] This is a structural feature of fibrinogen that needs more study before a final judgment can be rendered.

In the meantime, numerous other studies have been conducted on the terminal macrodomain corresponding to fragment D. As shown clearly in some electron micrographs (see Fig. 20–4), the terminal globule contains two well-defined modules.[58] Of course, it had been presumed long before these pictures that the terminal globule must contain two discrete domains because of the homology of the β and γ carboxy-terminal regions.[26, 59] Since then, further degradation studies coupled with microcalorimetry have subdivided each of these into two even smaller domains.[60, 61] A schematic depiction of a human fibrinogen molecule is presented in Figure 20–8. In keeping with our goal to relate structure and function at the atomic level, we refer to this drawing throughout the remainder of the chapter, bearing in mind its limitations and tentative aspects.

FIBRIN FORMATION

Fibrin formation is marked by the transition from a collection of soluble molecules (fibrinogen) to the extended polymeric network that forms the gel. The gel state results from the network's trapping bulk water and all the solutes and particles suspended therein (Fig. 20–9). Electron micrographs of fibrin show the constituent fibrous strands to be thick or thin and more or less branched, depending on the solution conditions during polymerization. If the strands are thick enough, staining reveals a uniformly banded pattern with a repeat distance of 225 Å, which is equivalent to half the length of a fibrinogen molecule (Fig. 20–10). Such observations, taken together with other considerations, long ago led to the reasonable conclusion that the fundamental polymerization events occur by a half-staggered molecule overlap.[62] It is interesting that fibrinogen itself can be packed into the same arrangement, even without the removal of the fibrinopeptides, merely by sedimentation into a glassy pellet in the ultracentrifuge.[63] Clearly, the shape of the molecules is conducive to a half-staggered overlap even when the molecules are merely crowded together.

Thrombin Action

Fibrinogen is converted into fibrin as a result of thrombin-cleaving peptides from the amino-terminal

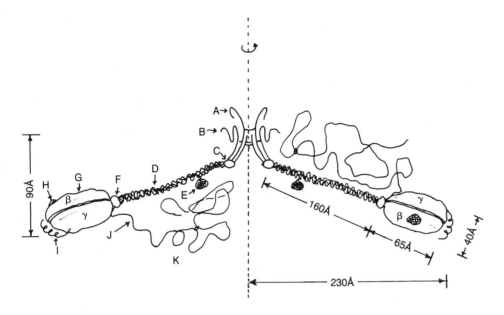

FIGURE 20–8. Diagrammatic depiction of a fibrinogen molecule. Key features identified include: A, fibrinopeptide A; B, fibrinopeptide B; C, first disulfide ring; D, coiled-coil connector; E, carbohydrate attachment site on γ chain; F, second disulfide ring; G, β chain; H, carbohydrate attachment site on β chain; I, γ-γ cross-linking site; J, plasmin attack points; K, α-chain protuberance. (From Doolittle, R. F.: Fibrinogen and fibrin. Reproduced, with permission, from the Annual Review of Biochemistry, Vol. 53, © 1984 by Annual Reviews Inc.)

ends of the α and β chains.[64] The released peptides are referred to as the fibrinopeptides A and B, respectively. In human fibrinogen the cleavages occur at arginyl-glycine bonds. Thrombin is a member of the trypsin serine protease family; it has a narrow specificity, almost always being restricted to particular arginyl linkages. In addition to fibrinogen, it cleaves certain other proteins involved in blood clotting, including factors V, VIII, and XIII and, when complexed with thrombomodulin, protein C.

The rates of release of the fibrinopeptides A and B can be markedly different, and in humans the fibrinopeptide A is released significantly faster than the fibrinopeptide B under typical physiological conditions.[65] Because the exposure of the glycyl-prolyl-argininyl segment corresponding to α chain residues 17 to 19 is the initiating feature of polymerization, only the release of the fibrinopeptide A is required for clot formation. As a result, certain snake venom enzymes (reptilase, for example) can clot fibrinogen even though they release only the fibrinopeptides A.[66] Thus, these three newly exposed residues, which we refer to from here on as Gly-Pro-Arg, constitute a conceptual "knob" that binds to a resident "hole" elsewhere in neighboring fibrin(ogen) molecules.[67, 68]

Actually, a number of different interactions must occur during the propagation of the fibers that form the gel network. The first of these involve the "knob-hole" interactions between individual molecules that have had at least one of their fibrinopeptides A removed. As the resulting dimers add more units, a second kind of interaction must occur in a more end-to-end fashion. These additions continue until the oligomers contain 18 to 20 units, a stage at which they are referred to as protofibrils.[69] Protofibrils are still in the solution phase; it is their aggregation with each other that effects gelation. Moreover, they may aggregate in both a lengthwise and a widthwise manner, depending on the solution conditions[70] and on whether or not the fibrinopeptides B have been released. The resulting fibrin has different properties depending on this progression, lengthwise propagation leading to finer fibers and transparent clots and lateral growth leading to coarser fibers and opaque clots.[71]

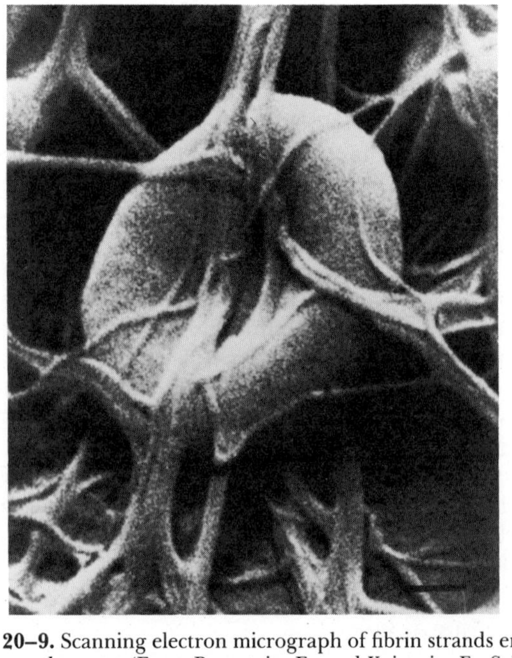

Initial Interaction of Fibrin Monomers

The removal of the fibrinopeptide A from the amino-terminus of the fibrinogen α chain gives rise to an entity denoted *fibrin monomer,* the spontaneous polymerization of which leads to fibrin.[72] Remarkably,

FIGURE 20–9. Scanning electron micrograph of fibrin strands entangling an erythrocyte. (From Bernstein, E., and Kairenin, E.: Science 173: cover photo, 1971. Copyright 1971 by the AAAS; with permission.)

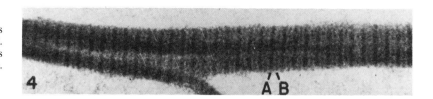

FIGURE 20–10. Negatively stained fibrin strands showing 225 Å repeated striations. (From Hall, C. E., and Slayter, H. S.: The fibrinogen molecule: Its size, shape and mode of polymerization. J. Biophys. Biochem. Cytol. 5:11, 1959; with permission.)

small peptides beginning with the sequence Gly-Pro-Arg are able to prevent the polymerization of fibrin monomers.[67] They do this by binding to complementary sites that are themselves always available and do not need to be uncovered by the action of thrombin. Equilibrium dialysis shows that each molecule of fibrinogen has two such sites, one per fragment D, which is to say one on each of the terminal domains.[68] Moreover, only full-size fragments D bind these peptides. Smaller fragments D produced in the absence of calcium ions and lacking the carboxy-terminal 109 residues of the γ chain do not bind Gly-Pro-Arg peptides.[59] Affinity-labeling studies have shown that tyrosine 363 is the only side chain labeled by bound peptides,[73, 74] and, as such, the "hole" must be close by that residue in a three-dimensional sense.

Interestingly, peptides beginning with Gly-His-Arg, the sequence exposed by the release of the fibrinopeptide B, also bind to fibrinogen, but they are not nearly as effective in preventing polymerization. The initial observation[68] was that Gly-His-Arg-Pro does not inhibit the association of fibrin monomers at all, but two recent reports claim this peptide is in fact effective under appropriate conditions.[75, 76] Previously, another study found that the Gly-His-Arg peptides are effective only in delaying clotting brought about by snake venom inhibitors that release the fibrinopeptide B.[77] There is general agreement, however, that Gly-His-Arg peptides can potentiate the action of Gly-Pro-Arg peptides.[78] The B-type peptides also bind to fragments D of all sizes and independent of the size of the γ chain. Further, binding is greatly enhanced by the presence of calcium ions.[79] This observation is at odds with the evidence that the high-affinity binding site resides in the γ chain portion of fragment D, and it may be that in the presence of calcium Gly-His-Arg peptides are actually binding to the Gly-Pro-Arg site.

Remarkably, peptides beginning with the sequence Gly-Pro-Arg are able to dissociate fibrin clots, so long as the clots have not been stabilized by factor XIII.[80] Further, the physical properties of clots exposed to these peptides change radically as the peptides diffuse into them.[81, 82] In spite of this impressive clot-preventing and gel-reversing power, peptides of this sort have not been used in clinical settings, presumably because they are cleared so rapidly from the circulation. Attempts to synthesize derivatives that bind to albumin and that, as a result, might have longer half-lives in vivo, have been only modestly successful.[83] Nonetheless, Gly-Pro-Arg peptides have proved useful in in vitro settings, where they can prevent clot formation during studies of other aspects of the coagulation scheme[84, 85] as well as in studies on fibrin formation itself.[86]

Calcium Effects

Evidence is mounting that the principal polymerization sites (the "holes" in the "knob-hole" interaction) are intimately associated with the calcium-binding sites on γ chains. The region (residues γ 300 to 350) contains a large number of aspartic acids, some of the negatively charged side chains of which likely contribute to the calcium-binding site and others to the pocket for binding the positive charges in the Gly-Pro-Arg "knob." Although fibrin can be formed in the absence of calcium ions, the gel structure is significantly weaker than that formed in its presence.[87]

Association of Protofibrils

Fibrin formation can be arrested at the protofibril stage by keeping the concentration of thrombin as the rate-limiting component and then adding an inhibitor of thrombin just before the onset of gelation.[88] The solution of rod-like oligomers can be passed over an appropriate gel filtration column to remove the inhibitor and most of the thrombin. If additional thrombin is then added, gelation occurs in the usual way.[88] Conditions can also be prescribed such that gelation occurs merely by the addition of physiological amounts of calcium ion or tiny amounts of zinc.[89]

Fibrin Stabilization

Although the forces involved in the polymerization process are non-covalent, fibrin clots formed under physiologic conditions are reinforced by the addition of covalent cross-links catalyzed by the calcium-dependent transglutaminase commonly known as factor XIII.[90] The enzyme, which occurs in both a plasma and a platelet form, circulates as a precursor and is itself activated by a thrombin-catalyzed cleavage. The activated form is referred to as factor XIIIa. Evidence suggests that the bulk of the circulating zymogen is bound to fibrinogen,[91] an association that ensures the availability of this relatively infrequent protein (Table 20–2) when polymerization occurs. The active enzyme ordinarily works on fibrin, introducing cross-links between specific lysine side chains and glutamine acceptors in neighboring molecules in the clot. The result of such a union is referred to as an ε-amino(γ-glutamyl)lysine isopeptide.

These isopeptide linkages occur in two different settings. In the first, the carboxy-terminal segments of γ chains in neighboring molecules are reciprocally linked.[92, 93] Virtually all units of the fibrin clot are joined in this fashion. In the second situation, α chains are linked into multimeric arrays.[94] Only a small fraction of molecules are ordinarily involved in this process. Cross-linked fibrin is considerably more stable than non–cross-linked, as reflected in its mechanical and elastic properties.[95–97] It is also considerably more resistant to fibrinolysis.[98]

Cross-linking also plays an important role in wound healing. Indeed, persons with genetically defective factor XIII do not always experience clotting problems, but their healing wounds tend to ooze.[99] In this regard, fibronectin can be cross-linked to fibrin, in which capacity it may serve as a bridge for invading fibroblasts destined to deposit collagen fibers.[100–102] This union is known to involve lysine donors from the fibrin α chain protuberances and fibronectin glutamine acceptor sites situated near its amino-termini.[103] Electron micrographs of fibronectin that has been cross-linked to fibrinogen by factor XIIIa show fully extended molecules bridged at their extremities,[104] another observation that argues against the notion of fibrinogen α chains being folded back upon the central domain.

Conformational Changes

In the simplest instance, one could imagine that fibrin might be indistinguishable from fibrinogen except for the absence of the fibrinopeptides and those surface groups hidden by the units being packed together. This being the case, fibrin might be expected to lack some immunological features present in fibrinogen merely because they were shielded by the packing arrangement. Conceivably, also, the newly exposed knobs in fibrin might occasionally protrude from the polymer and be detectable by suitable antibodies. Indeed, antibodies to both the Gly-Pro-Arg and Gly-His-Arg knobs have been obtained that react uniquely with fibrin.[105–107] Antibodies have also been obtained that can recognize fragments D that have been cross-linked by factor XIIIa.[108] In addition to these covalent differences between fibrinogen and fibrin, more subtle distinctions are likely possible as a result of conformational adjustments made during packing, and even though most of the molecule remains accessible to solvent, certain structural features may be covered or uncovered. Numerous immunochemical and labeling experiments have been conducted over the years in attempts to identify such shifting features and to measure the magnitude of the effect. The changes often remain elusive.[109] One potentially significant change involves γ chain residues 312 to 324, which have been reported to be a fibrin-specific epitope.[110] Because this is a region noted above as most likely to

be a part of the Gly-Pro-Arg binding pocket, its inaccessibility to antibodies in fibrinogen may well reflect adjustments made during polymerization.

Studies of this kind are of interest on two counts. First, they bear heavily on our understanding of exactly what happens when fibrinogen is transformed into fibrin. Second, it is of obvious utility in clinical settings to have tests that distinguish circulating fibrin from fibrinogen.

FIBRINOLYSIS

Fibrin clots are not meant to be permanent structures. Rather, they are temporary sealants that are ordinarily displaced as a part of the normal wound-healing process. The dismantling of the clot, whether it be the scaffolding at a wound site or a circulating thrombus, is primarily the role of plasmin; the conversion of plasminogen to plasmin sets the pace of dissolution. As described in Chapter 21, plasminogen occurs in the plasma in two different forms easily distinguished by their amino-termini: native Glu-plasminogen and a clipped form lacking 76 residues, Lys-plasminogen. Only the Lys- form binds to fibrinogen, and that quite weakly.[111] Both forms bind fibrin, but the Lys- form does so much more tightly, even though both have the five characteristic kringle domains[112] that confer unique binding properties. In either case it appears to be kringle 4 that has a high-affinity binding site for lysine.[113] Note that this binding site is not in the protease portion of the protein, although— perhaps not coincidentally—the enzyme also has a substrate-binding pocket that leads to preferential cleavage after lysine side chains.[114] The kringle lysine-binding site is utilized when plasminogen is purified by affinity chromatography,[115] and it is also the principal binding site for ε-aminocaproic acid (EACA), a well-known competitive inhibitor of fibrinolysis. Although a number of early studies had targeted lysines in fibrin as essential for lysis,[116, 117] it was Christenson who pointed out that carboxy-terminal lysines in proteolyzed fibrin must be most attractive to plasminogen, because only such lysines have the features inherent in EACA.[118] The happy result is that as plasmin degrades the fibrin clot, it provides more carboxy-terminal lysines that can attract additional plasminogen molecules.[119]

Plasminogen Activation

Plasminogen can be converted to plasmin either by limited proteolysis or by the binding action of certain bacterial activator proteins like streptokinase; physiologically, the most important process is limited proteolysis by tissue plasminogen activator (t-PA) released from damaged endothelial cells.[120] Should t-PA convert plasminogen to plasmin in the open circulation, the plasmin is promptly inactivated by α_2-antiplasmin.[121] Only when the activation takes place within the relatively safe confines of a clot does plasmin have free rein. To ensure this happening, t-PA itself contains kringle domains, one of which has been found to have a high-affinity binding site for lysine,[122, 123] and is likely responsible for the preferential binding of t-PA to lysines in fibrin.[124] It has been shown that t-PA on its own is not very effective in activating plasminogen, but fibrin and various fibrin breakdown products are able to increase the activation process by 50-fold.[125] Fibrinogen is wholly inactive in this capacity, so the activity must be attributed to some feature that is exposed during fibrin formation. The activating region has been localized to α chain residues 154 to 159,[126] another region found to be immunologically detectable in fibrin but not in fibrinogen.[127] Initially, it was presumed that the key residue was lysine 157, but in a puzzling and somewhat anticlimactic result, it was found that the lysine can be acetylated with impunity and that a number of other residues, including glutamate, can serve equally well in synthetic peptide analogues.[128]

Recombinant Activators

A determined effort is under way to construct more effective plasminogen activators by the use of recombinant DNA procedures. One popular strategy has been to combine mouse monoclonal antibodies specific for fibrin with a urokinase-type plasminogen activator.[129–131] Another approach is based on providing substitute kringles that may bind more tightly to fibrin.[132] These remarkable studies will doubtless claim more attention in the near future.

Physical Considerations

Whatever the exact mechanism of activation, the major problem to be confronted for dissolution is access to the inside of the clot. Although fibrin gels are relatively open meshworks that allow diffusion in and out, the fibrils themselves may be as much as a thousand molecules in diameter (see Fig. 20–9). Actually, there is a good deal of open space within the fibrils also, a consequence of the nodular structure of the individual units.[133] Even with an overlapping half-molecule stagger in which the terminal globules of one unit fit into the interglobular space of another, enough open space always remains for the "coiled coils" to remain exposed to solvent. Nonetheless, plasmin may be large enough to be excluded and may have to digest its way in from the outside. Theoretical studies have addressed the issue of the surface chemistry involved.[134, 135]

In any event, the coarser the fibers, the more accessible they are and the faster they are destroyed by plasmin.[136] Almost anything that leads to coarser clots facilitates lysis. For example, synthetic polymers used as plasma expanders induce coarser clots that are lysed much more rapidly than normal.[137, 138] Whether or not such clots are as effective in hemostasis may be another matter.

Differences in accessibility dictated by the nature of molecular packing in the clot may explain another apparent paradox about fibrinolysis. Aspirin has been reported to be directly involved in accelerating fibrinolysis, an effect attributable to the acetylation of lysines on fibrinogen.[139] Everything we have said heretofore might lead one to expect that any modification of lysines would slow the action of plasmin. If lysine modifications lead to coarser clots, however, the paradox might be resolved.

With regard to the actual dissolution of the fibrin clot, the mode of attack for plasmin is similar to the assault on fibrinogen described earlier. Again, the critical breakpoints are situated in the central regions of the "coiled coils" (Fig. 20–11), and, in a kind of reverse rendering of the polymerization process, solution occurs at the level of oligomers, long before the last of the individual units is cleaved.[140] The final core fragments are similar to those found when fibrinogen is digested with plasmin, except that cross-linked fibrin does not contain monomeric fragment D units but

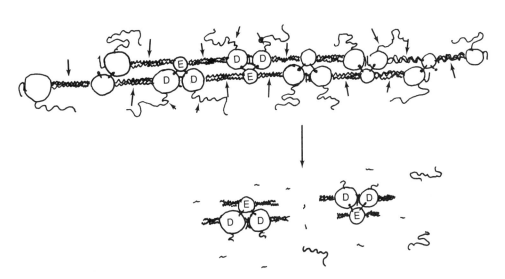

FIGURE 20–11. Destruction and solubilization of fibrin resulting from plasmin attack on central regions of coiled-coil connectors. (Adapted from Doolittle, R. F.: Fibrinogen and fibrin. *In* Bloom, A. L., and Thomas, D. P. [eds.]: Haemostasis and Thrombosis, 2nd ed. London, Churchill Livingstone, 1987, pp. 192–215; with permission.)

instead contains D-dimers resulting from the γ-γ cross-links. Furthermore, under physiologic conditions, these dimeric units remain bound to fragment E with its knobs still positioned in their complementary holes, the overall entity being called "D_2E."[141, 142] The fact that such an entity is not found when non–cross-linked fibrin is lysed is a reflection of the modest strength of interaction between the holes and knobs.

Breakdown Products as Inhibitors of Clotting

It has long been appreciated that fibrinogen and fibrin breakdown products can inhibit the spontaneous polymerization of fibrin monomers.[143] Indeed, fibrinogen itself can terminate growing fibrin oligomers once thrombin is cleared from the system, the lack of an exposed knob bringing the polymerization to a halt. Of the breakdown products, fragment D ought to be the most effective terminator because it has the necessary hole to participate in oligomer formation but lacks a knob to let the process continue. As might be expected, D-dimer is only about half as effective as fragment D in the inhibition of clotting.[144] The moiety D_2E should not be an effective inhibitor because all its sites are occupied, but an equilibrium between the D_2E form, on the one hand, and D_2 and free E, on the other, is likely. As a result, the transient D_2 can bind to growing fibrin units and be inhibitory under physiological conditions. Although some question may exist about just how important fibrin split products are in the self-limiting of clots under ordinary circumstances, fibrinogen split products are of great importance in some clinical settings. Thus, in the case of disseminated intravascular coagulation (DIC), plasmin is generated in disproportional amounts, and a massive destruction of fibrinogen ensues with a concomitant release of fragment D and resulting hemorrhage.[145] Certain snake venoms can produce a similar result by attacking fibrinogen directly.

FIBRINOGEN BIOSYNTHESIS

The principal—and perhaps only—site of fibrinogen biosynthesis in mammals is the liver. At one point it was thought that fibrinogen might also be made in megakaryocytes,[146, 147] but subsequent attempts to demonstrate the messenger RNAs in megakaryocyte cultures have not upheld the original reports.[148, 149] Apparently, all of the substantial amount of fibrinogen found in platelets is the result of sequestration.

The Regulatory Loop

The half-life of fibrinogen in the general circulation is less than 4 days, doubtless a reflection of its continuous conversion to fibrin and damage by other forms of limited proteolysis that leads to its removal from the circulation. Logically, one might expect fibrin and fibrinogen degradation products to play a role in the subsequent stimulation of fibrinogen biosynthesis, and numerous studies have been conducted to test that premise.[150–155] In most of these studies, the fragments D and E have been derived from in vitro digestion of fibrinogen by plasmin. As noted above, these fragments differ, to a degree, from the equivalent forms derived from fibrin, particularly cross-linked fibrin. Furthermore, some of these reports claim that *both* fragments D and E are effective stimulants of fibrinogen biosynthesis, a surprising observation in view of their completely different structures. It may be, of course, that there are two different receptors set to signal the need for more fibrinogen. In any event, the regulatory pathway is somewhat indirect in that the initial target cells are leukocytes, the monocyte in particular being most responsive.[150] These cells in turn release interleukin-6 (originally called hepatocyte-stimulating factor), which goes on to stimulate hepatocytes to manufacture fibrinogen and other proteins (Fig. 20–12). The intracellular linkage includes the involvement of protein kinase C[156] and hepatocyte nuclear factor (HNF-1), the latter binding directly to DNA.[157]

As is well known, fibrinogen is one of the "acute phase proteins," the biosynthesis of all of which is markedly increased in times of trauma and insult. The provocative stresses range from inflammation to pregnancy, and the responding proteins from α_1-antitrypsin to α_2-macroglobulin. Time-honored strategies for provoking the synthesis of acute phase proteins experimentally include the subdural administration of turpentine to laboratory rodents to effect localized inflammation, and the administration of snake venom enzymes to bring about massive degradation of fibrinogen. The first method was used by Bouma et al.[158] to increase mRNA levels sufficiently to show that the three chains of fibrinogen are made on separate messages. The latter method was used by Crabtree and Kant[159] in the first successful cloning of fibrinogen messages. It should be pointed out, also, that glucocorticoids have been used to stimulate fibrinogen biosynthesis in culture, and there must be hormonal involvements in vivo also.[160]

Gene Arrangement

Once the cDNAs for the three chains of fibrinogen were in hand, it was a straightforward matter to characterize the genes themselves. In mammals the three chains of fibrinogen are encoded by single-copy genes lying relatively near each other. In humans, the three genes encompass a 50-kilobase region on chromosome 4.[161] The α chain gene is situated between the γ chain and β chain genes. Interestingly, the β chain gene lies in the opposite orientation with its coding sequence on the other strand relative to the other two genes. Whether or not this inversion occurred at the time of the duplication that gave rise to the initial β chain is not known. In spite of this peculiar arrangement, all three genes are coordinately regu-

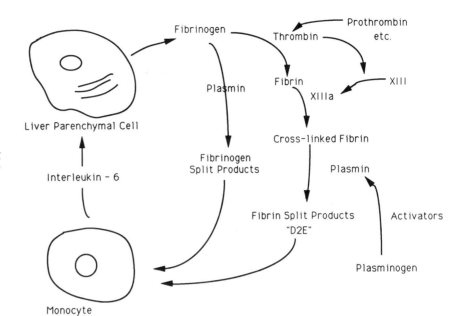

FIGURE 20–12. "Life cycle" of fibrin, outlining the regulation of its formation and destruction.

lated and made under control of the same signals. HNF-1 is known to bind to the promoters of both the α chain and β chain gene promoters.[157] In both instances the protein binds to a palindromic site upstream of the methionine start codons. The linkage from the receptors at the hepatocyte cell surface to the proteins that bind DNA may also involve glucocorticoids.[162]

All together, there are 20 introns in the three human fibrinogen genes: four in the α chain gene and eight each in the β chain and γ chain genes (see Figs. 20–5 and 20–6). Two of these are common to all three genes, a reflection of their common ancestry. The β and γ chain genes have an additional one in common, also. We will return to the consequences of intron distribution when we take up the subjects of minor and genetically defective forms of human fibrinogen.

Bioassembly of Fibrinogen

A number of logistical problems are associated with the assembly of a heterohexameric protein. The number of chains being made at any moment must be kept about the same, and they must find each other, form the appropriate disulfide bonds, and be processed properly before release into the circulation. In addition, although stimulation of the transcription of the genes may be coordinated, it must be remembered that α chains are half again as long as γ chains, and their translation ought to take proportionately longer. In fact, the balance seems to be met by maintaining a pool of free γ chains as homotrimers. The predicted driving force for this preassembly is the stability derived from the formation of "coiled coils."[18] Subsequently, an α chain displaces one of the γ chains, giving rise to a γ_2-α trimer.[163] Next, a β chain displaces another γ chain to give an α-β-γ half-molecule. There is not complete agreement on what happens next.

Although the half-molecules might be expected to simply join to give the hexamer, some recombinant studies have shown that various intermediates are also present, including those with the subunit composition $\alpha_2\beta_1\gamma_2$ and $\alpha_1\beta_1\gamma_2$.[164, 165] In any event, hexamers are eventually transported to the endoplasmic reticulum, where they are glycosylated, phosphorylated, and sulfated.

Post-translational Modifications

All three chains of fibrinogen are made in precursor forms with signal peptides that are cleaved during secretion into the endoplasmic reticulum.[166] Time-course studies indicate that the carbohydrate is added at somewhat different stages, the γ chain cluster being added before the β chain cluster.[167] Disulfide bonds are formed at an early stage, before the addition of phosphate or sulfates, the latter occurring after translocation but before secretion from the cell.[168] Interestingly, it is known from cDNA studies that the α chain contains a 15-residue carboxy-terminal extension that is not present in circulating fibrinogen.[43] Apparently this peptide is cleaved before or during secretion from the hepatocyte.

Fibrinogen contains both sulfate and phosphate groups that are added post-translationally. In many vertebrate species, but not primates, the fibrinopeptides B contain a sulfated tyrosine, a relatively uncommon residue in proteins. Interestingly, a minor form of fibrinogen that is the result of alternative splicing of the γ chain also has a sulfated tyrosine (see below).

Human fibrinogen contains partially phosphorylated serines at two different locations in the α chain: one at position 3 in the fibrinopeptide A, the other in the central region at position 345.[169] Fetal fibrinogen contains more phosphoserine than the adult form, perhaps the result of less extracellular dephosphory-lation rather than an increase in incorporation.[169]

Although phosphorylation is usually thought of as an intracellular process, the intimate association of fibrinogen and platelets may lead to specific extracellular phosphorylation.[170] Platelets have an ectokinase, and they release ATP during their activation, thereby providing the necessary wherewithal.[171] It has been shown that fibrinogen incubated with blood, radioactive ATP, and magnesium ions is indeed phosphorylated.[172] Moreover, it has been demonstrated that the fibers in fibrin gels formed from phosphorylated fibrinogen are altered, and subsequent fibrinolysis may be affected as well.[172]

Alternative Processing

Even though there is one gene for each of the three non-identical chains in human fibrinogen, two characteristic forms of the protein are ordinarily made. The second, which accounts for 5 to 10 per cent of the total fibrinogen, is distinguished by having a slightly longer version of the γ chain denoted γ′.[173] The mechanism accounting for the second form was first predicted on the basis of studies on a patient with a hereditary dysfibrinogenemia. Fibrinogen Paris I had an abnormality near the carboxy-terminus of the γ chain, and it was present in both the major and minor forms, indicating that both were the result of the same gene.[174] Indeed, the source of the γ′ chain is an alternative splicing during the maturation of the message.[175–177] In a predictable fraction of messages a splice of the last exon does not occur, a "readthrough" into the last intron occurring instead. The result is a γ chain in which the last four amino acids are replaced with a 20-residue alternate version. This sequence has a tyrosine that can be sulfated.[178] The γ′ fibrinogen forms fibrin in a normal way and is even cross-linked by factor XIII to produce γ-γ dimers.[174] It is not found in platelets, however, suggesting that the carboxy-terminus itself is involved in the sequestration process.

GENETICALLY DEFECTIVE FIBRINOGENS

Variant human fibrinogens have contributed much to our understanding of fibrinogen-fibrin biochemistry, in many instances providing important insights into structure-function relationships. Hundreds of such variants have already been identified, some because of their clinical consequences, many others where the clinical manifestation is mild or absent being found during routine screening, mostly revealed by long in vitro thrombin times. It is noteworthy that total afibrinogenemia is not automatically fatal, persons so afflicted often living into adulthood before some chance trauma overwhelms secondary hemostatic provisions.[179]

Technical problems are often involved in pinning down the molecular basis of a dysfibrinogenemia. In many cases the abnormal protein is made in diminished amounts. Moreover, the vast majority of persons found to have variant fibrinogens are heterozygotes.[180] The autosomal dominant nature of many dysfibrinogenemias is readily explained by the fact that even a small amount of a fibrinogen lacking either a knob or a hole (but not both, of course) can cap a growing fibrin polymer and inhibit clotting.

In principle, there ought to be as many kinds of genetically defective fibrinogen molecules as there are definable structural dependencies in the native molecule. Some may be strictly architectural, preventing proper folding and assembly, for example. Many are known in which the release of one or the other fibrinopeptides is inhibited, and many others in which the initial polymerization event is prevented. Still others may involve interactions with other components, including thrombin, plasmin(ogen), or t-PA.[181–183] Variants are now systematically catalogued,[180] and the subject is regularly reviewed.[184, 185] Here we highlight only a few of the more graphic and interesting (Table 20–3).[186–209]

The first variant fibrinogen to have its molecular basis identified was fibrinogen Detroit,* a case in which severely restricted fibrin formation was found to be correlated with the replacement of the arginine residue at α-19 by serine.[193] This is a classic case of a defective "knob." In the interval since that initial report, several other replacements have been found at that same position (see Table 20–3).

Other vulnerable locations are the peptide bonds attacked by thrombin. Interestingly, the arginine at α-16 is frequently replaced by histidine and the glycine at α-17 by cysteine (see Table 20–3). Unexpectedly, thrombin cleaves the bond in the former case, albeit at a much slower rate.[188] Some instances are also known in which the arginyl-glycine bond is unaffected, but substitution within the fibrinopeptide itself influences the binding of thrombin and leads to slow release.[186]

Of most interest are those variant fibrinogens that exhibit defective fibrin formation as a result of changes in their terminal domains. Thus, although the "knob" of the "knob-hole" interaction is well defined, the "hole" has not been identified with any precision. Amino acid replacements at γ chain residues 275, 292, 308, 310, 329, 330, and 375 all interfere with polymerization (Table 20–3), and all or most of these are assumed to be in the neighborhood of the binding pocket. One case is known in which a six-base pair deletion leads to the loss of γ chain residues 319 and 320 and also exhibits impaired polymerization.[198] Another interesting case involves anomalous carbohydrate attachment as the result of the replacement of residues twice-removed from asparagines. Several

---

*As in the case of variant human hemoglobins, variant fibrinogens are named after the city in which they were first found. When more than one variant is found in the same city, an appropriate number is appended.

TABLE 20–3. SOME GENETICALLY DEFECTIVE FIBRINOGENS

TYPE	DESIGNATION*	CHANGED RESIDUES	REFERENCE†
A. Variant fibrinopeptides	Lille	α7 D → N	186
	Rouen	α 12 G → V	187
B. Thrombin cleavage points	Petoskey‡	α16 R → H	188
	Metz‡	α16 R → C	189
	Seattle‡	β14 R → C	190
	Ise	β15 G → C	191
C. Central domain polymerization site (knob)	Kanazawa	α18 P → L	192
	Detroit	α19 R → S	193
	Munchen	α19 R → N	194
D. Terminal domain polymerization site (hole)	Bergamo II‡	γ275 R → H	195
	Osaka II	γ275 R → C	196
	Baltimore I	γ292 G → V	197
	Baltimore III	γ308 N → I	198
	Kyoto I	γ308 N → K	199
	Nagoya	γ329 Q → R	200
	Vlissinga	γ319-320 (deleted)	201
	Milano I	γ330 D → V	202
E. Defective cross-linking	Paris I	γ-C terminal insertion	203, 204
F. Carbohydrate obstruction	Asahi	γ310 M → T	205
	Caracas II	α434 S → N	206
	Pontoise	β335 A → T	207
G. Albumin obstruction	Nijmegen	β44 R → C	208
H. Secondary thrombin-binding site	New York	β9-72 (deleted)	209

*The designates with "‡" have been found in numerous other cities also.
†Numbers of references cited at end of chapter.

such variants have been found as a result of their defective polymerization (see Table 20–3).

A Didactic Case: Cysteine Changes

A good example of how genetic variants can be informative about a protein's structure is afforded by a class of variant fibrinogens with replacements involving cysteine. As noted in an earlier section, all the cysteine residues in fibrinogen are involved in disulfide bonds. This is true of most plasma proteins, of course, only a few of which have odd numbers of cysteines and a free sulfhydryl group as a result. Albumin is one of these exceptions, having 17 disulfide bonds and a single free cysteine.

If any of the cysteines in fibrinogen were to be replaced, its partner would be unpaired, and, depending on its location, might react with a molecule of free cysteine, with some other protein with a free sulfhydryl, or with another molecule like itself, or, conceivably, would maintain the free sulfhydryl. A similar situation would exist if any other amino acid in fibrinogen were replaced by a cysteine. In fact, both kinds of variant are known (see Table 20–3). In the case of fibrinogen New York, an entire exon amounting to 64 amino acids is absent from the β chain.[209] Amazingly, these fibrinogen molecules are still able to assemble into ordinary six-chained structures, even though the 64-residue β chain skein contains a cysteine residue that is ordinarily bound to one in the α chain. Apparently the unpaired cysteines at α-32 are able to find each other and form an additional bond between the two halves of the molecule. Other cases of change involve a cysteine in which a new disulfide bond occurs. In fibrinogen Metz the arginine at position α-16 is changed to cysteine, and, again, the two α chains in every fibrinogen molecule become linked by an additional disulfide.[210] In contrast, in fibrinogen Nijmegen, the arginine at β-44 is changed to cysteine, and the result is the formation of an external disulfide bond to the free cysteine in plasma albumin.[208] This observation is consistent with this portion of the β chain being highly exposed, it being common knowledge that one of the first bonds cleaved by plasmin is β-42-43.[211]

Albumin has also been found disulfide-bonded to fibrinogen IJmuiden, a case in which the arginine at β-14 is replaced with cysteine.[208] The same replacement was reported previously in fibrinogens Seattle and Christchurch II.[190] In contrast, replacement of the adjacent glycine by cysteine at β-15 does not lead to an attachment to albumin.[191] It may be that the new sulfhydryl in this case is capped with free cysteine, as is known to be the case in fibrinogen Osaka II.[196] In fibrinogen Osaka II the arginine at γ-275 is replaced with cysteine.

Site-Directed Mutagenesis

As valuable as naturally occurring variants have been, they may soon be overshadowed by site-directed mutagenesis experiments with recombinant fibrinogens expressed in recombinant systems. The first experiments in this area were limited to the expression of the individual chains,[212, 213] but recently a number of laboratories have succeeded in generating clottable fibrinogen in which all three non-identical chains have been assembled appropriately.[164, 165, 214]

As an example of the power of this approach, the portion of the γ chain that occurs in the terminal domain (γ 259 to 411) was expressed in *Escherichia coli* and mutants made in which cysteines 326 and 339 were omitted.[215] The goal was to find if the disulfide bond connecting these two residues in the native molecule is critical to calcium binding, as had been supposed by others. In fact, it was found that the mutant product bound radioactive calcium just as effectively as the recombinant native form, lending support to the finding noted earlier that the calcium-binding site involves only residues 311 to 336.[39]

MOLECULAR ECOLOGY OF FIBRINOGEN AND FIBRIN

Fibrinogen and fibrin and their breakdown products interact with a wide variety of proteins and cells. We have already touched upon involvements with thrombin, factor XIII, plasminogen, t-PA, and fibronectin and have alluded to binding to cell receptors that stimulate further synthesis. A few other proteins warrant mention, including thrombospondin and certain protease inhibitors, after which we can take up some interactions with cells and platelets. Let us review the list briefly.

Naturally, thrombin has a great affinity for fibrinogen. Less appreciated is the fact that thrombin also has a marked affinity for fibrin, a property that helps keep its action localized to the region of the clot.[216] We have already called attention to the fact that fibrin, but not fibrinogen, activates t-PA and binds plasminogen. In this game of point and counterpoint, inhibitors of plasmin and plasminogen activators associate with fibrinogen. For example, the serine protease inhibitor known as α$_1$-antitrypsin (a misnomer) is occasionally linked to fibrinogen by a disulfide bond,[217] and, more importantly, another inhibitor, α$_2$-antiplasmin, can be cross-linked by factor XIIIa into an acceptor site in the same general region of the fibrinogen molecule.[218] As in so much of extracellular biology, the regulatory theme that pervades the system is limited proteolysis and selective protease inhibition. Beyond that, many of the interactants are recruited in advance of their apparent need.

Thrombospondin

Thrombospondin is a large thrombin-sensitive glycoprotein that occurs in minute quantities in the circulating blood plasma but is released from activated platelets in significant amounts.[219, 220] It interacts with a number of proteins besides thrombin and has been found to be a plasmin inhibitor as well.[221] It also binds to fibrinogen and influences the nature of fibrin clots, perhaps by regulating the extent of fiber branching,[222, 223] and contributes to or stabilizes the adhesion of fibrinogen to activated platelets. The regions of fibrin(ogen) that are involved in this interaction have been found to include α chain residues 113 to 126 and β chain residues 243 to 252.[224] The first of these is situated in the middle region of the "coiled coils," whereas the second is a part of the terminal macrodomain (see Fig. 20–8).

The Interaction of Fibrinogen with Platelets

Fibrinogen is an essential cofactor in the adhesion of platelets to each other and to the endothelial lining of the circulatory system. A number of agents, including adenosine diphosphate, epinephrine, thrombin, and collagen, stimulate the exposure of fibrinogen receptors on the platelet surface. The primary receptor is the glycoprotein GPIIb-IIIa, an adhesion protein involved in the binding of other plasma proteins as well.[225] The cell-adhesion machinery appears to involve a combinatorial binding system that achieves its remarkable specificity by requiring two recognition components on every protein bound. One of these is the common tripeptidyl sequence Arg-Gly-Asp (RGD); the other, which imposes the bulk of the specificity, is peculiar to the protein bound.

Fibrinogen and fibrin both bind to platelets, but their plasmin degradation products do not.[226] This implies that the two components of a two-site recognition system become separated during the digestion. Consistent with this is the observation that α chains and γ chains both are involved in the binding.[227] The specificity-binding site has been localized to the carboxy-terminal 15 residues of the γ chain.[228] It will be recalled that this is the region of the molecule that first becomes cross-linked by factor XIII and that is presumed to be terminally situated in a spatial sense. As such, it is ideally located for bridge formation between platelets. The location of the alleged RGD site is more problematic. Human α chains contain two differently located RGD sequences, one at residues 95 to 97 and the other at 572 to 574. If it were supposed that the two γ chain sites are indeed located 450 Å apart at the extremes of the molecule, it might be anticipated that the α chain site would be situated terminally also, and not in the "coiled-coil" region, which encompasses residues 50 to 160 (see Fig. 20–8). As it happens, the site near the α chain carboxy-terminus (α 572 to 574) is not conserved from species to species, being absent in the rat, for example. This is not what one expects for an essential interaction site. Rat fibrinogen does have an RGD at positions α 280 to 282, however, as well as one in the coiled-coil region. Some investigators think that both RGD sites in human α chains contribute to the interaction.[228] Other work favors the notion that only the site near the carboxy-terminus is needed.[229] That at least one RGD site is essential to the interaction is borne out by the observation that trigamin, an RGD-containing peptide found in certain snake venoms, is a powerful inhibitor of the fibrinogen binding to platelets.[230]

Interactions with Other Cells

When provoked or damaged, the endothelial cells that line the vascular system also bind fibrinogen and fibrin.[231] Although there may be some subtle distinctions, the principal binding sites on fibrinogen appear to be the same as those involved in the binding to platelets.[229] If the underlying basement membrane is exposed, however, a high molecular weight protein called entactin becomes involved, reportedly binding to α and β chains but not γ chains.[232] Fibrin also binds to other cells of the circulatory system, including macrophages.[233] In this case, the central domain has been reported to be the principal site of interaction, specifically the Gly-Pro-Arg knob exposed by thrombin.[234] Fibronectin has also been implicated in the process.[233]

Interaction of Fibrinogen with Bacteria

Fibrinogen is unique among the plasma proteins in being able to "clump" certain strains of *Staphylococcus aureus*. The interactive site on fibrinogen has been localized to the carboxy-terminal segment of γ chains, precisely the region involved in fibrin cross-linking and, more relevant, the site required for binding to platelets.[235–237] That no other parts of fibrinogen are needed for clumping was dramatically demonstrated by construction of an artificial "clumper."[237] Thus, synthetic peptides corresponding to the terminal 15 residues of the γ chain can be coupled to carriers like albumin, and these constructs clump the bacteria in the complete absence of fibrinogen.

The question arises as to whether the phenomenon of "staph-clumping" is to the advantage of the bacterium or the host. On the one hand, it might be supposed that coating bacteria with fibrin, as opposed to fibrinogen, might lead to increased phagocytosis. On the other hand, fibrinogen coating might be part of an evasive strategy on the part of the bacterium. There is good reason to favor the latter. First, not all mammalian species have fibrinogens capable of clumping these bacteria, the carboxy-terminal sequences differing to the extent that no interactions occur, at least not with the strains tested. It seems more likely that the bacterium has been able to mimic the action of the platelet receptor than that the host has learned to bind the bacterium. If this were the case, the host could not change its site without compromising its ability to bind platelets. Staphylococci are also able to bind to fibrin thrombi, but in this case the interaction appears to be mediated by fibronectin, another protein with a binding site for these bacteria.[238] The fact that fibrinogen can "clump" these bacteria in vitro may be misleading. Experiments conducted under more physiologic conditions reveal that fibrinogen actually serves as a bridging molecule in the adherence of staphylococci to endothelial cells.[239]

Fibrinogen also binds to other bacteria, including many *Streptococcus* strains. The evidence in this realm strongly favors a protective action whereby phagocytosis of the coated bacterium is inhibited[240]; apparently these bacteria bind fibrinogen in order to avoid phagocytosis by host cells.[241] Preliminary experiments suggest that the β chain of fibrinogen contains the primary binding site.[241]

Finally, some pathogenic strains of *Bacteroides* have been found to bind fibrinogen specifically.[242] Surprisingly, different strains appear to bind to different parts of the molecule, the fragment D region in one case and the coiled-coil region in another.[242]

CONCLUDING REMARK

Fibrinogen is a highly differentiated protein. Although its primary functions are clot formation and platelet aggregation, it interacts with a wide variety of other proteins and cells. Its complex structure reflects these diverse actions. As much as possible, this chapter has tried to correlate structure and function by identifying those parts of the protein that are involved in polymerization, cross-linking, lysis, and binding to other proteins and cells. Some of these phenomena are better understood than others, and the reader must be cautious and not accept any claim uncritically. Fibrinogen is a protein shaped by natural selection to polymerize in various forms depending on conditions and is more or less vulnerable to lytic attack, depending on the assembled force of plasminogen and plasminogen activators arrayed against a counterforce of protease inhibitors. It is a molecule that can seal off wounds and prevent the invasion of some bacteria, while at the same time providing a safe haven for others. It is mysteriously self-regulating at several levels. Truly it is a protein for all seasons.

REFERENCES

1. Scheraga, H. A., and Laskowski, M., Jr.: The fibrinogen-fibrin conversion. Adv. Protein Chem. 12:1, 1957.
2. Doolittle, R. F.: Structural aspects of the fibrinogen-fibrin conversion. Adv. Protein Chem. 27:1, 1973.
3. Doolittle, R. F.: Fibrinogen and fibrin. *In* Bloom, A. L., and Thomas, D. P. (eds.): Haemostasis and Thrombosis, 2nd ed. London, Churchill Livingstone, 1987, pp. 192–215.
4. Bailey, K., Astbury, W. T., and Rudall, K. M.: Fibrinogen and fibrin as members of the keratin-myosin group. Nature 151:716, 1943.
5. Crick, F. H. C.: The packing of α-helices: Simple coiled-coils. Acta Crystallogr. 6:689, 1953.
6. Siegel, B. M., Mernan, J. P., and Scheraga, H. A.: The configuration of native and partially polymerized fibrinogen. Biochim. Biophys. Acta 11:329, 1953.
7. Shulman, S.: The size and shape of bovine fibrinogen studies of sedimentation, diffusion and viscosity. J. Am. Chem. Soc. 75:5846, 1953.
8. Hall, C. E., and Slayter, H. S.: The fibrinogen molecule: Its size, shape and mode of polymerization. J. Biophys. Biochem. Cytol. 5:11, 1959.

9. Cohen, C.: Invited discussion at 1960 Symposium on Protein Structure. J. Polymer Sci. 49:144, 1961.
10. Nussenzweig, V., Seligmann, M., Pelimont, J., and Grabar, P.: Les produits de degradation du fibrinogene humain par la plasmine. Ann. L'Institut Pasteur 100:377, 1961.
11. Marder, V. J., Shulman, N. R., and Carroll, W. R.: High molecular weight derivatives of human fibrinogen produced by plasmin. I. Physicochemical and immunological characterization. J. Biol. Chem. 244:2111, 1969.
12. Marder, V. J.: Physicochemical studies of intermediate and final products of plasmin digestion of human fibrinogen. Thromb. Diath. Haem. (Suppl.) 39:187, 1970.
13. Mills, D., and Karpatkin, S.: Heterogeneity of human fibrinogen: Possible relation to proteolysis by thrombin and plasmin as studied by SDS-polyacrylamide gel electrophoresis. Biochem. Biophys. Res. Commun. 40:206, 1970.
14. McKee, P. A., Rogers, L. A., Marler, E., and Hill, R. B.: The subunit polypeptides of human fibrinogen. Arch. Biochem. Biophys. 116:271, 1966.
15. Henschen, A.: Number and reactivity of disulfide bonds in fibrinogen and fibrin. Arkiv Kemi 22:355, 1964.
16. Tooney, N. M., and Cohen, C.: Microcrystals of a modified fibrinogen. Nature 237:23, 1972.
17. Rao, S. P. S., Poojary, M. D., Elliott, B. W., Jr., Melanson, L. A., Oriel, B., and Cohen, C.: Fibrinogen structure in projection at 18 Å resolution electron density by co-ordinated cryo-electron microscopy and X-ray crystallography. J. Mol. Biol. 222:89, 1991.
18. Doolittle, R. F.: Fibrinogen and fibrin. Ann. Rev. Biochem. 53:195, 1984.
19. Blombäck, B., Blombäck, M., Henschen, A., Hessel, B., Iwanaga, S., and Woods, K. R.: N-terminal disulfide knot of human fibrinogen. Nature 218:130, 1968.
20. Marder, V. J.: Identification and purification of fibrinogen degradation products produced by plasmin: Considerations on the structure of fibrinogen. Scand. J. Haem. (Suppl.) 13:21, 1971.
21. Kowalska-Loth, B., Gardlund, B., Egberg, N., and Blombäck, B.: Plasmic degradation products of human fibrinogen. II. Chemical and immunologic relation between Fragment E and N-DSK. Thromb. Res. 2:423, 1973.
22. Doolittle, R. F., Cassman, K. G., Cottrell, B. A., Friezner, S. J., and Takagi, T.: Amino acid sequence studies on the α-chain of human fibrinogen. The covalent structure of the α-chain portion of fragment D. Biochemistry 16:1710, 1977.
23. Doolittle, R. F., Goldbaum, D. M., and Doolittle, L. R.: Designation of sequences involved in the "coiled coil" interdomainal connector in fibrinogen: Construction of an atomic scale model. J. Mol. Biol. 120:311, 1978.
24. Henschen, A., and Lottspeich, F.: Amino acid sequence of human fibrin. Preliminary note on the γ-chain sequence. Hoppe-Seyler's Z. Physiol. Chem. 358:935, 1977.
25. Henschen, A., and Lottspeich, F.: Amino acid sequence of human fibrin. Preliminary note on the completion of the β-chain sequence. Hoppe-Seyler's Z. Physiol. Chem. 358:1643, 1977.
26. Watt, K. W. K., Takagi, T., and Doolittle, R. F.: Amino acid sequence of the β-chain of human fibrinogen: Homology with the γ-chain. Proc. Natl. Acad. Sci. USA 75:1731, 1978.
27. Doolittle, R. F., Watt, K. W. K., Cottrell, B. A., Strong, D. D., and Riley, M.: The amino acid sequence of the α-chain of human fibrinogen. Nature 280:464, 1979.
28. Townsend, R. R., Hilliker, E., Li, Y-T., Laine, R. A., Bell, W. R., and Lee, Y. C.: Carbohydrate structure of human fibrinogen. J. Biol. Chem. 257:9704, 1982.
29. Grieninger, G., Plant, P. W., and Kossoff, H. S.: Glycosylated A α chains in chicken fibrinogen. Biochemistry 23:5888, 1984.
30. Strong, D. D., Moore, M., Cottrell, B. A., Bohonus, V. L., Pontes, M., Evans, B., Riley, M., and Doolittle, R. F.: Lamprey fibrinogen γ chain: Cloning, cDNA sequencing and general characterization. Biochemistry 24:92, 1985.
31. Bohonus, V., Doolittle, R. F., Pontes, M., and Strong, D. D.: Complementary DNA sequence of lamprey fibrinogen β chain. Biochemistry 25:6512, 1986.
32. Doolittle, R. F., and Cottrell, B. A.: Lamprey fibrinogen B is a glycopeptide. Biochem. Biophys. Res. Commun. 60:1090, 1974.
33. Marguerie, G., Chagniel, G., and Suscillon, M.: The binding of calcium to bovine fibrinogen. Biochim. Biophys. Acta 490:94, 1977.
34. Purves, L. R., Lindsey, G. G., and Franks, J. J.: Role of calcium in the structure and interactions of fibrinogen. S. Afr. J. Sci. 74:202, 1978.
35. Marguerie, G., and Ardaillou, N.: Potential role of the A α chain in the binding of calcium to human fibrinogen. Biochim. Biophys. Acta 701:410, 1982.
36. Nieuwenhuizen, W., and Gravesen, M.: Anticoagulant and calcium-binding properties of high molecular weight derivatives of human fibrinogen, produced by plasmin (fragments X). Biochim. Biophys. Acta 668:81, 1981.
37. Haverkate, F., and Timan, G.: Protective effect of calcium in the plasmin degradation of fibrinogen and fibrin products D. Thromb. Res. 10:803, 1977.
38. Lawrie, J. S., and Kemp, G.: The presence of a Ca^{2+} bridge within the γ chain of human fibrinogen. Biochim. Biophys. Acta 577:415, 1979.
39. Dang, C. V., Ebert, R. F., and Bell, W. R.: Localization of a fibrinogen calcium binding site between γ-subunit positions 311 and 336 by terbium fluorescence. J. Biol. Chem. 260:9713, 1985.
40. Kant, J. A., Lord, S. T., and Crabtree, G. R.: Partial mRNA sequences for human A α, B β, and γ-fibrinogen chains: Evolutionary and functional implications. Proc. Natl. Acad. Sci. USA 80:3953, 1983.
41. Chung, D. W., Chan, W-Y., and Davie, E. W.: Characterization of a complementary deoxyribonucleic acid coding for the γ chain of human fibrinogen. Biochemistry 22:3250, 1983.
42. Chung, D. W., Que, B. G., Rixon, M. W., Mace, M., Jr., and Davie, E. W.: Characterization of complementary deoxyribonucleic acid and genomic deoxyribonucleic acid for the β chain of human fibrinogen. Biochemistry 22:3244, 1983.
43. Rixon, M. W., Chan, W-Y., Davie, E. W., and Chung, D. W.: Characterization of a complementary deoxyribonucleic acid coding for the α chain of human fibrinogen. Biochemistry 22:3237, 1983.
44. Crabtree, G. R., and Kant, J. A.: Molecular cloning of cDNA for the α, β and γ chains of rat fibrinogen. J. Biol. Chem. 257:7277, 1981.
45. Chung, D. W., Rixon, M. W., MacGillivray, R. T. A., and Davie, E. W.: Characterization of a cDNA clone coding for the β chain of bovine fibrinogen. Proc. Natl. Acad. Sci. USA 78:1466, 1981.
46. Weissbach, L., Oddoux, C., Procyk, R., and Grieninger, G.: The β chain of chicken fibrinogen contains an atypical thrombin cleavage site. Biochemistry 30:3290, 1991.
47. Weissbach, L., and Grieninger, G.: Bipartite mRNA for chicken α-fibrinogen potential encodes an amino acid sequence homologous to β- and γ-fibrinogens. Proc. Natl. Acad. Sci. USA 87:5198, 1990.
48. Pastori, R. L., Moskaitis, J. E., Smith, L. H., Jr., and Schoenberg, D. R.: Estrogen regulation of Xenopus laevis γ-fibrinogen gene expression. Biochemistry 29:2599, 1990.
49. Wang, Y. Z., Patterson, J., Gray, J. E., Yu, C., Cottrell, B. A., Shimizu, A., Graham, D., Riley, M., and Doolittle, R. F.: Complete sequence of the lamprey fibrinogen α chain. Biochemistry 28:9801, 1989.
50. Doolittle, R. F.: The structure and evolution of vertebrate fibrinogen. Ann. NY Acad. Sci. 408:315, 1983.
51. Huseby, R. M., Mosesson, M. W., and Murray, M.: Studies of the amino acid composition and conformation of human fibrinogen: Comparison of fractions I-4 and I-8. Physiol. Chem. Phys. 2:374, 1970.
52. Rudee, M. L., and Price, T. M.: Observation of the α-chain extensions of fibrinogen through a new electron microscope specimen preparation technique. Ultramicroscopy 7:193, 1981.

53. Price, T. M., Strong, D. D., Rudee, M. L., and Doolittle, R. F.: Shadow-cast electron microscopy of fibrinogen with antibody fragments bound to specific regions. Proc. Natl. Acad. Sci. USA 78:200, 1981.
54. Mosesson, M. W., Hainfeld, J., Wall, J., and Haschemeyer, R. H.: Identification and mass analysis of human fibrinogen molecules and their domains by scanning transmission electron microscopy. J. Mol. Biol. 153:695, 1981.
55. Erickson, H. P., and Fowler, W. E.: Electron microscopy of fibrinogen, its plasmic fragments and small polymers. Ann. NY Acad. Sci. 408:146, 1983.
56. Weisel, J. W., Stauffacher, C. V., Bullitt, E., and Cohen, C.: A model for fibrinogen: Domains and sequence. Science 230:1388, 1985.
57. Cierniewski, C. S., Plow, E. F., and Edgington, T. S.: Conformation of the carboxyterminal region of the A α chain of fibrinogen as elucidated by immunochemical analyses. Eur. J. Biochem. 141:489, 1984.
58. Williams, R. C.: Band patterns seen by electron microscopy in ordered arrays of bovine and human fibrinogen and fibrin after negative staining. Proc. Natl. Acad. Sci. USA 80:1570, 1983.
59. Doolittle, R. F., and Laudano, A. P.: Synthetic peptide probes and the location of fibrin polymerization sites. Protides Biol. Fluids 28:311, 1980.
60. Privalov, P. L., and Medved, L. V.: Domains in the fibrinogen molecule. J. Mol. Biol. 159:665, 1982.
61. Medved, L. V., Litinovich, S. V., and Privalov, P. L.: Domain organization of the terminal parts in the fibrinogen molecule. FEBS Lett. 202:298, 1986.
62. Ferry, J. D.: The mechanism of polymerization of fibrin. Proc. Natl. Acad. Sci. USA 38:355, 1952.
63. Stryer, L., Cohen, C., and Langridge, R.: Axial period of fibrinogen and fibrin. Nature 197:793, 1963.
64. Bailey, K., Bettelheim, F. R., Lorand, L., and Middlebrook, W. R.: Action of thrombin in the clotting of fibrinogen. Nature 167:233, 1951.
65. Blombäck, B., Hessel, B., Hogg, D., and Therkildsen, L.: A two-step fibrinogen-fibrin transition in blood coagulation. Nature 275:501, 1978.
66. Blombäck, B., Blombäck, M., and Nilsson, I. M.: Coagulation studies on reptilase, an extract of the venom from *Bothrops jararaca*. Thromb. Diath. Haem. 1:1, 1957.
67. Laudano, A. P., and Doolittle, R. F.: Synthetic peptide derivatives which bind to fibrinogen and prevent the polymerization of fibrin monomers. Proc. Natl. Acad. Sci. USA 75:3085, 1978.
68. Laudano, A. P., and Doolittle, R. F.: Studies on synthetic peptides that bind to fibrinogen and prevent fibrin polymerization. Structural requirements, numbers of binding sites and species differences. Biochemistry 19:1013, 1980.
69. Hantgan, R. R., and Hermans, J.: Assembly of fibrin. A light scattering study. J. Biol. Chem. 254:11272, 1979.
70. Weisel, J. W.: Fibrin assembly. Lateral aggregation and the role of the two pairs of fibrinopeptides. Biophys. J. 50:1079, 1986.
71. Ferry, J. D., and Morrison, P. R.: The conversion of human fibrinogen to fibrin under various conditions. J. Am. Chem. Soc. 69:380, 1947.
72. Donnelly, T. H., Laskowski, M., Jr., Notley, N., and Scheraga, H. A.: Equilibria in the fibrinogen-fibrin conversion. II. Reversibility of the polymerization steps. Arch. Biochem. Biophys. 56:369, 1955.
73. Shimizu, A., Nagel, G., and Doolittle, R. F.: Photoaffinity labeling of the primary fibrin polymerization site. I. Isolation and characterization of a labeled cyanogen bromide fragment corresponding to γ337–γ379. Proc. Natl. Acad. Sci. USA 89:2888, 1992.
74. Yamazumi, K., and Doolittle, R. F.: Photoaffinity labeling of the primary fibrin polymerization site. II. Localization of the label to tyrosine γ363. Proc. Natl. Acad. Sci. USA 89:2893, 1992.
75. Pandya, B. V., Gabriel, J. L., O'Brien, J., and Budzynski, A.

Z.: Polymerization site in the β chain of fibrin: Mapping of the B β 1-55 sequence. Biochemistry 30:162, 1991.
76. Hasegawa, N., and Sasaki, S.: Location of the binding site "b" for lateral polymerization of fibrin. Thromb. Res. 57:183, 1990.
77. Furlan, M., Rupp, C., and Beck, E. A.: Inhibition of fibrin polymerization by fragment D is affected by calcium, Gly-Pro-Arg and Gly-His-Arg. Biochim. Biophys. Acta 742:25, 1982.
78. Laudano, A. P., Cottrell, B. A., and Doolittle, R. F.: Synthetic peptides modeled on fibrin polymerization sites. Ann. NY Acad. Sci. 408:315, 1983.
79. Laudano, A. P., and Doolittle, R. F.: Influence of calcium ion on the binding of fibrin amino-terminal peptides to fibrinogen. Science 212:457, 1981.
80. Bale, M. D., Muller, M. F., and Ferry, J. D.: Effects of fibrinogen-binding tetrapeptides on mechanical properties of fine fibrin clots. Proc. Natl. Acad. Sci. USA 82:1410, 1985.
81. Schindlauer, G., Bale, M. D., and Ferry, J. D.: Interaction of fibrinogen-binding tetrapeptides with fibrin oligomers and fine fibrin clots. Biopolymers 25:1315, 1986.
82. Shimizu, A., Schindlauer, G., and Ferry, J. D.: Interaction of the fibrinogen-binding tetrapeptide Gly-Pro-Arg-Pro with fine clots and oligomers of α-fibrin; comparisons with α β-fibrin. Biopolymers 27:775, 1988.
83. Kuyas, C., and Doolittle, R. F.: Gly-Pro-Arg-Pro derivatives that bind to human plasma albumin and prevent fibrin formation. Thromb. Res. 43:485, 1986.
84. Harfenist, E. J., Guccione, M. A., Packham, M. A., and Mustard, J. F.: The use of the synthetic peptide, Gly-Pro-Arg-Pro, in the preparation of thrombin-degranulated rabbit platelets. Blood 59:952, 1982.
85. Almus, F. E., Rao, L. V. M., and Rapaport, S. I.: Functional properties of factor VIIA/tissue factor formed with purified tissue factor and with tissue factor expressed on cultured endothelial cells. Thromb. Haemost. 62:1067, 1989.
86. Mihalyi, E.: Clotting of fibrinogen. Calcium binding to fibrin during clotting and its dependence on release of fibrinopeptide B. Biochemistry 27:967, 1988.
87. Donovan, J. W., and Mihalyi, E.: Clotting of fibrinogen. I. Scanning calorimetric study of the effect of calcium. Biochemistry 24:3434, 1985.
88. Janmey, P. A., and Ferry, J. D.: Gel formation by fibrin oligomers without addition of monomers. Biopolymers 25:1337, 1986.
89. Marx, G.: Protofibrin clots induced by calcium and zinc. Biopolymers 26:911, 1987.
90. Curtis, C. G.: Plasma factor XIII. *In* Bloom, A. L., and Thomas, D. P. (eds): Haemostasis and Thrombosis, 2nd ed. London, Churchill-Livingstone, 1987, pp. 216–222.
91. Greenberg, C. S., and Shuman, M. A.: The zymogen forms of blood coagulation factor XIII bind specifically to fibrinogen. J. Biol. Chem. 257:6096, 1982.
92. Chen, R., and Doolittle, R. F.: Isolation, characterization and location of a donor-acceptor unit from crosslinked fibrin. Proc. Natl. Acad. Sci. USA 66:472, 1970.
93. Chen, R., and Doolittle, R. F.: γ- γ Cross-linking sites in human and bovine fibrin. Biochemistry 10:4486, 1971.
94. McKee, P. A., Mattock, P., and Hill, R. L.: Subunit structure of human fibrinogen, soluble fibrin, and cross-linked insoluble fibrin. Proc. Natl. Acad. Sci. USA 66:738, 1970.
95. Gerth, C., Roberts, W. W., and Ferry, J. D.: Rheology of fibrin clots. II. Linear viscoelastic behavior in shear creep. Biophys. Chem. 2:208, 1974.
96. Nelb, G. W., Kamykowski, G. W., and Ferry, J. D.: Kinetics of ligation of fibrin oligomers. J. Biol. Chem. 255:6398, 1980.
97. Bale, M. D., Janmey, P. A., and Ferry, J. D.: Kinetics of formation of fibrin oligomers. II. Size distributions of ligated oligomers. Biopolymers 21:2265, 1982.
98. Gaffney, P. J., and Whitaker, A. N.: Fibrin crosslinks and lysis rates. Thromb. Res. 14:85, 1979.
99. Duckert, F.: Documentation of the plasma factor XIII deficiency in man. Ann. NY Acad. Sci. 202:190, 1972.

100. Mosher, D. F.: Cross-linking of cold-insoluble globulin by fibrin-stabilizing factor. J. Biol. Chem. 250:6614, 1975.

101. Ruoslahti, E., and Vaheri, A.: Interaction of soluble fibroblast surface antigen with fibrinogen and fibrin. J. Exp. Med. 141:497, 1975.

102. Mosher, D. F., Schad, P. E., and Kleinman, H. K.: Cross-linking of fibronectin to collagen by blood coagulation factor XIII_a. J. Clin. Invest. 64:781, 1979.

103. Mosher, D. F., and Johnson, R. B.: Specificity of fibronectin-fibrin cross-linking. Ann. NY Acad. Sci. 408:583, 1983.

104. Erickson, H. P., Carrell, N., and McDonagh, J.: Fibronectin molecule visualized in electron microscopy: A long, thin, flexible strand. J. Cell Biol. 91:673, 1981.

105. Pacella, B. L., Jr., Hui, K. Y., Haber, E., and Matsueda, G. R.: Induction of fibrin-specific antibodies by immunization with synthetic peptides that correspond to amino termini of thrombin cleavage sites. Molec. Immunol. 20:521, 1983.

106. Hui, K. Y., Haber, E., and Matsueda, G. R.: Monoclonal antibodies to a synthetic fibrin-like peptide bind to human fibrin but not fibrinogen. Science 222:1129, 1983.

107. Scheefers-Borchel, U., Muller-Berghaus, G., Fuhge, P., Eberle, R., and Heimburger, N.: Discrimination between fibrin and fibrinogen by a monoclonal antibody against a synthetic peptide. Proc. Natl. Acad. Sci. USA 82:7091, 1985.

108. Wilner, G. D., Mudd, M. S., Hsieh, K-H., and Thomas, D. W.: Monoclonal antibodies to fibrinogen: Modulation of determinants expressed in fibrinogen by γ-chain cross-linking. Biochemistry 21:2687, 1982.

109. Procyk, R., Kudryk, B., Callender, S., and Blombäck, B.: Accessibility of epitopes on fibrin clots and fibrinogen gels. Blood 77:1469, 1991.

110. Schielen, W. J. G., Adams, H. P. H. M., van Leuven, K., Moskuilen, M., Tesser, G. I., and Nieuwenhuizen, W.: The sequence γ-(312–324) is a fibrin-specific epitope. Blood 77:2169, 1991.

111. Lucas, M. A., Fretto, L. J., and McKee, P. A.: The binding of human plasminogen to fibrin and fibrinogen. J. Biol. Chem. 258:4249, 1983.

112. Söttrup-Jensen, L., Claeys, H., Zajdel, M., Petersen, T. E., and Magnusson, S.: The primary structure of human plasminogen: Isolation of two lysine-binding fragments and one 'mini'-plasminogen (MW38000) by elastase-catalyzed-specific limited proteolysis. *In* Davidson, J. F., Rowan, R. M., Samama, M. M., and Desnoyers, P. C. (eds.): Progress in Chemical Fibrinolysis and Thrombolysis, Vol. 3. New York, Raven Press, 1978, pp. 191–209.

113. Rejante, M., Elliott, B. W., Jr., and Llinas, M.: A ¹H-NMR study of plasminogen kringle 4 interactions with intact and partially digested fibrinogen. Fibrinolysis 5:87, 1991.

114. Weinstein, M. J., and Doolittle, R. F.: Differential specificities of thrombin, plasmin and trypsin with regard to synthetic and natural substrates and inhibitors. Biochim. Biophys. Acta 258:577, 1972.

115. Deutsch, D. G., and Mertz, E. T.: Plasminogen: Purification from human plasma by affinity chromatography. Science 170:1095, 1970.

116. Radcliffe, R.: A critical role of lysine residues in the stimulation of tissue plasminogen activator by denatured proteins and fibrin clots. Biochim. Biophys. Acta 743:422, 1983.

117. Varadi, A., and Patthy, L.: β(Leu_{121}-Lys_{122}) segment of fibrinogen is in a region essential for plasminogen binding by fibrin fragment E. Biochemistry 23:2108, 1983.

118. Christensen, U.: C-terminal lysine residues of fibrinogen fragments essential for binding to plasminogen. FEBS Lett. 182:43, 1985.

119. Fleury, V., and Angles-Cano, E.: Characterization of the binding of plasminogen to fibrin surfaces: The role of carboxy-terminal lysines. Biochemistry 30:7630, 1991.

120. Rijken, D. C., Hoylaerts, M., and Collen, D.: Fibrinolytic properties of one-chain and two-chain human extrinsic (tissue-type) plasminogen activator. J. Biol. Chem. 257:2920, 1982.

121. Wiman, B., and Collen, D.: On the mechanism of reaction between human α₂-antiplasmin and plasmin. J. Biol. Chem. 254:9291, 1979.

122. Ichinose, A., Takio, K., and Fujikawa, K.: Localization of the binding site of tissue-type plasminogen activator to fibrin. J. Clin. Invest. 78:163, 1986.

123. Verheijen, J. H., Caspers, M. P. M., Chang, G. T. G., de Munk, G. A. W., Pouwels, P. H., and Enger-Valk, B. E.: Involvement of finger domain and kringle 2 domain of tissue-type plasminogen activator in fibrin binding and stimulation of activity by fibrin. EMBO J. 5:3525, 1986.

124. de Vos, A. M., Ultsch, M. H., Kelly, R. F., Padmanabhan, K., Tulinsky, A., Westbrook, M. L., and Kossiakoff, A. A.: Crystal structure of the kringle 2 domain of tissue plasminogen activator at 2.4-Å resolution. Biochemistry 31:270, 1992.

125. Nieuwenhuizen, W., Vermond, A., Voskuilen, M., Traas, D. W., and Verheijen, J. H.: Identification of a site in fibrin(ogen) which is involved in the acceleration of plasminogen activation by tissue-type plasminogen activator. Biochim. Biophys. Acta 748:86, 1983.

126. Voskuilen, M., Vermond, A., Veeneman, G. H., van Boom, J. H., Klasen, E. A., Zegers, N. D., and Nieuwenhuizen, W.: Fibrinogen lysine residue A α 157 plays a crucial role in the fibrin-induced acceleration of plasminogen activation, catalyzed by tissue-type plasminogen activator. J. Biol. Chem. 262:5944, 1987.

127. Schielen, W. J. G., Voskuilen, M., Tesser, G. I., and Nieuwenhuizen, W.: The sequence A α-(148-160) in fibrin, but not in fibrinogen, is accessible to monoclonal antibodies. Proc. Natl. Acad. Sci., USA 86:8951, 1989.

128. Schielen, W. J. G., Adams, H. P. H. M., Voskuilen, M., Tesser, G. J., and Nieuwenhuizen, W.: Structural requirements of position A α-157 in fibrinogen for the fibrin-induced rate enhancement of the activation of plasminogen by tissue-type plasminogen activator. Biochem. J. 276:655, 1991.

129. Vandamme, A.-M., Bulens, F., Bernar, H., Nelles, L., Lijnen, R. H., and Collen, D.: Construction and characterization of a recombinant murine monoclonal antibody directed against human fibrin fragment-D dimer. Eur. J. Biochem. 192:767, 1990.

130. Runge, M. S., Quertermous, T., Zavodny, P. J., Love, T. W., Bode, C., Freitag, M., Shaw, S.-Y., Huang, P. L., Chou, C.-C., Mullins, D., Schnee, J. M., Savard, C. E., Rothenberg, M. E., Newell, J., Matsueda, G. R., and Haber, E.: A recombinant chimeric plasminogen activator with high affinity for fibrin has increased thrombolytic potency *in vitro* and *in vivo*. Proc. Natl. Acad. Sci. USA 88:10337, 1991.

131. Laroche, Y., Demaeyer, M., Stassen, J.-M., Gansemans, Y., Demarsin, E., Matthyssens, G., Collen, D., and Holvoet, P.: Characterization of a recombinant single-chain molecule comprising the variable domains of a monoclonal antibody specific for human fibrin fragment D-dimer. J. Biol. Chem. 266:16343, 1991.

132. Langer-Safer, P. R., Ahern, T. J., Angus, L. B., Barone, K. M., Brenner, M. J., Horgan, P. G., Morris, G. E., Stoudemire, J. B., Timony, G. A., and Larsen, G. R.: Replacement of finger and growth factor domains of tissue plasminogen activator with plasminogen kringle 1. Biochemical and pharmacological characterization of a novel chimera containing a high affinity fibrin-binding domain linked to a heterologous protein. J. Biol. Chem. 266:3715, 1991.

133. Carr, M. E., Jr., and Hermans, J.: Size and density of fibrin fibers from turbidity. Macromolecules 11:46, 1978.

134. Brash, J. L., and ten Hove, P.: Transient adsorption of fibrinogen on foreign surfaces: Similar behavior in plasma and whole blood. J. Biomed. Mater. Res. 23:157, 1989.

135. van Oss, C. J.: Surface properties of fibrinogen and fibrin. J. Prot. Chem. 9:487, 1990.

136. Carr, M. E., Jr., and Hardin, C. L.: Large fibrin fibers enhance urokinase-induced plasmin digestion of plasma clots. Blood 70(Suppl. 1):400a, 1987.

137. Hunter, R. L., Bennett, B., and Check, I. J.: The effect of poloxamer 188 on the rate of in vitro thrombolysis mediated by t-PA and streptokinase. Fibrinolysis 4:117, 1990.

138. Carr, M. E., Jr., Powers, P. L., and Jones, M. R.: Effects of

poloxamer 188 on the assembly, structure and dissolution of fibrin clots. Thromb. Haemost. 66:565, 1991.

139. Bjornsson, T. D., Schneider, D. E., and Berger, H., Jr.: Aspirin acetylates fibrinogen and enhances fibrinolysis. Fibrinolytic effect is independent of changes in plasminogen activator levels. J. Pharmacol. Exp. Therap. 250:154, 1989.

140. Francis, C. W., Marder, V. J., and Barlow, G. H.: Plasmic degradation of crosslinked fibrin. J. Clin. Invest. 66:1033, 1980.

141. Hudry-Clergeon, G., Paturel, L., and Suscillon, M.: Identification d'un complexe (D-D) ... E dans les produits de dégradation de la fibrine bovine stabilisée par le facteur XIII. Path. Biol., Paris 22(Supp.):47, 1974.

142. Gaffney, P. J., and Joe, F.: The lysis of crosslinked human fibrin by plasmin yields initially a single molecular complex, D dimer-E. Thromb. Res. 15:673, 1979.

143. Latallo, Z. S., Fletcher, A. P., Alkjaersig, N., and Sherry, S.: Inhibition of fibrin polymerization by fibrinogen proteolysis products. Am. J. Physiol. 202:681, 1962.

144. Haverkate, F., Timan, G., and Nieuwenhuizen, W.: Anticlotting properties of fragments D from human fibrinogen and fibrin. Eur. J. Clin. Invest. 9:253, 1979.

145. Brozović, M.: Disseminated intravascular coagulation. In Bloom, A. L., and Thomas, D. P. (eds.): Haemostasis and Thrombosis, 2nd ed. London, Churchill Livingstone, 1987, pp. 535–541.

146. Leven, R., Schick, P. K., and Budzynski, A.: Fibrinogen biosynthesis in isolated guinea pig megakaryocytes. Blood 65:501, 1982.

147. Uzan, G., Kerbiriou, D., Stankovic, Z., Courtois, G., Crabtree, G., and Marguerie, G.: Fibrinogen expression in the megakaryocyte. Thromb. Haemost. 54:278, 1985 (abstract 01652).

148. Louache, F., Debili, N., Cramer, E., Breton-Gorius, J., and Vainchenker, W.: Fibrinogen is not synthesized by human megakaryocytes. Blood 77:311, 1991.

149. Lange, W., Luig, A., Dölken, G., Mertelsmann, R., and Kanz, L.: Fibrinogen γ-chain mRNA is not detected in human megakaryocytes. Blood 78:20, 1991.

150. Ritchie, D. G., Levy, B. A., Adams, M. A., and Fuller, G. M.: Regulation of fibrinogen synthesis by plasmin-derived fragments of fibrinogen and fibrin: An indirect feedback pathway. Proc. Natl. Acad. Sci. USA 79:1530, 1982.

151. Hatzfeld, J. A., Hatzfeld, A., and Maigne, J.: Fibrinogen and its fragment D stimulate proliferation of human hemopoietic cells in vitro. Proc. Natl. Acad. Sci. USA 79:6280, 1982.

152. Bell, W. R., Kessler, C. M., and Townsend, R. F.: Stimulation of fibrinogen biosynthesis by fibrinogen fragments D and E. Br. J. Haematol. 53:599, 1983.

153. Qureshi, G. D., Guzelian, P. S., Vennart, R. M., and Evans, H. J.: Stimulation of fibrinogen synthesis in cultured rat hepatocytes by fibrinogen fragment E. Biochim. Biophys. Acta 844:288, 1985.

154. LaDuca, F. M., Tinsley, L. A., Dang, C. V., and Bell, W. R.: Stimulation of fibrinogen synthesis in cultured rat hepatocytes by fibrinogen degradation product fragment D. Proc. Natl. Acad. Sci. USA 86:8788, 1989.

155. Wang, Y., and Fuller, G. M.: The putative role of fibrin fragments in the biosynthesis of fibrinogen by hepatoma cells. Biochem. Biophys. Res. Commun. 175:562, 1991.

156. Evans, E., Courtois, G. M., Kilian, P. L., Fuller, G. M., and Crabtree, G. R.: Induction of fibrinogen and a subset of acute phase response genes involves a novel monokine which is mimicked by phorbol esters. J. Biol. Chem. 262:10850, 1987.

157. Courtois, G., Baumhueter, S., and Crabtree, G. R.: Purified hepatocyte nuclear factor I interacts with a family of hepatocyte-specific promoters. Proc. Natl. Acad. Sci. USA 85:7937, 1988.

158. Bouma, H., III, Kwan, S.-W., and Fuller, G. M.: Radioimmunological identification of polysomes synthesizing fibrinogen polypeptide chains. Biochemistry 14:4787, 1975.

159. Crabtree, G. R., and Kant, J. A.: Coordinate accumulation of the mRNA for the α, β, and γ chains of fibrinogen after defibrination with Malayan pit viper venom. J. Biol. Chem. 257:7277, 1982.

160. Plant, P. W., and Grieninger, G.: Noncoordinate synthesis of the fibrinogen subunits in hepatocytes cultured under hormone-deficient conditions. J. Biol. Chem. 261:2331, 1986.

161. Kant, J., Fornace, A. J., Saxe, D., McBride, O. W., and Crabtree, G. R.: Organization and evolution of the human fibrinogen locus on chromosome four. Proc. Natl. Acad. Sci. USA 82:2344, 1985.

162. Otto, J. M., Grenett, H. E., and Fuller, G. M.: The coordinated regulation of fibrinogen gene transcription by hepatocyte-stimulating factor and dexamethasone. J. Cell Biol. 105:1067, 1987.

163. Yu, S., Sher, B., Kudryk, B., and Redman, C. M.: Fibrinogen precursors. Order of assembly of fibrinogen chains. J. Biol. Chem. 259:10574, 1984.

164. Roy, S. N., Procyk, R., Kudryk, B. J., and Redman, C. M.: Assembly and secretion of recombinant human fibrinogen. J. Biol. Chem. 266:4758, 1991.

165. Hartwig, R., and Danishefsky, K. J.: Studies on the assembly and secretion of fibrinogen. J. Biol. Chem. 266:6578, 1991.

166. Nickerson, J. M., and Fuller, G. M.: In vitro synthesis of rat fibrinogen: Identification of preA α, preB β, and pre γ polypeptides. Proc. Natl. Acad. Sci. USA 78:303, 1981.

167. Nickerson, J. M., and Fuller, G. M.: Modification of fibrinogen chains during synthesis: Glycosylation of B β and γ chains. Biochemistry 20:2818, 1981.

168. Kudryk, B., Okada, M., Redman, C. M., and Blombäck, B.: Biosynthesis of dog fibrinogen. Characterization of nascent fibrinogen in the rough endoplasmic reticulum. Eur. J. Biochem. 125:673, 1982.

169. Seydewitz, H. H., Kaiser, C., Rothweiler, H., and Witt, I.: The location of a second in vivo phosphorylation site in the A α-chain of human fibrinogen. Thromb. Res. 33:487, 1984.

170. Krust, B., Galabru, J., and Hovanessian, A. G.: Phosphorylation of the α-chain of fibrinogen by a platelet kinase activity enhanced by interferon. Biochem. Biophys. Res. Commun. 117:350, 1983.

171. Nauk, V. P., Kornecki, E., and Ehrlich, Y. H.: Phosphorylation and dephosphorylation of human platelet surface proteins by an ecto-protein kinase/phosphatase system. Biochim. Biophys. Acta 1092:256, 1991.

172. Martin, S. C., Forsberg, P-O., and Eriksson, S. D.: The effects of in vitro phosphorylation and dephosphorylation on the thrombin-induced gelation and plasmin degradation of fibrinogen. Thromb. Res. 61:243, 1991.

173. Wolfenstein-Todel, C., and Mosesson, M. W.: Human plasma fibrinogen heterogeneity: Evidence for an extended carboxyl-terminal sequence in a normal gamma chain variant (gamma'). Proc. Natl. Acad. Sci. USA 77:5069, 1980.

174. Wolfenstein-Todel, C., and Mosesson, M. W.: Carboxy-terminal amino acid sequence of a human fibrinogen γ-chain variant (γ'). Biochemistry 20:6146, 1981.

175. Crabtree, G. R., and Kant, J. A.: Organization of the rat gamma-fibrinogen gene: Alternative mRNA splice patterns produce the gamma A and gamma B (gamma') chains of fibrinogen. Cell 31:159, 1982.

176. Chung, D. W., and Davie, E. W.: γ and γ' chains of human fibrinogen are produced by alternative mRNA processing. Biochemistry 23:4232, 1984.

177. Fornace, A. J., Cummings, D. E., Comeau, C. M., Kant, J. A., and Crabtree, G. R.: Structure of the human γ-fibrinogen gene. Alternate mRNA splicing near the 3' end of the gene produces γA and γB forms of γ-fibrinogen. J. Biol. Chem. 259:12826, 1984.

178. Hirose, S., Oda, K., and Ikehara, Y.: Tyrosine O-sulfation of the fibrinogen γB chain in primary culture of rat hepatocytes. J. Biol. Chem. 263:7426, 1988.

179. Crabtree, G. R.: The molecular biology of fibrinogen. In Stamatoyannopoulos, G., Nienhuis, A. W., Leder, P., and Majerus, P. W. (eds.): Molecular Basis of Blood Diseases. Philadelphia, W. B. Saunders Company, 1985, pp. 631–655.

180. Ebert, R. F.: Index of Variant Human Fibrinogens. Boca Raton, FL, CRC Press, 1991.

181. Al-Mondhiry, H. A. B., Bilezikian, S. B., and Nossel H. L.: Fibrinogen "New York"—An abnormal fibrinogen associated with thromboembolism: Functional evaluation. Blood 45:607, 1975.

182. Soria, J., Soria, C., and Caen, J. P.: A new type of congenital dysfibrinogenaemia with defective fibrin lysis—Dusard syndrome: Possible relation to thrombosis. Br. J. Haematol. 53:575, 1983.

183. Ieko, M., Sawada, K.-I., Sakurama, S., Yamagishi, I., Isogawa, S., Nakagawa, S., Satoh, M., Tasukouchi, T., and Matsuda, M.: Fibrinogen Date: Congenital hypodysfibrinogenemia associated with decreased binding of tissue-plasminogen activator. Am J. Hematol. 37:228, 1991.

184. Southan, C.: Molecular and genetic abnormalities of fibrinogen. In Francis, J. L. (ed.): Fibrinogen, Fibrin Stabilisation, and Fibrinolysis. Chichester, England, Ellis Horwood, Ltd., 1988, pp. 65–99.

185. Matsuda, M., Yoshida, N., Terukina, S., Yamazumi, K., and Maekawa, H.: Molecular abnormalities of fibrinogen—The present status of structure elucidation. In Matsuda, M., Iwanaga, S., Takada, A., and Henschen, A. (eds.): Fibrinogen 4, Current Basic and Clinical Aspects. Amsterdam, Elsevier Science Publ., 1990, pp. 139–152.

186. Denninger, M. H., Finlayson, J. S., Raemer, L. A., Porquet-Gernez, A., Goudeman, M., and Menache, D.: Congenital dysfibrinogenaemia: Fibrinogen Lille. Thromb. Res. 13:453, 1978.

187. Kehl, M., Lottspeich, F., and Henschen, A.: Genetically abnormal fibrinogens releasing abnormal fibrinopeptides as characterised by high performance liquid chromatography. In Haverkate, F., Henschen, A., Nieuwenhuizen, W., and Straub, P. W. (eds.): Fibrinogen: Structure, Functional Aspects, Metabolism. Berlin, Walter de Gruyter, 1983, pp. 183–193.

188. Higgins, D. L., and Shafer, J. A.: Fibrinogen Petoskey, a dysfibrinogenemia characterized by replacement of Arg-A α 16 by a histidyl residue. Evidence for thrombin-catalyzed hydrolysis at a histidyl residue. J. Biol. Chem. 256:12013, 1981.

189. Soria, J., Soria, C., Samama, M., Henschen, A., and Southan, C.: Special report on fibrinogen Metz characterised by an amino acid substitution at the peptide bond split by thrombin. In Henschen, A., Graeff, H., and Lottspeich, F. (eds.): Fibrinogen, Recent Biochemical and Medical Aspects. Berlin, Walter de Gruyter, 1983, pp. 129–151.

190. Kaudewitz, H., Henschen, A., Pirkle, H., Heaton, D., Soria, J., and Soria, C.: Structure function relationships in abnormal fibrinogen with B β 14 Arg → Cys substitution; fibrinogens Seattle I and Christchurch II. Thromb. Haemost. 58:515, 1987 (abstract 1901).

191. Yoshida, N., Wada, H., Morita, K., Hirata, H., Matsuda, M., Yamazumi, K., Asakura, S., and Shirakawa, S.: A new congenital abnormal fibrinogen Ise characterized by the replacement of Bβ glycine-15 by cysteine. Blood 77:1958, 1991.

192. Uotani, C., Miyata, T., Kumabashiri, I., Asakura, H., Saito, M., Matsuda, T., Kajiyama, S., and Iwanaga, S.: Fibrinogen Kanazawa: A congenital dysfibrinogenaemia with delayed polymerization having a replacement of proline-18 by leucine in the A α-chain. Blood Coag. Fibrinol. 2:413, 1991.

193. Blombäck, M., Blombäck, B., Mammen, E. F., and Prasad, A. S.: Fibrinogen Detroit—A molecular defect in the N-terminal disulphide knot of human fibrinogen? Nature 218:134, 1968.

194. Southan, C., Henschen, A., and Lottspeich, F.: The search for molecular defects in abnormal fibrinogens. In Henschen, A., Graeff, H., and Lottspeich, F. (eds.): Fibrinogen—Recent Biochemical and Medical Aspects. Berlin, Walter de Gruyter, 1983, pp. 153–166.

195. Reber, P., Furlan, M., Henschen, A., Kaudewitz, H., Barbui, T., Hilgard, P., Nenci, G. G., Berrettini, M., and Beck, E. A.: Three abnormal fibrinogen variants with the same amino acid substitution (γ275 Arg → His): Fibrinogens Bergamo II, Essen and Perugia. Thromb. Haemost. 56:401, 1986.

196. Terukina, S., Matsuda, M., Hirata, H., Takeda, Y., Miyata, T., Takao, T., and Shimonishi, Y.: Substitution of γArg-275 by Cys in an abnormal fibrinogen, "Fibrinogen Osaka II." J. Biol. Chem. 263:13579, 1988.

197. Bantia, S., Mane, S. M., Bell, W. R., and Dang, C. V.: Fibrinogen Baltimore I: Polymerization defect associated with a γ²⁹² Gly → Val (GGC → GTC) mutation. Blood 76:2279, 1990.

198. Bantia, S., Bell, W. R., and Dang, C. V.: Polymerization defect of fibrinogen Baltimore III due to a gamma Asn³⁰⁸---Ile mutation. Blood 75:1659, 1990.

199. Yoshida, N., Terukina, S., Okuma, M., Moroi, M., Aoki, N., and Matsuda, M.: Characterization of an apparently lower molecular weight γ-chain variant in fibrinogen Kyoto I. J. Biol. Chem. 263:13848, 1988.

200. Miyata, T., Furukawa, K., Iwanaga, S., Takamatsu, J., and Saito, H.: Fibrinogen Nagoya, a replacement of glutamine-329 by arginine in the γ-chain that impairs the polymerization of fibrin monomer. J. Biochem. 105:10, 1989.

201. Koopman, J., Haverkate, F., Briët, E., and Lord, S. T.: A congenitally abnormal fibrinogen (Vlissingen) with a 6-base deletion in the γ-chain gene, causing defective calcium binding and impaired fibrin polymerization. J. Biol. Chem. 266:13456, 1991.

202. Reber, P., Furlan, M., Rupp, C., Kehl, M., Henschen, A., Mannucci, P. M., and Beck, E. A.: Characterization of fibrinogen Milano I: Amino acid exchange γ330 Asp → Val impairs fibrin polymerization. Blood 67:1751, 1986.

203. Budzynski, A. Z., Marder, V. J., Menache, D., and Guillin, M. C.: Defect in the gamma polypeptide chain of a congenital abnormal fibrinogen (Paris I). Nature 252:66, 1974.

204. Mosesson, M. W., Amrani, D. L., and Menache, D.: Studies of the structural abnormality of fibrinogen Paris I. J. Clin. Invest. 57:782, 1976.

205. Yamazumi, K., Shimura, K., Terukina, S., Takahashi, N., and Matsuda, M.: A γ methionine-310 to threonine substitution and consequent N-glycosylation at γ asparagine-308 identified in a congenital dysfibrinogenemia associated with post-traumatic bleeding, fibrinogen Asahi. J. Clin. Invest. 83:1590, 1989.

206. Maekawa, H., Yamazumi, K., Muramatsu, S., Kaneko, M., Hirata, H., Takahashi, N., de Bosch, N. B., Carvajal, Z., Ojeda, A., Arocha-Pinango, C. L., and Matsuda, M.: An A α Ser-434 to N-glycosylated Asn substitution in a dysfibrinogen, fibrinogen Caracas II, characterized by impaired fibrin gel formation. J. Biol. Chem. 266:11575, 1991.

207. Kaudewitz, H., Henschen, A., Soria, J., and Soria, C.: Fibrinogen Pontoise—a genetically abnormal fibrinogen with defective fibrin polymerization but normal fibrinopeptide release. In Lane, D. A., Henschen, A., and Jasani, M. K. (eds.): Fibrinogen-Fibrin Formation and Fibrinolysis, Vol. 4. Berlin, Walter de Gruyter, 1986, pp. 91–96.

208. Koopman, J., Haverkate, F., Grimbergen, J., Engesser, L., Nováková, I., Kerst, A., and Lord, S. T.: Formation of fibrinogen-albumin and fibrinogen-fibrinogen complexes in abnormal fibrinogens by disulfide bridges. Fibrinogen IJmuiden (B β Arg 14 → cys) and Nijmegen (B β Arg 44 → Cys). Proc. Natl. Acad. Sci. USA 89:3478, 1992.

209. Liu, C. Y., Koehn, J. A., and Morgan, F. J.: Characterization of fibrinogen New York I. J. Biol. Chem. 260:4390, 1985.

210. Mosesson, M. W., Siebenlist, K. R., Diorio, J. P., Hainfeld, J. F., Wall, J. S., Soria, J., Soria, C., and Samama, M.: Evidence that proximal NH₂-terminal portions of fibrinogen Metz (A α 16 Arg → Cys) A α chains are oriented in the same direction. In Müller-Berghaus, G., et al (eds.): Fibrinogen and Its Derivatives. Amsterdam, Elsevier Science Publ., 1986, pp. 3–15.

211. Takagi, T., and Doolittle, R. F.: Amino acid sequence studies on plasmin-derived fragments of human fibrinogen: Amino-terminal sequences of intermediate and terminal fragments. Biochemistry 14:940, 1975.

212. Lord, S. T.: Expression of a cloned human fibrinogen cDNA in Escherichia coli: Synthesis of an A alpha polypeptide. DNA 4:33, 1985.

213. Lord, S. T., Byrd, P. A., Hede, K. L., Wei, C., and Colby, T. J.: Analysis of fibrinogen A α-fusion proteins. Mutants which inhibit thrombin equivalently are not equally good substrates. J. Biol. Chem. 265:838, 1990.

214. Farrell, D. H., Mulvihill, E. R., Huang, S., Chung, D. W., and Davie, E. W.: Recombinant human fibrinogen and sulfation of the γ' chain. Biochemistry 30:9414, 1991.

215. Bolyard, M. G., and Lord, S. T.: Mutagenesis of human fibrinogen γ chain 259–411 synthesized in E. coli: Further characterization of the role of the disulfide bond Cys 326-Cys 339 in calcium binding. Biochem. Biophys. Res. Commun. 174:853, 1991.

216. Liu, C. Y., Nossel, H. L., and Kaplan, K. L.: The binding of thrombin by fibrin. J. Biol. Chem. 254:10421, 1979.

217. Laurell, C.-B., and Thulin, E.: Complexes in human plasma between α₁-antitrypsin and IgA, and α₁-antitrypsin and fibrinogen. Scand. J. Immunol. 4 (Suppl. 2):7, 1975.

218. Kimura, S., and Aoki, N.: Cross-linking site in fibrinogen for α₂-plasmin inhibitor. J. Biol. Chem. 261:15591, 1986.

219. Baenziger, N. L., Brodie, G. N., and Majerus, P. W.: A thrombin sensitive protein of human platelet membranes. Proc. Natl. Acad. Sci. USA 68:240, 1971.

220. Lawler, J. W., Slayter, H. S. L., and Coligan, J. E.: Isolation and characterization of high molecular weight glycoprotein from human platelets. J. Biol. Chem. 253:8609, 1978.

221. Hogg, P. J., Stenflo, J., and Mosher, D. F.: Thrombospondin is a slow tight-binding inhibitor of plasmin. Biochemistry 31:265, 1992.

222. Tuszynski, G. P., Srivastava, S., Switalska, I., Holt, J. C., Cierniewski, C. S., and Niewiarowski, S.: The interaction of human platelet thrombospondin with fibrinogen. J. Biol. Chem. 260:12240, 1985.

223. Bale, M. D., and Mosher, D. F.: Effects of thrombospondin on fibrin polymerization and structure. J. Biol. Chem. 261:862, 1986.

224. Bacon-Baguley, T., Ogilvie, M. L., Gartner, T. K., and Walz, D. A.: Thrombospondin binding to specific sequences within the A α- and B β-chains of fibrinogen. J. Biol. Chem. 265:2317, 1990.

225. Plow, E. F., Srouji, A. H., Meyer, D., Marguerie, G., and Ginsberg, M. H.: Evidence that three adhesive proteins interact with a common recognition site on activated platelets. J. Biol. Chem. 259:5388, 1984.

226. Holt, J. C., Mahmoud, M., and Gaffney, P. J.: The ability of fibrinogen fragments to support ADP-induced platelet aggregation. Thromb. Res. 16:427, 1979.

227. Hawiger, J., Timmons, S., Kloczewiak, M., Strong, D. D., and Doolittle, R. F.: γ and α chains of human fibrinogen possess sites reactive with human platelet receptors. Proc. Natl. Acad. Sci. USA 79:2068, 1982.

228. Hawiger, J., Kloczewiak, M., Bednarek, M. A., and Timmons, S.: Platelet receptor recognition domains on the α chain of human fibrinogen: Structure-function analysis. Biochemistry 28:2909, 1989.

229. Cheresh, D. A., Berliner, S. A., Vicente, V., and Ruggeri, Z. M.: Recognition of distinct adhesive sites on fibrinogen by related integrins on platelets and endothelial cells. Cell 58:945, 1989.

230. Huang, T-F., Holt, J. C., Lukasiewicz, H., and Niewiarowski, S.: Trigramin. A low molecular weight peptide inhibiting fibrinogen interaction with platelet receptors expressed on glycoprotein IIb-IIIa complex. J. Biol. Chem. 262:16157, 1987.

231. Cheresh, D. A.: Human endothelial cells synthesize and express an Arg-Gly-Asp–directed adhesion receptor involved in attachment to fibrinogen and von Willebrand factor. Proc. Natl. Acad. Sci. USA 84:6471, 1987.

232. Wu, C., and Chung, A. E.: Potential role of entactin in hemostasis. Specific interaction of entactin with fibrinogen A α and B β chains. J. Biol. Chem. 266:18802, 1991.

233. Blystone, S. D., Weston, L. K., and Kaplan, J. E.: Fibronectin dependent macrophage fibrin binding. Blood 78:2900, 1991.

234. Gonda, S. R., and Shainoff, J. R.: Adsorptive endocytosis of fibrin monomer by macrophages: Evidence of a receptor for the amino terminus of the fibrin α chain. Proc. Natl. Acad. Sci. USA 79:4565, 1982.

235. Duthie, E. S.: The action of fibrinogen on certain pathogenic cocci. J. Gen. Microbiol. 13:383, 1955.

236. Hawiger, J., Timmons, S., Strong, D. D., Cottrell, B. A., Riley, M., and Doolittle, R. F.: Identification of a region of human fibrinogen interacting with staphylococcal clumping factor. Biochemistry 21:1407, 1982.

237. Strong, D. D., Laudano, A. P., Hawiger, J., and Doolittle, R. F.: Isolation, characterization, and synthesis of peptides from human fibrinogen that block the staphylococcal clumping reaction and construction of a synthetic clumping particle. Biochemistry 21:1414, 1982.

238. Toy, P. T. C. Y., Lai, L.-W., Drake, T. A., and Sande, M. A.: Effect of fibronectin on adherence of Staphylococcus aureus to fibrin thrombi in vitro. Infect. Immun. 48:83, 1985.

239. Cheung, A. L., Krishnan, M., Jaffe, E. A., and Fischetti, V. A.: Fibrinogen acts as a bridging molecule in the adherence of Staphylococcus aureus to cultured human endothelial cells. J. Clin. Invest. 87:2236, 1991.

240. Poirier, T. P., Kehoe, M. A., Whitnack, E., Dockter, M. E., and Beachey, E. H.: Fibrinogen binding and resistance to phagocytosis of Streptococcus sanguis expressing cloned M protein of Streptococcus pyogenes. Infect. Immun. 57:29, 1989.

241. Traore, M. Y., Valentin-Weigand, P., Chhatwal, G. S., and Blobel, H.: Inhibitory effects of fibrinogen on phagocytic killing of streptococcal isolates from humans, cattle and horses. Vet. Microbiol. 28:295, 1991.

242. Lantz, M. S., Allen, R. D., Bounelis, P., Switalski, L. M., and Hook, M.: Bacteroides gingivalis and Bacteroides intermedius recognize different sites on human fibrinogen. J. Bacteriol. 172:716, 1990.

243. Hoeprich, P. D., and Doolittle, R. F.: Dimeric half-molecules of human fibrinogen are joined through disulfide bonds in an antiparallel orientation. Biochemistry 22:2049, 1983.

244. Bernstein, E., and Kairinen, E.: Science 173: cover photo, 1971.

245. Putnam, F. W.: Perspectives—Past, Present, and Future. In Putnam, F. W. (ed.): The Plasma Proteins, 2nd ed., Vol. 1. New York, Academic Press, 1975, pp. 1–55.

246. Putnam, F. W.: Alpha, beta, gamma, omega—the structure of the plasma proteins. In Putnam, F. W. (ed.): The Plasma Proteins, 2nd ed., Vol. 4. New York, Academic Press, 1984, pp. 45–166.

21

Fibrinolysis and the Control of Hemostasis

Désiré Collen and H. Roger Lijnen

INTRODUCTION

Mammalian blood contains an enzymatic system capable of dissolving blood clots. This system, called the fibrinolytic system, plays a role not only in the removal of fibrin from the vascular bed but also in other biological phenomena such as tissue repair, malignant transformation, macrophage function, ovulation, and embryo implantation. Most of the components of the fibrinolytic enzyme system were identified between 1930 and 1950.

The fibrinolytic system (Fig. 21–1) contains a proenzyme, plasminogen, which by the action of plasminogen activators is converted to the active enzyme plas-

min, which in turn digests fibrin to soluble degradation products. Inhibition of the fibrinolytic system occurs both at the level of the plasminogen activators, by plasminogen activator inhibitors (PAI-1 and PAI-2), and at the level of plasmin, mainly by α_2-antiplasmin. Some of the biochemical properties of the main components of the fibrinolytic system are summarized in Table 21–1 and are reviewed below.

The physiological plasminogen activators, tissue-type plasminogen activator (t-PA) and single-chain urokinase–type plasminogen activator (scu-PA), activate plasminogen preferentially at the fibrin surface. Plasmin, associated with the fibrin surface, is protected from rapid inhibition by α_2-antiplasmin and may thus

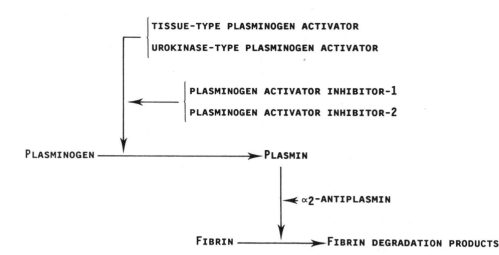

FIGURE 21–1. Schematic representation of the fibrinolytic system. The proenzyme plasminogen is activated to the active enzyme plasmin by tissue-type or urokinase-type plasminogen activator. Plasmin degrades fibrin into soluble fibrin degradation products. Inhibition of the fibrinolytic system may occur at the level of the plasminogen activators, by plasminogen activator inhibitors, or at the level of plasmin, mainly by α_2-antiplasmin.

efficiently degrade the fibrin of a thrombus.[1-3] These molecular interactions determining the fibrin specificity of fibrinolysis are illustrated in Figure 21–2 and are discussed below.

COMPONENTS OF THE FIBRINOLYTIC SYSTEM

Plasminogen

PHYSICOCHEMICAL PROPERTIES. Human plasminogen is a single-chain glycoprotein with a molecular weight of 92,000, present in plasma at a concentration of 1.5 to 2 μM. It was reported to consist of 790 amino acids with 24 disulfide bridges, and it contains five homologous triple-loop structures, or "kringles."[4] Subsequently, the cDNA sequence revealed the presence of an extra isoleucine at position 65, yielding a total of 791 amino acids in human plasminogen.[5] The primary structure of human plasminogen is schematically represented in Figure 21–3.

Native plasminogen has NH_2-terminal glutamic acid ("Glu-plasminogen") but is easily converted by limited plasmic digestion to modified forms with NH_2-terminal lysine, valine, or methionine,[6, 7] commonly designated "Lys-plasminogen." This conversion occurs by hydrolysis of the Arg 67–Met68, Lys 76–Lys77, or Lys 77–Val78 peptide bonds. Plasminogen is converted to

plasmin by cleavage of the Arg 560–Val 561 peptide bond.[8] The plasmin molecule is a two-chain trypsin-like serine proteinase with an active site composed of His 602, Asp 645, and Ser 740.[4] Activation of Glu-plasminogen in human plasma occurs primarily by direct cleavage of the Arg 560–Val 561 peptide bond without generation of Lys-plasminogen intermediates.[9]

The plasminogen molecule contains structures, called lysine-binding sites, that interact specifically with amino acids such as lysine and 6-aminohexanoic acid. These lysine-binding sites mediate the specific binding of plasminogen to fibrin and the interaction of plasmin with α_2-antiplasmin and play a crucial role in the regulation of fibrinolysis.[2, 3]

GENE STRUCTURE. A 2.7 kilobase (kb) insert of a cDNA clone for human plasminogen containing the complete coding region has been sequenced.[5] The coding region contains an amino-terminal sequence of 19 amino acids with the characteristics of a signal sequence and a mature protein sequence of 791 amino acids.[5]

The plasminogen gene was mapped to the long arm of chromosome 6 at band q26 or q27.[10] The gene for human plasminogen spans 52.5 kb of DNA and consists of 19 exons separated by 18 introns.[11] Each of the five kringles is encoded by two separate exons with a single intron in the middle of each structure. The

TABLE 21–1. SOME PROPERTIES OF THE MAIN COMPONENTS OF THE FIBRINOLYTIC SYSTEM

	M_r (kD)	CARBOHYDRATE CONTENT (%)	NUMBER OF AMINO ACIDS	PLASMA CONCENTRATION (mg/L)
Plasminogen	92	2	791 (790)*	200
t-PA	68	7	530 (527)*	0.005
scu-PA	54	7	411	0.008
α_2-Antiplasmin	70	13	452	70
PAI-1	52	ND	379	0.02
PAI-2	47, 60	ND	393	<0.005

t-PA = Tissue-type plasminogen activator; scu-PA = single-chain urokinase–type plasminogen activator, prourokinase; PAI-1 = plasminogen activator inhibitor-1; PAI-2 = plasminogen activator inhibitor-2; ND = not determined.
*The numbering of amino acid residues is usually based on these initially determined incorrect values.

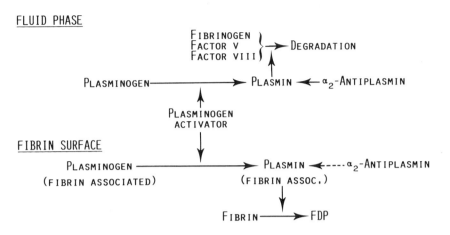

FIGURE 21–2. Molecular interactions determining the fibrin specificity of plasminogen activators. Non–fibrin-specific plasminogen activators (streptokinase, urokinase, APSAC) activate both plasminogen in the fluid phase and fibrin-associated plasminogen. Fibrin-specific plasminogen activators (t-PA and scu-PA) preferentially activate fibrin-associated plasminogen.

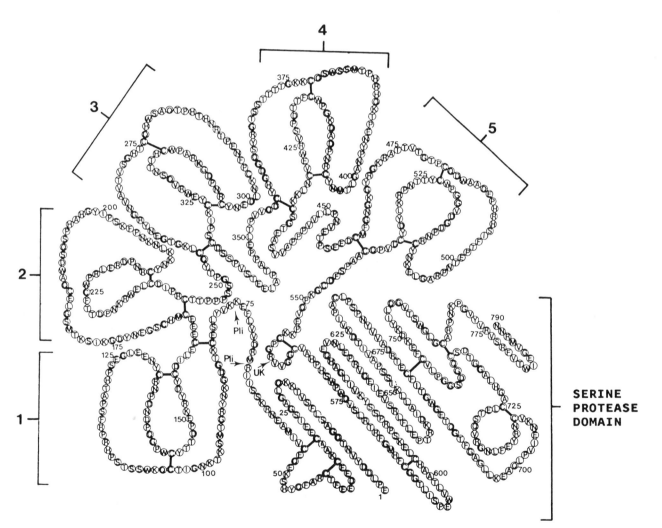

1-5 : KRINGLE DOMAINS

FIGURE 21–3. Schematic representation of the primary structure of plasminogen. Pli indicates the plasmic cleavage sites for conversion of Glu-plasminogen to Lys-plasminogen; UK indicates the cleavage site for plasminogen activators, yielding plasmin. The amino acids are represented by their single letter symbols, based on a total of 790 amino acids, and black bars indicate disulfide bonds.

gene organization for the light chain of plasminogen is similar to that of other serine proteases, such as t-PA, urokinase, and factor XII.[11] The gene coding for plasminogen is also closely related to that of apolipoprotein a.

POLYMORPHISM. The heterogeneity of plasminogen observed in human plasma[12] appears to be genetically controlled. Structural polymorphisms of human plasminogen have been described for the native protein[13] and for the desialylated protein.[14] Plasminogen is encoded by an autosomal gene with two common and a number (approximately 11) of rare alleles.[13-15] A nomenclature for the designation of plasminogen variant alleles has been proposed,[15] in which plasminogen variants are designated according to the relative direction of their pI in isoelectric focusing, relative to the two common types. The two common types found in all investigated races are designated PLG A (for more *acidic* pI) and PLG B (for more *basic* pI); the respective alleles are indicated by *PLG** A and *PLG** B. Rare variants with a more acidic pI than common PLG A or a more basic pI than common PLG B receive a numerical suffix for the relative direction of their pI shift.[15] The variants between common PLG A and PLG B are designated PLG M1, PLG M2, PLG M3, and so forth.[15]

The allele frequencies differ substantially in various racial groups but are fairly constant within one race.[16-19] In the European populations the distribution is roughly the following: common *PLG** A = 0.70, common *PLG** B = 0.28, and rare *PLG** = 0.020. The *PLG* B variant found in Japanese (allele frequency, 0.022) was shown to have a normal antigen level but reduced activity to approximately 40 per cent of normal.[20, 21] More recently the occurrence of a "silent" allele (*PLG*⁰) has been reported in a Swiss family.[22]

Several restriction fragment length polymorphisms (RFLP) have been described[10, 11] which may be useful in studying various normal and abnormal plasminogen genes.

Plasminogen Activators

Tissue-Type Plasminogen Activator (t-PA)

PHYSICOCHEMICAL PROPERTIES. Human t-PA is a serine proteinase with M_r about 70,000, composed of one polypeptide chain containing 527 amino acids with Ser as the NH_2-terminal amino acid[23]; its primary structure is schematically represented in Figure 21–4. It was subsequently shown that native t-PA contains an NH_2-terminal extension of three amino acids,[24] but in general the initial numbering system has been maintained. Limited plasmic hydrolysis of the Arg 275–Ile 276 peptide bond converts the molecule to a two-chain activator held together by one interchain disulfide bond. The t-PA molecule contains four domains: (1) a 47-residue-long (residues 4 to 50) amino-terminal region (F-domain), which is homologous with

the finger domains mediating the fibrin affinity of fibronectin; (2) residues 50 to 87 (E-domain), which are homologous with human epidermal growth factor; (3) two regions comprising residues 87 to 176 and 176 to 262 (K_1 and K_2 domains), which share a high degree of homology with the five kringles of plasminogen; and (4) a serine proteinase domain (residues 276 to 527) with the active site residues His 322, Asp 371, and Ser 478.

t-PA is a poor enzyme in the absence of fibrin, but fibrin strikingly enhances the activation rate of plasminogen. This has been explained by an increased affinity of fibrin-bound t-PA for plasminogen (lower K_m) without significant alteration of the catalytic rate constant (k_{cat}) of the enzyme.[25] Although different kinetic constants have been reported,[26] most authors agree that fibrin stimulates plasminogen activation by t-PA by at least two orders of magnitude.

GENE STRUCTURE. The gene coding for human t-PA has been localized to chromosome 8.[27-29] The localization of the t-PA gene (chromosome 8, bands 8.p.12 → q.11.2) coincides with a translocation breakpoint observed in myeloproliferative disorders.[29] The t-PA gene has been characterized in some detail.[30-32] A total of 36,594 base pairs (bp) has been sequenced, including 32,720 bp from the site of initiation of transcription to the polyadenylation site, in addition to 3530 bp of 5' and 344 bp of 3' flanking DNA. Thirteen introns (30,068 bp) divide the gene into 14 coding regions; the exons range in size from 43 to 914 bp and the introns from 111 to 14,257 bp. The transcription initiation site is an A residue with a "TATA box" nearby upstream (TATAAAAA at positions −22 to −29) and a "CAAT box" further upstream (CAATG at positions −112 to −116). The polyadenylation signal (AATAAA) is found at positions 32,688 to 32,693. The gene and 5' flanking region contain 28 copies of *Alu* repetitive DNA and a single *Kpn* I repeat.

The complete 2530 bp cDNA sequence of mature t-PA[23] contains a single reading frame, beginning with the ATG codon at nucleotides 85 to 87. This ATG probably serves as the site of translation initiation and is followed, 562 codons later, by a TGA termination triplet at nucleotides 1771 to 1773. The serine residue originally[23] designated the NH_2-terminal amino acid (disregarding the NH_2-terminal extension of three amino acids in native t-PA[24]) is preceded by 35 amino acids, 20 to 23 of which (residues −35 to −13) probably constitute a hydrophobic signal peptide involved in the secretion of t-PA. The remaining hydrophobic amino acids immediately preceding the start of mature t-PA (residues −14 to −1) may constitute a "pro" sequence similar to that found for serum albumin. The 3' untranslated region of 759 nucleotides contains the hexanucleotide AATAAA (positions 2496 to 2501) that precedes the site of polyadenylation in many eukaryotic messenger RNAs (mRNAs).

The t-PA gene is assembled by "exon shuffling," as suggested by the observation that the structural domains on the heavy chain (F, E, K_1, K_2) are encoded

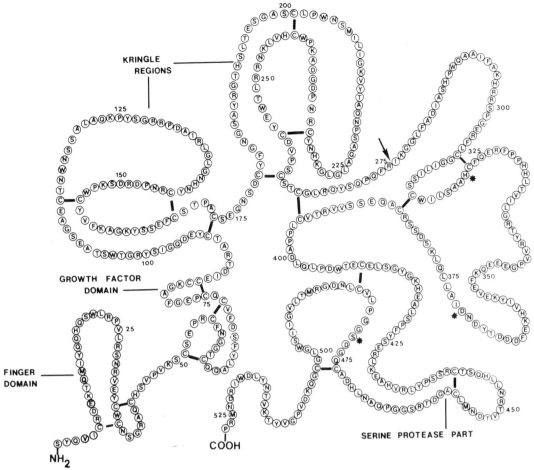

FIGURE 21–4. Schematic representation of the primary structure of t-PA. The amino acids are represented by their single letter symbols, and black bars indicate disulfide bonds. The active site residues His 322, Asp 371, and Ser 478 are indicated with an asterisk. The arrow indicates the plasmin cleavage site for conversion of single-chain t-PA to two-chain t-PA.

by a single exon or by two adjacent exons.[33] Because of the striking correlation between the intron-exon distribution of the gene and the putative domain structure of the protein, it was suggested that these domains would be autonomous, structural, and/or functional entities ("modules").[33, 34]

Urokinase-Type Plasminogen Activator (u-PA)

PHYSICOCHEMICAL PROPERTIES. scu-PA (prourokinase) is a single chain glycoprotein with M_r 54,000 containing 411 amino acids[35–37]; its primary structure is schematically represented in Figure 21–5. Upon limited hydrolysis by plasmin or kallikrein of the Lys 158–Ile[159] peptide bond, the molecule is converted to a two-chain derivative (tcu-PA, urokinase).[38] The NH₂-terminal chain contains a region homologous to human epidermal growth factor (E; residues 9 to 45) and one kringle region (K; residues 45 to 134). The catalytic center is located in the proteinase domain (residues 159 to 411) and is composed of His 204, Asp 255, and Ser 356. A low-M_r two-chain urokinase (M_r 33,000) can be generated by hydrolysis of the Lys 135–Lys 136 peptide bond with plasmin. A low-M_r scu-PA

with M_r 32,000 (scu-PA-32k) can be obtained by specific hydrolysis of the Glu 143–Leu 144 peptide bond in scu-PA by an unidentified protease.[39]

scu-PA has a very low reactivity toward low molecular weight synthetic substrates or active site inhibitors that are very reactive toward tcu-PA.[40, 41] In mixtures of purified scu-PA and plasminogen, both tcu-PA and plasmin are quickly generated.[42] The presence and magnitude of intrinsic plasminogen-activating potential in scu-PA are still controversial.[43–47]

GENE STRUCTURE. The cDNA of u-PA has been isolated and the nucleotide sequence determined.[37, 48] The cDNA sequence contains an open reading frame that starts with ATG at nucleotide positions 77 to 79 and extends for 1293 nucleotides until a TGA stop codon is reached at positions 1370 to 1372.[37] The open reading frame is preceded by at least 76 nucleotides of 5′-untranslated mRNA, very rich in G/C nucleotides (83 per cent). Beyond the termination codon, the complementary DNA (cDNA) extends for another 932 nucleotides. The sequence includes two AATAAAA polyadenylation signals (positions 2271 to 2276 and 2284 to 2289), preceding the polyadenylation site at position 2304.[37] The human u-PA gene is 6.4 kb long

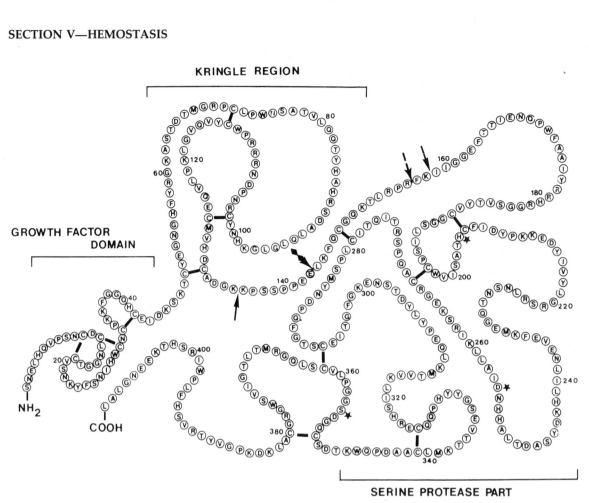

KRINGLE REGION

GROWTH FACTOR DOMAIN

SERINE PROTEASE PART

FIGURE 21–5. Schematic representation of the primary structure of scu-PA. The amino acids are represented by their single letter symbols, and black bars indicate disulfide bonds. The active site residues His 204, Asp 255, and Ser 356 are indicated with a star. The arrows indicate the plasmin cleavage sites for conversion of M_r 54,000 scu-PA to M_r 54,000 tcu-PA and of M_r 54,000 tcu-PA to M_r 33,000 tcu-PA (⟶), for conversion to inactive M_r 54,000 tcu-PA by thrombin (--⟶), and for conversion to M_r 32,000 scu-PA by an unidentified protease (◂▸).

and is located on chromosome 10.[27] It contains 11 exons,[49] and the intron-exon organization of the gene closely resembles that of the t-PA gene. However, exons III, VIII, and IX of t-PA are totally and exon IV is partially missing in the u-PA gene; this accounts for the absence of a finger domain and a second kringle in u-PA. Exon II of the u-PA gene codes for a signal peptide consisting of 20 amino acids; exons III and IV code for the growth factor domain and exons V and VI for the kringle region. The 5′ region of exon VII, which codes for the peptide connecting the light and the heavy chain, is 39 bp longer than the corresponding exon X of the t-PA gene. The 3′ region of exon VII and exons VIII to XI code for the heavy chain.

Streptokinase and Anisoylated Plasminogen-Streptokinase Activator Complex (APSAC)

Streptokinase is produced by several strains of hemolytic streptococci; it consists of a single polypeptide chain with M_r 47,000 to 50,000 and contains 414 amino acids.[50] Streptokinase cannot directly cleave peptide bonds, but it activates plasminogen to plasmin indi-

rectly, following a three-step mechanism.[51] In the first step, streptokinase forms an equimolar complex with plasminogen. This complex undergoes a conformational change, resulting in the exposure of an active site in the plasminogen moiety. In the second step, this active site catalyzes the activation of plasminogen to plasmin. In a third step, plasminogen-streptokinase molecules are converted to plasmin-streptokinase complex.[52] The active site residues in the plasmin-streptokinase complex are the same as those in the plasmin molecule. The main differences in the enzymatic properties of plasmin and the plasmin-streptokinase complex are found in their interaction with plasminogen and with α_2-antiplasmin. Plasmin, in contrast to its complex with streptokinase, is unable to activate plasminogen, whereas the plasmin(ogen)-streptokinase complex is virtually not inhibited by α_2-antiplasmin.[53]

Streptokinase disappears from the circulation with a half-life of approximately 20 minutes.[54] The level of antistreptokinase antibodies, which may result from previous infections with β-hemolytic streptococci, varies largely among individuals.[55] Because streptokinase is inactivated by interaction with antibodies, sufficient streptokinase must be infused to neutralize the antibodies. A few days after streptokinase administration, the antistreptokinase titer rises rapidly to 50 to 100 times the preinfusion value and remains high for 4 to 6 months, during which period renewed treatment is impractical.

APSAC was constructed with the aim to control the enzymatic activity of the plasmin(ogen)-streptokinase complex by a specific reversible chemical protection of its catalytic center (i.e., by titration with a p-anisoyl group).[56] APSAC is an equimolar non-covalent complex between human Lys-plasminogen and streptokinase, containing the titrated catalytic center and the lysine-binding sites of plasminogen. Reversible acylation of the catalytic center would thus not affect the weak fibrin-binding capacity of Lys-plasminogen in the complex.[56] Deacylation of APSAC, which uncovers the catalytic center, occurs both in the circulation and at the fibrin surface. A plasma half-life of 70 minutes was found for APSAC, compared with 25 minutes for the plasminogen-streptokinase complex formed in vivo after administration of streptokinase.[54] Patients with high streptokinase antibody titers do not respond to APSAC,[57] and APSAC causes a marked increase in the streptokinase antibody titer within 2 to 3 weeks, which persists for months.[54, 58]

Staphylokinase

Staphylokinase, a 36 amino acid protein produced by *Staphylococcus aureus*, was shown to have profibrinolytic properties more than four decades ago.[59] The gene coding for the bacterial protein has now been cloned and expressed in *Escherichia coli*[60, 61] and in *Bacillus subtilis*.[62] Staphylokinase, like streptokinase, forms a stoichiometric complex with plasminogen,[63] and the plasminogen-staphylokinase complex then activates plasminogen following Michaelis-Menten kinetics.[64, 65] In purified systems, α_2-antiplasmin rapidly inhibits the plasmin-staphylokinase complex, whereas addition of 6-aminohexanoic acid or of fibrin fragments induces a concentration-dependent reduction of the inhibition rate.[65]

Inhibitors of the Fibrinolytic System

Inhibition of the fibrinolytic system may occur at the level of plasmin or at the level of the plasminogen activators. α_2-Antiplasmin is the main physiological plasmin inhibitor in human plasma, whereas inhibition of the physiological plasminogen activators t-PA and u-PA occurs mainly by plasminogen activator inhibitor-1 (PAI-1) and plasminogen activator inhibitor-2 (PAI-2).

α_2-Antiplasmin

α_2-Antiplasmin is a single-chain glycoprotein with a molecular weight of 70,000 containing about 13 per cent carbohydrate. Based on its cDNA sequence,[66] the molecule consists of 452 amino acids and contains two disulfide bridges. α_2-Antiplasmin belongs to the serine proteinase inhibitor protein family (serpins), with reactive site peptide bond Arg 364–Met 365.[66] The concentration of the inhibitor in plasma is about 1 μM.

The inhibitor in normal plasma is heterogeneous and consists of functionally active and inactive material. Upon extensive activation of plasminogen in normal plasma, only about 70 per cent of the α_2-antiplasmin antigen forms a complex with plasmin; 30 per cent of the inhibitor-related antigen appears to be functionally inactive.[67] Human plasma indeed contains two forms of the inhibitor that differ in binding to plasminogen. The form that does not bind remains an active plasmin inhibitor but reacts more slowly with plasmin. This form lacks a 26 residue peptide from the COOH-terminal end of α_2-antiplasmin, which contains the plasminogen-binding site or complementary lysine-binding site.[68] Wiman et al.[69] measured the ratio of these forms in the plasma of pregnant women subjected to extensive plasmapheresis and concluded that the plasminogen-binding form of α_2-antiplasmin is primarily synthesized and that it becomes partly converted to the non–plasminogen-binding form in the circulating blood. α_2-Antiplasmin is cross-linked to the fibrin α chain when blood is clotted in the presence of calcium ions and activated coagulation factor XIII.[70] The fibrin-binding site involves the Gln residue in the second NH_2-terminal position of the inhibitor. The structure of α_2-antiplasmin is schematically shown in Figure 21–6.

α_2-Antiplasmin forms a 1:1 stoichiometric complex with plasmin that is devoid of protease or esterase

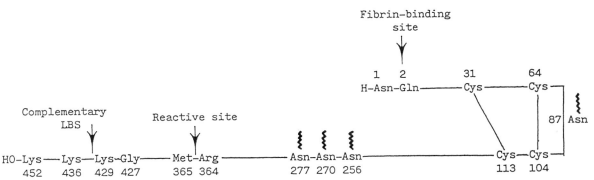

FIGURE 21–6. Schematic representation of the primary structure of α_2-antiplasmin. LBS indicates lysine-binding site; Asn indicates carbohydrate attached to Asn residues.

activity. The inhibition of plasmin (P) by α_2-antiplasmin (A) can be represented by two consecutive reactions: a fast, second-order reaction producing a reversible inactive complex (PA), which is followed by a slower first-order transition resulting in an irreversible complex (PA'). This model can be represented by

$$P + A \underset{k_{-1}}{\overset{k_1}{\rightleftarrows}} PA \overset{k_2}{\rightarrow} PA'$$

The second-order rate constant of the inhibition of plasmin by α_2-antiplasmin (k_1 = 2 to 4 $\times$ 10^7 M^{-1}s^{-1}) is among the fastest protein-protein reactions described.[71] This high inhibition rate depends upon the presence of a free lysine-binding site and active site in the plasmin molecule and of the plasminogen-binding site and the reactive site Arg 364–Met 365 in the inhibitor. The plasmin–α_2-antiplasmin complex is schematically represented in Figure 21–7. The half-life of plasmin molecules on the fibrin surface, which have both their lysine-binding sites and active center occupied, is estimated to be two to three orders of magnitude longer than that of free plasmin.[71]

The gene for human α_2-antiplasmin is located on chromosome 18.[72] The gene contains 10 exons and 9 introns distributed over approximately 16 kb of DNA.[73] The NH$_2$-terminal region of the protein, comprising the fibrin cross-linking site, is encoded by exon IV. Both the reactive site and the plasminogen-binding site are encoded by exon X. An RFLP, associated with the presence of two alleles, A and B, has been identified in the α_2-antiplasmin gene.[74] Allele B is the result of a 720 bp deletion in intron VIII. This RFLP is apparently caused by intrastrand recombination between *Alu* sequences.

Plasminogen Activator Inhibitors

PLASMINOGEN ACTIVATOR INHIBITOR-1 (PAI-1). PAI-1 was first identified in conditioned media of cultured human endothelial cells and rat hepatoma cells and subsequently in plasma, platelets, placenta, and conditioned media of fibrosarcoma cells and hepatocytes.[75] It is a single-chain glycoprotein with M$_r$ about 52,000 consisting of 379 amino acids. The PAI-1 gene is approximately 12.2 kb in length and consists of nine exons and eight introns. It has been mapped to chromosome 7, bands q21.3–q22.[76] The cDNA has been sequenced, revealing that PAI-1 is a member of the serine protease inhibitor (serpin) family. Its reactive site consists of Arg 346–Met 347.[77, 78]

In healthy individuals, highly variable plasma levels of both PAI activity and PAI-1 antigen have been observed. PAI activity ranges from 0.5 to 47 U/ml, with the majority of values (80 per cent) below 6 U/ml. PAI-1 antigen ranges between 6 ng/ml in 10 per cent of the plasmas and 85 ng/ml (geometric mean: 24 ng/ml).[79] PAI-1 levels are elevated in several disease states (see below, Pathophysiology of Fibrinolysis).

PAI-1 is stabilized by binding to a PAI-binding protein identified as S-protein, or vitronectin.[80] PAI-1 is the primary inhibitor of both t-PA and u-PA in human plasma.[81, 82] It reacts with single-chain and two-chain t-PA and with tcu-PA, but not with scu-PA or streptokinase. The second-order rate constant (k_1) for the inhibition of single-chain t-PA by PAI-1 is on the order of 10^7 M^{-1}s^{-1}, and inhibition of two-chain t-PA and tcu-PA is even somewhat more rapid (for references, cf. 75).

PAI-1 is very labile and is found in tissue culture fluid in a "latent" form that can be partly reactivated by treatment with denaturing agents such as urea,

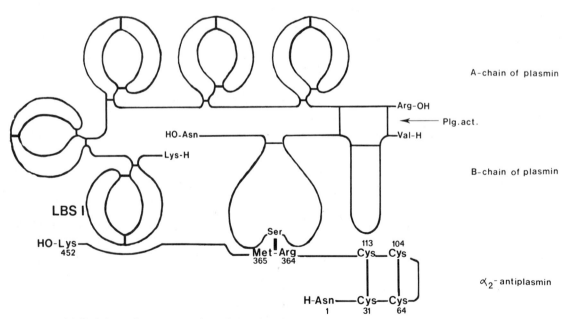

FIGURE 21–7. Schematic representation of the plasmin–α_2-antiplasmin complex. LBSI indicates the high-affinity lysine-binding site; Plg. act. indicates the site of cleavage by plasminogen activators.

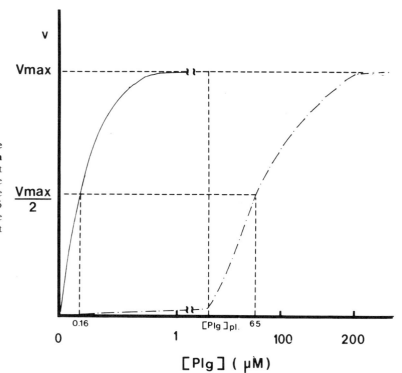

FIGURE 21–8. Influence of fibrin on the activation rate (v) of plasminogen (Plg) by tissue-type plasminogen activator. In the presence of fibrin the Michaelis constant equals 0.16 μM (—), compared with 65 μM in the absence of fibrin (—·—). This suggests that at the normal plasma concentration of plasminogen (Plg = 1.5 to 2 μM) no systemic plasminogen activation is to be expected, whereas in the presence of fibrin efficient activation can occur.

guanidine hydrochloride, and sodium dodecyl sulfate.[83] Production and/or release of PAI-1 from various cells is regulated by several stimuli, including thrombin, dexamethasone, endotoxin, interleukin-1, transforming growth factor β, and tumor necrosis factor (for references, cf. 75).

PLASMINOGEN ACTIVATOR INHIBITOR-2 (PAI-2). PAI-2 has been identified in human placenta and in pregnancy plasma; it is also secreted by leukocytes and by fibrosarcoma cells. It was purified from placenta, leukocytes, and U-937 cells. PAI-2 exists in two different forms with comparable inhibition properties: an intracellular non-glycosylated form with M_r 47,000 and pI 5.0 and a secreted glycosylated form with M_r 60,000 and pI 4.4 (for references, cf. 75). The cDNA has been sequenced[84–86]; PAI-2 is a serpin containing 393 amino acids with reactive site peptide bond Arg 358–Thr 359. The PAI-2 gene spans 16.5 kb of DNA and contains eight exons. A consensus sequence TATAAAA is found 22 bp 5′ of the proposed transcription initiation site. The PAI-2 gene is located on chromosome 18 q21-23. The structure of the gene is quite different from that of the PAI-1 gene but is similar to that of the chicken ovalbumin gene.[87]

PAI-2 inhibits tcu-PA with a second-order rate constant of 9×10^5 $M^{-1}s^{-1}$, which is about 10-fold slower than PAI-1. PAI-2 also efficiently inhibits two-chain t-PA ($k_1 = 2 \times 10^5$ $M^{-1}s^{-1}$), less efficiently single chain t-PA ($k_1 = 9 \times 10^3$ $M^{-1}s^{-1}$), and it does not inhibit scu-PA. Secretion of PAI-2 is regulated by endotoxin and by phorbol esters, which stimulate the gene transcription of PAI-2 more than 50-fold (for references, cf. 75).

Although PAI-2 in plasma occurs most frequently in association with pregnancy, it has occasionally been identified in men and in non-pregnant women.[88]

MECHANISMS OF FIBRIN-SPECIFIC FIBRINOLYSIS

The fibrin specificity of the physiological plasminogen activators t-PA and scu-PA has triggered great interest in the use of these agents for thrombolysis. Fibrin-specific fibrinolysis has also been observed with the bacterial protein staphylokinase.

Tissue-Type Plasminogen Activator (t-PA)

t-PA is a poor enzyme in the absence of fibrin, but the presence of fibrin strikingly enhances the activation rate of plasminogen.[25] The influence of fibrin on the activation rate of plasminogen by t-PA is schematically illustrated in Figure 21–8. In the presence of fibrin, the Michaelis constant equals 0.16 μM, compared with 65 μM in the absence of fibrin. The kinetic data of Hoylaerts et al.[25] support a mechanism in which fibrin provides a surface to which t-PA and plasminogen adsorb in a sequential and ordered way, yielding a cyclic ternary complex. Fibrin essentially increases the local plasminogen concentration by creating an additional interaction between t-PA and its substrate. The high affinity of t-PA for plasminogen in the presence of fibrin thus allows efficient activation on the fibrin clot, whereas plasminogen activation by t-PA in plasma is a comparatively inefficient process. Plasmin formed on the fibrin surface has both its lysine-binding sites and its active site occupied and is thus only slowly inactivated by α_2-antiplasmin (half-life of about 10 to 100 seconds); in contrast, free plasmin, when formed, is rapidly inhibited by α_2-antiplasmin (half-life of about 0.1 second).[71] The molecular interactions that regulate the fibrin specificity of t-PA are schematically illustrated in Figure 21–9. However, others have claimed that fibrin influences both the K_m and k_{cat} of the activation of plasminogen by t-PA.[26]

It was proposed that initial binding of t-PA to fibrin would be governed by the finger domain and that partial degradation of fibrin would result in enhanced binding of t-PA via kringle 2 to newly exposed COOH-terminal lysine residues.[89] This is in agreement with the observation that new t-PA binding sites with markedly lower (two to four orders of magnitude) dissociation constants are formed when fibrin is degraded by plasmin.[90] Thus, early fibrin digestion by plasmin may accelerate fibrinolysis by increasing the binding of both t-PA[89] and plasminogen.[91] Optimal binding of t-PA to partially plasmin-digested fibrin was shown to coincide with the generation of fibrin fragment X polymers,[92] whereas for interaction of plasminogen with fibrin the polymerized state of fragment X appears to be essential.[93] Optimal stimulation of t-PA–catalyzed plasminogen activation depends on modification by plasmin of fibrin to desA-fragment X-related moieties, and requires the presence of kringle domains 1 to 4 of plasminogen.[94] The fibrinolytic process thus seems to be triggered by and confined to fibrin.

Urokinase-Type Plasminogen Activator (u-PA)

tcu-PA has no fibrin specificity and activates fibrin-bound and circulating plasminogen relatively indiscriminately. Extensive plasminogen activation and depletion of α_2-antiplasmin may occur following treatment of patients with thromboembolic disease with tcu-PA, leading to degradation of several plasma proteins, including fibrinogen, factor V, and factor VIII (see Fig. 21–2).

scu-PA, in contrast to tcu-PA, has a significant fibrin specificity. Several hypotheses for the mechanism of plasminogen activation and fibrin specificity of clot lysis with scu-PA in a plasma milieu have been proposed. One hypothesis claims that scu-PA has some intrinsic plasminogen-activating potential which is counteracted by a competitive inhibitory mechanism in plasma, that is, reversed by fibrin.[42, 95] Alternatively, scu-PA was claimed to be inactive toward circulating native plasminogen (Glu-plasminogen) but active toward conformationally altered plasminogen (Lys-plasminogen) bound to partially digested fibrin.[96, 97] Third, scu-PA has been proposed to be a genuine proenzyme with negligible activity toward plasminogen,[46, 47] and fibrinolysis with scu-PA would thus depend entirely on generation of tcu-PA. The initial hypothesis that

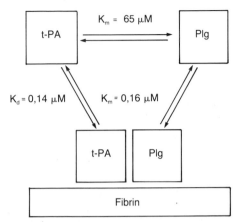

FIGURE 21–9. Schematic representation of the molecular interactions that regulate the fibrin-specific activation of the fibrinolytic system by tissue-type plasminogen activator. t-PA in circulating plasma has a low affinity for its substrate plasminogen (K_m = 65 μM), and no efficient plasminogen activation occurs. t-PA binds specifically to fibrin (K_d = 0.14 μM). The bimolecular t-PA–fibrin complex has a high affinity for plasminogen (K_m = 0.16 μM), compared with the low affinity of t-PA for plasminogen in the absence of fibrin. Plasminogen binds to the binary t-PA–fibrin complex and is activated to plasmin at the fibrin surface. This in loco–generated plasmin is protected from rapid inactivation by α_2-antiplasmin and degrades fibrin.

scu-PA would exert its fibrin-specific fibrinolytic action via binding to fibrin[98] has been abandoned.[42, 96]

The mechanism of plasminogen activation and fibrin specificity of scu-PA in in vitro plasma systems was recently reinvestigated by direct comparison of the relative catalytic efficiency and fibrinolytic potency of scu-PA, tcu-PA, and a plasmin-resistant mutant of scu-PA (scu-PA K158E) with the use of quantitative dose-effect relationships. Using plasmin-mediated fibrin clot lysis as the endpoint, scu-PA has a 2000-fold higher fibrinolytic potency than scu-PA K158E, but only a 2.5-fold lower potency than tcu-PA. This suggests that conversion of scu-PA to tcu-PA during clot lysis constitutes a primary positive feedback system.[43] Binding of plasminogen to fibrin or predigestion of fibrin by plasmin was found to result in relatively minor additional acceleration of fibrinolysis. Using an ELISA specific for two-chain forms of u-PA, it was shown that clot lysis with scu-PA in human plasma does not require extensive systemic conversion of scu-PA to tcu-PA. Systemic fibrinogen breakdown, however, occurs only secondarily to extensive systemic conversion of scu-PA to tcu-PA, resulting in a marked plasminogen activation and α_2-antiplasmin consumption.[99] Taken together, these data[43, 99] suggest that the clot selectivity of scu-PA may be mediated by preferential conversion of scu-PA to tcu-PA at the fibrin surface.

This mechanism of plasminogen activation and fibrin dissolution with scu-PA in a plasma milieu in vitro may, however, not be identical to its physiological mechanism of action. It was indeed found that plasmin-resistant mutants of scu-PA (i.e., scu-PA K158E) have only a threefold to fivefold lower in vivo thrombolytic potency than wild-type scu-PA,[100] suggesting that for in vivo thrombolysis, conversion of scu-PA to tcu-PA may play a less important role.

The molecular interactions that regulate the fibrin specificity of scu-PA remain to be further detailed. Because both M_r 54,000 scu-PA and scu-PA-32k induce very similar fibrin-specific clot lysis,[39, 101] the structures responsible for the fibrin specificity of scu-PA appear to be independent of the NH_2-terminal 143 amino acids of the protein.

Staphylokinase

Staphylokinase induces dose-dependent lysis of a ^{125}I-fibrin–labeled human plasma clot submerged in citrated human plasma without causing fibrinogenolysis.[64, 65] In animal models of venous thrombosis, staphylokinase was shown to be a potent thrombolytic agent, comparable to streptokinase.[102]

The following mechanism for the relatively fibrin-specific clot lysis with staphylokinase in a plasma milieu has been proposed.[64, 65] In plasma in the absence of fibrin, the plasminogen-staphylokinase complex is rapidly neutralized by α_2-antiplasmin, thus preventing systemic plasminogen activation. In the presence of fibrin, some of the plasminogen-staphylokinase complex binds via the lysine-binding sites of the plasminogen moiety to the clot. Its inhibition rate by α_2-antiplasmin is thereby reduced 130-fold (t½ prolonged from 0.26 to 35 seconds), thus allowing preferential plasminogen activation at the fibrin surface.[65]

PATHOPHYSIOLOGY OF FIBRINOLYSIS

The physiological importance of the fibrinolytic system is demonstrated by the association between abnormal fibrinolysis and a tendency toward bleeding or thrombosis. Impairment of fibrinolysis represents the most commonly observed hemostatic abnormality associated with thrombosis. It may be due to a defective synthesis and/or release of t-PA from the vessel wall, to a deficiency or functional defect in the plasminogen molecule, or to increased levels of inhibitors of t-PA or of plasmin. On the other hand, excessive fibrinolysis due to increased levels of t-PA or to α_2-antiplasmin deficiency may result in bleeding tendency.

α_2-Antiplasmin Deficiency and Bleeding

Congenital and Acquired α_2-Antiplasmin Deficiency

Koie et al. described the first case of homozygous α_2-antiplasmin deficiency in a patient who presented with a hemorrhagic diathesis.[104] Studies of family members indicated that this abnormality was inherited as an autosomal recessive gene.[105]

In contrast to the first published families with α_2-antiplasmin deficiency, which were discovered through a homozygous propositus with severe bleeding, several cases of heterozygosity have been described with no discernible bleeding symptoms. However, several heterozygotes in families with α_2-antiplasmin deficiency presented with mild bleeding tendencies (Table 21–2).[105-114] The α_2-antiplasmin levels in all heterozygotes described thus far are consistently between 40 and 60 per cent of normal. Antigen and activity levels usually correspond well, suggesting that the deficiency is due to decreased synthesis of a normal α_2-antiplasmin molecule. The bleeding tendency in these patients may be due to premature lysis of hemostatic plugs, because in the absence of α_2-antiplasmin, the half-life of plasmin molecules generated on the fibrin surface may be considerably prolonged.

Miura et al.[115, 116] have prepared genomic DNA from peripheral leukocytes of family members with reported congenital α_2-antiplasmin deficiency and se-

TABLE 21–2. CONGENITAL α_2-ANTIPLASMIN DEFICIENCY

REFERENCES	PROPOSITUS	α_2-ANTIPLASMIN LEVEL* (PER CENT OF NORMAL)	BLEEDING
Koie et al.[104, 105]	1 homozygote	0	Yes (severe)
	9 heterozygotes	±50	No
Kluft et al.[106, 107]	1 homozygote	2	Yes (severe)
	16 heterozygotes	50–60	6 Yes (mild)
			10 No
Yoshioka et al.[108]	3 homozygotes	1–2	Yes (severe)
	3 heterozygotes	±50	Yes (mild)
Knot et al.[109]	1 heterozygote	±50	Yes (mild)
Stormorken et al.[110]	1 heterozygote	41–47	No
Kordich et al.[111]	1 heterozygote	±50	Yes (severe)
Miles et al.[112]	2 homozygotes	<1	Yes
	5 heterozygotes	48 ± 12	2 Yes (mild)
			3 No
Kettle and Mayne[113]	1 homozygote	0	Yes
Leebeek et al.[114]	13 heterozygotes	±60	2 Yes (mild)

*Functional and antigenic levels correspond well.

quenced all the coding regions and the exon-intron boundaries of the gene. In this way, the molecular defect in the α_2-antiplasmin deficiency described by Koie et al. (α_2-antiplasmin Okinawa)[104, 105] has been identified as a trinucleotide deletion in exon VII, leading to deletion of Glu[137] in the protein.[115] The molecular defect in the α_2-antiplasmin deficiency described by Yoshioka et al. (α_2-antiplasmin Nara)[108] was identified as the insertion of a cytidine nucleotide at position 1438 in exon X. This leads to a shift in the reading frame of the mRNA, resulting in deletion of the COOH-terminal 12 amino acids of native α_2-antiplasmin and replacement with 178 unrelated amino acids.[116] It was suggested that these mutations lead to the deficiency by affecting the folding of the protein into the native configuration and thereby blocking its intracellular transport from the endoplasmic reticulum to the Golgi complex.[115]

Acquired alpha$_2$-antiplasmin deficiency associated with enhanced fibrinolysis has been reported in some conditions. In liver disease, especially in cirrhosis, increased fibrinolysis is a well-known phenomenon. The serum level of α_2-antiplasmin was found to be significantly decreased in cirrhosis and in several other liver diseases.[117–119] Teger-Nilsson et al.[117] reported a mean value of 73 ± 15 per cent for patients with cirrhosis compared with 100 ± 8 per cent in controls, whereas Williams[119] found levels of less than 50 per cent of normal in patients with liver disease. Decreased levels of α_2-antiplasmin may thus be an important factor in the increased fibrinolytic activity observed in patients with cirrhosis. Moreover, it is likely that the liver is the organ of synthesis or storage of α_2-antiplasmin.[120] Decreased levels of α_2-antiplasmin have also been found in patients with disseminated intravascular coagulation and/or fibrinolysis and in acute promyelocytic leukemia.[119, 121]

α_2-Antiplasmin levels may be significantly reduced in patients undergoing thrombolytic therapy, as a result of systemic activation of the fibrinolytic system. Following intravenous infusion of recombinant t-PA or streptokinase in patients with acute myocardial infarction, the decrease of α_2-antiplasmin was significantly greater in the streptokinase group.[122]

Dysfunctional α_2-Antiplasmin

An abnormal α_2-antiplasmin molecule (α_2-antiplasmin Enschede), associated with a serious bleeding tendency, has been found in two siblings in a Dutch family. These individuals had only 3 per cent of normal functional activity and 100 per cent of normal antigen levels.[123] Their apparently heterozygous parents had 50 per cent functional activity and 100 per cent antigen levels. The ability of the protein to bind reversibly to plasmin or plasminogen was not affected, but the abnormal α_2-antiplasmin was converted from an inhibitor of plasmin to a substrate. The molecular defect of α_2-antiplasmin Enschede consists of the insertion of an extra alanine residue (GCG insertion) somewhere between amino acid residues 353 and 357

(4 Ala residues), 7 to 10 positions on the NH$_2$-terminal side of the P$_1$ residue (Arg 364) in the reactive site of α_2-antiplasmin.[124]

Plasminogen Activator Inhibitor-1 and Thrombosis

The PAI-1 concentration in plasma is very low in healthy subjects (approximately 10 to 20 ng/ml), but it is increased in several diseases, including venous thromboembolism, obesity, sepsis, and coronary artery disease.

Mice transgenic for the human PAI-1 gene develop venous thrombosis at the tip of the tail within 3 days after birth, but no arterial thrombosis.[125] Furthermore, when endotoxin-treated rabbits, with a markedly increased plasma PAI-1 level, are infused with the defibrinogenating snake venom Ancrod, renal fibrin deposits are produced, whereas in normal rabbits Ancrod infusion causes hypofibrinogenemia without fibrin deposition.[126] These experiments suggest that increased PAI-1 levels may promote fibrin deposition in vivo.

Several cross-sectional studies of patients with ischemic heart disease, including angina pectoris and previous myocardial infarction, have consistently shown decreased fibrinolytic activity. The main mechanism for the fibrinolytic impairment seen in these patients is increased PAI-1 activity in plasma.[127–138] High PAI-1 activity constitutes an independent risk factor for myocardial reinfarction in young subjects,[133, 139] in whom PAI activity correlates with reinfarction within 3 years, but not with late reinfarction.[140] Furthermore, a clear correlation exists between the circadian variation in the time of onset of myocardial infarction, with the highest incidence at about 8 A.M., and the circadian rhythm of plasma PAI-1 activity, which is also highest early in the morning.[141] Elevated PAI-1 activity in plasma is better correlated with myocardial infarction than with angina pectoris or angiographically ascertained coronary artery disease.[130, 135, 142] To date, no clear correlation has been demonstrated between PAI-1 levels and the extent of coronary lesions.[127, 128, 130, 137, 143] A critical review of the relationship between impaired fibrinolytic activity and acute myocardial infarction has recently been published.[144]

It has been shown that insulin resistance is associated with increased PAI-1 concentration.[142, 145–148] A strong correlation ($r \approx 0.60$) between PAI-1 and insulin levels was observed in several populations, including normal subjects,[145] postmenopausal obese women,[146] android obesity,[147] type II diabetes,[148] and angina pectoris.[142] PAI-1 levels are also correlated with body mass index, waist to hip circumference ratio, plasma triglycerides, and apolipoprotein B, but this correlation disappears after adjustment for insulin levels. This association between insulin and PAI-1 is further substantiated by intervention studies aimed at decreasing insulin resistance and insulinemia in obese subjects: Fasting[145] and treatment with Metformin[149] induced a parallel decrease in plasma insulin, triglycerides, and PAI-1. Taken together, these studies suggest a direct link between insulin and PAI-1 levels, independent of other risk factors for atherothrombosis.

Genetic variation at a polymorphic locus of the PAI-1 gene is associated with differences in plasma PAI-1 levels.[150] Regulation of PAI-1 by triglycerides was also claimed to be genotype-specific.[150] Because regulation of PAI-1 at the transcriptional level is an important determinant of the PAI-1 concentration in plasma,[76, 151] identification of sequence variability in the gene that affects expression may be useful to identify individuals predisposed to thrombotic disease.[150]

Plasminogen Deficiency and Thrombosis

Two major types of plasminogen deficiency have been described. In type I deficiency, both plasminogen antigen and functional activity are reduced in parallel, suggesting reduced synthesis of a normally functioning plasminogen molecule (hypoplasminogenemia). In type II deficiency, plasminogen antigen levels are normal or only slightly reduced, whereas the activity is greatly reduced, suggesting an abnormally functioning plasminogen molecule (dysplasminogenemia).

Hypoplasminogenemia

Congenital plasminogen deficiency as a cause of thrombosis, characterized by a parallel decrease of functional and immunoreactive plasminogen, has been reported in only a few cases.[152-159] In these patients, other investigated hemostatic parameters were normal; thus, they apparently represent true isolated plasminogen deficiencies associated with severe thromboembolic complications.

Acquired plasminogen deficiency has been observed in several clinical conditions, including liver disease[160] and sepsis (25 to 45 per cent of normal activity).[161] Possible mechanisms for acquired plasminogen deficiency in severe liver disease include depressed hepatic synthesis of the protein, as well as increased consumption.[162] In the plasma of some septic patients, a low-M_r plasminogen-like molecule has been identified[161]; degradation of plasminogen into low-M_r plasminogen by leukocyte elastase has been suggested as a possible explanation for the reduced level.

Dysplasminogenemia

Abnormalities in the plasminogen molecule resulting in defective conversion to plasmin have been described by several authors (Table 21–3). Robbins[163] has proposed a classification of dysplasminogenemia in two types: type 1 dysplasminogenemia, with normal antigen level, and type 2 dysplasminogenemia-hypoplasminogenemia, with antigen level decreased to 60 to 70 per cent of normal. The molecular defect in the plasminogen molecule is an active site defect, which may be combined with charge mutation(s) or kinetic defects.

In 1978, Aoki et al.[164] identified a patient with recurrent thrombosis who had an abnormally low plasminogen activity (40 to 50 per cent of normal) but a normal level of plasminogen antigen. This antigen was shown to be a mixture of normal and abnormal molecules in approximately equal amounts. Studies on the patient's family members suggested that the molecular abnormality was inherited in an autosomal dominant pattern. One of the family members was a homozygote with virtually no plasminogen activity but normal antigen level. Miyata et al.[165] have shown that the absence of proteolytic activity in plasmin(ogen) Tochigi is due to a single amino acid substitution, Ala 600 to Thr, near the His residue of the active site. Characterization of the abnormal gene revealed that a

TABLE 21–3. CHARACTERIZATION OF DYSPLASMINOGENEMIAS

DESIGNATION	MOLECULAR DEFECT	ANTIGEN LEVEL	FUNCTIONAL LEVEL (PER CENT OF NORMAL)	THROMBOSIS Propositus	THROMBOSIS Relatives
Tochigi I[164, 165]	Ala 600 - - > Thr	Normal	40	Yes	No
Tochigi II[167]	Idem	Normal	50	No	No
Nagoya[167]	Idem	Normal	50	No	No
Tokyo[168]	Active site?	Normal	20–30	Yes	No
Paris I[169]	Active site?	Normal	45	Yes	No
Chicago I[172]	Lower affinity for activators	Normal	41	Yes	?
Chicago II[172]	Idem	Normal	88	Yes	?
Chicago III[173]	Lower affinity for activators + impaired cleavage of Arg 560–Val 561	Normal	80	Yes	?
Frankfurt I[174]	Active site	Low normal (78%)	37	Yes	?
Maywood I[175]	Low rate of plasmin generation	Low normal (70%)	26	Yes	?
Frankfurt II[176]	Idem	Low normal (66%)	63	Yes	No

guanosine in the GCT codon (coding for Ala 600) was replaced by an adenosine, resulting in the ACT codon (coding for Thr).[166] This Ala to Thr substitution in the plasmin light chain may affect the side chain of the Asp 645 or His 602 active site residues and thereby disturb the active site charge relay system, leading to loss of enzymatic activity. Two additional abnormal plasminogens with the same molecular defect (Ala 600 to Thr substitution), plasminogen Tochigi II and plasminogen Nagoya, have been identified in other members of the same family.[167] Two similar cases (normal plasminogen antigen level but 50 per cent reduced activity) with thrombotic complications have been reported, plasminogen Tokyo[168] and plasminogen Paris I.[169] This heterozygosity in plasminogen phenotype was found in about 4 per cent of a Japanese population but could not be identified in an American population.[170, 171] In all these cases the propositus was identified after suffering from thrombotic complications, but other family members with the same plasminogen abnormality have, in general, not presented with clinical symptoms of thrombosis.

Wohl and coworkers[172, 173] have characterized three human plasminogen variants (Chicago I, II, and III), identified in young males with a history of recurring deep vein thrombosis. Both plasminogens Chicago I and II have an activation defect characterized by a higher Michaelis constant and impaired plasminogen activator binding, whereas cleavage of the Arg 560–Val 561 peptide bond is normal.[172] Plasminogen Chicago III has both an impaired affinity for plasminogen activators, as evidenced by an increased Michaelis constant, and an impaired cleavage of the Arg 560–Val 561 peptide bond.[173] Plasminogen Frankfurt I (174) is characterized by an active site defect and a charge mutation. Plasminogen Maywood I[175] is characterized by a low rate of plasmin generation and has a low normal antigen level but a reduced activity level. All these dysplasminogenemias thus are characterized by a lowered ratio of functional to immunoreactive plasminogen. Plasminogen Frankfurt II[176] is also characterized by a low rate of plasmin generation and has reduced levels of both antigen and activity in an approximately 1:1 ratio.

Plasminogen Activator Deficiency and Thrombosis

Impairment of fibrinolysis due to deficient synthesis and/or release of t-PA from the vessel wall may be associated with a tendency to thrombosis. Clayton et al.[177] have measured several clinical and laboratory parameters preoperatively in women undergoing gynecological surgery and determined the occurrence of postoperative deep vein thrombosis. Of these parameters, a prolongation of the euglobulin clot lysis time was the most discriminating parameter, allowing a clinically useful separation between patients who subsequently developed deep vein thrombosis and those who did not. Similar results were reported by Rákóczi

et al.[178] Lowe et al.[179] proposed a simplified index, determined as the age in years plus (1.3 × % MW), with % MW defined as per cent mean weight for age, sex, and height. This index was validated in a prospective study on patients undergoing elective major gastrointestinal surgery.

Isacson and Nilsson[180] found a defective release of t-PA from the vessel wall during venous occlusion and/or a decreased t-PA content in walls of superficial veins in about 70 per cent of a large series of patients with idiopathic recurrent venous thrombosis. Korninger et al.[181] followed a group of 121 patients with a history of venous thrombosis and/or pulmonary embolism for approximately 5 years and observed a significantly lower recurrence rate in patients with a postocclusion euglobulin lysis time shorter than 60 minutes (4.8 per cent per year), compared with patients with a postocclusion euglobulin lysis time longer than 60 minutes (10.3 per cent per year). Several studies[182–184] have shown that a deficient fibrinolytic response may be caused by a deficient release of t-PA from the vessel wall or by an increased rate of neutralization. Juhan-Vague et al.[183] investigated 120 patients with spontaneous or recurrent deep vein thrombosis and observed three groups based on their reponse to venous occlusion. A poor fibrinolytic response (less than twofold increase) to venous occlusion occurred in 35 per cent of these patients, one quarter of them with deficient t-PA release and three quarters with normal t-PA release but increased levels of PAI-1.

Enhanced Plasminogen Activator Activity and Bleeding

Excessive fibrinolysis due to increased t-PA activity levels may be associated with a bleeding tendency. A life-long hemorrhagic disorder associated with enhanced fibrinolysis due to increased levels of circulating plasminogen activator has been described. No deficiency of any known inhibitor of fibrinolysis could be detected.[185] A similar case of (inherited) increased fibrinolytic potential due to an excess of t-PA was reported in a Spanish family.[186] Excessive fibrinolysis due to decreased PAI-1 levels has been reported in a few cases and was apparently associated with bleeding complications.[187, 188]

CLINICAL ASPECTS OF THROMBOLYSIS

Cardiovascular diseases, comprising acute myocardial infarction, stroke, and venous thromboembolism, are responsible for almost 50 per cent of deaths in the adult population. These conditions can lead not only to sudden death but also to long-term disability at large cost to society. The incidence of cardiovascular disease in the United States is currently estimated at 1.5 million patients per year with acute myocardial infarction, 1.5 million patients with stroke, and 0.5

million patients with deep vein thrombosis leading to pulmonary embolism.[189]

It is well established that in myocardial or cerebral infarction, the triggering event in the illness is not the atherosclerotic lesion of the blood vessel wall, but more so the obstruction of the artery by a thrombus or blood clot.[190, 191] Thus, the commonly encountered vascular diseases have, as their immediate underlying cause, thrombosis of critically situated blood vessels with loss of blood flow to vital organs.

One approach to the treatment of an established thrombosis consists of pharmacological dissolution of the blood clot via the intravenous infusion of plasminogen activators, which activates an enzyme system in our blood called the fibrinolytic system.

Thrombolytic agents, either approved for clinical use or under clinical investigation, include streptokinase, tcu-PA, APSAC, recombinant tissue-type plasminogen activator (rt-PA, produced either as single-chain alteplase or two-chain duteplase), and recombinant single-chain urokinase–type plasminogen activator (rscu-PA, prourokinase).[1]

Acute Myocardial Infarction

The recognition that thrombosis within the infarct-related coronary artery plays a major role in the pathogenesis of acute myocardial infarction[190] and the observation that early administration of thrombolytic agents results in recanalization of occluded coronary arteries[192] have provided the basis for the development of thrombolytic therapy in acute myocardial infarction. The hypothesis underlying this form of treatment is that coronary artery occlusion leads to ischemia and cell death, resulting in ventricular dysfunction and reduced life expectancy, and that timely recanalization prevents cell death, reduces infarct size, preserves myocardial function, and reduces early and late mortality. Clinical trials were therefore designed to (1) establish patterns of efficacy and safety for thrombolytic agents and (2) define the real impact of early thrombolytic therapy on mortality.

Mechanism of Clinical Benefit of Coronary Arterial Thrombolysis

Early coronary artery recanalization, within a time window that allows salvage of ischemic myocardium, most likely is a primary contributor to preservation of ventricular function and to reduction in mortality. The most rational treatment of patients with acute myocardial infarction is therefore likely to be thrombolytic therapy with agents or combinations that produce stable coronary artery recanalization as frequently and as rapidly as possible with an acceptable safety. Several observations suggest that late opening of an occluded coronary artery may also have some beneficial effect. Indeed, late reperfusion may limit left ventricular remodeling, improve the electrical stability of the heart, or provide collateral vessels to viable

myocardium.[193] Furthermore, adjunctive therapy with anticoagulant and/or antiplatelet agents may contribute to the efficacy of thrombolysis.[194]

Whatever the complexity of the mechanism by which thrombolytic therapy affects the survival of patients with acute myocardial infarction, several large-scale placebo-controlled trials with intravenous thrombolytic agents have established a significant reduction (of the order of 20 per cent or more) of both early and late mortality with streptokinase, APSAC, and rt-PA if administered within 4 to 6 hours. The life-threatening side effects, predominantly intracranial hemorrhage and other major bleeding, are not negligible but consistently less frequent than 1 per cent. Thus, these studies have been invaluable in demonstrating the beneficial effect of thrombolytic therapy on mortality, although, because of their simple design, they provide little or no information on the mechanisms by which this benefit is achieved.

Comparative Properties of Thrombolytic Agents

Comparative studies between streptokinase and rt-PA have shown a difference in efficacy for early coronary artery recanalization,[195] and this conclusion has been supported by results of several non-comparative studies with similar design and endpoints (for references, cf. 196). Coronary artery patency is present in approximately 22 per cent of patients within 90 minutes after the start of placebo infusion (usually heparin and occasionally aspirin), probably around 35 per cent after 24 to 48 hours, and around 65 per cent after 1 to 3 weeks. Streptokinase administration is associated with around 53 per cent patency at 90 minutes and 75 per cent after 1 to 3 weeks, whereas rt-PA, in combination with intravenous heparin, is associated with 75 per cent patency at 90 minutes, 85 per cent at 24 to 48 hours, and 81 per cent at 1 to 3 weeks.[197] Thus, early patency, measured around 90 minutes after the start of therapy, is significantly increased over placebo (22 per cent) with both streptokinase (53 per cent) and rt-PA (75 per cent), whereas the efficacy for coronary recanalization with rt-PA is about 50 per cent higher than with streptokinase. This difference between rt-PA and streptokinase is observed in patients with both early (<3 hours) and later (3 to 6 hours) initiation of thrombolytic therapy.[195, 197]

Two megatrials directly comparing streptokinase and rt-PA have not shown a difference in survival.[198, 199] This lack of correlation between initial efficacy and clinical outcome may have several explanations: (1) the protocols used in the megatrials may have blunted the differences in efficacy between thrombolytic agents and thereby the demonstration of potential differences in mortality; (2) delayed recanalization, which (following a catch-up phenomenon over several hours) occurs to a comparable extent with both streptokinase and t-PA, may be a major contributor to clinical benefit; or (3) there may be no direct correlation between early recanalization and clinical benefit, but other (unknown) mechanisms may be major contributors.

Under the first explanation, the higher initial efficacy of rt-PA for coronary recanalization, demonstrated in comparative efficacy studies with conjunctive intravenous heparin, might not have been obtained in the megatrials with delayed subcutaneous heparin. This hypothesis is supported by the results of several recent randomized trials with angiographic endpoints (Table 21–4), which have demonstrated that patency of the infarct-related coronary artery 7 hours to 5 days after thrombolytic therapy is significantly lower in patients treated with rt-PA without heparin than in patients given conjunctive immediate intravenous heparin.[201–203] Furthermore, in the absence of heparin, patency rates obtained with rt-PA are reduced to levels expected with streptokinase. Similar studies of the effect of heparin on the efficacy of streptokinase are unfortunately not available, although some effect of heparin might also be inferred from the observed clinical benefit.[204] These data suggest that in order to obtain high efficacy rates with rt-PA, concomitant use of intravenous heparin is required, whereas its beneficial effect in association with streptokinase is less well documented. Consequently, the omission of immediate intravenous heparin in the International t-PA/streptokinase mortality trial[198] and the ISIS-3 study[199] may have resulted in comparable efficacies for immediate and sustained coronary artery recanalization and may have accounted for the comparable clinical outcome.

Under the second hypothesis, recanalization following streptokinase, although initially slower, might catch up. The hypothesis that the frequency of early coronary artery recanalization compared with that of delayed recanalization is of only minor importance for the clinical outcome is essentially invalidated by the findings, in most studies, that mortality reduction is largest in patients treated early. Furthermore, the 65 per cent patency rate after 1 to 3 weeks in placebo-treated patients argues against a predominant role of late patency, in the absence of early patency, for clinical outcome.[197]

The hypothesis that there is no direct correlation between early recanalization and mortality reduction has not been adequately established by the International t-PA/SK Mortality Trial or by ISIS-3 because of uncertainty about the role of concomitant intravenous heparin. This hypothesis, which goes against a wealth of animal and human clinical data, could indeed be validated only by properly randomized studies of thrombolytic strategies with known differences in efficacy profiles for coronary recanalization. The obvious comparison would be between streptokinase and immediate aspirin, with or without intravenous heparin on the one hand, and 100 mg of alteplase with immediate intravenous heparin but with delayed administration of aspirin on the other hand. The streptokinase/aspirin combination has indeed been extensively validated for patency in angiographic studies (approximately 50 per cent at 90 minutes with a subsequent catch-up to be comparable after several hours with that obtained at 90 minutes with t-PA) and for safety and mortality reduction in ISIS-2. The alteplase/intravenous heparin combination with delayed aspirin (24 hours) has been extensively validated both for high early and delayed patency in TIMI-2A[205] and TIMI-2B[206] and for safety and clinical outcome in TIMI-2. Indeed, the TIMI-2 protocol, with its comparatively very low mortality, should at present be regarded as the "gold standard" for t-PA administration. The fact that the megatrials have consistently failed to use this well-validated therapeutic regimen in favor of alternative protocols with unknown efficacy and safety has undermined their scientific basis and invalidated any useful extrapolations to mechanisms of clinical benefit.

Questions Persisting After the rt-PA/Streptokinase Mortality Trial and the ISIS-3 Study

The aim of the International t-PA/SK Mortality Trial[198] was to compare the efficacy and safety of 100 mg of alteplase (Activase, Genentech) given over 3 hours with those of 1.5 million units streptokinase given over 1 hour, in approximately 20,000 patients with acute myocardial infarction treated with immediate aspirin and β blockade. In addition, the role of subcutaneous heparin, 12,500 units twice a day, started 12 hours after the onset of thrombolytic therapy, was evaluated. The primary endpoint, in-hospital mortality, was not significantly different between the strep-

TABLE 21–4. INFLUENCE OF HEPARIN ON CORONARY PATENCY FOLLOWING ALTEPLASE INFUSION

| HEPARIN | STUDY | ENDPOINT (TIME AFTER START OF THERAPY) | | | | ASPIRIN |
		90 min	7–14 hr	48–72 hr	48–120 hr	
With	Topol et al., 1989[200]	79 (50/63)				?
	Hsia et al., 1990[201]		82 (82/100)			No
	Bleich et al., 1990[202]			71 (30/42)		?
	ECSG, 1991[203]				83 (214/258)	Yes
Without	Topol et al., 1989[200]	79 (54/68)				?
	Hsia et al., 1990[201]		62 (48/93)			Yes
	Bleich et al., 1989[202]			43 (18/42)		?
	ECSG, 1991[203]				74 (181/244)	Yes
	P	0.83	<0.001	0.015	0.022	

TABLE 21–5. FREQUENCY OF CEREBRAL HEMORRHAGE IN THE TWO LARGE TRIALS COMPARING t-PA AND STREPTOKINASE IN PATIENTS WITH ACUTE MYOCARDIAL INFARCTION

	DEFINITION	STREPTOKINASE	t-PA	p
Int. Study/GISSI-2[198]	Definite hemorrhage	30/10,396 (0.3%)	44/10,372 (0.4%)	NS
ISIS-3[199]	"Probable" hemorrhage	39/12,848 (0.3%)	94/12,841 (0.7%)	<0.001
p		NS	0.003	

tokinase and rt-PA groups.[8] Although the aims and endpoints of the trial were simple and straightforward, the finding during the course of the study that the efficacy of rt-PA for coronary thrombolysis is strongly dependent on the conjunctive use of intravenous heparin (see above) has confused the issue.

The ISIS-3 study[199] compared the effects of 0.6 million units/kg (MU/kg) of duteplase (Prolysis, Burroughs-Wellcome) given over 4 hours, 1.5 MU of streptokinase over 1 hour, and 30 units of APSAC given as a bolus. Approximately 45,000 patients with acute myocardial infarction entered the study, and all were immediately treated with aspirin. In addition, the contribution of subcutaneous heparin, started 4 hours after thrombolytic therapy, was evaluated. The results indicated that early mortality was not significantly different with any of the thrombolytic agents, whereas the frequency of "probable" intracerebral hemorrhage was lower with streptokinase (0.3 per cent) than with duteplase (0.7 per cent) or APSAC (0.6 per cent) ($P < 0.00001$).

Irrespective of the problems associated with delayed subcutaneous heparin administration in ISIS-3, there are more serious questions concerning the dose of the duteplase rt-PA preparation used. Indeed, because both alteplase and duteplase are the translation product of the same cDNA (obtained from mRNA of the Bowes melanoma cell line), they could be expected to have identical biological properties. However, the production and/or purification process appears to have introduced some artifacts in the duteplase preparation, as suggested by the specific activity, determined by clot lysis assays, which is markedly lower for duteplase (approximately 300,000 IU/mg, based on data provided by Burroughs-Wellcome) than for alteplase (580,000 IU/mg, based on data provided by Genentech) and for the melanoma t-PA standard (500,000 IU/mg as established by the International Committee for Thrombosis and Haemostasis). In contrast, kinetic chromogenic substrate assays yield a specific activity for duteplase of approximately 500,000 IU/mg, comparable to that of the standard melanoma t-PA.

Extrapolation of the results obtained with duteplase in ISIS-3 to the standard use of 100 mg of alteplase is not obvious. A dose of duteplase of 0.6 M clot lysis units/kg body weight represents 2 mg/kg body weight. For the average 75 kg patient, this corresponds to a total dose of 45 million IU, or 150 mg. Based on the activity of both preparations in the standard clot lysis assay, the 45 MU dose of duteplase, given to the 75

kg patient in ISIS-3, appears to be somewhat underdosed relative to the 58 MU contained in 100 mg alteplase. However, based on the gravimetric amount of material given in ISIS-3, the average dose of 150 mg of duteplase is clearly overdosed relative to the 100 mg alteplase dose. In the absence of comparative studies between duteplase and alteplase, their equivalence remains enigmatic.

The frequency of intracranial bleeding in the International t-PA/SK Mortality Study[198] and in ISIS-3[199] (Table 21–5) deserves some comment. Indeed, the frequency of cerebral bleeding as defined in these studies was identical at 0.3 per cent in both streptokinase groups. The frequency of intracerebral bleeding with 100 mg of alteplase in the International t-PA/SK Mortality Trial was 0.4 per cent ($P = NS$), and with an average of 150 mg duteplase in ISIS-3 it was 0.7 per cent ($P < 0.001$). The difference in cerebral bleeding rates between these studies thus appears to be primarily, if not exclusively, due to a difference between duteplase and alteplase and not between alteplase and streptokinase. The TIMI-2 trial showed that 150 mg alteplase, given in combination with intravenous heparin, was associated with an intracerebral bleeding rate of 1.6 per cent.[206] This observation caused cessation of the testing of the 150 mg dose after several hundred patients and a worldwide reduction of the dose to 100 mg. In view of these earlier events, it is most surprising that the ISIS-3 trial, which was initially planned to enter 30,000 patients, was extended to 45,000 patients without a protocol change.

Is There a Correlation Between Efficacy for Early Coronary Recanalization and Clinical Outcome?

Because of the uncertainties concerning the efficacy of the treatment protocols used in the International t-PA/SK Mortality Study and the ISIS-3 trial, these studies cannot be heralded as the definitive tests of rt-PA versus streptokinase, nor as an indication that early and sustained recanalization does not primarily determine clinical outcome. In the absence of conclusive studies with mortality endpoints, comparing streptokinase with rt-PA in the presence of conjunctive immediate intravenous heparin, it might be of interest to review in-hospital mortality data of smaller comparative trials with rt-PA in combination with heparin against other non–fibrin-specific thrombolytic agents (streptokinase, urokinase, or APSAC) with presumed lower efficacy for coronary recanalization. The results of seven trials performed to date are summarized in Table 21–6. Cumulative in-hospital mortalities were 43 of 975 patients (4.4 per cent) randomly assigned to rt-PA and concomitant intravenous heparin and 71 of 972 patients (7.3 per cent) allocated to the non–fibrin-specific agents and intravenous heparin. Meta-analysis of the data yields an odds ratio for death with rt-PA versus the non–fibrin-specific agents of 0.59 (95 per cent CI: 0.41 to 0.87), $P = 0.0067$. It should be stressed that these results are derived from small studies that, although randomized, were not prospectively designed for mortality endpoints, and that final proof will need to be obtained from proper prospective clinical trials, using conjunctive intravenous heparin with rt-PA for maximal efficacy and delayed aspirin for reduced toxicity, as established in TIMI-2.

Because controversy continues on the relative impact of rt-PA and streptokinase on clinical outcome in patients with acute myocardial infarction, a major new comparative trial, the *Global Utilization of Streptokinase and T-PA for Occluded coronary arteries* (GUSTO) trial, is in progress. In this study with all patients given immediate aspirin, alteplase, given as a front-loaded dose over 90 minutes with concomitant intravenous heparin, will be compared with streptokinase with either concomitant intravenous or delayed subcutaneous heparin, and with the combination of streptokinase and rt-PA with immediate intravenous heparin. This mortality study will include a substudy with angiographic endpoints that is expected to allow correlation of recanalization data (early, intermediate, and late patency) with clinical outcome. It is assumed from pilot studies that the front-loaded rt-PA regimen as well as the combination therapy will induce very high early patency. The study may, therefore, finally establish the correlation or lack thereof between early and sustained recanalization and clinical outcome. However, data on the safety of the front-loaded t-PA

TABLE 21–6. IN-HOSPITAL MORTALITY IN RANDOMIZED STUDIES WITH rt-PA VERSUS SK, UK, OR APSAC IN PATIENTS WITH ACUTE MYOCARDIAL INFARCTION

STUDY	rt-PA	SK/UK/APSAC
ECSG-1[207]	3/64	3/65 (SK)
TIMI-I[208]	12/157	14/159 (SK)
White et al.[209]	5/135	10/135 (SK)
PAIMS[210]	4/86	7/85 (SK)
TAMI-5[211]	8/191	15/190 (UK)
GAUS[212]	6/124	5/121 (UK)
TAPS[213]	5/218	17/217 (APSAC)
	43/975 (4.4%)	71/972 (7.3%)

rt-PA = recombinant tissue-type plasminogen activator; SK = streptokinase; UK = urokinase; APSAC = anisoylated plasminogen-streptokinase activator complex.
Heterogeneity index: $X_2 = 4.76$; $P = 0.57$.
Odds ratio rt-PA: 0.59 (95 per cent CI: 0.41–0.87)
P value of the difference = 0.0067.

regimen with immediate intravenous heparin and immediate aspirin are limited. Again, the failure to include the TIMI-2 protocol with a well-validated efficacy/safety profile as one of the arms of the study is most unfortunate.

Should Thrombolytic Therapy with Alteplase be Tailored to the Patient?

Present treatment with alteplase involves a standard dose of 100 mg, usually in combination with intravenous heparin and 160 mg immediate "chewable" aspirin. The dose of alteplase was initially set at 150 mg to obtain maximal early coronary artery recanalization, but had to be reduced because of excess intracranial bleeding and was set at 100 mg given over 3 to 6 hours. The use of intravenous heparin appears to be necessary to obtain maximal and persistent coronary recanalization. Aspirin is usually given because it was shown in ISIS-2[214] to be beneficial by itself as well as in association with streptokinase. However, its beneficial effect on early recanalization with alteplase has not actually been demonstrated, whereas a marked interactive effect between aspirin and alteplase with respect to bleeding time prolongation and bleeding has been reported.[215–217] It is at least theoretically possible that concomitant aspirin might be useful with the relatively ineffective streptokinase, resulting in somewhat more than 50 per cent early patency, whereas it might not add to the 75 per cent early patency obtained with alteplase, as was suggested by the TIMI-2A[205] and HART[201] studies. In this case, delayed administration of aspirin, which does not affect the high initial and delayed coronary artery patency as demonstrated in TIMI-2,[206] would be preferable in order to maintain the potential effect on late reocclusion without causing a potentiation of the bleeding tendency during the infusion of alteplase.

Whatever the optimal administration scheme of aspirin with alteplase might be, the aggressive use of potent thrombolytic agents (e.g., 100 mg of alteplase) with conjunctive intravenous heparin and aspirin appears to confer optimal if not maximal benefit in patients with recent large infarcts in whom much myocardial salvage is still possible. This was suggested by the very low early mortality rates (<4 per cent in patients <70 years) in the TIMI-2,[206] ECSG-V,[218] and TAPS[213] studies. In more evolved infarcts or in older patients, the advantages of aggressive recanalization may be more limited or partially neutralized by an increased bleeding tendency, especially in combination with immediate aspirin. In these cases, a less aggressive thrombolytic strategy with a reduced dose of a more potent agent (e.g., 50 or possibly even 25 mg of alteplase with intravenous heparin) or with a full dose of a less potent agent (e.g., 1.5 MU streptokinase with immediate aspirin) might be preferable. Indeed, the equipotent doses of streptokinase and alteplase for coronary artery recanalization at 90 minutes appear to be 1.5 MU over 60 minutes and between 25 and 50 mg over 90 minutes, respectively.[219] It thus seems that a 50 mg dose of alteplase in combination with immediate intravenous heparin should be of comparable efficacy to streptokinase, but devoid of its hypotensive or allergic side effects, albeit at a much higher cost.

The recent International t-PA/SK Mortality Study and ISIS-3 trial have used a high dose of t-PA (100 mg of alteplase and on average 150 mg of duteplase, respectively), with immediate aspirin and delayed subcutaneous heparin in patients with acute myocardial infarction admitted into the trial up to 24 hours and without age limit. However, early intravenous heparin appears to be required for early, sustained recanalization with rt-PA, whereas immediate aspirin does not appear to increase the efficacy of alteplase but potentiates the effect of alteplase on bleeding. Thus, the clinical benefit of more rapid recanalization with rt-PA versus streptokinase probably was diluted (owing to inadequate anticoagulation and inclusion of patients with negligible salvageable myocardium), whereas all patients were exposed to a potentially increased bleeding risk from the combination of high dose t-PA with intravenous heparin and immediate aspirin.

Conclusions

Although the clinical benefit of thrombolytic therapy in patients with acute myocardial infarction is well established, more studies, both at the basic mechanistic and at the clinical outcome level, are required to define the optimal thrombolytic regimen in terms of both thrombolytic agent and conjunctive anticoagulant and/or antiplatelet agents. Indeed, thrombolytic therapy can no longer be considered a monotherapy with a single thrombolytic agent. At the present time, the only well-established advantage of treatment of patients with acute myocardial infarction with t-PA over streptokinase is that t-PA, when used with intravenous heparin, induces more rapid and more frequent early recanalization of the infarct-related coronary artery than does streptokinase combined with aspirin. However, notwithstanding a wealth of experimental and clinical data that early recanalization constitutes the major mechanism of benefit, there is at present no conclusive evidence from randomized clinical trials that, in the infarct population at large, this difference in efficacy will translate into a comparable difference in mortality outcome. Although this problem could most easily be solved by a prospective randomized clinical study comparing the streptokinase/aspirin protocol of ISIS-2 with the alteplase/heparin protocol of TIMI-2, this definitive test of t-PA versus streptokinase is still lacking.

Deep Vein Thrombosis

Six randomized controlled trials with streptokinase for deep venous thrombosis of the legs, in which phlebography was used, revealed that thrombolysis was achieved 3.7 times more often in streptokinase-treated patients than in heparin-treated patients ($P < 0.001$), but that bleeding was 2.9 times greater in the streptokinase group ($P < 0.04$).[220] Long-term venographic evaluation of thrombolytic versus anticoagulant therapy of deep vein thrombosis was reported in four randomized trials.[220–223] At 2 to 12 months after initial therapy, normal venograms were obtained in 52 per cent of 48 patients treated with streptokinase and in 16 per cent of 25 patients treated with heparin alone; the other patients had developed permanent collateral flow and/or incompetent venous valves. In a controlled study in 100 patients with a mean follow-up of 5.7 years, irreversible venous valve damage occurred despite thrombolytic therapy with streptokinase.[224] Other studies, however, have suggested a correlation between the reduction of postphlebitic syndrome and extent of clot lysis.[226, 227] Similarly, successful lysis of proximal vein thrombosis prevents the development of ulcerations.[228, 229] An ultra-high regimen of streptokinase (1.5 million IU per hour) maintained for 6 hours, and repeated if necessary for 1 to 5 days, was shown to induce total lysis in 41 per cent (35/86) and partial lysis in 45 per cent (39/86) of patients.[230] These results of the ultra-high intermittent regimen have been confirmed by other groups.[231–233]

The advantage of thrombolytic treatment must be weighed against the potential side effects. The risk of hemorrhage with streptokinase is three times that with heparin, with reported rates ranging from 8.0 to 25 per cent.[220] Intracranial bleeding is about twice as frequent as with heparin treatment and appears to increase with the duration of thrombolytic treatment.[234]

In a randomized trial with urokinase in venous thrombosis, the effectiveness of thrombolytic treatment was evaluated by a blinded comparison of phlebograms taken before and after treatment.[235] The effectiveness of intermittently administered urokinase (loading dose of 4400 IU/kg, maintenance dose of 1100 or 2200 IU/kg/hr for 12 hours) was compared with a continuous infusion of streptokinase. The urokinase administration was alternated with heparin every 12 hours for a total of 3 to 6 days. Despite the difference in the infusion schedules, the rate of moderate to marked venographic thrombolysis achieved at 3 days in both the higher-dose urokinase group (18 per cent) and in the lower-dose urokinase group (20 per cent) was equivalent to the rate of thrombolysis observed in the streptokinase group (20 per cent). However, systemic hemorrhagic complications were more frequent in streptokinase-treated patients. Experience with rt-PA in acute deep vein thrombosis is limited. rt-PA infused at a dose of 0.5 mg/kg over 4 hours produced lysis in approximately 60 per cent of patients; however, a lower dose results in a significantly smaller degree of lysis.[236–238] Increasing the dose of rt-PA to 100 and 50 mg over 8 hours on 2 subsequent days does not lead to improved results.[239] A continuous infusion of 0.75 to 1.75 mg rt-PA/kg/24 hours for 2 to 4 days may be a better therapeutic regimen, as was suggested in a study limited to a small number of patients.[240]

Pulmonary Embolism

The clinical utility of streptokinase and urokinase in submassive pulmonary embolism was extensively investigated.[241-244] Resolution of pulmonary emboli, improvement in cardiopulmonary hemodynamics, and reperfusion of the pulmonary vasculature occur more rapidly with streptokinase (250,000 IU loading followed by 100,000 IU/hr for 24 hours) or urokinase (4400 IU/kg loading dose and hourly maintenance dose for 12 or 24 hours) than with heparin or warfarin alone.[241, 245] The number of patients in these trials was, however, too small to demonstrate a significant reduction in mortality. Although thrombolytic therapy improved pulmonary gas exchange and capillary blood volume after 1 year follow-up, the clinical relevance of these findings is open to question.[245]

Bolus administration of urokinase (15,000 IU/kg body weight) in the right atrium in 14 patients with acute pulmonary embolism caused a decrease of the Miller angiographic index of 34 per cent at 12 hours.[246] These results have been confirmed in a large group of 161 patients.[247] Only 4 per cent of the patients experienced serious bleeding during the first 24 hours.

In the first trial of rt-PA in patients with severe pulmonary embolism, 50 mg was infused over 2 hours in 36 patients, followed, when necessary, by an additional 40 mg over 4 hours.[248] Pulmonary angiography revealed a 21 per cent improvement at 2 hours and 49 per cent at 6 hours, a significant decrease in pulmonary artery systolic pressure and in right ventricular diameter, and an increase in left ventricular diameter.[249] In a study in 34 patients with massive recent pulmonary embolism, rt-PA was given as a 10 mg bolus followed by 20 mg/hr for 2 hours either intravenously or into the pulmonary artery. A comparable improvement of the angiographic score of approximately 15 per cent was obtained in the two groups. Twenty-two patients were given a second infusion of 50 mg of rt-PA with an additional improvement in angiographic severity score of 38 per cent.[250]

A direct comparison between urokinase and rt-PA was made in 45 patients with pulmonary embolism.[251] The objective was to determine whether a fixed 2 hour dose of rt-PA conferred any advantage over a 24 hour urokinase regimen. By 2 hours, 82 per cent of rt-PA–treated patients showed clot lysis, compared with 48 per cent of urokinase-treated patients ($P = 0.008$). Improvement in lung scan reperfusion at 24 hours was similar in the two treatment groups.

Arterial Thromboembolism

Intravenous streptokinase clears 80 per cent of arterial occlusions treated within 12 hours and 60 per cent when treatment is delayed for up to 3 days.[252] In older obstructions, the success rate is much lower, whereas almost no lysis was obtained in thrombi older than 3 months.[253-256]

Local treatment with low-dose streptokinase or uro-kinase infused in the immediate vicinity of the clot is successful in about 50 to 80 per cent of patients, with sustained recanalization for 1 year in 50 per cent.[257-259] In 623 patients treated in 45 hospitals, in-hospital success rate was 50 per cent, but there were serious complications in 20 per cent, including leg amputation (16 per cent) and cerebrovascular accidents (1.4 per cent).[260] Furthermore, the mortality in this study was 2.3 per cent.

Pooled data of 14 trials with intrathrombotic infusion of streptokinase revealed a success rate of 67 per cent and a major complication rate of 19 per cent in 474 patients; with urokinase the corresponding figures are 81 per cent and 12 per cent in 162 patients.[261] In a follow-up study, 59 per cent of 77 patients who were successfully lysed with local urokinase treatment had a patent artery at 6 months.[262]

Experience with rt-PA in patients with thrombosed peripheral arteries and bypass grafts is limited to two studies. Sixty-five patients were treated for peripheral artery or bypass graft thrombosis with intra-arterial administration of 0.05 or 0.1 mg/kg/hr of rt-PA by Graor and al.[263, 264] The duration of infusion was 2 to 8 hours (mean duration, 5.25 hours). Sixty-one of 65 patients (94 per cent) had angiographically proven successful clot lysis. Following lysis, 76 per cent of patients required a secondary procedure (two percutaneous transluminal angioplasty and 20 surgical revision), and seven required anticoagulation to maintain patency. Infusion of rt-PA at a rate of 10 mg/hr into 50 thrombosed femoral and popliteal arteries produced recanalization in 43 of these patients.[265] Secondary angioplasty led to two reocclusions, and three patients experienced early rethrombosis.

Acute Thromboembolic Stroke

Stroke is the most common cause of local neurological disease in adults and probably the third most common cause of death in the adult population. Up to 85 per cent of strokes are caused by arterial thromboembolism.[266] The cerebral tissue zone with reversible ischemic paralysis of neurons and other structures surrounding an anoxic core may be salvaged within a narrow time window of 3 hours or perhaps more.[267] Because of the risk of secondary bleeding, however, there is considerable reticence regarding the use of anticoagulants in patients with stroke.

An overview of 20 patients with stroke in the carotid territory treated within 6 to 8 hours after onset of symptoms with intra-arterial urokinase (for 1 to 4 hours) or streptokinase (for 0.5 to 2 hours) has been recently published.[268] Arteriographically proven recanalization was complete in 15, partial in 3, and absent in 2 patients. In total, 10 of the 15 patients who had complete recanalization had a partial to nearly full functional recovery of the neurological deficits; 9 of these 10 patients were treated within 4 to 8 hours of symptom onset. Intracerebral bleeding in the basal ganglia without clinical deterioration was noted in 4 patients who experienced complete recanalization of the middle cerebral artery.

The outcome of another group of 22 patients with thromboembolic occlusion of the middle cerebral artery who received intra-arterial urokinase within a mean of 4.5 hours of symptoms was reported by Mori et al.[269] Complete (four) or partial (four) reperfusion was obtained in eight patients. The clinical symptoms improved considerably in patients with marked angiographic recanalization but was rather poor in two patients with minimal recanalization. In another study of 43 patients treated with variable dosages of streptokinase or urokinase, 19 reperfused and 14 survived.[270] Of the 24 non-recanalized patients, none survived.

A dose-finding study is underway to determine the optimal dose of rt-PA administered over 60 minutes.[271] In an NIH-sponsored multicenter trial, the incidence of bleeding and early outcome after rt-PA are being investigated.[272] Until larger studies are completed to define the efficacy and safety of thrombolytic drugs for acute ischemic stroke, the use of plasminogen activators must remain restricted to experimental protocols.

REFERENCES

1. Collen, D.: Plasminogen activators and thrombolytic therapy. ISI Atlas Sci: Pharmacology 3:116, 1988.
2. Wiman, B., and Collen, D.: Molecular mechanism of physiological fibrinolysis. Nature 272:549, 1978.
3. Collen, D.: On the regulation and control of fibrinolysis. Thromb. Haemost. 43:77, 1980.
4. Sottrup-Jensen, L., Petersen, T. E., and Magnusson, S.: Atlas of protein sequence and structure, Vol. 5, Suppl. 3. In Dayhoff, M. O (ed.). Washington, D.C., National Biomedical Research Foundation, 1978, p. 91.
5. Forsgren, M., Raden, B., Israelsson, M., Larsson, K., and Heden, L.O.: Molecular cloning and characterization of a full-length cDNA clone for human plasminogen. FEBS Lett 213:254, 1987.
6. Wallen, P., and Wiman, B.: Characterization of human plasminogen. I. On the relationship between different molecular forms of plasminogen demonstrated in plasma and found in purified preparations. Biochim. Biophys. Acta 221:20, 1970.
7. Wallen, P., and Wiman, B.: Characterization of human plasminogen. II. Separation and partial characterization of different molecular forms of human plasminogen. Biochim. Biophys. Acta 257:122, 1972.
8. Robbins, K. C., Summaria, L., Hsieh, B., and Shah, R. J.: The peptide chains of human plasmin. Mechanism of activation of human plasminogen to plasmin. J. Biol. Chem., 242:2333, 1967.
9. Holvoet, P., Lijnen, H. R., and Collen, D.: A monoclonal antibody specific for Lys-plasminogen. Application to the study of the activation pathways of plasminogen in vivo. J. Biol. Chem., 260:12106, 1985.
10. Murray, J. C., Buetow, K. H., Donovan, M., Hornung, S., Motulsky, A. G., Disteche, C., Dyer, K., Swisshelm, K., Anderson, J., Giblett, E., Sadler, E., Eddy, R., and Shows, T. B.: Linkage disequilibrium of plasminogen polymorphisms and assignment of the gene to human chromosome 6q26–6q27. Am. J. Hum. Genet. 40:338, 1987.
11. Petersen, T. E., Martzen, M. R., Ichinose, A., and Davie, E. W.: Characterization of the gene for human plasminogen, a key proenzyme in the fibrinolytic system. J. Biol. Chem. 265:6104, 1990.
12. Summaria, L., Arzadon, L., Bernabe, P., and Robbins, K. C.: Studies on the isolation of the multiple molecular forms of human plasminogen and plasmin by isoelectric focusing methods. J. Biochem. Biophys. 247:4691, 1972.
13. Hobart, M. J.: Genetic polymorphism of human plasminogen. Ann. Hum. Genet. 42:419, 1979.
14. Raum, D., Marcus, D., and Alper, C. A.: Genetic polymorphism of human plasminogen. Am. J. Hum. Genet., 32:681, 1980.
15. Skoda, U., Bertrams, J., Dykes, D., Eiberg, H., Hobart, M., Hummel, K., Kuehnl, P., Mauff, G., Nakamura, S., Nishimukai, H., Raum, D., Tokunaga, K., and Weidinger, S.: Proposal for the nomenclature of human plasminogen (PLG) polymorphism. Vox Sang. 51:244, 1986.
16. Nishimukai, H., Kera, Y., Sakata, K., and Yamasawa, K.: Three new variants in the plasminogen system. Hum. Hered. 32:130, 1982.
17. Nishimukai, H., Shinmyozu, K., and Tamaki, Y.: Polymorphism of plasminogen in healthy individuals and patients with cerebral infarction. Hum. Hered. 36:137, 1986.
18. Hitzeroth, H. W., Skoda, U., du Toit, E., and Mauff, G.: The plasminogen polymorphism in South African negro populations: Genetics and anthropogenetics. Hum. Genet. 74:341, 1986.
19. Dimo-Simonin, N., Brandt-Casadevall, C., and Gujer, H. R.: Gene frequencies of plasminogen in Switzerland. Hum. Hered. 35:343, 1985.
20. Kera, Y., Nishimukai, H., Yamasawa, K., and Komura, S.: Comparative study of phenotypes on activity and plasma concentration in the genetic system of plasminogen. Hum. Hered. 33:52, 1983.
21. Nishimukai, H., Kera, Y., Sakata, K., and Yamasawa, K.: Genetic polymorphism of plasminogen: A new basic variant (PLG B) and population study in Japanese. Vox Sang. 40:422, 1981.
22. Brandt-Casadevall, C., Dimo-Simonin, N., and Gujer, H. R.: A plasminogen silent allele detected in a Swiss family. Hum. Hered. 37:389, 1987.
23. Pennica, D., Holmes, W. E., Kohr, W. J., Harkins, R. N., Vehar, G. A., Ward, C. A., Bennett, W. F., Yelverton, E., Seeburg, P. H., Heyneker, H. L., Goeddel, D. V., and Collen, D.: Cloning and expression of human tissue-type plasminogen activator cDNA in E. coli. Nature 301:214, 1983.
24. Jörnvall, H., Pohl, G., Bergsdorf, N., and Wallen P.: Differential proteolysis and evidence for a residue exchange in tissue plasminogen activator suggest possible association between two types of protein microheterogeneity. FEBS Lett. 156:47, 1983.
25. Hoylaerts, M., Rijken, D. C., Lijnen, H. R., and Collen, D.: Kinetics of the activation of plasminogen by human tissue plasminogen activator. Role of fibrin. J. Biol. Chem. 257:2912, 1982.
26. Nieuwenhuizen, W., Voskuilen, M., Vermond, A., Hoegee-de Nobel, B., and Traas, D. W.: The influence of fibrin(ogen) fragments on the kinetic parameters of the tissue-type plasminogen-activator–mediated activation of different forms of plasminogen. Eur. J. Biochem. 174:163, 1988.
27. Rajput, B., Degen, S. F., Reich, E., Waller, E. K., Axelrod, J., Eddy, R. L., and Shows, T. B.: Chromosomal locations of human tissue plasminogen activator and urokinase genes. Science 230:672, 1985.
28. Verheijen, J. H., Visse, R., Wijnen, J. T., Chang, G. T. G., Kluft, C., and Meera Khan, P.: Assignment of the human tissue-type plasminogen activator gene (PLAT) to chromosome 8. Hum. Genet. 72:153, 1986.
29. Yang-Feng, T. L., Opdenakker, G., Volckaert, G., and Francke, U.: Human tissue-type plasminogen activator gene located near chromosomal breakpoint in myeloproliferative disorder. Am. J. Hum. Genet. 39:79, 1986.
30. Ny, T., Elgh, F., and Lund, B.: The structure of the human tissue-type plasminogen activator gene: Correlation of intron and exon structures to functional and structural domains. Proc. Natl. Acad. Sci. USA 81:5355, 1984.
31. Browne, M. J., Tyrrell, A. W. R., Chapman, C. G., Carrey, J.

E., Glover, D. M., Grosveld, F. G., Dodd, I., and Robinson, J. H.: Isolation of a human tissue-type plasminogen activator genomic DNA clone and its expression in mouse L cells. Gene 33:279, 1985.

32. Degen, S. J. F., Rajput, B., and Reich, E.: The human tissue plasminogen activator gene. J. Biol. Chem. 261:6972, 1986.

33. Patthy, L.: Evolution of the proteases of blood coagulation and fibrinolysis by assembly from modules. Cell 41:657, 1985.

34. Pannekoek, H., de Vries, C., and van Zonneveld, A. J.: Mutants of human tissue-type plasminogen activator (t-PA): Structural aspects and functional properties. Fibrinolysis 2:123, 1988.

35. Steffens, G. J., Günzler, W. A., Ötting, F., Frankus, E., and Flohé, L.: The complete amino acid sequence of low molecular mass urokinase from human urine. Hoppe-Seyler's Z. Physiol. Chem. 363:1043, 1982.

36. Günzler, W. A., Steffens, G. J., Ötting, F., Kim, S. M. A., Frankus, E., and Flohé, L.: The primary structure of high molecular mass urokinase from human urine. Hoppe-Seyler's Z. Physiol. Chem. 363:1155, 1982.

37. Holmes, W. E., Pennica, D., Blaber, M., Rey, M. W., Guenzler, W. A., Steffens, G. J., and Heyneker, H. L.: Cloning and expression of the gene for pro-urokinase in Escherichia coli. Biotechnology 3:923, 1985.

38. Günzler, W. A., Steffens, G. J., Ötting, F., Buse, C. T., and Flohé, L.: Structural relationship between human high and low molecular mass urokinase. Hoppe-Seyler's Z. Physiol. Chem. 363:133, 1982.

39. Stump, D. C., Lijnen, H. R., and Collen, D.: Purification and characterization of a novel low molecular weight form of single-chain urokinase-type plasminogen activator. J. Biol. Chem. 261:17120, 1986.

40. Wun, T. C., Schleuning, W. D., and Reich, E.: Isolation and characterization of urokinase from human plasma. J. Biol. Chem. 257:3276, 1982.

41. Nielsen, L. S., Hansen, J. G., Skriver, L., Wilson, E. L., Kaltoft, K., Zeuthen, J., and Danø, K.: Purification of zymogen to plasminogen activator from human glioblastoma cells by affinity chromatography with monoclonal antibody. Biochemistry 21:6410, 1982.

42. Lijnen, H. R., Zamarron, C., Blaber, M., Winkler, M. E., and Collen, D.: Activation of plasminogen by pro-urokinase. I. Mechanism. J. Biol. Chem. 261:1253, 1986.

43. Lijnen, H. R., Van Hoef, B., De Cock, F., and Collen, D.: The mechanism of plasminogen activation and fibrin dissolution by single chain urokinase-type plasminogen activator in a plasma milieu in vitro. Blood 73:1864, 1989.

44. Ellis, V., Scully, M. F., and Kakkar, V. V.: Plasminogen activation by single-chain urokinase in functional isolation. A kinetic study. J. Biol. Chem. 262:14998, 1987.

45. Petersen, L. C., Lund, L. R., Nielsen, L. S., Danø, K., and Skriver, L.: One-chain urokinase-type plasminogen activator from human sarcoma cells is a proenzyme with little or no intrinsic activity. J. Biol. Chem. 263:11189, 1988.

46. Husain, S. S.: Single-chain urokinase-type plasminogen activator does not possess measurable intrinsic amidolytic or plasminogen activator activities. Biochemistry 30:5797, 1991.

47. Manchanda, N., and Schwartz, B. S.: Single chain urokinase. Augmentation of enzymatic activity upon binding to monocytes. J. Biol. Chem. 266:14580, 1991.

48. Verde, P., Stoppelli, M. P., Galeffi, P., Di Nocera, P., and Blasi, F.: Identification and primary sequence of an unspliced human urokinase poly(A)+RNA. Proc. Natl. Acad. Sci. USA 81:4727, 1984.

49. Riccio, A., Grimaldi, G., Verde, P., Sebastio, G., Boast, S., and Blasi, F.: The human urokinase-plasminogen activator gene and its promoter. Nucleic Acids Res. 13:2759, 1985.

50. Jackson, K. W., and Tang, J.: Complete amino acid sequence of streptokinase and its homology with serine proteases. Biochemistry 21:6620, 1982.

51. Reddy, K. N. N.: Mechanism of activation of human plasminogen by streptokinase. In Kline, D. L., and Reddy, K.

N. N. (eds.): Fibrinolysis. Boca Raton, CRC Press, 1980, pp. 71–94.

52. Summaria, L., Wohl, R. C., Boreisha, I. G., and Robbins, K. C.: A virgin enzyme derived from human plasminogen. Specific cleavage of the arginyl-560-valyl peptide bond in the diisopropoxyphosphinyl virgin enzyme by plasminogen activators. Biochemistry 21:2056, 1982.

53. Cederholm-Williams, S. A., De Cock, F., Lijnen, H. R., and Collen, D.: Kinetics of the reactions between streptokinase, plasmin and α2-antiplasmin. Eur. J. Biochem. 100:125, 1979.

54. Staniforth, D. H., Smith, R. A. G., and Hibbs, M.: Streptokinase and anisoylated streptokinase plasminogen complex. Their action on haemostasis in human volunteers. Eur. J. Clin. Pharmacol. 24:751, 1983.

55. Verstraete, M., Vermylen, J., Amery, A., and Vermylen, C.: Thrombolytic therapy with streptokinase using a standard dosage scheme. Br. Med. J. 1:454, 1966.

56. Smith, R. A. G., Dupe, R. J., English, P. D., and Green, J.: Fibrinolysis with acyl-enzymes: A new approach to thrombolytic therapy. Nature 290:505, 1981.

57. Walker, I. D., Davidson, J. F., Rae, A. P., Hutton, I., and Lawrie, T. D. V.: Acylated streptokinase-plasminogen complex in patients with acute myocardial infarction. Thromb. Haemost. 51:204, 1984.

58. Prowse, C. V., Hornsey, V., Ruckley, C. V., and Boulton, F. E.: A comparison of acylated streptokinase-plasminogen complex and streptokinase in healthy volunteers. Thromb. Haemost. 47:132, 1982.

59. Lack, C. H.: Staphylokinase: An activator of plasma protease. Nature 161:559, 1948.

60. Sako, T., Sawaki, S., Sakurai, T., Ito, S., Yoshizawa, Y., and Kondo, I.: Cloning and expression of the staphylokinase gene of Staphylococcus aureus in Escherichia coli. Mol. Gen. Genet. 190:271, 1983.

61. Sako, T.: Overproduction of staphylokinase in Escherichia coli and its characterization. Eur. J. Biochem. 149:557, 1985.

62. Behnke, D., and Gerlach, D.: Cloning and expression in Escherichia coli, Bacillus subtilis and Streptococcus sanguis of a gene for staphylokinase—a bacterial plasminogen activator. Mol. Gen. Genet. 210:528, 1987.

63. Kowalska-Loth, B., and Zakrzewski, K.: The activation by staphylokinase of human plasminogen. Acta Biochim. Pol. 22:327, 1975.

64. Matsuo, O., Okada, K., Fukao, H., Tomioka, Y., Ueshima, S., Watanuki, M., and Sakai, M.: Thrombolytic properties of staphylokinase. Blood 76:925, 1990.

65. Lijnen, H. R., Van Hoef, B., De Cock, F., Okada, K., Ueshima, S., Matsuo, O., and Collen, D.: On the mechanism of fibrin-specific plasminogen activation by staphylokinase. J. Biol. Chem. 266:11826, 1991.

66. Holmes, W. E., Nelles, L., Lijnen, H. R., and Collen, D.: Primary structure of human α2-antiplasmin, a serine protease inhibitor (serpin). J. Biol. Chem. 262:1659, 1987.

67. Müllertz, S., and Clemmensen, I.: The primary inhibitor of plasmin in human plasma. Biochem. J. 159:545, 1976.

68. Sasaki, T., Morita, T., and Iwanaga, S.: Identification of the plasminogen-binding site of human α2-plasmin inhibitor. Thromb. Haemost. 50:170, 1983 (abstract).

69. Wiman, B., Nilsson, T., and Cedergren, B.: Studies on a form of α2-antiplasmin in plasma which does not interact with the lysine-binding sites in plasminogen. Thromb. Res. 28:193, 1982.

70. Ichinose, A., Tamaki, T., and Aoki, N.: Factor XIII-mediated cross-linking of NH2-terminal peptide of α2-plasmin inhibitor to fibrin. FEBS Lett. 153:369, 1983.

71. Wiman, B., and Collen, D.: On the kinetics of the reaction between human antiplasmin and plasmin. Eur. J. Biochem. 84:573, 1978.

72. Kato, A., Nakamura, Y., Miura, O., Hirosawa, S., Sumi, Y., and Aoki, N.: Assignment of the human alpha 2-plasmin inhibitor gene (PLI) to chromosome region 18p11.1-q11.2 by in situ hybridization. Cytogenet. Cell Genet. 47:209, 1988.

73. Hirosawa, S., Nakamura, Y., Miura, O., Sumi, Y., and Aoki,

N.: Organization of the human α₂-plasmin inhibitor gene. Proc. Natl. Acad. Sci. USA 85:6836, 1988.

74. Miura, O., Sugahara, Y., Nakamura, Y., Hirosawa, S., and Aoki, N.: Restriction fragment length polymorphism caused by a deletion involving *Alu* sequences within the human α₂-plasmin inhibitor gene. Biochemistry 28:4934, 1989.

75. Kruithof, E. K. O.: Plasminogen activator inhibitors—A review. Enzyme 40:113, 1988.

76. Klinger, K. W., Winqvist, R., Riccio, A., Andreasen, P. A., Sartorio, R., Nielsen, L. S., Stuart, N., Stanislovitis, P., Watkins, P., Douglas, R., Grzeschik, H. K., Alitalo, K., Blasi, F., and Danø, K.: Plasminogen activator inhibitor type 1 gene is located at region q21.3-q22 of chromosome 7 and genetically linked with cystic fibrosis. Proc. Natl. Acad. Sci. USA 84:8548, 1987.

77. Ny, T., Sawdey, M., Lawrence, D., Millan, J. L., Loskutoff, D. J.: Cloning and sequence of a cDNA coding for the human β-migrating endothelial-cell-type plasminogen activator inhibitor. Proc. Natl. Acad. Sci. USA 83:6776, 1986.

78. Pannekoek, H., Veerman, H., Lambers, H., Diergaarde, P., Verweij, C. L., van Zonneveld, A. J., and van Mourik, J. A.: Endothelial plasminogen activator inhibitor (PAI): A new member of the serpin gene family. EMBO J. 5:2539, 1986.

79. Kruithof, E. K. O., Gudinchet, A., and Bachmann, F.: Plasminogen activator inhibitor 1 and plasminogen activator inhibitor 2 in various disease states. Thromb. Haemost. 59:7, 1988.

80. Declerck, P. J., De Mol, M., Alessi, M. C., Baudner, S., Pâques, E. P., Preissner, K. T., Müller-Berghaus, G., and Collen, D.: Purification and characterization of a plasminogen activator inhibitor-1 binding protein from human plasma. Identification as a multimeric form of S protein (Vitronectin). J. Biol. Chem. 263:15454, 1988.

81. Kruithof, E. K. O., Tran-Thang, C., Ransijn, A., and Bachmann, F.: Demonstration of a fast-acting inhibitor of plasminogen activators in human plasma. Blood 64:907, 1984.

82. Juhan-Vague, I., Moerman, B., De Cock, F., Aillaud, M. F., and Collen, D.: Plasma levels of a specific inhibitor of tissue-type plasminogen activator (and urokinase) in normal and pathological conditions. Thromb. Res. 33:523, 1984.

83. Hekman, C. M., and Loskutoff, D. J.: Endothelial cells produce a latent inhibitor of plasminogen activators that can be activated by denaturants. J. Biol. Chem. 260:11581, 1985.

84. Schleuning, W. D., Medcalf, R. L., Hession, C., Rothenbühler, R., Shaw, A., and Kruithof, E. K. O.: Plasminogen activator inhibitor 2: Regulation of gene transcription during phorbol ester-mediated differentiation of U-937 human histiocytic lymphoma cells. Mol. Cell. Biol. 7:4564, 1987.

85. Ye, R. D., Wun, T. C., and Sadler, J. E.: cDNA cloning and expression in *Escherichia coli* of a plasminogen activator inhibitor from human placenta. J. Biol. Chem. 262:3718, 1987.

86. Webb, A. C., Collins, K. L., Snyder, S. E., Alexander, S. J., Rosenwasser, L. J., Eddy, R. L., Shows, T. B., and Auron, P. E.: Human monocyte Arg-serpin cDNA. Sequence, chromosomal assignment, and homology to plasminogen activator-inhibitor. J. Exp. Med. 166:77, 1987.

87. Ye, R. D., Ahern, S. M., Le Beau, M. M., Lebo, R. V., and Sadler, J. E.: Structure of the gene for human plasminogen activator inhibitor-2. The nearest mammalian homologue of chicken ovalbumin. J. Biol. Chem. 264:5495, 1989.

88. Lecander, I., and Astedt, B.: Occurrence of a specific plasminogen activator inhibitor of placental type, PAI-2, in men and non-pregnant women. Fibrinolysis 3:27, 1989.

89. van Zonneveld, A. J., Veerman, H., and Pannekoek, H.: On the interaction of the finger and kringle-2 domain of tissue-type plasminogen activator with fibrin. J. Biol. Chem. 261:14214, 1986.

90. Higgins, D. L., and Vehar, G. A.: Interaction of one-chain and two-chain tissue plasminogen activator with intact and plasmin-degraded fibrin. Biochemistry 26:7786, 1987.

91. Suenson, E., Lützen, O., and Thorsen, S.: Initial plasmin-degradation of fibrin as the basis of a positive feed-back mechanism in fibrinolysis. Eur. J. Biochem. 140:513, 1984.

92. de Vries, C., Veerman, H., and Pannekoek, H.: Identification of the domains of tissue-type plasminogen activator involved in the augmented binding to fibrin after limited digestion with plasmin. J. Biol. Chem. 264:12604, 1989.

93. Suenson, E., and Petersen, L. C.: Fibrin and plasminogen structures essential to stimulation of plasmin formation by tissue-type plasminogen activator. Biochim. Biophys. Acta 870:510, 1986.

94. Suenson, E., Bjerrum, P., Holm, A., Lind, B., Meldal, M., Selmer, J., and Petersen, L. C.: The role of fragment X polymers in the fibrin enhancement of tissue plasminogen activator-catalyzed plasmin formation. J. Biol. Chem. 265:22288, 1990.

95. Collen, D., Zamarron, C., Lijnen, H. R., and Hoylaerts, M.: Activation of plasminogen by pro-urokinase. II. Kinetics. J. Biol. Chem. 261:1259, 1986.

96. Pannell, R., and Gurewich, V.: Pro-urokinase: A study of its stability in plasma and of a mechanism for its selective fibrinolytic effect. Blood 67:1215, 1986.

97. Gurewich, V.: The sequential, complementary and synergistic activation of fibrin-bound plasminogen by tissue plasminogen activator and pro-urokinase. Fibrinolysis 3:59, 1989.

98. Husain, S. S., Gurewich, V., and Lipinski, B.: Purification and partial characterization of a single-chain high-molecular-weight form of urokinase from human urine. Arch. Biochem. Biophys. 220:31, 1983.

99. Declerck, P. J., Lijnen, H. R., Verstreken, M., Moreau, H., and Collen, D.: A monoclonal antibody specific for two chain urokinase-type plasminogen activator. Application to the study of the mechanism of clot lysis with single-chain urokinase-type plasminogen activator in plasma. Blood 75:1794, 1990.

100. Collen, D., Mao, J., Stassen, J. M., Broeze, R., Lijnen, H. R., Abercrombie, D., Puma, P., Almeda, S., and Vovis, G.: Thrombolytic properties of Lys-158 mutants of recombinant single chain urokinase-type plasminogen activator (scu-PA) in rabbits with jugular vein thrombosis. J. Vasc. Med. Biol. 1:46, 1989.

101. Lijnen, H. R., Nelles, L., Holmes, W., and Collen, D.: Biochemical and thrombolytic properties of a low molecular weight form (comprising Leu¹⁴⁴ through Leu⁴¹¹) of recombinant single-chain urokinase-type plasminogen activator. J. Biol. Chem. 263:5594, 1988.

102. Lijnen, H. R., Stassen, J. M., Vanlinthout, I., Fukao, H., Okada, K., Matsuo, O., and Collen, D.: Comparative fibrinolytic properties of staphylokinase and streptokinase in animal models of venous thrombosis. Thromb. Haemost. 66:468, 1991.

103. Sakai, M., Watanuki, M., and Matsuo, O.: Mechanism of fibrin-specific fibrinolysis by staphylokinase: Participation of α₂-plasmin inhibitor. Biochem. Biophys. Res. Comm. 162:830, 1989.

104. Koie, K., Ogata, K., Kamiya, T., Takamatsu, J., and Kohakura, M.: α₂-plasmin-inhibitor deficiency (Miyasato disease). Lancet 2:1334, 1978.

105. Aoki, N., Saito, H., Kamiya, T., Koie, K., Sakata, Y., and Kohakura, M.: Congenital deficiency of α₂-plasmin inhibitor associated with severe hemorrhagic tendency. J. Clin. Invest. 63:877, 1979.

106. Kluft, C., Vellenga, E., and Brommer, E. J. P.: Homozygous α₂-antiplasmin deficiency. Lancet 2:206, 1979.

107. Kluft, C., Vellenga, E., Brommer, E. J. P., and Wijngaards, G. A.: A familial hemorrhagic diathesis in a Dutch family: An inherited deficiency of α₂-antiplasmin. Blood 59:1169, 1982.

108. Yoshioka, A., Kamitsuji, H., Takase, T., Iida, Y., Tsukada, S., Mikami, S., and Fukui, H.: Congenital deficiency of α₂-plasmin inhibitor in three sisters. Haemostasis 11:176, 1982.

109. Knot, E. A. R., ten Cate, J. W., Lamping, R. J., and Gie, L. K.: α₂-Antiplasmin: Functional characterization and metabolism in a heterozygote deficient patient. Thromb. Haemost. 55:375, 1986.

110. Stormorken, H., Gogstad, G. O., and Brosstad, F.: Hereditary α₂-antiplasmin deficiency. Thromb. Res. 31:647, 1983.

111. Kordich, L., Feldman, L., Porterie, P., and Lago, O.: Severe

hemorrhagic tendency in heterozygous α_2-antiplasmin deficiency. Thromb. Res. 40:645, 1985.

112. Miles, L. A., Plow, E. F., Donnelly, K. J., Hougie, C., and Griffin, J. H.: A bleeding disorder due to deficiency of α_2-antiplasmin. Blood 59:1246, 1982.

113. Kettle, P., and Mayne, E. E.: A bleeding disorder due to deficiency of alpha 2-antiplasmin. J. Clin. Pathol. 38:428, 1985.

114. Leebeek, F. W., Stibbe, J., Knot, E. A., Kluft, C., Gomes, M. J., and Beudeker, M.: Mild haemostatic problems associated with congenital heterozygous alpha 2-antiplasmin deficiency. Thromb. Haemost. 59:96, 1988.

115. Miura, O., Sugahara, Y., and Aoki, N.: Hereditary α_2-plasmin inhibitor deficiency caused by a transport-deficient mutation (α_2-PI-Okinawa). Deletion of Glu[137] by a trinucleotide deletion blocks intracellular transport. J. Biol. Chem. 264:18213, 1989.

116. Miura, O., Hirosawa, S., Kato, A., and Aoki, N.: Molecular basis for congenital deficiency of α_2-plasmin inhibitor. A frameshift mutation leading to elongation of the deduced amino acid sequence. J. Clin. Invest. 83:1598, 1989.

117. Teger-Nilsson, A. C., Gyzander, E., Myrwold, E., Noppa, H., Olsson, R., and Wallmo, L.: Determination of fast-acting plasmin inhibitor (α_2-anti-plasmin) in plasma from patients with tendency to thrombosis and increased fibrinolysis. Haemostasis 7:155, 1978.

118. Aoki, N., and Yamanaka, T.: The α_2-plasmin inhibitor levels in liver diseases. Clin. Chim. Acta 84:99, 1978.

119. Williams, E. C.: Plasma alpha 2-antiplasmin activity. Role in the evaluation and management of fibrinolytic states and other bleeding disorders. Arch. Intern. Med. 149:1769, 1989.

120. Högstorp, H., Jacobsson, H., and Saldeen, T.: Effect of hepatectomy on the posttraumatic fibrinolysis inhibition and the primary fibrinolysis inhibitor in the rat. Thromb. Res. 18:361, 1980.

121. Avvisati, G., ten Cate, J. W., Sturk, A., Lamping, R., Petti, M. C., and Mandelli, F.: Acquired alpha-2-antiplasmin deficiency in acute promyelocytic leukaemia. Br. J. Haematol. 70:43, 1988.

122. Collen, D., Bounameaux, H., De Cock, F., Lijnen, H. R., and Verstraete, M.: Analysis of coagulation and fibrinolysis during intravenous infusion of recombinant human tissue-type plasminogen activator in patients with acute myocardial infarction. Circulation 73:511, 1986.

123. Nieuwenhuis, H. K., Kluft, C., Wijngaards, G., van Berkel, W., and Sixma, J. J.: Alpha 2-antiplasmin Enschede: An autosomal recessive hemorrhagic disorder caused by a dysfunctional alpha 2-antiplasmin molecule. Thromb. Haemost. 50:170, 1983 (abstract 528).

124. Holmes, W. E., Lijnen, H. R., Nelles, L., Kluft, C., Nieuwenhuis, H. K., Rijken, D. C., and Collen, D.: α_2-Antiplasmin Enschede: Alanine insertion and abolition of plasmin inhibitory activity. Science 238:209, 1987.

125. Erickson, L. A., Fici, G. J., Lund, J. E., Boyle, T. P., Polites, H. G., and Marotti, K. R.: Development of venous occlusions in mice transgenic for the plasminogen activator inhibitor-1 gene. Nature 346:74, 1990.

126. Krishnamurti, C., Barr, C. F., Hassett, M. A., Young, G. D., and Alving, B. M.: Plasminogen activator inhibitor: A regulator of ancrod-induced fibrin deposition in rabbits. Blood 69:798, 1987.

127. Páramo, J. A., Colucci, M., Collen, D., and Van de Werf, F.: Plasminogen activator inhibitor in the blood of patients with coronary artery disease. Br. Med. J. 291:573, 1985.

128. Mehta, J., Mehta, P., Lawson, D., and Saldeen, T.: Plasma tissue plasminogen activator inhibitor levels in coronary artery disease: Correlation with age and serum triglyceride concentrations. J. Am. Coll. Cardiol. 9:263, 1987.

129. Almér, L. O., and Öhlin, H.: Elevated levels of the rapid inhibitor of plasminogen activator (t-PAI) in acute myocardial infarction. Thromb. Res. 47:335, 1987.

130. Verheugt, F. W. A., ten Cate, J. W., Sturk, A., Imandt, L., Van Verhorst, P. M. J., Eenige, M. J., Verwey, W., and Roos, J. P.: Tissue plasminogen activator activity and inhibition in acute myocardial infarction and angiographically normal coronary arteries. Am. J. Cardiol. 59:1075, 1987.

131. Hamsten, A., Wiman, B., de Faire, U., and Blombäck, M.: Increased plasma levels of a rapid inhibitor of tissue plasminogen activator in young survivors of myocardial infarction. N. Engl. J. Med. 213:1557, 1985.

132. Hamsten, A., Blombäck, M., Wiman, B., Svensson, J., Szamosi, A., de Faire, U., and Mettinger, L.: Haemostatic function in myocardial infarction. Br. Heart J. 55:58, 1986.

133. Hamsten, A., de Faire, U., Walldius, G., Dahlen, G., Szamosi, A., Landou, C., Blombäck, M., and Wiman, B.: Plasminogen activator inhibitor in plasma: Risk factor for recurrent myocardial infarction. Lancet 2:3, 1987.

134. Nilsson, T. K., and Johnson, O.: The extrinsic fibrinolytic system in survivors of myocardial infarction. Thromb. Res. 48:621, 1987.

135. Aznar, J., Estellés, A., Tormo, G., Sapena, P., Tormo, V., Blanch, S., and Espana, F.: Plasminogen activator inhibitor activity and other fibrinolytic variables in patients with coronary artery disease. Br. Heart J. 59:535, 1988.

136. Francis, R. B., Jr., Kawanishi, D., Baruch, T., Mahrer, P., Rahimtoola, S., and Feinstein, D. I.: Impaired fibrinolysis in coronary artery disease. Am. Heart J. 115:776, 1988.

137. Huber, K., Rosc, D., Resch, I., Schuster, E., Glogar, D. H., Kaindl, F., and Binder, B. R.: Circadian fluctuations of plasminogen activator inhibitor and tissue plasminogen activator levels in plasma of patients with unstable coronary artery disease and acute myocardial infarction. Thromb. Haemost. 60:372, 1988.

138. Olofsson, B. O., Dahlen, G., and Nilsson, T. K.: Evidence for increased levels of plasminogen activator inhibitor and tissue plasminogen activator in plasma of patients with angiographically verified coronary artery disease. Eur. Heart J. 10:77, 1989.

139. Gram, J., Jespersen, J., Kluft, C., and Rijken, D. C.: On the usefulness of fibrinolysis variables in the characterization of a risk group for myocardial reinfarction. Acta Med. Scand. 221:149, 1987.

140. Wiman, B., and Hamsten, A.: The fibrinolytic enzyme system and its role in the etiology of thromboembolic disease. Sem. Thromb. Haemost. 16:207, 1990.

141. Muller, J. E., Stone, P. H., Turi, Z. G., Rutherford, J. D., Czeisler, C. A., Parker, C., Poole, W. K., Passamani, E., Roberts, R., and Robertson, T., et al.: Circadian variation in the frequency of onset of acute myocardial infarction. N. Engl. J. Med. 313:1315, 1985.

142. Juhan-Vague, I., Alessi, M. C., Joly, P., Thirion, X., Vague, P., Declerck, P. J., Serradimigni, A., and Collen, D.: Plasma plasminogen activator inhibitor-1 in angina pectoris. Influence of plasma insulin and acute-phase response. Arteriosclerosis 9:362, 1989.

143. Oseroff, A., Krishnamurti, C., Hassett, A., Tang, D., and Alving, B.: Plasminogen activator and plasminogen activator inhibitor activities in men with coronary artery disease. J. Lab. Clin. Med. 113:88, 1989.

144. Prins, M. H., and Hirsh, J.: A critical review of the relationship between impaired fibrinolysis and myocardial infarction. Am. Heart J. 122:545, 1991.

145. Vague, P., Juhan-Vague, I., Aillaud, M. F., Badier, C., Viard, R., Alessi, M. C., and Collen, D.: Correlation between blood fibrinolytic activity, plasminogen activator inhibitor level, plasma insulin level and relative body weight in normal and obese subjects. Metabolism 35:250, 1986.

146. Juhan-Vague, I., Vague, P., Alessi, M. C., Badier, C., Valadier, J., Aillaud, M. F., and Atlan, C.: Relationships between plasma insulin, triglyceride, body mass index, and plasminogen activator inhibitor-1. Diab. Metabol. 13:331, 1987.

147. Vague, P., Juhan-Vague, I., Chabert, V., Alessi, M. C., and Atlan, C.: Fat distribution and plasminogen activator inhibitor activity in nondiabetic obese women. Metabolism 38:913, 1989.

148. Juhan-Vague, I., Roul, C., Alessi, M. C., Ardissone, J. P., Heim, M., and Vague, P.: Increased plasminogen activator

inhibitor activity in non insulin dependent diabetic patients. Relationship with plasma insulin. Thromb. Haemost. 61:370, 1989.

149. Vague, P., Juhan-Vague, I., Alessi, M. C., Badier, C., and Valadier, J.: Metformin decreases the high plasminogen activator inhibition capacity, plasma insulin and triglyceride levels in non-diabetic obese subjects. Thromb. Haemost. 57:326, 1987.

150. Dawson, S., Hamsten, A., Wiman, B., Henney, A., and Humphries, S.: Genetic variation at the plasminogen activator inhibitor-1 locus is associated with altered levels of plasma plasminogen activator inhibitor-1 activity. Arteriosclerosis Thrombosis 11:183, 1991.

151. Riccio, A., Lund, L., Sartorio, R., Lania, A., Andreasen, P., Danø, K., and Blasi, F.: The regulatory region of the human plasminogen activator inhibitor type-1 gene. Nucleic Acids Res. 16:2805, 1988.

152. Hasegawa, D. K., Tyler, B. J., and Edson, J. R.: Thrombotic disease in three families with inherited plasminogen deficiency. Blood 60 (Suppl 1):213a, 1982 (abstract 780).

153. Ten Cate, J. W., Peters, M., and Büller, H.: Isolated plasminogen deficiency in a patient with recurrent thromboembolic complications. Thromb. Haemost. 50:59, 1983 (abstract 0166).

154. Lottenberg, R., Dolly, F. R., and Kitchens, C. S.: Recurring thromboembolic disease and pulmonary hypertension associated with severe hypoplasminogenemia. Am. J. Hematol. 19:181, 1985.

155. Mannucci, P. M., Kluft, C., Traas, D. W., Seveso, P., and D'Angelo, A.: Congenital plasminogen deficiency associated with venous thromboembolism: Therapeutic trial with stanozolol. Br. J. Haematol. 63:753, 1986.

156. Girolami, A., Marafioti, F., Rubertelli, M., and Cappellato, M. G.: Congenital heterozygous plasminogen deficiency associated with a severe thrombotic tendency. Acta Haematol. 75:54, 1986.

157. Hach-Wunderle, V., Scharrer, I., and Lottenberg, R.: Congenital deficiency of plasminogen and its relationship to venous thrombosis. Thromb. Haemost. 59:277, 1988.

158. Dolan, G., Greaves, M., Cooper, P., and Preston, F. E.: Thrombovascular disease and familial plasminogen deficiency: A report of three kindreds. Br. J. Haematol. 70:417, 1988.

159. Leebeek, F. W., Knot, E. A., ten Cate, J. W., and Traas, D. W.: Severe thrombotic tendency associated with a type I plasminogen deficiency. Am. J. Hematol. 30:32, 1989.

160. Davis, R. D., and Picoff, R. C.: Low plasminogen levels and liver disease. Am. J. Clin. Pathol. 59:661, 1969.

161. Kordich, L. C., Porterie, V. P., Lago, O., Bergonzelli, G. E., Sasseti, B., and Sanchez Avalos, J. C.: Mini-plasminogen like molecule in septic patients. Thromb. Res. 47:553, 1987.

162. Verstraete, M., Vermylen, J., and Collen, D.: Intravascular coagulation in liver disease. Ann. Rev. Med. 25:447, 1974.

163. Robbins, K. C.: Classification of abnormal plasminogens: Dysplasminogenemias. Semin. Thromb. Haemost. 16:217, 1990.

164. Aoki, N., Moroi, M., Sakata, Y., Yoshida, N., and Matsuda, M.: Abnormal plasminogen. A hereditary molecular abnormality found in a patient with recurrent thrombosis. J. Clin. Invest. 61:1186, 1978.

165. Miyata, T., Iwanaga, S., Sakata, Y., and Aoki, N.: Plasminogen Tochigi: Inactive plasmin resulting from replacement of alanine-600 by threonine in the active site. Proc. Natl. Acad. Sci. USA 79:6132, 1982.

166. Ichinose, A., Espling, E. S., Takamatsu, J., Saito, H., Shinmyozu, K., Maruyama, I., Petersen, T. E., and Davie, E. W.: Two types of abnormal genes for plasminogen in families with a predisposition for thrombosis. Proc. Natl. Acad. Sci. USA 88:115, 1991.

167. Miyata, T., Iwanaga, S., Sakata, Y., Aoki, N., Takamatsu, J., and Kamiya, T.: Plasminogens Tochigi II and Nagoya: Two additional molecular defects with Ala 600 → Thr replacement found in plasmin light chain variants. J. Biochem. 96:277, 1984.

168. Kazama, M., Tahara, C., Suzuki, Z., Gohchi, K., and Abe, T.: Abnormal plasminogen, a case of recurrent thrombosis. Thromb. Res. 21:517, 1981.

169. Soria, J., Soria, C., Bertrand, O., Dunn, F., Drouet, L., and Caen, J. P.: Plasminogen Paris I. Congenital abnormal plasminogen and its incidence in thrombosis. Thromb. Res. 32:229, 1983.

170. Aoki, N., Tateno, K., and Sakata, Y.: Differences of frequency distributions of plasminogen phenotypes between Japanese and American populations: New methods for the detection of plasminogen variants. Biochem. Genet. 22:871, 1984.

171. Nakamura, S., and Abe, K.: Genetic polymorphism of human plasminogen in the Japanese population: New plasminogen variants and relationship between plasminogen phenotypes and their biological activities. Hum. Genet. 60:57, 1982.

172. Wohl, R. C., Summaria, L., and Robbins, K. C.: Physiological activation of the human fibrinolytic system. Isolation and characterization of human plasminogen variants, Chicago I and Chicago II. J. Biol. Chem. 254:9063, 1979.

173. Wohl, R. C., Summaria, L., Chediak, J., Rosenfeld, S., and Robbins, K. C.: Human plasminogen variant Chicago III. Thromb. Haemost. 48:146, 1982.

174. Scharrer, I. M., Wohl, R. C., Hach, V., Sinio, L., Boreisha, I., and Robbins, K. C.: Investigation of a congenital abnormal plasminogen, Frankfurt I, and its relationship to thrombosis. Thromb. Haemostas. 55:396, 1986.

175. Robbins, K. C., and Godwin, J. E.: Abnormal fibrinogen, Maywood I. Thromb. Haemost. 62:83 (abstract 236), 1989.

176. Robbins, K. C., Boreisha, I. G., Hach-Wunderle, V., and Scharrer, I.: Congenital plasminogen deficiency with an abnormal plasminogen: Frankfurt II, dysplasminogenemia-hypoplasminogenemia. Fibrinolysis 5:145, 1991.

177. Clayton, K. J., Anderson, J. A., and McNicol, G. P.: Preoperative prediction of postoperative deep vein thrombosis. Br. Med. J. 2:910, 1976.

178. Rákóczi, I., Chamone, D., Collen, D., and Verstraete, M.: Prediction of postoperative leg-vein thrombosis in gynaecological patients. Lancet 1:509, 1978.

179. Lowe, G. D. O., McArdle, B. M., Carter, D. C., McLaren, D., Osborne, D. H., Smith, A., Forbes, C. D., and Prentice, C. R. M.: Prediction and selective prophylaxis of venous thrombosis in elective gastrointestinal surgery. Lancet 1:409, 1982.

180. Isacson, S., and Nilsson, I. M.: Defective fibrinolysis in blood and vein walls in recurrent "idiopathic" venous thrombosis. Acta Chir. Scand. 138:313, 1972.

181. Korninger, C., Lechner, K., Niessner, H., Gössinger, H., and Kundi, M.: Impaired fibrinolytic capacity predisposes for recurrence of venous thrombosis. Thromb. Haemost. 52:127, 1984.

182. Nilsson, I.M., Ljungner, H., and Tengborn, L.: Two different mechanisms in patients with venous thrombosis and defective fibrinolysis: Low concentration of plasminogen activator or increased concentration of plasminogen activator inhibitor. Br. Med. J. 290:1453, 1985.

183. Juhan-Vague, I., Valadier, J., Alessi, M. C., Aillaud, M. F., Ansaldi, J., Philip-Joet, C., Holvoet, P., Serradimigni, A., and Collen, D.: Deficient t-PA release and elevated PA inhibitor levels in patients with spontaneous or recurrent deep venous thrombosis. Thromb. Haemost. 57:67, 1987.

184. Jorgensen, M., and Bonnevie-Nielsen, V.: Increased concentration of the fast-acting plasminogen activator inhibitor in plasma associated with familial venous thrombosis. Br. J. Haematol. 65:175, 1987.

185. Booth, N. A., Bennett, B., Wijngaards, G., and Grieve, J. H. K.: A new life-long hemorrhagic disorder due to excess plasminogen activator. Blood 61:267, 1983.

186. Aznar, J., Estellés, A., Villa, V., Reganon, E., Espana, F., and Villa, P.: Inherited fibrinolytic disorder due to an enhanced plasminogen activator level. Thromb. Haemost. 52:196, 1984.

187. Schleef, R. R., Higgins, D. L., Pillemer, E., and Levitt, L. J.: Bleeding diathesis due to decreased functional activity of type 1 plasminogen activator inhibitor. J. Clin. Invest. 83:1747, 1989.

188. Diéval, J., Nguyen, G., Gross, S., Delobel, J., and Kruithof, E.

K. O.: A lifelong bleeding disorder associated with a deficiency of plasminogen activator inhibitor type 1. Blood 77:528, 1991.

189. United States Department of Health and Human Services: DHHS Publication No (PHS)85-1232. Hyattsville, MD, National Center for Health Statistics, 1984.

190. De Wood, M. A., Spores, J., Notske, R., Lowell, T., Mouser, T., Burroughs, R., Golden, M. S., and Lang, H. T.: Prevalence of total coronary occlusion during the early hours of transmural myocardial infarction. N. Engl. J. Med. 303:897, 1980.

191. Mohr, J. P., Caplan, L. R., Melski, J. W., Goldstein, R. J., Duncan, G. W., Kistler, J. P., Pessin, M. S., and Bleich, H. L.: The Harvard cooperative stroke registry: A prospective registry. Neurology 28:754, 1978.

192. Rentrop, K. P.: Thrombolytic therapy in patients with acute myocardial infarction. Circulation 71:627, 1985.

193. Braunwald, E.: Myocardial reperfusion, limitation of infarct size, reduction of left ventricular dysfunction, and improved survival. Should the paradigm be expanded? Circulation 79:441, 1989.

194. Gold, H. K.: Conjunctive antithrombotic and thrombolytic therapy for coronary-artery occlusion. N. Engl. J. Med. 323:1483, 1990.

195. Chesebro, J. H., Knatterud, G., and Braunwald, E.: Thrombolytic therapy. Correspondence. N. Engl. J. Med. 319:1544, 1988.

196. Collen, D.: Coronary thrombolysis: Streptokinase or recombinant tissue-type plasminogen activator? Ann. Intern. Med. 112:529, 1990.

197. Collen, D.: On the future of thrombolytic therapy in acute myocardial infarction. In Haber, E., and Braunwald, E. (eds.): Thrombolysis: Basic Contributions and Clinical Progress. St Louis, Mosby-Year Book, 1991, pp. 315–331.

198. The International Study Group: In-hospital mortality and clinical course of 20,891 patients with suspected acute myocardial infarction randomised between alteplase and streptokinase with or without heparin. Lancet 336:71, 1990.

199. ISIS-3 (Third International Study of Infarct Survival) Collaborative Group: ISIS-3: A randomized comparison of streptokinase vs. tissue plasminogen activator vs. anistreplase and of aspirin plus heparin vs. aspirin alone among 41,299 cases of suspected acute myocardial infarction. Lancet 339:753, 1992.

200. Topol, E. J., George, B. S., Kereiakes, D. J., Stump, D. C., Candela, R. J., Abbottsmith, C. W., Aronson, L., Pickel, A., Boswick, J. M., Lee, K. L., Ellis, S. G., Califf, R. M., and the TAMI Study Group: A randomized controlled trial of intravenous tissue plasminogen activator and early intravenous heparin in acute myocardial infarction. Circulation 79:281, 1989.

201. Hsia, J., Hamilton, W. P., Kleiman, N., Roberts, R., Chaitman, B. R., and Ross, A. M., for the Heparin-Aspirin Reperfusion Trial (HART) investigators: A comparison between heparin and low-dose aspirin as adjunctive therapy with tissue plasminogen activator for acute myocardial infarction. N. Engl. J. Med. 323:1433, 1990.

202. Bleich, S. D., Nichols, T. C., Schumacher, R. R., Cooke, D. H., Tate, D. A., and Teichman, S. L.: Effect of heparin on coronary arterial patency after thrombolysis with tissue plasminogen activator in acute myocardial infarction. Am. J. Cardiol. 66:1412, 1990.

203. de Bono, D. P., Simoons, M. L., Tijssen, J., Arnold, A. E., Betriu, A., Burgersdijk, C., Lopez Bescos, L., Mueller, E., Pfisterer, M., Van de Werf, F., Zÿlstra, F., Verstraete, M.: Effect of early intravenous heparin on coronary patency, infarct size, and bleeding complications after alteplase thrombolysis: Results of a randomised double blind European Cooperative Study Group trial. Br. Heart J. 67:122, 1992.

204. The SCATI (Studio sulla Calciparina nell'Angina e nella Trombosi Ventricolare nell'Infarto) Group: Randomised controlled trial of subcutaneous calcium-heparin in acute myocardial infarction. Lancet 2:182, 1989.

205. The TIMI Research Group: Immediate vs delayed catheterization and angioplasty following thrombolytic therapy for acute myocardial infarction. TIMI II A results. J. A. M. A. 260:2849, 1988.

206. The TIMI Study Group: Comparison of invasive and conservative strategies after treatment with intravenous tissue plasminogen activator in acute myocardial infarction. Results of the thrombolysis in myocardial infarction (TIMI) Phase II Trial. N. Engl. J. Med. 320:618, 1989.

207. Verstraete, M., Bernard, R., Bory, M., Brower, R. W., Collen, D., de Bono, D. P., Erbel, R., Huhmann, W., Lennane, R. J., Lubsen, J., Mathey, D., Meyer, J., Michels, H. R., Rutsch, W., Schartl, M., Schmidt, W., Uebis, R., and von Essen, R.: Randomized trial of intravenous recombinant tissue-type plasminogen activator versus intravenous streptokinase in acute myocardial infarction. Lancet 1:842, 1985.

208. The TIMI Study Group: The Thrombolysis in Myocardial Infarction (TIMI) trial: Phase I findings. N. Engl. J. Med. 312:932, 1985.

209. White, H. J., Rivers, J. T., Maslowski, A. H., Ormiston, J. A., Takayama, M., Hart, H. H., Sharpe, D. N., Whitlock, R. M. L., and Norris, R. M.: Effect of intravenous streptokinase as compared with that of tissue plasminogen activator on left ventricular function after first myocardial infarction. N. Engl. J. Med. 320:817, 1989.

210. Magnani, B., for the PAIMS Investigators: Plasminogen Activator Italian Multicenter Study (PAIMS). Comparison of intravenous recombinant single-chain human tissue-type plasminogen activator (rt-PA) with intravenous streptokinase in acute myocardial infarction. J. Am. Coll. Cardiol. 13:19, 1989.

211. Califf, R. M., Topol, E. J., Stack, R. S., Ellis, S. G., George, B. S., Kereiakes, D. J., Samaha, J. K., Worley, S. J., Anderson, J. L., Harrelson-Woodlief, L., Wall, T. C., Phillips, H. R., III, Abbottsmith, C. W., Candela, R. J., Flanagan, W. H., Sasahara, A. A., Mantell, S. J., and Lee, K. L., for the TAMI Study Group: Evaluation of combination thrombolytic therapy and timing of cardiac catheterization in acute myocardial infarction. Results of thrombolysis and angioplasty in myocardial infarction—phase 5 randomized trial. Circulation 83:1543, 1991.

212. Neuhaus, T. L., Tebbe, U., Gottwick, M., Weber, M. A. J., Feuerer, W., Niederer, W., Haerer, W., Praetorius, F., Grosser, K. D., Huhmann, W., Hoepp, H. W., Alber, B. G., Sheikhzadeh, A., and Schneider, B.: Intravenous recombinant tissue plasminogen activator (rt-PA) and urokinase in acute myocardial infarction: Results of the German activator urokinase study (GAUS). J. Am. Coll. Cardiol. 12:581, 1988.

213. Neuhaus, K.: The t-PA versus APSAC patency study (TAPS). Presented at the American college of cardiology meeting, Atlanta, GA, 1991.

214. ISIS-2 (Second International Study of Infarct Survival) Collaborative Group: Randomised trial of intravenous streptokinase, oral aspirin, both, or neither among 17,187 cases of suspected acute myocardial infarction: ISIS-2. Lancet 2:349, 1988.

215. Vaughan, D. E., Declerck, P. J., De Mol, M., and Collen, D.: Recombinant plasminogen activator inhibitor-1 reverses the bleeding tendency associated with combined administration of tissue-type plasminogen activator and aspirin in rabbits. J. Clin. Invest. 84:586, 1989.

216. Garabedian, H. D., Gold, H. K., Leinbach, R. C., Svizzero, T. A., Finkelstein, D. M., Guerrero, J. L., and Collen, D.: Correlation of bleeding with template bleeding times and hemostasis parameters during separate and combined administration of recombinant tissue-type plasminogen activator, aspirin and aprotinin in dogs. J. Am. Coll. Cardiol. 17:1213, 1991.

217. Gimple, L. W., Gold, H. K., Leinbach, R. C., Coller, B. S., Werner, W., Yasuda, T., Johns, J. A., Ziskind, A. A., Finkelstein, D., and Collen, D.: Correlation between template bleeding times and spontaneous bleeding during treatment of acute myocardial infarction with recombinant tissue-type plasminogen activator. Circulation 80:581, 1989.

218. Van de Werf, F., and Arnold, A. E. R.: Intravenous tissue plasminogen activator and size of infarct, left ventricular function, and survival in acute myocardial infarction. Br. Med. J. 297:1374, 1988.

219. Mueller, H. S., Rao, A. K., and Forman, S. A.: Thrombolysis in myocardial infarction (TIMI): Comparative studies of coronary reperfusion and systemic fibrinogenolysis with two forms of recombinant tissue-type plasminogen activator. J. Am. Coll. Cardiol. 10:479, 1987.

220. Goldhaber, S. Z., Buring, J. E., Lipnick, R. J., and Hennekens, C. H.: Pooled analysis of randomized trials of streptokinase and heparin in phlebographically documented acute deep venous thrombosis. Am. J. Med. 76:393, 1984.

221. Rösch, J., Dotter, C. T., Seaman, H. J., Porter, J. M., and Common, H. H.: Healing of deep venous thrombosis: Venographic findings in a randomized study comparing streptokinase and heparin. Am. J. Roentgenol. 127:553, 1976.

222. Kakkar, V. V., Howe, C. T., Laws, J. S., and Flanc, C.: Late results of treatment of deep vein thrombosis. Br. Med. J. 1:810, 1969.

223. Bieger, R., Boekhout-Mussert, R. J., Hohmann, F., and Loeliger, E. A.: Is streptokinase useful in the treatment of deep vein thrombosis? Acta Med. Scand. 199:81, 1976.

224. Elliot, M. S., Immelman, E. J., Jeffery, P., Benatar, S. R., Funston, M. R., Smith, J. A., Shepstone, B. J., Ferguson, A. D., Jacobs, P., Walker, W., and Louw, J. H.: A comparative randomized trial of heparin versus streptokinase in the treatment of acute proximal venous thrombosis: An interim report of a prospective trial. Br. J. Surg. 66:838, 1979.

225. Kakkar, V. V., and Lawrence, D.: Hemodynamic and clinical assessment after therapy for acute vein thrombosis. A prospective study. Am. J. Surg. 150:54, 1985.

226. Common, H. H., Seaman, A. J., Rösch, J., Porter, J. M., and Dotter, C. T.: Deep vein thrombosis treated with streptokinase or heparin. Follow-up of a randomized study. Angiology 27:645, 1976.

227. Arnesen, M., Høiseth, A., and Ly, B.: Streptokinase or heparin in the treatment of deep vein thrombosis. Acta Med. Scand. 211:65, 1982.

228. Widmer, L. K., Brandenberg, E., and Widmer, M. T.: Late sequelae of deep vein thrombosis. Int. Angiol. 1:31, 1982.

229. Eichlisberger, R., Widmer, M. T., Widmer, L. K., and Zemp, E.: Spätfolgen nach Becken-Bein-Venenthrombose. Basler Erfahrungen. Vasa (Suppl.) 20:95, 1987.

230. Martin, M., and Fiebach, B. J. O.: Die Streptokinase-Behandlung peripherer Arterien-und Venenverschlüsse unter besonderer Berücksichtigung der ultrahöhen Dosierung. Bern, Verlag H. Huber, 1985.

231. Lechler, E., Meyer-Börnecke, D., Winter, U. J., and Schulz, V.: Intermittent high dosage scheme of streptokinase/urokinase in fibrinolytic therapy. Thromb. Haemost. 54:272, 1985 (abstract 1613).

232. Theiss, W., Bauman, G., and Klein, G.: Fibrinolytische Behandlung tiefer Venenthrombosen mit Streptokinase in ultrahoher Dosierung. Dtsch. Med. Wochenschr. 112:668, 1987.

233. Koch, H. U.: Lysetherapie tiefer Phlebotrombosen mit ultrahochdosierter Streptokinase gefolgt von konventionell dosierter Urokinase. Med. Welt 39:245, 1988.

234. Conard, J., Samama, M., Milochevitch, R., Horellou, M. H., Chabrun, B., and Prestat, J.: Complications hémorragiques au cours de 98 traitements par la streptokinase. Place de la surveillance biologique. Nouv. Presse Méd. 8:1319, 1979.

235. van de Loo, J. C. W., Kriesmann, A., Trübestein, G., Knoch, K., de Swart, C. A. M., Asbeck, F., Marbet, G. A., Schmitt, H. E., Sewell, A. F., Duckert, F., Theiss, W., and Ritz, R.: Controlled multicenter pilot study of urokinase—heparin and streptokinase in deep vein thrombosis. Thromb. Haemost. 50:660, 1983.

236. Turpie, A. G. G., Jay, R. M., Carter, C. J., and Hirsh, J. A.: A randomized trial of recombinant tissue plasminogen activator for the treatment of proximal deep vein thrombosis. Circulation 72 (Suppl. III):193, 1985 (abstract 770).

237. Turpie, A. G. G.: Thrombolytic therapy in venous thromboembolism. In Sobel, B. E., Collen, D., Grossbard, E. B. (eds.): Tissue Plasminogen Activator in Thrombolytic Therapy. Basel, Marcel Dekker, 1987, pp. 131–146.

238. Turpie, A. G. G.: Thrombolysis in deep vein thrombosis. In Julian, D., Kübler, W., Norris, R. M., et al (eds.): Thrombolysis in Cardiovascular Disease. Basel, Marcel Dekker, 1989, pp. 397–408.

239. Verhaeghe, R., Besse, P., Bounameaux, H., and Marbet, G. A.: Multicenter pilot study of the efficacy and safety of systemic rt-PA administration in the treatment of deep vein thrombosis of the lower extremities and/or pelvis. Thromb. Res. 55:5, 1989.

240. Zimmermann, R., Horn, A., Harenberg, J., Diehm, C., Müller-Bühl, U., and Kübler, W.: Thrombolysetherapy der tiefen venösen Thrombose mit rt-PA. Klin. Wochenschr. 66 (Suppl. XII):137, 1988.

241. Urokinase Pulmonary Embolism Study Group: The Urokinase Pulmonary Embolism Trial (UPET). A national cooperative study. Circulation 47 (Suppl. 2):1, 1973.

242. Urokinase Pulmonary Embolism Trial Study Group: Urokinase-streptokinase embolism trial. Phase 2 results. J. A. M. A. 229:1606, 1974.

243. Groupe de Recherche Urokinase-Embolie Pulmonaire: Etude multicentrique sur deux protocoles d'urokinase dans l'embolie pulmonaire grave. Arch. Mal. Coeur 77:773, 1984.

244. François, G., Charbonnier, B., Raynaud, P., Garnier, L. F., Griguer, P., and Brochier, M.: Traitement de l'embolie pulmonaire aiguë par urokinase comparée à l'association plasminogène-urokinase. A propos de 67 cas. Arch. Mal. Coeur 79:435, 1986.

245. Sharma, G. V. R. K., O'Connell, D. J., Blelko, J. S., and Sasahara, A. A.: Thrombolytic therapy in deep vein thrombosis. In Paoletti, R., and Sherry, S. (eds.): Thrombosis and Urokinase. New York, Academic Press, 1977, p. 181.

246. Petitpretz, P., Simmoneau, G., Cerrina, J., Musset, D., Dreyfus, M., Vandenbroeck, M. D., and Duroux, P.: Effects of a single bolus of urokinase in patients with life-threatening pulmonary emboli: A descriptive trial. Circulation 70:861, 1984.

247. Stern, M., Meyer, G., and Sors, H.: Urokinase versus tissue plasminogen activator in pulmonary embolism. Lancet 2:691, 1988.

248. Goldhaber, S. Z., Markis, J. E., Meyerovitz, M. F., Kim, D. S., Dawley, D. L., Sasahara, A. A., Vaughan, D. E., Selwyn, A. P., Loscalzo, J., Kessler, C. M., Sharma, G. V. R. K., Grossbard, E. B., and Braunwald, E.: Acute pulmonary embolism treated with tissue plasminogen activator. Lancet 2:886, 1986.

249. Come, P. C., Kim, D., Parker, A., Goldhaber, S. Z., Braunwald, E., and Markis, J. E.: Early reversal of right ventricular dysfunction in patients with acute pulmonary embolism after treatment with intravenous tissue plasminogen activator. J. Am. Coll. Cardiol. 10:971, 1987.

250. Verstraete, M., Miller, G. A. H., Bounameaux, H., Charbonnier, B., Colle, J. P., Lecorf, G., Marbet, G. A., Mombaerts, P., and Olsson, C. G.: Intravenous and intrapulmonary recombinant tissue-type plasminogen activator in the treatment of acute massive pulmonary embolism. Circulation 77:353, 1988.

251. Goldhaber, S. Z., Kessler, C. M., Heit, J., Markis, J., Sharma, G. V. R. K., Dawley, D., Nagel, J. S., Meyerovitz, M., Kim, D., Vaughan, D. E., Parker, J. A., Tumeh, S. S., Drum, D., Loscalzo, J., Reagan, K., Selwyn, A. P., Anderson, J., and Braunwald, E.: Randomised controlled trial of recombinant tissue plasminogen activator versus urokinase in the treatment of acute pulmonary embolism. Lancet 2:293, 1988.

252. Amery, A., Deloof, W., Vermylen, J., and Verstraete, M.: Outcome of recent thromboembolic occlusions of limb arteries treated with streptokinase. Br. Med. J. 4:639, 1970.

253. Martin, M., Schoop, W., and Zeitler, E.: Streptokinase in chronic arterial occlusive disease. J. A. M. A. 211:1169, 1970.

254. Martin, M.: Thrombolytic therapy in arterial thromboembolism. Progr. Cardiovasc. Dis. 21:351, 1979.

255. Verstraete, M., Vermylen, J., and Donati, M. B.: The effect

of streptokinase infusion on chronic arterial occlusions and stenoses. Ann. Intern. Med. 74:377, 1971.

256. Fiessinger, J. N., Aiach, M., Lagneau, P., Husson, J. M., Cormier, J. M., and Housset, E.: Indications de la streptokinase dans les oblitérations artérielles des membres. Coeur Méd. Int. 15:453, 1976.

257. Gallus, A. S.: The use of antithrombotic drugs in artery disease. In Chesterman, C. N. (ed.): Clinics in Haematology. Thrombosis and the Vessel Wall, Vol. 15, No. 2. Philadelphia, W. B. Saunders Co., 1986, p. 509.

258. Graor, R. A., Risius, B., Young, J. R., Geisinger, M. A., Zelch, M. G., Smith, J. A. M., and Ruschhaupt, W. F.: Low-dose streptokinase for selective thrombolysis: Systemic effects and complications. Radiology 152:35, 1984.

259. McNamara, T. O., and Fisher, J. R.: Thrombolysis of peripheral arterial and graft occlusions: Improved results using high-dose urokinase. Am. J. Radiol. 144:769, 1985.

260. Ricotta, J. J., Green, R. M., and DeWeese, J. A.: Use and limitations of thrombolytic therapy in the treatment of peripheral arterial ischemia: Results of a multi-institutional questionnaire. J. Vasc. Surg. 6:45, 1987.

261. Graor, R. A., and Olin, J. W.: Regional thrombolysis in peripheral artery occlusions. In Julian, D., Kübler, W., Norris, R. M., Swam, H. J. C., Collen, D., and Verstraete, M. (eds.): Thrombolysis in Cardiovascular Disease. New York, Marcel Dekker, 1989, pp. 381–395.

262. McNamara, T. O., and Bomberger, R. A.: Factors affecting initial and 6 months patency rates after intraarterial thrombolysis with high dose urokinase. Am. J. Surg. 152:709, 1986.

263. Graor, R. A., Risius, B., Lucas, F. V., Young, J. R., Ruschhaupt, W. F., Beven, E. G., and Grossbard, E. B.: Thrombolysis with recombinant human tissue-type plasminogen activator in patients with peripheral artery and bypass graft occlusions. Circulation 74 (Suppl. I):I15, 1986.

264. Graor, R. A., Risius, B., Young, J. R., Denny, K., Beven, E. G., Geisinger, M. A., Hertzer, N. R., Krajewski, L. P., Lucas, F. V., O'Hara, P. J., Ruschhaupt, W. F., Winton, S., Zelch, M. G., and Grossbard, E. B.: Peripheral artery and bypass graft thrombolysis with recombinant human tissue-type plasminogen activator. J. Vasc. Surg. 3:115, 1986.

265. Verstraete, M., Hess, H., Mahler, F., Mietaschk, A., Roth, F. J., Schneider, E., Baert, A. L., and Verhaeghe, R.: Femoropopliteal artery thrombolysis with intra-arterial infusion of recombinant tissue-type plasminogen activator. Report of a pilot trial. Eur. J. Vasc. Surg. 2:155, 1988.

266. Mohr, J. P., Caplan, L. R., Melski, J. W., Goldstein, R. J., Duncan, G. W., Kistler, J. P., Pessin, M. S., and Bleich, H. L.: The Harvard cooperative stroke registry: A prospective registry. Neurology 28:754, 1978.

267. Lassen, N. A., and Astrup, J.: Ischemic penumbra. In Wood J. H. (ed.): Cerebral Blood Flow: Physiologic and Clinical Aspects. New York, McGraw-Hill, 1987, p. 458.

268. del Zoppo, G. J., Ferbert, A., Otis, S., Brueckmann, H., Hacke, W., Zyroff, J., Harker, L. A., and Zeumer, H.: Local intra-arterial fibrinolytic therapy in acute carotid territory stroke. Stroke 19:307, 1988.

269. Mori, E., Tabuchi, M., Yoshida, T., and Yamadori, A.: Intra-carotid urokinase with thromboembolic occlusion of the middle cerebral artery. Stroke 19:802, 1988.

270. Hacke, W., Zeumer, H., Ferbert, A., Brückmann, H., and del Zoppo, G. J.: Intra-arterial thrombolytic therapy improves outcome in patients with acute vertebrobasilar occlusive disease. Stroke 19:1216, 1988.

271. The t-PA Acute Stroke Study Group: An open multicenter study of the safety and efficacy of various doses of r-tPA in patients with acute stroke: Preliminary results. Stroke 19:134, 1988 (abstract 22).

272. Brott, T., Haley, E. C., Levy, D. E., Barsan, W. G., Reed, R. L., Olinger, C. P., and Marler, J. R.: Very early therapy for cerebral infarction with tissue plasminogen activator (tPA). Stroke 19:133, 1988 (abstract 20).

Platelets

Philip W. Majerus

INTRODUCTION

Platelets are small, discoid, anucleate cells 2 to 3 μm in diameter with a cell volume of approximately 10 fl. In man they circulate at a concentration of 250,000 ± 100,000 cells/μl of blood. The primary function of platelets is to prevent hemorrhage from defects in blood vessel walls by forming an aggregate at the site of injury. In addition to primary hemostasis, they also participate in reactions of blood coagulation, inflammation, and wound healing. In this chapter, I discuss the physiology and biochemistry of platelets, pointing out disease mechanisms as they apply to this discussion. Much has been learned recently, since platelets have become popular tools for cell biology research.

They contain receptors, have a secretion mechanism, are motile, and provide readily accessible human tissue for study.

Much of what is known about platelet function relates to participation of platelets in hemostasis, and, therefore, the pathophysiology of bleeding disorders due to platelet dysfunction is reasonably well understood. However, the greatest importance of platelets in human disease is their role in the pathogenesis of atherosclerosis and thrombosis. For example, in England in 1973, 33 patients died from bleeding disorders and 100,000 died from thrombosis.[1] Unfortunately, there is currently no definition of the abnormalities in platelet function that predispose to or cause these common disorders. Discovery of such abnormalities is the challenge of the future in platelet research.

BIOLOGY OF PLATELET PRODUCTION

Megakaryocyte Differentiation

Platelets are formed from large bone marrow cells called megakaryocytes by a remarkable and relatively poorly understood process. The stem cell that is the progenitor of megakaryocytes is morphologically unidentified and has been defined in experiments in which it has been cloned and differentiated in vitro, both in soft agar[2, 3] and by a plasma clot assay.[4–6] As megakaryocytes proliferate, they enlarge and undergo extensive DNA replication without mitosis.[7] The polyploid cells subsequently undergo endomitosis to form multilobed nuclei with 4 to 64 times the haploid amount of DNA[8] (Fig. 22–1), most commonly 16 or 32N. Why these cells are polyploid is completely obscure. Only after DNA replication has ceased do the cells begin to show cytoplasmic differentiation with production of the components that constitute the mature platelet. During this time, a number of platelet proteins appear, including fibrinogen,[9] coagulation factor V,[10] platelet factor 4,[11] platelet-derived growth factor,[12] von Willebrand factor (vWF),[13] and some platelet glycoproteins[14] (including glycoproteins Ib, IIb, and IIIa, which are discussed later).

With continued maturation the megakaryocyte cytoplasm develops an extensive membrane system termed *demarcation membranes*,[15, 16] formed by invagination of the plasma membrane. They communicate with the cell exterior, as shown by staining with extracellular tracers such as horseradish peroxidase. The mature megakaryocyte is located directly adjacent to bone marrow sinusoidal endothelial cells. As the extensive demarcation membrane system forms, mega-

karyocytes develop long filopodia (2.5 × 120 μm) that directly penetrate the endothelial cytoplasm and extend into the marrow capillaries.[17] These projections then fragment to produce mature platelets. Several thousand platelets are ultimately produced from the cytoplasm of a single mature megakaryocyte. Whether the ploidy of the parent cell has any influence on the number and/or quality of platelets produced is not clear. In rare instances, large fragments appear to break off, and even entire megakaryocytes can enter the circulation and lodge in pulmonary capillaries. In this way, a small percentage of platelet production occurs outside the marrow. In some disorders of bone marrow structure or function, increased numbers of megakaryocyte fragments circulate.

Thrombocytopoiesis

The production of platelets appears to be regulated by at least two humoral factors, thrombopoietin[18] and megakaryocyte colony-stimulating factor.[6] Thrombopoietin is a poorly characterized hormone that is thought to stimulate platelet production. It has been defined by the observation that plasma from animals rendered thrombocytopenic stimulates production of platelets in recipient animals, as measured by incorporation of radiolabeled amino acids into platelet proteins. The nature of this hormone is not further known, and because it has no activity in any in vitro assay, it has not been isolated. The other factor, megakaryocyte colony-stimulating factor, is also ill defined.[6, 19] This molecule stimulates the size and number of megakaryocyte colonies that grow in a clonogenic assay in a plasma clot.[20] The assay depends on the use of an antiplatelet glycoprotein antiserum that is used to identify megakaryocytes as cells containing platelet antigens. Serum from patients with aplastic anemia but not from normal subjects increases the number of colonies 10- to 20-fold. Sera that contain thrombopoietin activity are not active in this assay, indicating that these are separate moieties. The sites of production and factors controlling the production of these molecules that stimulate platelet production are unknown. Numerous cytokines have been reported to affect either thrombocytopoiesis or platelet number.[21] However, none of these factors meet the basic criteria to represent thrombopoietin as defined by Gerald Roth. Thrombopoietin is (1) lineage specific, (2) not toxic when administered in high doses, and (3) regulated by platelet numbers as described above. Thus, none of the cytokines is lineage specific and all are toxic in high dosage.

Platelet Homeostasis

In normal man, platelet numbers are maintained at a constant level. The total body platelet mass seems to determine platelet production rather than the circulating platelet number. Normally, approximately one

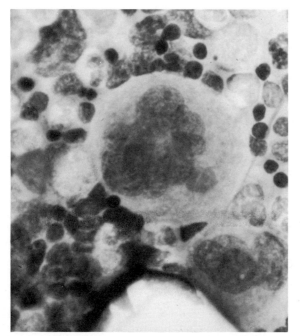

FIGURE 22–1. Human megakaryocyte stained with Wright's stain with two polyploid cells shown. (Original magnification, × 700.)

third of platelets are not circulating but remain in the splenic circulation. Thus, asplenic individuals have elevated circulating platelet counts. In disorders that result in splenomegaly, a larger fraction of platelets reside in the spleen, resulting in lower numbers of circulating platelets. However, the splenic platelets are available for mobilization, and patients with splenomegaly therefore often have decreased numbers of circulating platelets without altered hemostasis. Platelets are produced at a rate of approximately 40,000/μl of blood/day with a life span of 7 to 10 days.[8] Platelet consumption is by a combination of "senescence" and utilization in hemostatic reactions. Autologous platelet survival can be measured by radiolabeling cells in vitro with either ^{51}Cr or ^{111}In and reinfusing them.[22] Increased platelet consumption, as evidenced by decreased survival, has been reported in some patients with atherosclerosis or thrombosis; however, this parameter is not regularly associated with vascular disease, and its measurement in patients suspected of having vascular disease is of no practical value. In man, the time required for differentiation of megakaryocyte precursors to circulating platelets is 4 to 5 days. The best calculations estimate that the marrow can increase platelet production 5- to 10-fold in disease states, thereby maintaining normal platelet numbers despite increased consumption. Diseases associated with decreased platelet numbers result from either decreased production or increased destruction. These include decreased production due to marrow aplasia or infiltration and increased destruction due to autoimmune disorders in which antibody-mediated platelet destruction occurs. In general, spontaneous bleeding does not occur until platelet numbers are reduced to at least one tenth of normal.

A variety of disorders are associated with increased platelet numbers; these include so-called reactive thrombocytosis seen in patients with trauma, infections, iron deficiency, and cancer. Mechanisms for increased platelets in these cases are unknown. In myeloproliferative diseases with abnormal marrow function, such as myelofibrosis, polycythemia vera, chronic granulocytic leukemia, and primary thrombocytosis, elevated platelet numbers also occur and platelet function is often abnormal despite the increased numbers. Soft agar assays of progenitors of

megakaryocytes indicate that these patients produce many more megakaryocyte colonies than normal.[19] However, plasma of these patients does not contain megakaryocyte colony-stimulating factor, and the colonies are further stimulated by the addition of megakaryocyte colony-stimulating factor to culture medium. It is not clear whether these progenitors are able to proliferate without megakaryocyte colony-stimulating factor or whether some other environmental factor in bone marrow allows for excessive proliferation of megakaryocyte precursors.

Platelet Structure and Metabolism

The structure of human platelets is illustrated in Figure 22–2. These cells are free floating and discoid. They contain an intricate system of channels continuous with the plasma membrane that is similar to the demarcation system of the megakaryocyte. This is termed the *open canalicular system*.[23] The anatomy of the platelet is similar to that of a sponge, giving these cells an enormous surface area compared with a sphere of comparable size (i.e., approximately 20 μm^3 for a sphere versus 150 μm^3 for a platelet, as estimated from the density of cell surface lectin-binding sites[24]). Platelets have a dense tubular membrane system thought to be analogous to the sarcoplasmic reticulum of smooth muscle,[23] which serves to pump and release Ca^{2+}. They also contain at least three distinct types of secretory granules: dense, α, and lysosomes.[25] The α granules contain coagulation factors, such as fibrinogen, factor V,[26] high molecular weight kininogen, and von Willebrand factor (vWF) (Table 22–1). They also contain a number of other proteins and peptides whose functions are discussed later, including platelet-derived growth factor (PDGF), platelet factor 4, β thromboglobulin, thrombin-sensitive protein (thrombospondin, or TSP), and GMP-140. α Granules also contain low concentrations of all plasma proteins, suggesting import by fluid-phase endocytosis.[27]

Many of the proteins found in platelet α granules are packaged after synthesis in the precursor megakaryocyte. A number of α granule proteins have been shown to be synthesized de novo by megakaryocytes, including coagulation factor V,[10] platelet factor 4,[11]

TABLE 22–1. TYPES OF PROTEINS SECRETED BY PLATELET α GRANULES

MAJOR PLATELET PROTEIN (ALSO IN PLASMA)	UNIQUE TO PLATELETS	PLATELET CONTENT (<1% OF PLASMA CONTENT)
Coagulation factor V[1]	Platelet Factor IV[3]	α$_1$-Antitrypsin[6]
von Willebrand factor[2]	β-thromboglobulin[3]	α^2-Macroglobulin[6]
Fibrinogen[3]	Platelet-derived growth factor[4]	Fibronectin[7]
Lipoprotein-associated coagulation inhibitor[10]	TSP (thrombospondin)[5]	High molecular weight kininogen[8]
	GMP-140[11]	Histidine-rich glycoprotein[9]

[1]Chesney et al.: Proc. Natl. Acad. Sci. USA 78:5180, 1981.
[2]Zucker et al.: J. Lab. Clin. Med. 94:675, 1979.
[3]K. Kaplan et al.: Blood 53:604, 1979.
[4]D. Kaplan et al.: Blood 53:1043, 1979.
[5]Gerrard et al.: J. Clin. Invest. 66:102, 1980.
[6]Nachman et al.: J. Biol. Chem. 251:4514, 1976.
[7]Ginsberg et al.: Proc. Natl. Acad. Sci. USA 79:1049, 1980.
[8]Schmair et al.: J. Clin. Invest. 71:1477, 1983.
[9]Leung et al.: Blood 62:1016, 1983.
[10]Novotny et al.: Blood 72:2020, 1988.
[11]McEver: Thromb. Haemost. 66:80, 1991.

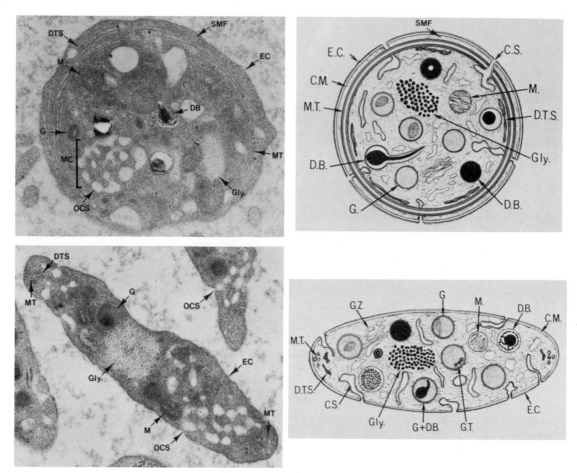

FIGURE 22–2. Platelet structure. The diagrams and electron micrographs of thin sections (original magnification, × 60,000) represent platelets cut in cross-section and in the equatorial plane. CM = Plasma membrane; CS,OCS = open canalicular membranes; DTS = dense tubular system; DB = dense body; EC = surface glycoproteins; Gly = glycogen granules; G = granules; MT = microtubules; M = mitochondria; SMF = microfilaments.

and vWF.[13] Other proteins contained in α granules, including immunoglobulin G (IgG), albumin, and fibrinogen, are taken up from plasma by a novel endocytotic mechanism.[28, 29] Fibronectin and high molecular weight kininogen may also be taken up by this mechanism, as their concentration in α granules exceeds that of plasma.[27] α Granule proteins are secreted in response to agonists except for GMP-140, which is an integral membrane protein that becomes a cell surface protein as α granule membranes fuse with plasma membranes during secretion. GMP-140 is a receptor for neutrophils and promotes their adhesion to platelets. The physiological roles for this phenomenon are uncertain.[30]

Although some α granule proteins are unique to platelets (i.e., PDGF and platelet factor 4), others are major plasma proteins (i.e., fibrinogen and coagulation factor V and lipoprotein-associated coagulation inhibitor). It is a mystery why these latter proteins are packaged in platelets when platelets circulate in a fluid that contains 5 to 10 times as much of these proteins. It has been suggested that agonist-induced secretion

from α granules may serve to elevate the local concentration of critical proteins in wounds.[31] A number of the plasma proteins contained in α granules, including histidine-rich glycoprotein,[32] fibronectin,[33] high molecular weight kininogen,[34] and α1 protease inhibitor,[35] have been proposed to be important in platelet physiology. Agonist-induced platelet secretion results in liberation of these molecules, although the meager quantities render any physiological importance problematical.

Another type of secretory granule in platelets is termed the *dense body*. This organelle contains Ca^{2+} and Mg^{2+} ions, adenosine triphosphate (ATP), adenosine diphosphate (ADP), and smaller amounts of other nucleotides, plus several vasoactive amines, particularly 5-hydroxytryptamine (serotonin). The third secretory granule is a lysosome-containing lysosomal enzyme similar to those found in other cells.

Platelets are anucleate and do not contain genomic DNA, although they contain mitochondria and small amounts of mRNA that has been amplified by polymerase chain reaction.[36] Platelets do not synthesize protein except possibly in mitochondria.[37] Platelets do carry out most reactions of carbohydrate[38] and lipid metabolism[39, 40] that occur in other cells.

PHYSIOLOGY OF PLATELET PLUG FORMATION

Platelet Adhesion to Foreign Surfaces

In the circulation, platelets are free-floating cells that do not adhere to each other or to vascular endothelium. When platelets are exposed to non-endothelial surfaces, they adhere, flatten, and spread on the surface. In this process platelet shape changes dramatically from a disc to a spiny sphere with long, fine filopodia that may be several times the length of a platelet. Presumably the excess surface membrane required to form the filopodia is obtained from the canalicular membrane system. Under pathological conditions of endothelial injury or wounds, the major non-endothelial surface to which platelets adhere is collagen fibrils. Experimental study of the adherence of platelets to collagen in vitro indicates that fibrillar collagen is required.[41] Collagen monomers or fragments of collagen chains do not support platelet adhesion. The platelet collagen receptor is a dimeric 110/150 kDa glycoprotein that was previously designated glycoprotein Ia/IIa but is now called VLA-2, as it is one of the integrins present on many cells.[42] No inherited abnormalities of this putative receptor have been found. In vivo collagen may not bind directly to platelets because a plasma protein, vWF, is required to support platelet adhesion to subendothelial surfaces. Among current hypotheses, the best is that vWF, under conditions of high flow and shear, first adheres to subendothelial collagen fibers, which leads to an alteration in the conformation of the vWF (or its receptor), allowing it to bind to a specific receptor site on platelets. Congenital lack of either vWF (von Willebrand's disease; see Chapter 19) or the platelet receptor (Bernard-Soulier syndrome; see von Willebrand Factor Receptor, page 766) leads to a hemorrhagic diathesis characterized by abnormal platelet adherence.[43] Because the extracellular matrix contains collagen fibers in most loci, platelets readily adhere to wound surfaces. Intact endothelium presumably has no such luminal collagen fibers. Whether other features of endothelial surface proteins are also important in the non-thrombogenicity of this tissue is unknown. Endothelial cells also produce an icosanoid mediator, prostacyclin, that further inhibits platelet adhesion.

Platelet Aggregation

Most of the platelets that accumulate at sites of injury do not adhere directly to subendothelial structures but rather to each other. The process of platelet-platelet adherence is termed aggregation and has properties distinct from adhesion. Platelet aggregation has been studied in vitro by measuring the aggregation of stirred suspensions of platelets by monitoring changes in optical density (Fig. 22–3). Platelet aggregation can be triggered experimentally by several potential physiological agonists, the most important of which are ADP and thrombin. Other potential agonists include epinephrine, thromboxane A_2, and platelet-activating factor (PAF).[44–46] In all systems studied, platelet aggregation requires both fibrinogen and ADP.[45] In the case of agonists such as thrombin and PAF that stimulate the secretion of platelet granule contents, ADP and fibrinogen are provided by their secretion. In vitro addition of ADP alone to a stirred platelet suspension causes aggregation only in the presence of added fibrinogen. Full aggregation and modest secretion (approximately one fourth of the α granules and dense bodies) occur in response to ADP only when thromboxane A_2 is formed. Thus, when platelets are taken from subjects who have ingested aspirin (thereby blocking cyclooxygenase and subsequent thromboxane production; see Production of Icosanoids, page 761), no secretion and only partial, reversible aggregation are observed with ADP (termed "first-phase" aggregation).

There are two general types of agonists for platelet aggregation[45]:

1. *Weak agonists,* such as ADP and epinephrine, cause aggregation only when thromboxane production occurs in the platelet. With these agonists, secretion follows and depends on platelet aggregation (i.e., if platelets are not stirred during the experiment to promote cell-cell contact, secretion does not occur). Furthermore, secretion is incomplete in response to these agonists.

2. *Strong agonists,* such as thrombin, collagen, and platelet-activating factor, cause secretion equally well with or without aggregation (i.e., the reaction is the same with or without stirring) and do not depend on thromboxane A_2 production. Thus, thrombin-induced aggregation and secretion occur even in aspirin-treated platelets. At low concentrations of strong agonists, secretion is both aggregation and thromboxane A_2 dependent. The molecular basis for these two apparently distinct mechanisms for platelet secretion is unknown.

Fibrinogen is required for platelet aggregation; it binds to receptors on activated platelets and appears to provide part of the mechanism linking platelets to each other.[46] Although vWF appears to link platelets to the subendothelial surface, fibrinogen links platelets to each other. It has been proposed that polymerization of fibrinogen (fibrin monomers) links one platelet to another. Fibrinogen alone does not support platelet aggregation, implying that fibrinogen receptors are not available on unstimulated cells.[47, 48] Addition of ADP makes fibrinogen-binding sites appear by a mechanism that has not been elucidated. Upon addition of ADP to platelets, aggregation appears to precede secretion, so that ADP does not act by causing α granule proteins to be secreted. Full ADP aggregation depends on thromboxane A_2 production.[49] There is a throm-

A

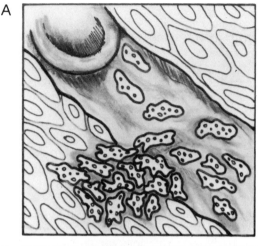

B

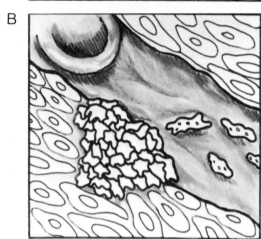

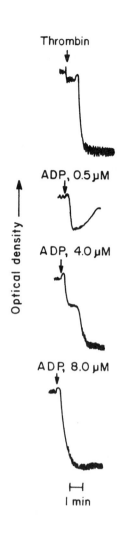

Thrombin

ADP, 0.5 μM

ADP, 4.0 μM

ADP, 8.0 μM

Optical density ——→

|—| 1 min

FIGURE 22–3. Platelet adhesion and aggregation. *A,* Platelets adhere to subendothelial structures at sites of vascular injury. *B,* Other platelets then aggregate to each other at the site to form a physical plug. The in vitro aggregation of platelets is determined by stirring platelet suspensions in a spectrophotometer and measuring aggregation as changes in optical density. As cells aggregate, optical density decreases. Strong agonists such as thrombin produce rapid, irreversible aggregation, as shown in the upper tracing on the right. ADP, 0.5 μM, produces transient, reversible aggregation; ADP, 4 μM, produces aggregation into phases, the second of which follows secretion; and ADP, 8 μM, produces rapid, irreversible aggregation.

THROMBOSPONDIN RECEPTORS

FIGURE 22–4. Domains of thrombospondin. A model of a thrombospondin subunit is depicted with sites of cellular receptors noted. See text for details. BBxB = Glycosoaminoglycan-binding site, where B is arginine or lysine and x is any amino acid. Amino acids involved in binding sites are indicated by the single-letter amino acid code. The small ovals indicate the binding sites for monoclonal antibodies.

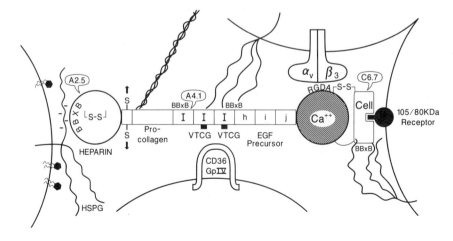

boxane A_2 receptor on platelets, but how this moiety, or thromboxane itself, enhances fibrinogen binding in the presence of ADP is unknown.

Other proteins have also been postulated to link fibrinogen or fibrin monomers to each other, including thrombospondin and fibronectin. Thrombospondin is an α granule protein that is secreted when platelets are activated.[50, 51] It is a 440 kDa trimeric protein that is disulfide linked[51] and that binds to the platelet surface after secretion.[52] This protein interacts with fibrinogen, and evidence suggests that thrombospondin may serve a bridging function between fibrinogen molecules on adjacent platelets.[53–55] The structure and various binding domains of thrombospondin are shown in Figure 22–4. This structure was elucidated by the use of monoclonal antibodies directed at epitopes from different parts of the molecule, proteolysis and isolation of peptides, and electron microscopy of the molecule decorated with antibody molecules. As noted in the figure, thrombospondin contains at least four cell-binding sites and is involved in adhesion of several other types of cells besides platelets.[56] One of these binds platelet GPIV via a VTCG motif, which is homologous to a malarial cell surface protein that provides a mechanism for malarial parasites to enter cells.[57] Antibody C6.7 binds to the carboxyl-terminal end of the molecule and blocks the aggregation of intact platelets. Studies with this antibody suggest that thrombospondin is required for platelet aggregation.[58, 59] However, the importance of thrombospondin in platelet aggregation is uncertain, because patients with congenital deficiency of α granules with less than 10 per cent of normal thrombospondin (gray platelet syndrome) do not have severely deranged platelet aggregation,[60] and thrombospondin binds a large number of other proteins.[61] Thus, the BBXB glycosaminoglycan-binding motifs[62] (where B = R/K) and the integrin-binding RGD motif[63] may not be involved in platelet function. Another proposed function for thrombospondin is that it binds to platelets and then to a plasma protein named *histidine-rich glycoprotein* to anchor this protein (a known heparin antagonist) to activated platelets. In this way, local coagulation reactions could be protected from inhibition by heparin.[64]

Although the measurement of platelet aggregation in vitro has been useful experimentally both in defining the requirements for aggregation and in classifying various hemorrhagic disorders, it is not a very useful test in medical practice. Abnormal platelet aggregation in vitro does not necessarily predict a clinically significant bleeding diathesis. The most direct demonstration of this point is that normal subjects who have taken aspirin have abnormal aggregation for several days thereafter without any significant bleeding disorder. Similarly, attempts to utilize "hyperaggregability" or hypersensitivity of platelets to in vitro stimuli as a predictor of future or current in vivo thrombotic events have been unsuccessful.

Physiological Generation of a Hemostatic Plug

After platelets adhere to collagen, the adherent platelets are presumably activated to secrete ADP, generate thromboxane A_2, and activate coagulation reactions leading to the production of thrombin. These agonists in turn recruit other platelets to aggregate, ultimately forming a physical plug that obstructs the wound surface. Upon this surface, a fibrin clot forms that contracts to seal the vessel wall or wound.

Platelet Secretion

Platelet secretion of α granules and dense body contents follows platelet aggregation by the agonists previously listed. There is also partial secretion of lysosomal enzymes. Strong agonists result in the secretion of 70 to 90 per cent of α granule and dense body contents. Secretion appears to be triggered by contraction of a circumferential band of microtubules that condenses the platelet granules into the center of the cell. There the granule membranes fuse with membranes of the surface-connected open canalicular membrane.[65] The secretion is analogous to squeezing water out of a sponge. The substances known to be secreted by platelets are listed in Table 22–1. The physiology of platelet motility required for shape change and secretion is discussed in the following section under clot retraction.

Platelet Contraction

After the platelet-fibrin hemostatic plug is formed, it decreases in volume by a process that depends on the contractile apparatus of the platelet. Platelet reactions that depend on the contractile system include filopodia formation, secretion, and clot retraction. The cytoskeleton of the platelet consists of actin filaments, microtubules (which are made up of tubulin), and a variety of associated proteins.[66] Platelets contain a smooth muscle–type contractile system. Actin, a 42 kDa protein, comprises approximately 15 per cent of soluble platelet protein.[67, 68] There are six separate genes for actin,[69, 70] producing different proteins in skeletal, cardiac, and various smooth muscle–containing cells, of which β and γ types are expressed in platelets.[68] Actin exists in two forms—as monomers, referred to as G-actin, and as a double-helical polymeric form, termed F-actin.[71] In unstimulated platelets, approximately 50 per cent of actin is F-actin.[72] Platelet myosin has a molecular weight of 460 kDa and consists of dimers of myosin heavy chains (200 kDa) and two types of light chains (20 kDa and 16 kDa).[71] The head of the myosin heavy chain contains the ATPase and actin-binding sites. The ATPase is active only when the 20 kDa light chain is phosphorylated.[73, 74] The phosphorylation of the light chain controls the contractile process, and it is catalyzed by myosin light chain kinase, a calcium ion and calmodulin-dependent enzyme.[75, 76] In unstimulated platelets, the myosin light chains are unphosphorylated. Upon activation by thrombin, they are phosphorylated within a few seconds, thereby initiating the contractile process. Most of the forces generated by contracting platelets are transmitted through the actin filaments, because actin, present at 100 times the concentration of myosin, comprises the majority of the mass of the cytoskeleton.[66] In fact, spreading and filopodia formation that occur in activated platelets may be accomplished by changes in actin polymerization independent of myosin reactions.

Study of the polymerization of actin has been facilitated by the recognition that actin filaments have a polarity that is demonstrated by adding heavy meromyosin to preparations of actin filaments. The myosin "decorates" the actin filaments in a characteristic way, producing an arrowhead-like structure with a pointed and a barbed end of the filament.[77] Actin filaments can grow by addition of monomers to either end of the filament, although growth is approximately fivefold faster at the barbed end, which is also the end that abuts the plasma membrane.[78, 79] In vitro, in physiological salts, the critical concentration of G-actin that leads to spontaneous polymerization is ~ 30 μM. The concentration of actin within platelets is ~ 10 times this concentration, suggesting that actin should be fully polymerized in unstimulated platelets. However, such is not the case, which indicates that platelets have a mechanism for preventing actin polymerization. Several regulating mechanisms have been proposed.[71] G-actin binds to profilin, a basic protein of 16 kDa in a 1:1 complex of relatively low affinity. Platelets contain sufficient profilin to bind approximately one half of the total actin in the cell, which is the proportion of G-actin in the unstimulated cells.[80] This complex may serve as an actin buffer such that when conditions favor rapid polymerization of actin, the complex dissociates and actin filaments can grow.[81, 82] PtdIns(4,5)P$_2$ binds profilin with high affinity ($K_d < 0.1$ μM) with a stoichiometry of 5 moles of PtdIns(4,5)P$_2$ per mole of profilin and thereby frees actin to polymerize.[83] It is possible that this function is served by the polyphosphorylated 3-phosphate–containing phosphatidylinositols in vivo (page 771). A second mechanism to inhibit polymerization is mediated by proteins that bind to the ends of actin filaments, thereby capping them and preventing further growth. Several proteins have been proposed as possible barbed-end capping proteins, including vinculin and α-actinin, but they have not been shown to act in this capacity in platelets.[67] Gelsolin, a 90 kDa protein found in platelets and leukocytes, is a barbed-end capping protein. However, gelsolin may act to regulate actin polymerization in stimulated rather than in resting cells, because this molecule requires μM calcium ions for activity.[84] In unstimulated platelets, the calcium ion concentration is ~ 0.1 μM, rising to several micromoles upon activation.

The state of actin polymerization in platelets has been measured experimentally in two ways. G-actin forms a 1:1 complex with DNase I, blocking its action on DNA. The proportion of G-actin in platelets can be measured as the DNase inhibitory activity in platelet lysates, and total actin is measured after actin filament depolymerization in guanidine.[72] A second method involves Triton detergent extraction of platelets, whereby the actin filaments remain as an insoluble residue that can be measured by subsequent sodium dodecyl sulfate (SDS) and polyacrylamide gel electrophoresis.[85] These methods have been used to demonstrate that actin filaments grow rapidly upon platelet activation to contain ~ 75 per cent total actin. The filaments appear to grow mainly from the barbed end, thereby pushing the membrane out into filapodia, with the pointed end pressing against the central circumferential band of microtubles, compressing the granules to the center of the cell. SDS gel electrophoresis of platelet Triton residues after thrombin activation indicates that a number of other proteins become rapidly associated with the actin network after platelet activation, including myosin, actin-binding protein, and a platelet membrane glycoprotein designated II$_b$/III$_a$ (discussed under Fibrinogen Receptor [Glycoprotein II$_b$/III$_a$], page 764). Whether actin is anchored directly to this membrane glycoprotein or via other putative actin-membrane–anchoring proteins such as ankyrin, vinculin, or α-actin remains to be elucidated. The function of actin-binding protein (a 270 kDa dimeric protein) in the control of actin polymerization is also unclear. Actin-binding protein tends to promote actin bundle formation and may also serve to crosslink actin filaments. The function of this protein may be modulated by proteolysis by a calcium ion–activated protease that occurs in platelets.[82, 84–86]

Once platelets are activated, they aggregate and secrete their granule contents. Coagulation reactions then occur on the platelet surface, and finally clot reaction occurs by action of myosin ATPase acting through actin filaments. The actin filaments are anchored to the membrane glycoprotein II$_b$/III$_a$ which, in turn, is linked to fibrin strands outside the cell. In this way platelet contraction can effectively diminish the volume of the much larger fibrin clot. A congenital disorder with defective clot retraction is Glanzmann's thrombasthenia (described under Fibrinogen Receptor [Glycoprotein II$_b$/III$_a$], page 765).

Role of Platelets in Coagulation Reactions

Over the past 10 to 20 years, the plasma coagulation factors have been identified, isolated, and characterized. The sequence of coagulation reactions that is most widely accepted is called the waterfall, or cascade, hypothesis.[87] However, the current scheme is quite different (see Chapter 18) in that the extrinsic system of factor VII and tissue factor is the initial stimulus that sets off the coagulation system.

Platelets potentially participate in a number of coagulation reactions. A major reaction that occurs on the platelet surface is the process of prothrombin activation. In this reaction, factor X_a catalyzes the conversion of prothrombin to thrombin in the presence of a cofactor, factor V_a.[88] This reaction occurs on a platelet surface receptor for factors X_a and V_a (see page 768).

A number of experiments have indicated that phospholipids and coagulation factor V_a can replace platelets in prothrombin activation in vitro. Additionally, phospholipid can substitute for platelets in various assays that measure the time required to clot activated plasma after addition of Ca^{2+}. For example, addition of Russell's viper venom to plasma activates factor X (all of the factor X in plasma), and the clotting time of such activated plasma can be shortened by addition of either platelets or phospholipids. Thus, it has been proposed that the entity in the platelet that promotes the conversion of prothrombin to thrombin is a phospholipoprotein on the platelet surface, which previously had been called platelet factor 3.[89] A variety of empirical tests have been devised to measure this substance, but none uses physiological amounts of the various components. In vivo, less than 1% of factor X is activated to factor X_a. At such low factor X_a concentrations, platelet surface prothrombin activation occurs 15- to 20-fold faster than that which occurs on an optimal phospholipid surface.[90–94] Once a prothrombinase complex is organized on its platelet receptor, it is protected from inactivation by plasma protease inhibitors.[90, 95] The anticoagulant heparin that acts by activating antithrombin III is unable to inhibit factor X_a once it is bound to the platelet surface. Thus, coagulation reactions, once started in the area of a hemostatic plug, are not blocked by heparin anticoagulation. This may explain the relative ineffectiveness of heparin in preventing arterial thromboses.

Platelets have other mechanisms that also protect ongoing surface coagulation reactions. Platelets secrete platelet factor 4, a 31 kDa tetrameric polypeptide that serves to bind heparin and thereby prevent its anticoagulant action.[96, 97] Similarly, thrombospondin, which is also secreted by platelets, binds to the platelet surface and then binds histidine-rich glycoprotein, which in turn binds heparin and blocks its anticoagulant effect.[64] Therefore, in the immediate platelet milieu, coagulation factors are protected from inhibition.

Prothrombin activation is readily studied in vitro, because all the prothrombin (1 μM) in plasma is activated during this process. Because a large amount of thrombin is formed, it is easily measured. Attempts

to define a role for platelets in the activation of factor X itself have been difficult, because such a small amount (<1 per cent) is activated during coagulation reactions in vitro. Thus, attempts to add factors IX_a, VIII_a, and X to platelets to demonstrate a specific platelet-catalyzed activation reaction have thus far been largely unsuccessful.[98] Similarly, it has not been possible to show convincingly that platelets participate in a physiological acceleration of the activation of factor XI, even though platelets have binding sites for both factors XI and XI_a.[99, 100] Deficiency of factor XII does not result in a bleeding disorder, suggesting that it is not required for factor XI activation. Patients who are factor XI deficient do bleed, and therefore it is clear that factor XI_a is important for hemostasis. The mechanism for the activation of factor XI in vivo remains to be elucidated but may involve thrombin as described (see Chapter 18). Platelets also contain factor XIII, the enzyme that cross-links fibrin clots. This moiety, however, is contained in the platelet cytoplasm and is not secreted when platelets are activated. Thus, it is difficult to envision a role for platelet factor XIII in hemostasis.

Production of Icosanoids

Platelets produce icosanoid mediators (oxygenated derivatives of arachidonic acid) in response to activation[101] (Fig. 22–5). Arachidonic acid (5,8,11,14-eicosatetraenoic acid) is the major polyunsaturated fatty acid in man. This fatty acid is essential because we are unable to desaturate fatty acids to form the 14 position double bond found in arachidonate. Dietary linoleate (9,12-octadecadienoic acid) is the major arachidonate precursor in man. Linoleate is converted to arachidonate in liver by desaturases, as shown in Table 22–2. Many cells that produce icosanoids, including platelets, lack desaturase enzymes and therefore depend on uptake from plasma for icosanoid precursor fatty acids.[102, 103] In unstimulated platelets, free arachidonate is present in only trace quantities compared with other long-chain fatty acids. Low free arachidonate levels prevent its metabolism by the unstimulated cell. These levels are maintained when arachidonate bound to albumin is added to platelets; arachidonate is esterified into phospholipids without the production of oxygenated metabolites. Other icosanoid precursor fatty acids are also readily incorporated into cellular phospholipids. In contrast, dietary fatty acids that are not icosanoid precursors, such as

TABLE 22–2. CONVERSION OF DIETARY LINOLEATE TO ARACHIDONATE

Fatty acid	18:2 linoleate	$\xrightarrow[\text{desaturase}]{\Delta 6}$	18:3	$\xrightarrow{+2C}$	20:3	$\xrightarrow[\text{desaturase}]{\Delta 5}$	20:4 arachidonate
Double bonds	9,12		6,9,12		8,11,14		5,8,11,14

Dietary linoleate is converted to the icosanoid precursor arachidonate in liver and some other tissues. Platelets and endothelial cells lack the desaturase enzymes. In essential fatty acid, deficiency-synthesized oleic acid 18:1 with a 9 position double bond is metabolized by this same pathway to produce 20:3 (5,8,11). This fatty acid is diagnostic of essential fatty acid deficiency.

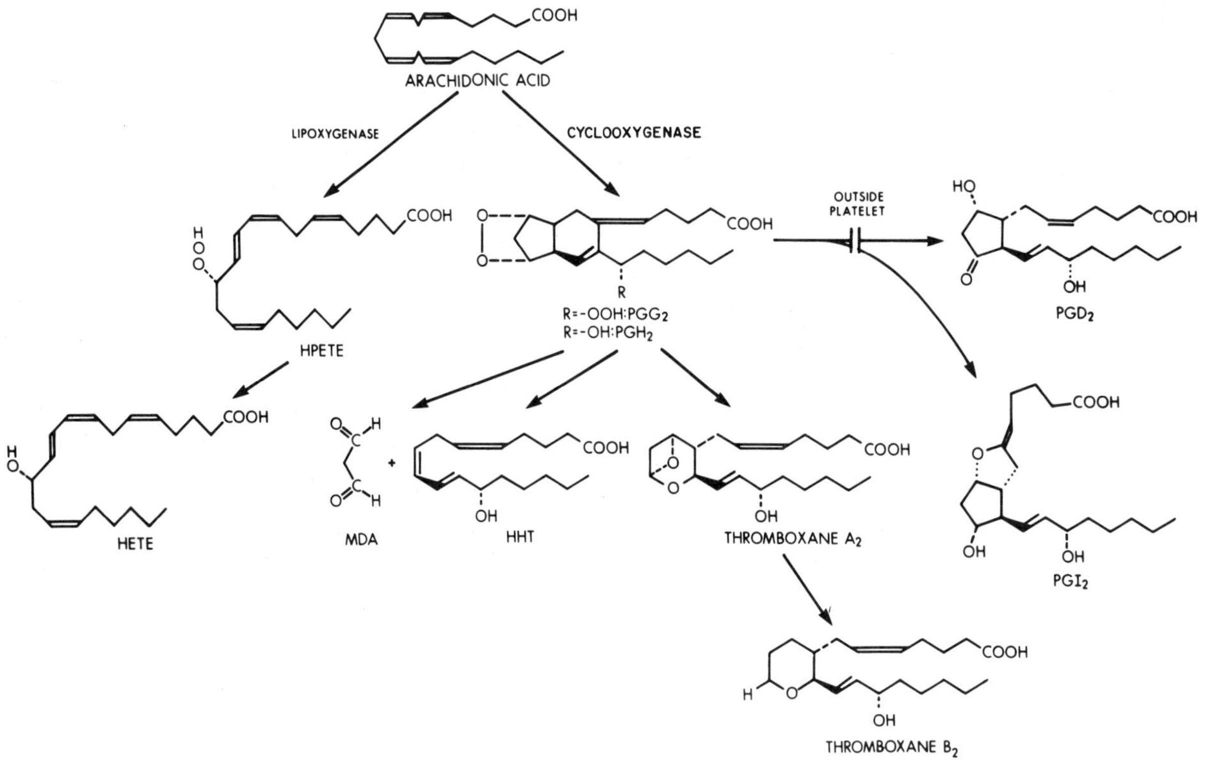

FIGURE 22–5. Arachidonate metabolism in platelets. Note that conversion of PGH$_2$ to PGI$_2$ and PGD$_2$ does not occur within platelets. The icosanoids listed can be divided into those that stimulate platelet aggregation (thromboxane A$_2$, PGH$_2$) and those that inhibit it (PGI$_2$, PGD$_2$).

palmitic, stearic, oleic, and linoleic acids, are esterified into platelet phospholipids at a relatively low rate.[104] As a result, significant pools of these fatty acids exist within the cell. These findings are explained by the fact that platelets contain a unique long-chain acyl-CoA synthetase that is specific for icosanoid precursor fatty acids.[105–107] This enzyme has a very high affinity for these fatty acids and prevents accumulation of free acids in unstimulated cells, ensuring sufficient substrate for icosanoid production. Human plasma contains less than 1 per cent of total free fatty acid as polyunsaturated fatty acids. Therefore, cells require a high-affinity uptake system. Most human cells contain the icosanoid precursor-specific acyl-CoA synthetase.[108]

Icosanoid synthesis requires free non-esterified arachidonate, because the oxygenating enzymes do not act on phospholipid-bound fatty acid. The quantity of icosanoid produced upon stimulation of the platelet depends on the nature of the stimulus as well as on the content of arachidonate in the platelets. Activation by agonists, such as ADP and epinephrine, results in liberation of only small amounts of arachidonate, whereas high concentrations of thrombin produce much larger amounts. The control of icosanoid production depends on lipase activity that liberates the fatty acid from phospholipids. This receptor-mediated pathway is discussed under Control of Icosanoid Production (page 772).

Arachidonate, once liberated from the stimulated

platelet, is either converted directly to icosanoids, as outlined in Figure 22–5, or liberated from the cell as free arachidonate, providing a potential substrate for adjacent cells to produce alternative icosanoid mediators.

Lipoxygenase Pathway

Platelets contain a cytosolic 12-lipoxygenase.[109, 110] The enzyme eliminates a proton at carbon 10 of arachidonate, leading to insertion of molecular oxygen at carbon 12 to form 12-hydroperoxy-arachidonate (12-HPETE).[111] Subsequently, 12-HPETE is converted to 12-HETE by a peroxidase enzyme. The role of these compounds (which are released from platelets) in platelet physiology remains unclear, because no specific inhibitors of their production are known, and no diseases have been associated with abnormal production of these compounds. A variety of effects of these substances have been noted in vitro. 12-HETE is chemotactic for neutrophils[112] and provides substrate to neutrophils to undergo further oxygenation to 5S, 12S, di-HETE,[113, 114] and 12,20-di-HETE.[115, 116] In platelets, 12-HPETE may stimulate the 12-lipoxygenase[117] and may also increase oxygenation of 5,8,11,14,17-eicosapentaenoic acid (EPA).[118] Both 12-HPETE and 12-HETE inhibit platelet aggregation in vitro.[119, 120]

Cyclooxygenase Pathway

Cyclooxygenase, a 72 kDa glycoprotein, is a membrane-bound enzyme that has been localized to the endoplasmic reticulum in fibroblasts[121] and to the dense tubular system in platelets.[122] Complementary DNAs (cDNAs) encoding cyclooxygenase have been isolated from a variety of tissues, including human platelets and a megakaryocyte precursor cell line.[123, 124] Cyclooxygenase is the first enzyme in a pathway leading to production of a variety of active mediators, including thromboxane A_2,[125] which is the most potent vasoconstrictor known (100 times the potency of angiotensin II) and an agonist that stimulates platelet aggregation and secretion.[126]

Cyclooxygenase catalyzes the abstraction of a proton at carbon 13 of arachidonate and related polyunsaturated fatty acids, which is followed by the insertion of two molecules of oxygen. In the case of arachidonate, the product is a cyclic endoperoxide PGG_2. The enzyme also catalyzes a second reaction in which PGG_2 is peroxidized to PGH_2.[127] In platelets these products are not secreted from cells under physiological conditions but are directly metabolized to other compounds. PGH_2 is converted to thromboxane A_2 by thromboxane synthase.[128] This compound is labile ($t1/2 = 30$ seconds in water) and degrades spontaneously to the inactive metabolite, thromboxane B_2. The latter compound is measured experimentally as evidence of platelet activation, either by radioimmunoassay or by radiochromatography. Thromboxane synthase also forms two other compounds from arachidonic acid in amounts approximately equal to thromboxane A_2. These are 12-L-hydroxy-5,8,10-heptadecatrienoic acid (HHT) and malonaldehyde. No function has been elucidated for these latter compounds, although malonaldehyde could act as a physiological cross-linking agent.

In other cells the cyclic endoperoxide, PGH_2, is the precursor of different icosanoids, including PGI_2 (discussed later), and the stable icosanoids PGE_2, PGD_2, and $PGF_2\alpha$. Formation of PGE_2 and PGD_2 is catalyzed by isomerase enzymes not present in platelets.[129, 130] Small amounts of these compounds can be formed by nonenzymatic breakdown of the labile endoperoxide, PGH_2. Thus, in platelets the major products (>90 per cent) of endoperoxide metabolism are thromboxane A_2, HHT, and malonaldehyde. However, PGD_2 is of interest because it is a potent inhibitor of platelet function. Albumin catalyzes production of PGD_2 from PGH_2.[131] This may be of physiological significance in preventing unwanted actions of PGH_2, as outlined in the following discussion. Platelets contain an enzyme that converts PGD_2 to 15-keto-PGD_2, an inactive metabolite.[132]

Aspirin in Platelet Function

Aspirin induces a mild hemostatic defect in man, as evidenced by prolongation of skin bleeding time and impaired platelet aggregation measured in vitro. The aspirin defect results from decreased thromboxane A_2 production. Aspirin inhibits icosanoid production by a unique mechanism; it acetylates cyclooxygenase covalently on a single serine residue (S/536).[133, 134] Aspirin inhibition of the enzyme is prevented by arachidonate in a competitive manner, suggesting that aspirin competes for the substrate-binding site. The inhibition is due to steric inhibition by the bulky acetyl group and not to inhibition of catalysis. Thus, mutant cyclooxygenase with S to A mutation at position 536 remains active, and substitution of bulky amino acids at this position inhibits activity.[135, 136] The covalent modification of the enzyme is permanent; therefore, the cell must synthesize new enzyme in order to recover the capacity of producing products. Because platelets are incapable of protein synthesis, the defect is permanent, lasting for the life of the platelet (7 to 10 days).[137] This results in a unique pharmacology of aspirin in platelets whereby the effect of repeated doses of the drug is cumulative as residual active enzyme is repeatedly exposed to aspirin. In the steady state (i.e., after several weeks of aspirin therapy), complete inactivation of platelet cyclooxygenase is achieved by extremely low doses of aspirin, much less than those required for other actions of the drug (<80 mg/day yields complete inactivation).[138–140] This has led to clinical trials of low-dose aspirin as an antithrombotic agent (discussed under Icosanoids, page 773). With this strategy, it is possible to block platelet cyclooxygenase selectively and not the same enzyme in other tissues. Recently, a second gene encoding a putative "inflammatory cyclooxygenase" has been discovered by molecular cloning at low stringency using the cDNA encoding the original or platelet cyclooxygenase. This cyclooxygenase is highly homologous to the above-described enzyme (especially around the S modified by aspirin). Its expression is induced by cytokines and inhibited by corticosteroids.[141–143]

Thromboxane Synthase Inhibition

Thromboxane synthase inhibitors are currently under investigation as potential antithrombotic agents.[144] These drugs, many of which are imidazole derivatives, have the theoretical advantage of blocking production of thromboxane A_2 in platelets while allowing continued production of cyclooxygenase products in other tissues. However, thromboxane synthase inhibitors allow accumulation of PGH_2, which is a potent platelet-aggregating agent itself. These drugs actually have little effect on platelet function in vitro.[145] If they have antithrombotic efficacy in vivo, they act by stimulating production of inhibitory icosanoids such as PGI_2 and PGD_2 (described under Icosanoids, page 774).

Cyclooxygenase Deficiency

"Aspirin-like" functional defects in subjects with mild bleeding are among the most common problems seen in clinical practice. It is extremely difficult to distinguish congenital cyclooxygenase deficiency from

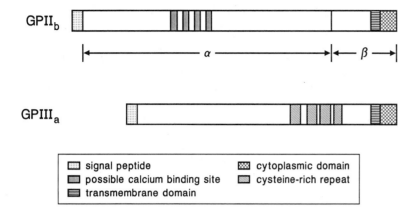

GPII_b

α β

GPIII_a

signal peptide   cytoplasmic domain
possible calcium binding site   cysteine-rich repeat
transmembrane domain

FIGURE 22–6. Model of structure of glycoprotein II_b/III_a. Amino-terminus on the left. The α and β chains of glycoprotein II_b are indicated.

prior aspirin ingestion, because the effects of aspirin persist for several days after the drug is ingested. Approximately 15 patients have been reported to have congenital cyclooxygenase deficiency.[146–149] This defect leads to a mild aspirin-like bleeding disorder characterized by a long skin bleeding time, easy bruising, and abnormal platelet aggregation in vitro. Serious hemorrhage has rarely been a problem in these patients. In none of the cases described to date is a pattern of inheritance demonstrated with multiple family members affected. In a few cases, radioimmunoassay of cyclooxygenase antigen indicates that true deficiency does exist.[150, 151] Measurement of cyclooxygenase antigen is currently the only certain way to diagnose cyclooxygenase deficiency.

It is not known whether cyclooxygenase deficiency affects only platelets or all tissues. In one case, cyclooxygenase in an excised vein was also found to be deficient, implying that prostacyclin production by blood vessels was also ablated. Despite deficiency of the antithrombotic icosanoid prostacyclin, this patient had no obvious thrombotic tendency. Cyclooxygenase deficiency in all tissues would imply that essential fatty acid deficiency,[152] which leads to multiple organ dysfunctions, including sterility and a renal concentrating defect, must be due to an inability to produce products of pathways other than cyclooxygenase.

PLATELET MEMBRANE RECEPTORS AND THEIR DISORDERS

Fibrinogen Receptor (Glycoprotein II_b/III_a)

On the basis of measurement of fibrinogen binding, there are approximately 45,000 fibrinogen receptors per platelet. This receptor has been isolated by immunoaffinity chromatography of a detergent-solubilized platelet membrane extract using monoclonal antibodies.[153, 154] It is a heterodimeric membrane glycoprotein and a member of the gene family of adhesive proteins called integrins[155, 156] (Fig. 22–6). The subunits are homologous but separate gene products designated glycoproteins II_b and III_a. Glycoprotein II_b is synthesized as a single polypeptide that is post-translationally cleaved into a heavy chain of 871 amino

acids and a disulfide-linked light chain of 137 amino acids.[157, 158] The heavy chain contains four repeated motifs homologous to calcium-binding domains of calmodulin.[158] Glycoprotein III_a consists of 762 amino acids with a single transmembrane domain near the carboxy-terminus. It contains four cysteine-rich repeats similar to the ligand-binding domains of other receptors such as the LDL receptor.[159, 160] The two chains form a calcium-dependent dimer in the membrane. They contain 15 per cent carbohydrate with a high content of mannose residues, suggesting the presence of both N-linked and high mannose oligosaccharide units.[154] The genes encoding these proteins are located together on chromosome 17q21–23.[159] The fibrinogen receptor, glycoprotein II_b/III_a, also links the extracellular fibrin matrix to the platelet contractile apparatus.[85] Hence, glycoprotein II_b/III_a links fibrinogen on the cell exterior with the contractile proteins of the cell interior. The former allows platelet aggregation[161] and the later clot retraction (Fig. 22–7). It also has been demonstrated that fibrinogen binds to isolated glycoprotein II_b/III_a,[162] and a photoactivatable derivative of fibrinogen becomes linked to this glycoprotein in ADP-activated platelets.[163] These data suggest that glycoprotein II_b/III_a is the fibrinogen receptor and is required for normal platelet aggregation. At least two sites in fibrinogen bind to the receptor. One is located at the carboxy-terminal end of the γ chain of fibrinogen[164] in the so-called fragment D domain. This was shown by demonstrating that the

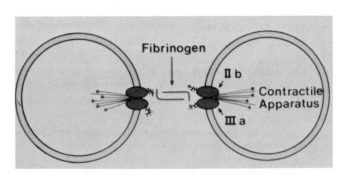

FIGURE 22–7. Model for the function of platelet membrane glycoprotein II_b/III_a. When platelets are activated, II_b/III_a binds contractile proteins on the cell interior and fibrinogen on the cell exterior.

binding of fibrinogen to platelets was blocked by low concentrations of a synthetic pentadecapeptide comprising residues 397 to 411 of the γ chain and by showing direct binding of fragment D of fibrinogen to solubilized glycoprotein II$_b$/III$_a$ in vitro.[165] Further cross-linking studies indicate that the fibrinogen peptide binds to a site on glycoprotein II$_b$ at amino acids 294 to 314.[166] Peptides from this region both inhibit platelet aggregation and binding of fibrinogen to platelets.[167, 168] The other site on fibrinogen is a pair of RGD sequences. The binding site for RGD is in glycoprotein III$_a$, and peptides containing RGD sequences inhibit fibrinogen binding to its receptor and thereby inhibit platelet aggregation. These peptides are under investigation as potential antithrombotic agents.[169]

Binding of fibrinogen to its receptor requires prior exposure of platelets to an agonist, and maximal binding occurs with the same concentrations of fibrinogen and calcium ions required for optimal platelet aggregation. It is unclear how agonists such as ADP lead to the development of fibrinogen-binding sites. No ADP receptor has been clearly defined, nor has it been shown that ADP binds to or alters the fibrinogen receptors directly.

Glanzmann's Thrombasthenia

One of the most common inherited disorders of platelet function is Glanzmann's thrombasthenia, a disorder due to the absence of the platelet fibrinogen receptor. The initial clue to the pathogenesis of this disorder was derived from study of an antibody obtained from the serum of a multiply transfused thrombasthenic patient.[170] This patient's antibody reacted with normal but not thrombasthenic platelets. The antibody arose from the fact that the patient was not tolerant to the normal fibrinogen receptor glycoprotein II$_b$/III$_a$.[171] It was later shown that the antibody precipitated glycoprotein II$_b$/III$_a$ and, most importantly, when added to normal platelets, induced a thrombasthenia-like functional defect in vitro. Direct binding studies of monoclonal antibodies to the fibrinogen receptor indicate absence of the receptor in patients with thrombasthenia with 50 per cent levels in obligate heterozygotes[153] (Fig. 22–8). Other monoclonal antibodies have been isolated that block platelet aggregation and fibrinogen binding to normal platelets.[172–175] Mutations that cause thrombasthenia have been found in both subunits. In the common Iraqi-Jewish disease, all six families studied had a common 11 base deletion in exon 12 of GPIII$_a$.[176] This results in a frameshift and protein termination just outside the membrane-spanning domain. In three of five Arab families studied, a 13 base deletion encompassing the splice acceptor site of exon 4 of GPII$_b$ causes a 6 amino acid deletion that includes a cysteine residue. The deletion must be critical to protein folding, as these patients have no detectable protein.[176] Definition of the mutations in patients with normal levels of glycoprotein II$_b$/III$_a$ but absent fibrinogen binding has fur-

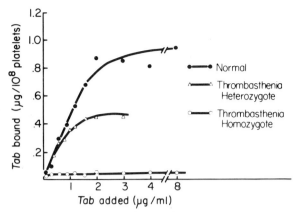

FIGURE 22–8. Binding of monoclonal antiglycoprotein II$_b$/III$_a$ (Tab) to normal and thrombasthenic platelets.

ther identified the binding domain. Thus mutation of D119 to Y in glycoprotein III$_a$ abolishes receptor function.[177] Similarly, mutation of R214 to Q in glycoprotein III$_a$ leads to loss of receptor function.[178]

The diagnosis of Glanzmann's thrombasthenia depends on the following criteria: (1) mucocutaneous bleeding, which is usually present from birth; (2) history of bleeding in sibs compatible with autosomal recessive inheritance; (3) normal platelet count and morphology with prolonged bleeding time,* absent clot retraction, absent platelet aggregation by ADP, epinephrine, collagen, and thrombin but normal aggregation by ristocetin in the presence of vWF.[179] The functional abnormalities in platelet aggregation and clot retraction are explained by the functions of the fibrinogen receptor protein.

Other proteins, including fibronectin,[180] vWF,[181–184] and thrombospondin,[178] bind to glycoprotein II$_b$/III$_a$. Binding of these molecules has been demonstrated using pure proteins and washed human platelets. The evidence that they bind to the same receptor site is that they compete with fibrinogen for binding, and binding is diminished or absent when platelets from thrombasthenic patients are used. These findings are of uncertain physiological significance. This is particularly true in the case of vWF, because patients with thrombasthenia do not have defective platelet adhesion, implying that adhesion mediated by vWF is through binding to a different receptor than glycoprotein II$_b$/III$_a$. In the presence of plasma, where high concentrations of fibrinogen are found, vWF does not bind to human platelets in the absence of ristocetin.[185]

The P1^{A1} antigen is a platelet-specific alloantigen present in 98 per cent of the population.[186] It is absent or reduced in patients with thrombasthenia, because the antigen resides on the III$_a$ subunit of glycoprotein II$_b$/III$_a$.[187] Individuals who lack P1^{A1} antigen but are otherwise normal have normal levels of glycoprotein II$_b$/III$_a$.[187] The P1^{A1} antigen is not required for normal

---

*Bleeding time is measured clinically by determining the time of bleeding after a standardized skin incision 5 mm long × 1 mm deep.

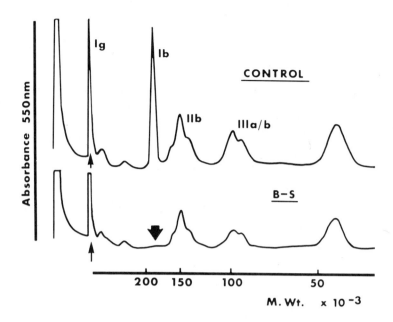

FIGURE 22–9. Sodium dodecyl sulfate polyacrylamide gel electrophoresis of normal *(top)* and Bernard-Soulier platelets. The gel was stained with periodic acid–Shiff reagent and was scanned by densitometry. Note the absence of glycoprotein I_b indicated by the heavy arrow.

function of the protein, and family studies of individuals carrying both thrombasthenia and $P1^{A1}$ gene mutations simultaneously indicate that the genes are inherited and segregate independently.[188] The $P1^{A1}$ antigen is due to a polymorphism in glycoprotein III_a $(L33 \rightarrow P)$[188a]; other rare polymorphisms also produce alloantigens.[188b]

von Willebrand Factor Receptor

A role for von Willebrand factor (vWF) in platelet function was elucidated fortuitously through studies of a toxic antibiotic, ristocetin, which caused thrombocytopenia.[189] Ristocetin was found to aggregate platelets in vitro in a reaction that required plasma vWF. Ristocetin does not aggregate platelets in plasma of patients with von Willebrand's disease, nor does it aggregate platelets from patients lacking the receptor for vWF. As with thrombasthenia, the elucidation of the vWF receptor has been greatly facilitated by studies of patients congenitally lacking this moiety who suffer from Bernard-Soulier syndrome. Binding studies using purified radiolabeled vWF have confirmed the presence of receptors for human vWF on platelets of normal individuals but not on platelets of Bernard-Soulier patients.[190–192] The vWF receptor is unique in that it does not bind its ligand unless the platelets are subjected to shear stress mediated by flow of blood. This is presumed to be due to a shear-induced conformation change in either vWF or the receptor.[193]

Nurden and Caen fractionated Bernard-Soulier platelet membrane proteins by electrophoresis in SDS and demonstrated a decrease in a major glycoprotein of M_r 155,000[194] (Fig. 22–9). This glycoprotein has been designated glycoprotein I or I_b; there are 25,000 molecules per normal platelet.[195] Studies using crossed immunoelectrophoresis of solubilized platelets clearly demonstrate that glycoprotein I_b is absent in most

Bernard-Soulier platelets.[196] Intermediate levels of the glycoprotein have been reported in obligate heterozygotes.[197, 198]

The vWF receptor is a complex structure that contains four polypeptides, designated glycoprotein $Ib\alpha(GPIb\alpha)$, glycoprotein $IB\beta(GPIb\beta)$, glycoprotein $IX(GPIX)$, and glycoprotein V (GPV) (Fig. 22–10). All four components of the receptor contain closely related leucine-rich repeat motifs that are highly conserved but of unknown function.[193] $GPIb\alpha$ and $GPIb\beta$ form a dimeric disulfide-linked heterodimer of 610 and 181 amino acids, respectively.[158, 193] GPIX and GPV form non-covalent complexes with the above proteins based on co-immunoprecipitation of all of the proteins by antisera against any one of them.[199] GPIX contains 160 amino acids[200] with a single transmembrane domain near the carboxy-terminus and is en-

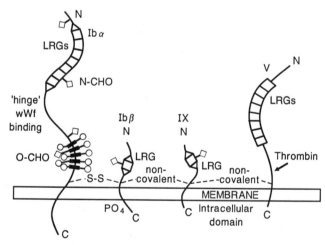

FIGURE 22–10. Model of von Willebrand factor receptor inserted into cell membrane (see text for details). LRG = Leucine-rich repeats; $Ib\alpha$ = glycoprotein $Ib\alpha$; $Ib\beta$ = glycoprotein $Ib\beta$; IX = glycoprotein IX; V = glycoprotein V.

coded by a gene on chromosome 3 that is apparently not linked to the genes for the other subunits of the receptor.[201] GPV (M_r 82,000) has been isolated but not yet cloned.[202, 203]

Bernard-Soulier Syndrome

In 1948 Bernard and Soulier reported a 5 month old infant with a history of spontaneous mucocutaneous bleeding beginning shortly after birth.[204] The patient had a prolonged bleeding time, and his platelets appeared abnormally large on peripheral blood smear. The patient had a sister who died of hemorrhage at the age of 3 years. Seventy patients with this syndrome have been reported, all with an autosomal recessive inheritance pattern. In most of these cases, the platelet aggregation defect or membrane glycoprotein deficiency has been demonstrated. The diagnosis is established by the finding of mucocutaneous bleeding, a family history compatible with autosomal recessive inheritance, and the following laboratory findings: decreased platelet count with giant platelets on blood smear (Fig. 22–11), normal clot retraction, absent platelet aggregation with vWF plus ristocetin, and normal platelet aggregation with physiological agonists. The degree of bleeding varies among patients even within a family, but most experience episodes severe enough to require transfusion. Unlike patients with coagulation factor abnormalities, these patients do not suffer from hemarthroses. The mechanism for formation of large platelets in the disease is unknown. Perhaps the lack of the vWF receptor affects the demarcation of platelets in the megakaryocyte.

Whether all four proteins are required for vWF receptor function awaits further definition of the mutations in Bernard-Soulier syndrome. Thus far, only mutations in glycoprotein I_b have been described. One is a frameshift that truncates the protein in half, deleting the transmembrane domain.[205] Another is a substitution of L57 to F. This is an informative mutation because it is within a conserved leucine repeat motif. The disease in the kindred is dominantly inherited, suggesting that receptors must interact in some way.[206] A third mutation in GPIbα substitutes G233 with V, but these patients do not have Bernard-Soulier syndrome. The patients have a von Willebrand disease–like syndrome, as their platelets bind plasma vWF abnormally without shear, producing thrombocytopenia.[207] Whether mutations in the other subunits of the vWF receptor lead to Bernard-Soulier syndrome awaits further study.

The antibiotic ristocetin is required for in vitro vWF binding and vWF-induced aggregation. Reports that platelet activation would allow binding of vWF without ristocetin do not measure the physiologically significant binding of vWF, as this binding is to glycoprotein II_b/III_a (described under Fibrinogen Receptor [Glycoprotein II_b/III_a], page 764). The requirement for ristocetin to demonstrate binding presumably reflects some conformational change induced in either vWF or the receptor that allows binding. Absence of either the vWF receptor in Bernard-Soulier syndrome or plasma vWF in von Willebrand's disease results in failure of platelet aggregation in platelet-rich plasma in the presence of ristocetin. Although ristocetin-induced aggregation is an in vitro phenomenon, it is the manifestation of a more physiological interaction of platelets with exposed subendothelial surfaces. Baumgartner and coworkers[208] measured this interaction by circulating anticoagulated blood through a perfusion chamber containing segments of rabbit aorta in which the subendothelium was exposed. The segments were fixed and examined microscopically, and the percentage of surface to which platelets became adherent was measured. Platelets from patients with Bernard-Soulier syndrome, like those from patients with von Willebrand's disease, show a decreased adherence to subendothelium.

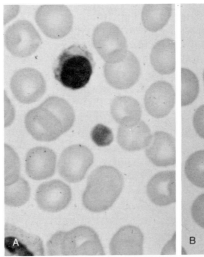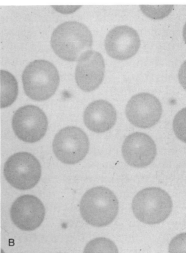

FIGURE 22–11. Peripheral blood smear from a patient with Bernard-Soulier syndrome (A) compared with that from a normal subject (B). Note giant platelet compared with a lymphocyte; normal film shows several normal platelets.

Thrombin Receptor

Platelets contain high-affinity binding sites for thrombin, and the binding of thrombin to these sites correlates with the activation of platelets by thrombin.[87] Thrombin receptors are specific for thrombin; they do not bind prothrombin or prethrombin II.[209] The latter has the same amino acid sequence as thrombin and lacks only a single internal cleavage that converts this single-chain precursor to the active enzyme. Thrombin inactivated with diisopropylfluorophosphate (DFP) also binds to the receptor but does not cause platelet activation. Thus, it has been postulated that platelet activation requires proteolysis of some membrane component. Although a number of putative thrombin substrates in the platelet membrane have been identified, in no case does the time course or the thrombin dependence of cleavage correlate with platelet activation.[210] Furthermore, the pattern of activation of platelets by thrombin does not suggest an enzymatic reaction but rather a ligand-receptor interaction, because small concentrations of thrombin result in rapid partial activation of platelets rather than slow complete activation, as might be predicted by turnover of a small amount of enzyme. The recent isolation of a cDNA encoding the thrombin receptor explains the properties described above. The receptor contains 425 amino acids with seven membrane-spanning domains similar to other receptors coupled to trimeric G proteins, such as adrenergic receptors.[211, 212] The receptor is activated by a novel mechanism wherein thrombin cleaves a single bond between R41/S42 to liberate a new amino-terminal sequence that serves as a tethered ligand to activate the receptor.[213] Synthetic peptides with this sequence are full thrombin agonists. It is not known how the peptide activates the receptor or which G protein, if any, is coupled to the response. No congenital abnormality of this receptor has yet been identified.

Factor Xa–Factor VA Receptor

Prothrombin activation occurs on the platelet surface. Platelets bind factor Xa with high affinity (K_d = 30 to 70 pM),[90–94, 214] and bound factor Xa catalyzes the activation of prothrombin 300,000 times faster than factor Xa in solution. Factor Xa binds to 200 to 300 sites on the platelet surface. The binding is specific for factor Xa, because neither the zymogen factor X nor other coagulation factors displace bound factor Xa. Factor Xa binding requires either exogenous factor Va or stimulation of the release reaction to release platelet factor V, which is then converted to factor VA.[91, 209] Human platelets contain ~0.3 μg factor V per 10^8 platelets,[215, 216] which when converted to factor Va is about 10 times the amount required to saturate the factor Xa–factor Va receptor sites.[214] Although factor Xa can bind to unstimulated platelets, no binding occurs in the absence of factor Va. Because factor Va is formed by thrombin, which also activates plate-

lets, it seems likely that physiological factor Xa binding occurs only when platelets are activated. Although platelets contain cytoplasmic proteases that can activate factor V, no evidence exists that they do so during platelet activation.[217] The fact that prothrombin activation normally occurs on the platelet surface is suggested by studies of patients with congenital factor V deficiency, because clinical severity correlates with platelet, rather than plasma, levels of factor V.[218]

The factor Xa receptor has not been isolated, so its protein nature can only be inferred. Factors Xa and Va appear to interact with each other in binding to platelets, as each stimulates the binding of the other.[219–221] Because factor Va can bind to platelets in the absence of factor Xa but not the converse, it appears that factor Va must bind to the platelet before factor Xa. A derivative of factor Xa that lacks the amino-terminal portion of the molecule is equivalent to factor Xa in its ability to interact with factor Va in solution and catalyze prothrombin activation, whereas its ability to bind to the human platelet factor Xa receptor is less than 10 per cent of native factor Xa. Thus, binding of factor Xa to platelets requires an interaction with platelet-bound factor Va, some platelet component, and a factor Xa domain at its amino-terminus.[219] The stoichiometry of binding is one factor Xa per factor Va.[220]

It has been assumed that the platelet components to which factors Xa and Va bind are negatively charged phospholipids, analogous to phospholipids used in in vitro coagulation assays. However, although they are required to accelerate prothrombin activation, there is no evidence that acidic phospholipids are exposed in the outer leaflet of the plasma membrane of platelets. Furthermore, phospholipids can substitute for platelets in prothrombin activation only when factor Xa is present in relatively high concentrations, and the affinity of phospholipid for factor Xa, even in the presence of factor Va, is much less than that of the platelet receptor. When platelets are damaged by vigorous stirring or by addition of calcium ionophore A23187, accelerated prothrombin activation can be demonstrated.[98] The factor Xa concentration dependence of this reaction suggests that it reflects phospholipids rather than the physiological platelet receptor.

Further evidence that the platelet receptor is not merely phospholipid is that a monoclonal antibody to factor Va blocks platelet-stimulated, but not phospholipid-stimulated, prothrombin activation.[218] A single patient with an abnormal platelet factor Xa receptor has been described,[214] who has 25 per cent of the normal number of factor Xa receptor sites and suffers from a moderately severe life-long bleeding disorder. In contrast, a patient who developed an autoantibody directed against acidic phospholipids has been described. This antibody blocks prothrombin activation in the presence of acidic phospholipids and has no effect on platelet surface prothrombin activation in vitro, and the patient has no bleeding diathesis.[222] Further characterization of the platelet factor Xa receptor has been hindered by the fact that so few of these moieties exist on the platelet. For example, a factor Xa receptor with a molecular weight of 100,000, has only 0.003 per cent of platelet membrane protein.

Icosanoid Receptors

Platelets appear to have three distinct icosanoid receptors—two inhibitory and one stimulatory. The inhibitory icosanoids act at a PGI_2/PGE_1 receptor and at a PGD_2 receptor.[223–225] These inhibitors block platelet function by stimulating adenylate cyclase and thereby elevating platelet cAMP levels. That platelets contain two distinct inhibitory receptors is indicated by direct ligand-binding studies. PGI_2 and PGE_1 both bind to platelets; they compete with each other but not with PGD_2, which also binds to platelets. PGD_2 binding is not inhibited by either PGI_2 or PGE_1. Experiments showing specific agonist desensitization also support the concept of separate PGI_2/PGE_1 and PGD_2 receptors; exposure of platelets to PGD_2 inhibits subsequent responses to PGD_2 but not to PGI_2 or PGE_1.[226, 227] Although distinct receptors are present, they appear to be coupled to the same adenylate cyclase molecules, because the increases in cAMP stimulated by these substances are not additive. PGI_2 is the most potent inhibitory icosanoid with 50 per cent of maximal inhibition of platelet function at about 1 nM. PGD_2 and PGE_1 are 50- and 25-fold less potent, respectively. Most patients with myeloproliferative disorders have relative refractoriness to PGD_2 and have reduced numbers of PGD_2 receptors.[228] Whether this defect contributes to the increased thromboses in these patients is uncertain. Responses to PGI_2 in these patients are normal.

The agonists for the stimulatory icosanoid receptor—cyclic endoperoxide PGH_2 and thromboxane A_2—are both labile, thereby precluding direct binding studies. However, selective PGH_2/thromboxane A_2 receptor antagonists such as 13-azaprostanoic acid have allowed demonstration of high-affinity binding sites on platelet membranes.[229] The platelet thromboxane A_2 receptor has been isolated by affinity chromatography,[230] and a cDNA encoding the receptor has been isolated from megakaryocyte cell line and placental cDNA libraries.[231] The receptor is composed of 343 amino acids and is a member of the seven membrane-spanning receptor family with distant homology to the rhodopsin and adrenergic receptors. Three unrelated patients with a mild, congenital "aspirin-like" bleeding disorder have been reported.[232–234] Platelets of affected individuals do not undergo secretion or second-wave aggregation in response to ADP and epinephrine. These platelets also fail to aggregate or undergo the release reaction in response to arachidonic acid, PGH_2, or cyclic endoperoxide analogues. Thromboxane A_2 formation from added arachidonate is normal, as determined by levels of thromboxane B_2. Rapid addition of arachidonate-stimulated platelet-rich plasma from normal subjects (which contains thromboxane A_2) fails to aggregate the platelets from affected patients, whereas arachidonate-stimulated platelets from patients aggregate aspirin-treated normal platelets. Thromboxane receptor antagonists could prove to be useful as antithrombotic agents.[235]

α-Adrenergic Receptor

Platelets are stimulated to aggregate by epinephrine, which is a relatively weak agonist. On the basis of studies with selective antagonists, the platelet adrenergic receptor is of the α_2 subtype. Because the levels of epinephrine achieved in man under conditions of stress are lower than those required for stimulation of platelet aggregation in vitro, the physiological significance of these receptors is uncertain. Patients with essential thrombocytosis have been reported to have decreased aggregation responses to epinephrine in vitro and decreased adrenergic receptors as demonstrated by direct binding studies.[236] Whether this defect contributes to the bleeding diathesis in these patients is uncertain.

STIMULUS-SECRETION COUPLING IN PLATELET ACTIVATION

The mechanism by which cells are activated when cell surface receptors are occupied by a ligand is a fundamental, unsolved problem. Platelets have been used extensively for studies of stimulus-response coupling, and much of what is currently known has been elucidated in these cells.

Role of Ca²⁺ in Platelet Activation

The current view of platelet activation by agonists involves several interrelated systems. Ca^{2+} fluxes are thought to mediate several reactions. In unstimulated platelets, the cytosolic Ca^{2+} concentration is estimated to be ~0.1 μM. When cells are maximally stimulated by thrombin or collagen, levels rise to 1 to 5 μM, as measured with the fluorescent indicator Quin-2.[237] Extracellular Ca^{2+} is not required for activation of human platelets. The source of Ca^{2+} is thought to be the platelet-dense tubular system, which is analogous to the sarcoplasmic reticulum in muscle. Upon activation, these membranes become permeable to Ca^{2+}, releasing it to the cytoplasm. It is then subsequently reaccumulated by a Ca^{2+}-transporting ATPase.[238] Platelet-dense granules also contain Ca^{2+}, which is secreted when platelets are activated. This Ca^{2+} is not thought to participate in platelet activation per se.[239]

The Ca^{2+} signal serves to trigger phosphatidylinositol breakdown (see Phosphoinositide-Derived Messengers in Platelet Activation, page 771), to initiate protein phosphorylation by a Ca^{2+}-dependent protein kinase (protein kinase C), and to activate myosin light chain kinase. The latter enzyme phosphorylates the myosin light chain, which is required for platelet contraction (see page 759). Other reactions that may be stimulated by Ca^{2+} include proteolysis by a Ca^{2+}-dependent protease that is found in the platelet cytosol and the glycogenolysis that occurs within seconds of platelet activation.[239]

Protein Phosphorylation

A second system of platelet activation involves protein phosphorylation reactions. When platelets are activated by thrombin, two major proteins are rapidly phosphorylated.[240] These are the myosin light chain and a 40 kDa protein, inositol 1,4,5-trisphosphate 5-phosphomonoesterase.[241] The latter phosphorylation is catalyzed by a ubiquitous protein kinase designated protein kinase C, which is the major protein kinase in platelets.[242] The enzyme is activated by acidic phospholipids, diglyceride, and Ca^{2+}. The lipids serve to increase the enzyme's affinity for Ca^{2+}, allowing activity to occur at lower Ca^{2+} concentrations. Protein kinase C also phosphorylates the myosin light chain, although at a different site and with a much slower time course than that catalyzed by myosin light chain kinase.[243, 244] Undoubtedly, there are yet undiscovered substrates for protein kinase C. Platelets also contain cAMP-dependent protein kinase, which presumably catalyzes a number of inhibitory platelet protein phosphorylations because elevation of cAMP inhibits platelet activation.

Platelets also contain large amounts of protein tyrosine phosphate.[245, 246] Thrombin, collagen, and other strong platelet agonists stimulate rapid tyrosine phosphorylation of a variety of platelet proteins.[247–249] Addition to vanadate, a protein tyrosine phosphatase inhibitor, to permeabilized platelets induces secretion and increased tyrosine phosphorylation.[250] The specific targets of tyrosine phosphorylation in platelets are unknown, as are the kinases and phosphatases that carry out these reactions. Platelets have been found to contain multiple different protein tyrosine phosphatases based on molecular cloning from a megakaryocyte cDNA library.[251, 252] Activation of receptors that are protein tyrosine kinases stimulates the formation of novel metabolites of phosphatidylinositol (described below) and is associated with formation of complexes between receptors and phosphatidylinositol 3-kinase. Thrombin stimulation of platelets is associated with formation of complexes containing phosphatidylinositol 3-kinase, even though this receptor is not a tyrosine kinase.[253] The role of these complexes in platelet activation is unknown.

Cyclic Adenosine Monophosphate

Agents that elevate cAMP levels inhibit platelet activation. cAMP blocks platelet function at a very early stage, because most platelet responses are inhibited, including aggregation, secretion, appearance of fibrinogen receptors, and phosphoinositide turnover.[239]

High cAMP levels stimulate calcium uptake by the platelet-dense tubular system, thereby diminishing any stimulatory Ca^{2+} signal.[254] cAMP may also inhibit the stimulatory phosphorylation reactions catalyzed by protein kinase C and myosin light chain kinase.[255] It may be that the rate and direction of change in Ca^{2+} concentration determine platelet activation rather than the actual level of Ca^{2+}. Degradation of polyphosphoinositides is partially resistant to inhibition by cAMP.[256, 257]

As in other cells, cAMP levels are controlled by a complex system. Adenylate cyclase that forms cAMP from ATP is essentially inactive in the absence of the stimulatory guanine-nucleotide–binding regulatory protein designated G_s (Fig. 22–12).[258] There is also an inhibitory guanine-nucleotide–binding protein designated G_i. Each of these proteins has α, β, and γ subunits, and they are activated by communication with receptors occupied by appropriate agonists. The β and γ subunits of G_s and G_i are the same. Guanosine triphosphate (GTP) binding to the stimulatory G protein leads to dissociation of the α from $\beta\gamma$ subunits, resolving free $G_s\alpha$, which activates adenylate cyclase. Conversely, dissociation of G_i releases free $\beta\gamma$, which, when present in excess, can bind $G_s\alpha$ and thereby lead to inhibition of adenylate cyclase. Some agents activate inhibitory receptors and others stimulatory receptors. GTP hydrolysis to guanosine diphosphate (GDP) results in reversal of activation of these proteins. Another enzyme that controls cAMP levels is cyclic nucleotide phosphodiesterase. Inhibition of this enzyme elevates cAMP and inhibits platelet function. Many inhibitors of platelet function act by raising cAMP levels, such as the adenylate cyclase stimulators PGE_1, PGI_2, and PGD_2, and the phosphodiesterase inhibitors, such as the antithrombotic agent dipyridamole. It has been difficult to prove that platelet agonists actually lower basal cAMP levels, although most can decrease pharmacologically elevated cAMP levels. Because cAMP turns over in platelets with a $t\frac{1}{2}$ of less than 1

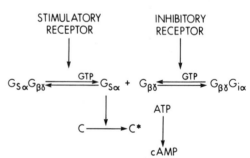

FIGURE 22–12. **Control of adenylate cyclase by guanine nucleotide–binding regulatory proteins.** The stimulatory GTP-binding protein has an α subunit that binds GTP when a stimulatory receptor is occupied. This subunit dissociates from the β and γ subunits and is free to stimulate the catalyst adenylate cyclase directly. When an inhibitory receptor is occupied, a different GTP-binding protein, G_i, is activated. In this case, GTP binds and $G_i\alpha$ dissociates. The $\beta\gamma$ subunits are the same as those of the stimulatory protein. These subunits can reassociate with $G_s\alpha$ and thereby inhibit adenylate cyclase.

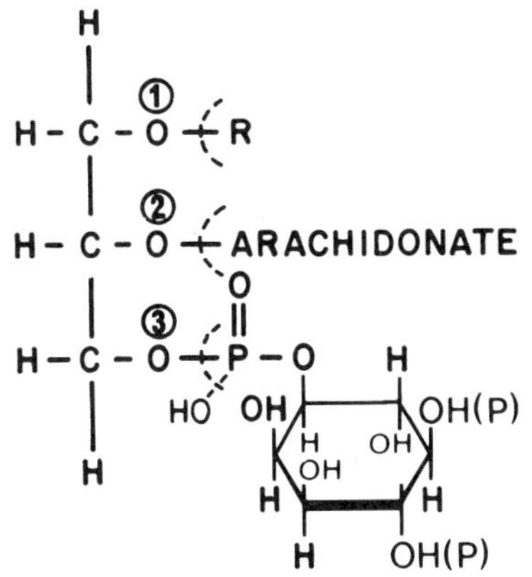

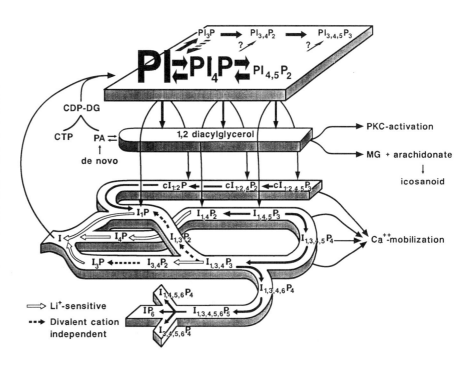

FIGURE 22–13. Phosphatidylinositol. This phospholipid and its phosphorylated forms serve as storehouses for messenger molecules. The P indicates the 4 and 5 positions, which contain phosphate groups in some molecules. When the molecule is broken by phospholipase C (reaction 1), inositol phosphates and diglyceride are the two products. Lipase reactions (reactions 2 and 3) subsequently liberate arachidonate from diglyceride.

Phosphoinositide-Derived Messengers in Platelet Activation

The phosphoinositides are minor phospholipids contained in all cells (Fig. 22–13). They serve as storage forms for messenger molecules. The responses of cells to external stimuli are mediated by a variety of messenger molecules. Three such molecules produced as a result of phosphoinositide metabolism are diglyceride, inositol trisphosphate, and arachidonic acid.[264] These substances have properties common to second messengers such as cAMP. Their production is initiated by specific agonists, they are potent activators of other cellular reactions, and they are rapidly degraded to inactive compounds.

Phosphoinositide Metabolism

Phosphoinositides are ubiquitous components of eukaryotic membranes. In platelets, phosphatidylinositol makes up about 5 to 7 per cent of phospholipids; phosphatidylinositol 4-phosphate, 1 per cent; and phosphatidylinositol 4,5-diphosphate, 0.4 per cent. The phosphoinositides are in equilibrium with each other through a "futile cycle" of kinases and phosphatases, as shown in Figure 22–14. Phosphoinositides undergo rapid breakdown in response to receptor-mediated cell activation.[264] All three phosphoinositides are degraded by a phospholipase C to form diglyceride and one of the inositol phosphates.[265] The inositol phosphates are produced in both cyclic and non-cyclic forms, as shown in Figure 22–14. Multiple phospholipase C enzymes occur in mammalian tissues, as deduced from direct protein isolation and molecular cloning studies.[266–268] It is not clear which isoforms are present in platelets. The different phospholipase C enzymes are coupled to receptors by different mech-

second,[259] perturbations in adenylate cyclase or phosphodiesterase can have rapid effects that may determine the threshold of platelets to activation, if not actually trigger the activation reaction. Most platelet agonists inhibit adenylate cyclase in cell-free preparations. These include ADP,[260] epinephrine,[261] and platelet-activating factor.[262] Thrombin inhibits adenylate cyclase as assayed in platelet membranes isolated after treatment of intact cells with thrombin.[263] It is not known how each of these agonists affects the system illustrated in Figure 22–12. Epinephrine presumably acts bound to an α_2 receptor that is coupled to a guanine-nucleotide inhibitory protein, as has been reported in other systems. The role of cGMP in platelet physiology remains to be elucidated.

FIGURE 22–14. Pathway for inositol phosphate metabolism. In the top level, PI indicates phosphatidylinositol; PI_4P, phosphatidylinositol 4-phosphate; PI_3P, phosphatidylinositol 3-phosphate; $PI_{3,4}P_2$, phosphatidylinositol 3,4-bisphosphate; $PI_{3,4,5}P_3$, phosphatidylinositol 3,4,5-trisphosphate; and $PI_{4,5}P_2$, phosphatidylinositol 4,5-bisphosphate. On the bottom level, I indicates inositol and P phosphate. The numbers preceding P refer to positions of phosphates on the inositol ring, and those following P, the number of phosphate groups. PA = Phosphatidic acid; CDP-DG = cytidine diphosphate diacylglycerol; PKC = protein kinase C; MG = 2 monoacylglycerol.

anisms. A novel trimeric G protein designated Gq couples one form of enzyme,[269-271] and another is activated by tyrosine kinase receptors.[267] The inositol phosphates are subsequently converted to a host of inositol phosphates, as shown in Figure 22–14, and subsequently degraded to inositol, which is used for resynthesis of phosphoinositides. The diglyceride is either hydrolyzed by lipases[272] to monoglyceride, which is further hydrolyzed to free arachidonate and glycerol, or it is phosphorylated by diglyceride kinase to form phosphatidic acid. Phosphatidic acid is then converted to phosphatidylinositol, completing the so-called phosphatidylinositol cycle.

Phosphatidylinositols containing phosphate esters in the 3 position of inositol represent a recently discovered pathway of phosphatidylinositol metabolism.[273] These include phosphatidylinositol 3-phosphate, phosphatidylinositol 3,4-bisphosphate, and phosphatidylinositol 3,4,5-trisphosphate (Fig. 22–14). Phosphatidylinositol 3-phosphate is present in cells under all conditions, whereas the polyphosphorylated 3-phosphate–containing phosphatidylinositols are formed transiently in response to agonists such as thrombin in the case of platelets. The functions of these compounds in signaling reactions are unknown, although the recent suggestion that they participate in cell motility by stimulating actin polymerization is intriguing.[274]

Inositol 1,4,5-Trisphosphate Formation and Calcium Mobilization

Polyphosphoinositides undergo agonist-induced hydrolysis, as evidenced by the transient appearance after thrombin treatment of platelets of inositol 1,4,5-trisphosphate (IP$_3$), inositol 1:2 cyclic 4,5-trisphosphate (cIP$_3$), and inositol 1,4-diphosphate (IP$_2$), which are products of phospholipase C action on polyphosphoinositides.[275, 276] IP$_2$, IP$_3$, and cIP$_3$ accumulate within a few seconds of stimulation, before major changes are seen in inositol 1-phosphate or inositol. Furthermore, polyphosphoinositide breakdown is the only platelet reaction that is not inhibited by elevated cAMP, suggesting that it is an early response in cell activation.[256, 257] IP$_3$ was first shown to mobilize Ca^{2+} in permeabilized pancreatic[277] and liver cells.[278] It also causes release of Ca^{2+} from isolated microsomes,[279] implying that the second messenger increases the permeability of the platelet-dense tubular system to Ca^{2+}. Both IP$_3$ and cIP$_3$ mobilize Ca^{2+} from permeabilized platelets.[280, 281] Hydrolysis of phosphatidylinositol by phospholipase C in vitro requires Ca^{2+}. IP$_3$ is the messenger for Ca^{2+} mobilization, and thus hydrolysis of phosphatidylinositol-4,5 diphosphate is Ca^{2+} independent. IP$_3$ induces calcium mobilization by binding to an IP$_3$-binding protein that serves as a calcium channel across membranes.[282, 283]

Diglyceride Accumulation and Protein Kinase C

Diglyceride levels rise transiently after stimulation of phosphoinositide turnover, thereby activating pro-tein kinase C. Nishizuka and coworkers found that a cyclic nucleotide–independent protein kinase previously identified in rat brain cytosol could be activated by anionic phospholipids in the presence of Ca^{2+}.[242] They also showed that micromolar amounts of diglyceride could dramatically lower the apparent K$_m$ for Ca^{2+} activation.[284] This finding implies that a control mechanism that increases diglyceride levels (namely, phosphatidylinositol breakdown) activates a cellular protein kinase without prior mobilization of Ca^{2+} or change in cAMP levels. In many tissues, including brain and platelets, 10 times as much protein kinase C activity is found as cAMP-dependent protein kinase.[284] There are multiple isoforms of protein kinase C, some of which are activated by fatty acids rather than diglyceride.[285, 286]

Castagna et al.[287] have shown that the tumor-promoting phorbol ester TPA (tetradecanoyl phorbol acetate) can substitute for diglyceride as an activator of protein kinase C at levels 1000-fold lower than diglyceride, leading to phosphorylation of several proteins in cells. Diglyceride is rapidly destroyed after its production, providing only a transient signal. In contrast to diglyceride, phorbol esters are not readily metabolized. This implies that a state of continued stimulation is deleterious. A synthetic diglyceride, 1-oleoyl-2-acetyl glycerol, which enters cells more readily than long-chain diacylglycerols, causes the same activation of protein kinase C as TPA and can be used in a similar manner. 1-oleoyl-2-acetyl glycerol and TPA can cause partial secretion by platelets without raising intracytoplasmic Ca^{2+}, as measured by the fluorescent Ca^{2+} binding dye Quin-2.[288] However, more recent studies using aequorin as a Ca^{2+} indicator suggest that intracellular Ca^{2+} may rise locally without being detected by Quin-2.[289] This suggests that secretion is a consequence of protein phosphorylation that may act synergistically with increasing Ca^{2+} concentration in platelets. This is further supported by experiments in which it was shown that subthreshhold amounts of a Ca^{2+} ionophore and the synthetic diglyceride or phorbol ester can result in synergistic platelet secretion.[290]

Control of Icosanoid Production

The enzymes that produce icosanoids appear to be continuously active in cells, and therefore the amounts of icosanoid produced after stimulation are determined by the amount of arachidonate (or other icosanoid precursor fatty acid) liberated. In platelets, approximately one half of released arachidonate is liberated from phosphoinositides, and the remainder is contributed by phosphatidylcholine. One mechanism for release of arachidonate uses a cytosolic phospholipase A$_2$ that is specific for icosanoid precursor fatty acids and has no homology to the secreted forms of phospholipase A$_2$ that have been studied extensively.[291] About 80 per cent of phosphatidylinositol molecules contain arachidonate at the sn-2 position. Hence, the bulk of the diglyceride produced by phospholipase C contains arachidonate, which is subsequently liberated by the sequential action of diglyceride and monoglyceride lipases.[272] In platelets, one third to two thirds of the diglyceride produced is degraded to arachidonate, depending on the stimulus, and the remainder is phosphorylated to phosphatidic acid. Control of the flow of diglyceride to hydrolysis versus conversion to phosphatidic acid may determine icosanoid production. Another controlling factor is the ability of cells to take up and esterify arachidonate into phospholipids (discussed under Production of Icosanoids, page 761). That this may be the case is suggested by experiments in cells lacking arachidonoyl-CoA synthase, wherein agonist-induced icosanoid production is diminished.[106]

In summary, current evidence suggests that phosphoinositide turnover serves as a signal-generating system, producing intracellular second messengers as well as liberating arachidonate for icosanoid production.

PLATELET–VESSEL WALL INTERACTIONS IN THE CONTROL OF HEMOSTASIS

Icosanoids

Icosanoid mediators transmit signals between platelets and cells of the vessel wall. When stimulated, platelets produce thromboxane A_2, which causes vasoconstriction of blood vessels, thereby promoting hemostasis. Conversely, endothelial cells produce PGI_2 or prostacyclin, which elevates platelet cAMP levels, thereby inhibiting platelet function; furthermore, it causes vasodilation. Thus, PGI_2 and thromboxane have opposite actions. On this basis it has been proposed that vascular homeostasis is determined by a balance of thromboxane A_2 (TxA_2) and PGI_2 and that the occurrence of thrombotic diseases might be influenced by factors that alter this balance (Fig. 22–15). This concept implies that aspirin might have paradoxical effects, because inhibition of endothelial PGI_2 by aspirin might actually promote thrombosis. Endothelial cells have receptors for thrombin, bradykinin, and histamine. Each of these agonists stimulates arachidonate release and conversion to PGI_2. An alternative source of substrate for PGI_2 is cyclic endoperoxides,

which are formed by platelets, as outlined in Figure 2–16. Endoperoxides may escape from platelets and be converted to PGI_2 by endothelium. The phenomenon of "endoperoxide steal" has been demonstrated in vitro[101]; its importance in vivo is uncertain, although it may explain the action of thromboxane synthetase inhibitors, as outlined in the following.

Early in vitro studies suggested that platelet cyclooxygenase is more sensitive to aspirin than cyclooxygenase in vascular tissue and that because of new enzyme synthesis by endothelium, vascular PGI_2 production was restored quickly after aspirin administration.[101] In this way it was proposed that there might be doses of aspirin at which a selective effect on platelet cyclooxygenase could be obtained. A large number of studies exploring this possibility indicate that although platelet cyclooxygenase is more sensitive to aspirin than that in the endothelium, even low doses of aspirin inhibit PGI_2 synthesis in part. High doses of aspirin, however, do not completely block PGI_2 production.

The concept of a balance between PGI_2 and thromboxane implies that PGI_2 is produced by normal endothelium. Several recent studies suggest that this is not the case. FitzGerald et al.[292, 293] estimate that circulating PGI_2 levels are ~3 pg/ml, which is 10-fold lower than the minimal amount that inhibits platelet function. It is possible, of course, that local concentrations of PGI_2 at sites of endothelial injury may reach higher, physiologically important concentrations. Follow-up of patients with rheumatoid arthritis treated with large doses of aspirin does not uncover an increase in thrombosis or atherosclerosis. Furthermore, patients with congenital cyclooxygenase deficiency, who may lack PGI_2, do not suffer from thrombotic episodes. Patients with atherosclerosis are not PGI_2 deficient but have higher than normal levels of urinary PGI_2 metabolites. Thus, there is no evidence that inhibition of PGI_2 production is an undesirable side effect of pharmacological inhibition of TxA_2 production. In fact, a number of clinical trials indicate that aspirin has a clinically useful antithrombotic effect. Meta-analysis has been used to evaluate the results of 25 trials of aspirin for prevention of death in myocardial infarction. This analysis showed that aspirin had no effect on non-vascular mortality but reduced vas-

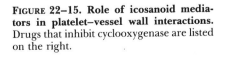

FIGURE 22–15. Role of icosanoid mediators in platelet–vessel wall interactions. Drugs that inhibit cyclooxygenase are listed on the right.

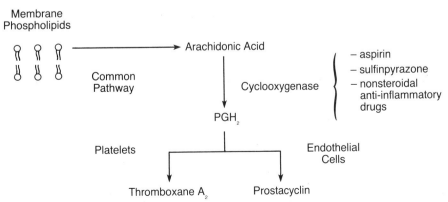

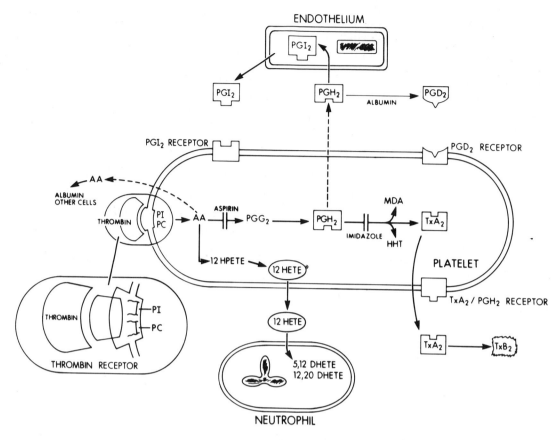

ARACHIDONATE METABOLISM IN PLATELETS

FIGURE 22–16. The pathways for liberation of arachidonate and its conversion to PGH₂ are shared by endothelial cells and platelets. PGH₂ is metabolized differently in the two cells to produce the aggregating agent thromboxane A₂ and the antiaggregating agent prostacyclin. Inhibition of cyclooxygenase by drugs can affect the production of both mediators.

cular mortality by 15 per cent and non-fatal vascular events (stroke, myocardial infarction) by 30 per cent. Low doses of 150 to 300 mg/day were effective.[294] An alternative antithrombotic therapy using selective inhibitors of thromboxane synthetase is also under investigation. Unfortunately, these drugs allow accumulation of cyclic endoperoxides (Fig. 22–16) in platelets, and the endoperoxides are themselves potent platelet-aggregating agents. In fact, these drugs may act primarily by stimulating the production of PGI₂ by endoperoxide steal and also by stimulating the conversion of PGH₂ to PGD₂ by albumin in plasma.

An alternative strategy to alter pathological vascular reactions mediated by icosanoids is the use of a diet with fatty acid eicosapentaenoic acid (5,8,11,14,17-EPA). EPA is the major polyunsaturated fatty acid of fish and other marine life. It is converted by vascular endothelium to PGI₃, which is an active prostacyclin, whereas the thromboxane metabolite of EPA, thromboxane A₃, is relatively inactive.[295] Additionally, cyclooxygenase metabolizes this fatty acid poorly, and it competes with arachidonate so that cells rich in EPA also produce decreased amounts of arachidonate-derived icosanoids. In fact, diets high in EPA result in decreased platelet function and prolonged skin bleed-

ing time. In leukocytes, similar findings are observed in production of leukotriene mediators. Small amounts of leukotrienes are formed, and those derived from EPA are relatively inactive.[296, 297] Epidemiological studies suggest that populations subsisting on a marine diet have a lower incidence of a number of diseases involving thrombosis. Experiments in NZB/NZW mice indicate that supplementation with EPA greatly ameliorates the autoimmune disorder that occurs in these animals.[298] These preliminary findings have created a wave of interest in dietary interventions involving supplementation with EPA. These supplements currently provide large sales for health-food stores.

Control of Thrombosis by Vascular Cells

Endothelial cells inhibit thrombosis by influencing both coagulation and fibrinolysis. Protein C is a vitamin K–dependent plasma protein described in Chapter 16. In vitro it is activated to protease that exhibits potent anticoagulant activity through the selected proteolysis of factors Va and VIIIa. The activation of protein C by thrombin, the only known physiological activator, is slow. Endothelial cells contain a cell surface protein designated thrombomodulin that acts as a cofactor for the activation of protein C, increasing the catalytic activity of thrombin by more than 1000-fold[299–303] (Fig. 22–17). This endothelial protein has the unique quality of converting thrombin from a coagulation factor to a major anticoagulant moiety. Thrombomodulin is localized to endothelial cells (and the syncytiotrophoblast of placenta, which is also exposed to blood).[304] When thrombin is generated in areas of vascular damage outside the vessel wall, procoagulant reactions occur, whereas inside the adjacent damaged vascular wall, thrombin is converted to an anticoagulant moiety, maintaining the fluidity of blood within the vascular channel. Thrombomodulin-stimulated protein C activation is modulated by coagulation factor Va, which is itself a substrate for activated protein C (APC).[305, 306] In the presence of factor Va, thrombomodulin activity is stimulated ~threefold.[307] Once APC is formed, the heavy chain of factor Va is degraded, and the remaining light chain serves to inhibit thrombomodulin activity. This is a feedback mechanism whereby factor Va promotes its own destruction, and once the anticoagulant function is destroyed, the residual light chain blocks further activation of protein C.

Vascular endothelium also contains heparin molecules,[308, 309] which greatly accelerate the inactivation of coagulation factors by antithrombin III (see Chapter 18). Another reaction important in inhibiting pathological thrombotic reactions is the production of tissue plasminogen activator by endothelial cells (see Chapter 21).

Platelet-Derived Growth Factor

Platelet-derived growth factor is a glycoprotein that has been isolated in two forms, one of 31 kDa, and the other of 28 kDa, which is smaller because of differences in glycosylation.[310] The two forms of PDGF have equivalent activity, and both are dimeric polypeptide chains linked by multiple interchain disulfide bridges. Human serum contains ~50 ng/ml of PDGF, whereas none is contained in plasma.[311] This growth factor appears to be the major growth-promoting component in serum. PDGF is contained in platelet α granules and is secreted at sites of platelet activation. In this way PDGF promotes wound healing, because it is a potent mitogen for cells of mesenchymal origin, including fibroblasts, glial cells, and smooth muscle cells.[312] When PDGF is added to plasma, it rapidly binds to $α_2$-macroglobulin.[313] This may serve as a clearance mechanism to prevent biologically active PDGF from entering the systemic circulation at sites of injury.

In addition to stimulating cell proliferation, PDGF is a potent chemotactic protein for inflammatory cells, including neutrophils and monocytes and certain other cells, such as smooth muscle cells and fibroblasts. PDGF attracts these cells to sites of injury, thereby furthering the repair process. The action of PDGF in wound healing may be its primary physiological function in vertebrates[314]; however, this molecule is also involved in atherogenesis.[315] In a number of models of atherosclerosis, it is clear that platelets are required for lesion development. This has led to the hypothesis that PDGF, when released intravascularly or into the vessel wall, leads to aberrant proliferation of smooth muscle cells, with formation of atherosclerotic lesions. For this reason, inhibitors of PDGF function are currently being sought.

PDGF stimulates target cells by binding to specific cell surface receptors.[316] Many responses follow rapidly, including enhancement of glycolysis, stimulation of amino acid transport, increased protein synthesis, increased turnover of phosphoinositides, and production of icosanoids.[310] Increased DNA synthesis and cell proliferation then occur. The plasma membrane receptor for PDGF has been identified as a 180 kDa glycoprotein.[317] This molecule has intrinsic and PDGF-stimulated protein tyrosine kinase activity. The PDGF

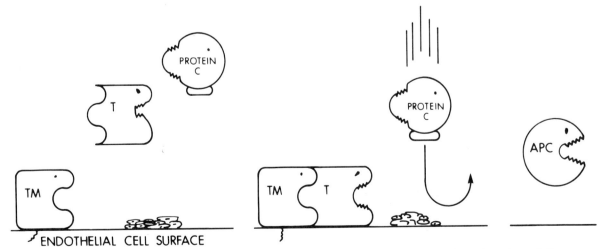

FIGURE 22–17. Mechanism of endothelial thrombomodulin-stimulated protein C activation. Thrombomodulin binds thrombin, which is postulated to result in a conformational change in thrombin that renders protein C a good substrate.

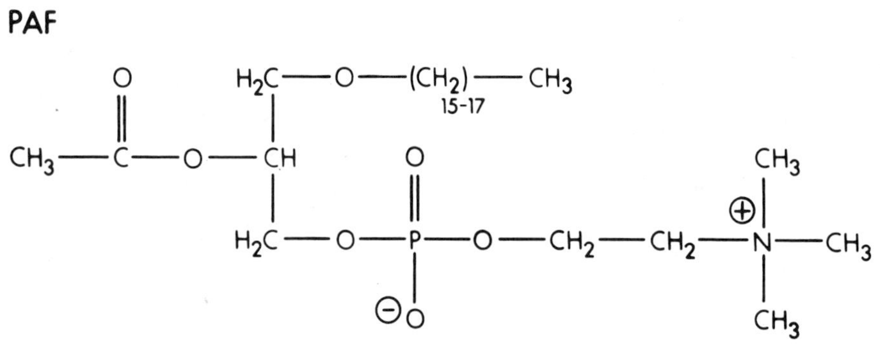

PAF

FIGURE 22–18. Structure of platelet-activating factor (PAF).

receptor kinase can also serve as a substrate for its own kinase activity and stimulates phosphorylation of other intracellular substrates. The mechanism by which tyrosine phosphorylation leads to cell proliferation has not been elucidated. The tyrosine-specific protein kinase activity of the PDGF receptor protein suggests a parallel to the biological activities observed in various retrovirus-transformed cells. Several retroviral transforming factors are tyrosine-specific protein kinases. The discovery that the α chain of PDGF is highly homologous to the retroviral transforming protein of the simian sarcoma virus[318, 319] has led to the development of the concept that normal growth factors may act as oncogenes (see Chapter 23).

Platelet-Activating Factor

Platelet-activating factor (PAF) is a potent lipid mediator produced by vascular endothelium[320, 321] and several other cell types, including stimulated neutrophils and macrophages.[322, 323] It was discovered as a product of IgE-sensitized rabbit basophils.[324] PAF administered parenterally to animals causes bronchoconstriction, vasodilation and hypotension, and neutrophil and platelet aggregation and secretion.[325] Obviously, the physiological function of this mediator does not include its access to the systemic circulation. Platelets have high-affinity receptors (K_d ~1 nM) for PAF,[326] and binding of PAF to these receptors correlates with the action of PAF on platelets. The PAF receptor contains 342 amino acids, has seven membrane-spanning domains, and shows homology of other such receptors.[327, 328] PAF is a strong platelet agonist, stimulating aggregation and secretion much like thrombin.[329, 330]

Endothelial cells produce PAF in response to thrombin[320, 321] and to leukotrienes,[331] implying receptor-mediated production. The PAF thus formed remains associated with the cells. At sites of vascular injury where thrombin is generated, PAF synthesized by endothelial cells may serve to activate platelets and leukocytes locally, causing them to adhere to sites of injury. Platelets themselves produce very small amounts of PAF in response to the Ca^{2+} ionophore A23187.[332, 333] Whether this is of physiological significance is uncertain, because thrombin-induced platelet activation does not result in PAF formation.[330]

Structure of Platelet-Activating Factor

PAF is 1-0-alkyl-2-acetyl-sn-glycerol-3-phosphoryl choline[334] (Fig. 22–18). The PAF produced by polymorphonuclear leukocytes contains primarily a 16-carbon–saturated alkyl moiety[335] in the 1 position, although 18-carbon PAF is very active and may be produced in other cells. The acetyl moiety is most important; fatty acids in the 2 position of four carbons or greater are inactive.[334] PAF is synthesized from 1-0 alkyl-2-lyso glycerol-3-phosphoryl choline and acetyl-CoA by an acetyl transferase enzyme.[336, 337] One potential rate-limiting step in PAF synthesis is the availability of lyso-PAF, implying that lipases may partially control production of PAF.[338, 339] In fact, hydrolysis of 1-alkyl-2-arachidonoyl-glycerol-3-phosphoryl choline by phospholipase A_2 could produce both lyso-PAF for PAF synthesis and free arachidonate for icosanoid production. When lyso-PAF is added to neutrophils, it is specifically reacylated with arachidonate, suggesting a link between PAF and arachidonate metabolism. In the case of platelets, PAF production is far less than that of thromboxane (picomoles versus nanomoles), and thus the coordinate production of PAF and thromboxane A_2 would be quantitatively insignificant with respect to thromboxane A_2. PAF production does not depend simply on provision of the lyso-PAF substrate. Addition of lyso-PAF to cells results mainly in acylation with arachidonic acid rather than production of PAF unless a stimulus such as thrombin is added. Stimulation of cells may activate the acetyl transferase reaction to control PAF production.[340, 341] The duration of PAF action is short, implying mechanisms for rapid inactivation of the mediator. Degradation of PAF to lyso-PAF is catalyzed by an acetyl hydrolase enzyme that is contained both in plasma[342] and in cells,[343] and the two forms of the enzyme appear distinct.[344] The role of PAF in human disease remains to be elucidated.

REFERENCES

1. Editorial. Lancet 2:133, 1973.
2. Metcalf, D., MacDonald, H. R., Odartchenko, N., and Sordat, B.: Growth of mouse megakaryocyte colonies in vitro. Proc. Natl. Acad. USA 72:1744, 1975.
3. Nakeff, A., and Daniels-McQueen, S.: In vitro colony assay for a new class megakaryocyte precursor: Colony forming unit megakaryocyte. Proc. Soc. Exp. Biol. Med. 151:587, 1976.

4. McLeod, D. L., Shreeve, M. M., and Axelrad, A. A.: Induction of megakaryocyte colonies with platelet formation in vitro. Nature 261:492, 1976.
5. Vainchenker, W., Bouquet, J., Guichard, J., and Breton-Gorius, J.: Megakaryocyte colony formation from human bone marrow precursors. Blood 54:940, 1979.
6. Mazur, E. M., Hoffman, R., and Bruno, E.: Regulation of human megakaryocytopoiesis. J. Clin. Invest. 68:733, 1981.
7. Ebbe, S., and Stohlman, F.: Megakaryocytopoiesis in the rat. Blood 26:20, 1965.
8. Penington, D. G.: Formation of platelets. In Dingle, J. T., and Gordon, J. L. (eds.): Platelets in Pathology and Biology 2. Amsterdam, Elsevier North Holland Biomedical Press, 1982, p. 19.
9. Mosesson, M. W., Homandberg, G. A., and Amrani, D. L.: Human platelet fibrinogen gamma chain structure. Blood 63:990, 1984.
10. Chiu, C. P., Schick, P., and Colman, R. W.: Biosynthesis of coagulation factor V in isolated guinea pig megakaryocytes. J. Clin. Invest. 75:339, 1985.
11. Ryo, R., Nakeff, A., Huang, S. S., Ginsberg, M., and Deuel, T. F.: Platelet factor 4 synthesis in a megakaryocyte enriched rabbit bone marrow culture. J. Cell Biol. 96:515, 1983.
12. Chernoff, A. R., Levine, R. F., and Goodman, D. S.: Origin of platelet derived growth factor in megakaryocytes in guinea pigs. J. Clin. Invest. 65:926, 1980.
13. Nachman, R. L., Levine, R. F., and Jaffe, E. A.: Synthesis of vWF in cultured guinea pig megakaryocytes. J. Clin. Invest. 60:914, 1977.
14. Rabellino, E. M., Levene, R. B., Leung, L. L. K., and Nachman, R. L.: Human megakaryocytes: II. Expression of platelet proteins in early marrow megakaryocytes. J. Exp. Med. 154:88, 1981.
15. Shaklai, M., and Tavassoli, M.: Demarcation membrane system in rat megakaryocyte and the mechanism of platelet formation: A membrane reorganization process. J. Ultrastruct. Res. 62:270, 1978.
16. Tavassoli, M.: Megacaryocyte-platelet axis and the process of platelet formation and release. Blood 55:537, 1980.
17. Radley, J. M., and Scurfield, G.: The mechanism of platelet release. Blood Cells 56:996, 1980.
18. Levin, J., and Evatt, B. L.: Humoral control of thrombopoiesis. Blood Cells 5:105, 1979.
19. Gerwitz, A. M., Bruno, E., Elwell, J., and Hoffman, R.: In vitro studies of megakaryocytopoiesis in thrombocytopenic disorders of man. Blood 61:384, 1983.
20. Hoffman, R., Yang, H. H., Stravenan, J., Bruno, E., and Spencer, C. D.: Purification and partial characterization of human megakaryocyte colony stimulating factor. Clin Res. 32:491a, 1984.
21. Gewirtz, A. M., and Poncz, M.: Megakaryocytopoiesis and platelet production. In Hoffman, R., Benz, E. J., Shattil, S. J., Furie, B., Cohen, H. J. (eds.): Hematology: Basic Principles and Practice. Livingston, NY, Churchill, 1991, pp. 1148–1157.
22. Heaton, W. A., Davis, H. H., Welsh, M. J., Mathias, C. J., Joist, H. J., Sherman, L. A., and Siegel, B. A.: Indium 111: A new radionuclide label for studying human platelet kinetics. Br. J. Haematol. 42:613, 1979.
23. White, J. G., and Gerrard, J. M.: Anatomy and structural organization of the platelet. In Colman, R. W., Hirsh, J., Marder, V. J., and Salzman, E. W. (eds.): Hemostasis and Thrombosis. Philadelphia, J. B. Lippincott Co., 1982, p. 343.
24. Feagler, J. R., Tillack, T. W., Chaplin, D. D., and Majerus, P. W.: The effects of thrombin of phytohemagglutinin receptor sites in human platelets. J. Cell Biol. 60:541, 1974.
25. Kaplan, K. L.: Platelet granule proteins: Localization and secretion. In Dingle, J. T., and Gordon, J. L. (eds.): Platelets in Pathology and Biology. Amsterdam, Elsevier/North Holland, 1981, p. 77.
26. Chesney, C. M., Pifer, D., and Colman, R. W.: Subcellular localization and secretion of factor V from human platelets. Proc. Natl. Acad. Sci. USA 78:5180, 1981.
27. George, J. N.: Platelet IgG: Its significance for the evaluation

28. Handagama, P. J., Shuman, M. A., and Bainton, D. F.: Incorporation of intravenously injected albumin, IgG, and fibrinogen into guinea pig megakaryocyte. J. Clin. Invest. 84:73, 1989.
29. Handgamma, P. J., Rappolee, D. A., Werb, Z., Levin, J., and Bainton, D. F.: Platelet α-granule fibrinogen, albumin, and immunoglobulin G are not synthesized by rat and mouse megakaryocytes. J. Clin. Invest. 86:1364, 1990.
30. McEver, R. P.: Leukocyte interactions mediated by selectins. Thromb. Haemost. 66:80, 1991.
31. Novotny, W. F., Girard, T. J., Miletich, J. P., and Broze, G. J.: Platelets secrete a coagulation inhibitor functionally and antigenically similar to the lipoprotein associated coagulation inhibitor. Blood 72:2020, 1988.
32. Leung, L. L. K., Harpel, P. C., Nachman, R. L., and Rabellino, E. M.: Histidine rich glycoprotein is present in human platelets and is released following thrombin stimulation. Blood 62:1016, 1983.
33. Ginsberg, M. H., Painter, R. G., Forsyth, J., Birdwell, C., and Plow, E. F.: Thrombin-increased expression of fibronectin antigen on the platelet surface. Proc. Natl. Acad. Sci USA 77:1049, 1980.
34. Schmaier, A. H., Zuckerberg, A., Silverman, C., Kuchibhotla, J., Tuszynski, G. P., and Colman, R. W.: High-molecular weight kininogen. A secreted platelet protein. J. Clin. Invest. 71:1477, 1983.
35. Nachman, R. L., and Harpel, P. C.: Platelet α₂ macroglobulin and α₁ antitrypsin. J. Biol. Chem. 251:4514, 1976.
36. Newman, P. J., Gorski, J., White, G. C., Gidwitz, S., Cretney, C. J., and Aster, R. H.: Enzymatic amplification of platelet-specific RNA using the polymerase chain reaction. J. Clin. Invest. 82:739, 1988.
37. Warshaw, A. L., Laster, L., and Shulman, N. R.: Protein synthesis by human platelets. J. Biol. Chem. 242:2094, 1967.
38. Akkerman, J. W. N.: Regulation of carbohydrate metabolism in platelets: A review. Thromb. Haemost. 39:712, 1979.
39. Majerus, P. W., Smith, M. B., and Clamon, G. H.: Lipid metabolism in human platelets. I. Evidence for a complete fatty acid synthesizing system. J. Clin. Invest. 48:156, 1969.
40. Lewis, N., and Majerus, P. W.: Lipid metabolism in human platelets. II. De novo phospholipid synthesis and the effect of thrombin on the pattern of synthesis. J. Clin. Invest. 48:2114, 1969.
41. Puett, D., Wasserman, B. K., Ford, J. D., and Cunningham, L. W.: Collagen mediated platelet aggregation: Effects of collagen modification involving the protein and carbohydrate moieties. J. Clin. Invest. 52:2495, 1973.
42. Hemler, M. E.: VLA proteins in the integrin family. Ann. Rev. Immunol. 8:365, 1990.
43. Baumgartner, H. R., Tshopp, T. B., and Weiss, H. J.: Platelet interaction with collagen fibrils in flowing blood. II. Impaired adhesion-aggregation in bleeding disorder. Thromb. Haemost. 37:17, 1977.
44. Gaarder, A., Jonsen, J., Laland, S., Hellem, A., and Owren, P. A.: ADP in red cells as a factor in the adhesiveness of human blood platelets. Nature 192:531, 1961.
45. Charo, I. F., Feinman, R. D., and Detwiler, T. C.: Interactions of platelet aggregation and secretion. J. Clin. Invest. 60:866, 1977.
46. Shattil, S. J., and Bennett, J. S.: Platelets and their membranes in hemostasis: Physiology and pathophysiology. Ann. Intern. Med. 94:108, 1980.
47. Bennett, J. S., and Vilaire, G.: Exposure of platelet fibrinogen receptors by ADP and epinephrine. J. Clin. Invest. 64:1393, 1979.
48. Marguerie, G. A., Plow, E. F., and Edgington, T. S.: Human platelets possess an inducible and saturable receptor for fibrinogen. J. Biol. Chem. 254:5357, 1979.
49. Bennett, J. S., Vilaire, G., and Burch, J. W.: A role for protaglandins and thromboxanes in the exposure of platelet fibrinogen receptors. J. Clin. Invest. 68:981, 1981.
50. Baenziger, N. L., Brodie, G. N., and Majerus, P. W.: Isolation

and properties of a thrombin-sensitive protein of human platelets. J. Biol. Chem. 247:2723, 1972.

51. Margossian, S. S., Lawler, J. W., and Slayter, H. S.: Physical characterization of platelet thrombospondin. J. Biol. Chem. 256:7495, 1981.

52. Phillips, D. R., Jennings, L. K., and Prasanna, H. R.: Ca⁺⁺ mediated association of glycoprotein-G (thrombin sensitive protein, thrombospondin) with human platelets. J. Biol. Chem. 255:11629, 1980.

53. Gartner, T. K., Gerrard, J. M., White, J. G., and Williams, D. C.: Fibrinogen is the receptor for the endogenous lectin of human platelets. Nature 289:688, 1981.

54. Jaffe, E. A., Leung, L. L. K., Nachman, R. L., Levin, R. I., and Mosher, D. F.: Thrombospondin is the endogenous lectin of human platelets. Nature 295:246, 1982.

55. Leung, L. L. K., and Nachman R. L.: Complex formation of platelet thrombospondin with fibrinogen. J. Clin. Invest. 70:542, 1982.

56. Frazier, W.: Structure and function of thrombospondins. Trends Glycosci. 4:152, 1992.

57. Oquendo, P., Hundt, E., Lawler, J., and Seed, B.: CD36 directly mediates cytoadherence of *Plasmodium falciparum* parasitized erythrocytes. Cell 58:95, 1989.

58. Dixit, V. M., Haverstick, D. M., O'Rouke, K. M., Hennessy, S. W., Grant, G. A., Santoro, S. A., and Frazier, W. A.: A monoclonal antibody against human thrombospondin inhibits platelet aggregation. Proc. Natl. Acad. Sci. USA 82:3472, 1985.

59. Galvin, N. J., Dixit, V. M., O'Rouke, K. M., Santoro, S. A., Grant, G. A., and Frazier, W. A.: Mapping of epitopes for monoclonal antibodies against human platelet thrombospondin with electron microscopy and high sensitivity amino acid sequencing. J. Cell Biol. 101:434, 1985.

60. Gerrard, J. M., Phillips, D. R., Rai, G. H. R., Plow, E. F., Walz, D. A., Ross, R., Harker, L. A., and White, J. G.: Biochemical studies of two patients with gray platelet syndrome. J. Clin. Invest. 66:102, 1980.

61. Mumby, S. M., Raugi, G. J., and Bornstein, P.: Interactions of thrombospondin with extracellular matrix proteins. J. Cell Biol. 98:646, 1984.

62. Cardin, A. D., and Weintraub, H. J. R.: Molecular modeling of protein-glycosaminoglycan interaction. Arteriosclerosis 9:21, 1989.

63. Lawler, J., and Hynes, R. O.: An integrin receptor on normal and thrombasthenic platelets that binds thrombospondin. Blood 74:2022, 1989.

64. Leung, L. L. K., Nachman, R. L., and Harpel, P. C.: Complex formation of platelet thrombospondin with histidine-rich glycoprotein. J. Clin. Invest. 73:5, 1984.

65. Stenberg, P. A., Shuman, M. A., Levine, S. P., and Bainton, D. F.: Redistribution of alpha-granules and their contents in thrombin-stimulated platelets. J. Cell Biol. 98:748, 1984.

66. Lin, S. E., and Stossel, T. P.: The micofilament network of the platelet. *In* Spaet, T. H. (ed.): Progress in Hemostasis and Thrombosis, Vol. 6. New York, Grune and Stratton, 1982, p. 63.

67. Fox, J. E., and Phillips, D. R.: Polymerization and organization of actin filaments within platelets. Semin. Hematol. 20:243, 1983.

68. Gordon, D. J., Boyer, J. L., and Korn, E. D.: Comparative biochemistry of non-muscle actins. J. Biol. Chem. 252:8300, 1977.

69. Vanderkerchkove, J., and Weber, K.: Comparisons of actins from calf thymus, bovine brain, and SV40-transformed mouse 3T3 cells with rabbit skeletal muscle actin. Eur. J. Biochem. 90:451, 1978.

70. Hanukoglu, I., Tanese, N., and Fuchs, E.: cDNA sequence of a human cytoplasmic actin. J. Mol. Biol. 163:673, 1983.

71. Korn, E. D.: Biochemistry of actomyosin-dependent cell motility (a review). Proc. Natl. Acad. Sci. USA 75:588, 1978.

72. Carlsson, L., Markey, F., Blikstad, I., Persson, T., and Lindberg, U.: Reorganization of actin in platelets stimulated by thrombin as measured by the DNAse I inhibition assay. Proc. Natl. Acad. Sci. USA 76:6376, 1979.

73. Adelstein, R. S., and Conti, M. A.: Phosphorylation of platelet myosin increases actin-activated ATPase activity. Nature 256:597, 1975.

74. Daniel, J. L., Molish, I. R., and Holmson, H.: Myosin phosphorylation in intact platelets. J. Biol. Chem. 256:7510, 1981.

75. Adelstein, R. S., and Eisenberg, E.: Regulation and kinetics of the actin-myosin-ATP interaction. Ann. Rev. Biochem. 49:921, 1980.

76. Adelstein, R. S., and Klee, C. B.: Purification and characterization of smooth muscle myosin light chain kinase. J. Biol. Chem. 256:7501, 1981.

77. Ishikawa, H., Bischoff, R., and Holtzer, H.: Formation of arrowhead complexes with heavy meromyosin in a variety of cell types. J. Cell Biol. 43:312, 1969.

78. Pollard, T. D., and Mooseker, M. S.: Direct measurement of actin polymerization rate constants by electron microscopy of actin filaments nucelated by isolated microvillous cores. J. Cell Biol. 88:654, 1981.

79. Tilney, L. G., Bonder, E. M., and DeRosier, D. J.: Actin filaments elongate from their membrane-associated ends. J. Cell Biol. 90:485, 1981.

80. Carlsson, L., Nystrom, L. E., Sundkvist, I., et al.: Actin polymerizability is influenced by profilin, a low MW protein in nonmuscle cells. J. Mol. Biol. 115:456, 1977.

81. Markey, F., Persson, T., and Lindberg, U.: Characterization of platelet extracts before and after stimulation with respect to the possible role of profilactin as microfilament precursor. Cell 23:145, 1981.

82. Fox, J. E. B., and Phillips, D. R.: Polymerization and organization of actin filaments within platelets. Semin. Hematol. 20:243, 1983.

83. Goldschmidt-Clermont, P. J., Machesky, L. M., Baldassare, J. J., and Pollard, T. D.: The actin-binding protein profilin binds to PIP₂ and inhibits its hydrolysis by phospholipase C. Science 247:1575, 1990.

84. Lind, S. E., Yin, H. L., and Stossel, T. P.: Human platelets contain gelsolin, a regulator of actin filament length. J. Clin. Invest. 69:1384, 1982.

85. Phillips, D. R., Jennings, L. K., and Edwards, H. H.: Identification of membrane proteins mediating the interaction of human platelets. J. Cell Biol. 86:77, 1980.

86. Fox, J. E. B., Reynolds, C. C., and Phillips, D. R.: Calcium-dependent proteolysis occurs during platelet aggregation. J. Biol. Chem. 258:9973, 1983.

87. Majerus, P. W., and Miletich, J. P.: Relationships between platelets and coagulation factors in hemostasis. Ann. Rev. Med. 29:41, 1978.

88. Milstone, J. H.: Thrombokinase as prime activator of prothrombin: Historical perspectives and present status. Fed. Proc. 63:742, 1964.

89. Marcus, A. J.: Recent advances in platelet lipid metabolism research. Ann. NY Acad. Sci. 201:102, 1972.

90. Miletich, J. P., Jackson, C. M., and Majerus, P. W.: Properties of the factor Xa binding site on human platelets. J. Biol. Chem. 253:6908, 1978.

91. Miletich, J. P., Jackson, C. M., and Majerus, P. W.: Interaction of coagulation factor Xa with human platelets. Proc. Natl. Acad. Sci. USA 74:4033, 1977.

92. Dahlback, B., and Stenflo, J.: Binding of bovine coagulation factor Xa to platelets. Biochemistry 17:4938, 1978.

93. Kane, W. H., Lindhout, M. L. J., Jackson, C. M., and Majerus, P. W.: Factor Va-dependent binding of factor Xa to human platelets. J. Biol. Chem. 255:1170, 1980.

94. Tracy, P. B., Peterson, J. M., Neshiem, M. E., McDuffie, F. C., and Mann, K. G.: Interaction of coagulation factor V and factor Va with platelets. J. Biol. Chem. 254:10354, 1979.

95. Teitel, J. M., and Rosenberg, R. D.: Protection of factor Xa from neutralization by the heparin-antithrombin complex. J. Clin. Invest. 71:1383, 1983.

96. Deuel, T. F., Keim, P. S., Farmer, M., and Heinrikson, R. L.: Amino acid sequence of human platelet factor 4. Proc. Natl. Acad. Sci. USA 74:2256, 1977.

97. Hermodson, M., Schmer, G., and Kurachi, K.: Isolation, crys-

tallization and primary amino acid sequence of platelet factor 4. J. Biol. Chem. 252:6276, 1977.

98. Hemker, H. C., van Rijn, J. L. M. L., Rosing, J., van Dieijen, G., Bevers, E. W., and Zwaal, R. F. S.: Platelet membrane involvement in blood coagulation. Blood Cells 9:303, 1983.

99. Walsh, P. N., and Griffin, J. H.: Contributions of human platelets to the proteolytic activation of blood coagulation factors XII and XI. Blood 57:106, 1981.

100. Sinha, D., Seaman, F. S., Koshy, A., Knight, L. C., and Walsh, P. N.: Blood coagulation factor XIa binds specifically to a site on activated human platelets distinct from that for factor XI. J. Clin. Invest. 78:1550, 1984.

101. Majerus, P. W.: Arachidonate metabolism in vascular disorders. J. Clin. Invest. 72:1521, 1983.

102. Needleman, S. W., Spector, A. A., and Hoak, J. C.: Enrichment of human platelet phospholipids with linoleic acid diminishes thromboxane release. Prostaglandins 124:607, 1982.

103. Kaduce, T. L., Hoak, J. C., and Fry, G. L.: Utilization of arachidonic and linoleic acids by cultured human endothelial cells. J. Clin. Invest. 68:1003, 1981.

104. Neufeld, E. J., Wilson, D. B., Sprecher, H., and Majerus, P. W.: High affinity esterification of eicosanoid precursor fatty acids by platelets. J. Clin. Invest. 72:214, 1983.

105. Wilson, D. B., Prescott, S. M., and Majerus, P. W.: Discovery of an arachidonoyl Coenzyme A synthetase in human platelets. J. Biol. Chem. 257:3510, 1982.

106. Neufeld, E. J., Bross, T. E., and Majerus, P. W.: A mutant $HSDM_1C_1$ fibrosarcoma line selected for defective eicosanoid precursor uptake lacks arachidonate-specific acyl-CoA synthetase. J. Biol. Chem. 259:1986, 1984.

107. Neufeld, E. J., Sprecher, H., Evans, R. W., and Majerus, P. W.: Fatty acid structural requirements for activity of arachidonoyl-CoA synthetase. J. Lipid Res. 25:288, 1984.

108. Laposata, M., Reich, E. L., and Majerus, P. W.: Arachidonoyl-CoA synthetase: Separation from non-specific acyl-CoA synthetase and distribution in various cells and tissues. J. Biol. Chem. 260:11016, 1985.

109. Hamberg, M., Svensson, J., and Samuelsson, B.: Prostaglandin endoperoxides. A new concept concerning the mode of action and release of prostaglandins. Proc. Natl. Acad. Sci. USA 71:3824, 1974.

110. Nugteren, D. H.: Arachidonate lipoxygenase in blood platelets. Biochim. Biophys. Acta 380:299, 1975.

111. Hamberg, M., and Hamberg, G.: On the mechanism of the oxygenation of arachidonic acid by human platelet lipoxygenase. Biochem. Biophys. Res. Commun. 95:1090, 1980.

112. Goetzl, E. J., and Sun, F. F.: Generation of unique monohydroxy eicosatetraenoic acids from arachidonic acid by human neutrophils. J. Exp. Med. 150:406, 1979.

113. Maclouf, J., Fruteau de Laclos, B., and Borgeat, P.: Stimulation of leukotriene biosynthesis in human blood leukocytes by platelet-derived 12-hydroperoxy-icosatetraenoic acid. Proc. Natl. Acad. Sci. USA 79:6042, 1982.

114. Marcus, A. J., Broekman, M. J., Safier, L. B., Ullman, H. L., Islam, N., Serhan, C. N., Rutherford, L. E., Korchak, H. M., and Weissman, G.: Formation of leukotrienes and other hydroxy acids during platelet-neutrophil interactions in vitro. Biochem. Biophys. Res. Commun. 109:130, 1982.

115. Marcus, A. J., Safier, L. B., Ullman, H. L., Broekman, M. J., Islam, N., Oglesby, T. D., and Gorman, R. R.: 12S,20-dihydroxyicosatetraenoic acid: A new icosanoid synthesized by neutrophils from 12S-hydroxyicosatetraenoic acid produced by thrombin- or collagen-stimulated platelets. Proc. Natl. Acad. Sci. USA 81:903, 1984.

116. Wong, P. Y.-K., Westlund, P., Hamberg, M., Granstrom, E., Chao, P. H.-W., and Samuelsson, B.: Omega-hydroxylation of 12-L-hydroxy-5,8,10,14-eicosatetraenoic acid in human polymorphonuclear leukocytes. J. Biol. Chem. 259:2683, 1984.

117. Siegel, M. J., McConnell, R. T., Abrahams, S. L., Porter, N. A., and Cuatrecasas, P.: Regulation of arachidonate metabolism via lipoxygenase and cyclooxygenase by 12-HPETE, the product of human platelet lipoxygenase. Biochem. Biophys. Res. Commun. 89:1273, 1979.

118. Morita, I., Takahashi, R., Saito, Y., and Murota, S.: Stimulation of eicosapentaenoic acid metabolism in washed human platelets by 12-hydroperoxyeicosatetraenoic acid. J. Biol. Chem. 258:10197, 1983.

119. Aharony, D., Smith, J. B., and Silver, M. J.: Regulation of arachidonate-induced platelet aggregation by lipoxygenase product, 12-hydroperoxyeicosatetraenoic acid. Biochim. Biophys. Acta 718:193, 1982.

120. Croset, M., and Lagarde, M.: Stereospecific inhibition of PGH_2-induced platelet aggregation by lipoxygenase products of icosaenoic acids. Biochem. Biophys. Res. Commun. 112:878, 1983.

121. Rollins, T. E., and Smith, W. L.: Subcellular localization of prostaglandin-forming cyclooxygenase in Swiss mouse 3T3 fibroblasts by electron microscopic immunocytochemistry. J. Biol. Chem. 255:4872, 1980.

122. Gerrard, J. M., White, J. G., Rao, G. H. R., and Townsend, D.: Localization of platelet prostaglandin production in the platelet dense tubular system. Am. J. Pathol. 83:283, 1976.

123. Funk, C. D., Funk, L. B., Kennedy, M. E., Pong, A. S., and Fitzgerald, G. A.: Human platelet/erythroleukemia cell prostaglandin G/H synthase:cDNA cloning, expression, and gene chromosomal assignment. FASEB J. 5:2304, 1991.

124. Takahashi, Y., Ueda, N., Yoshimoto, T., Yamamoto, S., Yokoyama, C., Miyata, A., Tanabe, T., Fuse, I., Hattori, A., and Shibata, A.: Immunoaffinity purification and cDNA cloning of human platelet prostaglandin endoperoxide synthase. Biochem. Biophys. Res. Communs. 182:433, 1992.

125. Hamberg, M., Svensson, J., and Samuelsson, B.: Thromboxanes: A new group of biologically active compounds derived from prostaglandin peroxides. Proc. Natl. Acad. Sci. USA 72:2994, 1975.

126. Samuelsson, B.: Prostaglandines, thromboxanes, and leukotrienes: Formation and biological rules. Harvey Lect. 75:1, 1981.

127. Roth, G. J., Machuga, E. T., and Strittmatter, P.: The heme-binding properties of prostaglandin synthetase from sheep vesicular gland. J. Biol. Chem. 256:10018, 1981.

128. Hammarstrom, S., and Falardeau, P.: Resolution of prostaglandin endoperoxide synthase and thromboxane synthase of human platelets. Proc. Natl. Acad. Sci. USA 74:3691, 1977.

129. Monen, P., Buytenhek, M., and Nugteren, D. H.: Purification of PGH-PGE isomerase from sheep vesicular glands. Meth. Enzymol. 86:84, 1982.

130. Shiemizu, T., Yamamoto, S., and Hayaishi, O.: Purification of PGH-PGD isomerase from rat brain. Meth. Enzymol. 86:73, 1982.

131. Watanabe, T., Narumiya, S., Shimizu, T., and Hayaishi, O.: Characterization of the biosynthetic pathway of prostaglandin D_2 in human platelet-rich plasma. J. Biol. Chem. 257:14847, 1982.

132. Watanabe, T., Shimizu, T., Narumiya, S., and Hayaishi, O.: NADP-linked 15-hydroxyprostaglandin dehydrogenase for prostaglandin D_2 in human blood platelets. Arch. Biochem. Biophys. 216:372, 1982.

133. Roth, G. J., Stanford, N., and Majerus, P. W.: The acetylation of prostaglandin synthetase by aspirin. Proc. Natl. Acad. Sci. USA 72:3073, 1975.

134. Roth, G. J., Machuga, E. T., and Ozols, J.: Isolation and covalent structure of the aspirin-modified, active-site region of prostaglandin synthetase. Biochemistry 22:4672, 1983.

135. DeWitt, D. L., El-Harith, E. A., Draimer, S. A., Andrews, M. J., Yao, E. F., Armstrong, R. L., and Smith, W. L.: The aspirin and heme-binding sites of ovine and murine prostaglandin endoperoxide synthases. J. Biol. Chem. 265:5192, 1990.

136. Shimokawa, T., and Smith, W. L.: Prostaglandin endoperoxide synthase: The aspirin acetylation region. J. Biol. Chem. 267:12387, 1992.

137. Burch, J. W., Stanford, N., and Majerus, P. W.: Inhibition of platelet prostaglandin cyclooxygenase by oral aspirin. J. Clin. Invest. 61:314, 1978.

138. Harter, H. R., Burch, J. W., Majerus, P. W., Stanford, N.,

Delmez, J. A., Anderson, C. G., and Weerts, C. A.: The prevention of thrombosis by low-dose aspirin. N. Engl. J. Med. 301:577, 1979.

139. Patrignani, P., Filabozzi, P., and Patrono, C.: Selective cumulative inhibition of platelet thromboxane production by low-dose aspirin in healthy subjects. J. Clin. Invest. 69:1366, 1982.

140. FitzGerald, G. A., Oates, J. A., Hawiger, J., Maas, R. L., Roberts, L. J., II, Lawson, S. A., and Brash, A. R.: Endogenous biosynthesis of prostacyclin and thromboxane and platelet function during chronic administration of aspirin in man. J. Clin. Invest. 71:676, 1983.

141. Xie, W., Chipman, J. G., Robertson, D. L., Erikson, R. L., and Simmons, D. L.: Expression of a mitogen-responsive gene encoding prostaglandin synthase is regulated by mRNA splicing. Proc. Natl. Acad. Sci. U.S.A. 88:2692, 1991.

142. Kujubu, D. A., Fletcher, B. S., Varnum, B. C., Lim, R. W., and Herschmann, H. R.: TIS10, a phorbol ester tumor promoter-inducable mRNA from Swiss 3T3 cells, encodes a novel prostaglandin synthase/cyclooxygenase homologue. J. Biol. Chem. 266:12866, 1991.

143. Obanion, M. K., Winn, V. D., and Young, D. A.: cDNA cloning and functional activity of a glucocorticoid-regulated inflammatory cyclooxygenase. Proc. Natl. Acad. Sci. U.S.A 89:4888, 1992.

144. Gorman, R. R.: Biology and biochemistry of thromboxane synthetase inhibitors. Adv. Prostaglandin Thromboxane Leukotriene Res. 11:235, 1983.

145. FitzGerald, G. A., Brash, A. R., Oates, J. A., and Pederson, A. K.: Endogenous prostacyclin biosynthesis and platelet function during selective inhibition of thromboxane synthetase in man. J. Clin. Invest. 72:1336, 1983.

146. Malmsten, C., Hamber, M., Svensson, J., and Samuelsson, B.: Physiological role of an endoperoxide in human platelets: Haemostatic defect due to platelet cyclooxygenase deficiency. Proc. Natl. Acad. Sci. USA 72:1466, 1975.

147. Weiss, H. J., and Lages, B. A.: Possible congenital defect in thromboxane synthetase. Lancet 1:760, 1977.

148. LaGarde, M., Byron, P. A., Vargaftig, B. B., and Dechavenue, M.: Impairment of platelet thromboxane A_2 generation and of the platelet release reaction in two patients with congenital deficiency of platelet cyclooxygenase. Br. J. Haematol. 38:251, 1978.

149. Pareti, F. I., Mannucci, P. M., and D'Angelo, A.: Congenital deficiency of thromboxane and prostacyclin. Lancet 1:898, 1980.

150. Roth, G. J., and Machuga, E. T.: Radioimmune assay of human platelet prostaglandin snythetase. J. Lab. Clin. Med. 99:187, 1982.

151. Roth, G. J.: Personal communication, 1985.

152. Laposata, M., Prescott, S. M., Bross, T. E., and Majerus, P. W.: Development and characterization of a tissue culture cell line with essential fatty acid deficiency. Proc. Natl. Acad. Sci. USA 79:7654, 1982.

153. McEver, R. P., Baenziger, N. L., and Majerus, P. W.: Isolation and quantitation of the platelet membrane glycoprotein defect in thrombasthenia using a monoclonal hybridoma antibody. J. Clin. Invest. 66:1311, 1980.

154. McEver, R. P., Baenziger, J. U., and Majerus, P. W.: Isolation and structural characterization of the polypeptide subunits of membrane glycoprotein IIb-IIIa from human platelets. Blood 59:80, 1982.

155. Hynes, R. O.: Integrins: Versatility, modulation, and signaling in cell adhesion. Cell 69:11, 1992.

156. Ruoslahti, E.: Integrins. J. Clin. Invest. 87:1, 1991.

157. Poncz, M., Eisman, R., Heidenreich, R., Silver, S. M., Vilaire, G., Surrey, S., Schwartz, E., and Bennett, J. S.: Structure of the platelet membrane glycoprotein IIb. J. Biol. Chem. 262:8476, 1987.

158. Kieffer, N., and Phillips, D. R.: Platelet membrane glycoproteins: Functions in cellular interactions. Annu. Rev. Cell Biol. 6:329, 1990.

159. Rosa, J.-P., Bray, P. F., Gayet, O., Johnston, G. I., Cook, R. G., Jackson, K. W., Shuman, M. A., and McEver, R. P.: Cloning of glycoprotein IIIa cDNA from human erythroleukemia cells and localization of the gene to chromosome 17. Blood 72:593, 1988.

160. Fitzgerald, L. A., Steiner, B., Rall, S. C., Lo, S. S., and Phillips, D. R.: Protein sequence of endothelial cell glycoprotein IIIa derived from a cDNA clone. Identity with platelet glycoprotein IIIa and similarity with "integrin." J. Biol. Chem. 262:3936, 1987.

161. Tollefsen, D. T., and Majerus, P. W.: Inhibition of human platelet aggregation by monovalent antifibrinogen antibody fragments. J. Clin. Invest. 55:1259, 1975.

162. Nachman, R. L., and Leung, L. L. K.: Complex formation of platelet membrane glycoproteins IIb-IIIa with fibrinogen. J. Clin. Invest. 69:263, 1982.

163. Bennett, J. S., Vilaire, G., and Cines, D. B.: Identification of the fibrinogen receptor on human platelets by photoaffinity labeling. J. Biol. Chem. 257:8049, 1982.

164. Kloczewiak, M., Timmons, S., Lukas, J., and Hawiger, J.: Platelet receptor recognition site on human fibrinogen. Biochemistry 23:1767, 1984.

165. Nachman, R. L., Leung, L. L. K., Kloczewiak, M., and Hawiger, J.: Complex formation to platelet membrane glycoprotein IIb-IIIa with fibrinogen D domain. J. Biol. Chem. 259:8584, 1984.

166. D'Souze, S. E., Ginsberg, M. H., Burke, T. A., and Plow, E. F.: The ligand binding site of the platelet integrin receptor GPIIb-IIIa is proximal to the second calcium binding domain of its α subunit. J. Biol. Chem. 265:3440, 1990.

167. D'Souze, S. E., Ginsberg, M. H., Matsueda, G. R., and Plow, E. F.: A discrete sequence in a platelet integrin is involved in ligand recognition. Nature 350:66, 1991.

168. Taylor, D. B., and Gartner, T. K.: A peptide corresponding to GPIIb 300–312, a presumptive fibrinogen γ chain binding site on the platelet integrin GP IIb/IIIa, inhibits the adhesion of platelets to at least four adhesive ligands. J. Biol. Chem. 167:11729, 1992.

169. Philips, D. R., Charo, I. F., and Scarborough, R. M.: GPIIb-IIIa: The responsive integrin. Cell 65:359, 1991.

170. Degos, L., Dautigny, A., Brouet, J. C., Colombani, M., Ardaillou, N., Caen, J. P., and Colombani, J.: A molecular defect in thrombasthenic platelets. J. Clin. Invest. 56:326, 1975.

171. Hagen, I., Nurden, A., Bjerrum, O. J., Solum, N. O., and Caen, J. P.: Immunochemical evidence for protein abnormalities in platelet from patients with Glanzmann's thrombasthenia and Bernard-Soulier syndrome. J. Clin. Invest. 65:722, 1980.

172. McEver, R. P., Bennett, E. B., and Martin, M. N.: Identification of two structurally and functionally distinct sites on human platelet membrane glyco protein IIb-IIIa using monoclonal antibodies. J. Biol. Chem. 258:5269, 1983.

173. Pidard, D., Montgomery, R. R., Bennett, J. S., and Kunicki, T. J.: Interaction of AP-2, a monoclonal antibody specific for the human glycoprotein IIb-IIIa complex, with intact platelets. J. Biol. Chem. 258:12582, 1983.

174. DiMinno, G., Thiagarajan, P., Perussia, B., Martinez, J., Shapiro, S., Trinchieri, G., and Murphy, S.: Exposure of platelet fibrinogen binding sites by collagen, arachidonate, and ADP: Inhibition by a monoclonal antibody to the glycoprotien IIb-IIIa complex. Blood 61:140, 1983.

175. Coller, B. S., Peershke, E. I., Scudder, L. E., and Sullivan, C. A.: A murine monoclonal antibody that completely blocks the binding of fibrinogen to platelets produces a thrombasthenic-like state in normal platelets and binds to glycoprotien IIb-IIIa. J. Clin. Invest. 72:325, 1983.

176. Newman, P. J., Seligsohn, U., Lyman, S., and Coller, B. S.: The molecular genetic basis of Glanzmann thrombasthenia in the Iraqi-Jewish and Arab populations in Israel. Proc. Natl. Acad. Sci. USA 88:3160, 1991.

177. Loftus, J. C., O'Toole, T. E., Plow, E. F., Glass, A., Frelinger, A. L., and Ginsberg, M. H.: A β_3 integrin mutation abolishes ligand binding and alters divalent cation-dependent conformation. Science 249:915, 1990.

178. Bajt, M. L., Ginsberg, M. H., Frelinger, A. L., Berndt, M. C., and Loftus, J. C.: A spontaneous mutation of integrin $\alpha_{IIb}\beta_3$

(GPIIb/IIIa) helps define a ligand binding site. J. Biol. Chem. 76:3789, 1992.

179. George, J. N., Nurden, A. T., and Phillips, D. R.: Molecular defects that cause abnormalities of platelet vessel wall interactions. N. Engl. J. Med. 311:1084, 1984.

180. Ginsberg, M. H., Forsyth, J., Lightsey, A., Chediak, J., and Plow, E. F.: Reduced surface expression and binding of fibronectin by thrombin-stimulated thrombasthenic platelets. J. Clin. Invest. 71:619, 1983.

181. Ruggeri, Z. M., Bader, R., and de Marco, L.: Glanzmann's thrombasthenia: Deficient binding of vWF to thrombin-stimulated platelets. Proc. Natl. Acad. Sci. USA 79:6038, 1982.

182. Ruggeri, Z. M., de Marco, L., Gatti, L., Bader, R., and Montogmery, R. F.: Platelets have more than one binding site for vWF. J. Clin. Invest. 72:1, 1983.

183. Fujimoto, T., and Hawiger, J.: ADP induces binding of vWF to human platelets. Nature 297:154, 1982.

184. Fujimoto, T., Ohara, S., and Hawiger, J.: Thrombin-induced exposure and PGI$_2$ inhibition of the receptor for factor VIII/vWF on human platelets. J. Clin. Invest. 69:1212, 1982.

185. Schullek, J., Jordan, J., and Mongomery, R. R.: Interaction of vWF with human platelets in plasma milieu. J. Clin. Invest. 73:421, 1984.

186. van Loghem, J. J., Jr., Dorfmeijer, H., and van der Hart, M.: Serological and genetic studies on a platelet antigen (ZW). Vox Sang. 4:161, 1959.

187. Kunicki, T. J., and Aster, R. H.: Deletion of the platelet-specific alloantigen Pl^{A1} from platelets in Glanzmann's thrombasthenia. J. Clin. Invest. 61:1225, 1978.

188. Kunicki, T. J., Picard, D., Cazenave, J. P., Nurden, A. J., and Caen, J. P.: Inheritance on the human platelet alloantigen Pl^{A1} in type one thrombasthenia. J. Clin. Invest. 67:717, 1981.

188a. Newman, P. J.: Platelet GPIIb–IIIa: Molecular variations and alloantigens. Thromb. Haemost. 66:111, 1991.

188b. Wang, R., Furihata, K., McFarland, J. G., Friedman, K., Aster, R. H., and Newman, P. J.: An amino acid polymorphism within the RGD binding domain of platelet membrane glycoprotein IIIa is responsible for the Pen^a/Pen^b alloantigen system. J. Clin. Invest. 90:2038, 1992.

189. Howard, M. A., and Firkin, B. G.: Ristocetin: A new tool in the investigation of platelet aggregation. Thromb. Diath. Haemorrh. 26:362, 1971.

190. Kao, K. J., Pizzo, S. V., and McKee, P. A.: Demonstration and characterization of specific binding sites for factor VIII/vWF on human platelets. J. Clin. Invest. 63:656, 1979.

191. Moake, J. L., Olson, J. D., Tang, S. S., Funicella, T., and Peterson, D. M.: Binding of radioiodinated human vWF to Bernard-Soulier, thrombasthenic, and von Willebrand's disease platelets. Thromb. Res. 19:21, 1980.

192. Ruan, C., Tobelem, G., McMichael, A. J., Drouet, L., Legrand, Y., Degos, L., Kieffer, L., Lee, H., and Caen, J. P.: Monoclonal antibody to human platelet glycoprotein. Br. J. Haematol. 49:511, 1981.

193. Roth, G. J.: Developing relationships: Arterial platelet adhesion, GPIb, and leucine-rich glycoproteins. Blood 77:5, 1991.

194. Nurden, A. T., and Caen, J. P.: Specific roles for platelet surface glycoproteins in platelet function. Nature 255:720, 1975.

195. Coller, B. S., Peerschke, E. I., Scudder, L. E., and Sullivan, C. A.: Studies with murine monoclonal antibody that abolishes ristocetin-induced binding of von Willebrand factor to platelets: Additional evidence in support of GP Ib as a platelet receptor for von Willebrand factor. Blood 61:97, 1983.

196. Nurden, A. T., Dupuis, D., Kunicki, T. J., and Caen, J. P.: Analysis of the glycoprotein and protein composition of Bernard-Soulier platelets by single and two-dimensional SDS-polyacrylamide gel electrophoresis. J. Clin. Invest. 67:1431, 1981.

197. Berndt, M. C., Gregory, C., Chong, B. H., Zola, H., and Castaldi, P. A.: Additional glycoprotein defects in Bernard-Soulier syndrome: Confirmation of genetic basis by parental analysis. Blood 62:800, 1983.

198. George, J. N., Reimann, T. A., Moake, J. L., Morgan, R. K., Cimo, P. A., and Sears, D. A.: Bernard-Soulier disease: A study of four patients and their parents. Br. J. Haematol. 48:459, 1981.

199. Modderman, P. W., Admiraal, L. G., Sonnenberg, A., and von dem Borne, A. E. G., Jr.: Glycoproteins V and Ib-IX form a noncovalent complex in the platelet membrane. J. Biol. Chem. 267:364, 1992.

200. Hickey, M. J., Williams, S. A., and Roth, G. J.: Human platelet glycoprotein IX: An adhesive prototype of leucine-rich glycoproteins with flank-center-flank structures. Proc. Natl. Acad. Sci. USA 86:6773, 1989.

201. Hickey, M. J., Deaven, L. L., and Roth, G. J.: Human platelet glycoprotein IX: Characterization of cDNA and localization of the gene to chromosome 3. FEBS Lett. 274:89, 1990.

202. Roth, G. J., Church, T. A., McMullen, B. A., and Williams, S. A.: Human platelet glycoprotein V: A surface leucine-rich glycoprotein related to adhesion. Biochem. Biophys. Res. Comm. 170:153, 1990.

203. Shimomura, T., Fujimura, K., Maehama, S., Takemoto, M., Oda, K., Fujkimoto, T., Oyama, R., Suzuki, M., Ichihara-Tanake, K., Titani, K., and Kuramoto, A.: Rapid purification and characterization of human platelet glycoprotein V: The amino acid sequence contains leucine-rich repetitive modules as in glycoprotein Ib. Blood 75:2349, 1990.

204. Bernard, J.: History of congenital hemorrhagic thrombocytopathic dystrophy. Blood Cells 9:179, 1983.

205. Ware, J., Russell, S. R., Vicente, V., Scharf, R. E., Tomer, A., McMill, R., and Ruggeri, Z. M.: Nonsense mutation in the glycoprotein Ibα coding sequence associated with Bernard-Soulier syndrome. Proc. Natl. Acad. Sci. USA 87:2026, 1990.

206. Miller, J. L., Lyle, V. A., and Cunningham, D.: Mutation of leucine-57 to phenylalanine in a platelet glycoprotein Ibα tandem repeat occurring in patients with an autosomal dominant variant of Bernard-Soulier syndrome. Blood 79:439, 1992.

207. Miller, J. L., Cunningham, D., Lyle, V. A., and Finch, C. N.: Mutation in the gene encoding the α chain of platelet glycoprotein Ib in platelet-type von Willebrand disease. Proc. Natl. Acad. Sci. USA 88:4761, 1991.

208. Weiss, H. J., Truitto, V. T., and Baumgartner, H. R.: Effect of shear rate on platelet interaction with subendothelium in citrated and native blood: I. Shear-rate dependent decrease of adhesion in von Willebrand's disease and the Bernard-Soulier syndrome. J. Lab. Clin. Med. 92:750, 1978.

209. Tollefsen, D., Jackson, C. M., and Majerus, P. W.: Binding of the products of prothrombin activation to human platelets. J. Clin. Invest. 56:241, 1975.

210. McGowan, E. B., Ding, A.-H., and Detwiler, T. C.: Correlation of thrombin-induced glycoprotein V hydrolysis and platelet activation. J. Biol. Chem. 258:11243, 1983.

211. Vu, T.-K. H., Hung, D. T., Wheaton, V. I., and Coughlin, S. R.: Molecular cloning of a functional thrombin receptor reveals a novel proteolytic mechanism of receptor activation. Cell 64:1057, 1991.

212. Coughlin, S. R., Vu, T.-K. H., Hung, D. T., and Wheaton, V. I.: Characterization of a functional thrombin receptor. J. Clin. Invest. 89:351, 1992.

213. Vu, T.-K. H., Wheaton, V. I., Hung, D. T., Charo, I. L., and Coughlin, S. R.: Domains specifying thrombin-receptor interaction. Nature 353:674, 1991.

214. Miletich, J. P., Kane, W. H., Hofmann, S. L., and Majerus, P. W.: Deficiency of factor Xa-factor Va binding sites on the platelets of a patient with a bleeding disorder. Blood 54:1015, 1979.

215. Kane, W. H., Lindhout, M. J., Jackson, C. M., and Majerus, P. W.: Factor Va-dependent binding of Factor Xa to human platelets. J. Biol. Chem. 255:1170, 1980.

216. Tracy, P. B., Eide, L. L., Bowie, J. W., and Mann, K. G.: Radioimmunoassay of factor V in human plasma and platelets. Blood 60:59, 1982.

217. Kane, W. H., Mruk, J. S., and Majerus, P. W.: Activation of

coagulation factor V by a platelet protease. J. Clin. Invest. 70:1092, 1982.

218. Miletich, J. P., Majerus, D. W., and Majerus, P. W.: Patients with congenital factor V deficiency have decreased factor Xa binding sites on their platelets. J. Clin. Invest. 62:824, 1978.

219. Kane, W. H., and Majerus, P. W.: The interaction of human coagulation factor Va with platelets. J. Biol. Chem. 257:3963, 1982.

220. Tracy, P. B., Nesheim, M. E., and Mann, K. G.: Factor Va-dependent factor Xa binding to unstimulated platelets. J. Biol. Chem. 256:743, 1981.

221. Higgins, D. L., and Mann, K. G.: The interaction of bovine factor V and factor V-derived peptides with phospholipid vesicles. J. Biol. Chem. 258:6503, 1983.

222. Thiagarajan, P., Shapiro, S. S., and De Marco, L.: Monoclonal immunoglobulin Mλ coagulation inhibitor with phospholipid specificity: Mechanism of a lupus anticoagulant. J. Clin. Invest. 66:397, 1980.

223. Siegl, A. M., Smith, J. B., and Silver, M. J.: Specific binding sites for prostaglandin D_2 on human platelets. Biochem. Biophys. Res. Commun. 90:291, 1979.

224. Siegl, A. M., Smith, J. B., Silver, M. J., Nicolaou, K. C., and Ahren, D.: Selective binding site for [^{3}H] prostacylin on platelets. J. Clin. Invest. 63:215, 1979.

225. Schafer, A. I., Cooper, B., O'Hara, D., and Handin, R. I.: Identification of platelet receptors for prostaglandin I_2 and D_2. J. Biol. Chem. 254:2914, 1979.

226. Cooper, B., Schafer, A. I., Puchalsky, D., and Handin, R. I.: Desensitization of prostaglandin-activated platelet adenylate cyclase. Prostaglandins 17:561, 1979.

227. Miller, O. V., and Gorman, R. R.: Evidence for distinct prostaglandin I_2 and D_2 receptors in human platelets. J. Pharmacol. Exp. Ther. 210:134, 1979.

228. Cerpes, B., and Ahern, D.: Characterization of the platelet PGD_2 receptor. J. Clin. Invest. 64:586, 1979.

229. Hung, S. G., Ghali, N. I., Venton, D. L., and Le Breton, G. C.: Specific binding of the thromboxane A_2 antagonist 13-azaprostanoic acid to human platelet membranes. Biochim. Biophys. Acta 728:171, 1983.

230. Ushikubi, F., Nakajima, M., Hirata, M., Okuma, M., Fujiwara, M., and Narumiya, S.: Purification of the thromboxane A_2/prostaglandin H_2 receptor from human blood platelets. J. Biol. Chem. 264:16496, 1989.

231. Hirata, M., Yasunori, H., Ushikubi, F., Yokota, Y., Kageyama, R., Nakanishi, S., and Narumiya, S.: Cloning and expression of a cDNA for a himan thromboxane A_2 receptor. Nature 349:617, 1991.

232. Wu, K. K., Le Breton, G. C., Tai, H.-H., and Chen, Y.-C.: Abnormal platelet response to thromboxane A_2. J. Clin. Invest. 67:1801, 1981.

233. Lages, B., Malmsten, C., Weiss, H. J., and Samuelsson, B.: Impaired platelet response to thromboxane-A_2 and defective calcium mobilization in a patient with a bleeding disorder. Blood 57:545, 1981.

234. Samama, M., Lecrubier, C., Conard, J., Hotchen, M., Breton-Gorius, J., Vargaftig, B., Chignard, M., Legarde, M., and Dechavanne, M.: Constitutional thrombocytopathy with subnormal response to thromboxane A_2. Br. J. Haematol. 48:293, 1981.

235. Gresele, P., Arnout, J., Janssens, W., Deckmyn, H., Lemmens, J., and Vermylen, J.: BM13.177, a selective blocker of platelet and vessel wall thromboxane receptors is active in man. Lancet 1:991, 1984.

236. Kaywin, P., McDonough, M., Insel, P. A., and Shattil, S. J.: Platelet function in essential thrombocythemia. N. Engl. J. Med. 299:505, 1978.

237. Rink, T. J., Smith, S. W., and Tsien, R. Y.: Cytoplasmic free Ca^{2+} in human platelets: Ca^{2+} thresholds and Ca-independent activation for shape-change and secretion. FEBS Lett. 148:21, 1982.

238. Cutler, L., Rodan, G., and Feinstein, M. B.: Cytochemical localization of adenylate cyclase and of calcium ion, magnesium ion-activated ATPases in the dense tubular system

239. Huang, E. M., and Detwiler, T. C.: Stimulus-response coupling mechanisms. In Phillips, D. R., and Shuman, J. A. (eds.): The Biochemistry of Platelets. New York, Academic Press, 1986, pp. 1–68.

240. Lyons, R. M., Stanford, N. L., and Majerus, P. W.: Thrombin-induced protein phosphorylation in human platelets. J. Clin. Invest. 56:924, 1975.

241. Connolly, T. M., Lawing, W. J., Jr., and Majerus, P. W.: Protein kinase C phosphorylates human platelet inositoltrisphosphate 5′-phosphomonoesterase increasing the phosphatase activity. Cell 46:951, 1986.

242. Takai, Y., Kishimoto, A., Iwasa, Y., Kawahara, Y., Mori, T., and Nishizuka, Y.: Calcium-dependent activation of multifunctional protein kinase by membrane phospholipids. J. Biol. Chem. 254:3692, 1979.

243. Naka, M., Nishikawa, M., Adelstein, R. S., and Hidaka, H.: Phorbol ester-induced activation of human platelets is associated with protein kinase C phosphorylation of myosin light chains. Nature 306:490, 1983.

244. Nishikawa, M., Sellers, J. R., Adelstein, R. S., and Hidaka, H.: Protein kinase C modulates in vitro phosphorylation of the smooth muscle heavy meromyosin by myosin light chain kinase. J. Biol. Chem. 259:8808, 1984.

245. Brugge, J., Cotton, P., Lustig, A., Yonemoto, W., Lipsich, L., Coussens, P., Barrett, J. N., Nonner, D., and Keane, R. W.: Characterization of the altered form of the c-src gene product in neuronal cells. Genes Dev. 1:287, 1987.

246. Golden, A., Nemeth, S. P., and Brugge, J. S.: Blood platelets express high levels of the pp66^{c-src}-specific tyrosine kinase activity. Proc. Natl. Acad. Sci. USA 83:852, 1986.

247. Ferrell, J. E. Jr., and Martin, S.: Platelet tyrosine-specific protein phosphorylation is regulated by thrombin. Mol. Cell. Biol. 8:3603, 1988.

248. Golden, A., and Brugge, J. S.: Thrombin treatment induces rapid changes in tyrosine phosphorylation in platelets. Proc. Natl. Acad. Sci. USA 86:901, 1989.

249. Nakamura, S., and Yamamura, H.: Thrombin and collagen induce repid phosphorylation of a common set of cellular proteins on tyrosine in human platelets. J. Biol. Chem. 263:7089, 1989.

250. Lerea, K. M., Tonks, N. K., Krebs, E. G., Fischer, E. H., and Glomset, J. A.: Vanadate and molybdate increase tyrosine phosphorylation in a 50-kilodalton protein and stimulate secretion in electropermeabilized platelets. Biochemistry 28:9286, 1989.

251. Gu, M., York, J. D., Warshawsky, I., and Majerus, P. W.: Identification, cloning, and expression of a cytosolic megakaryocyte protein-tyrosine-phosphatase with sequence homology to cytoskeletal protein 4.1. Proc. Natl. Acad. Sci. USA 88:5867, 1991.

252. Gu, M., Warshawsky, I., and Majerus, P. W.: Cloning and expression of a cytosolic megakaryocyte protein-tyrosine-phosphatase with sequence homology to retinaldehyde-binding protein and yeast SEC14p. Proc. Natl. Acad. Sci. USA 89:2980, 1992.

253. Mitchell, C. A., Jefferson, A. B., Bejeck, B. E., Brugge, J. S., Deuel, T. F., and Majerus, P. W.: Thrombin-stimulated immunoprecipitation of phosphatidylinositol 3-kinase from human platelets. Proc. Natl. Acad. Sci. USA 87:9396, 1990.

254. Feinstein, M. B., Egan, J. J., Shaafi, R. I., and White, J.: The cytoplasmic concentration of free calcium in platelets is controlled by stimulators of cyclic AMP production (PGD_2, PGE_1, forskolin). Biochem. Biophys. Res. Commun. 113:598, 1983.

255. Feinstein, M. B., Egan, J. J., and Opas, E. E.: Reversal of thrombin induced myosin phosphorylation and the assembly of cytoskeletal structure in platelets by the adenylate cyclase stimulants prostaglandin D_2 and forskolin. J. Biol. Chem. 258:1260, 1983.

256. Billah, M. M., and Lapetina, E. G.: Degradation of phosphatidylinositol 4,5-bisphosphate is insensitive to Ca^{++} mobili-

zation in stimulated platelets. Biochem. Biophys. Res. Commun. 109:1217, 1982.

257. Billah, M. M., and Lapetina, E. G.: Platelet-activating factor stimulates metabolism of phosphoinositides in horse platelets: Possible relationship to Ca++ mobilization during stimulation. Proc. Natl. Acad. Sci. USA 80:965, 1983.

258. Gilman, A. G.: G proteins and dual control of adenylate cyclase. Cell 36:577, 1984.

259. Walseth, T. F., Gander, J. E., Eide, S. J., Krick, T. P., and Goldberg, N. D.: 18O labeling of adenine nucleotide α-phosphoryls in platelets. Contribution of phosphodiesterase-catalyzed hydrolysis of cAMP. J. Biol. Chem. 258:1544, 1983.

260. Cooper, D. M. F., and Rodbell, M.: ADP is a potent inhibitor of human platelet membrane adenulate cyclase. Nature 282:517, 1979.

261. Steer, M. L., and Wood, A.: Regulation of human platelet adenylate cyclase by epinephrine, prostaglandin E1, and guanine nucleotides. Evidence for separate guanine nucleotide sites mediating stimulation and inhibition. J. Biol. Chem. 254:10791, 1979.

262. Haslam, R. J., and Vanderwal, M.: Inhibition of platelet adeynlate cyclase by 1-0-alkyl-2-0-acetyl-sn-glyceryl-3-phosphocholine (platelet activating factor). J. Biol. Chem. 257:6879, 1982.

263. Brodie, G. N., Baenziger, N. L., Chase, L. P., and Majerus, P. W.: The effects of thrombin on adenyl cyclase activity and a membrane protein from human platelets. J. Clin. Invest. 51:81, 1972.

264. Majerus, P. W., Neufeld, D. J., and Wilson, D. B.: Production of phosphoinositide-derived messengers. Cell 37:701, 1984.

265. Wilson, D. B., Bross, T. E., Hofmann, S. L., and Majerus, P. W.: Hydrolysis of polyphosphoinosidites by purified sheep seminal vesicle phospholipase C enzymes. J. Biol. Chem. 259:11718, 1984.

266. Bansal, V. S., and Majerus, P. W.: Phosphatidylinositol-derived precursors and signals. Annu. Rev. Cell Biol. 6:41, 1990.

267. Majerus, P. W., Ross, T. S., Cunningham, T. W., Caldwell, K. K., Jefferson, A. B., and Bansal, V. S.: Recent insights into phosphatidylinositol signaling. Cell 63:459, 1990.

268. Majerus, P. W.: Inositol phosphate biochemistry. Ann. Rev. Biochem. 61:225, 1992.

269. Pang, I. H., and Sternweis, P. C.: Purification of unique α subunits of GTP-binding regulatory proteins (G proteins) by affinity chromatography with immobilized βγ subunits. J. Biol. Chem. 265:18707, 1990.

270. Strathmann, M., and Simon, M. I.: G protein diversity: A distinct class of α subunits is present in vertebrates and invertebrates. Proc. Natl. Acad. Sci. USA 87:9113, 1990.

271. Taylor, S. J., Smith, J. A., and Exton, J. H.: Purification from bovine liver membranes of a guanine nucleotide-dependent activator of phosphoinositide-specific phospholipase C. J. Biol. Chem. 265:17150, 1990.

272. Prescott, S. M., and Majerus, P. W.: Characterization of 1,2-diacyl-glycerol hydrolysis in human platelets: Demonstration of an arachidonoyl-monoacylglycerol intermediate. J. Biol. Chem. 258:764, 1983.

273. Carpenter, C. L., and Cantley, L. C.: Phosphoinositide kinases. Biochemistry 29:11147, 1990.

274. Eberle, M., Traynor-Kaplan, A. E., Sklar, L. A., and Norgauer, J.: Is there a relationship between phosphatidylinositol trisphosphate and F-actin polymerization in human neutrophils? J. Biol. Chem. 265:16725, 1990.

275. Agranoff, B. W., Murthy, P., and Sequin, E. B.: Thrombin-induced phospho-diesteratic cleavage of phosphatidylinositol bisphosphate in platelets. J. Biol. Chem. 258:2076, 1983.

276. Ishii, H., Connolly, T. M., Bross, T. E., and Majerus, P. W.: Inositol cyclic trisphosphate (inositol 1:2-cyclic,4,5 trisphosphate) is formed upon thrombin stimulation of human platelets. Proc. Natl. Acad. Sci. USA 83:6397, 1986.

277. Streb, H., Irvine, R. F., Berridge, M. J., and Schulz, I.: Release of Ca2+ from a nonmitochondrial intracellular store in pancreatic acinar cells by inositol-1,4,5-tripsphophate. Nature 306:67, 1983.

278. Joseph, S. K., Thomas, A. P., Williams, R. J., Irvine, R. F., and Williamson, J. R.: myo-Inositol 1,4,5-trisphosphate: A second messenger from hormonal mobilization of intracellular Ca2+ in liver. J. Biol. Chem. 259:3077, 1984.

279. Prentki, M., Biden, T. J., Janjic, D., Irvine, R. F., Berridge, M. J., and Wollheim, C. B.: Rapid mobilization of Ca2+ from rat insulinoma microsomes by inositol-1,4,5-trisphosphate. Nature 309:562, 1984.

280. Wilson, D. B., Connolly, T. M., Bross, T. E., Majerus, P. W., Sherman, W. R., Tyler, A. N., Rubin, L. J., and Brown, J. E.: Isolation and characterization of the inositol cyclic phosphate products of polyphosphoinositide cleavage by phospholipase C: Physiological effects of permeabilized platelets in Limulus photoreceptor cells. J. Biol. Chem. 260:13496, 1985.

281. Brass, L. F., and Joseph, S. K.: A role for inositol triphosphate in intracellular Ca++ mobilization and granule secretion in platelets. J. Biol. Chem. 260:15172, 1985.

282. Supattapone, S., Worley, P. F., Baraban, J. M., and Snyder, S. H.: Solubilization, purification, and characterization of an inositol trisphosphate receptor. J. Biol. Chem. 263:1530, 1988.

283. Ferris, C. D., Huganir, R. L., Supattapone, S., and Snyder, S. H.: Purified inositol 1,4-5-trisphosphate receptor mediates calcium flux in reconstituted lipid vesicles. Nature 342:87, 1989.

284. Takai, Y., Kishimoto, A., Kikkawa, U., Mori, T., and Nishizuke, Y.: Unsaturated diacylglycerol as a possible messenger for the activation of calcium-activated, phospholipid-dependent protein kinase system. Biochem. Biophys. Res. Commun. 91:1218, 1979.

285. Knopf, J. L., Lee, M.-H., Sultzman, L. A., Kriz, R. W., Loomis, C. R., Hewick, R. M., and Bell, R. M.: Cloning and expression of multiple protein kinase C cDNA's. Cell 46:491, 1986.

286. Coussens, L., Parker, P. J., Rhee, L., Yang-Feng, T. L., Chen, E., Waterfield, M. D., Francke, U., and Ullrich, A.: Multiple distinct forms of bovine and human protein kinase C suggest diversity in cellular signalling pathways. Science 233:859, 1986.

287. Castagna, M., Takai, Y., Kaibuchi, K., Sano, K., Kikkawa, U., and Nishizuka, Y.: Direct activation of calcium-activated, phospholipid-dependent protein kinase by tumor-promoting phorbol esters. J. Biol. Chem. 257:7847, 1982.

288. Rink, T. J., Sanchez, R., and Hallam, T. S.: Diacylglycerol and PMA stimulate secretion without raising cytoplasm free calcium in human platelets. Nature 305:317, 1983.

289. Ware, J. A., Johnson, P. C., Smith, M., and Salzman, E. W.: Effect of common agonists of cytoplasmic ionized calcium concentration in platelets. J. Clin. Invest. 77:878, 1986.

290. Kaibuchi, K., Takai, Y., Sawamura, M., Hoshijmia, M., Fujikura, T., and Nishizuka, Y.: Synergistic functions of protein phosphorylation and calcium mobilization in platelet activation. J. Biol. Chem. 258:6701, 1983.

291. Clark, J. D., Lin, L., Kriz, R. W., Chakkodabylu, S. R., Sultzman, L. A., Lin, A. Y., Milona, N., and Knopf, J. L.: A novel arachidonic acid-selective cytosolic PLA2 contains a Ca-dependent translocation domain with homology to PKC and GAP. Cell 65:1043, 1991.

292. FitzGerald, G. A., Brash, A. R., Falardeau, P., and Oates, J. A.: Estimated rate of prostacyclin secretion into the circulation of normal man. J. Clin. Invest. 68:1271, 1981.

293. FitzGerald, G. A., Brash, A. R., Oates, J. A., and Pedersen, A. K.: Endogenous prostacyclin biosynthesis and platelet function during selective inhibition of thromboxane synthase in man. J. Clin. Invest. 71:1336, 1983.

294. Antiplatelet trialists collaboration. Secondary prevention of vascular disease by prolonged antiplatelet treatment. Br. Med. J. 296:320, 1988.

295. Needleman, P., Raz, A., Minkes, M. S., Ferrendelli, J. A., and Sprecher, H.: Triene prostaglandins: Prostacyclin and thromboxane biosynthesis and unique biological properties. Proc. Natl. Acad. Sci. USA 76:944, 1979.

296. Lee, T. H., Mencia Huerta, J. M., Shih, C., Corey, E. J., Lewis, R. A., and Austen, K. F.: Characterization and biologic

properties of 5,12-dihydroxy derivatives of eicosapentaenoic acid, including leukotriene B$_5$ and the double lipoxygenase product. J. Biol. Chem. 259:2383, 1984.

297. Prescott, S. M.: The effect of eicosapentaenoic acid on leukotriene B production by human neutrophils. J. Biol. Chem. 259:7615, 1984.

298. Prickett, J. D., Robinson, D. R., and Steinberg, A. D.: Dietary enrichment with polyunsaturated fatty acid eicosapentaenoic acid prevents proteinuria and prolongs survival in NZB X NZW F$_1$ mice. J. Clin. Invest. 68:556, 1981.

299. Esmon, C. T., and Owen, W. G.: Identification of an endothelial cell cofactor for thrombin-catalyzed activation of protein C. Proc. Natl. Acad. Sci. USA 78:2249, 1981.

300. Esmon, N. L., Owen, W. G., and Esmon, C. T.: Isolation of a membrane-bound cofactor for thrombin-catalyzed activation of protein C. J. Biol. Chem. 257:859, 1981.

301. Owen, W. G., and Esmon, C. T.: Functional properties of an endothelial cell cofactor for thrombin-catalyzed activation of protein C. J. Biol. Chem. 256:5532, 1981.

302. Salem, H. H., Maruyama, I., Ishii, H., and Majerus, P. W.: Isolation and characterization of thrombomodulin from human placenta. J. Biol. Chem. 259:12246, 1984.

303. Dittman, W. A., and Majerus, P. W.: Structure and function of thrombomodulin: A natural anticoagulant. Blood 74:1, 1990.

304. Maruyama, I., Bell, C. E., and Majerus, P. W.: Thrombomodulin is found on endothelium of arteries, veins, capillaries, lymphatics, and on syncytiotrophoblast of human placenta. J. Cell Biol. 101:363, 1985.

305. Salem, H. H., Broze, G. J., Miletich, J. P., and Majerus, P. W.: Human coagulation factor Va is a cofactor for the activation of protein C. Proc. Natl. Acad. Sci. USA 80:1584, 1983.

306. Salem, H. H., Esmon, N. L., Esmon, C. T., and Majerus, P. W.: The effects of thrombomodulin and coagulation factor Va-light chain on protein C activation in vitro. J. Clin. Invest. 73:968, 1984.

307. Maruyama, I., Salem, H. H., and Majerus, P. W.: Coagulation factor Va binds to human umbilical vein endothelial cells and accelerates protein C activation. J. Clin. Invest. 74:224, 1984.

308. Marcum, J. A., and Rosenberg, R. D.: Anticoagulantly active heparin molecules from vascular tissue. Biochemistry 33:1730, 1984.

309. Marcum, J. A., McKenney, J. B., and Rosenberg, R. D.: Acceleration of thrombin-antithrombin complex formation via heparin molecules bound to the endothelium. J. Clin. Invest. 74:341, 1984.

310. Deuel, T. F., and Huang, J. S.: Platelet derived growth factor structure, function and roles in normal transformed cells. J. Clin. Invest. 74:669, 1984.

311. Huang, J. S., Huang, S. S., and Deuel, T. F.: Human platelet-derived growth factor: Radioimmunoassay and discovery of a specific plasma-binding protein. J. Cell. Biol. 97:383, 1983.

312. Deuel, T. F., Kawahara, R. S., Mustoe, T. A., and Pierce, G. F.: Growth factors and wound healing: Platelet-derived growth factor as a model cytokine. Annu. Rev. Med. 42:567, 1991.

313. Huang, J. S., Huang, S. S., and Deuel, T. F.: Specific covalent binding of platelet-derived growth factor to human plasma α$_2$-macroglobulin. Proc. Natl. Acad. Sci. USA 81:342, 1984.

314. Deuel, T. F., Kawahara, R. S., Mustoe, T. A., and Pierce, A. F.: Growth factors and wound healing: PDGF as a model cytokine. Ann. Rev. Med. 42:567, 1991.

315. Ross, R., and Glomset, J.: The pathogenesis of atherosclerosis. N. Engl. J. Med. 296:369, 1976.

316. Huang, J. S., Huang, S. S., Kennedy, B., and Deuel, T. F.: Platelet-derived growth factor. Specific binding to target cells. J. Biol. Chem. 257:8130, 1982.

317. Williams, L. T.: Signal transduction by the PDGF receptor. Science 243:1564, 1989.

318. Waterfield, M. D., Scrace, G. T., Whittle, N., Stroobant, P., Johnsson, A., Wasteson, A., Westermark, B., Heldin, C.-H., Huang, J. S., and Deuel, T. F.: Platelet-derived growth

factor is structurally related to the putative transforming protein p28^{sis} of simian sarcoma virus. Nature 304:35, 1983.

319. Doolittle, R. F., Hunkapiller, M. W., Hood, L. E., Devare, S. G., Robbins, K. C., Aaronson, S. A., and Antoniades, H. N.: Simian sarcoma virus onc gene, v-sis, is derived from the gene encoding a platelet-derived growth factor. Science 221:275, 1983.

320. Prescott, S. M., Zimmerman, G. A., and McIntyre, T. M.: Human endothelial cells in culture produce platelet-activating factor (1-alkyl-2acetyl-sn-glycero-3-phosphocholine) when stimulated with thrombin. Proc. Natl. Acad. Sci. USA 81:3534, 1984.

321. Camussi, G., Aglietta, M., Malavasi, F., Tetta, C., Piscibello, W., Sanavio, W., and Bussolino, F.: The release of PAF from human endothelial cells in culture. J. Immunol. 131:2397, 1983.

322. Lynch, J. M., Lotner, G. Z., Betz, S. J., and Henson, P. M.: The release of a platelet-activating factor by stimulated rabbit neutrophils. J. Immunol. 123:1219, 1979.

323. Mencia-Huerta, J. M., and Benveniste, J.: Platelet-activating factor (PAF-acether) and macrophages. Cell. Immunol. 57:281, 1981.

324. Benveniste, J., Henson, P. M., and Cochrane, C. G.: Leukocyte-dependent histamine release from rabbit platelets: The role of IgE, basophils and a platelet-activating factor. J. Exp. Med. 136:1356, 1972.

325. Pinchard, R. N., McManus, L. M., Hanahan, D. J., and Halowen, M.: Immunopharmacology of PAF. In Newball H. H. (ed.): Immunopharmacology of the Lung. New York, Marcel Dekker, 1983, p. 73.

326. Hwang, S.-B., Lee, C.-S. C., Cheah, M. J., and Shen, T. Y.: Specific receptor sites for 1-0-alkyl-2-0-acetyl-sn-glycero-3-phosphocholine (platelet activating factor) on rabbit platelet and guinea pig smooth muscle membranes. Biochemistry 22:4756, 1983.

327. Hondo, Z. I., Nakamura, M., Mike, I., Minami, M., Watanabe, T., Seyama, Y., Okado, H., Toh, H., Ito, K., Miyamoto, T., and Shimizu, T.: Cloning by functional expression of platelet-activating factor receptor from guinea pig lung. Nature 49:342, 1991.

328. Ye, R. D., Prossnitz, E. R., Zou, A., and Cochrane, C. G.: Characterization of a human cDNA that encodes a functional receptor for platelet activating factor. Biochem. Biophys. Res. Commun. 180:105, 1991.

329. McManus, L. M., Hanahan, D. J., and Pinckard, R. N.: Human platelet stimulation of acetyl glyceryl ether phosphorylcholine. J. Clin. Invest. 67:903, 1981.

330. Marcus, A. J., Safier, L. B., Ullman, H. L., Wong, T. H., Broekman, J., Weksler, B. B., and Kaplan, K. L.: Effects of acetyl glyceryl ether phosphorylcholine in human platelet function in vitro. Blood 58:1027, 1981.

331. McIntyre, T. M., Zimmerman, G. A., and Prescott, S. M.: Leukotrienes C$_4$ and D$_4$ stimulate human endothelial cells to synthesize PAF and bind neutrophils. Proc. Natl. Acad. Sci. USA 83:2204, 1986.

332. Chignard, M., LeCouedic, J. P., Vargaftig, B. B., and Benveniste, J.: PAF secretion from platelets. Br. J. Haematol. 46:455, 1980.

333. Alam, I., Smith, J. B., and Silver, J. J.: Human and rabbit platelets form PAF in response to calcium ionophore. Thomb. Res. 30:71, 1983.

334. Demopoulos, C. A., Pinchard, R. N., and Hanahan, D. J.: Platelet-activating factor. Evidence of 1-0-alkyl-2-acetyl-sn-glyceryl-3-phosphorylcholine as the active component (a new class of lipid chemical mediators). J. Biol. Chem. 254:9355, 1979.

335. Clay, K. L., Murphy, R. C., Andres, J. L., Lynch, J., and Henson, P. M.: Structure elucidation of PAF derived from human neutrophils. Biochem. Biophys. Res. Commun. 121:815, 1984.

336. Wykle, R. L., Malone, B., and Snyder, F.: Enzymatic synthesis of 1-alkyl-2-acetyl-sn-glycero-3-phosphocholine, a hypotensive and platelet aggregating lipid. J. Biol. Chem. 255:10256, 1980.

337. Prescott, S. M., Zimmerman, G. A., and McIntyre, T. M.: Platelet activating factor. J. Biol. Chem. 265:17381, 1990.
338. Benveniste, J., Chignard, M., LeCouedic, J. P., and Vargaftig, B. B.: Biosynthesis of PAF. Thromb. Res. 25:375, 1982.
339. Chilton, F. H., O'Flaherty, J. T., Ellis, M. T., Swendsen, C. L., and Wykle, R. L.: Selection acylation of lyso-Paf by arachidonate in human neutrophils. J. Biol. Chem. 258:7268, 1983.
340. Ninio, E., Mencia-Heurta, J. M., and Benveniste, J.: Biosynthesis of PAF. Biochim. Biophys. Acta 751:298, 1983.
341. Albert, D. H., and Snyder, F.: Biosynthesis of PAF from 1-alkyl-2-acyl-sn-glycero-3-phosphocholine by rat alveolar macrophages. J. Biol. Chem. 258:97, 1983.
342. Blank, M. L., Hall, M. N. Cress, E. A., and Snyder, F.: Inactivation of PAF by a plasma hydrolase. Biochem. Biophys. Res. Commun. 113:666, 1983.
343. Blank, M. L., Lee, T., Fitzgerald, V., and Snyder, F.: A specific acetyl-hydrolase for PAF. J. Biol. Chem. 256:175, 1981.
344. Stafforini, D. M., Prescott, S. M., and McIntyre, T. M.: Human plasma platelet activating factor acetylhydrolase activity in human tissues and blood cells. Lipids 26:979, 1991.

SECTION VI

MOLECULAR ONCOLOGY

23

Molecular Aspects of Oncogenesis*

Jeffrey E. DeClue and Douglas R. Lowy

INTRODUCTION

The past 20 years have witnessed a veritable revolution in our understanding of cancer at the molecular level. Although many important questions remain, it is now possible to describe, at least in broad terms, the molecular mechanisms that regulate normal cell growth and how their breakdown ultimately leads to cancer.[1]

As more has been learned about the pathogenesis of cancer, it has become clear that specific molecular events underlie malignant progression. One important generalization is that the progression from normal cells to malignancy represents a multistep process, rather than arising directly as the result of a single change in a normal cell. This experimental finding correlates with the observation that many tumors develop following series of distinguishable stages, that malignant tumors are usually clonal, and that molecular analysis of tumors often reveals multiple genetic abnormalities. Another important paradigm is that in those instances when it has been possible to analyze tumor progression in detail, most of the steps have turned out to represent genetic changes. The vast majority of these genetic alterations have been found to involve one of two classes of genes: tumor-suppressor genes and proto-oncogenes. As their name implies, tumor-suppressor genes function to inhibit growth of the target cell. Proto-oncogenes, by contrast, stimulate growth of the target cell. Malignant tumors are therefore usually found to have lost the function of one or more tumor-suppressor genes and/or to possess increased activity of one or more proto-oncogenes.[2, 3] Point mutations, gene deletions, and chromosomal translocations often underlie these functional changes. Activated proto-oncogenes, whose capacity to induce morphological transformation of cultured cells is usually much greater than that of their normal versions, are often called transforming genes or oncogenes.

This chapter deals with three major themes: normal and abnormal cell growth, proto-oncogenes and their activation to oncogenes, and tumor-suppressor genes and their inactivation. The presentation seeks to emphasize general principles and therefore does not restrict its focus to the hematopoietic system. Our current picture of the molecular mechanisms that control growth and oncogenesis stems largely from work carried out in seemingly unrelated areas, such as tumor viruses, familial cancer, and the growth of cultured somatic cells and of yeast.

Tumor viruses have been intensively studied because their capacity to induce neoplastic disease in animals can often be correlated with their ability to alter the growth properties of cultured cells. Most tumor viruses contain genes known as viral oncogenes, which are necessary and sufficient for their growth-inducing potential. There are two major classes of tumor viruses: oncogenic retroviruses, which contain RNA as their genetic material, and DNA tumor viruses, whose genomes are DNA.[4, 5] Studies on both classes of tumor viruses have made significant contributions to our current understanding of molecular oncogenesis. The recognition that viral oncogenes could induce tumors provided an experimental basis for the hypothesis that a limited number of specific genes might be responsible for cancer. Tumor viruses also provided an experimental approach for analyzing the pathogenesis of neoplasia induced by the introduction of a limited number of well-defined genes.

Inquiry into the origin of retroviral oncogenes led to the discovery that normal cells contain proto-oncogenes.[6] Indeed, the first members of this class of cellular genes were identified by virtue of their close relationship to the oncogenes of retroviruses. This critically important observation helped to unify the thinking of investigators in various fields of cancer research. The relationship between viral oncogenes and their normal cellular counterparts formed the conceptual basis for studies in which tumor-derived transforming genes were identified by extracting DNA from tumor cells and introducing the DNA into recipient cells. As with retroviral oncogenes, the transforming genes identified in human tumors were modified versions of proto-oncogenes.

The analysis of certain familial cancers helped draw attention to the significance of tumor-suppressor genes in neoplasia.[7, 8] The genes responsible for several syndromes with a heritable predisposition to neoplasia have been found to encode proteins that ordinarily exert a negative effect on cell growth. In contrast to the genetically dominant oncogenes, which stimulate growth of the tumors in which they are found, it is through their loss of function that the tumor-suppressor genes contribute to uncontrolled proliferation of the target cells.[9]

DNA tumor virus oncogenes, which unlike retroviral oncogenes are virus-specific genes, have provided further insights into the biology of tumor-suppressor genes.[10] The cellular targets for oncoproteins encoded by DNA tumor viruses have been found in many instances to be the products of tumor-suppressor genes, which has provided novel approaches to probe the function and inactivation of these genes.

Studies begun on the cell-division cycle (CDC) in yeasts have provided a picture of the normal cell cycle and have led to the identification of critical genes involved in regulating cell growth.[11] One of the most intriguing aspects of these studies has been the recognition that many of these growth-control genes have been conserved through evolution and exist in mammalian species as well.[12] The evolutionary conservation of factors regulating cell growth underscores the principle that this type of control is a fundamental requirement for all life forms and cell types. Because cancer results from the failure to maintain normal growth control, this conservation of function means that elucidating the molecular basis of growth and its regulation in any organism may have relevance to human neoplasia.[12]

CANCER IS A DISEASE OF ABNORMAL GROWTH

Although molecular oncologists seek to define events and pathways that are of general importance in the development of cancer, it is clear that cancer is a collection of literally hundreds of distinct disease processes that can affect virtually any cell type. The unifying feature is that all types of cancer result from excessive, improperly regulated cell growth, ultimately at the expense of the organism.[13] To place abnormal growth in perspective, aspects of normal growth are briefly reviewed.

Normal Cell Growth

The Cell Cycle

When cells grow and divide, they must ensure that each progeny cell receives a full complement of DNA and a sufficient amount of other essential components (e.g., mitochondria, ribosomes) to be viable after separation. To accomplish this process, all growing eukaryotic cells cycle through a highly ordered series of events, which are commonly divided into four phases: G_1, S, G_2, and M (Fig. 23–1). DNA replication and histone protein synthesis are carried out during the S (synthetic) phase of the cell cycle, whereas the physical process of cell division occurs in the M (mitotic) phase. These two phases are separated by two gap (G) phases, with G_1 preceding S and G_2 preceding M. Higher eukaryotic cells that are growth-arrested in response to nutrient deprivation or differentiation are said to have entered the G_0 state, a period in which cells are no longer preparing for cell division or increasing their mass.

The entry into and exit from each phase of the cell cycle are tightly regulated. Elucidation of the mechanisms that underlie this regulation came initially from studies in lower eukaryotes, including genetic analysis of CDC mutants of yeasts.[14, 15] Compared with higher eukaryotes, yeasts have several important advantages as an experimental organism, including their short generation time, the ease with which mutant strains with stable phenotypes can be isolated, and the efficiency with which specific genes can be targeted for disruption and replacement.

Although many different genes are required for progression through the cell cycle, the $cdc2$ gene, whose activity is required for cells in G_1 to initiate the S phase as well as for their transition from G_2 to M, has a central role.[16] As first shown in the fission yeast *Schizosaccharomyces pombe*, the $cdc2$ gene encodes a serine/threonine–specific protein kinase of 34 kDa ($p34^{cdc2}$) that is itself regulated by phosphorylation at threonine and tyrosine residues.[17] The protein kinase

activity associated with $p34^{cdc2}$ accounts for the ability of this molecule to act as a biphasic regulator of the cell cycle.

The activity of $p34^{cdc2}$ is regulated by a group of evolutionarily conserved proteins called cyclins.[18] The products of the cyclin genes were first identified in developing invertebrates as proteins that accumulate at specific points in the cell cycle. Cyclins were subsequently shown to complex with $p34^{cdc2}$ and to regulate its activity and substrate specificity.[19] The "G_1-specific" cyclins, which are expressed in G_1, regulate the transition from G_1 to S, whereas the "mitotic" cyclins peak during G_2 and regulate the transition from G_2 to M. The complex formed between $p34^{cdc2}$ and the mitotic cyclins is subject to at least one additional level of control, because the complex must first be activated by dephosphorylation, which is mediated by a tyrosine-specific phosphatase.[20]

Mammalian cells regulate their cell cycle by analogous mechanisms, although the complexity of this regulation may be even greater than in yeast.[18, 21] Mammalian cells contain a $cdc2$ homologue that, in addition to its structural similarity, can functionally substitute in yeast for the yeast gene by providing the functions required at both the G_1-to-S and the G_2-to-M transitions.[11] Such conservation of function also implies conservation between yeast and human homologues of the molecules that associate with the $cdc2$ product and of the proteins it phosphorylates. As expected from this observation, mammalian cells contain genes that are structurally and functionally similar to the yeast cyclins. However, mammalian cells contain a greater number of cyclin genes, some of which do not appear to have distinct counterparts in yeast.[18, 22]

As discussed in the section on oncogenes, indirect evidence has implicated the abnormal regulation of some cyclins in the pathogenesis of several tumors, including those of hematopoietic origin.[18] The substrates for $p34^{cdc2}$ include the products of the proto-oncogenes c-*src* and c-*abl*, the SV40 large T antigen (which is the major oncoprotein of this DNA tumor virus), and the products of the tumor suppressor genes *p53* and *Rb*, which also argues for a potential link between cancer and the cell cycle.[23]

Extracellular Growth Signals: Positive and Negative

Multicellular eukaryotes are faced with the problem of maintaining a vast array of different cell types with the proper balance of growing and differentiated cells. The best studied mechanism for accomplishing this task is the production of soluble factors that act on a specific subset of cells by modulating their growth state.[24] These growth factors, cytokines, and hormones can have positive or negative effects on cell proliferation and may also induce differentiation of the target cells.[25] In some instances, removal of growth factors may place cells in a resting phase; in others, withdrawal from growth factor stimulation may lead to initiation of programmed cell death, termed apoptosis, which

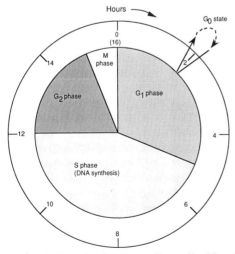

FIGURE 23–1. The cell cycle of a mammalian cell with a doubling time of 16 hours. The M (mitotic) phase, during which the physical separation of the chromosomes and cytoplasm occurs, is the shortest phase of the cycle. During G_1 the genome is diploid, while during G_2 it is tetraploid. The G_0, or resting state, is reached following growth factor deprivation, density-induced growth arrest, or terminal differentiation.

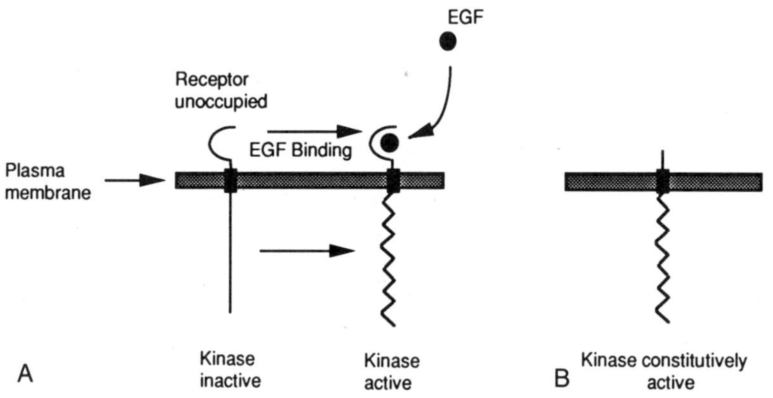

FIGURE 23–2. Regulated and constitutive activation of the EGF receptor. *A,* Binding of EGF to the extracellular region of the receptor produces a conformational change (and dimerization) that results in the activation of the intracellular kinase domain. *B,* Truncation of the *EGFR* gene (as is found in the case of v-*erbB*) results in loss of the ligand-binding domain, triggering a constitutive activation of the kinase.

occurs in embryonic development[26] and hematopoiesis.[27]

Nerve growth factor (NGF) and epidermal growth factor (EGF) were the first polypeptide factors to be identified.[28, 29] Subsequent work has led to the discovery of a large number of factors that, taken together, can regulate the growth of virtually all known cell types. By helping to maintain the delicate balance between differentiation and regeneration, these diffusible factors play a key role in normal growth control.

Mitogenic growth factors are required for cells in G_0 to re-enter the cell cycle and for cells in G_1 to commit to S phase.[24] The expression of many genes is altered by growth factor stimulation. These include the G_1 cyclins, a group of so-called "immediate early" and "early" response genes, which include at least three proto-oncogenes, c-*fos,* c-*jun,* and c-*myc.*[22, 30, 31] The induction of immediate early and early gene transcription occurs, respectively, within about 20 seconds and 2 minutes of growth factor treatment. Their induction does not require new protein synthesis, which serves to emphasize the efficiency with which the responding cell can transmit signals from the cell surface to the nucleus. Alterations in the regulated production of mitogenic factors or in the target cell that responds to them have been shown to contribute to a wide variety of neoplasms, as discussed in later sections of this chapter.

Application of a single growth factor is not sufficient to induce mitogenic stimulation of quiescent (G_0) mouse fibroblast cells such as BALB 3T3, which require a combination of at least two factors.[32] Certain growth factors, such as platelet-derived growth factor (PDGF) or fibroblast growth factor (FGF), are required to initiate re-entry into the cell cycle: These are called "competence" factors. Others, such as EGF or insulin-like growth factor type 1 (IGF-1), are called "progression" factors because they facilitate commitment to mitosis by driving the cell from G_1 to S. Although the requirement for more than one growth factor to initiate mitogenesis does not apply to all cells, it does seem to be relevant to at least some hematopoietic cells, including B cells and T cells.[33]

Receptors Transduce Extracellular Signals

The ability of target cells to respond to extracellular factors requires the expression of receptor proteins that can specifically bind to a given factor or group of factors. The extracellular factors are often referred to as ligands because their activities require that they bind to their cognate, cell-associated receptors. The receptors are the key to triggering a cell's response to a growth modulator because they serve as both a binding target for the ligand and a signaling switch for the cell.

In most cases, receptors are found at the cell surface; many contain an extracellular ligand-binding domain, a membrane-spanning region, and a cytoplasmic tail that allow for signal transduction from the exterior to the interior of the cell (Fig. 23–2A). The receptors for steroid and thyroid hormones are an important exception to this generalization.[34] These ligands can readily diffuse into cells, and their receptors are found inside the cell.

Many of the cell surface–associated receptors possess an intrinsic protein kinase activity that is activated by the binding of ligand to the receptor. Alternatively, the receptors may be non-covalently associated with a cytoplasmic kinase that is activated by ligand-receptor interaction.[35] Other receptors may alter protein phosphorylation in the opposite direction by regulating protein phosphatases.[36, 37] Still others associate with cellular enzymes or stimulate their activities via protein intermediates. The diversity of receptor types and the signals that they generate underscore the complex nature of growth regulation in a multicellular organism.

Signal-Transduction Pathways

In addition to their effects on cell growth, hormones and growth factors must modulate a wide variety of other processes in the target cell, including cellular metabolism, cytoskeletal changes, and gene expression. A further constraint is that these responses must occur within a short time. To carry out these diverse functions, cells have developed signal-transduction pathways through a variety of cellular intermediates that link the cell surface receptor to the cytoplasm and ultimately to the nucleus. The components of these pathways provide the amplification of the response to the ligand required to elicit the rapid, yet profound, changes in the state of the target cell. The fundamental nature of these signal-transduction pathways is underscored by the finding that most of the identified oncogenes represent gain-of-function mutants of components of these pathways.[38]

Following ligand binding, many growth factor receptors form dimers and undergo conformational changes that activate the receptor-associated protein kinase activity, which is required for receptor function. In almost all cases, the receptor kinase activity is specific for the phosphorylation of tyrosine residues; this tyrosine kinase activity is in contrast to most protein kinases, which phosphorylate serine and threonine residues. The activated receptors often phosphorylate themselves (at tyrosine residues) and then begin to associate with and phosphorylate cellular substrate proteins.

An entirely different set of responses to growth-modulating agents involves the ligand-stimulated production of "second messengers." These are small, often diffusible molecules such as cyclic nucleotides, sugar phosphates, ions, or lipid metabolites, which have diverse effects on cell metabolism. The second messengers are released in a regulated manner following the activation of receptor-associated or receptor-stimulated enzymes. Following their production, the second messengers bind to and activate specific intracellular target molecules, which constitutes the next step in the signal-transduction pathway. The EGF-induced activation of the enzyme phospholipase C-γ (PLC-γ) is an example of this process.[39] The tyrosine kinase activity of the activated EGF receptor phosphorylates PLC-γ on tyrosine, increasing the enzymatic activity of PLC-γ, which in turn cleaves membrane phosphatidylinositols to yield two classes of intracellular second messengers, diacylglycerol and inositol phosphates. Diacylglycerol is an activator of the serine/threonine–specific protein kinase C (PK-C), which is also activated by phorbol esters that are tumor promoters.[40] Release of inositol phosphate results in the elevation of intracellular calcium levels[41]; this calcium rise induces changes in a wide variety of metabolic pathways and cellular processes.

An alternative paradigm for the ligand-induced production of second messengers is provided by the G protein–coupled receptor family.[42] These hormone-binding receptors, typified by their seven membrane-spanning segments, do not themselves possess an enzymatic activity. Instead, these receptors exist at the cell surface as a complex with a heterotrimeric G protein (which is composed of three subunits, α, β, and γ).[43] The activity of the G protein is regulated by guanine nucleotide binding. Activation of the receptor induces the α subunit of the G protein to exchange GDP for GTP, which leads to the subunit's dissociating from the other two subunits and activating an effector enzyme. Effector enzymes whose activities are regu-

lated in these systems include adenylate cyclase and certain phospholipases.

Both the protein phosphorylation cascades and the production of second messengers described above contribute to changes in the growth state of the target cell. Their activation of cytoplasmic protein kinases such as PK-C, the c-*raf* proto-oncogene product, and cyclic AMP (cAMP)–dependent protein kinase (PK-A) is associated with the induction of specific changes in gene expression due at least in part to altered phosphorylation of nuclear transcriptional factors such as the *jun* proto-oncogene product. Thus, the changes triggered by binding of an extracellular ligand are relayed to the interior of the cell and ultimately affect gene expression.[44, 45]

Abnormal Cell Growth

Abrogation of Normal Growth Restraints

Cancer results from the ability of neoplastic cells to grow in inappropriate settings, as manifested by invasion and metastasis. Cell culture methods have made it possible to compare the in vitro growth properties of tumor-derived cells with those of non-cancerous cells. These comparisons have revealed that many "cancer-like" properties of the tumor cells are reflected in their in vitro growth characteristics. Furthermore, as methods became available to induce the in vitro transformation of cultured cells with tumor viruses, chemical carcinogens, and oncogenes, it became clear that in vitro transformed cells and cells derived from tumors share many properties that are distinct from those of normal cells. These observations imply that experimental studies of cultured cells can provide insight into mechanisms that underlie tumorigenesis.

Elucidation of the differences between normal and transformed cells has been obtained largely from the study of fibroblasts, which are easier to cultivate than many other cell types (Table 23–1). Normal fibroblasts and certain other cell types cultured in vitro exhibit particular requirements for growth, including the need for a substratum on which to adhere and grow (anchorage dependence). The adherent, normal cells form a monolayer of flat, non-refractile cells[46] whose growth ceases when the monolayer becomes confluent, a process referred to as contact inhibition or density-dependent inhibition.[47] Normal cells are also non-

TABLE 23–1. GROWTH CHARACTERISTICS OF NORMAL AND NEOPLASTIC CELLS

GROWTH CHARACTERISTICS	NORMAL CELLS	TUMOR CELLS
Density-dependent inhibition of growth	Present	Absent
Growth factor requirements	High	Low
Anchorage dependence	Present	Absent
Proliferative life span	Finite	Indefinite
Adhesiveness	High	Low
Morphology	Flat	Rounded

invasive in that they are unable to pass through a thick membranous structure such as a basement membrane.

These growth restraints are often lacking in tumor-derived or transformed cells (Table 23–1). In contrast to normal cells, many transformed or tumor-derived cells are capable of growth when placed in a semisolid agar suspension.[48] When allowed to grow on a substratum, transformed or tumor-derived cells may continue to divide and reach a much higher density than normal cells. The ability of transformed cells to overgrow a monolayer formed the basis for "focus" assays with tumor viruses and later with transfected oncogenes (Fig. 23–3); a focus of transformed cells arises when a cell in monolayer culture becomes transformed and overgrows the surrounding contact-inhibited cells.[49] The increased ability of transformed cells to invade and penetrate membranes is the basis for another in vitro assay. A further manifestation of the transformed phenotype is a distinctive change in the shape and appearance of cells, often referred to as morphological transformation. The transformed morphology (most obvious in fibroblasts and certain epithelial lines) is characterized by decreased adherence to the substratum and a rounded appearance of the cells, both of which make the cell appear more refractile in the light microscope.

Several biochemical alterations contribute to the rounded morphology and the decreased adhesiveness of transformed cells, including reduced expression of extracellular matrix proteins, such as fibronectin, which normally promote adhesion of cells to the substratum.[50] There is also disruption of the cytoskeleton and a reduction in focal adhesion plaques, which are areas of close apposition between the cellular cytoskeleton and the substratum. The microfilament system, which is composed of actin filament bundles, many of which terminate at the sites of focal adhesions, is particularly affected.[51]

Normal and transformed cells tend to progress through S, G_2, and M phases at similar rates, but the length of G_1 may be significantly shorter for transformed cells. Many transformed cells exhibit increased uptake of hexose sugars (especially glucose) and increased rates of glycolysis, both of which are necessary to sustain the rapid rate at which the cells progress through the cell cycle.

The biological differences between normal and transformed (or tumor-derived) cells can be assayed in vivo as well as in vitro. In contrast to normal cells, transformed cells are often capable of forming tumors in susceptible hosts. One widely used system tests the ability of inoculated cells to form tumors in nude (*nu/nu*) mice, whose genetic defect in thymic development impairs their cell-mediated immunity so that they do not reject cells from heterologous species, including human cells. Nude mice therefore provide a rapid assay system for the in vivo growth of non-syngeneic tumor cells without the risk of rejection that would occur in normal animals. Additional in vivo assays that can often distinguish transformed or tumor-derived cells from normal cells are based on the ability of the latter to induce angiogenesis or to metastasize in the experimental animal. These in vivo assays, in conjunction with in vitro transformation systems and molecular biological techniques, have permitted investigation of the role of specific molecules in many aspects of neoplasia.

Acquisition of Growth Factor Independence

Another hallmark of normal cells grown in vitro is their strict dependence on growth factors for continued proliferation. Many of these factors have now been identified, but it is still common for cells to be grown in animal serum, which contains a wide variety of incompletely defined polypeptide, steroid, and other growth-modulatory agents. Compared with normal cells, the growth of transformed or tumor-derived cells usually displays greatly reduced requirements for serum or growth factors. Often a tumor cell line of a given cell type survives and continues to divide in the absence of growth factors that are required for the growth of normal cells of the corresponding cell type.[24]

At least four mechanisms can account for the reduced dependence on serum or growth factors. In some instances, the tumor cell synthesizes one or more of the required growth factors. This "autocrine" production of ligand by the tumor cells continually activates the appropriate receptors, which abrogates the requirement for exogenous ligand.[52] In other cases, the number of receptors expressed in the tumor cells may be abnormally high, which endows lower concen-

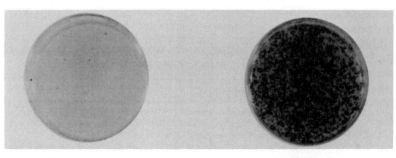

Control Dish　　　**Focal Transformation**

FIGURE 23–3. Assay for focal transformation in vitro. Established mouse fibroblasts grown in a monolayer culture in Petri dishes were either left untreated (control dish) or were subjected to transformation by the introduction of a viral transforming gene (focal transformation). Cells in the control dish are contact inhibited, whereas the transformed cells in the other dish continue to grow and form foci, visualized here by staining the cells in the dishes.

trations of ligand with greater activity. In still other instances, specific gain-of-function mutations involving oncogene products may be part of the normal cellular signal transduction machinery. These mutations result in the constitutive activation of signaling pathways, which would normally require activation by a ligand. The functional inactivation of tumor-suppressor gene products represents a fourth potential, but less well documented, mechanism for reduced dependence on serum and growth factors. Because these genes normally restrain cell growth, loss of their inhibitory activity may make certain signals sufficient to stimulate the growth of cells lacking these restraints, although these same signals would be insufficient to stimulate growth of normal cells.

Immortalization and Resistance to Differentiation

Even when all the requirements for their growth are provided, normal cells cultured in vitro are capable of only a limited number of doublings before they undergo a "crisis" period and begin to die. A small proportion of rodent cells survive the crisis period and give rise to established (or "immortalized") cell lines (e.g., the murine NIH 3T3 line). Established cells retain many properties of normal cells, but they can proliferate indefinitely without further crisis. Although it is very difficult to establish a human cell line in this way, many cell lines derived from human and animal tumors are found to be immortalized.

The molecular basis for immortalization has been intensively studied, because it relates to mechanisms that may regulate both carcinogenesis and aging. One conclusion from these studies is that immortalization of some cells can be achieved by increasing the activity of certain genes that stimulate growth (such as the *myc* oncogene) or decreasing the activity of some growth-inhibitory genes (such as the *p53* tumor-suppressor gene).[53] Thus, it is likely that immortalization of tumor cells reflects part of the overall change in their growth properties due to specific alterations in genes that regulate cell growth.

Differentiation represents another normal requirement of cells from complex, multicellular organisms, which demand a variety of differentiated cell types performing highly specialized functions. In many instances, fully differentiated cells are unable to proliferate. Such "terminal differentiation," which in erythroid cells and keratinocytes even includes loss of the nucleus, is obviously incompatible with the growth of tumor cells. Many tumors therefore arise from stem cell populations, with the most malignant tumors usually being composed of poorly differentiated, anaplastic cells that are blocked in their drive toward differentiation. Leukemias generally conform to this pattern, with the acute forms being much less able to express differentiated functions than the chronic forms.[54]

Tumor Progression: Mutations and Epigenetic Phenomena

Evidence from experimental and human cancer suggests that malignancy usually results only after a cell has undergone a series of genetic and perhaps some epigenetic changes.[1, 3, 12] In principle, each change should provide a selective growth advantage to the cell, compared with the progenitor cells lacking that change. This process results in the continual "progression" of the tumor, in which subsets of cells arise that have increasingly autonomous growth characteristics. Many of these changes are directly involved in increasing the rate of cell proliferation, whereas others may allow for the escape from an immune response directed against the incipient tumor cells. During the progression of the tumor, several mutational events may occur, such as those that allow for growth factor independence, reduced positional dependence of growth, and increased invasiveness. These altered growth properties may result from gain-of-function changes in proto-oncogenes, amplification (increased copy number) of these loci, or loss of function changes in tumor-suppressor genes.

Some tumor types may be associated with a consistent constellation of mutated genes, suggesting that each of these mutant genes serves an important and specific role in the tumor that cannot easily be duplicated by alterations in other genes. Certain in vitro cell transformation assays that depend on cooperation between more than one transforming gene appear to reflect analogous requirements, because only some combinations of genes induce transformation in these assay systems.[55] In oncogenic viruses that contain more than one viral oncogene, the oncogenes in combination in the virus can be shown to cooperate with one another by in vitro cell transformation assays or tumorigenesis assays in vivo.

In addition to genetic alterations, a separate type of change may occur that involves the altered expression of certain growth-regulating gene products. For example, there may be increased expression of cell surface receptors for a growth factor, which, as noted earlier, may enhance the sensitivity of the tumor cells to this factor. Such alterations are referred to as epigenetic because they do not involve a change in the genetic information in the cell but merely in the way in which the information is expressed.

Another common property of tumor cells during their progression to malignancy is genomic instability, including gross karyotypic changes and abnormalities.[56] These chromosomal changes may augment the genetic or epigenetic changes described above. For example, portions of chromosomes may be deleted, resulting in a loss of tumor-suppressor genes, whereas other portions may be duplicated, resulting in amplification of proto-oncogenes. Gene conversion events are also common; this process often represents another mode of gene amplification because it may result in a cell's being converted from heterozygosity for a mutant allele to homozygosity for the allele. The net result of these processes occurring together within the tumor cell population is the continuous progression of the tumor to a more oncogenic state.

ONCOGENES AND PROTO-ONCOGENES

Discovery and Definition of Oncogenes

The term *oncogene* originally referred to the ability of retroviruses to induce stable, tumorigenic changes in infected cells.[57] In the 1970s, the term came to refer more precisely to retroviral genes, which dramatically altered the growth properties of cells in which they were expressed. The essential feature of these genes is that they stimulate inappropriate growth of their target cells.[58] Oncogene expression can induce cellular transformation in vitro, as described in the previous section, or in vivo by causing neoplastic disease in target cells that express it. The term was also applied to the transforming genes of DNA tumor viruses.

Retroviruses are endogenous to chickens, mice, and many other species, and it was initially unclear whether viral oncogenes represented altered versions of viral replication genes or were composed of cell-derived genetic information. The recognition that retroviral oncogenes (collectively abbreviated v-*onc*) were derived from cellular genes (abbreviated c-*onc*) led to the normal cellular homologues of viral oncogenes being referred to as proto-oncogenes.[58] When altered versions of c-*onc* were identified in cancers, the term *oncogene* was expanded to include these genes as well. In this chapter and elsewhere, *oncogene* is now used even more broadly to include any gene whose ability to alter cell growth is similar to that of viral oncogenes. By this definition, a growth factor receptor whose activation stimulates cell growth is considered a proto-oncogene, and a constitutively active version of this receptor is termed an oncogene. Using this definition, close to 100 oncogenes have now been identified; most can be classified into groups, based on structural and functional criteria.[1]

DNA Tumor Viruses

Several groups of DNA-containing viruses have oncogenic potential (Table 23–2) (for review, see ref. 59). Genes that alter cell growth have been identified for Epstein-Barr virus,[60] but their precise role in tumorigenesis remains to be clarified. In a few cases, hepatitis B DNA has been found to integrate near host genes, such as c-*myc*, which are implicated in cell growth or differentiation, sometimes leading to expression of a fusion protein composed of a viral and a cellular gene.[61, 62] As discussed below, analogous alterations have been studied much more extensively with retroviruses.

The most revealing molecular and genetic analyses of the oncogenes encoded by DNA tumor viruses have been made for adenoviruses and papovaviruses, es-

TABLE 23–2. DNA VIRUSES ASSOCIATED WITH NATURALLY OCCURRING MALIGNANT TUMORS

VIRUS GROUP	VIRUS	TUMOR (HOST SPECIES)
Hepadenavirus	Hepatitis B	Hepatocellular carcinoma (humans, woodchuck)
Herpesvirus	Epstein-Barr virus	African Burkitt's lymphoma, nasopharyngeal carcinoma (humans)
	Marek's disease virus	T-cell lymphoma (chickens)
Papovaviruses, papillomavirus	Several HPV types (especially 5, 8, 16, 18, 31, 33)	Squamous cell carcinoma in cervical carcinoma and others (humans, rabbits, cows)
Polyoma/SV40	Polyoma	Various (mice)

pecially polyomavirus, SV40, and papillomaviruses (for reviews, see references 5 and 63 to 65). Papillomaviruses are classified as large papovaviruses (Table 23–2), but major structural and biological differences exist between the papillomaviruses and the small papovaviruses, such as SV40 and polyoma. The small papovaviruses and adenoviruses normally replicate through a lytic life cycle, which means that death of the host cell is associated with complete viral replication and the release of progeny virus. Cell transformation by these viruses therefore represents a form of incomplete (abortive) infection.

Some DNA tumor viruses, such as the papillomaviruses, induce tumors in their natural host, whereas others, such as SV40 and adenoviruses, induce tumors only in heterologous hosts. Tumorigenesis by these latter viruses results from abortive infection in a heterologous host. Integration of viral DNA into the host genome is often required for transformation by DNA tumor viruses, although papillomaviruses and Epstein-Barr virus are exceptions to this generalization. However, viral DNA integration into the genome of the host cell is not a normal part of the virus life cycle of DNA tumor viruses, in contrast to retroviruses.

Viral Transforming Genes

Molecular dissection of the genomes of the adenoviruses and papovaviruses has been combined with transformation assays to identify the genes responsible for their transforming function. This analysis has indicated that each virus contains at least two transforming genes. In every case, the genes are located within the viral genome's "early" region, so named because these genes, which encode non-structural viral proteins, are expressed soon after infection of the cell. These transforming genes have co-evolved with the virus and participate in virus replication, in contrast to retroviral oncogenes. Analysis of conditional mutants has shown that maintenance of the transformed phenotype depends on the continued activity of these genes.[5, 63–66]

The adenoviruses and papovaviruses can be infectious for resting cells, because they contain genes that, as part of the viral life cycle, induce DNA synthesis of resting cells. The normal roles for many of the transforming gene products include the induction of cellular DNA synthesis, initiation of viral DNA synthesis, and regulation of viral and cellular gene expression. Given that entry into S phase and control of gene expression represent major ways in which cell growth is controlled, it is perhaps not surprising that viral gene products which alter these functions can induce transformation.

The functional inactivation of the products of tumor-suppressor genes is an important mechanism by which the oncoproteins of the adenoviruses, small papovaviruses, and papillomaviruses induce transformation.[10, 66, 67] Analysis of these oncoproteins is therefore discussed in the section dealing with tumor-suppressor genes. Here the transforming genes are briefly introduced.

The two major transforming genes of adenoviruses are *E1A* and *E1B*, which encode nuclear proteins. The *E1A* products function as transcriptional transactivators, although they have not been demonstrated to bind DNA.[68] *E1A* can immortalize primary cells and cooperate with *E1B* in transformation.[69]

The SV40 early region encodes two gene products, designated small t and large T, of 17 kDa and 94 kDa, respectively. These proteins are encoded by a single primary RNA transcript that undergoes alternate splicing to yield messenger RNAs (mRNAs) that are specific for small t and large T. Genetic analysis has revealed that large T is the major transforming gene for cultured cells, although small t may enhance the transformed phenotype.[70] SV40 large T is localized in the cell nucleus. Polyomavirus is similar to SV40 in the size and structural organization of its genome. As with SV40, the early region of polyomavirus encodes two proteins from alternately spliced mRNAs; they are called small t and large T proteins, respectively, although they are structurally distinct from the SV40 proteins. An additional protein, designated middle T, is also encoded by this region of polyoma. Transformation of primary cells by polyoma requires the expression of both large T and middle T. Middle T can transform certain established cells, whereas large T can extend the life span of primary cells (immortalization) without morphologically transforming them.[71]

The genital human papillomavirus (HPV) types and the bovine papillomavirus type 1 (BPV) are the papillomaviruses that have been studied most intensively (for review, see reference 72). BPV, which induces large benign fibropapillomas, has two major transforming genes, *E5* and *E6*. *E5* encodes a 44 amino acid non-nuclear, membrane-associated protein. The *E6* product is a 16 kDa protein that is found, at least partially, in the nucleus.

Although the tumors induced by HPV are generally benign (warts), certain HPV (especially types 16 and 18) have also been implicated in malignancy, especially cervical cancer. Other genital HPV types, such as 6 and 11, that infect the cervix and other genital tissues are not associated with cervical malignancy (for review, see reference 66). This difference has led to viruses such as HPV6 and 11 being called "low risk" and those such as HPV16 and 18 being called "high risk." The genital HPVs contain two principal transforming genes, *E6* and *E7*, both of which encode nuclear proteins. DNA from high-risk HPVs can immortalize primary human epithelial cells, whereas DNA from low-risk HPV types are negative in such assays. Genetic analysis has shown that the *E6* and *E7* genes from a high-risk HPV type cooperate to induce immortalization.[73] The keratinocyte immortalization assay appears to measure a function related to the pathogenesis of HPV-associated cervical cancer, because non-mutated forms of *E6* and *E7* are preferentially retained and expressed in cervical carcinomas and in cell lines derived from them.[59]

Retroviruses

Classification

Retroviruses constitute the only group of RNA virus that induce cellular transformation or neoplasia. The oncogenic retroviruses can be divided into two broad classes. Some such as Moloney murine leukemia virus (Mo-MLV) and the avian leukosis viruses (ALV) do not possess a cell-derived viral oncogene (Fig. 23–4). These viruses tend to induce neoplastic disease only after a relatively long latency and do not usually induce focal transformation of cultured cells. The second class is known as the "acutely transforming" retroviruses (Fig. 23–4; Table 23–3). In susceptible hosts, these

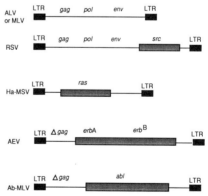

FIGURE 23–4. Genome structure of slowly and acutely transforming retroviruses, as they appear in the provirus form. The 5' end of the genome is shown on the left, and the 3' end is shown at the right. ALV and MLV represent weakly oncogenic leukosis viruses that have a full complement of replicative genes, but no v-*onc*. Rous sarcoma virus (RSV) also is replication competent but in addition encodes the v-*src* gene at the 3' end of the genome. Harvey murine sarcoma virus (Ha-MSV), avian erythroblastosis virus (AEV), and Abelson murine leukemia virus (Ab-MLV) represent replication-defective acutely transforming viruses in which most or all of the replicative genes have been replaced by v-*onc* sequences.

TABLE 23–3. SOME ACUTELY ONCOGENIC RETROVIRUSES, ONCOGENES, AND ONCOPROTEINS*

ONCOGENE	REPRESENTATIVE VIRUS	SPECIES	PROTEIN	FUNCTION
sis	Simian sarcoma virus	Monkey	p28$^{env\text{-}sis}$	Growth factor
src	Rous sarcoma virus	Chicken	p60^{src}	Tyrosine kinase
abl	Abelson leukemia virus	Mouse	p120$^{gag\text{-}abl}$	Tyrosine kinase
fps†	Fujinami sarcoma virus	Chicken	p140$^{gag\text{-}fps}$	Tyrosine kinase
fes†	Gardner-Arnstein feline sarcoma virus	Cat	p110$^{gag\text{-}fes}$	Tyrosine kinase
fms	McDonough feline sarcoma virus	Cat	p180$^{gag\text{-}fms}$	Tyrosine kinase
fgr	Gardner-Rasheed feline sarcoma virus	Cat	p70$^{gag\text{-}fgr}$	Tyrosine kinase
kit	Hardy-Zuckerman-4 feline sarcoma virus	Cat	p80$^{gag\text{-}kit}$	Tyrosine kinase
yes	Y73 sarcoma virus	Chicken	p90$^{gag\text{-}kit}$	Tyrosine kinase
ros	UR2 sarcoma virus	Chicken	p68$^{gag\text{-}ros}$	Tyrosine kinase
crk	Avian sarcoma virus CT10	Chicken	p47$^{gag\text{-}crk}$	SH2-SH3 adapter
raf	3611 murine sarcoma virus	Mouse	p75$^{gag\text{-}raf}$	Serine/threonine kinase
	Avian carcinoma virus MH2	Chicken	p100$^{gag\text{-}raf}$	Serine/threonine kinase
mos	Moloney sarcoma virus	Mouse	p37$^{env\text{-}mos}$	Serine/threonine kinase
Ha-*ras*	Harvey sarcoma virus	Rat	p21^{raH}	GTP binding
	Rasheed sarcoma virus	Rat	p29$^{gag\text{-}raH}$	GTP binding
Ki-*ras*	Kirsten sarcoma virus	Rat	p21^{rasK}	GTP binding
erbA	*Avian erythroblastosis virus*	*Chicken*	*p75$^{gag\text{-}erbA}$*	Thyroid hormone receptor
erbB	*Avian erythroblastosis virus*	*Chicken*	*p72^{erbB}*	Tyrosine kinase
rel	Reticuloendotheliosis virus	Turkey	p56$^{env\text{-}rel}$	Nuclear
fos	FBJ murine osteogenic sarcoma virus	Mouse	p55^{fos}	Nuclear
ski	Avian SK virus	Chicken	p110$^{gag\text{-}ski\text{-}gag}$	Nuclear
myc	Avian myelocytomatosis virus-29	Chicken	p110$^{gag\text{-}myc}$	Nuclear
jun	Avian sarcoma virus 17	Chicken	p55$^{gag\text{-}jun}$	Nuclear
myb	Avian myeloblastosis virus	Chicken	p45$^{gag\text{-}myb\text{-}env}$	Nuclear
ets	Avian erythroblastosis virus	Chicken	p135$^{gag\text{-}myb\text{-}ets}$	Nuclear

*In several cases, the same oncogene has been transduced by different viruses; only one example for most genes is given.

†*Fps* and *fes* are homologous genes of chicken and cat origin, respectively.

viruses typically can induce neoplasia in a matter of days or weeks and efficiently induce focal transformation of cultured cells. The critical difference between the two classes of viruses is that the acutely transforming retroviruses contain cell-derived oncogenes in addition to (or more often, in the place of) the replicative *gag, pol,* and *env* genes (Fig. 23–4). Examples of this type of virus include Rous sarcoma virus (RSV), avian erythroblastosis virus (AEV), Harvey murine sarcoma virus (Ha-MSV), and Abelson murine leukemia virus (Ab-MLV).

Retroviral Oncogenes

Most retroviral oncogenes represent gain-of-function mutants of their normal cellular homologues, which means that the v-*onc* and c-*onc* protein products tend to have many similarities. As gain-of-function mutants, the v-*onc* are excellent tools for elucidating many biological and biochemical aspects of their normal cellular counterparts. They also continue to be paradigms for how specific changes in the protein products of these genes may subvert their normal function and contribute to oncogenesis.

Many important advances in understanding oncogenes have come from the analysis of RSV (see Fig. 23–4), which was described in 1911.[74] The viral gene (called v-*src*) that accounted for the rapid induction of sarcomas by this virus was the first retroviral oncogene to be identified, although this did not happen for several decades. Identification of v-*src* was made pos-

sible largely through unique aspects of the composition of the RSV genome and by the development of cell and virus culture techniques that permitted investigators to examine pure virus strains and their interaction with relatively homogeneous populations of permissive host cells. Identification of retroviral oncogenes and certain cellular oncogenes also depended heavily on specific aspects of the retrovirus life cycle. Thus, to appreciate how these genes were identified, we shall briefly review the genetic organization and life cycle of retroviruses.

Retroviruses: Genome Structure and Replication

The retroviral genome forms a stable association with the cell by replicating through a DNA intermediate termed a provirus (Fig. 23–5).[4, 75, 76] As an integral part of retrovirus replication, the provirus is integrated into the cellular DNA and thus (irreversibly) forms part of the host cell genome. Proviral integration can occur throughout the host genome. Most retroviruses are not cytotoxic, although human immunodeficiency virus (HIV) is an important exception to this rule.

To undergo the complete replicative cycle, the retrovirus requires the products of three viral genes, designated *gag, pol,* and *env* (Fig. 23–5). The *gag* gene encodes the core proteins of the virion, *pol* the reverse transcriptase[77, 78] and associated activities that catalyze transcription of the viral RNA to the proviral DNA and mediate proviral integration, and *env* the virion

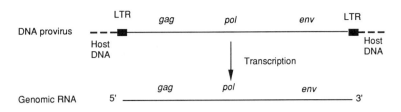

FIGURE 23–5. Expression of viral replicative genes from the integrated provirus of a weakly oncogenic retrovirus. The genomic RNA both serves as mRNA for *gag* and *pol* protein synthesis and also is packaged into virions. A second spliced mRNA (not shown) is used for translation of the *env* product.

envelope glycoprotein. These viral genes are not oncogenes. Their 5′ to 3′ order is *gag-pol-env*, both in the viral RNA genome and in the integrated provirus.

Certain sequences are duplicated at the 5′ and 3′ end of the provirus; the duplicated part of the provirus is called the long terminal repeat (LTR; Fig. 23–5).[79] Many of the viral elements that are required in *cis* are located within the LTR, including the major promoter/enhancer region of the provirus and the polyadenylation signal. Another important viral element that is required in *cis* is the *psi* sequence, which is found just 3′ of the 5′ LTR; *psi* specifies the efficient incorporation (or "packaging") of the viral RNA into virions during the late stages of the replicative cycle.

Acutely Transforming Retroviruses Contain Transforming Genes

Rous sarcoma virus is unique among the acutely transforming retroviruses in that most strains of this virus contain the three replicative genes (and therefore are replication competent), in addition to the transforming *src* gene at the 3′ end of the genome (see Fig. 23–4). The non-defectiveness of RSV facilitated the initial evidence that the highly oncogenic and transforming activities of RSV resided in sequences that were distinct from those required for viral replication.[80–82]

In contrast to RSV, the AEV, Ha-MSV, and Ab-MLV viruses bear large deletions in their replicative genes, portions of which are replaced by their respective oncogenes (*erbA* and *erbB*, *ras* or *abl*; see Fig. 23–4). These latter viruses are therefore replication defective, which means they are incapable of undergoing a full replicative cycle by themselves. However, they can be propagated through mixed infection with a replication-competent virus of the ALV or MLV type,[83] which can provide the replicative protein products in *trans*, allowing the viral RNA of the acutely oncogenic virus to be incorporated into virions and spread to new cells. Although the replication defectiveness of the acutely oncogenic viruses makes it unlikely for them to persist in the wild, they can be readily propagated in the laboratory.

Relationship of Retroviral Oncogenes to Proto-oncogenes

Discovery of Proto-oncogenes

The first clear evidence that v-*onc* were derived from cellular genes came from studies involving v-*src* of

RSV. Molecular hybridization studies showed that an RSV "*src*-specific" probe that lacked ALV sequences could hybridize to uninfected cellular DNA from chickens and from other species as well.[6, 84] Other evidence strongly suggested that the *src*-related sequences in cells had functional significance. When poorly oncogenic mutants of RSV that had deletions within v-*src* were injected into chickens, the viruses often reacquired the highly tumorigenic phenotype. This oncogenic change correlated with a recombinational event in the RSV genome; the v-*src* deletion had been repaired by the acquisition of cell-derived sequences that were almost identical to those in wild-type v-*src*.[85]

These experimental results meant that v-*src* and, by implication, other v-*onc* were derived from cellular genes that are conserved in evolution. Indeed, when similar analyses were performed using probes derived from the v-*onc* of other acutely transforming retroviruses, it was found that these genes, like *src*, had cellular homologues (for review, see reference 86). The evolutionary conservation of c-*src* and the other c-*onc* made it likely that this class of cellular genes carried out important normal functions in the cell but that these genes could be altered to give rise to dominant transforming genes. Because these cell-derived genes had oncogenic potential as retroviral oncogenes, the cellular homologues of retroviral oncogenes represented prime candidate genes to be involved in the pathogenesis of spontaneous tumors. Many, although not all, of the cellular genes that gave rise to viral oncogenes have subsequently been implicated in human tumors.

The Protein Products of Viral Oncogenes

Identification and analysis of v-*onc*–encoded proteins have provided enormous insight into how v-*onc* proteins transform cells and have contributed to elucidating the functions of their normal cellular homologues.

The v-*src* protein was the first retroviral oncoprotein to be identified, using sera from rabbits in which tumors had been induced with an RSV strain that was infectious for mammalian cells. The v-*src* gene product is a 60 kDa phosphoprotein designated pp60[v-*src*] (Table 23–3).[87] The sera also recognize the closely related 60 kDa c-*src* product pp60[c-*src*], which is found in normal cells. As antisera that recognized other v-*onc* proteins were developed, proteins related to these products were also identified in normal cells.

Biochemical analysis indicated that there are various

classes of viral oncoproteins (Table 23–3). The first insight into biochemical function was provided by pp60^{v-src}, which was shown to be a protein kinase,[88, 89] suggesting that it might transform cells via phosphorylation of critical substrates. The excitement generated by this observation was further enhanced by the subsequent finding that tyrosine is the amino acid phosphorylated on proteins by pp60^{v-src},[90] in contrast to previously described protein kinases, which phosphorylate proteins on serine and threonine residues. Normal cells contain very low levels of phosphotyrosine in their proteins (significantly less than 1 per cent of the total phosphoamino acids), and RSV transformation was associated with a 5- to 10-fold increase in cellular phosphotyrosine. These results therefore implied that cell transformation by v-src was mediated by altering the function of cellular substrate proteins that were phosphorylated on tyrosine by pp60^{v-src}.

A protein tyrosine kinase activity was also identified for the v-abl oncogene product of Ab-MLV, the v-erbB product of AEV, and several other v-onc products. Not all v-onc products with kinase activity are tyrosine kinases; the products of the v-mos and v-raf oncogenes are serine/threonine kinases (see Table 23–3). The protein kinase activities of these oncoproteins and of the v-onc proteins with tyrosine kinase activity are essential for their biological activity, because kinase-deficient mutants of these proteins are transformation defective.

Some v-onc products, although they are highly transforming, lack a detectable kinase activity and therefore transform cells via other mechanisms. Some, such as the Ras proteins, function through their ability to bind the guanine nucleotide GTP. The v-sis product is a growth factor (PDGF). Others, such as those encoded by v-myc, v-fos, v-jun, and v-myb, are nuclear proteins that are directly involved in the transcription of mRNA.

From c-onc to v-onc: Mutation and Overexpression

The demonstration that proto-oncogenes and their products may reside in normal cells raised two related issues: how normal cells are prevented from being transformed, and the nature of the differences between c-onc and v-onc. Comparisons between c-onc and v-onc have shown that almost all v-onc are highly transforming because they function as constitutively active versions of c-onc; both mutation and overexpression contribute to the conversion of normal cellular genes to the potent transforming genes found in retroviruses. These findings underlie the dominant paradigms of the field: that proto-oncogenes are normally involved in the regulation of cell growth and signal transduction, and that viral oncogenes disrupt the normal balance of growth control because they represent less regulated versions of these proto-oncogenes.[58, 86] Most proto-oncogenes, when overexpressed, are capable of inducing at least immortalization or partial transformation. However, except for

those v-onc that are identical to their cognate c-onc, v-onc are much more potent transforming genes than their normal cellular homologues.[91]

A wide variety of structural changes have been found to account for the mutational activation of v-onc. These include point mutation, which changes single amino acids (exemplified by the v-ras genes); deletion of the 5' end of the gene (v-raf); deletion of the 3' end of the gene (v-src); deletion of both 5' and 3' sequences (v-erbB); and fusion of c-onc sequences to portions of viral replicative genes, such as gag (v-abl). Often more than one of these changes have occurred in a given v-onc.

One common consequence of the changes is that their mutated protein products, in contrast to their normal counterparts, are more or less constitutively active. In the case of the protein kinases, these structural alterations remove negative regulatory regions that limit their activity. In the case of Ras proteins, which ordinarily shuttle between an active, GTP-bound conformation and an inactive, GDP-bound conformation, the mutations serve to maintain them in the active conformation. As these cases illustrate, the structural alterations found in the v-onc–encoded proteins enhance the function of the normal c-onc–encoded proteins, rather than investing the v-onc products with entirely new biochemical functions.

As noted earlier, the retroviral LTR acts as a strong promoter that contains multiple enhancer elements that result in a high level of expression for genes under their control. Thus, when a proto-oncogene is transduced and expressed from the viral LTR, its expression may greatly exceed the normal level of proto-oncogene expression, thereby overwhelming the delicate balance that controls normal cell proliferation.

Because expression from the viral LTR is constitutive, proto-oncogenes whose level of transcription is normally tightly regulated (e.g., fos and myc) by the cell cycle or other mechanisms are aberrantly expressed both temporally and quantitatively. Viral transduction of a proto-oncogene may be associated with loss of other steps at which gene expression may normally be regulated, such as mRNA stability and efficiency of translation. When retroviruses are inoculated into an organism, they may infect cell types in which the proto-oncogene that gave rise to their v-onc may not be expressed. Although many proto-oncogenes are expressed in virtually all cell types (e.g., c-ras), the expression of others is more restricted, so that their expression in inappropriate cells may be related to their activation. For example, transformation may result from expression of a transduced growth factor gene (e.g., v-sis) following viral infection of a cell that expresses the cognate receptor.

The relative contributions of different potential mechanisms to the activation of proto-oncogenes has been investigated in various ways. Molecular cloning techniques have been employed to isolate and determine the nucleotide sequence of the v-onc and their normal cellular homologues (for review, see reference 4). In addition to the obligatory loss of introns in the v-*onc*, these comparisons have revealed a high frequency of deletions and point mutations in v-*onc*. The contribution of these structural changes has then been determined by repairing the mutations, singly or in combination, and determining the activity of these genes. Also, the effects of overexpression have been tested by placing proto-oncogenes under the control of strong promoters, such as LTRs.[92] The development of transgenic mice has enabled investigators to assess the effect of v-*onc* expression in vivo, in a wide variety of different cell types, depending on the promoter used.[93]

Activation of Oncogenes by Insertional Mutagenesis

As noted in an earlier section, viruses of the ALV or Mo-MLV type, which lack cell-derived oncogenes, are still oncogenic, although they induce neoplasia more slowly than the acute transforming viruses. The same is true for the mouse mammary tumor virus (MMTV). The long latency between inoculation of these viruses into susceptible animals and the development of malignancy implied that several events, in addition to viral infection, might be required for a tumor to develop. The first mechanistic clues were provided by studies of ALV-induced bursal lymphomas in chickens.

When the integration sites of the ALV sequences were analyzed by Southern blotting experiments, primary and metastatic tumors in a given animal were all found to contain the same ALV integration site. By itself, this finding was not surprising, because it merely confirmed the clonal origin of the tumors. However, the ALV integration sites in bursal tumors from different animals indicated that the ALV sequences were integrated within the same region of cell DNA in most of the different tumors. Given the almost limitless number of potential integration sites in the host cell genome, finding a common integration site implied a selective growth advantage to the cells that contained this viral integration site.

Analysis of the viral DNA integration site in the tumor cells showed that it contained only a portion of the viral genome, with a large region deleted (Fig. 23–6). The sequences remaining in the tumor cells usually included an LTR but often contained little of the replicative genes. This result indicated that although inoculation of the virus was required to induce the lymphomas, neither the expression of viral genes nor viral replication was required for maintenance of the lymphomas.[94] It therefore seemed likely that the retrovirus integration itself might be acting as a mutagenic event, altering the expression of nearby gene (or genes) that might be involved in the regulation of cell growth. This prediction was fulfilled when it was determined that the common viral integration site was located within the c-*myc* proto-oncogene, the gene that had given rise to the v-*myc* oncogene of an acute transforming retrovirus.[95] The tumor cells were found to express an mRNA species that began at the viral

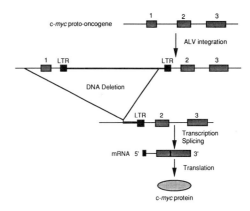

FIGURE 23–6. Activation of c-*myc* by proviral insertion in avian bursal lymphomas. Integration of the ALV provirus is usually followed by a deletion of the non-coding exon 1 of c-*myc* and most of the provirus. The 3' LTR then directs the production of an mRNA species encoding the normal c-*myc* protein. Because the expression of this mRNA lacks the normal control mechanisms that act on c-*myc*, an increase in the level of c-*myc*–encoded protein results.

LTR and encoded the normal protein-coding exons of c-*myc*, resulting in an increased level of the c-*myc* protein product, which in combination with other changes eventually led to the formation of the tumor.

This type of proto-oncogene activation, termed insertional mutagenesis, is not limited to the ALV-induced bursal lymphomas, nor is c-*myc* the only cellular target identified in this mechanism. In fact, many proto-oncogenes that gave rise to retroviral oncogenes were found to be targets for insertional mutagenesis by retroviruses that lacked their own v-*onc* (Table 23–4). In some cases, structural changes in the c-*onc* (e.g., deletions such as those discussed above)[96] were found in addition to the overexpression usually involved in the mechanism of insertional mutagenesis.

Despite the excitement of these discoveries, which linked oncogenesis by retroviruses lacking oncogenes to activation of proto-oncogenes, insertional mutagenesis in the region of known c-*onc* could not account for tumor induction by all of the slowly oncogenic retroviruses. For example, MMTV, a mammary tumor–inducing virus that lacked an oncogene, was not found to integrate its provirus near any of the known proto-oncogenes. However, the MMTV provirus did have common integration sites, which suggested that the target genes at these sites might represent novel proto-oncogenes that had not been identified as transduced retroviral oncogenes.

The *wnt-1* gene (formerly known as *int-1*), which is located at one of these common integration sites, was the first proto-oncogene discovered as a target for MMTV proviral insertion (Table 23–4).[97] Additional studies verified that *wnt-1* was conserved in evolution, had the biological properties of an oncogene in cell transformation experiments, and could induce mammary carcinomas when expressed as a transgene in mice.[98, 99] The expression of *wnt-1* is not detected in normal mammary tissue, and MMTV induces expression of the normal *wnt-1* product, which has many

TABLE 23—4. ONCOGENES ACTIVATED BY RETROVIRAL INTEGRATION

ONCOGENE	RETROVIRUS	NEOPLASM
myc	ALV	Avian bursal lymphomas
	MuLV and FeLV	Mouse and cat T-cell lymphomas
erbB	ALV	Avian erythroleukemias
wnt-1	MMTV	Mouse mammary carcinomas
wnt-3	MMTV	Mouse mammary carcinomas
int-2/FGF-3	MMTV	Mouse mammary carcinomas
int-3	MMTV	Mouse mammary carcinomas
Ha-ras	ALV	Avian nephroblastoma
Ki-ras	MuLV	Mouse bone marrow cell line
myb	MuLV	Mouse myeloid leukemias and plasmacytoid lymphosarcomas
	ALV	Avian bursal lymphomas
fms	MuLV	Mouse myeloid leukemias
mos	A particle	Mouse plasmacytomas
pim-1	MuLV	Mouse T-cell lymphomas
lck	MuLV	Mouse T-cell lymphomas
evi-1	MuLV	Mouse myeloid leukemias
interleukin-3	A particle	Mouse myelomonocytic leukemia
CSF-1	MuLV	Mouse monocyte tumor

features in common with peptide growth factors. In spite of its involvement in MMTV-induced tumors and its demonstrated oncogenic potential, wnt-1 has not been associated in humans with mammary cancer or with other tumors. On the other hand, wnt-1 represents the prototype of a multigene family whose members carry out important functions in normal development[100]; it is possible that other members of the wnt family that have been examined in less detail might participate in human tumors.

Several other common integration sites for the MMTV provirus in addition to wnt-1 have been mapped, including int-2 (also known as FGF-3),[101] wnt-3, and hst-1 (also known as FGF-4) (Table 23–4). Many MMTV-induced tumors have proviral integrations at two of these loci, most often at wnt-1 and int-2, and in transgenic animals these genes cooperate in the induction of mammary tumors.[102] Analysis of common integration sites with other slowly oncogenic retroviruses has led to the identification of other novel proto-oncogenes (see Table 23–4). For example, the lck proto-oncogene, whose sequence is similar to that of src, was discovered as the target for integration in a murine thymic tumor.[103] Thus, these studies of common viral integration sites have led to the identification of new oncogenes, in addition to explaining part of the mechanism of tumorigenesis by the slowly oncogenic retroviruses and underscoring the significance of oncogenes to cancer.

Tumor-Derived Oncogenes

Oncogenes have also been identified through analysis of human tumors. One approach has used gene-transfer techniques to test the ability of DNA from tumor cells to induce transformation similar to that of viral oncogenes.[2, 12] The other has involved the molecular analysis of specific cytogenetic abnormalities that are characteristic of certain human neoplasms, usually by identifying genes lying at or near chromosomal breakpoints.[56] As with insertional mutagenesis by retroviruses lacking oncogenes, both of these methods have implicated proto-oncogenes that were originally identified as the cellular homologues of retroviral oncogenes and have uncovered previously unidentified proto-oncogenes.

Cell transformation by DNA-mediated gene transfer was initially applied successfully to the DNA tumor viruses and to the proviral DNA of acutely transforming retroviruses.[104] One potential limitation of this approach for identifying dominant transforming genes in non–retrovirally induced tumors is the fact that eukaryotic genes tend to be extremely large, owing to the presence of long intronic sequences. This technique may therefore favor the identification of oncogenes encoded by relatively small segments of DNA, because a small gene has a greater chance of remaining intact during the gene-transfer process. On the other hand, the procedure can result in the artifactual "activation" of genes containing negative regulatory sequences at 5' or 3' ends, through the separation of these sequences from the rest of the gene.

When DNA extracted from chemically transformed murine cell lines was assayed by gene transfer, dominant-acting transforming sequences were detected by their ability to induce morphologically transformed cells among the recipient population.[105] Although DNA from non-transformed cells also gave rise to transformed foci, the frequency was much lower.[106] In either case, when DNA from the transformed recipient cells was extracted and subjected to a second round of gene transfer, the transforming gene was once again found to be passed on to the recipient cells.

DNA from certain cell lines derived from human tumors was also able to induce cell transformation.[107] The oncogenes discovered in these early cases turned out to be members of the ras gene family (Table 23–5): Ha-ras from a bladder tumor cell line[108, 109] and Ki-ras from a lung tumor line.[110] When the DNA sequence of the transforming human ras genes was compared with that of the normal proto-oncogene, point mutations were found to have occurred in the tumor-derived genes. These mutations, which affect only a limited number of amino acids, rendered the mutant ras genes much more active biologically. Furthermore, the mutations in the transforming human ras genes were similar to those that activated the retroviral ras oncogenes. These studies served to establish a closer relationship between c-onc, v-onc, and the biology of human cancer.

Many tumor-derived oncogenes have subsequently been isolated from a wide variety of human and animal tumors, several of which had not been previously identified as viral oncogenes (see Table 23–5). Some of these transforming genes carried activating muta-

TABLE 23–5. ONCOGENES IDENTIFIED BY GENE-TRANSFER TECHNIQUES

A. Tumor-Derived Oncogenes Detected by Gene Transfer

ONCOGENE	TUMOR	TYPE OF ALTERATION
Ha-*ras*, Ki-*ras*, and N-*ras*	Human and rodent carcinomas, sarcomas, neuroblastomas, leukemias, and lymphomas	Point mutation
neu	Rat neuroblastomas and glioblastomas	Point mutation
met	Chemically transformed human osteosarcoma cell line	Recombinant fusion protein
trk	Human colon carcinoma	Recombinant fusion protein

B. Proto-oncogenes Activated During the Gene Transfer Process

ONCOGENE	ACTIVATION MECHANISM
ret	Recombinant fusion proteins
ros	Recombinant fusion proteins
raf	Recombinant fusion proteins
B-*raf*	Recombinant fusion proteins
dbl	Recombinant fusion proteins
vav	Recombinant fusion proteins
hst	Aberrant gene expression
fgf-5	Aberrant gene expression
mas	Aberrant gene expression

tions that were present in the tumors from which the oncogenes were isolated. For example, the *neu* oncogene (also called *erbB-2*), which had the structure of a growth factor receptor, contained an activating point mutation in its transmembrane coding region.[111] Other cellular transforming genes were found to be activated as an artifact of the gene-transfer process itself; the mechanisms in these cases included deletion, gene fusion, and overexpression due to the loss of normal controlling sequences (see Table 23–5B).

Oncogenes have also been identified through molecular analysis of cytogenetic abnormalities in tumor cells. Genomic instability, generically referred to as aneuploidy, is a common characteristic of tumor cells. Frequent alterations include the loss or duplication of chromosomes, fragmentation of chromosomes, and translocation of portions of one chromosome to another (and vice versa in the case of reciprocal translocations). Specific karyotypic abnormalities have been noted in a high proportion of some tumor types. For example, chronic myelogenous leukemia (CML) is associated with the Philadelphia chromosome, which represents a translocation between chromosomes 9 and 22, and Burkitt's lymphoma is associated with a translocation between chromosome 8 and either chromosome 2, 14, or 22, which are sites of the immunoglobulin genes.

Molecular mapping of the sequences near the breakpoints that gave rise to the cytogenetic abnormalities in Burkitt's lymphomas indicated that the proto-oncogene c-*myc* mapped to the region of chromosome 8

that is translocated in the lymphomas. This form of lymphoma is therefore analogous to bursal lymphoma in chickens, in which c-*myc* is activated by ALV proviral insertion. In Burkitt's lymphoma, an increased level of c-*myc* expression was found in the tumor cells, owing to the *myc* coding sequences being placed under control of an immunoglobulin regulatory region (Fig. 23–7).[112, 113] Mutation within the first exon of the translocated c-*myc* gene contributed to the efficient transcription of c-*myc* coding sequences. A strikingly similar translocation involving c-*myc* was also found in murine plasmacytomas.[114]

The hypothesis that translocation involving proto-oncogenes contributes to tumor formation gained further support from the discovery that a distinct *abl* protein product with increased kinase activity was produced in the CML cells through the fusion of *abl* coding sequences, located near the breakpoint on chromosome 9, to another gene (called *bcr*) located at the breakpoint of chromosome 22.[115, 116] As discussed in greater detail in Chapter 24, the *bcr-abl* fusion protein is remarkably similar to the v-*abl* protein of A-MLV, in which activation of the kinase activity is associated with fusion of c-*abl* to viral *gag* sequences.

Examination of translocations in other tumors led to the identification of transforming genes that had not been found previously in retroviruses. *bcl-1* and *bcl-2* represent two such genes identified through analysis of the breakpoints in the t(11:14) and t(14:18) translocations in chronic lymphoid leukemia (CLL) and follicular lymphoma, respectively. As with c-*myc*

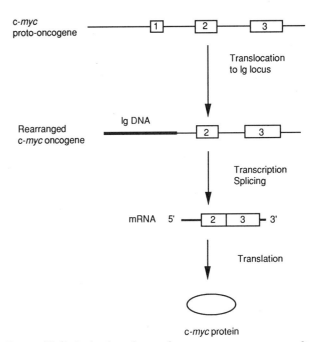

FIGURE 23–7. Activation of c-*myc* by rearrangement as a result of chromosomal translocation in Burkitt's lymphoma. Most tumors display a rearrangement as depicted in the second line: The promoter and first exon of c-*myc* (which is non-coding) are replaced by a portion of the immunoglobulin locus. The strong enhancer present in the immunoglobulin DNA results in the increased expression of normal c-*myc* mRNA and protein.

in Burkitt's lymphoma, bcl-1 and bcl-2 appear to have been activated by their translocation to an immunoglobulin enhancer located near the breakpoint on chromosome 14.[117] bcl-1 appears to represent a G1 cyclin[118]; it is located a greater distance from the breakpoint (up to 150 kb away) than most other genes identified through cytogenetic rearrangement. Transforming activity has been shown for bcl-2.[119] The potential involvement of several genes in T-cell tumors, including c-myc, has been identified through analysis of translocations that involve the T-cell receptor, located on chromosome 14.[56]

Amplification of Proto-oncogenes in Tumors

Gene amplification represents an additional way in which proto-oncogenes have been implicated in human cancer. This phenomenon, which represents an increase in the number of copies of a gene per cell, results in increased expression of the oncoprotein. Although gene amplification is not normally found in mammalian development or in somatic cells, situations in which selective pressure is exerted on cells (such as the development of drug resistance) can lead to amplification. As noted earlier, karyotypic abnormalities occur commonly during the progression of tumors. This tendency, coupled with selection for aggressively growing cells, may result in the amplification of genes that confer a growth advantage on cells. Amplified sequences can be found in chromosomes, often as homogeneous staining regions, or in small chromosomes lacking centromeres, termed "double minutes."

c-myc was the first proto-oncogene found to be amplified in human tumors, originally in the promyelocytic leukemia line HL-60.[120] A roughly 10-fold increase in the number of c-myc copies was shown to correlate with increased transcription of this gene. Subsequent work has identified amplifications of c-myc in breast, lung, and stomach cancers, among others (for review, see reference 121). The closely related N-myc gene was originally identified as a gene that underwent amplification in neuroblastomas. Significantly, amplification of N-myc in these tumors correlates strongly with a poor clinical prognosis.[122] Similarly, the L-myc gene was first identified by virtue of its amplification in lung carcinomas.

Other genes that are frequently found to be amplified in human cancers include the c-erbB/EGFR and the related neu/erbB-2 genes.[123, 124] c-erbB/EGFR, which encodes the EGF receptor, is frequently amplified in glioblastomas and squamous cell carcinomas, whereas neu/erbB-2 is amplified in a high percentage of breast and ovarian cancers. These amplifications are likely to contribute to the progression of these tumors, because overexpression of c-erbB or neu/c-erbB-2 can result in cell transformation in vitro, in a ligand-dependent manner for c-erbB[125] and apparently by a ligand-independent mechanism for neu/erbB-2.[126]

Functions of the Products of Proto-oncogenes and Oncogenes

The proto-oncogene products can be grouped into six major classes (Table 23–6), along with a few proteins whose function is less clear.[1, 3] In this section, the normal functions and biochemical properties of the proto-oncogene products, as well as the ways in which their oncogenic properties are unleashed, are considered.

Growth Factors

Because growth factors and their receptors normally regulate cell growth, it is perhaps not surprising that each of them represents a group of proteins encoded by proto-oncogenes (see Table 23–6). The first direct link between a growth factor and an oncogene was made in 1983, when analysis of the partial amino acid sequence of PDGF showed that it shared homology with the product encoded by the v-sis transforming gene of simian sarcoma virus (SSV).[127, 128] Further studies of PDGF have revealed that this growth factor is composed of two related polypeptides, A and B, which are encoded by different genes. Biologically active PDGF is a dimer that can consist of A-A, A-B, or B-B type molecules. The gene encoding the PDGF-B chain represents the cellular progenitor, c-sis, of v-sis. In fact, c-sis is transforming for those cells that are susceptible to transformation by v-sis, and no amino acid differences exist at the amino acid level between the mature PDGF-BB product and the v-sis product.

These findings implied that v-sis transforms cells by inducing the overproduction of a growth factor.[129] A further implication of this mechanism was that the target cells for transformation by v-sis must express PDGF receptors, because v-sis would transform cells by forming a constitutive autocrine loop in cells that expressed the appropriate receptors. This prediction has been borne out experimentally. Fibroblasts, which contain PDGF receptors, are efficiently transformed by SSV, whereas epithelial cells, which lack PDGF receptors, are resistant to transformation by SSV. Furthermore, when cells lacking endogenous PDGF receptors were induced to express these receptors (by gene-transfer techniques that introduced a cloned PDGF receptor gene under control of a strong promoter), they became susceptible to transformation by v-sis, which activated the tyrosine kinase activity of the PDGF receptors. These results also provided a clear mechanism for the restricted range of potential target cells for v-sis.

Autocrine production of other growth factor genes, in the absence of activating mutations, can also induce transformation of cells that express their cognate receptors. These include transforming growth factor α (TGFα) and members of the fibroblast growth factor α (fgf) and wnt families.[98, 130, 131] At least some of these factors can induce transformation when applied exogenously to cells, but the factors tend to be more

TABLE 23–6. FUNCTIONS OF ONCOGENE PRODUCTS

Class 1: Growth Factors

sis	PDGF β–chain growth factor
int-2	FGF-related growth factor
hst (KS3)	FGF-related growth factor
FGF-5	FGF-related growth factor
wnt-1	Growth and differentiation

Class 2: Growth Factor Receptors–Tyrosine Kinases

Ros	Membrane-associated receptor-like protein–tyrosine kinase
erbB	Truncated EGF receptor protein–tyrosine kinase
neu/erbB-2	Receptor-like protein–tyrosine kinase
fms	Mutant CSF-1 receptor protein–tyrosine kinase
met	Soluble truncated receptor-like protein–tyrosine kinase
trk	Soluble truncated NGF receptor protein–tyrosine kinase
kit (W locus)	Truncated stem-cell receptor protein–tyrosine kinase
sea	Membrane-associated truncated receptor-like protein–tyrosine kinase
ret	Truncated receptor-like protein–tyrosine kinase

Class 3: Cytoplasmic Protein–Tyrosine Kinases

src	Membrane-associated nonreceptor protein–tyrosine kinase
yes	Membrane-associated nonreceptor protein–tyrosine kinase
fgr	Nonreceptor protein–tyrosine kinase
lck	Membrane-associated nonreceptor protein–tyrosine kinase
fps/fes	Nonreceptor protein–tyrosine kinase
abl/bcr-abl	Nonreceptor protein–tyrosine kinase

Class 4: GTP-Binding Proteins

Ha-*ras*	Membrane-associated GTP-binding/GTPase
Ki-*ras*	Membrane-associated GTP-binding/GTPase
N-*ras*	Membrane-associated GTP-binding/GTPase
gsp	$G\alpha_s$ subunit of heterotrimeric G protein
gip	$G\alpha_i$ subunit of heterotrimeric G protein

Class 5: Protein-Serine/Threonine Kinases

raf/mil	Cytoplasmic protein–serine kinase
mos	Cytoplasmic protein–serine kinase (cytostatic factor)
pim-1	Cytoplasmic protein–serine kinase
cot	Cytoplasmic protein–serine kinase?

Class 6: Nuclear Transcription Factors

myc	Sequence-specific DNA-binding protein
N-*myc*	Sequence-specific DNA-binding protein
L-*myc*	Sequence-specific DNA-binding protein
myb	Sequence-specific DNA-binding protein
fos	Combines with c-*jun* product to form AP-1 transcription factor
jun	Sequence-specific DNA-binding protein; part of AP-1
rel	Related to NF-κB
ets	Sequence-specific DNA-binding protein
ski	Transcription factor?

Others/Unknown

mas	Angiotensin receptor
crk	SH2-SH3–containing protein that binds to and may regulate tyrosine-phosphorylated proteins
dbl	Guanine nucleotide exchange factor
bcl-2	Signal transducer?

active biologically when produced in an autocrine manner, which implies that they activate their receptors more efficiently by the autocrine than the paracrine route.

Although some cells are normally programmed to express a ligand and its cognate receptor in a controlled manner, the intercellular signaling function of polypeptide growth factors means that the ligand and its receptor are usually produced in different cells. This paracrine relationship between ligand and receptor may be altered in tumors to one of autocrine stimulation, leading to constitutive activation of the receptor. Autocrine production of the growth factor may occur as a primary event involving mutational activation of gene expression following insertional mutagenesis, gene amplification, or chromosomal translocation. It may also occur secondary to epigenetic changes in the regulation of growth factor expression, following activation of another oncogene, as occurs following *ras* gene activation.[132] Autocrine loops have been documented in human tumors; these include expression of PDGF and its receptor in sarcomas and gliomas, TGFα and the EGF receptor (the physiological receptor for TGFα) in carcinomas, basic FGF and its receptor in melanomas, and interleukin-3 (IL-3), which is activated in a t(5,14) translocation in some pre–B-cell acute lymphoblastic leukemias.[133–135] As additional ligands are identified, this mechanism may turn out to be even more common. Tumor cells may also produce secretory factors that contribute to invasion and metastasis.[136]

Growth Factor Receptors

The possible connection between retroviral oncogenes and growth factor receptor signaling systems was first suggested by biochemical studies carried out prior to recognition of the connection between PDGF and v-*sis*. Following identification of protein tyrosine kinase activity of the v-*src*– and v-*abl*–encoded proteins, EGF receptors were found to possess a protein tyrosine kinase activity that was induced when cells carrying these receptors were treated with EGF.[137, 138] Furthermore, when EGF receptors or PDGF receptors were activated by their ligand, the pattern of cellular proteins phosphorylated on tyrosine was similar to the pattern of those phosphorylated in v-*src* transformed cells.[139]

These results implied that a common mechanism might underlie stimulation of cell growth by diffusible polypeptide growth factors and transformation by certain v-*onc*. This possibility was confirmed by purification of human EGF receptors, which made it possible to determine the amino acid sequence for peptides from the receptor and to molecularly clone the *EGFR* gene.[140] Comparison of human *EGFR* coding sequence with those of viral oncogenes indicated that v-*erbB* of AEV was probably derived from the avian *EGFR* (leading to *EGFR* also being referred to as c-*erbB*). However, the v-*erbB* product differed structurally from the human EGF receptor. The EGF receptor contained a large extracellular ligand-binding domain at its N-terminus, a transmembrane domain, a cytoplasmic kinase domain, and a stretch of amino acids C-terminal to the kinase domain. The v-erbB product lacked most of the extracellular domain and some of the C-terminal amino acids, but it retained the transmembrane and kinase domains of the EGF receptor (see Fig. 23–2).

Because the extracellular domain of the EGF receptor serves as a ligand-dependent switch that activates the intracellular kinase domain, its absence from the v-erbB product suggested that the viral protein might possess a constitutive tyrosine protein kinase activity. Consistent with this hypothesis, v-erbB can transform cells in a ligand-independent manner, and the phosphotyrosine-containing proteins are similar in v-erbB–transformed cells and normal cells treated with EGF.[141] Furthermore, in a strain of chickens in which ALV induces erythroblastosis, rather than bursal lymphomas, the common ALV proviral integration site was determined to lie within the EGFR gene. In most of the birds with erythroblastosis, the proviral insertion results in constitutive expression of an EGFR product that lacks the extracellular domain and has unregulated kinase activity.[142]

Other v-onc have also turned out to encode modified versions of growth factor receptors (see Tables 23–3 and 23–6). These v-onc share a similar structural organization in that they encode membrane-spanning regions and intracellular kinase domains that possess the ability to phosphorylate substrate proteins at tyrosine residues. As is true of v-erbB, the mechanism of transformation by all of the receptor-like oncogenes is thought to involve the constitutive (unregulated) phosphorylation of cellular proteins, resulting in the activation of mitogenic signaling pathways within the cell.[38]

The proto-oncogene c-fms, which gave rise to the viral oncogene v-fms of the McDonough strain of feline sarcoma virus, was shown to encode the receptor for the hematopoietic growth factor colony-stimulating factor 1 (CSF-1).[143, 144] This identification was made following the demonstration, with antisera directed against the v-fms protein, that the c-fms product encoded a cell surface protein that was expressed predominantly in cells of the monocyte-macrophage lineage. Unlike the v-erbB product, the v-fms product retains its ligand-binding domain and is capable of binding CSF-1. Nevertheless, the tyrosine kinase of the v-fms product is constitutively active in the absence of ligand, although this activity can be further increased by exogenous ligand. A point mutation in the extracellular domain was found to be the most important genetic alteration in the conversion of c-fms to v-fms.[145] Overexpression of normal c-fms induces ligand-dependent transformation, but introducing this point mutation in c-fms constitutively activates its encoded kinase activity and renders the protein able to transform cells in the absence of ligand.

Several v-onc that encode receptor protein tyrosine kinases have been implicated in development and are discussed in greater detail in that section. These include v-kit, which is the v-onc of another feline sarcoma virus. v-kit is derived from the feline W gene[146, 147]; in mice, loss-of-function mutations of W are associated with anemia, coat color alteration, and defective gonadal development. Stem cell factor (SCF), which is the ligand for the c-kit product, has also been identified (for review, see reference 148). The c-ros proto-oncogene, which was transduced as the v-ros oncogene of an avian sarcoma virus UR2, has been shown to be closely related to the Drosophila sev gene, which is required for photoreceptor development in Drosophila.[149] The identity of other receptor-like genes that were initially recognized by gene-transfer experiments (see Table 23–5) has also been determined. These include met, which encodes the receptor for hepatic growth factor,[150] and trk, which encodes the high-affinity receptor for nerve growth factor.[151] The ligand for the neu/ErbB-2 product has also been described.[152]

Some growth factor receptors have been implicated in human cancers. As discussed in the section on growth factors, production of both ligand and receptor occurs in several types of tumors, allowing autocrine activation. Expression of the ligand is often associated with overexpression of its cognate receptor, as for TGFα and EGF receptors, because the high-level expression of both components is usually more potent than that of only one of them. It is therefore likely that the spontaneous tumors have coordinately selected for overexpression of both ligand and receptor. Co-expression of SCF and c-kit has been identified in small cell lung cancers, raising the possibility that their expression might contribute to the pathogenesis of this tumor.[153] Overexpression of neu/erbB-2 has also been described in breast cancers, where it appears to be associated with a poor prognosis in some studies.[123] Truncation of 5′ coding sequences from TAN-1, a homologue of the Drosophila notch gene, which encodes a receptor-like protein, has been identified in some patients with T-cell lymphoblastic lymphoma.[154] However, mutation of receptors has been documented comparatively rarely in human tumors, although this mechanism occurs frequently in experimental tumorigenesis.

In contrast to the above receptors, some membrane receptors that have been implicated in tumors do not encode tyrosine kinases. As discussed in greater detail in the next chapter, the erythropoietin (Epo) receptor is a member of this class. It can be mutated to induce Epo-independent transformation of appropriate hematopoietic target cells.[155] The Friend spleen focus forming virus (SFFV) is a replication-defective retrovirus that lacks a cell-derived oncogene but rapidly induces polyclonal splenic enlargement and can convert cell lines from Epo dependence to Epo independence. Further analysis has shown that the SFFV env protein, which is a truncated version of a full-length env protein, mimics the effects of Epo by binding to and activating the Epo receptor.[156] Although the events downstream from the Epo receptor have not been fully elucidated, there is evidence that non-receptor tyrosine kinases, as described in the next section, may participate in this process.[157]

The *mas* oncogene, which was identified as an artifactually created oncogene in gene transfer experiments, encodes a receptor of the seven-transmembrane region family.[158] Subsequent study has revealed that the *mas* product represents a mutated version of the receptor for serotonin 5HT1c[159]; stimulation of this receptor by serotonin normally activates PLC.

Cytoplasmic Protein Tyrosine Kinases

A large group of transforming oncogenes encode protein tyrosine kinases that lack membrane-spanning segments and thus are significantly different from the receptor-type kinases described above (see Table 23–6). Many of these transforming genes and the corresponding proto-oncogenes encode protein products that are associated with the inner surface of the cell plasma membrane, whereas others are predominantly cytoplasmic. Such non-receptor protein tyrosine kinases are encoded by several retroviral transforming genes, including v-*src*, v-*abl*, v-*fps/fes*, v-*fgr*, and v-*yes*. A relatively large number of cellular genes that were not transduced as viral oncogenes also encode non-receptor protein tyrosine kinases. Although many cellular substrates for these enzymes have been identified (for review, see references 1 and 160), to date it is still unclear which of these targets are responsible for the wide variety of changes induced by expression of the transforming proteins. It is likely, however, that a number of substrates are involved, because these proteins induce wide-ranging effects on cells.

Within the large gene family encoding protein tyrosine kinases, c-*src* is a member of a subfamily that includes c-*yes* and c-*fgr*, *lck*, *fyn*, *lyn*, *hck*, and *blk*.[161, 162] All members of the Src subfamily share several structural features (Fig. 23–8), including an amino-terminal membrane-binding domain, a heterogeneous region of about 70 amino acids, two non-catalytic, conserved, Src-homology domains (termed SH2 and SH3), the highly conserved kinase domain (which is considered SH1, comprises about 250 amino acids, and is present in the receptor tyrosine kinases as well), and a C-terminal regulatory region. Each of these regions plays a role in controlling the function of the proteins, as discussed below (reviewed in reference 160).

As with the oncogenic versions of receptor kinases, the transforming cytoplasmic protein tyrosine kinases, such as pp60[v-src], are constitutively active enzymes, in contrast to their normal cellular counterparts. Among the members of the Src subfamily, one consistent difference between the c-*onc*– and v-*onc*–encoded proteins is found downstream from the kinase region itself, at the extreme C-terminus of the protein. In the v-*onc*–encoded proteins, these C-terminal amino acids are replaced by other amino acids. Further analysis has shown that the last dozen C-terminal amino acids encode a region that negatively regulates the kinase activity. The most important feature of this region is a tyrosine residue conserved among many non-receptor tyrosine kinases (amino acid 527 of the c-*src* encoded protein). In the c-*onc* proteins, this tyrosine is normally phosphorylated in vivo by an Src-specific kinase, and its phosphorylation correlates with an inactive kinase. Dephosphorylation of tyrosine-527 in vitro stimulates the kinase activity of the c-*src*–encoded protein,[163] and mutants of c-*src* in which this codon is changed or deleted (as in v-*src*) display greatly increased transforming function.[164] Mutations in other sites of the v-*onc*–encoded proteins of this class also contribute to their full transforming activity.

Another tyrosine that is subject to phosphorylation is located in the middle of the kinase domain (residue 416 of the *src*-encoded protein). This tyrosine, which is found in all members of the protein tyrosine kinases, is phosphorylated, as a result of autophosphorylation, when the kinase is active.[165] In contrast to the C-terminal tyrosine, phosphorylation of this tyrosine increases the kinase activity of the protein.[164]

The N-terminal membrane-association domain, which specifies the addition of myristic acid and the ability of the protein to bind a plasma membrane receptor protein,[166] is essential for the ability of v-*src* to transform cells, implying that critical substrates for pp60[v-src] may be located at the plasma membrane.[167] The heterogeneous regions of the different proteins may be involved in the particular intracellular functions that the different members of the Src subfamily presumably carry out.

The SH2 and SH3 regions were originally recognized as regions of homology between v-*src*– and v-*fps/fes*–encoded proteins. Mutation in the SH2 coding region of the v-*fps/fes* gene could drastically alter its transforming function in a way that suggests that this

FIGURE 23–8. **Structural organization of the pp60**[c-src] **protein (533 amino acids).** The N-terminal 7 to 10 amino acids encode a myristylation domain. The unique region (which includes two sites of serine phosphorylation) varies considerably among the different members of the Src subfamily. The SH2 and SH3 domains direct associations of the protein with other cellular proteins and modulate the kinase activity. The kinase domain includes a lysine residue (K) at position 295 that is involved in the binding of ATP and an autophosphorylation site at tyrosine 416 that positively regulates the kinase activity. The C-terminal 19 amino acids of the protein include a tyrosine at position 527 that is phosphorylated and negatively regulates the kinase in vivo (these 19 amino acids are replaced by 12 unrelated amino acids in the v-*src* protein).

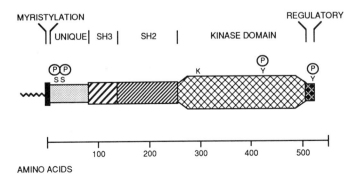

region of the protein might specify interactions of the v-*fps/fes*–encoded kinase with substrates or regulatory molecules.[168] In addition, the SH2 regions were evolutionarily conserved in many of the non-receptor tyrosine kinases, again suggesting a functional role for this domain.[169]

More recently, a large group of cellular proteins that are not tyrosine kinases have been found to contain SH2 and/or SH3 domains, including several enzymes that play a role in signal transduction.[170] These include PLC-γ, a subunit of phosphatidylinositol-3 (PI-3) kinase, and the GTPase-activating protein (GAP) that interacts with the proteins encoded by the *ras* gene family (see below). A large body of work has demonstrated that the SH2 regions are involved in protein-protein associations. In particular, these regions bind to phosphotyrosine residues in other proteins.[170]

The importance of SH2 regions in regulating protein-protein interactions has become clear through the analysis of membrane-spanning receptor tyrosine kinases.[171] Thus, when a receptor tyrosine kinase is activated by ligand binding and becomes autophosphorylated on tyrosine, SH2-containing proteins, such as PLC-γ, PI-3 kinase, and GAP, associate with the receptor by binding to the area containing the phosphotyrosine.[172] These proteins in turn become phosphorylated by the receptor and may dissociate and form complexes with other SH2-containing proteins.

The signal transduction enzymes mentioned above and the cytoplasmic kinases encoded by *c-src*, *c-yes*, and *fyn* are among the proteins that associate with receptors via this mechanism.[173] In this way, a network of protein-protein associations is built up, thus helping to define the cellular response to the input signal. These findings explain why many of the SH2-containing proteins are tyrosine phosphorylated following growth factor stimulation of cells or following transformation by tyrosine kinases such as pp60[v-src]. The role of SH3 regions is less clear; the fact that these domains have been found in cytoskeletal proteins such as α spectrin, myosin 1b, and a yeast actin-binding protein suggests that these elements may help mediate interactions between signaling molecules and the cytoskeleton.[170]

The v-*crk* gene of avian sarcoma virus CT10 is relevant to the oncogenic potential of interactions mediated by SH2 and SH3 domains. The v-*crk*–encoded protein requires only its SH2 and SH3 regions to function as a transforming gene.[174, 175] Although the v-*crk* product does not encode a kinase, v-*crk*–transformed cells contain elevated levels of phosphotyrosine, and the v-*crk* protein isolated from transformed cells is associated with protein tyrosine kinase activity.[176] Related genes, such as *nck* and *shc*, have also been identified. As with *crk*, they appear to encode SH2-SH3 domains that are not linked to any obvious catalytic activity, suggesting that they may function as "adaptor" proteins that interact with protein tyrosine kinases.[170] The presence of such adaptors suggests that transformation by v-*crk* may result from disruption of

a normal network of protein-protein associations regulated by SH2 and SH3 domains. Transformation by v-*crk* might also reflect alterations in the function of a protein tyrosine phosphatase (or phosphatases).

The functional consequence of SH2 interactions may be complex, as shown by analysis of the SH2 region of the c-*src* and v-*src* proteins. Experimental evidence suggests that the low enzymatic activity of pp60[c-src] is associated with the physical interaction between the SH2 region of pp60[c-src] and its C-terminal tail, through the phosphorylation of tyrosine 527 in pp60[c-src].[177] Mutations within the SH2 region tend to activate the biological and enzymatic activity of pp60[c-src], presumably by preventing the interaction between the SH2 region and the C-terminus of the protein.[178] However, if tyrosine 527 is mutated, as occurs in pp60[v-src], mutations within the SH2 region reduce its biological activity, presumably because they reduce the efficiency with which pp60[v-src] interacts with other proteins via its SH2 region. Furthermore, mutations in the SH2 region have been shown to produce a host cell–dependent transformation phenotype. Deletion of a single amino acid within a highly conserved motif in the v-*src* SH2 resulted in a protein that was highly transforming in chicken cells but was defective for rat cell transformation.[179] A similar phenotype resulted from a dipeptide insertion within the SH2 of the v-*fps* oncoprotein.[180]

Taken together, these results suggest a complicated role for the SH2 regions of the cytoplasmic protein tyrosine kinases, involving both modulation of the kinase activity and interaction with host cell substrate proteins. The latter of these functions is likely to be important for all SH2-containing proteins, as the highly conserved FLVRES amino acid motif found in all SH2-containing proteins has been shown to coordinate binding to phosphorylated tyrosine residues. Mutation of these residues in the case of the *abl* oncogene has demonstrated a correlation between binding to tyrosine phosphorylated proteins and transforming function.[181]

The structure of three different SH2 domains has been determined by nuclear magnetic resonance (NMR) and X-ray crystallography techniques[182–184]; in one case (the Src SH2), the structure was determined in the presence of bound phosphotyrosine-containing peptide.[184] These studies have revealed that SH2 domains of different proteins form a similar overall structure that is modular in nature and therefore ideal to be situated anywhere in a protein sequence without altering the overall protein structure. The most prominent feature of the SH2 domains is a deep pocket that comprises the phosphotyrosine recognition site. The specificity that underlies distinct SH2-phosphotyrosine interactions is most likely provided by the sequence of the amino acids that form the regions surrounding this pocket.

Non-receptor protein tyrosine kinases are believed to function in the physiological propagation of signals within the cell. Analysis of Src subfamily members has provided insights into how these molecules may function.[185] The product of the *lck* gene, p56[lck], which is expressed almost exclusively in T cells, has been shown to associate physically with the intracellular portions of the transmembrane cell surface glycoproteins CD4 (of T helper cells) and CD8 (of cytotoxic T cells). As with the Epo receptors, these receptors lack their own kinase domain. The CD4 and CD8 proteins serve as accessory molecules for the T-cell receptor and recognize elements of the major histocompatibility class (MHC) locus that are associated with antigens being presented to the T cells. These findings suggest that the binding of CD4 or CD8 to the MHC transmits a signal via alterations in the activity of the associated p56[lck]. This model for the function of p56[lck] also applies to the IL-2 receptor. Activation of this receptor by ligand results in the activation of p56[lck], which is physically associated with the receptor.[186, 187]

This model can be expanded in a general way to include the other members of the Src subfamily. Because the N-terminal heterogeneous domain that is involved in the association of p56[lck] with CD4, CD8, and the IL-2 receptor is divergent among the different Src subfamily members, they may form similar associations with membrane-spanning, signaling proteins that are likely to be unrelated in sequence. Recent experiments have demonstrated an association of the *fyn* product with the T-cell antigen receptor, and activation of the kinase activity of this molecule following stimulation of the receptor.[188] Similarly, the *blk*, *fyn*, and *lyn* products have been shown to become activated following stimulation of the B-cell antigen receptor.[189] These findings suggest a generalized role for the Src subfamily of kinases in which their specific role depends on the nature of the molecule (or molecules) with which they interact and the cell types in which they are expressed.

Tyrosine phosphorylation can be reversed by a specific class of phosphatases.[190] As with the protein tyrosine kinases, some of these phosphatases are transmembrane proteins that have a receptor-like structure, whereas others are cytoplasmic. One of the cytoplasmic phosphatases possesses two SH2 domains.[191] The tyrosine phosphatases are highly conserved in evolution, but their precise roles in the control of normal cellular processes and in oncogenesis remain to be clarified. It seems likely that they will contribute to both stimulation and inhibition of cell growth. Although their activity should attenuate the growth-promoting activity of tyrosine kinases, dephosphorylation of those tyro-

sines involved in negative regulation, such as tyrosine 527 of pp60[c-src], should have the opposite effect. One of the transmembrane phosphatases, CD45, participates in the activation of T cells by antigen. This activity of CD45 may be mediated by dephosphorylation of the C-terminal tyrosine of the *lck* protein, because this tyrosine is functionally analogous to tyrosine 527 of the *c-src*–encoded protein.[190]

Membrane-Associated G Proteins

The fourth major class of proto-oncogenes consists of membrane-associated guanine nucleotide–binding proteins (see Table 23–6). All of these proteins have in common the ability to bind and hydrolyze GTP. Because they are endowed with these properties, all members of this superfamily contain certain sequence motifs required for these functions.[192, 193] The proteins of this superfamily cycle between an active GTP-bound form and an inactive GDP-bound form. They respond to stimulatory input signals by binding GTP and then hydrolyze the GTP to GDP to attenuate the signal (Fig. 23–9). Rather than encoding their own enzymatic effector function, these proteins regulate the enzymatic activities of other proteins. They participate in a wide variety of cellular processes, including ribosomal translation function, signal transduction by a number of stimuli, trafficking of vesicles, and the control of growth and differentiation.

It is common to divide the G protein superfamily into three subfamilies: the prokaryotic and eukaryotic factors for translational initiation and elongation, the Ras-related (low molecular weight) GTP-binding proteins,[194] and the classic or "heterotrimeric" G proteins. Only members of the latter two subfamilies, particularly the Ras proteins, have been directly implicated in oncogenesis. Some evidence suggests that heterotrimeric G proteins may also participate in tumor formation.

The *ras* genes were first discovered as the v-Ha-*ras* and v-Ki-*ras* oncogenes of Ha-MSV and Ki-MSV, respectively. A third mammalian *ras* gene (N-*ras*) was identified through gene-transfer experiments. Activated *ras* genes have been detected in a large number of gene-transfer experiments from human and animal tumors.[195, 196]

The normal and oncogenic *ras* genes encode 21 kDa, membrane-associated proteins (p21[ras]), which bind GTP and GDP with high affinity.[197] The Ras

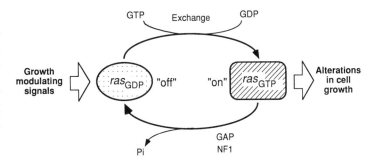

FIGURE 23–9. The activation/inactivation cycle of p21[ras] and its regulation by cellular factors. Input signals are transmitted through activated growth factor receptors, resulting in the activation of p21 by stimulating the release of GDP (exchange factors), inhibiting GTPase stimulators (GAP, NF1), or both. The binding of GTP to p21 allows for the molecule to present its effector domain in a conformation that can be recognized by both GTPase-stimulating proteins (GAP, NF1) and target (effector) molecules. The hydrolysis of GTP to GDP returns p21 to the inactive ("off") state.

proteins can hydrolyze the bound GTP to bound GDP: The GTP-bound protein is biologically active,[198] whereas the GDP-bound form is inactive. The proportion of GTP-bound protein rises in response to various extracellular signals, such as PDGF or serum treatment of fibroblasts or activation of the T-cell receptor in T cells (Fig. 23–9).[199–201] The biological importance of these changes in p21^{ras} activity is strongly supported by evidence, obtained with genes or antibodies that specifically interfere with p21^{ras} activity, that ras is essential for entry into S phase and for changes in gene expression induced by a variety of growth factors and protein tyrosine kinases.[202, 203] Even viral oncogenes that encode protein tyrosine kinases depend on endogenous Ras for mediating their oncogenic signals, because inhibition of Ras activity can inhibit transformation by v-src and related oncogenes.[204, 205] In Drosophila photoreceptor development, the sev gene, which encodes a receptor tyrosine kinase, activates Ras.[206] Taken together, these findings place Ras in signal-transduction pathways downstream from growth factors and protein tyrosine kinases.

As with other oncogenes, oncogenic ras genes represent gain-of-function mutants. The proportion of normal p21^{ras} in the active, GTP-bound state is tightly regulated, representing less than 5 per cent of p21^{ras} in unstimulated cells. By contrast, the activity of oncogenic ras mutants, which arise via point mutations involving particular codons, is constitutive because even in unstimulated cells the majority of their mutant proteins are found in the GTP-bound form.

The three mammalian ras genes encode closely related proteins, with alternate splicing of c-Ki-ras RNA giving rise to two products that differ at the C-terminus. As was the case for pp60^{v-src}, membrane association is critical for ras function: non–membrane-localized p21^{ras} is defective in transformation. Whereas membrane association in the src-encoded proteins is achieved via addition of lipid at the N-terminus, this function is carried out by the C-terminus in p21^{ras},[207] which undergoes a series of enzymatically controlled specific post-translational modifications (Fig. 23–10). These changes include the obligatory addition of a farnesyl residue (an intermediate of sterol metabolism) to p21^{ras} via a conserved cysteine located four amino acids from its C-terminus, followed by proteolytic cleavage of the three amino acids C-terminal to the farnesylated cysteine and carboxy methylation of the cysteine.[208–212] Except for one of the two c-Ki-ras–encoded products, one or two cysteines of the other p21^{ras} proteins, upstream from the farnesylated cysteine, are covalently linked to a palmitate residue. Each modification appears to be required for full biological activity of the protein.

As demonstrated from genetic analysis and X-ray crystallography, the majority of the Ras protein represents the catalytic region, which is responsible for the GTP-binding/hydrolysis activities and contains the amino acids implicated in p21^{ras} target function.[213] Oncogenic mutations are located within the catalytic region of the protein. The mutations most commonly

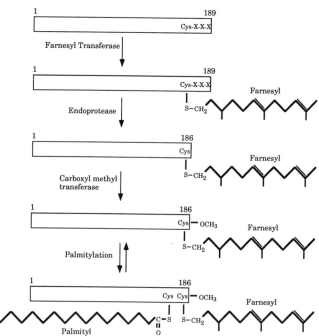

FIGURE 23–10. Post-translational processing of the mammalian Ras proteins. The primary translation product is a polypeptide of 189 amino acids (*top*). Processing begins with the addition of a 15-carbon farnesyl group to the cysteine residue of the C-X-X-X motif. This step can be inhibited by antagonists of the sterol biosynthetic pathway (e.g., lovastatin). Farnesylation is followed by proteolysis of the last three amino acids, and carboxymethylation of the C-terminal residue. Some, but not all, Ras proteins can undergo a reversible palmitylation at cysteine residue(s) located just N-terminal to the farnesylated cysteine (*bottom*). Each of these steps increases the hydrophobicity of the Ras protein and enhances binding to the membrane by Ras.

found in tumors involve codons 12, 13, and 61. Mutations at these residues impair the intrinsic GTPase activity and render the mutant Ras proteins resistant to negative regulation by the GAP- and NF-1-encoded proteins (see below).[192, 213] Ras can also be activated by mutations of residue 116 or 119, which increases the rate of guanine nucleotide dissociation from p21^{ras}.[214, 215]

The relatively small number of ras genes contrasts with the much greater number of growth factors and protein tyrosine kinases. Although the latter molecules tend to be expressed in a tissue-specific manner, the ras genes are widely expressed, which suggests that they may serve to transduce many different extracellular signals. Ras can couple to a variety of signaling systems. Mutational activation of ras genes in many different forms of cancer, including a variety of hematopoietic tumors,[216] is also consistent with the hypothesis that ras is involved in regulating the growth of many cell types.

The ras genes are even more highly conserved in evolution than many other proto-oncogenes, with homologues found in S. cerevisiae and S. pombe.[217, 218] RAS is required for S. cerevisiae to enter S phase, and S. cerevisiae lacking both of their RAS genes are non-viable. Mammalian ras can restore viability to yeast lacking their yeast *RAS* genes, and a mutant yeast *RAS* can induce transformation of mammalian cells, indicating that conservation of these genes is functional as well as structural. These findings suggested that determining the biological function of *RAS* in *S. cerevisiae*, using the power of yeast genetics, would be directly relevant to *ras* in higher eukaryotes. A primary function of *RAS* in *S. cerevisiae* was quickly determined. These proteins respond to the nutrient status of the cell and modulate the activity of adenylate cyclase, which produces cAMP and thereby regulates the activity of PK-A.[219] When this possible function for *ras* was tested in vertebrate systems, however, it was found that *ras* does not couple to adenylate cyclase in them.

Although analysis of *S. cerevisiae* has not identified the target effector of mammalian *ras* proteins, this system remains a highly useful model for understanding many aspects of *ras* function. As with other GTP-binding proteins, there are two major rate-limiting steps for Ras activity (see Fig. 23–9). One is the dissociation of bound GDP. This step leads to GTP binding because the intracellular concentration of GTP greatly exceeds that of GDP. The other step is GTP hydrolysis, which inactivates the protein.

Both steps have been shown to be enzymatically regulated in *S. cerevisiae*. Dissociation is mediated by *CDC25* (unrelated to *cdc25* of *S. pombe*), which is required for normal *RAS* function and has been shown to stimulate guanine nucleotide exchange on Ras protein in vitro.[220] Two *S. cerevisiae* genes, *IRA-1* and *IRA-2*, encode negative regulators of *RAS* that accelerate the intrinsic GTPase activity of Ras protein.[221] Loss of *IRA-1* or *IRA-2* results in higher *RAS* activity in the yeast.

Similar genes have been identified in higher eukaryotes. A *CDC25* homologue has recently been identified as being required for normal photoreceptor development in *Drosophila*, which is *ras* dependent.[222] This gene, *sos*, is located in the *ras* pathway, between the receptor tyrosine kinase gene *sev* and *ras*.[206] Mammalian homologues of *sos* and of yeast *CDC25* have also been described.[223, 224] Two different mammalian genes with homology to the *IRA* genes of *S. cerevisiae* have also been found. One encodes the 120 kDa protein called GAP, which was discovered prior to the *IRA* genes.[198] The other, *NF-1*, the gene responsible for the von Recklinghausen form of neurofibromatosis, is discussed in the section on tumor-suppressor genes. The protein encoded by *NF-1* has more extensive homology with the Ira proteins than with GAP. Both *GAP* and *NF-1* can substitute functionally for *IRA* in yeast (for review, see reference 225). GAP is a potent negative regulator of Ras protein in mammalian cells, and more limited evidence supports a similar function for the NF-1 protein.[226, 227]

The GAP and NF-1 products possess other characteristics that have made them candidate *ras* effector proteins, in addition to their negative regulatory role.[225] Although GAP and NF-1 accelerate the intrinsic GTPase activity of normal Ras protein, oncogenic Ras mutant proteins isolated from tumors are resistant

to this activity of GAP and NF-1. Indeed, the resistance to GAP and NF-1 correlates better than intrinsic GTPase activity with the oncogenic activity of these mutant Ras proteins.[225, 228] Although this correlation constitutes strong evidence that GAP and NF-1 are important negative regulators of normal p21[ras], the resistance of mutant *ras* proteins is not caused by failure of the mutant proteins to interact with GAP or NF-1. Rather, oncogenic *ras* proteins, when in the active, GTP-bound state, interact physically with the GAP and NF-1 proteins, as does normal p21[ras].[225, 229] Furthermore, GAP and NF-1 interact with the region of the *ras* protein that has been implicated in *ras* effector function.[228, 230] In a system in which Ras inhibits the opening of ion channels, this effect of Ras has been shown to depend on GAP,[231] and Ras-dependent transactivation of the polyomavirus enhancer can, under some conditions, depend on GAP.[232] The finding that GAP is a substrate for tyrosine phosphorylation by activated growth factor receptors and cytoplasmic protein tyrosine kinases may also support this model.[170] GAP and NF-1 remain prime candidate effectors for mammalian *ras*, but more direct experimental proof is needed to verify this model.[233]

An oncogene whose transforming activity may be related indirectly to *ras* transformation is the *dbl* oncogene, whose protein product functions as a guanine nucleotide exchange factor for certain Ras-related proteins. *dbl* is an artifactually created oncogene that was identified through gene-transfer experiments (see Table 23–5B); its possible role in tumors remains to be clarified.[234] Overexpression of the *dbl* proto-oncogene can transform established mouse fibroblasts, but the *dbl* oncogene, whose protein product represents an N-terminally truncated version of the normal protein, has much greater transforming activity. The *dbl* proto-oncogene represents the mammalian homologue of the *S. cerevisiae CDC24* gene, which encodes a guanine nucleotide release factor for the *CDC42* product, a member of the Rho subfamily of Ras-related proteins. Cdc42 is involved in the regulation of actin filaments and bud-site polarity. The truncated Dbl oncoprotein retains the guanine nucleotide–releasing activity that is specific for Rho proteins.[235] It has therefore been speculated that the Dbl oncoprotein may transform cells, although it is a constitutively active exchange factor for Rho proteins. Other mechanisms are possible, however, and it remains to be demonstrated that activated Rho proteins induce a phenotype similar to that of Dbl.

Genes encoding certain heterotrimeric G proteins have also been implicated in some tumors, although the evidence is much less extensive than for *ras* (see Table 23–6). As noted earlier, the heterotrimeric G proteins consist of three subunits, only one of which (the α subunit) actually binds and hydrolyzes GTP.[42, 192, 193, 236] The α subunits are approximately 40 kDa, and their activity is regulated, as with Ras proteins, by a guanine nucleotide activation cycle. The α subunits are further regulated by their association with the other subunits, termed β and γ, and by their appropriate receptor, which is invariably a member of the seven-transmembrane class. When the receptor becomes activated, the α subunit releases its bound GDP and binds GTP, dissociates from the β-γ complex, and binds to and activates a target effector molecule. Attenuation of the signal is achieved by hydrolysis of the α-bound GTP, dissociation from the effector, and rebinding to the β-γ receptor complex. An additional layer of complexity exists in this system, for in addition to the α subunits that activate the effector enzyme (G-α_s), inhibitory α subunits (G-α_i) can inhibit the same effector in a GTP-dependent manner.

The effector enzymes that respond to activated G-α subunits include adenylate cyclase, which catalyzes the formation of the second-messenger cAMP; cGMP phosphodiesterase, which functions in the retina to cleave cGMP in response to light stimulation; and PLC, which hydrolyzes phosphatidylinositol to release inositol phosphates and diacylglycerol. These enzymes all catalyze the formation of second messengers that in turn alter the activity of protein kinases and other molecules in the interior of the cell. The central position of the α subunits in pathways regulating the formation of second messengers implicated them as potential proto-oncogenes, and recently it has been shown that this may be the case.

The first indication of an altered G-α_s function in a human tumor was the finding that a group of human growth hormone–secreting pituitary adenomas had increased adenylate cyclase activity and that in purified membrane preparations from these cells, the cyclase activity was unresponsive to normal agonists.[237] Molecular cloning of the G-α subunits from these tumors revealed the presence of mutations that reduced GTP hydrolysis by G-α_s, resulting in a constitutive—that is, ligand-independent—stimulation of adenylate cyclase in the tumor cells.[238] A more recent survey of adrenal cortex and ovarian tumors led to the discovery of mutations in a G-α_i subunit in these tumors.[239] Strikingly, some of the mutations mapped to a residue analogous to that found to be mutated in G-α_s in the pituitary tumors, implying that the mutant G-α_s subunits might also have defective GTPase function.

Serine/Threonine Kinases

Although the vast majority of protein phosphorylation in the cell occurs at serine and threonine residues, to date only four genes encoding serine/threonine kinases have been unequivocally implicated as proto-oncogenes—*raf, mos, pim,* and *cot*—in contrast to the large number of proto-oncogenes that encode receptor and cytoplasmic tyrosine kinases (see Table 23–6). The genes *raf* and *mos* have been studied in greatest detail.

Many serine/threonine kinases are involved primarily in the regulation of metabolic pathways and processes whose relationship to cell growth may be indirect. Others, such as protein kinase C and the mitogen-activated protein (MAP) kinases, are associated with mitogen-associated signal transduction, but their role

in oncogenesis remains unclear.[240] These kinases and c-*raf* are part of a group of signal transducers, which also include the phosphatidylinositol 3′ (PI3) kinase, PLC-γ, and GAP, which are often phosphorylated and activated following activation of tyrosine protein kinases.[241]

The c-*raf* gene, which is widely expressed, is the progenitor of retroviral oncogenes present in avian and mammalian retroviruses (see Table 23–3). Two closely related cellular genes, designated A-*raf* and B-*raf*, have also been identified.[242] Their expression is more restricted than that of c-*raf*. Whereas the kinase activity of the v-*raf* product is constitutively high, the activity of the c-*raf* product is much lower. The v-*raf*–encoded protein lacks the N-terminus of the c-*raf* product (Fig. 23–11). Systematic deletion of the 5′ end of c-*raf* has demonstrated that the N-terminus of the c-*raf* protein encodes a negative regulatory domain, the removal of which activates its transforming activity and its kinase.[243]

The c-*raf* protein has been proposed to function in the transduction of mitogenic signals in normal cells,[242, 244] based on the finding that treatment of fibroblasts with a number of different growth factors, including EGF and PDGF, induces an increased phosphorylation of c-*raf* protein, as well as an increase in Raf kinase activity.[241, 245] Studies in lymphoid cells have yielded similar results when the cells were treated with hematopoietic growth factors such as IL-2, IL-3, granulocyte-macrophage colony-stimulating factor (GM-CSF), and CSF-1. Activation of the Raf kinase is associated with an increase in phosphoserines on Raf, even when Raf is stimulated by a membrane receptor with tyrosine kinase activity. This observation suggests that Raf is being regulated by another serine/threonine kinase and/or by autophosphorylation. Protein kinase C appears to account for Raf activation in at least some of these situations.[242] Stimulation of the Raf kinase by the T-cell receptor depends on PK-C. In

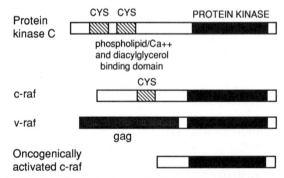

FIGURE 23–11. Structure of protein kinase C and the *raf*-encoded protein kinases. The amino-terminus of protein kinase C contains a calcium-binding domain with two cysteine-rich regions (CYS); binding of phospholipids to this region greatly reduces the calcium requirement for activation of the kinase. A similar structure is present in the c-*raf*–encoded protein, although at present the physiological activator of c-*raf* is unknown. Oncogenic forms of *raf* found in acutely transforming retroviruses (v-*raf*) or through transfection experiments (*bottom*) contain deletions of the amino-terminus.

addition, phorbol ester treatment, which stimulates PK-C, can regulate the Raf kinase in many cell types. Activation of the Raf kinase is associated with translocation of the protein from the cytosol to a perinuclear location, which presumably facilitates its ability to activate its downstream targets, including immediately early genes induced by mitogenic factors.[242]

The importance of the Raf protein in mitogenic signaling has recently been confirmed in established mouse fibroblasts through the use of a dominant inhibitory mutant of Raf, as well as by antisense *raf* RNA.[246] Expression of the mutant prevents activation of the Raf kinase, and cells expressing the mutant are unable to transduce the mitogenic signals of serum or phorbol ester or the transforming signals from an activated Ras protein. The latter result shows that Raf is required for transmission of the Ras signal, which is known to be required for the mitogenic activity of serum. Experiments with neutralizing Ras antibodies have shown that the transforming activity of v-*raf* does not require Ras, in contrast to the dependence of tyrosine protein kinases on Ras.[204] Taken together, these observations place Raf in the mitogenic signaling pathway, downstream from Ras.

The structure of the PK-C serine/threonine kinases is similar to that of the Raf family (Fig. 23–11).[40] PK-C can be activated physiologically by calcium and diacylglycerol and pharmacologically by phorbol esters such as TPA. PK-C has been implicated in mitogenic signaling, activation of PK-C is mitogenic for some cells, and Ras activity depends upon PK-C in some cell types. However, PK-C has not been identified as an oncogene. Although overexpression of PK-C has been reported to render mouse fibroblasts more susceptible to transformation by *ras*,[247] neither wild-type nor mutant PK-C appears to be capable of inducing bona fide cell transformation.[248]

The *mos* oncogene, originally identified as the transforming protein of Mo-MSV, is similar to *raf* in that it encodes a cytoplasmic serine/threonine kinase.[249] However, major differences exist between c-*mos* and c-*raf* with regard to their expression and to their protein products. Whereas the c-*raf* product is 672 amino acids in length, the c-*mos* gene encodes a much smaller protein of only 343 amino acids that lacks sequences analogous to the N-terminal regulatory domain of the c-*raf* protein. Furthermore, the v-*mos* protein product is structurally similar to the normal c-*mos*–encoded protein, and their kinase and biological activities are also similar. The mechanism of activation of *mos* therefore involves an increased expression of the normal kinase sequences, rather than truncation.

Expression of c-*mos* is highly restricted, its expression being limited mainly to the germ cells.[250] Elegant studies performed in *Xenopus* frog oocytes have shown that *mos* is required for the meiotic maturation of these cells, and that *mos* is a key component of "cytostatic factor," which keeps the mature oocyte arrested at the second meiotic prophase, awaiting fertilization.[251] These observations suggest that the *mos* kinase is involved in cell cycle regulation of the germ cells.

Inappropriate expression of *mos* in oncogenesis therefore probably results in abrogation of fundamental cell cycle control mechanisms.

The *pim*-1 gene was detected as a target for insertional mutagenesis in murine lymphomas. It resembles *mos* in that it is also a small gene (encoding a product of 313 amino acids) that is activated by altered expression rather than by structural mutation.[252]

Nuclear Proto-oncogenes: Regulators of Transcription

The nucleus represents the control center for many processes that take place within the cell. The regulation of cell growth by the nucleus occurs in two fundamental ways. Most importantly, the pattern of proteins expressed in the cell is determined by nuclear events that control gene transcription, RNA processing, and the transport of mature mRNA to the cytoplasm for translation.[44] In addition, DNA synthesis (S phase), as well as the events leading up to mitosis (M), are initiated in the nucleus in response to diverse signals emanating from the cytoplasm.

Extracellular signals that induce changes in gene expression exert most of these effects through altering gene transcription, although post-transcriptional changes may also play a role. The pattern of gene transcription is controlled principally by the action of transcription factors, which are a diverse class of proteins that influence the activity of the transcription complex for target genes. Transcription factors act in concert with each other to regulate gene expression.

Most transcription factors regulate expression of their target genes by interacting directly with specific DNA sequences located within the regulatory region of the gene. A typical transcription factor may be thought of as being composed of four functional regions (Fig. 23–12). One is a regulatory region, which permits the activity of the factor to be positively and negatively controlled. Another is the DNA-binding region, which permits the factor to interact preferentially with the specific DNA sequences in its target gene. Most transcription factors bind DNA as oligomers (usually as dimers), which typically form prior to DNA binding. This means that a transcription factor usually has a region that permits it to oligomerize with its appropriate partners. It is common for this region to enable a monomer to form heterodimers by binding to a range of related monomers encoded by other transcription factors, although some factors may form only homodimers. In some factors, this region is called a leucine zipper because of the arrangement of leucines within it.[253] The factor also has a signaling region, which contributes the activity of the factor to the transcription complex. The range of factors with which a monomer binds and the other factors present in the transcription complex offer variety and complexity in the effect a given factor may have on transcription of a particular target gene.

A subset of v-*onc*–encoded proteins is located in the nucleus. These include the proteins encoded by *myc*,

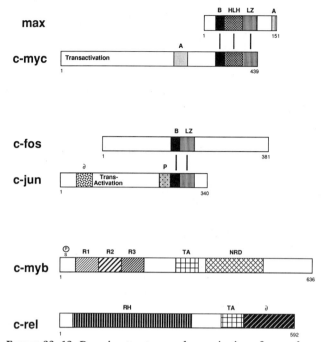

FIGURE 23–12. Domain structure and organization of several nuclear proto-oncogenes. *Top,* Structure of the c-*myc*–encoded protein and the associated Max protein. Vertical lines denote the presumed regions of association and DNA binding by Myc-Max heterodimers. Abbreviations: B = basic DNA-binding region; HLH = helix-loophelix domain; LZ = leucine-zipper domain; A = acidic region. Both the HLH and LZ domains may be involved in dimer formation by these proteins. *Upper middle,* Structure of the c-*fos*– and c-*jun*–encoded proteins. These proteins also contain basic (B) and leucinezipper (LZ) domains, which are thought to promote dimer formation and DNA binding in this case as well. The c-*jun* product contains two transactivation domains—a more N-terminal domain and a proline-rich (P) domain near the B/HLH region. Removal of a negative regulatory region (δ) of c-*jun* increases transformation by c-*jun* (δ is absent in v-*jun*). *Lower middle,* structure of the c-*myb* protein. A serine phosphorylation site for CK II is followed by three 52 amino acid repeat regions (R1, R2, R3) that specify DNA binding, a transactivation domain (TA), and a negative regulatory domain (NRD) toward the C-terminus. *Bottom,* Structure of the c-*rel*–encoded protein. A large N-terminal region of the protein comprises the *rel* homology (RH) domain, which is conserved among c-*rel*, NF-κB, and *dorsal* proteins. This domain includes regions specifying DNA binding, dimerization, nuclear localization, and binding to inhibitory regulator proteins. The transactivation domain (TA) is found near the C-terminus, followed by a region (δ) that is deleted in v-*rel*. Removal of the δ domain, which encodes a cytoplasmic retention signal (and partially overlaps with the TA domain), activates the transforming function of c-*rel*.

myb, jun, fos, erbA, ski, rel, and *ets* (see Table 23–6).[254–256] Several of these genes are treated in greater detail in Chapter 24 because of their involvement in hematopoietic tumors. Although the nuclear localization of these proteins suggests a diversity of potential functions, it is becoming clear that virtually all of these oncogene products act as regulators of transcription. This conclusion reflects the fundamental nature of transcriptional control in the regulation of cell growth. However, most of the relevant growth control genes whose transcription is regulated by these oncogenes remain to be identified. As described at the end of this section, evidence has also begun to implicate cell

cycle regulatory proteins, such as the cyclins, in oncogenesis.

The three well-characterized members of the *myc* family are c-*myc*, N-*myc*, and L-*myc*.[121] c-*myc* is a widely expressed early response gene whose transcription is induced within 1 to 2 minutes after growth-arrested cells are stimulated by serum or certain growth factors. It is likely that *myc* regulates the expression of genes in early G_1 that are required for entry into S phase.[257] In this regard, the mitogenic activity of the CSF-1 receptor, when expressed in quiescent fibroblasts, has been shown to depend on c-*myc* expression.[258]

The *myc* genes are aberrantly expressed in a wide range of malignant tumors, as noted earlier.[121] Although some activated *myc* genes contain mutations in their protein-coding sequences, increased (or inappropriate) expression accounts for most of their oncogenic properties. The v-*myc* product of the MC-29 avian retrovirus was the first v-*onc* product to be localized to the cell nucleus and the first to be shown to have DNA-binding properties,[259] but until recently its mechanism of action remained elusive.[260]

All of the *myc* genes encode similar phosphoproteins of approximately 60 kDa (Fig. 23–12).[261] The N-terminal domain of Myc contains a transcriptional transactivation domain. Further toward the C-terminus is a nuclear localization signal, followed by a series of domains that include a basic region, a helix-loop-helix (HLH) region, and a leucine zipper motif. The basic domain is involved with Myc binding to specific DNA sequences, whereas the HLH and zipper domains direct protein-protein interactions that are required for Myc to dimerize and function as a transcriptional transactivator. A second protein family of 21 to 22 kDa, named Max in humans and Myn in mice, can associate with the Myc proteins, via the HLH and zipper domains, to form heterodimers.[262–264] In contrast to Myc homodimers, which have little DNA-binding activity, the heterodimers bind DNA with greater affinity and function as potent transcriptional activators. Homodimers of Max are inactive in transcriptional activation because these proteins lack the activation domain found in the N-terminus of Myc.

Although the Myc proteins have a relatively short half-life and can be induced by the treatment of cells with certain mitogens, the Max proteins are much more stable. Thus, the cell can regulate the amount of transcriptionally active Myc-Max heterodimers in response to extracellular signals, with the concentration of c-*myc* (or L-*myc* or N-*myc*)–encoded protein in the cell determining its ability to function as transcriptionally active heterodimers.[265]

A dramatic example of convergence in the fields of molecular biology and molecular oncology was provided by studies on AP-1, *fos,* and *jun*.[255, 256] AP-1 was originally identified as a TPA-inducible DNA-binding activity that stimulated transcription of the simian virus 40 (SV40) enhancer. On further investigation, both of the major proteins present in purified AP-1 were found to be encoded by proto-oncogenes: c-*jun,* the progenitor of the v-*jun* transforming gene of avian sarcoma virus 17, and c-*fos,* the progenitor of the v-*fos* gene of the FBJ murine osteosarcoma virus.[266] Mutations in the v-*fos*–encoded protein leave it constitutively in the nucleus, whereas the nuclear localization of c-*fos* may depend on extracellular signals.[267] However, both c-*fos* and c-*jun* can be activated as transforming genes by overexpression of the non-mutated genes.

The c-*fos* and c-*jun* genes can be rapidly induced in a large number of different cell types by a variety of stimuli, including growth factors, and are thus immediate early response genes.[31, 268] Ras and Raf induce c-*fos* expression,[269, 270] and suppression of Jun or Fos activity inhibits transformation by Ras, which suggests that Fos and Jun are required for full transformation by oncogenes encoding non-nuclear proteins.[271, 272]

As with the other nuclear oncogenes, cells contain multiple *jun* and *fos*-related genes. All of the *fos* and *jun* genes encode proteins capable of dimerization and specific binding to the DNA sequence originally identified as the AP-1 binding site.[273] Structural analysis of the c-*jun*–encoded protein, which is 340 amino acids, revealed that its C-terminus contains a leucine zipper (for dimerization), a basic region (for specific DNA binding), and a proline-rich transactivation domain (see Fig. 23–12). The N-terminus of the protein contains a regulatory domain that is absent in the v-*jun* product. Phosphorylation of the N-terminal region, which is associated with increased DNA binding and transcriptional activity, can be induced by Ras in vivo[274] and by MAP kinases in vitro,[275] suggesting that this phosphorylation by upstream signals activates the Jun protein. Other data have raised the possibility that Jun activity may normally be inhibited by interaction between the N-terminus of Jun and a putative inhibitory molecule; by this model, activation of Jun by Src and Ras would be mediated by inactivation of the putative inhibitor.[276]

The c-*jun* proteins can form homodimers that are transcriptional activators or can associate with c-*fos* proteins to form heterodimers that transactivate at least as efficiently as the homodimers. The structure of the c-*fos* protein (381 amino acids) is similar, but not identical, to that of the c-*jun* product in that the protein contains the basic and zipper domains, but these domains are found in the middle of the *fos* protein (see Fig. 23–12). A major difference between the *fos*- and *jun*-encoded proteins is that the *fos* products are unable to form stable homodimers. Thus, transformation by the v-*fos*–encoded protein depends on the formation of heterodimers (via the zipper domains) with c-*jun* products to activate transcription. The Fos and Jun proteins also form heterodimers with the more distantly related transcription factors of the CREB (for cyclic AMP responsive element binding factors) family, whose DNA-binding sequence is similar, but not identical, to that of AP-1.[277, 278] This diversity of interactions presumably serves to finely tune the transcriptional activity of the target genes regulated by these factors.

The v-*myb* gene was first characterized as the transforming gene of avian myeloblastosis virus. The c-*myb* gene has also been activated by ALV and MLV proviral-mediated insertional mutagenesis. c-*myb* is a member of a multigene family encoding nuclear phosphoproteins with sequence-specific DNA-binding activity.[279] The expression of c-*myb* appears to be restricted to hematopoietic cells, especially cells of myeloid-macrophage lineage, and to brain. In contrast to many other oncogenes, v-*myb* is not transforming for fibroblasts, although it is a potent inducer of myeloid transformation.

The c-*myb*–encoded protein (see Fig. 23–12; 636 amino acids in length) is highly conserved, with a structural homologue being present in yeast. Transcriptional transactivation can be demonstrated by the c-*myb* product in yeast or mammalian cells.[280, 281] The N-terminal region of the c-*myb* product contains a site that is subject to phosphorylation by casein kinase II (CK II), followed by the DNA-binding domain. Interestingly, this CK II site is deleted in the v-*myb*–encoded protein and in the c-*myb* gene products activated by insertional mutagenesis, suggesting that phosphorylation of this site may regulate the DNA-binding activity of the normal protein.[279] Two transcriptional modulatory regions are C-terminal to the DNA-binding domain: a transactivation domain and a negative regulatory region. These regions may hold the key to the ability of *myb* both to increase cell proliferation and to prevent differentiation of hematopoietic cells.

rel represents yet another multigene family of transcriptional regulators with a member that was transduced as a retroviral oncogene. v-*rel* encodes the oncogene product of the Rev-T virus, which causes reticuloendotheliosis in turkeys and B-cell lymphomas in chickens.[282] The c-*rel* gene has a close homologue (for one half of the coding region) in the *Drosophila* gene *dorsal,* which controls the establishment of the dorsal-ventral axis in the developing embryo. The vertebrate c-*rel* gene is a member of the NF-κB gene family of transcription factors. The transcriptional activity of the proteins encoded by this gene family is regulated by their subcellular localization. Inactive *rel* proteins are sequestered in the cytoplasm by complexing with an inhibitory protein.[283] Their translocation to the nucleus is a prerequisite for their action as transcriptional regulatory factors. Once in the nucleus, it appears that *rel* proteins can both activate and repress transcription under appropriate circumstances. Compared with c-*rel,* the v-*rel* product lacks a large portion of the C-terminal, cytoplasmic-anchoring domain (see Fig. 23–12). On the basis of these findings, v-*rel* has been proposed to transform cells by altering either the regulation of c-*rel* or gene activation by c-*rel*/NF-κB complexes.[284]

In addition to transcription factors, inappropriate expression of certain G_1 cyclins, whose role in cell cycle control is described above, has been implicated in some tumors. Their overexpression may help override normal checkpoints of the cell cycle. The D_1 cyclin has been identified as being the most proximate gene on chromosome 11 in the bcl-1 t(11,14) translocation in patients with CLL.[118] This gene is also amplified and overexpressed in patients with breast cancer and squamous cell cancers of the head and neck.[285] It is overexpressed in parathyroid adenomas, in which analysis of the breakpoints of chromosome 11 inversions in the adenomas has shown that the D_1 coding sequence is juxtaposed to the regulatory region of the parathyroid hormone promoter.[286] A recently described common proviral integration site, vin-1, in murine retrovirus–induced T-cell leukemias of mice and rats leads to the constitutive expression of D_2 cyclin.[287] The cyclin A gene has been identified as the target for hepatitis B DNA integration in a hepatocellular carcinoma.[62]

Proto-oncogenes in Development

The evolutionary conservation of proto-oncogenes and their crucial role in normal cell growth suggested that they would participate in embryonic and postembryonic development. Many of these genes have been found to occupy roles in the processes that control development and cell differentiation.[288–291] An in-depth treatment of this topic is beyond the scope of this chapter, but a brief description is given of some approaches and a few specific examples.

The molecular identification of genes responsible for naturally occurring mutants represents one approach.[292] As discussed earlier, analysis of the v-kit oncogene led to identification of the genes at the white-spotting (W) and steel (Sl) loci of the mouse.[146–148] Mutations at either the W or Sl locus are associated with impaired development of hematopoietic, gonadal, and pigment cell lineages, and many naturally occurring mutant alleles at these genetic loci have been identified. Transplantation and coculture experiments involving hematopoietic stem cells and marrow stromal cells from W and Sl mutants indicated that the defect in W mutants is intrinsic to the hematopoietic stem cells, whereas the defect in Sl mutants lies in the stromal cells. These experiments therefore suggested that the Sl locus made a factor that stimulated growth of hematopoietic stem cells (and presumably of gonadal and pigment cell precursors as well). The phenotypic similarity between W and Sl mutants suggested that the W locus might be required for the stem cells to respond to the putative Sl factor.

The recognition that the c-kit–encoded protein had the structure of a receptor protein tyrosine kinase, combined with its tissue-specific expression, suggested that c-kit might represent the W gene. Analysis of different W mutants confirmed that the c-kit gene was mutated in each instance.[146, 147] The functional consequences of these mutations for the c-kit protein include impaired tyrosine kinase activity or failure to synthesize stable protein; these abnormalities have begun to provide insight into the molecular basis for the phenotypic differences associated with various W alleles.[293] The recognition that c-kit represented the gene at the W locus suggested that the putative factor made by the Sl locus might be the ligand for the c-kit–encoded protein. This hypothesis was confirmed by purification of the ligand (SCF) from cells whose culture fluid specifically stimulated cells expressing c-kit and by molecular cloning of the gene encoding SCF (for review, see reference 148). As the result of alternate RNA splicing, SCF is expressed as secreted and cell-associated forms; impairment of the cell-associated form is required for the Sl^- mutant phenotype.[294]

The deliberate functional inactivation of proto-oncogenes by gene targeting represents a more direct approach for the assessment of their roles in development.[290] Certain mouse stem cell lines, when implanted in pseudopregnant mice, can give rise to normal mice. Targeted disruption of a given allele in such cells can be achieved in vitro; implantation of these cells results in some mice whose germ cells carry one normal allele and one disrupted allele.[295] These mice can then be bred to each other to obtain progeny that are homozygous for the disrupted allele.

Targeted disruption has been achieved for several proto-oncogenes, including c-myb, wnt-1, c-abl, and c-src. c-myb, whose oncogenic activation is associated with hematopoietic tumors mainly of the myeloid and monocytic lineages, is normally expressed in brain and hematopoietic precursor cells. Embryos that are homozygous for a c-myb null allele show a significant reduction in various hematopoietic cell lineages and die in utero with severe anemia.[296] The appearance of the defect seems to correlate with the switching of hematopoiesis from the yolk sac to the fetal liver. Null mutants of the wnt-1 proto-oncogene have severe abnormalities of the developing central nervous system, which correlates with its expression in the developing neural tube.[297, 298]

The protein tyrosine kinases encoded by c-abl and c-src are ubiquitously expressed. Homozygous null alleles of either gene were not uniformly lethal in utero, although the animals are not normal. The mice that lack c-abl have a relatively restricted phenotype, limited primarily to thymic and splenic atrophy and a deficiency of T and B cells.[299] The major defect in the c-src null mice is limited to impaired osteoclast function, resulting in osteopetrosis, which is lethal for the mice when they are weaned.[300] The restricted nature of the defects associated with these null mutants has been interpreted as implying significant functional redundancy between certain non-receptor protein tyrosine kinases.

An additional approach involves the identification of close homologues of proto-oncogenes in simple species such as yeast (which have been discussed in earlier sections), Drosophila, and the nematode C. elegans, which are used as model systems to study developmental processes.[291, 301] After the gene is cloned, its chromosomal location can be readily identified, allowing investigators to determine if any known developmental defects have been mapped to the same region.[302] If none are, mutations in the cloned proto-oncogene homologue can be constructed and the gene returned to the genome, in place of or in addition to the normal copy of the gene. Serendipity represents a third way in which these associations have been made: Investigators studying a developmental pathway identify and clone the genes involved, and the search for homologies with known sequences sometimes uncovers similarities (or identities) with proto-oncogenes.

wnt-1 and *c-rel* are two proto-oncogenes whose homologues in *Drosophila* are known to have a role in development.[291] Mutants of the *wnt-1* homologue in *Drosophila* were originally identified as the alleles responsible for the wingless (*wg*) phenotype. The *wg* gene is essential for normal patterning in each developmental segment of the fly. The *wg* flies are therefore unable to undergo proper morphogenic development, implicating this proto-oncogene homologue as a regulator of this process. The gene producing the developmental defect *dorsal* is homologous to *c-rel*. The *dorsal* gene initiates a process that controls the establishment of dorsal-ventral polarity in the early *Drosophila* embryo. The *dorsal* gene is thought to function by influencing gene expression in the zygote, consistent with the function of the *c-rel* product described above in the section on nuclear oncogenes.

A pathway that is required for photoreceptor development of the R7 photoreceptor cell of the fly has revealed a signaling pathway whose order includes a paracrine-produced growth factor (encoded by the *boss* {*bride of sevenless*} gene), a receptor tyrosine kinase (encoded by the *sevenless* gene), putative guanine nucleotide exchange factor (encoded by the *sos* {*son of sevenless*} gene), and a *Drosophila ras* homologue, which is negatively regulated by a GAP-like gene (*gap-1*) (Fig. 23–13).[206, 222, 303, 304] A striking parallel has been described for the pathway controlling vulval development in the nematode *C. elegans*. The *let-60* gene of *C. elegans* encodes an allele of the *ras* gene, which normally functions downstream from a receptor tyrosine kinase (encoded by the *let-23* gene) required for normal vulval development.[305] The *sem-5* gene, which encodes an SH2-containing protein, is located on this pathway, between *let-23* and *ras*.[306]

TUMOR-SUPPRESSOR GENES

Identification of Tumor-Suppressor Genes

Tumor suppressors represent a class of genes that contribute to tumorigenesis through their inactivation (loss of function), in contrast to oncogenes.[8] This feature suggests that tumor-suppressor genes normally serve as negative regulators of cell growth.[307] These genes have been described in molecular terms only recently, and the molecular basis for their activity is less well understood than that of proto-oncogenes.[9]

One type of evidence for the existence of tumor-suppressor genes came from the analysis of somatic cell hybrids.[308] When tumorigenic cells were fused with normal cells, the hybrids were found to be non-tumorigenic, which implied that the tumor cells were lacking a function that could be replaced by the normal cells. Further analysis revealed that the tumor-suppressing activity could be localized to specific chromosomes. In some instances, hybrids made between two different tumor cell lines were non-tumorigenic, suggesting the existence of multiple recessive tumor-suppressor genes. Using microcell fusion, a refined technique by which single chromosomes can be transferred to recipient cells, it has been possible to identify specific regions of chromosomes that harbor tumor-suppressor genes. These techniques provided an experimental basis for the belief that cells contained tumor suppressors, but they did not lead directly to the identification of specific genes.[309]

Studies on the inheritance of familial cancers represented another approach that supported the notion that cells contained tumor-suppressor genes. The first of these studies focused on retinoblastoma; it was proposed that this form of cancer developed only after two independent loss-of-function mutations.[310] This hypothesis was based on comparative analysis of familial and sporadic cases of retinoblastoma (Fig. 23–14). In familial cases, approximately one half of the children in a family develop the disease, consistent with inheritance of a single, genetically dominant susceptibility allele, and many afflicted children develop independent primary tumors in each eye at an early age. In sporadic cases of retinoblastoma, patients develop only a single tumor, and the average age of onset is older than for familial cases. These characteristics suggested that the genetic basis for the familial form of the disease might be accounted for by inheritance of a defective allele in a critical gene, with retinoblastomas developing after mutational inactiva-

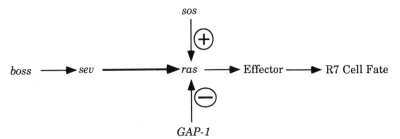

FIGURE 23–13. Role of the *ras* signaling pathway in the development of R7 photoreceptor cells in *D. melanogaster*. The product of the *boss* gene is a polypeptide growth modulator that binds specifically to the *sev*-encoded transmembrane protein tyrosine kinase. Binding of the *boss* product to *sev* is thought to result in the activation of Ras, either through the activation of the *sos*-encoded exchange factor, by inhibition of GAP-1, or both. Either of these mechanisms would increase the level of GTP-bound Ras. Elevated levels of Ras-GTP result in the stimulation of an unknown effector and produce the differentiation to an R7 cell fate.

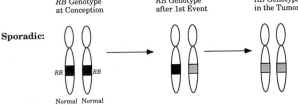

FIGURE 23–14. Development of retinoblastoma through the mutational inactivation of *RB* function. In the familial form of the disease, the patient inherits one mutant allele and one wild-type (normal) allele. Tumor formation arises after the remaining normal allele is inactivated by a gene-conversion event, resulting in a homozygous mutant genotype, or by a second independent somatic mutation. The sporadic form of the disease occurs when a somatic mutation of one of the normal *RB* alleles is followed by an inactivation of the second allele, again resulting in a tumor.

tion of the normal allele. In sporadic cases, each allele would be normal at birth, so two independent somatic mutations would be required to inactivate both alleles before a retinoblastoma would develop; two independent events are much less likely than a single one, accounting for the later onset and unilateral nature of the disease in sporadic cases.

Although this hypothesis was in fact correct, it could not predict the nature of the molecular defects involved in the development of retinoblastoma. For example, the mutations could have involved the activation of two different proto-oncogenes. Instead, subsequent studies have firmly established that both of the genetic lesions involved in retinoblastoma are mutations that inactivate alleles of the same cellular gene, designated *RB* (see Fig. 23–14).

The molecular identification of *RB* was accomplished by positional cloning.[311] This approach involves mapping the phenotype (such as retinoblastoma) to a particular chromosomal location through analysis of affected and unaffected family members, cloning the sequences in that region of the chromosome, and identifying a gene within the region in which mutations consistently correlate with the phenotype. The chromosomal localization of *RB* began with the observation that even normal cells from patients with familial retinoblastoma bore deletions in the q14 band of chromosome 13. A similar analysis of sporadic retinoblastoma patients revealed that the same region of chromosome 13 was frequently deleted in the tumor cells, but not the normal cells of these individuals.[312] The next step was identification of a gene in the 13q14 region (the gene encoding esterase D), which served as a linked genetic marker for susceptibility to retinoblastoma,[313] allowing an estimate of

its distance from the retinoblastoma susceptibility gene.

The actual identification of the *RB* gene was accomplished by molecular cloning of sequences from the 13q14 region that were absent in retinoblastoma patients. Then, DNA segments from adjacent regions of the chromosome and cDNAs were screened for evolutionary conservation and differential expression between normal retinal tissue and tumors.[314–316] These analyses led to the identification of *RB*, which encodes a 928 amino acid protein designated pRB. Retinoblastomas contain internal deletions within this gene, and retinoblastoma lines fail to express pRB.[317]

One of the novel findings arising from the search for the *RB* gene was the nature of the "second hit" at the *RB* locus. Rather than identifying a completely independent second mutation, investigators found that the normal allele was often replaced by a duplicated copy of the mutant allele, as a result of chromosomal non-disjunction, gene conversion, or mitotic recombination. This phenomenon is usually manifested as a loss of heterozygosity when adjacent chromosomal loci (e.g., esterase D) are assayed.[318] Evidence of loss of heterozygosity, usually by Southern blot analysis of restriction fragment length polymorphism (RFLP) in affected individuals, is now widely used in the mapping of other tumor-suppressor loci in a variety of tumor types.

As with many proto-oncogenes, *RB* appears to be expressed in all tissues. However, patients with familial retinoblastoma seem to be at increased risk of developing osteosarcomas, but not other tumors. In the general population, mutations in *RB* have been identified in most cases of small cell carcinoma and some carcinomas of the bladder and breast, in addition to retinoblastomas and osteosarcomas.[9] It remains to be determined what accounts for the association of only certain tumors with alterations in *RB*. Presumably, loss of *RB* function in these cell types has greater oncogenic potential than its loss in other cell types.

Gene isolation techniques similar to those just described for the isolation of *RB* are now widespread and have been successfully applied to isolate other tumor-suppressor genes. One such gene is *WT-1*, a candidate tumor-suppressor gene involved in Wilms' tumor. This type of nephroblastoma occurs sporadically and as a familial syndrome; about 7 per cent of cases are manifested as early-onset, bilateral tumors with an inherited component.[319] In contrast to retinoblastoma, a large body of evidence suggests that several genetic loci may be involved in the development of Wilms' tumor. One of these loci has been mapped to band 11p13, and positional cloning identified *WT-1* at this locus.

NF-1 disease is another dominantly inherited disorder, affecting about 1 in 3500 individuals. Approximately 50 per cent of cases appear to represent new mutations, which indicates that the locus has a high rate of spontaneous mutation. Patients with NF-1 disease are at increased risk of developing pheochromocytomas and a narrow group of malignant tumors that are classified as schwannomas or neurofibrosarcomas; these tumors are associated with mutation of the normal *NF-1* allele. Restriction fragment length polymorphism (RFLP) analysis localized *NF-1* to band 17q11.2. Molecular cloning of the *NF-1* gene was facilitated through identification of two patients with translocations involving this band.[320, 321] *NF-1* is very large, spanning more than 200 kb, which may contribute to its high spontaneous mutation rate.

Analysis of colorectal cancers has identified common cytogenetic abnormalities involving chromosomes 5q21 and 18q21.[322] Positional cloning at these loci has uncovered three different genes, one at 18q21, designated *DCC* (for deleted in colon cancer), and two at 5q21, designated *MCC* (for mutated in colon cancer) and *FAP* (for familial adenomatous polyposis).[323–325] These genes are inactivated in a variable proportion of colorectal cancers. Normal cells from patients with familial adenomatous polyposis, which is inherited as an autosomal dominant, have one mutant *FAP* allele. A mouse model of this disease has recently been identified; the dominantly inherited susceptibility of the mice to multiple intestinal neoplasia has been genetically localized to a germ line mutation in one allele of the murine *FAP* gene.[326]

In contrast to the elegant genetic analyses used to identify the tumor-suppressor genes discussed above, identification of *p53* as a tumor-suppressor gene occurred via a circuitous route.[327] Study of the *p53* gene began with the observation that a nuclear phosphoprotein of 53 kDa associates with the large T antigen of SV40 in cells transformed by this virus.[328] This association suggested that the p53 protein might play a role in transformation by large T, which led to purifying p53 and cloning the gene. When the resulting molecular clones encoding p53, which had been isolated from transformed cells, were tested for their biological activity, the *p53* gene was found to immortalize primary cells and functionally substitute for *myc* in *myc* + *ras* cotransformation assays of primary rodent fibroblasts.

Although these results therefore suggested that *p53* was a proto-oncogene, subsequent work showed that molecular clones of *p53* from normal tissues did not function in the transformation assay and that the earlier clones that had been used contained missense mutations in conserved regions of the gene. The nonmutated *p53* clones were actually found to suppress transformation of primary cells by *ras* and either *myc*, adenovirus *E1A*, or mutant *p53*.[329] These findings implied that normal *p53* was an inhibitor of cell growth and that the point mutations identified in *p53* isolated from tumors had functionally inactivated the gene. The designation of *p53* as a tumor-suppressor gene was firmly established by finding tumors in which *p53* alleles were absent or clearly inactive.[330] The oncogene-like activity of *p53* carrying point mutations has now been reinterpreted to mean that the mutant p53 protein inhibits the function of normal p53 protein; i.e., mutant *p53* is a dominant inhibitory mutant.

The *p53* gene is located on the short arm of chromosome 17, where loss of heterozygosity of markers has been associated with many different tumor types. In most instances, this loss of heterozygosity has been mapped to the *p53* gene, with point mutation of evolutionarily conserved codons being the most frequent genetic alteration. Of genes known to be involved in human cancer, *p53* is the most commonly altered, with abnormalities having been identified in tumors of the bladder, colon, liver, lung, brain, breast, and some leukemias, among others.[8, 331] In addition, the Li-Fraumeni syndrome, a dominantly inherited condition that predisposes affected individuals to several forms of malignancy, has been associated with inactivating germline point mutation of one *p53* allele.[332–334] The normal *p53* allele is inactivated in tumors that develop in these patients, as with *RB* in familial retinoblastoma.[335] Although patients with Li-Fraumini syndrome have a higher than expected incidence of several types of malignancy, including breast and brain tumors, it remains to be explained why the range of tumors in Li-Fraumini syndrome is much narrower than the many different tumor types in which *p53* mutations have been reported.

c-erbA and *rap1a/K-rev-1* are two other genes commonly regarded as tumor suppressors. The evidence for their functioning as tumor suppressors is more tenuous. *c-erbA* was first discovered as the cellular progenitor of *v-erbA* in AEV. As with *p53*, *c-erbA* was originally thought to be a proto-oncogene, but subsequent work has shown that *v-erbA* functions in erythroblastosis as a dominant interfering mutant that blocks the differentiation-inducing activity of *c-erbA* and other steroid hormone receptors.[336, 337] *K-rev-1* was identified in gene-transfer experiments as a complementary DNA (cDNA) clone that induced morphological reversion of a fibroblast line transformed by v-Ki-ras.[338] When the sequence of *K-rev-1* was determined, its encoded protein was found to have striking homology (greater than 50 per cent) to mammalian *ras*; in fact, the sequence had already been published as a gene (*rap1a* uncovered in a screen for *ras*-related genes.[339] *K-rev-1* can antagonize *ras* function in vitro, but it remains to be established whether or not this represents a physiological function of the protein.

Functions and Products of Tumor-Suppressor Genes

RB

RB encodes a 105 kDa nuclear phosphoprotein pRB.[340] The degree of phosphorylation of pRB fluctuates with the cell cycle, being high in *S* and reaching its lowest level during the interval between the end of *M* and the beginning of G_1. An important breakthrough in understanding pRB function came from the recognition that pRB binds to the oncoproteins of several DNA tumor viruses, including adenovirus E1A, SV40 large T, and E7 of certain HPV (Fig. 23–15.)[10, 67, 341] The biological activity of these oncoproteins

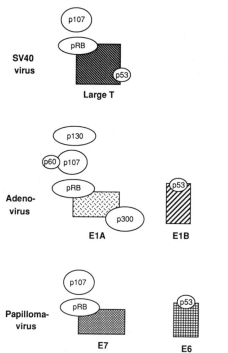

FIGURE 23–15. Formation of complexes between the products of DNA tumor virus oncogenes and cellular proteins. The large T antigen of SV40 binds the products of the *RB* and *p53* tumor-suppressor genes, as well as a less well characterized p107. The binding site for p107 is identical to that for pRB; the oncoprotein associates with these proteins at different stages of the cell cycle. In the case of the adenoviruses and the papillomaviruses, binding functions of pRB and p53 are encoded in different transforming proteins. Oncoproteins encoded by these viruses also form complexes with the 107 kDa protein. The E1A product of adenovirus also associates with the cyclin A gene product (p60) (via its association with p107) and with polypeptides of 130 and 300 kDa.

correlates with their ability to bind pRB, suggesting that binding functionally inactivates pRB as a repressor of cell growth. The observation that SV40 large T complexes preferentially with the hypophosphorylated form of pRB[342] implies that the growth-inhibitory function of pRB is limited to its hypophosphorylated forms. An antiproliferative function of pRB is suggested by the ability of an *RB* expression plasmid in quiescent cells to inhibit growth factor–stimulated expression of c-*fos*, an immediate early response gene.[343]

It is proposed that pRB inhibits growth by preventing cells from entering G_1, that only the hypophosphorylated form of pRB serves this suppressor function, and that phosphorylation of pRB inactivates this growth-suppression activity. The p34^{cdc2} kinase has been shown to phosphorylate pRB in vitro at sites that are also phosphorylated in vivo; an important function of this kinase may therefore be to relieve the negative influence of pRB.[344] It has been speculated that TGFβ may exert its antiproliferative function in part by inhibiting phosphorylation of pRB.[345]

The mechanism by which pRB affects cell growth is currently thought to involve the modulation of gene expression. Consistent with this idea, the underphos-

phorylated forms of pRB complex with E2F, a transcription factor whose activity is increased in response to mitogens.[346, 347] The binding of pRB to E1A, large T, or E7 results in the release of E2F.[348] These observations suggest that pRB inhibits growth by sequestering E2F (and perhaps other transcription factors that stimulate growth), thereby preventing E2F from regulating its target genes.

p53

The ubiquitous expression of p53, its potent growth-inhibitory activities, and its inactivation in a variety of tumors all suggested that this gene would serve an essential developmental function. Surprisingly, however, mice carrying disrupted null alleles of p53 develop normally, but p53-negative mice develop various tumors at an early age.[349] These experimental observations suggest that a major function of p53 may be to prevent the development of certain tumors.

Wild-type p53 is a nuclear protein that becomes phosphorylated during *S* phase.[327] It can be phosphorylated by the p34^{cdc2} kinase and by CK II in vitro, and it is tempting to speculate that the activity of p53 may be regulated by phosphorylation. The half-life of the wild-type protein is less than 30 minutes in most cell types. Most mutant versions of p53 display a much longer half-life and form a stable complex with the heat shock protein hsc70. Therefore, cells with mutant p53 often have much higher levels of the mutant protein than cells that contain only wild-type p53.

One striking feature of p53 is that a point mutation at one of many different codons can inactivate the growth-inhibitory activity of the wild-type gene.[331] The variety of point mutations that lead to this phenotype may account in part for the high frequency with which p53 is targeted for mutation in cancers. Many of these mutant alleles have growth-promoting effects in a *ras* cotransformation assay.[350]

Elucidation of biochemical aspects of p53 has provided a conceptual framework for understanding the altered functions of mutant p53, although the physiological targets of wild-type p53 remain unknown. A consensus DNA sequence has been identified to which oligomers (probably tetramers) of the wild-type protein can bind. Binding to this DNA sequence enables the wild-type protein to function as a transcriptional regulator from a synthetic promoter that contains this target sequence (Fig. 23–16).[351] Mutant p53 proteins that promote growth have lost the ability to bind the DNA and to regulate the promoter. However, these mutant proteins form oligomers with wild-type protein; in cotransfection experiments, such mutants can interfere with the ability of the wild-type gene to regulate the promoter. Normal and mutant forms of p53 form a tight complex with the *mdm-2* gene product, a putative transcription factor that can function as an oncoprotein.[352, 353] Overexpression of *mdm-2* can inhibit p53-mediated transactivation. These provocative observations suggest that *mdm-2* may be a physiological inactivator of growth inhibition by p53.

FIGURE 23–16. **Mutant p53 disrupts the function of wild-type p53.** *A,* Normal p53 proteins form oligomers that bind to the cellular DNA and alter transcription. *B,* The protein encoded by a mutant *p53* gene has a much longer half-life, so that the level of mutant protein greatly exceeds the level of wild-type protein in the cell. This protein can still form oligomers but no longer binds DNA. Thus, the product of mutant *p53* acts as a dominant negative, by blocking the function of the wild-type encoded protein. *C,* The presence of two mutant *p53* genes leaves the cell without normally functioning oligomeric complexes.

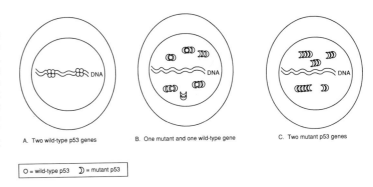

A. Two wild-type p53 genes   B. One mutant and one wild-type gene   C. Two mutant p53 genes

O = wild-type p53   D = mutant p53

Wilms' Tumor Gene (WT-1)

Sequence analysis of *WT-1* gene indicated that it was probably encoded by a regulator of transcription. The 439 amino acid *WT-1* product contains an N-terminal glutamine/proline–rich region that resembles a transcriptional regulatory domain, whereas its C-terminal region contains a series of four "zinc fingers," which are indicative of direct sequence-specific DNA-binding regions. The DNA-binding region of the *WT-1* protein is closely related to the corresponding region of the EGR-1 transcriptional activator, and the two proteins can bind the same DNA target sequences.[354] EGR-1 is encoded by an immediate early gene that is induced by mitogens, which argues that EGR-1 is a positive regulator of cell growth. These features suggest that the WT-1 protein interferes with the activity of EGR-1. Direct evidence for this model has been obtained by showing that WT-1 is a functional antagonist of EGR-1.[355] Suppression of transcription by WT-1 involves both its C-terminal DNA-binding region and its N-terminal transcriptional repression domain. Because expression of *WT-1* is normally limited to developing kidney and urogenital precursor cells, it is hypothesized that *WT-1* contributes to normal differentiation of these tissues by blocking the proliferative action of EGR-1 (or related proteins). This postulated role of *WT-1* is consistent with its functional inactivation being associated with Wilms' tumors.

Hormone Receptors: c-erbA and Retinoic Acid Receptors

The receptors for steroid hormones, thyroid hormones, retinoids, and vitamin D form a large family of transcriptional regulators that contain regions for hormone binding, sequence-specific DNA binding, dimerization, and transcriptional regulation.[34] When these receptors are activated following hormone binding, many of them induce differentiation rather than proliferation.

Triiodothyronine (T_3) is the steroid hormone ligand that activates the c-erbA–encoded protein.[356] As noted earlier, v-erbA can block differentiation of erythroid precursors. The finding that v-erbA could antagonize transcriptional regulation by c-erbA suggested that inhibition of c-erbA–dependent target genes accounted for inhibition of erythroid differentiation by v-erbA.[336]

This model was supported by the selective expression of c-erbA in erythroid cells and the demonstration that both c-erbA and v-erbA proteins can bind to the 5' regulatory region of the gene encoding carbonic anhydrase II, which is a frequently used marker of erythroid differentiation.[357] However, T_3 by itself is insufficient to regulate differentiation of erythroid cells in culture, and the DNA-binding domain of the v-erbA protein contains two mutations that are critical for its oncogenic activity and may alter the DNA-binding specificity of the v-erbA protein. The v-erbA protein can inhibit retinoic acid–inducible transcription by binding to DNA target sequences that also bind the retinoic acid receptor.[337] It therefore appears that v-erbA may function by antagonizing erythroid differentiation induced by T_3, retinoic acid, and possibly other steroid hormones.

NF-1

As noted in the section on the *ras* proto-oncogene, analysis of *NF-1* coding sequences revealed a region of homology with the GAP protein that regulates p21^{ras} and an even larger region of homology with the *S. cerevisiae* regulators of *ras, IRA-1,* and *IRA-2.*[358, 359] The GAP-related domain of *NF-1* was shown to encode a GTPase-activating function that could complement the loss of *IRA* function in *S. cerevisiae* and stimulate the GTPase activity of p21^{ras} in vitro.[360–362]

These results have suggested that the NF-1 protein (neurofibromin) might normally function as a negative regulator of p21^{ras} and that mutations at the *NF-1* locus abolish this activity, resulting in increased *ras* activity. This prediction has been fulfilled for malignant schwannoma cell lines derived from patients with NF-1 disease. Although the Ras protein in the cell lines was not mutated, an abnormally high proportion of Ras was found to be in the active, GTP-bound form.[226, 227] This finding was correlated with reduced to absent levels of neurofibromin and loss of GTPase activation. These cells were therefore analogous to mutants of *S. cerevisiae* lacking *IRA* function. The GAP-related domain of neurofibromin represents only about 10 per cent of this large protein; the functions of the remainder of the protein have yet to be determined.

FAP and MCC

The *FAP* and *MCC* genes are located near each other at chromosome 5q21. The *FAP* gene encodes a 2843 amino acid product whose sequence is related to structural proteins such as intermediate filaments. The gene is interrupted by mutations in patients with familial adenomatous polyposis coli, as well as in some sporadic cases of colorectal carcinoma.[323, 325] The majority of these mutations result in premature termination of the polypeptide chain.

MCC encodes a product of 839 amino acids.[324, 325] At least 15 per cent of sporadic colorectal tumors contain mutations in *MCC*.[363] The sequence of the *MCC* product also indicates a possible structural similarity to intermediate filament proteins, based on the appearance of potential "coiled-coil" domains separated by hinge regions. In fact, the *FAP* and *MCC* genes have some homology to each other, suggesting that they might have arisen via gene duplication.[325] One intriguing possibility is that the products of these genes might associate with each other as hetero-oligomers. Much work remains to be done in order to determine the roles of the *FAP* and *MCC* genes in colorectal cancer, as well as the biochemical function of their products.

DCC

The *DCC* gene at 18q21 is expressed in normal colonic mucosa, but is absent or expressed only at very low levels in colorectal carcinoma lines.[364] *DCC* encodes a 190 kDa transmembrane phosphoprotein that is related to cell adhesion molecules. The homology includes the presence of immunoglobulin-like repeats and fibronectin-related regions in the extracellular part of the protein. This structure suggests that the *DCC* product functions as a regulator of cell adhesion but also raises the possibility that it may be a receptor protein.

Oncoproteins of DNA Tumor Viruses

These tumor viruses and their viral transforming genes were introduced in the section on oncogenes and proto-oncogenes. As noted earlier, several oncoproteins of adenoviruses and papovaviruses inactivate the proteins encoded by tumor-suppressor genes. Analysis of these oncoproteins has helped to elucidate aspects of tumor-suppressor gene function.

Viral Proteins That Bind pRB

Analysis of adenovirus-transformed cells revealed that several cellular proteins bind E1A, as demonstrated in immunoprecipitation assays with E1A antibodies (see Fig. 23–15). The first of these cellular proteins to be identified was pRB, a finding that has had far-reaching ramifications.[10] It represented the first direct connection between an oncoprotein and the product of a tumor-suppressor gene. Because pRB was believed to inhibit cell growth, it seemed possible that pRB binding might contribute to the ability of E1A to stimulate cell growth. The most straight-forward interpretation was that the binding of pRB to E1A inactivates the normal inhibitory function of pRb.

SV40 large T[67] and the E7 proteins of HPV16 and 18 E7[341] also bind pRB. Mutagenic analysis of adeno, SV40, and HPV genes[365] showed that mutants encoding proteins that failed to bind pRB had severe defects in their transforming function, which strengthened the hypothesis that pRB binding was an important component of this activity. Furthermore, the E7 proteins of low-risk HPVs, which are less active in transformation assays than E7 from high-risk HPVs, have lower affinity for pRB. A single amino acid substitution in E7 from a low-risk HPV has been shown simultaneously to increase its transforming activity and affinity for pRB to levels similar to those of a high-risk E7.[366] Therefore, although papovaviruses, papillomaviruses, and adenoviruses are evolutionarily distinct, a striking convergence is that oncoproteins encoded by all of them bind pRB.

As discussed earlier, insight into the mechanism by which pRB functions was provided by finding that SV40 large T preferentially binds the underphosphorylated molecules of pRB.[342] This observation represented the first clue that the underphosphorylated form of pRb might be the active, inhibitory form and that phosphorylation of pRb might be a physiological mechanism for its inactivation.

The viral oncoproteins that bind pRB are multifunctional and form complexes with other proteins as well (see Fig. 23–15). Cellular proteins co-immunoprecipitated with E1A antibodies include p60, p107, p130, and p300 (the proteins are named according to their size in kDa). pRB has limited homology with p107.[367] The amino acid residues in E1A required for binding pRB are also required for binding p107 and p130. p60 is cyclin A; it binds to p107 rather than directly to E1A.[368] E1A mutants that fail to bind p300 are less active biologically than wild-type E1A. Large T and E7 also bind p107. In addition, E7 is phosphorylated by CK II, which is required for full biological activity.[365] Large T has several additional biochemical functions, such as ATPase activity and DNA binding (particularly to the origin of replication of SV40 and cellular replication forks), which are not required for its transforming function.

Viral Proteins That Bind p53

As discussed earlier, p53 was first identified as a protein that binds SV40 large T antigen[328] and was subsequently shown to bind the adenovirus 55 kDa E1B protein[369] and the E6 proteins of high-risk genital HPVs.[66] Whereas the intracellular levels of large T and E1B proteins are relatively high in cells transformed by these genes, cells transformed by HPV contain very small quantities of E6, which makes it unlikely that E6 functions merely by binding stoichiometric amounts of p53. Recent studies have shown that the half-life of p53 in a rabbit reticulocyte lysate is reduced by the addition of E6 of HPV 16 or 18 and that the presence of HPV 16 E6 markedly shortens the half-life of p53 in human keratinocytes.[370, 371] These results suggest that E6, in cooperation with cellular factors, induces the catalytic degradation of p53. E6-mediated degradation of p53 may have pathogenic significance, because it is not shared by the E6 proteins of low-risk HPVs, which are less transforming than E6 from high-risk HPVs. Furthermore, analysis of the status of the p53 and *RB* genes in cervical carcinoma cell lines argues that inactivation of p53 and pRB by HPV is important pathogenically; cell lines that contain HPV DNA (and therefore express E6 and E7) have wild-type p53 and *RB,* whereas these genes are mutated in lines that lack HPV.[372, 373]

Activation of Tyrosine Kinases

In contrast to the above oncoproteins, those encoded by two other transforming genes, middle T antigen of polyoma virus and E5 of bovine papillomavirus (BPV), appear to function by activating cellular protein tyrosine kinases. Middle T antigen has been shown to associate with and become phosphorylated by the product of the *c-src* proto-oncogene, pp60$^{c\text{-}src}$,[374] and with other members of the Src subfamily of protein tyrosine kinases. This association, which activates the kinase activity of pp60$^{c\text{-}src}$, occurs through an interaction at the C-terminus of pp60$^{c\text{-}src}$, where the negative regulatory site is located (for review, see reference 38). Indeed, these observations on the effects of middle T on pp60$^{c\text{-}src}$ provided the critical clue to the negative regulatory role of the C-terminal tyrosine 527 of pp60$^{c\text{-}src}$.

It is believed that the association of middle T relieves the normal negative regulation of the Src kinase through dephosphorylation of tyrosine 527. This hypothesis has been strengthened by the fact that mutants of middle T that are transformation defective fail to associate with pp60$^{c\text{-}src}$. Thus, the transforming ability of middle T probably results in the induction of mitogenic signals analogous to those generated by an activated kinase of the Src subfamily.

The BPV *E5* gene encodes a 44 amino acid product, which is the smallest known oncoprotein.[72] It can form homodimers via two cysteines. The protein cooperates with and activates EGF receptors and PDGF receptors in the absence of ligand.[375, 376] E5 has been shown, by immunoprecipitation, to form a complex with PDGF receptors, as well as with a 16 kDa protein that is a subunit of a vacuolar protein ATPase that functions in the acidification of subcellular compartments.[377] The role of the 16 kDa protein in transformation remains to be established.

CANCER: COLLABORATION AMONG GENES THAT REGULATE GROWTH

Most of the previous sections have focused on identifying genes that regulate cell growth and the diverse mechanisms by which alterations in a single gene may uncouple the cell from its normal growth controls and drive proliferation. As noted earlier, however, a wealth of evidence indicates that cancer in most instances represents a multistep process that results largely from a series of genetic changes rather than from a single genetic abnormality. It is theoretically possible that tumors arise following alterations in a random mixture of genes that regulate cell growth. However, analysis of experimentally induced tumors and of certain human tumors suggests that a pattern and order underlie the constellation of genetic changes that give rise to a particular tumor. This theme is also discussed in Chapter 24.

The observation that efficient transformation of primary rodent fibroblasts requires more than one oncogene has been noted earlier. Cotransfection of different mixtures of oncogenes in primary rodent cells has led to the general conclusion that efficient transformation by two oncogenes can usually be accomplished if one oncogene efficiently immortalizes cells and the other efficiently transforms established rodent cells.[55] Primary cells transfected with a single "transforming" gene are more likely to have a transformed phenotype if they are grown in the absence of surrounding normal cells. This finding is in agreement with the observation that normal cells, when mixed with transformed cells, can suppress the transformed phenotype in vitro and in vivo.[378, 379] The immortalizing oncogene may help override the inhibitory effect of the normal cells, which could be mediated by the release of growth-inhibitory cytokines from the normal cells. Support for this model has been provided by the finding that constitutive expression of c-myc can render keratinocytes resistant to the growth-inhibitory activity of TGF-β.[345]

In general, the "transforming" genes, such as *ras* or v-*src*, encode non-nuclear proteins, whereas the "immortalizing" genes, such as *myc* or mutant *p53*, encode nuclear proteins that regulate transcription. Consistent with this observation, some established, non-transformed rodent fibroblast cell lines that can be efficiently transformed by *ras* or v-*src* alone have been found to have mutant *p53* genes.[53]

The *bcl-2* gene, which is deregulated by translocation to an immunoglobulin heavy chain J chain in most follicular lymphomas, may represent an instructive exception to the rule that non-nuclear proteins lack immortalizing function. Although it encodes a non-nuclear protein, *bcl-2* can cooperate with *ras*, rather than with *myc*, to transform primary fibroblasts. However, *bcl-2* is "immortalizing" in that it can promote survival of hematopoietic cell lines deprived of growth factors.[380] Furthermore, *bcl-2* collaborates with c-*myc* to transform hematopoietic cells,[381] suggesting that results of studies carried out in fibroblasts may not apply to other cell types.

We have also noted that many DNA tumor viruses contain more than one oncogene, that the tumorigenic capacity of these viruses usually requires each of their oncogenes acting in concert, and that the encoded oncoproteins, such as adeno E1A, may be multifunctional. Retroviruses that carry two oncogenes also represent models for examining cooperation between oncogenes.[382] For example, mutational analysis of AEV (see Fig. 23–4) has shown that v-*erbB*, which encodes a constitutively active transmembrane receptor with protein tyrosine kinase activity, is necessary and sufficient for inducing erythroblastosis.[383] In contrast to tumors caused by wild-type AEV, those resulting from a mutant that lacks v-*erbA* are much less aggressive and include more differentiated cells that express hemoglobin.[384] Although v-*erbA* by itself is not oncogenic, these results demonstrate that it cooperates with v-*erbB*. In appropriate viral constructs, v-*src* and other v-*onc*'s that encode non-receptor protein tyrosine kinases can induce erythroblastosis; v-*erbA* can cooperate with these v-*onc*'s to increase the malignant potential of the tumors and to block the ability of the tumor cells to differentiate.[385]

The use of transgenic animals represents an extremely fruitful approach for studying experimental tumorigenesis in the intact organism. Analysis of the tumorigenic activity of the SV40 large T antigen in transgenic mice has demonstrated the critical role played by the promoter (for review, see reference 93). This oncogene can induce pancreatic, melanocytic, or lymphoid tumors if the promoter of the transgene is derived, respectively, from the pancreatic elastase gene, the tyrosinase gene, or the immunoglobulin heavy chain gene.[93]

The relative susceptibility of different strains of mice to tumorigenesis by specific oncogenes can also be probed by the analysis of transgenic mice. For example, mouse strains appear to vary markedly in the efficiency with which an activated *neu* oncogene can induce mammary tumors.[386, 387] The genetic basis for such differences in susceptibility can be explored by examining the differences between the transgenic animals derived from different strains.

Although it is possible to induce tumors with a single oncogene, the introduction of two different oncogenes as transgenes usually results in the formation of tumors with much greater efficiency than either transgene alone.[93] Furthermore, the latent period for tumor formation is shorter when two genes are used, and the tumors are often more malignant. As with in vitro transformation studies of primary rodent fibroblastic cells, *myc* and *ras* transgenes in mice have been shown to cooperate in the development of pre–B-cell lymphomas, mammary carcinomas, and hepatic malignancies, with the tumor type being determined largely by the promoter used.

Transgenes can also test the oncogenic potential of rearranged genes identified in tumors. As noted earlier, Burkitt's lymphomas often have a translocation that places the c-*myc* gene under the control of the enhancer from the immunoglobulin heavy chain gene. The oncogenic potential of such a chimeric gene has been documented by showing that when introduced as a transgene in mice, it results in B-cell or pre–B-cell tumors.[388] The tumors develop only after a long latency, implying that other genetic changes are required. Mutational activation of endogenous *ras* genes has been detected frequently in these tumors, as might be expected from the cooperation demonstrated between *myc* and *ras* in the development of B-cell tumors.

Molecular evidence from human cancers also supports the hypothesis that several genetic changes are required for malignancy. Alterations of several tumor suppressor genes (*FAP, DCC,* and *p53*) and at least one proto-oncogene (K-*ras*) have been implicated in the pathogenesis of colorectal tumors.[322] Inactivation of *FAP* is usually the first event, followed by activation of K-*ras* and inactivation of *DCC* and *p53*. Although these events do not occur in all colorectal tumors and probably do not happen in this precise order in every case, analysis of a large number of patients does suggest a general sequence of genetic alterations leading to malignancy. Pathologists have defined a discrete series of stages in the development of metastatic colorectal carcinoma, ranging from hyperproliferation of the epithelium to benign adenoma to carcinoma and the appearance of metastatic variants. Interestingly, the genetic changes detailed above appear to occur at defined stages of the tumor progression.[322]

The examples described in this section, derived from a variety of different systems, all point to the involvement of multiple genetic changes during the development of cancer. The epidemiology of cancer, in which the overall incidence shows a dramatic increase with the age of the individual, is in agreement with these findings.

FUTURE DIRECTIONS

The work described here represents the outcome of efforts aimed at understanding the molecular basis of normal and abnormal cell growth. It reflects the contributions of many fields of inquiry. Taken together, these studies have described a network of intracellular molecules that act in both a positive and a negative manner to control the growth of cells. Because all but the most terminally differentiated cells must respond to a variety of signals, many different players are needed to participate in the growth-control network. The result of this requirement is that more than 100 genes have been implicated as proto-oncogenes, and the list of potential tumor suppressors is growing as well.

One of the major problems of current research is to determine how multiple alterations in these different classes of genes result in different human neoplasms.[7] A more precise delineation of the cellular pathways through which these genes function and identification of the components with which their products interact are also needed. For example, the ligands for many receptor-like proteins encoded by proto-oncogenes remain unidentified, as do the critical substrates for the mitogenic signals transmitted by the protein kinases and the relevant genes regulated by nuclear transcription factors implicated in oncogenesis. It is also important to clarify the molecular mechanisms underlying progression to the metastatic phenotype.[389] The most fundamental challenge is to translate this enormous body of knowledge of normal and abnormal growth into more effective approaches to prevent and treat various forms of cancer. It seems reasonable to believe that elucidating the fundamental processes that lead to neoplastic disease represents a necessary step toward its eventual control.

REFERENCES

1. Bishop, J. M.: Molecular themes in oncogenesis. Cell 64:235, 1991.
2. Cooper, G. M.: Oncogenes. Boston, Jones and Bartlett Publishers, 1990.
3. Hunter, T.: Cooperation between oncogenes. Cell 64:249, 1991.
4. Weiss, R. A.: RNA Tumor Viruses, 2nd ed. Supplements and Appendices. Cold Spring Harbor, NY, Cold Spring Harbor Laboratory, 1985.
5. Tooze, J.: Molecular Biology of Tumor Viruses: DNA Tumor Viruses. Cold Spring Harbor, NY, Cold Spring Harbor Laboratory, 1981.
6. Stehelin, D., Varmus, H. E., Bishop, J. M., and Vogt, P. K.: DNA related to the transforming gene(s) of avian sarcoma viruses is present in normal avian DNA. Nature 260:170, 1976.
7. Cossman, J.: Molecular Genetics in Cancer Diagnosis. New York, Elsevier, 1990.
8. Marshall, C. J.: Tumor suppressor genes. Cell 64:313, 1991.
9. Weinberg, R. A.: Tumor suppressor genes. Science 254:1138, 1991.
10. Whyte, P., Buchkovich, K. J., Horowitz, J. M., Friend, S. H., Raybuck, M., Weinberg, R. A., and Harlow, E.: Association between an oncogene and an anti-oncogene: The adenovirus E1A proteins bind to the retinoblastoma gene product. Nature 334:124, 1988.
11. Nurse, P.: Universal control mechanism regulating onset of M-phase. Nature 344:503, 1990.
12. Weinberg, R. A.: Oncogenes and the molecular origins of cancer. Cold Spring Harbor, NY, Cold Spring Harbor Laboratory Press, 1989.
13. Carbone, M., and Levine, A. S.: Oncogenes, antioncogenes, and the regulation of cell growth. Trends Endocrinol Metab 2:248, 1990.
14. Hartwell, L. H.: *Saccharomyces cerevisiae* cell cycle. Bacteriol. Rev. 38:164, 1974.
15. Enoch, T., and Nurse, P.: Coupling M phase and S phase: Controls maintaining the dependence of mitosis on chromosome replication. Cell 65:921, 1991.
16. Pines J., and Hunter, T.: p34^{cdc2}: The S and M kinase? New Biologist 2:389, 1990.
17. Steele, R. E.: Protein-tyrosine phosphorylation: A glimmer of light in the darkness. Trends Biochem Genet 15:124, 1990.
18. Hunter, T., and Pines, J.: Cyclins and cancer. Cell 66:1071, 1991.
19. Draetta, G., Luca, F., Westendorf, J., Brizuela, L., Ruderman, J., and Beach, D.: *cdc2* Protein kinase is complexed with both cyclin A and B: Evidence for proteolytic inactivation of MPF. Cell 56:829, 1989.
20. Gautier, J., Solomon, M. J., Booher, R. N., Bazan, J. F., and Kirschner, M. W.: cdc25 is a specific tyrosine phosphatase that directly activates p34^{cdc2}. Cell 67:197, 1991.
21. Fang, F., and Newport, J. W.: Evidence that the G1-S and G2-M transitions are controlled by different cdc2 proteins in higher eukaryotes. Cell 66:731, 1991.
22. Matsushime, H., Roussel, M. F., Ashmun, R. A., and Sherr, C. J.: Colony stimulating factor 1 regulates novel cyclins during the G1 phase of the cell cycle. Cell 65:701, 1991.
23. Norbury, C., and Nurse, P.: Animal cell cycles and their control. Annu. Rev. Biochem. 61:441, 1992.
24. Aaronson, S. A.: Growth factors and cancer. Science 254:1146, 1991.
25. Cross, M., and Dexter, T. M.: Growth factors in development, transformation, and tumorigenesis. Cell 64:271, 1991.
26. Yuan, J., and Horvitz, H. R.: The caenorhabditis elegans genes *ced*-3 and *ced*-4 act cell autonomously to cause programmed cell death. Dev. Biol. 138:33, 1990.
27. Williams, G. T., Smith, C. A., Spooncer, E., Dexter, T. M., and Taylor, D. R.: Haemopoietic colony stimulating factors promote cell survival by supressing apoptosis. Nature 343:76, 1990.
28. Levi-Montalcini, R.: The nerve growth factor 35 years later. Science 237:1154, 1987.
29. Carpenter, G., and Cohen, S.: Epidermal growth factor. Ann. Rev. Biochem. 48:193, 1979.
30. Kelly, K., Cochran, B. H., Stiles, C. D., and Leder, P.: Cell-specific regulation of the c-*myc* gene by lymphocyte mitogens and platelet-derived growth factor. Cell 35:603, 1983.
31. Greenberg, M. E., and Ziff, E. B.: Stimulation of 3T3 cells induces transcription of the c-*fos* proto-oncogene. Nature 311:433, 1984.
32. Pardee, A. B.: G$_1$ events and regulation of cell proliferation. Science 246:603, 1989.
33. Crabtree, G. R.: Contingent genetic regulatory events in T lymphocyte activation. Science 243:355, 1989.
34. Green, S., and Chambon, P.: Nuclear receptors enhance our understanding of transcription regulation. Trends Genet. 4:309, 1988.
35. Ullrich, A., and Schlessinger, J.: Signal transduction by receptors with tyrosine kinase activity. Cell 61:203, 1990.
36. Hunter, T.: Protein-tyrosine phosphatases: The other side of the coin. Cell 58:1013, 1989.
37. Alexander, D. R.: The role of phosphatases in signal transduction. New Biologist 2:1049, 1990.
38. Cantley, L. C., Auger, K. R., Carpenter, C., Duckworth, B., Graziani, A., Kapeller, R., and Soltoff, S.: Oncogenes and signal transduction. Cell 64:281, 1991.
39. Nishibe, S., Wahl, M. I., Wedegaertner, P. B., Kim, J. J., Rhee, S. G., and Carpenter, G.: Selectivity of phospholipase-C phosphorylation by the epidermal growth factor receptor, the insulin receptor, and their cytoplasmic domains. Proc. Natl. Acad. Sci. USA 87:424, 1990.
40. Nishizuka, Y.: Studies and perspectives of protein kinase C. Science 233:305, 1986.
41. Berridge, M. J., and Irvine, R. F.: Inositol phosphates and cell signalling. Nature 341:197, 1989.
42. Collins, S., Caron, M. G., and Lefkowitz, R. J.: From ligand binding to gene expression: New insights into the regulation of G-protein–coupled receptors. Trends Biomed. Sci. 17:37, 1992.
43. Palczewski, K., and Benovic, J. L.: G-protein–coupled receptor kinases. Trends Biochem. Sci. 16:387, 1991.
44. Mitchell, P. J., and Tjian, R.: Transcriptional regulation in mammalian cells by sequence-specific DNA binding proteins. Science 245:371, 1989.
45. Schüle, R., and Evans, R. M.: Cross-coupling of signal transduction pathways: Zinc finger meets leucine zipper. Trends Genet. 7:377, 1991.
46. Abercrombie, M., and Heaysman, J. E. M.: Observations on the social behaviour of cells in tissue culture II. "Monolayering" of fibroblasts. Exp. Cell. Res. 6:293, 1954.
47. Holley, R. W., and Kiernan, J. A.: "Contact inhibition" of cell division in 3T3 cells. Proc. Natl. Acad. Sci. USA 60:300, 1968.
48. Macpherson, I., and Montagnier, L.: Agar suspension culture for the selective assay of cells transformed by polyoma virus. Virology 23:291, 1964.
49. Temin, H. M., and Rubin, H.: Characteristics of an assay for Rous sarcoma virus and Rous sarcoma cells in tissue culture. Virology 6:669, 1958.
50. Hynes, R. O.: Cell surface proteins and malignant transformation. Biochim. Biophys. Acta 458:73, 1976.

51. Pollack, R., Osborn, M., and Weber, K.: Patterns of organization of actin and myosin in normal and transformed cultured cells. Proc. Natl. Acad. Sci. USA 72:994, 1975.

52. Sporn, M. B., and Roberts, A. B.: Autocrine growth factors and cancer. Nature 313:745, 1985.

53. Harvey, D. M., and Levine, A. J.: p53 Alteration is a common event in the spontaneous immortalization of primary BALB/c murine embryo fibroblasts. Genes Dev. 5:2375, 1991.

54. Sawyers, C. L., Denny, C. T., and Witte, O. N.: Leukemia and the disruption of normal hematopoiesis. Cell 64:337, 1991.

55. Ruley, H. E.: Transforming collaborations between ras and nuclear oncogenes. Cancer Cells 2:258, 1990.

56. Solomon, E., Borrow, J., and Goddard, A. D.: Chromosome aberrations and cancer. Science 254:1153, 1991.

57. Todaro, G. J., and Huebner, R. J.: The viral oncogene hypothesis: New evidence. Proc. Natl. Acad. Sci. USA 69:1009, 1972.

58. Bishop, J. M.: Viral oncogenes. Cell 42:23, 1985.

59. zur Hausen, H.: Viruses in human cancers. Science 254:1167, 1991.

60. Kieff, E., and Liebowitz, D.: Epstein-Barr virus and its replication. In Fields, B. N., and Knipe, D. M. (eds.): Virology. New York, Raven Press, 1990, pp. 1889–1920.

61. Hsu, T.-Y., Möröy, T., Etiemble, J., Louise, A., Trépo, T. P., Tiollais, P., and Buendia, M.-A.: Activation of c-myc by Woodchuck hepatitis virus insertion in hepatocellular carcinoma. Cell 55:627, 1988.

62. Wang, J., Chenivesse, X., Henglein, B., and Brechot, C.: Hepatitis B virus integration in a cyclin A gene in a hepatocellular carcinoma. Nature 343:555, 1990.

63. Ginsburg, H. S. (ed.): The Adenoviruses. New York, Plenum Publishing Corporation, 1984.

64. Salzman, N. P. (ed.): The Papovaviridae: The Polyomaviruses. New York, Plenum Publishing Corporation, 1986.

65. Salzman, N. P., and Howley, P. M. (eds.): The Papovaviridae: The Papillomaviruses. New York, Plenum Publishing Corporation, 1987.

66. Werness, B. A., Münger, K., and Howley, P. M.: Role of the human papillomavirus oncoproteins in transformation and carcinogenic progression. In DeVita, V. T. (eds.): Important Advances in Oncology. Philadelphia, J. B. Lippincott, 1991, pp. 3–18.

67. DeCaprio, J. A., Ludlow, J. W., Figge, J., Shew, J.-Y., Huang, C.-M., Lee, W.-H., Marsilio, E., Paucha, E., and Livingston, D. M.: SV40 large tumor antigen forms a specific complex with the product of the retinoblastoma susceptibility gene. Cell 54:275, 1988.

68. Lillie, J. W., Loewenstein, P. M., Green, M. R., and Green, M.: Functional domains of adenovirus type 5 E1a proteins. Cell 50:1091, 1987.

69. Ruley, H. E.: Adenovirus region E1A enables viral and cellular transforming genes to transform primary cells in culture. Nature 304:602, 1983.

70. Livingston, D. M.: Review: The simian virus 40 large T antigen—a lot packed into a little. Mol. Biol. Med. 4:63, 1987.

71. Rassoulzadegan, M., Cowie, A., Carr, A., Glaichenhaus, N., Kamen, R., and Cuzin, F.: The role of individual polyoma virus early proteins in oncogenic transformation. Nature 300:713, 1982.

72. DiMaio, D.: Transforming activity of bovine and human papillomaviruses. Adv. Cancer Res. 56:133, 1991.

73. Barbosa, M. S., Vass, W. C., Lowy, D. R., and Schiller, J. T.: In vitro biological activities of the E6 and E7 genes vary among human papillomaviruses of different oncogenic potential. J. Virol. 65:292, 1991.

74. Rous, P.: Transmission of a malignant new growth by means of a cell-free filtrate. J.A.M.A. 56:198, 1911.

75. Varmus, H. E.: Form and function of retroviral proviruses. Science 216:812, 1982.

76. Varmus, H.: Retroviruses. Science 240:1427, 1988.

77. Baltimore, D.: Viral RNA-dependent DNA polymerase. Nature 226:1209, 1970.

78. Temin, H. M., and Mizutani, S.: RNA-dependent DNA polymerase in virions of Rous sarcoma virus. Nature 226:1211, 1970.

79. Temin, H. M.: Function of the retrovirus long terminal repeat. Cell 28:3, 1982.

80. Martin, G. S.: Rous sarcoma virus: A function required for the maintenance of the transformed state. Nature 227:1021, 1970.

81. Duesberg, P. H., and Vogt, P. K.: Differences between the ribonucleic acids of transforming and nontransforming avian tumor viruses. Proc. Natl. Acad. Sci. USA 67:1673, 1970.

82. Vogt, P. K.: Spontaneous segregation of nontransforming viruses from cloned sarcoma viruses. Virology 46:939, 1971.

83. Aaronson, S. A., Jainchill, J. L., and Todaro, G. J.: Murine sarcoma virus transformation of BALB/3T3 cells: Lack of dependence on murine leukemia virus. Proc. Natl. Acad. Sci. USA 66:1236, 1970.

84. Spector, D. H., Smith, K., Padgett, T., McCombe, P., Rulland-Dussoix, D., Moscovici, C., Varmus, H. E., and Bishop, J. M.: Uninfected avian cells contain RNA related to the transforming gene of avian sarcoma viruses. Cell 13:371, 1978.

85. Wang, L.-H., Galpern, C. C., Nadel, M., and Hanafusa, H.: Recombination between viral and cellular sequences generates transforming sarcoma virus. Proc. Natl. Acad. Sci. USA 75:5812, 1978.

86. Bishop, J. M., and Varmus, H. E.: Functions and origins of retroviral transforming genes. In Weiss, R., Teich, N., Varmus, H., and Coffin, J. (eds.): RNA Tumor Viruses. Cold Spring Harbor, NY, Cold Spring Harbor Laboratory, 1982, pp. 999–1108.

87. Brugge, J. S., and Erickson, R. L.: Identification of a transformation-specific antigen induced by an avian sarcoma virus. Nature 269:346, 1977.

88. Collett, M. S., and Erikson, R. L.: Protein kinase activity associated with the avian sarcoma virus src gene product. Proc. Natl. Acad. Sci. USA 75:2021, 1978.

89. Levinson, A. D., Opperman, H., Levintow, L., Varmus, H. E., and Bishop, J. M.: Evidence that the transforming gene of avian sarcoma virus encodes a protein kinase associated with a phosphoprotein. Cell 15:561, 1978.

90. Hunter, T., and Sefton, B. M.: Transforming gene product of Rous sarcoma virus phosphorylates tyrosine. Proc. Natl. Acad. Sci. USA 77:1311, 1980.

91. Parker, R. C., Varmus, H. E., and Bishop, J. M.: Expression of v-src and chicken c-src in rat cells demonstrates qualitative differences between pp60^{v-src} and pp60^{c-src}. Cell 37:131, 1984.

92. Velu, T. J., Vass, W. C., Lowy, D. R., and Tambourin, P. E.: Harvey murine sarcoma virus: Influence of coding and non-coding sequences on cell transformation in vitro and oncogenicity in vivo. J. Virol. 63:1384, 1989.

93. Adams, J. M., and Cory, S.: Transgenic models of tumor development. Science 254:1161, 1991.

94. Payne, G. S., Courtneidge, S. A., Crittenden, L. B., Fadly, A. M., Bishop, J. M., and Varmus, H. E.: Analysis of avian leukosis virus DNA and RNA in bursal tumors: Viral gene expression is not required for maintenance of the tumor state. Cell 23:311, 1981.

95. Hayward, W. S., Neel, B. G., and Astrin, S. M.: Activation of a cellular onc gene by promoter insertion in ALV-induced lymphoid leukosis. Nature 209:475, 1981.

96. Nilsen, T. W., Maroney, P. A., Goodwin, R. G., Rottman, F. M., Crittenden, L. B., Raines, M. A., and Kung, H.-J.: c-erbB Activation in ALV-induced erythroblastosis: Novel RNA processing and promoter insertion result in expression of an amino-truncated EGF receptor. Cell 41:719, 1985.

97. Nusse, R., and Varmus, H. E.: Many tumors induced by the mouse mammary tumor virus contain a provirus integrated in the same region of the host genome. Cell 31:99, 1982.

98. Brown, A. M. C., Wildin, R. S., Prendergast, T. J., and Varmus, H. E.: A retrovirus vector expressing the putative mammary oncogene int-1 causes partial transformation of a mammary epithelial cell line. Cell 46:1001, 1986.

99. Tsukamoto, A. S., Grosschedl, R., Guzman, R. C., Parslow, T., and Varmus, H. E.: Expression of the int-1 gene in transgenic mice is associated with mammary gland hyperplasia and adenocarcinomas in male and female mice. Cell 55:619, 1988.

100. Nusse, R., and Varmus, H. E.: Wnt genes. Cell 69:1073, 1992.

101. Peters, G., Brookes, S., Smith, R., and Dickson, C.: Tumorigenesis by mouse mammary tumor virus: Evidence for a common region for provirus integration in mammary tumors. Cell 33:369, 1983.

102. Kwan, H., Pecenka, V., Tsukamoto, A., et al.: Transgenes expressing the wnt-1 and int-2 proto-oncogenes cooperate during mammary carcinogenesis in doubly transgenic mice. Mol. Cell Biol. 12:147, 1992.

103. Voronova, A. F., and Sefton, B. M.: Expression of a new tyrosine protein kinase is stimulated by retrovirus promoter insertion. Nature 319:682, 1986.

104. Hill, H., and Hillova, J.: Production virale dans les fibroblasts de poule traites per l'acide desoxyribonucleique de cellules XC de rat transformees par le virus de Rous. Compt. Rend. Acad. Sci. 272:3094, 1971.

105. Shih, C., Shilo, B.-Z., Goldfarb, M. P., Dannenberg, A., and Weinberg, R. A.: Passage of phenotypes of chemically transformed cells via transfection of DNA and chromatin. Proc. Natl. Acad. Sci. USA 76:5714, 1979.

106. Cooper, G. M., Okenquist, S., and Silverman, L.: Transforming activity of DNA of chemically transformed and normal cells. Nature 284:418, 1980.

107. Krontiris, T. G., and Cooper, G. M.: Transforming activity of human tumor DNAs. Proc. Natl. Acad. Sci. USA 78:1181, 1981.

108. Parada, L. F., Tabin, C. J., Shih, C., and Weinberg, R. A.: Human EJ bladder carcinoma oncogene is homologue of Harvey sarcoma virus ras gene. Nature 297:474, 1982.

109. Santos, E., Tronick, S. R., Aaronson, S. A., Pulciani, S., and Barbacid, M.: T24 human bladder carcinoma oncogene is an activated form of the normal human homologue of BALB- and Harvey-MSV transforming genes. Nature 298:343, 1982.

110. Der, C. J., Krontiris, T. G., and Cooper, G. M.: Transforming genes of human bladder and lung carcinoma cell lines are homologous to the ras genes of Harvey and Kirsten sarcoma viruses. Proc. Natl. Acad. Sci. USA 79:3637, 1982.

111. Bargmann, C. I., Hung, M.-C., and Weinberg, R. A.: Multiple independent activations of the neu oncogene by a point mutation altering the transmembrane domain of p185. Cell 45:649, 1986.

112. Dalla-Favera, R., Bregni, M., Erikson, J., Patterson, D., Gallo, R. C., and Croce, C. M.: Human c-myc oncogene is located on the region of chromosome 8 that is translocated in Burkitt lymphoma cells. Proc. Natl. Acad. Sci. USA 79:7824, 1982.

113. Taub, R., Kirsch, I., Morton, C., Lenoir, G., Swan, D., Tronick, S., Aaronson, S., and Leder, P.: Translocation of the c-myc gene into the immunoglobin heavy chain locus in human Burkitt lymphoma and murine plasmacytoma cells. Proc. Natl. Acad. Sci. USA 79:7837, 1982.

114. Shen-Ong, G. L., Keath, E. J., Piccoli, S. P., and Cole, M. D.: Novel myc oncogene RNA from abortive immunoglobulin-gene recombination in mouse plasmacytomas. Cell 31:443, 1982.

115. Shtivelman, E., Lifshitz, B., Gale, R. P., and Canaani, E.: Fused transcript of abl and bcr genes in chronic myelogenous leukaemia. Nature 315:550, 1985.

116. Davis, R. L., Konopka, J. B., and Witte, O. N.: Activation of the c-abl oncogene by viral transduction or chromosomal translocation generates c-abl proteins with similar in vitro kinase properties. Mol. Cell. Biol. 5:204, 1985.

117. Finger, L. R., Harvey, R. C., Moore, R. C. A., Showe, L. C., and Croce, C. M.: A common mechanism of chromosomal translocation in T- and B-cell neoplasia. Science 234:982, 1986.

118. Withers, D. A., Harvey, R. C., Faust, J. B., Melnyk, O., Carey, K., and Meeker, T. C.: Characterization of a candidate bcl-1 gene. Mol. Cell Biol. 11:4846, 1991.

119. Reed, J. C., Cuddy, M., Slabiak, T., Croce, C. M., and Nowell, P. C.: Oncogenic potential of bcl-2 demonstrated by gene transfer. Nature 336:259, 1988.

120. Collins, S., and Groudine, M.: Amplification of endogenous myc-related DNA sequences in a human myeloid leukemia cell line. Nature 298:679, 1982.

121. DePinho, R. A., Schreiber-Agus, N., and Alt, F. W.: myc Family oncogenes in the development of normal and neoplastic cells. Adv. Cancer Res. 57:1, 1991.

122. Brodeur, G. M., Seeger, R. C., Schwab, M., Varmus, H. E., and Bishop, J. M.: Amplification of N-myc in untreated human neuroblastomas correlates with advanced disease stage. Science 224:1121, 1984.

123. Slamon, D. J., Godolphin, W., Jones, L. A., et al.: Studies of the HER-2/neu proto-oncogene in human breast and ovarian cancer. Science 244:707, 1989.

124. Hendler, F. J., Shum-Slu, A., Oechsli, M., Nanu, L., Richards, C. S., and Ozanne, B. W.: Increased EGF-R1 binding predicts a poor survival in squamous tumors. In Furth, M., and Greaves, M. (eds.): Cancer Cells 7: Molecular Diagnostics of Human Cancer. Cold Spring Harbor, NY, Cold Spring Harbor Laboratory, 1989, pp. 347–351.

125. Velu, T. J., Beguinot, L., Vass, W. C., Willingham, M. C., Merlino, G. T., Pastan, I., and Lowy, D. R.: Epidermal growth factor–dependent transformation by a human EGF receptor proto-oncogene. Science 238:1408, 1987.

126. Di Fiore, P. P., Pierce, J. H., Kraus, M. H., Segatto, O., King, C. R., and Aaronson, S. A.: erbB-2 is a potent oncogene when overexpressed in NIH/3T3 cells. Science 237:178, 1987.

127. Doolittle, R. F., Hunkapiller, M. W., Hood, L. E., Devare, S. G., Robbins, K. C., Aaronson, S. A., and Antoniades, H. N.: Simian sarcoma virus onc gene, v-sis, is derived from the gene (or genes) encoding a platelet-derived growth factor. Science 221:275, 1983.

128. Waterfield, M. D., Scrace, G. T., Whittle, N., et al.: Platelet-derived growth factor is structurally related to the putative transforming protein p28^{sis} of simian sarcoma virus. Nature 304:35, 1983.

129. Beckmann, M. P., Betsholtz, C., Heldin, C.-H., Westermark, B., Di Marco, E., Di Fiore, P. P., Robbins, K. C., and Aaronson, S. A.: Comparison of biological properties and transforming potential of human PDGF-A and PDGF-B chains. Science 241:1346, 1988.

130. Rosenthal, A., Lindquist, P. B., Bringman, T. S., Goeddel, D. V., and Derynck, R.: Expression in rat fibroblasts of a human transforming growth factor-α cDNA results in transformation. Cell 46:301, 1986.

131. Derynck, R.: Transforming growth factor α. Cell 54:593, 1988.

132. Shih, T. Y., Weeks, M. O., Young, H. A., and Scolnick, E. M.: p21 of Kirsten murine sarcoma virus is thermolabile in a viral mutant temperature sensitive for maintenance of transformation. J. Virol. 31:546, 1970.

133. Derynck, R., Goeddel, D. V., Ullrich, A., Gutterman, J. U., Williams, R. D., Bringman, T. S., and Berger, W. H.: Synthesis of messenger RNAs for transforming growth factors α and β and the epidermal growth factor receptor by human tumors. Cancer Res. 47:707, 1987.

134. Halaban, R., Kwon, B. S., Ghosh, S., Delli-Bovi, P., and Baird, A.: bFGF is an autocrine growth factor for human melanomas. Oncogene Res. 3:177, 1988.

135. Meeker, T. C., Hardy, D., Willman, C., Hogan, T., and Abrams, J.: Activation of the interleukin-3 gene by chromosome translocation in acute lymphocytic leukemia with eosinophilia. Blood 76:285, 1990.

136. Blood, C. H., and Zetter, B. R.: Tumor interactions with the vasculature; Angiogenesis and tumor metastasis. Biochim. Biophys. Acta 1032:89, 1990.

137. Ushiro, H., and Cohen, S.: Identification of phosphotyrosine as a product of epidermal growth factor–activated protein kinase in A431 cell membranes. J. Biol. Chem. 255:8363, 1980.

138. Hunter, T., and Cooper, J. A.: Epidermal growth factor

induces rapid tyrosine phosphorylation of proteins in A431 human tumor cells. Cell 24:741, 1981.

139. Cooper, J. A., Bowen-Pope, D. F., Raines, E., Ross, R., and Hunter, T.: Similar effects of platelet-derived growth factor and epidermal growth factor on the phosphorylation of tyrosine in cellular proteins. Cell 31:263, 1982.

140. Downward, J., Yarden, Y., Mayes, E., Scrace, G., Totty, N., Stockwell, P., Ullrich, A., Schlessinger, J., and Waterfield, M. D.: Close similarity of epidermal growth factor receptor and v-erb-B oncogene protein sequences. Nature 307:521, 1984.

141. Gilmore, T., DeClue, J. E., and Martin, G. S.: Protein phosphorylation at tyrosine is induced by the v-erbB gene product in vivo and in vitro. Cell 40:609, 1985.

142. Fung, Y.-K. T., Lewis, W. G., Crittenden, L. B., and Kung, H.-J.: Activation of the cellular oncogene c-erbB by LTR insertion: Molecular basis for induction of erythroblastosis by avian leukosis virus. Cell 33:357, 1983.

143. Sherr, C. J., Rettenmeier, C. W., Sacca, R., Roussel, M. F., Look, A. T., and Stanley, E. R.: The c-fms proto-oncogene product is related to the receptor for the mononuclear phagocyte growth factor, CSF-1. Cell 41:665, 1985.

144. Sherr, C. J.: Mitogenic response to colony-stimulating factor 1. Trends Genet. 7:398, 1991.

145. Roussel, M. F., Downing, J. R., Rettenmeer, C. W., and Sherr, C. J.: A point mutation in the extracellular domain of the human CSF-1 receptor (c-fms proto-oncogene product) activates its transforming potential. Cell 55:979, 1988.

146. Chabot, B., Stephenson, D. A., Chapman, V. M., Besmer, P., and Bernstein, A.: The proto-oncogene c-kit encoding a transmembrane tyrosine kinase receptor maps to the mouse W locus. Nature 335:88, 1988.

147. Geissler, E. N., Ryan, M. A., and Housman, D. E.: The dominant-white spotting (W) locus of the mouse encodes the c-kit proto-oncogene. Cell 55:185, 1988.

148. Witte, O. N.: Steel locus defines new multipotent growth factor. Cell 63:5, 1990.

149. Birchmeier, C., O'Neill, K., Riggs, M., and Wigler, M.: Characterization of the ROS1 cDNA from a human glioblastoma cell line. Proc. Natl. Acad. Sci. USA 87:4799, 1990.

150. Bottaro, D. P., Rubin, J. S., Faletto, D. L., Chan, A. M. L., Kmiecik, T. E., Vande Woude, G. F., and Aaronson, S. A.: Identification of the hepatocyte growth factor receptor as the c-met proto-oncogene product. Science 251:802, 1991.

151. Kaplan, D. R., Hempstead, B. L., Martin-Zanca, D., Chao, M. V., and Parada, L. F.: The trk proto-oncogene product—a signal transducing receptor for nerve growth factor. Science 252:554, 1991.

152. Wen, D., Peles, E., Cupples, R., et al.: Neu differentiation factor: A transmembrane glycoprotein containing an EGF domain and an immunoglobulin homology unit. Cell 69:559, 1992.

153. Hibi, K., Takahashi, T., Sekido, Y., Ueda, R., Hida, T., Ariyoshi, Y., Takagi, H., and Takahashi, T.: Coexpression of the stem cell factor and the c-kit genes in small-cell lung cancer. Oncogene 6:2291, 1991.

154. Ellisen, L. W., Bird, J., West, D. C., Soreng, A. L., Reynolds, T. C., Smith, S. D., and Sklar, J.: TAN-1, the human homolog of the drosophila notch gene, is broken by chromosomal translocations in T lymphoblastic neoplasms. Cell 66:649, 1991.

155. Yoshimura, A., Longmore, G., and Lodish, H. F.: Point mutation in the exoplasmic domain of the erythropoietin receptor resulting in hormone-independent activation and tumorigenicity. Nature 348:647, 1990.

156. Zon, L. I., Moreau, J.-F., Koo, J.-W., Mathey-Prevot, B., and D'Andrea, D. A.: The erythropoietin receptor transmembrane region is necessary for activation by the friend spleen focus-forming virus gp55 glycoprotein. Mol. Cell Biol. 12:2949, 1992.

157. Linnekin, D., Evans, G. A., D'Andrea, A., and Farrar, W. L.: Association of the erythropoietin receptor with protein tyrosine kinase activity. Proc. Natl. Acad. Sci. USA 89:6237, 1992.

158. Young, D., Waitches, G., Birchmeier, C., Fasano, O., and Wigler, M.: Isolation and characterization of a new cellular oncogene encoding a protein with multiple potential transmembrane domains. Cell 45:711, 1986.

159. Jackson, T. R., Blair, L. A. C., Marshall, J., Goedert, M., and Hanley, M. R.: The mas oncogene encodes an angiotensin receptor. Nature 335:437, 1988.

160. Parsons, J. T., and Weber, M. J.: Genetics of src: Structure and functional organization of a protein tyrosine kinase. Cur. Top. Microbiol. Immunol. 147:80, 1989.

161. Hanks, S. K., Quinn, A. M., and Hunter, T.: The protein kinase family: Conserved features and deduced phylogeny of the catalytic domains. Science 241:42, 1988.

162. Dymecki, S. M., Niederhuber, J. E., and Desiderio, S. V.: Specific expression of a tyrosine kinase gene, blk, in B lymphoid cells. Science 247:332, 1990.

163. Cooper, J. A., and King, C. S.: Dephosphorylation or antibody binding to the carboxy terminus stimulates pp60^{c-src}. Mol. Cell. Biol. 6:4467, 1986.

164. Kmiecik, T. E., and Shalloway, D.: Activation and suppression of pp60^{c-src} transforming ability by mutation of its primary sites of tyrosine phosphorylation. Cell 49:65, 1987.

165. Hanks, S. K., Quinn, A. M., and Hunter, T.: The protein kinase family: Conserved features and deduced phylogeny of the catalytic domains. Science 241:42, 1988.

166. Resh, M. D.: Membrane interactions of pp60v-src—a model for myristylated tyrosine protein kinases. Oncogene 5:1437, 1990.

167. Kamps, M. P., Buss, J. E., and Sefton, B. M.: Rous sarcoma virus transforming protein lacking myristic acid phosphorylates known polypeptide substrates without inducing transformation. Cell 45:105, 1986.

168. Sadowski, I., Stone, J. C., and Pawson, T.: A non-catalytic domain conserved among cytoplasmic protein-tyrosine kinases modifies the kinase function and transforming activity of fujinami sarcoma virus p30gag-fps. Mol. Cell Biol. 6:4396, 1986.

169. Pawson, T.: Non-catalytic domains of cytoplasmic protein-tyrosine kinases: Regulatory elements in signal transduction. Oncogene 3:491, 1988.

170. Koch, C. A., Anderson, D., Moran, M. F., Ellis, C., and Pawson, T.: SH2 and SH3 domains: Elements that control interactions of cytoplasmic signaling proteins. Science 252:668, 1991.

171. Heldin, C.-H.: SH2 domains: Elements that control protein interactions during signal transduction. Trends Biochem. Sci. 16:450, 1991.

172. Moran, M. F., Koch, C. A., Anderson, D., Ellis, C., England, L., Martin, G. S., and Pawson, T.: Src homology region 2 domains direct protein-protein interactions in signal transduction. Proc. Natl. Acad. Sci. USA 87:8622, 1990.

173. Kypta, R. M., Goldberg, Y., Ulug, E. T., and Courtneidge, S. A.: Association between the PDGF receptor and members of the src family of tyrosine kinases. Cell 62:481, 1990.

174. Mayer, B. J., Hamaguchi, M., and Hanafusa, H.: A novel viral oncogene with structural similarity to phospholipase C. Nature 332:272, 1988.

175. Matsuda, M., Mayer, B. J., and Hanafusa, H.: Identification of domains of the v-crk oncogene product sufficient for association with phosphotyrosine-containing proteins. Mol Cell Biol 11:1607, 1991.

176. Mayer, B. J., and Hanafusa, H.: Association of the v-crk oncogene product with phosphotyrosine-containing proteins and protein kinase activity. Proc. Natl. Acad. Sci. USA 87:2638, 1990.

177. Roussel, R. R., Brodeur, S. R., Shalloway, D., and Laudano, A. P.: Selective binding of activated pp60c-src by an immobilized synthetic phosphopeptide modeled on the carboxyl terminus of pp60c-src. Proc. Natl. Acad. Sci. USA 88:10696, 1991.

178. Hirai, H., and Varmus, H. E.: Site-directed mutagenesis of the SH2-coding and SH3-coding domains of c-src produces varied phenotypes, including oncogenic activation of p60^{c-src}. Mol. Cell. Biol. 10:1307, 1990.

179. Verderame, M. F., Kaplan, J. M., and Varmus, H. E.: A mutation in v-*src* that removes a single conserved residue in the SH-2 domain of pp60v-src restricts transformation in a host-dependent manner. J. Virol. 63:338, 1989.

180. DeClue, J. E., Sadowski, I., Martin, G. S., and Pawson, T.: A conserved domain regulates interactions of the v-*fps* protein-tyrosine kinase with the host cell. Proc. Natl. Acad. Sci. USA 84:9064, 1987.

181. Mayer, B. J., Jackson, P. K., Van Etten, R. A., and Baltimore, D.: Point mutations in the abl SH2 domain coordinately impair phosphotyrosine binding in vitro and transforming activity in vivo. Mol. Cell. Biol. 12:609, 1992.

182. Booker, G. W., Breeze, A. L., Downing, A. K., Panayotou, G., Gout, I., Waterfield, M. D., and Campbell, I. D.: Structure of an SH2 domain of the p85-alpha subunit of phosphatidylinositol-3-OH kinase. Nature 358:684, 1992.

183. Overduin, M., Rios, C. B., Mayer, B. J., Baltimore, D., and Cowburn, D.: Three-dimensional solution structure of the src homology 2 domain of c-abl. Cell 70:697, 1992.

184. Waksman, G., Kominos, D., Robertson, S. C., et al.: Crystal structure of the phosphotyrosine recognition domain SH2 of v-src complexed with tyrosine-phosphorylated peptides. Nature 358:646, 1992.

185. Sefton, B. M.: The *lck* tyrosine protein kinase. Oncogene 6:683, 1991.

186. Horak, I. D., Gress, R. E., Lucas, P. J., Horak, E. M., Waldmann, T. A., and Bolen, J. B.: T-lymphocyte interleukin 2-dependent tyrosine protein kinase signal transduction involves the activation of p56lck. Proc. Natl. Acad. Sci. USA 88:1996, 1991.

187. Hatakeyama, M., Kono, T., Kobayashi, N., Kawahara, A., Levin, S. D., Perlmutter, R. M., and Taniguchi, T.: Interaction of the IL-2 receptor with the src-family kinase p56lck: Identification of novel intermolecular association. Science 252:1523, 1991.

188. Samelson, L. E., Phillips, A. F., Luong, E. T., and Klausner, R. D.: Association of the fyn protein-tyrosine kinase with the T-cell antigen receptor. Proc. Natl. Acad. Sci. USA 87:4358, 1990.

189. Burkhardt, A. L., Brunswick, M., Bolen, J. B., and Mond, J. J.: Anti-immunoglobulin stimulation of B lymphocytes activates src-related protein-tyrosine kinases. Proc. Natl. Acad. Sci. USA 88:7410, 1991.

190. Fischer, E. H., Charbonneau, H., and Tonks, N. K.: Protein tyrosine phosphatases: A diverse family of intracellular and transmembrane enzymes. Science 253:401, 1991.

191. Shen, S. H., Bastien, L., Posner, B. I., and Chretien, P.: A protein-tyrosine phosphatase with sequence similarity to the SH2 domain of the protein-tyrosine kinases. Nature 352:736, 1991.

192. Bourne, H. R., Sanders, D. A., and McCormick, F.: The GTPase superfamily: A conserved switch for diverse cell functions. Nature 348:125, 1990.

193. Bourne, H. R., Sanders, D. A., and McCormick, F.: The GTPase superfamily: Conserved structure and molecular mechanism. Nature 349:117, 1991.

194. Hall, A.: The cellular functions of small GTP-binding proteins. Science 249:635, 1990.

195. Barbacid, M.: *ras* Genes. Ann. Rev. Biochem. 56:779, 1987.

196. Bos, J. L.: Ras oncogenes in human cancer: A review. Cancer Res. 49:4682, 1989.

197. Scolnick, E. M., Papageorge, A. G., and Shih, T. Y.: Guanine nucleotide–binding activity as an assay for *src* protein of rat-derived murine sarcoma viruses. Proc. Natl. Acad. Sci. USA 76:5355, 1979.

198. Trahey, M., and McCormick, F.: A cytoplasmic protein stimulates normal N-*ras* p21 GTPase, but does not affect oncogenic mutants. Science 238:542, 1987.

199. Satoh, T., Endo, M., Nakafuku, M., Nakamura, S., and Kaziro, Y.: Platelet-derived growth factor stimulates formation of active p21Ras.GTP complex in Swiss mouse 3T3 cells. Proc. Natl. Acad. Sci. USA 87:5993, 1990.

200. Gibbs, J. B., Marshall, M. S., Scolnick, E. M., Dixon, R. A. F., and Vogel, U. S.: Modulation of guanine nucleotides bound to ras in NIH3T3 cells by oncogenes, growth factors, and the GTPase activating protein (GAP). J. Biol. Chem. 265:20437, 1990.

201. Downward, J., Graves, J. D., Warne, P. H., Rayter, S., and Cantrell, D. A.: Stimulation of p21ras upon T-cell activation. Nature 346:719, 1990.

202. Mulcahy, L. S., Smith, M. R., and Stacey, D. W.: Requirements for *ras* proto-oncogene function during serum stimulated growth of NIH 3T3 cells. Nature 313:241, 1985.

203. Medema, R. H., Wubbolts, R., and Bos, J. L.: Two dominant inhibitory mutants of p21(ras) interfere with insulin-induced gene expression. Mol. Cell. Biol. 11:5963, 1991.

204. Smith, M. R., DeGudicibus, S. J., and Stacey, D. W.: Requirement for c-*ras* proteins during viral oncogene transformation. Nature 320:540, 1986.

205. Lowy, D. R., Zhang, K., DeClue, J. E., and Willumsen, B. M.: Regulation of p21^{ras} activity. Trends Genet. 7:346, 1991.

206. Simon, M. A., Bowtell, D. D. L., Dodson, G. S., Laverty, T. R., and Rubin, G. M.: Ras1 and a putative guanine nucleotide exchange factor perform crucial steps in signaling by the *sevenless* protein tyrosine kinase. Cell 67:701, 1991.

207. Willumsen, B. M., Christensen, A., Hubbert, N. L., Papageorge, A. G., and Lowy, D. R.: The p21 *ras* C-terminus is required for transformation and membrane association. Nature 310:583, 1984.

208. Hancock, J. F., Magee, A. I., Childs, J. E., and Marshall, C. J.: All *ras* proteins are polyisoprenylated but only some are palmitoylated. Cell 57:1167, 1989.

209. Hancock, J. F., Paterson, H., and Marshall, C. J.: A polybasic domain or palmitoylation is required in addition to the CAAX motif to localize p21Ras to the plasma membrane. Cell 63:133, 1990.

210. Hancock, J. F., Cadwallader, K., and Marshall, C. J.: Methylation and proteolysis are essential for efficient membrane binding of prenylated p21K-*ras*(B). EMBO J. 10:641, 1991.

211. Gibbs, J. B.: Ras C-terminal processing enzymes—new drug targets. Cell 65:1, 1991.

212. Kato, K., Der, C. J., and Buss, J. E.: Prenoids and palmitate: Lipids that control the biological activity of ras proteins. Semin. Cancer Biol. 3:179, 1992.

213. Wittinghofer, A., and Pai, E. F.: The structure of ras protein: A model for a universal molecular switch. Trends Biochem. Sci. 16:382, 1991.

214. Sigal, I. S., Gibbs, J. B., D'Alonzo, J. S., Temeles, G. L., Wolanski, B. S., Socher, S. H., and Scolnick, E. M.: Mutant *ras*-encoded proteins with altered nucleotide binding exert dominant biological effects. Proc. Natl. Acad. Sci. USA 83:952, 1986.

215. Walter, M., Clark, S. G., and Levinson, A. D.: The oncogenic activation of human p21-*ras* by a novel mechanism. Science 233:649, 1986.

216. Rodenhuis, S.: Ras and human tumors. Semin. Cancer Biol. 3:241, 1992.

217. Broach, J. R.: RAS genes in *Saccharomyces cerevisiae*—signal transduction in search of a pathway. Trends Genet. 7:28, 1991.

218. Powers, S.: Genetic analysis of *ras* homologs in yeasts. Semin. Cancer Biol. 3:209, 1992.

219. Toda, T., Uno, I., Ishikawa, T., et al.: In yeast, *RAS* proteins are controlling elements of adenylate cyclase. Cell 40:27, 1985.

220. Jones, S., Vignais, M. L., and Broach, J. R.: The CDC25 protein of *Saccharomyces cerevisiae* promotes exchange of guanine nucleotides bound to ras. Mol. Cell Biol. 11:2641, 1991.

221. Tanaka, K., Lin, B. K., Wood, D. R., and Tamanoi, F.: IRA2, an upstream negative regulator of RAS in yeast, is a RAS GTPase-activating protein. Proc. Natl. Acad. Sci. USA 88:468, 1991.

222. Fortini, M. E., Simon, M. A., and Rubin, G. M.: Signalling by the *sevenless* protein tyrosine kinase is mimicked by Ras1 activation. Nature 355:559, 1992.

223. Bowtell, D., Fu, P., Simon, M., and Senior, P.: Identification of murine homologs of the drosophila *son of sevenless* gene:

Potential activators of *ras*. Proc. Natl. Acad. Sci. USA 89:6511, 1992.

224. Martegani, E., Vanoni, M., Zippel, R., Coccetti, P., Brambilla, R., Ferrari, C., Sturani, E., and Alberghina, L.: Cloning by functional complementation of a mouse cDNA encoding a homologue of CDC25, a Saccharomyces-cerevisiae RAS activator. EMBO J. 11:2151, 1992.

225. Bollag, G., and McCormick, F.: Regulators and effectors of *ras* proteins. Annu. Rev. Cell Biol. 7:601, 1991.

226. DeClue, J. E., Papageorge, A. G., Fletcher, J. A., Diehl, S. R., Ratner, N., Vass, W. C., and Lowy, D. R.: Abnormal regulation of mammalian p21^ras contributes to malignant tumor growth in Von Recklinghausen (type-1) neurofibromatosis. Cell 69:265, 1992.

227. Basu, T. N., Gutmann, D. H., Fletcher, J. A., Glover, T. W., Collins, F. S., and Downward, J.: Aberrant regulation of ras proteins in malignant tumour cells from type-1 neurofibromatosis patients. Nature 356:713, 1992.

228. Adari, H., Lowy, D. R., Willumsen, B. M., Der, C. J., and McCormick, F.: Guanosine triphosphatase activating protein (GAP) interacts with the p21ras effector binding domain. Science 240:518, 1988.

229. Vogel, U. S., Dixon, R. A. F., Schaber, M. D., Diehl, R. E., Marshall, M. S., Scolnick, E. M., Sigal, I. S., and Gibbs, J. B.: Cloning of bovine GAP and its interaction with oncogenic *ras* p21. Nature 335:90, 1988.

230. Calès, C., Hancock, J. F., Marshall, C., and Hall, A.: The cytoplasmic protein GAP is implicated as the target for regulation by the *ras* gene product. Nature 332:548, 1988.

231. Martin, G. A., Yatani, A., Clark, R., Conroy, L., Polakis, P., Brown, A. M., and McCormick, F.: GAP domains responsible for ras p21-dependent inhibition of muscarinic atrial K^+ channel currents. Science 255:192, 1992.

232. Schweighoffer, F., Barlat, I., Chevallier-Multon, M. C., and Tocque, B.: Implication of GAP in ras-dependent transactivation of a polyoma enhancer sequence. Science 256:825, 1992.

233. Marshall, C. J.: How does p21 ras transform cells? Trends Genet. 7:91, 1991.

234. Eva, A., Vecchio, G., Rao, C. D., Tronick, S. R., and Aaronson, S. A.: The predicted *DBL* oncogene product defines a distinct class of transforming proteins. Proc. Natl. Acad. Sci. USA 85:2061, 1988.

235. Hart, M. J., Eva, A., Evans, T., Aaronson, S. A., and Cerione, R. A.: Catalysis of guanine nucleotide exchange on the CDC42Hs protein by the dbl oncogene products. Nature 354:311, 1991.

236. Kaziro, Y., Itoh, H., Kozasa, T., Nakafuku, M., and Satoh, T.: Structure and function of signal-transducing GTP-binding proteins. Annu. Rev. Biochem. 60:359, 1991.

237. Vallar, L., Spada, A., and Giannattasio, G.: Altered G_s and adenylate cyclase activity in human GH-secreting pituitary adenomas. Nature 330:566, 1987.

238. Landis, C. A., Masters, S. B., Spada, A., Pace, A. M., Bourne, H. R., and Vallar, L.: GTPase inhibiting mutations activate the α chain of G_s and stimulate adenylyl cyclase in human pituitary tumours. Nature 340:692, 1989.

239. Lyons, J., Landis, C. A., Harsh, G., et al.: Two G protein oncogenes in human endocrine tumors. Science 249:655, 1990.

240. Thomas, S. M., DeMarco, M., D'Arcangelo, G., Halegoua, S., and Brugge, J. S.: Ras is essential for nerve growth factor–induced and phorbol ester–induced tyrosine phosphorylation of MAP kinases. Cell 68:1031, 1992.

241. Morrison, D. K., Kaplan, D. R., Escobedo, J. A., Rapp, U. R., Roberts, T. M., and Williams, L. T.: Direct activation of the serine/threonine kinase activity of *raf*-1 through tyrosine phosphorylation by the PDGF receptor. Cell 58:649, 1989.

242. Rapp, U. R.: Role of raf-1 serinethreonine protein kinase in growth factor signal transduction. Oncogene 6:495, 1991.

243. Stanton, V. P., Jr., Nichols, D. W., Laudano, A. P., and Cooper, G. M.: Definition of the human *raf* amino-terminal regulatory region by deletion mutagenesis. Mol. Cell. Biol. 9:639, 1989.

244. Li, P., Wood, K., Mamon, H., Haser, W., and Roberts, T.: Raf-1: A kinase currently without a cause but not lacking in effects. Cell 64:479, 1991.

245. App, H., Hazan, R., Zilberstein, A., Ullrich, A., Schlessinger, J., and Rapp, U.: Epidermal growth factor (EGF) stimulates association and kinase activity of raf-1 with the EGF receptor. Mol. Cell Biol. 11:913, 1991.

246. Koch, W., Heidecker, G., Lloyd, P., and Rapp, U. R.: Raf-1 protein kinase is required for growth of induced NIH/3T3 cells. Nature 349:426, 1991.

247. Hsiao, W.-L. W., Housey, G. M., Johnson, M. D., and Weinstein, B. I.: Cells that overproduce protein kinase C are more susceptible to transformation by an activated H-*ras* oncogene. Mol. Cell Biol 9:2641, 1989.

248. Borner, C., Filipuzzi, I., Weinstein, I. B., and Imber, R.: Failure of wild-type or a mutant form of protein kinase C-α to transform fibroblasts. Nature 353:78, 1991.

249. Maxwell, S. A., and Arlinghaus, R. B.: Serine kinase activity associated with Moloney murine sarcoma virus-124–encoded p37^mos. Virology 143:321, 1985.

250. Goldman, D. S., Kiessling, A. A., Millette, C. F., and Cooper, G. M.: Expression of c-*mos* RNA in germ cells of male and female mice. Proc. Natl. Acad. Sci. USA 84:4509, 1987.

251. Sagata, N., Watanabe, N., Vande Woude, G. F., and Ikawa, Y.: The c-*mos* proto-oncogene product is a cytostatic factor responsible for meiotic arrest in vertebrate eggs. Nature 342:512, 1989.

252. Selten, G., Cuypers, H. T., Boelens, W., Robanus-Maandag, E., Verbeek, J., Domen, J., van Beveren, C., and Berns, A.: The primary structure of the putative oncogene *pim*-1 shows extensive homology with protein kinases. Cell 46:603, 1986.

253. Landschulz, W. H., Johnson, P. F., and McKnight, S. L.: The leucine zipper: A hypothetical structure common to a new class of DNA binding proteins. Science 240:1759, 1988.

254. Gutman, A., and Wasylyk, B.: Nuclear targets for transcription regulation by oncogenes. Trends Genet. 7:49, 1991.

255. Lewin, B.: Oncogenic conversion by regulatory changes in transcription factors. Cell 64:303, 1991.

256. Forrest, D., and Currane, T.: Cross signals: Oncogenic transcription factors. Curr. Opin. Genet. Dev. 2:19, 1992.

257. Penn, L. J. Z., Laufer, E. M., and Land, H.: C-MYC: Evidence for multiple regulatory functions. Cancer Biol. 1:69, 1990.

258. Roussel, M. F., Cleveland, J. L., Shurtleff, S. A., and Sherr, C. J.: Myc rescue of a mutant CSF-1 receptor impaired in mitogenic signalling. Nature 353:361, 1991.

259. Donner, P., Greisser-Wilke, I., and Moelling, K.: Nuclear localization and DNA binding of the transforming gene product of avian myelocytomatosis virus. Nature 296:262, 1982.

260. Lüscher, B., and Eisenman, R. N.: New light on myc and myb. Part I. Myc. Genes Devel. 4:2025, 1990.

261. Blackwood, E. M., Kretzner, L., and Eisenman, R. N.: Myc and max function as a nucleoprotein complex. Curr. Opin. Gent. Dev. 2:227, 1992.

262. Blackwood, E. M., and Eisenman, R. N.: Max: A helix-loop-helix zipper protein that forms a sequence-specific DNA-binding complex with myc. Science 251:1211, 1991.

263. Prendergast, G. C., Lawe, D., and Ziff, E. B.: Association of myn, the murine homology of max, with c-myc stimulates methylation-sensitive DNA binding and ras cotransformation. Cell 65:395, 1991.

264. Kato, G. J., Lee, W. M. F., Chen, L., and Dang, C. V.: Max: Functional domains and interaction with C-myc. Genes Devel. 6:81, 1992.

265. Cole, M. D.: Myc meets its max. Cell 65:715, 1991.

266. Chiu, R., Boyle, W. J., Meek, J., Smeal, T., Hunter, T., and Karin, M.: The c-*fos* protein interacts with c-*jun*/AP-1 to stimulate transcription of AP-1 responsive genes. Cell 54:541, 1988.

267. Roux, P., Blanchard, J.-M., Fernandez, A., Lamb, N., Jeanteur, P., and Pierchaczyk, M.: Nuclear localization of c-*fos* but not v-*fos* protein is controlled by extracellular signals. Cell 63:341, 1990.

268. Müller, R., Bravo, R., Burckhardt, J., and Curran, T.: Induc-

tion of c-*fos* gene and protein by growth factors precedes activation of c-*myc*. Nature 312:716, 1984.

269. Stacey, D. W., Watson, T., Kung, H.-F., and Curran, T.: Microinjection of transforming *ras* protein induces c-*fos* expression. Mol. Cell. Biol. 7:523, 1987.

270. Jamal, S., and Ziff, E.: Transactivation of C-fos and beta-actin genes by raf as a step in early response to transmembrane signals. Nature 344:463, 1990.

271. Ledwith, B. J., Manam, S., Kraynak, A. R., Nichols, W. W., and Bradley, M. O.: Antisense-Fos RNA causes partial reversion of the transformed phenotypes induced by the C-Ha-RAS oncogene. Mol. Cell Biol. 10:1545, 1990.

272. Smeal, T., Binetruy, B., Mercola, D. A., Birrer, M., and Karin, M.: Oncogenic and transcriptional cooperation with Ha-Ras requires phosphorylation of C-Jun on serine-63 and serine-73. Nature 354:494, 1991.

273. Bohmann, D., Bos, T. J., Admon, A., Nishimura, T., Vogt, P. K., and Tjian, R.: Human proto-oncogene c-*jun* encodes a DNA binding protein with structural and functional properties of transcription factor AP-1. Science 238:1386, 1987.

274. Binetruy, B., Smeal, T., and Karin, M.: Ha-*ras* augments c-*jun* activity and stimulates phosphorylation of its activation domain. Nature 351:122, 1991.

275. Pulverer, J., Kyriakis, J. M., Avruch, J., Nikolokaki, E., and Woodgett, J. R.: Phosphorylation of c-*jun* mediated by MAP kinases. Nature 353:670, 1991.

276. Baichwal, V. R., Park, A., and Tjian, R.: v-*src* and EJ *ras* alleviate repression of c-*jun* by a cell-specific inhibitor. Nature 352:165, 1991.

277. Hai, T., and Curran, T.: Cross-family dimerization of transcription factors Fos/Jun and ATF/CREB alters DNA-binding specificity. Proc. Natl. Acad. Sci. USA 88:3720, 1991.

278. Kovary, K., and Bravo, R.: Expression of different Jun and Fos proteins during the G0 to G1 transition in mouse fibroblasts: *In vitro* and *in vivo* associations. Mol. Cell Biol. 11:2451, 1991.

279. Lüscher, B., and Eisenman, R. N.: New light on myc and myb. Part II. Myb. Genes Devel. 4:2235, 1990.

280. Weston, K., and Bishop, J. M.: Transcriptional activation by the v-*myb* oncogene and its cellular progenitor, c-*myb*. Cell 58:85, 1989.

281. Klempnauer, K.-H., Arnold, H., and Biedenkapp, H.: Activation of transcription by v-*myb*: Evidence for two different mechanisms. Genes Dev. 3:1582, 1989.

282. Gilmore, T. D.: Malignant transformation by mutant rel proteins. Trends Genet. 7:318, 1991.

283. Davis, N., Ghosh, S., Simmons, D. L., Tempst, P., Liou, H.-C., Baltimore, D., and Bose, H. R. J.: Rel-associated pp40: An inhibitor of the Rel family of transcription factors. Science 253:1268, 1991.

284. Ballard, D. W., Walker, W. H., Doerre, S., Sista, P., Molitor, J. A., Dixon, E. P., Peffer, N. J., Hannink, M., and Greene, W. C.: The v-rel oncogene encodes a kB enhancer binding protein that inhibits NF-kB function. Cell 63:803, 1990.

285. Lammie, G. A., Vantl, V., Smith, R., Schuuring, E., Brookes, S., Michalides, R., Dickson, C., Arnold, A., and Peters, G.: D11S287, a putative oncogene on chromosome 11q13, is amplified and expressed in squamous cell and mammary carcinomas and linked to BCL-1. Oncogene 6:439, 1991.

286. Motokura, T., Bloom, T., Kim, H. G., Juppner, H., Ruderman, J. V., Kronenberg, H. M., and Arnold, A.: A novel cyclin encoded by a bcl1-linked candidate oncogene. Nature 350:512, 1991.

287. Hanna, Z., Jankowski, M., Tremblay, P., Xiaoyan, J., Milatovich, A., Francke, U., and Jolicoeur, P.: The Vin-1 gene, identified by provirus insertional mutagenesis, corresponds to the G1-phase cyclin D2. Oncogene (in press).

288. Adamson, E. D.: Oncogenes in development. Development 99:449, 1987.

289. Pawson, T., and Bernstein, A.: Receptor tyrosine kinases: Genetic evidence for their role in *Drosophila* and mouse development. Trends Genet. 6:350, 1990.

290. Forrester, L. M., Brunkow, M., and Bernstein, A.: Proto-oncogenes in mammalian development. Curr. Opin. Genet. Dev. 2:38, 1992.

291. Hoffman, F. M., Sternberg, P. W., and Herskowitz, I.: Learning about cancer genes through invertebrate genetics. Curr. Opin. Genet. Dev. 2:45, 1992.

292. Reith, A. D., and Bernstein, A.: Molecular basis of mouse developmental mutants. Genes Dev. 5:1115, 1991.

293. Nocka, K., Tan, J. C., Chiu, E., Chu, T. Y., Ray, P., Traktman, P., and Besmer, P.: Molecular bases of dominant negative and loss of function mutations at the murine c-*kit*/white spotting locus: $W^{37,}$ W^v, W^{41} and W. EMBO J. 9:1805, 1990.

294. Flanagan, J. G., Chan, D. C., and Leder, P.: Transmembrane form of the kit ligand growth factor is determined by alternative splicing and is missing in the SI(d) mutant. Cell 64:1025, 1991.

295. Capecchi, M. R.: Altering the genome by homologous recombination. Science 244:1288, 1989.

296. Mucenski, M. L., McLain, K., Kier, A. B., Swerdlow, S. H., Schreiner, C. M., Miller, T. A., Pietryga, D. W., Scott, W. J. J., and Potter, S. S.: A functional c-*myb* gene is required for normal murine fetal hepatic hematopoiesis. Cell 65:677, 1991.

297. McMahon, A. P., and Bradley, A.: The wnt-1 (int-1) proto-oncogene is required for development of a large region of the mouse brain. Cell 62:1073, 1990.

298. Thomas, K. R., and Capecchi, M. R.: Targeted disruption of the murine int-1 proto-oncogene resulting in severe abnormalities in midbrain and cerebellar development. Nature 346:847, 1990.

299. Tybulewicz, V. L. J., Crawford, C. E., Jackson, P. K., Bronsons, R. T., and Mulligan, R. C.: Neonatal lethality and lymphopenia in mice with a homozygous disruption of the c-*abl* proto-oncogene. Cell 65:1153, 1991.

300. Soriano, P., Montgomery, C., Geske, R., and Bradley, A.: Targeted disruption of the c-*src* proto-oncogene leads to osteopetrosis in mice. Cell 64:693, 1991.

301. Hoffmann, F. M.: *Drosophila abl* and genetic redundancy in signal transduction. Trends Genet. 7:351, 1991.

302. Bowen-Pope, D. F., Van Koppen, A., and Schatteman, G.: Is PDGF really important? Testing the Hypotheses. Trends Genet. 7:413, 1991.

303. Rubin, G. M.: Signal transduction and the fate of the R7 photoreceptor in *Drosophila*. Trends Genet. 7:372, 1991.

304. Gaul, U., Mardon, G., and Rubin, G. M.: A putative ras GTPase activating protein acts as a negative regulator of signaling by the sevenless receptor tyrosine kinase. Cell 68:1007, 1992.

305. Sternberg, P. W., and Horvitz, H. R.: Signal transduction during *C. elegans* vulval induction. Trends Genet. 7:366, 1991.

306. Clark, S. G., Stern, M. J., and Horvitz, H. R.: *C. elegans* cell-signalling gene sem-5 encodes a protein with SH2 and SH3 domains. Nature 356:340, 1992.

307. Boyd, J. A., and Barrett, J. C.: Tumor suppressor genes: Possible functions in the negative regulation of cell proliferation. Mol. Carcinog. 3:325, 1990.

308. Stanbridge, E. J.: Genetic regulation of tumorigenic expression in somatic cell hybrids. Adv. Viral Oncol. 6:83, 1987.

309. Harris, H.: The analysis of malignancy by cell fusion: The position in 1988. Cancer Res. 48:3302, 1988.

310. Knudson, A. G., Jr.: Mutation and cancer: Statistical study of retinoblastoma. Proc. Natl. Acad. Sci. USA 68:820, 1971.

311. Collins, F. S.: Positional cloning: Let's not call it reverse anymore. Nature Genet. 1:3, 1992.

312. Francke, U., and Kung, F.: Sporadic bilateral retinoblastoma and 13q chromosomal deletion. Med. Pediatr. Oncol. 2:379, 1976.

313. Sparkes, R. S., Murphree, A. L., Lingua, R. W., Sparkes, M. C., Field, L. L., Funderburk, S. J., and Benedict, W. F.: Gene for hereditary retinoblastoma assigned to human chromosome 13 by linkage to esterase D. Science 219:971, 1983.

314. Friend, S. H., Bernards, R., Rogelj, S., Weinberg, R. A., Rapaport, J. M., Albert, D. M., and Dryja, T. P.: A human

DNA segment with properties of the gene that predisposes to retinoblastoma and osteosarcoma. Nature 323:643, 1986.

315. Fung, Y.-K. T., Murphree, A. L., T'Ang, A., Qian, J., Hinrichs, S. H., and Benedict, W. F.: Structural evidence for the authenticity of the human retinoblastoma gene. Science 236:1657, 1987.

316. Lee, W.-H., Bookstein, R., Hong, F., Young, L.-J., Shew, J.-Y., and Lee, E. Y.-H. P.: Human retinoblastoma susceptibility gene: Cloning, identification, and sequence. Science 235:1394, 1987.

317. Horowitz, J. M., Park, S.-H., Bogenmann, E., Cheng, J.-C., Yandell, D. W., Kaye, F. J., Minna, J. D., Dryja, T. P., and Weinberg, R. A.: Frequent inactivation of the retinoblastoma anti-oncogene is restricted to a subset of human tumor cells. Proc. Natl. Acad. Sci. USA 87:2775, 1990.

318. Cavenee, W. K., Hansen, M. F., Nordenskjold, M., Kock, E., Maumenee, I., Squire, J., Phillips, R. A., and Gallie, B. L.: Genetic origins of mutations predisposing to retinoblastoma. Science 228:501, 1985.

319. Van Heyningen, V., and Hastie, N. D.: Wilms' tumour: Reconciling genetics and biology. Trends Genet. 8:16, 1992.

320. Wallace, M. R., Marchuk, D. A., Andersen, L. B., et al.: Type 1 neurofibromatosis gene: Identification of a large transcript disrupted in three NF1 patients. Science 249:181, 1990.

321. Cawthon, R. M., Weiss, R., Xu, G., et al.: A major segment of the neurofibromatosis type 1 gene: cDNA sequence, genomic structure, and point mutations. Cell 62:193, 1990.

322. Fearon, E. R., and Vogelstein, B.: A genetic model for colorectal tumorigenesis. Cell 61:759, 1990.

323. Groden, J., Thliveris, A., Samowitz, W., et al.: Identification and characterization of the familial adenomatous polyposis coli gene. Cell 66:589, 1991.

324. Kinzler, K. W., Nilbert, M. C., Vogelstein, B., et al.: Identification of a gene located at chromosome 5q21 that is mutated in colorectal cancers. Science 251:1366, 1991.

325. Kinzler, K. W., Nilbert, M. C., Su, L.-K., et al.: Identification of FAP locus genes from chromosome 5q21. Science 253:661, 1991.

326. Su, L.-K., Kinzler, K. W., Vogelstein, B., Preisinger, A. C., Moser, A. R., Luongo, C., Gould, K. A., and Dove, W. F.: Multiple intestinal neoplasia caused by a mutation in the murine homolog of the APC gene. Science 256:668, 1992.

327. Levine, A. J., Momand, J., and Finlay, C. A.: The p53 tumour suppressor gene. Nature 351:453, 1991.

328. Lane, D. P., and Crawford, L. V.: T antigen is bound to a host protein in SV40-transformed cells. Nature 278:261, 1979.

329. Finlay, C. A., Hinds, P. W., and Levine, A. J.: The p53 proto-oncogene can act as a suppressor of transformation. Cell 57:1083, 1989.

330. Mulligan, L. M., Matlashewski, G. J., Scrable, H. J., and Cavenee, W. K.: Mechanisms of p53 loss in human sarcomas. Proc. Natl. Acad. Sci. USA 87:5863, 1990.

331. Hollstein, M., Sidransky, D., Vogelstein, B., and Harris, C. C.: p53 mutations in human cancers. Science 253:49, 1991.

332. Malkin, D., Li, F. P., Strong, L. C., et al.: Germ line p53 mutations in a familial syndrome of breast cancer, sarcomas, and other neoplasms. Science 250:1233, 1990.

333. Srivastava, S. K., Zou, Z. Q., Pirollow, K., Blattner, W., and Chang, E. H.: Germ-line transmission of a mutated p53 gene in a cancer-prone family with Li-Fraumini syndrome. Nature 348:747, 1990.

334. Frebourg, T., Kassel, J., Lam, K. T., Gryka, M. A., Barbier, N., Andersen, T. I., Børresen, A.-L., and Friend, S. H.: Germ-line mutations of the p53 tumor suppressor gene in patients with high risk for cancer inactivate the p53 protein. Proc. Acad. Sci. USA 89:6413, 1992.

335. Srivastava, S., Tong, Y. A., Devadas, K., Zou, Z.-Q., Sykes, V. W., Chen, Y., Blattner, W. A., Pirollo, K., and Chang, E. H.: Detection of both mutant and wild-type p53 protein in normal skin fibroblasts and demonstration of a shared 'second hit' on p53 in diverse tumors from a cancer-prone family with Li-Fraumini syndrome. Oncogene 7:987, 1992.

336. Damm, K., Thompson, C. C., and Evans, R. M.: Protein

337. Sharif, M., and Privalsky, M. L.: v-erbA Oncogene function in neoplasia correlates with its ability to repress retinoic acid receptor action. Cell 66:885, 1991.

338. Kitayama, H., Sugimoto, Y., Matsuzaki, T., Ikawa, Y., and Noda, M.: A ras-related gene with transformation suppressor activity. Cell 56:77, 1989.

339. Pizon, V., Chardin, P., Lerosey, I. B. O., and Tavitian, A.: Human cDNAs rap1 and rap2 homologous to the Drosophila gene dras3 encode proteins closely related to ras in the "effector" region. Oncogene 3:201, 1988.

340. Lee, W.-H., Shew, J.-Y., Hong, F. D., Sery, T. W., Donoso, L. A., Young, L.-J., Bookstein, R., and Lee, E. Y.-H. P.: The retinoblastoma susceptibility gene encodes a nuclear phosphoprotein associated with DNA binding activity. Nature 319:642, 1987.

341. Dyson, N., Howley, P. M., Munger, K., and Harlow, E.: The human papilloma virus-16 E7 oncoprotein is able to bind to the retinoblastoma gene product. Science 243:934, 1989.

342. Ludlow, J. W., DeCaprio, J. A., Huang, C.-M., Lee, W.-H., Paucha, E., and Livingston, D. M.: SV40 large T antigen binds preferentially to an underphosphorylated member of the retinoblastoma susceptibility gene product family. Cell 56:57, 1989.

343. Robbins, P. D., Horowitz, J. M., and Mulligan, R. C.: Negative regulation of human c-fos expression by the retinoblastoma gene product. Nature 346:668, 1990.

344. Lin, B. T.-Y., Gruenwald, S., Morla, A. O., Lee, W.-H., and Wang, J. Y. J.: Retinoblastoma cancer suppressor gene product is a substrate of the cell cycle regulator cdc2 kinase. EMBO J. 10:857, 1991.

345. Pietenpol, J. A., Stein, R. A., Moran, E., et al.: Transforming growth factor beta 1 suppression of c-myc gene transcription: Role in inhibition of keratinocyte proliferation. Proc. Natl. Acad. Sci. USA 87:3758, 1990.

346. Chellappan, S. P., Hiebert, S., Mudryj, M., Horowitz, J. M., and Nevins, J. R.: The E2F transcription factor is a cellular target for the RB protein. Cell 65:1053, 1991.

347. Helin, K., Lees, J. A., Vidal, M., Dyson, N., Harlow, E., and Fattaey, A.: A cDNA encoding a PRB-binding protein with properties of the transcription factor E2F. Cell 70:337, 1992.

348. Chellappan, S., Kraus, V. B., Kroger, B., Munger, K., Howley, P. M., Phelps, W. C., and Nevins, J. R.: Andeovirus E1A, simian virus 40 tumor antigen, and human papillomavirus E7 protein share the capacity to disrupt the interaction between transcription factor E2F and the retinoblastoma gene product. Proc. Natl. Acad. Sci. USA 89:4549, 1992.

349. Donehower, L. A., Harvey, M., Slagle, B. L., McArthur, M. J., Montgomery, C. A., Butel, J. S., and Bradley, A.: Mice deficient for p53 are developmentally normal but susceptible to spontaneous tumours. Nature 356:215, 1992.

350. Hinds, P. W., Finlay, C. A., Quartin, R. S., Baker, S. J., Fearon, E. R., Vogelstein, B., and Levine, A. J.: Mutant p53 cDNAs from human colorectal carcinomas can cooperate with ras in transformation of primary rat cells. Cell Growth Diff. 1:571, 1990.

351. Kern, S. E., Pietenpol, J. A., Thiagalingam, S., Seymour, A., Kinzler, K. W., and Vogelstein, B.: Oncogenic forms of p53 inhibit p53-regulated gene expression. Science 256:827, 1992.

352. Fakharzadeh, S. S., Trusko, S. P., and George, D. L.: Tumorigenic potential associated with enhanced expression of a gene that is amplified in a mouse tumor cell line. EMBO J. 10:1565, 1991.

353. Momand, J., Zambetti, G. P., Olson, D. C., George, D., and Levine, A. J.: The mdm-2 oncogene product forms a complex with the p53 protein and inhibits p53-mediated transactivation. Cell 69:1237, 1992.

354. Rauscher, F. J. I., Morris, J. F., Tourney, O. E., Cook, D. M., and Curran, T.: Binding of the Wilms' tumor locus zinc finger protein to the EGF-1 consensus sequence. Science 250:1259, 1990.

355. Madden, S. L., Cook, D. M., Morris, J. F., Gashler, A.,

Sukhatme, V. P., and Rauscher, F. J., III: Transcriptional repression mediated by the WT1 Wilms tumor gene product. Science 253:1550, 1991.

356. Evans, R.: The steroid and thyroid hormone receptor superfamily. Science 240:889, 1988.

357. Disela, C., Glineur, C., Bugge, T., Sap, J., Stengl, G., Dodgson, J., Stunnenberg, H., Beug, H., and Zenke, M.: v-erbA Overexpression is required to extinguish c-erbA function in erythroid cell differentiation and regulation of the erbA target gene CAII. Genes Dev. 5:2033, 1991.

358. Xu, G. F., O'Connell, P., Viskochil, D., et al.: The neurofibromatosis type-1 gene encodes a protein related to GAP. Cell 62:599, 1990.

359. Marchuk, S. A., Saulino, A. M., Tavakkol, R., et al.: cDNA cloning of the type 1 neurofibromatosis gene: Complete sequence of the NF1 gene product. Genomics 11:931, 1991.

360. Ballester, R., Marchuk, D., Boguski, M., Saulino, A., Letcher, R., Wigler, M., and Collins, F.: The NF1 locus encodes a protein functionally related to mammalian GAP and yeast IRA proteins. Cell 63:851, 1990.

361. Martin, G. A., Viskochil, D., Bollag, G., et al.: The GAP-related domain of the neurofibromatosis type-1 gene product interacts with ras p21. Cell 63:843, 1990.

362. Xu, G. F., Lin, B., Tanaka, K., Dunn, D., Wood, D., Gesteland, R., White, R., Weiss, R., and Tamanoi, F.: The catalytic domain of the neurofibromatosis type-1 gene product stimulates ras GTPase and complements IRA mutants of S. cerevisiae. Cell 63:835, 1990.

363. Nishisho, I., Nakamura, Y., Miyoshi, Y., et al.: Mutations of chromosome 5q21 genes in FAP and colorectal cancer patients. Science 253:665, 1991.

364. Fearon, E., Cho, K., Nigro, J., et al.: Identification of a chromosome 18q gene that is altered in colorectal cancers. Science 247:49, 1990.

365. Barbosa, M. S., Edmonds, C., Fisher, C., Schiller, J. T., Lowy, D. R., and Vousden, K. H.: The region of the HPV E7 oncoprotein homologous to adenovirus E1A and SV40 large T-antigen contains separate domains for Rb binding and casein kinase-II phosphorylation. EMBO J. 9:153, 1990.

366. Heck, D. V., Yee, C. L., Howley, P. M., and Münger, K.: Efficiency of binding the retinoblastoma protein correlates with the transforming capacity of the E7 oncoproteins of the human papillomaviruses. Proc. Natl. Acad. Sci. USA 89:4442, 1992.

367. Ewen, M. E., Xing, Y. G., Lawrence, J. B., and Livingston, D. M.: Molecular cloning, chromosomal mapping, and expression of the cDNA for p107, a retinoblastoma gene product-related protein. Cell 66:1155, 1991.

368. Ewen, M. E., Xing, Y. G., Lawrence, J. B., and Livingston, D. M.: Molecular cloning, chromosomal mapping, and expression of the cDNA for p107, a retinoblastoma gene product-related protein. Cell 66:1155, 1991.

369. Sarnow, P., Ho, Y. S., Williams, J., and Levine, A. J.: Adenovirus E1B-58kd tumor antigen and SV40 large tumor antigen are physically associated with the same 54 kd cellular protein in transformed cells. Cell 28:387, 1982.

370. Scheffner, M., Werness, B. A., Huibregtse, J. M., Levine, A. J., and Howley, P. M.: The E6 oncoprotein encoded by human papillomavirus type-16 and type-18 promotes the degradation of p53. Cell 63:1129, 1990.

371. Hubbert, N. L., Sedman, S. A., and Schiller, J. T.: Human papillomavirus type 16 increases the degradation rate of p53 in human keratinocytes. J. Virol. 66:6237, 1992.

372. Scheffner, M., Munger, K., Byrne, J. C., and Howley, P. M.: The state of the p53 and retinoblastoma genes in human cervical carcinoma cell lines. Proc. Natl. Acad. Sci. USA 88:5523, 1991.

373. Wrede, D., Tidy, J. A., Crook, T., Lane, D., and Vousden, K.

H.: Expression of RB and p53 proteins in HPV-positive and HPV-negative cervical carcinoma cell lines. Mol. Carcinogen 4:171, 1991.

374. Courtneidge, S. A., and Smith, A. E.: Polyoma virus transforming protein associates with the product of the c-src cellular gene. Nature 303:435, 1983.

375. Martin, P., Vass, W. C., Schiller, J. T., Lowy, D. R., and Velu, T. J.: The bovine papillomavirus E5 transforming protein can stimulate the transforming activity of EGF and CSF-1 receptors. Cell 59:21, 1989.

376. Petti, L., Nilson, L. A., and Dimaio, D.: Activation of the platelet-derived growth factor receptor by the bovine papillomavirus-E5 transforming protein. EMBO J. 10:845, 1991.

377. Goldstein, D. J., Finbow, M. E., Andresson, T., Mclean, P., Smith, K., Bubb, V., and Schlegel, R.: Bovine papillomavirus-E5 oncoprotein binds to the 16K component of vacuolar H⁺-ATPases. Nature 352:347, 1991.

378. Dotto, G. P., Weinberg, R. A., and Ariza, A.: Malignant transformation of mouse primary keratinocytes by HaSV and its modulation by surrounding normal cells. Proc. Natl. Acad. Sci. USA 85:6389, 1988.

379. Stoker, A. W., Hatier, C., and Bissell, M. J.: The embryonic environment strongly attenuates v-src oncogenesis in mesenchymal and epithelial tissues but not in endothelia. J. Cell Biol. 111:217, 1990.

380. Nuñez, G., London, L., Hockenbery, D., Alexander, M., McDearn, J. P., and Korsmeyer, S. J.: Deregulated Bcl-2 gene expression selectively prolongs survival of growth factor-deprived hemopoietic cell lines. J. Immunol. 144:3602, 1990.

381. Vaux, D., Cory, S., and Adams, J.: BCL2 gene promotes haematopoietic cell survival and cooperates with c-myc to immortalize pre-B cells. Nature 335:440, 1988.

382. Palmieri, S.: Oncogene requirements for tumorigenicity: Cooperative effects between retroviral oncogenes. Curr. Top. Microbiol. Immunol. 148:43, 1989.

383. Graf, T., Ade, N., and Beug, H.: Temperature-sensitive mutant of avian erythroblastosis virus suggests a block of differentiation as mechanism of leukaemogenesis. Nature 257:496, 1978.

384. Graf, T., and Beug, H.: Role of the v-erbA and v-erb-B oncogenes of avian erythroblastosis virus in erythroid cell transformation. Cell 34:7, 1983.

385. Kahn, P., Frykberg, L., Brady, C., Stanley, I., Beug, H., Vennström, B., and Graf, T.: v-erbA cooperates with sarcoma oncogenes in leukemic cell transformation. Cell 45:349, 1986.

386. Muller, W. J., Sinn, E., Pattengale, P. K., Wallace, R., and Leder, P.: Single-step induction of mammary adenocarcinoma in transgenic mice bearing te activated c-neu oncogene. Cell 54:105, 1988.

387. Bouchard, L., Lamarre, L., Tremblay, P. J., and Jolicoeur, P.: Stoichastic appearance of mammary tumors in transgenic mice carrying the MMTV/c-neu oncogene. Cell 57:931, 1989.

388. Adams, J. M., Harris, A. W., Pinkert, C. A., Corcoran, L. M., Alexander, W. S., Cory, S., Palmiter, R. D., and Brinster, R. L.: The c-myc oncogene driven by immunoglobulin enhancers induces lymphoid malignancy in transgenic mice. Nature 318:533, 1985.

389. Liotta, L. A., Steeg, P. S., and Stetler-Stevenson, W. G.: Cancer metastasis and angiogenesis: An imbalance of positive and negative regulation. Cell 64:327, 1991.

ACKNOWLEDGMENTS: We thank Harold Varmus for many constructive suggestions and Laura Ricker for assistance in preparing the figures.

Mechanisms of Leukemogenesis

Owen N. Witte

INTRODUCTION

The goal of this chapter is to describe the range of mechanisms that have been identified to play a role in the causation of human and selected animal models of leukemia and lymphoma. The text is not intended to be comprehensive, but rather selective of those examples that are best defined or provocative. Because the literature on animal models for leukemia is so vast, examples have generally been chosen to complement or contrast with examples taken from human diseases.

This chapter centers on families of biochemical mechanisms rather than a disease-based organization (see Fig. 24–1 for a schematic overview). Certain leukemias are used to exemplify a variety of concepts. Knowledge of the clinical descriptions of various leu-kemias is assumed, as well as a basic understanding of cell growth control mechanisms, oncogenes, and tumor-suppressor genes, as presented in Chapter 23.

Leukemias and lymphomas must be considered in the light of the larger field of oncogenesis. The step-wise accumulation of genetic damage leading to a progressively malignant phenotype is a critical feature of leukemias, as it is for cancer in general. In almost every case a combination of genetic changes is found associated with the progression to frank leukemia in both human and animal models. Repeated association of changes in cancer genes with specific leukemias strengthens our belief that such mutations are crucial components of the disease.

Only recently have we begun to draw together the biochemical mechanisms that regulate cell growth.

_es_

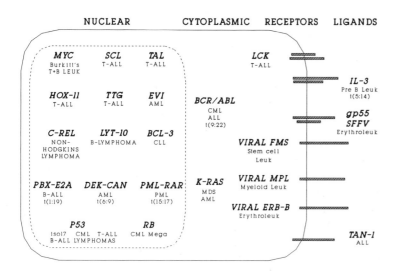

NUCLEAR   CYTOPLASMIC   RECEPTORS   LIGANDS

MYC Burkitt's T+B LEUK	*SCL* T-ALL	*TAL* T-ALL
HOX-11 T-ALL	*TTG* T-ALL	*EVI* AML
C-REL NON-HODGKINS LYMPHOMA	*LYT-10* B-LYMPHOMA	*BCL-3* CLL
PBX-E2A B-ALL t(1:19)	*DEK-CAN* AML t(6:9)	*PML-RAR* PML t(15:17)
P53 Isol7 CML T-ALL B-ALL LYMPHOMAS	*RB* CML Mega	

LCK T-ALL

BCR/ABL CML ALL t(9:22)

K-RAS MDS AML

VIRAL FMS Stem cell Leuk

VIRAL MPL Myeloid Leuk

VIRAL ERB-B Erythroleuk

IL-3 Pre B Leuk t(5:14)

gp55 SFFV Erythroleuk

TAN-1 ALL

FIGURE 24–1. Leukemia oncogenes.

Normal hematopoiesis is regulated by cell autonomous controls, as well as the influence of soluble and cell-bound growth factors. Signal transduction from the cytoplasm to the nucleus can be altered by changes in expression and the mutation of numerous proto-oncogenes. We consider changes in growth factor production, receptor expression and mutation, somatic mutations of cytoplasmic signaling components, and changes in transcription factor–derived oncogenes in separate sections. These divisions are used with the understanding that various combinations of mutations are usually required to produce a leukemia. A final section on cooperative oncogene effects in leukemogenesis presents selected examples of this important concept.

CELL SURFACE INTERACTIONS AS REGULATORS OF HEMATOPOIESIS AND PART OF THE LEUKEMOGENIC PROCESS

Peptide Growth and Differentiation Factors

The wealth of information defining the molecular structures of hematopoietic growth and differentiation factors and their receptors now dominates much of the field of experimental hematopoiesis.[1–3] Each factor and its cognate receptor can transmit a signal across the membrane. Some of the signals may be positive ones for growth, whereas others may suppress growth or favor differentiation. All types of additive, synergistic, or antagonistic combinations have been demonstrated in a wide range of cultured cells, as well as in animals.

Growth factors can interact in several ways with their receptors to generate an intracellular signal. Many factors are released as soluble molecules and travel through the blood stream or intercellular space to interact with receptors on other cells in a manner analogous to hormone or endocrine loops. Erythropoietin produced in the kidney must circulate to the bone marrow to affect red blood cell precursors. Some factors produced by stromal cells in the bone marrow, like interleukin(IL)-7 and granulocyte colony-stimulating factor (G-CSF), are released in soluble form and presumably function both within the local environment and after release into the general circulation.

Genes encoding other factors, such as macrophage (M)-CSF and Steel locus factor (SLF) (product of the Steel locus) produce a membrane-bound as well as a soluble form. This is usually accomplished by differential splicing to generate separate mRNAs that encode a transmembrane form expressed on the cell surface and a second form that contains a proteolytic cleavage site that results in release of a soluble molecule.[4–6] The action of the cell-bound molecule requires cell-cell contact. The soluble form could work locally or at a distance. The soluble form could act as an antagonist of the membrane-bound form by competing for the same receptor sites and blocking strong cell-cell contact.

The production of some factors, such as IL-2, can be stimulated by other factors or even by itself. One of the target cells responding to IL-2 is the same T lymphocyte triggered to produce the factor.[7–9] In such an autocrine production and response cycle, the factor could stimulate the cell by being released from the cell and binding back to an extracellular receptor, or possibly binding to the receptor while both are found within the endoplasmic reticulum or another internal membrane space. In either case, the local concentration of factor would be very high and the resulting growth stimulation potent. Factor released from the cell could, of course, stimulate neighboring cells, or distant cells if the concentration reached high enough levels.

Despite the large number of factors identified, relatively few examples of alteration of expression are correlated with definitive clonal overgrowth and leukemogenesis in humans. The specific activation of the IL-3 gene by the t(5:14) translocation in a subset of patients with acute pre–B-cell leukemias is well documented.[10] In this case the immunoglobulin heavy chain locus is joined to the promoter region of the IL-3 gene and results in an increase in expression and presumably an increase in factor level resulting in an autocrine loop. The precise role of this event along the pathway of leukemogenesis is not demonstrated.

Closely related studies in animal models suggest that such autocrine loops are unlikely to be sufficient explanations for the full leukemic phenotype. Forced expression of the IL-3 gene via retroviral vectors in mice results in a hyperplastic expansion of immature myeloid cells, but not a true malignancy. Similar studies on forced expression of GM-CSF or IL-7 in both in vitro and in vivo settings show that growth factor independence is a consequence of hyperexpression but is not consistently linked to malignant behavior of the cells.[11–13]

Other modes of activation of growth factor genes include the insertion of a retroviral provirus or a closely related intracellular mobile genetic element called an IAP (for intracisternal A particle) type of genome. The strong transcriptional enhancer activity of such genomes or their promoters can influence expression of neighboring genes. In a well-studied murine myelomonocytic tumor called WEHI-3, one activating mutation is the insertional activation of the IL-3 gene.[14] This results in an overexpression and autocrine stimulation of the cell. The full tumor phenotype requires additional changes, which are discussed in the section on co-operative oncogene effects in leukemia (see below).

Pseudoligand Stimulation of Receptors as Part of the Leukemic Process

The specificity of action of growth factors and their receptors is largely dictated by the distribution of the receptor. One of the most restricted of the hematopoietic receptors is that for erythropoietin (Epo), which is found on red blood cell precursors and megakaryocytes. The biological activity of the Friend murine leukemia virus complex depends on the distribution of the Epo receptor. This viral complex is composed of the replication-defective spleen focus forming virus (SFFV) and its replication-competent helper virus, called the Friend murine leukemia virus (F-MuLV). Together they efficiently cause erythroid hyperplasia in the spleen and marrow in susceptible mouse strains, followed by the outgrowth of highly leukemic erythroid tumors in many cases.[15]

Unlike most replication-defective, rapidly transforming retroviruses, the SFFV genome does not capture a cellular oncogene. The only gene product of SFFV is a glycoprotein of about 55,000 molecular weight (gp55), a truncated and mutated form of a retroviral envelope glycoprotein. The gp55 molecule is expressed from the integrated retroviral genome and processed by cellular pathways. This viral glycoprotein can bind to and stimulate the erythropoietin receptor by acting as a pseudoligand, which leads to an autocrine loop and hyperplasia.[16]

Does the early hyperplastic phase of the disease result from stimulation through the Epo receptor? One strategy to test this idea is to alter the receptor directly and test its potency to induce erythroid hyperplasia and malignant progression in a growth factor–independent fashion. Retroviral transplantation of a constitutively active form of the Epo receptor into growth factor–dependent cell lines or bone marrow implanted in vivo leads to hyperplasia with growth factor independence and later a malignant phenotype.[17] This strongly supports the idea that stimulation of the receptor alone is sufficient to account for the early effects of the Friend virus complex. It also suggests that the specificity of action of the Epo receptor may require intracellular components present in erythroid precursors, because the retroviral delivery system would be expected to gain access to multiple cell types but the biological response is highly restricted.

Mutations in Growth Factor Receptors Not Commonly Found in Association with Human Leukemias

Two large families of growth factor receptors have been described. One group is clearly related through their common enzymatic activity as tyrosine kinases[18] and includes the receptors for M-CSF, the product of the c-FMS proto-oncogene and receptor for the Steel factor (the product of c-KIT). Complexing of each receptor with its ligand leads to rapid autophosphorylation and transphosphorylation of cellular proteins. The presence of phosphotyrosine can help to trigger the assembly of multicomponent signaling complexes believed to be important in transmission of growth signals to the nucleus. The second group is called the cytokine receptor superfamily[19] and includes the receptors for IL-3, IL-4, IL-6, IL-7, GM-CSF, Epo, and others. Although it is not known precisely how these receptors transmit signals to the cell interior, stimulation with the appropriate ligand can again lead to the phosphorylation of tyrosine in cellular proteins. Presumably, members of the cytoplasmic tyrosine kinase group are activated by changes in the receptors.

One might imagine that an increase in receptor number alone could either lead to more sensitive signaling with a low level of cognate factor or increase the chance of ligand-independent stimulation through receptor oligomerization. Amplification of the HER-2/NEU tyrosine kinase receptor has been correlated with poor prognosis in metastatic breast carcinoma.[20] No comparable situations are commonly described for human leukemias.

Experimental animal models have documented a number of important mechanisms that alter growth factor receptors and lead to the development of leukemia. One of the best-described models is that of the avian erythroblastosis virus, or AEV. When inoculated into susceptible strains of chickens, AEV induces polyclonal hyperplasia of erythroid precursors. Other types of pathology, including fibrosarcomas, can also occur. A genetic analysis of this viral system has shown that two genes called v-erbA and v-erbB are required for the fully transformed phenotype.[21] The v-erbA gene is derived from the avian analogue of a member of the thyroid hormone receptor superfamily. The v-erbB gene is derived from the epidermal growth factor receptor gene. Several lines of evidence suggest that v-erbA arrests cell maturation, whereas v-erbB provides a strong mitogenic signal acting as a ligand-independent and constitutively active tyrosine kinase.[22, 23] In birds, the c-erbB gene likely plays a role in normal erythroid development,[24] as judged by its normal expression in red blood cell precursors. In mammals the epidermal growth factor (EGF) receptor does not appear to be expressed in hematopoietic cells.

The mechanism of activation of the c-erbB gene has been extensively studied in mammals as well as in birds. Activation of this family of receptors is initiated by ligand binding, followed by receptor dimerization and perhaps the formation of higher multimers.[18] This latter step appears to be important for the generation of the transmembrane signals necessary for autophosphorylation, and transphosphorylation of receptor molecules and cellular substrates. Mutations in both the extracellular domain and the intracellular kinase domain can lead to constitutive activation of the tyrosine kinase activity and correlate with transformation activity for this family of receptors. Genetic damage of even a very subtle nature, including single point mutations, has been shown to activate transforming potency. Some of these single point mutations may function through an increased tendency for the receptor to dimerize and transphosphorylate in a ligand-independent manner.

Activated forms of such receptors would be expected to have profound growth effects on a wide variety of blood cell types. When an activated form of c-FMS (the receptor for M-CSF) was introduced into murine bone marrow cells and reimplanted in vivo, a broad range of leukemias were induced, including some with characteristics of stem cell leukemias.[25] Surprisingly, no clear example of an activated tyrosine kinase transmembrane receptor acting as a dominant oncogene is available from the study of naturally occurring human leukemias. This may be due to the subtle nature of activating mutations, which would escape detection by screening techniques like DNA blotting methods or immunoblotting for protein products.

One perplexing connection has been made between the c-FMS oncogene and the myelodysplastic syndrome (MDS) associated with interstitial deletions of chromosome 5. The region of chromosome 5 deleted can vary over a large chromosomal distance but frequently includes a region that normally harbors an array of growth factor genes, including IL-3, IL-4, IL-5, IL-9, GM-CSF, and M-CSF. In addition, several growth factor receptors, including the PDGF receptor and the M-CSF receptor, often fall within the deleted region. MDS is usually thought of as a preleukemic

syndrome, in which marrow cellularity is increased but is accompanied by a failure to differentiate, resulting in low numbers of cells in the peripheral circulation. Development of myeloid leukemias, especially of the myelomonocytic type, occurs as a secondary event.[26]

It is not clear that deletion of any of the known regulator genes is critical in the development of MDS. It seems more likely that an unknown tumor-suppressor gene is affected by the deletion and accumulates additional mutations to inactivate its function on the second copy of chromosome 5. However, in some reports hemizygous and sometimes homozygous loss of the M-CSF receptor gene has been found.[27] The loss of function of this receptor may somehow blunt maturation and lead to the accumulation of blast cells, which acquire additional mutations during the outgrowth of a subsequent leukemia. It is difficult to reconcile the biology of MDS with the absence of this one receptor, but it provides an interesting avenue to pursue. Recent results have shown that the most commonly deleted region near 5q31.1 associated with myelodysplasia and leukemia contains the IRF-1 (interferon regulatory factor–1) gene. IRF-1 has properties of an antioncogene and is an excellent candidate for the critical gene in this group of hematopoietic disorders.[27a]

No clear examples of hyperexpression or alteration of the cytokine superfamily of receptors have been documented in association with a human leukemia. In addition to the activating mutations described for the erythropoietin receptor (see above), recent work has defined the transforming gene of the murine myeloproliferative leukemia virus as a truncated member of the cytokine superfamily of receptors.[28] The putative receptor gene, called MPL, was incorporated into a rapidly transforming but replication-defective retrovirus. Naturally recovered virus stocks contain a mixture of the transforming genome and a helper virus. Inoculation of this virus complex in mice results in an acute leukemia characterized by expansion of multiple lineages. The normal role for MPL cannot be discerned until its ligand is identified, but it is likely that this receptor regulates growth and maturation of immature stem and progenitor cells for the myeloerythroid lineages.

Changes in Cell Adhesion Properties as Part of the Leukemic Process

The complex processes of migration of cells from the bone marrow, selective adhesion, extravasation at sites of inflammation, and lymphoid tissue homing are regulated by specific protein-protein and protein-carbohydrate interactions.[29–31]

A number of studies have suggested that changes in the adhesive properties of leukemic cells compared with their normal counterparts may be important in the disease process. Studies on murine and human marrow have documented some specific interactions with stroma that regulate adhesion. Some molecules,

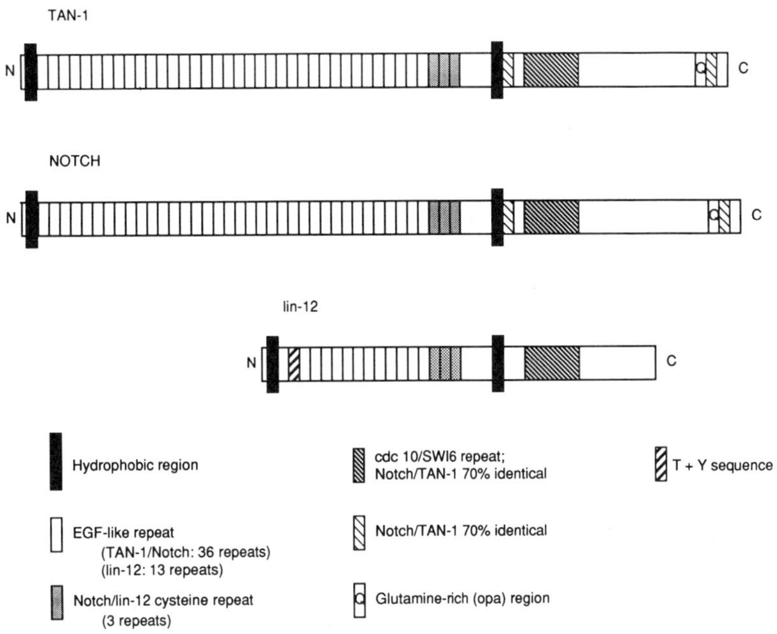

FIGURE 24–2. Schematic alignment of homologous domains in the amino acid sequences for the putative *notch*, *TAN-1*, and *lin-12* proteins. Homologous domains within the three protein sequences are shown and identified individually below. The hydrophobic domain at the N-terminus of all three protein sequences is the presumed signal peptide, and the hydrophobic region in the middle of the three proteins is the supposed transmembrane domain. (From Ellisen, L. W., Bird, J., West, D. C., Soreng, A. L., Reynolds, T. G., Smith, S. D., and Sklar, J.: *TAN-1*, the human homolog of the Drosophila *Notch* gene, is broken by chromosomal translocations in T-lymphoblastic neoplasms. Cell 66:649–661, 1991; with permission. Copyright by Cell Press.)

like hemonectin, bind specifically to cells in the granulocyte lineage.[32] Other studies have documented a role for fibronectin and the integrin VLA-4 in stem and multilineage progenitor cell adhesion.[33] Heparan sulfate has also been implicated in marrow adhesion for early progenitor cells.[34]

Loss of adhesion of progenitor cells from chronic myelogenous leukemia (CML) patients[35] and its reversal with interferon-α have been described.[36] Most of these studies have documented changes in the global property of adhesion to bone marrow stromal lines but have not defined specific changes in the level, structure, or function of the receptor-ligand partners that regulate the cell-cell interaction in question. The cytoadhesion molecule, LFA-3, is generally low in cells of patients with CML. Recently, the amount of LFA-3 has been shown to increase on CML progenitor cells in response to interferon.[37]

One interesting correlation between the action of the MYC oncogene and a change in a cell surface adhesion molecule has been investigated in B lymphoblastoid cells immortalized by Epstein-Barr virus (EBV). The natural history of Burkitt's lymphoma strongly supports the idea that the endemic form of the disease requires the synergistic action of a subset of EBV genes acting in concert with an activated form of the MYC oncogene.[38–40] The activation is usually associated with characteristic chromosome translocations in which transcriptional elements of an immunoglobulin gene are brought into continuity or proximity with the c-MYC gene (see further discussion below). An analogue of this synergy is seen when EBV-immortalized B-lymphoblastoid cell lines are transfected with c-MYC constructs under the control of a constitutive promoter. In some studies, such MYC-expressing lines acquire a more malignant phenotype,

including the ability to clone in soft agar and grow as tumors in nude mice.

Analysis of the EBV plus MYC lines showed a decrease in expression of LFA-1 (lymphoid function antigen number 1), a cell surface glycoprotein of the integrin family known to mediate adhesive properties of lymphocytes.[41] Cells from Burkitt's lymphomas also show a reduction in the expression of LFA-1. It is not clear how this change affects the malignant potential of lymphoid cells, but the finding raises the possibility that downstream effects of oncogenes can include changes in adhesive behavior that form a part of the leukemic phenotype.

A very different type of cell surface molecule has been recently implicated in T-cell leukemias associated with the t(7;9) chromosome translocation.[42] In this case the T-cell receptor β chain gene is rearranged into a specific portion of a cellular gene now called TAN-1 (translocation-associated notch homologue). The name is derived from the homology of the amino acid sequence deduced from the human complementary DNA (cDNA) to an integral cell membrane protein in *Drosophila* called notch (Fig. 24–2). A second gene called *delta*, expressed on a second cell type, encodes a binding partner for *notch*-expressing cells, and both codetermine specific cell fates.

All three proteins contain numerous epidermal growth factor (EGF)–like repeats in the extracellular domain that could function as cell-cell interaction motifs. Additional sequence motifs found within the intracellular portion of this family of molecules include homology to the cdc10/swi6 motif of yeast genes that regulate cell cycle start and cycle-regulated transcription events. These tantalizing homologies do not readily fit into an obvious mode of action, but the multiple extracellular EGF repeats suggest a cell-cell interaction strengthened by the potential multiplicity of binding sites.

The TAN-1 gene is expressed primarily in lymphoid tissues. The structural effect of the t(7;9) translocation is to truncate the TAN-1 gene product within the segment of EGF repeats.[42] This could inactivate the function of this copy of TAN-1, which might behave as a tumor-suppressor gene. This would require inactivation or loss of the other allele of TAN-1. In at least one case a loss of the nontranslocated chromosome 9 has been documented. Alternatively, the predicted truncated extracellular domain of TAN-1 could interrupt the function of the cell-bound form and change adhesive properties. Future work should detail the protein products of the normal and translocated alleles of TAN-1 and directly test their effects on lymphoid growth regulation. In either scenario, the demonstration that multiple cases show interruption of the TAN-1 gene within the same small region strongly supports an involvement in growth deregulation.

INTRACELLULAR SIGNALING MECHANISMS

Introduction

The pathways used to transmit signals from the cell surface to the nucleus to regulate cell division and differential gene expression are numerous. General families of signal transduction mechanisms, such as phosphorylation/dephosphorylation reactions, GTP-binding proteins and associated regulatory proteins, and small second messenger molecules like cAMP, Ca^{2+}, or specific phospholipids, have been defined.[43]

Some signaling components are uniquely expressed in one or a limited number of cell types and are presumed to be critically involved in a signaling function connected to a differentiated phenotype. For example, some members of the SRC family of tyrosine kinases are expressed only in single or closely derived lineages of hematopoietic cells (Table 24–1). The LCK gene product is found in T cells, HCK protein in monocytic and granulocytic cells, FGR protein in granulocytic cells, and BLK protein in B cells. Products of

other members of the SRC family, like FYN, are found in multiple hematopoietic lineages, including T, B, monocytic, and megakaryocytic cells. SRC protein is found in monocytes and in platelets and their precursors, as well as in many non-hematopoietic tissues.[44]

Restricted Expression and Malignant Potential of the p56[LCK] Gene

The p56[LCK] gene was first described as a member of the SRC family of tyrosine kinases activated by a retroviral insertion event in a murine T-cell–derived leukemia. Detailed analysis of its mode of activation showed that there were effects on both transcription and translation activation secondary to disruption of control sequences upstream of the first non-coding exon of the gene.[45] When the LCK gene is expressed in transgenic mice under the control of a lymphoid-specific promoter and enhancer, a direct correlation between higher level of expression and increased frequency of progression to leukemia was observed[46] (Fig. 24–3).

Activation of the LCK gene has been documented in some human T-cell leukemias in which control elements of the T-cell receptor β locus are joined by chromosome translocation to the LCK locus. This leads to activation of expression of the LCK gene as monitored at the RNA level.[47, 48]

Most activations of the SRC family of kinases associated with oncogenesis have documented the critical role of dephosphorylation of a carboxy-terminal tyrosine residue to leave the SRC kinase in the active state.[49] This is accomplished by a wide variety of deletion and substitution mutants within this region in naturally selected SRC variants or by site-directed mutagenesis. This leads to an increase in specific activity of the kinase. LCK can clearly be activated by such a mechanism in the laboratory.

Activation of LCK in leukemias has so far been associated only with an increase in expression of a non-mutated protein in T-cell tumors. This could be due to the trivial reason that specificity of expression has been dictated by promoters specific for T cells or that the original translocation occurred within the T-

TABLE 24–1. RELATIVE EXPRESSION OF *SRC* FAMILY MEMBERS IN SELECTED CELLS OF HEMOPOIETIC ORIGIN*

SRC FAMILY MEMBER	MOLECULAR WEIGHT (kDa)	CELL TYPE						
		T-Cell	B-Cell	NK Cell	Mast Cell	Monocyte	Granulocyte	Platelets
src	60–61	+	−	+	+	+	?	+
fyn	59–60	+	+	+	−	+	?	+
yes	62	+	−	+	+	?	?	+
lyn	55–58	+	+	+	+	+	?	+
lck	56	+	+	+	−	−	−	−
blk	55–58	−	+	−	−	−	−	−
hck	59–64	−	+	−	−	+	+	+
fgr	58	−	+	−	−	+	+	−

*The expression pattern and relative abundance of a given family member were determined by immune complex tyrosine protein kinase assays, alternative splicing of mRNA, or alternative start sites yielding multiple isozymes. (From Bolen, J: Personal communication; and Bolen, J. B., and Burkholdt, A. L.: Signal transduction by the SRC family of tyrosine protein kinases in hemopoietic cells. Cell Gr. Diff. 2:409–414, 1991; with permission.)

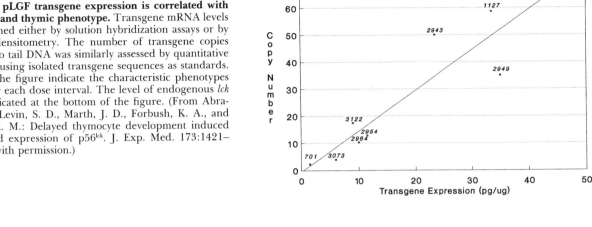

FIGURE 24–3. pLGF transgene expression is correlated with copy number and thymic phenotype. Transgene mRNA levels were determined either by solution hybridization assays or by quantitative densitometry. The number of transgene copies integrated into tail DNA was similarly assessed by quantitative densitometry using isolated transgene sequences as standards. Lines above the figure indicate the characteristic phenotypes observed over each dose interval. The level of endogenous *lck* mRNA is indicated at the bottom of the figure. (From Abraham, K. M., Levin, S. D., Marth, J. D., Forbush, K. A., and Perlmutter, R. M.: Delayed thymocyte development induced by augmented expression of p56^lck. J. Exp. Med. 173:1421–1432, 1991; with permission.)

cell lineage and hence the tumor arose within that cell type. Another consideration is that the mode of action of LCK and hence its oncogenic potency require the coexpression of a T-cell–specific product essential for the regulation or activation of LCK.

Three different T-cell signaling mechanisms have been shown to use unique membrane receptors in association with LCK as a signaling partner. The CD4 and CD8 molecules, which define the major subgroups of helper and cytotoxic killer T cells, have been shown to interact with LCK and likely signal through its tyrosine kinase.[50, 51] In addition, the IL-2 receptor system B chain forms an intermolecular complex with the LCK molecule through sequences within its kinase domain, and extracellular ligand binding triggers activation of the kinase activity of LCK.[52] Recently, a class of glycophospholipid (GPI)-linked lymphocyte surface molecules has been reported to associate specifically with LCK.[53] Cell types that lack the specific transmembrane or GPI receptor molecules might be relatively unaffected by higher doses of LCK kinase.

Viral Transduction and Chromosome Translocation Activating the ABL Tyrosine Kinase

The ABL oncogene was identified in the Abelson leukemia virus isolated from mice inoculated with the Moloney leukemia virus strain and simultaneously treated with corticosteroids to ablate the thymus. Moloney virus normally causes thymic-derived leukemias, and the steroid treatment protected most animals from developing leukemia. A few animals developed lymphosarcomas composed of immature B lymphoid–type cells that could be passaged to secondary animals.[54]

Abelson complex was shown to be a mixture of Moloney leukemia virus and the Abelson virus, which transduced a portion of the cellular ABL proto-oncogene. This results in a partial truncation of the amino-terminal portion of the cellular ABL protein and substitution with part of coding sequences of the GAG

(group antigen) gene in frame with the body of the ABL gene. The GAG-ABL gene product is responsible for all the transforming potentials of the Abelson complex. This protein harbors an intrinsic protein kinase activity that phosphorylates tyrosine residues and is critical for the transforming activity.[55]

The growth properties of a range of hematopoietic cell types can be affected by the Abelson virus complex.[54] Except for continuous fibroblast lines in vitro,[56] no examples of non-hematopoietic tissues transformed by Abelson virus have been reported. The reason for this specificity is not understood. The endogenous ABL gene is widely expressed in both hematopoietic and non-hematopoietic tissues,[57] and hence specificity of coupling to its signal transduction mechanisms would not likely be restricted. Some evidence, based on higher efficiency of lymphoid transformation by chimeric SRC/ABL constructs that retain the kinase domain of ABL, supports the idea that the ABL kinase is more effective at phosphorylation of critical hematopoietic target molecules.[58] The nature of such targets remains unclear.

The chromosomal location of the human ABL proto-oncogene homologue was shown to be on that portion of chromosome 9 commonly involved in the Philadelphia chromosome translocation t(9:22) associated with chronic myelogenous leukemia (CML) and some cases of acute lymphocytic (ALL) and acute myelogenous leukemia (AML).[59] With the use of probes to portions of the ABL gene, genomic fragments were isolated that defined a chromosomal breakpoint that crossed over into chromosome 22 sequences. Probes from this region could be used to define fragment length polymorphisms in other patients with CML and defined a breakpoint cluster region (bcr) for this disease on chromosome 22.[60] Demonstration of an 8.5 kb ABL-related mRNA and a 210,000 MW ABL tyrosine kinase form (P210) in CML cells correlated with an altered restriction map in the bcr region and the presence of the Philadelphia chromosome.[61, 62]

The Philadelphia chromosome results in a chimeric

gene structure that joins a 5' exon of the BCR gene to the majority of the ABL gene exons by messenger RNA (mRNA) splicing (Fig. 24–4). Almost all breakpoints on chromosome 22 in CML fall within a 5 to 6 kb region now defined as the M-bcr, for major bcr region. Several small exons of BCR within this M-bcr region are in the correct reading frame to form chimeric read-through translation products with the ABL gene segment.[61, 63] The breakpoints on chromosome 9 are not as restricted and can range over a 100 kb region. In all cases they fall 5' of the second or common acceptor exon of the ABL gene.

In patients with Ph[1]-positive ALL, the position of the breakpoint on chromosome 22 is much further 5', within the first intron of the BCR gene. This results in a distinctive chimeric mRNA of 7.0 kb and a smaller 185,000 to 190,000 MW BCR-ABL protein (P185 or P190 in various studies). The alternative BCR-ABL forms differ only in the contribution of BCR sequences (see Fig. 24–4). They both contain identical portions of the ABL gene.[64, 65]

Specific Effects of BCR on Transformation

The GAG-ABL form has three critical changes associated with greater kinase function and biological potency. The addition of the GAG gene with its myristylated amino-terminus affects cellular localization and is associated with enhanced transforming activity.[66] The transduction event results in deletion of the SH3 (SRC homology 3) domain, which is known to be a negative regulator of c-ABL activity.[67] A point mutation downstream of the kinase domain that synergizes with the SH3 deletion and GAG sequences affects transformation activity.[68]

Comparison of the alternative forms of the BCR-ABL gene products revealed that both kinase activity and biological potency of the P185 gene product were significantly increased over those of the P210 form.[69] Both forms show retention of the SH3 and SH2 domains, and no somatic mutations occur within the kinase region or elsewhere.[70] BCR sequences within the first exon of BCR (the portion retained in P185) are essential for transformation.[71] Replacement with other sequences, including GAG sequences, is not sufficient for transformation.

One plausible mechanism for the action of BCR sequences on the ABL kinase depends on a strong protein-protein interaction mediated by a high serine- and threonine-rich region encoded by the BCR first exon able to bind to the ABL SH2 domain. The binding requires phosphorylation on serine and threonine residues but does not require phosphotyrosine

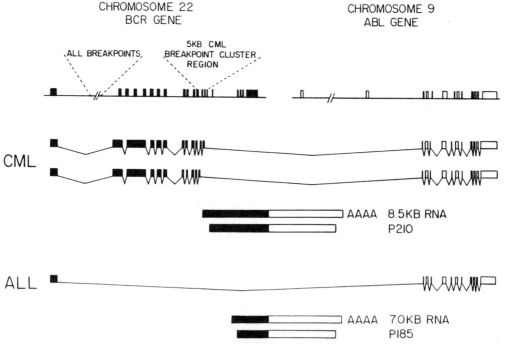

FIGURE 24–4. Production of the P210 and P185 proteins. The approximate genomic structures of the *BCR* and *ABL* genes are shown, with exonic sequences depicted by the open or blackened boxes. The two breakpoint cluster regions and the resulting chimeric RNA and protein products are identified. Translocation of the *ABL* oncogene to the CML breakpoint cluster region (bcr) in the middle of the *BCR* gene results in the expression of 8.5 kb *BCR-ABL* RNA and the P210 protein. *ABL* translocation to the ALL bcr in the 5' portion of the *BCR* gene results in the expression of the 7.0 kb BCR-ABL message and the P185 protein. (From Clark, S. S., Crist, W. M., and Witte, O. N.: Molecular pathogenesis of Rh-positive leukemias. Annu. Rev. Med. 40:113–122, 1989. Reproduced, with permission, from the Annual Review of Medicine, Vol. 40, © 1989 by Annual Reviews, Inc.)

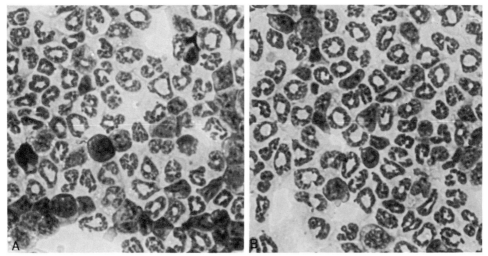

FIGURE 24–5. Morphology of cells from the spleen *(A)* and bone marrow *(B)* of mice presenting with BCR/ABL-induced granulocytosis. Cells were stained with Wright-Giemsa stain (×400).

as do other SH2-binding protein interactions.[72] Precisely how this SH2-binding activity results in alteration of kinase function and transformation is not clear.

The BCR protein is a broadly expressed phosphoprotein of 160,000 MW. The first exon of BCR has been shown to contain a unique type of serine and threonine protein kinase.[73] The role of this kinase activity in the activation of BCR-ABL may be to phosphorylate the region of the first BCR exon required for SH2 binding, but this remains to be directly tested.

The carboxy-terminal segment of BCR has been shown to function as a GTPase-activating protein (GAP) for a specific G protein family member called p21rac. In the P210 BCR-ABL product, the protein kinase of BCR would be linked to ABL, and the GAP portion of BCR could be expressed from the reciprocal translocation partner as an ABL (first exon)–BCR (GAP segment) chimera. As yet, no protein product of this type has been defined.[73a, 73b]

Biological Activities of the BCR-ABL Proteins

BCR-ABL forms engineered for expression from retroviral vectors can be introduced into bone marrow cell populations and selectively cultured on stromal layers that support growth of the early B-cell lineage. Both P210 and P185 result in outgrowths of immature B lineage progenitors or pre-B cells, many of which are initially weakly oncogenic, but after several months of in vitro passage acquire a malignant phenotype when transferred in vivo. The malignant potential of P185 is greater than that of P210, correlating with its greater kinase activity.[74]

The presence of the Philadelphia chromosome in multiple cell lineages within a single patient supports the concept that the primary leukemic cell is either the pluripotential hematopoietic stem cell or a multi-lineage progenitor. Introduction of P210 BCR-ABL

via retroviral vectors into murine bone marrow preparations enriched for stem cells and re-implantation into lethally irradiated animals can yield a range of leukemias. Some of the leukemias have the peripheral blood and marrow picture of the chronic phase of CML with dominance of mature and intermediate myeloid forms[75–77] (Fig. 24–5). Lymphoid leukemias and lymphomas and involvement of other lineages are also seen. Recent improvements in the protocol to generate the CML syndrome in multipotential cells have led to a higher efficiency of transfer of both the chronic phase leukemias and blast crisis development.[78, 78a] Results from transgene studies support the idea that BCR-ABL can affect a wide variety of hematopoietic cell types.[79, 80]

One correlation between higher kinase dosage and more aggressive growth is the occurrence of a second Philadelphia chromosome in CML. Although it is likely that additional genetic damage is required to progress to blast crisis, it is striking that the most common cytogenetic abnormality is a second Ph[1] chromosome. One acute phase patient has been observed with a splicing pattern that deletes the SH3 region of ABL and results in increased kinase activity.[81]

Point Mutations Activating the RAS Oncogene in Human Hematopoietic Disease

The RAS oncogenes are the prototypic transforming alleles of the guanine nucleotide–binding protein family. Activation of transforming activity for RAS is usually associated with specific point mutations that prolong the GTP-bound state and resist the function of the GTPase-activating protein[82] (see Chapter 23). Because these point mutations are so specific, it has been possible to combine the polymerase chain reaction technique with discriminating oligonucleotide probes to identify mutant RAS alleles in clinical materials.

A remarkable range of human tumors are associated with point mutations of members of the RAS family. In human hematopoietic disease there are several striking correlations. In various studies on myelodysplastic syndrome and human acute myelogenous leukemia, up to 40 per cent of the patients were found to have point mutations in the N-RAS allele. Patients with Philadelphia chromosome–negative CML are also frequently positive for RAS point mutations, but those with Philadelphia chromosome–positive CML almost never show such mutations.[83–85] Although other types of leukemias or cell lines derived from leukemias have been reported with RAS mutations, there is no striking pattern to assign a particular biological property to this molecular event.

TRANSCRIPTION FACTORS ACTING AS ONCOGENES IN THE CAUSATION OF HUMAN LEUKEMIAS

Many different types of transcription factors have been implicated in human leukemias and lymphomas (Table 24–2). Many participate in a particular type of chromosomal rearrangement associated with a specific pathology. The activation of the MYC gene in Burkitt's lymphoma by elements of the immunoglobulin genes' transcriptional control regions prompted searches for additional oncogene correlations (Fig. 24–6). The set of transcription factor oncogenes involved in leukemias now includes multiple members of the helix-loop-helix, homeobox, LIM domain, zinc finger, thyroid/steroid receptor, REL domain, and tumor-suppressor oncogene families. In most cases the molecular correlation has not proceeded to functional studies that demonstrate the actions of these putative oncogenes in cell culture or animal models. For this reason, only some examples selected from human leukemias are described in any detail, and when possible compared with information based on better developed animal systems.

Activation of the MYC Oncogene by a Wide Range of Mechanisms that Prolong Its Expression

The c-MYC product belongs to a family of proteins characterized by a set of sequence domains organized for both protein-protein and protein-DNA interactions.[86] The amino-terminal portion of the MYC family proteins is the most highly variable and likely works in the secondary or activating functions associated with the gene. Mutations within this region affect complex and incompletely understood functions, whose effects can be measured indirectly in various transformation assays.[87] The central portion contains a basic amino acid–rich region critical for DNA binding, next to a helix-loop-helix region important for protein-protein interactions. The carboxy-terminal portion contains a leucine zipper domain to mediate homodimeric or heterodimeric interactions.[88] A major advance in understanding MYC function comes from the demonstration that only when bound to a second protein, called MAX, does the heterodimer bind to a specific DNA target sequence (Fig. 24–7). The function of the MYC/MAX dimer appears to be regulated by the level of the MYC protein.[89–91] Recently, two groups[91a, 91b] have identified another partner for MAX, called MAD or MX1-1, which antagonizes the function of MYC by

TABLE 24–2. TRANSCRIPTIONAL REGULATORS NEAR CHROMOSOMAL BREAKPOINTS IN LEUKEMIA AND LYMPHOMA

TYPE	TRANSLOCATION	AFFECTED GENE	DISEASE
Basic helix-loop-helix proteins	t(8;14)(q24;q32)	c-MYC	Burkitt's lymphoma, BL-ALL
	t(2;8)(p12;q24)		
	t(8;22)(q24;q11)		
	t(8;14)(q24;q11)	c-MYC	Acute T-cell leukemia
	t(7;19)(q35;p13)	LYL-1	Acute T-cell leukemia
	t(1;14)(p32;q11)	TAL-1/SCL/TCL-5	Acute T-cell leukemia
	t(7;9)(q35;q34)	TAL-2	Acute T-cell leukemia
LIM proteins	t(11;14)(p15;q11)	Rhombotin 1/Ttg-1	Acute T-cell leukemia
	t(11;14)(p13;q11)	Rhombotin 2/Ttg-2	Acute T-cell leukemia
	t(7;11)(q35;p13)		
Homeodomain proteins	t(10;14)(q24;q11)	HOX-11	Acute T-cell leukemia
	t(7;10)(q35;q24)		
Rel family	t(14;19)(q32;q13.1)	BCL-3	Chronic B-cell leukemia
	t(10;14)(q24;q32)	LYT-10	B-cell lymphoma
Gene fusions	t(1;19)(q23;p13.3)	PBX-1 (1q23)	Acute pre–B-cell leukemia
		E2A(19p13.3)	
	t(15;17)(q21;q11–22)	PML(15q21)	Acute myeloid leukemia
		RAR(17q21)	
	t(6;9)(p23;q34)	CAN(6p23)	Acute myeloid leukemia
		DEK(9q34)	

Adapted from Rabbitts, T. H.: Translocations, master genes, and differences between the origins of acute and chronic leukemias. Cell 67:641, 1991; with permission. Copyright by Cell Press.

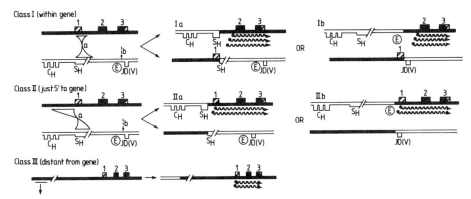

FIGURE 24–6. Three classes of exchange between c-*myc* and the IgH locus, defined by location of the c-*myc* breakpoints. The c-*myc* and IgH genes are in opposite transcriptional orientation, as indicated by placing them either above or below the bar. The IgH gene may be either switched or not, as indicated by the slashed S region. Recombination within the IgH locus is shown (a) within switch (S_H) regions or (b) between the enhancer (E) and the JD(V) gene, resulting in the alternative products shown to the right. Class II translocations have been somewhat arbitrarily defined as falling within approximately 9 kb upstream from exon 1, the position of the *Eco*RI site 5' to human c-*myc*. At least some class III translocations (shown on a reduced scale) may involve recombination within the V_H locus, but that is not shown here because none has been characterized at the molecular level. (From Cory, S.: Activation of cellular oncogenes in hematopoietic cells by chromosome translocation. Adv. Cancer Res. 47:189–234, 1986; with permission.)

both competing for MAX and binding at the same DNA target sequence. MAX can be thought of as a central partner with alternative regulators that have opposite effects at common DNA sites. MAD would be predicted to act as a negative or recessive oncogene.

The level of MYC in normal cells is regulated by a variety of mechanisms. In response to external stimuli like growth factor addition or the expression of certain cytoplasmic oncogenes, MYC mRNA dramatically increases from a low baseline. The response time for MYC is not as rapid as seen for the FOS or JUN oncogene mRNAs but usually occurs within a few hours. The primary mode of regulation appears to be at the level of transcriptional elongation,[92] with significant pause sites within the gene. Additional tight regulation comes from the normally rapid turnover of the mRNA and protein for MYC. The MYC protein autoregulates its own production under certain circumstances. Although conflicting data about autoregulation have come from examination of different cell culture and tumor models, in the case of transgenic mouse strains expressing either c-MYC or N-MYC there is a shut-off of endogenous genes only within the tissues that express the transgene. All of these

controls tend to keep the level of MYC within certain boundaries and regulate the duration of the high level of expression one sees on stimulation of quiescent cells into the cell cycle.[93, 94]

A wide variety of events can involve MYC in an oncogenic process. MYC was originally described as the critical oncogene in several independent strains of acute leukemia viruses of birds. In each case the coding sequences of MYC come under the control of the viral long terminal repeat (LTR), which functions as a constitutive strong promoter. In some cases MYC sequences are fused to viral sequences like the GAG gene. These viruses cause a variety of leukemias, predominantly of the myeloid and macrophage cell lineages.[94]

Another mechanism to activate and deregulate expression of MYC is seen in the insertional mutagenesis caused by the integration of the genome of the avian leukosis virus.[95] The proximity and orientation of the viral LTR to the MYC gene can be quite variable and may work by creating an LTR-MYC fusion message or by influencing the function of the endogenous MYC promoter through the enhancer component of the LTR.[96] In either case, this is a critical part of the pathway of development of leukosis in the chicken bursa. Similar insertional activation of the MYC gene has been documented in a variety of T-cell leukemias in mice, rats, and cats induced by long-latency leukemia viruses.[94]

Chromosome translocations are associated with the activation of MYC in human and murine B-cell lineage lymphoid tumors (see Fig. 24–6). Although the precise structure of the rearrangements and participating immunoglobulin gene heavy and light chain promoter and enhancer segments can vary considerably, the overall effect found in human Burkitt's lymphoma and murine plasmacytomas is the prolonged expression of the MYC gene.[38, 94]

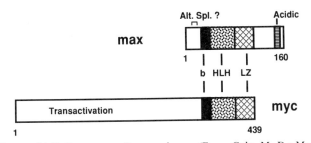

FIGURE 24–7. Structures of *myc* and *max*. (From Cole, M. D.: Myc meets its max. Cell 65:715–716, 1991; with permission. Copyright by Cell Press.)

The biology of endemic African Burkitt's lymphoma and its critical association with prior infection with EBV strongly support the conclusion that MYC is important in progression of the disease. The continued expression of selected EBV proteins suggests that they are critical components to the pathogenesis. For sporadic Burkitt's lymphoma, no clear viral antecedent like EBV is known. The distinctive pathology and epidemiology suggest different mechanisms, but the involvement of the MYC gene is almost universally found.

In many of the chromosome rearrangements involving MYC, the translocation breakpoint occurs within the first intron of the gene, leading to truncation of the first exon. Initially thought to be a non-coding exon, it has been recently shown that an alternative non-AUG codon from this exon can initiate translation and lead to a larger form of MYC protein with an amino-terminal extension. This larger form is expressed in normal cells and in tumor cells with rearrangements that do not truncate the first exon.[97] The role of the larger form has not been elucidated. It is interesting that a liver transcription factor named LAP, a member of the basic region/leucine zipper family, is antagonized by an alternative translation product called LIP that is produced from the same mRNA by utilizing alternative AUGs in the same reading frame.[98] The proteins vary at their amino-termini and compete with each other for effects on specific target genes.

Determining which specific genes are activated or repressed by MYC should help to explain its role in oncogenesis. A variety of potential target genes suppressed by MYC action have been identified, including cell surface molecules like LFA-1 in B-cell lineage lymphoblastoid lines[41] and certain histone genes normally expressed during erythroid cell differentiation.[99] Some genes, such as α-thymosin, are activated by MYC. It has not been established that such activities for MYC are critical for the creation of the transformed state.

The role of MYC as a primary determinant of DNA replication is even more complex and speculative. Actively replicating cells tend to express higher levels of MYC, and terminally differentiated cells tend not to express MYC, although there are notable exceptions to both statements. There is a good correlation of increased MYC expression with lessening of growth factor requirements, increased growth rate, shortening of the G_1 phase of the cell cycle, and block to terminal differentiation in a number of systems. The connection between these cellular phenotypes and MYC is not established. Because MYC is usually expressed well before the onset of S phase, it is unlikely that it plays a direct role in new DNA synthesis, but it could help to establish and regulate origins of replication, although reports of such activity remain controversial.[86, 94]

An alternative mode of action would be for MYC to interact with components of the cell cycle control complexes of various cyclins and associated kinases and regulators. Recently, a direct interaction between the amino-terminal domain of MYC and the retinoblastoma (RB) gene product has been described.[100] The MYC interaction domain appears to bind to the same sequences of RB as the papilloma virus transforming protein E7. Such cooperative effects would be critical during the G_1 phase of the cell cycle and help to regulate entry into the S phase. This is consistent with the timing of MYC expression and response of MYC to various growth factors that function during the G_1 phase of the cell cycle.

HLH Proteins Implicated in Human Leukemias

Additional non-random chromosome translocations have been shown to activate the expression of members of the helix-loop-helix (HLH) family of proteins in cases of T-cell acute lymphoblastic leukemia. Promoter and enhancer elements of several members of the T-cell receptor loci are juxtaposed to genes like LYL-1, TAL-1 (also called SCL or TCL-5 by different labs), and TAL-2.[101] Each of these is related to the HLH family of proteins implicated in developmental switches and transcriptional control. No demonstration of biological activity is yet available, and no test of the relative DNA-binding specificities of the new HLH members and how they relate to the development of the leukemia has yet been developed. Three members of the HLH family are associated with T-cell leukemias when expression of the gene is dictated by fusion with control elements of the T-cell receptor by chromosomal translocation or deletion. This finding suggests that a high level of expression affects common targets of action within T cells.

The TAL-1 (or SCL) gene was identified in the cells of patients with stem-cell or T-cell leukemia. The activation of the SCL gene occurred when a translocation brought the control elements of the T-cell receptor δ locus into the 5' untranslated region of the SCL gene. SCL is expressed in immature hematopoietic cells and is a good candidate for regulating some aspect of early blood cell development.[102, 103] The SCL locus appears transcriptionally complex with alternative promoters and splice variants.[104]

In addition to the translocation mechanism, an interstitial deletion mechanism has recently been identified in a few patients with T-cell ALL. This deletion activates SCL by creating a fusion transcript with a previously unknown gene called SIL.[105] Current evidence suggests that there is no joining of protein-coding information between the two genes. Interestingly, although neither SCL nor SIL is a member of the immunoglobulin family of genes, analysis of the germline sequences surrounding the interstitial deletion shows strong features of the heptamer, spacer, and nonamer sequences used by the immunoglobulin and T-cell receptor recombinase system. The recombined joints show evidence of non-templated nucleotides predicted from the action of terminal transferase.

No evidence exists that either of these genes recombines normally, but it is highly likely that these motifs and the recombinase system are used to generate both the translocation and deletion forms of SCL message found in T-cell leukemias.

Inappropriate Expression of Genes in the Causation of Human Leukemias and Lymphomas

The ability to use molecular probes to immunoglobulin and T-cell receptor gene family members to isolate new translocation breakpoint regions has led to the identification of multiple new candidate oncogenes in human leukemias and lymphomas. The cloning and sequencing of such candidate oncogenes show that many have homology to genes that function as primary regulators of development and usually as transcriptional control elements.

Members of the homeobox gene family were initially defined in insects as the master genes that regulate development of the body plan. Homeodomain-containing proteins have now been found in a wide variety of species, including mouse and man, and have been demonstrated to function in many developmental decisions.[106] Abnormal expression of such genes can affect the growth properties of hematopoietic cells and lead to leukemia. In the murine tumor cell line WEHI-3, a member of the homeobox gene family (HOX 2.6) is activated by insertion of a retrovirus-like genome.[107] The same cell line harbors an activated form of the IL-3 gene. A reconstruction experiment using retroviral vectors to deliver both genes simultaneously to bone marrow progenitors shows the rapid outgrowth of aggressive leukemias.[14] It remains to be determined if an activated growth factor gene is always required for a leukemogenic effect of a homeobox gene family member, but the idea that a growth-stimulus gene would synergize with a developmental regulatory gene is appealing.

Several laboratories have recently identified a homeobox-containing protein (HOX 11) at the site of a chromosome breakpoint in a type of human T-cell leukemia. The gene is transcriptionally activated by the proximity of elements of the T-cell receptor locus.[108–110] The HOX 11 gene is not normally expressed in the thymus. Its ectopic expression within the T-cell lineage could plausibly turn on a set of non–T-cell lineage genes, leading to growth deregulation, or act on genes normally expressed within T cells that have similar control sequences.

Alternative members of a new gene family called TTG or rhombotin 1 and 2 have been defined from chromosome breakpoints in human T-cell ALL patients.[111–113] Different elements of the T-cell receptor loci can be used to activate expression of these genes. The descriptive name of rhombotin comes from the expression pattern of the rhombotin 1 gene in the rhombomeres of the mouse hindbrain during embryonic development.[114] Each family member shows a strong homology with members of the LIM domain group of proteins. LIM denotes the LIN 11, ISL-1, and MEC 3 group of proteins. This group includes DNA-binding proteins and developmental regulators defined in *Caenorhabditis elegans*. Each shares a common cysteine-rich repeat domain that is repeated twice within the amino-terminal half of each protein. LIN 11 and MEC 3 also contain a homeobox domain segment believed to mediate their DNA-binding specificities.[115] The LIM domain may serve as a protein-protein dimerization motif. If this is the case, the rhombotin proteins could serve as abnormal binding partners for members of the LIN 11 or MEC 3 group of proteins and alter their function in either a positive or negative fashion.

Some direct experimental evidence for the action of rhombotin 1 as an oncogene comes from the production of T-cell tumors in mice carrying a transgene expressed under the influence of the T-cell–specific LCK gene promoter. Clones expressing high levels of transcript can develop aggressive tumors that originate in the thymus and metastasize to other lymphoid tissues. There is a 5- to 9-month latency before tumor development. During the preleukemic phase, T-cell development as monitored by composition of thymocyte populations appears to be normal.[116] This suggests that if genes like rhombotin work to deregulate the expression of sets of genes in the T-cell lineage as a part of the leukemic process, these perturbations are not severe enough to block normal development unless complemented by a secondary event.

The Zn Finger Class of Transcriptional Regulators as Oncogenes in Murine and Human Myeloid Leukemias

The Zn finger class of proteins has important roles as transcriptional regulators. One member of this group (EVI-1) was identified near common sites of retroviral integration in a murine model of myeloid leukemogenesis. The distance of the viral integration site from the coding sequences can be up to 100 kb.[117] Viral integration activates the expression of EVI-1, which is not normally expressed in hematopoietic tissues of mouse or man. EVI-1 protein is located in the nucleus and contains multiple Zn fingers organized into two predicted DNA-binding domains.[118] A screen of acute myeloid leukemias showed expression of EVI-1 in about 6 per cent of cases. Different myeloid phenotypes and degrees of aggressiveness were found among the positive cases. A variety of translocations, inversions, and deletions have been mapped near the EVI-1 locus at 3q26 when expression of EVI-1 was found. The structural changes have been mapped by pulse-field gel techniques and can be more than 150 kb away from the locus, either upstream or downstream of its transcriptional control region.[119] The position-independence and long-distance effects of such changes point out the importance of searching for key regulator genes near sites of chromosome

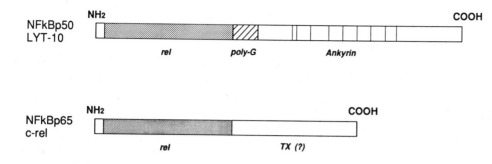

FIGURE 24–8. Schematic representation of the two subfamilies of NF-κB-rel molecules based on sequence homology and domain organization. (From Neri, A., Chang, C.-C., Lombardi, L., Salina, M., Corradini, P., Maiolo, A. T., Chaganti, R. S. K., Dalla-Favera, R.: B cell lymphoma-associated chromosomal translocation involves candidate oncogene *lyc*-10, homologous to NF-kappaB p50. Cell 67:1075–1087, 1991; with permission. Copyright by Cell Press.)

activity even if there is a lack of uniformity in the clinical biology or karyotypes.

Action of Oncogenic Members of the REL Family of Transcriptional Regulators and Their Inhibitors

The REV-T strain of avian retrovirus is replication defective and encodes a truncated and mutated version of the cellular REL gene, which causes rapidly progressive B lineage and myeloid-related leukemias in avian species.[120] The viral form lacks the transcriptional activation function of the cellular form. This fact and additional studies suggest that the viral form is most likely to cause its oncogenic effect by acting as a dominant negative effector to inhibit the action of the normal c-REL gene product.[121]

REL is the prototype of an intriguing family of transcriptional control genes[122] that includes developmental regulators like the *dorsal* gene of *Drosophila*, the members of the NFKB gene family (which control aspects of immunoglobulin and other cellular gene expression[123, 124]), and LYT-10, a putative proto-oncogene found at chromosomal breakpoints in certain human B-cell lymphomas.[125] The REL domain includes sequences important for DNA binding, nuclear localization, protein dimerization, and the sites for inhibitor binding.

The activity of REL-related transcription factors is regulated by interactions with other REL molecules, creating homodimers or heterodimers, and through the action of inhibitory molecules. These inhibitors can be encoded by separate genetic loci or synthesized as a part of REL precursor molecules.[123, 126, 127] Several examples of the group with self-contained inhibitor sequences have been defined. A precursor called p105 is organized with an amino-terminal REL domain, a central polyglycine region for proteolytic cleavage, and a carboxy-terminal domain with ankyrin repeats that inhibit the REL domain. Inhibition by an ankyrin repeat domain is also seen with a separately encoded protein called I-KB, which binds to and sequesters REL members in the cytoplasm.[128] Cleavage of p105 yields a p50 form from the amino-terminus; p50 can participate with other members of the REL family and possible inhibitors to modulate transcription of cellular genes. Other members of the REL family include c-REL itself and p65, which are not regulated by proteolytic cleavage and function as full-length molecules.

Several lines of evidence support involvement of members of the REL family and their inhibitors in the pathogenesis of some human leukemias and lymphomas. Fusion transcripts and amplifications have been found at the human c-REL locus in several non-Hodgkin's lymphomas.[129] The precise effects of such changes are difficult to predict but could act to increase the signals normally sent through the c-REL system or inhibit those signals via an imbalance of dimerization partners. A new member of the self-contained inhibitor class of REL proteins called LYT-10 has been defined in a small number of B-cell lymphoma patients[125] (Fig. 24–8). In these cases, a fusion transcript between the LYT-10 gene and the immunoglobulin α gene constant region is created. This results in the REL domain being separated from the inhibitor ankyrin domain, possibly leaving the REL function in an "on" configuration. Again it is difficult to predict if the growth stimulus associated with the cytogenetic event is working as an excess of REL signaling or through a dominant negative effect created by an imbalance of REL family subunits.

The opposite type of event has also been seen in the activation of the BCL-3 oncogene in chromosomal translocations found in some chronic lymphocytic leukemia patients.[130] BCL-3 encodes a segment of ankyrin repeats analogous to the inhibitor structures of I-KB and the p105 carboxy-terminal segment. Some in vitro evidence suggests that BCL-3 can work as an inhibitor of the p50 REL domain[131] (Baltimore, personal communication). Thus, both the increased expression of a REL-like domain (LYT-10) and the increased expression of a REL inhibitor (BCL-3) may contribute to the pathology of lymphoid tumors. It is not possible to describe any simple mechanism to reconcile these seemingly paradoxical events without considerably more information about the regulation of the REL family of transcription factors.

Chimeric Transcription Factor Exploitation of Functional Domains from Two Components to Create New Oncogenes

Several chromosomal translocations found in specific human leukemias form chimeric genes composed of exons from two genes known to encode transcriptional regulators or proteins with sequence features suggestive of such a function. The translocation breakpoints fall within intronic regions. This produces a primary transcript, which can be spliced to produce a mature mRNA form capable of being translated into a fusion protein. Such gene fusions include the PBX-E2A fusion in pre–B-cell ALL,[132–134] the DEK-CAN fusion found in a subset of myeloid leukemias,[135] and the PML-RAR fusion found in acute promyelocytic leukemia.[136–138] Some recent data suggest that other translocations, such as the t(8:21) found in cases of AML, also create a fusion message,[139–141] but the nature of the genes involved is not fully established. As in the case of the BCR-ABL gene fusion, the reciprocal translocation chromosomes are often retained, and their mRNA and protein products can be demonstrated in some instances. Their functional significance is not clear.

The oncogenic function of such chimeras might result either from the additive function of two components or from a unique synergy codependent on the molecular structure of two joined domains. This issue has been analyzed for MYB-ETS, the chimeric transcription factor–type oncogene of the E26 avian acute leukemia virus.[142] Both MYB and ETS are known to be transcriptional activators. Cellular MYB is essential for myeloid development and, when transduced into certain retroviral forms, can be a potent leukemogenic agent by itself. ETS is known to be a member of a gene family that has been implicated in some human chromosomal translocations[143] as well as other retrovirus-induced tumors.

In the case of the E26 virus, a 135-kDa fusion protein containing a portion of the viral GAG sequence is joined to MYB near its DNA-binding domain, followed by the MYB transactivation domain, followed by the ETS transactivation domain, and ending with the ETS DNA-binding domain. Creation of mutant forms of the virus in which the MYB and ETS domains are coexpressed in *trans* shows a dramatic loss of transforming activity compared with the *cis*-linked structure. Spontaneous mutations that recreate the fused MYB-ETS domain were frequently recovered and are highly transforming (Fig. 24–9). It is not possible to generalize this finding to all the other cases of chimeric transcription factors, but it raises the important concept that a fused gene product may acquire unique activities not found in the sum of its components.

One direct way to create a new specificity of action is to replace the DNA-binding domain of one transcription factor with another. Analysis of the 1:19 pre–B-cell ALL oncogene PBX-E2A shows this style of activation[133, 134] (Fig. 24–10). The E2A protein, which is involved in the regulation of immunoglobulin and other gene expression, has a transactivation domain followed by a leucine zipper, then a DNA-binding and helix-loop-helix motif. The translocation replaces the carboxy-terminal HLH portion of the E2A protein with the homeobox domain–containing portion of the PBX gene (initially referred to as PRL). One can imagine that the specificity of action is deter-

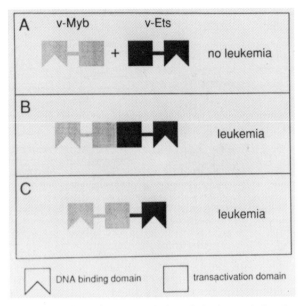

FIGURE 24–9. Schematic representation of virus-encoded Myb and Ets proteins and their leukemogenicity. *A*, Proteins encoded by myb/ets virus constructs. *B*, Protein encoded by the original E26 (myb-ets) virus. *C*, Protein encoded by a fusion-type variant lacking the Ets transactivation domain. (From Metz, T., and Graf, T.: Fusion of the nuclear oncoproteins v-Myb and v-Ets is required for the leukemogenicity of E26 virus. Cell 66:95–105, 1991; with permission. Copyright by Cell Press.)

mined by the new DNA-binding domain, but the degree of action is determined by the transactivation function or perhaps the creation of heterodimers through the leucine zipper domain.

Another potential mode of action for a chimeric oncogene is seen in the case of the PML-RAR product found in acute promyelocytic leukemia. In this case clinical biology and advances in treatment led the way to an understanding of the translocation product. Previous observations on certain AML-derived cell lines suggested that hormones like retinoic acid could induce some leukemias to differentiate to end-stage cells. A remarkably effective trial of all *trans*-retinoic acid on patients with the t(15:17) translocation and a diagnosis of acute promyelocytic leukemia stimulated a search for the connection between the hormone and the differential response of this type of leukemia.[144] Several groups showed that a member of the retinoic acid receptor family (a subgroup of the thyroid-steroid hormone receptor superfamily[145]) was located at the translocation breakpoint and disrupted by the translocation. A chimeric mRNA was created to join most of the coding sequences of the PML gene to the body of the RAR α-type receptor gene.[136–138] The predicted sequence of PML protein shows a very high cysteine and proline content. The cysteines are arranged and spaced similarly to other members of a subgroup of the metal binding or Zn finger domain group of transcriptional activators and DNA-binding proteins. The sequences of RAR α retained in the chimera include the DNA-binding domain and the hormone-responsive element.

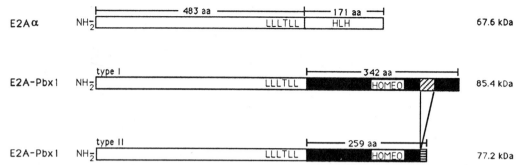

FIGURE 24–10. Linear representations of the proteins encoded by E2A.E12 and the E2A-pr1 mRNAs. As a consequence of translocation, the 171 amino acid carboxy-terminal portion of E2Aα, containing the helix-loop-helix motif (designated HLH), is replaced by 342 or 259 amino acids containing a homeobox (designated homeo) in the type I and type II E2A-pr1 fusion proteins, respectively (shown in the lower two diagrams). The translated sequence spliced in the type I transcript is cross-hatched, and the unique carboxyl-terminus in the type II protein, formed by translation in a second reading frame after excision of the intron, is designated by horizontal stripes. The designation LLLTLL represents a potential leucine zipper motif. The calculated molecular mass of the proteins is shown on the right. (From Kamps, M. P., Murre, C., Sun, X.-H., and Baltimore, D.: A new homeobox gene contributes the DNA binding domain of the t(1;19) translocation protein in pre-B ALL. Cell 60:547–555, 1990; with permission. Copyright by Cell Press.)

In functional studies, PML-RAR works as a weak retinoic acid–responsive transactivator. One attractive model for its function in the generation of the leukemic phenotype is that the chimeric gene product functions in a dominant negative mode over the normal RAR receptor at physiological concentrations of hormone.[146, 147] When supranormal dosages of retinoic acid are used, the chimeric receptor could now function in a positive manner, analogous to the wild type, and enhance differentiation. Further work is needed to exclude other possible modes of action for the chimeric receptor. Additional support for this type of mechanism comes from studies on the v-*erbA* oncogene, which was first identified in the avian erythroblastosis virus. Several types of data support the idea that v-*erbA* functions in a dominant negative fashion to prevent the action of not only its normal counterpart, the thyroid hormone receptor, but also related members of the steroid/thyroid superfamily such as the avian retinoic acid receptor.[148] Recently, a new chimeric oncogene encoded by the t(4;11) translocation associated with lymphoid leukemias has been described by two groups.[148a, 148b] The resulting mRNA encodes an over 400 kDa protein that includes sequences of a gene called ALL-1 or HRX with significant homology to the *Drosophila trithorax* gene, a transcriptional regulator of body plan. HRX (ALL-1) has sequence regions consistent with Zn++ finger DNA-binding domains.

PARTICIPATION OF GENES REGULATING PROGRAMMED CELL DEATH IN HUMAN LEUKEMIAS AND LYMPHOMAS

Cell death can be a specific developmental fate. The decision for specific cells to die can be an important signal for the growth and differentiation of other cells within a local environment.[149] Lymphoid cells of both the T- and B-cell lineages appear to use programmed cell death to regulate the numbers of immature precursor cells leaving the marrow and thymus, as well as balancing and selecting the peripheral pool of antigen-reactive cells in the lymph nodes and spleen.

Programmed cell death or apoptosis can be induced by positive mechanisms such as the addition of specific factors, cytotoxic drugs, monoclonal antibodies, or cell-cell contact, as well as negative mechanisms such as the withdrawal of specific growth factors. Apoptotic cell death is characterized by internal cell changes, including nuclear DNA fragmentation that precedes breakdown of the plasma membrane.

A new insight about the genesis of human B-cell follicular lymphoma and chronic lymphocytic leukemia with the t(14:18) or variant translocations involving chromosome 18 has come from the identification of the BCL-2 oncogene.[150–153] Follicular lymphoma is characterized by a relatively indolent proliferation of B-lymphoid cells with the characteristics of outer follicular zone cells surrounding the germinal centers in lymph nodes. The juxtaposition of the immunoglobulin heavy chain enhancer near the BCL-2 locus increases the mRNA level of the oncogene without disrupting its coding sequences.

Several lines of evidence strongly support the role of BCL-2 in the protection of cells from apoptosis. When growth factor–dependent cell lines are infected with constructs expressing BCL-2, they can withstand lengthy periods in the absence of growth factor and return to normal growth upon addition of the factor.[154] In contrast, control cell lines die within a few days. Animals rendered transgenic for BCL-2 under the control of immunoglobulin enhancer and promoter elements show complex phenotypes that include a relative hyperplasia of B lymphocytes (Fig. 24–11). Progression to malignant behavior occurs in concert with the activation of another oncogene, such as MYC.[155–157] These cells appear to represent functional B cells that are generally in a non-cycling state, are

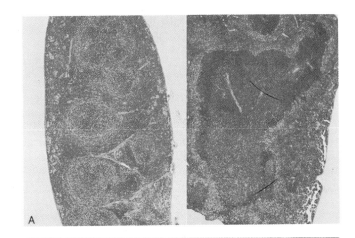

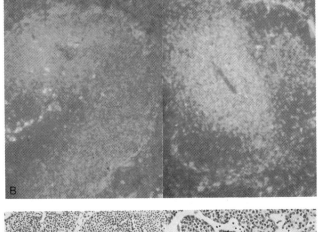

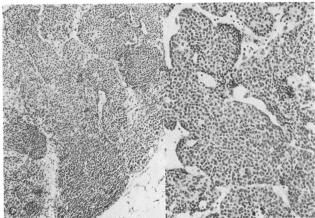

FIGURE 24–11. **Histology of normal and transgenic spleen and lymph node.** *A,* Sections of spleen from a normal littermate (left, ×50) and a 12-week-old M-23 transgenic line (right, ×42), stained with hematoxylin and eosin. *B,* Immunofluorescence photomicrographs of a frozen tissue section (5 μm) of spleen from an 8-week-old M-23 transgenic mouse. Anti-mouse IgM immunofluorescence is displayed on the left (×60) and anti-L3T4 immunofluorescence on the right (×60). *C,* Section of para-aortic lymph node from a 25-week-old M-23 transgenic mouse, stained with hematoxylin and eosin. The paracortical zone and medullary cords (left, ×100) are expanded by a mixed lymphocytic infiltrate of follicular center type cells, immunoblasts, and numerous plasma cells (right, ×240). (From McDonnell, T. J., Deane, N., Platt, F. M., Nunez, G., Jaeger, U., McKearn, J. P., and Korsmeyer, S. J.: *bcl*-2-immunoglobulin transgenic mice demonstrate extended B cell survival and follicular lymphoproliferation. Cell 57:79–88, 1989; with permission. Copyright by Cell Press.)

resistant to death in culture, can respond to antigenic stimuli, prolong B-cell memory, and potentiate autoimmune responses.[158, 159] It is postulated that inappropriate BCL-2 expression may prolong the life of cells normally destined for cell death as part of the maturation of different clones of immune cells within the lymph node or spleen.

The EBV may utilize BCL-2 to prolong the life of cells. The latent membrane protein of EBV, associated with transforming activity, can induce the expression of BCL-2 in B lymphocytes.[160] A variety of human leukemias and lymphomas, including chronic myelogenous leukemia and diffuse lymphomas that do not use specific translocation mechanisms to alter BCL-2, still express high levels of the BCL-2 protein.[161] The precise role of BCL-2 in such settings is difficult to decipher, but an increase in BCL-2 expression may be a common endpoint of different signaling pathways.

Examination of the expression of BCL-2 in normal tissues shows a strong correlation with those sites known or suspected of using apoptosis as a prominent control mechanism, such as T and B cells or tissues with long-lived cell types, including the nervous system.[162, 163] It seems likely that a complex phenotype-like protection from apoptosis is regulated by additional genes that may work in concert with BCL-2.

PROGRESSION OF LEUKEMIA INVOLVING COMBINATIONS OF ONCOGENES

Leukemias, like all cancers, are caused by a series of events that result in the progression of the malignant phenotype through selection of more aggressively growing subclones. There is no simple or consistent pattern to such progressive changes when either different leukemias or patients with the same clinical diagnosis are compared. The fundamental issue is whether certain combinations of oncogenes are synergistically leukemogenic in specific cell types.

The evolution of complex karyotypes during disease progression has been a useful way to dissect possible sequential oncogene changes. In chronic myelogenous leukemia, the Philadelphia chromosome with the BCR-ABL oncogene defines a specific disease state. During progression of the disease to the acute or blast crisis phase, a number of chromosomal changes are commonly observed, including duplication of Ph^1, isochromosome 17, trisomy 8, and trisomy 19.[164, 165] The additional dosage of BCR-ABL caused by a duplicated Ph^1 could plausibly increase the growth signal to the cell and force a more malignant phenotype. Variation in kinase dosage comparing P185 BCR-ABL with P210 BCR-ABL has been associated with a more rapid development of leukemia.[69] Similarly, an increase in chromosome number 8 or 19 increased the dosage of genes like c-MYC (on 8) or AXL and BCL-3 (on 19[130, 166]), but no direct evidence is available to link such a change to the phenotype.

A common secondary oncogene change seen in CML alters the p53 tumor-suppressor gene located on chromosome 17. Using a combination of cytogenetics, DNA blotting, DNA sequencing, and protein serological analyses, up to 25 to 30 per cent of CML patients with blast crisis show a loss of function of p53.[167, 168] This can be accomplished by the deletion of the gene or entire chromosome, mutations within the gene that create premature stop codons, or internal substitutions that destroy normal activity and function as dominant negative mutants (see Chapter 23). Almost all the cases of p53 mutation in CML occur in patients with myeloid type blast crisis. Mutations in p53 are also commonly found in a wide array of other hematopoietic tumors, including T- and B-cell–derived leukemias and lymphomas.[169–172]

Other types of tumor-suppressor genes may play a role in progression of CML. Recent studies have described the association of loss of expression of the retinoblastoma (RB) gene product with the rare megakaryocytic blast crisis of CML.[173] How this correlation will eventually relate to the growth regulation of different hematopoietic sublineages is not clear. Follicular lymphoma is another human disease in which stepwise damage to specific oncogenes was predicted from the evolution of chromosome changes during the course of the disease. Among patients with the t(14:18) which activates the BCL-2 oncogene, a subset progresses to a more acute lymphoma with poor prognosis. Some of these patients show additional translocations involving immunoglobulin loci that activate the expression of the c-MYC gene.[174, 175] This is analogous to the synergy between EBV and MYC translocations in the evolution of Burkitt's lymphoma. In addition, it resembles a situation observed with transgenic mice.[155–157]

These selected cases from human leukemia biology make the point that some combinations are favored but not essential for the progression of certain tumors. To more completely define a set of genes that could participate in the progression of specific types of leukemias, it is instructive to examine models of tumor progression initiated by specific retroviral or transgene expression of oncogenes.

The spleen focus-forming component of the Friend leukemia virus system, as discussed in a prior section, initiates disease by expressing a viral glycoprotein that mimics erythropoietin and stimulates proliferation of immature elements of the red cell lineage via the erythropoietin receptor. When animals develop transmissible leukemias, they show a remarkably high rate of loss of function of the cellular p53 gene through deletion, viral insertions, or point mutations.[15, 176] In addition, more than 30 per cent show activation of a proto-oncogene called SPI-1, which is a member of the ETS family of transcriptional regulators.[177–179] The selective pressure that regulates this specific combination of oncogene alterations is not clear.

An alternative approach to identify the multiple steps in tumor development is to establish animal models in which the probability of tumor development is high, but the latency is relatively long and can be accelerated by specific mutagenic events. Several groups have used mice transgenic for the MYC oncogene in such studies.[144, 180] The secondary activation of additional oncogenes is accomplished by infection with a replication-competent mouse leukemia virus that can integrate randomly and activate neighboring genes. The provirus can serve as a molecular tag to clone the surrounding chromosomal region and identify new transcripts that may harbor new oncogenes. Several new genes have been identified in this manner. They include members of the serine/threonine kinase family (PIM-1) and nuclear proteins with the characteristics of transcriptional regulators (BMI-1).[181, 182] Many tumors show activation of more than one gene and suggest that multiple events may be required for the eventual outgrowth of a malignant clone. What is striking is the high frequency with which some genes are activated in independent tumors. Given the large number of protein kinases in the murine genome, it is intriguing that PIM-1 is activated repetitively. This may reflect some specificity of retroviral insertion or again a specific synergy effective in lymphoid cells.

PRACTICAL IMPACT OF THE STUDY OF ONCOGENES ON THE DIAGNOSIS AND TREATMENT OF LEUKEMIA

The elucidation of specific genetic changes associated with human leukemias has complemented the development of new diagnostic techniques. Cytogenetic analysis by fluorescent in situ hybridization (FISH) on interphase cells increases the sensitivity of detection of specific chromosomal translocations where known oncogene probes are available. Different fluorochromes can be used to tag individual probes, and the relative proximity of two genes or chromosomal regions to each other can be tested. For example, the BCR and ABL genes can be co-localized in CML cells but not in normal peripheral blood or bone marrow cells[183] (Fig. 24–12). Translocations commonly found associated with Burkitt's lymphoma, follicular lymphoma, promyelocytic leukemias, and many others can be followed in this way. The FISH technique should also be very useful to detect any condition in which the normal number of a particular chromosome is changed, such as the trisomic or isochromosomic states found in blast crisis of CML.

Creation of tumor-associated restriction fragment length polymorphisms (RFLPs) can be monitored by restriction enzyme digestion and DNA blotting with specific oncogene probes. They aid in the determination of clonality and are useful for following individual patients for a change in the structure of a particular translocation. Such techniques are moderately sensitive and semiquantitative. Detection of a tumor-specific RFLP represented in about 5 to 10 per cent of the cells is routinely obtained. Although RFLP analysis by the DNA blot procedure is a bit more laborious and time consuming than FISH, the demonstration of a tumor-specific fragment is usually unambiguous.

The initial success of RFLP analysis for the detection of the Philadelphia chromosome was related to the relatively small genomic region on chromosome 22 (major bcr) within which most CML-associated translocations occur.[60] A limited set of restriction digests and a single probe can detect almost all CML-style BCR-ABL translocations. When the genomic bcr is greater than 10 to 20 kb in length, it becomes difficult to use standard RFLP analysis, unless a set of contiguous probes spanning the region is available. For those patients with Philadelphia chromosome–positive CML or ALL whose breakpoint on chromosome 22 falls within the 70 kb first intron of BCR, it is necessary to use a series of probes and several digests to confidently map the breakpoint RFLP.[184] Alternative techniques, such as pulse-field gels, can monitor changes over distances up to several hundred kilobases but are sufficiently complicated that routine use in clinical diagnosis seems unlikely.[185]

The ultrasensitive polymerase chain reaction (PCR) can be used to amplify any segment of DNA and detect length or sequence polymorphisms. This has proved very useful to detect small somatic mutations, such as those that occur during activation of the RAS oncogene, or in many cases of inactivation of the p53 gene.[169] This approach works best for small genes or specific regions of a larger gene.

RNA-based PCR depends on the initial conversion of mRNA to cDNA, which can then be amplified. This is an excellent technique to detect those translocations that join two different gene segments at the mRNA level if sequences on both sides of the junction are known.[186] The alternative BCR-ABL junctions in Ph[1] chromosome–positive leukemias, PML-RAR junctions in promyelocytic leukemia, and PBX-E2A in ALL can

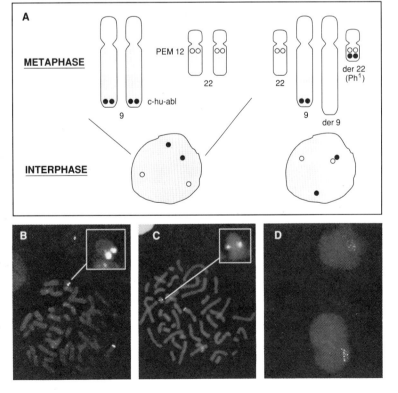

FIGURE 24–12. A, Hybridization patterns for normal and CML metaphase and interphase cells. Closed circles represent red signals from c-hu-abl (abl probe) and open circles represent green signals from PEM 12 (bcr probe). The left side of the figure shows a normal metaphase with c-hu-abl staining near the end of 9q and PEM 12 on proximal 22q. The corresponding interphase hybridization pattern shows random placement of all four signals. The right side of the figure shows a classic Ph[1] in CML. The bcr-abl fusion is represented by one set of red and green signals in close proximity in metaphase and interphase. B, The abl staining localized to telomeric region of a classic Ph[1] in a case of CML (CML-1) with 46,XY,t(9;22)(q34;q11). C, The abl staining is interstitial on the derivative 22 chromosome arising from an insertional event in a case of CML (CML-5) with 46,XY,ins(22;9)(q11;q34q34). D, Interphase cells from the K-562 cell line showing multiple abl signals localized to a region of the interphase nucleus. The same staining pattern was seen with bcr probe, indicating amplification of the bcr-abl fusion gene. (From Tkachuk, D. C., Westbrook, C. A., Andreeff, M., Donlon, T. A., Cleary, M. L., Suryanarayan, K., Homge, M., Redner, A., Gray, J., and Pinkel, D.: Detection of bcr-abl fusion in chronic myelogenous leukemia by in situ hybridization. Science 250:559–562, 1990; with permission. Copyright 1990 by the AAAS.)

all be readily detected in this manner. The extreme sensitivity of this method makes it especially valuable for the detection of minimal residual disease following therapy.[187, 188] As few as one leukemic cell per 100,000 nucleated cells can be detected in most studies. The long-term significance of therapeutic minimal residual disease at this level remains to be determined.

A few available examples show that specific therapies directed toward particular genetic changes can play a role in the treatment of human cancer. As discussed above, the precise mechanism of the retinoic acid effect on the chimeric PML-RAR oncoprotein is not known, but the clinical results are striking. Retinoic acid to induce differentiation and a clinical remission is now commonly used at many centers. Additional chemotherapy is necessary because most patients relapse from retinoic acid therapy alone.

It is easy to imagine that drugs that block the action of BCR-ABL, MYC, or BCL-2 might affect the growth properties of CML, Burkitt's lymphoma, or follicular lymphoma, respectively. Finding specific drugs that selectively impair the function of such proteins in the leukemia cells without undue toxicity to normal cells is a difficult and currently unrealized goal. Other conceivable strategies might be based on inhibition of the expression of specific mRNAs by ribozymes or anti-sense nucleic acids or on site-specific damage to the DNA template by triple helix formation. Many significant problems of drug design and delivery must be overcome if such novel therapeutic approaches have a chance to enter clinical practice. The realization that all leukemias are likely to be the result of sequential combinations of genetic changes complicates the search for effective targeted therapies because it might be necessary to target several genes or to choose the next appropriate target.

ACKNOWLEDGMENTS: I am grateful to my colleagues Bob Eisenman, Stan Korsmeyer, Jim Ihle, Roger Perlmutter, David Baltimore, Tim Hughes, Charles Sawyers, and especially Harold Varmus for many discussions and comments on the manuscript. The citations selected for this chapter represent a small fraction of the vast literature on human and experimental leukemia. In many cases recent reviews or articles were chosen over initial references to provide the interested reader with an overview of the subject. I hope those authors whose work was not directly cited will understand. Julia Shimaoka and Kris Vensel provided excellent and tireless assistance in preparing this manuscript. I gratefully acknowledge the support of the Howard Hughes Medical Institute and the National Cancer Institute for the work in my laboratory.

REFERENCES

1. Arai, K., Lee, F., Miyajima, A., Miyatake, S., Arai, N., and Yokota, T.: Cytokines: Coordinators of immune and inflammatory responses. Ann. Rev. Biochem. 59:783, 1990.
2. Nicola, N. A.: Hemopoietic cell growth factors and their receptors. Ann. Rev. Biochem. 58:45, 1989.
3. Cross, M., and Dexter, T. M.: Growth factors in development, transformation, and tumorigenesis. Cell 64:271, 1991.
4. Sherr, C. J., and Stanley, E. R.: Colony stimulating factor-1 (macrophage colony-stimulating factor). In Sporn, M. B., and Roberts, A. B. (eds.): Handbook of Experimental Pharmacology 95. New York, Springer-Verlag, 1990, p. 667.
5. Stein, J., Borzillo, G. V., and Rettenmier, C. W.: Direct stimulation of cells expressing receptors for macrophage colony-stimulating factor (CSF-1) by a plasma membrane-bound precursor of human CSF-1. Blood 76:1308, 1990.
6. Flanagan, J. G., Chan, D. C., and Leder, P.: Transmembrane form of the kit ligand growth factor is determined by alternative splicing and is missing in the S1^d mutant. Cell 64:1025, 1991.
7. Depper, J. M., Leonard, W. J., Drogula, C., Kronke, M., Waldmann, T. A., and Greene, W. C.: Interleukin 2 (IL-2) augments transcription of the IL-2 receptor gene. Proc. Natl. Acad. Sci. USA 82:4230, 1985.
8. Smith, K. A., and Cantrell, D. A.: Interleukin 2 regulates its own receptors. Proc. Natl. Acad. Sci. USA 82:864, 1985.
9. Meuer, S. C., Hussey, R. E., Cantrell, D. A., Hodgdon, J. C., Schlossman, S. F., Smith, K. A., and Reinherz, E. L.: Triggering of the T3-Ti antigen-receptor complex results in clonal T-cell proliferation through an interleukin 2-dependent autocrine pathway. Proc. Natl. Acad. Sci. USA 81:1509, 1984.
10. Meeker, T. C., Hardy, D., Willman, C., Hogan, T., and Abrams, J.: Activation of the interleukin-3 gene by chromosome translocation in acute lymphocytic leukemia with eosinophilia. Blood 76:285, 1990.
11. Chang, J. M., Metcalf, D., Lang, R. A., Gonda, T. J., and Johnson, G. R.: Nonneoplastic hematopoietic myeloproliferative syndrome induced by dysregulated multi-CSF (IL-3) expression. Blood 73:1487, 1989.
12. Johnson, G. R., Gonda, T. J., Metcalf, D., Hariharan, I. K., and Cory, S.: A lethal myeloproliferative syndrome in mice transplanted with bone marrow cells infected with a retrovirus expressing granulocyte-macrophage colony stimulating factor. EMBO J. 8:441, 1988.
13. Young, J. C., Gishizky, M. L., and Witte, O. N.: Hyperexpression of interleukin-7 is not necessary or sufficient for transformation of a pre-B lymphoid cell line. Mol. Cell. Biol. 11:854, 1991.
14. Perkins, A., Kongsuwan, K., Visvader, J., Adams, J. M., and Cory, S.: Homeobox gene expression plus autocrine growth factor production elicits myeloid leukaemia. Proc. Natl. Acad. Sci. USA 87:8398, 1990.
15. Ben-David, Y., and Bernstein, A.: Friend virus–induced erythroleukemia and the multistage nature of cancer. Cell 66:831, 1991.
16. Li, J.-P., D'Andrea, A. D., Lodish, H. F., and Baltimore, D.: Activation of cell growth by binding of Friend spleen focus-forming virus gp55 glycoprotein to the erythropoietin receptor. Nature 343:762, 1990.
17. Longmore, G. D., and Lodish, H. F.: An activating mutation in the murine erythropoietin receptor induces erythroleukemia in mice: A cytokine receptor superfamily oncogene. Cell 67:1089, 1991.
18. Ullrich, A., and Schlessinger, J.: Signal transduction by receptors with tyrosine kinase activity. Cell 61:203, 1990.
19. Cosman, D., Lyman, S. D., Idzerda, R. L., Beckmann, M. P., Park, L. S., Goodwin, R. G., and March, C. J.: A new cytokine receptor superfamily. Trends Biochem. Sci. 15:265, 1990.
20. Slamon, D. J., Clark, G. M., Wong, S. G., Levin, W. J., Ullrich, A., and McGuire, W. L.: Human breast cancer: Correlation of relapse and survival with amplification of the HER-2/neu oncogene. Science 235:177, 1987.
21. Graf, T., and Beug, H.: Role of the v-erbA and v-erbB oncogenes of avian erythroblastosis virus in erythroid cell transformation. Cell 34:7, 1983.
22. Zenke, M., Muñoz, A., Sap, J., Vennström, B., and Beug, H.: v-ervA oncogene activation entails the loss of hormone-dependent regulator activity of c-erbA. Cell 61:1035, 1990.
23. Hayman, M. J., and Enrietto, P. J.: Cell transformation by the

epidermal growth factor receptor and v-*erbB*. Cancer Cells 3:302, 1991.

24. Pain, B., Woods, C. M., Saez, J., Flickinger, T., Raines, M., Peyrol, S., Moscovici, C., Moscovici, M. G., Kung, H. J., Jurdic, P., Lazarides, E., and Samarut, J.: EGF-R as a hemopoietic growth factor receptor: The c-*erbB* product is present in chicken erythrocytic progenitors and controls their self-renewal. Cell 65:37, 1991.

25. Heard, J. M., Roussel, M. F., Rettenmier, C. W., and Sherr, C. J.: Multilineage hematopoietic disorders induced by transplantation of bone marrow cells expressing the v-*fms* oncogene. Cell 51:663, 1987.

26. Le Beau, M.: Deletions of chromosomes 5 in malignant myeloid disorders. *In* Witte, O. N. (ed.): Oncogenes in the Development of Leukaemia 15. Plainview, Cold Spring Harbor Laboratory Press, 1992, pp. 143–159.

27. Boutwood, J., Rack, K., Kelly, S., Madden, J., Sakaguchi, A. Y., Wang, L-M., Oscier, D. G., Buckle, V. J., and Wainscoat, J. S.: Loss of both CSF1R (FMS) alleles in patients with myelodysplasia and a chromosome 5 deletion. Proc. Natl. Acad. Sci. USA 88:6176, 1991.

27a. Willman, C. L., Sever, C. E., Pallavicini, M. G., Harada, H., Tanaka, N., Slovak, M. L., Yamamoto, H., Harada, K., Meeker, T. C., List, A. F., and Taniguchi, T.: Deletion of IRF-1, mapping to chromosome 5q31.1, in human leukemia and preleukemic myelodysplasia. Science 259:968, 1993.

28. Souyri, M., Vigon, I., Penciolelli, J.-F., Heard, J.-M., Tambourin, P., and Wendling, F.: A putative truncated cytokine receptor gene transduced by the myeloproliferative leukemia virus immortalizes hematopoietic progenitors. Cell 63:1137, 1990.

29. Stoolman, L. M.: Adhesion molecules controlling lymphocyte migration. Cell 56:907, 1989.

30. Osborn, L.: Leukocyte adhesion to endothelium in inflammation. Cell 62:3, 1990.

31. Ruoslahti, E.: Integrins. J. Clin. Invest. 87:1, 1991.

32. Campbell, A. D., Long, M. W., and Wicha, M. S.: Haemonectin, a bone marrow adhesion protein specific for cells of granulocyte lineage. Nature 329:744, 1987.

33. Williams, D. A., Rios, M., Stephens, C., and Patel, V. P.: Fibronectin and VLA-4 in haematopoietic stem cell–microenvironment interactions. Nature 352:438, 1991.

34. Gordon, M. Y., Riley, G. P., and Clarke, D.: Heparan sulfate is necessary for adhesive interactions between human early hemopoietic progenitor cells and the extracellular matrix of the marrow microenvironment. Leukemia 2:804, 1988.

35. Gordon, M. Y., Dowding, C. R., Riley, G. P., Goldman, J. M., and Greaves, M. F.: Altered adhesive interactions with marrow stroma of haematopoietic progenitor cells in chronic myeloid leukaemia. Nature 328:342, 1987.

36. Dowding, C., Guo, A.-P., Osterholz, J., Siczkowski, M., Goldman, J., and Gordon, M.: Interferon-α overrides the deficient adhesion of chronic myeloid leukemia primitive progenitor cells to bone marrow stromal cells. Blood 78:499, 1991.

37. Upadhyaya, G., Guba, S. C., Sih, S. A., Feinberg, A. P., Talpaz, M., Kantarjian, H. M., Deisseroth, A. B., and Emerson, S. G.: Interferon-alpha restores the deficient expression of the cytoadhesion molecule lymphocyte function antigen-3 by chronic myelogenous leukemia progenitor cells. J. Clin. Invest. 88:2131, 1991.

38. Klein, G.: Specific chromosomal translocations and the genesis of B-cell–derived tumors in mice and men. Cell 32:311, 1983.

39. Leder, P., Battey, J., Lenoir, G., Moulding, C., Murphy, W., Potter, H., Stewart, T., and Taub, R.: Translocations among antibody genes in human cancer. Science 222:765, 1983.

40. Cory, S.: Activation of cellular oncogenes in hematopoietic cells by chromosome translocation. Adv. Cancer Res. 47:189, 1986.

41. Inghirami, G., Grignani, F., Sternas, L., Lombardi, L., Knowles, D. M., and Dalla-Favera, R.: Down-regulation of LFA-1 adhesion receptors by C-*myc* oncogene in human B lymphoblastoid cells. Science 250:682, 1990.

42. Ellisen, L. W., Bird, J., West, D. C., Soreng, A. L., Reynolds, T. C., Smith, S. D., and Sklar, J.: *TAN-1*, the human homolog of the Drosophila *Notch* gene, is broken by chromosomal translocations in T lymphoblastic neoplasms. Cell 66:649, 1991.

43. Cantley, L. C., Auger, K. R., Carpenter, C., Duckworth, B., Graziani, A., Kapeller, R., and Soltoff, S.: Oncogenes and signal transduction. Cell 64:281, 1991.

44. Bolen, J. B.: Signal transduction by the SRC family of tyrosine protein kinases in hemopoietic cells. Cell Gr. Diff. 2:409, 1991.

45. Sefton, B. M.: The *lck* tyrosine protein kinase. Oncogene 6:683, 1991.

46. Abraham, K. M., Levin, S. D., Marth, J. D., Forbush, K. A., and Perlmutter, R. M.: Thymic tumorigenesis induced by overexpression of p56^{lck}. Proc. Natl. Acad. Sci. USA 88:3977, 1991.

47. Marth, J. D., Disteche, C., Pravtcheva, D., Ruddle, F., Krebs, E. G., and Perlmutter, R. M.: Localization of a lymphocyte-specific protein tyrosine kinase gene *(lck)* at a site of frequent chromosomal abnormalities in human lymphoma. Proc. Natl. Acad. Sci. USA 83:7400, 1986.

48. Tycko, B., Smith, S. D., and Sklar, J.: Chromosomal translocations joining LCK and TCRB loci in human T cell leukemia. J. Exp. Med. 174:867, 1991.

49. Hunter, T.: A tail of two *src*'s: Mutatis mutandis. Cell 49:1, 1987.

50. Rudd, C. E., Trevillyan, J. M., Dasgupta, J. D., Wong, L. L., and Schlossman, S. F.: The CD4 receptor is complexed in detergent lysates to a protein-tyrosine kinase (pp58) from human T lymphocytes. Proc. Natl. Acad. Sci. USA 85:5190, 1988.

51. Turner, J. M., Brodsky, M. H., Irving, B. A., Levin, S. D., Perlmutter, R. M., and Littman, D. R.: Interaction of the unique N-terminal region of tyrosine kinase p56^{lck} with cytoplasmic domains of CD4 and CD8 is mediated by cysteine motifs. Cell 60:755, 1990.

52. Hatakeyama, M., Kono, T., Kobayashi, N., Kawahara, A., Levin, S. D., Perlmutter, R. M., and Taniguchi, T.: Interaction of the IL-2 receptor with the *src*-family kinase p56^{lck}: Identification of novel intermolecular association. Science 252:1523, 1991.

53. Stefanová, I., Horejsí, V., Ansotegui, I. J., Knapp, W., and Stockinger, H.: GPI-anchored cell-surface molecules complexed to protein tyrosine kinases. Science 254:1016, 1991.

54. Rosenberg, N., and Witte, O. N.: The viral and cellular forms of the Abelson *(abl)* oncogene. Adv. Virus Res. 35:39, 1988.

55. Witte, O. N., Dasgupta, A., and Baltimore, D.: Abelson murine leukemia virus protein is phosphorylated in vitro to form phosphotyrosine. Nature 283:826, 1980.

56. Scher, C. D., and Siegler, R.: Direct transformation of 3T3 cells by Abelson murine leukemia virus. Nature 253:729, 1975.

57. Wang, J. Y. J., and Baltimore, D.: Cellular RNA homologous to the Abelson murine leukemia virus transforming gene: Expression and relationship to the viral sequence. Mol. Cell. Biol. 3:773, 1983.

58. Mathey-Prevot, B., and Baltimore, D.: Recombinants within the tyrosine kinase region v-*abl* and v-*src* identify a v-*abl* segment that confers lymphoid specificity. Mol. Cell. Biol. 8:234, 1988.

59. Heisterkamp, N., Groffen, J., Stephenson, J. R., Spurr, N. K., Goodfellow, P. N., Solomon, E., Carritt, B., and Bodmer, W. F.: Chromosomal localization of human cellular homologues of two viral oncogenes. Nature 299:747, 1982.

60. Groffen, J., Stephenson, J. R., Heisterkamp, N., de Klein, A., Bartram, C. R., and Grosveld, G.: Philadelphia chromosomal breakpoints are clustered within a limited region, bcr, on chromosome 22. Cell 36:93, 1984.

61. Shtivelman, E., Lifshitz, B., Gale, R. P., and Canaani, E.: Fused transcript of *abl* and *bcr* genes in chronic myelogenous leukaemia. Nature 315:550, 1985.

62. Konopka, J. B., Watanabe, S. M., and Witte, O. N.: An alteration of the human c-*abl* protein in K562 leukemia cells

unmasks associated tyrosine kinase activity. Cell 37:1035, 1984.

63. Shtivelman, E., Lifshitz, B., Gale, R. P., Roe, B. A., and Canaani, E.: Alternative splicing of RNAs transcribed from the human abl gene and from the bcr-abl fused gene. Cell 47:277, 1986.

64. Hermans, A., Heisterkamp, N., von Lindern, M., van Baal, S., Meijer, D., van der Plas, D., Wiedemann, L. M., Groffen, J., Bootsma, D., and Grosveld, G.: Unique fusion of bcr and c-abl genes in Philadelphia chromosome positive acute lymphoblastic leukemia. Cell 51:33, 1987.

65. Clark, S. S., McLaughlin, J., Crist, W. M., Champlin, R., and Witte, O. N.: Unique forms of the abl tyrosine kinase distinguish Ph1-positive CML from Ph1-positive ALL. Science 235:85, 1987.

66. Prywes, R., Foulkes, J. G., Rosenberg, N., and Baltimore, D.: Sequences of the A-MuLV protein needed for fibroblast and lymphoid cell transformation. Cell 34:569, 1983.

67. Van Etten, R. A., Jackson, P., and Baltimore, D.: The mouse type IV c-abl gene product is a nuclear protein, and activation of transforming ability is associated with cytoplasmic localization. Cell 58:669, 1989.

68. Shore, S. K., Bogart, S. L., and Reddy, E. P.: Activation of murine c-abl protooncogene: Effect of a point mutation on oncogenic activation. Proc. Natl. Acad. Sci. USA 87:6502, 1990.

69. Lugo, T. G., Pendergast, A., Muller, A. J., and Witte, O. N.: Tyrosine kinase activity and transformation potency of bcr-abl oncogene products. Science 247:1079, 1990.

70. Fainstein, E., Einat, M., Gokkel, E., Marcelle, C., Croce, C. M., Gale, R. P., and Canaani, E.: Nucleotide sequence analysis of human abl and bcr-abl cDNAs. Oncogene 4:1477, 1989.

71. Muller, A. J., Young, J. C., Pendergast, A.-M., Pondel, M., Littman, D. R., and Witte, O. N.: BCR first exon sequences specifically activate the BCR/ABL tyrosine kinase oncogene of Philadelphia chromosome-positive human leukemias. Mol. Cell. Biol. 11:1785, 1991.

72. Pendergast, A. M., Muller, A. J., Havlik, M. H., Maru, Y., and Witte, O. N.: BCR sequences essential for transformation by the BCR/ABL oncogene bind to the ABL SH2 regulatory domain in a non–phosphotyrosine-dependent manner. Cell 66:1, 1991.

73. Maru, Y. M., and Witte, O. N.: The BCR gene encodes a novel serine/threonine kinase activity within a single exon. Cell 67:459, 1991.

73a. Diekmann, D., Brill, S., Garrett, M. D., Totty, N., Hsuan, J., Monfries, C., Hall, C., Lim, L., and Hall, A.: BCR encodes a GTPase activating protein for p21rac. Nature 351:400, 1991.

73b. Melo, J. V., Gordon, D. E., Cross, N. C. P., and Goldman, J. M.: The ABL-BCR fusion gene is expressed in chronic myeloid leukemia. Blood 81:158, 1993.

74. McLaughlin, J., Chianese, E., and Witte, O. N.: Alternative forms of the BCR-ABL oncogene have quantitatively different potencies for stimulation of immature lymphoid cells. Mol. Cell. Biol. 9:1866, 1989.

75. Daley, G. Q., Van Etten, R. A., and Baltimore, D.: Induction of chronic myelogenous leukemia in mice by the P210bcr/abl gene of the Philadelphia chromosome. Science 247:824, 1990.

76. Kelliher, M. A., McLaughlin, J., Witte, O. N., and Rosenberg, N.: Induction of a chronic myelogenous leukemia-like syndrome in mice with v-abl and BCR/ABL. Proc. Natl. Acad. Sci. USA 87:6649, 1990.

77. Elefanty, A. G., Hariharan, I. K., and Cory, S.: bcr-abl, the hallmark of chronic myeloid leukaemia in man, induces multiple haemopoietic neoplasms in mice. EMBO J. 9:1069, 1990.

78. Daley, G. Q., Van Etten, R. A., and Baltimore, D.: Blast crisis in a murine model of chronic myelogenous leukemia. Proc. Natl. Acad. Sci. USA 88:11335, 1991.

78a. Gishizky, M. L., Johnson-White, J., and Witte, O. N.: Efficient transplantation of BCR/ABL induced CML-like syndrome in mice. Proc. Natl. Acad. Sci. USA 90:3755, 1993.

79. Heisterkamp, N., Jenster, G., ten Hoeve, J., Zovich, D., Pattengale, P. K., and Groffen, J.: Acute leukaemia in bcr/abl transgenic mice. Nature 344:251, 1990.

80. Hariharan, I. K., Harris, A. W., Crawford, M., Abud, H., Webb, E., Cory, S., and Adams, J. M.: A bcr-v-abl oncogene induces lymphomas in transgenic mice. Mol. Cell. Biol. 9:2798, 1989.

81. Soekarman, D., van Denderen, J., Hoefsloot, L., Moret, M., Meeuwsen, T., van Baal, J., Hagemeijer, A., and Grosveld, G.: A novel variant of the bcr-abl fusion product in Philadelphia chromosome–positive acute lymphoblastic leukemia. Leukemia 4:397, 1990.

82. Hall, A.: ras and GAP—Who's controlling whom? Cell 61:921, 1990.

83. Cogswell, P. C., Morgan, R., Dunn, M., Neubauer, A., Nelson, P., Poland-Johnston, N. K., Sandberg, A. A., and Liu, E.: Mutations of the Ras protooncogenes in chronic myelogenous leukemia: A high frequency of Ras mutations in bcr/abl rearrangement-negative chronic myelogenous leukemia. Blood 74:2629, 1989.

84. Janssen, J. W. G., Steenvoorden, A. C. M., Lyons, J., Anger, B., Böhlke, J. U., Bos, J. L., Seliger, H., and Bartram, C. R.: RAS gene mutations in acute and chronic myelocytic leukemias, chronic myeloproliferative disorders, and myelodysplastic syndromes. Proc. Natl. Acad. Sci. USA 84:9228, 1987.

85. van Kamp, H., de Pijper, C., Vries, M. V., Bos, J. L., Leeksma, C. H. W., Kerkhofs, H., Willemze, R., Fibbe, W. E., and Landegent, J. E.: Longitudinal analysis of point mutations of the N-ras proto-oncogene in patients with myelodysplasia using archived blood smears. Blood 79:1266, 1992.

86. Lüscher, B., and Eisenman, R. N.: New light on Myc and Myb. Part I. Myc. Genes Devel. 4:2025, 1990.

87. Stone, J., De Lange, T., Ramsya, G., Jakobovits, E., Bishop, J. M., Varmus, H., and Lee, W.: Definition of regions in human c-myc that are involved in transformation and nuclear localization. Mol. Cell. Biol. 7:1697, 1987.

88. Dang, C. V., McGuire, M., Buckmire, M., and Lee, W. M. F.: Involvement of the 'leucine zipper' region in the oligomerization and transforming activity of human c-myc protein. Nature 337:664, 1989.

89. Blackwood, E. M., and Eisenman, R. N.: Max: a helix-loop-helix zipper protein that forms a sequence-specific DNA-binding complex with Myc. Science 251:1211, 1991.

90. Prendergast, G. C., Lawe, D., and Ziff, E. B.: Assocation of Myn, the murine homolog of Max, with c-Myc stimulates methylation-sensitive DNA binding and Ras cotransformation. Cell 65:395, 1991.

91. Cole, M. D.: Myc meets its Max. Cell 65:715, 1991.

91a. Ayer, D. E., Kretzner, L., and Eisenman, R. N.: Mad: A heterodimeric partner for max that antagonizes Myc transcriptional activity. Cell 72:211, 1993.

91b. Zervos, A. S., Gyuris, J., and Brent, R.: Mxil, a protein that specifically interacts with Max to bind Myc-max recognition sites. Cell 72:223, 1993.

92. Bentley, D. L., and Groudine, M.: A block to elongation is largely responsible for decreased transcription of c-myc in differentiated HL60 cells. Nature 321:702, 1986.

93. Eisenman, R. N.: Nuclear oncogenes. In Weinberg, R. A. (ed.): Oncogenes and the Molecular Origins of Cancer. Plainview, Cold Spring Harbor Laboratory Press, 1989, p. 175.

94. Cole, M. D.: The myc oncogene: Its role in transformation and differentiation. Annu. Rev. Genet. 20:361, 1986.

95. Hayward, W. S., Neel, B. G., and Astrin, S. M.: Activation of a cellular onc gene by promoter insertion in ALV-induced lymphoid leukosis. Nature 290:475, 1981.

96. Payne, G., Bishop, J. M., and Varmus, H.: Multiple arrangements of proviral DNA and an activated cellular oncogene (c-myc) in bursal lymphomas. Nature 295:209, 1982.

97. Hann, S. R., King, M. W., Bentley, D. L., Anderson, C. W., and Eisenman, R. N.: A non-AUG translational initiation in c-myc exon 1 generates an N-terminally distinct protein whose synthesis is disrupted in Burkitt's lymphomas. Cell 52:185, 1988.

98. Descombes, P., and Schibler, U.: A liver-enriched transcriptional activator protein, LAP, and a transcriptional inhibitory protein, LIP, are translated from the same mRNA. Cell 67:569, 1991.

99. Cheng, G., and Skoultchi, A. I.: Rapid induction of polyadenylated H1 histone mRNAs in mouse erythroleukemia cells is regulated by c-*myc*. Mol. Cell. Biol. 9:2332, 1989.

100. Rustgi, A. K., Dyson, N., and Bernards, R.: Amino-terminal domains of c-*myc* and N-*myc* proteins mediate binding to the retinoblastoma gene product. Nature 352:541, 1991.

101. Rabbitts, T. H.: Translocations, master genes, and differences between the origins of acute and chronic leukemias. Cell 67:641, 1991.

102. Begley, G. C., Aplan, P. D., Denning, S. M., Haynes, B. F., Waldmann, T. A., and Kirsch, I. R.: The gene SCL is expressed during early hematopoiesis and encodes a differentiation-related DNA-binding motif. Proc. Natl. Acad. Sci. USA 86:10128, 1989.

103. Chen, Q., Cheng, J.-T., Tsai, L.-H., Schneider, N., Buchanan, G., Carroll, A., Crist, W., Ozanne, B., Siciliano, M. J., and Baer, R.: The *tal* gene undergoes chromosome translocation in T cell leukemia and potentially encodes a helix-loop-helix protein. EMBO J. 9:415, 1990.

104. Aplan, P. D., Begley, G. C., Bertness, V., Nussmeier, M. A., Ezquerra, A., Coligan, J., and Kirsch, I. R.: The SCL gene is formed from a transcriptionally complex locus. Mol. Cell. Biol. 10:6426, 1990.

105. Aplan, P. D., Lombardi, D. P., Ginsberg, A. M., Cossman, J., Bertness, V. L., and Kirsch, I. R.: Disruption of the human SCL locus by "illegitimate" V-(D)-J recombinase activity. Science 250:1426, 1990.

106. Scott, M. P., Tumkun, J. W., and Hartzell, G. W. I. I. I.: The structure and function of the homeodomain. Biochim. Biophys. Acta 989:25, 1989.

107. Blatt, C.: The betrayal of homeo box genes in normal development: The link to cancer. Cancer Cells 2:186, 1990.

108. Kennedy, M. A., Gonzalez-Sarmiento, R., Kees, U. R., Lampert, F., Dear, N., Boehm, T., and Rabbitts, T. H.: *HOX11*, a homeobox-containing T-cell oncogene on human chromosome 10q24. Proc. Natl. Acad. Sci. USA 88:8900, 1991.

109. Hatano, M., Roberts, C. W. M., Minden, M., Crist, W. M., and Korsmeyer, S. J.: Deregulation of a homeobox gene, HOX11, by the t(10;14) in T cell leukemia. Science 253:79, 1991.

110. Lu, M., Gong, Z., Shen, W., and Ho, A. D.: The *tcl*-3 proto-oncogene altered by chromosomal translocation in T-cell leukemia codes for a homeobox protein. EMBO J. 10:2905, 1991.

111. Boehm, T., Baer, R., Lavenir, I., Forster, A., Waters, J. J., Nacheva, E., and Rabbitts, T. H.: The mechanism of chromosomal translocation t(11;14) involving the T-cell receptor Cδ locus on human chromosome 14q11 and a transcribed region of chromosome 11p15. EMBO J. 7:385, 1988.

112. McGuire, E. A., Hockett, R. D., Pollock, K. M., Bartholdi, M. F., O'Brien, S. J., and Korsmeyer, S. J.: The t(11;14)(p15;q11) in a T-cell acute lymphoblastic leukemia cell line activates multiple transcripts, including *Ttg-1*, a gene encoding a potential zinc finger protein. Mol. Cell. Biol. 9:2124, 1989.

113. Boehm, T., Foroni, L., Kaneko, Y., Perutz, M. F., and Rabbitts, T. H.: The rhombotin family of cysteine-rich LIM-domain oncogenes: Distinct members are involved in T-cell translocations to human chromosomes 11p15 and 11p13. Proc. Natl. Acad. Sci. USA 88:4367, 1991.

114. Greenberg, J. M., Boehm, T., Sofroniew, M. V., Keynes, R. J., Barton, S. C., Norris, M. L., Surani, M. A., Spillantini, M.-G., and Rabbitts, T. H.: Segmental and developmental regulation of a presumptive T-cell oncogene in the central nervous system. Nature 344:158, 1990.

115. Rabbitts, T. H., and Boehm, T.: LIM domains. Nature 346:418, 1990.

116. McGuire, E. A., Sclar, G. M., Rintoul, C. E., and Korsmeyer, S. J.: Thymic overexpression of Ttg-1 in transgenic mice causes T cell acute lymphoblastic leukemia. Blood 78(Suppl.):78a, 1991.

117. Bartholomew, C., and Ihle, J. N.: Retroviral insertions 90 kb proximal to the *Evi*-1 myeloid transforming gene activate transcription from the normal promoter. Mol. Cell. Biol. 11:1820, 1991.

118. Matsugi, T., Morishita, K., and Ihle, J. N.: Identification, nuclear localization, and DNA-binding activity of the zinc finger protein encoded by the *Evi*-1 myeloid transforming gene. Mol. Cell. Biol. 10:1259, 1990.

119. Morishita, K., Parganas, E., Willman, C. L., Whittaker, M. H., Drabkin, H., Oval, J., Taetle, R., Valentine, M. B., and Ihle, J. N.: Activation of *Evi*-1 gene expression in human acute myelogenous leukemias by translocations spanning 300–400 kb on chromosome 3q26. Proc. Natl. Acad. Sci. USA 89:3937, 1992.

120. Gilmore, T. D.: Role of *rel* family genes in normal and malignant lymphoid cell growth. *In* Witte, O. N. (ed.): Oncogenes in the Development of Leukemia 15. Plainview, Cold Spring Harbor Laboratory Press, 1992, pp. 69–87.

121. Inoue, J.-I., Kerr, L. D., Ransone, L. J., Bengal, E., Hunter, T., and Verma, I. M.: c-rel activates but v-rel suppresses transcription from KB sites. Proc. Natl. Acad. Sci. USA 88:3715, 1991.

122. Gilmore, T. D.: NF-kappaB, KBF1, *dorsal*, and *rel*ated matters. Cell 62:841, 1990.

123. Ghosh, S., Gifford, A. M., Riviere, L. R., Tempst, P., Nolan, G. P., and Baltimore, D.: Cloning of the p50 DNA binding subunit of NF-kappaB: Homology to *rel* and *dorsal*. Cell 62:1019, 1990.

124. Kieran, M., Blank, V., Logeat, F., Vanderkerckhove, J., Lottspeich, F., Le Bail, O., Urban, M. B., Kourilsky, P., Baeuerle, P. A., and Israël, A.: The DNA binding subunit of NF-kappaB is identical to factor KBF1 and homologous to the *rel* oncogene product. Cell 62:1007, 1990.

125. Neri, A., Chang, C.-C., Lombardi, L., Salina, M., Corradini, P., Maiolo, A. T., Chaganti, R. S. K., and Dalla-Favera, R.: B cell lymphoma–associated chromosomal translocation involves candidate oncogene *lyt*-10, homologous to NF-kappaB p50. Cell 67:1075, 1991.

126. Davis, N., Ghosh, S., Simmons, D. L., Tempst, P., Liou, H.-C., Baltimore, D., and Bose, H. R., Jr.: Rel-associated pp40: An inhibitor of the Rel family of transcription factors. Science 253:1268, 1991.

127. Ballard, D. W., Walker, W. H., Doerre, S., Sista, P., Molitor, J. A., Dixon, E. P., Peffer, N. J., Hannink, M., and Greene, W. C.: The v-*rel* oncogene encodes a kB enhancer binding protein that inhibits NF-kB function. Cell 63:803, 1990.

128. Schmitz, M. L., Henkel, T., and Baeuerle, P. A.: Proteins controlling the nuclear uptake of NF-KB Rel and dorsal. Trends Cell Biol. 1:130, 1991.

129. Lu, D., Thompson, J. D., Gorski, G. K., Rice, N. R., Mayer, M. G., and Yunis, J. J.: Alterations at the *rel* locus in human lymphoma. Oncogene 6:1235, 1991.

130. Ohno, H., Takimoto, G., and McKeithan, T. W.: The candidate proto-oncogene *bcl*-3 is related to genes implicated in cell lineage determination and cell cycle control. Cell 60:991, 1990.

131. Hatada, E. N., Nieters, A., Wulczyn, F. G., Naumann, M., Meyer, R., Nucifora, G., McKeithan, T. W., and Scheidereit, C.: The ankyrin repeat domains of the NF-kappaB precursor p105 and the protooncogene *bcl*-3 act as specific inhibitors of NF-kappaB DNA binding. Proc. Natl. Acad. Sci. USA 89:2489, 1992.

132. Mellentin, J. D., Murre, C., Donlon, T. A., McCaw, P. S., Smith, S. D., Carroll, A. J., McDonald, M. E., Baltimore, D., and Cleary, M. L.: The gene for enhancer binding proteins E12/E47 lies at the t(1;19) breakpoint in acute leukemias. Science 246:379, 1989.

133. Kamps, M. P., Murre, C., Sun, X., and Baltimore, D.: A new homeobox gene contributes the DNA binding domain of the t(1;19) translocation protein in pre-B ALL. Cell 60:547, 1990.

134. Nourse, J., Mellentin, J. D., Galili, N., Wilkinson, J., Stan-

bridge, E., Smith, S. D., and Cleary, M. L.: Chromosomal translocation t(1;19) results in synthesis of a homeobox fusion mRNA that codes for a potential chimeric transcription factor. Cell 60:535, 1990.

135. von Lindern, M., Poustka, A., Lerach, H., and Grosveld, G.: The (6;9) chromosome translocation, associated with a specific subtype of acute nonlymphocytic leukemia, leads to aberrant transcription of a target gene on 9q34. Mol. Cell. Biol. 10:4016, 1990.

136. Borrow, J., Goddard, A. D., Sheer, D., and Solomon, E.: Molecular analysis of acute promyelocytic leukemia breakpoint cluster region on chromosome 17. Science 249:1577, 1990.

137. de Thé, H., Chomienne, C., Lanotte, M., Degos, L., and Dejean, A.: The t(15;17) translocation of acute promyelocytic leukemia fuses the retinoic acid receptor α gene to a novel transcribed locus. Nature 347:558, 1990.

138. Longo, L., Pandolfi, P. P., Biondi, A., Rambaldi, A., Mencarelli, A., Lo Coco, F., Diverio, D., Pegoraro, L., Avanzi, G., Tabilio, A., Zangrilli, D., Alcalay, M., Donti, E., Grignani, F., and Pelicci, P. G.: Rearrangements and aberrant expression of the retinoic acid receptor α gene in acute promyelocytic leukemias. J. Exp. Med. 172:1571, 1990.

139. Gao, J., Erickson, P., Gardiner, K., Le Beau, M. M., Diaz, M. O., Patterson, D., Rowley, J. D., and Drabkin, H. A.: Isolation of a yeast artificial chromosome spanning the 8;21 translocation breakpoint t(8;21)(q22;q22.3) in acute myelogenous leukemia. Proc. Natl. Acad. Sci. USA 88:4882, 1991.

140. Miyoshi, H., Shimizu, K., Kozu, T., Maseki, N., Kaneko, Y., and Ohki, M.: t(8;21) breakpoints on chromosome 21 in acute myeloid leukemia are clustered within a limited region of a single gene, AML1. Proc. Natl. Acad. Sci. USA 88:10431, 1991.

141. Ziemin-van der Poel, S., McCabe, N. R., Gill, H. J., Espinosa, R., III, Patel, Y., Harden, A., Rubinelli, P., Smith, S. D., LeBeau, M. M., Rowley, J. D., and Diaz, M. O.: Identification of a gene, MLL, that spans the breakpoint in 11q23 translocations associated with human leukemias. Proc. Natl. Acad. Sci. USA 88:10735, 1991.

142. Metz, T., and Graf, T.: Fusion of the nuclear oncoproteins v-Myb and v-Ets is required for the leukemogenicity of E26 virus. Cell 66:95, 1991.

143. Rovigatti, U., Watson, D. K., and Yunis, J. J.: Amplification and rearrangement of Hu-ets-1 in leukemia and lymphoma with involvement of 11q23. Science 232:398, 1986.

144. Berns, A.: Separating the wheat from the chaff. Curr. Bio. 1:28, 1991.

145. Evans, R. M.: The steroid and thyroid hormone receptor superfamily. Science 240:889, 1988.

146. Kakizuka, A., Miller, W. H. J., Umesono, K., Warrell, R. P. J., Frankel, S. R., Murty, V. V. V. S., Dmitrovsky, E., and Evans, R. M.: Chromosomal translocation t(15;17) in human acute promyelocytic leukemia fuses RARα with a novel putative transcription factor, PML. Cell 66:663, 1991.

147. de Thé, H., Lavau, C., Marchio, A., Chomienne, C., Degos, L., and Dejean, A.: The PML-RARα fusion mRNA generated by the t(15;17) translocation in acute promyelocytic leukemia encodes a functionally altered RAR. Cell 66:675, 1991.

148. Sharif, M., and Privalsky, M. L.: v-erbA oncogene function in neoplasia correlates with its ability to repress retinoic acid receptor action. Cell 66:885, 1991.

148a. Gu, Y., Nakamura, T., Alder, H., Prasad, R., Canaani, O., Cimino, G., Croce, C. M., and Canaani, E.: The t(4;11) chromosome translocation of human acute leukemias fuses the ALL-1 gene, related to Drosophila trithorax, to the AF-4 gene. Cell 71:701, 1992.

148b. Tkachuck, D. C., Kohler, S., and Cleary, M. L.: Involvement of a homolog of Drosophila trithorax by 11q23 chromosomal translocations in acute leukemias. Cell 71:691, 1992.

149. Willams, G. T.: Programmed cell death: Apoptosis and oncogenesis. Cell 65:1097, 1991.

150. Fukuhara, S., Rowley, J. D., Varrakojis, D., and Golomb, H.

M.: Chromosome abnormalities in poorly differentiated lymphocytic lymphoma. Cancer Res. 39:3119, 1979.

151. Tsujimoto, Y., Gorham, J., Cossman, J., Jaffe, E., and Croce, C. M.: The t(14;18) chromosome translocations involved in B-cell neoplasms result from mistakes in VDJ joining. Science 229:1390, 1985.

152. Bakhshi, A., Jensen, J. P., Goldman, P., Wright, J. J., McBride, O. W., Epstein, A. L., and Korsmeyer, S. J.: Cloning the chromosomal breakpoint to t(14;18) human lymphomas: Clustering around J_H on chromosome 14 and near a transcriptional unit on 18. Cell 41:899, 1985.

153. Cleary, M. L., and Sklar, J.: Nucleotide sequence of a t(14;18) chromosomal breakpoint in follicular lymphoma and demonstration of a breakpoint cluster region near a transcriptionally active locus on chromosome 18. Proc. Natl. Acad. Sci. USA 82:7439, 1985.

154. Vaux, D. L., Cory, S., and Adams, J. M.: Bcl-2 gene promotes haemopoietic cell survival and cooperates with c-myc to immortalize pre-B cells. Nature 335:440, 1988.

155. McDonnell, T. J., Deane, N., Platt, F. M., Nunez, G., Jaeger, U., McKearn, J. P., and Korsmeyer, S. J.: bcl-2-immunoglobulin transgenic mice demonstrate extended B cell survival and follicular lymphoproliferation. Cell 57:79, 1989.

156. McDonnell, T. J., and Korsmeyer, S. J.: Progression form lymphoid hyperplasia to high-grade malignant lymphoma in mice transgenic for the t(14;18). Nature 349:254, 1991.

157. Strasser, A., Harris, A. W., Bath, M. L., and Cory, S.: Novel primitive lymphoid tumours induced in transgenic mice by cooperation between myc and bcl-2. Nature 348:331, 1990.

158. Strasser, A., Whittingham, S., Vaux, D. L., Bath, M. L., Adams, J. M., Cory, S., and Harris, A. W.: Enforced BCL2 expression in B lymphoid cells prolongs antibody responses and elicits autoimmune disease. Proc. Natl. Acad. Sci. USA 88:8661, 1991.

159. Nuñez, G., Hockenbery, D., McDonnell, T. J., Sorensen, C. M., and Korsmeyer, S. J.: Bcl-2 maintains B cell memory. Nature 353:71, 1991.

160. Henderson, S., Rowe, M., Gregory, C., Croom-Carter, D., Wang, F., Longnecker, R., Kieff, E., and Rickinson, A.: Induction of bcl-2 expression by Epstein-Barr virus latent membrane protein 1 protects infected B cells from programmed cell death. Cell 65:1107, 1991.

161. Zutter, M., Hockenbery, D., Silverman, G. A., and Korsmeyer, S. J.: Immunolocalization of the Bcl-2 protein within hematopoietic neoplasms. Blood 78:1062, 1991.

162. Hockenbery, D. M., Zutter, M., Hickey, W., Nahm, M., and Korsmeyer, S. J.: BCL2 protein is topographically restricted in tissues characterized by apoptotic cell death. Proc. Natl. Acad. Sci. USA 88:6961, 1991.

163. Hockenbery, D., Nuñez, G., Milliman, C., Schreiber, R. D., and Korsmeyer, S.: Bcl-2, an inner mitochondrial membrane protein blocks programmed cell death. Nature 348:334, 1990.

164. Kurzrock, R., Gutterman, J. U., and Talpaz, M.: The molecular genetics of Philadelphia chromosome-positive leukemias. N. Engl. J. Med. 319:990, 1988.

165. Hagemeijer, A.: Chromosome abnormalities in CML. Baillière's Clin. Haematol. 1:963, 1987.

166. O'Bryan, J. P., Frye, R. A., Cogswell, P. C., Neubauer, A., Kitch, B., Prokop, C., Espinosa, R. I. I. I., Le Beau, M. M., Earp, H. S., and Liu, E. T.: axl, a transforming gene isolated from primary human myeloid leukemia cells, encodes a novel receptor tyrosine kinase. Mol. Cell. Biol. 11:5016, 1991.

167. Ahuja, H., Bar-Eli, M., Arlin, Z., Advani, S., Allen, S. L., Goldman, J., Snyder, D., Foti, A., and Cline, M.: The spectrum of molecular alterations in the evolution of chronic myelocytic leukemia. J. Clin. Invest. 87:2042, 1991.

168. Feinstein, E., Cimino, G., Gale, R. P., Alimena, G., Berthier, R., Kishi, K., Goldman, J., Zaccaria, A., Berrebi, A., and Canaani, E.: p53 in chronic myelogenous leukemia in acute phase. Proc. Natl. Acad. Sci. USA 88:6293, 1991.

169. Hollstein, M., Sidransky, D., Vogelstein, B., and Harris, C. C.: p53 mutations in human cancers. Science 253:49, 1991.

170. Farrell, P. J., Allan, G. J., Shanahan, F., Vousden, K. H., and Crook, T.: p53 is frequently mutated in Burkitt's lymphoma cell lines. EMBO J. 10:2879, 1991.

171. Gaidano, G., Ballerini, P., Gong, J. A., Inghirami, G., Neri, A., Newcomb, E. W., Magrath, I. T., Knowles, D. M., and Dalla-Favera, R.: p53 mutations in human lymphoid malignancies: Association with Burkitt lymphoma and chronic lymphocytic leukemia. Proc. Natl. Acad. Sci. USA 88:5413, 1991.

172. Cheng, J., and Haas, M.: Frequent mutations in the p53 tumor suppressor gene in human leukemia T-cell lines. Mol. Cell. Biol. 10:5502, 1990.

173. Towatari, M., Adachi, K., Kato, H., and Saito, H.: Absence of the human retinoblastoma gene product in the megakaryoblastic crisis of chronic myelogenous leukemia. Blood 78:2178, 1991.

174. Gauwerky, C. E., Haluska, F. G., Tsujimoto, Y., Nowell, P. C., and Croce, C. M.: Evolution of B-cell malignancy: Pre-B-cell leukemia resulting from MYC activation in a B-cell neoplasm with a rearranged *Bcl*-2 gene. Proc. Natl. Acad. Sci. USA 85:8548, 1988.

175. Koduru, P. R. K., and Offit, K.: Molecular structure of double reciprocal translocations: Significance in B-cell lymphomagenesis. Oncogene 6:145, 1991.

176. Munroe, D. G., Peacock, J. W., and Benchimol, S.: Inactivation of the cellular p53 gene is a common feature of Friend virus–induced erythroleukemia: Relationship of inactivation to dominant transforming alleles. Mol. Cell. Biol. 10:3307, 1990.

177. Moreau-Gachelin, F., Tavitian, A., and Tambourin, P.: Spi-1 is a putative oncogene in virally induced murine erythroleukaemias. Nature 331:277, 1988.

178. Moreau-Gachelin, F., Ray, D., Mattei, M.-G., Tambourin, P., and Tavitian, A.: The putative oncogene Spi-1: Murine chromosomal localization and transcriptional activation in murine acute erythroleukemias. Oncogene 4:1449, 1989.

179. Thompson, C. C., Brown, T. A., and McKnight, S. L.: Convergence of Ets- and notch-related structural motifs in a heteromeric DNA binding complex. Science 253:762, 1991.

180. Adams, J. M., and Cory, S.: Oncogene cooperation in leukemogenesis. *In* Witte, O. N. (ed.): Oncogenes in the Development of Leukaemia 15. Plainview, Cold Spring Harbor Laboratory Press, 1992, pp. 119–141.

181. van Lohuizen, M., Verbeek, S., Scheijen, B., Wientjens, E., van der Gulden, H., and Berns, A.: Identification of cooperating oncogenes in Eμ-*myc* transgenic mice by provirus tagging. Cell 65:737, 1991.

182. Haupt, Y., Alexander, W. S., Barri, G., Klinken, S. P., and Adams, J. M.: Novel zinc finger gene implicated as *myc* collaborator by retrovirally accelerated lymphomagenesis in Eμ-*myc* transgenic mice. Cell 65:753, 1991.

183. Tkachuk, D. C., Westbrook, C. A., Andreeff, M., Donlon, T. A., Cleary, M. L., Suryanarayan, K., Homge, M., Redner, A., Gray, J., and Pinkel, D.: Detection of *bcr-abl* fusion in chronic myelogeneous leukemia by in situ hybridization. Science 250:559, 1990.

184. Denny, C. T., Shah, N., Ogden, S., Willman, C., McConnell, T., Crist, W., Carroll, A., and Witte, O. N.: Localization of preferential sites of rearrangement within the BCR gene in Philadelphia chromosome positive acute lymphoblastic leukemia. Proc. Natl. Acad. Sci. USA 86:4254, 1989.

185. Hooberman, A. L., Rubin, C. M., Barton, K. P., and Westbrook, C. A.: Detection of the Philadelphia chromosome in acute lymphoblastic leukemia by pulsed-field gel electrophoresis. Blood 74:1101, 1989.

186. Kawasaki, E. S., Clark, S. S., Coyne, M. Y., Smith, S. D., Champlin, R., Witte, O. N., and McCormick, F. P.: Diagnosis of chronic myeloid and acute lymphocytic leukemias by detection of leukemia-specific mRNA sequences amplified in vitro. Proc. Natl. Acad. Sci. USA 85:5698, 1988.

187. Hughes, T. P., Ambrosetti, A., Barbu, V., Bartram, C., Battista, R., Biondi, A., Chiamenti, A., Cimino, G., Ernst, P., Frassoni, F., Gasparini, P., Gentilini, I., Gluckman, E., Grosveld, G., Guerrasio, A., Hegewich, S., Janssen, J. W. G., Keating, A., Lo Coco, F., Martiat, P., Martinelli, G., Mills, K., Morgan, G., Nadali, G., Pelicci, P. G., Perona, G., Pignatti, P. F., Richard, P., Saglio, G., Trabetti, E., Turco, A., Veneri, D., Zaccaria, A., Zander, A., and Goldman, J. M.: Clinical value of PCR in diagnosis and follow-up of leukaemia and lymphoma: Report of the Third Workshop of the Molecular Biology/BMT Study Group. Leukemia 5:448, 1991.

188. Crescenzi, M., Seto, M., Herzig, G. P., Weiss, P. D., Griffith, R. C., and Korsmeyer, S. J.: Thermostable DNA polymerase chain amplification of t(14;18) chromosome breakpoints and detection of minimal residual disease. Proc. Natl. Acad. Sci. USA 85:4869, 1988.

SECTION VII

VIRUSES

25

The Molecular and Biological Properties of the Human Immunodeficiency Virus*

Malcolm A. Martin

INTRODUCTION

During the late 1970s and early 1980s, physicians in several large American cities began seeing previously healthy male patients who presented with symptoms of immune dysfunction. This new and unusual syndrome was characterized by generalized lymphadenopathy, opportunistic infections (most typically *Pneumocystis carinii* pneumonia, mucosal candidiasis, and disseminated cytomegalovirus [CMV] infections), and Kaposi's sarcoma. In June 1981, the disease was first brought to the attention of the general medical community when the Centers for Disease Control described five Los Angeles area men with severely impaired immune systems in the *Morbidity and Mortality Weekly Report*.[1] This notification was soon followed by several reports[2-4] describing immunocompromised homosexual men or intravenous drug users with T lymphocytes that responded poorly to antigen and mitogen stimulation in functional assays. Within several months it became clear that an immunodeficiency

disease was also affecting other groups, including recent Haitian immigrants, hemophiliacs, transfusion recipients, and sexual partners and/or children of members of the different risk groups.

The epidemiological pattern that emerged suggested that the new disease was acquired from contaminated blood or following sexual intercourse with an infected person. Between late 1981 and early 1983, numerous microbial agents were proposed as the cause of the acquired immunodeficiency syndrome (AIDS), as the disease was soon called. A strong case was made for herpesviruses, particularly CMVs, which were known to replicate efficiently in human lymphocytes and were frequently present in clinical specimens collected from AIDS patients.[4, 5] Other groups proposed a retroviral cause based on the presence of antibodies specific for human T-cell leukemia virus type-1 (HTLV-1) in some AIDS patients.[6-10] In 1983, scientists at the Pasteur Institute isolated a retrovirus from the lymph nodes of an asymptomatic individual who presented with generalized lymphadenopathy of unknown origin.[11] During its growth in vitro, the lymphadenopathy-associated virus, or LAV as it was named, generated progeny virions containing reverse transcriptase and possessing electron microscopic features typical of retroviruses. Unlike the previously described and intensively studied retroviruses of diverse vertebrate origin, LAV was highly cytopathic during its replication in human peripheral blood lymphocytes, specifically killing the CD4-positive lymphocytes in the culture.[12, 13] Other groups isolated similar T-cell cytopathic viruses from peripheral blood lymphocytes of AIDS patients in 1984[14, 15] and obtained strong serological evidence that linked exposure to LAV-like retroviruses and immunodeficient individuals from the various groups at risk.[16–18] This new retrovirus, which was etiologically associated with AIDS in the United States, Europe, and central Africa, was named human immunodeficiency virus, or HIV[19] (and subsequently HIV-1). In 1986, a related but immunologically distinct human retrovirus (now called HIV-2) was recovered from individuals residing in West Africa and was also shown to cause AIDS.[20, 21]

HIV MOLECULAR BIOLOGY: CLINICAL PERSPECTIVES

Although there has been a veritable explosion of new information pertaining to the organization of the HIV genome, the regulation of viral gene expression, the function of many of the viral proteins, and the isolation and detection of virus in infected persons, our understanding of how HIV replicates and spreads in vivo or induces disease in infected individuals is quite rudimentary. A major impediment has been the lack of an animal model to study the immunodeficiency induced by HIV-1. Virtually all current knowledge pertaining to virus replication and pathogenesis derives from tissue culture infections or has been inferred from analyses of clinical specimens collected from seropositive individuals. Unfortunately, the microenvironments typical of lymph nodes (microglia in the central nervous system, Langerhans cells of the skin, and unstimulated, CD4-positive mononuclear cells circulating in the peripheral blood) are difficult, if not impossible, to duplicate in the tissue culture flask.

Studies of HIV replication in vivo were initially hampered by the unavailability of assays sensitive enough to detect extremely low levels of virions, viral nucleic acids, or viral proteins. However, several important and fundamental questions pertaining to the different stages of clinical disease can now be addressed using the tools of modern molecular biology. For example, it is still unclear what type (or types) of HIV inocula (cell-free virus particles or infected cells) usually initiate the "flu-like" primary HIV infection; where in the body (peripheral blood, lymphoid tissue, tissue dendritic cell, bone marrow) the in vivo infection is initially established; and whether the CD4-positive mononuclear cell target is in an activated or resting state. The interplay of the different arms of the immune system in restricting the primary exposure to HIV, as well as studies ascertaining when or if components of the humoral or cell-mediated response become irreversibly compromised, need to be rigorously pursued. The extent of virus replication and the tissue location of virus particles/virus-producing cells during the asymptomatic phase of HIV infection are now amenable to vigorous investigation. Similarly, the mechanisms responsible for sustaining the low-level production of relatively non-cytopathic virions and their dissemination to peripheral tissues, such as the central nervous system during clinical latency, deserve close scrutiny.

The factors responsible for clinical progression to AIDS remain largely unknown. The elevated production of intracellular and extracellular virus, the changing cytopathicity and tropism of HIV, and the precipitous loss of CD4 cells (the ultimate hallmark of the severe immune dysfunction) must be diligently evaluated at the virological, immunological, and molecular levels. Similarly, related questions concerning direct and indirect effects of HIV proteins on the function of T lymphocytes, tissue macrophages, and microglia; programmed cell death; and chronic stimulation of the immune system should be carefully investigated. Advances in molecular biology now allow a more exhaustive examination of these issues, which are critical for understanding the clinical aspects of HIV infection.

CLASSIFICATION AND ORGANIZATION OF HIV GENOMES

Progress in unraveling the structure and function of the numerous HIV genes during the past decade has been nothing less than spectacular. This was helped to a considerable extent by the development and use of continuous human leukemia cell lines that could be acutely infected with HIV and undergo rapid cytopathic infection and other cell systems that chronically release lower levels of virus while exhibiting little, if any, cytopathicity.[14, 22–24] The efficient production of virus particles permitted the isolation of HIV genomic RNA, which was used to generate sensitive complementary DNA (cDNA) probes. Molecular clones of proviral DNA were quickly obtained, and the sequences of full-length cloned proviruses were reported by several groups in early 1985.[25–31] Analyses of nucleotide sequence data indicated that HIV-1 indeed had a genomic organization similar to that of other replication-competent retroviruses (Fig. 25–1). However, in addition to the group-specific antigen (*gag*), polymerase (*pol*), and envelope (*env*) genes, which encode the structural proteins of other well-studied retroviral particles,[32, 33] the HIV genome contained several additional open reading frames with functions that were then unknown.

Retroviruses are members of a larger group of related eukaryotic retrotransposable elements[34–37] that have the capacity to generate DNA copies of their RNA intermediates with the enzyme reverse transcriptase. Sequence information from geographically diverse HIV-1 isolates permitted a more precise as-

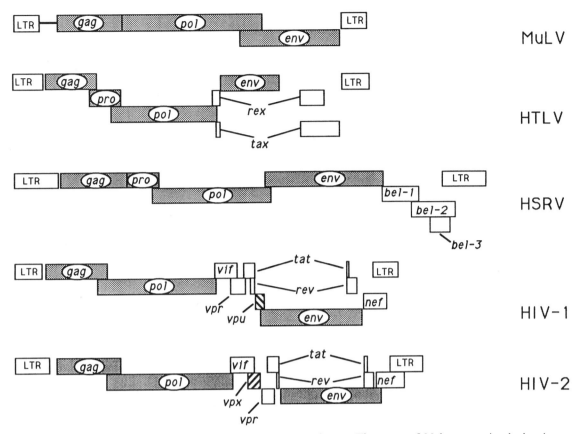

FIGURE 25–1. Genomic organization of mammalian retroviruses. The genes of Moloney murine leukemia virus (MuLV), human T-cell leukemia virus type I (HTLV), human spumavirus (HSRV), and human immunodeficiency virus type 1 (HIV-1) and type 2 (HIV-2), derived from nucleotide sequences of molecular clones,[25, 27, 30, 32, 51, 578–580] are depicted as they are arranged in their respective proviral DNAs. The position of the protease (pro) open reading frame is shown when it differs from that of the *pol* gene. The sizes of the different proviral DNAs are shown in proportion to the 9.7 kb HIV provirus.

sessment of their evolution and phylogenetic relationship to other retroviruses (Fig. 25–2). When portions of retroviral *pol* and *gag* genes were examined, five major viral subfamilies became evident: (1) the spumaviruses; (2) mammalian C-type oncoviruses; (3) the BLV/HTLV leukemia viruses; (4) a heterogeneous group including Rous sarcoma and the A, B, and D-type viruses; and (5) lentiviruses, including HIV-1 and HIV-2 and closely related simian viruses.[38] As their name suggests, lentiviruses cause a slow, unremitting disease in sheep, horses, and cattle, affecting various lineages of hematopoietic cells, particularly lymphocytes and differentiated macrophages. Although the original electron microscopic studies of HIV-1 revealed 100- to 120-nm particles containing a bullet-shaped cylindrical core, morphological features similar to those previously described for visna virus,[12, 39–42] the nucleotide sequence analyses were required to place HIV-1 securely in the lentivirus subfamily.[38] These analyses of human and simian immunodeficiency virus (SIV) genomes also indicated that HIV-2 is more closely related to the SIVs than to HIV-1.[43–46]

In contrast to previously sequenced retroviruses such as Rous sarcoma and Moloney murine leukemia viruses, the HIV genome contains multiple and, in some cases, overlapping open reading frames (see Fig. 25–1).[25, 27, 30, 47] The structures of retroviral genomes are known to differ from one another with respect to whether translational access to the *pol* gene was through ribosomal frameshifting[48] or suppression of a termination codon[49] and whether the virus-encoded protease occupied a reading frame separate from *gag* and *pol*.[50–52] Although an extra open reading frame, now known to encode a superantigen, was identified within the 3' long terminal repeat (LTR) of mouse mammary tumor virus proviral DNA,[53, 53a, 53b] the existence of additional, functionally important retroviral genes was generally unappreciated until shortly before the isolation of HIV-1. The sequencing of HTLV-I proviral DNA revealed the presence of three short, overlapping open reading frames, located between the *env* gene and the 3' LTR,[51] one of which encoded a transactivator of transcription, the Tax protein.[54–56] Although all of the known human retroviruses contain several additional genes, this chapter focuses on the genetics and molecular biology of only HIV-1 and HIV-2; the HTLVs are described in detail in Chapter 26. Despite the similarity of their genomic organization, the two human immunodeficiency viruses can be readily distinguished from one another on the basis

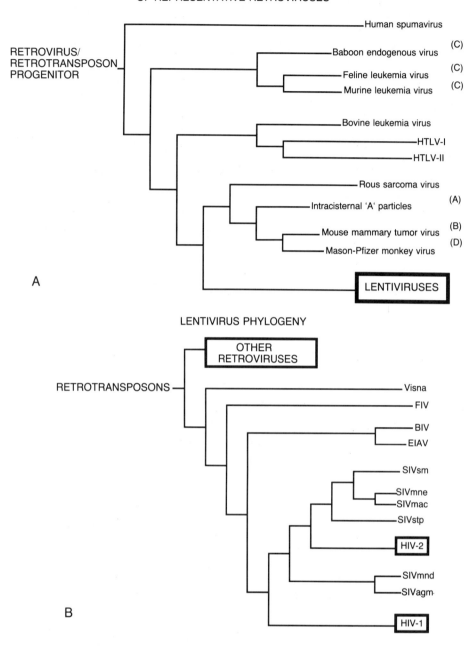

PHYLOGENETIC RELATIONSHIPS (RT)
OF REPRESENTATIVE RETROVIRUSES

RETROVIRUS/
RETROTRANSPOSON
PROGENITOR

Human spumavirus

Baboon endogenous virus (C)

Feline leukemia virus (C)

Murine leukemia virus (C)

Bovine leukemia virus

HTLV-I

HTLV-II

Rous sarcoma virus

Intracisternal 'A' particles (A)

Mouse mammary tumor virus (B)

Mason-Pfizer monkey virus (D)

LENTIVIRUSES

A

LENTIVIRUS PHYLOGENY

RETROTRANSPOSONS

OTHER
RETROVIRUSES

Visna

FIV

BIV

EIAV

SIVsm

SIVmne

SIVmac

SIVstp

HIV-2

SIVmnd

SIVagm

HIV-1

B

FIGURE 25–2. Phylogenetic relationships of representative retroviruses. *A*, Different retrovirus subfamilies were related to one another based on sequences encoding reverse transcriptase.[38] The letters in parentheses refer to different retrovirus morphologic types. *B*, The relationship of the nonprimate lentiviruses to themselves and to the primate lentivirus group is based on reverse transcriptase[38]; the relationships between the primate lentiviruses are based on *gag* sequences.[581] FIV = Feline immunodeficiency virus; BIV = bovine immunodeficiency virus; EIAV = equine infectious anemia virus; SIV_{sm} = simian immunodeficiency virus, sooty mangabey; SIV_{mne} = simian immunodeficiency virus, pig-tailed macaque; SIV_{mac} = simian immunodeficiency virus, rhesus macaque; SIV_{stp} = simian immunodeficiency virus, stump-tailed macaque; SIV_{mnd} = simian immunodeficiency virus, mandrill; and SIV_{agm} = simian immunodeficiency virus, African green monkey. (Adapted from Doolittle, R. F., Feng, D. F., McClure, M. A., and Johnson, M. S.: Retrovirus phylogeny and evolution. Curr. Top. Microbiol. Immunol. 157:1, 1990; and Khan, A. S., et al.: A highly divergent simian immunodeficiency virus [SIV_{stm}] recovered from stored stump-tailed macaque tissues. J. Virol. 65:7061, 1991; with permission.)

of a single unique open reading frame: HIV-1 contains the *vpu* gene[57, 58] and HIV-2 encodes the *vpx* gene product (see Fig. 25–1).[59, 60, 580]

VIRUS REPLICATION: OVERVIEW

As is the case for other replication-competent retroviruses, the overall goal of the HIV replicative cycle (Fig. 25–3) is to produce progeny particles containing (1) two copies of the 9.2 kilobase (kb) RNA genome encased within a protective nucleocapsid consisting of Gag proteins; (2) enzymes (protease, reverse transcriptase/RNase H, and integrase); and (3) an outer lipoprotein membrane and associated viral envelope glycoproteins. Infections initiated by cell-free enveloped viruses typically begin with the binding of particles to a receptor associated with the plasma membrane of susceptible cells. For both HIV-1 and HIV-2, the receptor used for this adsorption step is the CD4 molecule, present on the surface of the helper/inducer subset of T lymphocytes.[61–63] Adsorbed viral particles lacking envelope glycoproteins enter the cytoplasm of infected cells and, following partial uncoating, initiate the reverse transcription of the viral genome. As is the case for other retroelements,[64–68] the double-stranded DNA reverse transcript most likely is transported to the nucleus as a component of a nucleoprotein structure containing Gag and Pol proteins, which

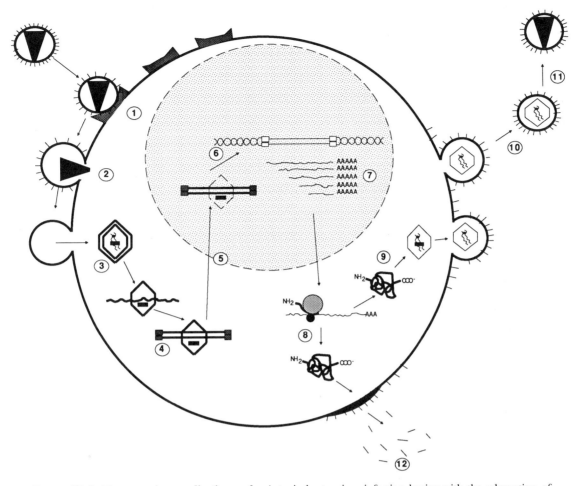

FIGURE 25–3. The retrovirus replicative cycle. A typical retrovirus infection begins with the adsorption of cell-free virions to receptors (step 1) on the surface of susceptible cells. In the case of HIV, virus entry (step 2) is a pH-independent process that follows the fusion of virus and cellular membranes and results in the partial uncoating (step 3) of incoming virions. Reverse transcription occurs within subviral particles in the cytoplasm of infected cells (step 4), and the double-stranded DNA product is transported to the nucleus (step 5), where integration into chromosomal DNA (step 6) is mediated by the virus-encoded integrase *(black bar)*, a component of a subviral nucleoprotein complex. The integrated viral DNA serves as a template for DNA-dependent RNA polymerase and leads to the production of mRNAs (step 7) that are translated into viral proteins in the cytoplasm of infected cells (step 8). Envelope (step 8) and Gag plus Gag/Pol (step 9) polyproteins are transported via independent pathways to the plasma membrane, where progeny virus particles begin "budding" from cells and are released as immature particles (step 10). Subsequent proteolysis by the virion-encoded protease generates mature particles (step 11) containing a characteristic condensed core *(upper right)*. Non-virion–associated gp 120 envelope protein is also released from cells (step 12).

mediates the integration of full-length linear molecules of HIV DNA into the chromosome of the infected cell. These "early" steps in the retrovirus replicative cycle very likely require the participation of cellular factors for their successful completion. The mechanism responsible for the resistance of certain mouse cells to exogenous murine leukemia virus infection (associated with the Fv-1 resistance determinant located on mouse chromosome 4[69–71]) may in fact reflect the presence of alternative forms of a cell factor(or factors) involved in virus uncoating. In virtually all retroviral systems examined, integration of the linear DNA reverse transcription product is required for the efficient production of viral gene products.[72–74] The subsequent translation of viral mRNAs in the cytoplasm of productively infected cells results in the

trafficking of Gag/Gag-Pol polyproteins and envelope glycoproteins via *independent* pathways to the plasma membrane, where the process of virion assembly is initiated. As is the case for other retroviruses, newly released HIV particles must undergo additional maturation, primarily via a series of proteolytic digestions of Gag and Pol precursor proteins, to attain their full infectious potential.

Although both HIV-1 and HIV-2 follow this general strategy, some of the steps in the replicative cycle and/or virus-encoded gene products deserve special mention: (1) Unlike many enveloped viruses, HIV and several other retroviruses enter their host cells by a pH-independent fusion mechanism and not by receptor-mediated endocytosis.[75–77] The *direct* fusion of input virions with the plasma membrane of infected cells has in fact been documented by electron microscopy.[77] (2) At least two of the "accessory" gene products encoded by HIV (Tat and Rev) are RNA-binding, regulatory proteins that interact with regions of viral RNA that form unique secondary structures. The Tat and Rev proteins modulate steady-state levels of viral mRNA and the amounts of unspliced or singly spliced cytoplasmic mRNAs, respectively. (3) During its evolution, HIV has incorporated several elements into its genome that do not encode a protein product (so-called *cis*-acting elements), but nonetheless are needed for the balanced and coordinated production of viral gene products (Fig. 25–4). In addition to sequences found in other replication-competent retroviruses that are required for reverse transcription (the primer binding site [**pbs**] and the polypurine tract [**PPT**]), packaging (the **psi** site), ribosomal frameshifting (**FS**), and polyadenylation (**PA**), the HIV genome has acquired binding motifs (**TAR** and **RRE**) for its two transactivating proteins as well as elements responsible for the nuclear retention and instability (**IR**) of unspliced/partially spliced mRNAs. (4) Several of the HIV accessory proteins (Vif, Vpr, Vpu and Nef) are not *absolutely* required for replication in cultured human T cells. Infectivity may be affected up to several thousand-fold, depending on the accessory gene mutated and the infected cell studied. (5) Many of the HIV-encoded proteins are initially synthesized as polyprotein precursor molecules, whereas others undergo little or no processing or modification following translation (Fig. 25–5). Pulse-chase experiments have revealed precursor/product relationships of some of these viral gene products. (6) For many retroviruses, the principal determinants of tropism reside in the external envelope glycoprotein and the LTR.[78–82] Although changes in the LTR may modulate the efficiency of replication in a variety of T-cell types, the *main* determinant of HIV host range resides in the envelope glycoproteins.

THE MOLECULAR BIOLOGY OF HIV REPLICATION

With the exception of the chimpanzee, which develops an asymptomatic virus infection,[83, 84] no other animal is susceptible to HIV-1. Consequently, nearly all molecular and biological studies of HIV have been limited to tissue culture systems and, in many instances, have relied on approaches or reagents not readily applicable to HIV infections in vivo. These include (1) transient *transfections* of mammalian epithelial cell lines with LTR-driven reporter genes or subgenomic proviral DNA constructs; (2) the isolation of transcriptional regulatory factors from non-lymphoid cells and the subsequent characterization of their effects on HIV LTR-driven gene activity in the same non-lymphoid cells; (3) side-by-side comparisons of CD4-positive human T lymphocytes *infected* with wild-type HIV preparations with epithelial cells transiently *transfected* with full-length clones of HIV proviral DNA; (4) HIV infections of primary lymphocyte or macrophage cultures, established from cells obtained from healthy donors, and their comparison with virus infections of continuous human leukemia cell lines; and (5) infectivity studies using tissue culture–adapted variants of HIV rather than the slowly replicating, non-cytopathic virus present in infected individuals. Nonetheless, much of the published literature is relevant to the general strategy of HIV replication; some of the mechanistic insights that have emerged are being used to rationally develop antiviral drugs.

The HIV LTR

Retroviral LTR elements represent a useful starting point for understanding the complex interplay be-

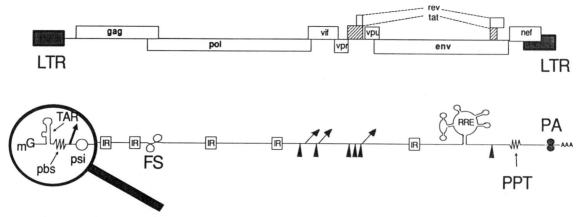

FIGURE 25–4. *Cis*-acting elements associated with the HIV-1 genome. The *cis* elements present in HIV-1 genomic RNA have been aligned with a map *(top)* depicting the virus genomic organization. mG = the methyl capped terminal G residue at 5′ terminus of viral RNA; TAR = Tat-responsive stem-bulge-loop structure; pbs = binding site for the tRNALys primer; *psi* = major packaging site; IR = RNA instability/nuclear retention elements; FS = frameshift motif; RRE = Rev-responsive element; PPT = polypurine tract, the initiation sequence for second-strand DNA synthesis; PA = polyadenylation signal; arrowheads = splice acceptors; arrows = splice donors.

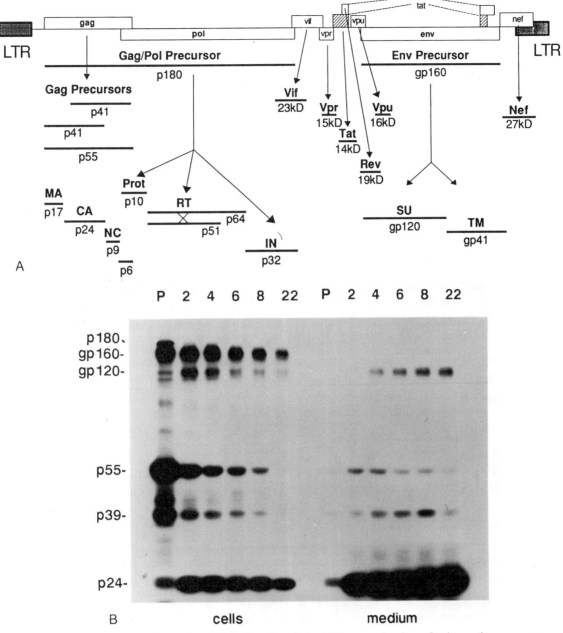

FIGURE 25–5. HIV-encoded proteins. *A,* The location of the HIV genes, the sizes of primary (in some cases polyproteins) translation products, and the processed mature viral proteins are indicated. *B,* A pulse-chase labeling experiment illustrating precursor-product relationships of the viral-encoded structural proteins. HeLa cells were pulse labeled for 30 minutes with ^{35}S-methionine, 2 days following transfection with an infectious molecular clone of HIV, and then maintained in complete medium for the indicated times (hours). Samples of the cell lysates and supernatant medium (containing released virions) were immunoprecipitated with the serum from an AIDS patient, and the resultant proteins were resolved by polyacrylamide gel electrophoresis. Note that increasing amounts of gp120 and p24 appear in the medium as the amounts of intracellular gp160 and p55 Gag precursor proteins diminish. No gp160 is detected in the medium. p180 = The Gag/Pol precursor polyprotein; gp160 = the envelope precursor polyprotein; gp120 = the mature glycosylated surface (SU) envelope protein; p55 = the Gag precursor polyprotein; p39 = a Gag precursor polyprotein; p24 = processed Gag capsid (CA) protein. The first lane in the two panels depicts the radioactivity incorporated during the 30-minute pulse (P) period, and the other five show the distribution of the label at the indicated times (hours) after the pulse.

tween HIV and their major host cells, human CD4-positive mononuclear cells. LTRs are generated during the process of reverse transcription[85–87] and serve a multitude of functions during the replicative cycle

(Fig. 25–6). DNA or RNA sequences mapping to the R region of the LTR participate directly in the process of reverse transcription by forming intermolecular DNA-RNA hybrid "bridges" that link short nascent

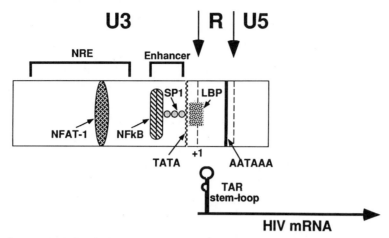

FIGURE 25–6. Structure of the HIV-1 long terminal repeat (LTR). The HIV-1 LTR, a duplicated 630+ bp component of integrated proviral DNA, is subdivided into regions associated with termini of the viral RNA genome. The R (repeat) region is defined as a 96 bp nt repeat present at the 3′ and 5′ termini of HIV-1 genomic RNA; U5 is defined as an 84 nt segment located adjacent to the R region at the 5′ end of the viral genome; and U3 is a 454 nt segment situated adjacent to the R region at the 3′ end of the viral RNA. The "enhancer" domain contains three Sp1 binding elements and two NF-κB binding motifs. The transcription start site is located at map position "+1," which is defined as the border between U3 and R. The negative regulatory element (NRE) is situated between positions −410 and −157 and contains a binding site for the nuclear factor of activated T cells (NFAT-1). The TATA site is positioned 22 bp upstream of the transcription initiation site. LBP = Leader binding protein; TAR = Tat transactivation response region; AATAAA = polyadenylation signal. An HIV RNA transcript, which is initiated at the first nucleotide within the R region (designated "+1") and contains the TAR element near its 5′ terminus, is shown at the bottom.

single-stranded DNA molecules and the untranscribed genomic RNA template.[88–90] LTR sequences located at the termini of the unintegrated viral DNA molecules (see Fig. 25–1) mediate their precise and efficient integration into the chromosomal DNA of the host cell.[91, 92] Other sequences located in the LTR contribute to the packaging of progeny RNA genomes during the assembly process.[93]

A major function of the retroviral LTR is the regulation of viral RNA production subsequent to the integration of the viral DNA.[94–97] The promoter/enhancer elements, needed for efficient transcriptional initiation, are located within the U3 region and function in the context of the 5′ LTR (see Fig. 25–6). The polyadenylation signal (AATAAA) and addition sites are also positioned in the R region but are active only as components of the 3′ LTR. The regulation of eukaryotic (and animal virus) gene activity involves the interaction of cellular proteins with transcriptional promoters, a process that determines both basal and induced levels of expression. Some of these regulatory proteins are constitutively produced, whereas others are synthesized in specific cells only following "induction" or "activation." One class of constitutively expressed transcription factors, which include TFIIA, TFIIB, TFIID, TFIIE, and TFIIF, interact with RNA polymerase II (Pol II) to form an active transcription initiation complex.[98–100] These "initiation factors" bind to the TATA element, which, in the HIV LTR, is located −29 to −24 nucleotides (nt) upstream of the transcriptional start site (see Fig. 25–6). A second class of eukaryotic transcriptional regulatory proteins interacts with DNA motifs located upstream of the TATA element. This latter group of DNA-binding proteins (e.g., Sp1, ATF, CTF) presum-

ably modulate RNA synthesis via their "activation" domains (hence their name, transcriptional transactivators) and interact with the Pol II initiation complex during or after its assembly.[101–105] A final class of regulatory factors, the so-called coactivator proteins, may augment transcriptional activity by linking DNA-binding transactivators with proteins associated with the Pol II initiation complex.[106–109]

Like other eukaryotic promoters, the HIV LTR contains its own ensemble of DNA elements to which transcriptional regulatory factors bind. Some of these were identified from mutagenesis studies of LTR-driven reporter gene constructs, some were found following gel-retardation or DNA footprinting experiments, and others were discovered from searches of nucleotide sequence data bases (Table 25–1). The LTR elements depicted in Figure 25–6 have all been shown to bind proteins isolated from human cells or to participate in a functionally relevant step related to HIV expression, or both; only they are discussed further.

The Sp1 and TATA motifs bind cellular proteins that are constitutively expressed in most eukaryotic cells and are critical for basal levels of HIV gene expression. Sp1, isolated originally from HeLa cells, was shown to bind to the multiple GGGCGG motifs (GC box) associated with the 21 base pair (bp) repeats in SV40 DNA and to activate both early and late SV40 transcription in vitro.[110–114] The Sp1-binding sites are frequently present in tandem arrays upstream of the transcription initiation site of many eukaryotic genes and may be adjacent to DNA motifs that interact with other known transcription factors.[115] Highly purified preparations of Sp1 bind to sequences in the HIV LTR mapping between positions −43 and −83, a

TABLE 25–1. TRANSCRIPTION FACTOR BINDING SITES IN THE HIV LTR

| FACTOR | CONSENSUS SEQUENCE OF BINDING SITE | HIV BINDING SITES | | PROPERTIES/FUNCTION | SOURCE OF FACTOR | REFERENCE |
		Number	Location			
Ap-1	$^G/_C$TGACT$^C/_A$A	2	−350 to −345	DNA binding	H9 cells	160, 164
TRE/ERE, Coup	GGTCA...TCA$^C/_T$C	1	−356 to −323	DNA binding	Activated Jurkat cells	165
NFAT	−290 to −263 in IL-2 enhancer	1	−254 to −216	DNA binding	Activated T lymphocytes	163
USF	GGCCACTGTGACC	1	−179 to −159	DNA binding	HeLa cells	116
NF-κB	GGGACTTTCC	2	−109 to −79	DNA binding; basal and TAT-activated transcription	T cells; B cells	120, 148–150
Sp-1	GGGCGG	3	−79 to −30	DNA binding; basal and TAT-activated transcription	HeLa and T cells	116–119
TATA	ATATAA	1	−27 to −23	DNA binding; basal and TAT-activated transcription	HeLa cells	166, 167
LBP	TCTGG or CCAGA	2	−58 to −16 −16 to +27	DNA binding; stimulation and repression of transcription	HeLa and Jurkat cells	168, 169
UBP-1	CTCTCTGG	1	−13 to +28	DNA binding	HeLa cells	170
CTF/NFI	CCAAT	1	+40 to +45	DNA binding	HeLa cells	168

region containing three Sp1-binding sites.[116, 117] Functional analyses of HIV LTR driven reporter constructs indicate that mutations of individual or pairs of Sp1 sites had little, if any, effect on the basal or Tat-transactivated levels of expression.[118] Mutation of all three HIV Sp1 sites, however, markedly reduced the response to Tat.[118, 119] The role of the Sp1 elements during HIV production is somewhat variable depending on the cell type infected.[120–122] Mutations that functionally inactivate all three Sp1 motifs completely abrogated replicative capacity in Jurkat cells, delayed progeny virus production in CEM and H9 cells, and had little effect on infectivity in peripheral blood lymphocytes (PBLs).

In the HIV-1 LTR, the two NF-κB motifs, together with the three Sp1 sites, are considered to function as the principal *enhancers* of transcription (see Fig. 25–6). NF-κB was originally described as a factor, induced by lipopolysaccharide or phorbol esters in mature B cells, that bound to the enhancer for the κ light chain gene and activated its transcription.[123, 124] Subsequent work has shown that a variety of immunologically relevant genes, including interleukin (IL)-2, β-interferon, granulocyte-macrophage colony-stimulating factor (GM-CSF), tumor necrosis factor (TNF)-α, IL-2 receptor α chain, T-cell receptor β chain, and class I major histocompatibility complex (MHC), can be activated or inhibited (IL-6) by NF-κB[125–132]; many of these genes contain the upstream canonical NF-κB–binding site (GGGACTTTCC). It is therefore not surprising that primate lentiviruses, which may reside for many years in the T cells and/or macrophages of their infected hosts, include the NF-κB–binding motif upstream of their respective transcriptional start sites.

It has recently been reported that NF-κB is a member of a large family of transcriptionally important proteins, which include the c-*rel* protein and the *dorsal*

gene product of *Drosophila,* a regulator of pattern development.[133–137] NF-κB "binding activity" was originally identified as a heterodimeric protein consisting of 50 kDa and 65 kDa subunits.[138] Because different members of the c-Rel family may contribute to the formation of NF-κB, a heterogeneous population of heterodimers with different functional specificities constitute this group of eukaryotic regulatory proteins. NF-κB heterodimers have been identified in the cytoplasm of many cells complexed to a member of a family of inhibitory proteins known as IkB.[139–141] Experiments carried out in vitro show that phosphorylation of the IkB moiety of the IkB/NF-κB complex leads to its dissociation from NF-κB and a concomitant translocation of "free" NF-κB from the cytoplasm to the nucleus, where it can function to regulate RNA synthesis.[142] NF-κB activation is therefore post-transcriptional and depends on a variety of stimuli that induce protein kinase A or protein kinase C to phosphorylate the 40 kDa species of IkB.[141, 142] Inducers of NF-κB include T-cell activators such as mitogens, antigens, and cytokines as well as agents known specifically to stimulate NF-κB, such as lipopolysaccharides, phorbol esters, calcium ionophores, and the HTLV-I Tax protein.[130, 131, 143–147]

Activated human T lymphocytes and T-cell lines contain factors that bind to the HIV NF-κB sites and stimulate both the basal and Tat-induced levels of chloramphenicol acetyl transferase (CAT) synthesis as monitored in transient transfection assays.[148–150] Mutations of the two NF-κB–binding sites abolish the response of the HIV LTR to T-cell activators in these reporter gene systems. In contrast, when the NF-κB motifs were mutated or deleted in the context of wild-type HIV, little, if any, effect was noted during subsequent virus infection of human T-cell lines or phytohemaglutinin (PHA)–activated peripheral blood lymphocytes.[120] In an infected individual, however, the HIV NF-κB elements very likely facilitate the response to activation signals. HIV-1 cannot replicate in resting T lymphocytes.[151-154] Following T-cell activation, however, the block to infection is relieved, and NF-κB binding to its cognate site in the integrated provirus induces the synthesis of the "earliest" viral gene products (regulatory proteins) required for the initiation of the replicative cycle.

Early studies of HIV LTR-directed expression of reporter genes suggested that a large domain (-410 to -157) within U3, designated the *Negative Regulatory Element* (or NRE; see Fig. 25–6), might "silence" viral gene activity.[155-157] The NRE inhibitory effect was inferred from a series of nested deletions extending from the 5' end of the LTR, which successively eliminated putative binding sites for transcriptionally relevant factors and was associated with increases in basal and Tat-induced levels of transcription in Jurkat cells. Factors have been purified from human T-cell lines that bind to HIV NRE; one of these, a 50 kDa protein, also binds to a transcriptional suppressor element located upstream of the IL-2 receptor α-chain gene.[158-160] Despite reports that (1) target the negative effect of the HIV Nef protein to NRE[161] and (2) suggest that mutations localized to the NRE result in augmented virus replication in monocytes/macrophages,[162] there is a paucity of convincing evidence that the NRE plays a significant role in the HIV life cycle. Of note are studies showing that a stimulatory factor present in activated T cells (NFAT), which binds to the IL-2 enhancer, also reacts with the NRE domain of the HIV LTR.[163] Confounding this observation, however, was the unexpected finding that the NFAT-binding site in the HIV LTR has no homology with the NFAT motif associated with the IL-2 gene. As noted in Table 25–1, the R region of the HIV LTR, situated *downstream* of the transcription start site, contains cognate binding sites for at least three cellular factors that potentially regulate RNA synthesis during productive infection.

Gene products encoded by several heterologous animal viruses are also capable of transactivating the HIV LTR.[156, 171-175] Although this effect has been touted by some as indicating a role of these viruses in disease progression, the co-infection of human T cells by HIV and other viruses has been difficult to document in seropositive individuals. On the basis of tropism for CD4-positive human mononuclear cells, agents capable of directly or indirectly transactivating the HIV LTR would include human T-cell leukemia virus (HTLV)-I, human cytomegalovirus (HCMV), human herpes virus type 6 (HHV6), and possibly human adenoviruses.[176] In the case of HTLV-I, it has been proposed that the elevated levels of NF-κB induced by the viral-encoded Tax protein[130, 131] activate HIV replication by binding to the two NF-κB motifs in its LTR.

HIV-Encoded Regulatory Proteins

Tat

Although the mechanism underlying Tat transactivation of HIV LTR-directed expression is hotly debated, it is universally agreed that the major effect of Tat is to increase the steady-state levels of viral RNA. When the *tat* gene of an infectious molecular proviral clone of HIV is mutagenized, no detectable progeny virions are produced.[177, 178] HIV-1 Tat is a nuclear protein[179, 180] with 86 to 101 residues (depending on the isolate), encoded by two exons. A shorter 72 amino acid "single-exon Tat protein" possesses all of the functional properties of the full-length Tat, as measured in tissue culture infections or LTR-driven reporter gene experiments.[177, 181-183] The termination codon following the first Tat exon is highly conserved[184] among different HIV-1 isolates, suggesting possible unique roles for the "one exon" and "two exon" Tat proteins during different phases of productive infection in vivo.

As previously noted, RNA synthesis in eukaryotic cells is modulated by transcription activator proteins that bind to DNA motifs located upstream of their respective promoters. Visna virus, another member of the lentivirus subfamily, encodes a DNA-binding transcriptional transactivator that interacts with Ap-1 sites located in its LTR upstream of the viral promoter.[185] HTLV-I/HTLV-II and the human spumaviruses encode their own transactivating proteins designated Tax and Bel-1, respectively (see Fig. 25–1), which interact (indirectly, in the case of Tax) with LTR elements also situated upstream of the transcriptional start site[186-188] (see Chapter 26). In contrast, the immediate target of primate lentiviral transcriptional activators, including HIV Tat, maps to sequences *downstream* of the start site for viral RNA synthesis.[155] This unusually located transactivation response region, or TAR element (see Fig. 25–6), in fact, lacks several properties usually associated with transactivators of eukaryotic *pol* II mediated transcription: It is inactive when present (1) in an inverted orientation; (2) 5' to the promoter; or (3) downstream of the transcription termination site (U5 region of the 3' LTR).[155, 182, 189-193] These unusual properties were subsequently reconciled when it was demonstrated that the TAR-binding site did not function as a component of DNA, but as an element situated at the 5' terminus of *all* viral mRNAs (see Fig. 25–6).[194]

HIV-1 TAR was originally thought to encompass the first 57 nt of nascent HIV transcripts and had the capacity to fold into a stable stem-loop structure. Subsequent work has shown that the minimal TAR element (mapping between bases $+19$ and $+42$) consists of two short stems, a U-rich bulge, and a G-rich loop (Fig. 25–7).[189-192, 195-197] Interestingly, the TAR element associated with HIV-2 is a double stem-loop structure, each possessing the U-rich bulge and G-rich loop.[198] Sequences located in both the pentanucleotide loop and the trinucleotide bulge of the HIV-1 TAR are critical for Tat function.[192, 195-197] Purified preparations of Tat bind to TAR RNA at a ratio of 1:1 and with high affinity (12 μM).[199] Tat binds to wild-type or "loop" mutants of TAR but *not* to TAR elements containing alterations affecting the bulge region.[166, 189, 190, 196, 200-202] Modification of the invariant "bulge" U_{+22} nucleotide and elimination of the base pairs immediately above and below the bulge (see Fig. 25–7) significantly reduces

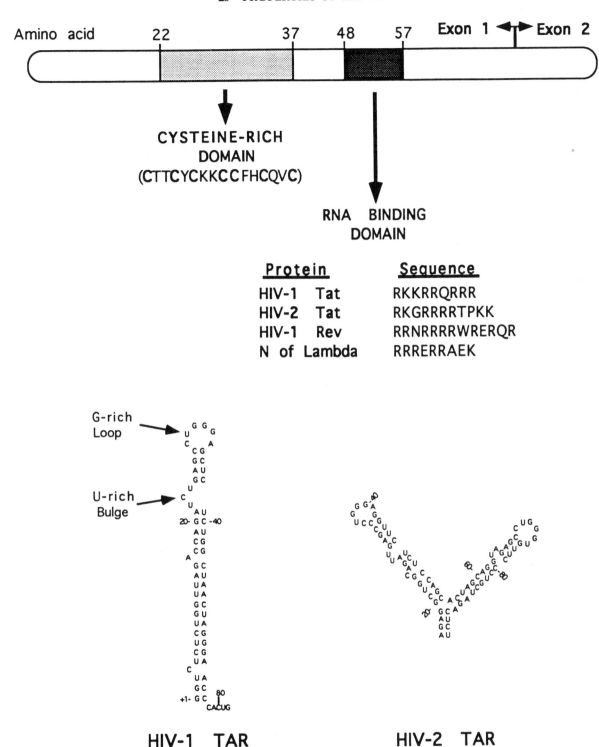

FIGURE 25–7. Tat and its response element TAR. Schematic representation of the HIV-1 Tat protein *(top)* with the cysteine-rich activating and RNA-binding domains indicated. The portions of the Tat protein encoded by its two exons are indicated as well as arginine-rich motifs, present in other proteins thought to be involved in RNA binding.[210] The stem-bulge-loop configurations of HIV-1 and HIV-2 TAR elements are shown at the bottom.

the binding of Tat.[202] It has also been shown that Tat binds to synthetic oligoribonucleotide structures containing as few as one to three unpaired bases.[203, 204]

The failure of TAR "loop mutants" to support increased LTR-directed expression despite their capacity to bind Tat in vitro raised the possibility that cellular proteins might be required to interact with the loop or other regions of TAR to stabilize the Tat-

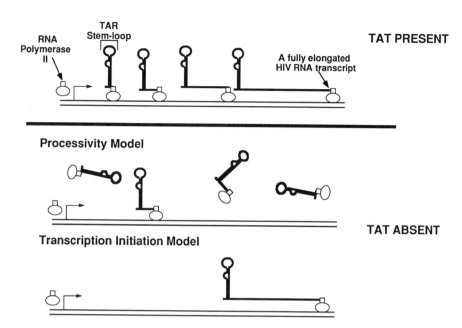

TAT PRESENT

TAT ABSENT

FIGURE 25–8. Models of Tat transactivation. In the presence of Tat *(top)*, the transcription initiation complex, containing RNA polymerase II, is assembled at the transcription start site *(bent arrow)* and produces many RNA transcripts containing the stem-bulge-loop TAR structure at their 5' termini. According to the processivity model *(middle)* for Tat transactivation, the initiation of RNA synthesis is normal and does not require Tat. In the absence of Tat, however, the elongation of normally initiated nascent transcripts proceeds poorly. Newly synthesized HIV mRNAs are prematurely terminated, released from the template, and degraded. In the transcription initiation model *(bottom)* of Tat transactivation, Tat participates in the assembly of the initiation complex, and in its absence, only a limited number of viral transcripts are produced.

TAR complex and/or to increase the specificity of complex formation. A 68 kDa loop-binding protein, originally identified following UV cross-linking to TAR RNA, in fact fails to interact with most TAR "loop mutants" and cooperatively interacts with Tat to modestly stimulate in vitro HIV LTR-directed transcription.[205, 206] In addition, a 185 kDa protein that binds to the lower TAR stem and a 44 kDa protein that interacts with the upper stem connecting the bulge to the loop have also been reported.[207, 208]

Wild-type and mutagenized Tat proteins have been exhaustively analyzed for their ability to bind to TAR or to transactivate HIV LTR-regulated reporter genes, or both. The RNA binding domain of the Tat protein has been mapped to a lysine-arginine–rich region between residues 48 to 57 (see Fig. 25–7); peptides containing this segment bind to the TAR bulge region with somewhat less affinity and specificity than do purified preparations of Tat.[209] This highly basic domain of Tat has similarities to the binding region present in the HIV Rev transactivator protein (see below) and is also found in a larger family of arginine-rich RNA-binding proteins.[210] A nuclear localization signal (GRKKR) also overlaps this RNA-binding region of Tat.[180, 211] The transcription activation domain of Tat has been more difficult to map and encompasses the amino-terminal 48 residues containing (1) highly acidic amino acids (residues 1 to 21); (2) cysteine-rich amino acids (7 cysteines/16 residues; position 22 to 37); and (3) a segment highly conserved among different HIV isolates (amino acids 41 to 47) (see Fig. 25–7). Site-directed mutagenesis in these portions of the Tat protein drastically reduces transactivation activity.[166, 211]

The HIV Tat protein was originally described as a regulator of *both* RNA and protein production[179, 183, 212, 213] based on the results of CAT assays in which the Tat-induced levels of protein synthesis, measured as CAT enzyme activity, were always greater than the observed increases in RNA production. This apparent duality of function was subsequently shown to reflect the relatively long half-life of CAT protein compared with the stability of CAT RNA; when the synthesis rather than the accumulation of CAT was monitored, the effects of Tat transactivation on RNA and protein synthesis were indistinguishable.[214]

Although the mechanism(or mechanisms) underlying Tat transactivation has engendered considerable debate, there is general agreement on two points: (1) Tat increases steady-state levels of HIV LTR-directed transcripts; and (2) the promoter proximal positioning of Tat (via its interaction with TAR) is required for transcriptional transactivation. Two models have been invoked to explain the elevated levels of viral RNA synthesized in the presence of Tat (Fig. 25–8). One proposes that Tat acts at the step of transcription initiation. The other model suggests that in the absence of Tat, transcription initiation is normal; in this second model, Tat acts at a postinitiation step to facilitate transcriptional elongation.

The elongation/processivity model evolved from the observed accumulation in transfected monkey kidney cells of short RNA transcripts (~59 nt), which were converted to larger RNA species following the addition of Tat.[191] When it was subsequently demonstrated that the elimination of sequences (mapping to the TAR region) purportedly responsible for premature transcriptional termination failed to relieve the observed block, the model was modified. Instead, it was proposed that in the absence of Tat, HIV LTR-directed transcription terminated randomly at multiple sites prior to the synthesis of full-length RNA, owing to inefficient elongation.[189, 192, 215] Because prematurely released nascent transcripts were unstable and rapidly degraded, only the 59 nt TAR RNA stem-loops could be detected, presumably because they represented the major nuclease resistant product.[192] In in vitro transcription experiments, Tat relieved a block in the production of "long" TAR-containing RNAs.[205, 216] All of these experiments buttress the elongation/processivity model in which Tat is viewed as a general elongation factor that becomes a component of the assembled transcription complex by virtue of its association with TAR and functions to generate full-length viral mRNAs.

In the transcription initiation model, Tat behaves like a conventional eukaryotic transactivator/coactivator of transcription and participates in the assembly of the initiation complex. Three lines of evidence support this mechanism of Tat function:

1. Deletion mutagenesis of the HIV LTR has shown that the upstream enhancer elements NF-κB and Sp1 are required for Tat transactivation.[120, 150] When both sets of binding motifs are removed from the HIV LTR, responsiveness to Tat is lost, a result implying that Tat interacts directly or indirectly with cellular transcription factors to increase steady state levels of HIV RNA. This cooperativity is analogous to the reported interactions of other viral transactivators with cellular regulatory proteins such as VP16 of herpes simplex virus (HSV) type 1 with Oct-1, the E2 protein of bovine papillomavirus type 1 with Sp1, and the E1A protein of adenovirus with TFIID during the formation of the initiation complex.[217–220]

2. In nuclear run-on assays, Tat induced a 15-fold increase in the density of transcripts within 80 nt of the start site as well as a substantial augmentation of RNAs mapping further downstream.[221, 222] In this experimental setting, Tat was responsible for an increase in transcription initiation.

3. Chimeric proteins, consisting of Tat fused to peptides containing known binding sites for RNA (R17 and Rev) or DNA (c-jun and Gal 4), conferred new targets onto Tat and, by implication, demonstrated that transactivation could occur when Tat is recruited to the initiation complex during its assembly.[223–227] Most important, transactivation was observed in the absence of TAR and whether Tat was bound to DNA or RNA.

The mechanistic differences between the two models of Tat transactivation may be more apparent than real. Both models posit Tat affecting the "quality" of the assembled transcription complex. Advocates of Tat as a transcription initiation factor propose that Tat binds to TAR merely to deploy it in the general vicinity of the initiation complex, where it could "bend backward" or even be released from TAR to interact with the complex. The role of TAR (and TAR-binding proteins) in this process would be merely to deliver Tat to the promoter, where it could provide a missing function or displace a factor that inhibits efficient transcription. In the processivity model, Tat would be incorporated into a partially assembled transcription complex following the polymerization of the first 60+ nt of HIV RNA (to generate the TAR stem-loop), thereby promoting the elongation of short nascent transcripts.

During transactivation it is quite likely that Tat cooperatively binds to transcription factors, and its interaction with TAR requires the participation of other cellular proteins. In this regard, Tat transactivation is markedly reduced in rodent cells compared with human cells. Stable human-rodent cell hybrids containing human chromosome 12, however, support high levels of Tat responsiveness, suggesting the existence of a Tat cofactor (or cofactors) in human cells.[228, 229]

Possible extracellular roles for Tat have been suggested from studies showing that Tat is taken up by cultured cells, enters the nucleus, and transactivates genes linked to the HIV LTR.[230] Tat purified from *Escherichia coli* has also been reported to inhibit antigen-induced, but not mitogen-induced, proliferation of peripheral blood mononuclear cells.[231] In a similar vein, low concentrations of Tat exhibit a modest stimulatory effect on a tissue culture model of AIDS–Kaposi sarcoma cells.[232] The significance of these extracellular Tat activities in HIV-infected individuals is currently unclear.

Rev

During studies of certain *tat* mutants, it was noted that *tat* cDNAs supplied in *trans* failed to completely correct the original mutant phenotype. Although the high steady-state levels of the multiply spliced mRNAs were restored in the nucleus and cytoplasm, the unspliced/partially spliced transcripts and their encoded proteins were markedly reduced or absent in the cytoplasm. The defect observed was later shown to reflect the absence of a second HIV-encoded regulatory protein (Rev), which had been simultaneously inactivated by the mutation initially thought to affect only *tat*.[233] Subsequent studies demonstrated that the Rev protein acts post-transcriptionally to facilitate the transport of unspliced *gag/pol* and singly spliced *vif*, *vpr*, and *vpu/env* mRNAs from the nucleus to the cytoplasm of infected cells.[234–237] In the absence of Rev, these classes of HIV transcripts fail to accumulate in the cytoplasm and virus does not replicate.[212–233] Rev-responsive transcripts all contain a *cis*-acting element that is required for Rev activation (Fig. 25–9). This element (*rev responsive element*, or RRE) has been mapped to a 200+ nt segment of the *env* gene.[235, 237, 238]

In eukaryotic cells, nascent RNA transcripts undergo additional modification (or modifications) prior to their translation. Capping/methylation, polyadenylation, and splicing occur concomitant with, or shortly after, the synthesis of the primary transcripts and precede the export of messenger RNAs (mRNAs) from the nucleus to the cytoplasm, where translation occurs. Consequently, nascent transcripts must interact in a highly ordered fashion with multiple RNA-binding proteins involved in these processing steps.

The genomes of replication-competent retroviruses must undergo differential splicing to generate viral structural and regulatory proteins; the coordinated expression of completely spliced, partially spliced, and unspliced mRNAs is required for this process. In

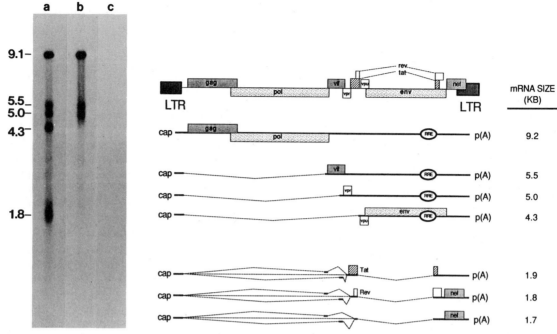

FIGURE 25–9. HIV RNA transcripts present in productively infected cells. A Northern blot analysis *(left)* in which poly(A)⁺ RNA, prepared from HIV-1–infected human PBLs and immobilized on a nitocellulose membrane following electrophoresis through 1 per cent formaldehyde agarose gels, was hybridized to labeled LTR (lane a), Vif (lane b), and control plasmid (lane c) DNA probes. The LTR probe would be expected to react with all classes of HIV mRNA, whereas the Vif probe would hybridize only to the 9.2 kb *gag/pol* and 5.5 kb *vif* mRNAs as diagrammed on the right. The structure of different HIV-1 RNA transcripts is shown on the right. The location of coding sequences and position of the Rev-responsive element (RRE), present in mRNAs encoding viral structural proteins, are indicated. The dashed lines connect splice donors and acceptors; alternative forms of Tat, Rev, and Nev mRNAs, some of which contain short upstream non-coding exons, are shown at the bottom. (Left side of figure with permission from Rabson, A. B., et al.: Transcription of novel open reading frames of the AIDS retrovirus during infection of lymphocytes. Science 229:1388, 1985. Copyright 1985 by the AAAS.)

contrast, the splicing of cellular transcripts is usually rapid and complete; the export of incompletely spliced cellular mRNAs is an infrequent occurrence.[239–241] If an individual splice donor or acceptor site for a particular cellular transcript is mutagenized, the splicing reaction may be arrested at an early step and the RNA becomes sequestered in the nucleus and ultimately degraded. Such eukaryotic RNAs "committed" to or engaged in splicing are ignored by the nuclear machinery responsible for export to the cytoplasm. It has been suggested that murine and avian retroviruses regulate the synthesis of unspliced *gag/pol* and single-spliced *env* mRNAs by incorporating "suboptimal" splice sites into their genomes. Interestingly, the substitution of "strong" splice sites for weak ones in these retroviral genomic RNAs results in the overproduction of the proteins encoded by spliced mRNAs and the generation of replication-incompetent particles.[242–244]

HIV-1 encodes the Rev protein to regulate the expression and utilization of the unspliced 9.2 kb *gag/pol* and the singly spliced 5.5 kb *vif*, 5.0 kb *vpr*, and 4.3 kb *vpu/env* mRNAs in the cytoplasm of infected cells (see Fig. 25–9). During virus production, the multiply spliced class of HIV-1 transcripts, which range between 1.7 and 2.0 kb in size and encode the Tat, Rev, and Nef proteins, are the first detectable

viral mRNAs synthesized. The delayed production of the unspliced and partially spliced HIV transcripts has led to the proposal that primate lentiviral gene expression is temporally regulated.[245]

Polymerase chain reaction (PCR) analyses have demonstrated the presence of more than 30 different HIV transcripts in virus-producing cells.[246–251] Many of these mRNAs are members of the heterogeneous 1.7 to 2.0 kb multiply spliced class encoding important regulatory proteins, and several contain very short (50 and 74 bp) upstream non-coding exons, possibly present to increase transcript stability (see Fig. 25–9). Nef mRNA is the initial and most abundant multiply spliced transcript produced during infection.[246] The functional significance of the plethora of multiply spliced mRNA species encoding the same viral protein (e.g., three *tat*, six *rev*, and three *nef* transcripts[248]), as well as the delineation of the hierarchy of HIV splice site usage, is at present unclear and under intensive investigation.

In contrast to many prokaryotic transcripts, eukaryotic mRNAs usually direct the synthesis of a single protein. Efficient translation in eukaryotic cells generally relies on a "scanning" mechanism by which ribosomes bind near the 5′ end of a messenger RNA and begin translation at the first AUG codon when it

REV PROTEIN

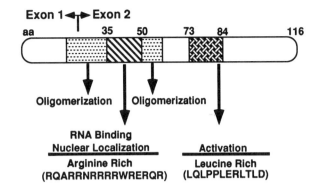

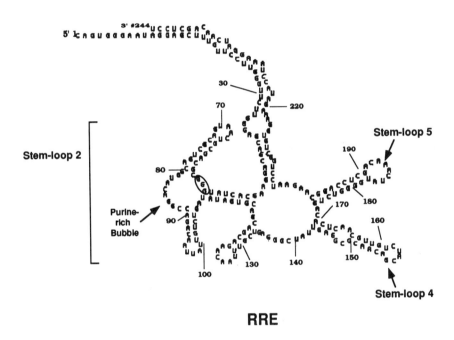

RRE

FIGURE 25–10. Rev and its response element, RRE. A schematic representation of the HIV-1 Rev protein with RNA-binding, activation, and oligomerization domains is shown at the top. The proposed structure of the RRE[237] is presented at the bottom with the targets of HIV-1 Rev (stem-loop 2) and HTLV I Rex (stem-loops 4 and 5) indicated. The "bulged" G residues are circled.

is present in a suitable context; most proteins are initiated from the first AUG, and it is uncommon to use more than one initiation site within a given mRNA.[252] Some animal viruses, however, have been shown to express more than one protein from a single transcript.[252] In the case of HIV-1, PCR analyses have shown that all of the *env* mRNAs contain an intact *vpu* open reading frame upstream of the *env* coding sequences. The efficient expression of Env is, in fact, dependent on "leaky" scanning and bypassing of the initiation codon for the Vpu protein, which is situated in a weak consensus context for efficient translation.[249, 253] The substitution of the HIV-1 *tat* initiation codon, with its strong context for translation initiation, for the weak *vpu* initiation site markedly reduces *env* expression. Because the *rev* AUG is also considered to exist in a "weak" context, *rev* mRNAs, which contain *nef* coding sequences downstream, may also be bicistronic and direct the synthesis of Nef.

HIV Rev is a 19 kDa nuclear phosphoprotein con-

taining 116 amino acid residues. Like Tat, Rev is encoded by two exons and contains two functional domains: one for RNA binding or oligomerization and a second that is the effector for transactivation (Fig. 25–10).[256, 259] However, unlike *tat*, *both* coding exons of *rev* are required for function; a singly spliced mRNA encodes a 25 residue non-functional Rev protein.[248, 260] As noted earlier (Fig. 25–7), the arginine-rich region of Rev (residues 35 to 50) shares homology with Tat as well as a larger family of arginine-rich RNA-binding proteins;[210] like the RNA-binding region of Tat, this domain of Rev also contains a nuclear localization signal. Regions of Rev abutting this binding domain participate in the formation of Rev oligomers, which generate large tube-like structures that may "coat" the viral RNA.[261, 262]

The Rev effector domain is leucine rich (mapping between residues 73 and 84) and is highly conserved among different lentiviral Rev proteins. This region of HIV Rev is related to a large family of repeating

Leu-Leu motifs (only a single copy is found in HIV Rev) present in a number of soluble or membrane-bound proteins, including the U2 snRNP protein and yeast adenylate cyclase.[263] Unlike the leucine repeats found in some eukaryotic transcription factors, the Rev leucine-rich domain appears to mediate protein-protein interactions. Mutants mapping to this region of Rev are able to bind to the RRE but are functionally inactive. They interfere with the transactivation mediated by wild-type Rev, exerting a so-called trans-dominant effect in assays for Rev function.[257, 259, 264]

The RRE is a complex RNA structure containing multiple stem-loops branching from a large central loop (see Fig. 25–10). The RRE must be present within a Rev-responsive transcript and in the sense orientation for Rev responsiveness.[238, 265] As shown in Figure 25–9, the RRE is spliced out of the mRNAs encoding Tat, Rev, and Nef. Nuclease protection, chemical modification, and mutagenesis studies indicate that Rev interacts with a 60 + nt portion of the RRE, designated stem-loop 2, required for Rev activity (see Fig. 25–10).[256, 266–270] This region of RRE binds Rev even when isolated from the complete RRE and mediates Rev activity in functional assays.[271] The determinants for high-affinity binding of Rev to RRE reside in the central purine-rich "bubble" in stem-loop 2 (see Fig. 25–10), which contains bulged G nucleotides capable of forming unique RNA structures.[256, 261, 272–275] Although high concentrations of purified Rev have been reported to form tubular oligomeric structures in the absence of RNA, it has been proposed that Rev initially makes contact with nucleotides in the RRE loop 2 bubble, thereby generating a nucleation point for the polymerization of additional Rev molecules.[261, 262] HTLV-I is evolutionarily and biologically distinct from HIV, yet encodes a transactivating protein, Rex, which can functionally substitute for HIV Rev (see Chapter 26). In contrast to Rev, Rex binds to stem-loops 4 and 5 of the HIV-1 RRE (see Fig. 25–10) rather than to stem-loop 2.[276, 277]

Rev-deficient HIV mutants are unable to synthesize the Gag, Pol, and Env viral structural proteins and are therefore not infectious. Although the steady-state levels of viral RNA are normal in cells infected with Rev mutants, gag/pol, env, vif, and vpr mRNAs are markedly reduced, and the multiply spliced tat, rev, and nef mRNAs are overrepresented.[212, 233, 235, 237] This pattern of RNA expression suggested that Rev might function as a regulator of splicing. It was subsequently appreciated, however, that the ratios of unspliced (or singly spliced) to multiply spliced viral transcripts in the nucleus did not change in the presence or absence of Rev[235, 237]; instead, the Rev defect was associated with an excess of the 1.7 to 2.0 kb multiply spliced RNA only in the cytoplasmic compartment. Because Rev did not regulate the amounts of unspliced cytoplasmic HIV mRNAs simply by inhibiting splicing of viral transcripts, it was then proposed that Rev controlled the transport of unspliced HIV mRNAs from the nucleus to the cytoplasm.

As noted earlier, the nuclear export of unspliced viral mRNAs is a critical step in retrovirus replication. The nuclei of eukaryotic cells contain factors that interfere with the transport of certain RNAs to the cytoplasm. For example, the C1 and C2 ribonucleoproteins that bind to sequences downstream of the polyadenylation site of nascent RNA transcripts appear to be responsible for the nuclear retention of certain hnRNPs.[278] Similarly, prolonged association of splicing factors with retroviral splice donor and acceptor sites—which are known to be "suboptimal"[242–244]—and the commitment of such "stalled" complexes for the splicing reaction may also contribute to the sequestration of HIV transcripts in the nucleus. In this regard, the presence of even a single suboptimal splice site in an RRE-containing globin transcript has been shown to block its transport to the cytoplasm unless Rev is supplied in trans.[279] Furthermore, the gag, pol, and env regions of the HIV genome contain sequences (designated IR in Figure 25–4) that severely inhibit the expression of covalently linked reporter genes by altering RNA transport to the cytoplasm or decreasing RNA stability.[238, 280, 281] Rev is able to reverse these effects, provided that the RRE is present in such transcripts. The role of Rev in mediating the transport of unspliced viral RNA to the cytoplasm may actually represent a more general regulatory process in eukaryotic cells. By recognizing elements on unspliced transcripts that are intrinsically sequestered in the nucleus, Rev-like proteins function to facilitate transport and utilization of these mRNAs. It has been proposed that the incorporation of transcripts containing the RRE into a rod-like Rev filament may dissociate RNA from binding proteins responsible for nuclear retention.[261]

Two recent reports have suggested that in addition to regulating the intracellular distribution of viral RNA, Rev may be required for the efficient translation of HIV proteins.[282, 283] In the absence of Rev, viral mRNAs, although detectable in the cytoplasm of transfected HeLa or human B cells, were excluded from polyribosomes. In the presence of Rev, HIV mRNA became polysome associated. Any mechanistic link between the RNA splicing/transport and putative translation functions of Rev awaits further analysis.

Nef

The Nef gene, present only in primate lentiviruses, overlaps approximately one half of the 3' LTR (Fig. 25–5) and encodes a 27 kDa membrane-associated and myristylated phosphoprotein. Because Nef, like the HIV Tat and Rev proteins, is encoded by multiply spliced 1.7 to 2.0 kb mRNAs, it was originally considered to be a viral regulatory protein needed for a critical step during the early phase of the replicative cycle. Nef is indeed the first RNA transcript detected in HIV-infected human T-cell lines[246] but is dispensable for virus replication in tissue culture systems. Early reports suggested that Nef downregulated virus replication by affecting a target in the NRE, which restricted transcription directed by the HIV LTR.[161, 284–286] Subsequent studies have failed to confirm these results.[287] It has also been suggested that

Nef was related to G-proteins such as *ras,* possessing GTP-binding and GTPase activities, and therefore might function as a modulator of intracellular second messenger signaling pathways.[288] Subsequent work has not corroborated these biochemical properties.[289–291]

In contrast to these conflicting reports, the deletion of the Nef gene has a profound effect in the SIV/rhesus macaque animal model system. Nef has been shown to be required for (1) the maintenance of large numbers of circulating mononuclear cells containing SIV proviral DNA and (2) the development of immunodeficiency.[292] Monkeys inoculated with *Nef*-deleted virus developed excellent antibody responses but produced no detectable circulating virus. These results imply that Nef plays a critical role in initiating and sustaining SIV infection in vivo. In its absence, virus replication and spread are severely compromised. Although very low levels of progeny virus production were adequate to elicit antibody production in animals inoculated with *nef*-deleted SIV, they were unable to induce disease. The elucidation of the as yet undermined Nef function has obvious implications for primate lentivirus pathogenesis.

An interesting and confirmed property attributed to Nef is its capacity to inhibit the cell surface expression of CD4.[288] The Nef-induced CD4 downregulation in human T, B, and macrophage lines is not associated with reduced steady-state levels of CD4 RNA or protein and occurs via a protein kinase C–independent mechanism.[293]

HIV-Encoded Structural and Other Non-Regulatory Proteins

Gag

Most enveloped virus particles consist of a nucleocapsid core surrounded by an outer lipoprotein shell or envelope. The retrovirus core is encoded by the *gag* (group specific *antigen*) gene, which, in the case of HIV, directs the synthesis of the 55 kDa Gag precursor. This polyprotein (also known as p55) is released from cells as a component of the immature virus particle and is ultimately cleaved by the HIV protease into the mature 17 kDa matrix (MA), 24 kDa capsid (CA), and 15 kDa nucleocapsid (NC) virion proteins (see Fig. 25–5).[294–298] The last is subsequently processed to form the p9 and p6 proteins. As noted previously, the mRNA for p55 is the unspliced 9.2 kb transcript (see Fig. 25–9) that requires Rev for its expression in the cytoplasm. Retroviral Gag proteins have three principal functions during virus assembly: (1) forming the structural inner framework of the virion; (2) encapsidation of the viral genome; and (3) the acquisition of a lipid bilayer and associated glycoproteins during particle release. These processes require that *gag* gene products participate in protein/protein, protein/RNA, and protein/lipid interactions. As is the case for other replication-com-petent retroviruses, the HIV-1 Gag proteins are critical for virus assembly and release, virion stability, and many of the early steps (steps 3 to 6 in Fig. 25–3) in the subsequent replication cycle, including uncoating, reverse transcription, and integration.[64, 299–305]

The HIV p55 Gag precursor rapidly oligomerizes following its translation and is targeted to the plasma membrane, where particle assembly is initiated. *Trans*-dominant HIV-1 *gag* mutants have been reported that interfere with the production of infectious virions, presumably by directing wild-type p55 monomers into non-functional multimeric structures.[306] Retroviruses differ in the mechanisms used for particle assembly. Lentiviruses and the C-type oncoretroviruses assemble progeny virions *only* at the plasma membrane. In contrast, B- and D-type retrovirus particles are formed in the cytoplasm and are subsequently transported to the plasma membrane, where they are released from the cell. However, particle formation by all types of retrotransposable elements is a self-assembly process[307–310]; in the case of HIV-1, particles have been generated in vaccinia, baculovirus, and SV40 expression systems.[311–315] Only the Gag precursor polypeptide is needed for particle formation[310, 311, 316, 317]; there is no requirement for genomic RNA or the envelope, reverse transcriptase, or protease proteins[309, 317–323] (Fig. 25–11). However, *infectious* virions are produced only at those sites on the plasma membrane where nucleoprotein structures, consisting of oligomerized Gag and Gag/Pol precursors plus two molecules of genomic RNA, directly interact with envelope glycoprotein multimers. Proteolytic processing by the viral-encoded protease (PR) subsequent to budding (step 11 in Fig. 25–3) results in a condensation of the immature nucleoid into the cone-shaped core characteristic of mature HIV particles (Fig. 25–12). In many retroviral systems, particularly HIV-1, *non—virion-associated* Gag (and Env) proteins may be released from cells in large quantities and mistakenly identified and titered as components of infectious particles.

The MA domain of p55 is responsible for transporting the oligomerized Gag polyprotein to the cell surface and for initiating the extrusion of the plasma membrane during the early steps of budding. These processes depend on the addition of myristic acid to an amino-terminal glycine residue of the retroviral Gag polyprotein.[324–327] When this glycine of the HIV p17 MA is mutagenized, budding as well as the release of particles fails to occur,[320] reconfirming the importance of myristic acid–mediated association of Gag precursor oligomers with the cell membrane. Following budding and virion maturation, the MA protein of HIV forms an inner shell, detected by immuno-electron microscopy, which is interposed between the glycoprotein envelope and virus core.[328]

The encapsidation of viral genomic RNA is an important step in the production of infectious HIV particles. Like other retroviruses, HIV does not suppress cellular RNA synthesis and has therefore evolved a process for selectively packaging the small fraction of intracellular RNA consisting of unspliced viral

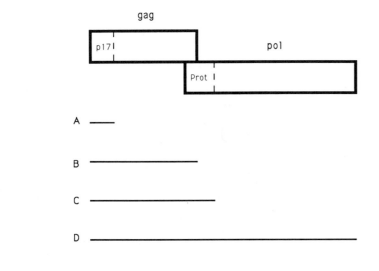

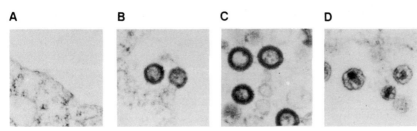

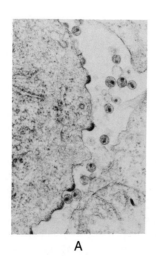
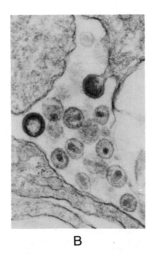
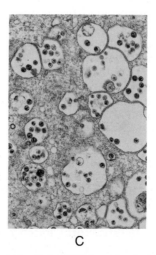

FIGURE 25–11. Requirements for HIV-1 particle formation. DNA segments, isolated from an infectious molecular clone of HIV-1 and encoding p17 Gag (fragment A), p55 Gag precursor (fragment B), p55 Gag plus protease (fragment C), and p55 plus the Gag/Pol fusion protein (fragment D), were incorporated into recombinant vaccinia viruses. HeLa cells, infected with the vaccinia recombinants containing HIV segments A, B, C, or D, were examined by electron microscopy (insets A–D). Note that expression of the p17 MA protein failed to generate detectable particles, whereas cells exposed to the HIV *gag* or *gag* + *pol* gene segments (segments B, C, and D) directed the synthesis of particles. Note that only the *gag/pol* segment D produced particles containing a condensed nucleoid structure. (Adapted from Ross, E. K., et al.: Maturation of human immunodeficiency virus particles assembled from the *gag* precursor protein requires in situ processing by *gag-pol* protease. AIDS Res. Hum. Retroviruses 7:475, 1991; with permission.)

RNA. This is the function of the NC domain of the Gag precursor polyprotein, which is responsible for incorporating two copies of viral RNA into the assembling virion.[329, 330] Because subgenomic spliced retroviral mRNAs and genomic RNA possess indistinguishable 5′ and 3′ termini, it was proposed that preferential packaging of full-length RNA was directed by a *cis* element, designated *psi* (see Fig. 25–4), located in intronic sequences absent from processed transcripts.[331, 332] Such sequences have been mapped 3′ to the major splice donor near the 5′ terminus of avian, murine, and human retroviral genomes, including HIV. Mutation of the HIV-1 *psi* site markedly reduces RNA packaging and virus infectivity.[333–335] Dimerization of retroviral genomic RNA may occur prior to or concomitant with its incorporation into the multimerized Gag precursor. The annealing of the two RNA molecules utilizes a unique 5′ to 5′ linkage[336]

FIGURE 25–12. Electron micrographs of HIV-1–infected human mononuclear cells. *A*, An HIV-1 productively infected T cell with budding structures at the plasma membrane and extracellular virus particles containing the characteristic bullet-shaped core (52,000×). *B*, Higher power micrograph showing HIV-1 particles (1) in the process of budding, (2) with an uncondensed core, and (3) with a processed bullet-shaped nucleoid (108,000×). *C*, Particles located within intracytoplasmic vacuoles in an HIV-1 productively infected monocyte-derived macrophage (25,000×). (These photomicrographs were kindly provided by Dr. Jan Orenstein.)

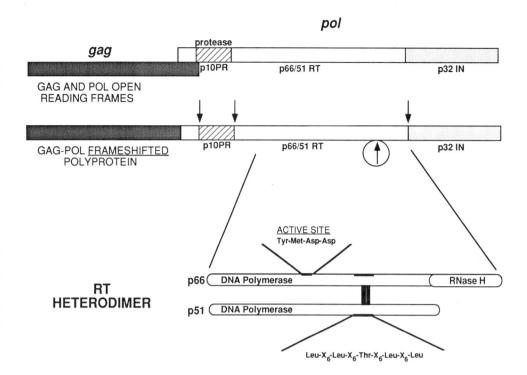

FIGURE 25–13. Derivation of the HIV-1 reverse transcriptase. The overlapping *gag* and *pol* opening reading frames are shown at the top, and the frame-shifted Gag-Pol precursor protein in the middle. The indicated *pol* gene products are proteolytically processed from the frame-shifted Gag/Pol polyprotein precursor (*downward-pointing arrows*). Following the formation of the p66 reverse transcriptase homo-dimer, proteolytic digestion by the HIV p10 protease (*upward-pointing arrow in circle*) releases a 15 kDa RNase H–related product from one of the p66 subunits to generate the p66/p51 heterodimer depicted at the bottom. The location of the active site for DNA polymerization (Tyr-Met-Asp-Asp), a leucine-rich putative intersubunit linker, and the RNase H domain of RT are shown.

and requires an approximately 100 nt domain of HIV that includes the *psi* element.[337–338] The dimerization reaction in vitro is accelerated by purified HIV NC protein and is observed only with preparations of "sense" RNA.

The HIV-1 NC protein, like its homologue in other retroviruses, contains tandem repeats of invariantly spaced cysteine and histidine residues of the sequence $C-X_2-C-X_4-H-X_4-C$.[302, 339–342] This sequence is referred to as a cysteine array, or Cys-His box, and is required for the packaging of retroviral genomic RNA during virion assembly.[302, 340, 342, 343] The NC cysteine array is the functional equivalent of the zinc finger motif originally described for the gene 32 single-stranded DNA-binding protein of T4 phage.[344] It has recently been demonstrated that purified HIV-1 NC binds zinc and other metal ions in vitro, and purified virions contain stably associated zinc.[345–347] Mutation of the two HIV-1 Cys-His boxes reduces the packaging of viral RNA to 2 to 20 per cent of wild-type virus and completely abolishes infectivity.[348]

A curiosity of HIV *gag* expression in human cells is that substantial amounts of the p55 Gag polyprotein are processed intracellularly.[349] This production of cell-associated p24 CA protein can be partially blocked by inhibitors of the HIV protease. The release of such non–virion-associated processed CA from virus-producing cells undoubtedly contributes to the p24 antigenemia characteristic of the late stages of HIV infection in vivo.

Pol

The *pol* gene is the most highly conserved region of the HIV genome. As is the case for other replication-competent retroviruses, the *pol* gene encodes four enzymatic activities (protease, reverse transcriptase, RNase H, and integrase) needed for several early events that occur during productive infection. None of the Pol proteins contain an initiator methionine residue; all are derived by enzymatic cleavage of a 180 kDa Gag-Pol fusion protein that can be produced only by a ribosomal frameshifting mechanism (Fig. 25–13). The ratio of Gag to Gag-Pol proteins in retrovirus-producing cells is tightly regulated and is usually in the range of 10 to 20:1,[48, 350–352] undoubtedly reflecting the relative inefficiency of the frameshifting process. In the HIV genome, the *gag* and *pol* reading frames overlap for 241 nt; the frameshift to the *pol* reading frame is − 1 relative to *gag*. If the requirement for frameshifting in the HIV genome is eliminated by the insertion of a single nucleotide, the Gag-Pol precursor is overexpressed. This results in the intracellular proteolytic processing of the Gag and Gag-Pol polyproteins by the abundant amounts of viral protease arising from the "in-frame" Gag-Pol precursor, the release of free p24 and reverse transcriptase from cells, and no production of progeny virions.[353] The switch from the *gag* to the HIV-1 *pol* reading frame occurs during translation of a run of uracil residues and is less dependent than other retroviral frameshift events on downstream RNA secondary structure.[351, 354] Like p55 Gag, the N-terminus of the Gag-Pol fusion protein is myristoylated and targeted to the plasma membrane, where it also interacts with envelope glycoprotein multimers during the budding process. Because the frameshift to the *pol* reading frame of HIV-1 occurs downstream of the second Cys-His box, it is likely that the Gag-Pol precursor also coordinates zinc ions and binds to genomic RNA.

PROTEASE (PR). The sequence encoding the retroviral protease is always located between the *gag* and *pol* genes; in the HIV genome, it is physically part of the *pol* open reading frame (see Fig. 25–1). The proteolytic digestion of the Gag and Pol precursors is required to generate infectious virions, a process that occurs following particle release (step 11, Fig. 25–3). PR mutants of HIV-1, generated by transfection, lack the bullet-shaped core characteristic of mature virions (see Fig. 25–12) and are not infectious.[355, 356] Retroviral PRs are members of the aspartic protease family of cellular proteases because they contain the conserved Asp-Thr(Ser)-Gly sequence at their active site.[357–359] However, because they are less than half the size of cellular aspartic proteases (HIV PR is only 99 amino acids in length), it was hypothesized that retroviral PRs functioned as dimers, with each monomer contributing the conserved sequence to the active site. Biochemical studies have indeed shown that enzymatically active retroviral PRs are dimeric molecules.[360, 361] Crystallography of HIV-1 PR indicates that it possesses the twofold symmetry of a dimer and that the substrate-binding site is located within a cleft formed between the two monomers.[362–369] Like cellular aspartic proteases, the HIV PR dimer also contains "flaps" that overhang the binding site and may stabilize the substrate within the cleft. Structural studies of this type may prove useful for constructing inhibitors of HIV PR.

The HIV and other retroviral PRs are spontaneously cleaved from their respective Gag-Pol precursors subsequent to budding from infected cells or following their expression in bacteria and yeast.[296, 370–372] This reaction requires low pH[361] and high concentrations of the Gag-Pol precursor,[373] conditions obviously achievable within newly released particles. When mutant HIV proviruses, engineered to synthesize a linked PR dimer, are transfected into cells, the autocatalytic processing of PR intracellularly is extremely rapid, resulting in the premature processing of Gag and Gag-Pol polyproteins and no production of progeny particles.[374]

The PR cleavage sites in the Gag and Gag-Pol precursors of HIV are not identical. The proteolytic processing of model proteins and substrate analogues by the HIV PR indicates that the binding cleft can accommodate a peptide 6 to 7 residues long; synthetic peptides of this size are cleaved in vitro.[363, 368, 375] Although the PR cleavage sites are quite diverse, the amino acid upstream of the target peptide bond is usually hydrophobic and unbranched at the β carbon (such as Phe, Tyr, Leu, and Met).[376] The cleavage of different scissile bonds within the p55 polyprotein by HIV PR is highly ordered; processing at the amino-terminus of p15 NC is the most rapid in vitro, whereas the cleavage converting p25 to p24 CA is the slowest (see Fig. 25–5).[377, 378]

REVERSE TRANSCRIPTASE (RT). The second *pol* gene product, RT, possesses the enzymatic activity enabling retroviruses to convert their RNA genomes into proviral DNA, the template integrated into chromosomal DNA and used for mRNA synthesis. Although it has been extensively studied and used as a soluble enzyme in vitro, RT activity is invariably particle associated during retroviral infections and intracellular retrotransposition.[64, 379] Unlike the monomeric 84 kDa Moloney murine leukemia virus (MuLV) RT,[380] the mature HIV-1 RT is a heterodimer consisting of 66 and 51 kDa subunits that are colinear at their N-termini (see Fig. 25–13).[381, 382] The p66/p51 heterodimer is the RT species present in purified virions and generated in bacterial expression systems.[370, 371, 383–385] Retroviral RTs have three enzymatic activities: (1) RNA-directed DNA polymerase (for "negative"-strand DNA synthesis); (2) RNase H (for the degradation of the genomic RNA present in DNA/RNA hybrid intermediates); and (3) DNA-directed DNA polymerase (for second or "positive"-strand DNA synthesis to generate a double-stranded DNA substrate for integration). As is true for other DNA polymerases, reverse transcription is primer dependent; retroviruses employ specific tRNAs for this function. HIV and the other lentivirus RTs utilize tRNA^{Lys}, which binds to the primer-binding site (pbs in Fig. 25–4) to initiate negative-strand DNA synthesis. The primer tRNA^{Lys} also preferentially binds to the HIV RT via interactions mediated by its anticodon loop and has been reported to induce conformational changes in the enzyme.[386]

The 560 residue p66 subunit of HIV-1 RT contains all of the sequence information needed for enzymatic activity: an N-terminal 166 amino acid polymerase domain and a C-terminal approximately 120 amino acid RNase H domain.[385, 387–391] These two regions of p66 are linked to one another by a protease-sensitive "tether" containing leucine zipper–like motifs (Leu-X$_6$-Leu-X$_6$-Thr-X$_6$-Leu-X$_6$-Leu) (see Fig. 25–13) that may stabilize its binding to the p51 subunit.[382, 392, 393] The proteolytic cleavage (by the HIV PR) of the RNase H domain from one subunit of the p66 homodimer generates a functional RT heterodimer. Even though each subunit possesses an intact active site for the DNA polymerization reaction (Tyr-Met-Asp-Asp), both monomeric forms of the HIV RT are enzymatically inert.[394] The processed p66/p51 heterodimer has 10 times more polymerizing activity than the p66 homodimer, reflecting the possible steric hindrance of an extra 15 kDa RNase H domain; a p51 homodimer has virtually no measurable RT activity.[385, 395–398] In reconstitution experiments, wild-type p51 cannot restore polymerizing activity to a heterodimer in which the active site for DNA polymerization in the 66 kDa subunit has been mutagenized.[399] The recent elucidation of the crystallographic structure of the HIV RT indicates that the p66/p51 heterodimer is an asymmetrical structure containing single active DNA-polymerizing, RNase H, and tRNA-binding sites.[568] The 66kDa subunit contains a prominent cleft, extending from the polymerizing to the RNase H active sites, which could accommodate a DNA-RNA hybrid intermediate. The p51 subunit does not form a polymerizing cleft, and the two aspartic acid residues constituting its active site are buried within the molecule, thereby explaining the results of reconstitution experiments.[399]

RNA viruses are more genetically variable than viruses with DNA genomes owing to the error-prone nature of RNA polymerases.[400] Much of the genetic variability associated with retroviruses is attributed to the infidelity of reverse transcription, which utilizes an enzyme devoid of 3' to 5' exonuclease activity needed for proofreading and correcting misincorporated nucleotides. In addition, recombination, copy-choice template switches, and catalysis by mutant polymerases all contribute to the high level of sequence diversity characteristic of retroviruses, and of lentiviruses in particular. In most assays monitoring the fidelity of reverse transcription in vitro, the HIV-1 RT was found to be less accurate than MuLV or avian myeloblastosis virus (AMV) RTs.[401] This lack of fidelity by the HIV-1 RT affects the copying of *both* RNA and DNA templates; the error rate was 1 per 6000 nt polymerized, compared with at least a fivefold lower rate with MuLV RT.[402] This may reflect the capacity of the HIV-1 RT to continue polymerization beyond a point of nucleotide mismatch compared with the MuLV and AMV RTs.[403] The misincorporation frequencies derived from in vitro assays may only partially explain the HIV-1 genomic variability observed in vivo, where a variety of selective forces may confer growth or survival advantages on existing or newly emerging viral variants. Of interest in this regard is the reported in vivo mutation rate of one base per genome per replicative cycle for HIV-1 (approximately 9200 nt).[404]

The intrinsic genetic variability of HIV-1 provides a mechanism to explain the development of 3'-azido-3'-deoxythymidine (AZT) resistance observed in individuals following prolonged (6 to 18 months) antiviral therapy.[405] Mutations affecting two regions of the HIV-1 RT (involving amino acid residues 67, 70, 215, and 219) were observed only after the institution of AZT treatment and were associated with isolates that exhibited reduced sensitivity to the drug.[406, 407] From the crystallographic data, these revertant changes cluster in a portion of the molecule where the interaction of RT with the RNA template might be affected.[568] In vitro, the degree of AZT resistance can be correlated with amino acid substitutions in the RT; partially resistant isolates have subsets of the four mutations. The picture is not as clear-cut in vivo because of the presence of genotypic mixtures of HIV with variable sensitivities to AZT.

The RNase H activity associated with the HIV-1 RT degrades the genomic template during DNA synthesis and removes primer RNAs by an endonucleolytic cleavage mechanism. On the basis of amino acid homology to *E. coli* RNase H and the region of the MuLV RT encoding RNase H, the HIV-1 RNase H domain was positioned at the C-terminus of the 66 kDa (and absent from the 51 kDa) RT subunit (see Fig. 25–13).[388, 391, 408, 409] Mutagenesis studies have partially confirmed this modular organization of the HIV RT, with distinct polymerase and RNase H domains, although several mutations affect *both* enzymatic activities, suggesting extensive overlap of the two func-

tions.[387, 410] One RNase H point mutant with "wild-type" polymerizing activity was unable to reinitiate DNA synthesis at natural "pause" sites on an *RNA* template containing *gag* sequences, yet had no difficulty continuing nascent strand extension when the same site was present in a DNA template.[411] This result points to a subtle but tightly linked interdependence between RNase H and polymerizing activities during reverse transcription. Biochemical studies as well as the recently reported three-dimensional structures of the HIV-1 RT and its RNase H domain in fact suggest that RNA-primed DNA synthesis is associated with cleavage of the RNA template by RNase H 15 to 18 nt *downstream* of the polymerization site.[412, 568, 569]

INTEGRASE. The proteolytic cleavage of the C-terminal portion of the HIV-1 Gag-Pol polyprotein by PR releases the 32 kDa integrase (IN) protein (see Fig. 25–13) that mediates the insertion of a DNA copy of the viral genome into the host cell DNA. Unintegrated, flush-ended linear viral DNA is the immediate precursor to integrated proviral DNA.[65, 413] In all retroviral systems, integration proceeds in four steps (Fig. 25–14): (1) IN removes two nucleotides from the 3' termini of both strands of full-length viral DNA, generating a pre-integration substrate with 3'-recessed ends; (2) IN induces a staggered (five bases for HIV[414–416]) cleavage of the cellular "target"; (3) in a strand-transfer reaction, the 3' recessed ends of viral DNA are joined to the 5' "overhanging" termini of the cleaved cellular DNA; and (4) cellular repair synthesis is responsible for a gap-filling reaction.[65, 415, 417–421] As a result of the staggered cleavage of the cellular DNA, the integrated HIV provirus is flanked by a 5 bp direct repeat and terminates with the dinucleotides 5'-TG and CA-3' (see line E, Fig. 25–14). In the MuLV system, IN activity is associated with a subviral 160S structure, which may be involved in the transport of a nucleoprotein complex, containing linear viral DNA and Gag protein,[64] from the cytoplasm to the nucleus and/or participates in the different phases of the integration reaction. The recent development of in vitro assays to monitor IN activity makes it possible to screen for agents that block this critical step in the HIV life cycle.[65, 421–426]

As is the case for other *pol* gene mutants, alterations of IN have little, if any, effect on replication directed by proviral DNA in transfection assays. However, IN-deficient MuLV is approximately 300-fold less infectious than wild-type virus, and IN-negative HIV mutants produce *no* infectious progeny following infection of human lymphocyte cultures.[323, 427] Because the unintegrated DNA that accumulated in cells infected by the prototype lentivirus, visna, was attributed to its failure to integrate into host cell chromosomal DNA,[427a] the high levels of unintegrated HIV DNA in virus-producing, non-dividing macrophage cultures were similarly interpreted and led to proposals suggesting that HIV did not integrate into cells of this lineage. However, the recently demonstrated physical association of HIV DNA with the high molecular weight fraction of macrophage DNA suggests that IN function is also re-

INTEGRATION OF HIV DNA

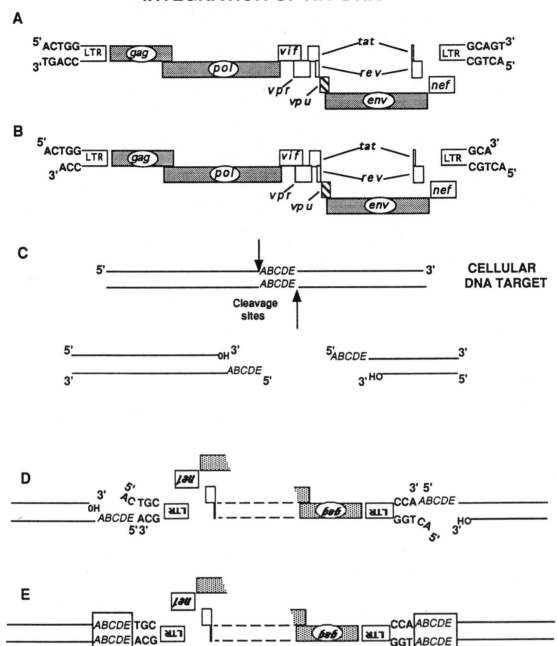

FIGURE 25–14. Integration of HIV-1 DNA. Two nucleotides are removed from the 3' ends of each strand of full-length viral DNA by the HIV integrase (A and B), and 5 bp staggered cuts are made in the cellular DNA target (C). The recessed ends of the viral DNA are then joined to the protruding termini of the digested cellular DNA (D), and the remaining "gap" is filled in by cellular repair enzymes (E). The 5 bp "target site duplication" in cellular DNA is boxed.

quired in these non-dividing cells.[428] Assays evaluating the infectivity of IN-negative mutants in this system will provide the definitive answer to the role of IN during HIV replication of monocytes/macrophages.

Env

The HIV envelope plays a major role in the virus life cycle. It contains the determinants that (1) interact with the CD4 cell surface receptor, (2) mediate the fusion of particles with the plasma membrane during virus entry, and (3) specify the tropism for cells of the lymphocytic or macrophage lineages. In addition, the HIV Env proteins contain epitopes that elicit immune responses that are of importance from both diagnostic and vaccine development perspectives.

The synthesis of the HIV envelope is directed by the partially spliced 4.3 kb Vpu/Env bicistronic mRNA

THE HIV-1 ENVELOPE

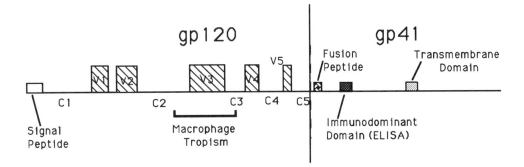

FIGURE 25–15. Functional organization of the HIV-1 envelope. The conserved (C1 to C5) and variable (V1 to V5) regions of gp120 are shown, as well as other functionally important domains of gp120 and gp41.

(see Fig. 25–9) and occurs on polyribosomes associated with the rough endoplasmic reticulum (ER). The 160 kDa envelope polyprotein precursor (gp160) is anchored to cell membranes by a hydrophobic spanning region in its C-terminal half (destined to be the mature transmembrane [TM] envelope glycoprotein gp41 following cleavage) (Fig. 25–15). gp160 rapidly undergoes glycosylation and oligomerization in the ER and is subsequently transported to the Golgi, where, like other retroviral envelope precursor proteins, it is processed by cellular enzymes to the 120 kDa surface (SU) glycoprotein (gp120) and gp41 TM subunits present on progeny virions.[429–436] Cleavage of gp160, following a characteristic Lys-Arg dipeptide motif at residue 510, is required for infectivity because it exposes the hydrophobic N-terminus of gp41 needed for the initiation of the fusion reaction with the plasma membrane of a susceptible cell.[437–439] Subsequent to this cleavage, gp120 and gp41 are not covalently linked by disulfide bonds but form a weak association with one another that is critical for their coordinate transport from the Golgi to the cell surface.[440] When both the principal and an upstream alternative gp120/gp41 cleavage sites are mutagenized, the unprocessed gp160 is incorporated into virus particles, but the virions are not infectious.[441]

The production of the HIV envelope glycoproteins is quite inefficient; only 10 to 15 per cent of the gp160 initially synthesized during virus infection of PBLs is converted to gp120 and gp41 (Fig. 25–16).[436] The

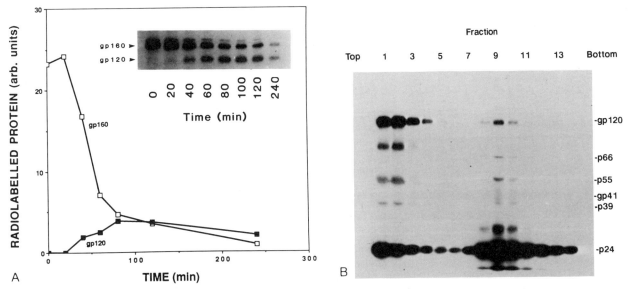

FIGURE 25–16. HIV-1 gp120 production is extremely inefficient. A, The amounts of cell-associated gp160 (□) and gp120 (■) present in HIV-1–infected human peripheral blood lymphocytes at the indicated times following 30 minutes of labeling with ³⁵S-methionine in a pulse-chase experiment are shown autoradiographically (inset) and plotted following densitometric analysis. B, ³⁵S-methionine–labeled (overnight labeling) virus present in the medium of HeLa cells, transfected with an infectious molecular clone of HIV proviral DNA, was centrifuged for 16 hr through a 10 to 60 per cent (w/v) sucrose gradient. Individual fractions were collected, immunoprecipitated with serum from an AIDS patient, and analyzed by SDS polyacrylamide gel electrophoresis. Under these conditions of centrifugation, virus particles band in fractions 8 to 10 (density = 1.18 gm/ml). Note the large amounts of non–virion-associated p24 and gp120 present in gradient fractions 1 to 4 and the virion-associated p66 RT present in fraction 9.

remainder is transported to (and degraded in) lysosomes. In addition, nearly 90 per cent of the gp120 released from cells is not associated with gp41 or virus particles (see the sucrose gradient analysis in Fig. 25–16). Not only does the release of this "free" gp120 further compromise infectious virion production but has led to the proposal that its binding to uninfected CD4-positive cells may lead to autocytolysis and depletion of this T-cell subset in AIDS patients.[443]

The primary translation product of the 480+ residue gp120 is approximately 60 kDa but doubles in size as a consequence of extensive N-linked (Asn-X-Ser/Thr) glycosylations. As shown in Figure 25–15, gp120 contains interspersed conserved (C1 to C5) and variable (V1 to V5) domains.[444] HIV-1 isolates of diverse geographic origin may exhibit greater than 85 per cent amino acid identity within conserved domains of gp120, whereas only 20 to 30 per cent of the residues may be conserved within hypervariable regions.[184, 445] This "plasticity" of the HIV *env* gene is graphically illustrated in Figure 25–17; the tissue culture propagation of an uncloned macrophage-tropic HIV-1 isolate in activated PBLs, subsequent to successive passages in primary human macrophages, results in major structural alterations in gp120. In contrast,

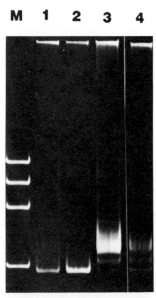

FIGURE 25–17. Selection of host-range variants of HIV-1 occurs in a tissue culture system. A segment of the *env* gene (located between the second constant [C2] and fifth constant [C5] domains [see Fig. 25–15]) from the uncloned macrophage-tropic isolate HIV$_{Ada}$) was analyzed by: (1) reverse transcription/PCR; (2) *Bgl* II digestion of the amplified DNA; and (3) polyacrylamide gel electrophoresis. The amplified and *Bgl* II digested envelope products detected following the 11th and 12th successive passage of HIV$_{Ada}$ in primary macrophage cultures are shown in lanes 1 and 2, respectively. In the 13th and 14th passages, HIV$_{Ada}$ was successively propagated in peripheral blood lymphocytes (lane 3) and then back into primary macrophages (lane 4). Note that the lower amplified DNA species present during the earlier passages in macrophages (lanes 1 and 2) is replaced by a prominent and slowly migrating *env* fragment following only a single additional passage in lymphocytes (lane 3). The rapidly migrating *env* species reappears when the HIV$_{Ada}$ progeny from lymphocytes is used to infect the macrophage culture (lane 4). Size markers were included in the "M" lane.

the cysteines present in the gp120s of different isolates are highly conserved. Eighteen cysteine residues are present in all of the HIV-1 isolates sequenced to date and form nine disulfide bonds that link different regions of gp120 to one another; *none* of the disulfide bonds joins gp120 to gp41.[440] The gp120s of different HIV-1 isolates also contain more than 20 N-linked glycosylation sites, 13 of which are invariant. All 24 sites associated with the HIV-1$_{IIIB}$ isolate are utilized and linked to complex or hybrid/high mannose–type oligosaccharides.[440]

The tropism of HIV and SIV for CD4-positive T lymphocytes is due to the specific interaction of their respective external envelope glycoproteins with the CD4 protein, the first retroviral receptor protein identified.[151, 446, 447] CD4 is located on the surface of T lymphocytes, where its normal function is to interact with class II MHC molecules in class II MHC-restricted T-cell responses. The expression of a human CD4 cDNA clone in normally CD4-negative human cells, such as HeLa and Raji cells, confers susceptibility to HIV infection.[448] However, the surface expression of human CD4 is necessary but insufficient for HIV infectivity: Mouse cells expressing human CD4 bind HIV but fail to support viral entry.[448] In vitro mutagenesis and antibody-blocking studies have localized the CD4-binding function to the C3 and C4 domains of gp120,[437, 449] although more recent reports suggest that the interactive region may be more discontinuous.[450, 451]

CD4 is a 55 kDa member of the immunoglobulin (Ig) superfamily, consisting of a highly charged cytoplasmic domain, a single hydrophobic membrane-spanning domain, and four extracellular Ig-like domains.[452] The high-affinity CD4-binding site for gp120 ($K_m = 10^{-9}$)[449, 453] has been localized to a small segment of the N-terminal extracellular domain, analogous to the second complementarity-determining region (CDR-2) loop of an Ig κ chain variable domain.[454–456] In addition, a second region of CD4 (CDR-3), distinct from the primary gp120 binding site, is required for virus-induced syncytium formation and HIV infectivity.[443, 457, 458] Cell adhesion molecules such as LFA-1 also appear to play a role in HIV-induced syncytia formation, but not the binding of gp120 to CD4 or the cell-to-cell transmission of virus.[459, 460]

The binding of virions to their cellular receptor is only the first of several steps occurring during the initiation of a virus infection. The enveloped ortho- and paramyxoviruses encode specialized structural proteins that mediate the fusion of viral and cellular membranes. The N-terminus of the gp41 TM protein serves this function for HIV. It contains a stretch of 28 hydrophobic amino acids, including the conserved Phe-Leu-Gly-Phe-Leu-Gly motif associated with the fusogenic regions of other viral TM envelope proteins.[461] Mutations within this region of gp41 greatly reduce or block syncytium formation and result in the production of non-infectious progeny virions.[439, 462–464] The fusion function in HIV is not limited to gp41. The V3 loop of gp120 (see Fig. 25–15), which elicits isolate-specific neutralizing antibodies, has also been shown to modulate the virus-cell fusion reaction. Mutations in the ascending and descending stems, as well as those affecting the Gly-Pro-Gly-Arg crown of the V3 loop, suppress syncytium formation without perturbing the processing, transport, and CD4-binding properties of gp120.[465–467]

The interaction of HIV with human mononuclear cells bearing surface CD4 initiates a chain of events culminating in pH-independent virus entry.[75, 77] As noted above, the binding of virions to the high-affinity site on CD4 is merely the first step in this process. An increasing body of data, including studies using a soluble form of CD4 (sCD4), indicates that, in addition to the initial binding, subsequent gp120/CD4 interaction is required for both the fusion reaction and virus entry. Low concentrations of sCD4 reversibly inhibit the infection induced by laboratory strains of HIV by competing with CD4 receptor molecules for binding to virus particles; treatment of virus preparations with high concentrations of sCD4 induces an irreversible dissociation of gp120 from HIV particles, thereby rendering them non-infectious.[453, 468–470] In other experiments, the incubation of HIV-infected *cells* with sCD4 led to increased binding of antibodies to the V3 loop of cell-associated gp120, as well as augmented proteolytic cleavage of the loop by thrombin; both results suggested that the bound sCD4 altered the conformation of gp120 expressed on the cell surface.[471] This putative sCD4-induced gp120 conformational change was accompanied by the release of gp120/CD4 complexes from cells and increased antibody reactivity to epitopes on gp41. All of these findings suggest that the post-binding interaction of gp120 with CD4 is critical for inducing conformational changes necessary for the exposure of the fusogenic N-terminus of gp41. The recently reported augmentation of SIV and HIV-2 infectivity following incubation with sCD4 supports such a model.[472–474]

sCD4 and Ig chimeras of sCD4 have been rapidly introduced into clinical trials because of their ability to effectively inhibit syncytia formation and HIV infectivity in tissue culture systems.[475–480] Unfortunately, sCD4 therapy of HIV-infected individuals has had little, if any, effect on the levels of p24 antigenemia or viremia.[481–483] The failure of sCD4 in vivo appears to reflect the relative resistance (~100-fold) of primary HIV isolates to CD4 neutralization, compared with laboratory strains of virus.[481] A recent study attributes this difference to the reduced binding of sCD4 to virus recently isolated from infected individuals, and to a resistance to the sCD4-induced shedding of gp120 from non–tissue culture-adapted strains of HIV.[484] The high concentration of CD4 present on circulating mononuclear cells very likely competes effectively with sCD4 for binding to gp120, contributing to the failure of sCD4 therapy.

Tissue macrophages are major HIV targets in the brain, spinal cord, lung, skin, and lymph nodes of infected individuals. The commonly studied HIV isolates (e.g., HIV-1$_{IIIB}$, HIV-1$_{Lai}$, and HIV-1$_{SF-2}$) readily infect activated human PBLs and T-cell lines such as

H9 and CEM but replicate poorly, if at all, in primary human monocytes/macrophages. In contrast, the host range of macrophage-tropic strains of HIV is usually limited to PBLs and cells of the monocyte/macrophage lineages; continuous T-cell lines are usually refractory to infection by this class of HIV, typically isolated from asymptomatic individuals.[485–489] With the passage of time, the virus present in an infected person gradually changes, and cytopathic isolates capable of inducing syncytia (Fig. 25–18) and infecting PBLs and T-cell lines (but not macrophages) become more prevalent. These host range properties are specified by *env* determinants that mediate virus adsorption and entry and are independent of the HIV LTR.[490, 491] Analyses of several HIV isolates have shown that the determinants of macrophage tropism reside in a region of gp120 that includes the V3 loop (see Fig.

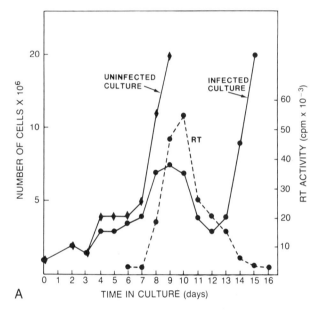

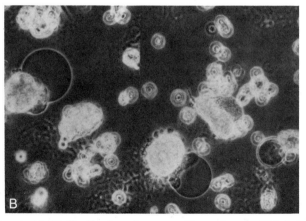

FIGURE 25–18. Replication of a cytopathic strain of HIV-1 in T-cell lines induces syncytia and causes cell death. *A*, The kinetics of HIV-1 infection of CEM cells inoculated at a multiplicity of infection of approximately 1×10^{-3}. Cell viability in the virus and mock infected cells was determined by ^{3}H-thymidine uptake. *B*, Typical ballooning syncytia visualized by light microscopy on day 8 of infection. (The photomicrograph was kindly provided by Dr. Thomas Folks.)

25–15).[492–494] In one study, the substitution of a 20 amino acid, V3 loop segment from the macrophage-tropic isolate HIV-1$_{BaL}$ conferred tropism for monocytes/macrophages to the T-cell tropic isolate HIV-1$_{HXB2}$.[492] Another report showed that in addition to V3, amino acids located in the V2 domain of gp120 were needed for the conversion of the closely related T-cell tropic virus HIV$_{NL4-3}$.[495] The V3 regions of macrophage-tropic HIV isolates from patients appear to be very heterogeneous, and a consensus sequence of this gp120 domain has recently been reported.[495a] Although it is not currently understood how the V3 domain regulates tropism for monocytes/macrophages, there is general agreement that interaction with the high-affinity binding region of CD4 is *not* involved. Instead, it is likely that the V3 region actively participates in post-binding events that alter the conformation of gp120; distinct gp120 V3 loops may be required for fusing HIV to different lineages of CD4-positive cells.

HIV Env glycoproteins are quite immunogenic, eliciting the antibodies detected in a variety of assays used for serologic screening.[429, 496] The most immunodominant region of the envelope has been mapped to a seven amino acid peptide located in the extracellular domain of gp41 that reacts with 100 per cent of sera from HIV-infected individuals.[497, 498] Antibodies directed to this gp41 epitope are of diagnostic importance only, exhibiting no demonstrable virus-neutralizing activity. In contrast, gp120 elicits two types of neutralizing antibodies that may be relevant for vaccine development. Type (isolate)-specific antibodies appear following the initial exposure to HIV in recently infected persons or are synthesized in mice, rabbits, goats, and chimpanzees following immunization with virus, intact gp120, or its peptide subunits.[499–503] HIV type-specific antibodies (1) bind with high affinity to linear epitopes situated in the V3 loop, (2) do *not* block the interaction of gp120 with CD4, and (3) inhibit syncytia formation and virus entry.[504–508] Type-specific antibodies characteristically neutralize only a single HIV isolate; amino acid changes introduced into the V3 loop and/or certain other regions of gp120 allow such variants to escape from neutralization. The second type of neutralizing antibody elicited by gp120 appears months to years following a primary HIV infection and can neutralize a large number of different virus isolates.[509–513] This broad neutralizing activity is directed to discontinuous conformational epitopes in gp120, rather than only the V3 loop, and may also interfere with binding to CD4.

A major effort has been mounted to rapidly develop an effective HIV vaccine. Some human volunteers inoculated with preparations of gp120 and gp160, produced in baculovirus or vaccinia virus expression systems, have developed low levels of type-specific neutralizing antibodies that rapidly fall to the undetectable range within months of vaccination. This response is very similar to that observed in small animals and chimpanzees that have been inoculated with the same vaccine candidates as well as with gp120

purified from virus particles, gp120 peptides, and combinations thereof. The presence of cross-neutralizing antibodies in *infected* individuals and their absence in immunized human volunteers and vaccinated animals suggest that they are induced in response to the sustained, low-level exposure to a gp120 epitope or epitopes located on virus-producing cells, progeny virions, or a combination of both. An attenuated vaccine similar to that recently reported for SIV and based on such gp120 conformational determinants could lead to protection against a broad range of HIV isolates.[513a]

Vif

The *vif* (*v*irus *i*nfectivity *f*actor) gene, present in all lentiviruses except equine infectious anemia virus,[514] overlaps the *pol* and *vpr* genes of HIV-1 (see Fig. 25–5A) and is expressed as an unmodified 23 kDa basic protein in productively infected cells from a singly spliced 5.5 kb mRNA. In contrast to the Gag, Pol, Env, and Vpu proteins, relatively small amounts of intracellular Vif are synthesized, and none is detected in the tissue culture medium or associated with progeny virions. It was originally reported that the phenotype of *vif*-negative mutants depended on the target cell used for infection and whether the inoculum was cell-free virus particles or HIV-producing cells.[515–517] More recent studies indicate that the infectivity of *vif*-minus virus depends on the cells in which the mutant virions are assembled. For example, *vif*-defective HIVs produced in COS, SupT1, and Jurkat cells are able to establish a spreading infection in several cell lines, whereas H9, CEM, and human PBLs lack a cellular factor (a putative Vif "surrogate") required for successful infection by *vif*-negative virus.[517a, 517b] Biochemical studies indicate that Vif plays *no* role in the packaging of genomic RNA or the release of progeny virions. Available data indicate that the *vif* function is required for some very early steps in the virus life cycle.

Vpu

The signature of the HIV-1 family of primate lentiviruses is the presence of the *vpu* gene; it is absent from HIV-2 and all SIVs examined to date. Vpu is a small integral membrane phosphoprotein (81 amino acid residues) that is produced at intracellular levels comparable to those of Gag proteins in virus-infected cells.[57, 518–520] Like Vif, the Vpu protein has not been detected in virus particles. Vpu mutants are defective in the release of viral proteins and progeny virions; the intracellular synthesis and processing of HIV-1 proteins are unaffected. The recent demonstration that Vpu and the Env precursor polyprotein are expressed from the same bicistronic 4.3 kb mRNA (see Fig. 25–9) has focused attention on the possible functional interaction of Vpu and gp160.[249] A characteristic feature of HIV-1 infection is the "downregulation" of surface CD4 expression, a phenomenon associated with the formation of intracellular gp160/CD4 complexes that are retained in the ER.[24, 521, 522] It has recently been demonstrated that Vpu interferes with gp160/CD4 complex formation by inducing the degradation of CD4 in the ER via a non-lysosomal pathway.[523, 523a] Vpu can therefore be considered a regulator of gp120 production, because it modulates the formation of gp160/CD4 complexes, a dead-end process that sequesters both proteins in the ER and prevents their transport to the cell surface.

NATURAL HISTORY OF HIV IN VIVO

During the past decade, advances in virology, cell biology, immunology, and molecular biology have led to a greater understanding of clinical HIV infections. HIV is transmitted from person to person in blood and blood products, semen, and vaginal secretions but not in purified or processed biological products such as gamma globulin.[524, 525] An increasingly important mode of virus transmission, particularly in underdeveloped countries, is from mother to infant, most likely during labor and delivery. Partner studies indicate that infected individuals with severe immune dysfunction and high levels of circulating virus are more likely to transmit HIV than are asymptomatic persons.[526, 527] The probability of transmission for different types of interpersonal contacts has been reported to be 1 per 3 to 4 for mother to infant, 1 per 100 to 500 for a single anal receptive sexual contact, 1 per 500 to 1000 for a single male-to-female vaginal sexual contact, 1 per 1000 to 1500 for a single female-to-male vaginal sexual contact, and 3 to 4 per 1000 for a single percutaneous exposure to HIV infected blood.[528–531a]

A primary HIV infection frequently causes an acute self-limited viral syndrome that may be accompanied by fever, lymphadenopathy, pharyngitis, rash, and gastrointestinal and occasionally neurological symptoms.[532, 533] Virus has been isolated from peripheral blood mononuclear cells (PBMCs), plasma, and the cerebrospinal fluid of individuals recently infected with HIV.[533–535] Relatively high titers (10^1 to 10^4 tissue culture infectious units per milliliter of plasma) of circulating infectious virus have been measured at times that coincide with symptoms of the febrile illness.[536, 537] The HIV viremia rapidly falls coincident with the emergence of antibodies to Gag and Env proteins, 2 to 4 weeks following the onset of symptoms.[538–540] In some individuals this immunological response effectively reduces the plasma virus load to a level at which cell-free HIV is not recoverable from the plasma until much later in the clinical course. It has been repeatedly reported that the virus isolated from asymptomatic seropositive individuals usually replicates only to low titers, is not syncytia inducing, and is tropic only for PBMCs (and not continuous T-cell lines).[489, 541, 542] This apparently is *not* the phenotype of the HIV associated with primary infection. In fact, the biological properties of virus recovered from a recently infected person appeared to be indistinguishable from those of HIV isolated from the individual transmitting that infection: both samples replicated to high titers and induced syncytia in PBMCs as well as in the two T-cell lines, H9 and Hut 78.[537]

The relatively asymptomatic clinical course following initial exposure to HIV has been a long-standing and perplexing aspect of HIV infections in vivo. The duration of the clinically latent state is unpredictable, but it has been estimated to last up to 8 to 10 years in seropositive adults.[543, 544] This phase of viral infection is characterized by extremely low numbers of HIV-infected CD4-positive cells (1 per 50,000) in the peripheral blood, the absence of detectable plasma viremia, and levels of CD4-positive cells greater than 400/mm^3.[527, 545–547] The lack of significant virus production during this period has led to proposals of HIV latency based primarily on the herpes simplex virus (HSV) paradigm, in which dormant HSV genomes reside in dorsal root ganglia until they are activated to initiate new rounds of replication.

Some models of HIV latency have invoked a complex interplay of viral and cellular regulatory factors that block the transition from the "early" to the "late" pattern of viral transcription: The synthesis of Tat, Rev, and Nef is normal, but none of the viral structural proteins (and no progeny virions) are produced.[548] This model of latency evolved from numerous reports of CD4-positive T-cell lines that have survived an acute HIV infection yet remain capable of being induced to express viral RNA and protein.[549] Although such systems have proved invaluable for investigations of cytokine induction of virus or the activation of the HIV LTR by other physiologically relevant factors, these "survivor" cell lines have invariably been shown to contain copies of "damaged" integrated proviral DNA that have been mutated (or selected for) during the preceding tissue culture infection.[550] In general, the expression of the proviruses in these cells is not being repressed by some "effector of latency" but is compromised by mutations affecting viral regulatory and structural genes. There is a paucity of evidence associating this type of viral latency with the benign clinical course that follows recovery from the primary HIV infection. Recent reports demonstrating high levels of cells productively infected with HIV in lymph nodes, adenoid, and tonsillar tissue of asymptomatic, seropositive individuals provides strong evidence for viral persistence, not viral latency.[551, 551a, 551b] These results focus attention on lymphoid organs as sites for sustaining continuous virus production throughout the many years of infection and as targets for the deleterious effects of HIV and/or its ensemble of gene products.

With the exception of certain lentiviral infections of monocytes/macrophages, the replication of retroviruses is blocked in non-dividing cells.[552, 553] Therefore, a case for viral "latency" can legitimately be made for HIV infections of unstimulated CD4-positive T lymphocytes in the peripheral blood or in lymphoid organs. Resting PBLs in culture have been shown to be refractory to virus infection unless they are stimulated with mitogens and propagated in the presence of

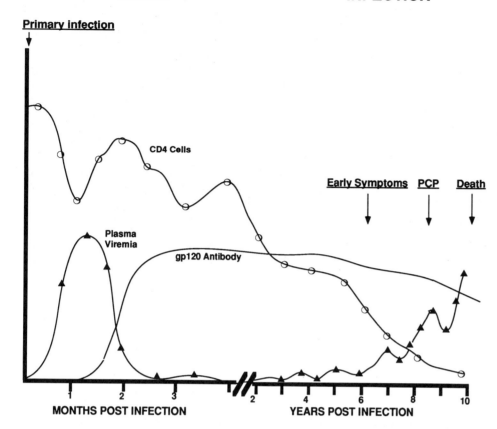

FIGURE 25–19. Schematic representation of an in vivo HIV infection.

IL-2.[151, 153, 154] Although some controversy exists regarding whether the reverse transcription or integration step of the HIV-replicative cycle is inhibited in unstimulated T lymphocytes, there is general agreement that no viral proteins or progeny virions are produced.[554, 555] Activation of resting PBLs up to 14 days following an initial abortive infection can still resurrect a productive infection.[556] Under these circumstances and during this time frame, an HIV infection could be considered "latent."

A persistence model for HIV infection in vivo assumes that virus production in a seropositive individual is continuous from the moment of primary infection. During the many years of asymptomatic HIV production, virus is subjected to a variety of selective influences, particularly those emanating from the immune system. Alterations affecting the different regions of gp120, especially the principal neutralization domain V3, may facilitate evasion from host immune surveillance for many years and, as noted previously, influence tropic/cytopathic properties, which are also specified by this region of the viral envelope. Initial investigations of HIV-1 sequence heterogeneity reported high levels of genetic variability among viral DNA samples obtained from a single infected individual and suggested that the HIV genome was extremely unstable during all phases of in vivo infection.[557] More recent analyses, however, suggest that sequence variability in vivo may actually be less extensive than

initially reported and depend on the clinical state of the patient, the CD4 cell levels, and the complexity of the original infecting inoculum.[558–560]

Perhaps the most mystifying and as yet unanswered question about AIDS and HIV-induced pathogenesis concerns the identification of factors that drive an asymptomatic in vivo infection to a fulminant and fatal immunodeficiency. It is now clear that during clinical latency the virus load is quite substantial, even though the number of circulating infected CD4-positive T lymphocytes and the levels of virus in the plasma are vanishingly low. Studies demonstrating that cell-to-cell transmission of HIV is much more efficient (~1000-fold) for initiating de novo viral infections than cell-free virus inocula[561, 562, 562a] are particularly relevant in this regard, because the former would be ideally suited for lymphoid organs, in which cell concentrations approaching 10^8/ml favor cell-to-cell spread.

A likely scenario of the HIV-1 life cycle in vivo (Fig. 25–19) very likely begins with the transmission of *infected cells* to a new host. An ensuing primary HIV infection would be established by cell-to-cell virus transmission in lymphoid tissue[551b] and give rise to a febrile illness accompanied by a plasma viremia. The acute phase virus, able to replicate to high titers and possibly induce syncytia in a variety of T-cell lines in vitro,[537] elicits a rapid and vigorous immune response that effectively eliminates cell-free virions from the plasma, thereby aborting the primary infection. Immunological pressure, which can be sustained for years, selects slowly growing, low-titer, non-cytopathic HIV variants that are largely confined to lymphoid organs or tissue macrophages.[551a] The latter represent a potentially important reservoir for the maintenance of the persistently infected state because of two unique aspects of HIV replication in cultured primary macrophages: Progeny virions accumulate intracellularly in cytoplasmic vacuoles (see Fig. 25–12), and relatively little gp120 is expressed on the surface of these infected cells.[563, 564] In the case of HIV-infected microglial cells, the cerebrospinal fluid (CSF) represents an additional barrier against immune recognition. Slowly growing, macrophage-tropic variants can be recovered from infected persons during all phases of the in vivo infection and may therefore represent the stable biological form of HIV that survives in nature. The rapidly replicating, highly cytopathic viruses that gradually emerge much later in the clinical course are very likely derivatives of macrophage-tropic viruses, and their appearance may herald disease progression. Unfortunately, the lack of an animal model precludes a definitive verification of this important point.

What, then, can be said about the role of HIV proteins in the development of disease? Some examples of the harmful effects of individual viral proteins on cell viability are worthy of mention. Expression of the gp160 Env precursor *alone* has been shown to cause extensive killing of CD4-positive Jurkat and U937 cells owing to the formation of intracellular gp160/CD4 complexes.[570] Further analysis has shown that nuclear pores and adjoining perinuclear spaces in the affected cells were filled with gp160 aggregates and were unable to transport proteins containing a nuclear transfer signal into the nucleus.[571] Two HIV proteins, Vpu and Nef, have been reported to block the cell surface expression of CD4[288, 293, 523]; Vpu induces CD4 degradation via a non-lysosomal pathway, thereby effecting the concomitant disruption of CD4/gp160 complexes in the ER.[523a] Anecdotal reports have suggested that the constitutive expression of Nef may lead to decreased viability of cells in culture and intrauterine/perinatal deaths of transgenic mice bearing the *nef* gene. It is not clear whether these Nef-associated effects involve CD4 or other critical cell functions.[571a]

Rather than implicating a particularly "toxic" HIV protein, a large body of work now points to "virus load" as the major determinant of viral pathogenicity. The virus load (measured by the number of PBMCs needed for virus isolation) in rhesus macaques inoculated with SIV containing a deleted *nef* gene is at least 100-fold lower than in animals exposed to wild-type virus.[292] The monkeys injected with the Nef-deficient SIV failed to develop disease, and their plasma contained no detectable circulating CA antigen. The experience with chimpanzees inoculated with HIV-1 also supports the linkage of lentivirus load with disease induction. Although virus can be recovered from infected chimpanzees following the cocultivation of their PBMCs and human PBLs and although high antibody levels directed against HIV-1 p24 and gp120 rapidly

appear following exposure to the virus, no CA antigen or free virions have been detected in samples of plasma, and disease manifestations are minimal.[572] The converse has been reported for an SIV variant ($SIV_{SMM[PBj-14]}$) that produces an acute and fulminant virus infection associated with very high levels of plasma viremia: accumulation of infected lymphocytes in gastrointestinal lymphoid tissues, protracted diarrhea presumably due to excess cytokine production, and death 7 to 13 days following inoculation.[573] The association of plasma viremia and the symptomatic phase of HIV infection in man are also in agreement with these findings.

Because precedents for replication-incompetent retroviral variants (such as Friend spleen focus-forming virus or derivatives of feline leukemia virus) capable of causing disease already exist,[565–567] an alternative explanation for clinical progression would be the emergence of a uniquely mutated, defective form of HIV that induces the progressive, irreversible, and terminal immunodeficiency associated with AIDS.

The unremitting nature of the HIV-1 infection in vivo coupled with the steady increase in the virus load and the appearance of more cytopathic virus variants over time (see Fig. 25–19) would support the use of antiviral drugs early in the clinical course. Many of the agents currently available or in clinical trial are directed against *pol* gene products and include the nucleotide RT inhibitors (such as AZT) and the less toxic non-nucleotide RT inhibitors,[574–576] as well as compounds that block the HIV protease.[577] Unfortunately, as noted earlier, HIV-1 variants resistant to these types of antiviral drugs invariably emerge, sometimes as rapidly as weeks to months following the initiation of therapy. The appearance of drug-resistant virus in asymptomatic individuals attests to the vigor of the underlying infection, even during clinical latency, and suggests that substantial numbers of CD4-positive cells are being eliminated during all phases of the in vivo infection. Furthermore the clinical effectiveness of sCD4 has been disappointing to date, and more "experimental" therapies such as anti-sense and ribozyme approaches are still in the early stages of development. Current strategies anticipate the appearance of drug-resistant variants and are directed to long-term treatment with a combination of agents that simultaneously target multiple viral proteins or steps in the replicative cycle, or both.

REFERENCES

1. Centers for Disease Control: Pneumocystis pneumonia—Los Angeles. M.M.W.R. 30:250, 1981.
2. Gottlieb, M. S., Schroff, R., Schanker, H. M., Weisman, J. D., Fan, P. T., Wolf, R. A., and Saxon, A.: *Pneumocystis carinii* pneumonia and mucosal candidiasis in previously healthy homosexual men: Evidence of a new acquired cellular immunodeficiency. N. Engl. J. Med. 305:1425, 1981.
3. Masur, H., Michelis, M. A., Green, J. B., Onorato, I., Stouwe, R. A., Holzman, R. S., Wormser, G., Brettman, L., Lange, M., Murry, H. W., and Cunningham-Rundles, S.: An outbreak of community-acquired *Pneumocystis carinii* pneumonia: Initial manifestation of cellular immune dysfunction. N. Engl. J. Med. 305:1431, 1981.

4. Seigal, F. P., Lopez, C., Hammer, G. S., Brown, A. E., Kornfeld, S. J., Gold, J., Hassett, J., Hirschman, S. Z., Cunningham-Rundles, C., Adelsberg, B. R., Parham, D. M., Siegal, M., Cunningham-Rundles, S., and Armstrong, D.: Severe acquired immunodeficiency in male homosexuals, manifested by chronic perianal ulcerative herpes simplex lesions. N. Engl. J. Med. 305:1439, 1981.

5. Quinnan, G. V., Masur, H., Rook, A. H., Armstrong, G., Frederick, W. R., Epstein, J., Manischewitz, J. F., Macher, A. M., Jackson, L., Ames, J., Smith, H. A., Parker, M., Pearson, G. R., Parrillo, J., Mitchell, C., and Straus, S. E.: Herpesvirus infections in the acquired immune deficiency syndrome. J.A.M.A. 252:72, 1984.

6. Jaffe, H. W., Francis, D. P., McLane, M. F., Cabradilla, C., Curran, J. W., Kilbourne, B. W., Lawrence, D. N., Haverkos, H. W., Spira, T. J., Dodd, R. Y., Gold, J., Armstrong, D., Ley, A., Groopman, J., Mullins, J., Lee, T. H., and Essex, M.: Transfusion-associated AIDS: Serological evidence of human T-cell leukemia virus infection of donors. Science 223:1309, 1984.

7. Gelmann, E. P., Popovic, M., Blayney, D., Masur, H., Sidhu, G., Stahl, R. E., and Gallo, R. C.: Proviral DNA of a retrovirus, human T-cell leukemia virus, in two patients with AIDS. Science 220:862, 1983.

8. Essex, M., McLane, M. F., Lee, T. H., Falk, L., Howe, C. W. S., Mullins, J. I., Cabradilla, C., and Francis, D. P.: Antibodies to cell membrane antigens associated with human T-cell leukemia virus in patients with AIDS. Science 220:859, 1983.

9. Gallo, R. C., Sarin, P. S., Gelmann, E. P., Robert-Guroff, M., Richardson, E., Kalyanaraman, V. S., Mann, D., Sidhu, G. D., Stahl, R. E., Zolla-Pazner, S., Leibowitch, J., and Popovic, M.: Isolation of Human T-cell leukemia virus in acquired immune deficiency syndrome (AIDS). Science 220:865, 1983.

10. Schupbach, J., Sarngadharan, M. G., and Gallo, R. C.: Antigens on HTLV-infected cells recognized by leukemia and AIDS sera are related to HTLV viral glycoprotein. Science 224:607, 1984.

11. Barré-Sinoussi, F., Chermann, J. C., Rey, F., Nugeyre, M. T., Chamaret, S., Gruest, J., Dauguet, C., Axler-Blin, C., Vézinet-Brun, F., Rouzioux, C., Rozenbaum, W., and Montagnier, L.: Isolation of a T-lymphotropic retrovirus from a patient at risk for acquired immune deficiency syndrome (AIDS). Science 220:868, 1983.

12. Montagnier, L., Chermann, J., Barré-Sinoussi, F., Chamaret, S., Gruest, J., Nugeyre, M. T., Rey, F., Dauguet, C., Axler-Blin, C., Brun-Vizenet, F., Rouzioux, C., Saimot, G. A., Rozenbaum, W., Gluckman, J. C., Klatzmann, D., Vilmer, E., Griscelli, C., Foyer-Gazengel, C., and Brunet, J. P.: A new human T-lymphotropic retrovirus: Characterization and possible role in lymphadenopathy and acquired immune deficiency syndromes. In Gallo, R. C., Essex, M. E., and Gross, L. (eds.): Human T-Cell Leukemia/Lymphoma Virus. Cold Spring Harbor, NY, Cold Spring Harbor Laboratory, 1984, pp. 363–379.

13. Gallo, R. C., Salahuddin, S. Z., Popovic, M., Shearer, G. M., Kaplan, M., Haynes, B. F., Palker, T. J., Redfield, R., Oleske, J., Safai, B., White, G., Foster, P., and Markham, P. D.: Frequent detection and isolation of cytopathic retroviruses (HTLV-III) from patients with AIDS and at risk for AIDS. Science 224:500, 1984.

14. Popovic, M., Sarngadharan, M. G., Read, E., and Gallo, R. C.: Detection, isolation, and continuous production of cytopathic retroviruses (HTLV-III) from patients with AIDS and pre-AIDS. Science 224:497, 1984.

15. Levy, J. A., Hoffman, A. D., Kramer, S. M., Landis, J. A., Shimabukuro, J. M., and Oshiro, L. S.: Isolation of lymphocytopathic retroviruses from San Francisco patients with AIDS. Science 225:840, 1984.

16. Schupbach, J., Popovic, M., Gilden, R. V., Gonda, M. A., Sarngadharan, M. G., and Gallo, R. C.: Serological analysis of a subgroup of human T-lymphotropic retroviruses (HTLV-III) associated with AIDS. Science 224:503, 1984.

17. Sarngadharan, M. G., Popovic, M., Bruch, L., Schupbach, J., and Gallo, R. C.: Antibodies reactive with human T-lymphotropic retroviruses (HTLV III) in the serum of patients with AIDS. Science 224:506, 1984.

18. Vilmer, E., Barre-Sinoussi, F., Rouzioux, C., Gazengel, C., Brun-Vezinet, F., Dauguet, C., Fischer, A., Manigne, P., Chermann, J. C., Griscelli, C., and Montagnier, L. Isolation of a new lymphotropic retrovirus from two siblings with haemophilia B, one with AIDS. Lancet 7:753, 1984.

19. Coffin, J., Haase, A., Levy, J. A., Montagnier, L., Oroszlan, S., Teich, N., Temin, H., Toyoshima, K., Varmus, H., Vogt, P., and Weiss, R.: Human immunodeficiency viruses. Science 232:697, 1986.

20. Clavel, F., Guetard, D., Brun-Vezinet, F., Chamaret, S., Rey, M. A., Santos-Ferreira, M. O., Laurent, A. G., Dauguet, C., Katlama, C., and Rouzioux, C.: Isolation of a new human retrovirus from West African patients with AIDS. Science 233:343, 1987.

21. Clavel, F., Mansinho, K., Chamaret, S., Guetard, D., Vavier, V., Nina, J., Santos-Ferreira, M. O., Champalimaud, J. L., and Montagnier, L.: Human immunodeficiency virus type 2 infection associated with AIDS in West Africa. N. Engl. J. Med. 316:1180, 1987.

22. Dalgleish, A. G., Beverly, P. C., Clapham, P. R., Crawford, D. H., Greaves, M. F., and Weiss, R. A.: The CD4 (T4) antigen is an essential component of the receptor for the AIDS retrovirus. Nature 312:763, 1984.

23. Folks, T., Benn, S., Rabson, A., Theodore, T., Hoggan, M. D., Martin, M., Lightfoote, M., and Sell, K.: Characterization of a continuous T-cell line susceptible to the cytopathic effects of the acquired immunodeficiency syndrome (AIDS)–associated retrovirus. Proc. Natl. Acad. Sci. USA 82:4539, 1985.

24. Hoxie, J. A., Alpers, J. D., Rackowski, J. I., Huebner, K., Haggarty, B. S., Cedarbaum, A. J., and Reed, J. C.: Alterations in T4 (CD4) protein and mRNA synthesis in cells infected with HIV. Science 234:1123, 1986.

25. Wain-Hobson, S., Sonigo, P., Danos, O., Cole, S., and Alizon, M.: Nucleotide sequence of the AIDS virus, LAV. Cell 40:9, 1985.

26. Alizon, M., Sonigo, P., Barre-Sinoussi, F., Chermann, J., Tiollais, P., Montagnier, L., and Wain-Hobson, S.: Molecular cloning of lymphadenopathy-associated virus. Nature 312:757, 1984.

27. Sanchez-Pescador, R., Power, M. D., Barr, P. J., Steimer, K. S., Stempien, M. M., Brown-Shimer, S. L., Gee, W. W., Renard, A., Randolph, A., Levy, J., Dino, D., and Luciw, P.: Nucleotide sequence and expression of an AIDS-associated retrovirus (ARV-2). Science 227:484, 1985.

28. Luciw, P. A., Potter, S. J., Steimer, K., and Dina, D.: Molecular cloning of AIDS-associated retrovirus. Nature 312:760, 1984.

29. Hahn, B. H., Shaw, G. M., Arya, S. K., Popovic, M., Gallo, R. C., and Wong-Staal, F.: Molecular cloning and characterization of the HTLV-III virus associated with AIDS. Nature 312:166, 1984.

30. Ratner, L., Haseltine, W., Patarca, R., Livak, K. J., Starcich, B., Josephs, S. F., Doran, E. R., Rafalski, J. A., Whitehorn, E. A., Baumeister, K., Ivanoff, L., Petteway, S. R., Pearson, M. L., Lautenberger, J. A., Papas, T. S., Ghrayeb, J., Chang, N. T., Gallo, R. C., and Wong-Staal, F.: Complete nucleotide sequence of the AIDS virus, HTLV-III. Nature 313:277, 1985.

31. Shaw, G. M., Hahn, B. H., Arya, S. K., Groopman, J. E., Gallo, R. C., and Wong-Staal, F.: Molecular characterization of human T-cell leukemia (lymphotropic) virus type III in the AIDS. Science 226:1165, 1984.

32. Shinnick, T. M., Lerner, R. A., and Sutcliffe, J. G.: Nucleotide sequence of Moloney murine leukemia virus. Nature 293:543, 1981.

33. Schwartz, D. E., Tizard, R., and Gilbert, W.: Nucleotide sequence of Rous sarcoma virus. Cell 32:853, 1983.

34. Rogers, J. H.: The origin and evolution of retroposons. Int. Rev. Cytol. 93:188, 1985.

35. Doolittle, R. F., Feng, D. F., Johnson, M. S., and McClure, M.

A.: Origins and evolutionary relationships of retroviruses. Q. Rev. Biol. 64:1, 1989.

36. Weiner, A. M., Deininger, P. L., and Efstratiadis, A.: Nonviral retroposons: Genes, pseudogenes, and transposable elements generated by the reverse flow of genetic information. Ann. Rev. Biochem. 55:631, 1986.

37. Xiong, Y., and Eickbush, T. H.: Origin and evolution of retroelements based upon their reverse transcriptase sequences. EMBO J. 9:3353, 1990.

38. Doolittle, R. F., Feng, D. F., McClure, M. A., and Johnson, M. S.: Retrovirus phylogeny and evolution. Curr. Top. Microbiol. Immunol. 157:1, 1990.

39. Gonda, M. A., Wong-Staal, F., Gallo, R. C., Clements, J. E., Narayan, O., and Gilden, R. V.: Sequence homology and morphologic similarity of HTLV-III and visna virus, a pathogenic lentivirus. Science 227:173, 1985.

40. Gelderblom, H. R., Ozel, M., Gheysen, D., et al.: Morphogenesis and fine structure of lentiviruses. In Schellekens H., and Horzinek, M. (eds.): Animal Models in AIDS. Amsterdam, Elsevier, 1990, pp. 1–26.

41. Gelderblom, H. R., Hausmann, E. H. S., Ozel, M., Pauli, G., and Koch, M. A.: Fine structure of human immunodeficiency virus (HIV) and immunolocalization of structural proteins. Virology 156:171, 1987.

42. Gelderblom, H. R.: Assembly and morphology of HIV: Potential effect of structure on viral function. AIDS 5:617, 1991.

43. Hirsch, V. M., Olmsted, R. A., Murphey-Corb, M., Purcell, R. H., and Johnson, P. R.: An African primate lentivirus (SIV$_{sm}$) closely related to HIV-2. Nature 339:389, 1989.

44. Gojobori, T., Moriyama, E. N., Ina, Y., Ikeo, K., Miura, T., Tsujimoto, H., Masanori, H., and Yokoyama, S.: Evolutionary origin of human and simian immunodeficiency viruses. Proc. Natl. Acad. Sci. USA 87:4108, 1990.

45. Smith, T. F., Srinivasan, A., Schochetman, G., Marcus, M., and Myers, G.: The phylogenetic history of immunodeficiency viruses. Nature 333:573, 1988.

46. Miura, T., Sakuragi, J., Kawamura, M., Fukasawa, M., Moriyama, E. N., Gojobori, T., Ishikawa, K., Mingle, J. A., Nettey, V. B., Akari, H., Enami, M., Tsujimoto, H., and Hayami, M.: Establishment of a phylogenetic survey system for AIDS-related lentiviruses and demonstration of a new HIV-2 subgroup. AIDS 4:1257, 1990.

47. Muesing, M. A., Smith, D. H., Cabradilla, C. D., Benton, C. V., Lasky, L. A., and Capon, D. J.: Nucleic acid structure and expression of the human AIDS/lymphadenopathy. Nature 313:450, 1985.

48. Jacks, T., and Varmus, H. E.: Expression of the Rous sarcoma virus pol gene by ribosomal frameshifting. Science 230:1237, 1985.

49. Yoshinaka, Y., Katoh, I., Copeland, T. D., and Oroszian, S.: Murine leukemia virus protease is encoded by the gag-pol gene and is synthesized through suppression of an amber termination codon. Proc. Natl. Acad. Sci. USA 82:1618, 1985.

50. Power, M. D., Marx, P. A., Bryant, M. L., Gardner, M. B., Barr, P. J., and Luciw, P. A.: Nucleotide sequence of SRV-1, a type D simian acquired immune deficiency syndrome retrovirus. Science 231:1567, 1986.

51. Seiki, M., Hattori, S., Hirayama, Y., and Yoshida, M.: Human adult T-cell leukemia virus: Complete nucleotide sequence of the pro-virus genome integrated in leukemia cell DNA. Proc. Natl. Acad. Sci. USA 80:3618, 1983.

52. Moore, R., Dixon, M., Smith, R., Peters, G., and Dickson, C.: Complete nucleotide sequence of a milk-transmitted mouse mammary tumor virus: Two frameshift suppression events are required for translation of gag and pol. J. Virol. 61:480, 1987.

53. Dickson, C., and Peters, G.: Protein-coding potential of mouse mammary tumor virus genome RNA as examined by in vitro translation. J. Virol. 37:36, 1981.

53a. Marrack, P., Kushner, E., and Kappler, J.: A maternally inherited superantigen encoded by mammary tumor virus. Nature 349:524, 1991.

53b. Frankel, W. N., Rudy, C., Coffin, J. M., and Huber, B. T.: Linkage of Mls genes to endogenous mammary tumour viruses of inbred mice. Nature 349:526, 1991.

54. Haseltine, W. A., Sodroski, J., Patarca, R., Briggs, D., Perkins, D., and Wong-Staal, F.: Structure of 3′ terminal region of type II human T lymphotropic virus: Evidence of new coding region. Science 225:419, 1984.

55. Nagashima, K., Yoshida, M., and Seiki, M.: A single species of pX mRNA of human T-cell leukemia virus type I encodes trans-activator p40x and two other phosphoproteins. J. Virol. 60:394, 1986.

56. Chen, I. S., Slamon, D. J., Rosenblatt, J. D., Shah, N. P., Quan, S. G., and Wachsman, W.: The x gene is essential for HTLV replication. Science 229:54, 1985.

57. Strebel, K., Klimkait, T., and Martin, M. A.: A novel gene of HIV-1, vpu, and its 19-kilodalton product. Science 241:1221, 1988.

58. Cohen, E. A., Terwilliger, E. F., Sodroski, J. G., and Haseltine, W. A.: Identification of a protein encoded by the vpu gene of HIV-1. Nature 334:532, 1988.

59. Kappes, J. C., Morrow, C. D., Lee, S., Jameson, B. A., Kent, S. B., Hood, L. E., Shaw, G. M., and Hahn, B. H.: Identification of a novel retroviral gene unique to human immunodeficiency virus type 2 and simian immunodeficiency. J. Virol. 62:3501, 1988.

60. Henderson, L. E., Sowder, R. C., Copeland, T. D., Benveniste, R. E., and Oroszlan, S.: Isolation and characterization of a novel protein (X-ORF product) from SIV and HIV-2. Science 241:199, 1988.

61. Engleman, E. G., Benike, C., Glickman, E., and Evans, R. L.: Antibodies to membrane structures that distinguish suppressor/cytotoxic and helper T lymphocyte subpopulations block the mixed leukocyte reaction in man. J. Exp. Med. 154:193, 1981.

62. Reinherz, E. L., and Schlossman, S. F.: The differentiation and function of human T cells. Cell 19:821, 1980.

63. Reinherz, E. L., Kung, P. C., Goldstein, G., and Schlossman, S. F.: Separation of functional subsets of human T cells by a monoclonal antibody. Proc. Natl. Acad. Sci. USA 76:4061, 1979.

64. Bowerman, B., Brown, P. O., Bishop, J. M., and Varmus, H. E.: A nucleoprotein complex mediates the integration of retroviral DNA. Genes Dev. 3:469, 1989.

65. Brown, P. O., Bowerman, B., Varmus, H. E., and Bishop, J. M.: Correct integration of retroviral DNA in vitro. Cell 49:347, 1987.

66. Fuetterer, J., and Hohn, T.: Involvement of nucleocapsids in reverse transcription: A general phenomenon? Trends Biochem. Sci. 12:92, 1987.

67. Fujiwara, T., and Mizuuchi, K.: Retroviral DNA integration: Structure of an integration intermediate. Cell 54:497, 1988.

68. Garfinkel, D. J., Boeke, J. D., and Fink, G. R.: Ty element transposition: Reverse transcriptase and virus-like particles. Cell 42:507, 1985.

69. Rommelaere, J., Donis-Keller, H., and Hopkins, N.: RNA sequencing provides evidence for allelism of determinants of the N-, B-, or NB-tropism of murine leukemia viruses. Cell 16:43, 1979.

70. Ou, C., Boone, L. R., Koh, C. K., Tennant, R. W., and Yang, W. K.: Nucleotide sequences of gag-pol regions that determine the Fv-1 host range property of BALB/c N-tropic and B-tropic murine leukemia viruses. J. Virol. 48:779, 1983.

71. Rowe, W. P., and Sato, H.: Genetic mapping of the Fv-1 locus of the mouse. Science 180:640, 1973.

72. Hippenmeyer, P. J., and Grandgenett, D. P.: Requirement of the avian retrovirus pp32 DNA binding protein domain for replication. Virology 137:358, 1984.

73. Donehower, L. A., and Varmus, H. E.: A mutant murine leukemia virus with a single missense codon in pol is defective in a function affecting integration. Proc. Natl. Acad. Sci. USA 81:6461, 1984.

74. Panganiban, A. T., and Temin, H. M.: The retrovirus pol gene encodes a product required for DNA integration: Identification of a retrovirus int locus. Proc. Natl. Acad. Sci. USA 81:7885, 1984.

75. McClure, M. O., Sommerfelt, M. A., Marsh, M., and Weiss, R. A.: The pH independence of mammalian retrovirus infection. J. Gen. Virol. 71:767, 1990.

76. McClure, M. O., Marsh, M., and Weiss, R. A.: Human immunodeficiency virus infection of CD-4-bearing cells occurs by a pH-independent mechanism. EMBO J. 7:513, 1988.

77. Stein, B. S., Gowda, S. D., Lifson, J. D., Penhallow, R. C., Bensch, K. G., and Engelman, E. G.: pH-independent HIV entry into CD4-positive T cells via virus envelope fusion to the plasma membrane. Cell 49:659, 1989.

78. Holland, C. A., Hartley, J. W., Rowe, W. P., and Hopkins, N.: At least four viral genes contribute to the leukemogenicity of murine retrovirus MCF 247 in AKR mice. J. Virol. 53:158, 1985.

79. Oliff, A., Signorelli, K., and Collins, L.: The envelope gene and long terminal repeat sequences contribute to the pathogenic phenotype of helper-independent Friend viruses. J. Virol. 53:788, 1984.

80. Rosen, C. A., Haseltine, W. A., Lenz, J., Ruprecht, R., and Cloyd, M. W.: Tissue selectivity of murine leukemia virus infection is determined by long terminal repeat sequences. J. Virol. 55:862, 1985.

81. Li, Y., Golemis, E., Hartley, J. W., and Hopkins, N.: Disease specificity of nondefective Friend and Moloney murine leukemia viruses is controlled by a small number of nucleotides. J. Virol. 61:693, 1987.

82. Bosze, Z., Thiesen, H., and Charnay, P.: A transcriptional enhancer with specificity for erythroid cells is located in the long terminal repeat of the Friend murine leukemia virus. EMBO J. 5:1615, 1986.

83. Nara, P., Hatch, W., Kessler, J., Kelliher, J., and Carter, S.: The biology of human immunodeficiency virus-1 III$_B$ infection in the chimpanzee: In vivo and in vitro correlations. J. Med. Primatol. 18:343, 1989.

84. Fultz, P. N., McClure, H. M., Swenson, R. B., McGrath, C. R., Brodie, A., Getchell, J. P., Jensen, F. C., Anderson, D. C., Broderson, J. R., and Francis, D. P.: Persistent infection of chimpanzees with human T-lymphotropic virus type III/lymphadenopathy-associated virus: A potential model for acquired immunodeficiency syndrome. J. Virol. 58:116, 1986.

85. Varmus, H. E., Heasley, S., Kung, H., Oppermann, H., Smith, V. C., Bishop, J. M., and Shank, P. R.: Kinetics of synthesis, structure and purification of avian sarcoma virus-specific DNA made in the cytoplasm of acutely infected cells. J. Mol. Biol. 120:55, 1978.

86. Shank, P. R., Hughes, S. H., Kung, H., Majors, J. E., Quintrell, N., Guntaka, R. V., Bishop, J. M., and Varmus, H. E.: Mapping unintegrated avian sarcoma virus DNA: Termini of linear DNA bear 300 nucleotides present once or twice in two species of circular DNA. Cell 15:1383, 1978.

87. Hsu, T. W., Sabran, J. L., Mark, G. E., Guntaka, R. V., and Taylor, J. M.: Analysis of unintegrated avian RNA tumor virus double-stranded DNA intermediates. J. Virol. 28:810, 1978.

88. Stoll, E., Billeter, M. A., Palmenberg, A., and Weissmann, C.: Avian myeloblastosis virus RNA is terminally redundant: Implications for the mechanism of retrovirus replication. Cell 12:57, 1977.

89. Coffin, J. M., and Haseltine, W. A.: Terminal redundancy and the origin of replication of Rous sarcoma virus RNA. Proc. Natl. Acad. Sci. 74:1908, 1977.

90. Collett, M. S., and Faras, A. J.: Avian retrovirus RNA-directed DNA synthesis: Transcription at the 5′ terminus of the viral genome and the functional role for the viral terminal redundancy. Virology 86:297, 1975.

91. Colicelli, J., and Goff, S. P.: Mutants and pseudorevertants of Moloney murine leukemia virus with alterations at the integration site. Cell 42:573, 1985.

92. Panganiban, A. T., and Temin, H. M.: The terminal nucleotides of retrovirus DNA are required for integration but not virus production. Nature 306:155, 1983.

93. Murphy, J. E., and Goff, S. E.: Construction and analysis of deletion mutations in the U5 region of Moloney murine leukemia virus: Effects on RNA packaging and reverse transcription. J. Virol. 63:319, 1989.

94. Sealey, L., and Chalkley, R.: At least two nuclear proteins bind specifically to the Rous sarcoma virus long terminal repeat enhancer. Mol. Cell. Biol. 7:787, 1987.

95. Speck, N. A., and Baltimore, D.: Six distinct nuclear factors interact with the 75-base-pair repeat of the Moloney murine leukemia virus enhancer. Mol. Cell. Biol. 7:1101, 1987.

96. Cordingley, M. G., Riegel, A. T., and Hager, G. L.: Steroid-dependent interaction of transcription factors with the inducible promoter of mouse mammary tumor virus in vivo. Cell 48:261, 1987.

97. Fujisawa, J., Seiki, M., Sato, M., and Toshida, M.: A transcriptional enhancer sequence of HTLV-1 is responsible for trans-activation mediated by p40x of HTLV-1. EMBO J. 5:713, 1986.

98. Buratowski, S., Hahn, S., Guarente, L., and Sharp, P. A.: Five intermediate complexes in transcription initiation by RNA polymerase II. Cell 56:549, 1989.

99. Reinberg, D., and Roeder, R. G.: Factors involved in specific transcription by mammalian RNA polymerase II. Purification and functional analysis of initiation factors IIB and IIE. J. Biol. Chem. 262:3310, 1987.

100. Reinberg, D., Horikoshi, M., and Roeder, R.: Factors involved in specific transcription in mammalian RNA polymerase II. Functional analysis of initiation factors IIA and IID and identification of a new factor downstream of the initiation site. J. Biol. Chem. 262:3322, 1987.

101. Lee, K. A., Hai, T., Sivaraman, L., Thimmappaya, B., Hurst, H. C., Jones, N. C., and Green, M. R.: A cellular protein, activating transcription factor, activates transcription of multiple E1A-inducible adenovirus early promoters. Proc. Natl. Acad. Sci. USA 84:8355, 1987.

102. Ma, J., and Ptashne, M.: Deletion analysis of GAL4 defines two transcriptional activating segments. Cell 48:847, 1987.

103. Courey, A. J., and Tjian, R.: Analysis of Sp1 in vivo reveals multiple transcriptional domains, including a novel glutamine-rich activation motif. Cell 55:887, 1988.

104. Mermod, N., O'Neill, E. A., Kelly, T. J., and Tjian, R.: The proline-rich transcriptional activator of CTF/NF-1 is distinct from the replication and DNA binding domain. Cell 58:741, 1989.

105. Ptashne, M.: How eukaryotic transcriptional activators work. Nature 335:683, 1988.

106. Berger, S. L., Cress, W. D., Cress, A., Triezenberg, S. J., and Guarente, L.: Selective inhibition of activated but not basal transcription by the acidic activation domain of VP16: Evidence for transcriptional adaptors. Cell 61:1199, 1990.

107. Hoey, T., Dynlacht, B. D., Peterson, M. G., Pugh, B. F., and Tjian, R.: Isolation and characterization of the Drosophila gene encoding the TATA box binding protein, TFIID. Cell 61:1179, 1990.

108. Kelleher, R. J., Flanagan, P. M., and Kornberg, R. D.: A novel mediator between activator proteins and the RNA polymerase II transcription apparatus. Cell 61:1209, 1990.

109. Pugh, B. F., and Tjian, R.: Mechanism of transcriptional activation by Sp1: Evidence for coactivators. Cell 61:1187, 1990.

110. Dynan, W. S., Sazer, S., and Tjian, R.: Transcription factor Sp1 recognizes a DNA sequence in the mouse dihydrofolate reductase promoter. Nature 319:246, 1986.

111. Dynan, W. S., and Tjian, R.: Isolation of transcription factors that discriminate between different promoters recognized by RNA polymerase II. Cell 32:669, 1983.

112. Dynan, W. S., and Tjian, R.: The promoter-specific transcription factor SP1 binds to upstream sequences in the SV40 early promoter. Cell 35:79, 1983.

113. Gidoni, D., Dynan, W. S., and Tjian, R.: Multiple specific contacts between a mammalian transcription factor and its cognate promoters. Nature 312:409, 1984.

114. Gidoni, D., Kadonga, J. T., Barrera-Saldana, H., Takahashi, K., Chambon, P., and Tjian, R.: Bidirectional SV40 transcription mediated by tandem SP1 binding interactions. Science 230:511, 1985.

115. Jones, K. A., Yamamoto, K. R., and Tjian, R.: Two distinct transcription factors bind to the HSV thymidine kinase promoter *in vitro*. Cell 42:559, 1985.
116. Garcia, J. A., Wu, F. K., Mitsuyasu, R., and Gaynor, R. B.: Interactions of cellular proteins involved in the transcriptional regulation of the human immunodeficiency virus. EMBO J. 6:3761, 1987.
117. Jones, K. A., Kadonga, J. T., Luciw, P. A., and Tjian, R.: Activation of the AIDS retrovirus promoter by the cellular transcription factor, Sp1. Science 232:755, 1986.
118. Harrish, D., Garcia, J., Wu, F., Mitsuyasu, R., Gonzalez, J., and Gaynor, R.: Role of SP1-binding domains in In vivo transcriptional regulation of the human immunodeficiency virus type 1 long terminal repeat. J. Virol. 63:2585, 1989.
119. Berkhout, B., and Jeang, K.: Functional roles for the TATA promoter and enhancers in basal and tat-induced expression of the human immunodeficiency virus type 1 long terminal repeat. J. Virol. 66:139, 1992.
120. Leonard, J., Parrott, C., Buckler-White, A. J., Turner, W., Ross, E. K., Martin, M. A., and Rabson, A. B.: The NF-κB binding sites in the human immunodeficiency virus type 1 long terminal repeat are not required for virus infectivity. J. Virol. 63:4919, 1989.
121. Parrott, C., Seidner, T., Duh, E., Leonard, J., Theodore, T. S., Buckler-White, A., Martin, M. A., and Rabson, A. B.: Variable role of the long terminal repeat Sp1-binding sites in human immunodeficiency virus replication in T lymphocytes. J. Virol. 65:1414, 1991.
122. Ross, E. K., Buckler-White, A. J., Rabson, A. B., Englund, G., and Martin, M. A.: Contribution of NF-κB and Sp1 binding motifs to the replicative capacity of human immunodeficiency virus type 1: Distinct patterns of viral growth are determined by T-cell types. J. Virol. 65:4350, 1991.
123. Queen, C., and Baltimore, D.: Immunoglobulin gene transcription is activated by downstream sequence elements. Cell 33:741, 1983.
124. Sen, R., and Baltimore, D.: Multiple nuclear factors interact with the immunoglobulin enhancer sequence. Cell 46:705, 1986.
125. Hoyos, B., Ballard, D. W., Bohnlein, E., Siekevitz, M., and Greene, W. C.: Kappa B-specific DNA binding proteins: Role in the regulation of human interleukin-2 gene expression. Science 244:457, 1989.
126. Visvanathan, K. V., and Goodbourn, S.: Double-stranded RNA activates binding of NF-κB to an inducible element in the human β-interferon promoter. EMBO J. 4:1129, 1989.
127. Lenardo, M. J., Fan, C. M., Maniatis, T., and Baltimore, D.: The involvement of NF-κB in β-interferon gene regulation reveals its role as widely inducible mediator of signal transduction. Cell 57:287, 1989.
128. Schreck, R., and Baeuerle, P. A.: NF-κB as inducible transcriptional activator of the granulocyte-macrophage colony-stimulating factor gene. Mol. Cell. Biol. 10:1281, 1990.
129. Shakhov, A. N., Collart, M. A., Vassalli, P., Nedospasov, S. A., and Jongeneel, C. V.: κB-type enhancers are involved in lipopolysaccharide-mediated transcriptional activation of the tumor necrosis factor alpha gene in primary macrophages. J. Exp. Med. 171:35, 1990.
130. Ballard, D. W., Bohnlein, E., Lowenthal, J. W., Wano, Y., Franza, B. R., and Greene, W. C.: HTLV-1 Tax induces cellular proteins that activate the κB element in the IL-2 receptor alpha gene. Science 241:1652, 1988.
131. Leung, K., and Nabel, G. J.: HTLV-1 transactivator induces interleukin-2 receptor expression through an NF-κB-like factor. Nature 333:776, 1988.
132. Israel, A., Yano, O., Logeat, F., Kieran, M., and Kourilsky, P.: Two purified factors bind to the same sequence in the enhancer of mouse MHC class I genes: One of them is a positive regulator induced upon differentiation of teratocarcinoma cells. Nucleic Acids Res. 17:5245, 1989.
133. Gilmore, T. D.: NF-κB, KBF1, *dorsal,* and *rel*ated matters. Cell 62:841, 1990.
134. Bours, V., Villalobos, J., Burd, P. R., Kelly, K., and Siebenlist, U.: Cloning of a mitogen-inducible gene encoding a κB DNA-binding protein with homology to the *rel* oncogene and to cell-cycle motifs. Nature 348:76, 1990.
135. Ghosh, S., Gifford, A. M., Riviere, L. R., Tempst, P., Nolan, G. P., and Baltimore, D.: Cloning of the p50 DNA binding subunit of NF-κB: Homology to *rel* and *dorsal.* Cell 62:1019, 1990.
136. Kieran, M., Blank, V., Logeat, F., Vandekerckhove, J., Lottspeich, F., LeBall, O., Urban, M. B., Kourilsky, P., Bauerle, A., and Israel, A.: The DNA binding subunit of NF-κB is identical to factor KBF1 and homologous to the *rel* oncogene product. Cell 62:1007, 1990.
137. Meyer, R., Hatada, E. N., Hohmann, H., Halker, M., Bartsch, C., Rothlisberger, U., Lahm, H., Schleger, E. J., van Loon, A. P., and Scheidereit, C.: Cloning of the DNA-binding subunit of human nuclear factor κB: The level of its mRNA is strongly regulated by phorbol ester or tumor necrosis factor α. Proc. Natl. Acad. Sci. USA 88:966, 1991.
138. Baeuerle, P. A., and Baltimore, D.: A 65 kD subunit of active NF-κB is required for inhibition of NF-κB. Genes Dev. 3:1689, 1989.
139. Baeuerle, P. A., and Baltimore, D.: Activation of DNA-binding activity in an apparently cytoplasmic precursor of the NF-κB transcription factor. Cell 53:211, 1988.
140. Inoue, J., Kerr, L. D., Kakizuka, A., and Verma, I. M.: IκBγ, a 70 kd protein identical to the C-terminal half of p110 NF-κB: A new member of the IκB family. Cell 68:1109, 1992.
141. Kerr, L. D., Inoue, J., Davis, N., Link, E., Baeuerle, P. A., Bose, H. R., and Verma, I. M.: The rel-associated pp40 protein prevents DNA binding of rel and NF-κB: Relationship with IκBβ and regulation by phosphorylation. Genes Dev. 5:1464, 1991.
142. Ghosh, S., and Baltimore, D.: Activation *in vitro* of NF-κB by phosphorylation of its inhibitor IκB. Nature 344:678, 1990.
143. Osborn, L., Kunkel, S., and Nabel, G. J.: Tumor necrosis factor α and interleukin-1 stimulate the human immunodeficiency virus enhancer by activation of the nuclear factor κB. Proc. Natl. Acad. Sci. USA 86:2336, 1989.
144. Sen, R., and Baltimore, D.: Inducibility of κ immunoglobulin enhancer-binding protein NF-κB by a post-translational mechanism. Cell 47:921, 1986.
145. Novak, T. J., Chen, D., and Rothenberg, E. V.: Interleukin-1 synergy with phosphoinositide pathway agonists for induction of interleukin-2 gene expression: Molecular basis of costimulation. Mol. Cell. Biol. 10:6325, 1990.
146. Haas, J. G., Baeuerle, P. A., Riethmuller, G., and Ziegler-Heitbrock, H. W. L.: Molecular mechanisms in down-regulation of tumor necrosis factor expression. Proc. Natl. Acad. Sci. USA 87:9563, 1990.
147. Hazan, U., Thomas, D., Alcami, J., Bachelerie, F., Israel, N., Yessel, H., Virelizier, J., and Arenzana-Siesdedos, F.: Stimulation of a human T-cell clone with anti-CD3 or tumor necrosis factor induces NF-κB translocation but not human immunodeficiency virus 1 enhancer-dependent transcription. Immunology 87:7861, 1990.
148. Kawakami, K., Scheidereit, C., and Roeder, R. G.: Identification and purification of a human immunoglobulin-enhancer-binding protein (NF-κB) that activates transcription from a human immunodeficiency virus type 1 promotor *in vitro*. Proc. Natl. Acad. Sci. USA 85:4700, 1988.
149. Nabel, G., and Baltimore, D.: An inducible transcription factor activates expression of human immunodeficiency virus in T cells. Nature 326:711, 1987.
150. Franza, B. R., Josephs, S. F., Gilman, M. Z., Ryan, W., and Clarkson, B.: Characterization of cellular proteins recognizing the HIV enhancer using a microscale DNA-affinity precipitation assay. Nature 330:391, 1987.
151. McDougal, J. S., Mawle, A., Cort, S. P., Nicholson, J. K., Cross, G. D., Scheppler-Campbell, J. A., Hicks, D., and Sligh, J.: Cellular tropism of the human retrovirus HTLV-III/LAV I. Role of T cell activation and expression of the T4 antigen. J. Immunol. 135:3151, 1985.
152. Folks, T., Kelly, J., Benn, S., Kinter, A., Justement, J., Gold, J., Redfield, R., Sell, K. W., and Fauci, A. S.: Susceptibility

of normal human lymphocytes to infection with HTLV-III/LAV. J. Immunol. 136:4049, 1986.

153. Zagury, D., Bernard, J., Leonard, R., Cheynier, R., Feldman, M., Sarin, P. S., and Gallo, R. C.: Long term cultures of HTLV-III infected cells: A model of cytopathology of T cell depletion in AIDS. Science 231:850, 1986.

154. Gowda, S. D., Stein, B. S., Mohagheghpour, N., Benike, C. J., and Engleman, E. G.: Evidence that T cell activation is required for HIV-1 entry in CD4 lymphocytes. J. Immunol. 142:773, 1989.

155. Rosen, C. A., Sodroski, J. G., and Haseltine, W. A.: The location of cis-acting regulatory sequences in the human T cell lymphotropic virus type III (HTLV-III/LAV) long terminal repeat. Cell 41:813, 1985.

156. Siekevitz, M., Josephs, S. F., Dukovich, M., Peffer, N., Wong-Staal, F., and Greene, F. C.: Activation of the HIV-1 LTR by T cell mitogens and the trans-activator protein of HTLV-1. Science 238:1575, 1987.

157. Bohan, C. A., Robinson, R. A., Luciw, P. A., and Srinivasan, A.: Mutational analysis of sodium butyrate inducible elements in the human immunodeficiency virus type 1 long terminal repeat. Virology 172:573, 1989.

158. Orchard, K., Perkins, N., Chapman, C., Harris, J., Emery, V., Goodwin, G., Latchman, D., and Collins, M.: A novel T-cell protein which recognizes a palindromic sequence in the negative regulatory element of the human immunodeficiency virus long terminal repeat. J. Virol. 64:3234, 1990.

159. Smith, M. R., and Greene, W. C.: The same 50-kDa cellular protein binds to the negative regulatory elements of the interleukin-2 receptor α-chain gene and the HIV-1 LTR. Proc. Natl. Acad. Sci. USA 86:8526, 1989.

160. Yamamoto, K., Mori, S., Okamoto, T., Shimotohno, K., and Kyogoku, Y.: Identification of transcriptional suppressor proteins that bind to the negative regulatory element of the human immunodeficiency virus type 1. Nucl. Acids Res. 19:6107, 1991.

161. Ahmad, N., and Venkatesan, S.: Nef protein of HIV-1 is a transcriptional repressor of HIV-1 LTR. Science 241:1481, 1988.

162. Lu, Y., Touzjian, N., Stenzel, M., Dorfman, T., Sodroski, J. G., and Haseltine, W. A.: Identification of cis-acting repressive sequences within the negative regulatory element of human immunodeficiency virus type 1. J. Virol. 64:5226, 1990.

163. Shaw, J., Utz, P. J., Durand, D. B., Toole, J. J., Emmel, E. A., and Crabtree, G. R.: Identification of a putative regulator of early T cell activation genes. Science 241:202, 1988.

164. Franza, B. R., Rauscher, F. J., Josephs, S. F., and Curran, T.: The Fos complex and Fos-related antigens recognize sequence elements that contain AP-1 binding sites. Science 239:1150, 1988.

165. Cooney, A. J., Tsai, S. Y., O'Malley, B. W., and Tsai, M.: Chicken ovalbumin upstream promoter transcription factor binds to a negative regulatory region in the human immunodeficiency virus type 1 long terminal repeat. J. Virol. 65:2853, 1991.

166. Garcia, J. A., Harrich, D., Soultanakis, E., Wu, F., Mitsuyasu, R., and Gaynor, R. B.: Human immunodeficiency virus type 1 LTR TATA and TAR region sequences required for transcriptional regulation. EMBO J. 8:765, 1989.

167. Nakajima, N., Horikoshi, M., and Roeder, R. G.: Factors involved in specific transcription by mammalian RNA polymerase II: Purification, genetic specificity, and TATA box-promoter interactions of TFIID. Mol. Cell. Biol. 8:4028, 1988.

168. Jones, K. A., Luciw, P. A., and Duchange, N.: Structural arrangements of transcription control domains within the 5'-untranslated leader regions of the HIV-1 and HIV-2 promoters. Genes Dev. 2:1101, 1988.

169. Kato, H., Horikoshi, M., and Roeder, R. G.: Repression of HIV-1 transcription by a cellular protein. Science 251:1476, 1991.

170. Wu, F. K., Garcia, J. A., Harrich, D., and Gaynor, R. B.: Purification of the human immunodeficiency virus type 1

171. Nelson, J. A., Reynolds-Kohler, C., Oldstone, M. B., and Wiley, C. A.: HIV and HCMV coinfect brain cells in patients with AIDS. Virology 165:286, 1988.

172. Gendelman, H. E., Phelps, W., Frigenbaum, L., Ostrove, J. M., Adachi, A., Howley, P. M., Khoury, G., Ginsberg, H. S., and Martin, M. A.: Trans-activation of the human immunodeficiency virus long terminal repeat sequence by DNA viruses. Proc. Natl. Acad. Sci. USA 83:9759, 1986.

173. Mosca, J. D., Bednarik, D. P., Raj, N. B., Rosen, C. A., Sodroski, J. G., Haseltine, W. A., and Pitha, P. M.: Herpes simplex virus type-1 can reactivate transcription of latent human immunodeficiency virus. Nature (London) 325:67, 1987.

174. Davis, M. G., Kenney, S. C., Kamine, J., Pagano, J. S., and Huang, E. S.: Immediate-early gene region of human cytomegalovirus trans-activates the promoter of human immunodeficiency virus. Proc. Natl. Acad. Sci. USA 84:8642, 1987.

175. Lusso, P., Ensoli, B., Markham, P. D., Ablashi, D. V., Salahuddin, S. Z., Tschachler, E., Wong-Staal, F., and Gallo, R. C.: Productive dual infection of human CD4+ T lymphocytes by HIV-1 and HHV-6. Nature 337:370, 1989.

176. Nelson, J. A., Ghazal, P., and Wiley, C. A.: Role of opportunistic viral infections in AIDS. AIDS 4:1, 1990.

177. Dayton, A., Sodroski, J. G., Rosen, C. A., Goh, W. C., and Haseltine, W. A.: The trans-activator gene of the human T-cell lymphotropic virus type III is required for replication. Cell 44:941, 1986.

178. Fisher, A. G., Feinberg, M. B., Josephs, S. F., Harper, M. E., Marselle, L. M., Reyes, G., Gonda, M. A., Aldovini, A., Debouk, C., Gallo, R. C., and Wong-Staal, F.: The trans-activator gene of HTLV-III is essential for virus replication. Nature 320:367, 1986.

179. Wright, C. M., Felber, B. K., Paskalis, H., and Pavlakis, G. N.: Expression and characterization of the trans-activator of the HTLV-III/LAV virus. Science 234:988, 1986.

180. Hauber, J., Perkins, A., Heimer, E. P., and Cullen, B. R.: Trans-activation of human immunodeficiency virus gene expression is mediated by nuclear events. Proc. Natl. Acad. Sci. USA 84:6364, 1987.

181. Sodroski, J. G., Patarca, R., Rosen, C. A., Wong-Staal, F., and Haseltine, W. A.: Location of the trans-activating region on the genome of human T-cell lymphotropic virus type III. Science 229:74, 1985.

182. Muesing, M. A., Smith, D. H., and Capon, D. J.: Regulation of mRNA accumulation by a human immunodeficiency virus trans-activator protein. Cell 48:691, 1987.

183. Cullen, B. R.: Trans-activation of human immunodeficiency virus occurs via a bimodal mechanism. Cell 46:973, 1986.

184. Myers, G., Rabson, A. B., Josephs, S. F., and Wong-Staal, F.: Human Retroviruses and AIDS 1988. Los Alamos, NM, Los Alamos National Laboratory, 1988, pp. 1–353.

185. Hess, J. L., Small, J. A., and Clements, J. E.: Sequences in the visna virus long terminal repeat that control transcriptional activity and respond to viral trans-activation: Involvement of AP-1 sites in basal activity and trans-activation. J. Virol. 63:3001, 1989.

186. Keller, A., Partin, K. M., Lochelt, M., Bannert, H., Flugel, R. M., and Cullen, B. R.: Characterization of the transcriptional trans activator of human foamy retrovirus. J. Virol. 65:2589, 1991.

187. Brady, J., Jeang, K., Duvall, J., and Khoury, G. K.: Identification of p40x-responsive regulatory sequences within the human T-cell leukemia virus type I long terminal repeat. J. Virol. 61:2175, 1987.

188. Paskalis, H., Felber, B. K., and Paulakis, G. N.: Cis-acting sequences responsible for transcriptional activation of human T-cell leukemia virus type I constitute a conditional enhancer. Proc. Natl. Acad. Sci. USA 83:6558, 1986.

189. Hauber, J., and Cullen, B. R.: Mutational analysis of the trans-activation-responsive region of the human immunodefi-

ciency virus type I long terminal repeat. J. Virol. 62:673, 1988.

190. Jakobovits, A., Smith, D. H., Jakobovits, E. B., and Capon, D. J.: A discrete element 3′ of human immunodeficiency virus 1 (HIV-1) and HIV-2 mRNA initiation sites mediates transcriptional activation by an HIV *trans* activator. Mol. Cell. Biol. 8:2555, 1988.

191. Kao, S. Y., Calman, A. F., Luciw, P. A., and Peterlin, B. M.: Anti-termination of transcription within the long terminal repeat of HIV-1 by tat gene product. Nature 330:489, 1987.

192. Selby, M. J., Bain, E. S., Luciw, P. A., and Peterlin, B. M.: Structure, sequence, and position of the stem-loop in tar determine transcriptional elongation by tat through the HIV-1 long terminal repeat. Genes Dev. 3:547, 1989.

193. Peterlin, B. M., Luciw, P. A., Barr, P. J., and Walker, M. D.: Elevated levels of mRNA can account for the *trans*-activation of human immunodeficiency virus. Proc. Natl. Acad. Sci. USA 83:9734, 1986.

194. Berkhout, B., Silverman, R. H., and Jeang, K. T.: Tat *trans*-activates the human immunodeficiency virus through a nascent RNA target. Cell 59:273, 1989.

195. Berkhout, B., and Jeang, K.: *Trans*-activation of human immunodeficiency virus type 1 is sequence specific for both the single-stranded bulge and loop of the trans-acting-responsive hairpin: A quantitative analysis. J. Virol. 63:5501, 1989.

196. Feng, S., and Holland, E. C.: HIV-1 tat *trans*-activation requires the loop sequence within tar. Nature 334:165, 1988.

197. Roy, S., Parkin, N. T., Rosen, C., Itovitch, J., and Sonenberg, N.: Structural requirements for trans activation of human immunodeficiency virus type 1 long terminal repeat-directed gene expression by tat: Importance of base pairing, loop sequence, and bulges in the tat-responsive sequence. J. Virol. 64:1402, 1990.

198. Emerman, M., Guyader, M., Montagnier, L., Baltimore, D., and Muesing, M. A.: The specificity of the human immunodeficiency virus type 2 transactivator is different from that of human immunodeficiency virus type 1. EMBO J. 6:3755, 1987.

199. Dingwall, C., Ernberg, I., Gait, M. J., Green, S. M., Heaphy, S., Karn, J., Lowe, A. D., Singh, M., and Skinner, M. A.: HIV-1 tat protein stimulates transcription by binding to a U-rich bulge in the stem of the TAR RNA structure. EMBO J. 9:4145, 1990.

200. Dingwall, C., Ernberg, I., Gait, M. J., Green, S. M., Heaphy, S., Karn, J., Lowe, A. D., Singh, M., Skinner, M. A., and Valerio, R.: Human immunodeficiency virus 1 tat protein binds *trans*-activation-responsive region. Proc. Natl. Acad. Sci. USA 86:6925, 1989.

201. Roy, S., Delling, U., Chen, C. H., Rosen, C. A., and Sonenberg, N.: A bulge structure in HIV-1 TAR is required for Tat binding and Tat-mediated *trans*-activation. Genes Dev. 4:1365, 1990.

202. Weeks, K. M., Ampe, C., Schultz, S. C., Steitz, T. A., and Crothers, D. M.: Fragments of the HIV-1 Tat protein specifically bind TAR RNA. Science 249:1281, 1990.

203. Weeks, K. M., and Crothers, D. M.: RNA recognition by Tat-derived peptides: Interaction in the major groove? Cell 66:577, 1991.

204. Roy, S., Agy, M., Hovanessian, A. G., Sonenberg, N., and Katze, M. G.: The integrity of the stem structure of human immunodeficiency virus type 1 Tat-responsive sequence RNA is required for interaction with the interferon-induced 68,000-M_r protein kinase. J. Virol. 65:632, 1991.

205. Marciniak, R. A., Calnan, B. J., Frankel, A. D., and Sharp, P.: HIV-1 Tat protein *trans*-activates transcription in vitro. Cell 63:791, 1990.

206. Marciniak, R. A., Garcia-Blanco, M. A., and Sharp, P. A.: Identification and characterization of a HeLa nuclear protein that specifically binds to the *trans*-activation-response element of human immunodeficiency virus. Proc. Natl. Acad. Sci. 87:3624, 1990.

207. Gaynor, R., Soultanakis, E., Kuwabara, M., Garcia, J., and Sigman, D. S.: Specific binding of a HeLa cell nuclear protein to RNA sequences in the human immunodeficiency virus *trans*-activating region. Proc. Natl. Acad. Sci. USA 86:4858, 1989.

208. Gatignol, A., Buckler-White, A., Berkhout, B., and Jeang, K.: Characterization of a human TAR RNA-binding protein that activates the HIV-1 LTR. Science 251:1597, 1991.

209. Cordingley, M. G., LaFemina, R. L., Callahan, P. L., Condra, J. H., Sardana, V. V., Graham, D. J., Nguyen, T. M., LeCrow, K., Gotlib, L., Schlabach, A. J., and Colonno, R. J.: Sequence-specific interaction of Tat protein and Tat peptides with the transactivation-responsive sequence element of human immunodeficiency virus type 1 in vitro. Proc. Natl. Acad. Sci. USA 87:8985, 1990.

210. Lazinski, D., Grzadzielska, E., and Das, A.: Sequence-specific recognition of RNA hairpins by bacteriophage antiterminators requires a conserved arginine-rich motif. Cell 59:207, 1989.

211. Ruben, S., Perkins, A., Purcell, R., Joung, K., Sia, R., Burghoff, R., Haseltine, W. A., and Rosen, C. A.: Structural and functional characterization of human immunodeficiency virus *tat* protein. J. Virol. 63:1, 1989.

212. Feinberg, M. B., Jarrett, R. F., Aldovini, A., Gallo, R. C., and Wong-Staal, F.: HTLV-III expression and production involve complex regulation at the levels of splicing and translation of viral RNA. Cell 46:807, 1986.

213. Rosen, C. A., Sodroski, J. G., Goh, W. C., Dayton, A. I., Lippke, J., and Haseltine, W. A.: Post-transcriptional regulation accounts for the *trans*-activation of the human T-lymphotropic virus type III. Nature 319:555, 1986.

214. Rice, A. P., and Mathews, M. B.: Transcriptional but not translational regulation of HIV-1 by the *tat* gene product. Nature 332:551, 1988.

215. Feinberg, M. B., Baltimore, D., and Frankel, A. D.: The role of Tat in the immunodeficiency virus life cycle indicates a primary effect on transcriptional elongation. Proc. Natl. Acad. Sci. 88:4045, 1991.

216. Marciniak, R. A., and Sharp, P. A.: HIV-1 Tat protein promotes formation of more-processive elongation complexes. EMBO J. 10:4189, 1991.

217. Horikoshi, N., Maguire, K., Kralli, A., Maldonado, E., Reinberg, D., and Weinmann, R.: Direct interaction between adenovirus E1A protein and the TATA box binding transcription factor IID. Proc. Natl. Acad. Sci. USA 88:5124, 1991.

218. Li, R., Knight, J. D., Jackson, S. P., Tjian, R., and Botchan, M. R.: Direct interaction between Sp1 and the BPV enhancer E2 protein mediates synergistic activation of transcription. Cell 65:493, 1991.

219. Stern, S., Tanaka, M., and Herr, W.: The Oct-1 homeodomain directs formation of a multiprotein-DNA complex with the HSV transactivator VP16. Nature 341:624, 1989.

220. Gerster, T., and Roeder, R. G.: A herpesvirus *trans*-activating protein interacts with transcription factor OTF-1 and other cellular proteins. Proc. Natl. Acad. Sci. USA 85:6347, 1988.

221. Laspia, M. F., Rice, A. P., and Mathews, M. B.: HIV-1 Tat protein increases transcriptional initiation and stabilizes elongation. Cell 59:283, 1989.

222. Laspia, M. F., Rice, A. P., and Mathews, M. B.: Synergy between HIV-1 Tat and adenovirus Ela is principally due to stabilization of transcriptional elongation. Genes Dev. 4:2397, 1990.

223. Southgate, C. D., and Green, M. R.: The HIV-1 Tat protein activates transcription from an upstream DNA-binding site: Implications for Tat function. Genes Dev. 5:2496, 1991.

224. Berkhout, B., Gatignol, A., Rabson, A. B., and Jeang, K.: TAR-independent activation of the HIV-1 LTR: Evidence that Tat requires specific regions of the promoter. Cell 62:757, 1990.

225. Selby, M. J., and Peterlin, B. M.: Trans-activation by HIV-1 Tat via a heterologous RNA binding protein. Cell 62:769, 1990.

226. Southgate, C., Zapp, M. L., and Green, M. R.: Activation of transcription by HIV-1 Tat protein tethered to nascent RNA through another protein. Nature 345:640, 1990.

227. Subramanian, T., Govindarajan, R., and Chinnadurai, G.: Heterologous basic domain substitutions in the HIV-1 Tat protein reveal an arginine-rich motif required for transactivation. EMBO J. 10:2311, 1991.

228. Hart, C. E., Ou, C., Galphin, J. C., Moore, L. T., Bachler, L. T., Wasmuth, J. J., Petteway, S. R., and Schochetman, G.: Human chromosome 12 is required for HIV-1 expression in human-hamster hybrid cells. Science 246:488, 1989.

229. Newstein, M., Stanbridge, E. J., Casey, G., and Shank, P. R.: Human chromosome 12 encodes a species-specific factor, which increases human immunodeficiency virus type 1 Tat-mediated trans-activation in rodent cells. J. Virol. 64:4565, 1990.

230. Frankel, A. D., and Pabo, C. O.: Cellular uptake of the Tat protein from human immunodeficiency virus. Cell 55:1189, 1988.

231. Viscidi, R. P., Mayur, K., Lederman, H. M., and Frankel, A. D.: Inhibition of antigen-induced lymphocyte proliferation by Tat protein from HIV-1. Science 246:1606, 1989.

232. Ensoli, B., Barillari, G., Salahuddin, S. Z., Gallo, R. C., and Wong-Staal, F.: Tat protein of HIV-1 stimulates growth of cells derived from Kaposi's sarcoma lesions of AIDS patients. Nature 345:84, 1990.

233. Sodroski, J., Goh, W. C., Rosen, C. A., Dayton, A., Terwilliger, E., and Haseltine, W. A.: A second post-transcriptional activator gene required for HTLV-3 replication. Nature 321:412, 1986.

234. Emerman, M., Vazeux, R., and Peden, K.: The rev gene product of the human immunodeficiency virus affects envelope-specific RNA localization. Cell 57:1155, 1989.

235. Felber, B. K., Hadzopoulou-Cladaras, M., Cladaras, C., Copeland, T., and Pavlakis, G. N.: Rev protein of human immunodeficiency virus type 1 affects the stability and transport of the viral mRNA. Proc. Natl. Acad. Sci. USA 86:1495, 1989.

236. Hammarskjold, M., Heimer, J., Hammarskjold, B., Sangwan, I., Albert, L., and Rekosh, D.: Regulation of human immunodeficiency virus env expression by the rev gene product. J. Virol. 63:1959, 1989.

237. Malim, M. H., Hauber, J., Le, S., Maizel, J. V., and Cullen, B. R.: The HIV-1 Rev trans-activator acts through a structured target sequence to activate nuclear export of unspliced viral mRNA. Nature 338:254, 1989.

238. Rosen, C. A., Terwillinger, E., Dayton, A., Sodroski, J. G., and Haseltine, W. A.: Intragenic cis-acting art gene-responsive sequences of the human immunodeficiency virus. Proc. Natl. Acad. Sci. USA 85:2071, 1988.

239. Gruss, P., Lai, C. J., Dhar, R., and Khoury, G.: Splicing as a requirement for biogenesis of functional 16S mRNA of simian virus 40. Proc. Natl. Acad. Sci. USA 76:4317, 1979.

240. Gruss, P.: Rescue of a splicing defective mutant by insertion of an heterologous intron. Nature 286:634, 1980.

241. Lai, C. J., and Khoury, G.: Deletion mutants of simian virus 40 defective in biosynthesis of late viral mRNA. Proc. Natl. Acad. Sci. USA 76:71, 1979.

242. Arrigo, S., and Beemon, K.: Regulation of Rous sarcoma virus RNA splicing and stability. Mol. Cell. Biol. 8:4858, 1988.

243. Katz, R. A., Kotler, M., and Skalka, A. M.: cis-Acting intron mutations that affect the efficiency of avian retroviral RNA splicing: Implications for mechanisms of control. J. Virol. 62:2686, 1988.

244. Miller, C. K., Embretson, J. E., and Temin, H. M.: Transforming viruses spontaneously arise from nontransforming reticuloendotheliosis virus strain T-derived viruses as a result of increased accumulation of spliced viral RNA. J. Virol. 62:1219, 1988.

245. Kim, S., Byrn, R., Groopman, J., and Baltimore, D.: Temporal aspects of DNA and RNA synthesis during human immunodeficiency virus infection: Evidence for differential gene expression. J. Virol. 63:3708, 1989.

246. Guatelli, J. C., Gingeras, T. R., and Richman, D.: Alternative splice acceptor utilization during human immunodeficiency virus type 1 infection of cultured cells. J. Virol. 64:4093, 1990.

247. Robert-Guroff, M., Popovic, M., Gartner, S., Markham, P., Gallo, R. C., and Reitz, M. S.: Structure and expression of tat-, rev-, and nef-specific transcripts of human immunodeficiency virus type 1 in infected lymphocytes and macrophages. J. Virol. 64:3391, 1990.

248. Schwartz, S., Felber, B. K., Benko, D. M., Fenyo, E. M., and Pavlakis, G. N.: Cloning and functional analysis of multiply spliced mRNA species of human immunodeficiency virus type 1. J. Virol. 64:2519, 1990.

249. Schwartz, S., Felber, B. K., Fenyo, E. M., and Pavlakis, G. N.: Env and Vpu proteins of human immunodeficiency virus type 1 are produced from multiple bicistronic mRNAs. J. Virol. 64:5448, 1990.

250. Schwartz, S., Felber, B. K., and Pavlakis, G. N.: Expression of human immunodeficiency virus type-1 vif and vpr mRNAs is Rev-dependent and regulated by splicing. Virology 183:677, 1991.

251. Furtado, M. R., Balachandran, R., Gupta, P., and Wolinsky, S. M.: Analysis of alternatively spliced human immunodeficiency virus type-1 mRNA species, one of which encodes a novel TAT-ENV fusion protein. Virology 185:258, 1991.

252. Kozak, M.: An analysis of vertebrate mRNA sequences: Initiations of translational control. J. Cell. Biol. 115:887, 1991.

253. Schwartz, S., Felber, B. K., and Pavlakis, G. N.: Mechanism of translation of monocistronic and multicistronic human immunodeficiency virus type 1 mRNAs. Mol. Cell. Biol. 12:207, 1992.

254. Malim, M. H., Bohnlein, S., Fenrick, R., Le, S., Maizel, J. V., and Cullen, B. R.: Functional comparison of the Rev trans-activators encoded by different primate immunodeficiency virus species. Proc. Natl. Acad. Sci. USA 86:8222, 1989.

255. Cochrane, A. W., Perkins, A., and Rosen, C. A.: Identification of sequences important in the nucleolar localization of human immunodeficiency virus Rev: Relevance of nucleolar localization to function. J. Virol. 64:881, 1990.

256. Malim, M., Tiley, L., McCarn, D., Rusche, J., Hauber, J., and Cullen, B.: HIV-1 structural gene expression requires binding of the Rev trans-activator to its RNA target sequence. Cell 60:675, 1990.

257. Malim, M. H., Bohnlein, S., Hauber, J., and Cullen, B. R.: Functional dissection of the HIV-1 rev trans-activator—derivation of a trans-dominant repressor of rev function. Cell 58:205, 1989.

258. Olsen, H. S., Cochrane, A. W., Dillon, P. J., Nalin, C. M., and Rosen, C. A.: Interaction of the human immunodeficiency virus type 1 Rev protein with a structured region in env mRNA is dependent on multimer formation mediated through a basic stretch of amino acids. Genes Dev. 4:1357, 1990.

259. Mermer, B., Felber, B. K., Campbell, M., and Pavlakis, G. N.: Identification of trans-dominant HIV-1 rev protein mutants by direct transfer of bacterially produced proteins into human cells. Nucl. Acids Res. 18:2037, 1990.

260. Sadaie, M. R., Rappaport, J., Benter, T., Josephs, S. F., Willis, R., and Wong-Staal, F.: Missense mutations in an infectious human immunodeficiency viral genome: Functional mapping of tat and identification of the rev splice acceptor. Proc. Natl. Acad. Sci. USA 85:9224, 1988.

261. Heaphy, S., Finch, J. T., Gait, M. J., Karn, J., and Singh, M.: Human immunodeficiency virus type 1 regulator of virion expression, rev, forms nucleoprotein filaments after binding to a purine-rich "bubble" located within the rev-responsive region of viral mRNAs. Proc. Natl. Acad. Sci. USA 88:7366, 1991.

262. Wingfield, P. T., Stahl, S. J., Payton, M. A., Venkatesan, S., Misra, M., and Steven, A. C.: HIV-1 Rev expressed in recombinant Escherichia coli: Purification, polymerization, and conformational properties. Biochemistry 30:7527, 1991.

263. Fresco, L. D., Harper, D. S., and Keene, J. D.: Leucine periodicity of U2 small nuclear ribonucleoprotein particle (snRNP) A' protein is implicated in snRNP assembly via protein-protein interactions. Mol. Cell. Biol. 11:1578, 1991.

264. Venkatesh, L. K., and Chinnadurai, G.: Mutants in a conserved region near the carboxy-terminus of HIV-1 Rev identify

265. Hadzopoulou-Cladaras, M., Felber, B. K., Cladaras, C., Athanassopoulos, A., Tse, A., and Pavlakis, G. N.: The *rev (trs/art)* protein of human immunodeficiency virus type 1 affects viral mRNA and protein expression via a *cis*-acting sequence in the *env* region. J. Virol. 63:1265, 1989.

266. Dayton, E. T., Powell, D. M., and Dayton, A. I.: Functional analysis of CAR, the target sequence for the Rev protein of HIV-1. Science 246:1625, 1989.

267. Heaphy, S., Dingwall, C., Ernberg, I., Gait, M. J., Green, S. M., Karn, J., Lowe, A. D., Singh, M., and Skinner, M. A.: HIV-1 regulator of virion expression (Rev) binds to an RNA stem-loop structure located in the Rev-response element region. Cell 60:685, 1990.

268. Holland, S. M., Ahmad, N., Maitra, R. K., Wingfield, P., and Venkatesan, S.: Human immunodeficiency virus Rev protein recognizes a target sequence in Rev-responsive element RNA within the context of RNA secondary structure. J. Virol. 64:5966, 1990.

269. Kjems, J., Brown, M., Chang, D. D., and Sharp, P. A.: Structural analysis of the interaction between the human immunodeficiency virus Rev protein and the Rev response element. Proc. Natl. Acad. Sci. 88:683, 1991.

270. Olsen, H. S., Nelbock, P., Cochrane, A. W., and Rosen, C. A.: Secondary structure is the major determinant for interaction of HIV rev protein with RNA. Science 247:845, 1990.

271. Huang, X., Hope, T. J., Bond, B. L., McDonald, D., Grahl, K., and Parslow, T. G.: Minimal Rev-response element for type 1 human immunodeficiency virus. J. Virol. 65:2131, 1991.

272. Holland, S. M., Chavez, M., Gerstberger, S., and Venkatesan, S.: A specific sequence with a bulged guanosine residue(s) in a stem-bulge-stem structure of Rev-responsive element RNA is required for *trans* activation by human immunodeficiency virus type 1 Rev. J. Virol. 66:3699, 1992.

273. Bartel, D., Zapp, M., Green, M., and Szostak, J. W.: HIV-1 Rev regulation involves recognition of non-Watson-Crick base pairs in viral RNA. Cell 67:529, 1991.

274. Dayton, E., Powell, D., and Dayton, A.: Functional analysis of CAR, the target sequence for the Rev protein of HIV-1. Science 246:1625, 1989.

275. Kjems, J., Frankel, A. D., and Sharp, P. A.: Specific regulation of mRNA splicing in vitro by a peptide from HIV-1 Rev. Cell 67:169, 1991.

276. Hanly, S. M., Rimsky, L. T., Malim, M. H., Kim, J. H., Hauber, J., Dodon, M. D., Le, S.-Y., Maizel, J. V., Cullen, B. R., and Greene, W. C.: Comparative analysis of the HTLV-I Rex and HIV-1 Rev *trans*-regulatory proteins and their RNA response elements. Genes Dev. 3:1534, 1989.

277. Solomin, L., Felber, B. K., and Pavlakis, G. N.: Different sites of interaction for Rev, Tev, and Rex proteins within the Rev-responsive element of human immunodeficiency virus type 1. J. Virol. 64:6010, 1990.

278. Wilusz, J., Feig, D. I., and Shenk, T.: The C proteins of heterogeneous nuclear ribonucleoprotein complexes interact with RNA sequences downstream of polyadenylation cleavage sites. Mol. Cell. Biol. 8:4477, 1988.

279. Chang, D. D., and Sharp, P. A.: Regulation by HIV Rev depends upon recognition of splice sites. Cell 59:1989, 1989.

280. Maldarelli, F., Martin, M. A., and Strebel, K.: Identification of posttranscriptionally active inhibitory sequences in human immunodeficiency virus type 1 RNA: Novel level of gene regulation. J. Virol. 65:5732, 1991.

281. Schwartz, S., Felber, B. K., and Pavlakis, G. N.: Distinct RNA sequences in the *gag* region of human immunodeficiency virus type 1 decrease RNA stability and inhibit expression in the absence of Rev protein. J. Virol. 66:150, 1992.

282. Arrigo, S., and Chen, I. S.: Rev is necessary for translation but not cytoplasmic accumulation of HIV-1 *vif*, *vpr*, and *env/vpu* 2 RNAs. Genes Dev. 5:808, 1991.

283. D'Agostino, D. M., Felber, B. K., Harrison, J. E., and Pavlakis, G. N.: The Rev protein of human immunodeficiency virus type 1 promotes polysomal association and translation of *gag/pol* and *vpu/env* mRNAs. Mol. Cell. Biol. 12:1375, 1992.

284. Cheng-Mayer, C., Iannello, P., Shaw, K., Luciw, P. A., and Levy, J. A.: Differential effects of Nef on HIV replication: Implications for viral pathogenesis in the host. Science 246:1629, 1989.

285. Luciw, P. A., Cheng-Mayer, C., and Levy, J. A.: Mutational analysis of the human immunodeficiency virus: The orf-B region down-regulates virus replication. Proc. Natl. Acad. Sci. USA 84:1434, 1987.

286. Niederman, T. M., Thielan, B. J., and Ratner, L.: Human immunodeficiency virus type 1 negative factor is a transcriptional silencer. Proc. Natl. Acad. Sci. USA 86:1128, 1989.

287. Kim, S., Ikeuchi, K., Byrn, R., Groopman, J., and Baltimore, D.: Lack of a negative influence on viral growth by the *nef* gene of human immunodeficiency virus type 1. Proc. Natl. Acad. Sci. USA 86:9544, 1989.

288. Guy, B., Kieny, M. P., Riviere, Y., Peuch, C. L., Dott, K., Girard, M., Montagnier, L., and Lecocq, J. P.: HIV F/3'orf encodes a phosphorylated GTP-binding protein resembling an oncogene product. Nature 330:266, 1987.

289. Nebreda, A. R., Bryan, T., Segade, F., Wingfield, P., Venkatesan, S., and Santos, E.: Biochemical and biological comparison of HIV-1 Nef and *ras* gene products. Virology 183:151, 1991.

290. Matsuura, Y., Maekawa, M., Hattori, S., Ikegami, N., Hayashi, A., Yamazaki, S., Morita, C., and Takebe, Y.: Purification and characterization of human immunodeficiency virus type 1 *nef* gene product expressed by a recombinant baculovirus. Virology 184:580, 1991.

291. Kaminchik, J., Bashan, N., Pinchasi, D., Amit, B., Sarver, N., Johnston, M. I., Fischer, M., Yavin, Z., Gorecki, M., and Panet, A.: Expression and biochemical characterization of human immunodeficiency virus type 1 *nef* gene product. J. Virol. 64:3447, 1990.

292. Kestler, H. W., Ringler, D. J., Mori, K., Panicali, D. L., Sehgal, P. K., Daniel, M. D., and Desrosiers, R. C.: Importance of the *nef* gene for maintenance of high virus loads and for development of AIDS. Cell 65:651, 1991.

293. Garcia, J. V., and Miller, D.: Serine phosphorylation-independent downregulation of cell-surface CD4 by *nef*. Nature 350:508, 1991.

294. Chassagne, J., Verrelle, P., Dionet, C., Clavel, F., Barre-Sinoussi, F., Chermann, J. C., Montagnier, L., Gluckman, J. C., and Klatzmann, D.: A monoclonal antibody against LAV *gag* precursor: Use for viral protein analysis and antigenic expression in infected cells. J. Immunol. 136:1442, 1988.

295. Henderson, L. E., Copeland, T. D., Sowder, R. C., Schultz, A. M., and Oroszlan, S.: Analysis of proteins and peptides purified from sucrose gradient banded HTLV-III. UCLA Symp. Mol. Cell. Biol. 71:135, 1988.

296. Kramer, R. A., Schaber, M. D., Skalka, A. M., Ganguly, K., Wong-Staal, F., and Reddy, E. P.: HTLV-III gag protein is processed in yeast cells by the virus *pol*-protease. Science 231:1580, 1986.

297. Mervis, R. J., Ahmad, N., Lillehoj, E. P., Raum, M. G., Salazar, F. H., Chan, H. W., and Venkatesan, S.: The *gag* gene products of human immunodeficiency virus type 1: Alignment within the *gag* open reading frame, identification of posttranslational modifications, and evidence for alternative Gag precursors. J. Virol. 62:3993, 1988.

298. Veronese, F. diM., Copeland, T. D., Oroszian, S., Gallo, R. C., and Sarngadharan, M. G.: Biochemical and immunological analysis of human immunodeficiency virus *gag* gene products. J. Virol. 62:795, 1988.

299. Crawford, S., and Goff, S. P.: Mutations in *Gag* proteins p12 and p15 of Moloney murine leukemia virus block early stages of infection. J. Virol. 49:909, 1984.

300. Hsu, H. W., Schwartzenberg, P., and Goff, S.: Point mutations in the p30 domain of the *gag* gene of Moloney leukemia virus. Virology 142:211, 1985.

301. Meric, C., and Spahr, P.: Rous sarcoma virus nucleic acid-binding protein p12 is necessary for viral 70S RNA dimer formation and packaging. J. Virol. 60:450, 1986.

302. Meric, C., and Goff, S.: Characterization of Moloney murine leukemia virus mutants with single-amino-acid substitutions in the Cys-His box of the nucleocapsid protein. J. Virol. 63:1558, 1989.

303. Prats, A. C., Sarih, L., Gabus, C., Litvak, S., Keith, G., and Darlix, J.: Small finger protein of avian and murine retroviruses has nucleic acid annealing activity and positions the replication primer tRNA onto genomic RNA. EMBO J. 7:1777, 1988.

304. Schultz, A. M., and Rein, A.: Unmyristylated Moloney murine leukemia virus Pr65^{gag} is excluded from virus assembly and maturation events. J. Virol. 63:2370, 1989.

305. Schwartzberg, P., Colicelli, J., Gordon, M. L., and Goff, S.: Mutations in the gag gene of Moloney murine leukemia virus: Effects on production of virions and reverse transcriptase. J. Virol. 49:918, 1984.

306. Trono, D., Feinberg, M. G., and Baltimore, D.: HIV-1 Gag mutants can dominantly interfere with the replication of the wild-type virus. Cell 59:113, 1989.

307. Garfinkel, D. J., Boeke, J. D., and Fink, G. R.: Ty element transposition: Reverse transcriptase and virus-like particles. Cell 42:507, 1985.

308. Kawai, S., and Hanafusa, H.: Isolation of defective mutant of avian sarcoma virus. Proc. Natl. Acad. Sci. USA 70:3493, 1973.

309. Levin, J. G., Grimley, P. M., Ramseur, J. M., and Berezesky, I. K.: Deficiency of 60 to 70S RNA in murine leukemia virus particles assembled in cells treated with actinomycin D. J. Virol. 14:152, 1974.

310. Shields, A., Witte, O. N., Rothenberg, E., and Baltimore, D.: High frequency of aberrant expression of Moloney murine leukemia virus in clonal infections. Cell 14:601, 1978.

311. Ross, E. K., Fuerst, T. R., Orenstein, J. M., O'Neill, T., Martin, M. A., and Venkatesan, S.: Maturation of human immunodeficiency virus particles assembled from the gag precursor protein requires in situ processing by gag-pol protease. AIDS Res. Hum. Ret. 7:475, 1991.

312. Smith, A. J., Cho, M. I., Hammarskjold, M. L., and Rekosh, D.: Human immunodeficiency virus type 1 Pr55gag and Pr160gag-pol expressed from a simian virus 40 late replacement vector are efficiently processed and assembled into viruslike particles. J. Virol. 64:2743, 1990.

313. Gheyson, D., Jacobs, E., deForesta, F., Thiriat, C., Francotte, M., Thines, D., and DeWilde, M.: Assembly and release of HIV-1 precursor Pr55^{gag} virus-like particles from recombinant baculovirus-infected cells. Cell 59:103, 1989.

314. Karacostas, V., Nagashima, K., Gonda, M. A., and Moss, B.: Human immunodeficiency virus-like particles produced by a vaccinia virus expression vector. Proc. Natl. Acad. Sci. USA 86:8964, 1989.

315. Shioda, T., and Shibuta, H.: Production of human immunodeficiency virus (HIV)-like particles from cells infected with recombinant vaccinia viruses carrying the gag gene of HIV. Virology 175:139, 1990.

316. Gheyson, D., Jacobs, E., deForesta, F., Thiriart, C., Francotte, M., Thines, D., and DeWilde, M.: Assembly and release of HIV-1 precursor Pr55gag virus-like particles from recombinant baculovirus-infected insect cells. Cell 59:103, 1989.

317. Ramsay, G., and Hayman, M. J.: Analysis of cells transformed by defective leukemia virus OK10: Production of noninfectious particles and synthesis of Pr76gag and an additional 200,000-dalton protein. Virology 106:71, 1980.

318. Crawford, S., and Goff, S. P.: A deletion mutation in the 5' part of the pol gene of Moloney murine leukemia virus blocks proteolytic processing of the gag and pol polyproteins. J. Virol. 53:899, 1985.

319. Eisenman, R. N., Mason, W. S., and Linial, M.: Synthesis and processing of polymerase proteins of wild-type and mutant avian retroviruses. J. Virol. 36:62, 1980.

320. Gottlinger, H. G., Sodroski, J. G., and Haseltine, W. A.: Role of capsid precursor processing and myristylation in morphogenesis and infectivity of human immunodeficiency virus type 1. Proc. Natl. Acad. Sci. USA 86:5781, 1989.

321. Linial, M., Fenno, J., Burnette, W. N., and Rohrschneider, L.: Synthesis and processing of viral glycoproteins in two nonconditional mutants of Rous sarcoma virus. J. Virol. 36:280, 1980.

322. Linial, M., Medeiros, E., and Hayward, W. S.: An avian oncovirus mutant (SE 21Qlb) deficient in genomic RNA: Biological and biochemical characterization. Cell 15:1371, 1978.

323. Schwartzberg, P., Colicelli, J., and Goff, S. P.: Construction and analysis of deletion mutations in the pol gene of Moloney murine leukemia virus: A new viral function required for productive infection. Cell 37:1043, 1984.

324. Rhee, S. S., and Hunter, E.: Myristylation is required for intracellular transport but not for assembly of D-type retrovirus capsids. J. Virol. 61:1045, 1987.

325. Rein, A., McClure, M. R., Rice, N. R., Luftig, R. B., and Schultz, A. M.: Myristylation site in Pr65^{gag} is essential for virus particle formation by Moloney murine leukemia virus. Proc. Natl. Acad. Sci. USA 83:7246, 1986.

326. Schultz, A. M., and Oroszlan, S.: In vivo modification of retroviral gag gene-encoded polyproteins by myristic acid. J. Virol. 46:355, 1983.

327. Henderson, L. E., Krutzch, H. C., and Oroszlan, S.: Myristyl amino termination acylation of murine retroviral proteins: A new posttranslational protein modification. Proc. Natl. Acad. Sci. USA 80:339, 1983.

328. Gelderblom, H. R., Hausmann, E. H., Ozel, M., Pauli, G., and Koch, M. A.: Fine structure of human immunodeficiency virus (HIV) and immunolocalization of structural proteins. Virology 156:171, 1987.

329. Luban, J., and Goff, S. P.: Binding of human immunodeficiency virus type 1 (HIV-1) RNA to recombinant HIV-1 gag polyprotein. J. Virol. 65:3203, 1991.

330. Karpel, R. L., Henderson, L. E., and Oroszlan, S.: Interactions of retroviral structural proteins with single-stranded nucleic acids. J. Biol. Chem. 262:4961, 1987.

331. Watanabe, S., and Temin, H. M.: Encapsidation sequences for spleen necrosis virus, an avian retrovirus, are between the 5' long terminal repeat and the start of the gag gene. Proc. Natl. Acad. Sci. USA 79:5986, 1982.

332. Mann, R., Mulligan, R. C., and Baltimore, D.: Construction of a retrovirus packaging mutant and its use to produce helper-free defective retrovirus. Cell 33:153, 1983.

333. Aldovini, A., and Young, R.: Mutations of RNA and protein sequences involved in human immunodeficiency virus type 1 packaging result in production of noninfectious virus. J. Virol. 64:1920, 1990.

334. Clavel, F., and Orenstein, J. M.: A mutant of human immunodeficiency virus with reduced RNA packaging and abnormal particle morphology. J. Virol. 64:5230, 1990.

335. Lever, A., Gottlinger, H., Haseltine, W., and Sodroski, J.: Identification of a sequence required for efficient packaging of human immunodeficiency virus type 1 RNA into virions. J. Virol. 63:4085, 1989.

336. Kung, H. J., Hu, S., Bender, W., Bailey, J. M., Davidson, N., Nicolson, M. O., and McAllister, R. M.: RD-114, baboon, and woolly monkey viral RNAs compared in size and structure. Cell 7:609, 1976.

337. Darlix, J., Gabus, C., Nugeyre, M., Clavel, F., and Barre-Sinoussi, F.: Cis elements and trans-acting factors involved in the RNA dimerization of the human immunodeficiency virus HIV-1. J. Mol. Biol. 216:689, 1990.

338. Marquet, R., Baudin, F., Gabus, C., Darlix, J., Mougel, M., Ehresmann, C., and Ehresmann, B.: Dimerization of human immunodeficiency virus (type 1) RNA: Stimulation by cations and possible mechanism. Nucl. Acids Res. 19:2349, 1991.

339. Fu, X., Katz, R. A., Skalka, A. M., and Leis, J.: Site-directed mutagenesis of the avian retrovirus nucleocapsid protein. J. Biol. Chem. 263:2140, 1988.

340. Gorelick, R. J., Henderson, J. E., Hanser, J. P., and Rein, A.: Point mutants of Moloney murine leukemia virus that fail to package viral RNA: Evidence for specific RNA recognition by a "zinc finger-like" protein sequence. Proc. Natl. Acad. Sci. USA 85:8420, 1988.

341. Henderson, L. E., Copeland, T. D., Sowder, R. C., Smythers, G. W., and Oroszlan, S.: Primary structure of the low-molecular-weight nucleic acid binding proteins of murine leukemia viruses. J. Biol. Chem. 256:8400, 1981.

342. Meric, C., Gouilloud, E., and Spahr, P.: Mutations in Rous sarcoma virus nucleocapsid protein p12 (NC): Deletions of Cys-His boxes. J. Virol. 62:3328, 1988.

343. Xiangdong, F., Katz, R. A., Skalka, A. M., and Leis, J.: Site-directed mutagenesis of the avian retrovirus nucleocapsid protein. J. Biol. Chem. 263:2140, 1988.

344. Giedroc, D. P., Keating, D. M., Williams, K. R., Konisgberg, W. H., and Coleman, J. E.: Gene 32 protein, the single-stranded DNA binding protein from bacteriophage T4, is a zinc metalloprotein. Biochemistry 83:8452, 1986.

345. Bess, J. W., Powell, P. J., Issaq, H. J., Schumack, L. J., Grimes, M. K., Henderson, L. E., and Arthur, L. O.: Tightly bound zinc in human immunodeficiency virus type 1, human T-cell leukemia virus type I, and other retroviruses. J. Virol. 66:840, 1992.

346. South, T. L., Blake, P. R., Sowder, R. C., Arthur, L. O., Henderson, L. E., and Summers, M. F.: The nucleocapsid protein isolated from HIV-1 particles binds zinc and forms retroviral-type zinc fingers. Biochemistry 29:7786, 1990.

347. Fitzgerald, D. W., and Coleman, J. E.: Physicochemical properties of cloned nucleocapsid protein from HIV interactions with metal ions. Biochemistry 30:5195, 1991.

348. Gorelick, R. J., Nigida, S. M., Bess, J. W., Arthur, L. O., Henderson, L. E., and Rein, A.: Noninfectious human immunodeficiency virus type 1 mutants deficient in genomic RNA. J. Virol. 64:3207, 1990.

349. Kaplan, A. H., and Swanstrom, R.: Human immunodeficiency virus type 1 Gag proteins are processed in two cellular compartments. Proc. Natl. Acad. Sci. USA 88:4528, 1991.

350. Jacks, T., Townsley, K., and Varmus, H. E.: Two efficient ribosomal frameshifting events are required for synthesis of mouse mammary tumor virus gag-related polyproteins. Proc. Natl. Acad. Sci. USA 84:4298, 1987.

351. Jacks, T., Power, M. D., Marsiarz, F. R., Luciw, P. A., Barr, P. J., and Varmus, H. E.: Characterization of ribosomal frameshifting in HIV-1 gag-pol expression. Nature 331:280, 1988.

352. Jamjoon, G. A., Naso, R. B., and Arlinghaus, R. B.: Further characterization of intracellular precursor polyproteins of Rauscher leukemia virus. Virology 78:11, 1977.

353. Park, J., and Morrow, C. D.: Overexpression of the gag-pol precursor from human immunodeficiency virus type 1 proviral genomes results in efficient proteolytic processing in the absence of virion production. J. Virol. 65:5111, 1991.

354. Wilson, W., Braddock, M., Adams, S. E., Rathjen, P. D., Kingsman, S. M., and Kingsman, A. J.: HIV expression strategies: Ribosomal frameshifting is directed by a short sequence in both mammalian and yeast systems. Cell 55:1159, 1988.

355. Peng, C., Ho, B. K., Chang, T. W., and Chang, N. T.: Role of human immunodeficiency virus type 1-specific protease in core protein maturation and viral infectivity. J. Virol. 63:2550, 1989.

356. Kohl, N. E., Emini, E. A., Schleif, W. A., Davis, L. J., Heimbach, J. C., Dixon, R. A., Scolnick, E. M., and Sigal, I. S.: Active immunodeficiency virus protease is required for viral infectivity. Proc. Natl. Acad. Sci. USA 85:4686, 1988.

357. Toh, H., Kikuno, R., Hayashida, H., Miyata, T., Kugimiya, W., Inouye, S., Yuki, S., and Saigo, K.: Close structural resemblance between putative polymerase of a Drosophila transposable genetic element 17.6 and pol gene product of Moloney murine leukaemia virus. EMBO J. 4:1267, 1985.

358. Loeb, D. D., Hutchison, C. A., Edgell, M. H., Farmerie, W. G., and Swanstrom, R.: Mutational analysis of human immunodeficiency virus type 1 protease suggests functional homology with aspartic proteinases. J. Virol. 63:111, 1989.

359. Skalka, A.: Retroviral proteases: First glimpses at the anatomy of a processing machine. Cell 56:911, 1989.

360. Hansen, J., Billich, S., Schulze, T., Sukrow, S., and Moelling, K.: Partial purification and substrate analysis of bacterially expressed HIV protease by means of monoclonal antibody. EMBO J. 7:1785, 1988.

361. Kotler, M., Danho, W., Katz, R. A., Leis, J., and Skalka, A. M.: Avian retroviral protease and cellular aspartic proteases are distinguished by activities on peptide substrates. J. Biol. Chem. 264:3428, 1989.

362. Lapatto, R., Blundell, T., Hemmings, A., Overington, J., Wilderspin, A., Wood, S., Merson, J. R., Whittle, P. J., and Danley, D. E.: X-ray analysis of HIV-1 proteinase at 2.7 Å resolution confirms structural homology among retroviral enzymes. Nature (London) 342:299, 1989.

363. Miller, M., Schneider, J., Sathyanarayana, B. K., Toth, M. V., Marshall, G. R., Clawson, L., Selk, L., Kent, S. B., and Wlodawer, A.: Structure of complex of synthetic HIV-1 protease with a substrate-based inhibitor at 2.3 Å resolution. Science 246:1149, 1989.

364. Navia, M. A., Fitzgerald, P. M., McKeever, B. M., Leu, C., Heimbach, J. C., Herber, W. K., Sigal, I. S., Darke, P. L., and Springer, J. P.: Three-dimensional structure of aspartyl protease from human immunodeficiency virus HIV-1. Nature (London) 337:615, 1989.

365. Miller, M., Jaskolski, M., Mohana-Rao, J. K., Leis, J., and Wlodawer, A.: Crystal structure of a retroviral protease proves relationship to aspartic protease family. Nature 337:576, 1989.

366. Weber, I. T., Miller, M., Jaskolski, M., Leis, J., Skalka, M., and Wlodawer, A.: Molecular modeling of the HIV-1 protease and its substrate binding site. Science 243:928, 1989.

367. Wlodawer, A., Miller, M., Jaskolski, M., Sathyanarayana, K., Baldwin, E., Weber, I. T., Selk, L. M., Clawson, L., Schneider, J., and Kent, S. B.: Conserved folding in retroviral proteases: Crystal structure of a synthetic HIV-1 protease. Science 245:616, 1989.

368. Erickson, J., Neidhart, D. J., VanDrie, J., Kempf, D. J., Wang, X. C., Norbeck, D. W., Plattner, J. J., Rittenhouse, J. W., Turon, M., Wideburg, N., Kohlbrenner, W. E., Simmer, R., Helfrich, R., Paul, D. A., and Knigge, M.: Design, activity, and 2.8 Å crystal structure of a C_2 symmetric inhibitor complexed to HIV-1 protease. Science 249:527, 1990.

369. Fitzgerald, P. M., McKeever, B. M., VanMiddlesworth, J. F., Springer, J. P., Heimbach, J. C., Leu, C., Herber, W. K., Dixon, R. A., and Darke, P. L.: Crystallographic analysis of a complex between human immunodeficiency virus type 1 protease and acetyl-pepstatin at 2.0Å resolution. J. Biol. Chem. 265:14209, 1990.

370. Mous, J., Heimer, E. P., and LeGrice, S. F.: Processing protease and reverse transcriptase from human immunodeficiency virus type I polyprotein in Escherichia coli. J. Virol. 62:1433, 1988.

371. Farmerie, W. G., Loeb, D. D., Casavant, N. C., Hutchinson, C. A., Edgell, M. H., and Swanstrom, R.: Expression and processing of the AIDS virus reverse transcriptase in Escherichia coli. Science 236:305, 1987.

372. Debouck, D., Gorniak, J. G., Strickler, J. E., Meek, T. D., Metcalf, B. W., and Rosenberg, M.: Human immunodeficiency virus protease expressed in Escherichia coli exhibits autoprocessing and specific maturation of the gag precursor. Proc. Natl. Acad. Sci. USA 84:8903, 1987.

373. Krausslich, H.-G., Schneider, H., Zybarth, G., Carter, C. A., and Wimmer, E.: Processing of in vitro-synthesized gag precursor proteins of human immunodeficiency virus (HIV) type 1 by HIV proteinase generated in Escherichia coli. J. Virol. 62:4393, 1988.

374. Krausslich, H.-G.: Human immunodeficiency virus proteinase dimer as component of the viral polyprotein prevents particle assembly and viral infectivity. Proc. Natl. Acad. Sci. USA 88:3213, 1991.

375. Billich, S., Knoop, M., Hansen, J., Strop, P., Sedlacek, J., Mertz, R., and Moelling, K.: Synthetic peptides as substrates and inhibitors of human immune deficiency virus-1 protease. J. Biol. Chem. 263:17905, 1988.

376. Pettit, S. C., Simsic, J., Loeb, D. D., Everitt, L., Hutchison, C. A., and Swanstrom, R.: Analysis of retroviral protease cleavage sites reveals two types of cleavage sites and the structural

requirements of the P1 amino acid. J. Biol. Chem. 266:14539, 1991.

377. Tritch, R. J., Cheng, Y. E., Yin, F. H., and Erickson-Viitanen, S.: Mutagenesis of protease cleavage sites in the human immunodeficiency virus type 1 gag polyprotein. J. Virol. 65:922, 1991.

378. Erickson-Viitanen, S., Manfredi, J., Viitanen, P., Tribe, D. E., Tritch, R., Hutchison, C. A., Loeb, D. D., and Swanstrom, R.: Cleavage of HIV-1 gag polyprotein synthesized in vitro: Sequential cleavage by the viral protease. AIDS Res. Hum. Retroviruses 5:577, 1989.

379. Boeke, J. D., Garfinkel, D. J., Styles, C. A., and Fink, G. R.: Ty elements transpose through an RNA intermediate. Cell 40:490, 1985.

380. Verma, I. M.: Studies on reverse transcriptase of RNA tumor viruses. III. Properties of purified Moloney murine leukemia virus DNA polymerase and associated RNase H. J. Virol. 15:843, 1975.

381. Chandra, A., Gerber, T., and Chandra, P.: Biochemical heterogeneity of reverse transcriptase purified from the AIDS virus, HTLV-III. FEBS Lett. 197:84, 1986.

382. Muller, B., Restle, T., Weiss, S., Gautel, M., Sczakiel, G., and Goody, R. S.: Co-expression of the subunits of the heterodimer of HIV-1 reverse transcriptase in Escherichia coli. J. Biol. Chem. 264:13975, 1989.

383. Lightfoote, M., Coligan, J., Folks, T., Fauci, A., Martin, M., and Venkatesan, S.: Structural characterization of reverse transcriptase and endonuclease polypeptides of the acquired immunodeficiency syndrome retrovirus. J. Virol. 60:771, 1986.

384. Veronese, F. diM., Copeland, T. D., DeVico, A. L., Rahman, R., Oroszlan, S., Gallo, R. C., and Sarngadharan, M. G.: Characterization of highly immunogenic p66/p51 as the reverse transcriptase of HTLV-III/LAV. Science 231:1289, 1986.

385. Hansen, J., Schulze, T., Mellert, W., and Moelling, K.: Identification and characterization of HIV-specific RNase H by monoclonal antibody. EMBO J. 7:239, 1988.

386. Barat, C., Lullien, V., Schatz, O., Keith, G., Nugeyre, M. T., Gruninger-Leitch, F., Barre-Sinoussi, F., LeGrice, S. F., and Darlix, J. L.: HIV-1 reverse transcriptase specifically interacts with the anticodon domain of its cognate primer tRNA. EMBO J. 8:3279, 1989.

387. Prasad, V. R., and Goff, S. P.: Linker insertion mutagenesis of the human immunodeficiency virus reverse transcriptase expressed in bacteria: Definition of the minimal polymerase domain. Proc. Natl. Acad. Sci. USA 86:3104, 1989.

388. Johnson, M. S., McClure, M. A., Feng, D., Gray, J., and Doolittle, R. F.: Computer analysis of retroviral pol genes: Assignment of enzymatic functions to specific sequences and homologies with nonviral enzymes. Proc. Natl. Acad. Sci. USA 83:7648, 1986.

389. Hizi, A., Barber, A., and Hughes, S. H.: Effects of small insertions on the RNA-dependent DNA polymerase activity of HIV-1 reverse transcriptase. Virology 170:326, 1989.

390. Larder, B., Purifoy, D., Powell, K., and Darby, G.: AIDS virus reverse transcriptase defined by high level expression in Escherichia coli. EMBO J. 6:3133, 1987.

391. Tanese, N., and Goff, S. P.: Domain structure of the Moloney murine leukemia virus reverse transcriptase: Mutational analyses and separate expression of the DNA polymerase and RNase H activities. Proc. Natl. Acad. Sci. USA 85:1777, 1988.

392. Ferris, A. L., Hizi, A., Showalter, S. D., Pichuantes, S., Babe, L., Craik, C. S., and Hughes, S. H.: Immunologic and proteolytic analysis of HIV-1 reverse transcriptase structure. Virology 175:456, 1990.

393. Baillon, J. G., Nashed, N. T., Kumar, A., Wilson, S. H., and Jerina, D. M.: A leucine zipper-like motif may mediate HIV reverse transcriptase subunit binding. New Biol. 3:1015, 1991.

394. Restle, T., Muller, B., and Goody, R. S.: Dimerization of human immunodeficiency virus type 1 reverse transcriptase. J. Biol. Chem. 265:8986, 1990.

395. Becerra, S. P., Kumar, A., Lewis, M. S., Widen, S. G., Abbotts, J., Karawya, E. M., Hughes, S. H., Shiloach, J., and Wilson, S. H.: Protein-protein interactions of HIV-1 reverse transcriptase: Implication of central and C-terminal regions in subunit binding. Biochemistry 30:11707, 1991.

396. Lowe, D. M., Atiken, A., Bradley, C., Darby, G. K., Larder, B. A., Powell, K. L., Purifoy, D. J., Tisdale, M., and Stammers, D. K.: HIV-1 reverse transcriptase: Crystallization and analysis of domain structure by limited proteolysis. Biochemistry 27:8884, 1988.

397. Tisdale, M., Ertl, P., Larder, B. A., Purifoy, D. J., Darby, G., and Powell, K. L.: Characterization of human immunodeficiency virus type I reverse transcriptase by using monoclonal antibodies: Role of the C terminus in antibody reactivity and enzyme function. J. Virol. 62:3662, 1988.

398. Hizi, A., McGill, C., and Hughes, S. H.: Expression of soluble, enzymatically active, human immunodeficiency virus reverse transcriptase in Escherichia coli and analysis of mutants. Proc. Natl. Acad. Sci. USA 85:1218, 1988.

399. LeGrice, S. F., Naas, T., Wohlgensinger, B., and Schatz, O.: Subunit-selective mutagenesis indicates minimal polymerase activity in heterodimer-associated p51 HIV-1 reverse transcriptase. EMBO J. 10:3905, 1991.

400. Steinhauer, D. A., and Holland, J. J.: Rapid evolution of RNA viruses. Ann. Rev. Microbiol. 41:409, 1987.

401. Preston, B. D., Poiesz, B. J., and Loeb, L. A.: Fidelity of HIV-1 reverse transcriptase. Science 242:1168, 1988.

402. Ji, J., and Loeb, L. A.: Fidelity of HIV-1 reverse transcriptase copying RNA in vitro. Biochemistry 31:954, 1992.

403. Ricchetti, M., and Buc, H.: Reverse transcriptases and genomic variability: The accuracy of DNA replication is enzyme specific and sequence dependent. EMBO J. 9:1583, 1990.

404. Goodenow, M., Huet, T., Saurin, W., Kwok, S., Sninsky, J., and Wain-Hobson, S.: HIV-1 isolates are rapidly evolving quasispecies: Evidence for viral mixtures and preferred nucleotide substitutions. J. Acquir. Immune Defic. Syndr. 2:344, 1989.

405. Larder, B. A., Darby, G., and Richman, D. D.: HIV with reduced sensitivity to zidovudine (AZT) isolated during prolonged therapy. Science 243:1731, 1989.

406. Richman, D. D., Guatelli, J. C., Grimes, J., Tsiatis, A., and Gingeras, T.: Detection of mutations associated with zidovudine resistance in human immunodeficiency virus by use of the polymerase chain reaction. J. Infect. Dis. 164:1075, 1991.

407. Larder, B. A., and Kemp, S. D.: Multiple mutations in HIV-1 reverse transcriptase confer high-level resistance to zidovudine (AZT). Science 246:1155, 1989.

408. Repaske, R., Hartley, J. W., Kavlick, M. F., O'Neill, R. R., and Austin, J. B.: Inhibition of RNase H activity and viral replication by single mutations in the 3' region of Moloney murine leukemia virus reverse transcriptase. J. Virol. 63:1460, 1989.

409. Mizrahi, V., Lazarus, G. M., Miles, L. M., Meyers, C. A., and Debouck, C.: Recombinant HIV-1 reverse transcriptase: Purification, primary structure, and polymerase/ribonuclease H activities. Arch. Biochem. Biophys. 273:347, 1989.

410. Schatz, O., Cromme, F. V., Gruninger-Leitch, F., and LeGrice, S. F.: Point mutations in conserved amino acid residues within the C-terminal domain of HIV-1 reverse transcriptase specifically repress RNase H function. FEBS Lett. 257:311, 1989.

411. Mizrahi, V., Usdin, M. T., Harington, A., and Dudding, L. R.: Site-directed mutagenesis of the conserved Asp-443 and Asp-498 carboxy-terminal residues of HIV-1 reverse transcriptase. Nucl. Acids Res. 18:5359, 1990.

412. Davies, J. F., Hostomska, Z., Hostomsky, Z., Jordan, S. R., and Matthews, D. A.: Crystal structure of the ribonuclease H domain of HIV-1 reverse transcriptase. Science 252:88, 1991.

413. Colicelli, J., and Goff, S. P.: Sequence and spacing requirements of a retrovirus integration site. J. Mol. Biol. 199:47, 1988.

414. Bushman, F. D., Fujiwara, T., and Craigie, R.: Retroviral DNA

integration directed by HIV integration protein *in vitro.* Science 249:1555, 1990.

415. Ellison, V., Abrams, H., Roe, T., Lifson, J., and Brown, P.: Human immunodeficiency virus integration in a cell-free system. J. Virol. 64:2711, 1990.

416. Vink, C., Groenink, M., Elgersma, Y., Fouchier, R. A., Tersmette, M., and Plasterk, R. H.: Analysis of the junctions between human immunodeficiency virus type 1 proviral DNA and human DNA. J. Virol. 64:5626, 1990.

417. Brown, P. O., Bowerman, B., Varmus, H. E., and Bishop, J. M.: Retroviral integration: Structure of the initial covalent product and its precursor, and a role for the viral IN protein. Proc. Natl. Acad. Sci. USA 86:2525, 1989.

418. Farnet, C. M., and Haseltine, W. A.: Integration of human immunodeficiency virus type 1 DNA *in vitro.* Proc. Natl. Acad. Sci. USA 87:4164, 1990.

419. Grandgenett, D. P., and Vora, A. C.: Site specific nicking at the avian retrovirus LTR circle junction by the viral pp32 DNA endonuclease. Nucl. Acids Res. 13:6205, 1985.

420. Roth, M. J., Schwartzberg, P. L., and Goff, S. P.: Structure of the termini of DNA intermediates in the integration of retroviral DNA. Dependence on IN function and terminal DNA sequence. Cell 58:47, 1989.

421. Leavitt, A. D., Rose, R. B., and Varmus, H. E.: Both substrate and target oligonucleotide sequences affect in vitro integration mediated by human immunodeficiency virus type 1 integrase protein produced in *Saccharomyces cerevisiae.* J. Virol. 66:2359, 1992.

422. Bushman, F. D., and Craigie, R.: Activities of human immunodeficiency virus (HIV) integration protein *in vitro:* Special cleavage and integration of HIV DNA. Proc. Natl. Acad. Sci. USA 88:1339, 1991.

423. Fujiwara, T., and Craigie, R.: Integration of mini-retroviral DNA: A cell-free reaction for biochemical analysis of retroviral integration. Proc. Natl. Acad. Sci. USA 86:3065, 1989.

424. Katz, R. A., Merkel, G., Kulkosky, J., Leis, J., and Skalka, A. M.: The avian retroviral IN protein is both necessary and sufficient for integrative recombination *in vitro.* Cell 63:87, 1990.

425. Sherman, P. A., and Fyfe, J. A.: Human immunodeficiency virus integration protein expressed in *Escherichia coli* possesses selective DNA cleaving activity. Proc. Natl. Acad. Sci. USA 87:5119, 1990.

426. Vink, C., vanGent, D. C., Elgersma, Y., and Plasterk, R. H.: Human immunodeficiency virus integrase protein requires a subterminal position of its viral DNA recognition sequence for efficient cleavage. J. Virol. 65:4636, 1991.

427. Stevenson, M., Haggerty, S., Lamonica, C. A., Meier, C. M., Welch, S., and Wasiak, A. J.: Integration is not necessary for expression of human immunodeficiency virus type 1 protein products. J. Virol. 64:2421, 1990.

427a. Harris, J. D., Blum, H., Scott, J., Traynor, B., Ventura, P., and Haase, A.: Slow virus visna: Reproduction *in vitro* of virus from extrachromosomal DNA. Proc. Natl. Acad. Sci. USA 81:7212, 1984.

428. Weinberg, J. B., Matthews, T. J., Cullen, B. R., and Malim, M. H.: Productive human immunodeficiency virus type 1 (HIV-1) infection of nonproliferating human monocytes. J. Exper. Med. 174:1477, 1991.

429. Allan, J. S., Coligan, J. E., Barin, F., McLane, M. F., Sodroski, J. G., Rosen, C. A., Haseltine, W. A., Lee, T. H., and Essex, M.: Major glycoprotein antigens that induce antibodies in AIDS patients are encoded by HTLV-III. Science 228:1091, 1985.

430. Dewar, R. L., Vasudevachari, M. B., Natarajan, V., and Salzman, N. P.: Biosynthesis and processing of human immunodeficiency virus type 1 envelope glycoproteins: Effects of monensin on glycosylation and transport. J. Virol. 63:2452, 1989.

431. Earl, P. L., Doms, R. W., and Moss, B.: Oligomeric structure of the human immunodeficiency virus type 1 envelope glycoprotein. Proc. Natl. Acad. Sci. USA 87:648, 1990.

432. Earl, P. L., Moss, B., and Doms, R. W.: Folding, interaction, with GRP78-BiP, assembly, and transport of the human

immunodeficiency virus type 1 envelope protein. J. Virol. 65:2047, 1991.

433. Geyer, H., Holschbach, C., Hunsmann, G., and Schneiden, J.: Carbohydrates of human immunodeficiency virus. J. Biol. Chem. 263:11, 760, 1988.

434. Stein, B. S., and Engleman, E. G.: Intracellular processing of the gp160 HIV-1 envelope precursor. J. Biol. Chem. 265:2640, 1990.

435. Veronese, F. diM., DeVico, A. L., Copeland, T. D., Oroszlan, S., Gallo, R. C., and Sarngadharan, M. G.: Characterization of gp41 as the transmembrane protein coded by the HTLV-III/LAV envelope gene. Science 229:1402, 1985.

436. Willey, R. L., Bonifacino, J. S., Potts, B. J., Martin, M. A., and Klausner, R. D.: Biosynthesis, cleavage, and degradation of the human immunodeficiency virus type 1 envelope glycoprotein gp160. Proc. Natl. Acad. Sci. USA 85:9580, 1988.

437. Kowalski, M., Potz, J., Basiripour, L., Dorfman, T., Goh, W. C., Terwilliger, E., Dayton, A., Rosen, C., Haseltine, W., and Sodroski, J.: Functional regions of the envelope glycoprotein of human immunodeficiency virus type 1. Science 237:1351, 1987.

438. McCune, J. M., Rabin, L. B., Feinberg, M. B., Lieberman, M., Kosek, J. C., Reyes, G. R., and Weissman, I. L.: Endoproteolytic cleavage of gp160 is required for the activation of human immunodeficiency virus. Cell 53:55, 1988.

439. Felser, J. M., Klimkait, T., and Silver, J.: A syncytia assay for human immunodeficiency virus type 1 (HIV-1) envelope protein and its use in studying HIV-1 mutations. Virology 170:566, 1989.

440. Leonard, C. K., Spellman, M. W., Riddle, L., Harris, R. J., Thomas, J. N., and Gregory, T. J.: Assignment of intrachain disulfide bonds and characterization of potential glycosylation sites of the type 1 recombinant human immunodeficiency virus envelope glycoprotein (gp120) expressed in Chinese hamster ovary cells. J. Biol. Chem. 265:10373, 1990.

441. Willey, R. L., Klimkait, T., Frucht, D. M., Bonifacino, J. S., and Martin, M. A.: Mutations within the human immunodeficiency virus type 1 gp160 envelope glycoprotein alter its intracellular transport and processing. Virology 184:319, 1991.

442. Willey, R. L., Bonifacino, J. S., Potts, B. J., Martin, M. A., and Klausner, R. D.: Biosynthesis, cleavage, and degradation of the human immunodeficiency virus type 1 envelope glycoprotein gp160. Proc. Natl. Acad. Sci. USA 85:9580, 1988.

443. Siliciano, R. F., Lawton, T., Knall, C., Karr, R. W., Berman, P., Gregory, T., and Reinherz, E. L.: Analysis of host-virus interactions in AIDS with anti-gp120 T cell clones: Effect of HIV sequence variation and a mechanism for CD4+ cell depletion. Cell 54:561, 1988.

444. Modrow, S., Hahn, B. H., Shaw, G. M., Gallo, R. C., Wong-Staal, F., and Wolf, H.: Computer-assisted analysis of envelope protein sequences of seven human immunodeficiency virus isolates: Prediction of antigenic epitopes in conserved and variable regions. J. Virol. 61:570, 1987.

445. Willey, R. L., Rutledge, R. A., Dias, S., Folks, T., Theodore, T., Buckler, C. E., and Martin, M. A.: Identification of conserved and divergent domains within the envelope gene of the acquired immunodeficiency syndrome retrovirus. Proc. Natl. Acad. Sci. USA 83:5038, 1986.

446. Dalgleish, A. G., Beverly, P. C., Clapham, P. R., Crawford, D. H., Greaves, M. F., and Weiss, R. A.: The CD4 (T4) antigen is an essential component of the receptor for the AIDS retrovirus. Nature 312:763, 1984.

447. Klatzmann, D., Champagne, E., Chameret, S., Gruest, J., Guetard, D., Hercend, T., Gluckman, J., and Montagnier, L.: T-lymphocyte T4 molecule behaves as the receptor for human retrovirus LAV. Nature 312:767, 1984.

448. Maddon, P. J., Dalgleish, A. G., McDougal, J. S., Clapham, P. R., Weiss, R. A., and Axel, R.: The T4 gene encodes the AIDS virus receptor and is expressed in the immune system and the brain. Cell 47:333, 1986.

449. Lasky, L. A., Nakamura, G., Smith, D. H., Fennie, C., Shimasaki, C., Patzer, E., Berman, P., Gregory, T., and Capon, D. J.: Delineation of a region of the human immunodeficiency

virus type 1 gp120 glycoprotein critical for interaction with the CD4 receptor. Cell 50:975, 1987.

450. Cordonnier, A., Riviere, Y., Montagnier, L., and Emerman, M.: Effects of mutations in hyperconserved regions of the extracellular glycoprotein of human immunodeficiency virus type 1 on receptor binding. J. Virol. 63:4464, 1989.

451. Olshevsky, U., Helseth, E., Furman, C., Li, J., Haseltine, W., and Sodroski, J.: Identification of individual human immunodeficiency virus type 1 gp120 amino acids important for CD4 receptor binding. J. Virol. 64:5701, 1990.

452. Maddon, P. J., Moleneaux, S. M., Maddon, D. E., Zimmerman, K. A., Godfrey, M., Alt, F. W., Chess, L., and Axel, R.: Structure and expression of the human and mouse T4 genes. Proc. Natl. Acad. Sci. USA 84:9155, 1987.

453. Moore, J. P., McKeating, J. A., Norton, W. A., and Sattentau, Q. J.: Direct measurement of soluble CD4 binding to human immunodeficiency virus type 1 virions: gp120 dissociation and its implications for virus-cell binding and fusion reactions and their neutralization by soluble CD4. J. Virol. 65:1133, 1991.

454. Clayton, L. K., Hussey, R. E., Steinbridge, R., Ramachandran, H., Hussain, Y., and Reinherz, E. L.: Substitution of murine for human CD4 residues identifies amino acids critical for HIV-gp120 binding. Nature (London) 335:363, 1988.

455. Arthos, J., Deen, K. C., Chaikin, M. A., Fornwald, J. A., Sathe, G., Sattentau, Q. J., Clapham, P. R., Weiss, R. A., McDougal, J. S., Pietropaolo, C., Axel, R., Truneh, A., Maddon, P. J., and Sweet, R. W.: Identification of the residues in human CD4 critical for the binding of HIV. Cell 57:469, 1989.

456. Ryu, S., Kwong, P. D., Truneh, A., Porter, T. G., Arthos, J., Rosenberg, M., Dai, X., Xuong, N., Axel, R., Sweet, R. W., and Hendrickson, W. A.: Crystal structure of an HIV-binding recombinant fragment of human CD4. Nature (London) 348:419, 1990.

457. Truneh, A., Buck, D., Cassatt, D. R., Juszczak, R., Kassis, S., Ryu, S. E., Healey, D., Sweet, R., and Sattentau, Q.: A region in domain 1 of CD4 distinct from the primary gp120 binding site is involved in HIV infection and virus-mediated fusion. J. Biol. Chem. 266:5942, 1991.

458. Healey, D., Dianda, L., Moore, J. P., McDougal, J. S., Moore, M. J., Estess, P., Buck, D., Kwong, P. D., Beverley, P. C., and Sattentau, Q. J.: Novel anti-CD4 monoclonal antibodies separate human immunodeficiency virus infection and fusion of CD4 cells from virus binding. J. Exp. Med. 172:1233, 1990.

459. Hildreth, J. E., and Orentas, R. J.: Involvement of a leukocyte adhesion receptor (LFA-1) in HIV-induced syncytium formation. Science 244:1075, 1989.

460. Pantaleo, G., Butini, L., Graziosi, C., Poli, G., Schnittman, S., Greenhouse, J. J., Gallin, J. I., and Fauci, A. S.: Human immunodeficiency virus (HIV) infection in CD4+ T lymphocytes genetically deficient in LFA-1: LFA-1 is required for HIV-mediated cell fusion but not for viral transmission. J. Exp. Med. 173:511, 1991.

461. Gallaher, W. R.: Detection of a fusion peptide sequence in the transmembrane protein of human immunodeficiency virus. Cell 50:327, 1987.

462. Kowalski, M., Bergeron, L., Dorfman, T., Haseltine, W., and Sodroski, J.: Attenuation of human immunodeficiency virus type 1 cytopathic effect by a mutation affecting the transmembrane envelope glycoprotein. J. Virol. 65:281, 1991.

463. Freed, E. O., Myers, D. J., and Risser, R.: Characterization of the fusion domain of the human immunodeficiency virus type 1 envelope glycoprotein gp41. Proc. Natl. Acad. Sci. USA 87:4650, 1990.

464. Helseth, E., Olshevsky, U., Gabuzda, D., Ardman, B., Haseltine, W., and Sodroski, J.: Changes in the transmembrane region of the HIV-1 gp41 envelope glycoprotein affect membrane fusion. J. Virol. 64:5764, 1990.

465. Bergeron, L., Sullivan, N., and Sodroski, J.: Target cell-specific determinants of membrane fusion within the human immunodeficiency virus type 1 gp120 third variable region and gp41 amino terminus. J. Virol. 66:2389, 1992.

466. Grimaila, R. J., Fuller, B. A., Rennert, P. D., Nelson, M. B.,

Hammarskjold, M., Potts, B., Murray, M., Putney, S. D., and Gray, G.: Mutations in the principal neutralization determinant of human immunodeficiency virus type 1 affect syncytium formation, virus infectivity, growth kinetics, and neutralization. J. Virol. 66:1875, 1992.

467. Freed, E. O., and Risser, R.: Identification of conserved residues in the human immunodeficiency virus type 1 principal neutralizing determinant that are involved in fusion. AIDS Res. Hum. Retroviruses 7:807, 1991.

468. Byrn, R. A., Sekigawa, I., Chamow, S. M., Johnson, J. S., Gregory, T. J., Capon, D. J., and Groopman, J. E.: Characterization of in vitro inhibition of human immunodeficiency virus by purified recombinant CD4. J. Virol. 63:4370, 1989.

469. Kirsh, R., Hart, T. K., Ellens, H., Miller, J., Petteway, S. R., Lambert, D. M., Leary, J., and Bugelski, P. J.: Morphometric analysis of recombinant soluble CD4 mediated release of the envelope glycoprotein gp120 from HIV-1. AIDS Res. Hum. Retroviruses 6:1209, 1990.

470. Moore, J. P., McKeating, J. A., Weiss, R. A., and Sattentau, Q. J.: Dissociation of gp120 from HIV-1 virions induced by soluble CD4. Science 250:1139, 1990.

471. Sattentau, Q. J., and Moore, J. P.: Conformational changes induced in the human immunodeficiency virus envelope glycoprotein by soluble CD4 binding. J. Exp. Med. 174:407, 1991.

472. Allan, J. S., Strauss, J., and Buck, D. W.: Enhancement of SIV infection with soluble receptor molecules. Science 247:1084, 1990.

473. Sekigawa, I., Chamow, S. M., Groopman, J. E., and Byrn, R. A.: CD4 immunoadhesin, but not recombinant soluble CD4, blocks syncytium formation by human immunodeficiency virus type 2-infected cells. J. Virol. 64:5194, 1990.

474. Werner, A., Winskowsky, G., and Kurth, R.: Soluble CD4 enhances simian immunodeficiency virus SIV$_{agm}$ infection. J. Virol. 64:6252, 1990.

475. Capon, D. J., Chamow, S. M., Mordenti, J., Marsters, S. A., Gregory, T., Mitsuya, H., Byrn, R. A., Lucas, C., Wurm, F. M., Groopman, J. E., and Smith, D. H.: Designing CD4 immunoadhesins for AIDS therapy. Nature (London) 337:525, 1989.

476. Clapham, P. R., Weber, J. N., Whitby, D., McIntosh, K., Dalgleish, A. G., Maddon, P. J., Deen, K. C., Sweet, R. W., and Weiss, R. A.: Soluble CD4 blocks the infectivity of diverse strains of HIV and SIV for T cells and monocytes but not for brain and muscle cells. Nature (London) 337:368, 1989.

477. Deen, K. C., McDougal, J. S., Inacker, R., Folena-Wasserman, G., Arthos, J., Rosenberg, J., Maddon, P. J., Axel, R., and Sweet, R. W.: A soluble form of CD4 (T4) protein inhibits AIDS virus infection. Nature (London) 331:82, 1988.

478. Hussey, R. E., Richardson, N. E., Kowalski, M., Brown, N. R., Chang, H. C., Siliciano, R. F., Dorfman, T., Walker, B., Sodroski, J., and Reinherz, E. L.: A soluble CD4 protein selectively inhibits HIV replication and syncytium formation. Nature (London) 331:78, 1988.

479. Smith, D. H., Byrn, R. A., Marsters, S. A., Gregory, T., Groopman, J. E., and Capon, D. J.: Blocking of HIV-1 infectivity by a soluble secreted form of the CD4 antigen. Science 238:1704, 1987.

480. Traunecker, A., Luke, W., and Karjaleinen, K.: Soluble CD4 molecules neutralise human immunodeficiency virus type 1. Nature (London) 331:84, 1988.

481. Daar, E. S., Li, X. L., Moudgil, T., and Ho, D. D.: High concentrations of recombinant soluble CD4 are required to neutralize primary HIV-1 isolates. Proc. Natl. Acad. Sci. USA 87:6574, 1990.

482. Kahn, J. O., Allan, J. D., Hodges, T. L., Kaplan, L. D., Arri, C. J., Fitch, H. F., Izu, A. E., Mordenti, J., Sherwin, S. A., Groopman, J. E., and Volberding, P. A.: The safety and pharmacokinetics of recombinant soluble CD4 (rCD4) in subjects with the acquired immunodeficiency syndrome (AIDS) and AIDS-related complex. Ann. Intern. Med. 112:254, 1990.

483. Schooley, R. T., Merigan, T. C., Gaut, P., Hirsch, M. S., Holodniy, M., Flynn, T., Liu, S., Byington, R. E., Henochowica, S., Gubish, E., Spriggs, D., Kufe, D., Schindler, J., Dawson, A., Thomas, D., Hanson, D., Letwin, B., Liu, T., Gulinello, J., Kennedy, S., Fisher, R., and Ho, D. D.: A phase I/II escalating dose trial of recombinant soluble CD4 therapy in patients with AIDS or AIDS-related complex. Ann. Intern. Med. 112:247, 1990.

484. Moore, J. P., McKeating, J. A., Huang, Y., Ashkenazi, A., and Ho, D. D.: Virions of primary human immunodeficiency virus type 1 isolates resistant to soluble CD. J. Virol. 66:235, 1992.

485. Gartner, S., Markovits, P., Markovitz, D. M., Kaplan, M. H., Gallo, R. C., and Popovic, M.: The role of mononuclear phagocytes in HTLV-III/LAV infection. Science 233:215, 1986.

486. Collman, R., Hassan, N. F., Walker, R., Godfrey, B., Cutilli, J., Hastings, J. C., Friedman, H., Douglas, S. D., and Nathanson, N.: Infection of monocyte-derived macrophages with human immunodeficiency virus type 1: Monocyte-tropic and lymphocyte-tropic strains of HIV-1 show distinctive patterns of replication in a panel of cell types. J. Exp. Med. 170:1149, 1989.

487. Cheng-Mayer, C., Weiss, C., Seto, D., and Levy, J. A.: Isolates of human immunodeficiency virus type 1 from the brain may constitute a special group of the AIDS virus. Proc. Natl. Acad. Sci. 86:8575, 1989.

488. Cheng-Mayer, C., Quiroga, M., Tung, J. W., Dina, D., and Levy, J. A.: Viral determinants of HIV-1 T cell/macrophage tropism, cytopathicity, and CD4 antigen modulation. J. Virol. 64:4390, 1990.

489. Schuitemaker, H., Kootstra, N., DeGoede, F., DeWolf, F., Miedema, F., and Tersmette, M.: Monocytotropic human immunodeficiency virus 1 (HIV-1) variants detectable in all stages of HIV infection are predominantly lacking T-cell line tropism and syncytium-inducing ability in primary T-cell culture. J. Virol. 65:356, 1990.

490. Pomerantz, R. J., Feinberg, M. G., Andino, R., and Baltimore, D.: The long terminal repeat is not a major determinant of the cellular tropism of human immunodeficiency virus type 1. J. Virol. 65:1041, 1991.

491. O'Brien, W. A., Koyanagi, Y., Namazie, A., Zhao, J., Diagne, A., Idler, K., Zack, J. A., and Chen, I. S.: HIV-1 tropism for mononuclear phagocytes can be determined by regions of hp120 outside the CD4-binding domain. Nature 348:69, 1990.

492. Hwang, S. S., Boyle, T. J., Lyerly, H. K., and Cullen, B. R.: Identification of the envelope V3 loop as the primary determinant of cell tropism in HIV-1. Science 253:71, 1991.

493. Shioda, T., Levy, J. A., and Cheng-Mayer, C.: Macrophage and T-cell line tropisms of HIV-1 are determined by specific regions of the envelope gp120 gene. Nature (London) 349:167, 1991.

494. Westervelt, P., Gendelman, H. E., and Ratner, L.: Identification of a determinant within the HIV-1 surface envelope glycoprotein critical for productive infection of cultured primary monocytes. Proc. Natl. Acad. Sci. 88:3097, 1991.

495. Westervelt, P., Trowbridge, D. B., Epstein, L. G., Blumberg, B. M., Li, Y., Hahn, B. H., Shaw, G. M., Price, R. W., and Ratner, L.: Macrophage tropism determinants of human immunodeficiency virus type 1 in vivo. J. Virol. 66:2577, 1991.

495a. Chesebro, B., Wehrly, K., Nishio, J., and Perryman, S.: Macrophage-tropic human immunodeficiency virus isolates from different patients exhibit unusual V3 envelope sequence homogeneity in comparison with T-cell–tropic isolates: Definition of critical amino acids involved in cell tropism. J. Virol. 66:6547, 1992.

496. Barin, F., McLane, M. F., Allan, J. S., and Lee, T. H.: Virus envelope protein of HTLV-III represents major target antigen for antibodies in AIDS patients. Science 228:1094, 1985.

497. Gnann, J. W., Nelson, J. A., and Oldstone, M. B.: Fine mapping of an immunodominant domain in the transmembrane glycoprotein of human immunodeficiency virus. J. Virol. 61:2639, 1987.

498. Kennedy, R. C., Henkel, R. D., Pauletti, D., Allan, J. S., Lee, T. H., Essex, M., and Dreesman, G. R.: Antiserum to a synthetic peptide recognizes the HTLV-III envelope glycoprotein. Science 231:1556, 1986.

499. Weiss, R. A., Clapham, P. R., Weber, J. N., Dalgleish, A. G., Lasky, L. A., and Berman, P. W.: Variable and conserved neutralization antigens of human immunodeficiency virus type 1. Nature 324:572, 1986.

500. Arthur, L. O., Pyle, S. W., Nara, P. L., Bess, J. W., Gonda, M. A., Kelliher, J. C., Gilden, R. V., Robey, W. G., Bolognesi, D. P., Gallo, R. C., and Fischinger, P. J.: Serological responses in chimpanzees inoculated with human immunodeficiency virus glycoprotein (gp120) subunit vaccine. Proc. Natl. Acad. Sci. USA 84:8583, 1987.

501. Nara, P. L., Robey, W. G., Pyle, S. W., Hatch, W. C., Dunlop, N. M., Bess, J. W., Kelliher, J. C., Arthur, L. O., and Fischinger, P. J.: Purified envelope glycoproteins from human immunodeficiency virus type 1 variants induce individual, type-specific neutralizing antibodies. J. Virol. 62:2622, 1988.

502. Matthews, T., Langlois, A., Robey, W., Chang, N., Gallo, R., Fischinger, P., and Bolognesi, D.: Restricted neutralization of divergent human T-lymphotropic virus type III isolated by antibodies to the major envelope glycoprotein. Proc. Natl. Acad. Sci. USA 83:9709, 1986.

503. Putney, S., Matthews, T., Robey, W. G., Lynn, D., Robert-Guroff, M., Mueller, W., Langlois, A., Ghrayeb, J., Petteway, S., Weinhold, K., Fischinger, P., Wong-Staal, F., Gallo, R. C., and Bolognesi, D.: HTLV-III/LAV-neutralizing antibodies to an E. coli-produced fragment of the virus envelope. Science 234:1392, 1986.

504. Rusche, J. R., Javaherian, K., McDanal, C., Petro, J., Lynn, D. L., Grimaila, R., Langlois, A., Gallo, R. C., Arthur, L. O., Fischinger, P. J., Bolognesi, D. P., Putney, S. D., and Matthews, T. J.: Antibodies that inhibit fusion of human immunodeficiency virus-infected cells bind a 24-amino acid sequence of the viral envelope, gp120. Proc. Natl. Acad. Sci. USA 85:3198, 1988.

505. Linsley, P., Ledbetter, J., Thomas, E., and Hu, S.: Effects of anti-gp120 monoclonal antibodies on CD4 receptor binding by the env protein of human immunodeficiency virus type 1. J. Virol. 62:3695, 1988.

506. McKeating, J., Gow, J., Goudsmit, J., Pearl, L., Mulder, C., and Weiss, R.: Characterization of HIV-1 neutralization escape mutants. AIDS 3:777, 1989.

507. Nara, P., Robey, W., Arthur, L., Asher, D., Wolff, A., Gibbs, C., Gajdusek, D. C., and Fischinger, P.: Persistent infection of chimpanzees with human immunodeficiency virus: Serological responses and properties of reisolated viruses. J. Virol. 61:3173, 1987.

508. Skinner, M., Langlois, A., McDanal, C., McDougal, J. S., Bolognesi, D., and Matthews, T.: Characteristics of a neutralizing monoclonal antibody to the HIV envelope glycoprotein. J. Virol. 62:4195, 1988.

509. Profy, A., Salisas, P., Eckler, L., Dunlop, N., Nara, P., and Putney, S.: Epitopes recognized by the neutralizing antibodies of an HIV-1-infected individual. J. Immunol. 144:4641, 1990.

510. Weiss, R., Clapham, P., Cheingsong-Popov, R., Dalgleish, A., Carne, C., Weller, I., and Tedder, R.: Neutralization of human T-lymphotropic virus type III by sera of AIDS and AIDS-risk patients. Nature (London) 316:69, 1985.

511. Steimer, K. S., Scandella, C. J., Skiles, P. V., and Haigwood, N. L.: Neutralization of divergent HIV-1 isolates by conformation-dependent human antibodies to Gp120. Science 254:105, 1991.

512. Berkower, I., Smith, G. E., Giri, C., and Murphy, D.: Human immunodeficiency virus: Predominance of a group-specific neutralizing epitope that persists despite genetic variation. J. Exp. Med. 170:1681, 1989.

513. Thali, M., Olshevsky, U., Furman, C., Gabuzda, D., Posner, M., and Sodroski, J.: Characterization of a discontinuous

human immunodeficiency virus type 1 gp120 epitope recognized by a broadly reactive neutralizing human monoclonal antibody. J. Virol. 65:6188, 1991.

513a. Daniel, M. D. Kirchhoff, F., Czajak, S. C., Sehgal, P. K., and Desrosiers, R. C.: Protective effects of a live attenuated SIV vaccine with a deletion in the *nef* gene. Science 258:1938, 1992.

514. Kawakami, T., Sherman, L., Dahlberg, J., Gazit, A., Yaniv, A., Tronick, S. R., and Aaronson, S. A.: Nucleotide sequence analysis of equine infectious anemia virus proviral DNA. Virology 158:300, 1987.

515. Fisher, A. G., Ensoli, B., Ivanoff, L., Chamberlain, M., Petteway, S., Ratner, L., Gallo, R. C., and Wong-Staal, F.: The sor gene of HIV-1 is required for efficient virus transmission *in vitro*. Science 237:888, 1987.

516. Strebel, K.: The HIV "A" *(sor)* gene product is essential for virus infectivity. Nature 328:728, 1987.

517. Sodroski, J., Goh, W. C., Rosen, C., Tartar, A., Portetelle, D., Burny, A., and Haseltine, W. A.: Replicative and cytopathic potential of HTLV-III/LAV with sor gene deletions. Science 231:1549, 1986.

517a. Gabuzda, D. H., Lawrence, K., Langhoff, E., Terwilliger, E., Dorfman, T., Haseltine, W. A., and Sodroski, J.: Role of *vif* in replication of human immunodeficiency virus type 1 in CD4$^+$ T lymphocytes. J. Virol. 66:6489, 1992.

517b. Sakai, H., Shibata, R., Sakuragi, J., Sakuragi, S., Kawamura, M., and Adachi, A.: Cell-dependent requirement of human immunodeficiency virus type 1 *vif* protein for maturation of virus particles. J. Virol. 67:1663, 1993.

518. Terwilliger, E. F., Cohen, E. A., Lu, Y. C., Sodroski, J. G., and Haseltine, W. A.: Functional role of human immunodeficiency virus type 1 vpu. Proc. Natl. Acad. Sci. USA 86:5163, 1989.

519. Klimkait, T., Strebel, K., Hoggan, M. D., Martin, M. A., and Orenstein, J. M.: The human immunodeficiency virus type 1-specific protein *vpu* is required for efficient virus maturation and release. J. Virol. 64:621, 1990.

520. Strebel, K., Klimkait, T., Maldarelli, F., and Martin, M. A.: Molecular and biochemical analyses of human immunodeficiency virus type 1 *vpu* protein. J. Virol. 63:3784, 1989.

521. Crise, B., Buonocore, L., and Rose, J. K.: CD4 is retained in the endoplasmic reticulum by the human immunodeficiency virus type 1 glycoprotein precursor. J. Virol. 64:5585, 1990.

522. Stevenson, M., Zhang, X., and Volsky, D. J.: Downregulation of cell surface molecules during noncytopathic infection of T cells with human immunodeficiency. J. Virol. 61:3741, 1987.

523. Willey, R. L., Maldarelli, F., Martin, M. A., and Strebel, K.: Human immunodeficiency virus type 1 Vpu protein regulates the formation of intracellular gp160-CD4 complexes. J. Virol. 66:226, 1992.

523a. Willey, R. L., Maldarelli, L. F., Martin, M. A., and Strebel, K.: Human immunodeficiency virus type 1 Vpu protein induces rapid degradation of CD4. J. Virol. 66:7193, 1992.

524. Goedert, J. J., and Blattner, W. A.: AIDS: Etiology, Diagnosis, Treatment, and Prevention, 2nd ed. Philadelphia, J. B. Lippincott, 1988.

525. Blanche, S., Rouzioux, C., Moscato, M. G., Veber, F., Mayaux, M., Jacomet, C., Tricoire, J., Deville, A., Vial, M., Firtion, G., deCrepy, A., Douard, D., Robin, M., Courpotin, C., Ciraru-Vigneron, N., LeDeist, F., and Griscelli, C.: A prospective study of infants born to women seropositive for human immunodeficiency virus type 1. N. Engl. J. Med. 320:1643, 1989.

526. Goedert, J. J., Eyster, M. E., Biggar, R. J., Salahuddin, S. Z., Sarin, P. S., and Blattner, W. A.: Heterosexual transmission of human immunodeficiency virus: Association with severe depletion of T-helper lymphocytes in men with hemophilia. AIDS Res. Hum. Retroviruses 3:335, 1987.

527. Ho, D. D., Moudgil, T., and Alam, M.: Quantitation of human immunodeficiency virus type 1 in the blood of infected persons. N. Engl. J. Med. 321:1621, 1989.

528. Goedert, J. J., Drummond, J. E., Minkoff, H. L., Stevens, R., Blattner, W. A., Mendez, H., Robert-Guroff, M., Holman,

S., Rubinstein, A., Willoughby, A., and Landesman, S. H.: Mother-to-infant transmission of human immunodeficiency virus type 1: Association with prematurity or low anti-gp120. Lancet 2:1351, 1989.

529. Padian, N., Marquis, L., Frances, D. P., Anderson, R. E., Rutherford, G. W., O'Malley, P. M., and Winkelstein, W.: Male to female transmission of human immunodeficiency virus. J.A.M.A. 258:788, 1987.

530. CDC: Update: Human immunodeficiency virus infections in health-care workers exposed to blood of infected patients. M. M. W. R. 36:285, 1987.

531. Blattner, W. A.: HIV epidemiology: Past, present, and future. FASEB J. 5:2340, 1991.

531a. Tokars, J. I., Marcus, R., Culver, D. H., Schable, C. A., McKibben, P. S., Baudea, C. I., and Bell, D. M.: Surveillance of HIV infection and zidovudine use among health care workers after occupational exposure to HIV infected blood. Ann. Intern. Med. 118:913, 1993.

532. Cooper, D. A., Gold, J., MacLean, P., Donovan, B., Finlayson, R., Barnes, T. G., Michelmore, H. M., Brooke, P., and Penny, R.: Definition of a clinical illness associated with seroconversion. Lancet 1:537, 1985.

533. Ho, D. D., Sarngadharan, M. G., Resnick, L., Dimarzo-Veronese, F., Rota, T. R., and Hirsch, M. S.: Primary human T-lymphotropic virus type III infection. Ann. Intern. Med. 103:880, 1985.

534. Gaines, H., von Sydow, A. J., Sonnerborg, A., Chiodi, F., Ehrnst, A., Strannegard, O., and Asjo, B.: HIV antigenaemia and virus isolation from plasma during primary HIV infection. Lancet 1:1317, 1987.

535. Goudsmit, J, deWolf, F., and Paul, D. A.: Expression of human immunodeficiency virus antigen (HIV-Ag) in serum and cerebrospinal fluid during acute and chronic infection. Lancet 2:177, 1986.

536. Daar, E. S., Moudgil, T., Meyer, R. D., and Ho, D. D.: Transient high levels of viremia in patients with primary human immunodeficiency virus type 1 infection. N. Engl. J. Med. 324:961, 1991.

537. Clark, S. J., Michael, S. S., Decker, W. D., Campbell-Hill, S., Roberson, J. L., Veldkamp, P. J., Kappes, J. C., Hahn, B. H., and Shaw, G. M.: High titers of cytopathic virus in plasma of patients with symptomatic primary HIV-1 infection. N. Engl. J. Med. 324:954, 1991.

538. Gaines, H., vonSydow, M., Sonnerborg, A., Albert, J., Czajkowski, J., Pehrson, P. O., Chiodi, F., Moberg, L., Fenyo, E. M., Asjo, B., and Forsgren, M.: Antibody response in primary human immunodeficiency virus infection. Lancet 1:1249, 1987.

539. Sinicco, A., Palestro, G., Caramello, P., Giacobbi, D., Giuliani, G., Paggi, G., Sciandra, M., and Gioannini, P.: Acute HIV-1 infection: Clinical and biological study of 12 patients. J. Acquir. Immune Defic. Syndr. 3:260, 1990.

540. Cooper, D. A., Imrie, A. A., and Penny, R.: Antibody response to human immunodeficiency virus after primary infection. J. Infect. Dis. 155:1113, 1987.

541. Tersmette, M., Gruters, R. A., deWolf, F., deGoede, R. E., Lange, J. M., Schellekens, P. T., Goudsmit, J., Huisman, H. G., and Miedema, F.: Evidence for a role of virulent human immunodeficiency virus (HIV) variants in the pathogenesis of acquired immunodeficiency syndrome: Studies on sequential HIV isolates. J. Virol. 63:2118, 1989.

542. Fenyo, E. M., Morfeldt-Manson, L., Chiodi, F., Lind, B., von Gegerfelt, A., Albert, J., Olausson, E., and Asjo, B.: Distinct replicative and cytopathic characteristics of human immunodeficiency virus isolates. J. Virol. 62:4414, 1988.

543. Ward, J. W., Holmberg, S. D., Allen, J. R., Cohn, D. L., Critchley, S. E., Kleinman, S. H., Lenes, B. A., Ravenholt, O., Davis, J. R., Quinn, M. G., and Jaffe, H. W.: Transmission of human immunodeficiency virus by blood transfusions screened as negative for HIV. N. Engl. J. Med. 318:473, 1988.

544. Curran, J. W., Jaffe, H. W., Hardy, A. M., Morgan, W. M., Selik, R. M., and Dondero, T. J.: Epidemiology of HIV

infection and AIDS in the United States. Science 239:610, 1988.

545. Schnittman, S. M., Psallidopoulos, M. C., Lane, H. C., Thompson, L., Baseler, M., Massari, F., Fox, C. H., Salzman, N. P., and Fauci, A. S.: The reservoir for HIV-1 in human peripheral blood is a T cell that maintains expression of CD4. Science 245:305, 1989.

546. CDC: Classification system for human T lymphotropic virus type III/lymphadenopathy associated virus. Ann. Intern. Med. 105:234, 1986.

547. Schnittman, S. M., Greenhouse, J. J., Psallidopoulos, M. C., Baseler, M., Salzman, N. P., Fauci, A. S., and Lane, H. C.: Increasing viral burden in CD4+ T cells from patients with human immunodeficiency virus (HIV) infection reflects rapidly progressive immunosuppression and clinical disease. Ann. Intern. Med. 113:438, 1990.

548. Pomerantz, R. J., Trono, D., Feinberg, M. B., and Baltimore, D.: Cells nonproductively infected with HIV-1 exhibit an aberrant pattern of viral RNA expression: A molecular model for latency. Cell 61:1271, 1990.

549. Folks, T., Justement, J., Kinter, A., Dinarello, C. A., and Fauci, A. S.: Cytokine induced expression of HIV-1 in a chronically-infected promonocyte cell line. Science 238:800, 1987.

550. Folks, T. M., Powell, D., Lightfoote, M., Koenig, S., Fauci, A. S., Benn, S., Rabson, A., Daugherty, D., Gendelman, H. E., Hoggan, M. D., Venkatesan, S., and Martin, M. A.: Biological and biochemical characterization of a cloned Leu-3 cell surviving infection with the acquired immune deficiency syndrome retrovirus. J. Exp. Med. 164:280, 1986.

551. Pantaleo, G., Graziosi, C., Butini, L., Pizzo, P. A., Schnittman, S. M., Kotler, D. P., and Fauci, A. S.: Lymphoid organs function as major reservoirs for human immunodeficiency virus. Proc. Natl. Acad. Sci. USA 88:9838, 1991.

551a. Pantaleo, G., Graziosi, C., Demarest, J. F., Butini, L., Montroni, M., Fox, C. H., Orenstein, J. M., Kotler, D. P., and Fauci, A. S.: HIV infection is active and progressive in lymphoid tissue during the clinically latent stage of disease. Nature 362:355, 1993.

551b. Embretson, J., Zupancic, M., Ribas, J. L., Burke, A., Racz, P., Tenner-Racz, K., and Haase, A. T.: Massive covert infection of helper T lymphocytes and macrophages by HIV during the incubation period of AIDS. Nature 362:359, 1993.

552. Fritsch, E. F., and Temin, H. M.: Inhibition of viral DNA synthesis in stationary chicken embryo fibroblasts infected with avian retroviruses. J. Virol. 24:461, 1977.

553. Varmus, H. E., Padgett, T., Heasley, S., Simon, G., and Bishop, J. M.: Cellular functions are required for the synthesis and integration of avian sarcoma virus-specific DNA. Cell 11:307, 1977.

554. Stevenson, M., Stanwick, T. L., Dempsey, M. P., and Lamonica, C. A.: HIV-1 replication is controlled at the level of T cell activation and proviral integration. EMBO J. 9:1551, 1990.

555. Zack, J. A., Cann, A. J., Lugo, J. P., and Chen, I. S.: HIV-1 production from infected peripheral blood T cells after HTLV-I induced mitogenic stimulation. Science 240:1026, 1988.

556. Zack, J. A., Arrigo, S. J., Weitsman, S. T., Go, A. S., Haislip, A., and Chen, I. S.: HIV-1 entry into quiescent primary lymphocytes: Molecular analysis reveals a labile, latent viral structure. Cell 61:213, 1990.

557. Meyerhans, A., Cheynier, R., Albert, J., Seth, M., Kwok, J., Sninsky, L., Morfeldt-Manson, L., Asjo, B., and Wain-Hobson, S.: Temporal fluctuations in HIV quasispecies in vivo are not reflected by sequential HIV isolations. Cell 58:901, 1989.

558. Simmonds, P., Balfe, P., Ludlam, C. A., Bishop, J. O., and Brown, A. J.: Analysis of sequence diversity in hypervariable regions of the external glycoprotein of human immunodeficiency virus type 1. J. Virol. 64:5840, 1990.

559. McNearney, T., Westervelt, P., Thielan, B. J., Trowbridge, D. B., Garcia, J., Whittier, R., and Ratner, L.: Limited sequence heterogeneity among biologically distinct human immunodeficiency virus type 1 isolates from individuals involved in a clustered infectious outbreak. Proc. Natl. Acad. Sci. USA 87:1917, 1990.

560. Kleim, J. P., Ackermann, A., Brackmann, H. H., Gahr, M., and Schneweis, K. E.: Epidemiologically closely related viruses from hemophilia B patients display high homology in two hypervariable regions of the HIV-1 env gene. AIDS Res. Hum. Retroviruses 7:417, 1991.

561. Sato, H., Orenstein, J., Dimitrov, D., and Martin, M. A.: Cell-to-cell spread of HIV-1 occurs within minutes and may not involve the participation of virus particles. Virology 186:712, 1992.

562. Li, P., and Burrell, C. J.: Synthesis of human immunodeficiency virus DNA in a cell-to-cell transmission model. AIDS Res. Hum. Retroviruses 8:253, 1992.

562a. Dimitrov, D. S., Willey, R. L., Sato, H., Chang, L. J., Blumenthal, R., and Martin, M. A.: Quantitation of human immunodeficiency virus type 1 infection kinetics. J. Virol. 67:2182, 1993.

563. Orenstein, J. M., Meltzer, M. S., Phipps, T., and Gendelman, H. E.: Cytoplasmic assembly and accumulation of human immunodeficiency virus types 1 and 2 in recombinant human colony-stimulating factor-1-treated human monocytes: An ultrastructural study. J. Virol. 62:2578, 1988.

564. Potts, B. J., Maury, W., and Martin, M. A.: Replication of HIV-1 in primary monocyte cultures. Virology 175:465, 1990.

565. Overbaugh, J., Donahue, P. R., Quackenbush, S. L., Hoover, E. A., and Mullins, J. I.: Molecular cloning of a feline leukemia virus that induces fatal immunodeficiency disease in cats. Science 239:906, 1988.

566. Li, J., Bestwick, R. K., Spiro, C., and Kabat, D.: The membrane glycoprotein of Friend spleen focus-forming virus: Evidence that the cell surface component is required for pathogenesis and that it binds to a receptor. J. Virol. 61:2782, 1987.

567. Aziz, D. C., Hanna, Z., and Jolicoeur, P.: Severe immunodeficiency disease induced by a defective murine leukaemia virus. Nature 338:505, 1989.

568. Kohlstaedt, L. A., Wang, J., Friedman, J. M., Rice, P. A., and Steitz, T. A.: Crystal structure at 3.5 Å resolution of HIV-1 reverse transcriptase complexed with an inhibitor. Science 256:1783, 1992.

569. Furfine, E. S., and Reardon, J. E.: Reverse transcriptase RNase H from the human immunodeficiency virus. J. Biol. Chem. 266:406, 1991.

570. Koga, Y., Sasaki, M., Yoshida, H., Wigzell, H., Kimura, G., and Nomoto, K.: Cytopathic effect determined by the amount of CD4 molecules in human cell lines expressing envelope glycoprotein of HIV. J. Immunol. 144:94, 1990.

571. Koga, Y., Sasaki, M., Yoshida, H., Oh-Tsu, M., Kimura, G., and Nomoto, K.: Disturbance of nuclear transport of proteins in CD4+ cells expressing gp160 of human immunodeficiency virus. J. Virol. 65:5609, 1991.

571a. Skowronski, J., Parks, D., and Mariani, R.: Altered T cell activation and development in transgenic mice expressing the HIV-1 nef gene. EMBO J. 12:703, 1993.

572. Nara, P., Hatch, W., Kessler, J., Kelliher, J., and Carter, S.: The biology of human immunodeficiency virus-1 IIIB infection in the chimpanzee: In vivo and in vitro correlations. J. Med. Primatol. 18:343, 1989.

573. Fultz, P. N., McClure, H. M., Anderson, D. C., and Switzer, W. M.: Identification and biologic characterization of an acutely lethal variant of simian immunodeficiency virus from sooty mangabeys. AIDS Res. Hum. Retroviruses 5:397, 1989.

574. Mitsuya, H., Weinhold, K. J., Furman, F. A., St. Clair, M. H., Lehrman, S. N., Gallo, R. C., Bolognesi, D., Barry, D. W., and Broder, S.: 3'-Azido-3'-deoxythymidine (BW A509U): An antiviral agent that inhibits the infectivity and cytopathic effect of human T-lymphotropic virus type III/lymphadenopathy-associated virus in vitro. Proc. Natl. Acad. Sci. USA 82:7096, 1985.

575. Pauwels, R., Andries, K., Desmyter, J., Schols, D., Kukla, M. J., Breslin, H. J., Raeymaeckers, A., Van Gelder, J., Woestenborghs, R., Heykants, J., Schellekens, K., Janssen, M. A.

C., De Clercq, E., and Janssen, P. A. J.: Potent and selective inhibition of HIV-1 replication *in vitro* by a novel series of TIBO derivatives. Nature 343:470, 1990.

576. Merluzzi, V. J., Hargrave, K. D., Labadia, M., Grozinger, K., Skoog, M., Wu, J. C., Shih, C.-K., Eckner, K., Hattox, S., Adams, J., Rosenthal, A. S., Faanes, R., Eckner, R. J., Koup, R. A., and Sullivan, J. L.: Inhibition of HIV-1 replication by a nonnucleoside reverse transcriptase inhibitor. Science 250:1411, 1990.

577. Roberts, N. A., Martin, J. A., Kinchington, D., Broadhurst, A. V., Craing, J. C., Duncan, I. B., Galpin, S. A., Handa, B. K., Kay, J., Krohn, A., Lambert, R. W., Merrett, J. H., Mills, J. S., Parkes, K. E. B., Redshaw, S., Ritchie, A. J., Taylor, D. L., Thomas, G. J., and Machin, P. J.: Rational design of peptide-based HIV proteinase inhibitors. Science 248:358, 1990.

578. Maurer, B., Bannert, H., Darai, G., and Flugel, R. M.: Analysis of the primary structure of the long terminal repeat and the *gag* and *pol* genes of the human spumaretrovirus. J. Virol. 62:1590, 1988.

579. Flugel, R. M., Rethwilm, A., Maurer, B., and Darai, G.: Nucleotide sequence analysis of the *env* gene and its flanking regions of the human spumaretrovirus reveals two novel genes. EMBO J. 6:2077, 1987.

580. Guyader, M., Emerman, M., Sonigo, P., Clavel, F., Montagnier, L., and Alizon, M.: Genome organization and transactivation of the human immunodeficiency virus type 2. Nature 326:662, 1987.

581. Khan, A., Galvin, T. A., Lowenstine, L. J., Jennings, M. B., Gardner, M. B., and Buckler, C. E.: A highly divergent simian immunodeficiency virus (SIV_{stm}) recovered from stored stump-tailed macaque tissues. J. Virol. 65:7061, 1991.

Viral Pathogenesis of Hematological Disorders

Introduction

Neal S. Young

This chapter consists of portraits of members of three virus families—the Parvoviridae, Retroviridae, and Herpesviridae—that cause blood diseases. These microorganisms have been chosen because they cause important human diseases and also illustrate the extraordinary diversity of interactions between viruses and humans, pathogenic associations that result from complex yet relatively well understood molecular, cellular, and immunological processes.

In practice, research in virology is so splintered that underlying principles about viruses often are either simplistic or obscure. Viruses are defined by their dependence on host cells for propagation, but otherwise they are extremely different one from another. Some general features of animal viruses—physical structure, genetic organization, replication strategy, regulation of gene expression—bear directly on relevant aspects of human clinical infections, especially cytopathology, host range and tissue tropism, and the host immune response. "Black boxes" have encased important aspects of virus biology: the mechanisms underlying virus entry, tissue specificity, cytotoxicity, latency, and subtle effects on host cell function. Refractory to investigation until recently, these processes are now clearly accessible to experimentation. Some principles of virology and the impetus for this chapter are made explicit by way of introduction.

Viruses show great diversity in their strategies for propagation. One example of the range is the difference in sheer quantity of genetic material between, for example, a parvovirus, consisting of 5 kb of DNA and a few genes, through cytomegalovirus, with about 200 kb of DNA and more than 100 genes, to poxviruses of 300 kb of DNA. Functionally, the dependence of virus replication on the host cell has fostered extraordinary complexity in the regulation of their own genes and interactions with cellular genes, including such remarkable features as translation from overlapping reading frames, bidirectional transcription, multiple functions for single proteins, integration into host chromosomes, and complex mechanisms for the maintenance of latency.

Viruses can have very different effects on host cells. B19 parvovirus is clearly toxic to its host cell, the erythroid progenitor. Its close cousin, adeno-associated virus, has little apparent effect on cells in culture and produces no disease in humans. DNA viruses like adenovirus and SV40 and RNA viruses like human T-cell lymphotropic virus type 1 (HTLV-1) can transform cells and promote or create a malignant phenotype. Cell death and cancer are obvious sequelae of virus infection. Much more subtle effects may result from virus infections that slow cell growth or inhibit cellular "luxury" functions. For example, the only cytopathic effect of infection of murine anterior pituitary gland cells by lymphochoriomeningitis virus is inhibition of hormone secretion.

Host factors help determine viral disease. Most viral infections of humans are asymptomatic. Devastating syndromes have been characterized for individuals (herpes simplex encephalitis), kindreds (Epstein-Barr virus and X-linked lymphoproliferative disease), and populations (cytomegalovirus in the neonate, mumps in adult men, varicella in the immunosuppressed, measles in Pacific islanders). The most important determinants probably relate to defects in the host immune response, exemplified in this chapter by the permissive effect on parvovirus infection of defective antibody production and on cytomegalovirus disease of diminished T cells. In contrast and probably more commonly, other viral diseases may result from the host immune response, from the "cytokine flu" symptoms of the common cold to virus-triggered, T cell–mediated autoimmune disease in animal models and humans (demyelination in the nervous system, diabetes, and probably also post-hepatitis aplastic anemia).

Experiments drive understanding. Virology is an empirical science, and detailed understanding of viruses and virus diseases depends on the types of experiments that can be performed. Early observations of naturally ill and purposely inoculated animals and humans demonstrated the infectivity of cell-free extracts, aspects of contagion, and histopathological alterations of virus infection. Until relatively recently, virology was dominated by biochemistry and especially immunology: Antisera and specific antibodies allowed strain typing, neutralization assays, and the study of individual structural proteins. Antibody-based techniques were less helpful in studying intracellular events, which in our own era have been resolved by molecular biological approaches to replication and gene expression, cell receptors, and protein trafficking.

Excellent discussions of these subjects and bibliographies of the extensive literature are contained in current textbooks[1] and monographs.[2–5]

A. B19 PARVOVIRUS*

Neal S. Young

The B19 parvovirus is the only known member of an important virus family to cause disease in humans. Illnesses due to B19 parvovirus infection range from a relatively innocuous rash of childhood to fatal fetal infection. Although it was discovered only 20 years ago, many aspects of B19 parvovirus are well understood or should soon be so; this chapter emphasizes virus structure, replication strategy, gene expression, antigenicity, tissue tropism, pathogenesis, and host immune response.

Yvonne Cossart, a virologist working in London in the mid-1970s, discovered B19 parvovirus while investigating laboratory assays for hepatitis B.[6] She used an immunoelectrophoretic technique in which sera from blood bank donors, serving as a source of antigen, were reacted with samples from patients with hepatitis, used as a source of antibody. In comparison with more specific assays, she noted a number of apparently false-positive reactions. When she excised the precipitin lines from the agarose and examined them by electron microscopy, she noted particles typical in appearance of parvoviruses (Fig. 26–1). (One viremic blood bank donor's serum had been encoded "B19"—there are no parvoviruses A or B1 to 18!)

Using the same assay system, British colleagues found antibodies in a high proportion of normal adults.[7] Subsequently, evidence of acute infection, immunoglobulin M (IgM) or viral antigen, was seroepidemiologically linked to transient aplastic crisis of sickle cell anemia[8] and fifth disease in normal children.[9] The genetic material of the particles present in acute phase sera could be characterized as single-stranded DNA, allowing classification of the agent as a proper member of the Parvoviridae family,[10, 11] and in the mid-1980s the virus was cloned by Cotmore and Tattersall at Yale[12] and sequenced by Astell's laboratory in Vancouver.[13] About the same time, B19 parvovirus was first cultivated in vitro using human bone marrow cells by Ozawa and colleagues at the National Institutes of Health.[14] Human erythroid progenitors remain the most convenient productive tissue culture system, and inoculation of these cells has allowed a description of the virus' molecular biology. Expression of B19 parvovirus capsid proteins using recombinant technology has been useful for development of clinical assays for specific parvovirus antibodies, and engineered capsids should be suitable for a human vaccine.[15]

Although the rash due to acute parvovirus infection in children is a minor illness, B19 is not always so benign: aplastic crisis and persistent infection can terminate fatally, and the arthropathy that follows infection in adult women may have substantial morbidity. Because of the relative unavailability of clinical assays and the low index of suspicion, the full spectrum of B19 parvovirus illness is probably still not known. Parvoviruses are intrinsically worthy of study, but in

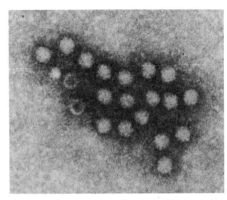

FIGURE 26–1. Electron micrograph of B19 parvovirus particles showing icosahedral symmetry and empty capsids, both characteristic of members of the *Parvoviridae* family. (Courtesy of Dr. A. Field.)

addition the clarity of our understanding of the interactions among pathogenic virus, target cell, and host immune system makes them an excellent model for understanding viral disease in the hematopoietic system. For fuller discussions of the Parvoviridae, the reader is referred to textbooks of virology[16, 17] and monographs[18, 19] and, for B19 parvovirus, to several recent comprehensive reviews.[20–23]

EPIDEMIOLOGY

The B19 parvovirus is the cause of a common infection in humans. IgG antibody specific for the virus, which appears in the first 2 weeks after inoculation and persists for life,[24–26] is the most convenient marker of past exposure. About 50 per cent of adults have IgG antibody to B19 parvovirus; the proportion increases to more than 90 per cent in the elderly.[27] An annual seroconversion rate of 1.5 per cent was estimated from studies of serial samples from women of childbearing age.[28] Thus, most individuals acquire immunity during childhood, but susceptibility continues for others throughout adult life. Seroprevalence of IgG antibody is similarly high worldwide,[21, 29, 30] except among some isolated Brazilian[31] and African[32] tribal populations.

Fifth disease is seasonal, with peak occurrence in spring and summer. Both fifth disease and transient aplastic crisis appear to cycle in approximately 3- to 4-year periods. Epidemics of fifth disease in normal children and clusters of transient aplastic crisis in patients with underlying hemolysis occur concurrently, but they frequently are recognized and treated by different physician specialists.[33] Although IgG antibody to B19 parvovirus is common, viral antigen is detected very rarely in normal persons: Only one of 24,000 blood donors contained a high titer of virus in one purposeful screen.[34]

B19 parvovirus is excreted from the nasopharynx, and the major route of transmission is probably through the upper airway.[25] There is little evidence of virus excretion in feces or urine.[25] In epidemics the attack rate is high: Between 10 and 60 per cent of susceptible school children develop fifth disease in school outbreaks,[28, 32, 35] and for school and day-care personnel, parvovirus infections occurred in 20 to 30 per cent.[36] Sibling-to-sibling transfer is probably a major path of transmission.[28] Although viremia is rare, B19 parvovirus can be transmitted in transfused blood products, especially pooled coagulation factor concentrates.[37] Parvoviruses, including B19, are very heat resistant and can withstand the usual thermal treatment to destroy viral infectivity. Parvovirus has been transmitted by dry- and steam-heated products,[38] but hemophiliacs who received factor VIII concentrate that had been heated to 80°C for 72 hours had a lower rate of seroconversion than those who received unheated concentrate.[39] Nosocomial transmission from infected patients to medical staff can occur[40] but is probably infrequent.

THE PARVOVIRUSES

The *Parvoviridae*—small, single-stranded DNA viruses—are common animal pathogens. Feline panleukopenia virus was one of the first viruses experimentally demonstrated to cause disease in animals; this virus infects cat hematopoietic and lymphocytic cells and causes often fatal neutropenia.[41, 42] The canine, mink, and feline parvoviruses are similar enough to one another at the nucleotide and amino acid level to be grouped as host range variants.[43] These parvoviruses are striking for the recent development of tropism for some species, like mink and dogs, and their host-dependent behavior. Canine parvovirus suddenly appeared among dogs worldwide in the panzootic of 1978,[43] and more recently the virus spread to isolated wolf populations in Michigan's upper peninsula. There are interesting examples of the variety of clinical syndromes resulting from infection by animal parvoviruses in different hosts. Feline panleukopenia virus causes congenital ataxia in kittens owing to a remarkably specific attack on cells of the developing fetal cerebellum.[44] Canine parvovirus is notorious for myocarditis in puppies, which is rare in kittens, whereas feline panleukopenia virus often kills cats as a result of marrow myeloid hypoplasia and neutropenia, which do not usually occur in dogs.[43, 45] Tropism for bone marrow hematopoietic progenitors may be a general feature of parvovirus biology: Minute virus of mice suppresses murine progenitor and stem cells[46]; Aleutian disease virus replicates in mink lymphocytes[47]; and a chicken marrow aplasia agent also has characteristics of a parvovirus.[48]

Physical Features

Parvoviruses are defined by their size, symmetry, and genetic material. *Parvum* is Latin for "small," and the parvoviruses are among the smallest viruses, usually 15 to 28 nm in diameter. In the electron microscope, they show icosahedral symmetry; the specific arrangement of viral proteins in the capsid has been determined by x-ray crystallography, described below. The absence of a lipid envelope contributes to the high heat stability of parvoviruses, a major factor in their extremely contagious behavior. Each parvovirus capsid contains a single copy of the viral genome, composed of about 5000 bases of single-stranded DNA (Fig. 26–2). (For convenient reference, the entire genome is equated to 100 map units.) Parvoviruses have molecular weights ranging from 1.55 to 1.97 × 10^6, about half of which represents DNA; their buoyant density in cesium chloride density gradients ranges from 1.36 to 1.43 g/ml, the less dense particles representing empty capsids.

Genomic Organization

Most vertebrate parvoviruses share a similar genomic organization, with the capsid proteins encoded by genes on the right side of the genome and nonstructural proteins by genes on the left side. At both ends of the genome are terminal repeat sequences, palindromes of variable length and symmetry according to the species of virus (Fig. 26–3). These inverted repeat elements serve as the double-stranded matrix needed to initiate DNA synthesis, and they are therefore required for virus propagation.[49, 50] Somewhat surprisingly, the terminal repeats also appear to be necessary and sufficient for other virus functions, including not only replication but also packaging of DNA.[51, 52] B19 has the longest terminal repeats among

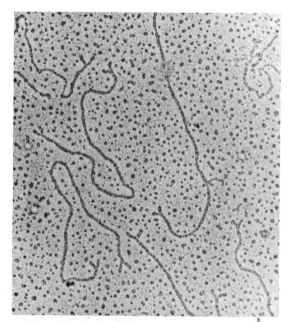

FIGURE 26–2. Electron micrograph of B19 parvovirus DNA, annealed in vitro and showing terminal hairpin structures. (Courtesy of Dr. B. J. Cohen.)

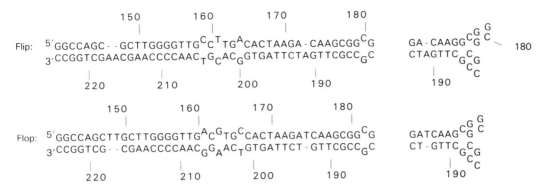

FIGURE 26–3. Schematic of the palindromic nucleotide sequences that form the terminal hairpin structures of B19 parvovirus; alternative conformations are shown. (Adapted from Deiss, V., Tratschin, J.-D., Weitz, M., and Siegl, G.: Cloning of the human parvovirus B19 genome and structural analysis of its palindromic termini. Virology 175: 247–254, 1990; with permission.)

the parvoviruses, 365 nucleotides (nt) rivaled only by human adeno-associated virus and bovine parvovirus. In both B19 parvovirus and adeno-associated virus, the 5' and 3' ends are of identical sequence.[50] The length, the presence of several long direct repeat sequences, the high content of guanosine-cytosine pairs, and the resulting strong secondary structure of the B19 parvovirus terminal repeat sequences have made them resistant to molecular cloning in bacteria until the recent achievement of full length cloning of a (presumably) infectious virus.[53]

Non-structural Protein

The gene for non-structural protein is fairly homologous among the parvoviruses, consistent with its required role in virus propagation.[13] Non-structural protein is generally restricted to the nucleus and binds to DNA.[54] Nickase, helicase, and endonuclease activities have been assigned to non-structural protein of adeno-associated virus,[55] but the non-structural protein genes do not share homology with known cellular toxins or pore-forming proteins. Parvovirus non-structural proteins are pleiotropic: They are required for parvovirus replication,[56] including resolution of the terminal hairpin structures[57]; they are needed for RNA transcription[58]; they function as enhancer elements for the parvovirus structural gene promoter[59] and their own promoter[60]; they are required for excision of the parvoviral genome from transfecting plasmid[61]; and they may "lead" the DNA strand into the preformed capsid.[62] The non-structural proteins also cause host cell death[63, 64]; they can suppress heterologous promoter function[65]; and they are the mediators of parvovirus "oncosuppressive" effects in a variety of cell culture systems.[66, 67] Mutation and deletion analyses of the non-structural protein gene have not allowed separation or assignment of the protein's functions to specific regions, and multiple activities can be abolished with an appropriate single amino acid substitution.[68] Non-structural protein gene expression precedes capsid protein gene expression and DNA synthesis for B19 parvovirus[69] (and minute

virus of mice,[70]), corresponding to the early and late events of virus replication for many other viruses.

Structural Proteins

The two or three capsid proteins are derived from overlapping reading frames and thus share substantial amino acid identity; for example, in B19 parvovirus, the minor capsid protein sequence differs from that of the major capsid protein by an additional 227 amino acids at its amino-terminus. By convention, the longest and least abundant minor capsid species is denoted VP1, and the shorter major capsid protein is denoted VP2 (or VP3). The B19 virion is composed of 60 capsid proteins, 5 to 10 per cent of which are VP1 and the remainder VP2. For animal parvoviruses, tissue tropism[71, 72] and host range specificity[73] have been mapped to a few nucleotides within the capsid genes. The canine/feline differences are located on the virus surface in exposed loop regions and may affect binding.[74] For murine parvovirus, tissue tropism (for fibroblast or lymphocyte) is determined in the nucleus,[75] suggesting multiple functional effects for the structural as well as non-structural proteins.

With the recent solution at the atomic level of the structure of canine parvovirus, the three-dimensional organization of capsid proteins has been determined in detail[76] (Fig. 26–4). The central structural motif of eight β-pleated sheets is similar to that of many other DNA and RNA viruses of the same size and symmetry. An unusual feature is the large protrusion on the threefold axes. The threefold axis forms a spike on the surface made up of VP2 loop regions that are important as antigen recognition sites for neutralizing antibodies. There are deep canyons about the fivefold axes which may represent, by analogy with other viruses, binding sites for receptors[77]; alternatively, viral attachment protein might be a spike projection or a disordered loop extending from the surface[78] (see below).

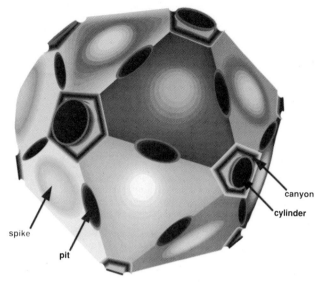

FIGURE 26–4. Schematic of the surface structure of canine parvovirus.

Taxonomy

The classification of Parvoviridae is based on morphology and functional characteristics. The family is divided into three genuses. The insect parvoviruses occupy one genus, called Densovirus. Most vertebrate disease-causing parvoviruses are autonomous parvoviruses (genus Parvovirus), meaning that they replicate in the absence of helper virus. Adeno-associated viruses occupy the third genus, Dependovirus, and require coinfection of target cells with adenovirus or herpesviruses for replication. The adeno-associated viruses infect human tissue culture cells and also human beings, but they appear to be entirely nonpathogenic.[79] Adeno-associated viruses remain latent in the absence of helper virus, and in some cell lines they have the remarkable property of site-specific integration into chromosome 19.[80] Autonomous parvoviruses may have evolved from a defective parvovirus, originally a cellular transposon that functioned by interfering with viral infections.[81] (Perhaps consistent with this theory is the rather strange discovery that human herpesvirus 6 carries a portion of the nonstructural protein gene of adeno-associated virus.[82]) Sequence homology suggests that B19 parvovirus, minute virus of mice, and adeno-associated virus are equally different from each other and presumably separated at about the same evolutionary point in time.[13] B19 parvovirus behaves like an autonomous parvovirus and is now classified in the Parvovirus genus, but its genomic organization and extremely limited tissue host range suggest a close relationship also to the adeno-associated viruses.

B19 PARVOVIRUS

B19 in Cell Culture

B19 parvovirus is extraordinarily trophic for human erythroid cells. Viral replication occurs at high levels only in erythroid progenitor cells,[14] and replicative double-stranded DNA forms can be detected in the bone marrow of infected patients.[83] In tissue culture, B19 parvovirus has been propagated in the erythroid cells of human bone marrow[84] and fetal liver,[85, 86] in cultured cells from a patient with erythroleukemia,[87] and, most recently, in a human megakaryocytoblastoid cell line derived from a patient with leukemia and called UT-7.[88]

Erythroid colony formation by the late erythroid progenitor cell, the colony-forming unit–erythrocyte (CFU-E), and the more primitive erythroid progenitor, the burst-forming unit (BFU-E), is strongly inhibited by virus, whereas myelopoiesis, granulocyte-macrophage colony formation by the CFU-GM progenitor, is unaffected even by high concentrations of virus.[89–91] Susceptibility of marrow cells increases with erythroid differentiation,[92] and in all culture systems virus propagation depends on the presence of erythropoietin. For the UT-7 cell line, adaptation to growth over months in erythropoietin is required before virus can be propagated,[88] suggesting that cell susceptibility to virus is related to the hormone's sustained effects on erythroid differentiation and not to more transient alterations in cell metabolism. In these chronically infected cells, virus is latent, although not integrated into the genome; cell synchronization induces virus replication, transcription, and protein production.[93]

B19 parvovirus is directly cytotoxic to the host cell and induces characteristic light[84] and electron[94] microscopic morphological changes in erythroid precursors. The virus' cytopathic effect is manifest as giant pronormoblasts, first recognized by Owren in 1948 in the bone marrow of patients with transient aplastic crisis[95] and reproduced by tissue culture infection.[84] Giant pronormoblasts are early erythroid cells with a diameter of about 25 to 32 μm, nuclear inclusions or multiple nucleoli, and cytoplasmic vacuolization; these cells are scattered throughout the aspirate smear of infected bone marrow and are striking for their disproportionate size (Fig. 26–5). The number of giant pronormoblasts in a specimen roughly corresponds to the virus content, but giant pronormoblasts themselves may not contain detectable B19 viral capsid proteins. More mature erythroid cells are absent from infected tissue culture or clinical specimens. There may be subtle dysplastic alterations in myeloid and megakaryocytic cells. Infected late erythroid progenitors from tissue culture inoculations show cytopathic ultrastructural changes on electron microscopy, including characteristic margination of chromatin, pseudopod formation, vacuolization, and viral particles in lacunae within the chromatin (Fig. 26–6).

Virus toxicity is the result of expression of the single non-structural protein of the virus. Cotransfection of the non-structural protein gene and a selectable gene (for antibiotic resistance) into certain non-permissive cells abrogates colony formation of these cells in selective medium.[64] On the other hand, cell lines can express the parvovirus capsid proteins without any effect on cell proliferation.[96] Limited expression of the

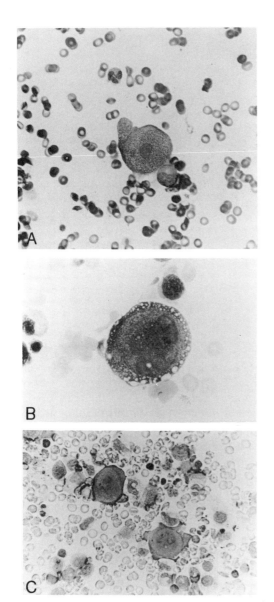

FIGURE 26–5. *A–C*, Giant pronormoblasts in B19 parvovirus–infected bone marrow erythroid progenitor culture.

non-structural protein gene may explain inhibition of myelopoiesis and megakaryocytopoiesis in patients in the absence of virus replication in these cells. In vitro, B19 parvovirus depresses megakaryocytic colony formation; although replication of virus is not detectable by DNA analysis, there is low-level RNA expression in these cells, and mutations within the non-structural protein gene abrogate the inhibitory effect of virus on platelet progenitors.[97]

DNA Structure and Replication

Replication of parvovirus single-stranded DNA is initiated from brief, short double-stranded regions contained in self-annealing, terminal hairpin structures (see Fig. 26–2). For B19 parvovirus DNA, which is 5.6 kb in total length, DNA synthesis proceeds from

the long palindromes to produce high molecular weight intermediates through a rolling hairpin model.[98] Parvovirus DNA replicative intermediates correspond to duplexes equivalent to twofold or fourfold the original single-stranded template.[14] High molecular weight replicative intermediates can be detected directly by Southern analysis (of DNA extracted under low salt conditions) or after restriction enzyme digestion (of DNA extracted with normal salt concentration); asymmetrical fragments are obtained after *Bam*HI digestion, resulting in characteristic doublets on electrophoresis and hybridization (Fig. 26–7). DNA analysis thus allows determination of both presence and propagation of parvovirus in tissue culture and clinical samples.

Late events in parvovirus DNA replication include exonuclease cleavage of the large DNA intermediates, resolution of the hairpin structures, and packaging of the newly synthesized DNA single strands into capsids. Binding of cellular proteins and parvovirus non-structural proteins to DNA is involved in these processes for animal parvoviruses and in adeno-associated virus, but the mechanics of these events have not been determined for B19 parvovirus in erythroid target cells.

RNA Synthesis

Although the scheme of DNA replication of B19 parvovirus is broadly similar to that of other autonomous parvoviruses, the pattern of transcription for B19 parvovirus sets it apart from most of the other Parvoviridae (Fig. 26–8). B19 parvovirus transcription is unusual in several important features: (1) the large number of transcripts, (2) the extent of splicing and the large size of the introns removed, (3) failure to coterminate all transcripts at the far right side of the genome, (4) the use of unusual polyadenylation signals for termination of transcripts in the middle of the genome, and (5) the use of a single strong promoter at the far left side (at map unit 6, thus termed P_6, with an accompanying leader sequence to initiate transcription of all RNA species (Fig. 26–9). Because the TATA box in the middle of the genome does not represent a functional promoter, in either bone marrow targets or transfected cells,[99, 100] B19 parvovirus is denied the use of multiple promoters and enhancer elements to regulate transcript abundance.

Tissue Tropism of B19 Parvovirus

Permissivity, the ability of some cells to support B19 parvovirus propagation, may be tied to messenger RNA (mRNA) processing. In permissive erythroid progenitor cells, the major RNA species that accumulate not surprisingly encode the capsid proteins.[100] The non-structural protein gene transcript, the only unspliced RNA species, is relatively sparse in erythroid cells propagating parvovirus. In contrast, when the

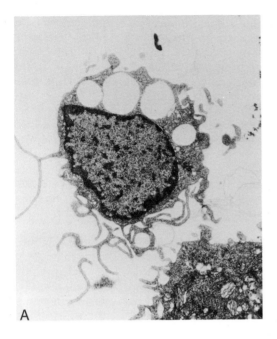

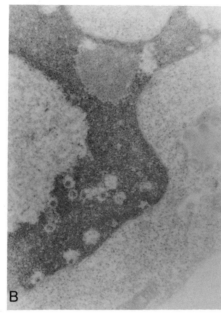

FIGURE 26–6. *A* and *B*, Electron micrograph of an early erythroid precursor infected with B19 parvovirus in vitro, showing margination of nuclear chromatin, vacuolization, and pseudopod formation in the cytoplasm. Virus particles are present in lacunae within the marginated chromatin.

B19 parvovirus genome is transfected into non-permissive cells, the pattern of RNA transcription is altered so that the non-structural protein transcript is overrepresented.[101] A functional "block" in virus transcription in these non-permissive cells can be localized to the middle of the parvovirus genome by RNase protection experiments, and, conversely, removal of about a kilobase of sequence from this region increases read-through transcription from the far right side of the genome[101] (Fig. 26–10). Attenuator sequences located downstream of parvovirus promoters have been demonstrated for rodent parvoviruses,[102] and these results with B19 parvovirus suggest the possibility that during evolution of the virus a functional attenuator for the middle promoter was retained while the promoter activity itself was lost. Unique or abundant cellular transcription factors present in erythroid cells could explain the ability of the virus to propagate in these hematopoietic cells. Predominant transcription of the non-structural protein gene, corresponding to abortive infection, in non-permissive cells would explain virus reduction of megakaryocytic progenitor numbers in vitro, and platelets and white cell levels in infected persons, in the absence of the ability of the virus to productively infect these cells.

The presence of only one promoter and the extensive use of splicing suggest that much of the molecular regulation of B19 parvovirus occurs at the level of RNA. The control of the relative quantities of the minor and major capsid proteins, which are derived

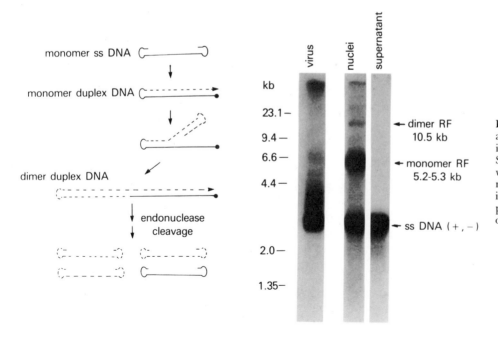

FIGURE 26–7. Restriction enzyme analysis of DNA from erythroid cells infected with B19 parvovirus. On this Southern analysis, high molecular weight replicating monomers and dimers are present in the nuclei but not in the cytosol or in cytoplasm or supernatant of cultures, which contain only virions.

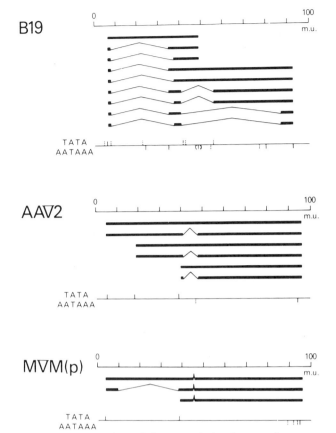

FIGURE 26–8. Comparison of the transcriptional maps of representative parvovirus species. There is no middle promoter in the B19 parvovirus genome.

from overlapping sequences on the right side of the genome, is modulated by multiple upstream AUG codons that are present before the authentic transcription initiation codon; these spurious triplets reduce the efficiency of translation. The upstream AUG codons are removed by splicing of the VP2 RNA, greatly improving translation of the major capsid protein.[103]

Determination of B19 tissue tropism by RNA processing would be a unique mechanism among the parvoviruses. B19 parvovirus might also be blocked at cell entry in non-permissive cells; however, the virus appears to enter megakaryocytes[97] and macrophages (our unpublished data), yet replication does not occur in these cells. Virtually nothing is known about the cell surface receptor for B19 parvovirus or about parvovirus receptors in general. In the case of minute virus of mice, host cell permissivity toward viral strains tropic for fibroblasts or lymphocytes is unrelated to cell entry; replication proceeds to the dimer stage, but no further, in non-permissive cells,[104] implicating an intranuclear factor required for completion of the processing of DNA to infectious monomers. Porcine parvovirus permissivity also is restricted intracellularly, not at the cell membrane.[105] (In contrast, *species* specificity is determined by binding to host cell surface receptors.[74]).

CLINICAL SYNDROMES

Fifth Disease

Acute infection with B19 parvovirus causes the childhood exanthem fifth disease (erythema infectiosum).[33, 106, 107] Children with fifth disease are usually not very ill. The characteristic rash—the "slapped cheek" facial erythema and a lacy, reticular, evanescent maculopapular eruption over the trunk and proximal extremities (Fig. 26–11)—combined with its contagious character, allows recognition of parvovirus infection in the individual patient and of the epidemic in the community. Adults with fifth disease more often suffer joint pains or frank arthritis, alone or in combination with a rash, than do affected children, and symptoms that mimic rheumatoid arthritis[108, 109] or fibromyalgia[110] can occasionally persist for months and even years. Acute parvovirus infection in adults often is asymptomatic or produces only a non-specific flu-like illness.[111]

Transient Aplastic Crisis

This was the first human parvoviral illness identified; the clear clinical relationship between acute virus infection and a specific form of marrow failure led to hematological interest in this pathogen. In persons with underlying hemolysis, acute B19 infection causes transient aplastic crisis, an abrupt cessation of erythropoiesis characterized by reticulocytopenia, absent erythroid precursors in the bone marrow, and precipitous worsening of anemia. The aregenerative quality of anemic crisis was recognized very early from observations on hereditary spherocytosis in large Scandinavian kindreds,[112] later appreciated also for other persons with underlying hemolysis.[113] Owren introduced the term *aplastic crisis* and stressed the relationship of anemic crisis to preceding infection and the temporary quality of red cell failure.[95] Transient aplastic crisis occurs as a unique event in the life of patients with a variety of forms of underlying hemolysis, not only sickle cell disease but also erythrocyte membrane defects, enzymopathies, and thalassemias. Transient aplastic crisis can also occur under conditions of erythroid stress, such as hemorrhage and iron deficiency, and following bone marrow transplantation.[114] In retrospect, parvovirus infection was almost certainly responsible for cases of transient erythropoietic failure that were blamed on kwashiorkor,[115, 116] folic acid deficiency,[117, 118] some drugs (especially immunosuppressive agents), and bacterial infections.[119, 120] It is not accidental that many of the reported cases of aplastic crisis occurred in hospitalized patients, as the virus can be transmitted nosocomially.[121, 122] Parvovirus infection was likely responsible for cases of aplastic anemia (5/6 of which occurred in sickle cell patients and were restricted to anemia only) that once were imputed to glue sniffing.[123]

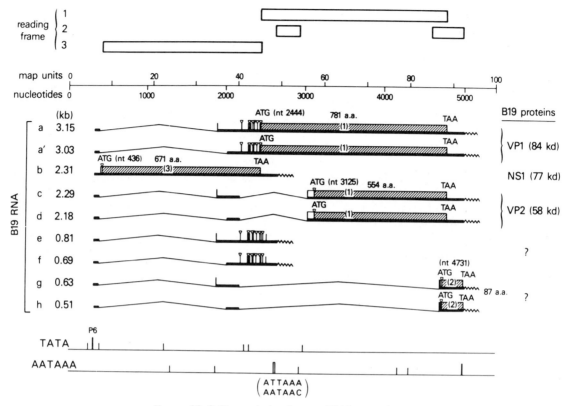

FIGURE 26–9. Transcriptional map of B19 parvovirus.

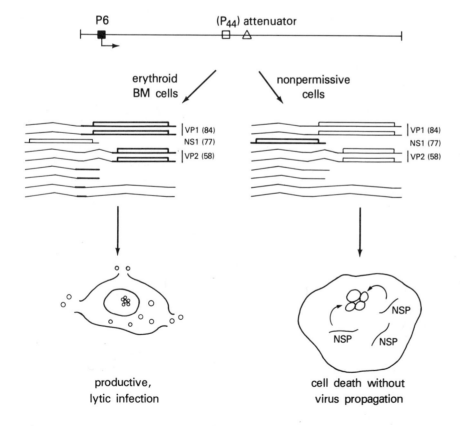

FIGURE 26–10. Transcription is related to permissivity of B19 parvovirus. Permissive cells allow full-length transcription of both the non-structural and the capsid gene RNAs. Capsid RNAs are the predominant RNA species in erythroid cells. Non-permissive cells have a functional transcriptional block in the middle of the genome that results in relative overexpression of non-structural protein RNA and cell death without viral propagation.

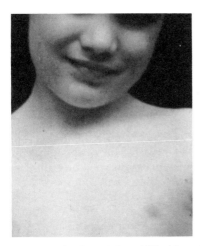

FIGURE 26–11. "Slapped cheek" rash in a child with typical erythema infectiosum. (Courtesy of Dr. M. J. Anderson.)

Although suffering from an ultimately self-limited illness, the patient with an aplastic crisis may be acutely and profoundly ill. Symptoms can include not only the dyspnea and fatigue of worsened anemia but also extreme lassitude, confusion, and congestive heart failure; death can occur. Aplastic crisis may be the first evidence of hereditary spherocytosis in a patient with compensated hemolysis.[124, 125] Transient aplastic crisis,[126–128] as well as experimental parvovirus infection in humans,[129] is often associated with variable degrees of neutropenia and thrombocytopenia. Some cases of idiopathic thrombocytopenic purpura and Henoch-Schönlein purpura[130, 131] have apparently followed acute parvovirus infection. Rarely, transient aplastic crisis may be complicated by bone marrow necrosis.[132, 133] Typical transient aplastic crisis is readily treated by blood transfusion. Atypically, transient pancytopenia[134–136] and a case of typical severe aplastic anemia[137] have been reported to follow acute parvovirus infection. Pancytopenia with hemophagocytosis, which can occur after many different viral infections, also has been noted after parvovirus infection.[138] More tenuously linked are cases of idiopathic thrombocytopenic purpura[131, 139] because both this syndrome and IgM antibody to parvovirus are not uncommon in pediatric populations.

Community-acquired aplastic crisis is almost always due to parvovirus infection.[140–143] B19 parvovirus infection should be the presumptive diagnosis in transient aplastic crisis and should be sought in any patient with anemia due to an abrupt cessation of erythropoiesis. (Transient erythroblastopenia of childhood, temporary failure of red cell production in very young, hematologically normal children, is not associated with B19 parvovirus seroconversion.[144, 145]) Patients with transient aplastic crisis are often viremic at presentation, with concentrations of viral genomes as high as 10^{14}/ml as determined by DNA dot-blot hybridization of serum.[146, 147] IgM antibody appears during the first week of convalescence and is a specific indicator of recent infection.[148] Testing for IgG antibody is not helpful, as IgG to parvovirus is present in about 50 per cent of the adult population, and IgG may not be present in early serum specimens in transient aplastic crisis. Both IgG and IgM antibody to parvovirus can be measured in capture immunoassays.[7]

Hydrops Fetalis Due to B19 Parvovirus

In utero infection is a cause of nonimmune hydrops fetalis, in which death occurs as a result of severe anemia[149, 150] (Fig. 26–12). Hydropic infants born of mothers infected with parvovirus show leukoerythroblastosis, iron deposition in the liver, and viral cytopathic alterations of erythroblasts in the liver; virus has been demonstrated by DNA hybridization and protein immunoblot, mainly in the liver.[151, 152] The risk of a fatal outcome for the fetus is probably greatest if infection occurs during the first two trimesters; although the probability of stillbirth has not been quantitated, it almost certainly is low. In a prospective British study of 190 seropositive women, there was significant excess fetal loss during the second trimester, and the risk of fetal death due to B19 parvovirus was estimated at 9 per cent, with a transplacental transmission rate of 33 per cent.[153] Similar findings came from a retrospective American study.[150] Both series showed that normal infants were born even when the umbilical cord blood tested positive for specific IgM antibody. An increased risk of spontaneous abortion during the first trimester is being investigated in several large epidemiological surveys;

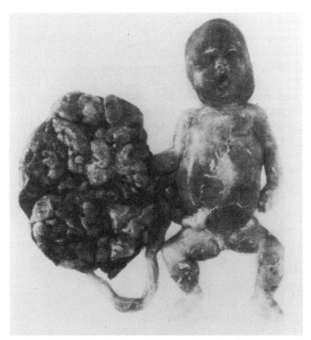

FIGURE 26–12. Hydropic fetus and placenta after intrauterine B19 parvovirus infection. (From Caul, O.E., Usher, J.M., and Burton, A.P.: Intrauterine infection with human parvovirus B19: A light and electron microscopy study. J. Med. Virol. 24:55–66, 1988. Copyright © 1988. Reprinted by permission of Wiley-Liss, a Division of John Wiley and Sons, Inc.)

a preliminary estimate is that about 5 per cent of infected women suffer spontaneous fetal abortions.[154] No congenital physical malformations have been associated with intrauterine parvovirus infection, either prospectively or in retrospective analysis of banked fetal tissue, although viral infection of myocardial cells was shown by in situ hybridization at autopsy of one hydropic infant[155] and immune thrombocytopenia was observed in another viremic newborn.[156]

Although the overall risk of a poor outcome to pregnancy is probably low, the concern of the potentially exposed pregnant mother is not. Parvovirus infection is very contagious. Pregnant women are commonly exposed to fifth disease through other children in the household, at schools and day-care centers, and by contact with nursing and medical personnel. About half of the pregnant population has acquired protective immunity, as determined by assay for IgG antibody to parvovirus. Evidence of seroconversion should be sought in exposed women who entered pregnancy lacking antiparvovirus antibodies. Hydrops can be detected by ultrasonography, and suspected hydrops has been treated with intrauterine red blood cell transfusion.[157] The utility of this type of intervention, or of the administration of commercial immunoglobulins containing antiparvovirus antibodies, needs to be determined.

Congenital Infection

Parvovirus infection of the fetus need not be fatal but may persist after birth.[156, 158] We have studied an infant born with chronic anemia and susceptible to frequent infections; there was a history of maternal exposure to parvovirus during pregnancy and hydrops at birth.[159] Congenital infection is distinctive among parvovirus syndromes in the low level of viral infection: Virus can be detected in the bone marrow by gene amplification but does not circulate. Presumably, infection early in ontogeny allows very efficient suppression of red cell production. Our case terminated fatally, and virus was present in other tissues obtained at autopsy, including thymus, brain, heart, liver, and spleen, suggesting the possibility of parvovirus effects on other organ systems after in utero infection. Exposure of the fetal immune system to virus early in pregnancy would be predicted to result in tolerance to the capsid proteins and absence of an antibody response despite continued virus production.

Persistent Infection

Patients with persistent B19 parvovirus infection have pure red cell aplasia. Persistently infected patients have failed to mount a neutralizing antibody response to the virus, and they lack the immune complex–mediated symptoms of fifth disease—fever, rash, and polyarthralgia/polyarthritis. Persistent parvovirus infection and pure red cell aplasia have been documented in four patient populations: congenital immunodeficiency (Nezelof's syndrome),[83, 160] children with lymphoblastic leukemia in remission on chemotherapy,[161] patients with the acquired immunodeficiency syndrome (AIDS),[162] and recipients of solid organ transplants (our unpublished observations). However, defective antibody production occurs also in other diseases associated with pure red cell aplasia, like chronic lymphocytic leukemia and malignancies treated with cytotoxic drugs, and some of these cases may also represent occult viral infection (as parvovirus infection likely was unrecognized previously in AIDS[163] and leukemia[164]).

The anemia is severe and the patients are dependent on erythrocyte transfusions. There may be associated neutropenia. The bone marrow should contain some giant pronormoblasts, the cytopathic sign of parvovirus infection, although these are infrequent. The anemia may be intermittent, with periods of relapse associated with viremia and remission with spontaneous disappearance of virus from the circulation, possibly due to depletion of the erythroid target cell population. The diagnosis is established by detection of B19 parvovirus genome in the serum, blood, or bone marrow cells by dot-blot hybridization; polymerase chain reaction amplification of viral DNA may be necessary in rare cases.[165] Antibody testing is not useful in the diagnosis of persistent infection (see below). It should be stressed that persistent parvovirus infection may be the dominant manifestation of some inherited immunodeficient states, although multiple immune system defects are apparent once directed testing of T- and B-cell function is performed.

Effective therapy consists of infusion of commercial immunoglobulin preparations, which are a good source of neutralizing antibodies because most of the adult population has been exposed to the virus. One patient with congenital immunodeficiency was cured by a 10-day course followed by intermittent injections until virus disappeared from his serum.[162] Patients with AIDS respond to a 5- to 10-day course but may relapse some months later; they respond to a second course.[162] In an occasional patient, virus may disappear from the circulation yet anemia may persist.[166] Patients with AIDS have had very high virus serum concentrations, orders of magnitude greater than in other patients with chronic parvovirus infection.[162] Measurement of serum virus is helpful in predicting relapse and may assist in determining optimal treatment regimens.

IMMUNE RESPONSE

Normal Response

Both virus-specific IgM and IgG antibodies are made following experimental[129] and natural[148] B19 parvovirus infection. Following intranasal inoculation of volunteers, virus can first be detected at days 5 to 6 and levels peak at days 8 to 9 (Fig. 26–13). Virus is rarely detected in patients with clinical fifth disease because the manifestations are secondary to immune complex formation, and patients therefore present to medical attention after the period of viremia has passed. IgM antibody to virus appears about 10 to 12 days after experimental inoculation; IgM antibody may be present in patients with transient aplastic crisis at the time of reticulocyte nadir and during the subsequent 10 days. IgG antibody appears in normal volunteers about 2 weeks after inoculation; in patients with transient aplastic crisis, IgG is not present at the time of reticulocyte depression but appears and rises rapidly with recovery. IgM antibody may be found in serum samples for several months after exposure.[24] IgG presumably persists for life and protects against a second infection. IgA antibodies to B19 parvovirus can also be detected and presumably play a role in protection against infection by the natural naso-oropharyngeal route.[167] In acute infection, the period of viremia is brief, usually 1 to 3 days, and virus titers can be extremely high (10^{11} to 10^{14} genome copies/ml).[146, 147] In persistent infection, virus can be demonstrated in serum samples obtained months apart; the viral titer is often lower (10^6 genome copies/ml), although AIDS patients may have serum concentrations as high as in an acute infection.

The pattern of disease that follows parvovirus infection is the result of balance between virus, marrow target cell, and the immune response (Fig. 26–14). Bone marrow depression in parvovirus infection occurs during the early viremic phase and under normal conditions is terminated by a neutralizing antibody response. The immune response produces the clinical manifestations of rash and joint pains, which occur during the period of antibody formation and are immune complex mediated (fifth disease symptoms can be precipitated by treatment of persistent infection with immunoglobulin). In patients with hyperactive erythropoiesis, larger amounts of virus may be produced and the immune response may be weak, perhaps resulting in relatively greater quantities of antigen to antibody and little immune complex formation (rash and joint pains are very rare in patients with transient aplastic crisis[128]). In both persistent infection in children and adults and in utero infection, failure to mount a neutralizing antibody response allows parvovirus to persist and cause chronic anemia.[165]

The humoral response appears to be dominant in controlling human parvovirus infection: Not only does normal recovery from infection correlate with the appearance of circulating specific antivirus antibody, but also administration of commercial immunoglobulins can cure or ameliorate persistent parvovirus infection in immunodeficient patients. Although patients with persistent parvovirus infection suffer T-cell as well as B-cell immune deficits, and a cellular component to the normal immune response to parvovirus must exist, attempts to measure lymphocyte proliferation in response to free parvovirus antigen have been unsuccessful.[168] A cellular immune response has been easier to demonstrate for other parvoviruses. T-cell responses are important in limiting rat parvovirus infection[169]; delayed hypersensitivity to canine virus can be passively transferred by lymphocytes exposed to virus in vitro, and T cells proliferate and secrete

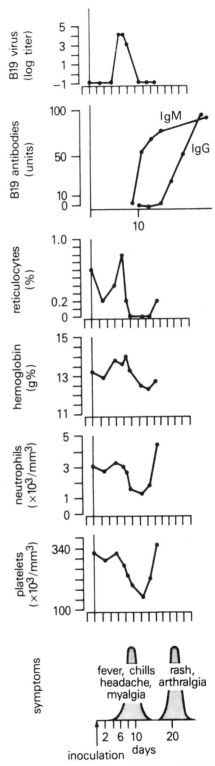

FIGURE 26–13. Virological, immunological, and clinical course after B19 infection in a normal host. (Adapted from Anderson, M. J., Higgins, P. G., Davis, L. R., et al.: Experimental parvoviral infection in humans. J. Infect. Dis. 152:251–265, 1985; with permission of the University of Chicago Press.)

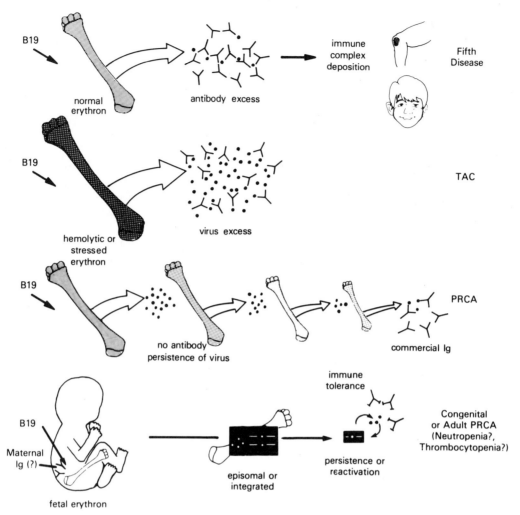

FIGURE 26–14. Pathogenesis of human diseases caused by B19 parvovirus. TAC = transient aplastic crisis; PRCA = pure red cell aplasia.

interleukin-2 in response to soluble viral antigen and T-cell epitopes map to the major capsid protein[170]; for Aleutian disease virus, lymphocyte responses probably represent pathological phenomena.[171, 172] Finally, many animal parvoviruses infect lymphocytes in vivo and replicate in lymphocytes and macrophages in vitro, including minute virus of mice,[173] porcine parvovirus,[174] feline panleukopenia virus,[175] and Aleutian disease virus.[176]

B-Cell Neutralizing Epitopes

Several regions containing neutralizing epitopes have been localized to linear sequences of B19 parvovirus: one region at the amino-terminus of VP2 at amino acids 38 to 87[177] and six others distributed within the carboxyl-terminal half of VP2 (amino acids 253 to 272, 309 to 330, 328 to 344, 359 to 382, 449 to 468, and 491 to 515[178, 179]). Neutralizing epitopes are also found in the unique region of VP1.[180] Some of the neutralizing epitopes of VP2, by analogy with the three-dimensional structure of canine parvovirus,[76]

would correspond to external loops of the protein present on the virus surface as major protrusions or spikes[180] (Fig. 26–15). Anti-VP2 antibodies directed against sequences in the β barrel central core structure are produced in animals immunized with VP2-only–containing empty capsids, but these antibodies fail to neutralize virus activity.[15, 181] Addition of VP1 to the capsid has two effects: It allows presentation of the spike to the immune system and adds its own intrinsic neutralizing sequences. Antisera raised to the unique region of VP1, 227 amino acids at the amino-terminus, do precipitate empty capsids and virions, indicating that the unique region is expressed on the virus surface, and these antibodies also neutralize virus activity.[180] Both anti-VP2 and anti-VP1 specificities are present in normal human convalescent antisera, and sera that predominate in either one or the other specificity both effectively neutralize virus; however, VP1 is the major antigen recognized on immunoblot by late convalescent phase antiserum or in commercial immunoglobulin preparations.[168]

Only a limited number of linear epitopes have been detected, but the majority of monoclonal antibodies

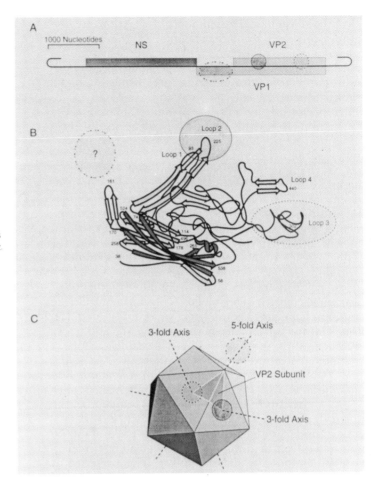

FIGURE 26–15. Some neutralizing epitopes of B19 parvovirus superimposed after alignment by homology on the atomic structure of canine parvovirus.

that neutralize B19 parvovirus do not recognize peptide sequences within the capsid proteins and presumably bind to conformationally determined epitopes.[177] The structure of B19 parvovirus may be more dynamic than suggested by the static picture presented in x-ray crystallography. Although VP2 contains neutralizing epitopes, these are not presented to the immune system in VP2-only empty capsids,[15] suggesting that the conformation of some VP2 determinants, particularly those on the prominent spike, is altered by insertion of one or two VP1 molecules per 60 protein subunit capsids.[181] A further alteration probably occurs with insertion of DNA into empty capsids containing both proteins, as many monoclonal antibodies raised to virions and screened by ELISA fail to recognize VP1 plus VP2 empty capsids in the same test (Yoshimoto, Rosenfeld, Kennedy, and Young, unpublished data).

Antibody Defect in Persistent Infection

Persistent B19 parvovirus infection is the result of failure to produce effective neutralizing antibodies by the immunosuppressed host. Antibodies to parvovirus, as determined in immunoassays or ELISA, are not present in most patients, but a pattern of antibody response suggestive of early infection (IgM antibody

and IgG antibody directed to the major capsid protein) may be found in patients with congenital immunodeficiency.[168] A poor reaction on immunoblot testing is a consistent finding and correlates with poor neutralizing activity for the virus in erythroid colony assays.[168] These results suggest that the linear epitopes detected by immunoblotting are functionally very important, and the clinical findings in persistent infection are analogous to animal data showing dependence of a neutralizing antibody response on presentation of specific epitopes, particularly from the amino-terminal region of the minor capsid protein. Perhaps because of the limited epitopes presented to the immune system by B19 parvovirus, the congenital immunodeficiency states associated with persistent infection may be clinically subtle, with susceptibility restricted largely to parvovirus.

Passive Immunity and Vaccine Development

Antibodies play a dominant role in the normal immune response to parvovirus, and antibodies are protective in both passive and active immunizations. Convalescent antiserum can protect puppies against canine parvovirus infection,[182] and commercial immunoglobulin from normal donors can cure or ameliorate persistent B19 parvovirus infection in immunosuppressed human patients.[160, 162] Human convalescent phase antisera[168] and commercial immunoglobulin preparations[183] contain neutralizing antibodies to parvovirus, as assessed in vitro using erythroid colony systems.

Parvovirus infection can be prevented in animals by vaccination. A human vaccine would be useful, at a minimum, to prevent transient aplastic crisis in persons with hemolysis and to protect the fetus in seronegative pregnant women. Universal vaccination might be more efficient and would eliminate the risk of chronic red cell aplasia with acquired immunosuppression as well as the wide range of parvovirus-related illnesses, the full spectrum of which is unknown. Effective vaccines have been produced for animals using attenuated or fixed virus preparations, including feline,[184] canine,[43] and porcine[185] parvoviruses. Antisera raised against peptide fragments of canine parvovirus, determined to contain neutralizing epitopes, have also been protective in a dog model.[186] Prospects for a B19 parvovirus vaccine are also good, although the immunogen almost certainly will be a recombinant capsid rather than attenuated or killed virus, owing to the difficulty of propagating B19 parvovirus in tissue culture and the potential danger of inadvertently modifying its tissue range for the worse by in vitro selection. Recombinant B19 parvovirus capsids produced in baculovirus are suitable to induce neutralizing antibodies in inoculated animals,[15] even in the absence of adjuvant.[187] The presence of VP1 protein in the capsid immunogen appears critical for the production of antibodies that neutralize virus activity in vitro: Capsids with supernormal VP1 content are more efficient in inducing neutralizing activity in immunized animals, and neutralization correlates with anti-VP1 reactivity on immunoblot.[187]

The basic biology of B19 parvovirus is well understood and directly relevant to human diseases caused by this agent. B19 parvovirus is cytotoxic to human erythroid target cells, but serious disease results only if the host's erythroid marrow is stressed or immunity is inadequate. The antibody response limits virus propagation in the human host, and a very limited number of viral epitopes presented to the immune system may allow the virus to elude some genetically deficient immune systems. Development of recombinant empty capsids should provide a basis for vaccination and prevention of parvovirus disease.

PROSPECTS

Outstanding and interesting questions about the B19 virus remain. What is the exact molecular basis of altered transcription in erythroid cells and its relation to tissue tropism? What is the mechanism of cell death induced by non-structural protein? What is the cell surface receptor for parvovirus? How is virus uncoated? Does virus persist in non-erythroid cells? Does the virus kill cells outside the bone marrow? The history of virology suggests that the answers to these questions will have implications not only for B19 parvovirus but for normal cell function as well.

REFERENCES

1. Fields, B. N., Knipe, D. M., Chanoek, R. M., Hirsch, M. S., Melnick, J. L., Monath, T. P., and Rolzman, B. (eds.): Virology. New York, Raven Press, 1990.
2. Notleins, A. L., and Oldstone, M. B. A. (eds.): Concepts in Viral Pathogenesis. New York, Springer-Verlag, 1984.
3. Notleins, A. L., and Oldstone, M. B. A. (eds.): Concepts in Viral Pathogenesis II. New York, Springer-Verlag, 1986.
4. Notleins, A. L., and Oldstone, M. B. A. (eds.): Concepts in Viral Pathogenesis III. New York, Springer-Verlag, 1989.
5. Young, N. S. (ed.): Viruses and the Bone Marrow. New York, Marcel Dekker, 1993.
6. Cossart, Y. E., Field, A. M., Cant, B., et al.: Parvovirus-like particles in human sera. Lancet 1:72, 1975.
7. Cohen, B. J., Mortimer, P. P., and Pereira, M. S.: Diagnostic assays with monoclonal antibodies for the human serum parvovirus-like virus (SPLV). J. Hyg. 91:113, 1983.
8. Pattison, J. R., Jones, S. E., Hodgson, J., et al.: Parvovirus infections and hypoplastic crisis in sickle cell anemia. Lancet 1:664, 1981.
9. Anderson, M. J., Jones, S. E., Fisher-Hoch, S. P., Lewis, E., Hall, S. M., Bartlett, C. LR., Cohen, B. J., Mortimer, P. P., and Pereira, M. S.: Human parvovirus, the cause of erythema infectiosum (fifth disease)? Lancet 1:1378, 1983.
10. Clewley, J. P.: Biochemical characterization of a human parvovirus. J. Gen. Virol. 65:241, 1984.
11. Summers, J., Jones, S. E., and Anderson, M. J.: Characterization of the genome of the agent of erythrocyte aplasia permits its classification as a human parvovirus. J. Gen. Virol. 64:2527, 1983.
12. Cotmore, S. F., and Tattersall, P.: Characterization and molecular cloning of a human parvovirus genome. Science 226:1161, 1984.
13. Shade, R. O., Blundell, M. C., Cotmore, S. F., Tattersall, P., and Astell, C. R.: Nucleotide sequence and genome organization of human parvovirus B19 isolated from the serum of a child during aplastic crisis. J. Virol. 58:921, 1986.
14. Ozawa, K., Kurtzman, G., and Young, N. S.: Replication of the B19 parvovirus in human bone marrow cultures. Science 233:883, 1986.
15. Kajigaya, S., Fujii, H., Field, A. M., Rosenfeld, S., Anderson, L. J., Shimada, T., and Young, N. S.: Self-assembled B19 parvovirus capsids, produced in a baculovirus system, are antigenically and immunologically similar to native virions. Proc. Natl. Acad. Sci. USA 88:4646, 1991.
16. Berns, K. I.: Parvoviridae and their replication. In Fields, B. M., et al. (eds.): Virology. New York, Raven Press, 1990, pp. 1743–1764.
17. Pattison, J.R.: Parvoviruses. In Fields, B. M., et al. (eds.): Virology. New York, Raven Press, 1990, pp. 1765–1786.
18. Berns, K. I. (ed.): The Parvoviruses. New York, Plenum, 1984.
19. Pattison, J. R. (ed.): Parvoviruses and Human Disease. Boca Raton, CRC Press, 1988.
20. Anderson, L. J.: Human parvoviruses. J. Infect. Dis. 161:603, 1990.
21. Anderson, L. J., and Torok, T. J.: The clinical spectrum of human parvovirus B19 infections. Curr. Clin. Top. Infect. Dis. 11:267, 1991.
22. Anderson, M. J.: Paroviruses as agents of human disease. Prog. Med. Virol. 34:55, 1987.
23. Young, N.: Hematologic and hematopoietic consequences of B19 parvovirus infection. Semin. Hematol. 25:159, 1988.
24. Anderson, L. J., Tsou, C., Parker, R. A., Chorba, T. L., Wulff, H., Tattersall, P., and Mortimer, P. P.: Detection of antibodies and antigens of human parvovirus B19 by enzyme-linked immunosorbent assay. J. Clin. Microbiol. 24:522, 1986.
25. Anderson, M. J., Higgins, P. G., Davis, L. R., et al.: Experi-

mental parvoviral infection in humans. J. Infect. Dis. 152:257, 1985.

26. Yaegashi, N., Shiraishi, H., Tada, K., Yajima, A., and Sugamura, K.: Enzyme-linked immunosorbent assay for IgG and IgM antibodies against human parvovirus B19: Use of monoclonal antibodies and viral antigen propagated in vitro. J. Virol. Methods 26:171, 1989.

27. Cohen, B. J., and Buckley, M. M.: The prevalence of antibody to human parvovirus B19 in England and Wales. J. Med. Microbiol. 25:151, 1988.

28. Koch, W. C., and Adler, S. P.: Human parvovirus B19 infections in women of childbearing age and within families. Pediatr. Infect. Dis. J. 8:83, 1989.

29. Nascimento, J. P., Buckley, M. M., Brown, K. E., and Cohen, B. J.: The prevalence of antibody to human parvovirus B19 in Rio de Janeiro, Brazil. Rev. Inst. Med. Trop. Sao Paulo 32:41, 1990.

30. Nunoue, T., Okochi, K., Mortimer, P. P., and Cohen, B. J.: Human parvovirus (B19) and erythema infectiosum. J. Pediatr. 107:38, 1985.

31. de Freitas, R. B., Wong, D., Boswell, F., de Miranda, M. F., Linhares, A. C., Shirley, J., and Desselberger, U.: Prevalence of human parvovirus (B19) and rubellavirus infections in urban and remote rural areas in northern Brazil. J. Med. Virol. 32:203, 1990.

32. Schwarz, L., Gurtler, L. G., Zoulek, G., Deinhardt, F., and Roggendorf, M.: Seroprevalence of human parvovirus B19 infection. Int. J. Med. Microbiol. 271:231, 1989.

33. Chorba, T. L., Coccia, P., Holman, R. C., Tattersall, P., Anderson, L. J., Sudman, J., Young, N. S., Kurczynski, E., Saarinen, U. M., Moir, R., Lawrence, D. N., Jason, J. M., and Evatt, B.: Role of parvovirus B19 in aplastic crisis and erythema infectiosum (fifth disease). J. Infect. Dis. 154:383, 1986.

34. Cohen, B. J., Field, A. M., Gudnadottir, S., Beard, S., and Barbara, J. A.: Blood donor screening for parvovirus B19. J. Virol. Methods 30:223, 1990.

35. Plummer, A. F., Hammond, W. G., and Forward, K.: An erythema infectiosum–like illness caused by human parvovirus infection. N. Engl. J. Med. 313:74, 1985.

36. Gillespie, S. M., Cartter, M. L., Asch, S., Rokos, J. B., Gary, G. W., Tsou, C. J., Hall, D. B., Anderson, L. J., and Hurwitz, E. S.: Occupational risk of human parvovirus B19 infection for school and day-care personnel during an outbreak of erythema infectiosum. J.A.M.A. 263:2061, 1990.

37. Mortimer, P. P., Luban, N. L. C., Kelleher, J. F., and Cohen, B. J.: Transmission of serum parvovirus-like virus by clotting-factor concentrates. Lancet 2:482, 1983.

38. Bartolomei Corsi, O., Azzi, A., Morfini, M., Fanci, R., and Rossi Ferrini, P.: Human parvovirus infection in hemophiliacs first infused with treated clotting factor concentrates. J. Med. Virol. 25:165, 1988.

39. Williams, M. D., Beddall, A. C., Pasi, K. J., Mortimer, P. P., and Hill, F. G. H.: Transmission of human parvovirus B19 by coagulation factor concentrates. Vox Sang. 58:177, 1990.

40. Bell, L. M., Naides, S. J., Stoffman, P., Hodinka, R. L., and Plotkin, S. A.: Human parvovirus B19 infection among hospital staff members after contact with infected patients. N. Engl. J. Med. 321:485, 1989.

41. Kurtzman, G.: Feline panleucopenia virus. In Young, N.S. (ed.): Viruses and the Bone Marrow. New York, Marcel Dekker, 1993, p. 119.

42. Kurtzman, G. J., Platanias, L., Lustig, L., Frickhofen, N., and Young, N. S.: Feline parvovirus propagates in cat bone marrow cultures and inhibits hematopoietic colony formation in vitro. Blood 74:71, 1989.

43. Parrish, C. R.: Emergence, natural history, and variation of canine, mink, and feline parvoviruses. Adv. Virus Res. 38:403, 1990.

44. Kilham, L., and Margolis, G.: Viral etiology of spontaneous ataxia of cats. Am. J. Pathol. 48:991, 1966.

45. Macartney, L., McCandlish, I. A. P., Thompson, H., and Cornwell, J. J. C.: Canine parvovirus enteritis 1: Clinical,

haematological and pathological features of experimental infection. Vet. Rec. 115:201, 1984.

46. Segovia, J. C., Real, A., Bueren, J. A., and Almendral, J. M.: In vitro myelosuppressive effects of the parvovirus minute virus of mice (MVMi) on hematopoietic stem and committed progenitor cells. Blood 77:980, 1991.

47. Mori, S., Wolfinbarger, J. B., Miyazawa, M., and Bloom, M. E.: Replication of Aleutian mink disease parvovirus in lymphoid tissues of adult mink: Involvement of follicular dendritic cells and macrophages. J. Virol. 65:952, 1991.

48. Goryo, M., Sugimura, H., Matsumoto, S., Umemura, T., and Itakura, C.: Isolation of an agent inducing chicken anemia. Avian Pathol. 14:483, 1985.

49. Berns, K. I. Parvovirus replication. Microbiol. Rev. 54:316, 1990.

50. Tattersall, P., and Cotmore, S. F.: Reproduction of autonomous parvovirus DNA. In Tijssen, P., (ed.): Handbook of Parvoviruses, Vol. 1. Boca Raton, CRC Press, 1990, pp. 123–140.

51. McLaughlin, S. K., Collis, P., Hermonat, P. L., and Muzyczka, N.: Adeno-associated virus general transduction vectors: Analysis of proviral structures. J. Virol. 62:1963, 1988.

52. Srivastava, C. H., Samulski, R. J., Lu, L., Larsen, S. H., and Srivastava, A.: Construction of a recombinant human parvovirus B19: Adeno-associated virus 2 (AAV) DNA inverted terminal repeats are functional in an AAV-B19 hybrid virus. Proc. Natl. Acad. Sci. USA 86:8078, 1989.

53. Deiss, V., Tratschin, J.-D., Weitz, M., and Siegl, G.: Cloning of the human parvovirus B19 genome and structural analysis of its palindromic termini. Virology 175:247, 1990.

54. Cotmore, S. F., and Tattersall, P.: The NS-1 polypeptide of minute virus of mice is covalently attached to the 5′ termini of duplex replicative-form DNA and progeny single strands. J. Virol. 62:851, 1988.

55. Im, D.S., and Muzyczka, N.: The AAV origin binding protein Rep68 is an ATP-dependent site-specific endonuclease with DNA helicase activity. Cell 61:447, 1990.

56. Tratschin, J.-D., Tal, J., and Carter, B. J.: Negative and positive regulation in trans of gene expression from adeno-associated virus vectors in mammalian cells by a viral rep gene product. Mol. Cell. Biol. 6:2884, 1986.

57. Synder, R. O., Im, D. S., and Muzyczka, N.: Evidence for covalent attachment of the adeno-associated virus (AAV) rep protein to the ends of the AAV genome. J. Virol. 64:6204, 1990.

58. Doerig, C., Hirt, B., Antonietti, J.-P., and Beard, P.: Nonstructural protein of parvoviruses B19 and minute virus of mice controls transcription. J. Virol. 64:387, 1990.

59. Rhode, S. L.: trans-Activation of parvovirus P38 promoter by the 76k noncapsid protein. J. Virol. 55:886, 1985.

60. Hanson, N. D., and Rhode, S. L. III: Parvovirus NS1 stimulates P4 expression by interaction with the terminal repeats and through DNA amplification. J. Virol. 65:4325, 1991.

61. Rhode, S. L.: Both excision and replication of cloned autonomous parvovirus DNA require the NS1 (rep) protein. Virology 63:4249, 1989.

62. Cotmore, S. F., and Tattersall, P.: A genome-linked copy of the NS-1 polypeptide is located on the outside of infectious parvovirus particles. J. Virol. 63:3902, 1989.

63. Caillet-Fauquet, P., Perros, M., Branderburger, A., Spegelaere, P., and Rommelaere, J.: Programmed killing of human cells by means of an inducible clone of parvoviral genes encoding non-structural proteins. EMBO J. 9:2989, 1990.

64. Ozawa, K., Ayub, J., Kajigaya, S., Shimada, T., and Young, N.S.: The gene encoding the nonstructural protein of B19 (human) parvovirus may be lethal in transfected cells. J. Virol. 62:2884, 1988.

65. Labow, M. A., Graf, L. H., Jr., and Berns, K. I.: Adeno-associated virus gene expression inhibits celluar transformation by heterologous genes. Mol. Cell. Biol. 7:1320, 1987.

66. Khleif, S. N., Myers, T., Carter, B. J., and Trempe, J. P.: Inhibition of cellular transformation by the adeno-associated virus rep gene. Virology 181:738, 1991.

67. Rommelaere, J., and Tattersall, P.: Oncosuppression by par-

voviruses. *In* Tijssen, P. (ed.): Handbook of Parvoviruses, Vol. 2. Boca Raton, CRC Press, 1990, pp. 41–57.

68. Li, X., and Rhode S. L. III: Mutation of lysine 405 to serine in the parvovirus H-1 NS1 abolishes its functions for viral DNA replication, late promoter trans activation, and cytotoxicity. J. Virol. 64:4654, 1990.

69. Shimomura, S., Wong, S., Komatsu, N., Kajigaya, S., and Young, N. S.: Early and late gene expression in UT-7 cells infected with B19 parvovirus. Virology (in press).

70. Clemens, K. E., and Pintel, D. J.: The two transcriptional units of the autonomous parvovirus minute virus of mice are transcribed in a temporal order. J. Virol. 62:1448, 1988.

71. Antonietti, J. P., Shali, R., Beard, P., and Hirt, B.: Characterization of the cell type-specific determinant in the genome of minute virus of mice. J. Virol. 62:552, 1988.

72. Ball-Goodrich, L. J., Moir, R. D., and Tattersall, P.: Parvoviral target cell specificity: Acquisition of fibrotropism by a mutant of the lymphotropic strain of minute virus of mice involves multiple amino acid substitutions within the capsid. Virology 184:175, 1991.

73. Parrish, C. R., Aquadro, C. F., and Carmichael, L. E.: Canine host range and a specific epitope map along with variant sequences in the capsid protein gene of canine parvovirus and related feline, mink and raccoon parvoviruses. Virology 166:293, 1988.

74. Parrish, C. R.: Mapping specific functions in the capsid structure of canine parvovirus and feline panleukopenia virus using infectious plasmid clones. Virology 183:195, 1991.

75. Spalholz, B. A., and Tattersall, P.: Interaction of minute virus of mice with differentiated cells: Strain-dependent target cell specificity is mediated by intracellular factors. J. Virol. 46:937, 1983.

76. Tsao, J., Chapman, M. S., Agbandje, M., Keller, W., Smith, K., Wu, H., Luo, M., Smith, T. J., Rossmann, M. G., Compans, R. W., and Parrish. C. R.: The three-dimensional structure of canine parvovirus and its functional implications. Science 251:1456, 1991.

77. Rossmann, M. G.: The canyon hypothesis. Viral Immunol. 2:143, 1989.

78. Bass, D. M., and Greenberg, H. B.: Strategies for the identification of icosahedral virus receptors. J. Clin. Invest. 89:3, 1992.

79. Berns, K. I., and Bohenzky, R. A.: Adeno-associated viruses: An update. Adv. Virus Res. 32:243, 1987.

80. Kotin, R. M., Siniscalco, M., Samulski, R. J., Zhu, X., Hunter, L., Laughlin, C. A., McLaughlin, S., Muzyczka, N., Rocchi, M., and Berns, K. I.: Site-specific integration by adeno-associated virus. Proc. Natl. Acad. Sci. USA 87:2211, 1990.

81. Fisher, R. E., and Mayor, H. D.: The evolution of defective and autonomous parvoviruses. J. Theor. Biol. 149:429, 1991.

82. Thomson, B. J., Efstathiou, S., and Honess, R. W.: Acquisition of the human adeno-associated virus type-2 rep gene by human herpesvirus type-6. Nature 351:78, 1991.

83. Kurtzman, G., Ozawa, K., Hanson, G. R., Cohen, B., Oseas, R., and Young, N.: Chronic bone marrow failure due to persistent B19 parvovirus infection. N. Engl. J. Med. 317:287, 1987.

84. Ozawa, K., Kurtzman, G., and Young, N.: Productive infection by B19 parvovirus of human erythroid bone marrow cells in vitro. Blood 70:384, 1987.

85. Brown, K. E., Mori, J., Cohen, B. J., and Field, A. M.: In vitro propagation of parvovirus B19 in primary foetal liver cultures. J. Gen. Virol. 72(Pt 3):741, 1991.

86. Yaegashi, N., Shiraishi, H., Takeshita, T., Nakamura, M., Yajima, A., and Sugamura, K.: Propagation of human parvovirus B19 in primary culture of erythroid lineage cells derived from fetal liver. J. Virol. 63:2422, 1989.

87. Takahashi, T., Ozawa, K., Mitani, K., Miyazono, K., Asano, S., and Takaku, F.: B19 parvovirus replicates in erythroid leukemic cells in vitro [letter]. J. Infect. Dis. 160:548, 1989.

88. Shimomura, S., Komatsu, N., Frickhofen, N., Anderson, S., Kajigaya, S., and Young, N.S.: First continuous propagation of B19 parvovirus in a cell line. Blood 79:18, 1992.

89. Mortimer, P. P., Humphries, R K., Moore, J. G., Purcell, R. H., and Young, N. S.: A human parvovirus-like virus inhibits hematopoietic colony formation in vitro. Nature 302:426, 1983.

90. Srivastava, A., and Lu, L.: Replication of B19 parvovirus in highly enriched hematopoietic progenitor cells from normal human bone marrow. J. Virol. 62:3059, 1988.

91. Takahashi, M., Koike, T., and Moriyama, Y.: Inhibition of erythropoiesis by human parvovirus-containing serum from a patient with hereditary spherocytosis in aplastic crisis. Scand. J. Haematol. 37:118, 1986.

92. Takahashi, T., Ozawa, K., Takahashi, K., Asano, S., and Takaku, F.: Susceptibility of human erythropoietic cells to B19 parvovirus in vitro increases with differentiation. Blood 75:603, 1990.

93. Joss, D. V., Barrett, A. J., Kendra, J. R., Lucas, C. F., and Desai, S.: Hypertension and convulsions in children receiving cyclosporin A [letter]. Lancet 1:906, 1982.

94. Young, N. S., Harrison, M., Moore, J. G., Mortimer, P. P., and Humphries, R.K.: Direct demonstration of the human parvovirus in erythroid progenitor cells infected in vitro. J. Clin. Invest. 74:2024, 1984.

95. Owren, P. A.: Congenital hemolytic jaundice: The pathogenesis of the "hemolytic crisis." Blood 3:231, 1948.

96. Kajigaya, S., Shimada, T., Fujita, S., and Young, N. S.: A genetically engineered cell line that produces empty capsids of B19 (human) parvovirus. Proc. Natl. Acad. Sci. USA 86:7601, 1989.

97. Srivastava, A., Bruno, E., Briddell, R., Cooper, R., Srivastava, C., van Besien, K., and Hoffman, R.: Parvovirus B19-induced perturbation of human megakaryocytopoiesis in vitro. Blood 76:1997, 1990.

98. Astell, C. R.: Terminal hairpins of parvovirus genomes and their role in DNA replication. *In* Tijssen, P. (ed.): Handbook of Parvoviruses, Vol. 1. Boca Raton, CRC Press, 1990, pp. 59–79.

99. Liu, J. M., Fujii, H., Green, S. W., Komatsu, N., Young, N. S., and Shimada, T.: Indiscriminate activity from the B19 parvovirus P6 promoter in nonpermissive cells. Virology 182:361, 1991.

100. Ozawa, K., Ayub, J., Yu-Shu, H., Kurtzman, G., Shimada, T., and Young, N.: Novel transcription map for the B19 (human) pathogenic parvovirus. J. Virol. 61:2395, 1987.

101. Liu, J., Green, S., Shimada, T., and Young, N. S.: A block in full-length transcript maturation in cells nonpermissive for B19 parvovirus. J. Virol. 66:4686, 1992.

102. Krauskopf, A., Resnekov, O., and Aloni, Y.: A cis downstream element participates in regulation of in vitro transcription initiation from the P38 promoter of minute virus to mice. J. Virol. 64:354, 1990.

103. Ozawa, K., Ayub, J., and Young, N. S.: Translational regulation of B19 parvovirus capsid protein production by multiple upstream AUG triplets. J. Biol. Chem. 263:10922, 1988.

104. Spalholz, B. A., and Tattersall, P.: Interaction of minute virus of mice with differentiated cells: Strain-dependent target cell specificity is mediated by intracellular factors. J. Virol. 46:937, 1983.

105. Oraveerakul, K., Choi, C.-S., and Molitor, T. W.: Restriction of porcine parvovirus replication in nonpermissive cells. J. Virol. 66:715, 1992.

106. Ager, E. A., Chin, T. D. Y., and Poland, J. D.: Epidemic erythema infectiosum. N. Engl. J. Med. 275:1326, 1966.

107. Balfour H. H., Jr.: Erythema infectiosum (fifth disease): Clinical review and description of 91 cases seen in an epidemic. Clin. Pediatr. 8:721, 1969.

108. Reid, D. M., Reid, T. M. S., Rennie, J. A. N., Brown, T., and Eastmond, C. J.: Human parvovirus-associated arthritis: A clinical and laboratory description. Lancet 1:422, 1985.

109. White, D. G., Woolf, A. D., Mortimer, P. P., Cohen, B. J., Blake, D. R., and Bacon, P. A.: Human parvovirus arthropathy. Lancet 1:419, 1985.

110. Leventhal, L. J., Naides, S. J., and Freundlich, B.: Fibromyalgia and parvovirus infection. Arthritis Rheum. 34:1319, 1991.

111. Woolf, A. D., Campion, G. V., Chishick, A., Wise, S., Cohen,

B. J., Klouda, P. T., Caul, O., and Dieppe, P. A.: Clinical manifestation of human parvovirus B19 in adults. Arch. Intern. Med. 149:1153, 1989.

112. Lyngar, E.: Samtidig optreden av anemisk kriser hos 3 barn i en familie med hemolytisk ikterus. Nord. Med. 14:1246, 1942.

113. Gasser, C.: Aplasia of erythropoiesis. Acute and chronic erythroblastopenias or pure (red cell) aplastic anaemias in childhood. Pediatr. Clin. N. Am. 4:445, 1987.

114. Weiland, H. T., Salimans, M. M. M., Fibbe, W. E., Kluin, P. M., and Cohen, B. J.: Prolonged parvovirus B19 infection with severe anaemia in a bone marrow transplant recipient [letter]. Br. J. Haematol. 710:300, 1989.

115. Kho, L.-K.: Erythroblastopenia with giant pro-erythroblasts in kwashiorkor. Blood 12:171, 1957.

116. Zucker, J. M., Tchernia, G., Vuylsteke, P., Becart-Michael, R., Giorgi, R., and Blot, J.: Acute and transitory erythroblastopenia in kwashiorkor under treatment. Nouv. Rev. Fr. Hematol. Blood Cells 11:131, 1971.

117. Alperin, J. B.: Folic acid deficiency complicating sickle cell anemia. Arch. Intern. Med. 120:398, 1967.

118. Pierce, L. E., and Rath, C. E.: Evidence for folic acid deficiency in the genesis of anemic sickle cell crisis. Blood 20:19, 1962.

119. Choremis, C. B., Megas, H. A., Liaromati, A. A., and Michael, S. C.: Aplastic crisis in the course of infectious diseases. Report of 10 cases. Helv. Paediatr. Acta 2:134, 1961.

120. Jootar, S., Srichaikul, R., and Atichartakaran, V.: Pure red cell aplasia in Thailand: Report of twenty four cases. Southeast Asian J. Trop. Med. Pub. Health 16:291, 1985.

121. Evans, J. P. M., Rossiter, M. A., Kumaran, T. O., Marsh, G. W., and Mortimer, P. P.: Human parvovirus aplasia: Case due to cross infection in a ward [letter]. Br. Med. J. 288:681, 1985.

122. Shneerson, J. M., Mortimer, P. P., and Vandervelde, E. M.: Febrile illness due to a parvovirus. Br. Med. J. 280:1580, 1980.

123. Powars, D.: Aplastic anemia secondary to glue sniffing. N. Engl. J. Med. 273:700, 1965.

124. Lefrère, J.-J., Courouçé, A.-M., Bertrand, Y., Girot, R., and Soulier, J.-P.: Human parvovirus and aplastic crisis in chronic hemolytic anemias: A study of 24 observations. Am. J. Hematol. 23:271, 1986.

125. McLellan, N. J., and Rutter, N.: Hereditary spherocytosis in sisters unmasked by parvovirus infection. Postgrad. Med. J. 63:49, 1987.

126. Doran, H. M., and Teall, A. J.: Neutropenia accompanying erythroid aplasia in human parvovirus infection [letter]. Br. J. Haematol. 69:287, 1988.

127. Kurtzman, G., Gascon, P., Caras, M., Cohen, B., and Young, N.: B19 parvovirus replicates in circulating cells of acutely infected patients. Blood 71:1448, 1988.

128. Nunoue, T., Koike, T., Koike, R., Sanada, M., Tsukada, T., Mortimer, P. P., and Cohen, B. J.: Infection with human parvovirus (B19), aplasia of the bone marrow and a rash in hereditary spherocytosis. J. Infect. 14:67, 1987.

129. Anderson, M. J., Higgins, P. G., Davis, L. R., Williams, J. S., Jones, S. E., Kidd, I. M., Pattison, J. R., and Tyrrell, D. A. J.: Experimental parvoviral infection in humans. J. Infect. Dis. 152:257, 1985.

130. Lefrère, J. J.: Peripheral thrombocytopenia in human parvovirus infection [letter]. J. Clin. Pathol. 40:469, 1987.

131. Lefrère, J. J., Courouçé, A. M., and Kaplan, C.: Parvovirus and idiopathic thrombocytopenic purpura [letter]. Lancet 1:279, 1989.

132. Conrad, M. E., Studdard, H., and Anderson, L. J.: Case report: Aplastic crisis in sickle cell disorders: Bone marrow necrosis and human parvovirus infection. Am. J. Med. Sci. 295:212, 1988.

133. Pardoll, D. M., Rodeheffer, R. J., Smith, R. R. L., and Charache, S.: Aplastic crisis due to extensive bone marrow necrosis in sickle cell disease. Arch. Intern. Med. 142:2223, 1982.

134. Frickhofen, N., Raghavachar, A., Heit, W., Heimpel, H., and Cohen, B. J.: Human parvovirus infection [letter]. N. Engl. J. Med. 314:646, 1986.

135. Hanada, T., Koike, K., Takeya, T., Nagasawa, T., Matsunaga, Y., and Takita, H.: Human parvovirus B19-induced transient pancytopenia in a child with hereditary spherocytosis. Br. J. Haematol. 70:113, 1988.

136. Saunders, P. W. G., Reid, M. M., and Cohen, B. J.: Human parvovirus induced cytopenias: A report of five cases [letter]. Br. J. Haematol. 63:407, 1986.

137. Hamon, M. D., Newland, A. C., and Anderson, M. J.: Severe aplastic anaemia after parvovirus infection in the absence of underlying haemolytic anaemia [letter]. J. Clin. Pathol. 41:1242, 1988.

138. Boruchoff, E. S., Woda, A. B., Pihan, A. G., Durbin, A. W., Burnstein, D., and Blacklow, R. N.: Parvovirus B19-associated hemophagocytic syndrome. Arch. Intern. Med. 150:897, 1990.

139. Lefrère, J. J., and Got, D.: Peripheral thrombocytopenia in human parvovirus infection [letter]. J. Clin. Pathol. 40:469, 1987.

140. Anderson, M. J., Davis, L. R., Hodgson, S. E., Jones, L., Murtaza, J. R., Pattison, C. E., and White, J. M.: Occurrence of infection with a parvovirus-like agent in children with sickle cell anaemia during a two-year period. J. Clin. Pathol. 35:744, 1982.

141. Kelleher J. F., Jr., Luban, N. L. C., Cohen, B. J., and Mortimer, P. P.: Human serum parvovirus as the cause of aplastic crisis in sickle cell disease. Am. J. Dis. Child. 138:401, 1984.

142. Rao, K. R. P., Patel, A. R., Anderson, M. J., Hodgson, J., Jones, S. E., and Pattison, J. R.: Infection with parvovirus-like virus and aplastic crisis in chronic hemolytic anemia. Ann. Intern. Med. 98:930, 1983.

143. Serjeant, G. R., Topley, J. M., Mason, K., Serjeant, B. E., Pattison, J. R., Jones, S. E., and Mohamed, R.: Outbreak of aplastic crises in sickle cell anaemia associated with parvovirus-like agent. Lancet 2:595, 1981.

144. Wodzinski, M. A., and Lilleyman, J. S.: Transient erythroblastopenia of childhood due to human parvovirus B19 infection. Br. J. Haematol. 73:127, 1989.

145. Young, N. S., Mortimer, P. P., Moore, J. G., and Humphries, R. K.: Characterization of a virus that causes transient aplastic crisis. J. Clin. Invest. 73:224, 1984.

146. Anderson, M. J., Jones, S. E., and Minson, A. C.: Diagnosis of human parvovirus infection by dot-blot hybridization using cloned viral DNA. J. Med. Virol. 15:163, 1985.

147. Clewley, J. P.: Detection of human parvovirus using a molecularly cloned probe. J. Med. Virol. 15:173, 1985.

148. Saarinen, U. M., Chorba, T. L., Tattersall, P., Young, N. S., Anderson, L. J., Palmer, E., and Coccia, P. F.: Human parvovirus B19-induced epidemic acute red cell aplasia in patients with hereditary hemolytic anemia. Blood 67:1411, 1986.

149. Leads from the MMWR: Risks associated with human parvovirus B19 infection. J.A.M.A. 261:1406, 1989.

150. Anderson, L. J., and Hurwitz, E. S.: Human parvovirus B19 and pregnancy. Clin. Perinatol. 15:273, 1988.

151. Anand, A., Gray, E. S., Brown, T., Clewley, J. P., and Cohen, B. J.: Human parvovirus infection in pregnancy and hydrops fetalis. N. Engl. J. Med. 316:183, 1987.

152. Cotmore, S. F., McKie, V. C., Anderson, L. J., Astell, C. R., and Tattersall, P.: Identification of the major structural and nonstructural proteins encoded by human parvovirus B19 and mapping of their genes by procaryotic expression of isolated genomic fragments. J. Virol. 60:548, 1986.

153. Public Health Laboratory Service Working Party on Fifth Disease: Prospective study of human parvovirus (B19) infection in pregnancy. Br. Med. J. 300:1166, 1990.

154. Rodis, J. F., Quinn, D. L., Gary, G. W., Jr., and Anderson, L. J.: Management and outcomes of pregnancies complicated by human B19 parvovirus infection: A prospective study. Am. J. Obstet. Gynecol. 163 (4 pt 1):1168, 1990.

155. Porter, H. J., Quantrill, A. M., and Fleming, K. A.: B19 parvovirus infection of myocardial cells [letter]. Lancet 1:535, 1988.

156. Wright, I. M., Williams, M. L., and Cohen, B. J.: Congenital parvovirus infection. Arch. Dis. Child. 66:253, 1991.

157. Schwarz, T. F., Roggendorf, M., Hottentrager, B., Deinhardt, F., Enders, G., Gloning, K. P., Schramm, T., and Hansmann, M.: Human parvovirus B19 infection in pregnancy [letter]. Lancet 2:566, 1988.

158. Belloy, M., Morinet, F., Blondin, G., Couroucé, A. M., Peyrol, Y., and Vilmer, E.: Erythroid hypoplasia due to chronic infection with parvovirus B19. N. Engl. J. Med. 322:633, 1990.

159. Brown, K. E., Antunez de Mayolo, J. J., Bellanti, J. A., Vetro, S. W., Green, S. W., Fitzpatrick, S. B., Gutierrez, P., Eglinton, G. S., and Young, N. S.: Congenital infection with B19 parvovirus: Pure red cell aplasia and immunodeficiency. Pediatrics (submitted for publication).

160. Kurtzman, G., Frickhofen, N., Kimball, J., Jenkins, D. W., Nienhuis, A. W., and Young, N. S.: Pure red-cell aplasia of 10 years' duration due to persistent parvovirus B19 infection and its cure with immunoglobulin therapy. N. Engl. J. Med. 321:519, 1989.

161. Kurtzman, G., Cohen, B., Myers, P., Amanullah, A., and Young, N.: Persistent B19 parvovirus infection as a cause of severe anemia in children with acute lymphocytic leukemia in remission. Lancet 2:1159, 1988.

162. Frickhofen, N., Abkowitz, J., Safford, M., Berry, J. M., Antunez-de-Mayolo, J., Astrow, A., Cohen, R., Halperin, I., King, L., Mintzer, D., Cohen, B., and Young, N. S.: Persistent parvovirus infection in patients infected with human immunodeficiency virus-1: A treatable cause of anemia in AIDS. Ann. Intern. Med. 113:926, 1990.

163. Berner, Y. N., Green, L., and Handzel, Z. T.: Erythroblastopenia in acquired immunodeficiency syndrome (AIDS) [letter]. Acta Haematol. 70:273, 1983.

164. Sallan, S. E., and Buchanan, G. R.: Selective erythroid aplasia during therapy for acute lymphoblastic leukemia. Pediatrics 59:895, 1977.

165. Frickhofen, N., and Young, N. S.: Persistent parvovirus B19 infections in humans. Microbiol. Pathogen. 7:319, 1989.

166. Bowman, C. A., Cohen, B. J., Norfolk, D. R., and Lacey, C. J. N.: Red cell aplasia associated with human parvovirus B19 and HIV infection: Failure to respond clinically to intravenous immunoglobulin [letter]. AIDS 4: 1038, 1990.

167. Erdman, D. D., Usher, M. J., Tsou, C., Caul, E. O., Gary, G. W., Kajigaya, S., Young, N. S., and Anderson, L. J.: Human parvovirus B19 specific IgG, IgA, and IgM antibodies and DNA in serum specimens from persons with erythema infectiosum. J. Med. Virol. 35:110, 1991.

168. Kurtzman, G., Cohen, R., Field, A. M., Oseas, R., Blaese, R. M., and Young, N.: The immune response to B19 parvovirus infection and an antibody defect in persistent viral infection. J. Clin. Invest. 84:1114, 1989.

169. Jacoby, R. O., Johnson, E. A., Paturzo, F. X., Gaertner, D. J., Brandsma, J. L., and Smith, A. L.: Persistent rat parvovirus infection in individually housed rats. Arch. Virol. 117:193, 1991.

170. Rimmelzwaan, G. F., Van der Heijden, R. W. J., Tijhaar, E., Poelen, M. C. M., Carlson, J., Osterhaus, A. D. M. E., and UytdeHaag, F. G. C. M.: Establishment and characterization of canine parvovirus-specific murine CD4+ T cell clones and their use for the delineation of T cell epitopes. J. Gen. Virol. 71:1095, 1990.

171. Alexandersen, S., Bloom, M. E., and Perryman, S.: Nucleotide sequence and genomic organization of Aleutian mink disease parvovirus (ADV): Sequence comparisons between a nonpathogenic and a pathogenic strain. J. Virol. 62:2903, 1988.

172. An, S. H., and Wilkie, B. N.: Mitogen- and viral antigen–induced transformation of lymphocytes from normal mink and from mink with progressive or nonprogressive Aleutian disease. Infect. Immun. 34:111, 1981.

173. Tattersall, P., and Bratton, J.: Reciprocal productive and restrictive virus-cell interactions of immunosuppressive and prototype strains of minute virus of mice. J. Virol. 46:944, 1983.

174. Harding, M. J., and Molitor, T.: Porcine parvovirus: Replication and inhibition of selected cellular functions of swine alveolar macrophages and peripheral blood lymphocytes. Arch. Virol. 101:105, 1988.

175. Carlson, J. H., Scott, F. W., and Duncan, J. R.: Feline panleukopenia III: Development of lesions in the lymphoid tissue. Vet. Pathol. 15:383, 1978.

176. Porter, D. D., and Larsen, A. E.: Mink parvovirus infections. In Tijssen, P. (ed.): Handbook of Parvoviruses, Vol. 2. Boca Raton, CRC Press, 1990, pp. 87–101.

177. Yoshimoto, K., Rosenfeld, S., Frickhofen, N., Kennedy, D., Kajigaya, S., and Young, N. S.: A second neutralizing epitope of B19 parvovirus implicates the spike region in the immune response. J. Virol. 65:7056, 1991.

178. Sato, H., Hirata, J., Furukawa, M., Kuroda, N., Shiraki, H., Maeda, Y., and Okochi, K.: Identification of the region including the epitope for a monoclonal antibody which can neutralize human parvovirus B19. J. Virol. 65:1667, 1991.

179. Sato, H., Hirata, J., Kuroda, N., Shiraki, H., Maeda, Y., and Okochi, K.: Identification and mapping of neutralizing epitopes of human parvovirus B19 by using human antibodies. J. Virol. 65:5845, 1991.

180. Rosenfeld, S. R., Yoshimoto, K., Anderson, S., Kajigaya, S., Young, N. S., Warrener, P., Bonsal, G., and Collett, M.: The unique region of the minor capsid protein of human parvovirus B19 is exposed on the virion surface. J. Clin. Invest. 1992.

181. Rosenfeld, S. J., Kajigaya, S., Young, N. S., Ayub, J., and Saxinger, C.: Fine structure epitope mapping of B19 parvovirus empty capsids. Immunology (submitted for publication).

182. Meunier, P. C., Cooper, B. J., Appel, M. J. G., Lanieu, M. E., and Slauson, D. O.: Pathogenesis of canine parvovirus enteritis: Sequential virus distribution and passive immunization studies. Vet. Path. 22:617, 1985.

183. Takahashi, M., Koike, T., Moriyama, Y., and Shibata, A.: Neutralizing activity of immunoglobulin preparation against erythropoietic suppression of human parvovirus [letter]. Am. J. Hematol. 37:68, 1991.

184. Davis, E. V., Gregory, G. G., and Beckenhauer, W. H.: Infectious feline panleukopenia. Developmental report of a tissue culture origin formalin-inactivated vaccine. Vet. Med./Small Animal Clin. 65:237, 1970.

185. Pye, D., Bates, J., Edwards, S. J., and Hollingworth, J.: Development of a vaccine preventing parvovirus-induced reproductive failure in pigs. Aust. Vet. J. 67:179, 1979.

186. Rimmelzwaan, G. F., Carlson, J., UytdeHaag, F. G., and Osterhaus, A. D.: A synthetic peptide derived from the amino acid sequence of canine parvovirus structural proteins which defines a B cell epitope and elicits antiviral antibody in BALB c mice. J. Gen. Virol. 71:2741, 1990.

187. Bansal, G. P., Hatfield, J., Dunn, F. E., Warrener, P., Young, J. F., Top, F. H., Collett, M. C., Anderson, S., Rosenfeld, S., Kajigaya, S., and Young, N. S.: Immunogenicity studies of recombinant human parvovirus B19 proteins. In Brown, F., Chanock, R. M., Ginsberg, H. S., and Lerner, R. A.: Vaccines 92. Cold Spring Harbor, N.Y., Cold Spring Harbor Press, 1992, p. 315.

188. Caul, O. E., Usher, J. M., and Burton, A. P.: Intrauterine infection with human parvovirus B19: A light and electron microscopy study. J. Med. Virol. 24:55, 1988.

B. RETROVIRUSES (HTLVs)

Mitsuaki Yoshida

INTRODUCTION TO RETROVIRUSES

General Descriptions

Retroviruses constitute a unique family of RNA viruses that contain reverse transcriptase, which, upon infection, transcribes genomic RNA into DNA. The cores of the viral particles contain, in addition to genomic RNA, Gag protein and reverse transcriptase. Enveloping the core is a membrane, similar to the plasma membrane of host cells, on which viral Env (envelope) glycoprotein is exposed. The interaction of Env protein with a receptor on a target cell is required for infection. Upon infection, the RNA genome is reverse-transcribed into DNA, which is then integrated into host cell DNA by covalent linkage to form proviral DNA. The proviral genomes can be maintained in infected cells as cellular DNA sequences with or without viral replication.

Rous sarcoma virus was found in transmissible sarcomas of chickens in 1910. Since then, retroviruses have been isolated from many species of animals, and those from mice and chickens have been investigated extensively. The viruses may be transmitted in two ways: horizontally from host to host by replication and infection (exogenous viruses) and vertically to successive generations of hosts by transmission of proviral genomes through germ cells (endogenous viruses). Of wide interest because of their tumorigenic properties, studies of retroviruses have led to the discovery of oncogenes. Retroviruses have also been of interest in connection with autoimmune and neurological diseases.

Viral Replication

The viral particle contains two copies of a single-stranded, positive RNA, which is dimerized in the 5' region. After incorporation of a viral particle by a cell, the reverse transcriptase in the viral core reverse-transcribes the genomic RNA to complementary DNA (cDNA) (Fig. 26–16). The cDNA is then converted to double-stranded DNA and integrated into the host's chromosomal DNA. The integrated DNA, or "provirus," has a repeating sequence (LTR) at both ends, which contains many elements essential to viral gene expression and replication. Details of the mechanism of replication have been presented elsewhere.[1]

Integrated proviruses are transcribed by the cellular machinery, integration itself being necessary for retroviral gene expression and replication. A subpopulation of the viral transcripts is spliced into subgenomic mRNA, and both spliced and unspliced RNAs are translated into viral proteins. Unspliced genomic RNA and viral proteins are assembled at specific sites under the plasma membrane, and the particles are released from cells by budding. Generally, retroviral replication is not especially harmful to cells, and infected cells can commonly be used to establish virus-producing cell lines. The integrated proviruses are stable and are transmitted to daughter cells independent of proviral genome expression.

Retroviruses can infect a wide range of cellular types in vitro. The receptors for a few retroviruses have been identified as membrane proteins,[2, 3] and their expression in many types of cells is consistent with the wide spectrum of cells susceptible to retroviral infection. The receptors for most retroviruses have not, however, been identified. In contrast to the broad specificity of retroviral infection, retroviruses are able to induce tumors in relatively few tissues.

Genomic Structures

All retroviruses can be placed in one of two groups: those that carry and those that do not carry host-derived oncogenes (Fig. 26–17). Retroviruses not carrying oncogenes are generally competent in replication and have *gag*, *pol*, and *env* genes in their genomes. Some of these viruses induce leukemia or lymphoma after a long period of latency and are thus called chronic leukemia viruses. For a long time, the mechanism by which retroviruses lacking oncogenes could induce tumors was unknown, but it is now established that LTRs at the proviral termini can activate expression of adjacent cellular genes. When a provirus is, by chance, integrated in the vicinity of a proto-oncogene, the normal regulation of the cellular/retro-oncogene expression can be disrupted, leading to abnormal expression and tumorigenesis. The promoter-insertion mechanism operates in a variety of tumor systems: *myc* activation by avian leukemia virus (ALV) in B-cell lymphoma,[4] *erbB* activation by ALV in chicken erythroblastosis,[5] and *Wnt*-1 and *int*2 activation by mouse mammary tumor virus (MMTV) in mouse mammary tumors.[6] Because LTR can function as an enhancer, integration of the provirus into certain regions, as opposed to specific sequences, is sufficient for activation of a cellular proto-oncogene.[7] Because proviral integration is not site specific, repeated integration through viral replication is usually required before the provirus appears in a tumorigenic site, which explains the long latent period between infection and tumorigenesis.

The second group of retroviruses carry an oncogene acquired from a cellular proto-oncogene.[1] In the acquisition of this oncogene, a portion of the RNA comprising the *gag*, *pol*, and *env* genes is deleted. Consequently, acute sarcoma/leukemia viruses are generally replication defective, and they must infect cells in company with a chronic leukemia virus that acts as a "helper" in replication. One exception is Rous

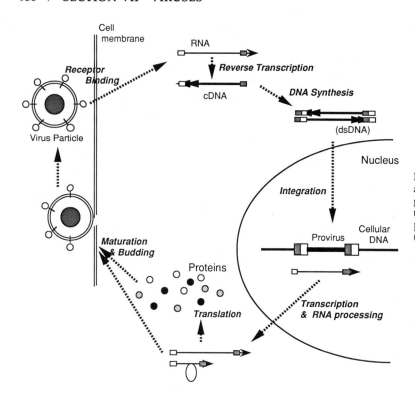

FIGURE 26–16. Replication cycle of retroviruses. Open and closed boxes at the termini of the RNA and proviral genomes represent the U5 and U3 sequences, respectively, and the fused sequences at the termini of the proviral genome represent the long terminal repeats (LTRs).

sarcoma virus, which has the oncogene *src* inserted between *env* and the 3′ LTR. The acute leukemia viruses transform cells using the protein encoded by the viral oncogene. Thus, cellular transformation requires viral gene expression, but as it does not require viral replication or site-specific integration, tumor development is rapidly induced. The tissue specificity of retroviral tumorigenesis is restricted by either the class of oncogene in the viral genome or the promoter activity of the integrated LTR, as well as the nature of the viral receptors on the host's cells.

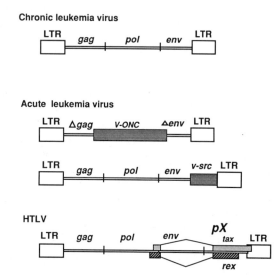

FIGURE 26–17. Genomic structure of retroviruses as illustrated by their proviral DNAs. The open boxes are the LTRs, and closed boxes represent the viral oncogenes (v-*onc*), which, with the exception of those in human T-cell leukemia virus–1 (HTLV-1), have been acquired from cellular DNA.

HUMAN RETROVIRUSES

Introduction

Retroviruses have been isolated from a variety of animals, but only recently have they been isolated from humans. The human T-cell leukemia virus (HTLV), human immunodeficiency virus (HIV; see Chapter 25), human endogenous viruses, and human foamy viruses are distributed among four groups of retroviruses. Here we review the replication of and pathology associated with the HTLV and related viruses. With some exceptions, observations on HTLV-1 are applicable to other members of the HTLV group.

HTLVs and Diseases

Human T-cell leukemia virus type I (HTLV-1) is a causative factor in adult T-cell leukemia (ATL).[8] ATL was first described in 1977 in Japan[9] as a unique T-cell malignancy (see below under Pathogenesis). The clustering of patients with this disease in Kyushu and Shikoku in southwestern Japan strongly suggested an association with viral infection. The human retrovirus HTLV was reported in the United States in 1980 upon characterization of reverse transcriptase in cultured T cells established from a T-cell lymphoma. Establishment of a T-cell line using cells from an ATL patient was achieved independently in Japan by co-cultivation of cord-blood lymphocytes and peripheral lymphocytes from an ATL patient.[11, 12] In these cultures, retrovirus-like particles were detected at the peripheries of T cells. Furthermore, the sera of ATL patients were found to contain antibodies that reacted specifically with the cell line established from the ATL patient.[13] These in vitro observations, combined with epidemiological studies,[14, 15] suggested that a *human retrovirus* existed in association with ATL. Direct proof of the presence of a retrovirus in ATL patients and its relationship to the patients' antibodies was obtained through characterization of the viral genome[16] and seroepidemiological surveys.[13, 17] Because the viral genome has an extra sequence, pX, in addition to the *gag, pol,* and *env* genes, HTLV was classified as a distinct type of retrovirus (see Fig. 26–17).[18]

After characterization of HTLV, another virus, HTLV-2, immunologically similar to the known HTLV (HTLV-1) retrovirus, was isolated from a patient with hairy T-cell leukemia.[19, 20] Identical over about 60 per cent of their genomic sequences,[21] HTLV-1 and HTLV-2 are clearly distinct. HTLV-2 is frequently isolated from intravenous drug abusers and persons infected with HIV,[22] but HTLV-2 has been found in only three patients with hairy T-cell leukemia. Thus, its association with this disease may be fortuitous.

A virus similar to HTLV-1, simian T-cell leukemia virus (STLV), was isolated from various species of non-human primates,[23, 24] including the Japanese macaque, African green monkey, pig-tailed macaque, gorilla, and chimpanzee. The STLVs share 90 to 95 per cent identity of genomic sequence with HTLV-1 and also are very similar to each other.[25] In some colonies of Japanese macaques, 60 to 70 per cent of all monkeys are STLV positive, whereas in other, sometimes neighboring, colonies, virtually all animals are STLV negative. Although the virus is widely distributed in monkeys, no typically leukemic animals have been observed. A causal connection between STLV and disease remains to be established despite a few cases of a leukemia-like disease that have been noted in STLV-infected monkeys.[26]

Another member of the HTLV group is bovine leukemia virus (BLV).[27] This virus infects and replicates in B cells of cows and induces B-cell lymphoma. BLV also infects lymphocytes of sheep and induces leukemia after a short latent interval.

Epidemiology

Nearly all ATL patients have circulating antibodies to HTLV-1 proteins.[13] These antibodies are easily detected by indirect immunostaining of cells infected with HTLV-1, by enzyme-linked immunosorbent assay (ELISA), particle-agglutination assay, or Western blotting. HTLV-1 antibodies are also detectable in some healthy adults[14, 15]; these asymptomatic, seropositive persons are defined as carriers of the virus. HTLV-1 can be isolated from such individuals through the establishment of infected cell lines.[28] With use of the polymerase chain reaction (PCR), HTLV-1 DNA sequences in circulating lymphocytes can be detected in nearly all seropositive people. Thus, antibodies to HTLV-1 proteins are reliable indicators of HTLV-1 infection and replication.

GEOGRAPHICAL CLUSTERING. HTLV-1 antibodies are now recognized in 5 to 15 per cent of adults clustered in southwestern Japan,[14] the Caribbean islands and South America,[15] central Africa,[29] and Papua New Guinea and the Solomon Islands in Melanesia[30] (Fig. 26–18A and B). The prevalence of healthy, seropositive adults varies significantly from district to district and even from village to village within areas of endemicity. For example, in a given isolated island in Kyushu, Japan, 30 to 40 per cent of people over 40 years of age might be infected, whereas on a neighboring island, the prevalence may be far lower.[31] Significantly, ATL and HTLV-1–associated myelopathy/tropical spastic paraparesis (HAM/TSP) (see below) are also clustered, overlapping HTLV-1 in distribution. ATL patients and healthy carriers are found sporadically all over the world, but most patients live in or have moved from an area of endemicity. These epidemiological findings indicate a close association of HTLV-1 with ATL and HAM/TSP. In the case of ATL, it has been proposed that infection by HTLV-1 early in life is important to the later development of leukemia.

AGE-DEPENDENT PREVALENCE. The prevalence of virus carriers increases with age after 20, reaching a maximum in people between 40 and 60 years of age. The prevalence is significantly (1.6 times) higher in women than in men (Fig. 26–19). The increase in prevalence of seropositivity with advancing age among women is attributed to sexual transmission of HTLV-1 from husbands to wives. Conversely, the results indicate that HTLV-1 transmission from wives to husbands is infrequent. The reason for the age-dependent increase of antibody prevalence among men is not clear.

FAMILIAL AGGREGATION. Familial aggregation, noted in studies of antibody prevalence, was thought to indicate a genetic predisposition to HTLV-1 infection. Today this aggregation is understood to be the result of viral transmission from husband to wife and mother to child.

GENOMIC STABILITY. Molecular analyses demonstrated that the viral genome is well conserved in Japan and the Caribbean area.[32] The viral isolates from Africa may vary more. Retroviral genomes are thought to be less unstable than those of other viruses owing to the necessity of reverse transcription. Thus, the discovery of stability, surprising as it was to retrovirologists, now stands in sharp contrast to the highly labile genome of HIV. Recently, it has been reported that viral isolates from Papua New Guinea vary significantly in genomic sequence.[30] Such variation may provide insights into the origin of HTLV-1. Why this virus is clustered in such widely separated regions is unknown; perhaps an explanation lies in the mode of viral transmission and host-related factors that affect responses to infection (see below).

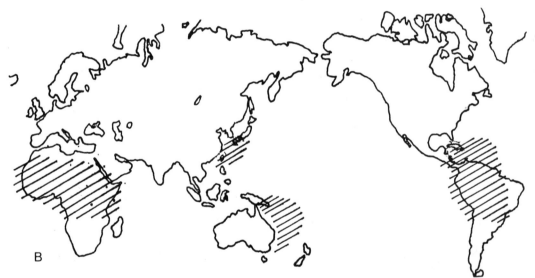

FIGURE 26–18. Geographical distribution of HTLV-1 and adult T-cell leukemia (ATL) in Japan (A) and the world (B). The viruses isolated from these regions are very similar.

Infection by and Expression of HTLV-1

In Vitro Infection and Transformation

Cell-free viral particles of HTLV-1 show extremely low infectivity in vitro and usually cannot establish an infection in vitro. However, co-cultivation with virus-producing cells can result in transmission of HTLV-1 to a variety of human cells,[11, 12] including T and B lymphocytes, fibroblasts, and epithelial cells, as well as cells from monkeys, rats,[33] rabbits,[34] and hamsters (but, curiously, not mice) (Fig. 26–20). In infected cells, the provirus is integrated into random sites in the chromosomal DNA, and most of the viral genes are successfully expressed. HTLV-1 infection in culture usu-

ally induces the fusion of many infected cells to form syncytia.

Only T cells with the CD4+ marker are frequently immortalized upon infection of peripheral blood cells with HTLV-1.[11, 12, 35] Immortalized cells express high levels of the α chain of interleukin (IL)-2R[36] and proliferate in an IL-2–dependent fashion. The phenotypes expressed by cells immortalized in vitro mimic those of leukemic cells in vivo (see below).[37, 38] Immortalization by HTLV-1 appears unique to HTLVs; animal retroviruses that do not carry an oncogene do not immortalize or transform cells in vitro. Similar immortalization of T cells by HTLV-2 and STLV has been reported. Thus, immortalization seems to be a general property conferred upon T cells by HTLVs

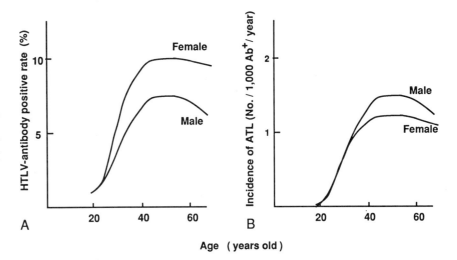

FIGURE 26–19. Schematic illustration of prevalence of seropositivity (A) and of ATL (B) as a function of age. Seropositivity to HTLV-1 and prevalence of ATL rise in parallel, but the ratios of the prevalences differ between males and females. The seropositive rate for people under 20 years of age is not zero.

and, accordingly, a contribution of the pX gene to this effect has been proposed.

In Vivo Transmission

In contrast to the broad range of cell types that can be infected in vitro by HTLV-1, the cells of both ATL patients and asymptomatic viral carriers infected in vivo are almost exclusively CD4+ T cells (see Fig. 26–20). Interestingly, HTLV-infected cells, irrespective of whether or not they are leukemic, do not express, even as RNA, viral information at significant levels. That these cells can express viral genes after several hours' culture in vitro[39] demonstrates that latency in vivo is not a function of a defect in the integrated provirus. As shown by reverse-PCR on mRNA, more

than 99 per cent of infected cells fail to express viral genes in vivo.[40] It was previously suspected that viral gene suppression is linked to the lack of replication of infected T cells in peripheral blood. However, no significant viral expression is demonstrable in either enlarged lymph nodes or skin lesions in which some populations of malignant cells are dividing.[46]

Viral transmission can occur through (1) blood transfusion, (2) the sharing of contaminated needles by intravenous drug abusers, (3) nursing of infants by infected mothers, and (4) sexual relations (Fig. 26–21).

BLOOD TRANSFUSION. Retrospective studies of blood transfusions showed that 60 to 70 per cent of recipients of fresh seropositive blood were infected with HTLV-1.[41] Surprisingly, no recipients of fresh seropositive plasma were infected, indicating that the transfer of infected cells from donor to recipient is required for viral transmission. HTLV-1 infection acquired through transfusion seems not to induce ATL (see Sexual Transmission, below) but does induce HAM/TSP.[42] Therefore, rejection of HTLV-1–positive blood can protect against both HTLV-1 infection and development of HAM/TSP.

INTRAVENOUS DRUG ABUSE. In some areas of the United States and Jamaica,[43] HTLV antibodies have been detected in up to 20 per cent of abusers of intravenous drugs. The high prevalence is a result of the sharing of unsterilized needles and is frequently associated with HIV infection as well. Surprisingly, studies of DNA using PCR indicated that a large proportion of the viruses were, in fact, HTLV-2, a finding that might aid in defining the area of endemicity of HTLV-2.

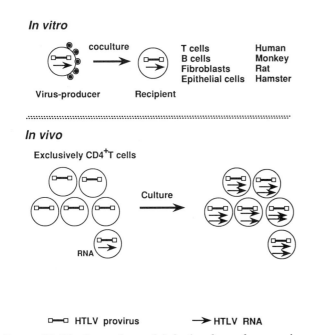

FIGURE 26–20. Comparison of infection by and expression of HTLV-1 in vivo and in vitro. Transmission in vitro requires cocultivation with virus-producing cells. Infected cells in vivo are mostly CD4+ T cells that do not express the viral genome.

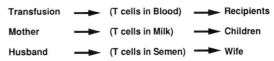

FIGURE 26–21. Transmission of HTLV-1 over three major pathways. In these pathways, transfer of infected, living cells into recipients is essential to efficient viral transmission.

MOTHER TO CHILD. Viral transmission from mother to child was originally suggested by epidemiological evidence: Most mothers of seropositive children were carriers of the virus, and about 30 per cent of the children of seropositive mothers were themselves seropositive.[44, 45] Neonatal infection was initially suspected, but surveys of lymphocytes in cord bloods from a large number of children born to seropositive mothers have excluded this possibility. Instead, breast milk was found to be a likely source of transmissible virus.[45, 115] Milk from seropositive mothers given to adult marmosets leads to the appearance of antibodies in these monkeys. Avoidance of breast-feeding by seropositive mothers drastically reduced the seroconversion rates of their children (see below).

SEXUAL TRANSMISSION. Wives with seropositive husbands are usually seropositive. Conversely, the husbands of seropositive wives show the same frequency of seropositivity as do men of the region under study. On these grounds, it seems that the virus can be transmitted from husband to wife but not from wife to husband.[31, 47] Infected T cells are present in semen from infected men and probably transmit the virus from man to woman.

Despite the 1.6 per cent higher rate of seropositivity in women, the sex-specific incidence of ATL does not mirror this difference: HTLV-1 infections sexually transmitted to women do not appear to lead to disease development.

Molecular Biology of HTLV-1 Gene Expression

The HTLV-1 Genome

The HTLV-1 proviral genome was cloned from leukemic cell DNA acquired from an ATL patient,[48] and the complete nucleotide sequence was determined.[18] The proviral genome is 9032 bp long and contains, in common with other retroviruses, *gag, pol,* and *env* genes and 3' and 5' LTRs. The presence of a so-called pX region on the 3' side of the *env* gene distinguishes the HTLV-1 genome from those of other retroviruses (see Fig. 26–17). In recognition of this distinction, HTLV-1 is placed into a distinct group of pX-bearing retroviruses that includes HTLV-2, STLV, and BLV. The pX sequence is not, like retroviral oncogenes, of cellular origin, but is a virus-specific sequence essential to replication.

Retroviral LTRs regulate viral gene expression and replication. The pX region of HTLV contains additional, overlapping regulatory genes (Fig. 26–22): *tax, rex,* and a gene whose function remains unknown. The products of the genes are p40*tax*,[49–51] p27*rex*[52, 61] and p21*x*.[46, 52, 61] The Tax protein, or p40*tax*, is a *trans*-activator of proviral transcriptional initiation[53–56] and is essential to viral gene expression and replication. The Tax protein also *trans*-activates transcription of some cellular genes whose functions are associated with T-cell proliferation (see below).[57] The second

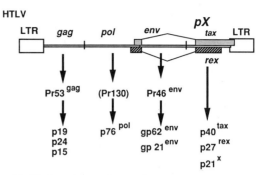

FIGURE 26–22. Protein products of HTLV-1. Gag, Pol, and Env proteins are processed from precursors, and the pX proteins are encoded by overlapping genes in the pX sequence.

protein, p27*rex*, is a *trans*-acting modulator of RNA processing, which induces unspliced *gag* and *env* mRNAs.[58, 59] Without *rex*-gene function, all HTLV-1 transcripts are doubly spliced into an mRNA encoding Tax and Rex proteins,[60] effectively preventing production of viral structural proteins. Thus, Rex is also essential for HTLV-1 gene expression and replication. The protein of unknown function, p21*x*,[61] is composed of the same sequence as the C-terminal portion of p27*rex*. The regulatory system in HTLVs is unique, operating at the levels of transcription and RNA processing and exerting control of both qualitative and quantitative aspects of gene expression.

Transcription

Retroviral LTR sequences lie at both termini of the integrated proviral genome and contain elements for efficient transcriptional initiation and termination. The elements include a TATA box, a transcriptional enhancer, and a poly(A) signal, all of which consist of short nucleotide sequences. As these elements are recognized by cellular transcriptional factors for RNA polymerase II, expression of the retrovirus depends upon the cellular machinery of the host.

In addition to LTR-associated regulators, HTLV-1 contains the *tax* gene, which acts in *trans* to stimulate viral transcription.[53–56] *Trans*-activation of the LTR by the Tax protein increases viral gene expression more than 200-fold. This *trans*-activation requires a transcriptional enhancer in the LTR, which is composed of three direct repeats of a 21 bp sequence[62–64] containing a cyclic AMP (cAMP)–responsive element (CRE) (Fig. 26–23).

Tax is a protein containing a zinc finger motif,[65] but it does not bind directly to the 21 bp sequence. It has been proposed that Tax interacts with a cellular protein that then binds to the enhancer to mediate *trans*-activation. Candidates for this role include several Tax-responsive element-binding proteins (TREBs), the coding sequences of which have been isolated and cloned as cDNA,[66, 67] activating transcription factor (ATF),[68] and others.[69] All of the proteins in question have in common a leucine zipper structure, a domain of basic amino acids, and several possible phosphorylation sites, features similar to those conserved in the

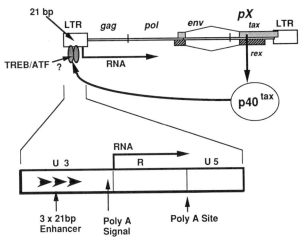

FIGURE 26–23. Tax *trans*-activates transcription of the viral genome. The essential element in *trans*-activation is the viral enhancer, which consists of three direct repeats of the 21 bp sequence.

transcription factor CREB (cAMP-responsive element-binding protein) and the oncogenes c-*fos* and c-*jun*.[70] The proteins form homodimers or heterodimers through the leucine zipper structures and bind to specific DNA sequences CRE, AP-1, or 21 bp enhancer, through the basic amino acid domain. As is the case in formation of the heterodimer Fos-Jun, TREB7 (CREB-BP1 or ATF2) can interact with c-Jun,[71] and TREB5 (hXBP1) is reported to interact with c-Fos protein.[72] TREB7 was found to mediate transcriptional activation by adenovirus E1A,[73, 74] but there is no direct evidence for involvement of these enhancer-binding proteins in Tax *trans*-activation. Nevertheless, because synthesis of new protein is not required,[75] pre-existing transcription factor is expected to play a role in Tax-mediated *trans*-activation.

Tax activates cellular as well as viral genes (see Fig. 26–27).[18, 19] The responsive cellular genes include those for IL-2,[57] the α chain of the IL-2 receptor (IL-Rα),[57] and granulocyte-macrophage colony-stimulating factor (GM-CSF),[76] the proto-oncogenes c-*fos*[77] and c-*jun*,[78] and the genes for parathyroid hormone—related protein (PTHrP)[79] and major histocompatibility complex (MHC) class I antigen.[80] Activation has been demonstrated directly as induction of the endogenous cellular genes and as expression of the CAT gene linked to the promoter/enhancer of these cellular genes. In addition, it has been reported that Tax suppresses the gene for DNA polymerase β.[38]

The binding site for NF-κB is involved in activation of the IL-2Rα gene, and Tax expression is reported to induce NF-κB–like activity.[81, 82] The transcription factor NF-κB p50 is produced upon processing of its precursor, p105,[83] and becomes active in DNA binding and transcriptional activation. However, p50 forms complexes with factors p65 and i-κB and is retained in the cytoplasm.[84–86] The inactive complexes must be dissociated by cellular factors before p50 can enter the nucleus and react with enhancer DNA.[86] The mechanism of Tax-mediated activation of the NF-κB site is unknown, but studies employing fusion proteins (Tax

with DNA-binding protein) strongly suggest that Tax should associate with the enhancer DNA to elicit *trans*-activation.[87] The NF-κB site differs throughout in sequence from that of the 21 bp enhancer of the viral enhancer; thus Tax activates two structurally unrelated enhancers of transcription. The significance of *trans*-activation of cellular genes is discussed under Mechanism of Viral Involvement.

RNA Processing

Despite the potency of *trans*-activation by Tax, HTLV-1 replication is highly restricted in vivo. This restriction is, in part, a function of the *rex* gene, the second pX gene.[59, 60] For replication of HTLV-1, three species of HTLV-1 mRNA are required: genomic (unspliced) RNA as *gag* and *pol* mRNA; a 4.2 kb, singly spliced, subgenomic RNA as *env* mRNA; and a 2.1 kb, doubly spliced mRNA for the expression of Tax and Rex proteins. A certain balance of expression of these three unspliced and spliced mRNAs is essential to efficient HTLV replication.[88] The process differs from that involved in expression of host-cell mRNA, in which splicing is not a means of regulation and is controlled post-transcriptionally by p27[rex] (Fig. 26–24).

A defect in the proviral *rex* gene leads to production of completely spliced *tax/rex* mRNA,[60] whereas expression of additional *rex* genes complements the defect, inducing production of *gag* and *env* mRNAs. Clearly, Rex protein is required for the expression of unspliced mRNA and production of viral structural proteins, and therefore, Rex is essential to viral replication. In

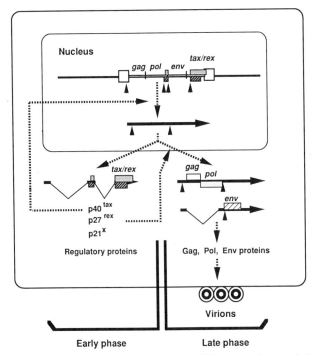

FIGURE 26–24. Processing of HTLV-1 RNA transcripts and the effects of Tax and Rex upon it. Tax activates transcription of the genome to RNA, and Rex induces production of *gag* and *env* mRNA while inhibiting production of *tax/rex* mRNA.

return, the activity of Rex reduces the level of spliced mRNA that encodes regulatory proteins, a reduction resulting in a lower level of Tax protein and, eventually, viral transcription. Thus, Rex produces a *trans*-acting positive signal for the expression of viral structural proteins but a negative signal for total viral gene expression. In short, Rex exerts feedback control of viral gene expression. Because Tax and Rex are encoded by a single species of spliced mRNA, activation by Tax is always followed by the negative effect of Rex.

The mechanism by which Rex functions is not clearly understood. Rex requires a *cis*-acting element (RxRE) consisting of 205 nt located in the 3' region of the viral RNA.[89] The unique secondary structure of this element allows Rex protein to bind to it. Human immunodeficiency virus (HIV) has a gene, *rev*, strikingly similar in function to *rex* in HTLV-1.[90] In the HIV system, Rev binds to RvRE, which is unique in secondary structure[92] and is found in the *env* coding sequence.[91] The binding of Rev is thought to activate transport of unspliced RNA to the cytoplasm.[93] Surprisingly, Rex can also interact with HIV RvRE to regulate HIV-gene expression,[94] indicating that similar mechanisms are involved in the regulation of RNA processing by HTLV-1's Rex and HIV-1's Rev.

HTLV-1's Rex seems not to exert its influence through simple activation of nuclear transport. First, Rex can induce production of some unspliced RNA constructs even in the nucleus.[95] Second, the action of Rex is affected by mutations in the splicing signals that do not contribute to nuclear transport of RNA.[96] These observations suggest that some process or processes operating in the nucleus prior to transport may be the target of Rex regulation. Confusing the issue is the fact that the effect of Rex may vary according to the RNA construct used in the analysis.

Significance of trans-acting Regulation

The combination of the two regulatory genes *tax* and *rex* produces time-dependent positive and negative regulations: Tax regulates viral transcription, then Rex modulates expression of subgenomic mRNA species at the level of RNA processing and, finally, represses the expression of Tax. This unique regulatory system operates in members of the HTLV group and seems important for the replication and survival of them all.

The initial genetic expression of HTLV produces Tax, which *trans*-activates transcription, causing the proviral DNA in a cell to further enhance its own expression. Accumulated Rex protein induces expression of unspliced mRNA, leading to an abundance of mRNA molecules and maximum preparation of the virus for a burst of replicative activity, all before the infected cells express viral antigens, which are targets of the host's immune response, and before the negative regulation by Rex becomes effective. Because of sequential regulation by Tax and Rex, viral replication is transient (Fig. 26–25) and infected cells can escape

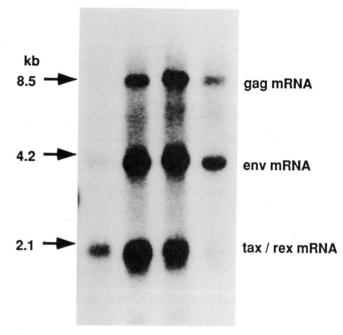

Time after transfection

10   16   26   52 hours

kb
8.5 →   gag mRNA
4.2 →   env mRNA
2.1 →   tax / rex mRNA

FIGURE 26–25. **Demonstration of transient expression of the HTLV-1 genome.** Intact provirus was transfected into cells, and RNA expressed in the cells was analyzed by RNA blotting.

the host's immunological defenses. It is not known what cellular factors are needed to sustain long periods of latency.

Some cell lines infected with HTLV-1 in vitro do express the viral genes efficiently.[10, 11, 16] These established cell lines usually contain multiple copies (generally 10 or so) of defective proviruses,[32] in some of which expression of Tax is insensitive to suppression by Rex. Thus, defective Tax/Rex regulation accounts for why cultured cell lines contain many defective proviruses and express viral antigens. Other retroviruses do not have the equivalent of the *tax/rex* gene, and regulation of their genetic expression is affected by unknown mechanisms.

Pathogenesis

Adult T-cell Leukemia (ATL)

CLINICAL FEATURES. The onset of ATL occurs in individuals between 20 and 70 years of age, with the peak rate of onset at 40 to 60 years of age (see Fig. 26–19).[97] The male/female ratio of incidence of ATL is 1.4:1. Symptoms of ATL vary from patient to patient. Typical manifestations of ATL are skin lesions; enlargement of lymph nodes, liver, and/or spleen; and infiltration of leukemic cells into the lungs and other organs.[97] Laboratory findings include antibodies to HTLV-1 proteins, an increased level of serum LDH, and hypercalcemia.

In addition to the typical, acute form of ATL, smoldering, chronic, and acute (lymphoma-associated) types of ATL have been recognized.[97] In smoldering ATL, patients commonly have from 1 to several per cent of morphologically abnormal T cells in their peripheral blood, but they do not show other signs of severe illness and are thus thought to be in an early stage of ATL development. The abnormal cells are not aggressively malignant but are HTLV-1 infected and clonally expanded. Patients with chronic ATL have rather high levels of HTLV-1–infected leukemic cells but can maintain stable phenotypes for some time. Their leukemic cells also carry clonally integrated HTLV-1 proviruses. The acute form or acute phase of ATL is aggressive and resistant to treatment, and most patients die within 6 months of its onset.

ATL Cells. Leukemic cells are T cells with the CD4+ phenotype and, usually, a highly lobulated nucleus (Fig. 26–26). These cells always carry integrated HTLV-1 proviruses, and the site of integration is monoclonal in a given ATL patient.[8] In 70 to 80 per cent of cases of ATL examined, one copy of the complete provirus was integrated into each leukemic cell. Occasionally, one or two copies of defective provirus are integrated into the DNA of a single cell. Preservation of the pX region, even in defective proviruses,[98] is thought to reflect the important role of pX in tumorigenesis.

The leukemic cells express a high level of IL-2Rα on their surfaces. Production of PTHrP, IL-1β, or GM-CSF by tumor cells has also been reported. In almost all cases, leukemic cells carry aberrant chromosomes, and there are frequently multiple abnormalities, such as trisomy of chromosome 7,[99] and 14q11,[100] 14q32,[101] and 6/q15 translocations, in a single cell. No single abnormality common to all cells was identified in systematic studies in Japan. The translocation 14q32 was found in 25 per cent of ATL patients[100]; other abnormalities appeared less frequently.

Cause of ATL. The role of HTLV-1 in the development of ATL has been demonstrated by seroepidemiological, molecular biological, and experimental studies: (1) ATL and HTLV-1 are identical in geographical distribution, and most ATL patients are infected with HTLV-1. (2) Leukemic cells from ATL patients are infected with HTLV-1 and show monoclonal integration of proviral DNA, indicating that leukemic cells originate from a single HTLV-1–infected cell and, thus, that HTLV-1 plays a causative role in leukemogenesis.[8] (3) Infection by HTLV-1 can immortalize T cells in vitro. The phenotypes of immortalized T cells are very similar to those of leukemic cells,[11, 16] indicating that the transforming capacity of HTLV-1 plays a critical role in leukemogenesis.

It is estimated that there are approximately 1 million carriers of HTLV-1 in Japan, and that about 500 cases of ATL arise each year. About 2 to 5 per cent of all carriers of HTLV-1 are thought to develop ATL during their lifetimes. No significant difference in incidence of ATL was found in two endemic areas of Japan, Kyushu (south) and Hokkaido (north), suggesting that no other exogenous factor is involved in development of ATL.

Although the vast majority of cases of ATL are associated with HTLV-1 infection, a form of ATL seemingly unrelated to HTLV-1 infection has been described.[102] Patients with this disease are phenotypically indistinguishable clinically and hematologically from patients with typical ATL, but they lack HTLV-1 antibodies and their leukemic cells carry no HTLV-1 proviral DNA. The causative factor in this disease has not been identified.

Mechanism of Viral Involvement. ATL cells have clonally integrated HTLV-1 proviruses. However, no common site of integration has been observed among ATL patients,[103] and HTLV-1's role in leukemogenesis is independent of its integration site. In this feature, HTLV-1 differs from the chronic retroviruses in tumor cells of other animals, in which integration was commonly adjacent to a proto-oncogene (see above). As *cis*-activation of a human cellular gene by an LTR of an integrated HTLV-1 provirus is not involved in production of ATL, a *trans*-acting function of HTLV-1 is postulated in leukemogenesis.

Molecular biological studies of HTLV-1-gene expression identified two *trans*-acting functions of *tax* and *rex* (see above). The *trans*-activating effect of Tax on transcription of the viral genome is thought to correspond to the *trans*-acting function of the proviral integration sites. Consistent with this suspicion is the ability of Tax to activate cellular genes in addition to viral genes (Fig. 26–27).[18, 19] The cellular genes so activated include those for IL-2, IL-2Rα, GM-CSF, c-Fos, c-Jun, PTHrP, and MHC class I antigen. The induced synthesis of IL-2, IL-2Rα, c-Fos, and c-Jun suggest induction of cellular proliferation and may explain the continuous abnormal growth of infected T cells. Expression of the *tax* gene in primary lymphocytes could immortalize T cells in an IL-2–dependent fashion.[104] Recently, the transforming capacity of Tax on rodent fibroblasts was demonstrated using colony

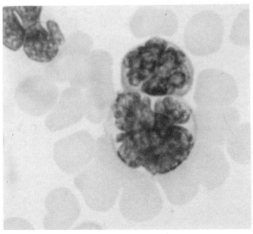

FIGURE 26–26. Typical morphology of leukemic T cells (center) from a patient with ATL. Peripheral blood cells were stained with Giemsa solution; the highly lobulated nucleus is characteristic.

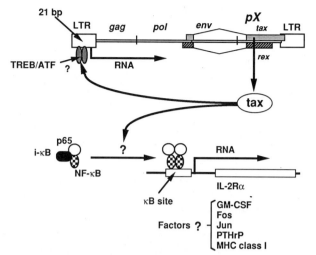

FIGURE 26–27. Tax protein *trans*-activates cellular genes. The *trans*-activation of the IL-2Rα promoter requires the NF-κB site; activation of this promoter thus seems different from that associated with a viral LTR.

formation of NIH3T3 and rat-cell lines in soft agar suspension.[105] Tax was also shown to interact with the c-*ras* gene in cellular transformation of rat embryonic cells.[106] Furthermore, transgenic mice carrying the *tax* gene developed mesenchymal tumors.[114] Although the significance of this transformation is unclear, the results imply a tumor-promoting ability of Tax protein. Collectively, these observations suggest that infection of activated T cells with HTLV-1 initiates abnormal proliferation through *trans*-activation of the *tax* gene and that this molecular mechanism operates in the early stage of ATL development.[107]

PROBLEMS IN LEUKEMOGENIC TRANSFORMATION. Viral activation of genes for growth factors, growth factor receptors, and cellular proto-oncogenes can account for induction of abnormal proliferation of HTLV-1–infected T cells and transformation of murine cells in vitro. However, cells immortalized in vitro differ from leukemic cells in vivo. For example, infected cells in vivo do not produce significant amounts of Tax protein, but they do express IL-2Rα and proliferate abnormally. Furthermore, were Tax the

instigator of abnormal cellular growth, the affected cells should be randomly selected, as they are in asymptomatic carriers of HTLV-1; proviral integration in leukemic cells in vivo is, however, always monoclonal. Therefore, the presence of Tax may be sufficient to explain carrier states but not the development of leukemic cells. Perhaps a second and possibly even a third genetic alteration is involved in production of acute ATL (Fig. 26–28). There is no evidence that these alterations need be related to viral function. The idea that further alteration is necessary is consistent with the long delay in ATL development after HTLV-1 infection early in life.

Another explanation of leukemogenic transformation does involve viral function. Antibodies to HTLV-1 proteins are present throughout infection, indicating continuous expression of viral antigens. A small population of infected cells was shown by PCR to express viral mRNA.[40] Perhaps the low level of Tax in a small cell population selects for a particular cell that enjoys an advantage in growth over other infected cells, and, consequently, clonal selection for leukemogenesis depends on viral function.

HAM/TSP and Other Diseases

During epidemiological screening for HTLV-1 antibodies, some populations of patients with neural disease were found to be strongly antibody positive. These patients had a slowly progressive myelopathy known in tropical zones as tropical spastic paraparesis (TSP)[108, 109] and in endemic areas of Japan as HTLV-1–associated myelopathy (HAM).[110, 111]

The unique phenotypes of HAM/TSP stem from chronic, symmetrical, bilateral involvement of the pyramidal tracts, at mainly the thoracic level of the spinal cord, and include progressive spastic paresis with spastic bladder and minimal sensory deficits. HTLV-1–infected T cells infiltrate into the spinal fluid and cord.[111] Patients respond in some measure to steroid treatment.

Patients with HAM/TSP frequently have titers of HTLV-1 antibodies that are 10 times higher than those of asymptomatic carriers or ATL patients. Because

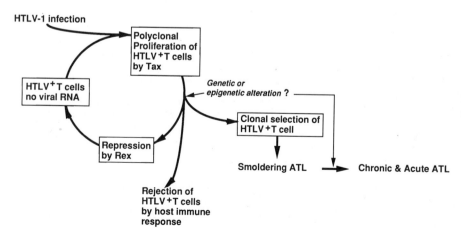

FIGURE 26–28. Phase transition of HTLV-1–infected T cells from the carrier state to malignant ATL. Polyclonal proliferation of HTLV-1–infected T cells leads to immunological rejection by the host, to a latent phase of viral expression, or to clonal selection for leukemogenesis. The clonal selection of infected cells might be influenced by Tax, mutation of one or more cellular genes, or one or more host-specific, epigenetic factors.

Japanese patients have certain common HLA types, an association of HAM/TSP with particular HLA types has been proposed.[112] Asymptomatic members of families of HAM/TSP patients who have the same HLA haplotypes also have high titers of HTLV-1 antibodies. Thus, the HLA types are associated with strong immune responses to HTLV-1 infection. Despite their immunological reaction to HTLV-1 infection, most HAM/TSP patients harbor much larger populations of infected cells than do HTLV-1 carriers at large,[113] an observation attributed to infection of activated T cells. It would be of value to confirm these findings in an endemic area other than Japan.

It is not known how HTLV-1 induces HAM/TSP. Transfusion of seropositive blood can lead to HAM/TSP after an average interval of 2 years.[42] Recently developed procedures for screening for seropositive blood have greatly reduced the risk of acquiring HAM/TSP through transfusion.

Through induction of immunodeficiency, HTLV-1 infection is associated with many diseases other than ATL and HAM/TSP: chronic lung diseases, monoclonal gammopathy, chronic renal failure, strongyloidiasis, nonspecific dermatomycosis, and HTLV-1–associated lymphadenitis and uveitis. Further systematic studies are required to elucidate the exact relationships of these diseases with HTLV-1 infection.

Prevention of HTLV-1 Infection

Infection by HTLV-1 induces production of antibodies to the viral proteins and can be diagnosed by the presence of these antibodies. To this end, assay kits for ELISA, western blotting, and particle agglutination are used for diagnosis. Extracts of HTLV-1–infected cells are used in commercially available kits, and, recently, assays employing recombinant proteins have also been developed. Each system has its advantages and disadvantages, but results can be checked by Western blotting or indirect immunostaining of infected cells, although both of these methods also require further improvement.

Transfusion of seropositive blood results in transmission of HTLV-1 to two thirds of the recipients,[41] but, with the introduction of HTLV-1 screening systems in blood banks, seropositive blood is now routinely rejected in Japan, viral transmission through transfusion has been greatly reduced, and transfusion-related HAM/TSP has been effectively prevented. Application of these systems to populations in all endemic areas is important to prevention of HTLV-1 infection.

The major, natural route of viral transmission is from mother to child via infected T cells in breast milk.[45, 115] Curiously, mothers with high levels of antibodies to Tax protein transmit the virus to their offspring at a higher rate than do those with low titers of Tax antibodies.[116] Tax is the activator of viral gene expression; thus, the high titer of antibody might be thought to prevent viral replication, yet just the opposite is observed. It is possible that efficient replica-

tion of HTLV-1 stimulates antibody production at high levels but that the antibodies do not, in fact, significantly inhibit viral replication.

Given that breast milk is the major source of infection, avoidance of breast-feeding should prevent infection of children. This possibility is being tested using seropositive mothers in Nagasaki City, Japan. By consent, pregnant women are surveyed for HTLV-1 antibodies; those who are seropositive are asked not to breast-feed their infants. The trial is still in progress, but preliminary results indicate a drastic reduction in the incidence of seropositive children, from about 30 per cent to just a few per cent. The early success of this trial provides direct evidence for viral transmission through milk and suggests the possibility of eliminating ATL within a few generations.

Unfortunately, not all children of seropositive mothers who did not breast-feed remained seronegative. These few cases might reflect protocol violation, but studies of animal models do suggest other pathways of viral transmission. For example, when female rats were infected with HTLV-1 by injection of cells infected in vitro, they transmitted the virus to their pups; even some pups that were transferred to uninfected foster mothers immediately after birth were infected. Although preliminary, these findings suggest that neonatal infection or some other means of transmission bears intensive study in the interests of completely preventing viral transmission from mother to child.

Additional problems are involved in studying viral transmission from mother to child. Recent studies of children of seropositive mothers indicate that some of them carry HTLV-1 proviral DNA but have no circulating antibodies to HTLV-1 when they are over 6 months of age and no longer carry maternal antibodies to HTLV-1.[117] These observations are based on results of PCR, which is capable of detecting even one molecule of HTLV-1 DNA, and further analyses are required for confirmation. Nonetheless, these findings imply the existence of unknown mechanisms of viral infection and response by the host that may involve unique immunological properties of the host, a level of gene expression too low to result in an immunological response, or insufficient numbers of proviral copies to induce antibody production.

Epidemiological studies have established that HTLV-1 infects individuals at an early age through breast milk. Within 6 to 12 months of birth, one quarter to one third of children born to seropositive mothers develop antibodies to HTLV-1. A dramatic increase in age-specific rates of seropositivity is observed only in those over 20 years old. Sexual transmission of HTLV-1 from husband to wife may account for a portion of this increase but cannot explain the increase in men. No other means of horizontal transmission has been described. Further investigations of these phenomena are essential to comprehend HTLV-1 viral infection, replication, and pathogenesis in all their complexity. Only then might complete prevention of HTLV-1 infection be attainable.

REFERENCES

1. Weiss, R., Teich, N., Varmus, H., and Coffin, J. (eds.): RNA Tumor Viruses. Cold Spring, Cold Spring Harbor Laboratory, 1985.

2. Johann, S. V., Gibbons, J. J., and O'Hara, B.: GLVR1, a receptor for Gibbon ape leukemia virus, is homologous to a phosphate permease of Neurospora crassa and is expressed at high levels in the brain and thymus. J. Virol. 66:1635, 1992.

3. Dalgleish, A. G., Beverly, C. L., Calpman, P. R., Crawford, D. H., Greaves, M. F., and Weiss, R. A.: The CD4 antigen is an essential component of the receptor for the AIDS retrovirus. Nature 312:763, 1985.

4. Hayward, W. S., Neel, B. G., and Astrin, S.: Activation of a cellular oncogene by promoter insertion in ALV-induced lymphoid leukosis. Nature 290:475, 1981.

5. Fung, Y. K., Lewis, W. G., Crittenden, L. B., and Kung, H. J.: Activation of the cellular oncogene c-erb B by LTR insertion: Molecular basis for induction of erythroblastosis by avian leukosis virus. Cell 33:375, 1983.

6. Nusse, R., and Varmus, H. E.: Many tumors induced by the mouse mammary tumor virus contain a provirus integrated in the same region of the host genome. Cell 31:99, 1982.

7. Chatis, P. A., Holland, C. A., Hartley, J. W., Rowe, W. P., and Hopkins, N.: Role for the 3' end of the genome in determining disease specificities of Friend and Moloney leukemia viruses. Proc. Natl. Acad. Sci. USA. 80:4408, 1983.

8. Yoshida, M., Seiki, M., Yamaguchi K., and Takatsuki, K.: Monoclonal integration of HTLV in all primary tumors of adult T-cell leukemia suggests causative role of HTLV in the disease. Proc. Natl. Acad. Sci. USA 81:2534, 1984.

9. Uchiyama, T., Yodoi, J., Sagawa, K., Takatsuki, K., and Uchino, H.: Adult T cell leukemia: Clinical and hematological features of 16 cases. Blood 50:481, 1977.

10. Poiesz, B. J., Ruscetti, F. W., Gazdar, A. F., Bunn, P. A., Minna, J. D., and Gallo, R. C.: Detection and isolation of type C retrovirus particles from fresh and cultured lymphocytes of a patient with cutaneous T-cell lymphoma. Proc. Natl. Acad. Sci. USA 77:7415, 1980.

11. Miyoshi, I., Kubonishi, I., Yoshimoto, S., Akagi, T., Ohtsuki, Y., Shiraishi, Y., Nagata, K., and Hinuma, Y.: Type C virus particles in a cord T cell line derived by cocultivating normal human cord leukocytes and human leukemic T cells. Nature 294:770, 1981.

12. Miyoshi, I., Kubonishi, I., Sumida, M., Hiraki, S., Kimura, I., Miyamoto, K., and Sato, J.: A novel T cell line derived from adult T cell leukemia. Jpn. J. Cancer Res. (Gann) 71:155, 1980.

13. Hinuma, Y., Nagata, K., Misaka, M., Nakai, M., Matsumoto, T., Kinoshita, K., Shirakawa, S., and Miyoshi, I.: Adult T cell leukemia: Antigen in an ATL cell line and detection of antibodies to the antigen in human sera. Proc. Natl. Acad. Sci. USA 78:6476, 1981.

14. Hinuma, Y., Komoda, H., Chosa, T., Kondo, T., Kohara, M., Takenaka, T., Kikuchi, M., Ichimaru, M., Yunoki, K., Sato, I., Matsuo, R., Takiuchi, Y., Uchino, H., and Hamaoka, M.: Antibodies to adult T-cell leukemia-virus-associated antigen (ATLA) in sera from patients with ATL and controls in Japan: A nation-wide sero-epidemiologic study. Int. J. Cancer 29:631, 1982.

15. Blattner, W., Kalyanaraman, V. S., Robert-Guroff, M., Lister, T. A., Galton, D. A., Sarin, P. S., Crawford, M. H., Catovsky, D., Greaves, M., and Gallo, R. C.: The human type C retrovirus, HTLV in blacks from the Caribbean region, and relationship to adult T-cell leukemia/lymphoma. Int. J. Cancer 30:257, 1982.

16. Yoshida, M., Miyoshi, I., and Hinuma, Y.: Isolation and characterization of retrovirus from cell lines of human adult T cell leukemia and its implication in the disease. Proc. Natl. Acad. Sci. USA 79:2031, 1982.

17. Kalyanaraman, V. S., Sarngadharan, M. G., Nakao, Y., Ito, Y., Aoki, T., and Gallo, R. C.: Natural antibodies to the structural protein (p24) of the human T cell leukemia (lymphoma) retrovirus found in sera of leukemia patients in Japan. Proc. Natl. Acad. Sci. USA 79:1653, 1982.

18. Seiki, M., Hattori, S., Hirayama, Y., and Yoshida, M.: Human adult T cell leukemia virus: Complete nucleotide sequence of the provirus genome integrated in leukemia cell DNA. Proc. Natl. Acad. Sci. USA 80:3618, 1983.

19. Kalyanaraman, V. S., Sarngadharan, M. G., Robert-Guroff, M., Miyoshi, I., Blayney, D., Golde, D., and Gallo, R. C.: A new subtype of human T cell leukemia virus (HTLV-II) associated with a T cell variant of hairy T cell leukemia. Science 218:571, 1982.

20. Chen, I. S. Y., McLaghlin, J., Gasson, J. C., Clark, S. C., and Golde, D. W.: Molecular characterization of genome of a novel human T cell leukemia virus. Nature 305:502, 1983.

21. Shimotohno, K., Golde, D. W., Miwa, M., Sugimura, T., and Chen, I. S. Y.: Nucleotide sequence analysis of the long terminal repeat of human T-cell leukemia virus type II. Proc. Natl. Acad. Sci. USA 81:1079, 1984.

22. Lee, H., Swanson, P., Shorty, V. S., Zack, J. A., Rosenblatt, J. D., and Chen, I. S. Y.: High rate of HTLV-II infection in seropositive IV drug abusers in New Orleans. Science 244:471, 1989.

23. Miyoshi, I., Yoshimoto, S., Fujishita, M., Ohtsuki, Y., Taguchi, H., Shiraishi, Y., Akagi, T., and Minezawa, M.: Isolation in culture of a type C virus from Japanese monkey seropositive to adult T cell leukemia-associated antigens. Jpn. J. Cancer Res. (Gann) 74:323, 1983.

24. Ishikawa, K., Fukusawa, M., Tsujimoto, H., Else, J. G., Ishakia, M., Ubhi, N. K., Ishida, T., Takenaka, O., Kawamoto, Y., and Shotake, T.: Serological survey and virus isolation of simian T cell leukemia/T-lymphotropic virus type I(STLV01) in non human primates in their native countries. Int. J. Cancer 40:233, 1987.

25. Komuro, A., Watanabe, T., Miyoshi, I., Hayami, M., Tsujimoto, H., Seiki, M., and Yoshida, M.: Detection and characterization of simian retroviruses homologous to human T-cell leukemia virus type I. Virology 138:373, 1984.

26. Tsujimoto, H., Seiki, M., Nakamura, H., Watanabe, T., Sakakibara, I., Sasagawa, A., Honjo, S., Hayami, M., and Yoshida, M.: Adult T-cell leukemia-like disease in monkey naturally infected with simian retrovirus related to human T-cell leukemia virus type I. Jpn. J. Cancer Res. (Gann) 76:911, 1985.

27. Sagata, N., Yasunaga, T., Tsuzuku-Kawamura, J., Ohishi, K., Ogawa, Y., and Ikawa, Y.: Complete nucleotide sequence of the genome of bovine leukemia virus. Its evolutionary relationship. Proc. Natl. Acad. Sci. USA 82:677, 1985.

28. Gotoh, Y., Sugamura, K., and Hinuma, Y.: Healthy carriers of a human retrovirus, adult T cell leukemia virus (ATLV): Demonstration by clonal culture of ATLV carrying T cells from peripheral blood. Proc. Natl. Acad. Sci. USA 79:4780, 1982.

29. Ratner, L., Josephs, S. F., Starcich, B., Hahn, B., Shaw, G. M., Gallo, R. C., and Wong-Staal, F.: Nucleotide sequence analysis of a variant of human T cell leukemia virus (HTLV-Ib) provirus with a deletion in pX-I. J. Virol. 54:781, 1985.

30. Yanagihara, R., Nerurkar, V. R., and Ajdukiewicz, A. B.: Comparison between strains of human T lymphotropic virus type I isolated from inhabitants of the Solomon islands and Papua New Guinea. J. Infect. Dis. 164:443, 1991.

31. Tajima, K., Tominaga, S., Suchi, T., Kawagoe, T., Komoda, H., Hinuma, Y., Oda, T., and Fujita, K.: Epidemiological analysis of the distribution of antibody to adult T cell leukemia virus associated antigen: Possible horizontal transmission of adult T cell leukemia virus. Jpn. J. Cancer Res. (Gann) 73:893, 1982.

32. Watanabe, T.: HTLV type I (U.S. isolate) and ATLV (Japanese isolate) are the same species of human retrovirus. Virology 133:238, 1984.

33. Tateno, M., Kondo, N., Itoh, T., Chubachi, T., Togashi, T., and Yoshiki, T.: Rat lymphoid cell lines with human T cell leukemia virus production. I. Biological and serological characterization. J. Exp. Med. 159:1105, 1984.

34. Miyoshi, I., Yoshimoto, S., Taguchi, H., Kubonishi, I., Fujish-

ita, M., Ohtsuki, Y., Shiraishi, Y., and Akagi, T.: Transformation of rabbit lymphocytes with adult T cell leukemia virus. Gann (Jpn. J. Cancer Res.) 74:1, 1983.

35. Popovic, M., Lange-Wantzin, G., Sarin, P. S., Mann, D., and Gallo, R. C.: Transformation of human umbilical cord blood T cells by human T cell leukemia/lymphoma virus. Proc. Natl. Acad. Sci. USA 80:5402, 1983.

36. Wano, Y., Uchiyama, T., Fukui, K., Maeda, M., Uchino, H., and Yodoi, J.: Characterization of human interleukin 2 receptor (Tac antigen) in normal and leukemic T cells. Coexpression of normal and aberrant receptors on HUT 102 cells. J. Immunol. 132:3005, 1984.

37. Hattori, T., Uchiyama, T., Tobinai, K., Takatsuki, K., and Uchino, H.: Surface phenotype of Japanese adult T-cell leukemia cells characterized by monoclonal antibodies. Blood 58:645, 1981.

38. Jeang, K. T., Widen, S. G., Semmens, O. J., and Wilson, S. H.: HTLV-1 trans-activator protein, Tax, is a trans-repressor of the human β-polymerase. Science 247:1082, 1990.

39. Hinuma, Y., Gotoh, Y., Sugamura, K., Nagata, K., Goto, T., Nakai, M., Kamada, N., Matsumoto, T., and Kinoshita, K.: A retrovirus associated with human adult T cell leukemia: In vitro activation. Jpn. J. Cancer Res. (Gann) 73:341, 1982.

40. Kinoshita, T., Shimoyama, M., Tobinai, K., Ito, M., Ito, S., Ikeda, S., Tajima, K., Shimotohno, K., and Sugimura, T.: Detection of mRNA for the tax$_1$/rex$_1$ gene of human T cell leukemia virus type I in fresh peripheral blood mononuclear cells of adult T-cell leukemia patients and viral carriers by using the polymerase chain reaction. Proc. Natl. Acad. Sci. USA 86:5620, 1989.

41. Okochi, K., Sato, H., and Hinuma, Y.: A retrospective study of transmission of adult T cell leukemia virus by blood transfusion: Seroconversion in recipients. Vox Sang. 46:245, 1983.

42. Osame, M., Izumo, S., Tagata, A., Matsumoto, M., Matsumoto, T., Sonoda, S., Tara, M., and Shibata, Y.: Blood transfusion and HTLV-1 associated myelopathy. Lancet 2:104, 1986.

43. Robert-Guroff, M., Weiss, S. H., Giron, J. A., Jennings, A. M., Ginzgurg, H. M., Margolis, I. B., Blattner, W. A., and Gallo, R. C.: Prevalence of antibodies to HTLV-I, -II and -III in intravenous drug abusers from an AIDS endemic region. J.A.M.A. 255:3133, 1986.

44. Kusuhara, K., Sonoda, S., Takahashi, K., Tokunaga, K., Fukushige, J., and Ueda, K.: Mother to child transmission of human T cell leukemia virus type I (HTLV-I): A fifteen year follow up in Okinawa. Int. J. Cancer 40:755, 1987.

45. Hino, S., Yamaguchi, K., Katamine, S., Sugiyama, H., Amagasaki, T., Kinoshita, K., Yoshida, Y., Doi, H., Tsuji, Y., and Miyamoto, T.: Mother to child transmission of human T cell leukemia virus type I. Jpn. J. Cancer Res. (Gann) 76:474, 1985.

46. Yoshida, M.: Expression of the HTLV-1 genome and its association with a unique T-cell malignancy. Biochim. Biophys. Acta 970:145, 1987.

47. Seiki, M., Hattori, S., and Yoshida, M.: Human adult T-cell leukemia virus: Molecular cloning of the provirus DNA and the unique terminal structure. Proc. Natl. Acad. Sci. USA 79:6899, 1982.

48. Kiyokawa, T., Seiki, M., Imagawa, K., Shimizu, F., and Yoshida, M.: Identification of a protein (p40x) encoded by a unique sequence *pX* of human T-cell leukemia virus type I. Gann (Jpn. J. Cancer Res.) 75:747, 1984.

49. Haseltine, W. A., Sodroski, J., Patarca, R., Briggs, D., Perkins, D., and Wong-Staal, F.: Structure of 3' terminal region of type II human T lymphotropic virus: Evidence for new coding region. Science 225:419, 1984.

50. Lee, T. H., Coligan, J. E., Sodroski, J., Haseltine, W. A., Salahuddin, S. Z., Wong-Staal, F., Gallo, R. C., and Essex, M.: Antigens encoded by the 3' terminal region of human T cell leukemia virus: Evidence for a functional gene flanked by the env gene and 3'LTR. Science 226:57, 1984.

51. Slamon, D. J., Press, M. F., Souza, L. M., Cline, M. J., Golde, D. W., Gasson, J. C., and Chen, I. S. Y.: Studies of the putative transforming protein of the type I human T cell leukemia virus. Science 228:1427, 1985.

52. Kiyokawa, T., Seiki, M., Iwashita, S., Imagawa, K., Shimizu, F., and Yoshida, M.: P27x-III and p21x-III, proteins encoded by the pX sequence of human T-cell leukemia virus type I. Proc. Natl. Acad. Sci. USA 82:8359, 1985.

53. Sodroski, J. G., Rosen, C. A., and Haseltine, W. A.: Trans-acting transcriptional activation of the long terminal repeat of human T lymphotropic viruses in infected cells. Science 225:381, 1984.

54. Fujisawa, J., Seiki, M., Kiyokawa, T., and Yoshida, M.: Functional activation of long terminal repeat of human T-cell leukemia virus type I by trans-activator. Proc. Natl. Acad. Sci. USA 82:2277, 1985.

55. Felber, B. K., Paskalis, H., Kleinman-Ewing, C., Wong-Staal, F., and Pavlakis, G. N.: The pX protein of HTLV-1 is a transcriptional activator of its long terminal repeats. Science 229:675, 1985.

56. Chen, I. S. Y., Slamon, D. J., Rosenblatt, J. D., Shah, N. P., Quan, S. G., and Wachsman, W.: The x gene is essential for HTLV replication. Science 229:54, 1985.

57. Inoue, J., Seiki, M., Taniguchi, T., Tsuru, S., and Yoshida, M.: Induction of interleukin 2 receptor gene expression by p40x encoded by human T-cell leukemia virus type I. EMBO J. 5:2883, 1986.

58. Inoue, J., Seiki, M., and Yoshida, M.: The second pX product p27x-III of HTLV-1 is required for gag gene expression. FEBS Lett. 209:187, 1986.

59. Inoue, J., Yoshida, M., and Seiki, M.: Transcriptional (p40x) and post-transcriptional (p27x-III) regulators are required for the expression and replication of human T cell leukemia virus type I genes. Proc. Natl. Acad. Sci. USA 84:3635, 1987.

60. Hidaka, M., Inoue, M., Yoshida, M., and Seiki, M.: Post-transcriptional regulator (rex) of HTLV-1 initiates expression of viral structural proteins but suppresses expression of regulatory proteins. EMBO J. 7:519, 1988.

61. Nagashima, K., Yoshida, M., and Seiki, M.: A single species of pX mRNA of HTLV-1 encodes trans-activator p40x and two other phosphoproteins. J. Virol. 60:394, 1986.

62. Fujisawa, J., Seiki, M., Sato, M., and Yoshida, M.: A transcriptional enhancer of HTLV-1 is responsible for trans-activation mediated by p40x of HTLV-1. EMBO J. 5:713, 1986.

63. Shimotohno, K., Takano, M., Teruuchi, T., and Miwa, M.: Requirement of multiple copies of a 21-nucleotide sequence in the U3 regions of human T-cell leukemia virus type I and type II long terminal repeats for trans-acting activation of transcription. Proc. Natl. Acad. Sci. USA 83:8112, 1986.

64. Fujisawa, J., Toita, M., and Yoshida, M.: A unique enhancer element for the transactivator (p40tax) of human T cell leukemia virus type 1 from cAMP and TPA-responsive elements. J. Virol. 63:3234, 1989.

65. Seiki, M., Hikikoshi, A., Taniguchi, T., and Yoshida, M.: Expression of the pX gene of HTLV-1: General splicing mechanism in the HTLV family. Science 228:1532, 1985.

66. Yoshimura, T., Fujisawa, J., and Yoshida, M.: Multiple cDNA clones encoding nuclear proteins that bind to the tax-dependent enhancer of HTLV-1: All contain a leucine zipper structure and basic amino acid domain. EMBO J. 9:2537, 1989.

67. Maekawa, T., Sakura, H., Kanei, C., Sudo, T., Yoshimura, T., Fujisawa, J., Yoshida, M., and Ishii, S.: Leucine zipper structure of the protein CRE-BP1 binding to the cyclic AMP response element in brain. EMBO J. 8:2023, 1989.

68. Hai, T., Liu, F., Coukos, W.J., and Green, M.R.: Transcription factor ATF cDNA clones: An extensive family of leucine zipper proteins able to selectively form DNA-binding heterodimers. Genes Dev. 3:2083, 1989.

69. Tsujimoto, A., Nyuunoya, H., Morita, T., Sato, T., and Shimotohno, K.: Isolation of cDNAs for DNA binding proteins which specifically bind to a tax-responsive element in the long terminal repeat of human T cell leukemia virus type I. J. Virol. 65:1420, 1991.

70. Landshulz, W.H., Johnson, P. F., and McKnight, S.L.: The

leucine zipper: A hypothetical structure common to a new class of DNA binding proteins. Science 240:1759, 1988.

71. Maguire, K., Shi, X.P., Horikoshi, N., Rappaport, J., Rosenberg, M., and Weinmann, R.: Interaction between adenovirus E1A and members of the AP-1 family of cellular transcription factors. Oncogene 6:1417, 1991.

72. Ono, S. J., Bazik, V., Levi, B. Z., Ozato, K., and Strominger, J. L.: Transcription of subset of human class II major histocompatibility complex genes is regulated by a nucleoprotein complex that contains c-fos or an antigenically related protein. Proc. Natl. Acad. Sci. USA 88:4304, 1991.

73. Liu, F., and Green, M. R.: A specific member of the ATF transcription factor family can mediate transcription activation by adenovirus Ela protein. Cell 61:1217, 1990.

74. Maekawa, T., Matsuda, S., Fujisawa, J.-I., Yoshida, M., and Ishii, S.: Cyclic AMP response element-binding protein, CRE-BP1, mediates the E1A-induced but not the Tax induced *trans*-activation. Oncogene 6:627, 1991.

75. Jeang, K. T., Shank, P. R., and Kumar, A.: Transcriptional activation of homologous viral long terminal repeats by the human immunodeficiency virus type 1 or the human T-cell leukemia virus type 1 that occurs in the absence of de novo protein synthesis. Proc. Natl. Acad. Sci. USA 85:8291, 1988.

76. Miyatake, S., Seiki, M., Malefijt, R. D., Heike, T., Fujisawa, J., Takebe, Y., Nishida, J., Shlomai, J., Yokota, T., Yoshida, M., Arai, K., and Arai, N.: Activation of T cell-derived lymphokine genes in T cells and fibroblasts: Effects of human T cell leukemia virus type I p40^{tax} protein and bovine papilloma virus encoded E2 protein. Nucleic Acid Res. 16:6547, 1988.

77. Fujii, M., Sassone-Corsi, P., and Verma, I. M.: C-fos promoter trans-activation by the tax$_1$ protein of human T-cell leukemia virus type I. Proc. Natl. Acad. Sci. USA 85:8526, 1988.

78. Fujii, M., Niki, T., Mori, T., Matsuda, T., Matsui, M., Nomura, N., and Seiki, M.: HTLV-1 Tax induces expression of various immediate early serum responsive genes. Oncogene 6:1023, 1991.

79. Watanabe, T., Yamaguchi, K., Takatsuki, K., Osame, M., and Yoshida, M.: Constitutive expression of parathyroid hormone-related protein (PTHrP) gene in HTLV-1 carriers and adult T cell leukemia patients which can be trans-activated by HTLV-1 tax gene. J. Exp. Med. 172:759, 1990.

80. Sawada, M., Suzumura, A., Yoshida, M., and Marunouchi, T.: Human T-cell leukemia virus type I *trans* activator induces class I major histocompatibility complex antigen expression in glial cells. J. Virol. 64:4002, 1990.

81. Leung, K., and Nabel, G. J.: HTLV-1 transactivator induces interleukin-2 receptor expression through an NF-κB-like factor. Nature (London) 333:776, 1988.

82. Lowenthal, J. W., Böhnlein, E., Ballard, D. W., and Greene, W.: Regulation of interleukin 2 receptor a subunit (Tac or CD25 antigen) gene expression: Binding of inducible nuclear proteins to discrete promoter sequences correlates with transcriptional activation. Proc. Natl. Acad. Sci. USA 85:4468, 1988.

83. Fan, C.-M., and Maniatis, T.: Generation of p50 subunit of NF-κB by processing of p105 through an ATP-dependent pathway. Nature 354:395, 1991.

84. Baeuerle, P. A., and Baltimore, D.: Activation of DNA-binding activity in an apparently cytoplasmic precursor of the NF-κB transcription factor. Cell 53:211, 1988.

85. Baeuerle, P. A., and Baltimore, D.: I kappa-B: A specific inhibition of the NF-κB transcription factor. Science 242:540, 1988.

86. Blank, V., Kourilsky, P., and Israel, A.: Cytoplasmic retention, DNA binding and processing of the NF-κB procursor are controlled by a small region in its C-terminus. EMBO J. 10:4159, 1991.

87. Fujisawa, J., Toita, M., Yoshimura, T., and Yoshida, M.: The indirect association of human T-cell leukemia virus *tax* fusion protein with DNA results in transcriptional activation. J. Virol. 65:4525, 1991.

88. Yoshida, M., and Seiki, M.: Molecular biology of HTLV-1: Biological significance of viral genes in its replication and leukemogenesis. *In* Gallo, R. C., and Wong-Staal, F. (eds.): Retrovirus Biology and Human Disease. New York, Marcel Dekker, 1989, pp. 161–186.

89. Toyoshima, H., Itoh, M., Inoue, J., Seiki, M., Takaku, F., and Yoshida, M.: Secondary structure of the HTLV-1 rex responsive element is essential for rex regulation of RNA processing and transport of unspliced RNAs. J. Virol. 64:2825, 1990.

90. Feinberg, M. B., Jarrett, R. F., Aldovini, A., Gallo, R. C., and Wong-Staal, F.: HTLV-III expression and production involve complex regulation at the levels of splicing and translation of viral RNA. Cell 46:807, 1986.

91. Zapp, M. L., and Green, M. R.: Sequence-specific RNA binding by the HIV-1 Rev protein. Nature 342:714, 1989.

92. Malim, M. H., Hauber, J., Fenrick, R., and Cullen, B. R.: Immunodeficiency virus rev trans-activator modulates the expression of the viral regulatory genes. Nature 335:181, 1988.

93. Malim, M. H., Hauber, J., Le, S.-Y., Maizel, J. V., and Cullen, B. R.: The HIV-1 rev trans-activator acts through a structured target sequence to activate nuclear export of unspliced viral mRNA. Nature 338:254, 1989.

94. Rimsky, L., Hauber, J., Dukovich, M., Malim, M. H., Langlois, A., Cullen, B. K., and Greene, W. C.: Functional replacement of the HIV-1 rev protein by the HTLV-1 rex protein. Nature 335:738, 1988.

95. Inoue, J., Itoh, M., Akizawa, T., Toyoshima, H., and Yoshida, M.: HTLV-1 Rex protein accumulates unspliced RNA in the nucleus as well as in cytoplasm. Oncogene 6:1753, 1991.

96. Knight, D. M., Flomerfelt, F. A., and Gyrayab, J.: Expression of art/trs protein of HIV and study of its role in viral envelope synthesis. Science 236:837, 1987.

97. Takatsuki, K., Yamaguchi, K., Kawano, F., Hattori, T., Nishimura, H., Tsuda, H., Sanada, I., Nakada, K., and Itai, Y.: Clinical diversity in adult T-cell leukemia/lymphoma. Cancer Res. 45 (Suppl.):4644, 1985.

98. Yoshida, M., Seiki, M., Hattori, S., and Watanabe, T.: Genome structure of human T cell leukemia virus and its involvement in the development of adult T-cell leukemia. *In* Human T-cell Leukemia/Lymphoma Virus. Cold Spring, N.Y., Cold Spring Harbor Laboratory, 1984, pp. 141–148.

99. Ueshima, T., Fukuhara, S., Hattori, T., Uchiyama, T., Takatsuku, K., and Uchino, H.: Chromosome studies in adult T cell leukemia in Japan: Significance of trisomy 7. Blood 58:420, 1981.

100. Sadamori, N., Nishino, K., Kusano, M., Tomonaga, Y., Tagawa, M., Yao, E., Sasagawa, I., Nakamura, H., and Ichimaru, M.: Significance of chromosome 14 anomaly at band 14q11 in Japanese patients with adult T cell leukemia. Cancer 58:2244, 1986.

101. Miyamoto, K., Tomita, N., Ishii, A., Nonaka, H., Kondo, T., Tanaka, T., and Katasjima, K.: Chromosome abnormalities of leukemia cells in adult patients with T cell leukemia. J. Natl. Cancer Inst. 73:353, 1984.

102. Shimoyama, M., Shimotohno, K., Miwa, M., et al.: Adult T-cell leukemia/lymphoma not associated with human T-cell leukemia virus type I. Proc. Natl. Acad. Sci. USA 83:4524, 1986.

103. Seiki, M., Eddy, R., Shows, T. B., and Yoshida, M.: Nonspecific integration of the HTLV provirus genome into adult T-cell leukemia cells. Nature 309:640, 1984.

104. Grassman, R., Dengler, C., Muller-Fleckenstein, I., Fleckenstein, B., McGuire, K., Dokhelar, M., Sodroski, J., and Haseltine, W.: Transformation to continuous growth of primary human T lymphocytes by human T cell leukemia virus type I X-region genes transduced by a *Herpesvirus saimiri* vector. Proc. Natl. Acad. Sci. USA 86:3351, 1989.

105. Tanaka, A., Takahashi, C., Yamaoka, S., Nosaka, T., Maki, M., and Hatanaka, M.: Oncogenic transformation by the tax gene of human T cell leukemia virus type I in vitro. Proc. Natl. Acad. Sci. USA 87:1071, 1990.

106. Willems, L., Heremans, H., Chen, G., Portetelle, D., Billiau, A., Burny, A., and Kettmenn, R.: Cooperation between

bovine leukemia virus transactivator and Haras oncogene product in cellular transformation. EMBO J. 9:1577, 1990.

107. Yoshida, M., and Seiki, M.: Recent advances in the molecular biology of HTLV-1: Trans-activation of viral and cellular genes. Annu. Rev. Immunol. 5:541, 1987.

108. Gessain, A., Barin, F., Vernant, J. C., Gout, O., Maurs, L., Calender, A., and De The, G.: Antibodies to human T lymphotropic virus type 1 in patients with tropical spastic paraparesis. Lancet 2:407, 1985.

109. Rodgers-Johnson, P., Gajdusek, D. C., Morgan, O., Zaninovic, V., Sarin, P., and Graham, D. S.: HTLV-1 and HTLV-III antibodies and tropical spastic paraparesis. Lancet 2:1247, 1985.

110. Osame, M., Matsumoto, M., Usuku, K., Izumo, S., Ijichi, N., Amitani, H., Tara, M., and Igata, A.: Chronic progressive myelopathy associated with elevated antibodies to human T-lymphotropic virus type 1 and adult T-cell leukemia-like cells. Ann. Neurol. 21:117, 1987.

111. Osame, M., Usuku, K., Izumo, S., Ijichi, N., Amitani, H., Igata, A., Matsumoto, M., and Tara, M.: HTLV-1 associated myelopathy, a new clinical entity. Lancet 1:1031, 1986.

112. Usuku, K., Sonoda, S., Osame, M., Yashiki, S., Takahashi, K., Matsumoto, M., Sawada, T., Tsuji, K., Tara, M., and Igata, A.: HLA haplotype-linked high immune responsiveness against HTLV-1 in HTLV-1-associated myelopathy: Com-

parison with adult T-cell leukemia/lymphoma. Ann. Neurol. 23:143, 1988.

113. Yoshida, M., Osame, M., Kawai, H., Toita, M., Kuwasaki, N., Nishida, Y., Hiraki, Y., Takahashi, K., Nomura, K., Sonoda, S., Eiraku, N., Ijichi, S., and Usuku, K.: Increased replication of HTLV-1 in HTLV-1-associated myelopathy. Ann. Neurol. 26:331, 1989.

114. Nerenberg, M., Hinrichs, S. H., Reynolds, R. K., Khoury, G., and Jay, G.: The tat gene of human T lymphotropic virus type I induces mesenchymal tumors in transgenic mice. Science 237:1324, 1987.

115. Kinoshita, K., Amagasaki, T., Hino, S., Dio, H., Yamanouchi, K., Ban, N., Momita, S., Ikeda, S., Kamihira, S., Ichimaru, M., Katamine, S., Miyamoto, T., Tsuji, Y., Ishimaru, T., Yamabe, T., Ito, M., Kamura, S., and Tsuda, T.: Milk-borne transmission of HTLV-1 from carrier mothers to their children. Jpn. J. Cancer Res. (Gann) 78:674, 1987.

116. Hino, S., Doi, H., Yoshikumi, H., Sugiyama, H., Ishimaru, T., Yamabe, T., Tsuji, Y., and Miyamoto, T.: HTLV-1 carrier mothers with high titer antibody are at high risk as a source of infection. Jpn. J. Cancer Res. (Gann) 78:1156, 1986.

117. Saito, S., Ando, Y., Furuki, K., Kakimoto, K., Tanigawa, T., Moriyama, I., Ichijo, M., Nakamura, M., Ohtani, K., and Sugamua, K.: Detection of HTLV-I genome in sero-negative infants born to HTLV-I seropositive mothers by polymerase chain reaction. Jpn. J. Cancer Res. (Gann) 80:808, 1989.

C. HERPESVIRUSES

Bill Sugden

Herpesviruses cause a variety of diseases in animals and people. Chickenpox and infectious mononucleosis can arise soon after infection, whereas herpetic cold sores, retinitis in immunocompromised patients, and Burkitt's lymphoma can arise years after people are first infected with these viruses. These varied diseases reflect disparate virus-host relationships. The outcome of an infection with a given herpesvirus depends on the cell tropism of that virus, on the molecular details of its life cycle, and on the host's immune response to the infecting virus. In addition, the ability to prevent herpesviral diseases or to intervene in ongoing infections also requires an appreciation of each virus's life cycle in cells and the organism's reaction to that infection. This appreciation has led to a vaccine that prevents a herpesvirus-induced lymphoma in chickens and to antiviral drugs that are effective in the treatment of some herpesviral diseases in people. Additional successful therapies will flow only from an increased understanding of the modus operandi of these viruses as cellular parasites and the host's responses to them.

Herpesviruses take their less than salubrious-sounding name (meaning "creeping, slimy liquid") from lesions that some of them induce. They constitute a large family of viruses with members capable of infecting species from channel catfish to man. Members share similarities in virion structure: The virus particles are enveloped and contain glycoproteins within this lipid coat. The envelope covers an amorphous layer termed either the tegument or matrix, which itself covers an icosahedral structure of 162 protein

capsomers. This structure houses a DNA genome as the kernel of these viruses. Their DNA genomes are all duplex, linear molecules that range in length from 134,000 bp for channel catfish virus[1] to 230,000 bp for human cytomegalovirus (HCMV).[2] The latter virus is, therefore, currently distinguished as having the largest genome of any known virus.

The family of Herpesviridae has been divided into three subfamilies on the basis of their differing biological properties.[3] The α-herpesviruses usually have a broad host range and usually are neurotropic; they include human herpes simplex viruses types 1 and 2 (HSV-1 and HSV-2) and human varicella-zoster virus (VZV). The β-herpesviruses have a restricted host range and a protracted replicative cycle. For example, the β-herpesvirus HCMV can be clinically identified by its efficient propagation only in human fibroblast strains and its plaques requiring 7 to 14 days to form in these cells. By way of contrast, HSV-1 yields plaques in a variety of cells in 2 to 3 days. The α-herpesviruses are characterized both by their having a limited host range and by their infecting lymphoid cells in vivo and in cell culture. Epstein-Barr virus (EBV) is a member of this subfamily in the human. HCMV and EBV are herpesviruses that are described in detail*

---

*Several excellent reviews have served as general sources for this description. They are Ho, M.: Cytomegalovirus Biology and Infection, 2nd ed. (New York, Plenum Medical Book Company, 1991); Kieff, E., and Liebowitz, D.: Epstein-Barr virus and its replication, and Miller, G.: Epstein-Barr virus biology, pathogenesis, and medical aspects, both in Fields, B. N., and Knipe, D.M. (eds.): Virology (New York, Raven Press), 1990, pp. 1889–1920 and 1921–1958.

because they both are human pathogens and infect hematopoietic cells in vivo and in vitro.

STRUCTURAL PROPERTIES OF HERPESVIRUSES

The large size of the viral DNA indicates that herpesviruses encode much information. Many of their genes are devoted to the regulation of and coding for structural proteins of the viral particle. This complexity of viral information is consistent with the complexity of the large structure of the viral particles. The particles range in size from 150 to 300 nm, which is just below the edge of visibility in a light microscope. They are pleomorphic, and stocks of HCMV, for example, contain an array of particles, some of which lack envelopes and some of which lack DNA.[4] The infectious particles in such a stock are presumed to be fully enveloped and must contain viral DNA; the DNA alone can be infectious.[5] The size and density of herpesviral particles make them extremely difficult to purify because intact and fragmented cellular membrane-bound organelles copurify with them. Therefore, it can never be assumed that a "purified" sample of virus is free of cellular contaminants. This lack of purity obviously makes analyses of viral components difficult. This difficulty is minimized in studies of HSV-1, in part because this virus replicates to high titers (10^9 infectious units or 10^{11} particles per milliliter of cell culture fluid) in cell culture so that viral particles can predominate over cellular debris. The well-studied structure derived for the HSV-1 particle has served as a paradigm for that of other herpesviruses, and often features of the latter's particles are assumed to be identical with those established for HSV-1.

Particles of herpesviruses are surrounded by lipid envelopes derived from the cells in which the viruses assemble. Herpesviruses encode an array of glycoproteins that are embedded in these lipid bilayers and that have been of particular interest, both as targets for the humoral immune response and as potentially required viral ligands for the cellular receptors that mediate viral binding and entry into cells. The glycoproteins in viral envelopes can be detected by labeling their sugar moieties in partially purified viral preparations.[6] They can elicit neutralizing antibodies in immunized animals[7] and in infected human beings.[8] One glycoprotein encoded by EBV, gp340, serves not only to elicit neutralizing antibodies[9] and a cellular immune response,[10] but also to bind a cellular glycoprotein, CD21, which is a receptor for the C3d component of complement and for EBV.[11, 12] The glycoprotein gp340 of EBV is currently being tested as a vaccine for EBV.[13]

Beneath the herpesviral envelopes is found an amorphous layer of material termed the tegument or matrix. This portion of the viral particle contains specific proteins. For example, the tegument of HCMV contains a polypeptide of 33 kDa that can bind either the Fc moiety of human immunoglobulin or β_2-microglobulin[14] (Fig. 26–29). The tegument covers the

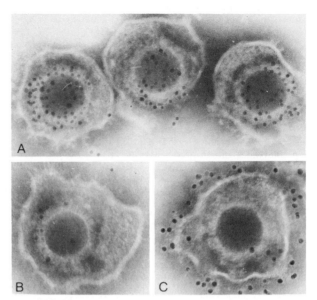

FIGURE 26–29. Electron microscopic detection of specific viral antigens localizes them to specific regions of human cytomegalovirus (HCMV) particles. The virion envelope, the amorphous tegument within it, and the nucleocapsid that houses the viral DNA are clearly visible. The antigens are detected by coupling antibodies to them with colloidal gold, which is electron dense. A viral antigen that binds the Fc portion of immunoglobulin proteins is localized to the tegument in A; this viral antigen does not efficiently bind the Fab portion of immunoglobulin in B; a viral glycoprotein is localized to the virion envelope in C. (From Stannard, L. M., and Hardie, D. R.: An Fc receptor for human immunoglobulin G is located within the tegument of human cytomegalovirus. J. Virol. 65: 3411–3415, 1991; with permission.)

core or nucleocapsid, which is icosahedral in shape and is composed of 162 subunits or capsomers. Although several proteins form these subunits, a single major polypeptide within the HCMV nucleocapsid accounts for 90 per cent of its mass.[2, 15]

The nucleocapsids house the polyamine-coated DNA genomes of herpesviruses.[16] These linear, double-stranded molecules encode between 100 and 200 genes. As the structures of viral particles of herpesviruses are related, so too are their DNAs. Homologues for 30 open reading frames (ORFs) in HCMV are found in EBV.[2] In addition, related tracts of ORFs have been identified in these two viral genomes, which, however, display different relative orientations (Fig. 26–30).[17] This clustering of related genes affirms the relatedness of HCMV and EBV DNAs and is consistent with their having evolved from a common ancestor.[2]

The structures of EBV DNA molecules for a given strain display quite limited heterogeneities. Regions of this DNA that are highly repetitious in sequence may contain different numbers of the repeats (see Fig. 26–30).[18] The structures of HCMV DNA molecules for a given strain, however, exhibit a striking, defined heterogeneity. HCMV DNA from a cloned viral stock is composed of four variants or isomers that arise in the infected host cell. The HCMV DNA molecule contains two pairs of inverted repeats, with one member of each pair at the ends of the linear molecules and the

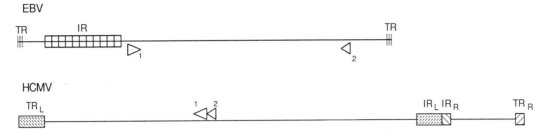

FIGURE 26–30. The viral genomes of Epstein-Barr virus (EBV) and HCMV are depicted as they would be isolated from viral particles. They are linear duplex DNAs of approximately 170,000 bp and 230,000 bp, respectively. The DNA of EBV has multiple, variable copies of a terminal repeat (TR) at its ends and multiple, variable copies of an unrelated internal repeat (IR). Only one isomer of EBV DNA is found in virions, although different molecules will have different numbers of these repeats. The DNA of HCMV has two stretches of unique DNA sequences. The long unique sequence is flanked by the left terminal repeat (Tr_L) and its inverted copy, the left internal repeat (IR_L). The short unique sequence is flanked by the right internal repeat (IR_R) and its inverted copy, the right terminal repeat (TR_R). Homologous recombination between TR_L and IR_L would invert the orientation of the long unique sequence relative to that shown; similarly, homologous recombination between IR_R and TR_R would invert the orientation of the short unique sequence. These recombination events would be one possible mechanism by which the four isomers of HCMV DNA found in virions arise. The distant but clear evolutionary relatedness of EBV and HCMV is exemplified by regions of similar DNA sequences 1 and 2, which are juxtaposed in HCMV but are separated by 92,000 bp in EBV and in which the orientation of sequence 1 relative to that of 2 differs between these two herpesviruses. (From Kouzarides, T., Bankier, A. T., Satchwell, S. C., Weston, K., Tomlinson, P., and Barrell, B. G.: Large-scale rearrangement of homologous regions in the genomes of HCMV and EBV. Virology 157:397–413, 1987; with permission.)

other member of each pair juxtaposed internally (Fig. 26–30). Recombination between the pairs of the inverted repeats yields the isomers found in stocks of HCMV and of other herpesviruses (e.g., HSV-1, HSV-2, and VZV). Not all herpesviruses generate different isomers of their DNAs (e.g., EBV), and if isomerization plays a role in the life cycle of those that do, that role is elusive. For example, mutants of HSV-1 that do not isomerize their DNAs replicate well in cell culture.[19]

LATENT AND LYTIC INFECTIONS BY HERPESVIRUSES

Herpesviruses can infect their human hosts latently. This form of infection, in fact, is pathognomonic for this family of viruses. Latent infections are defined operationally. This means that the virus cannot be detected in an infectious form in the host much of the time, but occasionally it can. As molecular analyses of latent infections have advanced, this operational definition has had to be qualified, but it remains an approximate description of how some herpesviruses fare in their human hosts. Latent infections occur after primary infections in which the introduced virus is amplified by infecting cells of the host lytically: that is, the virus infects some cells, progeny virus is produced, the cells die and lyse, and progeny virus is released. This initial lytic or productive infection is eventually limited by the host's immune response. Latent infections may ensue.

These two types of infection have in vitro counterparts. HCMV infects human fibroblast strains lytically; EBV infects human B lymphocytes latently and induces them to proliferate, and only rarely do these latently infected B lymphoblasts convert spontaneously

to support a productive infection. It may seem odd that a latent infection takes place in cell culture in the absence of an immune response. For EBV, however, the initial productive infection of the host may well occur in nonlymphoid cells.[20] Infection of B lymphocytes in vitro would, therefore, reflect a virus–host cell relationship that is primarily latent in the patient, too.

INFECTION BY HCMV IN CELL CULTURE

HCMV infects early-passage human fibroblast strains efficiently in culture. A candidate for a receptor for HCMV has been found.[21] Presumably, the virus binds to this molecule, gains entry into the cell, and wends its way to the nucleus, in which the nucleocapsid has been detected within minutes of exposure of cells to virus.[22] The viral information is now at the site in which it can be expressed, but, as with most animal DNA viruses, the expression of HCMV genes is well regulated. Some of this regulation may be achieved by the virus particle's bringing with it viral proteins that affect viral gene expression, as does HSV-1,[23, 24] but such putative HCMV proteins have not yet been identified.[25, 26] Cellular transcription factors surely participate in the regulation of expression of the first set of HCMV genes to be expressed in infected cells. This set, which is dubbed α, or immediate early, genes, is transcribed from distinct regions of HCMV DNA.[27, 28] Much work has been done on the *cis*-acting signals, which affect the transcription of one cluster of HCMV immediate early genes[29–31]; this indicates that several cellular transcription factors can bind to and regulate these genes. Products of the immediate early genes of HCMV themselves perform regulatory functions. They can increase the expression from viral promoters[32, 33] or decrease it.[34] They contribute to the viral life cycle both by downregulating their own expression[34] and by inducing expression of the next two temporal sets of viral genes termed β, or early, and γ, or late, genes.[35, 36] Products of the early genes contribute to the machinery required to synthesize viral DNA, and products of the late genes include virion structural proteins.[2]

The protracted course of the life cycle of HCMV in fibroblasts is not readily explained by transcriptional controls of the sets of viral genes expressed sequentially. Similar controls are found in α-herpesviruses, which can rapidly complete their life cycles. A post-transcriptional control for processing viral RNAs late in infection may retard the life cycle of HCMV.[37] In addition, a mechanism for regulating translation of some possible HCMV mRNAs has been posited to affect the life cycle of this β-herpesvirus.[38, 39]

Once the early RNAs of HCMV are transcribed and translated, viral DNA synthesis begins. Little is known about the mechanics of this process, but four genes of HCMV have been identified as homologues of HSV-1 genes that are known to encode proteins that participate in viral DNA synthesis.[2] In addition, a stretch of viral DNA has been identified in HCMV DNA that is complex in structure and that supports replication when inserted into plasmid vectors and introduced into HCMV-infected cells.[40] The identification of this putative origin of viral DNA synthesis should allow an elucidation of the intermediates that would define the pathway by which HCMV replicates its DNA.

With the onset of viral DNA synthesis, the last stages of the productive cycle of HCMV take place. Virions are assembled in the nucleus and encapsidate newly synthesized DNA. They presumably obtain their envelope by deriving it from that of the nucleus, as has been suggested for HSV-1: HSV-1 is often observed to be fully enveloped while still in the cytoplasm of the infected cell.[41] The productively infected cells die and release virus. It is not clear whether cell lysis is the general means by which herpesviruses exit the cell. It is possible that they also use secretory pathways to escape from the cell prior to its lysis.[42]

The study of a productive infection of human fibroblasts by HCMV in cell culture forms the basis of our understanding of this virus–host cell relationship at a molecular level. Yet it can provide only a limited appreciation of the complexity of infection of human hosts by HCMV. Another window on this complexity is provided by the identification of a variety of viral genes that have no obvious role in infections in cell culture but are likely to provide a selective advantage to HCMV in its human host. For example, the sequencing of the DNA of HCMV indicates that it encodes 54 ORFs or exons for glycoproteins.[2] It encodes a gene related to class I histocompatibility genes, which can bind β$_2$ microglobulin and may help HCMV-infected cells to escape a T-cell–mediated immune response.[43] It also encodes three genes whose products are related to the rhodopsin family of receptors, all of which transduce signals via coupling to G

proteins.[44] These examples indicate that HCMV maintains a spectacular array of genes that are likely to benefit its infection in vivo but may not aid it in cell culture.

INFECTION BY EBV IN CELL CULTURE

Whereas infection of fibroblast strains by HCMV yields a productive outcome for the virus, infection of B lymphocytes by EBV in general is non-productive. This difference is only heightened on consideration of the fates of the two host cells. Human fibroblast strains have a limited life span in culture of 50 to 100 cell divisions. HCMV replicates best in those fibroblasts that have been in culture for only a few generations and that divide rapidly. These proliferating cells are killed by HCMV. EBV, on the other hand, infects non-proliferating, primary B lymphocytes that exhibit no proliferative capacity in culture. Upon infection with EBV, these cells are induced to proliferate and efficiently yield progeny capable of proliferating indefinitely in cell culture; that is, EBV "immortalizes" infected B lymphocytes efficiently. These immortalized cells, however, only rarely yield progeny virus.[45, 46]

As the outcome of infection by EBV differs so strikingly from that of HCMV, so do many but not all of the events that occur during that process. EBV binds to a cellular receptor CD21[11, 47] and is internalized into cell vacuoles in which nucleocapsids are released from their envelopes.[48] The nucleocapsids migrate to the nucleus, where the viral DNA is circularized and transcribed. It is not known whether EBV brings into the cells proteins that affect transcription of its DNA. It is known that, during the first 72 hours after infection, viral RNA synthesis from one strand occurs from one promoter termed Wp and then switches to a second termed Cp[49] (Fig. 26–31). By 72 to 96 hours after infection, products from a third promoter on the other strand can be detected. These primary transcripts range from 3 to 100 kb in size, and some are multiply spliced.[50–52] These transcripts are translated into 10 or 11 proteins (reviewed in reference 53), whereas the remaining 90 or so ORFs of EBV are not expressed. By the time those viral genes characteristic of the latent phase of the viral life cycle are expressed, dramatic changes in the host cell also occur. These dramatic changes are induced by the actions of some or all of the latent viral genes. The small resting B lymphocyte swells to a lymphoblast, expresses new cellular antigens,[54, 55] and traverses the cell cycle. The circularized EBV DNA now replicates in synchrony with the cell DNA.[56] To do so requires a plasmid origin of replication, *oriP*, one viral protein, Epstein-Barr nuclear antigen 1 (EBNA-1) (see Fig. 26–31), and additional cellular enzymes needed for DNA synthesis.[57–60] This B lymphoblast now proliferates efficiently, maintains EBV DNA as a plasmid that expresses a small subset of its genes, and efficiently yields progeny that over time are found to be immortalized.

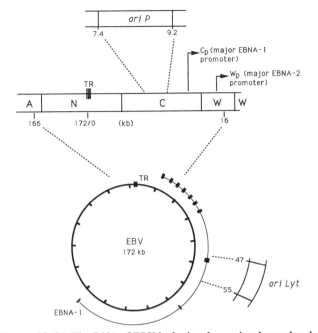

FIGURE 26–31. The DNA of EBV is depicted as a circular molecule as it would be found in cells immortalized by infection in vitro or in lymphoma cells isolated from patients. The linear molecule shown here has been circularized by ligation of the terminal repeats (TR). The hatch marks on this circle denote 10,000 bp intervals. The expanded diagram at the top of the figure depicts important *cis*-acting signals that affect EBV in the cell immortalized in vitro. The origin of plasmid DNA replication, *oriP*, lies between TR and two promoters, Cp and Wp, which direct clockwise transcription. Early after infection, these transcripts originate from Wp and later from Cp. Primary clockwise transcripts from these promoters often are quite long and are differentially spliced to yield multiple, distinct mRNAs. One primary transcript is shown that, once spliced and exported to the cytoplasm, could encode EBNA-1. Its exons are represented by thick lines, and its introns, which are removed by splicing, are shown as thin lines. The structure of such a primary transcript can be deduced only from isolated cDNA clones that are composed of the exons. Additional RNAs are encoded by EBV in immortalized cells, which are not depicted here (reviewed in reference 52). The origin of DNA replication used during the lytic phase (*oriLyt*) of EBV's life cycle maps approximately 40,000 bp away from *oriP*.

Were EBV to immortalize only infected B lymphocytes, the result of the infection, although it might be of profound importance for a human host, would be a dead end for the virus. EBV also undergoes a productive infection in these immortalized cells, albeit quite inefficiently. Between 0.1 and 0.001 per cent of cells in different clones of EBV-immortalized B lymphoblasts spontaneously convert to support a productive infection in each cell generation.[46] The immediate cause of this conversion is not known, but an early subsequent event is the induction of a viral gene, BZLF-1, which is a transcriptional activator that induces several viral genes that collectively regulate expression of the remaining 90 or so ORFs of EBV.[61–63] From this stage on, the ensuing lytic phase of EBV's life cycle can be likened to the latter stages of HCMV's productive infection of fibroblasts. The early genes of EBV are expressed, some of which encode enzymes necessary for viral DNA synthesis.[64]

The late genes are subsequently expressed; some of these encode virion structural proteins.[64] Concomitant with the expression of late genes, EBV DNA is synthesized. This synthesis is distinct from that occurring during the latent phase of the viral life cycle. An origin different from *oriP* is used for lytic DNA synthesis, termed *oriLyt*, which yields large concatemeric structures, presumably via a rolling circle mechanism.[65] These concatemeric DNAs are cleaved and packaged into viral nucleocapsids in the nucleus. The assembly of complete virions and their exit from their host cells are presumed to mimic those processes of HCMV in fibroblasts.

INFECTIONS IN THE HUMAN HOST

It is important in considering pathogenesis by herpesviruses in general to appreciate their possible dual life styles. We can expect that some symptoms of a particular viral infection result from cell lysis and the immune response to it; some symptoms of another infection result from latent infection and changes in the latently infected host cell. We shall use our understanding of the lytic and latent phases of viral life cycles gleaned from studies in cell culture to analyze the molecular bases of blood diseases associated with HCMV and EBV.

HCMV as a Pathogen: Early History

As with most animal viruses, the history of HCMV is short. Scattered observations of human tissues that may have been infected by HCMV and displayed characteristic structures now interpreted to be cytomegalic inclusions have been reported since the beginning of the twentieth century.[66] The advent of cell culture in the 1940s provided the essential vehicle that led to the isolation of HCMV in the middle 1950s.[67] Since its isolation, much work has gone into mapping the prevalence of the virus and use of various approaches to associate it with specific human diseases. The vast majority of infections with HCMV are benign. Ferreting out which ones under what conditions lead to disease has been difficult and continues today.

Clinical Manifestations of HCMV Infections

Most people in the world are eventually infected by HCMV, as determined by their antibodies to HCMV-associated antigens. People in affluent countries tend to be infected later in life than those in Third World countries, but more than half of all screened populations are infected by age 50.[66] Historically, the first syndrome associated with HCMV infections was cytomegalic inclusion disease (CID). CID occurred in certain fatal infections in which affected tissues contained large cells with polymorphic inclusions in their nuclei (Fig. 26–32). A search for the causative agent for CID

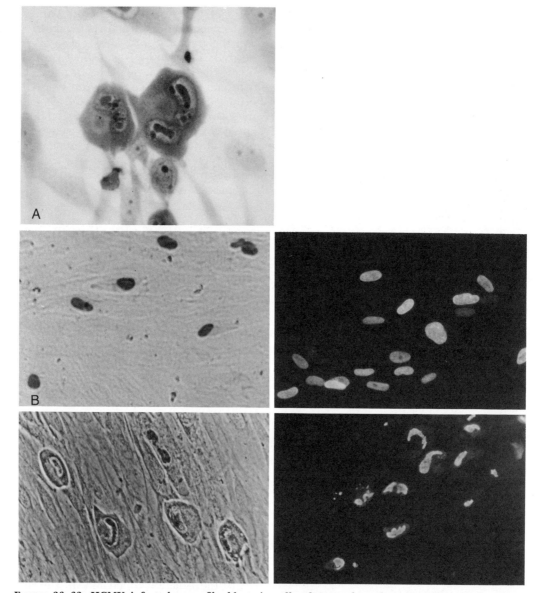

FIGURE 26–32. HCMV infects human fibroblasts in cell culture and produces inclusion bodies late in infection that are pathognomonic for cytomegalic inclusion disease in vivo. Simian CMV infects established monkey epithelial cells and produces similar inclusion bodies in them. In *A*, monkey epithelial cells infected with simian CMV are fixed and stained with hematoxylin and eosin to reveal the cytomegalic inclusion bodies within their nuclei. In *B*, a strain of human fibroblasts is infected with HCMV. The upper two panels show infected cells fixed and stained with monoclonal antibodies to an immediate-early protein of HCMV; that on the upper left is visualized with a horseradish peroxidase (HRP)–mediated reaction and that on the upper right by immunofluorescence. The nuclei of the infected cells are uniformly stained. The lower two panels show infected cells fixed and stained with monoclonal antibodies to a late protein of HCMV; that on the lower left is visualized with HRP and that on the lower right with immunofluorescence. The nuclei are not uniformly stained; rather, the staining is compartmentalized to the inclusion bodies within the nuclei and indicate that cytomegalic inclusions contain viral proteins expressed late in the viral life cycle. These analyses were performed by Dr. A. Lakeman of the University of Alabama with monoclonal antibodies developed by Dr. W. Britt from the University of Alabama.

led to the isolation of HCMV.[67] Intranuclear inclusions caused by HCMV result from synthesis and compartmentalization of late viral gene products and are therefore indicative of productive infection. Although most infections by HCMV are clinically silent, some result in disease.

Primary infections during pregnancy with HCMV are associated with several sequelae, including mental retardation of the child. The magnitude of this problem has been addressed in England by a 7-year prospective study of more than 10,000 women.[68] Fifty-eight per cent of the women were seropositive when first tested; 0.75 per cent of those studied had primary infections during their pregnancies, and 20 per cent of their children had congenital infections. Twelve per cent of the congenitally infected children by 4 years of age became severely retarded, although they displayed no gross problems at birth. These data indicate that in similar populations approximately 1 to 2 per 10,000 live births can be expected to develop mental retardation as a result of primary infection with HCMV.[68] This prospective study is also informative in indicating that primary infection at any time during pregnancy increases the risk of inducing mental retardation.[68]

Infection with HCMV also leads to interstitial pneumonitis, both upon primary infection and upon reactivation. In most cases this pneumonitis arises in immunocompromised patients—either those who have received immunosuppressive therapy or those who are immunocompromised by other means, such as acquired immunodeficiency syndrome (AIDS). HCMV-associated pneumonitis may be difficult to diagnose. It can present as does pneumonitis caused by gram-negative bacteria; in addition, HCMV and gram-negative bacteria may simultaneously contribute to a pneumonitis.[66] It is therefore important to detect HCMV rapidly and accurately. Various methods are now used,[69] and it seems likely that they will improve in sensitivity as the polymerase chain reaction (PCR) is applied to detect HCMV routinely.

HCMV-associated pneumonitis is often fatal. In one study of bone marrow recipients, 84 per cent of those who developed pneumonitis died.[70] This extraordinarily high rate may reflect the association between graft-versus-host disease (GVHD) and HCMV infection,[71] in which GVHD itself would be a major contributor to mortality.

Primary infection with HCMV in the normal population can cause a mononucleosis-like syndrome.[72] This mononucleosis is characterized by high fever, mild lymphocytosis, some atypical lymphocytes, and mild hepatitis.[66] It is usually distinguished from the more common EBV-associated mononucleosis by being negative for heterophile antibodies (antibodies to foreign antigens such as horse red blood cells). HCMV-associated mononucleosis also occurs as a result of transfusions. Early studies found a high incidence of this transfusion-related mononucleosis.[73] Two recent studies indicate, however, that now, when seronegative recipients are transfused with blood from seropositive donors, the risk of seroconverting is on the order of 1 per cent per unit of blood transfused.[74, 75] Current rates of transfusion-related mononucleosis are presumably correspondingly lower than those found earlier. Only 20 per cent of graft recipients who are seronegative and immunosuppressed and who receive both transfusions and a kidney from seropositive donors have been found to develop HCMV-associated mononucleosis in a recent survey.[75a]

Current Understanding of HCMV-Associated Mononucleosis

Mononucleosis is the predominant blood disease associated with HCMV. The evidence that HCMV causes it is correlative but strong. The disease follows immediately upon infection, as evidenced by seroconversion. What is not clear is what virus–host cell relationships take place in the patient to cause the syndrome. Specifically, what cells are infected? What is the outcome of these infections? What is the immune response to these infections?

Human T cells, once they are stimulated to proliferate, can be productively infected by HCMV in cell culture.[76] Peripheral blood cells isolated from seropositive normal donors contain a few T cells and monocytes that express HCMV immediate early RNAs as monitored by in situ nucleic acid hybridization.[77] Importantly, similar studies in patients infected with human immunodeficiency virus (HIV) indicate that productive infections also occur in these cells.[77] It therefore seems possible that HCMV-associated mononucleosis results from a productive infection of mononuclear cells in the blood. This hypothesis is consistent with the immunosuppression detected in patients with this mononucleosis.[78]

Those proliferating T cells that are CD8 positive (CD8 +) support replication of HCMV most efficiently in cell culture,[76] and the atypical lymphocytes found in HCMV-associated mononucleosis are predominantly CD8 +.[79] These two observations are consistent with a scenario in which HCMV infects mononuclear cells in vivo, and an immune response develops in which CD8 + T cells are induced to proliferate. Some of these proliferating CD8 + T cells may be infected, but they eventually function to kill the HCMV-infected cells. (CD8 + T cells in general act as cytotoxic affector cells.)

Two hypotheses must be tested: that HCMV-associated mononucleosis results from productive infections of mononuclear cells and that CD8 + cells are the predominant atypical lymphocytes in this disease because they are amplified to kill the HCMV-infected cells. Until these theories are substantiated or refuted and replaced by valid models, our understanding of HCMV-associated mononucleosis will remain rudimentary.

Treatment of HCMV-Associated Diseases

HCMV-associated mononucleosis in adults is often treated to ameliorate the high fevers it may cause. However, HCMV-associated diseases in immunocompromised patients usually require immediate intervention. The associated pneumonitis is often fatal, and an HCMV-associated retinitis in AIDS patients is usually progressive. Each of these diseases apparently reflects productive infection by HCMV. The most effective treatment to date is to limit the productive infection by inhibiting viral DNA replication. One of the four genes of HCMV that are homologues of HSV-1 genes involved in DNA replication encodes a DNA polymerase[2] that is inhibited by the nucleoside analogue ganciclovir 9-(1,3-dihydroxy-2-propoxymethyl)guanine once it is phosphorylated by cellular kinases.[80] Treatment of HCMV-associated retinitis with ganciclovir is remarkably effective.[81] Treatment of HCMV-associated pneumonitis with ganciclovir is apparently less effective[82] but can be improved when combined with immunoglobulin in bone marrow recipients.[83, 84] This combined therapy needs to be tested in controlled studies of different populations of patients to determine if it is generally effective for HCMV-associated pneumonitis.

The use of ganciclovir has at least two attendant problems. First, cellular DNA polymerases are also inhibited by phosphorylated forms of ganciclovir[80] so that, as higher doses of the inhibitor are used, more uninfected cells are affected deleteriously. Second, prolonged use of ganciclovir selects for mutants of HCMV that are resistant to it.[85] A solution to these problems should evolve as HCMV is studied further and targets for antiviral therapy other than the DNA polymerase are identified.

EBV as a Pathogen: Early History

Not only is EBV's history brief, but so too is the medical community's recognition of some of the diseases with which it is associated. Its discovery, however, is a marvelous tale.[86] Dennis Burkitt[87] identified a formerly unrecognized childhood tumor prevalent in East Africa in the mid-1950s and from his clever investigations postulated that it was caused by a vector-borne virus.[88] Epstein and his colleagues developed means to propagate cells from these childhood tumors (now known as Burkitt's lymphomas), which had to be flown from East Africa to England for their studies, and they identified in rare cells in these cultures a new virus—Epstein-Barr virus.[89] Soon after the identification of EBV, acute observation and serendipity were coupled by the Henles, who noted that a laboratory colleague seroconverted to express antibodies to EBV upon developing infectious mononucleosis.[90] This finding paved the way for retrospective and prospective epidemiological surveys that have established EBV as the causative agent of the heterophile-positive form of infectious mononucleosis.[91, 92]

Clinical Manifestations of EBV Infections

Most infections with EBV are clinically silent. In less affluent peoples of the world, children are usually infected without subsequent disease during the first few years of their lives after the protection from maternally acquired antibodies has waned. In more affluent peoples, many are first infected as adolescents. In these individuals primary infection can result in heterophile-positive infectious mononucleosis. Patients usually present with sore throats, fevers that last for two to three weeks, and a lingering malaise. During the acute phase of infectious mononucleosis, EBV-infected B lymphocytes can be detected in the peripheral blood; in extreme cases up to 20 per cent of these cells have been found to be infected.[93] Some of these

infected cells are proliferating[94] and constitute a portion of the atypical lymphocytes characteristic of infectious mononucleosis.[95] EBV-infected, proliferating B lymphocytes secrete immunoglobulins[96] that presumably are the source of the heterophile antibodies. T lymphocytes proliferate in response to EBV-infected cells and also contribute to the atypical lymphocytes. The large number of proliferating lymphocytes, including both EBV-infected lymphocytes and responding T cells, may contribute to the generalized lymphadenopathy and the frequent splenomegaly associated with infectious mononucleosis. In most cases the acute phase of the disease passes within three weeks. During convalescence, the number of atypical cells declines to undetectable levels in the blood, and the infection in a few of these cells is latent. However, people often excrete EBV in their saliva for long times after recovering from infectious mononucleosis.[97, 98]

Young children in some regions of the world, including East Africa and New Guinea, in which malaria is endemic, can develop Burkitt's lymphoma 7 to 48 months after infection by EBV.[99] The tumor is often recognized clinically as a mass of the jaw and usually has colonized several additional sites when diagnosed. These additional sites may include the orbit and the abdomen, but not often the bone marrow.[100] Burkitt's lymphoma not necessarily associated with EBV or malaria also occurs throughout the world at about 1 per one million children per year, or 1 per cent of the frequency of Burkitt's lymphoma in East Africa and New Guinea. It does not usually present as a mass of the jaw and often involves the bone marrow.[100]

In EBV-positive Burkitt's lymphoma, the tumor mass grows rapidly and contains proliferating cells with mitotic figures. The tumor cells express at least one viral gene product, EBNA-1,[101, 102] and usually contain multiple copies of the viral genome present as plasmids.[103] The tumor cell expresses immunoglobulin on its surface and has been judged monoclonal both by its expression of a single X-linked glucose-6-phosphate dehydrogenase isozyme in heterozygous females[104] and by its expression of surface immunoglobulin with a single specificity.[105] The tumor cell can be propagated readily in cell culture and often over time expresses all those viral genes characteristic of the latent phase of EBV's life cycle in addition to EBNA-1.[106] Burkitt's lymphoma tumor cells, be they of East African origin or not, usually display a striking and characteristic karyotype. They contain a chromosomal translocation that juxtaposes one of the three immunoglobulin loci with the c-myc locus.[107, 108] This rearrangement leads to the expression only of the translocated c-myc allele at a level similar to that of nonrearranged c-myc in B lymphoblasts immortalized by EBV in vitro.[109]

EBV is also causally associated with B-cell lymphomas in immunocompromised hosts. Patients can be congenitally immunodeficient, such as those males who have an X-linked lymphoproliferative syndrome (XLP)[110]; or they can be immunosuppressed, such as graft recipients[111, 112]; or they can be immunocompromised with AIDS.[113] In all these cases the EBV-associated lymphomas express EBV antigens, are polyclonal, and lack the characteristic chromosomal translocations between immunoglobulin loci and that of c-myc.

Non-lymphoid diseases are also associated with EBV. Some AIDS patients develop oral hairy leukoplakia, which represents a productive infection of mucosal epithelial cells by EBV.[114] The affected tissue consists of stratified squamous epithelium. EBV is not detected in the basal layer of this tissue, but in the upper layers the BZLF-1 gene of EBV is expressed, and amplified viral DNA can be detected.[115]

In some regions of the world, including China, Hong Kong, Taiwan, and areas in which Burkitt's lymphoma is endemic, infection of epithelial cells in the postnasal space with EBV is associated with nasopharyngeal carcinoma.[116] This tumor is common in these regions; between 50,000 and 100,000 new cases develop each year. EBNA-1 is expressed in the tumor cells,[117, 118] which contain multiple copies of viral plasmid DNAs.[119] That the tumor cells proliferate in vivo to kill the host while maintaining multiple viral genomes indicates that this disease represents predominantly a latent infection. A prospective seroepidemiological study indicates that antibodies of the immunoglobulin A (IgA) class to EBV-associated early antigens constitute a major risk factor for the development of nasopharyngeal carcinoma.[120] This finding, therefore, causally associates EBV with nasopharyngeal carcinoma.

Molecular and Cellular Analyses of EBV-Associated B-Lymphoid Diseases

How does infection of B lymphocytes by one virus lead to such differing results—a self-limiting proliferation, infectious mononucleosis, or a rapidly dividing Burkitt's lymphoma—in human hosts? Only a partial answer exists for this question, but it is nonetheless instructive, because it illustrates routes by which EBV contributes to diseases of the blood.

First, it is clear that, although different strains of EBV exist, no one strain has been peculiarly associated with one disease or another.[121] Second, in infectious mononucleosis, although many infected B lymphocytes are induced to proliferate in vivo[94] and continue to proliferate upon explantation into cell culture,[122] an effective cytotoxic response to these infected cells has been documented.[123–125] Viral targets for this response include many genes of EBV, other than EBNA-1, characteristic of latent infection. This response in vivo leads to a dramatic diminution of infected B lymphocytes in the peripheral blood of convalescing patients, although most people once infected with EBV retain some small number of infected cells in their blood. These persisting, EBV-positive cells can be detected long after convalescence by culturing explanted lymphoid cells in the presence of cyclosporine to inhibit a cytotoxic response to the proliferating, infected cells[125a]

or by introducing them into SCID mice (mice inbred to display a particular severe combined immunodeficiency), in which they grow as polyclonal tumors that kill the host.[126]

The importance of an effective, cell-mediated response to EBV-infected cells in rendering infectious mononucleosis "self-limiting" can also be inferred from the course of primary infections in immunocompromised hosts. EBV-seronegative bone marrow recipients, for example, can develop polyclonal EBV-associated lymphomas of donor origin 2 to 3 months after receiving grafts from EBV-seropositive donors.[127] It also seems likely that the persistence of EBV-infected cells in the healthy host is important to stimulate the immune response constitutively to limit frequent reinfections throughout life. Many people excrete EBV in their saliva, and thus we can expect to be reinoculated with it frequently.[97]

Given the above description of infection of EBV and a host's response to it, what differs in the infection of children destined to develop Burkitt's lymphoma? A prospective seroepidemiological survey has found that children with abnormally high titers of antibodies to EBV late proteins have an increased risk of developing Burkitt's lymphoma compared with matched controls.[99] This finding is consistent with high-risk children having a particularly robust infection with EBV. Most children in regions in which Burkitt's lymphoma is endemic have chronic malaria,[128, 129] and it has been shown that malaria induces a T-cell immunosuppression such that a host no longer efficiently kills its own EBV-infected B lymphocytes.[130, 131] Thus, it appears that those destined to develop Burkitt's lymphoma have both a robust infection with EBV and an impaired immune response that only inefficiently limits the infected, proliferating cells.

Several known molecular alterations occur in a clone of EBV-infected cells that develops into a tumor. (See Chapter 24 for a detailed account of chromosomal translocations in cancers.) Although it is not known when they happen, it is simplest to envision that they occur after infection in a rare cell among the large population of cells induced to proliferate by EBV. One of three immunoglobulin loci is juxtaposed to the c-myc locus[108] in more than 90 per cent of cases, and mutations occur in the tumor-suppressor gene termed p53 in 40 to 75 per cent of the cases studied.[132, 133] These mutations usually are followed by subsequent events that inactivate the expression of the wild-type allele.[132, 133] These mutations, because of their ubiquity, can be assumed to provide the mutant cell a selective advantage in vivo. One such hypothetical advantage might be to allow the EBV-infected cell to continue to proliferate in the absence of expression of some of the EBV genes required for immortalization.[134, 135] If the growth-promoting functions of these viral genes were substituted by those of cellular genes, the cells would have a selective advantage, because the viral gene products are targets for T-cell–mediated cytotoxicity and would no longer need to be expressed. EBNA-1, which is required to maintain the viral DNA as a plasmid in proliferating cells,[58, 59] has not been found to be such a target and is found to be expressed in recently explanted Burkitt's lymphomas.[106] Whether this hypothesized advantage proves correct or not, it is clear that several rare events must occur in one clone of cells for it to evolve into a Burkitt's lymphoma. Only in those regions of the world in which chronic malaria and early infection with EBV overlap is the frequency of these rare events high enough to yield the one case of Burkitt's lymphoma per 10,000 children characteristic of these regions.

Treatment of EBV-Associated Lymphoid Diseases

The symptoms of EBV-associated infectious mononucleosis are usually mild and treated with bed rest. Infrequent cases that are complicated by respiratory obstruction or hemolytic anemia are treated with corticosteroids.[135a] Those rare cases that progress to splenic rupture are treated surgically. In other instances of EBV infections antiviral therapy may be used. For example, one antiviral therapy for EBV is directed against the lytic phase of its life cycle. The compound, acyclovir (9-[(2-hydroxyethoxy)methyl] guanine), once phosphorylated in the cell, is recognized by EBV's DNA polymerase, incorporated into a growing DNA chain, and terminates that chain.[136] In immunosuppressed patients who develop a syndrome similar to infectious mononucleosis in which the proliferating B lymphocytes are karyotypically normal, treatment with acyclovir is successful in resolving the disease.[137] The usefulness of acyclovir in treating additional EBV-associated lymphoid diseases is being studied now.

Lymphomas associated with EBV in general and Burkitt's lymphoma in particular cannot now be treated only with antiviral therapies. The one viral gene consistently expressed in tumor cells is EBNA-1. No therapies designed to inhibit its function have been developed. Burkitt's lymphomas are currently treated with combined chemotherapies and, if the initial tumor mass requires it, radiation therapy.[100] Responses to these therapies in African cases are high,[100] with 60 to 90 per cent 2-year tumor-free rates depending on the extent of the tumor at the time of treatment.

Our appreciation for the mechanism by which EBV immortalizes B lymphocytes at a molecular level is growing rapidly. The viral proteins involved are being identified and functionally characterized now. It seems likely that new families of antiviral drugs will be developed that can limit non-malignant EBV-induced lymphoproliferations. As these drugs are developed, the concomitant directed research may also contribute to antiviral therapies applicable to EBV-associated malignancies.

REFERENCES

1. Davison A.: Channel catfish virus: A new type of herpesvirus. Virology 186:9, 1992.

2. Chee, M. S., Bankier, A. T., Beck, S., Bohni, R., Brown, C. M., Cerny, R., Horsnell, T., Hutchison, C. A. III, Kouzarides, T., Martignetti, J. A., Preddie, E., Satchwell, S. C., Tomlinson, P., Weston, K. M., and Barrell, B. G.: Analysis of the protein-coding content of the sequence of human cytomegalovirus strain AD169. Curr. Top. Microbiol. Immunol. 154:125, 1990.

3. Roizman, B., Carmichael, L. E., Deinhardt, F., de-The, G., Nahmias, A. J., Plowright, W., Rapp, F., Sheldrick, P., Takahashi, M., and Wolf, K.: Herpesviridae: Definition, provisional nomenclature and taxonomy. Intervirology 16:201, 1981.

4. Stinski, M. F.: Human cytomegalovirus: Glycoproteins associated with virions and dense bodies. J. Virol. 19:594, 1976.

5. Lakeman, A. D., and Osborn, J. E.: Size of infectious DNA from human and murine cytomegalovirus. J. Virol. 30:414, 1979.

6. Farrar, G. H., and Oram, J. D.: Characterization of the human cytomegalovirus envelope glycoproteins. J. Gen. Virol. 65:1991, 1984.

7. Rasmussen, L., Nelson, M., Neff, M., and Merigan, T. C., Jr.: Characterization of two different human cytomegalovirus glycoproteins which are targets for virus neutralizing antibody. Virology 163:308, 1988.

8. Matsumoto, Y., Sugano, T., Miyamoto, C., and Masuho, Y.: Generation of hybridomas producing human monoclonal antibodies against human cytomegalovirus. Biochem. Biophys. Res. Commun. 137:273, 1986.

9. Yao, Q. Y., Rowe, M., Morgan, A. J., Sam, C. K., Prasad, U., Dang, H., Zeng, Y., and Rickinson, A. B.: Salivary and serum IgA antibodies to the Epstein-Barr virus glycoprotein gp340: Incidence and potential for virus neutralization. Int. J. Cancer 48:45, 1991.

10. Wallace, L. E., Wright, J., Ulaeto, D. O., Morgan, A. J., and Rickinson, A. B.: Identification of two T-cell epitopes on the candidate Epstein-Barr virus vaccine glycoprotein gp340 recognized by CD4+ T-cell clones. J. Virol. 65:3821, 1991.

11. Fingeroth, J. D., Weis, J. J., Tedder, T. F., Strominger, J. L., Biro, P. A., and Fearon, D. T.: Epstein-Barr virus receptor of human B lymphocytes is the C3d receptor CR2. Proc. Natl. Acad. Sci. USA 81:4510, 1984.

12. Nemerow, G. R., Mold, C., Schwend, V. K., Tollefson, V., and Cooper, N. R.: Identification of gp350 as the viral glycoprotein mediating attachment of Epstein-Barr virus (EBV) to the EBV/C3d receptor of B cells: Sequence homology of gp350 and C3 complement fragment C3d. J. Virol. 61:1416, 1987.

13. Morgan, A. J., Allison, A. C., Finerty, S., Scullion, F. T., Byars, N. E., and Epstein, M. A.: Validation of a first-generation Epstein-Barr virus vaccine preparation suitable for human use. J. Med. Virol. 29:74, 1989.

14. Stannard, L. M., and Hardie, D. R.: An Fc receptor for human immunoglobulin G is located within the tegument of human cytomegalovirus. J. Virol. 65:3411, 1991.

15. Gibson, W.: Protein counterparts of human and simian cytomegaloviruses. Virology 128:391, 1983.

16. Gibson, W., and Roizman, B.: Compartmentalization of spermine and spermidine in the herpes simplex virion. Proc. Natl. Acad. Sci. USA 68:2818, 1971.

17. Kouzarides, T., Bankier, A. T., Satchwell, S. C., Weston, K., Tomlinson, P., and Barrell, B. G.: Large-scale rearrangement of homologous regions in the genomes of HCMV and EBV. Virology 157:397, 1987.

18. Kintner, C., and Sugden, B.: Conservation and progressive methylation of Epstein-Barr viral DNA sequences in transformed cells. J. Virol. 38:305, 1981.

19. Jenkins, F. J., and Roizman, B.: Herpes simplex virus 1 recombinants with noninverting genomes frozen in different isomeric arrangements are capable of independent replication. J. Virol. 59:494, 1986.

20. Sixbey, J. W.: Epstein-Barr virus and epithelial cells. In Klein, G. (ed.): Advances in Viral Oncology, Vol. 8. New York, Raven Press, 1989, pp. 187–202.

21. Taylor, H. P., and Cooper, N. R.: The human cytomegalovirus

receptor on fibroblasts is a 30-kD membrane protein. J. Virol. 64:2484, 1990.

22. Smith, J. D., and De Harven, E.: Herpes simplex virus and human cytomegalovirus replication in WI-38 cells. II. An ultrastructural study of viral penetration. J. Virol. 14:945, 1974.

23. Batterson, W., Furlong, D., and Roizman, B.: Molecular genetics of herpes simplex virus VIII. Further characterization of a temperature-sensitive mutant defective in release of viral DNA and in other stages of the viral reproductive cycle. J. Virol. 45:397, 1983.

24. Preston, C. M., Frame, M. C., and Campbell, M. E. M.: A complex formed between cell components and an HSV structural polypeptide binds to a viral immediate early gene regulatory DNA sequence. Cell 52:425, 1988.

25. Stinski, M. F., and Roehr, T. J.: Activation of the major immediate early gene of human cytomegalovirus by cis-acting elements in the promoter-regulatory sequence and by virus-specific trans-acting components. J. Virol. 55:431, 1985.

26. Spaete, R. R., and Mocarski, E. S.: Regulation of cytomegalovirus gene expression: α and β promoters are *trans* activated by viral functions in permissive human fibroblasts. J. Virol. 56:135, 1985.

27. Wathen, M. W., and Stinski, M. F.: Temporal patterns of human cytomegalovirus transcription: Mapping the viral RNAs synthesized at immediate early, early, and late times after infection. J. Virol. 41:462, 1982.

28. Weston, K.: An enhancer element in the short unique region of human cytomegalovirus regulates the production of a group of abundant immediate early transcripts. Virology 162:406, 1988.

29. Thomsen, D. R., Stenberg, R. M., Goins, W. F., and Stinski, M. F.: Promoter-regulatory region of the major immediate early gene of human cytomegalovirus. Proc. Natl. Acad. Sci. USA 81:659, 1984.

30. Hennighausen, L., and Fleckenstein, B.: Nuclear factor 1 interacts with five DNA elements in the promoter region of the human cytomegalovirus major immediate early gene. EMBO J. 5:1367, 1986.

31. Ghazal, P., and Nelson, J. A.: Enhancement of RNA polymerase II initiation complexes by a novel DNA control domain downstream from the CAP site of the cytomegalovirus major immediate-early promoter. J. Virol. 65:2299, 1991.

32. Cherrington, J. M., and Mocarski, E. S.: Human cytomegalovirus ie1 transactivates the α promoter-enhancer via an 18-base-pair repeat element. J. Virol. 63:1435, 1989.

33. Malone, C. L., Vesole, D. H., and Stinski, M. F.: Transactivation of a human cytomegalovirus early promoter by gene products from immediate-early gene IE2 and augmentation by IE1: Mutational analysis of the viral proteins. J. Virol. 64:1498, 1990.

34. Pizzorno, M., O'Hare, P., Sha, L., La Femina, R. L., and Hayward, G. S.: Transactivation and autoregulation of gene expression by the immediate-early region 2 gene products of human cytomegalovirus. J. Virol. 62:1167, 1988.

35. Staprans, S. I., Rabert, D. K., and Spector, D. H.: Identification of sequence requirements and trans-acting functions necessary for regulated expression of a human cytomegalovirus early gene. J. Virol. 62:3463, 1988.

36. Depto, A. S., and Stenberg, R. M.: Regulated expression of the human cytomegalovirus pp65 gene: Octamer sequence in the promoter is required for activation by viral gene products. J. Virol. 63:1232, 1989.

37. Goins, W. F., and Stinski, M. F.: Expression of a human cytomegalovirus late gene is posttranscriptionally regulated by a 3'-end-processing event occurring exclusively late after infection. Mol. Cell. Biol. 6:4202, 1986.

38. Geballe, A. P., Spaete, R. R., and Mocarski, E. S.: A cis-acting element within the 5' leader of a cytomegalovirus (beta) transcript determines kinetic class. Cell 46:865, 1986.

39. Geballe, A. P., and Mocarski, E. S.: Translational control of cytomegalovirus gene expression is mediated by upstream AUG codons. J. Virol. 62:3334, 1988.

40. Anders, D. G., and Punturieri, S. M.: Multicomponent origin of cytomegalovirus lytic-phase DNA replication. J. Virol. 65:931, 1991.

41. Schwartz, J., and Roizman, B.: Concerning the egress of herpes simplex virus from infected cells: Electron and light microscope observations. Virology 38:42, 1969.

42. Johnson, D. C., and Spear, P. G.: Monersin inhibits the processing of herpes simplex virus glycoproteins, their transport to the cell surface, and the egress of virions from infected cells. J. Virol. 43:1102, 1982.

43. Brawne, H., Smith, G., Beck, S., and Minson, T.: A complex between the MHC class I homologue encoded by human cytomegalovirus and β₂ microglobulin. Nature 347:770, 1990.

44. Chee, M. S., Satchwell, S. C., Preddie, E., Weston, K. M., and Barrell, B. G.: Human cytomegalovirus encodes three G protein-coupled receptor homologues. Nature 344:774, 1990.

45. Wilson, G., and Miller, G.: Recovery of Epstein-Barr virus from non-producer neonatal human lymphoid cell transformants. Virology 95:351, 1979.

46. Sugden, B.: Expression of virus-associated functions in cells transformed in vitro by Epstein-Barr virus: Epstein-Barr virus cell surface antigen and virus-release from transformed cells. *In* Purtillo, D. T. (ed.): Immune Deficiency and Cancer. New York, Plenum Medical Book Co., 1984, pp. 165–177.

47. Nemerow, G. R., Wolfert, R., McNaughton, M. E., and Cooper N. R.: Identification and characterization of the Epstein-Barr virus receptor on human B lymphocytes and its relationship to the C3d complement receptor (CR2). J. Virol. 55:347, 1985.

48. Nemerow, G. R., and Cooper, N. R.: Early events in the infection of human B lymphocytes by Epstein-Barr virus: The internalization process. Virology 132:186, 1984.

49. Woisetschlaeger, M., Yandava, C. N., Furmanski, L. A., Strominger, J. L., and Speck, S. H.: Promoter switching in Epstein-Barr virus during the initial stages of infection of B-lymphocytes. Proc. Natl. Acad. Sci. USA 87:1725, 1990.

50. Bodescot, M., and Perricaudet, M.: Epstein-Barr virus mRNAs produced by alternative splicing. Nucleic Acids Res. 14:7103, 1986.

51. Laux, G., Perricaudet, M., and Farrell, P.: A spliced Epstein-Barr virus gene expressed in immortalized lymphocytes is created by circularization of the linear viral genome. EMBO J. 7:769, 1988.

52. Speck, S. H., and Strominger, J. L.: Transcription of Epstein-Barr virus in latently infected, growth-transformed lymphocytes. *In* Klein, G. (ed.): Advances in Viral Oncology, Vol. 8. New York, Raven Press, 1989, pp. 133–150.

53. Kieff, E., and Liebowitz, D.: Epstein-Barr virus and its replication. *In* Fields, B. N., and Knipe, D. M. (eds.): Virology, 2nd ed. New York, Raven Press, 1990, pp. 1889–1920.

54. Kintner, C., and Sugden, B.: Identification of antigenic determinants unique to the surfaces of cells transformed by Epstein-Barr virus. Nature 294:458, 1981.

55. Gregory, G. D., Kirchgens, C., Edwards, C. F., Young, L. S., Rowe, M., Forster, A., Rabbitts, T. H., and Rickinson, A. B.: Epstein-Barr virus-transformed human precursor B cell lines: Altered growth phenotype of lines with germline or rearranged but non-expressed heavy chain genes. Eur. J. Immunol. 17:1199, 1987.

56. Adams, A., Pozos, T. C., and Purvey, H. V.: Replication of latent Epstein-Barr virus genomes in normal and malignant lymphoid cells. Int. J. Cancer 44:560, 1989.

57. Yates, J., Warren, N., Reisman, D., and Sugden, B.: A *cis*-acting element from the Epstein-Barr viral genome that permits stable replication of recombinant plasmids in latently infected cells. Proc. Natl. Acad. Sci. USA 81:3806, 1984.

58. Yates, J. L., Warren, N., and Sugden, B.: Stable replication of plasmids derived from Epstein-Barr virus in various mammalian cells. Nature 313:812, 1985.

59. Lupton, S., and Levine, A. J.: Mapping genetic elements of Epstein-Barr virus that facilitate extrachromosomal persist-

ence of Epstein-Barr virus-derived plasmids in human cells. Mol. Cell. Biol. 5:2533, 1985.

60. Gahn, T. A., and Schildkraut, C. L.: The Epstein-Barr virus origin of plasmid replication, *oriP*, contains both the initiation and termination sites of DNA replication. Cell 58:527, 1989.

61. Countryman, J., and Miller, G.: Activation of expression of latent Epstein-Barr herpesvirus after gene transfer with a small cloned subfragment of heterogeneous viral DNA. Proc. Natl. Acad. Sci. USA 82:4085, 1985.

62. Grogan, E., Jenson, H., Countryman, J., Heston, L., Gradoville, L., and Miller, G.: Transfection of a rearranged viral DNA fragment, WZ het, stably converts latent Epstein-Barr viral infection to productive infection in lymphoid cells. Proc. Natl. Acad. Sci. USA 84:1332, 1987.

63. Takada, K., Shimizu, N., Sakuma, S., and Ono, Y.: Transactivation of the latent Epstein-Barr virus (EBV) genome after transfection of the EBV DNA fragment. J. Virol. 57:1016, 1986.

64. Baer, R., Bankier, A. T., Biggin, M. D., Deininger, P. L., Farrell, P. J., Gibson, T. J., Hatfull, G., Hudson, G. S., Satchwell, S. C., Seguin, C., Tuffnell, P. S., and Barrell, B. G.: DNA sequence and expression of the B95-8 Epstein-Barr virus genome. Nature (London) 310:207, 1984.

65. Hammerschmidt, W., and Sugden, B.: Identification and characterization of oriLyt, a lytic origin of DNA replication of Epstein-Barr virus. Cell 55:427, 1988.

66. Ho, M.: Cytomegalovirus, 2nd ed. New York, Plenum Medical Book Co., 1991.

67. Weller, T. H.: Cytomegalovirus: The difficult years. J. Infect. Dis. 122:532, 1970.

68. Griffiths, P. D., and Baboonian, C.: A prospective study of primary cytomegalovirus infection during pregnancy: Final report. Br. J. Obstet. Gynecol. 91:307, 1984.

69. Paradis, I. L., Grgurich, W. F., Dummer, J. S., Dekker, A., and Dauber, J. H.: Rapid detection of cytomegalovirus pneumonia from lung lavage cells. Am. Rev. Respir. Dis. 138:697, 1988.

70. Meyers, J. D., Flournoy, N., and Thomas, E. D.: Risk factors for cytomegalovirus infection after human marrow transplantation. J. Infect. Dis. 153:478, 1986.

71. Neiman, P. E., Reeves, W., Ray, G., Flournoy, N., Lerner, K. G., Sale, G. E., and Thomas, E. D.: A prospective analysis of interstitial pneumonia and opportunistic viral infection among recipients of allogeneic bone marrow grafts. J. Infect. Dis. 136:754, 1977.

72. Klemola, E., von Essen, R., Henle, G., and Henle, W.: Infectious-mononucleosis-like disease with negative heterophil agglutination test. Clinical features in relation to Epstein-Barr virus and cytomegalovirus antibodies. J. Infect. Dis. 121:608, 1970.

73. Lang, D. J., and Hanshaw, J. B.: Cytomegalovirus infection and the postperfusion syndrome (recognition of primary infections in four patients). N. Engl. J. Med. 280:1145, 1969.

74. Wilhelm, J. A., Matter, L., and Schopfer, K.: The risk of transmitting cytomegalovirus to patients receiving blood transfusions. J. Infect. Dis. 154:169, 1986.

75. Preiksaitis, J. K., Brown, L., and McKenzie, M.: The risk of cytomegalovirus infection in seronegative transfusion recipients not receiving exogenous immunosuppression. J. Infect. Dis. 157:523, 1988.

75a. Weir, M. R., Henry, M. L., Blackmore, M., Smith, J., First, M. R., Irwin, B., Shen, S., Genemans, G., Alexander, J. W., Corry, R. J., Nghiem, D. D., Ferguson, R. M., Kittur, D., Shield, C. F., III, Sommer, B. G., and Williams, G. M.: Incidence and morbidity of cytomegalovirus disease associated with a seronegative recipient receiving seropositive donor-specific transfusion, and living-related donor transplantation. Transplantation 45:111, 1988.

76. Braun, R. W., and Reiser, H. C.: Replication of human cytomegalovirus in human peripheral blood T cells. J. Virol. 60:29, 1986.

77. Nelson, J. A., Gnann, J. W., Jr., and Ghazal, P.: Regulation and tissue-specific expression of human cytomegalovirus. Curr. Top. Microbiol. Immunol. 154:75, 1990.

78. Carney, W. P., Iacoviello, V., and Hirsch, M. S.: Functional properties of T lymphocytes and their subsets in cytomegalovirus mononucleosis. J. Immunol. 130:390, 1983.

79. Felsenstein, D., Carney, W. P., Iacoviello, V. R., and Hirsch, M. S.: Phenotypic properties of atypical lymphocytes in cytomegalovirus-induced mononucleosis. J. Infect. Dis. 152:198, 1985.

80. Mar, E. C., Chiou, J. F., Cheng, Y. C., and Huang, E. S.: Inhibition of cellular DNA polymerase alpha and human cytomegalovirus-induced DNA polymerase by the triphosphates of 9-(2-hydroxyethoxymethyl)guanine and 9-(1,3-dihydroxy-2-propoxymethyl)guanine. J. Virol. 53:776, 1985.

81. Mills, J., Jacobson, M. A., O'Donnell, J. J., Cederberg, D., and Holland, G. N.: Treatment of cytomegalovirus retinitis in patients with AIDS. Rev. Infect. Dis. 10 (Suppl.) 3:S522, 1988.

82. Erice, A., Jordan, M. C., Chace, B. A., Fletcher, C., Chinnock, B. J., and Balfour, H. H., Jr.: Ganciclovir treatment of cytomegalovirus disease in transplant recipients and other immunocompromised hosts. J. A. M. A. 257:3082, 1987.

83. Emanuel, D., Cunningham, I., Jules-Elysee, K., Brockstein, J. A., Kernan, N. A., Laver, J., Stover, D., White, D. A., Fels, A., Polsky, B., Castro-Malaspina, H., Peppard, J. R., Bartus, P., Hammerling, U., and O'Reilly, R. J.: Cytomegalovirus pneumonia after bone marrow transplantation successfully treated with the combination of ganciclovir and high-dose intravenous immune globulin. Ann. Intern. Med. 109:777, 1988.

84. Reed, E. C., Bowden, R. A., Dandliker, P. S., Lilleby, K. E., and Meyers, J. D.: Treatment of cytomegalovirus pneumonia with ganciclovir and intravenous cytomegalovirus immunoglobulin in patients with bone marrow transplants. Ann. Intern. Med. 109:783, 1988.

85. Erice, A., Chou, S., Biron, K. K., Stanat, S. C., Balfour, H. H., Jr., and Jordan, M. C.: Progressive disease due to ganciclovir-resistant cytomegalovirus in immunocompromised patients. N. Engl. J. Med. 320:289, 1989.

86. Epstein, M. A.: Historical background; Burkitt's lymphoma and Epstein-Barr virus. IARC Sci. Pub. no. 60. Lyon, IARC Press, 1985, pp. 17–27.

87. Burkitt, D.: A sarcoma involving the jaws in African children. Br. J. Surg. 46:218, 1958.

88. Burkitt, D.: Determining the climatic limitations of a children's cancer common in Africa. Br. Med. J. 2:1019, 1962.

89. Epstein, M. A., Achong, B. G., and Barr, Y. M.: Virus particles in cultured lymphoblasts from Burkitt's lymphoma. Lancet 1:702, 1964.

90. Henle, G., Henle, W., and Diehl, V.: Relation of Burkitt's tumor-associated herpes-type virus to infectious mononucleosis. Proc. Natl. Acad. Sci. USA 59:94, 1968.

91. Niederman, J. C., McCollum, R. W., Henle, G., and Henle, W.: Infectious mononucleosis. J. A. M. A. 203:205, 1968.

92. Evans, A. S.: The transmission of EB viral infections. *In* Hooks, J. J., and Jordan, G. W. (eds.): Viral Infections in Oral Medicine. New York, Elsevier North Holland, 1982, pp. 211–225.

93. Robinson, J. E., Smith, D., and Niederman, J.: Plasmacytic differentiation of circulating Epstein-Barr virus-infected B lymphocytes during acute infectious mononucleosis. J. Exp. Med. 153:235, 1981.

94. Robinson, J., Smith, D., and Niederman, J.: Mitotic EBNA-positive lymphocytes in peripheral blood during infectious mononucleosis. Nature 287:334, 1980.

95. Giuliano, V. J., Jasin, H. E., and Ziff, M.: The nature of the atypical lymphocyte in infectious mononucleosis. Clin. Immunol. Immunopathol. 3:90, 1974.

96. Bird, A. G., and Britton, S.: A new approach to the study of human B lymphocyte function using an indirect plaque assay and a direct B cell activator. Immunol. Rev. 45:41, 1979.

97. Miller, G., Niederman, J. C., and Andrews, L.-L.: Prolonged

oropharyngeal excretion of Epstein-Barr virus after infectious mononucleosis. N. Engl. J. Med. 288:229, 1973.

98. Niederman, J. C., Miller, G., Pearson, H. A., Pagano, J. S., and Dowaliby, J. M.: Infectious mononucleosis. Epstein-Barr-virus shedding in saliva and the oropharynx. N. Engl. J. Med. 294:1355, 1976.

99. de-Thé, G., Geser, A., Day, N. E., Tukei, P. M., Williams, E. H., Beri, D. P., Smith, P. G., Dean, A. G., Bornkamm, G. W., Feorino, P., and Henle, W.: Epidemiological evidence for causal relationship between Epstein-Barr virus and Burkitt's lymphoma from Ugandan prospective study. Nature 274:756, 1978.

100. Magrath, I. T.: Malignant non-Hodgkin's lymphomas. In Pizzo, P. A., and Poplach, D. G. (eds.): Principles and Practice of Pediatric Oncology. Philadelphia, J. B. Lippincott, 1989, pp. 415–456.

101. Lindahl, T., Klein, G., Reedman, B. M., Johansson, B., and Singh, S.: Relationship between Epstein-Barr virus (EBV) DNA and the EBV-determined nuclear antigen (EBNA) in Burkitt lymphoma biopsies and other lymphoproliferative malignancies. Int. J. Cancer 13:764, 1974.

102. Gregory, C. D., Rowe, M., and Rickinson, A. B.: Different Epstein-Barr virus–B cell interactions in phenotypically distinct clones of a Burkitt's lymphoma cell line. J. Gen. Virol. 71:1481, 1990.

103. Lindahl, T., Adams, A., Bjursell, G., Bornkamm, G. W., Kaschka-Dierich, C., and Jehn, U.: Covalently closed circular duplex DNA of Epstein-Barr virus in a human lymphoid cell line. J. Mol. Biol. 102:511, 1976.

104. Fialkow, P. J., Klein, G., Gartler, S. M., and Clifford, P.: Clonal origin for individual Burkitt tumors. Lancet 1:384, 1970.

105. Gunven, P., Klein, G., Klein, E., Norin, T., and Singh, S.: Surface immunoglobulins on Burkitt's lymphoma biopsy cells from 91 patients. Int. J. Cancer 25:711, 1980.

106. Rowe, M., Rowe, D. T., Gregory, C. D., Young, L. S., Farrell, P. J., Rupani, H., and Rickinson, A. B.: Differences in B cell growth phenotype reflect novel patterns of Epstein-Barr virus latent gene expression in Burkitt's lymphoma cells. EMBO J. 6:2743, 1987.

107. Zech, L., Haglund, U., Nilsson, K., and Klein, G.: Characteristic chromosomal abnormalities in biopsies and lymphoid-cell lines from patients with Burkitt and non-Burkitt lymphomas. Int. J. Cancer 17:47, 1976.

108. Klein, G.: Specific chromosomal translocations and the genesis of B-cell-derived tumors in mice and men. Cell 32:311, 1983.

109. Spencer, C. A., and Groudine, M.: Control of c-myc regulation in normal and neoplastic cells. Adv. Cancer Res. 56:1, 1991.

110. Purtilo, D. T., Sakamoto, K., Saemundsen, A. K., Sullivan, J. L., Synnerholm, A. C., Anvret, M., Pritchard, J., Sloper, C., Sieff, C., Pincott, J., Pachman, L., Rich, K., Cruzi, F., Cornet, J. A., Collins, R., Barnes, N., Knight, J., Sandstedt, B., and Klein, G.: Documentation of Epstein-Barr virus infection in immunodeficient patients with life-threatening lymphoproliferative diseases by clinical, virological, and immunopathological studies. Cancer Res. 41:4226, 1981.

111. Crawford, D. H., Thomas, J. A., Janossy, G., Sweny, P., Fernando, O. N., Moorhead, J. F., and Thompson, J. H.: Epstein Barr virus nuclear antigen positive lymphoma after cyclosporin A treatment in patients with renal allograft. Lancet i:1355, 1980.

112. Hanto, D. W., Frizzera, G., Purtilo, D. T., Sakamoto, K., Sullivan, J. L., Saemundsen, A. K., Klein, G., Simmons, R. L., and Najarian, J. S.: Clinical spectrum of lymphoproliferative disorders in renal transplant recipients and evidence for the role of the Epstein-Barr virus. Cancer Res. 41:4253, 1981.

113. Ernberg, I.: Epstein-Barr virus and acquired immunodeficiency syndrome. In Klein G. (ed.): Advances in Viral Oncology, Vol. 8. New York, Raven Press, 1989, pp. 203–217.

114. Greenspan, J. S., Greenspan, D., Lennette, E. T., Abrams, D. I., Conant, M. A., Peterson, V., and Freese, U. K.: Replication of Epstein-Barr virus within the epithelial cells of oral

"hairy" leukoplakia, an AIDS-associated lesion. N. Engl. J. Med. 313:1564, 1985.

115. Young, L. S., Lau, R., Rowe, M., Niedobitek, G., Packham, G., Shanahan, F., Rowe, D. T., Greenspan, D., Greenspan, J. S., Rickinson, A. B., and Farrell, P. J.: Differentiation-associated expression of the Epstein-Barr virus BZLF1 trans-activator protein in oral hairy leukoplakia. J. Virol. 65:2868, 1991.

116. Klein, G., Giovanella, B. C., Lindahl, T., Fialkow, P. J., Singh, S., and Stehlin, J. S.: Direct evidence for the presence of Epstein-Barr virus DNA and nuclear antigen in malignant epithelial cells from patients with poorly differentiated carcinoma of the nasopharynx. Proc. Natl. Acad. Sci. USA 71:4737, 1974.

117. Tugwood, J. D., Lau, W.-H., Sai-Ki, O., Tsao, S.-Y., Martin, W. M. C., Shiu, W., Desgranges, C., Jones, P. H., and Arrand, J. R.: Epstein-Barr virus-specific transcription in normal and malignant nasopharyngeal biopsies and in lymphocytes from healthy donors and infectious mononucleosis patients. J. Gen. Virol. 68:1081, 1987.

118. Young, L.S., Dawson, C. W., Clark, D., Rupani, H., Busson, P., Tursz, T., Johnson, A., and Rickinson, A. B.: Epstein-Barr virus gene expression in nasopharyngeal carcinoma. J. Gen. Virol. 69:1051, 1988.

119. Kaschka-Dierich, C., Adams, A., Lindahl, T., Bornkamm, G. W., Bjursell, G., and Klein, G.: Intracellular forms of Epstein-Barr virus DNA in human tumour cells in vivo. Nature 260:302, 1976.

120. Zeng, Y., Zhang, L. G., Wu, Y. C., Huang, Y. S., Huang, N. Q., Li, J. Y., Wang, Y. B., Jiang, M. K., Fang, Z., and Meng, N. N.: Prospective studies on nasopharyngeal carcinoma in Epstein-Barr virus IgA/VCA antibody-positive persons in Wuzhou City, China. Int. J. Cancer 36:545, 1985.

121. Sugden, B.: Comparison of Epstein-Barr viral DNAs in Burkitt lymphoma biopsy cells and in cells clonally transformed in vitro. Proc. Natl. Acad. Sci. USA 74:4651, 1977.

122. Hinuma, Y., and Katsuki, T.: Colonies of EBNA-positive cells in soft agar from peripheral leukocytes of infectious mononucleosis patients. Int. J. Cancer 21:426, 1978.

123. Svedmyr, E., and Jondal, M.: Cytotoxic effector cells specific for B cell lines transformed by Epstein-Barr virus are present in patients with infectious mononucleosis. Proc. Natl. Acad. Sci. USA 72:1622, 1975.

124. Murray, R. J., Kurilla, M. G., Griffin, H. M., Brooks, J. M., Mackett, M., Arrand, J. R., Rowe, M., Burrows, S. R., Moss, D. J., Kieff, E., and Rickinson, A. B.: Human cytotoxic T-cell responses against Epstein-Barr virus nuclear antigens demonstrated by using recombinant vaccinia viruses. Proc. Natl. Acad. Sci. USA 87:2906, 1990.

125. Burrows, S. R., Sculley, T. B., Misko, I. S., Schmidt, C., and Moss, D. J.: An Epstein-Barr virus-specific cytotoxic T cell epitope in EBV nuclear antigen 3 (EBNA 3). J. Exp. Med. 171:345, 1990.

125a. Yao, Q. Y., Rickinson, A. B., and Epstein, M. A.: A re-examination of the Epstein-Barr virus carrier state in healthy seropositive individuals. Int. J. Cancer 35:35, 1985.

126. Mosier, D. E., Baird, S. M., Kirven, M. B., Gulizia, R. J., Wilson, D. B., Kubayashi, R., Picchio, G., Garnier, J. L., Sullivan, J. L., and Kipps, T. J.: EBV-associated B-cell lymphomas following transfer of human peripheral blood lymphocytes to mice with severe combined immune deficiency. Curr. Top. Microbiol. Immunol. 166:317, 1990.

127. Schubach, W. H., Hackman, R., Neiman, P. E., Miller, G., and Thomas, E. D.: A monoclonal immunoblastic sarcoma in donor cells bearing Epstein-Barr virus genomes following allogeneic marrow grafting for acute lymphoblastic leukemia. Blood 60:180, 1982.

128. Morrow, R. H., Kisuule, A., Pike, M. C., and Smith, P. G.: Burkitt's lymphoma in the Mengo districts of Uganda: Epidemiologic features and their relationship to malaria. J. Natl. Cancer Inst. 56:479, 1976.

129. Facer, C. A., and Playfair, J. H. L.: Malaria, Epstein-Barr virus, and the genesis of lymphomas. Adv. Cancer Res. 53:33, 1989.

130. Moss, D. J., Burrows, S. R., Castelino, D. J., Kiane, R. G., Pope, J. H., Rickinson, A. B., Alpers, M. P., and Heywood, P. F.: A comparison of Epstein-Barr virus-specific T-cell immunity in malaria-endemic and -nonendemic regions of Papua New Guinea. Int. J. Cancer 31:727, 1983.

131. Whittle, H. C., Brown, J., Marsh, K., Greenwood, B. M., Seidelin, P., Tighe, H., and Wedderburn, L.: T-cell control of Epstein-Barr virus-infected B cells is lost during *P. falciparum* malaria. Nature 312:449, 1984.

132. Gaidano, G., Ballerini, P., Gong, J. Z., Inghirami, G., Neri, A., Newcomb, E. W., Magrath, I. T., Knowles, D. M., and Dalla-Favera, R.: p53 Mutations in human lymphoid malignancies: Association with Burkitt lymphoma and chronic lymphocytic leukemia. Proc. Natl. Acad. Sci. USA 88:5413, 1991.

133. Farrell, P. J., Allan, G. J., Shanahan, F., Vousden, K. H., and Crook, T.: p53 Is frequently mutated in Burkitt's lymphoma cell lines. EMBO J. 10:2879, 1991.

134. Hammerschmidt, W., and Sugden, B.: Genetic analysis of immortalizing functions of Epstein-Barr virus in human B-lymphocytes. Nature 340:393, 1989.

135. Cohen, J. I., Wang, F., Mannick, J., and Kieff, E.: Epstein-Barr virus nuclear protein 2 is a key determinant of lymphocyte transformation. Proc. Natl. Acad. Sci. USA 86:9558, 1989.

135a. Miller, G.: Epstein-Barr virus biology, pathogenesis, and medical aspects. *In* Fields, B. N., and Knipe, D. M. (eds.): Virology. New York, Raven Press, 1990, pp. 1921–1958.

136. Colby, B. M., Shaw, J. E., Elion, G. B., and Pagano, J. S.: Effect of acyclovir [9-(2-hydroxyethoxymethyl)guanine] on Epstein-Barr virus DNA replication. J. Virol. 34:560, 1980.

137. Hanto, D. W., Frizzera, G., Gajl-Peczalska, K. J., Balfour, H. H., Jr., Simmons, R. L., and Najarian, J. S.: Acyclovir therapy of Epstein-Barr virus-induced posttransplant lymphoproliferative diseases. Transplant. Proc. 17:89, 1985.

INDEX

Note: Page numbers in *italics* refer to illustrations; page numbers followed by t refer to tables; page numbers followed by f refer to footnotes.

ISBN 0-7216-4735-9